西医经典名著集成

克氏外科学
SABISTON
TEXTBOOK OF
SURGERY

The BIOLOGICAL BASIS of MODERN SURGICAL PRACTICE

TOWNSEND

BEAUCHAMP · EVERS · MATTOX

20TH EDITION

第20版（影印中文导读版）

编译委员会主任委员　陈孝平　刘玉村

下册

 湖南科学技术出版社

CONTENTS 目 录

ESOPHAGUS

第九篇　食管

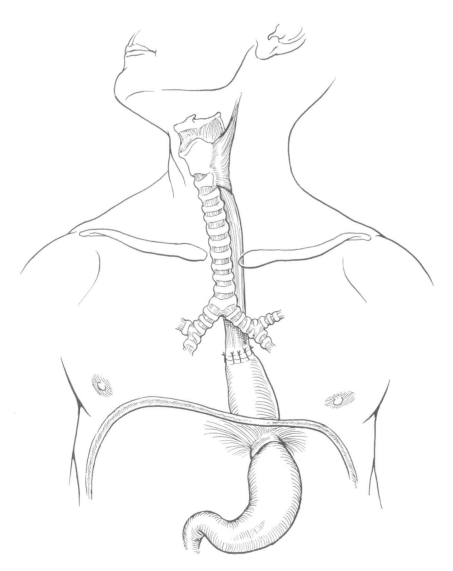

41 CHAPTER

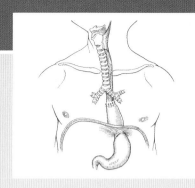

Esophagus

Jonathan D. Spicer, Rajeev Dhupar, Jae Y. Kim, Boris Sepesi,
Wayne Hofstetter

第四十一章　食管疾病

中文导读

　　本章共分为5节：①食管运动功能障碍；②食管憩室；③胃食管反流性疾病；④获得性食管良性疾病；⑤食管肿瘤。

　　第一节通过介绍评价食管运动功能的芝加哥分类方法，从食管运动机制切入详细介绍了原发性食管运动障碍的5种主要类型（失弛缓症、弥漫性食管痉挛、胡桃夹食管、高压性食管下段括约肌和无效食管蠕动）的诊断方法和处理原则，以及继发性食管运动障碍不同于前者的评估方法和治疗原则。

　　第二节介绍了食管憩室的不同分类方法及相应临床症状和治疗方法。传统上根据憩室发生部位将食管憩室分为3种类型：咽食管憩室（Zenker憩室）、食管中段憩室和膈上食管憩室。根据组成憩室壁的食管组织层次不同分为真性憩室（由黏膜、黏膜下层和黏膜基层等食管壁全层组成）和假性憩室（由黏膜和黏膜下层组成）。分别介绍了各种类型憩室的发病机制

和药物治疗、手术治疗的适应证。

　　第三节介绍胃食管反流是最常见的食管良性疾病，因胃内容物经食管下段括约肌反流进入食管而产生进行性加重的烧心症状。部分病人通过采用以质子泵抑制药为代表的药物治疗和改变生活方式的保守治疗能够有效控制病情进展，而对于保守治疗无效或已存在并发症的病人则需行手术治疗，并以图示方法介绍了经典胃底折叠术不同术式的具体手术方法。

　　第四节介绍了食管穿孔、食管腐蚀伤、食管异物、良性气管食管瘘和Schatzki环等常见疾病。分别介绍了每种疾病的发病机制、关键诊断方法和治疗原则。以食管穿孔为例强调了及时诊断和合适治疗是改善预后的关键。

第五节以食管癌TNM分期为核心，系统性阐述了食管癌治疗策略的历史演进和现状，通过详细讲解目前临床所采用的第7版食管癌TNM分期中的改变内容及其对食管癌治疗方法选择的影响，强调了治疗前准确临床分期对于指导食管癌个体化治疗方案选择和改善预后、提高病人生活质量的关键作用。以早期表浅肿瘤为对象，介绍了内镜治疗方法（消融治疗、冷冻治疗、内镜下食管黏膜切除）和食管切除术的适应证和各自优缺点。以局部进展期肿瘤为对象介绍了食管切除术、化学治疗、放射治疗等综合治疗方法的适应证，并归纳总结了目前相关临床试验的结果，全方面展现了目前食管癌治疗领域的现状和未来发展趋势。

〔赵　波〕

An organ that spans the distance of neck to stomach, the esophagus for all of its tube-like simplicity is in actuality a complex and relatively durable organ. It traverses the outside world and passes through precious territory in the mediastinum. The esophagus functions within areas that transition through pressure changes ranging from atmospheric to vacuum. Yet, the precision of a normal esophagus is virtually unrecognized. We swallow without effort, pain, or thought; but introduce disease within the organ, and we incur various degrees of malady, some quite severe and invariably chronic. We have yet to come up with perfect solutions for most of the dysfunction that is described in the forthcoming section, and replacement of the esophagus at this point is accomplished only by substitution of tissues rather than a renewal. Ultimately, among the "fixes" that are described, nothing functions as well as the original healthy organ. This leaves us and the future generation of esophagologists with the opportunity for innovation and much needed improvement. Our hope is that this chapter serves as an introduction to the esophagus and its various forms of function and dysfunction. One could literally spend a lifetime delving into each of these areas.

DIAGNOSIS AND MANAGEMENT OF ESOPHAGEAL MOTILITY DISORDERS

Diagnosis

Esophageal motility disorders constitute a relatively rare group of conditions, the underlying causes of which remain poorly understood. Patients with these conditions will present with a variety of symptoms including dysphagia, chest pain, heartburn, regurgitation, and weight loss. By definition, esophageal motility disorders are diagnosed when manometric findings exceed two standard deviations from normal. Unfortunately, symptom severity does not always correlate well with manometry, which is of critical importance in planning for surgical intervention in these generally complicated patients. Esophageal motility disorders are probably best classified by the Chicago classification, which was derived from data obtained by high-resolution manometry (HRM) with esophageal pressure topography (Table 41-1).[1] Because this classification is purely based on differentiating patterns of manometric findings, the exact clinical utility of this classification remains under investigation. Nevertheless, the findings from these ultramodern diagnostic modalities correlate well with those from conventional, water-perfused manometry. From a practical standpoint, the primary difference between HRM and conventional manometry is that in HRM, the pressure sensors are no more than 1 cm apart rather than every 3 to 5 cm. Up to 36 sensors can be found distributed radially and longitudinally, allowing a three-dimensional spatial pressure map to be drawn during deglutition. The graphical representation of this is what is referred to as esophageal pressure topography.

Whereas manometry is diagnostic for patients with named esophageal motility disorders, their presenting complaints are frequently vague and nonspecific. Hence, a complete workup including careful exclusion of other organ systems (cardiac, respiratory, peptic ulcer disease, and pancreaticobiliary disease) as the source of symptoms is paramount. In addition, attention to systemic symptoms of connective tissue disorders such as scleroderma is key as the surgical management of such patients requires specific modifications to avoid disastrous outcomes. With respect to the esophageal portion of the workup, a barium esophagram continues to be a highly useful road map to guide further investigations. When the esophagus is thought to be the cause of the patient's symptoms, upper endoscopy is necessary to rule out mucosal abnormalities and to provide improved visualization of the defects in question (stricture, hernia, diverticulum, esophagitis, masses). A computed tomography (CT) scan of the chest and abdomen is not uniformly required but may be helpful, particularly when there is suspicion of an extrinsic cause for the presenting symptoms. The addition of pH testing in the context of a documented esophageal motility disorder is necessary only when the motility disorder is thought to be the result of end-stage gastroesophageal reflux disease (GERD) as a means of documenting this.

Classically, esophageal motility disorders have been classified into primary and secondary causes. Primary disorders fall into five categories of motor disorders: achalasia, diffuse esophageal spasm (DES), nutcracker (jackhammer) esophagus, hypertensive lower esophageal sphincter (LES), and ineffective esophageal motility (IEM). Secondary conditions result from progressive damage induced by an underlying collagen vascular or neuromuscular disorder; they include scleroderma, dermatomyositis, polymyositis, lupus erythematosus, Chagas disease, and myasthenia gravis. Whereas such a classification is rooted in the basic etiology of this collection of diseases, it does not help much with interpreting manometric results, nor is it helpful as a guide to treatment strategies. For this reason, we suggest an anatomic approach to

TABLE 41-1 The Chicago Classification of Esophageal Motility

CRITERIA	
Achalasia and Esophagogastric Junction Outflow Obstruction	
Type I achalasia (classic)	Median IRP >15 mm Hg; 100% failed peristalsis (DCI <100 mm Hg•s •cm); premature contractions with DCI <450 mm Hg•s •cm satisfy criteria for failed peristalsis
Type II achalasia (with esophageal compression)	Median IRP >15 mm Hg; 100% failed peristalsis, panesophageal pressurization with ≥20% of swallows
Type III achalasia (spastic achalasia)	Median IRP >15 mm Hg; no normal peristalsis, spastic contractions with DCI >450 mm Hg•s •cm with ≥20% of swallows
Esophagogastric junction outflow obstruction (achalasia in evolution)	Median IRP >15 mm Hg; sufficient evidence of peristalsis such that criteria for types I-III are not met
Major Disorders of Peristalsis	
Absent contractility	Normal median IRP, 100% failed peristalsis
Distal esophageal spasm	Normal median IRP; ≥20% premature contractions with DCI >450 mm Hg•s•cm
Hypercontractile esophagus (jackhammer)	At least 2 swallows with DCI >8000 mm Hg•cm •s
Minor Disorders of Peristalsis	
Ineffective esophageal motility	≥50% ineffective swallows
Fragmented peristalsis	≥50% fragmented contractions with DCI >450 mm Hg•cm
Normal esophageal motility	None of the above criteria are met
Integrated relaxation pressure (IRP) is the mean of the 4 seconds of maximal deglutitive relaxation in the 10-second window beginning at the upper esophageal sphincter relaxation referenced to gastric pressure; distal contractile integral (DCI) is the amplitude × duration × length (mm Hg•s •cm) of the distal esophageal contraction exceeding 20 mm Hg from the transition zone to the proximal margin of the lower esophageal sphincter.	

Data from Roman S, Gyawali CP, Xiao Y, et al: The Chicago classification of motility disorders. *Gastrointest Endosc Clin N Am* 24:545–561, 2014.

classifying esophageal motility disorders based on involvement of the esophageal body or LES as this is the basis for understanding basic esophageal manometry and often the key to guide surgical therapy.

Motility Disorders of the Esophageal Body
Diffuse Esophageal Spasm

DES is a poorly understood hypermotility disorder of the esophagus. Under the Chicago classification, this would now be called distal esophageal spasm. Although it is manifested in a similar fashion to achalasia, it is five times less common. It is seen most often in women and is often found in patients with multiple medical complaints. The cause of the neuromuscular physiology

is unclear. The basic pathology is related to a motor abnormality of the esophageal body that is most notable in the lower two thirds of the esophagus. Muscular hypertrophy and degeneration of the branches of the vagus nerve in the esophagus have been observed. As a result, the esophageal contractions are repetitive, simultaneous, and of high amplitude.

The clinical presentation of DES is typically that of chest pain and dysphagia. These symptoms may be related to eating or exertion and may mimic those of angina. Patients will complain of a squeezing pressure in the chest that may radiate to the jaw, arms, and upper back. The symptoms are often pronounced during times of heightened emotional stress. Regurgitation of esophageal contents and saliva is common but acid reflux is not. However, acid reflux can aggravate the symptoms, as can cold liquids. Other functional gastrointestinal complaints, such as irritable bowel syndrome and pyloric spasm, may accompany DES, whereas other gastrointestinal problems, such as gallstones, peptic ulcer disease, and pancreatitis, all trigger DES.

The diagnosis of DES is made by radiographic and manometric studies. The classic picture of the corkscrew esophagus or pseudodiverticulosis on an esophagram is caused by the presence of tertiary contractions and indicates advanced disease. A distal bird beak narrowing of the esophagus and normal peristalsis can also be noted. The classic manometry findings in DES are simultaneous multipeaked contractions of high amplitude (>120 mm Hg) or long duration (>2.5 seconds). These erratic contractions occur after more than 10% of wet swallows. Because of the spontaneous contractions and intermittent normal peristalsis, standard manometry may not be enough to identify DES. Correlation of subjective complaints with evidence of spasm (induced by a vagomimetic drug, bethanechol) on manometric tracings is also convincing evidence of this capricious disease.

The treatment for DES is far from ideal as symptom relief is often partial. Today, the mainstay of treatment for DES is nonsurgical, and pharmacologic or endoscopic intervention is preferred. All patients are evaluated for psychiatric conditions, including depression, psychosomatic complaints, and anxiety. Control of these disorders and reassurance of the esophageal nature of the chest pain that the patient is experiencing is often therapeutic in and of itself. If dysphagia is a component of a patient's symptoms, steps must be taken to eliminate trigger foods or drinks from the diet. Similarly, if reflux is a component, acid suppression medications are helpful. Nitrates, calcium channel blockers, sedatives, and anticholinergics may be effective in some cases, but the relative efficacy of these medicines is not known. Peppermint may also provide temporary symptomatic relief. Bougie dilation of the esophagus up to 50 or 60 Fr provides relief for severe dysphagia and is 70% to 80% effective. Botulinum toxin injections have also been tried with some success, but the results are not sustainable.

Surgery is indicated for patients with incapacitating chest pain or dysphagia who have failed to respond to medical and endoscopic therapy or in the presence of a pulsion diverticulum of the thoracic esophagus. A long esophagomyotomy is performed through a left thoracotomy or a video-assisted technique through the abdomen or left side of the chest. Esophageal manometry is a useful tool to guide the extent of the myotomy. Some surgeons advocate extending the myotomy up into the thoracic inlet, but most agree that the proximal extent generally should be high enough to encompass the entire length of the abnormal motility, as determined by manometric measurements. The distal extent of the myotomy is extended down onto the LES, but the need to include the stomach is not agreed on uniformly. A Dor fundoplication is recommended to provide reflux protection as the surgery itself interrupts the phrenoesophageal ligament and encourages reflux. Results of the long esophagomyotomy for DES are variable, but it is reported to provide relief of symptoms in up to 80% of patients.

Nutcracker Esophagus

Recognized in the late 1970s as a distinct entity and known as hypercontractile esophagus in the Chicago classification, nutcracker or jackhammer esophagus is a disorder characterized by excessive contractility. It is described as an esophagus with hypertensive peristalsis or high-amplitude peristaltic contractions. It is seen in patients of all ages, with equal gender predilection, and is the most common of all esophageal hypermotility disorders. Like DES, the pathophysiologic process is not well understood. It is associated with hypertrophic musculature that results in high-amplitude contractions of the esophagus and is the most painful of all esophageal motility disorders.

Patients with nutcracker esophagus present in a similar fashion to those with DES and frequently complain of chest pain and dysphagia. Odynophagia is also noted, but regurgitation and reflux are uncommon. An esophagram may or may not reveal any abnormalities, depending on how well "behaved" the esophagus is during the examination. The Chicago classification characterizes the diagnosis of nutcracker esophagus as the subjective complaint of chest pain with at least one swallow showing a distal contractile integral greater than 8000 mm Hg•s•cm with single or multipeaked contractions on HRM. The LES pressure is normal, and relaxation occurs with each wet swallow (Fig. 41-1). Ambulatory monitoring can help distinguish this disorder from DES. This is of critical importance because a subset of DES patients with dysphagia can be helped with esophagomyotomy, but surgery is of questionable value in patients with a nutcracker esophagus.

The treatment of nutcracker esophagus is medical. Calcium channel blockers, nitrates, and antispasmodics may offer temporary relief during acute spasms. Bougie dilation may offer some temporary relief of severe discomfort but has no long-term benefits. Patients with nutcracker esophagus may have triggers and are counseled to avoid caffeine, cold, and hot foods.

Motility Disorders of the Lower Esophageal Sphincter
Hypertensive Lower Esophageal Sphincter

Hypertensive LES was first described as a distinct entity by Code and colleagues.[2] According to the Chicago classification, this entity has been renamed esophagogastric junction (EGJ) outflow obstruction and is defined as a median integrated relaxation pressure greater than 15 mm Hg (hypertensive, poorly relaxing sphincter). Thought by some to be achalasia in evolution, the diagnosis differs by evidence of effective peristalsis that is not present in classic achalasia. Hypertensive LES may be observed in patients presenting with dysphagia, chest pain, and manometric findings of an elevated LES. Patients with hypertensive LES will infrequently present with acid reflux and regurgitation. The diagnosis is made by manometry. Conventional manometry will demonstrate LES pressures above normal (>26 mm Hg), and relaxation will be incomplete but may not be consistently abnormal. Motility of the esophageal body may be hyperperistaltic or normal. An esophagram may show narrowing at the gastroesophageal junction (GEJ) with delayed flow and abnormalities of esophageal contraction; however, these are nonspecific findings. About 50% of the time, peristalsis in the esophageal body is normal. In

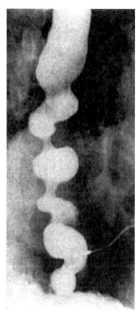

FIGURE 41-1 Barium esophagram of diffuse esophageal spasm. (Adapted from Peters JH, DeMeester TR: Esophagus and diaphragmatic hernia. In Schwartz SI, Fischer JE, Spencer FC, et al, editors: *Principles of surgery*, ed 7, New York, 1998, McGraw-Hill.)

the remainder, abnormal contractions are noted to be hypertensive peristaltic or simultaneous waveforms. The pathogenesis is not well understood.

The treatment of hypertensive LES is with endoscopic and surgical intervention. Botox injections alleviate symptoms temporarily, and hydrostatic balloon dilation may provide long-term symptomatic relief. Surgery is indicated for patients who fail to respond to interventional treatments and those with significant symptoms. A laparoscopic modified Heller esophagomyotomy is the operation of choice. In patients with normal esophageal motility, a partial antireflux procedure (e.g., Dor or Toupet fundoplication) is added. Recently, some have advocated the use of per-oral endoscopic myotomy for such patients (discussed further in the section on achalasia).[3]

Motility Disorders Affecting Both Body and Lower Esophageal Sphincter
Achalasia

The literal meaning of the term *achalasia* is "failure to relax." It is the best understood of all esophageal motility disorders. The incidence is 6/100,000 persons/year, with a predilection to affect young women. Its pathogenesis is presumed to be idiopathic or infectious neurogenic degeneration. Severe emotional stress, trauma, drastic weight reduction, and Chagas disease (parasitic infection with *Trypanosoma cruzi*) have also been implicated. Regardless of the cause, the muscles of the esophagus and LES are affected. Prevailing theories support the model that the destruction of the nerves to the LES is the primary pathologic process and that degeneration of the neuromuscular function of the body of the esophagus is secondary. This degeneration results in hypertension of the LES and failure of the LES to relax on pharyngeal swallowing as well as pressurization of the esophagus, esophageal dilation, and resultant loss of progressive peristalsis.

Vigorous (or spastic/type III) achalasia is seen in a subset of patients presenting with chest pain. In these patients, the LES is hypertensive and fails to relax, as seen in achalasia. Furthermore, the contractions of the esophageal body continue to be simultaneous and nonperistaltic. However, the amplitude of the contractions in response to swallowing is normal or high, which is inconsistent with classic achalasia (Fig. 41-2). It is postulated that patients in the early phases of achalasia may not have abnormalities in the esophageal body that are seen in later stages of the disease. Patients presenting with vigorous achalasia may be in this early phase and will go on to develop abnormal esophageal body contractions predicated on the presence of outflow obstruction of the esophagus.

Achalasia is also known to be a premalignant condition of the esophagus. During a 20-year period, a patient will have up to an 8% chance for development of carcinoma. Squamous cell carcinoma is the most common type identified and is thought to be the result of long-standing retained undigested fermenting food in the body of the esophagus, causing mucosal irritation. If the histology is adenocarcinoma, it tends to appear in the middle third of the esophagus, below the air-fluid level, where the mucosal irritation is the greatest. In contrast to these theories of carcinogenesis, it appears that even in patients with treated achalasia, there is an ongoing cancer incidence risk. Although no specific surveillance program for patients with treated achalasia has yet been endorsed by any of the gastroenterology societies, long-term surveillance is strongly recommended to monitor for recurrent achalasia and cancer.

The classic triad of presenting symptoms of achalasia consists of dysphagia, regurgitation, and weight loss. Heartburn, postprandial choking, and nocturnal coughing are commonly seen. The dysphagia that patients experience often begins with liquids and progresses to solids. Most patients describe eating as a laborious process during which they must pay special attention to the process. They eat slowly and use large volumes of water to help wash the food down into the stomach. As the water builds up pressure, retrosternal chest pain is experienced and can be severe until the LES opens, which provides quick relief. Regurgitation of undigested, foul-smelling food is common, and with progressive disease, aspiration can become life-threatening. Pneumonia, lung abscess, and bronchiectasis often result from long-standing achalasia. The dysphagia progresses slowly during years, and patients adapt their lifestyle to accommodate the inconveniences that accompany this disease. Patients often do not seek medical attention until their symptoms are advanced and will present with marked distention of the esophagus.

The diagnosis of achalasia is usually made from an esophagram and a motility study. The findings may vary, depending on the degree to which the disease has advanced. The esophagram will often show a dilated esophagus with a distal narrowing referred to as the classic bird's beak appearance of the barium-filled esophagus (Fig. 41-3). Sphincter spasm and delayed emptying through the LES as well as dilation of the esophageal body are observed. A lack of peristaltic waves in the body and failure of relaxation of the LES (the sine qua non of this disease) are noted. Lack of a gastric air bubble is a common finding on the upright portion of the esophagram and is a result of the tight LES not allowing air to pass easily into the stomach. In the more advanced stage of disease, massive esophageal dilation, tortuosity, and sigmoidal esophagus (megaesophagus) are seen (Fig. 41-4).

Manometry is the "gold standard" test for diagnosis and will help differentiate other potential esophageal motility disorders. In typical achalasia (type I), the manometry tracings show five classic findings, two abnormalities of the LES and three of the esophageal body. The LES will be hypertensive, with pressures usually higher than 35 mm Hg (integrated relaxation pressure >15 mm Hg), but more important, it will fail to relax with deglutition. The body of the esophagus will have a pressure above baseline (pressurization of the esophagus) from incomplete air evacuation, simultaneous mirrored contractions with no evidence of progressive

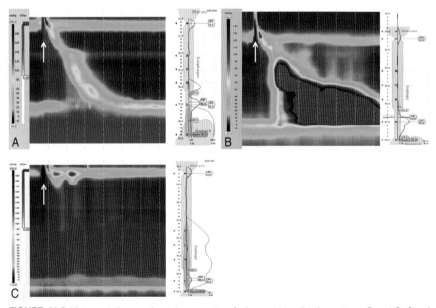

FIGURE 41-2 High-resolution esophageal manometry. **A,** A normal swallowing pattern. **B** and **C,** Classic (type I) achalasia and atypical spastic or vigorous achalasia (type III). The *arrows* denote initiation of swallowing.

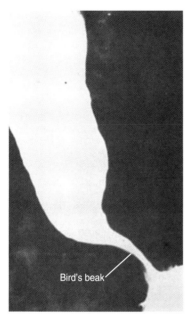

FIGURE 41-3 Barium swallow showing achalasia. (Adapted from Dalton CB: Esophageal motility disorders. In Pearson FG, Cooper JD, Deslauriers J, et al, editors: *Esophageal surgery*, ed 2, New York, 2002, Churchill Livingstone.)

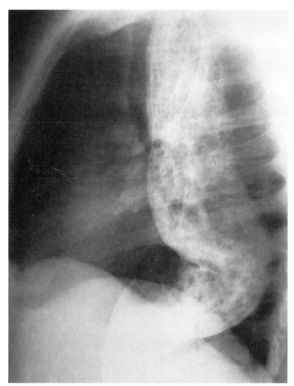

FIGURE 41-4 Barium swallow showing megaesophagus. (From Orringer MB: Disorders of esophageal motility. In Sabiston DC, editor: *Textbook of surgery*, ed 15, Philadelphia, 1997, WB Saunders.)

peristalsis, and low-amplitude waveforms indicating a lack of muscle tone. These five findings provide a diagnosis of achalasia. Endoscopy is performed to evaluate the mucosa for evidence of esophagitis or cancer.

There are surgical and nonsurgical treatment options for patients with achalasia; all are directed toward relieving the obstruction caused by the LES. Because none of them are able to address the issue of decreased motility in the esophageal body, they are all palliative treatments. Nonsurgical treatment options include medications and endoscopic interventions but usually are only a short-term solution to a lifelong problem. In the early stage of the disease, medical treatment with sublingual nitroglycerin, nitrates, or calcium channel blockers may offer hours of relief from chest pressure before or after a meal. Pneumatic dilation has been shown to provide excellent relief of symptoms although frequently requiring multiple interventions and with a risk of esophageal perforation of less than 4%. Injection of botulinum toxin (Botox) directly into the LES blocks acetylcholine release, prevents smooth muscle contraction, and effectively relaxes the LES. With repeated treatments, Botox may offer symptomatic relief for years, but symptoms recur more than 50% of the time within 6 months.

Surgical esophagomyotomy offers excellent results that are durable. The current technique is a modification of the Heller myotomy that was described originally through a laparotomy in 1913. Various changes have been made to the originally described procedure, but the modified laparoscopic Heller myotomy is now the operation of choice. It is done open or with video or robotic assistance. The decision to perform an antireflux procedure remains controversial. Most patients who have undergone a myotomy will experience some amount of reflux, either symptomatic or not. The addition of a partial antireflux procedure, such as a Toupet or Dor fundoplication, will restore a barrier to reflux and decrease postoperative symptoms.

Currently, per-oral endoscopic myotomy is being investigated as a natural orifice approach to perform the myotomy. With use of an operating endoscope, the mucosa of the esophagus is divided around the mid to distal third, and a submucosal tunnel is created. Through this tunnel, the muscular layer of the distal esophagus, LES, and cardia is visualized and divided, effectively performing an endoscopic myotomy. Although concern for the lack of an antireflux procedure and the possibility of debilitating reflux remains, results thus far have been encouraging.[4] This is a promising new technique, but it remains to be seen whether it is superior to laparoscopic Heller myotomy and the excellent long-term results reported in multiple large series of surgically treated patients.

Esophagectomy is considered in any symptomatic patient with a tortuous esophagus (megaesophagus), sigmoid esophagus, failure of more than one myotomy, or reflux stricture that is not amenable to dilation. Less than 60% of patients undergoing repeated myotomy benefit from surgery, and fundoplication for treatment of reflux strictures has even more dismal results. In addition to definitively treating the end-stage achalasia patient, esophageal resection also eliminates the risk for carcinoma in the resected area. A transhiatal esophagectomy with or without preservation of the vagus nerve offers a good long-term result. However, in the setting of megaesophagus, a total esophagectomy incorporating a transthoracic dissection may be safest, given the difficulty in palpating the borders of the esophagus through a transhiatal approach.

Results of medical, interventional, and surgical procedures all point to surgery as the safest and most effective treatment of achalasia. In comparing balloon dilation to Botox injections, remission of symptoms occurred in 89% versus 38% of patients at 1 year, respectively. Studies done to compare balloon dilation versus surgery have shown perforation rates of 4% and 1% and mortality rates of 0.5% and 0.2%, respectively. Results were considered excellent in 60% of patients undergoing balloon dilation and in 85% of those undergoing surgery. However, more recently in a randomized controlled trial of the European Achalasia Trial Investigators,[5] pneumatic dilation was found to be equivalent to laparoscopic Heller myotomy and Dor fundoplication with therapeutic success rates of 86% versus 90% at 2 years. Perforation occurred in 4% of the patients during pneumatic dilations and mucosal tears occurred in 12% during laparoscopic Heller myotomy, but all were repaired intraoperatively. Patients in the pneumatic dilation cohort had a 25% rate of redilation to achieve treatment success. Clinicians need to remain wary and vigilant with achalasia patients, even after "successful" intervention. Continued asymptomatic outflow obstruction will lead to dilation. Close monitoring of these patients is appropriate.

Ineffective Esophageal Motility

IEM was first recognized as a distinct motility disturbance by Castell in 2000. It is defined as a contraction abnormality of the distal esophagus and is usually associated with GERD. It may be secondary to inflammatory injury of the esophageal body because of increased exposure to gastric contents. Dampened motility of the esophageal body leads to poor acid clearance in the lower esophagus. Once altered motility is present, the condition appears to be irreversible.

The symptoms of IEM are mixed, but patients usually present with symptoms of reflux and dysphagia. Heartburn, chest pain, and regurgitation are noted. Diagnosis is made by manometry. IEM is defined by greater than 50% of swallows being deemed ineffective (distal contractile integral <450 mm Hg). A barium esophagram demonstrates nonspecific abnormalities of esophageal contraction but will not further distinguish IEM from other motor disorders.

The best treatment of IEM is prevention, which is associated with effective treatment of GERD. Once altered motility occurs, it appears to be irreversible. Similarly, scleroderma may be manifested manometrically as IEM and is best treated by addressing the underlying condition. In cases in which the motility disorder has become irreversible and intractable, the surgical approach must be tailored to the manometric findings. However, great caution must be taken in approaching surgical therapy in this cohort of patients as the likelihood of a favorable result remains low.

DIVERTICULAR DISORDERS

It is now well established that most diverticula are a result of a primary motor disturbance or an abnormality of the upper esophageal sphincter or LES. Diverticula were originally classified according to their location, and as a convention, these are classifications to which we still adhere. The three most common sites of occurrence are pharyngoesophageal (Zenker), parabronchial (midesophageal), and epiphrenic (supradiaphragmatic). True diverticula involve all layers of the esophageal wall, including mucosa, submucosa, and muscularis. A false diverticulum consists of mucosa and submucosa only. Pulsion diverticula are false diverticula that occur because of elevated intraluminal pressures generated from abnormal motility disorders. These forces cause the mucosa and submucosa to herniate through the esophageal musculature. Both a Zenker diverticulum and an epiphrenic diverticu-

lum fall under the category of false pulsion diverticula. Traction, or true, diverticula result from external inflammatory mediastinal lymph nodes adhering to the esophagus as they heal and contract, pulling the esophagus during the process. Over time, the esophageal wall herniates, forming an outpouching, and a diverticulum ensues. These are more common in the midesophageal region around the carinal lymph nodes.

Pharyngoesophageal (Zenker) Diverticulum

Originally described by Zenker and von Ziemssen,[6] the pharyngoesophageal diverticulum (Zenker diverticulum) is the most common esophageal diverticulum found today (Fig. 41-5). It is usually manifested in older patients in the seventh decade of life and has been postulated to be a result of loss of tissue elasticity and muscle tone with age. It is specifically found herniating from Killian's triangle, between the oblique fibers of the thyropharyngeus muscle and the horizontal fibers of the cricopharyngeus muscle. As the diverticulum enlarges, the mucosal and submucosal layers dissect down the left side of the esophagus into the superior mediastinum, posteriorly along the prevertebral space. Zenker diverticulum is often referred to as cricopharyngeal achalasia and is managed accordingly.

Until the Zenker diverticulum begins to enlarge, patients are often initially asymptomatic. Commonly, patients complain of a sticking in the throat. A nagging cough, excessive salivation, and intermittent dysphagia often are signs of progressive disease. As the sac increases in size, regurgitation of foul-smelling, undigested material is common. Halitosis, voice changes, retrosternal pain, and respiratory infections are especially common in older adults. The most serious complication from an untreated Zenker diverticulum is aspiration pneumonia or lung abscess. In an older patient, this can be morbid and sometimes fatal.

Diagnosis is made by barium esophagram. At the level of the cricothyroid cartilage, the diverticulum can be seen filled with barium resting posteriorly alongside the esophagus (the "cricopharyngeal bar"). Lateral views are critical because this is usually a posterior structure. Neither esophageal manometry nor endoscopy is needed to diagnose Zenker diverticulum.

Surgical or endoscopic repair of a Zenker diverticulum is the gold standard of treatment. Traditionally, an open repair through the left side of the neck was advocated. However, endoscopic exclusion has gained popularity in many centers. Two types of open repair are performed, resection and surgical fixation of the diverticulum. The diverticulectomy and diverticulopexy are performed through an incision in the left side of the neck. In all cases, a myotomy of the proximal and distal thyropharyngeus and cricopharyngeus muscles is performed. In cases of a small diverticulum (<2 cm), a myotomy alone is often sufficient. In most patients with good tissue or a large sac (>5 cm), excision of the sac is indicated. Should a diverticulopexy be performed, it is important to suture the diverticulum to the posterior pharynx as opposed to the prevertebral fascia to allow free vertical movement of the pharynx during deglutition. The postoperative stay is approximately 2 or 3 days, during which the patient remains unable to eat or to drink.

An alternative to open surgical repair is the endoscopic Dohlman procedure, which has become more popular. Endoscopic division of the common wall between the esophagus and diverticulum using a laser, electrocautery, or stapler device has been similarly successful. Because of the configuration of the inline stapling device, this approach has been advocated for larger diverticula. The risk for an incomplete myotomy increases with

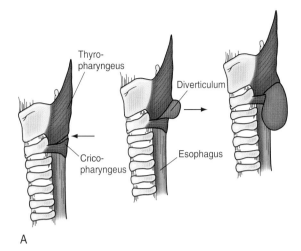

A

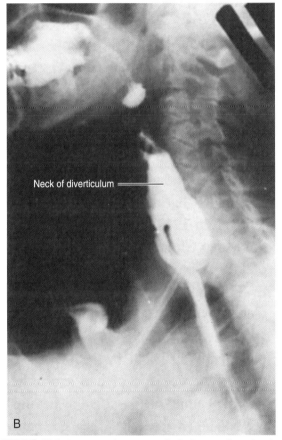

Neck of diverticulum ————————

B

FIGURE 41-5 **A,** Zenker diverticulum. **B,** Barium swallow showing Zenker diverticulum. (Adapted from Trastek VF, Deschamps C: Esophageal diverticula. In Shields TW, Locicero J III, Ponn RB, editors: *General thoracic surgery*, ed 5, Philadelphia, 1999, Lippincott Williams & Wilkins.)

diverticula smaller than 3 cm. This method divides the distal cricopharyngeus muscle while obliterating the sac. The esophagus and diverticulum ultimately form a common channel. The technique requires maximal extension of the neck and can be difficult to perform in older patients with cervical stenosis. For this reason, many have advocated the use of the needle knife by flexible endoscopy to perform the myotomy. Overall, the postoperative course

is slightly shorter for transoral approaches, with patients taking liquids the following day and requiring only a single overnight hospital stay. Thus, these techniques have gained favor and are advocated for patients with diverticula between 2 and 5 cm.

The results of open repair versus endoscopic repair have been well studied.[7] For diverticula 3 cm or smaller, surgical repair is superior to endoscopic repair in eliminating symptoms. For any diverticulum larger than 3 cm, the results are the same. Both the hospital stay and length of inanition are shorter with an endoscopic procedure. Regardless of the method of repair, patients do well and the results are excellent.

Midesophageal Diverticula

Midesophageal diverticula were first described in the 19th century. Historically, inflamed mediastinal lymph nodes from an infection with tuberculosis accounted for most cases. Infections with histoplasmosis and resultant fibrosing mediastinitis have now become more common. Inflammation of the lymph nodes exerts traction on the wall of the esophagus and leads to the formation of a true diverticulum in the midesophagus. This continues to be an important mechanism for these traction diverticula, but it is now believed that some may also be caused by a primary motility disorder, such as achalasia, DES, or other esophageal motility disorders.

Most patients with a midesophageal diverticulum are asymptomatic. They are often incidentally found during a workup for some other complaint (Fig. 41-6). Dysphagia, chest pain, and regurgitation can be present and are usually indicative of an underlying primary motility disorder. Patients presenting with a chronic cough are under suspicion for development of a bronchoesophageal fistula. Rarely, hemoptysis can be a presenting symptom, indicating infectious erosion of lymph nodes into major vasculature and the bronchial tree. In this case, the diverticulum is an incidental finding of lesser importance.

The diagnosis of the anatomic structure as well as of the size and location of an esophageal diverticulum is made through barium esophagram. Midesophageal diverticula typically are on the right because of the overabundance of structures in the midthoracic region of the left side of the chest. A CT scan is helpful to identify any mediastinal lymphadenopathy and may help lateralize the sac. Endoscopy is important to rule out mucosal abnormalities, including cancer that may be hidden in the sac. In addition, endoscopy may aid in identifying a fistula. Manometric studies are undertaken in all patients, symptomatic or not, to identify a primary motor disorder. Treatment is guided by the results of the manometric findings.

Determining the cause for midesophageal diverticula is critical for guiding treatment. In asymptomatic patients who have inflamed mediastinal lymph nodes, treatment of the underlying cause is the management of choice. If the diverticulum is smaller than 2 cm, it can be observed. If patients progress to become symptomatic or if the diverticulum is 2 cm or larger, surgical intervention is indicated. Usually, midesophageal diverticula have a wide mouth and rest close to the spine. Therefore, a diverticulopexy can be performed, whereby the diverticulum is suspended from the thoracic vertebral fascia. In patients with severe chest pain or dysphagia and a documented motor abnormality, a long esophagomyotomy is also indicated.

Epiphrenic Diverticula

Epiphrenic diverticula are found adjacent to the diaphragm in the distal third of the esophagus, within 10 cm of the GEJ. They are

MIDESOPHAGEAL TRACTION DIVERTICULUM

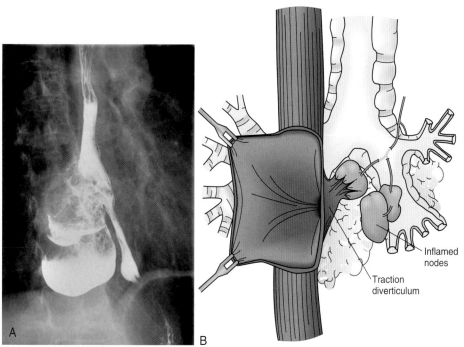

Inflamed
nodes

Traction
diverticulum

A

B

FIGURE 41-6 A, Barium esophagram demonstrating a giant midesophageal diverticulum. (Courtesy Dr. Lorenzo E. Ferri). **B,** Midesophageal diverticulum. (Adapted from Peters JH, DeMeester TR: Esophagus and diaphragmatic hernia. In Schwartz SI, Fischer JE, Spencer FC, et al, editors: *Principles of surgery*, ed 7, New York, 1998, McGraw-Hill.)

most often related to thickened distal esophageal musculature or increased intraluminal pressure. They are pulsion, or false, diverticula that are often associated with DES, achalasia, or IEM disorders. In patients in whom a motility abnormality cannot be identified, a congenital (Ehlers-Danlos syndrome) or traumatic cause is considered. As with midesophageal diverticula, epiphrenic diverticula are more common on the right side and tend to be wide-mouthed.

Most patients with epiphrenic diverticula present asymptomatically. They may present with dysphagia or chest pain, which is indicative of a motility disturbance. The diagnosis is often made during the workup for a motility disorder, and the diverticulum is found incidentally. Other symptoms, such as regurgitation, epigastric pain, anorexia, weight loss, chronic cough, and halitosis, are indicative of an advanced motility abnormality resulting in a sizable epiphrenic diverticulum.

A barium esophagram is the best diagnostic tool to detect an epiphrenic diverticulum (Fig. 41-7). The size, position, and proximity of the diverticulum to the diaphragm can all be clearly delineated. The underlying motility disorder is often identified as well; however, manometric studies need to be undertaken to evaluate the overall motility of the esophageal body and LES. Endoscopy is performed to evaluate for mucosal lesions, including esophagitis, Barrett esophagus, and cancer.

The treatment of an epiphrenic diverticulum is similar to that of a midesophageal diverticulum. These types of diverticula also have a wide mouth and rest close to the spine. Small (<2 cm) diverticula can also be suspended from the vertebral fascia and need not be excised. If a diverticulopexy is performed, a myotomy

is begun at the neck of the diverticulum and extended onto the LES. If a diverticulectomy is pursued, a vertical stapling device is placed across the neck and the diverticulum is excised. It is essential during this process to have an esophageal bougie in place to avoid narrowing the esophageal lumen while stapling. The muscle is closed over the excision site, and a long myotomy is performed on the opposite esophageal wall, extending from the level of the diverticulum onto the LES. If a large hiatal hernia is also present, the diverticulum is excised, a myotomy performed, and the hiatal hernia repaired. Failure to repair the hernia results in a high incidence of postoperative reflux. It is essential to relieve outflow obstruction in patients with diverticula; failure to do so can result in significant complications of leak or recurrence.

GASTROESOPHAGEAL REFLUX DISEASE

GERD is the most common benign condition of the esophagus, affecting millions of people worldwide. It occurs when there is retrograde flow of gastric contents through the LES that most commonly is manifested as "heartburn." The disease is characterized by progressive worsening of heartburn symptoms until they are frequent, persistent, and troublesome and possibly result in primary or secondary complications. Some of these complications include strictures, ulcers, metaplasia, dysplasia, carcinoma, and pulmonary disease (asthma, fibrosis).

The treatment of GERD has evolved significantly in the last several decades with the improved efficacy of antisecretory medications and refinement of surgical procedures. For many, the

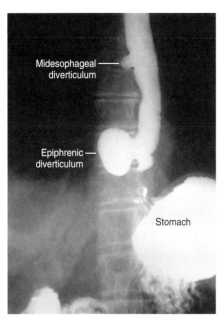

FIGURE 41-7 Barium swallow showing mid and distal esophageal diverticula. (Adapted from Pearson FG, Cooper JD, Deslauriers J, et al: *Esophageal surgery*, ed 2, New York, 2002, Churchill Livingstone.)

symptoms can be managed with medication and lifestyle modification alone. However, some people will experience symptoms that are refractory to these treatments or complications that are not medically treatable and require surgical intervention. The following sections explore the workup and surgical management of GERD in the context of failed medical management.

Medical Management

Although some patients wish to have antireflux surgery to avoid taking medication, most referrals to a surgeon are because of uncontrolled, persistent symptoms of heartburn or regurgitation despite medication. Commonly, patients will have tried proton pump inhibitors (PPIs) once daily and have progressed to twice daily. Frequently, patients will have tried several brands of PPI and have mixed multiple antacid medications. Cessation of PPIs will often result in heartburn or regurgitation that is prohibitive to normal function. However, to appropriately select patients who will have successful surgical intervention, it is critical to ensure that maximal medical therapy has been attempted and has failed with time. Patients for whom medical therapy never relieved symptoms or who demonstrate atypical symptoms should be further investigated for other causes before surgery is offered. It has been observed that the patients with the greatest likelihood of successful surgical therapy are those who have typical symptoms and good response to antisecretory therapy.[8]

Lifestyle modifications will rarely eliminate GERD symptoms, but they can decrease severity and duration and result in greater efficacy of medication. The modifications include weight loss (if overweight), smoking cessation, elimination of inciting foods, smaller and more frequent meals, and elimination of constipation. Medical therapy is usually maximal with twice-daily PPI therapy.

Workup

There are several components to the workup for surgical management of GERD that will promote successful selection of therapy.

They allow tailoring of the surgical procedure to the patient's needs and avoidance of unanticipated events during surgery. The standard studies include pH test, esophageal motility test, video esophagram, and endoscopy with biopsy. Additional tests may include gastric emptying study or CT scan.

Because gastric contents are acidic, measurement of pH acts as a surrogate for reflux. Not only will it document exposure of the lower esophagus to gastric refluxate, but it will also correlate symptoms with this exposure. The test is performed by placing a disposable probe in the distal esophagus (commonly by endoscopy) and allowing a remote recorder to collect data for 24 to 48 hours. It is critical to document abnormal refluxate exposure because other disease processes can have GERD-like symptoms. In addition, several studies have correlated abnormal pH testing with successful surgical outcomes.[9] The patient should be off of antisecretory and antacid medications at the time of testing (usually cease medications 5 days to 2 weeks prior).

Esophageal motility testing allows the surgeon to evaluate if contractions are strong and effective, if there is a motility disorder, and sometimes if there is an incompetent LES. Not only is this important in distinguishing GERD from other disorders (such as achalasia or scleroderma), but it can allow tailoring of surgery for patients with coexistent GERD and motility disorder. For example, a patient with mildly impaired motility in the setting of positive pH testing might be suited to a floppy or partial fundoplication procedure rather than a full wrap. Often, patients with long-standing GERD will have esophageal dysmotility, and they must be counseled about postoperative dysphagia after fundoplication. Patients with severe dysmotility should be considered for further workup or nonsurgical therapy.

Video esophagography shows both structure and function. It will diagnose abnormalities that would modify surgical treatment, such as strictures, masses, hiatal hernia, foreshortened esophagus, or diverticula. Functionally, video esophagography confirms reflux and correlates it with symptoms and can be suggestive of motility disorders or achalasia. It is considered the "road map" before surgery, can be obtained immediately after surgery, and is useful in long-term follow-up.

Finally, endoscopy allows the surgeon to evaluate the shape and course of the esophagus, to evaluate for signs of reflux such as esophagitis and metaplasia, and to rule out masses and strictures as a cause of symptoms. A particularly dilated and tortuous esophagus can be indicative of motility disorders, and hiatal hernias not seen on esophagram can be seen on retroflexed views in the stomach. Biopsy of abnormal findings will evaluate for metaplasia, dysplasia, and carcinoma, which might alter plans for surgery and surveillance.

If there are inconsistencies between the findings on workup and the patient's symptoms, it is important to revise the diagnosis, to continue investigation, or to obtain second opinions. Surgical procedures when the diagnosis is incorrect can result in additional new symptoms without resolution of the initial complaint, leading to a dissatisfying outcome. Adjunct studies to consider include CT scan of the chest and abdomen, small bowel follow-through, gastric emptying study, and colonoscopy.

Surgical Therapy

Several operations termed "antireflux" procedures have been developed over the years as surgeons have tailored them to symptoms of patients. This section will not discuss transthoracic approaches because these are rarely indicated as primary procedures for reflux. Rather, it outlines the basic concepts of the most commonly performed transabdominal fundoplication procedure and some variations.

After it is verified that the patient's symptoms are due to reflux (see earlier) and the patient is deemed a safe surgical candidate, the surgeon has several options. Regardless of the procedure chosen, the basic tenets of antireflux surgery remain constant: (1) preserve natural tissue planes and linings, (2) identify and preserve both vagus nerves, (3) identify the true EGJ for placement of the wrap, (4) have sufficient length of intra-abdominal esophagus, and (5) reestablish the angle of His.

The Nissen fundoplication, first described in the 1950s, has become a standard in antireflux surgery (Fig. 41-8A). Conceptually, it is the re-creation of a sphincter around the EGJ, done by wrapping the fundus around the esophagus. Whether by laparoscopy or laparotomy, the procedure is the same. The gastrohepatic ligament is incised until the phrenoesophageal ligament is visualized, with care taken to avoid replaced hepatic arteries. The esophagus is circumferentially mobilized, with great care to preserve both vagus nerves and the peritoneal lining along the crura. Short gastric vessels are taken, and the gastrosplenic ligament is mobilized to meet the dissection along the left crus, with care taken to remain far from the splenic hilum. Any hiatal hernia will require dissection in the mediastinum to bring down sufficient esophageal length. The fat pad is then mobilized from the anterior stomach or esophagus to visualize the true EGJ and to be able to exclude both vagus nerves from the wrap.

With sufficient esophageal and gastric mobilization as well as exposure of the true EGJ, the fundic tip along the line of the short gastrics can be passed posterior to the esophagus (excluding the vagus nerves in the fat pad) to create the wrap. A "shoeshine maneuver" ensures adequate mobility and lack of tension. A 50 to 54 Fr bougie is usually in the esophagus while the stomach is then sutured to the anterior esophagus. After the bougie is removed, the diaphragmatic hiatus is assessed and is closed with suture anterior and posterior to the esophagus, ensuring not to kink or impinge too heavily on the esophagus. Usually, the passage of instruments easily through the hiatus ensures that it is not too tight. An nasogastric tube should be inserted overnight for decompression.

Some surgeons have advocated the use of mesh at the hiatus as "reinforcement" or if there is excessive tension at the crural closure. Mesh is not usually necessary if the natural linings are preserved along the crus. If there is tension on closure, this can be overcome by inducing a left-sided pneumothorax with a small amount of carbon dioxide insufflation, which will relax the left diaphragm and usually allows tension-free closure. Relaxing incisions on the diaphragm have also been described.

The wrap can be individualized to the patient's symptoms. Full 360-degree wraps are particularly important when reflux causes respiratory compromise, such as the lung transplant population. A floppy wrap, whereby there is space for the passage of an instrument between the stomach and esophagus, will result in less dysphagia but may create a less competent valve. A partial or near Nissen, with a wrap of 300 or 320 degrees, will allow some ability to belch and possibly to vomit and will lessen symptoms of dysphagia and bloat.

Variations on this classic procedure exist that allow an operation to be individualized to the patient's needs. Toupet fundoplication involves posterior partial wrap of 180 to 270 degrees, with additional tacking sutures to fix the stomach to the crura in the abdomen (Fig. 41-8B). Dor fundoplication is most commonly used in the setting of esophageal myotomy but consists of an anterior 180-degree wrap (Fig. 41-8C). A newer device named LINX can be used in patients with minimal or no hiatal hernia.[10] It is a series of magnetic beads that are placed around the EGJ that will stretch with slight pressure in the esophagus, thereby mimicking the natural LES. Long-term results of this device are not available, but short-term efficacy is promising.

A consideration for patients with bile or gastric reflux, obesity, diabetes, or esophageal dysmotility is Roux-en-Y reconstruction.[11] A near-esophagojejunostomy (with small gastric pouch) allows the passage of almost all gastric and biliary contents far downstream from the esophagus, thereby preventing symptoms related to reflux. In this population, there will be additional benefits of impact on obesity and diabetes. This is also an option in revisional surgery, in which there is a lot of scarring or the integrity of the vagus nerves is questionable.

Finally, the patient undergoing fundoplication in whom there is less than adequate intra-abdominal esophagus may require partial gastric tubularization, or Collis gastroplasty (Fig. 41-8D-F). This involves stapling the fundus of the stomach with a bougie in the esophagus to create a few centimeters of additional length around which the stomach can be wrapped. Both transthoracic and transabdominal approaches have been described, and although this technically difficult maneuver should be approached with caution, it is imperative to realize when it should be done.

Complicated GERD

Long-standing reflux will cause complications to the esophagus, which require management that extends beyond antireflux surgery. In the patient with esophagitis, biopsy specimens from endoscopy can reveal medically treatable problems, such as candidiasis or eosinophilic infiltrative processes. Often, these patients can have relief of symptoms without surgical intervention, and surgical intervention may not relieve their symptoms. All strictures should be biopsied to rule out malignant processes and can frequently be managed with dilation if they are benign. Metaplastic changes (Barrett esophagus) should be biopsied in four quadrants every centimeter to evaluate for dysplasia and cancer. Fundoplication procedures can still be performed in this setting, but surveillance must continue at regular intervals because regression is rare (Table 41-2).[12]

Some patients with heartburn or dysphagia will have partial or complete intrathoracic stomach. The workup and surgical therapy for these patients can be significantly different from that for standard GERD, depending on the degree of hiatal herniation. Small hernias where the GEJ is above the diaphragmatic hiatus can be manifested with classic GERD symptoms, and the workup and therapy can be the same. When there is a moderate to large hiatal hernia, consideration must be given to the degree of symptoms related to the mechanical component versus the reflux. This can be a confusing picture because patients often have symptoms from both, but if the main complaints are dysphagia, food sticking, early satiety, regurgitation, and vomiting, the mechanical component may be the dominant pathologic process. This is particularly true of nearly total intrathoracic stomach. Workup may include pulmonary function tests because of compromised lung function and thorough cardiac evaluation because of overlapping symptoms. Manometry testing is often not possible with large hernias.

During reduction of the hernia, the esophagus might be foreshortened, and the options of gastropexy versus fundoplication or Collis gastroplasty/fundoplication will have to be weighed. With dominant mechanical symptoms, patients have relief with return

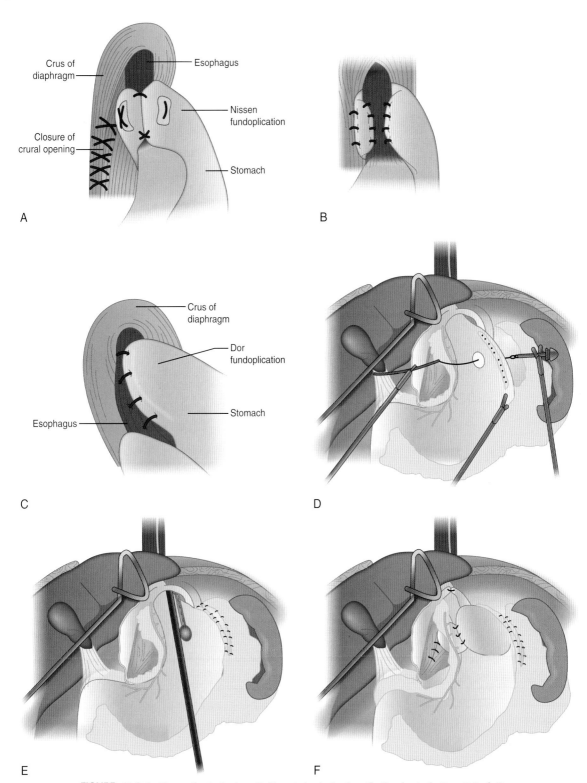

FIGURE 41-8 A, Nissen fundoplication. B, Toupet fundoplication. C, Dor fundoplication. D-F, Collis gastroplasty.

TABLE 41-2 **American Gastroenterological Association Guidelines for Surveillance After Fundoplication for Barrett Esophagus**

VARIABLE	SCORE
Age >75 years	1
Tachycardia (>100 beats/min)	1
Leukocytosis (>10,000 white blood cells/mL)	1
Pleural effusion	1
Fever (>38.5° C)	2
Noncontained leak (barium swallow or CT scan)	2
Respiratory compromise (respiratory rate >30, increasing oxygen requirement, or mechanical ventilation)	2
Time to diagnosis >24 hours	2
Presence of cancer	3
Hypotension	3

of the stomach to the abdominal cavity with gastropexy. However, they may subsequently suffer from reflux symptoms and require antisecretory medication thereafter. Most patients would likely benefit from a partial or floppy fundoplication procedure, keeping in mind that esophageal motility will likely be unknown.

ACQUIRED BENIGN DISORDERS OF THE ESOPHAGUS

Acquired Esophageal Disease

Perforation

Esophageal perforation is a potentially lethal condition that can have poor outcomes if there is a delay in diagnosis or improper treatment. Most series have reported overall mortality between 20% and 30%, frequently with strong correlations to etiology and interval from event to intervention.[13] The most commonly recognized cause is iatrogenic perforation during endoscopy, with others being forceful retching (Boerhaave syndrome), traumatic injury, foreign body ingestion, and tumor perforation. It is generally regarded that better outcomes are possible if the intervention is within 24 hours of the event, and poor outcomes are associated with cancer-related perforations. The key to management and patient survival is early recognition with timely diagnosis and therapy.

Suspicion of esophageal perforation begins with symptoms of epigastric or chest pain, neck or throat pain, and dysphagia. Physical examination findings might include crepitus on the chest, neck, or face; neck swelling; epigastric tenderness; nasal voice; or sometimes normal examination findings. Other early evidence might include a chest radiograph with mediastinal or cervical air, free abdominal air, or pleural effusion. A CT scan may show mediastinal air and periesophageal air or fluid. Of course, the mechanism of injury can be the greatest clue that would initiate further workup.

Once there is suspicion, the diagnostic workup must proceed on the basis of the index of suspicion. Barium esophagram is the standard for diagnosis (Fig. 41-9), but CT scan with oral administration of contrast material is sometimes acceptable if the diagnosis is clear. If the results of these studies are normal but the level of suspicion is high, patients may require evaluation by direct laryngoscopy or endoscopy, depending on the clinical

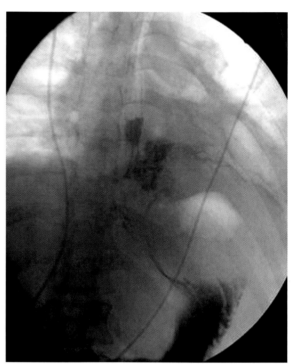

FIGURE 41-9 Barium esophagram demonstrating an esophageal perforation.

TABLE 41-3 **Pittsburgh Esophageal Perforation Score**

SCORE	<3	3-5	>5
Morbidity (%)	53	65	81
Mortality (%)	2	6	27
Duration of stay (days)	10	16	28

circumstance. Of note, procedural evaluation can convert a small or partial perforation into a more clinically significant process, so caution must be used with these procedures. Once the diagnosis is made, there are several therapeutic options that must be considered on an individual basis by a team of experienced surgeons as the subtleties of management preclude algorithmic treatment. Determining severity of injury to prognosticate morbidity and mortality can be done with a clinical severity score proposed by the Pittsburgh group (Table 41-3).[14] This score has been correlated with lower morbidity, lower mortality, and shorter hospital stay and can be used to guide treatment.

The principles of management after diagnosis include (1) treatment of contamination, (2) wide local drainage, (3) source control, and (4) enteral feeding access. In the circumstance of small perforations with contained leaks and no fluid collections in the mediastinum or chest, contamination might be minimal. In general, though, perforation is treated with broad-spectrum antibiotics, including antifungals, with duration that will vary on the basis of control of infection and the patient's condition. Drainage of the area with chest tubes is most common, with the number, location, and duration to vary by the degree of leak. In select cases, radiologically guided drains can be used as well.

Video-assisted thoracoscopic surgery or open thoracic washout with decortication may be necessary, depending on the duration of the leak and amount of pleural space soiling.

Source control will also depend on the patient's condition, the severity and location of perforation, and the surgeon's experience. Endoluminal therapy with covered stents has become more widely popularized and can give good results when it is used in the appropriate patient population. Although the criteria are still debated, stents can be considered in patients with early, small perforations, with minimal contamination in a location amenable to stenting.[15] Surgical control would be considered the gold standard, with approach depending on the location of the leak.[16] In general, high perforations are approached through a left-sided neck incision, midesophageal through a right thoracotomy, and distal esophageal through a left thoracotomy or laparotomy. Radiographic studies that demonstrate a right- or left-sided leak may modify the approach. Minimally invasive approaches are reasonable, depending on the surgeon's preference.

After the area of perforation is identified, assessment continues with myotomy to expose the injury, débridement of devitalized tissues, assessment of extent of injury, and considerations for repair. Any sign of obstruction (achalasia, stricture, tumor) must be remedied at the time of the initial operation, else the perforation will not heal. Small injuries with healthy tissues can be repaired primarily in two layers with tissue flap coverage (intercostal muscle, pericardial fat, pleura, omentum), but extensive injuries with devitalized areas can be managed with controlled fistulization by T-tube. Very large or devitalized defects will require esophageal exclusion with creation of a cervical esophagostomy and gastrostomy tube, with plans for future reconstruction by esophagectomy with gastric, colon, or small bowel conduit. Gastrostomy and jejunostomy tubes at the first operation can provide decompression and drainage near the perforation as well as enteral access for nutrition.

Caustic Ingestion

The majority of caustic ingestion is accidental small-volume drinking of household products by young children. In adults, it is more commonly a suicide attempt with large volumes, and therefore more extensive injury is usually present. The injury pattern can vary from short-segment superficial injury to full-thickness necrosis of the proximal gastrointestinal tract. There are many factors that affect the extent of injury (pH, volume, duration of exposure), and the evaluation and management after the ingestion are challenging and require experience and sound judgment.

The initial evaluation should involve a surgeon immediately. Physical examination findings of upper airway compromise (dyspnea, drooling, stridor, hoarseness) will likely require endotracheal intubation. However, this should be done with bronchoscopic guidance and preparation to perform cricothyroidotomy as there is danger of inability to secure a safe airway or iatrogenic perforation. Nasogastric and orogastric tubes should not be inserted blindly. Subsequent evaluation should include radiographic studies to guide the first procedure, ideally a CT scan of chest and abdomen with intravenous and oral administration of contrast material, followed by a barium swallow study.

Evaluation continues in the operating room. With rare exception, most patients should have an endoscopic evaluation of the degree and extent of injury. It is recommended that this be done early in the hospital course as the risk of perforation increases after 48 hours. Pediatric endoscopes are useful to minimize insufflation and mechanical stresses. The traditional teaching is that

TABLE 41-4 Classification Scheme for Caustic Ingestion	
ENDOSCOPIC FINDING	GRADE
Normal	0
Superficial edema/erythema	1
Mucosal/submucosal ulceration	2
Superficial edema/erythema	2A
Deep or circumferential	2B
Transmural ulcerations with necrosis	3
Focal necrosis	3A
Extensive necrosis	3B
Perforation	4

endoscopy should not proceed past an area of circumferential injury; however, an experienced endoscopist can cautiously proceed to complete the evaluation if it is thought that management will change with additional information. It is important to note location and degree of injury at all locations because subsequent evaluations are frequently necessary (Table 41-4).

All patients should be treated with broad-spectrum antibiotics. Depending on the clinical course, patients may benefit from repeated endoscopy 48 to 72 hours after the event to assess for signs of worsening injury. Of paramount importance is frequent clinical reassessment as deterioration at any time should prompt resumption of workup and surgical intervention as indicated. Surgical intervention can vary from endoscopy only to placement of gastrostomy or jejunostomy tubes or esophagectomy, gastrectomy, and small bowel resection with proximal diversion and feeding tube. Reconstruction can be complicated, sometimes requiring several months of recovery and the use of colon or small bowel conduits. In the long term, patients may develop strictures that require repeated dilation or eventual resection, fistulas that require surgical interventions, or esophageal cancer (>1000 times increased risk). The use of routine corticosteroids is no longer advocated. Early dilation, esophageal stents, and other adjunctive measures must be considered on a case-by-case basis.

Foreign Body Ingestion, Benign Tracheoesophageal Fistula, and Schatzki Ring

The patient with foreign body ingestion can require technical expertise to prevent iatrogenic perforation. If the object is lodged in the esophagus, careful endoscopy under general anesthesia is preferred. Forceful pushing to move the object into the stomach can result in perforation. Full relaxation, lubrication with water, and gentle pressure can sometimes be enough. Bringing the object proximally requires special large endoscopic graspers, nets, or lassoes along with patience and full visualization as the object is removed to prevent injury in the esophagus and oropharynx. Over-tubes are frequently useful in this setting, as is rigid esophagoscopy. If the object is not retrievable, laparoscopy or laparotomy with gastrotomy may be necessary. Evaluation of the full gastrointestinal tract is recommended with radiographs and CT scan before an intervention. Inpatient psychiatric evaluation and occasionally involuntary commitment are needed for the patient's safety.

Benign tracheoesophageal fistula can be seen in patients with multiple procedures or foreign objects in the upper mediastinum. A classic example of benign tracheoesophageal fistula is in the patient with endotracheal tube (or tracheostomy) and nasogastric tube. It is manifested most commonly with recurrent or persistent respiratory infection and bilious or salivary contents emanating from the tracheostomy. CT scan and barium swallow can be helpful in determining the diagnosis. Further evaluation is done with bronchoscopy and endoscopy, ensuring that bronchoscopy is performed such that the entire airway is evaluated; the tracheostomy may have to be temporarily removed during the endoscopy. If tracheoesophageal fistula is identified, treatment principles are (1) discontinuation of the causative agent, (2) consideration of exclusion of the fistula by stent or diversion, and finally (3) repair or delayed healing. In a stable patient, definitive repair may preclude the need for temporary exclusion or diversion. If the fistula was caused by a tracheostomy balloon, a longer or cuffless tracheostomy will be required. Antibiotics are usually employed as well. Enteral access and gastric decompression can be achieved with gastrostomy and jejunostomy tubes. Repair can be undertaken when the patient is medically suitable by either thoracotomy or cervical approach with resection of the fistula, possible primary repair or resection, and vascularized tissue interposition. Attempts at definitive repair in a compromised patient are not optimal. Delayed healing can occur if the offending agents are removed and diversion is successful. Esophageal stents can occasionally be used in this setting as well, although this must be determined on a case-by-case basis.

A Schatzki ring is a concentric, nonmalignant, fibrous thickening and narrowing of the GEJ with squamous epithelium above and columnar cells below (Fig. 41-10). The cause is unknown, with correlations to reflux disease and hiatal hernia that are still debated. Presence of a ring is not pathologic, but these can be seen in patients suffering from dysphagia or obstruction. In the symptomatic patient, whether the diagnosis is by esophagram or endoscopy, treatment is usually with dilation (bougie or balloon). The area should always be biopsied to rule out malignancy. Repeated dilation is often necessary and is a reasonable way to manage symptomatic rings as there are few permanent surgical

options. Persistent strictures should always raise suspicion for malignant disease.

ESOPHAGEAL NEOPLASMS AND DIAGNOSTIC APPROACHES TO ESOPHAGEAL CANCER

Epidemiology

Approximately 17,000 cases of esophageal cancer occur annually in the United States and about 480,000 cases occur worldwide.[17] Unfortunately, esophageal cancer typically is manifested at an advanced stage, and the majority of patients ultimately die of their disease. Worldwide, squamous cell carcinoma (SCC) is the most common histology, but in the United States, adenocarcinoma is more frequent. During the last 20 years, the incidence of adenocarcinoma has risen dramatically in Western countries with a concomitant decline in the incidence of SCC (Fig. 41-11).[18] This appears to be a true increase in incidence of adenocarcinoma rather than overdiagnosis as the overall stage distribution has not significantly shifted during this time. Other types of esophageal tumors, including mesenchymal tumors, neuroendocrine cancers, and benign tumors, are much more rare.

Tobacco and alcohol are strong risk factors for SCC, and they have a synergistic effect on risk. The disease is four times more prevalent in men, and race also appears to be a factor. The incidence of SCC is much higher among African Americans compared with their white counterparts, even after adjusting for socioeconomic status and tobacco and alcohol use. Worldwide, parts of the Middle East, central Asia, and China have the highest rates of SCC, after adjusting for tobacco and alcohol use, indicating that there may be some genetic predisposition or other environmental factors. The recognition of the importance of human papillomavirus (HPV) in the pathogenesis of SCC in other organs has spurred an interest in its role in esophageal SCC. Currently, it appears that HPV-related SCC represents only a small subset of esophageal SCC. For those tumors that are HPV related, the

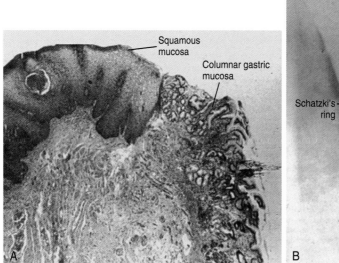
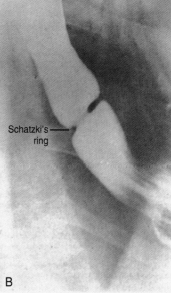

FIGURE 41-10 A, Histology of a Schatzki ring. **B,** Barium esophagram of a Schatzki ring. (**A** and **B,** Adapted from Wilkins EW Jr: Rings and webs. In Pearson FG, Cooper JD, Deslauriers J, et al, editors: *Esophageal surgery,* ed 2, New York, 2002, Churchill Livingstone.)

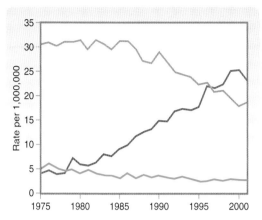

FIGURE 41-11 Trends in incidence of esophageal cancer histologic types (1975-2001). *Red line,* adenocarcinoma; *blue line,* squamous cell carcinoma; *green line,* not otherwise specified. (From Pohl H, Welch HG: The role of overdiagnosis and reclassification in the marked increase of esophageal adenocarcinoma incidence. *J Natl Cancer Inst* 97:142–146, 2005).

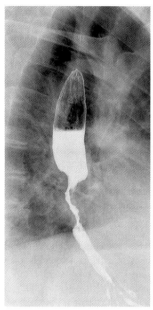

FIGURE 41-12 Barium esophagram demonstrating advanced carcinoma with abrupt, irregular narrowing in the distal esophagus, with more proximal dilation and air-fluid level.

clinical implications of HPV association are unclear. SCC is associated with certain intrinsic disorders of the esophagus, such as Plummer-Vinson syndrome and achalasia. Other hereditary cancer syndromes associated with esophageal SCC include tylosis and Fanconi anemia. Patients with a history of caustic ingestion are at significantly increased risk for SCC.

During the last 30 years, the incidence of esophageal adenocarcinoma has risen faster than any other cancer in the United States. It is now the most common histologic type of esophageal cancer in the United States. It is still relatively rare among African Americans and Asian Americans. Adenocarcinoma typically arises in the setting of Barrett esophagus. In addition to GERD, smoking and obesity are risk factors for adenocarcinoma. As with SCC, there is a male predominance. There are also familial forms of Barrett esophagus that increase the risk of adenocarcinoma.

SCC may arise in any part of the esophagus, but the majority of cases arise in the proximal and middle esophagus. In contrast, the majority of adenocarcinomas arise in the distal esophagus or GEJ. Under current American Joint Committee on Cancer (AJCC) and National Comprehensive Cancer Network staging guidelines, GEJ adenocarcinomas are staged and classified as esophageal cancers, with the exception of Siewert III tumors (tumors with an epicenter 2 to 5 cm below the GEJ).[19,20]

The majority of esophageal cancers are symptomatic at the time of diagnosis. Dysphagia is the most common symptom at presentation, with 74% of patients reporting difficulty in swallowing.[21] Often, patients will report progressive dysphagia, beginning with an initial episode after eating solid food. After the initial episode of dysphagia, many patients will adapt by chewing more thoroughly, avoiding hard foods, or drinking liquids with swallows. Thus, it is only after the dysphagia has worsened significantly that patients seek medical attention, by which point the majority have weight loss. Many patients with adenocarcinoma will endorse a long history of reflux symptoms including heartburn and regurgitation. Other associated findings may include fatigue, retrosternal pain, and anemia. Locally advanced tumors may be manifested with laryngeal nerve involvement causing hoarseness or with tracheoesophageal fistula. A careful physical examination should be performed with particular attention to cervical and supraclavicular lymph nodes. Early-stage tumors are often asymptomatic and are sometimes discovered during endoscopy done for Barrett esophagus.

Diagnosis and Staging

Barium esophagram may demonstrate irregular narrowing or ulceration (Fig. 41-12). The classic "apple-core" filling defect is seen only if there is symmetrical, circumferential narrowing. Instead, there is often an asymmetrical bulge seen with an infiltrative appearance.

The diagnosis of esophageal cancer is almost always made by endoscopic biopsy. Endoscopy should be performed in any patient with dysphagia, even if the barium esophagram is suggestive of a motility disorder. Classically, esophageal cancers appear as friable, ulcerated masses, but the endoscopic appearance can be varied. Early-stage tumors may appear as ulcerations or small nodules. More advanced tumors are more likely to be friable masses but may also appear as strictures or ulcerations. In many cases, the initial endoscopist may not recognize the presence of cancer and a single biopsy may not be diagnostic. Therefore, multiple biopsies should be performed for any suspicious lesions. During endoscopy, the location of the tumor relative to the incisors and GEJ should be noted, as well as the length of the tumor and degree of obstruction. The most proximal extent and circumferential extent of any Barrett esophagus should also be noted according to the Prague criteria. For small tumors or nodules, an experienced endoscopist should perform endoscopic mucosal resection (EMR) to provide a specimen that accurately assesses depth of invasion.

Once a diagnosis of esophageal cancer is made, accurate staging is essential to guide appropriate therapy and to predict prognosis. The most recent, seventh edition AJCC staging system acknowledged differences in the biology of adenocarcinoma and SCC by creating separate stage groupings for the two histologic types (Tables 41-5 to 41-7). The seventh edition staging classifies GEJ tumors as esophageal cancers as long as the tumor epicenter is within 5 cm of the GEJ. Tumor location also affects stage for SCC but not for adenocarcinoma (Fig. 41-13). The cervical esophagus begins at the hypopharynx and extends to the thoracic inlet, which is the level of the sternal notch. On endoscopy, this corresponds to approximately 15 to 20 cm from the incisors. The upper thoracic esophagus begins at the thoracic inlet and extends to the azygos vein. This is approximately 20 to 25 cm from the incisors. Midthoracic tumors arise from the lower border of the azygos vein to the inferior pulmonary vein. This is approximately 25 to 30 cm from the incisors. Lower tumors arise distal to the lower border of the inferior pulmonary vein to the GEJ. This is usually more than 30 cm from the incisors. Tumor grade is included in stage classification for earlier stage tumors.

Another major change in the staging system was the shift in nodal staging. The previous staging system classified celiac nodes as metastatic (M1a) for tumors of the lower esophagus, whereas cervical nodes were considered M1a for tumors of the upper thoracic esophagus. In the current system, all these nodes are considered regional regardless of the location of the primary tumor. Furthermore, nodal stage is based on the total number of involved nodes.

The depth of invasion of the tumor defines the T stage (Fig. 41-14). High-grade dysplasia encompasses all noninvasive neoplastic epithelium that was formerly classified as carcinoma in situ. T1a tumors invade the muscularis mucosa, whereas T1b tumors invade into the submucosa. T2 tumors invade the muscularis propria, and T3 tumors invade the adventitia but not

surrounding structures. T4a tumors invade adjacent structures that are usually resectable (diaphragm and pericardium). T4b tumors invade adjacent structures that are typically unresectable (trachea and aorta).

Small, superficial lesions that are evaluated by an experienced endoscopist may be resected by EMR without additional staging. In this setting, EMR provides adequate staging for depth of penetration (T stage) and may provide additional information about the risk of nodal metastasis. Endoscopic ultrasound (EUS) has less accuracy for superficial disease and will seldom obviate the need

TABLE 41-6 Stage Groupings for Esophageal Adenocarcinoma

STAGE	T	N	M	G
0	HGD	0	0	1
IA	1	0	0	1-2
IB	1	0	0	3
	2	0	0	1-2
IIA	2	0	0	3
IIB	3	0	0	Any
	1-2	1	0	Any
IIIA	1-2	2	0	Any
	3	1	0	Any
	4a	0	0	Any
IIIB	3	2	0	Any
IIIC	4a	1-2	0	Any
	4b	Any	0	Any
	Any	3	0	Any
IV	Any	Any	1	Any

From Edge S, Byrd DR, Compton CR, et al, editors: *AJCC cancer staging manual*, ed 7, New York, 2010, Springer-Verlag.
T, tumor status; *N*, lymph node status; *M*, metastasis; *G*, grade; *HGD*, high-grade dysplasia.

TABLE 41-5 Esophageal Carcinoma Stage Classifications

Primary Tumor (T)

TX	Tumor cannot be assessed
T0	No evidence of tumor
Tis	High-grade dysplasia
T1	Tumor invades the muscularis mucosa (T1a) or submucosa (T1b)
T2	Tumor invades into but not beyond the muscularis propria
T3	Tumor invades the adventitia
T4a	Tumor invades adjacent structures that are usually resectable (diaphragm and pericardium)
T4b	Tumor invades unresectable structures

Regional Lymph Nodes (N)

NX	Regional lymph nodes cannot be assessed
N0	No regional lymph node metastasis
N1	Metastasis in 1-2 regional lymph nodes
N2	Metastasis in 3-6 regional lymph nodes
N3	Metastasis in >7 regional lymph nodes

Distant Metastasis (M)

M0	No distant metastasis
M1	Distant metastasis

Histologic Grade

GX	Grade cannot be assessed—stage grouping as G1
G1	Well differentiated
G2	Moderately differentiated
G3	Poorly differentiated
G4	Undifferentiated—stage grouping as G3 squamous

TABLE 41-7 Stage Groupings for Esophageal Squamous Cell Carcinoma

STAGE	T	N	M	G	LOCATION
0	HGD	0	0	1	Any
IA	1	0	0	1	Any
IB	1	0	0	2-3	Any
	2-3	0	0	1	Lower
IIA	2-3	0	0	1	Upper, middle
	2-3	0	0	2-3	Lower
IIB	2-3	0	0		Upper, middle
	1-2	1	0	Any	Any
IIIA	1-2	2	0	Any	Any
	3	1	0	Any	Any
	4a	0	0	Any	Any
IIIB	3	2	0	Any	Any
IIIC	4a	1-2	0	Any	Any
	4b	Any	0	Any	Any
	Any	3	0	Any	Any
IV	Any	Any	1	Any	Any

From Edge S, Byrd DR, Compton CR, et al, editors: *AJCC cancer staging manual*, ed 7, New York, 2010, Springer-Verlag.
T, tumor status; *N*, lymph node status; *M*, metastasis; *G*, grade; *HGD*, high-grade dysplasia.

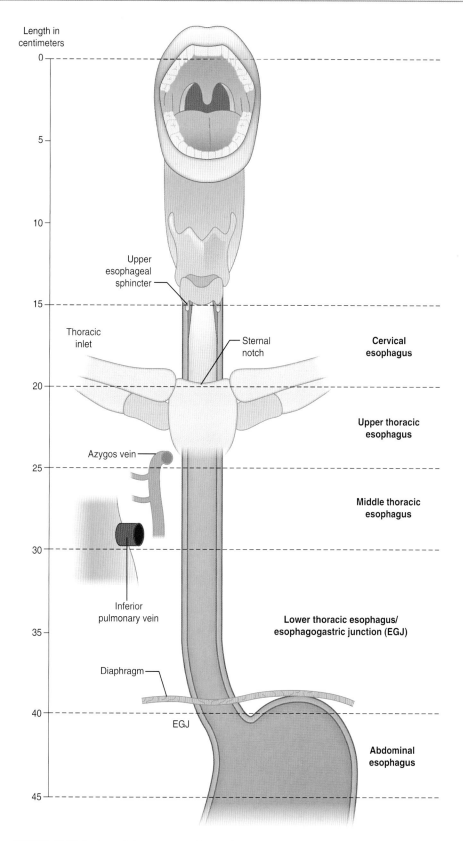

FIGURE 41-13 Regions of the esophagus. The cervical esophagus extends from the upper esophageal sphincter to the thoracic inlet. The upper thoracic esophagus extends from the thoracic inlet to the azygos vein. The midthoracic esophagus extends from the lower border of the azygos vein to the inferior pulmonary vein. The lower thoracic esophagus extends from the lower border of the inferior pulmonary vein to the gastroesophageal junction.

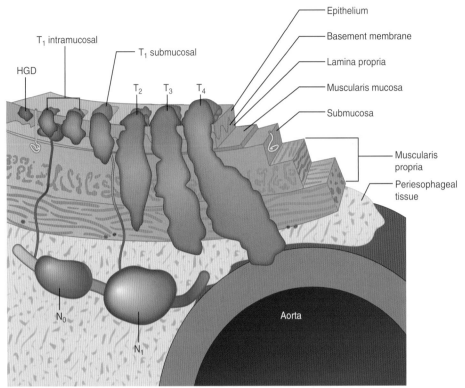

FIGURE 41-14 Tumor classification for esophageal carcinoma as defined by depth of invasion. *HGD*, high-grade dysplasia.

for EMR.[22,23] For T1a tumors resected by EMR, the risk of lymph node metastasis is very low, and additional staging studies are not required.

Most tumors, however, will be manifested as larger lesions. For these, we recommend further staging with a contrast-enhanced CT scan of the chest and abdomen and positron emission tomography (PET)/CT to evaluate for distant metastatic disease. If there is no evidence of distant metastatic disease, EUS should be performed to assess T stage and regional lymph nodes. Obtaining the PET/CT scan before EUS has several advantages. The PET/CT scan may demonstrate distant metastatic disease, eliminating the need for the patient to undergo EUS. The PET/CT scan may also identify a suspicious lymph node that can be specifically examined and sampled during the EUS procedure (Fig. 41-15). EUS is superior to CT or PET for assessment of both T and N stage. It is highly accurate for celiac nodal status with a sensitivity of 85% and specificity of 96%.[24] The accuracy rate is slightly lower for other regional lymph nodes because it is often impossible to biopsy peritumoral lymph nodes without traversing the tumor. Obstructing lesions may preclude EUS assessment. In these cases, dilation to perform EUS is associated with a risk of perforation. These risks must be weighed against the benefits of obtaining additional staging information. Most tumors with such tight stenoses are locally advanced and should likely be treated with multimodality therapy. Although EUS provides information about invasion of adjacent structures, bronchoscopy should also be performed for tumors above the carina to assess for direct tracheal invasion.

Appropriate staging is critical for treatment decisions. Superficial, T1a tumors can usually be treated with EMR. Locally

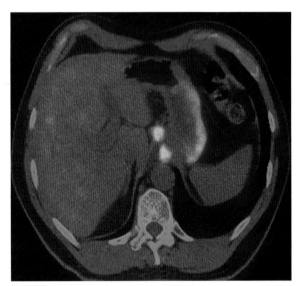

FIGURE 41-15 Fused transaxial PET/CT image demonstrating increased FDG activity in a gastroesophageal junction tumor and celiac lymphadenopathy.

advanced tumors (T3 tumors or T2 tumors with nodal involvement) require multimodality therapy. Stage IV disease requires systemic or palliative therapy. Without accurate staging, patients are likely to be either undertreated or overtreated, leading to decreased survival and quality of life.

Benign Tumors of the Esophagus

Benign tumors of the esophagus are less common than esophageal cancer. Among benign lesions, tumors of the submucosa and muscularis propria occur more frequently than mucosal tumors. Most of these lesions are asymptomatic and are identified incidentally on endoscopy. Barium esophagram characteristically demonstrates a smooth defect in the lumen.

Benign mucosal tumors include granular cell tumors and fibrovascular polyps. Granular cell tumors may be found in a variety of locations, including the skin, respiratory tract, gastrointestinal tract, breast, and tongue. Within the gastrointestinal tract, the distal third of the esophagus is the most common location. They appear as bulging lesions with a normal-appearing mucosa. Up to 11% of patients may have multiple lesions.[25] On EUS, lesions typically have regular borders and arise within the first and second sonographic layers. Because these lesions are usually covered by a layer of normal squamous epithelium, standard biopsies may be nondiagnostic. Tunneled biopsies will reveal eosinophilic granules. The tumors stain positive for S100, and it has been proposed that they arise from Schwann cells. Granular cell tumors are largely benign lesions, with only 1% to 2% having been described as malignant. Atypical features on EUS, large size (>2 cm), and presence of symptoms are reasonable indications for excision. Endoscopic resection is a valuable tool for these lesions when diagnosis is in question and for lesions smaller than 3 cm.[26]

Fibrovascular polyps are a heterogeneous group of soft tissue tumors most often found in the cervical esophagus at or near the cricopharyngeus. They appear cylindrical or elongated, with a stalk. Symptoms are rare, but large tumors may cause dysphagia and some may even prolapse into the hypopharynx, causing airway obstruction. Even large tumors can usually be resected endoscopically after securing the airway.

Squamous papillomas most often occur in the distal esophagus and are usually associated with some underlying inflammation. They appear as colorless, exophytic projections. Complete excision is warranted to rule out carcinoma and can usually be performed endoscopically.[27]

Benign submucosal tumors include lipomas, hemangiomas, and neural tumors. Lipomas have a characteristic, homogeneous, hyperechoic, smooth appearance on EUS. Symptoms are rare even with large tumors. Resection is seldom warranted. Hemangiomas typically appear as a purple or reddish nodule. EUS will demonstrate a smooth, hypoechoic, submucosal mass. Most tumors are asymptomatic. Lesions causing either dysphagia or bleeding can usually be treated endoscopically. Neural tumors including neurofibromas and schwannomas are rare in the esophagus. The majority are benign, with a handful of case reports on malignant esophageal schwannoma.[28] Symptomatic tumors can usually be resected by enucleation. Large tumors may require esophagectomy.

Leiomyomas are the most common benign tumors of the esophagus. They have a 2:1 male predominance. Although they are usually asymptomatic, large tumors may cause dysphagia or discomfort (Fig. 41-16). The tumors arise in the muscularis propria and are usually found in the mid to distal esophagus. Like most other benign esophageal tumors, they will demonstrate a smooth filling defect on barium esophagram. The endoscopic appearance is a round protrusion into the lumen of the esophagus with smooth, normal mucosa. On EUS, leiomyomas are hypoechoic, have regular borders, and arise from the muscularis mucosa, submucosa, or muscularis propria. Small, asymptomatic lesions with this appearance may be safely observed without

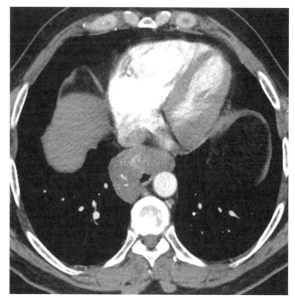

FIGURE 41-16 CT image of an 8-cm leiomyoma that was causing dysphagia. The lesion was enucleated thoracoscopically, and the patient's dysphagia resolved.

biopsy. Symptomatic lesions may be enucleated, and even large lesions can usually be removed with a minimally invasive approach.[29] One must keep in mind the differential diagnosis of a larger submucosal smooth tumor, including leiomyosarcoma, gastrointestinal stromal tumor (GIST), and leiomyoma.

Other Malignant Tumors of the Esophagus

Although SCC and adenocarcinoma represent the overwhelming majority of esophageal cancers, a variety of other malignant histologic types may be encountered. Small cell carcinomas of the esophagus account for 0.6% of esophageal cancers.[30] These tumors have the same aggressive phenotype and histologic appearance of other poorly differentiated neuroendocrine cancers. The tumors typically are manifested at an advanced stage, but stage-specific survival may be comparable to that of non–small cell esophageal carcinomas. Long-term survival is possible in earlier stage tumors treated with surgery. Neoadjuvant therapy appears to improve survival as well.

Primary melanoma of the esophagus is even rarer than small cell carcinoma, accounting for 0.1% to 0.2% of esophageal malignant neoplasms.[31] Similar to small cell carcinoma, most tumors are manifested at a late stage, and prognosis is generally poor.

GISTs and sarcomas of the esophagus are far less common than benign leiomyomas. GISTs have similar appearance to leiomyomas but can be distinguished histologically by CD117 stain positivity. Although well-differentiated leiomyosarcomas may be difficult to distinguish from leiomyomas, higher grade sarcomas often erode through the mucosa and will appear as an ulcerated or exophytic mass on endoscopy. EUS may show more irregular borders or a heterogeneous appearance that is uncharacteristic for leiomyoma. Local resection of small GISTs may be reasonable if negative margins can be achieved, but because of the propensity of the tumors to recur locally, formal esophagectomy should be performed for larger tumors.[32] Imatinib should be considered for any GIST larger than 3 cm or with other high-risk features. Imatinib may also be considered in the neoadjuvant setting for locally advanced tumors. In general, esophagectomy is the treatment of choice for leiomyosarcomas. Other sarcomas of the esophagus have been reported but are much more rare. Lymph node metastasis is an unusual event in these mesenchymal tumors.

Approach to Early-Stage Esophageal Cancer

In the last 10 years, there has been a significant shift in the way early-stage esophageal cancers are treated.[33] Improved endoscopic technology as well as a better understanding of the biology of early-stage tumors has led to the increased use of endoscopic therapies for the diagnosis, staging, and treatment of early-stage esophageal cancers. It is likely that surgery will play a smaller role for superficial cancers as endoscopic and ablative therapies continue to evolve and biomarkers of prognosis are refined. Given the changing nature of these treatments, multidisciplinary care with surgeons, gastroenterologists, and pathologists is essential to providing patients with the best long-term outcomes.

High-Grade Dysplasia and Superficial Cancers

Dysplasia arising in Barrett esophagus is characterized by cytologic malignant changes including atypical nuclei, increased mitoses, and lack of surface maturation. High-grade dysplasia is distinguished from low-grade dysplasia by more prominent cytologic or architectural derangements. As long as the cells are confined to the epithelium without invasion of the basement membrane, the pathology should be described as dysplasia regardless of the degree of abnormality. This encompasses what was previously referred to as carcinoma in situ. Historically, esophagectomy was often recommended for patients with high-grade dysplasia for a number of reasons. In the past, endoscopic biopsies were relatively inaccurate, and up to 50% of patients who underwent esophagectomy for high-grade dysplasia were found to have invasive cancer in the surgical specimen. Also, therapies to reverse or to halt the progression of dysplasia to invasive cancer were unavailable. Although esophagectomy had very high rates of cure for high-grade dysplasia, it was associated with significant morbidity.

Overtreatment has also been a concern. Despite the data that many patients with high-grade dysplasia have invasive cancer found on esophagectomy, there is evidence from other groups reporting that only a minority of patients with flat high-grade dysplasia develop invasive cancer on follow-up endoscopy.[34] Some of the conflict may be due to interobserver variation in the

diagnosis of high-grade dysplasia versus invasive adenocarcinoma on biopsy specimens and the practice of diligent search for cancer at some institutions. Any biopsy specimens with high-grade dysplasia or invasive adenocarcinoma should be reviewed by a specialty pathologist experienced with Barrett esophagus and esophageal cancer. In contrast to the high rates of cancer development in patients with high-grade dysplasia, the incidence of cancer with nondysplastic Barrett esophagus appears to be low. The largest study of endoscopic surveillance in patients with Barrett esophagus found that the annual risk for development of cancer was 0.39% in patients with no dysplasia versus 0.77% in patients with low-grade dysplasia.[35]

The Seattle biopsy protocol is still widely accepted for mapping of Barrett esophagus with high-grade dysplasia. This involves four-quadrant biopsies at 1-cm intervals along the entire length of Barrett esophagus in addition to targeted biopsies of all visible lesions. Emerging endoscopic imaging techniques increase the sensitivity for detection of dysplasia. Many specialty centers routinely use high-resolution endoscopy and some sort of chromoendoscopy or simulated chromoendoscopy, such as narrow-band imaging (Olympus), to evaluate Barrett esophagus. Narrow-band imaging uses light filters to allow more narrow wavelengths of light. The wavelengths penetrate only superficially and are absorbed well by hemoglobin, better revealing irregular mucosal vascular patterns (Fig. 41-17). Additional technologies include autofluorescence endoscopy, confocal endomicroscopy, and optical coherence tomography. These techniques hold promise for even greater resolution but require more specialized training and equipment compared with the relatively user-friendly technology of high-resolution endoscopy and narrow-band imaging.

Therapeutics

Ablation. Various endoscopic ablative and resection techniques have been developed that have largely supplanted the role of esophagectomy for high-grade dysplasia. The most commonly used technology today is radiofrequency ablation (RFA). RFA is much more effective than photodynamic therapy with a lower stricture (and overall complication) rate. RFA may be delivered with a circumferential balloon or an electrical plate using a bipolar electrode that transmits radiofrequency energy, which generates heat and destroys superficial tissue. The treated mucosa is replaced by neosquamous mucosa. The standard ablation program uses two

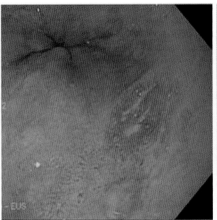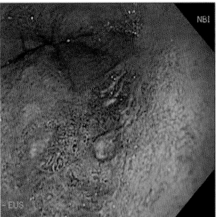

FIGURE 41-17 Traditional, white light view of Barrett esophagus with high-grade dysplasia *(left)* and narrow-band imaging of the same area *(right)*.

double pulses of 12 J/cm^2. The balloon is then repositioned distally, and the procedure is repeated until the entire segment of Barrett esophagus is treated. If there are areas of residual Barrett esophagus on follow-up endoscopy, those segments may be treated with more focal ablation.

Multiple studies have demonstrated the effectiveness of RFA for eradicating Barrett esophagus and dysplasia. In the Ablation of Intestinal Metaplasia (AIM-II) trial, 81% of patients with high-grade dysplasia and 90% of patients with low-grade dysplasia had eradication of dysplasia.[36] Only 4% of patients had their dysplasia progress to a higher grade of dysplasia or cancer. In a multicenter European trial of 136 patients randomly assigned to RFA versus surveillance, 1.5% of patients treated with ablation progressed to cancer versus 8.8% in the surveillance arm.[37] RFA was able to eradicate dysplasia in 93% of patients.

Cryotherapy. Cryotherapy is an alternative ablative technique that uses extreme cold rather than heat to destroy tissue. There have been no head-to-head comparisons between cryotherapy and RFA, but reports indicate similar efficacy to RFA.[38] Cryotherapy is generally well tolerated with little pain and low stricture rates. One advantage of cryotherapy compared with RFA is that cryotherapy does not require a probe to be in contact with the tissue. However, a decompression tube is required to prevent overdistention of the stomach and intestine with gas.

Regardless of what ablation technology is used, patients should have close surveillance and long-term acid suppression after ablation. A repeated endoscopy should be performed 3 months after ablative therapy, preferably with high-resolution endoscopy and some form of chromoendoscopy. Many patients will require more than one ablation session to eradicate all Barrett esophagus. There is also a small risk that areas of Barrett epithelium could be hidden beneath areas of the new squamous epithelium, known as buried glands. Malignancy can arise within these buried glands, and these cancers may be more difficult to identify during endoscopy. The clinical significance of this phenomenon is unknown, and the incidence of malignancy developing within these areas of buried glands appears to be very low.[39] Nevertheless, the potential implications of unrecognized incomplete eradication justifies future surveillance of ablated patients. After eradication of Barrett esophagus, fundoplication may also be considered for the treatment of reflux, although studies have not conclusively demonstrated effectiveness of antireflux surgery for prevention of esophageal cancer.

Endoscopic mucosal resection. One limitation of ablative therapies is the limited depth of penetration. Another disadvantage is the lack of definitive pathologic analysis. Therefore, patients with nodular or raised Barrett esophagus or other abnormalities suggestive of superficial invasive cancer should undergo EMR rather than ablation. EMR provides larger specimens to accurately determine the depth of invasion. EMR resects the full thickness of the mucosa, down into the submucosa (Fig. 41-18). Therefore, it is a good therapeutic option for superficial lesions with a low risk of nodal metastases. Depending on the size of the lesion, degree of differentiation, and lymphovascular invasion, the overall risk of nodal metastasis for lesions confined to the mucosa (T1a) ranges from less than 2% to more than 15% (Table 41-8).[40] For selected T1a lesions, EMR is highly effective (Fig. 41-19).[41] Although EMR can technically remove lesions involving the submucosa (T1b), the risk of lymph node involvement increases with depth of submucosal invasion. Therefore, EMR is generally not considered adequate for tumors involving the submucosa. Lesions involving only the most superficial third of the submucosa (SM1) have relatively low rates of nodal metastases, typically reported as less than 30%. On the other hand, lesions involving the deepest third of the submucosa (SM3) may have nodal involvement in more than 50% of cases.[42] T1b cancers with squamous cell histology also appear to have a higher risk of nodal metastasis compared with adenocarcinoma (45% versus 26%).[43] Thorough and accurate pathologic assessment is critical to formulating treatment plans. In patients who are poor surgical candidates, EMR of SM1 adenocarcinomas with low-risk features may be a reasonable treatment option. Likewise, for patients who are good surgical candidates, esophagectomy is a reasonable option for T1a lesions with high-risk features. EUS has low accuracy for assessing T stage for superficial tumors, so patients with suspected T1 lesions should have EMR performed by a qualified endoscopist to obtain accurate staging. Complications of EMR include bleeding, stricture, pain, and perforation. The stricture risk is increased for patients requiring circumferential resection. Although EMR may be performed for the entire segment of Barrett esophagus, complication rates are lower if EMR is focused on specific areas combined with ablation for residual Barrett esophagus.

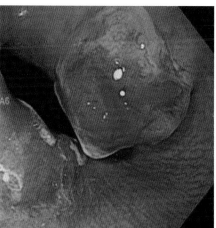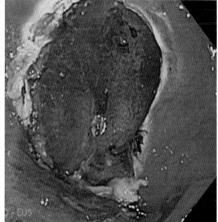

FIGURE 41-18 A superficial T1a adenocarcinoma arising in the setting of Barrett esophagus *(left)* and submucosal defect after endoscopic mucosal resection *(right)*.

TABLE 41-8 Nomogram for Prediction of Lymph Node Metastases in Early-Stage Esophageal Cancer

VARIABLE		POINTS
Size, per cm		+ 1 (per cm)
Depth		
T1a		+ 0
T1b		+ 2
Differentiation		
Well		+ 0
Moderate		+ 3
Poor		+ 3
Lymphovascular invasion		+ 6

RISK CATEGORY	POINTS	PREDICTED RISK OF LYMPH NODE METASTASES (%)
Low	0-1	≤2
Moderate	2-4	3-6
High	5+	≥7

Adapted from Lee L, Ronellenfitsch U, Hofstetter WL, et al: Predicting lymph node metastases in early esophageal adenocarcinoma using a simple scoring system. *J Am Coll Surg* 217:191–199, 2013.

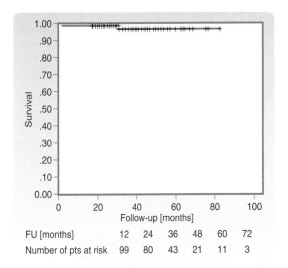

FU [months]	12	24	36	48	60	72
Number of pts at risk	99	80	43	21	11	3

FIGURE 41-19 Survival curve of patients undergoing endoscopic mucosal resection for low-risk, superficial esophageal adenocarcinoma. (From Ell C, May A, Pech O, et al: Curative endoscopic resection of early esophageal adenocarcinomas [Barrett's cancer]. *Gastrointest Endosc* 65:3–10, 2007.)

EMR may be performed with a submucosal lifting technique, which raises the target lesion by injecting fluid into the submucosa beneath the lesion. This allows the lesion to be suctioned more easily into a cap, creating a pseudopolyp, allowing resection with a snare. Another technique uses suction to raise the lesion, allowing a band to be placed at the base of the pseudopolyp that is created and then using a snare to resect. One drawback of EMR is that larger lesions are typically removed piecemeal. Reports describe the efficacy of endoscopic submucosal dissection using an endoscopic needle knife that allows greater submucosal dissection and en bloc resection of larger lesions.[44] The safety of this technique outside a few specialized centers is unknown.

Surveillance is an important component of the treatment for superficial esophageal cancers. Patients should receive high-dose acid suppression therapy with a PPI to help EMR and ablation sites to heal. Many patients require multiple procedures to completely eradicate Barrett epithelium. Short-interval follow-up endoscopy should be performed 3 months after endoscopic treatment is completed. Any residual Barrett epithelium may be focally ablated at that time. Surveillance endoscopies should be performed frequently (i.e., every 3 months) for the first year after endoscopic treatment for high-grade dysplasia or intramucosal cancer, after which time the frequency of endoscopic surveillance may be spaced out. For superficial lesions treated endoscopically, radiologic imaging, such as fluorodeoxyglucose (FDG) PET, has no value.

Esophagectomy. The role of esophagectomy as a single-modality treatment for esophageal cancer is diminishing. Most tumors are found after symptoms develop, at which point they are usually locally advanced or metastatic. Locally advanced tumors should be treated with multimodality therapy. Asymptomatic tumors are usually found during surveillance for Barrett esophagus. These are typically superficial and can be treated with EMR with lower complication rates than with esophagectomy. This leaves a relatively narrow subset of tumors that are treated appropriately with surgery only. As discussed earlier, T1b tumors have significant risk for nodal metastasis and in general should be treated with esophagectomy. High-risk T1a lesions (larger tumors or lesions with lymphovascular invasion) could also be considered for esophagectomy. Extensive, multifocal lesions and ulcerated tumors may also be difficult to eradicate endoscopically and would be appropriate candidates for esophagectomy.

An area of controversy is the optimal treatment for clinical T2N0 tumors. Esophagectomy with an adequate lymphadenectomy would be expected to confer an overall 5-year survival of anywhere between 40% and 65% for a pathologic T2N0 cancer, depending on histology, grade, and location of tumor.[20] Unfortunately, a clinical stage of T2N0 is inaccurate in the majority of cases, and many patients are found to have node-positive disease on final pathology after esophagectomy. Clinical T2N0 patients were included in the CROSS trial, which compared neoadjuvant chemoradiation followed by surgery versus surgery alone for esophageal and GEJ cancer. Although the trial demonstrated a survival benefit for the neoadjuvant chemoradiation arm, clinical T2N0 patients represented only a small subset of the study cohort, and it is unclear how much benefit these patients in particular received.[45] It is clear that many patients with clinical T2N0 disease are understaged, but retrospective analyses indicate that there may not be a survival advantage for neoadjuvant therapy in this group.[46] One management strategy may be to selectively offer neoadjuvant therapy to patients with clinical T2N0 disease based on other high-risk factors, such as long T2N0 tumors. Similarly, an equal number of patients with cT2N0 are actually overstaged, so liberal use of diagnostic EMR is appropriate.

The advent of EMR also influences the type of esophagectomy that should be performed in early-stage esophageal cancer. Because of the potential for decreased complication and improved physiologic outcomes, vagal-sparing esophagectomy has been advocated by some for intramucosal adenocarcinoma and high-grade dysplasia. However, most low-risk lesions are now resected by EMR. Because standard lymphadenectomy is not performed as part of vagal-sparing esophagectomy, it is not appropriate for the majority of patients who are undergoing surgery for higher risk lesions. Minimally invasive esophagectomy is also a technique that is gaining favor. Long-term survival has not been directly compared with open esophagectomy in a prospective fashion, but one small, randomized trial reported reduced postoperative complications with a minimally invasive approach.[56]

Patients have increasing options for the treatment of early-stage esophageal cancers. Care needs to be individualized so patients may make informed decisions, balancing the effectiveness of therapies with their risks and impact on quality of life.

Locally Advanced Esophageal Cancer

Despite improved awareness of the increasing trend in esophageal adenocarcinoma and more frequent detection of early esophageal adenocarcinoma on surveillance endoscopies, the majority of patients with esophageal cancer still present with locally advanced or metastatic disease. Usually, it is not until patients experience dysphagia, which generally signifies transmural tumor involvement (T3), that an esophageal cancer is diagnosed. In this setting, the probability of lymph node metastases reaches 80%, so the majority of patients present with clinical stage T3N1-3 according to the seventh edition (AJCC) of esophageal cancer staging. It should be stressed that the seventh edition of esophageal cancer staging is based on the pathology specimen from patients treated with surgical therapy alone, and therefore its utility in the clinical pretreatment setting in the era of multimodality therapy is arguably limited. However, compared with the sixth edition, which grouped all patients with positive nodal disease into N1 status, current staging recognized the prognostic value in the number of metastatic lymph nodes and grouped patients into three categories: N1 (one to three positive nodes), N2 (four to six positive nodes), and N3 (seven or more positive nodes). The anatomic location of the regional nodal disease relative to the primary tumor is no longer considered an important factor; however, in clinical practice, nodal disease location continues to influence treatment decisions. This confusion is partly due to the lack of consensus and definition of which nodal stations represent regional versus distant metastatic disease. In the era of multimodality therapy and selective surgery, the rigorous definition of locally advanced esophageal cancer is necessary to guide pretreatment therapeutic decisions before committing to either aggressive locoregional therapy or initiating systemic treatment.

For esophageal adenocarcinoma, mostly located in the distal esophagus or GEJ, we consider nodal disease located in the area from the celiac axis up to the paratracheal region to represent regional disease; nodal disease located outside of these boundaries is regarded as distant disease. For esophageal SCC, which mostly arises in the mid or proximal esophagus, periesophageal cervical lymphadenopathy is still considered a regional disease. Whereas the current staging system takes the tumor differentiation into account, it is mainly the disease burden that dictates the decisions about the treatment strategy, and therapeutic decisions are best discussed in a multidisciplinary setting.

The Evolution and Principles of Multimodality Therapy for Locally Advanced Esophageal Carcinoma

Surgical resection of the esophagus was the mainstay of esophageal cancer treatment in the past. However, we have learned that even the most radical resections with extensive lymph node dissections are not adequate to cure locoregionally advanced disease in the majority of cases. Distant recurrence or metastatic disease continues to be the main cause of death in patients with esophageal cancer.

Our understanding and treatment of esophageal cancer have evolved significantly during the last 100 years. The initial recognition that a localized esophageal cancer may be cured with surgical resection dates back to the first successful esophagectomy performed by Franz Torek in 1913. Despite rather poor perioperative outcomes at that time, surgery became a supplement to radiation as the treatment of choice for localized esophageal cancer in the early 20th century. Over time, more extensive en bloc esophageal resections and lymphadenectomy became favored with the hope that radical resection of disease would result in a cure more frequently. However, similar to Halstead's radical mastectomy, we have learned that whereas extended esophagectomy may lead to better locoregional control, it fails to achieve cure in patients destined to die of metastatic disease. Today, technical aspects of esophagectomy are still passionately debated as the technologic advances enable us to perform these procedures safely even with less invasive or robotically assisted techniques. From an oncologic standpoint, however, surgical therapy has its limits in what it can contribute to the cure rate of esophageal cancer. Moreover, there continues to be a tremendous variability in the performance of surgical resection of the esophagus among surgeons, with some favoring transthoracic and some transabdominal approaches with varied extents of lymph node dissections. This lack of procedural standardization confounds the analysis of esophageal cancer treatment outcomes.

Increased understanding of cancer biology led to the development of nonsurgical treatment strategies for solid organ malignant neoplasms, including esophageal carcinoma. Chemotherapy was combined concomitantly with radiation therapy to improve the local-regional efficacy and potentially for systemic effect. Intuitively, this strategy targets both local disease and systemic micrometastases. The demonstrated efficacy of this treatment paradigm subsequently stimulated interest in combining surgery, radiation, and chemotherapy to maximize the treatment effect. The combination of these treatment modalities became the focus of several clinical trials investigating the role and timing of each method.

Treatment Modalities Used in Locally Advanced Esophageal Cancer

Radiation therapy. Radiation was employed as the first treatment modality for esophageal cancer. Early experiences with radium bougies and external beam radiation demonstrated esophageal tumor regression with occasional complete tumor responses. With the evolution of surgical care, radiation became a part of a multidisciplinary approach to esophageal cancer therapy with the goal of sterilizing areas within or around the operative field. Early randomized trials of neoadjuvant radiation administered doses of 20 to 40 Gy before resection in an attempt to decrease local recurrence and to improve survival rates. With one exception, all of these trials included patients with SCC only, and none of the trials demonstrated significant benefits of adding radiation therapy to resection.

Although the lower radiation doses (20 to 40 Gy) may have been inadequate, clinicians were wary of combining higher dose radiation before surgery, given the toxicity risks (note that radiation delivery and particles used in therapy were very different in the past compared with current therapy). Nonetheless, high rates of locoregional recurrence after surgery led to the consideration of adjuvant radiation therapy for esophageal cancer. The rationale for this approach was the ability to deliver higher doses (40 to

60 Gy) of radiation postoperatively without worsening perioperative complications. Postoperative radiation therapy for esophageal cancer appeared to be potentially beneficial in several trials, although the data are conflicting and subject to selection bias.

Chemotherapy. The cause of death from esophageal cancer is mainly due to metastatic disease. Intuitively, systemic chemotherapy has the potential to target micrometastatic deposits. Even in the setting of a seemingly localized disease, it usually downstages marginally resectable tumors, allowing improved complete (R0) resection rates, and decreases the incidence of locoregional recurrence.[47] The synergistic effect of chemotherapy with radiation strengthens the argument for its use. Importantly, when it is administered preoperatively, the biologic response can be evaluated and quantified pathologically in terms of pathologic tumor histoviability, and the degree of this response has been correlated as an indicator of outcome. Current chemotherapeutic regimens are based on platinum compounds (cisplatin and carboplatin) in combination with 5-fluorouracil or taxanes as a doublet. In several prospective randomized trials, researchers compared chemotherapy followed by surgery with surgery alone for both esophageal adenocarcinoma and SCC (Table 41-9).[48] The landmark trial by Roth and colleagues demonstrated longer median survival durations in patients with major or complete response to chemotherapy, which highlighted the biologic diversity of esophageal cancers and their varied susceptibility to chemotherapy.[49] One of the largest randomized trials using chemotherapy and surgery versus surgery alone in esophageal cancer patients was the North American Intergroup Trial (INT 0113).[50] This trial did not demonstrate better survival with chemotherapy plus surgery than with surgery alone in either histologic type. However, inaccurate staging, response evaluation, and high toxicity rates leading to a low surgical incidence confound the results of the study. Contrary to the INT 0113 trial, a phase 3 study run by the Medical Research Council (MRC) in the United Kingdom consisting of chemotherapy plus surgery versus surgery alone in locally advanced esophageal cancer demonstrated survival benefit of chemotherapy.[51] The largest trial of its kind, the MRC trial included 802 patients randomized to receive chemotherapy plus esophagectomy versus esophagectomy alone. The survival benefit of chemotherapy persisted at the updated median follow-up duration of 6 years, with 5-year survival rates of 23% with chemotherapy plus surgery

and 17% with surgery alone ($P = .03$). Both adenocarcinoma and SCC patients experienced benefit. Another commonly referenced trial that demonstrated survival advantage and better R0 resection rate of neoadjuvant chemotherapy and surgery over surgery alone was the MRC Adjuvant Gastric Infusional Chemotherapy (MAGIC) trial by Cunningham and colleagues.[52] The majority of the enrolled patients had gastric carcinoma, with only a subgroup having esophageal or GEJ tumors.

In the adjuvant setting, the results of chemotherapy have not been convincing. The majority of trials were in the esophageal SCC setting, such as a phase 3 multicenter Japan Clinical Oncology Group trial (JCOG 9204), or JCOG 9907, which randomized 330 patients comparing the effects of neoadjuvant (164 patients) and adjuvant (166 patients) chemotherapy for stage II and stage III esophageal SCC.[53] Patients received the same two cycles of cisplatin and 5-fluorouracil as in JCOG 9204 before or after radical resection. The interim analysis demonstrated a significantly better ($P = .044$) median progression-free survival duration in the neoadjuvant group (3 years) than in the adjuvant group (2 years) and the difference in estimated 5-year overall survival rate of 60% versus 38% in the neoadjuvant and adjuvant arms, respectively ($P = .013$). On the basis of these findings, it was recommended to terminate the trial. The limitations of this study included disproportionate compliance with therapy between the two groups, omission of postoperative chemotherapy in patients with pN0 disease based on the JCOG 9204 results, and premature termination of the trial. In adenocarcinoma histology, the effects of adjuvant chemotherapy on survival after R0 resection was studied in a phase 2 Eastern Cooperative Oncology Group trial (E8296).[54] The median 2-year overall survival rate was 60%, which appeared to be better than that in historical controls. Similarly, Ferri and colleagues demonstrated a greater than 60% 3-year overall survival, with a preponderance of stage III patients (AJCC sixth edition), treated with perioperative docetaxel, cisplatin, and 5-fluorouracil.[55]

Chemoradiation alone. Chemoradiation may be administered in a preoperative or postoperative setting, as definitive bimodality therapy, or as part of trimodality therapy when combined with surgery. Concomitant administration of chemotherapy and radiation has a synergistic effect with increased tumor cytotoxicity at low doses. The validity of chemoradiation use for all locations

TABLE 41-9 **Randomized Trials Comparing Chemotherapy and Surgery versus Surgery Alone**

TRIAL	N	HISTOLOGY	CHEMOTHERAPY	R0 (%)	SURVIVAL
MRC		SCC, ADC	Cisplatin, 5-FU		Median (months)
CT	400			60	17
Sx	402			54	13
RTOG 8911		SCC, ADC	Cisplatin, 5-FU		Median (months)
CT	213			63	14.9
Sx	227			59	16.1
MAGIC		ADC	Epirubicin, cisplatin, 5-FU	NA	5 years (%)
CT	250				36*
Sx	253				23
FFCD		ADC	Cisplatin, 5-FU		5 years (%)
CT	113			84	38*
Sx	111			74	24

Adapted from Cools-Lartigue J, Spicer J, Ferri LE: Current status of management of malignant disease: Current management of esophageal cancer. *J Gastrointest Surg* 19:964–972, 2015.

ADC, adenocarcinoma; *CT*, chemotherapy; *5-FU*, 5-fluorouracil; *SCC*, squamous cell carcinoma; *Sx*, surgery.
*$P < .05$.

of esophageal cancer is based on encouraging results of definitive chemoradiation for cervical esophageal SCC. Randomized trials of chemoradiation versus radiation alone include RTOG 85-01 by Herskovic and colleagues, which established that a group of patients with esophageal SCC or adenocarcinoma could be cured with bimodality therapy alone. To improve on the favorable outcomes observed in the RTOG 85-01 trial, researchers attempted to increase locoregional disease control rates in the subsequent Intergroup 0123/RTOG 94-05 trial by modifying the intensity of radiation therapy to high-dose 64.8 Gy given concurrently with chemotherapy. Unfortunately, at a median follow-up duration of 16 months, the survival and locoregional disease control rates with the higher radiation dose did not differ significantly from those in the RTOG 85-01 trial, but the toxicity and treatment-related deaths were worse in the high-dose radiation therapy group. This study established that 50.4 Gy of radiation used concomitantly with chemotherapy is both a neoadjuvant and potentially definitive dose.[56]

Chemoradiation and surgery. When used alone, each cancer treatment modality has its limitations, ranging from inadequate therapeutic effect to excessive toxicity. The synergistic effect of chemoradiation combined with surgical resection maximizes the chances of effectively treating both locoregional disease and potential undetectable metastases (Table 41-10). Early clinical trials testing a trimodality treatment paradigm did not demonstrate a survival advantage over surgery alone. Many of these trials were underpowered and mixed SCC and esophageal adenocarcinoma histology as well as varied radiation and chemotherapy regimens. Some trials suffered from poor patient accrual or inconsistent surgical outcomes. The most notable and frequently quoted trial that compared chemoradiation followed by surgery with surgery alone for esophageal and EGJ cancer was the Chemoradiotherapy for Oesophageal Cancer Followed by Surgery Study (CROSS).[57] This trial enrolled an impressive 368 patients during a 4-year period, and 366 patients were included in the final analysis. The surgery-alone group consisted of 188 patients, whereas 178 underwent chemoradiation followed by surgery. The majority (75%) of the patients had adenocarcinoma, and 22% had SCC. The chemoradiation regimen consisted of a 5-week course of carboplatin and paclitaxel administered concurrently with radiation therapy at a dose of 41.4 Gy given in 23 fractions 5 days a week. Esophagectomy was performed within 4 to 6 weeks in the treatment group and immediately after randomization in the control group. The completeness (R0) of resection was higher in the trimodality group than in the surgery-alone group (92% versus 69%; $P < .001$). Patients with SCC experienced complete pathologic response (ypT0N0M0) significantly more than patients with adenocarcinoma (49% versus 29%; $P < .001$). Expectedly, nodal positivity was higher in patients with surgery alone compared with the trimodality group (75% versus 31%; $P < .001$). At a median follow-up duration of 45 months, patients receiving the trimodality therapy had significantly longer median overall survival

TABLE 41-10 Randomized Trials Comparing Chemoradiation and Surgery versus Surgery Alone

TRIAL	N	HISTOLOGY	CHEMOTHERAPY	RT (Gy)	pCR (%)	R0 (%)	SURVIVAL
Walsh		ADC	Cisplatin, 5-FU	40	25	NA	3 years (%)
CT-RT-Sx	58						32*
Sx	55						6
Bosset		SCC	Cisplatin	37	26	NA	Median (months)
CT-RT-Sx	143						18.6
Sx	149						18.6
Urba		SCC, ADC	Cisplatin, 5-FU, vinblastine	45	28	90	3 years (%)
CT-RT-Sx	50					90	30*
Sx	50						16
Lee		SCC	Cisplatin, 5FU	45.6	43		Median (months)
CT-RT-Sx	51					100	27.3
Sx	50					87.5	28.2
Burmeister		SCC, ADC	Cisplatin, 5-FU	35	16		Median (months)
CT-RT-Sx	128					80*	22.2
Sx	128					59	19.3
Tepper		SCC, ADC	Cisplatin, 5-FU	50.4	33	NR	5 years (%)
CT-RT-Sx	30						39*
Sx	26						16
CROSS		SCC, ADC	Carboplatin, paclitaxel	41.4	29		5 years (%)
CT-RT-Sx	178					92*	47*
Sx	188					69	34
Mariette		SCC, ADC	Cisplatin, 5-FU	45	33.3		3 years (%)
CT-RT-Sx	98					93.8	47.5
Sx	97					92.1	53

Adapted from Cools-Lartigue J, Spicer J, Ferri LE: Current status of management of malignant disease: Current management of esophageal cancer. *J Gastrointest Surg* 19:964–972, 2015.
ADC, adenocarcinoma; *CT,* chemotherapy; *5-FU,* 5-fluorouracil; *NA,* not available; *NR,* not reported; *pCR,* pathologic complete response; *RT,* radiotherapy; *SCC,* squamous cell carcinoma; *Sx,* surgery.
*$P > .05$.

duration (49.4 months) than did patients undergoing surgery alone (24 months; hazard ratio [HR], 0.65; 95% confidence interval [CI], 0.49-0.87; P = .003). The estimated 5-year survival rate in the trimodality therapy group was 47% compared with 34% (HR, 0.65; 95% CI, 0.49-0.87; P = .003) in the surgery group. Interestingly, trimodality therapy did not significantly benefit patients with adenocarcinoma histology (HR, 0.74; 95% CI, 0.53-1.02; P = .07), and inexplicably it benefited patients with clinically node-negative disease (HR, 0.42; 95% CI, 0.23-0.74; P = .003) but not those with node-positive disease (HR, 0.80; 95% CI, 0.57-1.13; P = .21).

The Role of Surgery in Trimodality Therapy and Salvage Surgery

Subsequent to the CROSS trial report, many Western centers adopted the trimodality therapy as the standard of care for the treatment of esophageal carcinoma. However, this trial still left many questions unanswered about the treatment strategy for locoregional esophageal carcinoma. Whereas we have observed that neoadjuvant chemoradiation improves R0 resection and locoregional recurrence rates and results in pathologic complete responses in many patients, other subgroups of patients clearly derive no benefit from neoadjuvant therapy over surgery alone. Equally, patients who are "cured" by neoadjuvant chemoradiation derive no additional survival benefit from further surgical extirpation of the esophagus. We are currently unable to identify these groups of patients and must search for simple, reproducible, and validated surrogate markers predictive of treatment outcome. So far, only histopathologic tumor response after neoadjuvant therapy has emerged as a predictor of survival in esophageal cancer patients.[58] Surgical resection and evaluation of histopathologic tumor response will therefore continue to play a role in the treatment of esophageal cancer in upcoming years.

Nevertheless, both randomized trials comparing preoperative chemotherapy versus preoperative chemoradiation failed to show a significant difference between the two treatment approaches (Table 41-11).[59,60] Indeed, the latest meta-analysis inclusive of 24 trials and 4188 patients focusing on survival after neoadjuvant chemotherapy or chemoradiotherapy for resectable esophageal carcinoma provided strong evidence for survival benefit of multimodality therapy versus surgery alone.[61] The ideal preoperative treatment regimen, however, has yet to be determined, with no clear benefit of neoadjuvant chemoradiation over chemotherapy having been demonstrated.

Some authors have debated the value of surgery after bimodality therapy. Two trials of chemoradiation versus chemoradiation

and surgery suggested that there was no advantage to surgical resection. However, both these trials had unacceptably high perioperative mortality rates.[62,63] Murphy and colleagues[64] subsequently showed that surgical resection and tumor differentiation were the only independent predictors of survival in a retrospective analysis. Clearly, impeccable perioperative outcomes are necessary to demonstrate oncologic benefit of surgical therapy. Hence, one strategy is to use esophageal resection selectively, only in the setting of disease persistence or recurrence after definitive chemoradiation. This treatment paradigm was the focus of the RTOG 0246 phase 2 trial by Swisher and colleagues.[65] The study was designed to detect improvement in 1-year survival from 60% to 77.5% in patients undergoing selective or salvage esophagectomy. More than 70% of enrolled patients had T3 or N1 disease stage. Forty-one patients were included in the analysis, of whom 21 (51%) underwent salvage esophagectomy because of residual or recurrent disease; one patient requested resection. Patients with complete clinical response after definitive chemoradiation had overall survival of 53%, with clinical incomplete response of 33% and clinical incomplete response salvaged by surgery of 41%. Salvage esophagectomy after definitive chemoradiation is a feasible treatment strategy and seems to provide additional survival benefit in patients with incomplete clinical response after definitive chemoradiation.

Surveillance

Patients who have received definitive chemoradiation therapy (bimodality therapy) for esophageal cancer continue to suffer from the fear that the disease may reappear again either as locoregional or distant metastatic recurrence. The purpose behind the periodic surveillance of patients who completed definitive bimodality therapy is to potentially implement salvage therapy for locoregional failure. Evidence-based surveillance algorithms are not available; however, most providers observe patients every 3 to 6 months with clinical examination and a variety of imaging or endoscopy studies. This strategy is often costly and anxiety-provoking for patients, and it may not change the ultimate outcome for the patient. Considering the fact that more than 98% of local recurrences occur in the first 36 months, most authors suggest vigilant surveillance during this time after bimodality therapy to potentially catch recurrences early enough to render salvage surgery a feasible strategy.

Palliative Options for Esophageal Carcinoma

Patients with poor performance status or distant metastatic disease at the time of diagnosis are not candidates for aggressive

TABLE 41-11   Randomized Trials Comparing Chemoradiation and Surgery versus Chemotherapy and Surgery

TRIAL	N	HISTOLOGY	CHEMOTHERAPY	CHEMORADIOTHERAPY	pCR (%)	R0 (%)	SURVIVAL
Stahl		ADC	Cisplatin, 5-FU	Induction: cisplatin, 5-FU			3 years (%)
CT-RT	60			Concurrent: cisplatin, etoposide	15.6*	72	47.4
CT	59			(30 Gy)	2	69	27.7
Burmeister		ADC	Cisplatin, 5-FU	Cisplatin			Median (months)
CT-RT	39			5-FU (35 Gy)	31*	84.6	32
CT	36				8	80.5	29

Adapted from Cools-Lartigue J, Spicer J, Ferri LE: Current status of management of malignant disease: Current management of esophageal cancer. *J Gastrointest Surg* 19:964–972, 2015.
ADC, adenocarcinoma; *CT*, chemotherapy; *5-FU*, 5-fluorouracil; *pCR*, pathologic complete response; *RT*, radiotherapy.
*P < .05.

locoregional therapy. The goal of treatment in these circumstances is either to palliate existing symptoms or potentially to avoid future complications related to the disease extent. Metastatic esophageal carcinoma may be manifested with a variety of symptoms, depending on the disease spread; however, dysphagia, odynophagia, chest pain, fatigue, and weight loss are likely to be among the most common symptoms. Palliative treatment is always individualized on the basis of a patient's physiologic status, symptoms, disease extent, and wishes. Options for palliation range from best supportive care for symptom control to the use of chemotherapy or radiation, esophageal stent placement, and enteral nutrition support. With advancements in image-guided percutaneous and endoscopic procedures, surgical procedures for palliation of esophageal carcinoma have become exceedingly rare.

This concise review of achalasia gives a thorough overview of the evolution of the cause and pathogenesis of this disease.

Yammamoto S, Kawahara K, Maekawa T: Minimally invasive esophagectomy for stage I and II esophageal cancer. *Ann Thorac Surg* 80:2070–2075, 2005.

This is one of the largest series of esophageal cancer patients undergoing a minimally invasive procedure to treat early-stage disease. It has become an important study, suggesting that minimally invasive surgery may be a viable option in these patients.

SUMMARY

Multimodality therapy using a combination of neoadjuvant chemotherapy with or without radiation followed by surgery is presently regarded as the standard of care for either locally advanced esophageal adenocarcinoma or SCC. Whereas some patients benefit from this aggressive locoregional treatment strategy, the majority of patients continue to develop distant metastatic disease, which is presently incurable. As the search for molecular predictors and targeted therapies for this cancer continues, we will have to rigorously test novel agents to determine their places in the therapeutic armamentarium. Standardized perioperative care in well-designed clinical trials will be imperative so the potential therapeutic benefit of surgery is not offset by unacceptably high perioperative mortality rates. The heterogeneity of esophageal adenocarcinoma will require novel treatment strategies to improve personalized treatment outcomes of this cancer.

SELECTED REFERENCES

Banki F, Mason RJ, DeMeester SR: Vagal-sparing esophagectomy: A more physiologic alternative. *Ann Surg* 236:324–335, 2002.

This was the first paper to document physiologic outcomes of vagal-sparing esophagectomy in detail (the surgery was first described by Akiyama).

Gu Y, Swisher SG, Ajani JA, et al: The number of lymph nodes with metastasis predicts survival in patients with esophageal cancer or esophagogastric junction adenocarcinoma who receive preoperative chemoradiotherapy. *Cancer* 106:1017–1025, 2006.

This paper discusses the notion that in addition to location and response to neoadjuvant therapy, the number of lymph nodes may be one of the most significant predictors of outcome.

Orringer MB, Sloan H: Esophagectomy without thoracotomy. *J Thorac Cardiovasc Surg* 76:643–654, 1978.

This landmark paper was the first to describe the transhiatal esophagectomy and to document the outcomes in detail.

Park W, Vaezi MF: Cause and pathogenesis of achalasia: The current understanding. *Am J Gastroenterol* 101:202–203, 2006.

REFERENCES

1. Kahrilas PJ, Bredenoord AJ, Fox M, et al: The Chicago Classification of esophageal motility disorders, v3.0. *Neurogastroenterol Motil* 27:160–174, 2015.
2. Code CF, Schlegel JF, Kelley ML, Jr, et al: Hypertensive gastroesophageal sphincter. *Proc Staff Meet Mayo Clin* 35:391–399, 1960.
3. Stavropoulos SN, Desilets DJ, Fuchs KH, et al: Per-oral endoscopic myotomy white paper summary. *Surg Endosc* 28:2005–2019, 2014.
4. Inoue H, Sato H, Ikeda H, et al: Per-oral endoscopic myotomy: A series of 500 patients. *J Am Coll Surg* 221:256–264, 2015.
5. Boeckxstaens GE, Annese V, des Varannes SB, et al: Pneumatic dilation versus laparoscopic Heller's myotomy for idiopathic achalasia. *N Engl J Med* 364:1807–1816, 2011.
6. Zenker FA, von Ziemssen HW: Krankheiten des Oesophagus. *Leipzig* 1867.
7. Bonavina L, Bona D, Abraham M, et al: Long-term results of endosurgical and open surgical approach for Zenker diverticulum. *World J Gastroenterol* 13:2586–2589, 2007.
8. Campos GM, Peters JH, DeMeester TR, et al: Multivariate analysis of factors predicting outcome after laparoscopic Nissen fundoplication. *J Gastrointest Surg* 3:292–300, 1999.
9. Richter JE, Pandolfino JE, Vela MF, et al: Utilization of wireless pH monitoring technologies: A summary of the proceedings from the esophageal diagnostic working group. *Dis Esophagus* 26:755–765, 2013.
10. Ganz RA, Peters JH, Horgan S, et al: Esophageal sphincter device for gastroesophageal reflux disease. *N Engl J Med* 368:719–727, 2013.
11. Awais O, Luketich JD, Reddy N, et al: Roux-en-Y near esophagojejunostomy for failed antireflux operations: Outcomes in more than 100 patients. *Ann Thorac Surg* 98:1905–1911, discussion 1911–1913, 2014.
12. Kahrilas PJ, Shaheen NJ, Vaezi MF, et al: American Gastroenterological Association Medical Position Statement on the management of gastroesophageal reflux disease. *Gastroenterology* 135:1383–1391, 1391.e1–5, 2008.
13. Skinner DB, Little AG, DeMeester TR: Management of esophageal perforation. *Am J Surg* 139:760–764, 1980.
14. Abbas G, Schuchert MJ, Pettiford BL, et al: Contemporaneous management of esophageal perforation. *Surgery* 146:749–755, discussion 755–756, 2009.

15. Sepesi B, Raymond DP, Peters JH: Esophageal perforation: Surgical, endoscopic and medical management strategies. *Curr Opin Gastroenterol* 26:379–383, 2010.

16. Rice R, Dubose JJ, Spicer JD, et al: Perforated esophageal intervention focus (PERF) study: A multi-center study of contemporary management. *J Thorac Cardiovasc Surg* 2015. [in press].

17. Siegel RL, Miller KD, Jemal A: Cancer statistics, 2015. *CA Cancer J Clin* 65:5–29, 2015.

18. Pohl H, Welch HG: The role of overdiagnosis and reclassification in the marked increase of esophageal adenocarcinoma incidence. *J Natl Cancer Inst* 97:142–146, 2005.

19. Strong VE, D'Amico TA, Kleinberg L, et al: Impact of the 7th Edition AJCC staging classification on the NCCN clinical practice guidelines in oncology for gastric and esophageal cancers. *J Natl Compr Canc Netw* 11:60–66, 2013.

20. Rice TW, Rusch VW, Ishwaran H, et al: Cancer of the esophagus and esophagogastric junction: Data-driven staging for the seventh edition of the American Joint Committee on Cancer/International Union Against Cancer Cancer Staging Manuals. *Cancer* 116:3763–3773, 2010.

21. Daly JM, Fry WA, Little AG, et al: Esophageal cancer: Results of an American College of Surgeons Patient Care Evaluation Study. *J Am Coll Surg* 190:562–572, discussion 572–573, 2000.

22. Pouw RE, Heldoorn N, Alvarez Herrero L, et al: Do we still need EUS in the workup of patients with early esophageal neoplasia? A retrospective analysis of 131 cases. *Gastrointest Endosc* 73:662–668, 2011.

23. Dhupar R, Rice RD, Correa AM, et al: Endoscopic ultrasound estimates for tumor depth at the gastroesophageal junction are inaccurate: Implications for the liberal use of endoscopic resection. *Ann Thorac Surg* 2015. [Epub ahead of print].

24. van Vliet EP, Heijenbrok-Kal MH, Hunink MG, et al: Staging investigations for oesophageal cancer: A meta-analysis. *Br J Cancer* 98:547–557, 2008.

25. Orlowska J, Pachlewski J, Gugulski A, et al: A conservative approach to granular cell tumors of the esophagus: Four case reports and literature review. *Am J Gastroenterol* 88:311–315, 1993.

26. Chen WS, Zheng XL, Jin L, et al: Novel diagnosis and treatment of esophageal granular cell tumor: Report of 14 cases and review of the literature. *Ann Thorac Surg* 97:296–302, 2014.

27. Carr NJ, Monihan JM, Sobin LH: Squamous cell papilloma of the esophagus: A clinicopathologic and follow-up study of 25 cases. *Am J Gastroenterol* 89:245–248, 1994.

28. Murase K, Hino A, Ozeki Y, et al: Malignant schwannoma of the esophagus with lymph node metastasis: Literature review of schwannoma of the esophagus. *J Gastroenterol* 36:772–777, 2001.

29. Bonavina L, Segalin A, Rosati R, et al: Surgical therapy of esophageal leiomyoma. *J Am Coll Surg* 181:257–262, 1995.

30. Kukar M, Groman A, Malhotra U, et al: Small cell carcinoma of the esophagus: A SEER database analysis. *Ann Surg Oncol* 20:4239–4244, 2013.

31. Hu YM, Yan JD, Gao Y, et al: Primary malignant melanoma of esophagus: A case report and review of literature. *Int J Clin Exp Pathol* 7:8176–8180, 2014.

32. Lott S, Schmieder M, Mayer B, et al: Gastrointestinal stromal tumors of the esophagus: Evaluation of a pooled case series

33. Berry MF, Zeyer-Brunner J, Castleberry AW, et al: Treatment modalities for T1N0 esophageal cancers: A comparative analysis of local therapy versus surgical resection. *J Thorac Oncol* 8:796–802, 2013.

34. Schnell TG, Sontag SJ, Chejfec G, et al: Long-term nonsurgical management of Barrett's esophagus with high-grade dysplasia. *Gastroenterology* 120:1607–1619, 2001.

35. de Jonge PJ, van Blankenstein M, Looman CW, et al: Risk of malignant progression in patients with Barrett's oesophagus: A Dutch nationwide cohort study. *Gut* 59:1030–1036, 2010.

36. Shaheen NJ, Sharma P, Overholt BF, et al: Radiofrequency ablation in Barrett's esophagus with dysplasia. *N Engl J Med* 360:2277–2288, 2009.

37. Phoa KN, van Vilsteren FG, Weusten BL, et al: Radiofrequency ablation vs endoscopic surveillance for patients with Barrett esophagus and low-grade dysplasia: A randomized clinical trial. *JAMA* 311:1209–1217, 2014.

38. Shaheen NJ, Greenwald BD, Peery AF, et al: Safety and efficacy of endoscopic spray cryotherapy for Barrett's esophagus with high-grade dysplasia. *Gastrointest Endosc* 71:680–685, 2010.

39. Gray NA, Odze RD, Spechler SJ: Buried metaplasia after endoscopic ablation of Barrett's esophagus: A systematic review. *Am J Gastroenterol* 106:1899–1908, quiz 1909, 2011.

40. Lee L, Ronellenfitsch U, Hofstetter WL, et al: Predicting lymph node metastases in early esophageal adenocarcinoma using a simple scoring system. *J Am Coll Surg* 217:191–199, 2013.

41. Ell C, May A, Pech O, et al: Curative endoscopic resection of early esophageal adenocarcinomas (Barrett's cancer). *Gastrointest Endosc* 65:3–10, 2007.

42. Shimada H, Nabeya Y, Matsubara H, et al: Prediction of lymph node status in patients with superficial esophageal carcinoma: Analysis of 160 surgically resected cancers. *Am J Surg* 191:250–254, 2006.

43. Gockel I, Sgourakis G, Lyros O, et al: Risk of lymph node metastasis in submucosal esophageal cancer: A review of surgically resected patients. *Expert Rev Gastroenterol Hepatol* 5:371–384, 2011.

44. Hirasawa K, Kokawa A, Oka H, et al: Superficial adenocarcinoma of the esophagogastric junction: Long-term results of endoscopic submucosal dissection. *Gastrointest Endosc* 72:960–966, 2010.

45. van Hagen P, Hulshof MC, van Lanschot JJ, et al: Preoperative chemoradiotherapy for esophageal or junctional cancer. *N Engl J Med* 366:2074–2084, 2012.

46. Speicher PJ, Ganapathi AM, Englum BR, et al: Induction therapy does not improve survival for clinical stage T2N0 esophageal cancer. *J Thorac Oncol* 9:1195–1201, 2014.

47. Ajani JA, Roth JA, Ryan B, et al: Evaluation of pre- and postoperative chemotherapy for resectable adenocarcinoma of the esophagus or gastroesophageal junction. *J Clin Oncol* 8:1231–1238, 1990.

48. Cools-Lartigue J, Spicer J, Ferri LE: Current status of management of malignant disease: Current management of esophageal cancer. *J Gastrointest Surg* 19:964–972, 2015.

49. Roth JA, Pass HI, Flanagan MM, et al: Randomized clinical trial of preoperative and postoperative adjuvant chemotherapy with cisplatin, vindesine, and bleomycin for carcinoma

of the esophagus. *J Thorac Cardiovasc Surg* 96:242–248, 1988.

50. Kelsen DP, Winter KA, Gunderson LL, et al: Long-term results of RTOG trial 8911 (USA Intergroup 113): A random assignment trial comparison of chemotherapy followed by surgery compared with surgery alone for esophageal cancer. *J Clin Oncol* 25:3719–3725, 2007.

51. Medical Research Council Oesophageal Cancer Working Group: Surgical resection with or without preoperative chemotherapy in oesophageal cancer: A randomised controlled trial. *Lancet* 359:1727–1733, 2002.

52. Cunningham D, Allum WH, Stenning SP, et al: Perioperative chemotherapy versus surgery alone for resectable gastroesophageal cancer. *N Engl J Med* 355:11–20, 2006.

53. Ando N, Kato H, Igaki H, et al: A randomized trial comparing postoperative adjuvant chemotherapy with cisplatin and 5-fluorouracil versus preoperative chemotherapy for localized advanced squamous cell carcinoma of the thoracic esophagus (JCOG9907). *Ann Surg Oncol* 19:68–74, 2012.

54. Armanios M, Xu R, Forastiere AA, et al: Adjuvant chemotherapy for resected adenocarcinoma of the esophagus, gastro-esophageal junction, and cardia: Phase II trial (E8296) of the Eastern Cooperative Oncology Group. *J Clin Oncol* 22:4495–4499, 2004.

55. Ferri LE, Ades S, Alcindor T, et al: Perioperative docetaxel, cisplatin, and 5-fluorouracil (DCF) for locally advanced esophageal and gastric adenocarcinoma: A multicenter phase II trial. *Ann Oncol* 23:1512–1517, 2012.

56. Minsky BD, Pajak TF, Ginsberg RJ, et al: INT 0123 (Radiation Therapy Oncology Group 94-05) phase III trial of combined-modality therapy for esophageal cancer: High-dose versus standard-dose radiation therapy. *J Clin Oncol* 20:1167–1174, 2002.

57. Shapiro J, van Lanschot JJ, Hulshof MC, et al: Neoadjuvant chemoradiotherapy plus surgery versus surgery alone for oesophageal or junctional cancer (CROSS): Long-term results of a randomised controlled trial. *Lancet Oncol* 16:1090–1098, 2015.

58. Francis AM, Sepesi B, Correa AM, et al: The influence of histopathologic tumor viability on long-term survival and recurrence rates following neoadjuvant therapy for esophageal adenocarcinoma. *Ann Surg* 258:500–507, 2013.

59. Stahl M, Walz MK, Stuschke M, et al: Phase III comparison of preoperative chemotherapy compared with chemoradiotherapy in patients with locally advanced adenocarcinoma of the esophagogastric junction. *J Clin Oncol* 27:851–856, 2009.

60. Burmeister BH, Thomas JM, Burmeister EA, et al: Is concurrent radiation therapy required in patients receiving preoperative chemotherapy for adenocarcinoma of the oesophagus? A randomised phase II trial. *Eur J Cancer* 47:354–360, 2011.

61. Sjoquist KM, Burmeister BH, Smithers BM, et al: Survival after neoadjuvant chemotherapy or chemoradiotherapy for resectable oesophageal carcinoma: An updated meta-analysis. *Lancet Oncol* 12:681–692, 2011.

62. Bedenne L, Michel P, Bouche O, et al: Chemoradiation followed by surgery compared with chemoradiation alone in squamous cancer of the esophagus: FFCD 9102. *J Clin Oncol* 25:1160–1168, 2007.

63. Stahl M, Stuschke M, Lehmann N, et al: Chemoradiation with and without surgery in patients with locally advanced squamous cell carcinoma of the esophagus. *J Clin Oncol* 23:2310–2317, 2005.

64. Murphy CC, Correa AM, Ajani JA, et al: Surgery is an essential component of multimodality therapy for patients with locally advanced esophageal adenocarcinoma. *J Gastrointest Surg* 17:1359–1369, 2013.

65. Swisher SG, Winter KA, Komaki RU, et al: A phase II study of a paclitaxel-based chemoradiation regimen with selective surgical salvage for resectable locoregionally advanced esophageal cancer: Initial reporting of RTOG 0246. *Int J Radiat Oncol Biol Phys* 82:1967–1972, 2012.

42 | CHAPTER

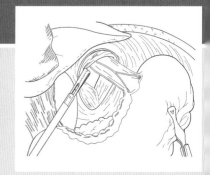

Gastroesophageal Reflux Disease and Hiatal Hernia

Robert B. Yates, Brant K. Oelschlager, Carlos A. Pellegrini

第四十二章　胃食管反流病与食管裂孔疝

中文导读

　　本章共分3节：①胃食管反流性疾病；②食管裂孔疝；③总结。

　　第一节主要介绍了胃食管反流性疾病（gastro-esophageal reflux disease，GERD）的病理生理学、临床表现、诊断方法及治疗。GERD发生的原因主要与食管下括约肌自身抗反流机制失效有关。其典型症状为胸骨后不适、反酸和胃灼热感。动态pH和阻抗监测、食管测压、食管胃镜及钡餐有助于GERD的诊断。GERD的内科保守治疗主要为服用质子泵抑制药（proton pump inhibitor，PPI）药物。如长期服用PPI效果不佳则可考虑抗反流手术。本节还介绍了GERD治疗最新进展EsophyX和LINX装置。

　　第二节主要介绍了食管裂孔疝（paraesophageal hernia，PEH）的病理生理学基础、临床症状、术前评估、手术修复等内容。促进PEH形成的两个关键事件是食管裂孔处膈肌脚的扩大和膈食管膜的拉伸。PEH的最常见症状包括气短、胸骨后烧灼感、间歇性腹胀、腹痛等。钡餐、胃镜、食管测压为常用术前评估手段。动态pH监测便于复发病人的评估。目前大多数PEH修补术都可通过腹腔镜手术进行。含4个关键步骤：①还纳疝内容物；②完全切除疝囊；③充分游离远端食管至少3 cm；④抗反流操作。

　　第三节总结了在腹腔镜手术时代，GERD和PEH的手术治疗已变得越来越普遍，且并发症越来越少发生。根据临床症状、对药物治疗的反应及术前检查评估有助于医生精心挑选病人。

〔朱　珉〕

Gastroesophageal reflux disease (GERD) is the most common benign medical condition of the stomach and esophagus. In patients with GERD who experience persistent life-limiting symptoms despite maximal medical therapy, antireflux surgery should be strongly considered. The application of laparoscopy to antireflux surgery has decreased perioperative morbidity, hospital length of stay, and cost compared with open operations. Conceptually, laparoscopic antireflux surgery (LARS) is straightforward; however, the correct construction of a fundoplication requires significant operative experience and skills in complex laparoscopy. In patients who present with late complications of antireflux surgery, including recurrent GERD and dysphagia, reoperative antireflux surgery can be effectively performed. Compared with first-time operations, however, reoperative antireflux surgery is technically more challenging, is associated with higher risk of perioperative complications, and results in less durable symptom improvement. Consequently, surgeons should have a higher threshold for performing reoperative antireflux surgery, and reoperations should be performed by experienced, high-volume gastroesophageal surgeons. To decrease perioperative risk and to maximize long-term relief of GERD symptoms, surgeons must be familiar with all aspects of preoperative evaluation and operative management of patients with GERD.

Hernias at the esophageal hiatus span the spectrum from a small sliding hiatal hernia to a large paraesophageal hernia (PEH). Similarly, the symptoms of PEH can vary from mild gastroesophageal obstructive symptoms to severe, acute complications, including gastric volvulus, which requires immediate intervention. The repair of a large PEH is challenging, but when it is performed at high-volume centers by experienced surgeons, hiatal hernia and PEH can be repaired safely and provide patients with long-lasting control of gastroesophageal symptoms.

GASTROESOPHAGEAL REFLUX DISEASE

Pathophysiology

Endogenous antireflux mechanisms include the lower esophageal sphincter (LES) and spontaneous esophageal clearance. GERD results from the failure of these endogenous antireflux mechanisms.

The LES has the primary role of preventing reflux of gastric contents into the esophagus. Rather than a distinct anatomic structure, the LES is a zone of high pressure located in the lower end of the esophagus. The LES can be identified with esophageal manometry.

The LES is made up of four anatomic structures:
1. The *intrinsic musculature of the distal esophagus* is in a state of tonic contraction. Within 500 milliseconds of the initiation of a swallow, these muscle fibers relax to allow passage of liquid or food into the stomach, and then they return to a state of tonic contraction.
2. *Sling fibers of the gastric cardia* are oriented diagonally from the cardia-fundus junction to the lesser curve of the stomach. Located at the same anatomic depth as the circular muscle fibers of the esophagus, the sling fibers contribute significantly to the high-pressure zone of the LES (Fig. 42-1).
3. The *crura of the diaphragm* surround the esophagus as it passes through the esophageal hiatus. During inspiration, when intrathoracic pressure decreases relative to intra-abdominal pressure, the anteroposterior diameter of the crural opening is decreased, compressing the esophagus and increasing the measured pressure at the LES. Because of this fluctuation in LES

pressure, it is important to measure the LES pressure at mid-expiration or end-expiration.
4. When the gastroesophageal junction (GEJ) is firmly anchored in the abdominal cavity, *increased intra-abdominal pressure* is transmitted to the GEJ, which increases the pressure on the distal esophagus and prevents spontaneous reflux of gastric contents.

Gastroesophageal reflux (GER) occurs when intragastric pressure is greater than the high-pressure zone of the distal esophagus. This can develop under two conditions: the LES resting pressure is too low (i.e., hypotensive LES); and the LES relaxes in the absence of peristaltic contraction of the esophagus (i.e., spontaneous LES relaxation). Hypotensive LES is frequently associated with hiatal hernia because of displacement of the GEJ into the posterior mediastinum. However, hypotensive LES can occur in its normal anatomic position, and even small changes in the high-pressure zone can compromise its effectiveness. Consequently, it is important to recognize that GER is a normal physiologic process that occurs even in the setting of a normal LES. The distinction between physiologic reflux (i.e., GER) and pathologic reflux (i.e., GERD) hinges on the total amount of esophageal acid exposure, the patient's symptoms, and the presence of mucosal damage of the esophagus.

Hiatal hernias are often associated with GERD because their abnormal anatomy compromises the efficacy of the LES. Hiatal hernias are classified into four types (I to IV). Type I hiatal hernia (Fig. 42-2A), also called a sliding hiatal hernia, is the most common. A type I hernia is present when the GEJ migrates cephalad into the posterior mediastinum. This occurs because of laxity of the phrenoesophageal membrane, a continuation of the endoabdominal peritoneum that reflects onto the esophagus at the hiatus (Fig. 42-3). A small sliding hernia does not necessarily imply an incompetent LES, but the larger its size, the greater the risk for abnormal GER. Furthermore, the presence of a type I sliding hiatal hernia alone does not constitute an indication for operative repair. In fact, many patients with small type I hiatal hernias do not have symptoms and do not require treatment.

Hiatal hernia types II to IV, also referred to as PEH, are frequently associated with gastroesophageal obstructive symptoms (e.g., dysphagia, early satiety, and epigastric pain). However, they can also be associated with GERD. A type II hernia (Fig. 42-2B) occurs when the GEJ is anchored in the abdomen, and the gastric fundus migrates into the mediastinum through the hiatal defect. A type III hernia (Fig. 42-2C) is characterized by both the GEJ and fundus located in the mediastinum. Finally, a type IV hernia occurs when any visceral structure (e.g., colon, spleen, pancreas, or small bowel) migrates cephalad to the esophageal hiatus and is located in the mediastinum. For more information on PEH, refer to the last section of this chapter.

Clinical Presentation
Typical Symptoms of GERD
The prevalence of symptoms among 1000 patients with GERD is presented in Table 42-1. Heartburn, regurgitation, and water brash are the three typical esophageal symptoms of GERD. Heartburn and regurgitation are the most common presenting symptoms. Heartburn is specific to GERD and described as an epigastric or retrosternal caustic or stinging sensation. Typically, it does not radiate to the back and is not described as a pressure sensation, which are more characteristic of pancreatitis and acute coronary syndrome, respectively. It is important to ask the patient about his or her symptoms in detail to differentiate typical heartburn

from symptoms of peptic ulcer disease, cholelithiasis, or coronary artery disease.

The presence of regurgitation often indicates progression of GERD. In severe cases, patients will be unable to bend over without experiencing an episode of regurgitation. Regurgitation of gastric contents to the oropharynx and mouth can produce a sour taste that patients will describe as either acid or bile. This phenomenon is referred to as water brash. In patients who report regurgitation as a frequent symptom, it is important to distinguish between regurgitation of undigested food and regurgitation of digested food. Regurgitation of undigested food is not common

in GERD and suggests the presence of a different pathologic process, such as an esophageal diverticulum or achalasia.

Extraesophageal Symptoms of GERD

Extraesophageal symptoms of GERD arise from the respiratory tract and include both laryngeal and pulmonary symptoms (Box 42-1). Two mechanisms may lead to extraesophageal symptoms of GERD. First, proximal esophageal reflux and microaspiration

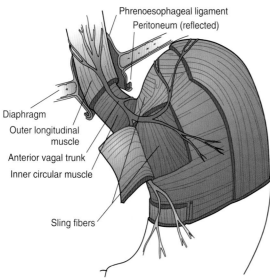

FIGURE 42-1 Schematic drawing of the muscle layers at the gastroesophageal junction. The intrinsic muscle of the esophagus, diaphragm, and sling fibers contribute to lower esophageal sphincter pressure. The circular muscle fibers of the esophagus are at the same depth as the sling fibers of the cardia.

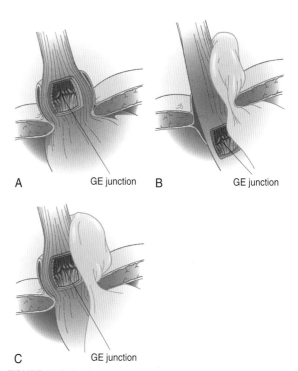

FIGURE 42-2 The three types of hiatal hernia. **A,** Type I is also called a sliding hernia. **B,** Type II is known as a rolling hernia. **C,** Type III is referred to as a mixed hernia. *GE,* gastroesophageal.

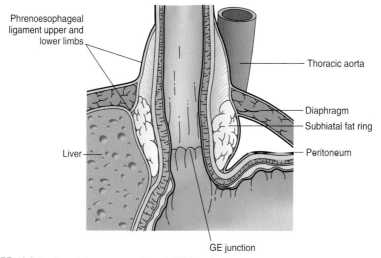

FIGURE 42-3 Section of the gastroesophageal (GE) junction demonstrates the relationship of the peritoneum to the phrenoesophageal membrane. The phrenoesophageal membrane continues as a separate structure into the posterior mediastinum. The parietal peritoneum continues as the visceral peritoneum as it reflects onto the stomach.

of gastroduodenal contents cause direct caustic injury to the larynx and lower respiratory tract; this is the most common mechanism. Second, distal esophageal acid exposure triggers a vagal nerve reflex that results in bronchospasm and cough. The latter mechanism is due to the common vagal innervation of the trachea and esophagus.

Unlike typical GERD symptoms (i.e., heartburn and regurgitation), extraesophageal symptoms of reflux are not specific to GERD. Before LARS is performed, it is necessary to determine whether a patient's extraesophageal symptoms are due to abnormal GER or a primary laryngeal, bronchial, or pulmonary cause. This can be challenging. A lack of response of extraesophageal symptoms to proton pump inhibitor (PPI) therapy cannot reliably refute GERD as the cause of these symptoms. Although PPI therapy can improve or completely resolve *typical* GERD symptoms, patients with *extraesophageal symptoms* experience variable response to medical treatment. This may be explained by recent evidence suggesting that acid is not the only underlying caustic agent resulting in laryngeal and pulmonary injury.[1] PPI therapy will suppress gastric acid production, but microaspiration of nonacid refluxate, which contains caustic bile salts and pepsin, can cause ongoing injury and symptoms. Therefore, in patients with extraesophageal symptoms of GERD, a mechanical barrier to reflux (i.e., esophagogastric fundoplication) may be necessary to prevent ongoing laryngeal, tracheal, or bronchial injury.

In patients who present with abnormal GER and bothersome extraesophageal symptoms, a thorough evaluation must be completed to rule out a primary disorder of the upper or lower respiratory tract. This should be completed whether or not typical GERD symptoms are also present. At the University of Washington Center for Esophageal and Gastric Surgery, we frequently refer patients with GERD and extraesophageal symptoms to a laryngologist or a pulmonologist to determine if a nongastrointestinal condition is causing these symptoms. If a nonreflux cause of the extraesophageal symptoms cannot be identified, then proceeding with an antireflux operation is acceptable. We counsel these patients a 70% likelihood of improvement in extraesophageal symptoms after LARS.[2] If a patient's laryngeal or pulmonary symptoms are not due to abnormal GER, an antireflux operation is not performed.

Pulmonary Disease, GERD, and Antireflux Surgery

Increasing evidence suggests that GERD is a contributing factor to the pathophysiologic mechanism of several pulmonary diseases. In their extensive review, Bowrey and colleagues[3] examined medical and surgical antireflux therapy in patients with GERD and asthma. In these patients, the use of antisecretory medications is associated with improved respiratory symptoms in only 25% to 50% of patients with GERD-induced asthma. Furthermore, less than 15% of these patients experience objective improvement in pulmonary function. One explanation for these results is that most of these studies lasted 3 months or less, which is potentially too short to see any improvement in pulmonary function. In addition, in several trials, gastric acid secretion was incompletely blocked by acid suppression therapy, and patients experienced ongoing GERD.

In patients with asthma and GERD, antireflux surgery appears to be more effective than medical therapy at managing pulmonary symptoms. Antireflux surgery is associated with improvement in respiratory symptoms in nearly 90% of children and 70% of adults with asthma and GERD. Several randomized trials have compared histamine 2 receptor antagonists and antireflux surgery in the management of GERD-associated asthma. Compared with patients treated with antisecretory medications, patients treated with antireflux surgery were more likely to experience relief of asthma symptoms, to discontinue systemic steroid therapy, and to improve peak expiratory flow rate.

Idiopathic pulmonary fibrosis (IPF) is a severe, chronic, and progressive lung disease that generally results in death within 5 years of diagnosis. Proximal esophageal reflux with microaspiration of acid and nonacid gastric contents has been implicated as one possible cause of alveolar epithelial injury that can lead to IPF. The incidence of GERD in patients with IPF has been reported to be as high as 94%.[4] Because typical symptoms of GERD are not sensitive for abnormal reflux in patients with IPF, the threshold for testing patients with IPF for GERD should be low.

Medical treatment of GERD in patients with IPF is associated with longer survival and slower pulmonary decline.[5] Whereas this is promising, PPI therapy does not prevent reflux of nonacid gastroduodenal contents, which may contribute to ongoing pulmonary injury in some patients. Therefore, in IPF patients with significant GERD, the argument could be made that a mechanical

TABLE 42-1 Prevalence of Symptoms Occurring More Frequently Than Once per Week in 1000 Patients With GERD	
SYMPTOM	PREVALENCE (%)
Heartburn	80
Regurgitation	54
Abdominal pain	29
Cough	27
Dysphagia for solids	23
Hoarseness	21
Belching	15
Bloating	15
Aspiration	14
Wheezing	7
Globus	4

BOX 42-1 Extraesophageal Symptoms of GERD

Laryngeal Symptoms of Reflux
Hoarseness or dysphonia
Throat clearing
Throat pain
Globus
Choking
Postnasal drip
Laryngeal and tracheal stenosis
Laryngospasm
Contact ulcers

Pulmonary Symptoms of Reflux
Cough
Shortness of breath
Wheezing
Pulmonary disease (asthma, idiopathic pulmonary fibrosis, chronic bronchitis, and others)

barrier to both acid and nonacid reflux (i.e., LARS) is more appropriate than PPI therapy. Although very little literature exists on LARS in patients with IPF, it appears to be safe and to provide effective control of distal esophageal acid exposure, and it may mitigate decline in pulmonary function.[6] At the time of this publication, a National Institutes of Health–funded multicenter prospectively randomized trial in patients with IPF and GERD is comparing LARS with PPI therapy. The results of this study may profoundly affect the management of these patients.

Physical Examination

Except in patients with severely advanced disease, the physical examination rarely contributes to confirmation of the diagnosis of GERD. In such patients, several observations may suggest the presence of GERD. For example, a patient who constantly drinks water during the interview may be facilitating esophageal clearance, which can suggest frequent reflux. Other patients with advanced disease will sit leaning forward and carry out the interview with their lungs inflated to almost vital capacity. This maneuver flattens the diaphragm, narrows the anteroposterior diameter of the hiatus, and increases the LES pressure to counteract GER. Patients who have severe proximal esophageal reflux and regurgitation of gastric contents into the mouth may develop erosion of their dentition (revealing yellow teeth caused by the loss of dentin), injected oropharyngeal mucosa, or signs of chronic sinusitis.

Although physical examination findings are generally not specific for GERD, the physical examination may be helpful in determining the presence of other disease processes. For example, supraclavicular lymphadenopathy in a patient with heartburn and dysphagia may suggest esophageal or gastric cancer. Similarly, if the patient's retrosternal pain is reproducible with palpation, a musculoskeletal source of the pain should be investigated. Short of these extreme presentations, the physical examination is generally not helpful in confirming or excluding GER as a pathologic entity.

Preoperative Diagnostic Testing

Frequently, the diagnosis of GERD is based on the presence of typical symptoms and improvement in those symptoms with PPI therapy. However, when a surgeon evaluates a patient for antireflux surgery, four diagnostic tests are useful to establish the diagnosis of GERD and to identify abnormalities in gastroesophageal anatomy and function that may have an impact on the performance of LARS.

Ambulatory pH and Impedance Monitoring

Ambulatory pH monitoring quantifies distal esophageal acid exposure and is the "gold standard" test to diagnose GERD. A 24-hour pH monitoring is conducted with a thin catheter that is passed into the esophagus through the patient's nares. The simplest catheter is a dual-probe pH catheter, which contains two solid-state electrodes that are spaced 10 cm apart and detect fluctuations in pH between 2 and 7. To ensure valid study results, the distal electrode must be placed 5 cm proximal to the LES; the location of the LES is identified on esophageal manometry (see next section). Alternatively, 48-hour ambulatory pH monitoring can be performed using an endoscopically placed wireless pH monitor.

Ambulatory pH monitoring generates a large amount of data concerning esophageal acid exposure, including total number of reflux episodes (pH < 4), longest episode of reflux, number of episodes lasting longer than 5 minutes, and percentage of time spent in reflux in the upright and supine positions. A formula assigns each of these data points a relative weight according to its capacity to cause esophageal injury, and the composite DeMeester score is calculated. Abnormal distal esophageal acid exposure is defined by a DeMeester score of 14.7 or higher.

In addition to these objective data, the patient can keep track of reflux-related symptoms by pressing a button on an electronic data recorder. During the interpretation of the pH study, symptom index and symptom-associated probability are calculated on the basis of the temporal relationship between the symptom event and episodes of distal esophageal acid exposure (Fig. 42-4). A symptom episode that occurs within 2 minutes of a reflux episode is defined as a close temporal relationship and suggests but does not confirm a cause and effect relationship between GER and the patient's symptoms. When interpreting these studies, it should be remembered that patients often do not maintain their normal activities and eating patterns when they have the catheter in place. Consequently, their symptoms may not be as prevalent during the study period. Whereas the decision to perform LARS should not hinge on symptom correlation, it can help predict symptom improvement after LARS.[7]

Esophageal impedance monitoring identifies episodes of nonacid reflux. Similar to 24-hour pH monitoring, esophageal impedance is performed with a thin, flexible catheter placed through the patient's nares into the esophagus. Impedance catheters use electrodes placed at 1-cm intervals to detect changes in the resistance to flow of an electrical current (i.e., impedance). Impedance increases in the presence of air and decreases in the presence of a liquid bolus. Therefore, this technology can detect both gas and liquid movement in the esophagus.

Some impedance catheters also have one or more pH sensors, allowing the simultaneous detection of acid and nonacid reflux. When pH-impedance catheters are used, it is possible to determine the direction of movement of esophageal acid exposures and therefore to differentiate between an antegrade event (as in a swallow) and a retrograde event (as in GER). There also exists a

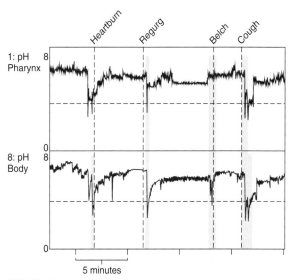

FIGURE 42-4 A 1-hour segment from a 24-hour ambulatory pH study. Time is marked on the x-axis, and pH is marked on the y-axis. Symptom events are marked along the top of the tracing. (Courtesy University of Washington Center for Esophageal and Gastric Surgery, Seattle.)

specialized pH-impedance catheter with a very proximal pH sensor that detects pharyngeal acid reflux. This catheter can be useful in the evaluation of patients with extraesophageal symptoms, such as cough, throat clearing, hoarseness, and wheezing. One disadvantage of impedance technology, however, is that the automated analytic software is very sensitive and tends to overestimate the number of nonacid reflux episodes, mandating that these studies be manually reviewed and edited, which can be time-consuming.

Combined impedance-pH monitoring has been shown to identify reflux episodes with greater sensitivity than pH testing alone.[8] Although there is no consensus on whether impedance-pH testing should be performed on or off acid suppression therapy, our practice is to perform all impedance-pH testing off acid suppression. Furthermore, how impedance-pH monitoring should guide the management of GERD is unknown. Patel and colleagues[9] attempted to determine the parameters on esophageal impedance-pH monitoring that predict response of GERD symptoms to both medical and surgical treatment. They showed that acid exposure time, and not the number of nonacid reflux events, best predicted symptom improvement with both medical and surgical therapy. Although the addition of impedance monitoring increased the sensitivity of the study, nonacid reflux measurements alone were unable to accurately predict symptom response to medical or surgical therapy for GERD.

Esophageal Manometry

Esophageal manometry is the most effective way to assess function of the esophageal body and the LES. Standard esophageal manometry provides linear tracings of pressure waves of the esophageal body and LES (Fig. 42-5). High-resolution esophageal manometry gathers data using a 32-channel flexible catheter with pressure-sensing devices arranged at 1-cm intervals, placed into the esophagus through the nares; the study is conducted in approximately 15 minutes, during which time the patient performs 10 swallows. A color-contour plot is generated and shows the response of the upper esophageal sphincter and LES as well as of the esophageal body; time is on the x-axis, esophageal length is on the y-axis, and pressure is represented by a color scale (Fig. 42-6). In patients undergoing evaluation for GERD, esophageal manometry can exclude achalasia and identify patients with ineffective esophageal body peristalsis. Repeated exposure of the esophagus to gastric reflux can lead to esophageal motility disorders; in one study, 25% of patients with mild esophagitis demonstrated esophageal dysmotility, whereas 48% of patients with severe esophagitis had impaired motility on manometry.[10] In patients with significant esophageal dysmotility who are undergoing LARS, the surgeon should consider a partial fundoplication to decrease the likelihood of postoperative dysphagia. A full discussion of the implications of esophageal dysmotility on the type of fundoplication is presented in a later section of this chapter. Esophageal manometry also measures the LES resting pressure and assesses the LES for appropriate relaxation with deglutition. Because the LES is the major barrier to GER, a defective LES is common in patients with GERD.

Esophagogastroduodenoscopy

Endoscopy is an essential step in the evaluation of patients with GERD who are being considered for LARS. The esophagus should be examined for evidence of mucosal injury due to GER, including ulcerations, peptic strictures, and Barrett esophagus. Esophagitis can be reported according to several scoring systems, including

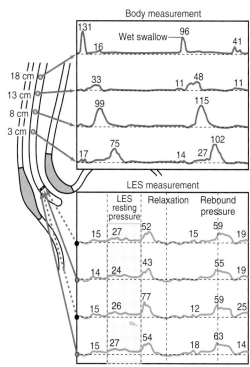

FIGURE 42-5 Representative linear tracings from standard esophageal manometry. A wet swallow initiates both esophageal peristalsis and lower esophageal sphincter (LES) relaxation.

the Savary-Miller and Los Angeles (LA) classifications.[11] Both peptic strictures and LA class C and D esophagitis can be considered pathognomonic for GERD. Consequently, ambulatory pH monitoring is unnecessary in these patients. However, because of significant interobserver variability in LA class A and B esophagitis, these forms of mild esophagitis cannot be considered reliable markers of GERD.[12] As such, patients found to have LA class A and B esophagitis should undergo pH testing to confirm abnormal distal esophageal acid exposure.

Endoscopic evaluation should also include an assessment of the GEJ flap valve. To do this, the endoscope is retroflexed 180 degrees in the stomach to visualize the GEJ from below. The flap valve is graded 1 to 4, according to the length of the valve and how tightly it adheres to the endoscope. The endoscopist should make note of the presence of a hiatal hernia, and the hernia should be measured in both cranial-caudal and lateral dimensions. In patients who are being evaluated for persistent or recurrent gastroesophageal symptoms after an antireflux operation or PEH repair, it is recommended that the surgeon who is evaluating the patient perform the endoscopy. This allows the operating surgeon to correlate endoscopic findings with the patient's symptoms and data obtained on 24-hour pH monitoring, esophageal manometry, and upper gastrointestinal (UGI) series to determine if a functional or anatomic abnormality exists that can be corrected with reoperation.

Barium Esophagram

Barium esophagram provides a detailed anatomic evaluation of the esophagus and stomach that is useful during preoperative evaluation of patients with GERD. Of particular importance are the presence, size, and anatomic characteristics of a hiatal hernia

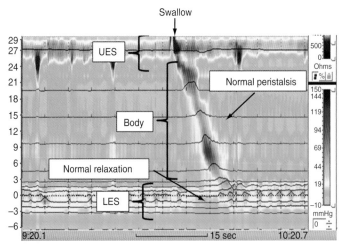

FIGURE 42-6 High-resolution esophageal manometry. The initiation of a swallow is associated with simultaneous relaxation of the upper esophageal sphincter (UES) and lower esophageal sphincter (LES) and onset of peristalsis in the esophageal body.

or PEH (Fig. 42-7). For example, a GEJ that is fixed in the posterior mediastinum on esophagography can suggest a more difficult operation that may require a more extensive intrathoracic esophageal mobilization. Despite its ability to identify episodes of GER, which can occur spontaneously or in response to positioning of the patient during the study, barium esophagram cannot confirm or refute the diagnosis of GERD. On occasion, patients presenting to the surgical clinic for evaluation of GERD may have already undergone computed tomography scan of the chest or abdomen to evaluate atypical symptoms of GERD (e.g., chest or abdominal pain). Horizontal images as well as coronal and sagittal reconstructions can provide information concerning the anatomic relationship of the stomach and esophagus to other abdominal and thoracic structures. However, we still prefer to obtain a barium esophagram as computed tomography scan frequently fails to identify important anatomic and functional gastroesophageal disease.

Additional gastroesophageal conditions that can be identified on barium esophagram are esophageal diverticula, tumors, peptic strictures, achalasia, dysmotility, and gastroparesis. If any one of these is found in a patient undergoing evaluation for GERD, LARS should be delayed until appropriate evaluation of the unexpected findings is completed.

Additional Preoperative Considerations
Dysphagia
Patients with GERD will occasionally experience dysphagia. The causes of dysphagia are listed in Box 42-2. In patients with GERD, the most common cause of dysphagia is a reflux-associated inflammatory process of the esophageal wall. This inflammation can be manifested as a Schatzki ring, a diffuse distal esophageal inflammation, or a peptic stricture. Although relatively rare since the widespread adoption of PPI therapy, peptic strictures are pathognomonic for long-standing reflux and develop from the chronic mucosal inflammation that occurs with GERD. When strictures result in significant dysphagia, patients can experience weight loss and protein-calorie malnutrition. In addition, strictures can be associated with esophageal shortening, which makes obtaining adequate intra-abdominal esophageal length at the time of opera-

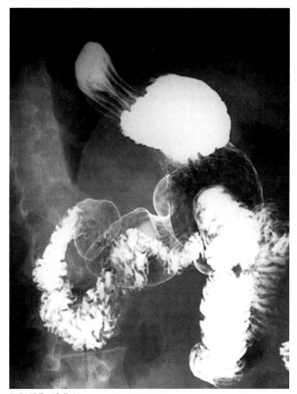

FIGURE 42-7 Upper gastrointestinal series demonstrating a large hiatal hernia. The rugal folds of the stomach clearly transgress the shadow of the left hemidiaphragm.

tion more difficult (see "Intraoperative Management of Short Esophagus").

In patients with peptic strictures, it can be challenging to document abnormal GER on ambulatory pH monitoring because the presence of a tight stricture may prevent reflux of acid, resulting in a false-negative pH study. In patients with typical GERD symptoms and a peptic stricture, it is reasonable to forego ambulatory pH monitoring because the presence of a peptic stricture is considered pathognomonic for severe GER. If pH monitoring is performed, it is ideally completed after dilation of the stricture to increase the validity of the test. Importantly, because they are associated with long-standing GER, peptic strictures should be biopsied to rule out intestinal metaplasia, dysplasia, and malignancy.

The majority of peptic strictures are effectively treated with dilation and PPI therapy. Successful dilation can be performed with either a balloon dilator or Savary dilator, and no strong data exist to support the superiority of one dilation technique over another. Refractory peptic strictures are defined as strictures that recur despite dilation and PPI therapy. Although rare, refractory strictures can pose a significant challenge to surgeons and gastroenterologists. In these patients, LARS should strongly be considered. For patients who are unfit for or do not wish to undergo an operation, steroid injections of the stricture have been shown to result in fewer dilations.[13]

Another cause of dysphagia in patients with GERD is a Schatzki ring. Similar to peptic strictures, these are located in the distal esophagus. However, Schatzki rings are submucosal fibrotic bands (as opposed to mucosal strictures). Typically, peptic strictures and Schatzki rings can be differentiated on endoscopy. Both should be dilated to relieve obstruction, but Schatzki rings develop in the submucosal space, so in the absence of other endoscopically identified mucosal abnormalities, biopsies do not need to be performed. Furthermore, Schatzki rings are not pathognomonic for GERD, so abnormal distal esophageal acid exposure must be documented on ambulatory pH monitoring to confirm the presence of abnormal GER before LARS is performed.

Dysphagia in patients with GERD may not have a clear anatomic cause, and mild dysphagia in these patients may simply be due to the esophageal inflammation that results from persistent GER. This type of dysphagia tends to resolve after abnormal reflux is controlled. In patients who present with dysphagia and GERD, other causes of dysphagia must be excluded, including tumors, diverticula, and esophageal motor disorders. Although these conditions are much less common than peptic stricture and Schatzki ring, they require dramatically different treatments. In patients who report simultaneous onset of dysphagia to liquids and solids, one must have a high suspicion for a neuromuscular or autoimmune disorder as the etiology. Finally, some patients with severe GERD experience dysphagia without exhibiting an anatomic or physiologic abnormality of the esophagus. This is believed to be caused by inflammation associated with reflux, and we have found that such patients typically experience improvement in dysphagia after LARS.

Obesity

Obesity is a significant risk factor for the development of GERD. Compared with patients of normal weight, obese patients have increased intra-abdominal pressure, decreased LES pressure, and more frequent transient LES relaxations. Obese patients with GERD present a particular challenge to surgeons. Whereas it is clear that LARS can be performed safely in obese patients, the literature is mixed on the ability of LARS to provide long-term control of GERD-related symptoms. In appropriately selected patients, laparoscopic Roux-en-Y gastric bypass is the most durable method of weight loss and control of obesity-related comorbidities, including GERD. In severely obese patients with GERD, serious consideration should be given to performing a laparoscopic Roux-en-Y gastric bypass instead of a fundoplication. Ultimately, the decision to pursue gastric bypass instead of fundoplication must include a careful balance of the patient's interest in bariatric surgery, presence of other medical comorbidities, and availability of a surgeon to perform the operation.

Partial versus Complete Fundoplication

Antireflux operations include partial posterior (180-and 270-degree), partial anterior (90- and 180-degree), and 360-degree esophagogastric fundoplications. In the field of antireflux surgery, there has been a long-standing debate about which fundoplication provides superior control of GERD symptoms while mitigating postoperative side effects (e.g., dysphagia and gas-bloat). Furthermore, studies have attempted to determine whether the type of fundoplication performed should be tailored to the patient's preoperative esophageal motility and symptoms.

In patients with GERD and esophageal dysmotility, it has been suggested that partial fundoplication should be performed because of concern that a Nissen fundoplication will lead to greater postoperative dysphagia. Booth and colleagues[14] completed a randomized controlled trial to compare laparoscopic Nissen fundoplication with Toupet fundoplication in patients who were stratified on the basis of preoperative manometry. At 1 year postoperatively, there were no differences between Nissen and Toupet groups for heartburn and regurgitation. Dysphagia was more frequent in patients who underwent Nissen fundoplication. However, when a Nissen fundoplication was constructed, patients with normal and impaired esophageal motility experienced similar rates of postoperative dysphagia. Similarly, we have shown that a Nissen fundoplication can be performed in patients with ineffective esophageal motility without an increase in development of dysphagia.[15]

Fein and Seyfried[16] reviewed nine randomized trials that evaluated laparoscopic anterior, partial posterior, and total fundoplications in the management of GERD. Anterior fundoplication was associated with greater risk of recurrent GERD symptoms. In several studies, Nissen fundoplication was associated with increased postoperative dysphagia, but these patients required minimal treatment and no reoperations. In randomized trials, no difference in gas-bloat symptoms was seen between Nissen and Toupet fundoplications. However, more gas-bloat was reported in nonrandomized trials.

Shan and colleagues[17] reviewed 32 studies, including 9 randomized controlled trials, that compared laparoscopic Nissen fundoplication with laparoscopic Toupet fundoplication. No differences

---

BOX 42-2   Potential Causes of Dysphagia in Patients Undergoing Evaluation for GERD

Esophageal Obstruction
Peptic strictures
Schatzki ring
Malignant neoplasm
Benign neoplasm
Foreign body

Esophageal Motility Disorders
Diffuse esophageal spasm
Hypercontractile ("Jackhammer") esophagus
Ineffective esophageal motility
Achalasia

were noted between groups concerning patient satisfaction with the operation or perioperative morbidity and mortality. In 24 studies that assessed postoperative dysphagia, no difference was noted between fundoplication types when esophageal motility was normal. However, in patients with abnormal esophageal motility, laparoscopic Nissen fundoplication was associated with greater rates of dysphagia. An additional analysis was performed that assessed for dysphagia in patients with normal motility who underwent a Nissen fundoplication and patients with abnormal motility who underwent a Toupet fundoplication. In this comparison, the patients who underwent a Nissen fundoplication reported more dysphagia. Finally, this meta-analysis found increased rates of postoperative gas-bloat and inability to belch in patients who underwent Nissen fundoplication. This review would suggest that Toupet fundoplication is the treatment of choice, leading to effective GERD symptom control and fewer postoperative side effects.

Despite numerous randomized clinical trials and two meta-analyses, there still remains conflicting evidence about the fundoplication that provides the most durable control of reflux and the best side-effect profile. The reason for this is likely to be the heterogeneity of these studies in terms of patient characteristics, patient selection, and operative technique. For example, in the studies evaluated by Fein and Seyfried,[16] four different bougie sizes are used (34 Fr to 60 Fr), fixation of the stomach to the esophagus and hiatus is inconsistent among surgeons, and division of the short gastric vessels is not always performed. Currently, the only consistent finding in these studies is that anterior fundoplications provide less durable control of GERD than posterior partial and total fundoplications. Otherwise, surgeons should perform the fundoplication that they are most comfortable performing and not tailor fundoplication type to esophageal dysmotility.

Barrett Esophagus

In some patients, long-standing acid (and perhaps alkaline) reflux is associated with a histologic change of the distal esophageal mucosa from its normal squamous epithelium to a columnar configuration. This histologic alteration is called intestinal metaplasia or Barrett esophagus. On endoscopic evaluation, Barrett esophagus appears as velvety-red "tongues" of mucosa that extend cephalad from the GEJ. Based on endoscopic measurements, it can be classified into long segment ($\geq$3 cm) and short segment (<3 cm). If Barrett esophagus is suspected on the basis of endoscopic appearance of the esophageal mucosa, multiple biopsy specimens should be taken to histologically establish the diagnosis and to determine the presence of dysplasia. When dysplasia is present, there is an increased risk for development of adenocarcinoma. Although the incidence of adenocarcinoma in patients with Barrett esophagus is about 40 times greater than that in the general population, the overall incidence of cancer in these patients is still very low.

Because Barrett esophagus is the result of repeated injury of the mucosa due to GER, it would be expected that an antireflux operation might cause regression of intestinal metaplasia or decrease the rate of dysplasia and cancer. However, the evidence in the literature is not conclusive. Studies have reported regression of intestinal metaplasia in up to 55% of patients after antireflux surgery.[18] At the University of Washington, we have seen regression in 55% of patients with short-segment Barrett esophagus (<3 cm). Just as important, patients with Barrett esophagus experienced excellent long-term clinical relief of GERD symptoms.

Rossi and colleagues[19] compared the efficacy of Nissen fundo-

plication and medical therapy in the regression of low-grade dysplasia in patients with Barrett esophagus. At 18 months after therapy with high-dose PPIs or laparoscopic Nissen fundoplication, 12 of 19 patients (63%) in the medical arm and 15 of 16 (94%) in the surgery arm had regression from low-grade dysplasia to Barrett esophagus ($P = .03$). Despite these promising results, the pathologic findings on preoperative endoscopy should still dictate postoperative endoscopic surveillance.

Treatment of Gastroesophageal Reflux Disease
Medical Management

For patients who present with typical symptoms of GERD, an 8-week course of PPI therapy is recommended.[20] However, before empirically prescribing a PPI, it is necessary to ensure that the patient does not have symptoms that may indicate the presence of a gastroesophageal malignant neoplasm or other non-GERD diagnosis, including rapidly progressive dysphagia, regurgitation of undigested food, anemia, extraesophageal symptoms of GERD, and weight loss. If the symptoms improve with PPI therapy, the trial is considered both diagnostic and therapeutic. If the symptoms persist after a trial of medical therapy, a more extensive evaluation, as described earlier, is indicated. Although lifestyle modification has been advocated before or as an adjunct to medical therapy, the efficacy of such changes in the treatment of esophagitis has not been proved.[21]

PPIs have revolutionized the pharmacologic treatment of GERD. As one of the most widely prescribed drugs worldwide, the annual expenditure on PPI therapy has reached approximately $24 billion.[22] These drugs stop gastric acid production by irreversibly binding the proton pump in the parietal cells of the stomach. The maximal pharmacologic effect occurs approximately 4 days after initiation of therapy, and the effect lasts for the life of the parietal cell. For this reason, patients must stop PPI therapy 1 week before ambulatory pH monitoring to avoid a false-negative test result.

PPIs are well tolerated medications. Immediate side effects of PPI therapy are relatively rare and generally mild, including headache, abdominal pain, flatulence, constipation, and diarrhea. This relatively safe side-effect profile and their effectiveness at controlling GERD symptoms have led to overprescription of these medications in both the outpatient and inpatient settings.[23] Although there are published evidence-based recommendations that might limit this practice of overprescription, including on-demand dosing and step-down therapy, clinicians frequently do not follow these guidelines.

Despite their short-term safety, there has been concern about the long-term effects of PPI use since their initial preclinical trials.[24] The most concerning long-term complication of PPI use is hypergastrinemia leading to enterochromaffin cell hyperplasia and ultimately carcinoid tumors. The first case of neuroendocrine tumor of the stomach in a patient with 15-year history of PPI use has just been published,[25] so it seems that the true risk of this is exceptionally low. However, additional associations have recently been made between PPI use and enteric infections, antiplatelet medication interactions, bone fractures, nutritional deficiencies, and community-acquired pneumonia.[23] Importantly, however, no cause and effect relationship has been established, and patients prescribed PPI therapy have more comorbid conditions than the general population, which may explain some of these associations. Therefore, until further studies better elucidate PPI as a contributing factor to these conditions, the results of these studies should be interpreted with caution.

Surgical Management

For patients who exhibit elevated distal esophageal acid exposure and persistent typical GERD symptoms despite maximal medical therapy, antireflux surgery should be strongly considered. The application of laparoscopy to antireflux surgery has decreased patient morbidity and hospital length of stay. Furthermore, several studies have shown that LARS is cost-effective compared with prolonged PPI therapy.[12] In patients who experience absolutely no improvement in their symptoms with the use of PPIs, the diagnosis of GERD should be questioned, and surgeons must carefully consider alternative causes before offering surgical treatment. In patients with extraesophageal symptoms of GERD that do not improve with PPI therapy, consultation with an otolaryngologist or pulmonologist should be considered to determine if a primary laryngeal, bronchial, or pulmonary cause of the symptoms is present. Endoscopic evidence of severe esophageal injury (e.g., ulcerations, peptic strictures, and Barrett esophagus) can be considered evidence of abnormal distal esophageal acid exposure and may make ambulatory pH monitoring unnecessary in patients who exhibit these findings; however, endoscopic findings should not be considered an indication for operative therapy by themselves.

Operative technique. We perform all laparoscopic antireflux operations with the patient in low lithotomy position. This provides the surgeon improved ergonomics by standing between the patient's legs; the assistant stands at the patient's left. In addition, the patient is placed in steep reverse Trendelenburg position, which allows improved visualization of the esophageal hiatus. The patient is appropriately padded to prevent pressure ulcers and neuropathies. Preoperative antibiotics are administered to reduce the risk of surgical site infection, and subcutaneous heparin and sequential compression devices are used to reduce the risk of venous thromboembolic events.

Access to the abdomen is obtained with a Veress needle at Palmer's point in the left upper quadrant of the abdomen. Three additional trocars are placed. The surgeon operates through the two most cephalad ports, and the assistant operates through the two caudad ports. A Nathanson liver retractor does not require a trocar and is placed through a small epigastric incision (Fig. 42-8).

We begin our dissection at the left crus by dividing the phrenogastric membrane and then enter the lesser sac at the level of the inferior edge of the spleen. This allows early ligation of the short gastric vessels and mobilization of the gastric fundus (Fig. 42-9). After the fundus is mobilized, the phrenoesophageal membrane is divided to expose the entire length of the left crus (Fig. 42-10).

Right crural dissection is then performed. The gastrohepatic ligament is divided, and the right phrenoesophageal membrane is opened to expose the right crus (Fig. 42-11). A retroesophageal window is created. Care is taken to preserve the anterior and posterior vagus nerves during this mobilization. A Penrose drain is placed around the esophagus to facilitate the posterior mediastinal dissection and to assist with creation of the fundoplication.

The esophagus is mobilized in the posterior mediastinum to obtain a minimum of 3 cm of intra-abdominal esophagus. Then, the crura are approximated posteriorly with permanent sutures (Fig. 42-12). The esophagus should maintain a straight orientation without angulation, and a 52 Fr bougie should easily pass beyond the esophageal hiatus and into the stomach. At this point, the fundoplication is created.

Creation of a 360-degree fundoplication. The most common technical failure in performing a Nissen fundoplication is failure to create appropriate fundoplication anatomy. The description that follows clearly explains our method of performing a correct, effective, and reproducible Nissen fundoplication. To maintain appropriate orientation of the fundus during the creation of the fundoplication, the posterior aspect of the fundus is marked with a suture 3 cm distal to the GEJ and 2 cm off the greater curvature (Fig. 42-13). The posterior fundus is then passed behind the esophagus from the patient's left to right. The anterior fundus on the left side of the esophagus is then grasped 2 cm from the greater curvature and 3 cm from the GEJ, and both portions of the fundus are positioned on the anterior aspect of the esophagus. It is of paramount importance that the two points at which the fundus is grasped are equidistant from the greater curvature (Fig. 42-14). Creation of the fundoplication in this manner decreases the chance of constructing the fundoplication with the body of the stomach, which creates a redundant posterior aspect of the wrap that can impinge on the distal esophagus and cause dysphagia. With use of three or four interrupted permanent sutures, the fundoplication is created to a length of 2.5 to 3 cm. Similar to the crural repair, the completed fundoplication should allow the easy passage of a 52 Fr bougie. After removal of the bougie, the wrap is anchored to the esophagus and crura (Fig. 42-14, *inset*) to help prevent herniation into the mediastinum and slipping of the fundoplication over the body of the stomach. The suture line of the fundoplication should lie parallel to the right anterior aspect of the esophagus.

Creation of a partial fundoplication. There are several types of partial fundoplications. The most commonly performed is the Toupet fundoplication. In this operation, the gastric and esophageal dissections as well as the repair of the crura are the same as for a 360-degree fundoplication. In addition, the fundoplication must be created with the fundus, not the body, of the stomach. The key difference is that the stomach is wrapped 180 to 270 degrees (compared with 360 degrees) around the posterior aspect of the esophagus (Fig. 42-15*A* and *C*). On both sides of the esophagus, the most cephalad sutures of the fundoplication incorporate the fundus, crus, and esophagus; the remaining sutures anchor the fundus to either the crura or the esophagus.

If an anterior fundoplication is to be performed (e.g., Thal or Dor), there is no need to disrupt the posterior attachments of the

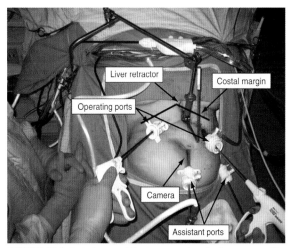

FIGURE 42-8 Port placement for laparoscopic antireflux surgery. The surgeon operates through the two cephalad ports, and the assistant operates through the two caudad ports.

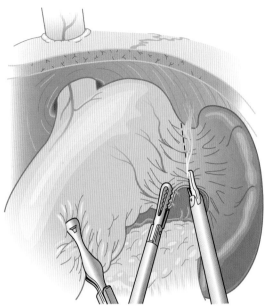

FIGURE 42-9 In the left crus approach to the esophageal hiatus, the fundus of the stomach is mobilized early during the operation to provide early visualization of the spleen, which helps prevent splenic injury.

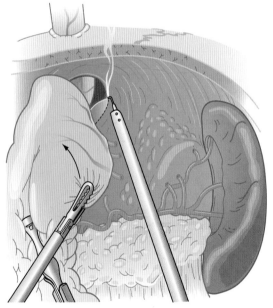

FIGURE 42-10 After the fundus has been mobilized, the phrenoesophageal membrane is incised at the left crus, with care taken to avoid injury to the esophagus, posterior vagus nerve, and aorta.

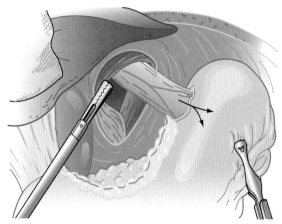

FIGURE 42-11 The phrenoesophageal membrane is incised at the right crus to complete the exposure of the hiatus. Performing the dissection immediately adjacent to the crura decreases the likelihood of injury to adjacent structures.

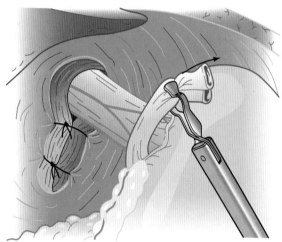

FIGURE 42-12 Posterior crural closure is performed with heavy permanent suture. Note how the peritoneum overlying the crura is incorporated into the closure. The exposure is facilitated by displacement of the esophagus anteriorly and to the left.

esophagus, and the fundus is folded over the anterior aspect of the esophagus and anchored to the hiatus and esophagus (Fig. 42-15*B*).

Intraoperative management of short esophagus. Normal esophageal length exists when the GEJ rests at or below the esophageal hiatus. As the GEJ becomes displaced cephalad to the esophageal hiatus, the esophagus effectively shortens. At the time of LARS, a minimum of 3 cm of intra-abdominal esophagus

should be obtained. When the GEJ is mildly displaced cephalad to the GEJ, adequate intra-abdominal esophageal length can be obtained with distal esophageal mobilization in the posterior mediastinum. However, if the GEJ migrates high into the posterior mediastinum, as occurs with a large hiatal hernia or PEH, the effective length of the esophagus can decrease significantly. Furthermore, this process causes adhesions to develop between the esophagus and the mediastinum that anchor the contracted esophagus in the chest. When this occurs, extensive mobilization of the esophagus must be undertaken, sometimes to the level of the inferior pulmonary veins. However, even in the case of a large hiatal hernia or PEH, mediastinal dissection alone can return the GEJ to the abdominal cavity.

In some cases, despite extensive mediastinal mobilization of the esophagus, intra-abdominal esophageal length still appears inadequate. In these rare cases, a unilateral vagotomy can result in an additional 1 to 2 cm of esophageal length, and division of both vagus nerves typically yields 3 to 4 cm of additional esopha-

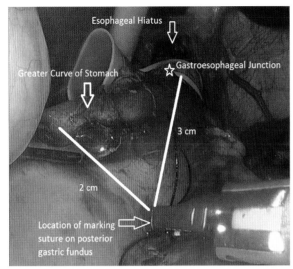

FIGURE 42-13 A posterior gastric marking suture is helpful to ensure proper geometric configuration of the fundoplication. With the greater curvature of the stomach rotated to the patient's right, the posterior stomach is exposed, and a marking stitch is placed on the posterior fundus 3 cm from the gastroesophageal junction and 2 cm from the greater curvature of the stomach.

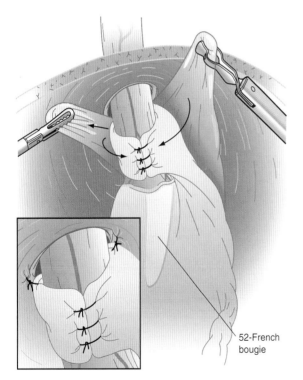

FIGURE 42-14 Creation of a 360-degree Nissen fundoplication. The anterior and posterior fundus must be grasped equidistant from the greater curvature posterior to the esophagus. After placement of the first suture of the fundoplication, a 52 Fr bougie is passed into the stomach, and the fundoplication is completed. With the bougie removed from the patient, the fundoplication is secured to the diaphragm with right and left coronal sutures *(inset)* and a single posterior suture (not shown).

gus. Many surgeons hesitate to electively transect the vagus nerves because of concern for the development of postoperative delayed gastric emptying. However, we have shown this not to be the case. In our study of 102 patients who underwent reoperative LARS ($n = 50$) or PEH repair ($n = 52$), we performed a vagotomy in 30 patients (29%) to increase intra-abdominal esophageal length after extensive mediastinal mobilization.[26] Compared with patients who did not undergo vagotomy, patients who underwent vagotomy reported similar severity of abdominal pain, bloating, diarrhea, and early satiety.

Finally, if adequate intra-abdominal esophageal length cannot be accomplished with these techniques, a stapled wedge gastroplasty may be performed (Fig. 42-16). Since the widespread adoption of laparoscopy in the management of GERD and PEH, wedge gastroplasty has generally supplanted the traditional Collis gastroplasty that used a double-staple technique (circular and linear stapler). However, we have found this technique unnecessary in all but a very small number of patients.

Postoperative Care and Recovery

Except when the patient's comorbid medical conditions dictate otherwise, postoperatively patients are admitted to a general surgical ward without cardiac or pulmonary monitoring. Patients are given a clear liquid diet the evening of the operation and are advanced to a full liquid diet on postoperative day 1. Discharge requirements include tolerance of a diet to maintain hydration and nutrition, adequate pain control with oral analgesics, and ability to void without a Foley catheter. After discharge from the hospital, patients can slowly introduce soft foods into their diet, and they should expect to resume a diet without limitations in about 4 to 6 weeks.

Clinical Outcomes of Antireflux Surgery

The success of antireflux surgery can be measured by relief of symptoms, improvement in esophageal acid exposure, complications, and failures. Several randomized trials with long-term follow-up have compared medical and surgical therapy for GERD (Table 42-2). LARS is a safe operation that provides durable improvement in typical symptoms of GERD that are refractory to medical management.

Spechler and colleagues[27] found that surgical therapy results in good symptom control after 10-year follow-up. Although 62% of patients in the surgical group were taking antisecretory medications at long-term follow-up, GERD symptoms were not the indication for this medication use in all patients, and reflux symptoms did not change significantly when these patients stopped taking these medications.

Lundell and colleagues[28] randomized patients with erosive esophagitis into surgical or medical therapy. Treatment failure was defined as moderate or severe symptoms of heartburn, regurgitation, dysphagia, or odynophagia; recommencement of PPI therapy; reoperation; or grade 2 esophagitis. At 7-year follow-up, fewer treatment failures were seen in patients managed with fundoplication than with omeprazole (33% versus 53%; $P = .002$). In patients who did not respond to the initial dose of omeprazole, dose escalation was completed; however, surgical intervention remained superior. Patients treated with fundoplication experienced more obstructive and gas-bloat symptoms (e.g., dysphagia, flatulence, inability to belch) compared with the medically treated cohort. At 12-year follow-up, the durability of these results remained; patients who underwent fundoplication had fewer treatment failures compared with patients treated with medical

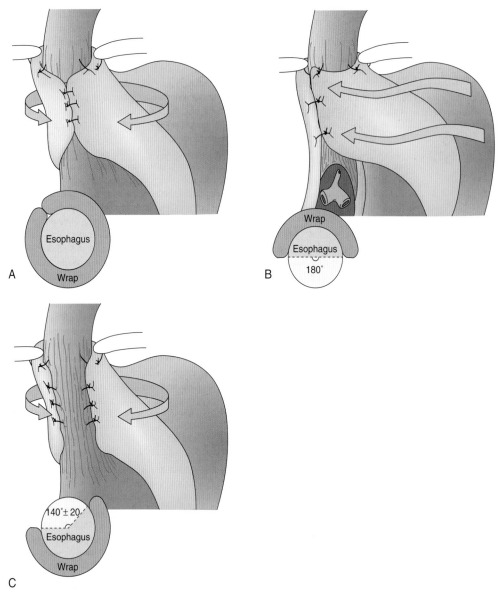

FIGURE 42-15 Three types of fundoplication. **A,** A 360-degree fundoplication. **B,** Partial anterior fundoplication. **C,** Partial posterior fundoplication.

therapy (47% versus 55%; P = .022).[29]

During the past 25 years, the experience of surgeons with LARS has increased dramatically. With increased experience, the durability of symptom improvement has increased, and perioperative complications have decreased. This is especially true in high-volume centers. In one single-institution study that observed 100 patients for 10 years after LARS, 90% of patients remained free of GERD symptoms.[30] We published our experience in a cohort of 288 patients undergoing LARS. With median follow-up of more than 5 years, symptom improvement was 90% for heartburn and 92% for regurgitation.[31] These results confirm that LARS can provide excellent durable relief of GERD when patients are appropriately selected and excellent technique is employed.

Operative Complications and Side Effects of Antireflux Surgery

LARS is a safe operation when it is performed by experienced surgeons. Using the American College of Surgeons National Surgical Quality Improvement Program, Niebisch and colleagues[32] reviewed more than 7500 patients who underwent laparoscopic fundoplication between 2005 and 2009. Overall, 30-day mortality was rare (0.19%). In patients older than 70 years, mortality was statistically significantly higher (0.8%; P < .0001). Complications were also more frequent in older patients (2.2% in patients <50 years and 7.8% in patients >70 years; P < .0001) and in patients with higher American Society of Anesthesiologists classification (2% in class 2 and 14% in class 4).

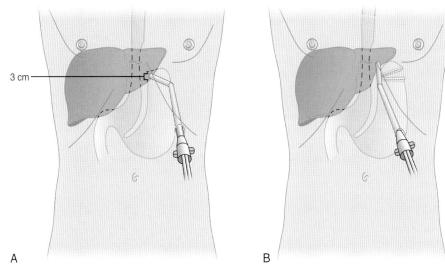

A   B

FIGURE 42-16 Laparoscopic stapled wedge gastroplasty for esophageal lengthening. **A,** With a 48 Fr bougie placed beyond the gastroesophageal junction and into the stomach, a linear stapler is used to transect the fundus perpendicular to the bougie approximately 3 to 4 cm distal to the angle of His. **B,** A second linear stapler is used to resect the portion of gastric fundus parallel to the bougie.

TABLE 42-2   Randomized Controlled Trials Comparing Surgical and Medical Therapies for GERD

STUDY	STUDY GROUPS	FOLLOW-UP	OUTCOME
Anvari et al,[46] 2011	PPI, n = 52 ARS, n = 52	3 years	ARS and PPI provided equal symptom control, ARS provided more heartburn-free days
Grant et al,[47] 2008	PPI, n = 179 ARS, n = 178	1 year	Reflux score: PPI, 73; ARS, 85; P < .05
Lundell et al,[29] 2009	Omeprazole, n = 71 ARS, n = 53	12 years	Treatment failure: Omeprazole, 55%; ARS, 47%; P = .022
Lundell et al,[28] 2007	Omeprazole, n = 119 ARS, n = 99	7 years	Treatment failure: Omeprazole, 53%; ARS, 33%; P = .002

ARS, antireflux surgery; *PPI,* proton pump inhibitor.

TABLE 42-3   Complications in 400 Laparoscopic Antireflux Procedures at the University of Washington

COMPLICATION	NO. OF PATIENTS (%)
Postoperative ileus	28 (7)
Pneumothorax	13 (3)
Urinary retention	9 (2)
Dysphagia	9 (2)
Other minor complications	8 (2)
Liver trauma	2 (0.5)
Acute herniation	1 (0.25)
Perforated viscus	1 (0.25)
Death	1 (0.25)
Total	72 (17.25)

Complications of LARS are typically minor and not related specifically to antireflux surgery; they include urinary retention, wound infection, venous thrombosis, and ileus. Complications that are specific to antireflux surgery include pneumothorax, gastric or esophageal injury, and splenic or liver injury. In addition, LARS can result in postoperative side effects, including bloating and dysphagia. Complications in 400 patients who have undergone LARS at the University of Washington are listed in Table 42-3.

Operative Complications

Pneumothorax. Pneumothorax is one of the most common intraoperative complications, yet it is reported to occur in less than 2% of patients.[33] Although postoperative chest radiographs are not obtained in all patients, pneumothorax should rarely be missed as intraoperative identification of pleural violation that causes pneumothorax should be identified. The pleural violation results in intrathoracic infusion of carbon dioxide, which is absorbed rapidly. Because no underlying lung injury exists, the lung will reexpand without incident. When violation of the pleura is identified intraoperatively, the pleura should be closed with a suture, and a postoperative radiograph should be obtained. If a pneumothorax is identified on this radiograph, the patient may be maintained on oxygen therapy to facilitate its resolution. Unless the patient experiences shortness of breath or persistent oxygen therapy to maintain normal hemoglobin oxygenation saturation, no further radiographs are obtained.

Gastric and esophageal injuries. Gastric and esophageal injuries have been reported to occur in approximately 1% of patients undergoing LARS.[33] Typically, these injuries result from overaggressive manipulation of these organs or at the time the bougie is passed into the stomach. Gastric and esophageal injuries are more likely to occur in reoperative cases and should be rare during initial operations. If they are identified at the time of operation, these injuries can be repaired with suture (more commonly) or stapler (if the injury involves the stomach) without sequelae. If the injury is not identified intraoperatively, the patient will likely need a second operation to repair the viscus, unless the leak is small and contained.

Splenic and liver injuries or bleeding. The incidence of splenic parenchymal injury that results in bleeding is about 2.3% in population-based studies; major liver injury is rarely reported.[34] Whereas splenic bleeding is relatively uncommon, in rare cases, it can require splenectomy. Most commonly, splenic parenchymal injury occurs during mobilization of the fundus and greater curvature of the stomach. For this reason, we prefer beginning laparoscopic Nissen fundoplication with the "left crus approach" to provide early and direct visualization of the short gastric vessels and the spleen. As described in the operative technique section, the left crus approach begins by dividing the phrenogastric ligament and the short gastric vessels, which provides the advantage of a direct and early view of the short gastric vessels and spleen. Care must be taken during mobilization of the fundus to avoid excessive traction on the splenogastric ligament. A second type of injury that can occur to the spleen is a partial splenic infarction. This injury typically occurs during transection of the short gastric vessels and inadvertent coagulation of superior pole branch of the main splenic artery.[34] Partial splenic infarction rarely causes any symptoms. Finally, lacerations and subcapsular hematomas of the left lateral section of the liver can be avoided by carefully retracting it out of the operative field with a fixed retractor.

Side Effects

Bloating. The normal act of air swallowing is the main factor leading to gastric distention, and the physiologic mechanism for venting this air is belching. Gastric belching occurs through vagus nerve–mediated transient LES relaxation. After antireflux surgery, patients experience fewer transient LES relaxations and therefore decreased belching. Consequently, patients can experience abdominal bloating. Kessing and colleagues[35] investigated the impact of gas-related symptoms on the objective and subjective outcomes of both Nissen and Toupet fundoplications. Interestingly, they demonstrated that preoperative belching and air swallowing were not predictive of postoperative gas-related symptoms, including bloating. They concluded that gas-related symptoms are, in part, due to gastrointestinal hypersensitivity to gaseous distention. In this study, all patients experienced postoperative normalization of esophageal acid exposure. However, these authors found that patients who developed postoperative gas symptoms were less satisfied with LARS compared with patients who did not experience these symptoms.

During the early postoperative period, patients who report persistent nausea and demonstrate inadequate intake of a liquid diet should undergo abdominal radiography. If significant gastric distention is identified, a nasogastric tube can safely be placed to decompress the stomach for 24 hours. Few patients require further intervention for gastric bloating.

Dysphagia. It is expected that patients will experience mild, temporary dysphagia during the first 2 to 4 weeks postoperatively. This is thought to be a result of postoperative edema at the fundoplication and esophageal hiatus. In the majority of these patients, this dysphagia spontaneously resolves. A second but less common cause of dysphagia in the early postoperative period is

the presence of a hematoma of the stomach or esophageal wall that develops during the placement of the sutures to create the fundoplication. Although this may create more severe dysphagia, it typically resolves in several days. In both these situations, surgeons should ensure that the patient can maintain nutrition and hydration on a liquid or soft diet; however, additional interventions are rarely needed. If the patient cannot tolerate liquids, a UGI series should be obtained to ensure that no anatomic abnormality, such as an early hiatal hernia, exists. Assuming that there is no early recurrent hiatal hernia and the patient can tolerate liquids, patience should be employed for 3 months. If the patient cannot maintain hydration or dysphagia persists beyond 3 months, a UGI series should be obtained to ensure no anatomic abnormality that could explain the dysphagia. If the UGI series demonstrates an appropriately positioned fundoplication below the diaphragm, esophagogastroduodenoscopy with empirical dilation of the GEJ should be performed.

Failed Antireflux Surgery

Patients who have undergone antireflux surgery may present back to the physician with recurrent, persistent, or completely new foregut symptoms. The most common symptoms of failed LARS are typical symptoms of GERD (i.e., heartburn, regurgitation, and water brash sensation) and dysphagia. During the first 2 months after the operation, most symptoms, particularly when they are mild, are of little significance, and the majority of these will abate with time. One large retrospective review of more than 1700 patients who underwent antireflux surgery found that only 5.6% of patients ultimately required a reoperation for symptoms of recurrent GERD or dysphagia.[36] Persistent symptoms should be investigated by the surgeon to evaluate for functional and anatomic problems associated with the fundoplication or the hiatal closure. Anatomic problems after a fundoplication that can cause symptoms include persistent or recurrent hiatal hernia, slipped fundoplication, and incorrectly constructed fundoplication.

All patients who present with recurrent or persistent symptoms of GERD should be evaluated with esophageal manometry and ambulatory pH study. If the pH study demonstrates elevated distal esophageal acid exposure, an esophagram and upper endoscopy should be performed. Once the diagnosis of persistent or recurrent GERD is made, PPI therapy should be instituted. Most of these patients experience resolution of their symptoms with resumption of PPI therapy. If the patient's symptoms are not effectively managed by medical therapy, reoperation should be performed to create an effective antireflux valve.

The late development of dysphagia after LARS suggests esophageal obstruction. In this setting, esophageal obstruction most frequently results from a recurrent hiatal hernia or a slipped fundoplication. A UGI series and esophagogastroduodenoscopy should be the initial studies obtained in these patients. If a clear anatomic abnormality is visualized (Fig. 42-17), reoperation can be performed without further investigation. If concurrent GERD symptoms are present, ambulatory pH testing and manometry should be performed. To achieve resolution of symptoms, reoperation is almost always necessary in these patients.

Some patients experience no improvement or even worsened symptoms after initial LARS. In these patients, one ought to examine the indication for the original procedure and the technique of the operation as these are the two most important factors associated with success or failure. An incorrectly constructed fundoplication (generally created out of the body of the stomach and

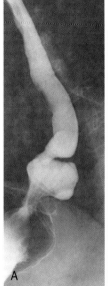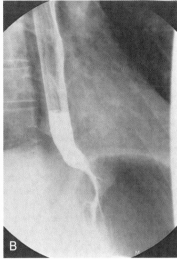

FIGURE 42-17 An upper gastrointestinal series provides invaluable anatomic information in patients with persistent or recurrent postoperative symptoms. **A,** Upper gastrointestinal series demonstrating a 360-degree fundoplication that has both slipped down around the stomach and herniated into the mediastinum. **B,** Normal anatomic appearance of 360-degree fundoplication. Note the smooth tapering of the distal esophagus.

not the fundus) can do nothing to prevent GER and cause new-onset gastroesophageal obstructive symptoms. Failure to completely excise the sac of a hiatal hernia or PEH frequently leads to an early recurrence of hiatal hernia. In our experience, patients who present with persistent symptoms or early recurrence of symptoms after LARS typically require operative management. After appropriate evaluation with pH testing, manometry, UGI series, and esophagogastroduodenoscopy, the patient should undergo operative correction of the anatomic problem with creation of an appropriately constructed fundoplication.

It is important to understand that reoperative antireflux surgery comes with higher stakes than first-time antireflux surgery. Tissues are less pliable, making it more challenging for surgeons to construct an effective antireflux valve. In addition, adhesions and less visible tissue planes contribute to increased rates of intraoperative injury of the stomach and esophagus. Consequently, we have a higher threshold to perform reoperative antireflux surgery. With the exceptions described before, we reserve reoperation for patients with significant symptoms despite maximal nonoperative management.

Novel Therapies for GERD

Despite the fact that LARS provides durable symptom relief with an excellent safety profile, the last decade has seen a drive to develop new therapies for GERD. These therapies have focused on augmenting the LES by modalities such as radiofrequency energy (Mederi Therapeutics Inc, Greenwich, Conn), injection of inert biopolymers (Enteryx; Boston Scientific, Natick, Mass), creation of gastroplications (EndoCinch, Bard, Warwick, RI; EsophyX, EndoGastric Solutions, Redmond, Wash; Plicator, NDO Surgical, Mansfield, Mass), and implantation of a magnetic sphincter augmentation device (LINX, Torax Medical, Shoreview,

Minn). The two most studied therapies that are currently available clinically are the endoscopic suturing device used to complete transoral incisionless fundoplication (TIF), EsophyX, and the only implantable magnetic sphincter augmentation device (MSAD), LINX.

EsophyX

EsophyX is a flexible, multichannel endoluminal device that uses fasteners to construct a full-thickness gastric plication and to create an antireflux valve at the GEJ. The endoluminal fundoplication can be created up to 4 cm in length and 270 degrees. The procedure is performed under general anesthesia; the device is inserted over a gastroscope, and because multiple fasteners are loaded on the end of the device, the entire antireflux valve can be created during a single device insertion.

Since the initial studies evaluating the safety of TIF were published in 2008, additional investigation has demonstrated that TIF improves GERD-related quality of life, results in patient satisfaction with GERD symptom control, is associated with reduced PPI use, and is associated with few side effects.[37] However, whereas it appears that TIF is associated with significant *reduction* in acid exposure and improvement in GERD symptoms, *normalization* of esophageal acid exposure and complete cessation of PPI use have not been demonstrated in these short-term studies. In a long-term (3-year) follow-up study, Muls and colleagues[38] demonstrated similar results. Patients reported durable improvement in GERD-related quality of life and significant reduction in PPI use; however, 48% of patients had normalization of pH study results. Furthermore, 12 of 66 patients required revisional procedures (11 redo TIF and 1 Nissen) because of inadequate control of GERD symptoms associated with esophagitis (92%), PPI use (83%), and Hill grade III or IV antireflux valve (92%).

LINX

LINX is an MSAD that consists of a string of magnetic beads that is positioned around the distal esophagus to increase LES resting pressure to counteract GER. During peristaltic swallows, the propagated food bolus separates the beads, opening the GEJ and allowing the bolus to pass into the stomach, after which the beads return to their original position.

Several characteristics of the MSAD make it attractive. First, it can be sized to the esophagus of the individual patient, which creates LES augmentation to prevent pathologic GER but permits the passage of a food bolus and allows the patient to belch. Second, unlike springs and elastics, magnetic forces are inversely proportional to the distance between them, allowing easier passage of larger food boluses. In addition, magnetic forces do not decay over time, so the antireflux effects should not diminish with the age of the device. Third, the device can be placed laparoscopically, and the placement of the device is reproducible, eliminating the variability that can occur among surgeons with the creation of a fundoplication.

Two studies have evaluated the short-term outcomes comparing MSAD with Nissen fundoplication. These studies demonstrate that MSAD controls typical and extraesophageal symptoms as effectively as Nissen fundoplication but with greater rate of early postoperative dysphagia that resolves with endoscopic dilation. Louie and colleagues[39] retrospectively compared 34 patients who underwent MSAD with 32 patients who underwent Nissen fundoplication. Operative time was shorter for MSAD compared with Nissen fundoplication (73 versus 118 minutes; $P = .001$). At mean postoperative follow-up of 6 months for MSAD and 10 months for Nissen fundoplication, both groups reported significantly improved typical and extraesophageal symptoms of GERD. Objectively, both groups experienced normalization of DeMeester score and total percentage time of pH below 4. However, patients who underwent MSAD experienced significantly more total esophageal acid exposure and higher DeMeester scores than patients who underwent Nissen fundoplication. Furthermore, 44% of patients who underwent MSAD had a DeMeester score above 14.7 (threshold for normal). The total number of reflux episodes was higher for MSAD than for Nissen fundoplication (60.1 versus 21.5; $P = .002$), and the majority of these reflux episodes were postprandial. This exemplifies the trade-off that is seen with MSAD; patients experience greater ability to belch in the postprandial state but experience decreased control of reflux. It also suggests that MSAD is a more "physiologic" antireflux procedure that allows postprandial gastric venting yet is not associated with worse GERD symptoms.

At 6 weeks postoperatively, dysphagia was more severe in Nissen patients; however, by 6 months, swallowing returned to baseline in both groups. Incidence of other side effects (including gas-bloat) was similar between groups; however, patients who underwent MSAD were significantly more likely to be able to belch than patients who underwent Nissen fundoplication.

Sheu and colleagues[40] found similar results in comparing MSAD with Nissen fundoplication in a case-controlled study of 12 patients. MSAD was performed in less operative time (64 versus 90 minutes; $P < .001$), and neither group experienced any morbidity, mortality, or readmission during the first 30 days postoperatively. At mean postoperative follow-up of 7 months, both groups experienced resolution of both typical and extraesophageal symptoms of GERD, and symptom resolution was similar between the groups (MSAD 75% versus Nissen fundoplication 83%; $P = .99$). Patients undergoing Nissen fundoplication experienced significantly more gas-bloat symptoms. There was no difference in the rate of overall postoperative dysphagia (MSAD 83% versus Nissen fundoplication 58%; $P = .37$); however, endoscopic dilation for the management of dysphagia was more frequent in patients who underwent MSAD (50% versus 0%; $P = .014$). No routine objective postoperative testing for GERD was completed; two patients underwent postoperative pH testing for recurrent symptoms, but both demonstrated normal esophageal acid exposure.

Postoperative rates of dysphagia appear similar between MSAD and Nissen fundoplication; however, the need for dilation is more frequent with MSAD. The fact that dysphagia associated with MSAD improves with dilation suggests that the cause of the dysphagia is not from the placement of an undersized device. An alternative explanation is that a fibrous band develops around the MSAD. This fixed ring resists passage of food. Dilation disrupts this scar tissue and relieves dysphagia. This mechanism is supported by the time course for dysphagia between the two groups; patients undergoing Nissen fundoplication experience early dysphagia that resolves without intervention (probably because of edema at the fundoplication), whereas patients undergoing MSAD develop dysphagia relatively later postoperatively, it is progressive, and it resolves only after dilation.

Because LINX is a medical device approved by the U.S. Food and Drug Administration (FDA), all adverse events related to LINX must be reported to the FDA's safety database. Lipham and colleagues[41] reviewed the FDA database and all published surgical literature on the safety of LINX. Between 2007 and 2013, 1048 patients underwent LINX implantation. There were no intraoperative complications; however, one patient experienced an immediate postoperative respiratory arrest that was deemed unrelated to the device itself. The overall readmission rate was 1.4%, and all but one readmission occurred within 90 days postoperatively. Reasons for readmission included dysphagia, pain, nausea, and vomiting. Esophageal dilation was performed in 5.6% of patients; the majority of these were completed within 90 days postoperatively, and no further interventions were required.

Device removal has occurred in 3.6% of patients. Indications for removal were persistent dysphagia (most common), odynophagia, recurrent GERD and desire to undergo fundoplication, nausea or emesis, and need for magnetic resonance imaging. There have been no reported complications with device removal, and the operative technique appears uncomplicated.[42] One instance of device erosion into the esophageal lumen was managed with endoscopic removal of the exposed portion of the device, and the patient subsequently underwent laparoscopic removal of the remainder of the MSAD. The patient experienced no further clinical sequelae. No reported cases of device migration have been reported.

PARAESOPHAGEAL HERNIA

The anatomic definitions of PEH are discussed in a previous section and can be reviewed in Figure 42-2. PEH is frequently associated with obstructive symptoms and, less frequently, typical symptoms of GERD. On occasion, a PEH is identified incidentally on imaging performed for another purpose, and the patient's PEH is asymptomatic. Indication for operative repair of PEH is based on the size of the hernia and the presence and severity of symptoms. To prevent acute gastric volvulus and gastric strangulation, a case can be made for operative repair of a large but minimally symptomatic PEH. Otherwise, the presence of a small asymptomatic hiatal hernia or PEH does not constitute an indication for operative correction.

Pathophysiology

The two key events that facilitate the formation of a PEH are the widening of the diaphragmatic crura at the esophageal hiatus and stretching of the phrenoesophageal membrane. As the hernia enlarges, the phrenoesophageal membrane balloons into the posterior mediastinum like a parachute. After repeated episodes of the viscera entering the hernia sac, adhesions develop between the wall of the sac and the surrounding thoracic structures, thus preventing the herniated abdominal contents from returning to their normal position in the peritoneal cavity. The most common structure to herniate through the esophageal hiatus is the fundus of the stomach; however, the entire stomach as well as other abdominal organs including spleen, colon, pancreas, small bowel, and omentum can migrate into the chest.

Gastric volvulus develops because of laxity in the stomach's peritoneal attachments and subsequent rotation of the gastric fundus on the organoaxial or mesenteric axis of the stomach. The frequency with which this occurs is a matter of debate. Historically, surgeons believed that a large PEH would inevitably volvulize, become incarcerated, and result in gastric strangulation; the mere presence of a PEH was an indication for operative repair. However, more recent evidence suggests that the risk for acute strangulation is approximately 1% per year.[43] We recommend operative repair of completely asymptomatic large hernias only in young (<60 years) and otherwise healthy patients.

Clinical Presentation

The most common symptoms attributed to PEH are gastroesophageal obstructive symptoms, including dysphagia, odynophagia, and early satiety. Intermittent epigastric and chest pain can develop secondary to visceral torsion and distention, which leads to ischemia of the hernia contents. Spontaneous reduction then provides relief of these symptoms. Gastrointestinal bleeding can result from mucosal ischemia or mechanical ulceration of the gastric mucosa. Respiratory symptoms, primarily shortness of breath, can be explained by the mass effect of the hernia contents in the chest. Finally, heartburn and regurgitation are also reported by patients with PEH. These symptoms can be present individually or in combination. Because the symptoms of PEH are diverse and nonspecific, the diagnosis of PEH is often made only after performance of a barium esophagram or UGI endoscopy.

Preoperative Evaluation

The clinical investigations obtained in patients with PEH are similar to those of patients undergoing workup for GERD. A barium esophagogram provides the operating surgeon the most accurate image of the gastroesophageal anatomy (Fig. 42-18). Endoscopy evaluates the gastric and esophageal mucosa for Barrett esophagus and mechanical gastric mucosal erosions (i.e., Cameron ulcers) that can result in gastrointestinal blood loss. Manometry is necessary to determine the motor function of the esophageal body, which can affect the type of antireflux operation performed at the time of PEH repair. Even if a large PEH prevents the passage of the manometry catheter through the LES, it is generally possible to determine the degree of esophageal peristalsis. Finally, in patients with typical symptoms of GERD, ambulatory pH monitoring is indicated to document the presence of abnormal distal esophageal acid exposure. Although the results of ambulatory pH monitoring rarely change the decision for operative repair of PEH, preoperative documentation of GERD is particularly useful as a baseline for comparison in patients who have recurrent symptoms postoperatively.

Operative Repair

PEH can be repaired through the left side of the chest or the abdomen and with open or minimally invasive techniques. Laparoscopy has decreased perioperative morbidity associated with elective PEH repair, and most PEH repairs are currently performed by a laparoscopic approach. This is of particular importance because PEH occurs frequently in older patients with multiple medical comorbidities. Regardless of the operative approach, there are four key steps to PEH repair: (1) reduction of the hernia contents to the abdominal cavity; (2) complete excision of the hernia sac from the posterior mediastinum; (3) mobilization of the distal esophagus to achieve a minimum of 3 cm of intraabdominal esophageal length; and (4) an antireflux operation.

Our preferred approach is laparoscopic PEH repair. Only in the very rare patient have we found the need to perform either an open abdominal operation or a thoracotomy. Patient positioning and trocar placement for laparoscopic PEH repair are the same as for LARS. However, several important variations in operative technique must be made because of the unique anatomy of PEH.

The operation begins by reducing the hernia contents to the abdominal cavity using gentle traction and only to the extent that the contents can be easily reduced. Frequently, however, the hernia contents cannot be fully reduced because adhesions develop between the hernia sac and the posterior mediastinum. This pre-

vents clear visualization of the left crus. Consequently, we divide the short gastric vessels to mobilize the fundus of the stomach and safely expose the left crus.

Once the left crus is exposed, it is necessary to enter the posterior mediastinum outside the hernia sac, which will facilitate complete excision of the hernia sac from the chest. This plane lies between the phrenoesophageal membrane and the left crus. Visualization of the muscle fibers of the left crus is confirmation that the surgeon is in the correct plane. At this point, the peritoneal sac should be divided anteriorly, parallel to the left crus. Further dissection of the sac from its mediastinal attachments will free the stomach and allow it to be delivered into the peritoneal cavity. During this mobilization, the surgeon and assistant must avoid vigorous traction on the sac, which is still attached to the esophagus and can result in esophageal tears. After the hernia contents are returned to the peritoneal cavity, the hernia sac must be transected circumferentially at the hiatus.

The most challenging aspect of the sac dissection is encountered during the mobilization of the posterior sac. The esophagus and posterior vagus nerve are intimately associated with the sac posteriorly and can be easily injured during this dissection. A lighted bougie helps identify the exact location of the esophagus. Once the esophagus is clearly identified, the bougie should be pulled back to avoid unnecessarily thinning the esophageal wall and maximizing the posterior mediastinal space to facilitate further dissection. After the sac is freed at the hiatus, a concerted effort is made to remove as much of the hernia sac from the mediastinum as possible. However, the pleura, esophagus, pericardium, aorta, and inferior pulmonary veins are intimately related to the hernia sac, and these vital structures may be injured during this dissection. The surgeon's desire to remove the entire sac must be tempered by the possibility of injuring these vital

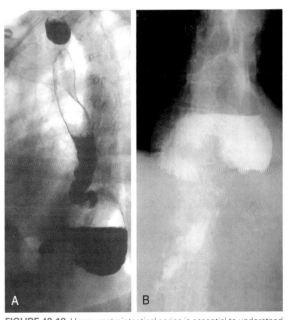

FIGURE 42-18 Upper gastrointestinal series is essential to understand the anatomy of a paraesophageal hernia. **A,** Oblique view demonstrating a distended stomach with an air-fluid level anterior to the esophagus and well into the mediastinum. **B,** Anteroposterior view demonstrating complete organoaxial volvulus with a completely intrathoracic stomach and the pylorus at the hiatus.

structures. Once the sac is excised from the mediastinum, the esophagus is further mobilized to obtain a minimum of 3 cm of intra-abdominal length. Then, the crura are reapproximated with interrupted nonabsorbable suture.

Tension-free closure of the esophageal hiatus is a key step in the repair of PEH. In some patients, lack of pliability of the diaphragmatic crura makes a tension-free closure of the hiatus impossible. In our experience, the size of the hernia does not accurately predict the ability to close the hiatus without tension. However, scarred and poorly pliable crura are frequently encountered during repair of recurrent hiatal hernias. If a tension-free closure is not possible, two options are available: (1) close the hiatus under tension and reinforce the closure with biologic mesh; and (2) perform a diaphragmatic relaxing incision to allow primary tension-free closure of the hiatus and reinforce the relaxing incision and hiatal closure with biologic mesh. Importantly, permanent synthetic mesh should never be used at the esophageal hiatus as it is associated with esophageal erosion and stenosis.

If the hiatus can be closed primarily but under some tension, biologic mesh should be placed to reinforce this closure. To do this, a 7 × 10-cm piece of biologic mesh is cut into the shape of a horseshoe. The mesh is then placed at the hiatus. This can be done in a U configuration, with the base overlying the posterior hiatal closure, or in a C configuration, with the base overlying the right crus and limbs of the mesh lying anterior and posterior to the esophagus. The C configuration has the advantage of reinforcing the anterior and posterior hiatus. The orientation of the mesh placement should be according to the surgeon's preference. The mesh is sutured to the diaphragm, and fibrin glue is used to reinforce the mesh placement (Fig. 42-19).

Several studies have investigated the use of mesh to reinforce hiatal closure in PEH repair (Table 42-4). A multi-institutional randomized clinical trial compared primary hiatal closure and reinforcement of primary closure with biologic mesh. At 6 months of follow-up, hiatal hernia recurrence rate was significantly lower when the hiatus was reinforced with biologic mesh compared with primary closure alone (9% versus 24%; P = .04).[44] However, at 5-year follow-up, there was no significant difference in hiatal hernia recurrence rates between patients with and without mesh.[45] This suggests that biologic mesh reinforcement of the hiatal closure in PEH repair decreases early but not late recurrent hiatal hernias. In this randomized trial using biologic mesh, there were no mesh-related complications.

On occasion, the pliability of the crura is so poor that the hiatus cannot be closed primarily. In this situation, a crural relaxing incision is performed to facilitate closure. Relaxing incisions have been described on the right and left crura. We prefer to perform a relaxing incision on the right crus (Fig. 42-20) and to patch the defect with a U-shaped biologic mesh, as described before. In very few patients, when the hiatus will not close with

a right-sided relaxing incision, a left-sided relaxing incision is performed, which facilitates medialization of the left crus and primary closure. In our experience, coverage of the left-sided relaxing incision with biologic mesh is associated with the development of diaphragmatic hernias and need for reoperation. Therefore, we now patch this defect with permanent synthetic polytetrafluoroethylene mesh (Fig. 42-21). We have not encountered any complications with permanent mesh placement in this location.

After the hiatus is closed, an antireflux procedure is performed. A Nissen fundoplication is performed in all patients except those with severely ineffective motility or aperistaltic esophagus. In such patients, a Toupet fundoplication is performed. Although the need for an antireflux procedure is controversial, many patients with PEH have abnormal reflux, and the fundoplication will seal the hiatus, preventing access by other viscera. Postoperative care is the same as for patients who have undergone LARS.

Acute Gastric Volvulus and Strangulation

A relatively rare occurrence, acute gastric volvulus is a clinical emergency. Patients present with sudden onset of chest or epigastric pain associated with retching without the production of emesis. The development of fever, tachycardia, and leukocytosis suggests gastric strangulation and impending perforation. Gastric volvulus is necessary but not sufficient for gastric ischemia to develop. More often, patients present with subacute or chronic recurrent gastric volvulus, which causes gastroesophageal obstructive symptoms but never results in gastric ischemia.

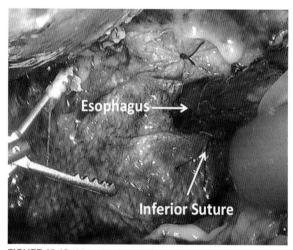

FIGURE 42-19 When the closure of the esophageal hiatus is met with mild to moderate tension, we place a 7 × 10-cm piece of biologic mesh to reinforce the hiatal closure.

TABLE 42-4	Studies of Biologic Mesh in Patients Undergoing Paraesophageal Hernia Repair				
STUDY	STUDY DESIGN	ARMS		MEDIAN FOLLOW-UP	RECURRENCE
Oelschlager et al,[45] 2011	RCT	Surgisis, n = 26; no mesh, n = 34		59 months	Surgisis, 54%; no mesh, 59%; P = .7
Oelschlager et al,[48] 2006	RCT	Surgisis, n = 51; no mesh, n = 57		6 months	Surgisis, 9%; no mesh, 24%; P = .04
Ringley et al,[49] 2006	Retrospective	Alloderm, n = 22; no mesh, n = 22		7 months	Alloderm, 0%; no mesh, 9%; P < .05
Jacobs et al,[50] 2007	Retrospective	Surgisis, n = 127; no mesh, n = 93		38 months	Surgisis, 3%; no mesh, 20%; P < .01

RCT, randomized controlled trial.

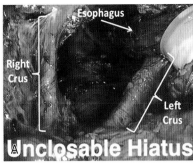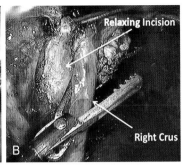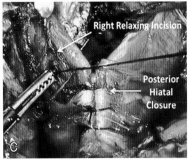

FIGURE 42-20 When poorly pliable crura prevent primary closure of the esophageal hiatus (*left*), a relaxing incision is placed on the right crus (*middle*) to facilitate closure (*right*).

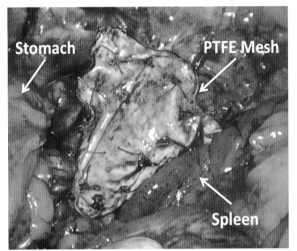

FIGURE 42-21 When bilateral relaxing incisions are necessary to facilitate hiatal closure, the left-sided relaxing incision is covered with permanent mesh to prevent the development of a diaphragmatic hernia. *PTFE*, polytetrafluoroethylene.

Initial management of acute gastric volvulus should include placement of a nasogastric tube for gastric decompression. If bedside placement of a nasogastric tube is not possible, esophagoscopy can facilitate gastric decompression and nasogastric tube placement. On occasion, endoscopic reduction of volvulus is possible. Endoscopy also allows assessment of the gastric mucosa; if gastric ischemia is present, emergent operation is indicated.

The operative management of acute gastric volvulus should follow the same tenets as for PEH repair. In otherwise healthy patients, a formal laparoscopic PEH repair should be performed. In high operative risk patients who may not tolerate a prolonged general anesthetic necessary for PEH repair, consideration should be given to laparoscopic reduction of the gastric volvulus and anterior abdominal wall gastropexy.

SUMMARY

Operative treatment of GERD and PEH has become more common in the era of laparoscopic procedures. Careful selection of patients based on symptom assessment, response to medical therapy, and preoperative testing will optimize chances for effective and durable postoperative control of symptoms. Complications of LARS and

repair of PEH are rare and generally can be managed without reoperation. When reoperation is necessary for operative failures, it should be performed by high-volume surgeons.

SELECTED REFERENCES

Jobe BA, Richter JE, Hoppo T, et al: Preoperative diagnostic workup before antireflux surgery: An evidence and experience based consensus of the Esophageal Diagnostic Advisory Panel. *J Am Coll Surg* 217:586–597, 2013.

A consensus statement from experienced surgeons and gastroenterologists in the field of GERD on the preoperative diagnostic testing of patients with GERD.

Niebisch S, Fleming FJ, Galey KM, et al: Perioperative risk of laparoscopic fundoplication: Safer than previously reported—analysis of the American College of Surgeons National Surgical Quality Improvement Program 2005-2009. *J Am Coll Surg* 215:61–68, 2012.

An observational study of more than 7500 patients who underwent laparoscopic fundoplication demonstrating a 30-day mortality and morbidity of 0.18% and 3.8%, respectively.

Oelschlager BK, Pellegrini CA, Hunter JG, et al: Biologic mesh to prevent recurrence after laparoscopic paraesophageal hernia repair: Long-term follow-up from a multicenter, prospective, randomized trial. *J Am Coll Surg* 213:461–468, 2011.

Long-term follow-up to a randomized trial evaluating the effectiveness of biologic mesh reinforcement of the esophageal hiatus at the time of paraesophageal hernia repair.

Oelschlager BK, Petersen RP, Brunt LM, et al: Laparoscopic paraesophageal hernia repair: Defining long-term clinical and anatomic outcomes. *J Gastrointest Surg* 16:453–459, 2012.

A multicenter randomized trial that evaluated the symptomatic response to laparoscopic paraesophageal hernia repair as well as the relationship between recurrent symptoms and recurrent hiatal hernia.

Richenbacher N, Kotter T, Kochen MM, et al: Fundoplication versus medical management of gastroesophageal reflux disease: A systemic review and meta-analysis. *Surg Endosc* 28:143–155, 2014.

Meta-analysis of trials comparing surgical fundoplication with medical management of GERD.

Smith CD: Antireflux surgery. *Surg Clin North Am* 88:943–958, 2008.

Comprehensive review of the diagnostic workup, patient selection criteria, surgical technique, and postoperative management for patients with GERD.

Soper NJ, Teitelbaum EN: Laparoscopic paraesophageal hernia repair: Current controversies. *Surg Laparosc Endosc Percutan Tech* 23:442–445, 2013.

Review of laparoscopic paraesophageal hernia repair operative technique and discussion of controversies in repair, including use of mesh cruroplasty and performance of esophagogastric fundoplication.

Wileman SM, McCann S, Grant AM, et al: Medical versus surgical management for gastro-oesophageal reflux disease (GORD) in adults. *Cochrane Database Syst Rev* (3):CD003243, 2010.

Comprehensive review of major studies investigating whether medical or surgical management is the most clinically and cost-effective treatment for patients with GERD.

Worrell SG, Greene CL, DeMeester TR: The state of surgical treatment of gastroesophageal reflux disease after five decades. *J Am Coll Surg* 219:819–830, 2014.

A clear, concise, and thorough description of the approach to the surgical management of patients with GERD, including selection of the appropriate operation and avoidance of operative technical pitfalls.

REFERENCES

1. Mainie I, Tutuian R, Shay S, et al: Acid and non-acid reflux in patients with persistent symptoms despite acid suppressive therapy: A multicentre study using combined ambulatory impedance-pH monitoring. *Gut* 55:1398–1402, 2006.
2. Worrell SG, DeMeester SR, Greene CL, et al: Pharyngeal pH monitoring better predicts a successful outcome for extraesophageal reflux symptoms after antireflux surgery. *Surg Endosc* 27:4113–4118, 2013.
3. Bowrey DJ, Peters JH, DeMeester TR: Gastroesophageal reflux disease in asthma: Effects of medical and surgical antireflux therapy on asthma control. *Ann Surg* 231:161–172, 2000.
4. Raghu G, Freudenberger TD, Yang S, et al: High prevalence of abnormal acid gastro-oesophageal reflux in idiopathic pulmonary fibrosis. *Eur Respir J* 27:136–142, 2006.
5. Lee JS, Ryu JH, Elicker BM, et al: Gastroesophageal reflux therapy is associated with longer survival in patients with idiopathic pulmonary fibrosis. *Am J Respir Crit Care Med* 184:1390–1394, 2011.
6. Raghu G, Yang ST-Y, Spada C, et al: Sole treatment of acid gastroesophageal reflux in idiopathic pulmonary fibrosis: A case series. *Chest* 129:794–800, 2006.
7. Campos GMR, Peters JH, DeMeester TR, et al: Multivariate analysis of factors predicting outcome after laparoscopic Nissen fundoplication. *J Gastrointest Surg* 3:292–300, 1999.
8. Bredenoord AJ, Weusten BL, Timmer R, et al: Addition of esophageal impedance monitoring to pH monitoring increases the yield of symptom association analysis in patients off PPI therapy. *Am J Gastroenterol* 101:453–459, 2006.
9. Patel A, Sayuk GS, Gyawali CP: Parameters on esophageal pH-impedance monitoring that predict outcomes of patients with gastroesophageal reflux disease. *Clin Gastroenterol Hepatol* 13:884–891, 2015.
10. Kahrilas PJ, Dodds WJ, Hogan WJ, et al: Esophageal peristaltic dysfunction in peptic esophagitis. *Gastroenterology* 91:897–904, 1986.
11. Armstrong D: Endoscopic evaluation of gastro-esophageal reflux disease. *Yale J Biol Med* 72:93–100, 1999.
12. Epstein D, Bojke L, Sculpher MJ, et al: Laparoscopic fundoplication compared with medical management for gastro-oesophageal reflux disease: Cost effectiveness study. *BMJ* 339:b2576, 2009.
13. Wong RK, Hanson DG, Waring PJ, et al: ENT manifestations of gastroesophageal reflux. *Am J Gastroenterol* 95(Suppl):S15–S22, 2000.
14. Booth MI, Stratford J, Jones L, et al: Randomized clinical trial of laparoscopic total (Nissen) versus posterior partial (Toupet) fundoplication for gastro-oesophageal reflux disease based on preoperative oesophageal manometry. *Br J Surg* 95:57–63, 2008.
15. Oleynikov D, Eubanks TR, Oelschlager BK, et al: Total fundoplication is the operation of choice for patients with gastroesophageal reflux and defective peristalsis. *Surg Endosc* 16:909–913, 2002.
16. Fein M, Seyfried F: Is there a role for anything other than a Nissen's operation? *J Gastrointest Surg* 14(Suppl 1):S67–S74, 2010.
17. Shan CX, Zhang W, Zheng XM, et al: Evidence-based appraisal in laparoscopic Nissen and Toupet fundoplications for gastroesophageal reflux disease. *World J Gastroenterol* 16:3063–3071, 2010.
18. Kaufman JA, Houghland JE, Quiroga E, et al: Long-term outcomes of laparoscopic antireflux surgery for gastroesophageal reflux disease (GERD)–related airway disorder. *Surg Endosc* 20:1824–1830, 2006.
19. Rossi M, Barreca M, de Bortoli N, et al: Efficacy of Nissen fundoplication versus medical therapy in the regression of low-grade dysplasia in patients with Barrett esophagus: A prospective study. *Ann Surg* 243:58–63, 2006.
20. Katz PO, Gerson LB, Vela MF: Guidelines for the diagnosis and management of gastroesophageal reflux disease. *Am J Gastroenterol* 108:308–328, quiz 329, 2013.
21. Finley K, Giannamore M, Bennett M, et al: Assessing the impact of lifestyle modification education on knowledge and behavior changes in gastroesophageal reflux disease patients on proton pump inhibitors. *J Am Pharm Assoc* 49:544–548, 2009.
22. Ali T, Roberts DN, Tierney WM: Long-term safety concerns with proton pump inhibitors. *Am J Med* 122:896–903, 2009.
23. Heidelbaugh JJ, Kim AH, Chang R, et al: Overutilization of proton-pump inhibitors: What the clinician needs to know. *Ther Adv Gastroenterol* 5:219–232, 2012.

24. Havu N: Enterochromaffin-like cell carcinoids of gastric mucosa in rats after life-long inhibition of gastric secretion. *Digestion* 35(Suppl 1):42–55, 1986.
25. Jianu CS, Lange OJ, Viset T, et al: Gastric neuroendocrine carcinoma after long-term use of proton pump inhibitor. *Scand J Gastroenterol* 47:64–67, 2012.
26. Oelschlager BK, Yamamoto K, Woltman T, et al: Vagotomy during hiatal hernia repair: A benign esophageal lengthening procedure. *J Gastrointest Surg* 12:1155–1162, 2008.
27. Spechler SJ, Lee E, Ahnen D, et al: Long-term outcome of medical and surgical therapies for gastroesophageal reflux disease: Follow-up of a randomized controlled trial. *JAMA* 285:2331–2338, 2001.
28. Lundell L, Miettinen P, Myrvold HE, et al: Seven-year follow-up of a randomized clinical trial comparing proton-pump inhibition with surgical therapy for reflux oesophagitis. *Br J Surg* 94:198–203, 2007.
29. Lundell L, Miettinen P, Myrvold HE, et al: Comparison of outcomes twelve years after antireflux surgery or omeprazole maintenance therapy for reflux esophagitis. *Clin Gastroenterol Hepatol* 7:1292–1298, 2009.
30. Dallemagne B, Weerts J, Markiewicz S, et al: Clinical results of laparoscopic fundoplication at ten years after surgery. *Surg Endosc* 20:159–165, 2006.
31. Oelschlager BK, Eubanks TR, Oleynikov D, et al: Symptomatic and physiologic outcomes after operative treatment for extraesophageal reflux. *Surg Endosc* 16:1032–1036, 2002.
32. Niebisch S, Fleming FJ, Galey KM, et al: Perioperative risk of laparoscopic fundoplication: Safer than previously reported—analysis of the American College of Surgeons National Surgical Quality Improvement Program 2005 to 2009. *J Am Coll Surg* 215:61–68, discussion 68–69, 2012.
33. Bizekis C, Kent M, Luketich J: Complications after surgery for gastroesophageal reflux disease. *Thorac Surg Clin* 16:99–108, 2006.
34. Odabasi M, Abuoglu HH, Arslan C, et al: Asymptomatic partial splenic infarction in laparoscopic floppy Nissen fundoplication and brief literature review. *Int Surg* 99:291–294, 2014.
35. Kessing BF, Broeders JA, Vinke N, et al: Gas-related symptoms after antireflux surgery. *Surg Endosc* 27:3739–3747, 2013.
36. Lamb PJ, Myers JC, Jamieson GG, et al: Long-term outcomes of revisional surgery following laparoscopic fundoplication. *Br J Surg* 96:391–397, 2009.
37. Bell RCW, Mavrelis PG, Barnes WE, et al: A prospective multicenter registry of patients with chronic gastroesophageal reflux disease receiving transoral incisionless fundoplication. *J Am Coll Surg* 215:794–809, 2012.
38. Muls V, Eckardt AJ, Marchese M, et al: Three-year results of a multicenter prospective study of transoral incisionless fundoplication. *Surg Innov* 20:321–330, 2013.
39. Louie BE, Farivar AS, Shultz D, et al: Short-term outcomes using magnetic sphincter augmentation versus Nissen fundoplication for medically resistant gastroesophageal reflux disease. *Ann Thorac Surg* 98:498–504, discussion 504–505, 2014.
40. Sheu EG, Nau P, Nath B, et al: A comparative trial of laparoscopic magnetic sphincter augmentation and Nissen fundoplication. *Surg Endosc* 29:505–509, 2015.
41. Lipham JC, DeMeester TR, Ganz RA, et al: The LINX reflux management system: Confirmed safety and efficacy now at 4 years. *Surg Endosc* 26:2944–2949, 2012.
42. Harnsberger CR, Broderick RC, Fuchs HF, et al: Magnetic lower esophageal sphincter augmentation device removal. *Surg Endosc* 29:984–986, 2015.
43. Stylopoulos N, Gazelle GS, Rattner DW: Paraesophageal hernias: Operation or observation? *Ann Surg* 236:492–500, discussion 500–501, 2002.
44. Oelschlager BK, Pellegrini CA, Hunter J, et al: Biologic prosthesis reduces recurrence after laparoscopic paraesophageal hernia repair: A multicenter, prospective, randomized trial. *Ann Surg* 244:481–490, 2006.
45. Oelschlager BK, Pellegrini CA, Hunter JG, et al: Biologic prosthesis to prevent recurrence after laparoscopic paraesophageal hernia repair: Long-term follow-up from a multicenter, prospective, randomized trial. *J Am Coll Surg* 213:461–468, 2011.
46. Anvari M, Allen C, Marshall J, et al: A randomized controlled trial of laparoscopic Nissen fundoplication versus proton pump inhibitors for the treatment of patients with chronic gastroesophageal reflux disease (GERD): 3-year outcomes. *Surg Endosc* 25:2547–2554, 2011.
47. Grant AM, Wileman SM, Ramsay CR, et al: Minimal access surgery compared with medical management for chronic gastro-oesophageal reflux disease: UK collaborative randomised trial. *BMJ* 337:a2664, 2008.
48. Oelschlager BK, Pellegrini CA, Hunter J, et al: Biologic prosthesis reduces recurrence after laparoscopic paraesophageal hernia repair: A multicenter, prospective, randomized trial. *Ann Surg* 244:481–490, 2006.
49. Ringley CD, Bochkarev V, Ahmed SI, et al: Laparoscopic hiatal hernia repair with human acellular dermal matrix patch: Our initial experience. *Am J Surg* 192:767–772, 2006.
50. Jacobs M, Gomez E, Plasencia G, et al: Use of Surgisis mesh in laparoscopic repair of hiatal hernias. *Surg Laparosc Endosc Percutan Tech* 17:365–368, 2007.

SECTION X

ABDOMEN

第十篇　腹部

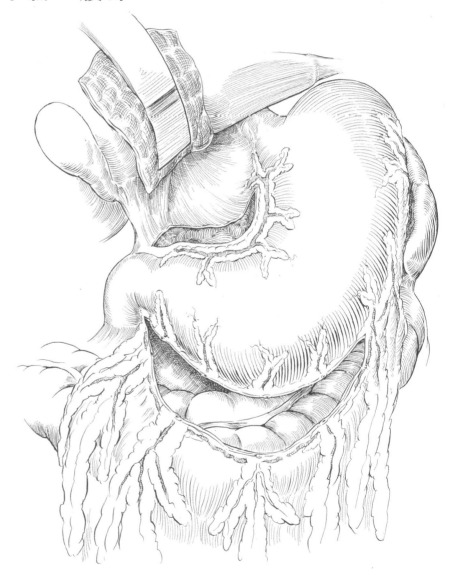

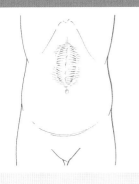

Abdominal Wall, Umbilicus, Peritoneum, Mesenteries, Omentum, and Retroperitoneum

Richard H. Turnage, Jason Mizell, Brian Badgwell

第四十三章　腹壁、脐、腹膜、肠系膜、网膜与腹膜后腔

中文导读

本章共分4节：①腹壁和脐；②腹膜和腹膜腔；③肠系膜和网膜；④腹膜后腔。

第一节从胚胎学开始介绍腹壁及脐由胚胎早期至胚胎形成过程中，腹壁各部分的融合变化。从解剖学介绍腹壁九层组成部分，包括皮肤、皮下组织、浅筋膜、腹外斜肌、腹内斜肌、腹横肌、腹横筋膜、腹膜外脂肪组织及腹膜。同时也描述了腹壁的血液供应及神经分布。从先天性和后天获得性的角度，针对腹壁畸形中的脐疝、脐膨出、腹裂、腹直肌分离、前腹壁疝等疾病进行介绍。另外也介绍了腹壁恶性肿瘤，包括硬纤维瘤、腹壁肉瘤以及腹壁转移瘤。最后阐述了关于涉及腹壁的腹内疾病的症状。

第二节首先从解剖学介绍了腹膜的构成及毗邻，以及腹膜腔的分隔；从生理学介绍了腹膜的功能，特别是腹膜针对感染的反应。针对腹膜疾病，进行了分

类的介绍，包括腹水、腹膜炎、腹膜恶性肿瘤等。重点介绍了腹水，从病理生理学和病因学开始，包括临床表现及诊断、肝硬化腹水、乳糜腹水的治疗。腹膜炎是本节的另一个重点内容，包括自发性细菌性腹膜炎、结核性腹膜炎、慢性门诊腹膜透析相关性腹膜炎等。最后还介绍了腹膜恶性肿瘤，主要对腹膜假性黏液瘤、恶性腹膜间皮瘤进行了描述。

第三节由胚胎学和解剖学开始作为引导，从起源和发育开始描述，同时介绍了大网膜及肠系膜的生理功能。具体到网膜疾病，介绍了包括大网膜囊肿、大网膜扭转和梗死、大网膜肿瘤、大网膜移植和转位。肠系膜疾病中，对肠系膜囊肿、急性肠系膜淋巴结炎、硬化性肠系膜炎重点进行了诊断相关的描述；对

于肠系膜相关疝，特别是结肠系膜（或十二指肠旁）疝进行了详细介绍，包括不同两种类型的诊断和手术治疗方式。最后还将肠系膜恶性肿瘤，特别是肠系膜和腹腔内硬纤维瘤的内容进行了描述。

　　第四节从解剖学上解释了腹膜后腔的定义，介绍了腹膜后手术入路的适用手术类型。对于腹膜后疾病，重点介绍了腹膜后脓肿的分类、治疗方法，腹膜后血肿的诱因及对应的处理方式，同时也描述了腹膜后纤维化，这种少见的炎症性疾病。最后阐述了腹膜后恶性肿瘤，特别是腹膜后肉瘤的内容。

〔胡俊波〕

ABDOMINAL WALL AND UMBILICUS

Embryology

The abdominal wall begins to develop in the earliest stages of embryonic differentiation from the lateral plate of the embryonic mesoderm. At this stage, the embryo consists of three principal layers—an outer protective layer termed the *ectoderm;* an inner nutritive layer, the *endoderm;* and the *mesoderm.*

The mesoderm becomes divided by clefts on each side of the lateral plate that ultimately develop into somatic and splanchnic layers. The splanchnic layer with its underlying endoderm contributes to the formation of the viscera by differentiating into muscle, blood vessels, lymphatics, and connective tissues of the alimentary tract. The somatic layer contributes to the development of the abdominal wall. Proliferation of mesodermal cells in the embryonic abdominal wall results in the formation of an inverted U-shaped tube that in its early stages communicates freely with the extraembryonic coelom.

As the embryo enlarges and the abdominal wall components grow toward one another, the ventral open area, bounded by the edge of the amnion, becomes smaller. This results in the development of the umbilical cord as a tubular structure containing the omphalomesenteric duct, allantois, and fetal blood vessels, which pass to and from the placenta. By the end of the third month of gestation, the body wall has closed, except at the umbilical ring. Because the alimentary tract increases in length more rapidly than the coelomic cavity increases in volume, much of the developing gut protrudes through the umbilical ring to lie within the umbilical cord. As the coelomic cavity enlarges to accommodate the intestine, the intestine returns to the peritoneal cavity so that only the omphalomesenteric duct, allantois, and fetal blood vessels pass through the shrinking umbilical ring. At birth, blood no longer courses through the umbilical vessels, and the omphalomesenteric duct has been reduced to a fibrous cord that no longer communicates with the intestine. After division of the umbilical cord, the umbilical ring heals rapidly by scarring.

Anatomy

There are nine layers to the abdominal wall: skin, subcutaneous tissue, superficial fascia, external oblique muscle, internal oblique muscle, transversus abdominis muscle, transversalis fascia, preperitoneal adipose and areolar tissue, and peritoneum (Fig. 43-1).

Subcutaneous Tissues

The subcutaneous tissue consists of Camper and Scarpa fasciae. Camper fascia is the more superficial adipose layer that contains the bulk of the subcutaneous fat, whereas Scarpa fascia is a deeper, denser layer of fibrous connective tissue contiguous with the fascia lata of the thigh. Approximation of Scarpa fascia aids in the alignment of the skin after surgical incisions in the lower abdomen.

Muscle and Investing Fasciae

The muscles of the anterolateral abdominal wall include the external and internal oblique and transversus abdominis. These flat muscles enclose much of the circumference of the torso and give rise anteriorly to a broad flat aponeurosis investing the rectus abdominis muscles, termed the *rectus sheath.* The external oblique muscles are the largest and thickest of the flat abdominal wall muscles. They originate from the lower seven ribs and course in a superolateral to inferomedial direction. The most posterior of the fibers run vertically downward to insert into the anterior half of the iliac crest. At the midclavicular line, the muscle fibers give rise to a flat, strong aponeurosis that passes anteriorly to the rectus sheath to insert medially into the linea alba (Fig. 43-2). The lower portion of the external oblique aponeurosis is rolled posteriorly and superiorly on itself to form a groove on which the spermatic cord lies. This portion of the external oblique aponeurosis extends from the anterior superior iliac spine to the pubic tubercle and is termed the *inguinal* or *Poupart ligament.* The inguinal ligament is the lower free edge of the external oblique aponeurosis posterior to which pass the femoral artery, vein, and nerve and the iliacus, psoas major, and pectineus muscles. A femoral hernia passes posterior to the inguinal ligament, whereas an inguinal hernia passes anterior and superior to this ligament. The shelving edge of the inguinal ligament is used in various repairs of inguinal hernia, including the Bassini and the Lichtenstein tension-free repairs (see Chapter 44).

The internal oblique muscle originates from the iliopsoas fascia beneath the lateral half of the inguinal ligament, from the anterior two thirds of the iliac crest and lumbodorsal fascia. Its fibers course in a direction opposite to those of the external oblique, that is, inferolateral to superomedial. The uppermost fibers insert into the lower five ribs and their cartilages (Fig. 43-3; see Fig. 43-2A). The central fibers form an aponeurosis at the semilunar line, which, above the semicircular line (of Douglas), is divided

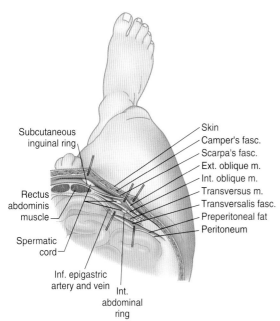

FIGURE 43-1 The nine layers of the anterolateral abdominal wall. (From Thorek P: *Anatomy in surgery*, ed 2, Philadelphia, 1962, JB Lippincott, p 358.)

into anterior and posterior lamellae that envelop the rectus abdominis muscle. Below the semicircular line, the aponeurosis of the internal oblique muscle courses anteriorly to the rectus abdominis muscle as part of the anterior rectus sheath. The lowermost fibers of the internal oblique muscle pursue an inferomedial course, paralleling that of the spermatic cord, to insert between the symphysis pubis and pubic tubercle. Some of the lower muscle fascicles accompany the spermatic cord into the scrotum as the cremasteric muscle.

The transversus abdominis muscle is the smallest of the muscles of the anterolateral abdominal wall. It arises from the lower six costal cartilages, spines of the lumbar vertebrae, iliac crest, and iliopsoas fascia beneath the lateral third of the inguinal ligament. The fibers course transversely to give rise to a flat aponeurotic sheet that passes posterior to the rectus abdominis muscle above the semicircular line and anterior to the muscle below it (Fig. 43-4). The inferiormost fibers of the transversus abdominis originating from the iliopsoas fascia pass inferomedially along with the lower fibers of the internal oblique muscle. These fibers form the aponeurotic arch of the transversus abdominis muscle, which lies superior to Hesselbach triangle and is an important anatomic landmark in the repair of inguinal hernias, particularly the Bassini operation and Cooper ligament repairs. Hesselbach triangle is the site of direct inguinal hernias and is bordered by the inguinal ligament inferiorly, lateral margin of the rectus sheath medially, and inferior epigastric vessels laterally. The floor of this triangle is composed of transversalis fascia.

The transversalis fascia covers the deep surface of the transversus abdominis muscle and, with its various extensions, forms a complete fascial envelope around the abdominal cavity (Fig. 43-5; see Fig. 43-4B). This fascial layer is regionally named for the muscles that it covers, for example, iliopsoas fascia, obturator fascia, and inferior fascia of the respiratory diaphragm. The trans-

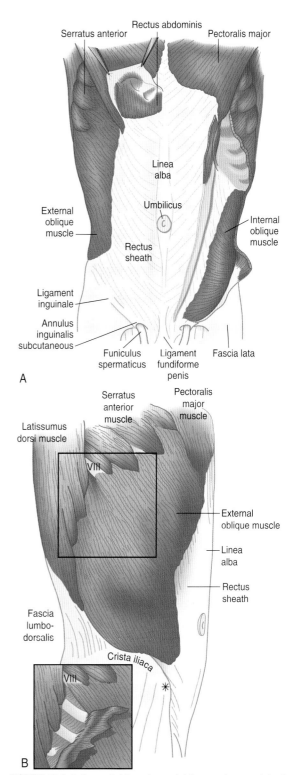

FIGURE 43-2 **A,** External oblique, internal oblique, and rectus abdominis muscles and anterior rectus sheath. **B,** Lateral view of the external oblique muscle and its aponeurosis as it enters the anterior rectus sheath. *Inset,* Origin of the external oblique muscle fibers from the lower ribs and their costal cartilages. (From McVay C: *Anson and McVay's surgical anatomy*, ed 6, Philadelphia, 1984, WB Saunders, pp 477–478.)

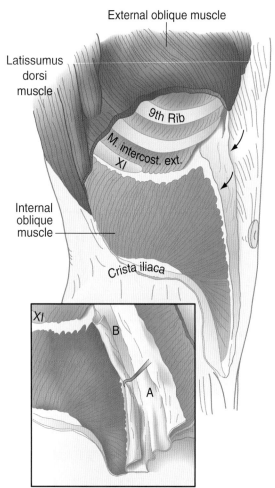

External oblique muscle

Latissumus dorsi muscle

9th Rib

M. intercost. ext.

XI

Internal oblique muscle

Crista iliaca

XI

B

A

FIGURE 43-3 Lateral view of the internal oblique muscle. The external oblique muscle has been removed to show the underlying internal oblique muscle originating from the lower ribs and costal cartilages. (From McVay C: *Anson and McVay's surgical anatomy,* ed 6, Philadelphia, 1984, WB Saunders, p 479.)

versalis fascia binds together the muscle and aponeurotic fascicles into a continuous layer and reinforces weak areas where the aponeurotic fibers are sparse. This layer is responsible for the structural integrity of the abdominal wall, and by definition, a hernia results from a defect in the transversalis fascia.

The rectus abdominis muscles are paired muscles that appear as long, flat, triangular ribbons wider at their origin on the anterior surfaces of the fifth, sixth, and seventh costal cartilages and the xiphoid process than at their insertion on the pubic crest and pubic symphysis. Each muscle is composed of long parallel fascicles interrupted by three to five tendinous inscriptions (Fig. 43-5), which attach the rectus abdominis muscle to the anterior rectus sheath. There is no similar attachment to the posterior rectus sheath. These muscles lie adjacent to each other, separated only by the linea alba. In addition to supporting the abdominal wall and protecting its contents, contraction of these powerful muscles flexes the vertebral column.

The rectus abdominis muscles are contained within the rectus sheath, which is derived from the aponeuroses of the three flat abdominal muscles. Superior to the semicircular line, this fascial sheath completely envelops the rectus abdominis muscle, with the external oblique and anterior lamella of the internal oblique aponeuroses passing anterior to the rectus abdominis and aponeuroses from the posterior lamella of the internal oblique muscle, transversus abdominis muscle, and transversalis fascia passing posterior to the rectus muscle. Below the semicircular line, all these fascial layers pass anterior to the rectus abdominis muscle, except the transversalis fascia. In this location, the posterior aspect of the rectus abdominis muscle is covered only by transversalis fascia, preperitoneal areolar tissue, and peritoneum.

The rectus abdominis muscles are held closely in apposition near the anterior midline by the linea alba. The linea alba consists of a band of dense, crisscrossed fibers of the aponeuroses of the broad abdominal muscles that extends from the xiphoid to the pubic symphysis. It is much wider above the umbilicus than below, thus facilitating the placement of surgical incisions in the midline without entering the right or left rectus sheath.

Preperitoneal Space and Peritoneum

The preperitoneal space lies between the transversalis fascia and parietal peritoneum and contains adipose and areolar tissue. Coursing through the preperitoneal space are the following:
- Inferior epigastric artery and vein
- Medial umbilical ligaments, which are the vestiges of the fetal umbilical arteries
- Median umbilical ligament, which is a midline fibrous remnant of the fetal allantoic stalk or urachus
- Falciform ligament of the liver, extending from the umbilicus to the liver

The round ligament, or ligamentum teres, is contained within the free margin of the falciform ligament and represents the obliterated umbilical vein, coursing from the umbilicus to the left branch of the portal vein (Fig. 43-6). The parietal peritoneum is the innermost layer of the abdominal wall. It consists of a thin layer of dense, irregular connective tissue covered on its inner surface by a single layer of squamous mesothelium. The peritoneum is covered in more depth later in the chapter.

Vessels and Nerves of the Abdominal Wall
Vascular Supply

The anterolateral abdominal wall receives its arterial supply from the last six intercostals and four lumbar arteries, superior and inferior epigastric arteries, and deep circumflex iliac arteries (Fig. 43-7). The trunks of the intercostal and lumbar arteries together with the intercostal, iliohypogastric, and ilioinguinal nerves course between the transversus abdominis and internal oblique muscles. The distalmost extensions of these vessels pierce the lateral margins of the rectus sheath at various levels and communicate freely with branches of the superior and inferior epigastric arteries. The superior epigastric artery, one of the terminal branches of the internal mammary artery, reaches the posterior surface of the rectus abdominis muscle through the costoxiphoid space in the diaphragm. It descends within the rectus sheath to anastomose with branches of the inferior epigastric artery. The inferior epigastric artery, derived from the external iliac artery just proximal to the inguinal ligament, courses through the preperitoneal areolar tissue to enter the lateral rectus sheath at the semilunar line of Douglas. The deep circumflex iliac artery, arising from the lateral aspect of the external iliac artery near the origin of the inferior epigastric artery, gives rise to an ascending branch that penetrates the abdominal wall musculature just above the iliac crest, near the

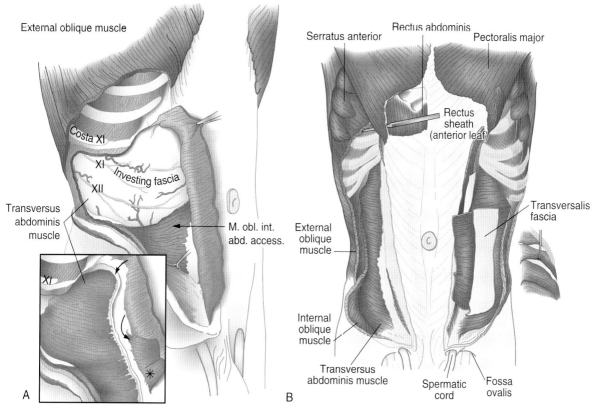

FIGURE 43-4 A, Anterolateral view of the investing fascia of the transversus abdominis muscle and the muscle itself with the fascia removed *(inset)*. The external and internal oblique muscles have been removed. Also note the appearance of the intercostal nerves lying between the fascia of the transversus abdominis muscle and internal oblique muscle. **B,** Anterior view of the transversus abdominis muscle *(left)* and the transversalis fascia *(right)*. Note that the transversalis fascia is shown by reflecting the overlying transversus abdominis muscle medially. (From McVay C: *Anson and McVay's surgical anatomy,* ed 6, Philadelphia, 1984, WB Saunders, pp 480–481.)

anterior superior iliac spine.

The venous drainage of the anterior abdominal wall follows a relatively simple pattern in which the superficial veins above the umbilicus empty into the superior vena cava by way of the internal mammary, intercostal, and long thoracic veins. The veins inferior to the umbilicus—the superficial epigastric, circumflex iliac, and pudendal veins—converge toward the saphenous opening in the groin to enter the saphenous vein and become a tributary to the inferior vena cava (Fig. 43-8). The numerous anastomoses between the infraumbilical and supraumbilical venous systems provide collateral pathways whereby venous return to the heart may bypass an obstruction of the superior or inferior vena cava. The paraumbilical vein, which passes from the left branch of the portal vein along the ligamentum teres to the umbilicus, provides important communication between the veins of the superficial abdominal wall and portal system in patients with portal venous obstruction. In this setting, portal blood flow is diverted away from the higher pressure portal system through the paraumbilical veins to the lower pressure veins of the anterior abdominal wall. The dilated superficial paraumbilical veins in this setting are termed *caput medusae.*

The lymphatic supply of the abdominal wall follows a pattern similar to the venous drainage. Those lymphatic vessels arising from the supraumbilical region drain into the axillary lymph nodes, whereas those arising from the infraumbilical region drain toward the superficial inguinal lymph nodes. The lymphatic vessels from the liver course along the ligamentum teres to the umbilicus to communicate with the lymphatics of the anterior abdominal wall. It is from this pathway that carcinoma in the liver may spread to involve the anterior abdominal wall at the umbilicus (Sister Mary Joseph node or nodule).

Innervation

The anterior rami of the thoracic nerves follow a curvilinear course forward in the intercostal spaces toward the midline of the body (see Fig. 43-7). The upper six thoracic nerves end near the sternum as anterior cutaneous sensory branches. Thoracic nerves 7 to 12 pass behind the costal cartilages and lower ribs to enter a plane between the internal oblique muscle and the transversus abdominis. The seventh and eighth nerves course slightly upward or horizontally to reach the epigastrium, whereas the lower nerves have an increasingly caudal trajectory. As these nerves course medially, they provide motor branches to the abdominal wall musculature. Medially, they perforate the rectus sheath to provide

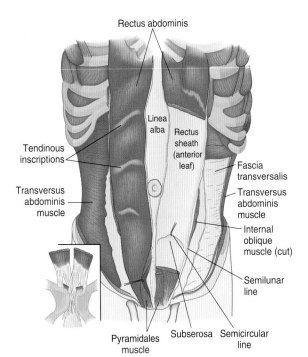

FIGURE 43-5 Rectus abdominis muscle and contents of the rectus sheath. Note the semicircular line, below which the posterior rectus sheath is absent; the rectus abdominis muscle overlies the transversalis fascia, preperitoneal areolar tissue, and peritoneum. (From McVay C: *Anson and McVay's surgical anatomy*, ed 6, Philadelphia, 1984, WB Saunders, p 482.)

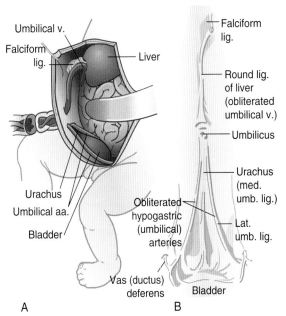

FIGURE 43-6 Umbilicus. **A,** In the fetus, the umbilical vein superiorly and the two umbilical arteries and urachus inferiorly radiate from the umbilicus. **B,** View of the umbilicus from within the peritoneal cavity showing the round ligament of the liver (derived from the obliterated umbilical vein) superiorly and the median umbilical ligament (derived from the obliterated urachus) and medial umbilical ligaments (also called the lateral umbilical ligaments, derived from the obliterated umbilical arteries). (From Thorek P: *Anatomy in surgery*, ed 2, Philadelphia, 1962, JB Lippincott, p 375.)

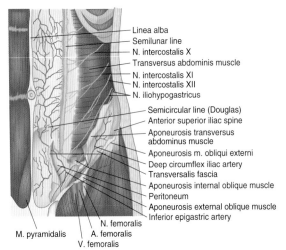

FIGURE 43-7 Arteries and nerves of the anterolateral abdominal wall. (From McVay C: *Anson and McVay's surgical anatomy*, ed 6, Philadelphia, 1984, WB Saunders, p 501.)

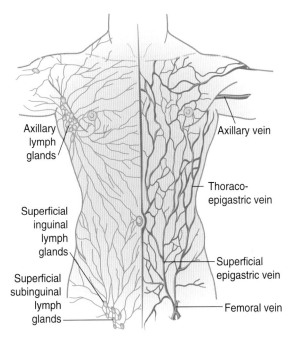

FIGURE 43-8 Venous and lymphatic drainage of the anterolateral abdominal wall. (From Thorek P: *Anatomy in surgery*, ed 2, Philadelphia, 1962, JB Lippincott, p 345.)

sensory innervation to the anterior abdominal wall. The anterior ramus of the 10th thoracic nerve reaches the skin at the level of the umbilicus, and the 12th thoracic nerve innervates the skin of the hypogastrium.

The ilioinguinal and iliohypogastric nerves often arise in common from the anterior rami of the 12th thoracic and first lumbar nerves to provide sensory innervation to the hypogastrium and lower abdominal wall. The iliohypogastric nerve runs parallel to the 12th thoracic nerve to pierce the transversus abdominis muscle near the iliac crest. After coursing between the transversus abdominis muscle and internal oblique for a short distance, the nerve pierces the internal oblique to travel under the external oblique fascia toward the external inguinal ring. It emerges through the superior crus of the external inguinal ring to provide sensory innervation to the anterior abdominal wall in the hypogastrium. The ilioinguinal nerve courses parallel to the iliohypogastric nerve but closer to the inguinal ligament than the iliohypogastric nerve. Unlike the iliohypogastric nerve, the ilioinguinal nerve courses with the spermatic cord to emerge from the external inguinal ring, with its terminal branches providing sensory innervation to the skin of the inguinal region and scrotum or labium. The ilioinguinal nerve, iliohypogastric nerve, and genital branch of the genitofemoral nerve are commonly encountered during the performance of inguinal herniorrhaphy.

Abnormalities of the Abdominal Wall

These can be congenital or acquired.

Congenital Abnormalities

Umbilical hernias. Umbilical hernias may be classified into three distinct forms: omphalocele and gastroschisis, infantile umbilical hernia, and acquired umbilical hernia.

Omphalocele. An omphalocele is a funnel-shaped defect in the central abdomen through which the viscera protrude into the base of the umbilical cord. It is caused by failure of the abdominal wall musculature to unite in the midline during fetal development. The umbilical vessels may be splayed over the viscera or pushed to one side. In larger defects, the liver and spleen may lie within the cord, along with a major portion of the bowel. There is no skin covering these defects, only peritoneum and, more superficially, amnion. Of infants who are born with an omphalocele, 50% to 60% will have concomitant congenital anomalies of the skeleton, gastrointestinal (GI) tract, nervous system, genitourinary system, or cardiopulmonary system.

Gastroschisis. Gastroschisis is another congenital defect of the abdominal wall in which the umbilical membrane has ruptured in utero, allowing the intestine to herniate outside the abdominal cavity. The defect is almost always to the right of the umbilical cord, and the intestine is not covered with skin or amnion. Typically, the intestine has not undergone complete mesenteric rotation and fixation; hence, the infant is at risk for mesenteric volvulus, with resultant intestinal ischemia and necrosis. Concomitant congenital anomalies occur in about 10% of these patients. Both omphalocele and gastroschisis are discussed in greater detail in Chapter 66.

Infantile umbilical hernia. The infantile umbilical hernia appears within a few days or weeks after the stump of the umbilical cord has sloughed. It is caused by a weakness in the adhesion between the scarred remnants of the umbilical cord and umbilical ring. In contrast to omphalocele, the infantile umbilical hernia is covered by skin. In general, these small hernias occur in the superior margin of the umbilical ring. They are easily reducible and become prominent when the infant cries. Most of these hernias resolve within the first 24 months of life, and complications such as strangulation are rare. Operative repair is indicated for those children in whom the hernia persists beyond the age of 3 or 4 years. This condition and its management are discussed further in Chapters 44 and 66.

Acquired umbilical hernia. In this condition, an umbilical hernia develops at a time remote from closure of the umbilical ring. This hernia occurs most commonly at the upper margin of the umbilicus and results from weakening of the cicatricial tissue that normally closes the umbilical ring. This weakening can be caused by excessive stretching of the abdominal wall, which may occur with pregnancy, vigorous labor, or ascites. In contrast to infantile umbilical hernias, acquired umbilical hernias do not spontaneously resolve but gradually increase in size. The dense fibrous ring at the neck of this hernia makes strangulation of herniated intestine or omentum an important complication.

Abnormalities resulting from persistence of the omphalomesenteric duct. During fetal development, the midgut communicates widely with the yolk sac through the vitelline or omphalomesenteric duct. As the abdominal wall components approximate one another, the omphalomesenteric duct narrows and comes to lie within the umbilical cord. Over time, communication between the yolk sac and intestine becomes obliterated, and the intestine resides free within the peritoneal cavity. Persistence of part or all of the omphalomesenteric duct results in a variety of abnormalities related to the intestine and abdominal wall (Fig. 43-9).

Persistence of the intestinal end of the omphalomesenteric duct results in Meckel's diverticulum. These true diverticula arise from the antimesenteric border of the small intestine, most often the ileum. A rule of 2s is often applied to these lesions in that they are found in approximately 2% of the population, are within 2 feet of the ileocecal valve, are often 2 inches in length, and contain 2 types of ectopic mucosa (gastric and pancreatic). Meckel's diverticula may be complicated by inflammation, perforation, hemorrhage, or obstruction. GI bleeding is caused by peptic ulceration of adjacent intestinal mucosa from hydrochloric acid secreted by

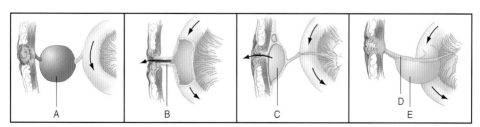

FIGURE 43-9 Abnormalities resulting from persistence of the omphalomesenteric duct. **A,** Omphalomesenteric duct cyst. **B,** Persistent omphalomesenteric duct with an enterocutaneous fistula. **C,** Omphalomesenteric duct cyst and sinus. **D,** Fibrous cord between the small intestine and the posterior surface of the umbilicus. **E,** Meckel's diverticulum. (From McVay C: *Anson and McVay's surgical anatomy*, ed 6, Philadelphia, 1984, WB Saunders, p 576.)

ectopic parietal cells within the diverticulum. Intestinal obstruction associated with Meckel's diverticulum is usually caused by intussusception or volvulus around an abnormal fibrous connection between the diverticulum and posterior aspect of the umbilicus. These lesions are discussed in Chapter 49.

The omphalomesenteric duct may remain patent throughout its course, thus producing an enterocutaneous fistula between the distal small intestine and umbilicus. This condition is manifested with the passage of meconium and mucus from the umbilicus in the first few days of life. Because of the risk for mesenteric volvulus around a persistent omphalomesenteric duct, these lesions are promptly treated with laparotomy and excision of the fistulous track. Persistence of the distal end of the omphalomesenteric duct results in an umbilical polyp, which is a small excrescence of omphalomesenteric ductal mucosa at the umbilicus. Such polyps resemble umbilical granulomas except that they do not disappear after silver nitrate cauterization. Their presence suggests that a persistent omphalomesenteric duct or umbilical sinus may be present, and hence they are most appropriately treated by excision of the mucosal remnant and underlying omphalomesenteric duct or umbilical sinus, if present. Umbilical sinuses result from the persistence of the distal omphalomesenteric duct. The morphology of the sinus track can be delineated by a sinogram. Treatment involves excision of the sinus. Finally, the accumulation of mucus in a portion of a persistent omphalomesenteric duct may result in the formation of a cyst, which may be associated with the intestine or umbilicus by a fibrous band. Treatment consists of excision of the cyst and associated persistent omphalomesenteric duct.

Abnormalities resulting from persistence of the allantois. The allantois is the cranialmost component of the embryologic ventral cloaca. The intra-abdominal portion is termed the *urachus* and connects the urinary bladder with the umbilicus, whereas the extra-abdominal allantois is contained within the umbilical cord. At the end of gestation, the urachus is converted into a fibrous cord that courses between the extraperitoneal urinary bladder and umbilicus as the median umbilical ligament. Persistence of part or all of the urachus may result in the formation of a vesicocutaneous fistula, with the appearance of urine at the umbilicus, an extraperitoneal urachal cyst presenting as a lower abdominal mass, or a urachal sinus with the drainage of a small amount of mucus. Because of the risk of complications including transformation into malignancy, treatment is excision of the urachal remnant with closure of the bladder, if necessary.

Acquired Abnormalities

Diastasis recti. Diastasis recti refers to a thinning of the linea alba in the epigastrium and is manifested as a smooth midline protrusion of the anterior abdominal wall. The transversalis fascia is intact, and hence this is not a hernia. There are no identifiable fascial margins and no risk for intestinal strangulation. The presence of diastasis recti may be particularly noticeable to the patient on straining or when lifting the head from the pillow. Appropriate treatment consists of reassurance of the patient and family about the innocuous nature of this condition.

Anterior abdominal wall hernias. Epigastric hernias occur at sites through which vessels and nerves perforate the linea alba to course into the subcutaneum. Through these openings, extraperitoneal areolar tissue and, at times, peritoneum may herniate into the subcutaneous tissue. Although these hernias are often small, they may produce significant localized pain and tenderness because of direct pressure of the hernia sac and its contents on

the nerves emerging through the same fascial opening. Spigelian hernias occur through the fascia in the region of the semilunar line and are manifested with localized pain and tenderness. The hernia sac is only rarely palpable because it is often small and tends to remain beneath the external oblique aponeurosis. Ultrasonography of the abdominal wall or computed tomography (CT) with thin cuts through the abdomen, after careful marking of the suspected site, should be diagnostic. Treatment consists of simple operative closure of the fascial defect. These hernias are discussed in Chapter 44.

Rectus sheath hematoma. Rectus sheath hematoma is an uncommon condition characterized by acute abdominal pain and the appearance of an abdominal wall mass. It is more common in women than in men and in older than in younger individuals. A review of 126 patients with rectus sheath hematomas treated at the Mayo Clinic found that almost 70% were receiving anticoagulants at the time of diagnosis. A history of nonsurgical abdominal wall trauma or injury is common (48%), as is the presence of a cough (29%).[1] In young women, rectus sheath hematomas have been associated with pregnancy.

Patients with rectus sheath hematomas usually present with the sudden onset of abdominal pain, which may be severe and is often exacerbated by movements requiring contraction of the abdominal wall. Physical examination will demonstrate tenderness over the rectus sheath, often with voluntary guarding. An abdominal wall mass may be noted in some patients, 63% in the Mayo Clinic series. Abdominal wall ecchymosis, including periumbilical ecchymosis (Cullen sign) and blue discoloration in the flanks (Grey Turner sign), may be present if there is a delay from the onset of symptoms to presentation. The pain and tenderness associated with this process may be severe enough to suggest peritonitis. In those cases in which the hematoma expands into the perivesical and preperitoneal spaces, the hematocrit level may fall, although hemodynamic instability is uncommon.

Ultrasonography or CT will confirm the presence of the hematoma and localize it to the abdominal wall in almost all cases. Usually, these patients may be managed successfully with rest and analgesics and, if necessary, blood transfusion. In the Mayo Clinic series, almost 90% of patients were managed successfully in this manner. In general, coagulopathies are corrected, although continued anticoagulation of selected patients may be prudent, depending on the indications for anticoagulation and seriousness of the bleeding. Progression of the hematoma may necessitate angiographic embolization of the bleeding vessel or, uncommonly, operative evacuation of the hematoma and hemostasis.

Malignant Neoplasms of the Abdominal Wall

The most common primary malignant neoplasms of the abdominal wall are desmoid tumors and sarcomas. Although it is unusual, a variety of common cancers may metastasize through the blood stream to the soft tissue of the abdominal wall, where they are manifested as soft tissue masses. Metastatic melanoma, in particular, may be manifested in this manner. Finally, transperitoneal seeding of the abdominal wall by intra-abdominal malignant neoplasms may complicate transabdominal biopsies or operative procedures.

Desmoid Tumor

Desmoid tumor, also known as *fibromatosis*, *aggressive fibromatosis*, or *desmoid-type fibromatosis*, is an uncommon neoplasm that occurs sporadically or as part of an inherited syndrome, most notably familial adenomatous polyposis (FAP) and Gardner syndrome, an autosomal dominant syndrome of GI adenomatous polyps or adenocarcinoma, osteomas, and skin and soft tissue tumors. These tumors arise from fibroaponeurotic tissue and typically are manifested as a slowly growing mass. Although they lack metastatic potential, they can be multifocal as well as locally aggressive and invasive, with a high propensity for recurrence.

Desmoid tumors are typically classified by location as extra-abdominal or extremity desmoids (i.e., those tumors occurring in the proximal extremities or limb girdle), abdominal wall tumors, and intra-abdominal desmoids (see "Mesenteric and Intra-abdominal Desmoid Tumors"), which involve the mesentery, pelvis, or bowel wall. The frequency of desmoid tumors in the general population is 2.4 to 4.3 cases/million; this risk increases 1000-fold in patients with FAP.[2,3] The majority of desmoid tumors are sporadic, typically in young women during pregnancy or within a year of childbirth. Oral contraceptive use has also been associated with the occurrence of these tumors. These associations, combined with the detection of estrogen receptors within the tumor, suggest a regulatory role for estrogen in this disease.

Patients with a desmoid tumor present with an asymptomatic mass or with symptoms related to mass effect from the tumor. There is often a temporal association between the discovery of the tumor and an antecedent history of abdominal trauma or operation.[3] Imaging (CT or magnetic resonance imaging [MRI]) is necessary to delineate the extent of tumor involvement fully, but otherwise there is no need to perform staging for metastatic disease. On CT, a desmoid tumor appears as a homogeneous mass arising from the soft tissue of the abdominal wall (Fig. 43-10). A desmoid tumor will appear as a homogeneous and isointense mass compared with muscle on T1-weighted MRI images, whereas T2-weighted images demonstrate greater heterogeneity and a signal slightly less intense than fat.

Biopsy is required to establish the diagnosis. Core needle biopsy or incisional biopsy will demonstrate a tumor composed of bundles of spindle cells and an abundant fibrous stroma. The center of the tumor is often acellular, whereas the periphery contains most of the fibroblasts. The histology can be similar to that of a low-grade fibrosarcoma, but diagnosis is usually not difficult because the fibroblasts are highly differentiated and lack the mitotic activity found in malignancy. Immunohistochemistry can help clarify difficult diagnoses; the tumors typically stain positive for β-catenin, actin, and vimentin and stain negative for cytokeratin and S-100.

Resection of the tumor with a wide margin of normal tissue was historically considered the optimal treatment. The extent of this resection will often require abdominal wall reconstruction with local tissue flaps or mesh prostheses. The completeness of resection is an important prognostic factor; Stojadinovic and colleagues[4] have reported that 68% of desmoid tumors resected with a positive margin recur within 5 years, compared with none of the tumors in which the resection margin was free of disease.

Recently, however, an approach to postpone surgery for patients with desmoid tumors, particularly for those patients who would require surgery with considerable risk of morbidity and loss of function, has gained acceptance.[5] This approach, centered on an initial observation period for all patients, was based on contemporary data that contradicted the relevance of negative surgical margins and was further supported by high recurrence rates despite optimal local treatment.[6,7] Patients undergoing observation require close follow-up to identify tumor growth early and must agree to frequent imaging. Studies suggest that approximately 50% of patients will not progress at short-term follow-up, with spontaneous regression occurring in up to 10%.[5,8,9] A conservative approach to selection of patients for surgery in desmoid-type fibromatosis is becoming the new standard of care, with further research needed in identifying select subgroups that would benefit from surgery.[10,11]

Abdominal wall desmoids are responsive to radiation therapy, although the treatment effect is slow and may be progressive for several years. Radiotherapy alone is an acceptable treatment option for patients with unresectable desmoid tumors or tumors for which resection will be associated with high morbidity risks or major functional loss. A retrospective review from the M.D. Anderson Cancer Center has reported 10-year recurrence rates of 38% for surgery alone (27% for those with negative margins), 25% for combined surgery and radiation, and 24% for radiation therapy alone.[6] It was also concluded that radiation therapy can assuage the adverse effect of positive margins on local tumor recurrence. Similar large studies have reported local control rates of approximately 80% with radiotherapy alone, rates that are consistently equivalent with or even superior to surgery alone.[12]

Adjuvant radiation therapy is controversial; most centers reserve this modality for patients with positive margins or close margins because of critical structures. The use of neoadjuvant radiation therapy is less well accepted than adjuvant radiation therapy because of the slow response times, often 1 year or more, with the potential for making subsequent abdominal wall reconstruction more difficult, and few studies demonstrated a clear benefit.

Estrogen receptor antagonists, nonsteroidal anti-inflammatory drugs, and systemic chemotherapy have been used successfully in the treatment of patients with locally advanced, recurrent, or unresectable desmoid tumors. The use of these agents in an adjuvant or neoadjuvant setting is not well studied, and they would be best used in the setting of a clinical trial.

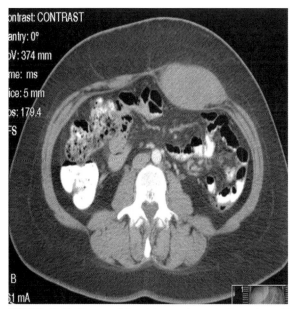

FIGURE 43-10 CT scan of the abdomen demonstrating a desmoid tumor arising within the left rectus sheath. The tumor appears as a homogeneous soft tissue mass.

The detection of estrogen receptors on desmoid tumors and the association with pregnancy and oral contraceptives provide some support for the use of antiestrogens, such as tamoxifen. Clinical improvement has been reported in 43% of patients receiving antiestrogens, although the response rate varies among studies. Tumor responses to antiestrogens are slow in onset but often last for several years.[13,14] Most reports of nonsteroidal anti-inflammatory drug treatment use sulindac, but indomethacin has also been used. A study using combination high-dose tamoxifen and sulindac recommended this regimen as initial treatment for FAP-associated desmoid tumors.[15]

Various cytotoxic chemotherapy regimens have been used in the treatment of patients with inoperable desmoids. Methotrexate with vinblastine, doxorubicin-based therapy, and ifosfamide-based regimens have been reported, with positive responses in 20% to 40% of patients.[13,16] For desmoids with rapid growth, medical oncologists may recommend therapies typically used for sarcomas, such as doxorubicin and dacarbazine. Reports have also suggested imatinib, a tyrosine kinase inhibitor, as another effective treatment option for patients with these tumors.[17]

Abdominal Wall Sarcoma

Abdominal wall sarcomas are classified as truncal sarcomas, including the chest and abdominal wall, and account for 10% to 20% of sarcomas overall. In general, sarcomas are rare, and abdominal wall sarcomas are exceedingly rare. Similar to desmoid tumors, these neoplasms most often are manifested as a painless mass, although as many as one third of patients with abdominal wall sarcomas will have pain at the site of the tumor. Pertinent history, such as a history of retinoblastoma, FAP, neurofibromatosis, radiation therapy, or Li-Fraumeni syndrome, should be sought. The differential diagnosis includes many common conditions, such as lipomas, hematomas, ventral hernias, endometriosis, and inflammatory processes, such as needle site granulomas in diabetics. Histologic subtypes include liposarcoma, fibrosarcoma, leiomyosarcoma, rhabdomyosarcoma, and malignant fibrous histiocytoma.

Axial imaging with MRI or CT will provide important information about the location and extent of the tumor as well as involvement of contiguous structures. Chest CT should be included to rule out metastatic disease. Definitive diagnosis requires biopsy, which may be performed with a core needle or by incision. The accuracy of core needle biopsy is consistently reported as more than 90% and can be performed under CT guidance for deep lesions. If an incisional biopsy is performed, it is optimally done by the surgeon who will perform the definitive resection; it should be oriented in the same plane as the underlying muscle to minimize unnecessary tissue loss during the definitive procedure and to facilitate reconstruction. No attempt is made to develop tissue flaps around the lesion, and hemostasis is meticulous to avoid dissemination of the tumor along the tissue planes by a postoperative hematoma.

Definitive treatment of abdominal wall sarcomas is resection with tumor-free margins; most surgeons attempt to obtain at least a 2-cm margin around the tumor. The extent of resection and associated morbidity must be balanced, however, as metastatic disease and not local recurrence represents the greatest risk of death. Lymph node metastases are rare (2% to 3%). Reconstruction of the abdominal wall defect may be accomplished primarily with myocutaneous flaps or with prosthetic meshes, depending on the site and extent of resection. Response rates with radiation and chemotherapy are generally low, although specific response rates depend on histology and grade.

Soft tissue sarcomas are discussed in greater detail in Chapter 31.

Metastatic Disease

Metastases to the abdominal wall may occur by direct seeding of the abdominal wall during biopsy or resection of an intra-abdominal malignant neoplasm or by hematogenous spread of an advanced tumor. The risk of tumor implantation at the port site after laparoscopic colon resection for adenocarcinoma is 0.9% and has been shown in randomized controlled trials to be no different from the risk of tumor recurrence in the wound after open colon resections.[18] Wound implantation with tumor can have particular relevance during cytoreductive surgery with hyperthermic intra-peritoneal chemotherapy applied to the treatment of a peritoneal surface malignant neoplasm. Patients undergoing cytoreductive surgery have typically received prior surgery with abdominal wall scar or tumor formation and often require abdominal wall resection with complex reconstruction.

The most common tumors that metastasize to soft tissue are lung, colon, melanoma, and renal cell tumors. Although metastases to soft tissue are unusual, the abdominal wall is the site of such recurrence in approximately 20% of cases.[19] Similar to desmoid tumors or sarcomas, metastases to the abdominal wall are manifested as a painless mass. Immunohistochemistry staining of the tumor may allow specific identification of the type of primary tumor and facilitate differentiation from primary sarcomas of the abdominal wall. The Sister Mary Joseph nodule is often described and seldom seen; it is a palpable nodule in the region of the umbilicus representing metastatic abdominal or pelvic cancer.

Symptoms of Intra-abdominal Disease Referred to the Abdominal Wall

Abdominal pain may be categorized as visceral, somatoparietal, and referred. Visceral pain is caused by stimulation of visceral nociceptors by inflammation, distention, or ischemia. The pain is dull in nature and poorly localized to the epigastrium, periumbilical regions, or hypogastrium, depending on the embryonic origin of the organ involved. Inflammation of the stomach, duodenum, and biliary tract (derivatives of the embryonic foregut) localizes visceral pain to the epigastrium. Stimulation of nociceptors in midgut-derived organs (small intestine, appendix, right colon, proximal transverse colon) causes the sensation of pain in the periumbilical region, whereas inflammation or distention of hindgut-derived organs (distal transverse colon, left colon, rectum) causes hypogastric pain. The pain is felt in the midline because these organs transmit sympathetic sensory afferents to both sides of the spinal cord. The pain is poorly localized because the innervation of most viscera is multisegmental and contains fewer nerve receptors than highly sensitive organs such as the skin. The pain is often characterized as cramping, burning, or gnawing and may be accompanied by secondary autonomic effects, such as sweating, restlessness, nausea, vomiting, perspiration, and pallor.

Somatoparietal pain arises from inflammation of the parietal peritoneum; it is more intense and more precisely localized than visceral pain. The nerve impulses mediating parietal pain travel within the somatosensory spinal nerves and reach the spinal cord in the peripheral nerves corresponding to the cutaneous dermatomes from the T6 to the L1 region. Lateralization of parietal pain is possible because only one side of the nervous system innervates a given part of the parietal peritoneum.

The difference between visceral and somatoparietal pain is well illustrated by the pain associated with acute appendicitis, in which the early, vague, periumbilical visceral pain is followed by the localized somatoparietal pain at McBurney point. The visceral pain is produced by distention and inflammation of the appendix, whereas the localized somatoparietal pain in the right lower quadrant of the abdomen is caused by extension of the inflammation to the parietal peritoneum.

Referred pain is felt in anatomic regions remote from the diseased organ. This phenomenon is caused by convergence of visceral afferent neurons innervating an injured or inflamed organ with somatic afferent fibers arising from another anatomic region. This occurs within the spinal cord at the level of second-order neurons. Well-known examples of referred pain include shoulder pain on irritation of the diaphragm, scapular pain associated with acute biliary tract disease, and testicular or labial pain caused by retroperitoneal inflammation.

PERITONEUM AND PERITONEAL CAVITY

Anatomy

The peritoneum consists of a single sheet of simple squamous epithelium of mesodermal origin, termed *mesothelium,* lying on a thin connective tissue stroma. The surface area is 1.0 to 1.7 m^2, approximately that of the total body surface area. In males, the peritoneal cavity is sealed, whereas in females, it is open to the exterior through the ostia of the fallopian tubes. The peritoneal membrane is divided into parietal and visceral components. The parietal peritoneum covers the anterior, lateral, and posterior abdominal wall surfaces and the inferior surface of the diaphragm and the pelvis. The visceral peritoneum covers most of the surface of the intraperitoneal organs (i.e., stomach, jejunum, ileum, transverse colon, liver, spleen) and the anterior aspect of the retroperitoneal organs (i.e., duodenum, left and right colon, pancreas, kidneys, adrenal glands).

The peritoneal cavity is subdivided into interconnected compartments or spaces by 11 ligaments and mesenteries. The peritoneal ligaments or mesenteries include the coronary, gastrohepatic,

hepatoduodenal, falciform, gastrocolic, duodenocolic, gastrosplenic, splenorenal, and phrenicocolic ligaments and the transverse mesocolon and small bowel mesentery (Fig. 43-11). These structures partition the abdomen into nine potential spaces: right and left subphrenic, subhepatic, supramesenteric and inframesenteric, right and left paracolic gutters, pelvis, and lesser space. These ligaments, mesenteries, and peritoneal spaces direct the circulation of fluid in the peritoneal cavity and thus may be useful in predicting the route of spread of infectious and malignant diseases. For example, perforation of the duodenum from peptic ulcer disease may result in the movement of fluid (and the development of abscesses) in the subhepatic space, right paracolic gutter, and pelvis. The blood supply to the visceral peritoneum is derived from the splanchnic blood vessels, whereas the parietal peritoneum is supplied by branches of the intercostal, subcostal, lumbar, and iliac vessels. The innervation of the visceral and parietal peritoneum is discussed earlier.

Physiology

The peritoneum is a bidirectional, semipermeable membrane that controls the amount of fluid in the peritoneal cavity, promotes the sequestration and removal of bacteria from the peritoneal cavity, and facilitates the migration of inflammatory cells from the microvasculature into the peritoneal cavity. Normally, the peritoneal cavity contains less than 100 mL of sterile serous fluid. Microvilli on the apical surface of the peritoneal mesothelium markedly increase the surface area and promote the rapid absorption of fluid from the peritoneal cavity into the lymphatics and portal and systemic circulations. The amount of fluid in the peritoneal cavity may increase to many liters in some diseases, such as cirrhosis, nephrotic syndrome, and peritoneal carcinomatosis.

The circulation of fluid in the peritoneal cavity is driven in part by the movement of the diaphragm. Intercellular pores in the peritoneum covering the inferior surface of the diaphragm (termed *stomata*) communicate with lymphatic pools in the diaphragm. Lymph flows from these diaphragmatic lymphatic channels through subpleural lymphatics to the regional lymph nodes and

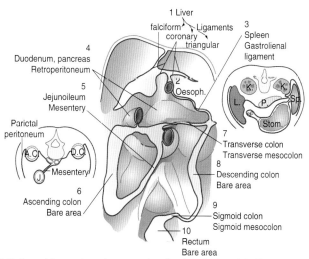

FIGURE 43-11 Peritoneal ligaments and mesenteric reflections in the adult. These attachments partition the abdomen into nine potential spaces: right and left subphrenic, subhepatic, supramesenteric, and inframesenteric spaces; and right and left paracolic gutters, pelvis, and omental bursa *(inset, right).* (From McVay C: *Anson and McVay's surgical anatomy,* ed 6, Philadelphia, 1984, WB Saunders, p 589.)

ultimately the thoracic duct. Relaxation of the diaphragm during exhalation opens the stomata, and the negative intrathoracic pressure draws fluid and particles, including bacteria, into the stomata. Contraction of the diaphragm during inhalation propels the lymph through the mediastinal lymphatic channels into the thoracic duct. It is postulated that this so-called diaphragmatic pump drives the movement of peritoneal fluid in a cephalad direction toward the diaphragm and into the thoracic lymphatic vessels. This circulatory pattern of peritoneal fluid toward the diaphragm and into the central lymphatic channels is consistent with the rapid appearance of sepsis in patients with generalized intra-abdominal infections as well as the perihepatitis of Fitz-Hugh–Curtis syndrome in patients with acute salpingitis.

The peritoneum and peritoneal cavity respond to infection in five ways:

1. Bacteria are rapidly removed from the peritoneal cavity through the diaphragmatic stomata and lymphatics.
2. Peritoneal macrophages release proinflammatory mediators that promote the migration of leukocytes into the peritoneal cavity from the surrounding microvasculature.
3. Degranulation of peritoneal mast cells releases histamine and other vasoactive products, causing local vasodilation and the extravasation of protein-rich fluid containing complement and immunoglobulins into the peritoneal space.
4. Protein in the peritoneal fluid opsonizes bacteria, which, along with activation of the complement cascade, promotes neutrophil- and macrophage-mediated bacterial phagocytosis and destruction.
5. Bacteria become sequestered within fibrin matrices, thereby promoting abscess formation and limiting the generalized spread of the infection.

Peritoneal Disorders
Ascites

Pathophysiology and cause. Ascites is the pathologic accumulation of fluid in the peritoneal cavity. The principal causes of ascites formation and their pathophysiologic bases are listed in Box 43-1. Cirrhosis is the most common cause of ascites in the United States, accounting for approximately 85% of cases. Ascites is the most common complication of cirrhosis, with approximately 50% of compensated cirrhotic patients developing ascites within 10 years of diagnosis. The onset of ascites is an important prognostic factor for poor outcome in patients with cirrhosis because of its association with the occurrence of spontaneous bacterial peritonitis, renal failure, worsened quality of life, and increased likelihood of death within 2 to 5 years.

In cirrhotic patients, the two principal factors underlying the formation of ascites in cirrhotic patients are renal sodium and water retention and portal hypertension. Renal sodium retention is driven by activation of the renin-angiotensin-aldosterone and sympathetic nervous systems, which cause proximal and distal renal tubule sodium reabsorption. It is postulated that the abnormal release of nitric oxide within the splanchnic circulation causes vasodilation and a decrease in the effective circulating blood volume. Renin, aldosterone, and other hormones are generated as a counterregulatory mechanism to restore the effective circulating blood volume to normal. Portal hypertension is produced by postsinusoidal vascular obstruction from the deposition of collagen in the cirrhotic liver. Increased hydrostatic pressure within the hepatic sinusoids and splanchnic vasculature drives the extravasation of fluid from the microvasculature into the extracellular compartment. Ascites results when the capacity of the lymphatic

---

BOX 43-1 Principal Causes of Ascites Formation Categorized According to Underlying Pathophysiology

Portal Hypertension
Cirrhosis
Noncirrhotic
- Prehepatic portal venous obstruction
  - Chronic mesenteric venous thrombosis
  - Multiple hepatic metastases
- Posthepatic venous obstruction: Budd-Chiari syndrome

Cardiac
Congestive heart failure
Chronic pericardial tamponade
Constrictive pericarditis

Malignant Disease
Peritoneal carcinomatosis
- Primary peritoneal malignant neoplasms
  - Primary peritoneal mesothelioma
  - Serous carcinoma
- Metastatic carcinoma
  - Gastrointestinal carcinomas (e.g., gastric, colonic, pancreatic cancer)
  - Genitourinary carcinomas (e.g., ovarian cancer)
Retroperitoneal obstruction of lymphatic channels
- Lymphoma
- Lymph node metastases (e.g., testicular cancer, melanoma)

Obstruction of the lymphatic channels at the base of the mesentery
- Gastrointestinal carcinoid tumors

Miscellaneous
Bile ascites
- Iatrogenic after operations of the liver or biliary tract
- Traumatic after injuries to the liver or biliary tract
Pancreatic ascites
- Acute pancreatitis
- Pancreatic pseudocyst
Chylous ascites
- Disruptions of retroperitoneal lymphatic channels
  - Iatrogenic during retroperitoneal dissections: retroperitoneal lymphadenectomy, abdominal aortic aneurysmorrhaphy
  - Blunt or penetrating trauma
- Malignant disease
  - Obstruction of retroperitoneal lymphatic channels
  - Obstruction of lymphatic channels at the base of the mesentery
- Congenital lymphatic abnormalities
Primary lymphatic hypoplasia
Peritoneal infections
- Tuberculous peritonitis
- Myxedema
- Nephrotic syndrome
- Serositis in connective tissue disease

system to return this fluid to the systemic circulation is overwhelmed. Studies have reviewed the pathophysiologic mechanism underlying fluid retention, hyponatremia, and ascites formation that characterize patients with cirrhosis.[20,21]

Obstruction of the portal or hepatic venous blood flow in the absence of cirrhosis (e.g., portal vein thrombosis or Budd-Chiari syndrome, respectively) also causes ascites formation by increasing hydrostatic pressure within the splanchnic microvasculature. A similar pressure-based mechanism contributes to ascites formation in patients with heart failure, although the release of vasopressin and renin-angiotensin-aldosterone also promotes sodium and water retention in these patients. Patients with malignant neoplasms develop ascites by one of three mechanisms:

1. Multiple hepatic metastases cause portal hypertension by narrowing or occluding branches of the portal venous system.
2. Malignant cells scattered throughout the peritoneal cavity release protein-rich fluid into the peritoneal cavity, as in peritoneal carcinomatosis.
3. Obstruction of retroperitoneal lymphatics by a tumor, such as lymphoma, causes rupture of major lymphatic channels and the leakage of chyle into the peritoneal cavity.

Finally, ascites may result from the leakage of pancreatic fluid, bile, or lymph into the peritoneal cavity after an iatrogenic or inflammatory disruption of a major pancreatic, bile, or lymphatic duct.

Clinical presentation and diagnosis. The diagnosis of ascites is made on the basis of the medical history and appearance of the abdomen. Obviously, risk factors for hepatitis or cirrhosis are sought, as is evidence of cardiac disease, renal disease, or malignant disease. A full bulging abdomen with dullness of the flanks on percussion is suggestive of the presence of ascites. Approximately 1.5 liters of fluid must be present before dullness can be detected by percussion. Physical evidence of cirrhosis is also sought, such as palmar erythema, dilated abdominal wall collateral veins, and multiple spider angiomas. Patients with cardiac ascites have impressive jugular venous distention and other evidence of congestive heart failure.

Ascitic fluid analysis. Paracentesis with ascitic fluid analysis is the most rapid and cost-effective method of determining the cause of ascites and should be performed for patients with new-onset ascites. Another important indication for early paracentesis in a patient with ascites is the occurrence of signs and symptoms of infection, such as abdominal pain or tenderness, fever, encephalopathy, hypotension, renal failure, acidosis, or leukocytosis. Paracentesis can be performed safely in most patients, including those with cirrhosis and mild coagulopathy. It is usually performed in the lower abdomen, with the left lower quadrant preferred to the right. Ultrasound guidance may be useful in obese patients and in those with a history of laparotomy. Runyon[22] has suggested that only ongoing disseminated intravascular coagulation or clinically evident fibrinolysis is a contraindication to paracentesis in patients with ascites. In this study, no cases of hemoperitoneum, death, or infection after more than 229 paracenteses performed in 125 cirrhotic patients were reported; abdominal hematomas occurred in 2% of cases, with only 50% of these requiring blood transfusion.

Examination of the ascitic fluid begins with its gross appearance. Normal ascitic fluid is slightly yellow and transparent. The presence of more than 5000 leukocytes/mm³ will cause the fluid to be cloudy, whereas ascitic fluid specimens with fewer than 1000 cells/mm³ are almost clear. Blood in the ascitic fluid may be caused by a traumatic tap, in which case the fluid may be blood

streaked and will often clot unless it is immediately transferred to a tube containing an anticoagulant. Nontraumatic blood-tinged ascitic fluid does not clot because the required factors have been depleted by previous clotting in the peritoneal cavity. Lipid in the ascitic fluid, such as that which accompanies chylous ascites, causes the fluid to appear opalescent, ranging from cloudy to completely opaque. If it is placed in the refrigerator for 48 to 72 hours, the lipids usually layer out.

The most valuable laboratory tests on ascitic fluid are the cell count, differential, and determination of ascitic fluid albumin and total protein concentrations. Studies vary, but most state that a normal total leukocyte count is between 100 and 300 cell/mm³ in uncomplicated cirrhotic ascites, and approximately 50% of these cells are neutrophils. An increased polymorphonuclear neutrophil count (>250 cells/mm³) suggests an acute inflammatory process, the most common of which is spontaneous bacterial peritonitis.

The serum-ascites albumin gradient (SAAG) is the most reliable method to differentiate causes of ascites due to portal hypertension from those not due to portal hypertension. The SAAG is calculated by measuring the albumin concentration of serum and ascitic fluid specimens and subtracting the ascitic fluid value from the serum value. If the SAAG is 1.1 g/dL or more, the patient has portal hypertension; a SAAG of less than 1.1 g/dL is consistent with the absence of portal hypertension. Examples of high- and low-gradient causes of ascites are shown in Table 43-1. The accuracy of this measurement in predicting the presence or absence of portal hypertension is approximately 97%.[23]

Treatment of ascites in cirrhotic patients. The standard treatment protocol for patients with ascites caused by portal hypertension (as opposed to patients with a SAAG of <1.1 g/dL) is a stepwise approach beginning with sodium restriction, diuretic therapy, and paracentesis.[20,21,24,25] The initial goal of medical therapy is to induce a state in which renal sodium excretion exceeds sodium intake, a situation that will reduce the extracellular volume and improve ascites. A reasonable dietary sodium restriction for most cirrhotic patients with ascites is 88 mEq (2 g) per day. The patient's compliance may be assessed by measuring the 24-hour urinary sodium excretion. Patients who are compliant with their dietary restriction and excrete more than 78 mmol/day of sodium in their urine lose weight. However, most patients will require a combination of sodium restriction and diuretics.

TABLE 43-1 Classification of Ascites by Serum-Ascites Albumin Gradient	
HIGH GRADIENT (≥1.1 g/dL)	**LOW GRADIENT (<1.1 g/dL)**
Cirrhosis	Peritoneal carcinomatosis
Alcoholic hepatitis	Tuberculous peritonitis
Cardiac failure	Pancreatic ascites
Massive liver metastases	Biliary ascites
Fulminant hepatic failure	Nephrotic syndrome
Budd-Chiari syndrome	Postoperative lymphatic leak
Portal vein thrombosis	Serositis in connective tissue diseases
Myxedema	

From Runyon B: Ascites: spontaneous bacterial peritonitis. In Sleisenger MH, Feldman M, Friedman LS, editors: *Sleisenger and Fordtran's gastrointestinal and liver disease: Pathophysiology, diagnosis, management,* ed 7, Philadelphia, 2002, WB Saunders, p 1523.

Spironolactone and furosemide, when given in a dosing ratio of 100:40, will promote natriuresis while maintaining normokalemia. In general, spironolactone (100 mg/day) and furosemide (40 mg/day) are begun initially. If this regimen is ineffective in increasing urinary sodium excretion and decreasing body weight, the dosages of these drugs may be increased while maintaining the 100:40 ratio.

Large-volume paracentesis, in which more than 5 liters of ascites fluid is removed from the peritoneal cavity, may be useful for patients with ascites that has been unresponsive to sodium restriction and diuretic treatment; this occurs in less than 10% of patients. The intravenous infusion of albumin (6 to 8 g/liter of ascitic fluid removed) at the time of paracentesis will minimize the symptoms of intravascular volume depletion and renal insufficiency, which may accompany the removal of more than 5 liters of ascitic fluid. The continuation of diuretics and salt restriction will prevent or delay the reaccumulation of ascites after paracentesis. Others have suggested that weekly albumin administration, independent of large-volume paracentesis, may be a useful adjunct to salt restriction and diuretic therapy in patients with refractory ascites. Transjugular intrahepatic portosystemic shunt and, ultimately, hepatic transplantation have been used to manage ascites refractory to simpler, less invasive options. These modalities are discussed in Chapter 53.

Chylous ascites. Chylous ascites is the collection of chyle in the peritoneal cavity and may result from one of three principal mechanisms: (1) obstruction of major lymphatic channels at the base of the mesentery or the cisterna chyli, with exudation of chyle from dilated mesenteric lymphatics; (2) direct leakage of chyle through a lymphoperitoneal fistula caused by abnormal or injured retroperitoneal lymphatic vessels; and (3) exudation of chyle through the walls of retroperitoneal megalymphatics, without a visible fistula or thoracic duct obstruction.

In adults, the most common cause of chylous ascites is an intra-abdominal malignant neoplasm obstructing the lymphatic channels at the base of the mesentery or in the retroperitoneum. Lymphoma is the most common malignant neoplasm associated with chylous ascites, although chylous ascites has also been associated with ovarian, colon, renal, prostate, pancreatic, and gastric malignant neoplasms. Carcinoid tumors may cause chylous ascites by obstructing the lymphatics at the base of the mesentery through direct invasion and the dense fibrosis characteristic of this neoplasm. Chylous ascites may also result from injury of the retroperitoneal lymphatics during surgical procedures, such as operations on the abdominal aorta and retroperitoneal lymph node dissections. Blunt and penetrating traumatic injuries are also important causes of chylous ascites, particularly in children. Chylous ascites in children may be caused by congenital lymphatic abnormalities, such as primary lymphatic hypoplasia, resulting in lower extremity lymphedema, chylothorax, and chylous ascites.

Patients with chylous ascites most often present with painless abdominal distention. Malnutrition and dyspnea occur in approximately 50% of cases. Paracentesis yields a characteristic milky fluid with a high protein and fat content. The SAAG will be less than 1.1 mg/dL, and the triglyceride level will be higher than that of plasma, often two to eight times higher than that of plasma. CT, lymphoscintigraphy, and lymphangiography may provide information about the site of obstruction, although the last two modalities are rarely available.

Although large studies are lacking on ideal practices, management of patients with chylous ascites includes the maintenance or improvement of nutrition, reduction in the rate of chyle formation, and correction of the underlying disease process. Most patients will be successfully treated with either a high-protein, low-fat diet and diuretics or fasting with total parenteral nutrition with or without somatostatin. A low-fat, medium-chain triglyceride diet combined with diuretics has been used successfully to treat adults with chylous ascites complicating retroperitoneal lymph node dissections. It is postulated that reducing the intake of long-chain triglycerides will reduce the rate of chyle flow because their metabolites are transported through the splanchnic lymphatics as chylomicrons. In contrast, medium-chain triglycerides are directly absorbed by enterocytes and transported to the liver through the splanchnic blood vessels as free fatty acids and glycerol. Paracentesis may temporarily relieve the dyspnea and abdominal discomfort associated with chylous ascites; however, repeated paracentesis leads to hypoproteinemia and malnutrition. Experience with peritoneovenous shunts to treat chylous ascites has generally been disappointing. Surgical exploration of the abdomen and retroperitoneum is generally reserved for patients who fail to improve with nonoperative management. In rare cases, the application of fibrin glue has been a beneficial adjunct to surgical exploration of the retroperitoneum.

Peritonitis

Peritonitis is inflammation of the peritoneum and peritoneal cavity, usually caused by a localized or generalized infection. Primary peritonitis results from bacterial, chlamydial, fungal, or mycobacterial infection in the absence of perforation of the GI tract, whereas secondary peritonitis occurs in the setting of GI perforation. Frequent causes of secondary bacterial peritonitis include peptic ulcer disease, acute appendicitis, colonic diverticulitis, and pelvic inflammatory disease.

Spontaneous bacterial peritonitis. Spontaneous bacterial peritonitis (SBP) is defined as a bacterial infection of ascitic fluid in the absence of an intra-abdominal source of infection, such as visceral perforation, abscess, acute pancreatitis, or cholecystitis. Although it is usually associated with cirrhosis, SBP may also occur in patients with nephrotic syndrome and, less commonly, congestive heart failure. It is extremely rare for patients with ascitic fluid containing a high protein concentration to develop SBP, such as those with peritoneal carcinomatosis. The most common pathogens in adults with SBP are the aerobic enteric flora *Escherichia coli* and *Klebsiella pneumoniae*. In children with nephrogenic or hepatogenic ascites, group A streptococcus, *Staphylococcus aureus*, and *Streptococcus pneumoniae* are common isolates. SBP is seldom produced by anaerobic microorganisms because of their incapacity to translocate to the intestinal mucosa and because of the high volume of oxygen in the intestinal wall and in the tissues that surround it.[26-30]

Bacterial translocation from the GI tract is thought to be an important step in the pathogenesis of SBP. Impaired GI motility in cirrhotics is thought to alter normal gut microflora, and impaired local and systemic immune function prevents the effective clearance of translocated bacteria from the mesenteric lymphatics and bloodstream. A low protein concentration in ascitic fluid prevents effective opsonization of bacteria and hence clearance by macrophages and neutrophils.

The diagnosis of SBP is made initially by demonstrating more than 250 neutrophils/mm³ of ascitic fluid in a clinical setting consistent with this diagnosis, that is, abdominal pain, fever, or leukocytosis in a patient with low-protein ascites. In addition, cultured fluid can be only monomicrobial as polymicrobial infections, particularly with gram-negative enteric organisms, raise the suspicion of secondary peritonitis. It is unusual to document bacterascites on Gram staining of ascitic fluid, and delay of appropriate antibiotic management until the ascitic fluid cultures grow bacterial isolates risks the development of overwhelming infection and death. Bedside screening of ascitic fluid for leukocyte esterase, using colorimetric leukocyte esterase reagent strips, has been used to shorten the time from paracentesis to treatment, although its widespread use remains controversial.[31,32]

Broad-spectrum antibiotics, such as a third-generation cephalosporin, are started immediately in patients suspected of having ascitic fluid infection. These agents cover approximately 95% of the flora most commonly associated with SBP and are the antibiotics of choice for patients thought to have SBP.[33,34] The spectrum of the antibiotic coverage may be narrowed once the results of antibiotic sensitivity tests are known. Repeated paracentesis with ascitic fluid analysis is not needed when there is typical rapid improvement in response to antibiotic therapy. If the setting, symptoms, ascitic fluid analysis, and response to therapy are atypical, repeated paracentesis may be helpful for detecting secondary peritonitis. The immediate mortality risk caused by SBP is low, particularly if it is recognized and treated expeditiously. However, the development of other complications of hepatic failure, including GI hemorrhage and hepatorenal syndrome, contributes to the death of many of these patients during the hospitalization in which SBP is detected. The occurrence of SBP is an important landmark in the natural history of cirrhosis, with 1- and 2-year survival rates of approximately 30% and 20%, respectively. Several studies, including a randomized controlled trial, have shown that plasma expansion with albumin improves circulatory function and reduces the risk for hepatorenal syndrome and hospital mortality in patients with SBP.[35]

Tuberculous peritonitis. Tuberculosis is common in impoverished areas of the world and is encountered with increasing frequency in the United States and other developed countries because of factors such as HIV infection and increasing use of immunosuppressive medications. Others have described an association between peritoneal tuberculosis and alcoholic cirrhosis and chronic renal failure.[36] Peritoneal tuberculosis is the sixth most common site of extrapulmonary tuberculosis, after lymphatic, genitourinary, bone and joint, miliary, and meningeal. Most cases result from reactivation of latent peritoneal disease that had been previously established hematogenously from a primary pulmonary focus. Only approximately 17% of cases are associated with active pulmonary disease.

The illness often is manifested insidiously, with patients having had symptoms for several weeks to months at the time of presentation. Its clinical presentation mimics inflammatory conditions such as Crohn's disease and malignant diseases, so obtaining a diagnosis can be problematic at times. Abdominal swelling caused by ascites formation is the most common symptom, occurring in more than 80% of cases. Similarly, most patients complain of a nonlocalized, vague abdominal pain. Constitutional symptoms such as low-grade fever and night sweats, weight loss, anorexia, and malaise are reported in approximately 60% of patients. The concomitant presence of other chronic conditions, such as uremia, cirrhosis, and AIDS, makes these symptoms difficult to interpret. Abdominal tenderness is present on palpation in approximately 50% of patients with peritoneal tuberculosis.[36] A positive tuberculin skin test response is present in most cases, whereas only approximately 50% of these patients will have an abnormal chest radiograph. The ascitic fluid SAAG is less than 1.1 g/dL, consis-

tent with a high protein concentration in the ascitic fluid. Microscopic examination of the ascites shows erythrocytes and an increased number of leukocytes, most of which are lymphocytes. Measurement of ascitic fluid adenosine deaminase activity, even in the presence of cirrhosis, and polymerase chain reaction assays have been used as noninvasive and rapid tests for tuberculous peritonitis. Ascitic fluid adenosine deaminase activity, in particular, appears to be highly sensitive and specific for tuberculous peritonitis.

Abdominal imaging with ultrasound or CT may suggest the diagnosis but lacks the sensitivity and specificity to be diagnostic. Ultrasound may demonstrate the presence of echogenic material in the ascitic fluid, seen as fine mobile strands or particulate matter. CT will demonstrate the thickened and nodular mesentery with mesenteric lymphadenopathy and omental thickening.

The diagnosis is made by laparoscopy with directed biopsy of the peritoneum. In more than 90% of cases, laparoscopy demonstrates a number of whitish nodules (<5 mm) scattered over the visceral and parietal peritoneum; histologic examination demonstrates caseating granulomas. Multiple adhesions are commonly present between the abdominal organs and parietal peritoneum. The gross appearance of the peritoneal cavity is similar to that of peritoneal carcinomatosis, sarcoidosis, and Crohn's disease, thus reiterating the importance of biopsy. Blind percutaneous peritoneal biopsy has a much lower yield than directed biopsy, and laparotomy with peritoneal biopsy is reserved for cases in which laparoscopy has been nondiagnostic or cannot be safely performed. Microscopic examination of ascitic fluid for acid-fast bacilli identifies the organism in less than 3% of cases, and culture results are positive in less than 20% of cases. Furthermore, the diagnostic usefulness of mycobacterial cultures is further limited by the time it may take for the cultures to yield definitive information, up to 8 weeks.

Treatment of peritoneal tuberculosis consists of antituberculous drugs. Drug regimens useful in treating pulmonary tuberculosis are also effective for peritoneal disease; a commonly used and effective regimen is isoniazid and rifampin daily for 9 months. The presence of associated alcoholic cirrhosis may complicate the use of these agents because of hepatotoxicity.

Peritonitis associated with chronic ambulatory peritoneal dialysis. In the United States, approximately 6% of patients with chronic renal failure undergo peritoneal dialysis. Peritonitis is one of the most common complications of chronic ambulatory peritoneal dialysis, occurring with an incidence of approximately one episode every 1 to 3 years. A study of all patients undergoing peritoneal dialysis in Scotland between 1999 and 2002 found that one episode of peritonitis occurred in every 19.2 months of peritoneal dialysis. Importantly, refractory or recurrent peritonitis was the most common cause of technical failure, accounting for 43% of all cases of technique failure.[37]

Patients present with abdominal pain, fever, and cloudy peritoneal dialysate containing more than 100 leukocytes/mm³, with more than 50% of the cells being neutrophils. Gram staining detects organisms only in approximately 10% to 40% of cases. Approximately 75% of infections are caused by gram-positive organisms, with *Staphylococcus epidermidis* accounting for 30% to 50% of cases. *S. aureus,* gram-negative bacilli, and fungi are also important causes of dialysis-associated peritonitis.[37]

Peritoneal dialysis–associated peritonitis is treated by the intraperitoneal administration of antibiotics, usually a first-generation cephalosporin. Overall, 75% of infections are cured by culture-directed antibiotic therapy. The cure rate for peritonitis using antibiotics without catheter removal varies according to the causative organism; one study showed rates of 90% with coagulase-negative staphylococcus compared with rates of 66%, 56%, and 0% for *S. aureus,* gram-negative bacilli, and fungi, respectively.[37] Recurrent or persistent peritonitis requires removal of the dialysis catheter and resumption of hemodialysis.

Malignant Neoplasms of the Peritoneum

Primary malignant neoplasms of the peritoneum are rare; these include malignant mesothelioma, primary peritoneal carcinoma, and sarcomas (e.g., angiosarcoma). Most malignant neoplasms that involve the peritoneum are transperitoneal metastases originating from carcinomas of the GI tract (especially the stomach, colon, and pancreas), the genitourinary tract (usually, ovarian), or, more rarely, an extra-abdominal site (e.g., breast). When metastatic cancer deposits diffusely coat the visceral and parietal peritoneum, these peritoneal metastases are referred to as *carcinomatosis.*

Pseudomyxoma peritonei. Pseudomyxoma peritonei describes mucinous ascites arising from a ruptured ovarian or appendiceal adenocarcinoma. In this disease, the peritoneum becomes coated with a mucus-secreting tumor that fills the peritoneal cavity with tenacious semisolid mucus and large, loculated cystic masses. Although the term *pseudomyxoma peritonei* is often used to describe any condition with accumulation of intraperitoneal mucin or mucinous ascites, here we focus on pseudomyxoma peritonei resulting from ruptured epithelial neoplasms of the appendix. The pathologic classification of appendiceal epithelial tumors can be confusing as there are differing classification systems. It is easier to consider these as tumors that extend along a spectrum from benign mucinous cystadenoma (also referred to as disseminated peritoneal adenomucinosis) to malignant cystadenocarcinoma, similar to the adenoma to carcinoma sequence in colorectal cancer.[38] The histology of appendiceal tumors is an important predictor of survival; adenomucinosis has the best survival rate (75% at 5 years) and peritoneal mucinous carcinomatosis the worst (14% at 5 years).[39]

Pseudomyxoma peritonei occurs most commonly in patients who are 40 to 50 years of age and occurs with equal frequency in men and women. Patients are often asymptomatic until late in the course of their disease. On presentation, they will often describe a global deterioration in their health long before the diagnosis is made. Symptoms of abdominal pain and distention and nonspecific complaints are common. Physical examination may reveal a new hernia, ascites, distended abdomen with non-shifting dullness, and, occasionally, a palpable abdominal mass.

CT of the chest, abdomen, and pelvis may provide important information about the diagnosis and the ability to resect the tumor completely or to perform an adequate cytoreduction, which is often limited by involvement of the small bowel or porta hepatis by tumor. Preoperative colonoscopy will differentiate a mucinous neoplasm of the appendix from that arising from the colon. The diagnosis is often made at laparotomy, when the surgeon is presented with a peritoneal cavity containing tenacious semisolid mucus and large, loculated cystic masses. If the surgeon is unprepared to perform a definitive procedure, the best approach is to establish the diagnosis by the least invasive procedure possible and to relieve symptoms of intestinal obstruction, if present. The patient can then be referred to a center experienced in the management of these patients.

The current treatment of patients with pseudomyxoma peritonei involves resection of as much of the tumor as possible (cyto-

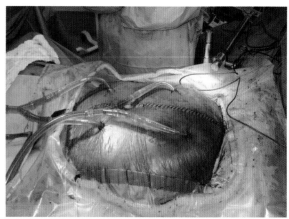

FIGURE 43-12 Placement of peritoneal catheters during the performance of intraperitoneal hyperthermic chemotherapy using the closed technique for chemotherapy administration.

reduction) and intraperitoneal heated chemotherapy (IPHC). Operative management includes omentectomy, stripping of involved peritoneum, resection of involved organs, and appendectomy, if not previously performed. There should be no residual tumor nodules larger than 2 mm in diameter after resection to facilitate penetration of the chemotherapy into any residual disease. In general, a right hemicolectomy is performed for these tumors, although a review of 501 patients with mucinous tumors of the appendix has suggested that this is unnecessary if the resection margin at appendectomy is negative.[40] IPHC can be performed by an open technique, in which the abdomen is left open to ensure adequate chemotherapy distribution throughout the peritoneal cavity, or a closed technique, in which the abdomen is closed after inflow and outflow cannulas are placed. The latter allows easier maintenance of hyperthermia (Fig. 43-12). There are many variations of surgical technique and chemotherapy administration, but one commonly used technique has been reported extensively by Stewart and associates.[41]

Cytoreduction with IPHC is associated with improved survival for patients with pseudomyxoma peritonei compared with historical controls. Before cytoreduction and IPHC, most studies reported long-term survival rates of 20% to 30% for patients with this disease undergoing serial debulking of the tumor with systemic chemotherapy. Gonzalez-Moreno and Sugarbaker[40] have reported 10-year survival rates of 55% in 501 patients undergoing cytoreduction and IPHC. Unfortunately, there are not likely to be any randomized controlled trials for this technique, given the infrequency with which this disease is encountered and the improved survival rates reported with IPHC compared with historical treatment with surgery alone. Furthermore, reported experiences are complicated by the use of various chemotherapy regimens, surgical techniques, and preoperative and intraoperative staging protocols.[42] At centers with experience in this technique, 30-day mortality rates are 2% to 3%, with 25% to 35% of patients developing a complication. The most common postoperative complications are prolonged ileus and pulmonary complications, although bleeding, intra-abdominal infections, enterocutaneous fistula, pancreatitis, and bone marrow suppression have also been reported.

Malignant peritoneal mesothelioma. The most common primary malignant peritoneal neoplasm is malignant mesothelioma, which results from malignant transformation of the simple squamoid epithelium covering the peritoneal cavity. Peritoneal mesothelioma is rare, with approximately 400 new cases per year, with a slight male predominance and a median age at presentation of approximately 50 years.[43] As with mesothelioma of the pleura, most patients with peritoneal mesothelioma will have had exposure to asbestos.

Most patients present with abdominal pain and weight loss. Ascites is common and often intractable. The omentum may become diffusely involved with tumor and present as an epigastric mass. CT demonstrates mesenteric thickening, peritoneal studding, hemorrhage within the tumor, and ascites. At laparotomy, the ascitic fluid ranges from a serous transudate to a viscous fluid rich in mucopolysaccharides. The neoplasm tends to involve all peritoneal surfaces, producing masses and plaques of tumor that are hard and white. In contrast to pseudomyxoma peritonei, local invasion of intra-abdominal organs, such as the liver, intestine, bladder, and abdominal wall, can occur, and encasement of bowel can create a malignant bowel obstruction. In some cases, it may be difficult to differentiate malignant peritoneal mesothelioma from diffuse peritoneal carcinomatosis arising from an intra-abdominal organ such as the stomach, pancreas, colon, or ovary. Careful examination of the pattern of spread and histologic examination of the biopsy specimen will often allow this distinction to be made. Furthermore, malignant peritoneal mesothelioma will generally remain confined to the abdomen, whereas advanced-stage intra-abdominal carcinomas frequently have pulmonary and other extra-abdominal metastases. Extension of the mesothelioma into one or both pleural cavities is more likely than hematogenous dissemination. Levy and colleagues[44] have reviewed the pathologic and radiographic features of peritoneal malignant neoplasms.

Complete surgical resection is difficult because of the extent of disease. Historically, operative management consisted of debulking of the tumor and enteroenterostomies to bypass areas of actual or impending intestinal obstruction. Systemic chemotherapy and abdominal radiation have been tried, without significant improvement in survival. Radiation therapy alone, whether by open-field techniques, intraperitoneal instillation of radioactive agents, or external beam irradiation, has had limited success and substantial associated morbidity.

As with pseudomyxoma peritonei, combined-modality approaches using surgery and IPHC may offer substantial improvements compared with historical controls. There have been several retrospective series using this technique, with median survival rates of 30 to 60 months and even 5-year survival rates of up to 50%. In light of these findings and the rarity of the disease, a multi-institutional data registry from eight institutions was created, including 405 patients treated with cytoreductive surgery and perioperative intraperitoneal chemotherapy.[45] Chemotherapeutic regimens varied (cisplatin, mitomycin, and doxorubicin were most commonly used), as did the timing and administration of the chemotherapy. The morbidity rate was 46%, and the mortality rate was 2%. Median survival was impressive at 53 months. The 3- and 5-year survival rates were 60% and 47%, respectively, offering significant improvement over what was previously considered a preterminal condition.

MESENTERY AND OMENTUM

Embryology and Anatomy

The greater and lesser omenta are complex peritoneal folds that pass from the stomach to the liver, transverse colon, spleen, bile duct, pancreas, and diaphragm. They originate from the dorsal and ventral midline mesenteries of the embryonic gut. In the very early stages of development, the alimentary canal traverses the future coelomic cavity as a straight tube, suspended posteriorly by an uninterrupted dorsal mesentery and anteriorly by a ventral mesentery in the cranial portion of its extent. The embryonic stomach rotates 90 degrees on its longitudinal axis so that the lesser curvature faces to the right and the greater curvature to the left. Much of the embryonic ventral mesentery is resorbed; however, the portion extending from the fissure of the ligamentum venosum and porta hepatis to the proximal duodenum and lesser curvature of the stomach (gastrohepatic ligament) persists as the lesser omentum. The right border of the lesser omentum is a free edge that forms the anterior border of the opening into the lesser sac, termed the *foramen of Winslow*. Between the layers of the lesser omentum, and at its right border, are the common hepatic duct, portal vein, and hepatic artery.

The embryonic dorsal mesogastrium grows as a sheet of peritoneum extending from the greater curvature of the stomach over the anterior surface of the small intestine. After passing inferiorly almost to the pelvis, the peritoneal membrane turns up on itself to pass upward to a line of attachment on the transverse colon slightly above that of the transverse mesocolon. Fat is laid down in this omental apron and provides an insulating layer of protection of the abdominal viscera.

Early in its development, the small intestine elongates to form an anteriorly oriented intestinal loop, which then rotates counterclockwise so that the cecum and ascending colon move to the right side of the peritoneal cavity, and the descending colon assumes a vertical position on the left wall of the peritoneal cavity. The jejunum and ileum are supported by the peritoneum-covered dorsal mesentery carrying the mesenteric blood vessels and lymphatics. The posterior line of attachment of the mesentery extends obliquely from the duodenojejunal junction at the left side of the second lumbar vertebra toward the right iliac fossa to terminate anterior to the sacroiliac articulation.

Physiology

The omentum and intestinal mesentery are rich in lymphatics and blood vessels. The omentum contains areas with high concentrations of macrophages, which may aid in the removal of foreign material and bacteria. Furthermore, the omentum becomes densely adherent to intraperitoneal sites of inflammation, often preventing diffuse peritonitis during cases of intestinal gangrene or perforation, such as acute diverticulitis or acute appendicitis.

Diseases of the Omentum
Omental Cysts

Omental cysts are unilocular or multilocular cysts containing serous fluid that are thought to arise from congenital or acquired obstruction of omental lymphatic channels. They are lined by a lymphatic endothelium similar to that of cystic lymphangiomas. These lesions are most common in children and young adults, in whom small cysts are usually asymptomatic and discovered incidentally; larger cysts are manifested as a palpable abdominal mass. Uncomplicated cysts usually lie in the lower midabdomen and are freely movable, smooth, and nontender. Complications are more common in children and include torsion, infection, and rupture.

Plain radiographs of the abdomen may show a well-circumscribed soft tissue density in the midabdomen, and contrast studies of the intestine may show displacement of intestinal loops and extrinsic compression on adjacent bowel. Ultrasound or CT will show a fluid-filled, complex, cystic mass with internal septations. The differential diagnosis of these lesions includes cysts and solid tumors of the mesentery, peritoneum, and retroperitoneum, including desmoid tumors. Ultimately, the diagnosis is made by excision of the cyst and histologic examination of the wall. Local excision, either laparoscopically or open, is curative.

Omental Torsion and Infarction

Torsion of the greater omentum is defined as the axial twisting of the omentum along its long axis. If the twist is tight enough or the venous obstruction is of sufficient duration, arterial inflow will become compromised, leading to infarction and necrosis. Omental torsion is classified as primary when no coexisting causative condition is identified or secondary when the torsion occurs in association with a causative condition, such as a hernia, tumor, or adhesion. Primary omental torsion usually involves the right side of the omentum.

Omental torsion occurs twice as often in men as in women and is most frequent in patients in their fourth or fifth decade of life. Patients present with the acute onset of severe abdominal pain localized to the right side of the abdomen in 80% of patients. Nausea and vomiting may be present but are not predominant findings. The patient's temperature is usually normal, and palpation of the abdomen demonstrates localized abdominal tenderness with guarding, suggesting peritonitis. A mass may be palpable if the involved omentum is sufficiently large.

The differential diagnosis includes any disease associated with right-sided abdominal pain and tenderness, most notably acute appendicitis, acute cholecystitis, and torsion of an ovarian cyst. CT often demonstrates an omental mass with signs of inflammation. Usually, the patient's clinical presentation justifies laparotomy or laparoscopy, at which time a segment of the omentum appears congested and acutely inflamed. Serosanguineous fluid is often present in the peritoneal cavity. Treatment consists of resection of the involved omentum and correction of any related condition.

Omental Neoplasms

Primary malignant neoplasms of the omentum are extremely rare and are usually of soft tissue origin. The omentum is usually invaded by metastatic tumor that has spread transperitoneally from an intra-abdominal carcinoma.

Omental Grafts and Transpositions

The arterial and venous blood supplies to the greater omentum are derived from omental branches of the right and left gastroepiploic arteries, which course along the greater curvature of the stomach. Division of the right or left gastroepiploic artery and vasa recta along the greater curvature of the stomach, with mobilization of the omentum from the transverse colon, allows the development of a vascularized omental pedicle flap. This graft may be used to cover chest and mediastinal wounds after chest wall resections and to prevent the small intestine from entering the pelvis after abdominal perineal resection, thus preventing radiation enteritis during radiation therapy for rectal carcinoma. Finally, the formation of dense adhesions between the omentum and sites of perforation or inflammation facilitates its use as a patch for duodenal perforations from ulcer disease (Graham patch; Fig. 43-13).

Diseases of the Mesentery
Mesenteric Cysts

The most common non-neoplastic mesenteric cysts are termed *mesothelial cysts* on the basis of the ultrastructure of the cells lining

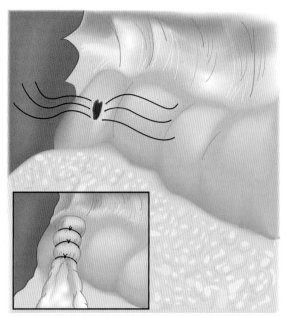

FIGURE 43-13 Closure of a perforated duodenal ulcer with an omental (Graham) patch. (From Graham RR: The treatment of perforated duodenal ulcers. *Surg Gynecol Obstet* 64:235–238, 1937.)

the cyst. The cysts contain chyle or a clear serous fluid and may occur in the mesentery of the small intestine (60%) or colon (40%). These cysts usually occur in adults, with a mean age of 45 years, and are twice as common in women as in men. Depending on the size of the cyst, patients may present with complaints of abdominal pain, fever, and emesis. A midabdominal mass may be palpable on examination of the abdomen. The diagnosis can usually be made preoperatively with ultrasonography or CT. Enucleation of the cyst at laparotomy is curative and can generally be accomplished because the mesenteric blood vessels and intestinal wall are usually not adherent to the cyst wall. Internal drainage of the cyst into the peritoneal cavity has also been successfully used in the treatment of very large cysts. Aspiration alone has a high rate of cyst recurrence. In those cases in which the cyst is not completely excised, the contents of the cyst and the internal architecture of the cyst wall must be carefully inspected and the cyst wall examined histologically to rule out a non-neoplastic cause.

Acute Mesenteric Lymphadenitis

Acute mesenteric lymphadenitis is a syndrome of acute right lower quadrant abdominal pain associated with mesenteric lymph node enlargement and a normal appendix. In general, the diagnosis is made on exploration of the abdomen of a patient suspected of having acute appendicitis, at which time a normal appendix and enlarged mesenteric lymph nodes are discovered. This syndrome occurs most commonly in children and young adults, with equal frequency in males and females.

Numerous causative agents have been implicated in the pathobiology of acute mesenteric lymphadenitis, including viral, bacterial, parasitic, and fungal infections. *Yersinia enterocolitica* in particular has been associated with this syndrome in children. Culture and histologic examination of the enlarged lymph nodes, stool culture, and antibody titers have been used to identify causative agents but are not routinely used in the treatment of these patients.

The symptom complex associated with acute mesenteric lymphadenitis is similar to that of acute appendicitis; it includes the acute onset of periumbilical pain, which shifts to the right lower quadrant over time. Physical examination demonstrates right lower quadrant tenderness, with abdominal wall muscle rigidity and rebound tenderness. Nausea, vomiting, and anorexia may also be present but are not dominant symptoms. In general, the patient's temperature and white blood cell count are normal or only slightly elevated.

The diagnosis is made at the time of operation for presumed acute appendicitis, at which time a normal-appearing appendix is found, with enlarged mesenteric lymph nodes. Excision of an enlarged lymph node with culture and nodal histology may provide information about the cause but is not routinely used.

Sclerosing Mesenteritis

Sclerosing mesenteritis is a rare inflammatory disease of the mesentery characterized histologically by sclerosing fibrosis, fat necrosis with lipid-laden macrophages, chronic inflammation with germinal centers, and focal calcification. Early in the course of the disease, sclerosing mesenteritis has a loose myxomatous appearance that progresses to chronic inflammation and dense sclerosis. This condition is characterized grossly by marked thickening of the mesentery of the small intestine, with irregular areas of discoloration suggesting fat necrosis. There may also be multiple discrete nodules on the mesentery, or the disease may appear as a single matted mass. The process most often involves the root of the small bowel mesentery and frequently encompasses the mesenteric vessels. It affects the small bowel by retraction and shortening of the mesentery without invasion. In advanced cases, mesenteric venous and lymphatic obstruction may be present. The mesocolon may also be affected but less frequently than the small bowel mesentery.[44]

Sclerosing mesenteritis is twice as common in men as in women and usually occurs in the fifth decade of life. Most patients are asymptomatic, and the diagnosis is discovered incidentally on imaging for an unrelated condition. When symptoms are present, abdominal pain or symptoms of intestinal obstruction with nausea, vomiting, and abdominal distention are most common. An abdominal mass is palpable in more than 50% of patients. Laboratory studies are usually normal, except that the erythrocyte sedimentation rate and C-reactive protein levels may be elevated.

The differential diagnosis of sclerosing mesenteritis includes a heterogeneous group of conditions that alter the density of the mesenteric fat, including inflammatory and neoplastic causes. Differentiation from peritoneal carcinomatosis, carcinoid tumor, and mesenteric and retroperitoneal sarcomas is particularly important. The CT characteristics of sclerosing mesenteritis are well described[46,47] and include the following:

- A fatty mass arising from the base of the mesentery that has well-delineated margins separating it from normal mesentery, a feature described as a *tumoral pseudocapsule*
- The presence of normal adipose tissue surrounding mesenteric vessels, termed *fat ring sign*
- The presence of normal mesenteric vessels coursing through the fatty mass, without evidence of vascular involvement or deviation
- An intra-abdominal mass that displaces adjacent bowel loops without invading them

Laparotomy or laparoscopy with biopsy of the involved mesentery remains necessary for definitive diagnosis.

Most patients with mesenteric panniculitis experience spontaneous resolution of their symptoms. If patients do not improve, corticosteroids and other anti-inflammatory and immunosuppressive agents have been reported to be successful in improving the symptoms and radiographic findings. Operative management is indicated only for patients in whom there is confusion about the diagnosis and for treatment of intestinal obstruction.

Intra-abdominal (Internal) Hernias
Internal Hernias Caused by Developmental Defects
There are three general mechanisms whereby developmental abnormalities result in the formation of internal hernias: (1) abnormal retroperitoneal fixation of the mesentery resulting in anomalous positioning of the intestine (e.g., mesocolic or paraduodenal hernia); (2) abnormally large internal foramina or fossae (e.g., foramen of Winslow, supravesical hernia); and (3) incomplete mesenteric surfaces with the presence of an abnormal opening through which the intestine herniates (e.g., mesenteric hernia).

The anatomic and radiographic features of acquired and congenital internal hernias have been reviewed by Martin and associates.[48]

Mesocolic (paraduodenal) hernias. Mesocolic hernias are unusual congenital hernias in which the small intestine herniates behind the mesocolon. They result from abnormal rotation of the midgut and have been categorized as right or left. A right mesocolic hernia occurs when the prearterial limb of the midgut loop fails to rotate around the superior mesenteric artery. This results in most of the small intestine remaining to the right of the superior mesenteric artery. Normal counterclockwise rotation of the cecum and proximal colon into the right side of the abdomen and fixation to the posterolateral peritoneum cause the small intestine to become trapped behind the mesentery of the right side of the colon. The ileocolic, right colic, and middle colic vessels lie within the anterior wall of the sac, and the superior mesenteric artery courses along the medial border of the neck of the hernia (Fig. 43-14A).

Left mesocolic hernias are thought to be caused by in utero herniation of the small intestine between the inferior mesenteric vein and posterior parietal attachments of the descending mesocolon to the retroperitoneum. The inferior mesenteric artery and vein are integral components of the hernia sac (Fig. 43-14B). Approximately 75% of mesocolic hernias occur on the left side.

Patients with paraduodenal hernias usually present with symptoms of acute or chronic small bowel obstruction. Barium radiographs will demonstrate displacement of the small intestine to the left or right side of the abdomen. CT with intravenous administration of contrast material may demonstrate displacement of the mesenteric vessels and evidence of intestinal obstruction, if present.

The operative treatment of patients with a right mesocolic hernia involves incision of the lateral peritoneal reflections along the right colon, with reflection of the right colon and cecum to the left. The entire gut then assumes a position simulating that of nonrotation of the prearterial and postarterial segments of the midgut. Opening the neck of the hernia will injure the superior mesenteric vessels and fails to free the herniated bowel (Fig. 43-14C).

The operative treatment of patients with a left mesocolic hernia consists of incision of the peritoneal attachments and adhesions

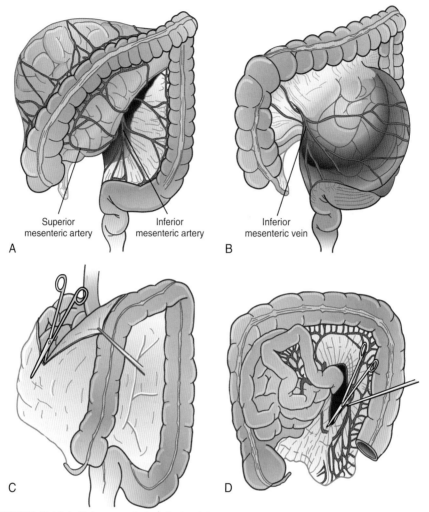

FIGURE 43-14 A, Right mesocolic (paraduodenal) hernia. Note that the anterior wall of a right mesocolic hernia is the ascending mesocolon. The hernia orifice lies to the right of the midline, and the superior mesenteric artery and ileocolic artery course along the anterior border of the hernia neck. **B,** Left mesocolic (paraduodenal) hernia. The hernia orifice is to the left of the midline, and the herniated intestine lies behind the anterior wall of the descending mesocolon. **C,** A right mesocolic hernia is repaired by division of the lateral peritoneal attachments of the ascending colon, reflecting it toward the left side of the abdomen. The small and large intestine then assume a position simulating that of nonrotation of the prearterial and postarterial segments of the midgut. Opening the neck of the hernia will injure the superior mesenteric vessels and fail to free the herniated bowel. **D,** A left mesocolic hernia is reduced by incising the hernia sac along an avascular plane immediately to the right of the inferior mesenteric vessels. (**A, B,** From Brigham RA, d'Avis JC: Paraduodenal hernia. In Nyhus LM, Condon RE, editors: *Hernia,* ed 3, Philadelphia, 1989, JB Lippincott, pp 484–485. **C, D,** From Brigham R, Fallon WF, Saunders JR, et al: Paraduodenal hernia: Diagnosis and surgical management. *Surg* 96:498–502, 1984.)

along the right side of the inferior mesenteric vein, with reduction of the herniated small intestine from beneath the inferior mesenteric vein. The vein is then allowed to return to its normal position on the left side of the base of the mesentery of the small intestine. The neck of the hernia may be closed by suturing the peritoneum adjacent to the vein to the retroperitoneum (Fig. 43-14D).

Mesenteric hernias. Mesenteric hernias occur when the intestine herniates through an abnormal orifice in the mesentery of the small intestine or colon. The most common location for these hernias is near the ileocolic junction, although defects in the sigmoid mesocolon have also been described. Patients present with intestinal obstruction resulting from compression of the loops of bowel at the neck of the hernia or torsion of the herniated segment. Treatment involves reduction of the hernia and closure of the mesenteric defect.

Acquired Internal Hernias

Acquired internal hernias result from the creation of abnormal mesenteric defects after operative procedures or trauma. These usually result from inadequate closure (or dehiscence) of mesenteric defects created during the performance of gastrojejunostomy, colostomy, ileostomy, or bowel resection. The creation of a small space allows the herniation of the small intestine through the mesenteric rent and development of intestinal obstruction. Depending on the type of surgery performed, variation exists in routine closure of the mesenteric defect. For instance, herniation after laparoscopic colectomy is uncommon (approximately 1%), so the defect is usually not closed. However, hernia rates after laparoscopic Roux-en-Y gastric bypass (i.e., Peterson hernia) are reported as high as 9%, so the defect is usually closed.[49] Treatment of these patients is operative reduction of the hernia and closure of the peritoneal defect.

Malignant Neoplasms of the Mesentery

Similar to the peritoneum and omentum, the most common neoplasm involving the mesentery is metastatic disease from an intra-abdominal adenocarcinoma. This may result from the direct invasion of the primary tumor (or its lymphatic metastases) into the mesentery or from the transperitoneal spread of the malignant neoplasm into the mesentery. Distortion and fixation of the mesentery by the tumor itself or by the resultant desmoplastic reaction, as in carcinoid tumors of the GI tract, may cause intestinal obstruction. The most common primary malignant neoplasm of the mesentery is a desmoid tumor.

Mesenteric and Intra-abdominal Desmoid Tumors

Mesenteric desmoids account for less than 10% of sporadic desmoid tumors, although they are reported to occur in 10% to 15% of patients with FAP. In this group of patients, 70% of the desmoid tumors are intra-abdominal, and 50% to 75% of these involve the mesentery.[2,3] The association between desmoid tumor and FAP is particularly strong in the subset of patients with Gardner syndrome. Patients with FAP and a family history of desmoid tumors have a 25% chance for development of a desmoid tumor. Several studies have shown intra-abdominal surgery to be a significant risk factor (as high as a threefold risk) for development of desmoids.[50] Levy and coworkers[46] have reviewed the pathologic and radiographic findings of these uncommon tumors.

Intra-abdominal desmoids are more lethal than those that occur at other anatomic sites because of the possibility of bowel obstruction or ischemia. Resection is less frequently possible, involves greater risk to critical structures, and may be associated with causing more aggressive growth and progression in these tumors. Intra-abdominal desmoid tumors are also more often multiple than those at other anatomic sites. Resection of mesenteric desmoids may require sacrifice of significant lengths of intestine, thus leaving the patient with an inadequate absorptive surface to maintain adequate nutrition. Finally, ureteral involvement of the tumor may require resection with reconstruction.

Although mesenteric desmoid tumors tend to be aggressive, there is considerable variability in their growth rate during the course of the disease. In fact, the biology of intra-abdominal desmoid tumors may be characterized by initial rapid growth followed by stability or even regression. Mesenteric desmoid tumors, by virtue of their relationship to vital structures and ability to infiltrate adjacent organs, may cause significant local complications, including intestinal obstruction, ischemia and perforation, hydronephrosis, and even aortic rupture, requiring operative management. Despite these complications, the overall 10-year survival rate for patients with intra-abdominal desmoid tumors is 60% to 70%.[51]

Establishing the rate of growth can be helpful in determining the optimal treatment of intra-abdominal desmoid tumors. The American Society of Clinical Oncology and Society of Surgical Oncologists have reviewed the current role of risk-reducing surgery in common hereditary cancer syndromes.[52] These recommendations, in addition to practice parameters from the Standards Task Force of the American Society of Colon and Rectal Surgeons, suggest that surgery should be reserved for small tumors with a well-defined and a clearly resectable margin.[53] Reported recurrence rates for intra-abdominal desmoids are higher than for other sites and range from 57% to 86%, although surgery can be curative in select patients.[51] Small bowel transplantation has been described for otherwise unresectable lesions.

Given the high likelihood of recurrence and prolonged survival, even in the setting of advanced disease, some have suggested that a trial of watchful waiting, along with minimally toxic agents such as sulindac and antiestrogen therapy, may be the best strategy, particularly in patients with minimal symptoms. In this nascent era of target-specific biologic therapy, clinical response to imatinib by patients with heavily treated desmoid tumor has been reported. Imatinib mesylate, specifically designed to inhibit the Bcr-Abl tyrosine kinase rendered constitutive by the Philadelphia chromosome translocation in chronic myeloid leukemia, also inhibits the tyrosine kinase receptor for platelet-derived growth factor and c-kit. The observation that patients with desmoid tumors have partial tumor response and arrest of disease progression while receiving oral imatinib offers an alternative to surgical resection of desmoid tumors arising in the mesentery.[17]

RETROPERITONEUM

Anatomy

The retroperitoneal space lies between the peritoneum and posterior parietal wall of the abdominal cavity, extending from the diaphragm to the pelvic floor. This space contains the contiguous lumbar and iliac fossae. The lumbar fossa extends from the 12th thoracic vertebra and lateral lumbocostal arch superiorly to the base of the sacrum, iliac crest, and iliolumbar ligament inferiorly. The floor of the space is formed by the fascia overlying the quadratus lumborum and psoas major muscles. This space contains varying amounts of fatty areolar tissue and the adrenal glands, kidneys, ascending and descending colon, and duodenum. It is also traversed by the ureter, renal vessels, gonadal vessels, inferior vena cava, and aorta. The iliac fossa is contiguous with the lumbar fossa superiorly, lateral and anterior preperitoneal spaces of the abdominal wall, and pelvis inferiorly. The iliacus muscle with its investing fascia is the floor of the iliac fossa, which contains the iliac vessels, ureter, genitofemoral nerve, gonadal vessels, and iliac lymph nodes.

Operative Approaches

The aorta, vena cava, iliac vessels, kidneys, and adrenal glands may be approached operatively through the retroperitoneal space. Specific operative procedures performed through the retroperitoneum include extirpative procedures, such as adrenalectomy and nephrectomy, and aortic aneurysmorrhaphy and renal transplantation. The advantages to this approach over a transabdominal approach are as follows: less postoperative ileus, facilitating a more rapid resumption of diet and earlier discharge from the hospital; no intra-abdominal adhesions, thus reducing the likelihood of subsequent small bowel obstruction; less intraoperative evaporative fluid losses, with less dramatic intravascular fluid shifts; and fewer respiratory complications, such as atelectasis and pneumonia.

Retroperitoneal Disorders

Retroperitoneal Abscesses

Retroperitoneal abscesses may be classified as primary if the infection results from hematogenous spread or secondary if it is related to an infection in an adjacent organ. The conditions associated with the development of retroperitoneal abscesses are shown in Table 43-2; the anatomic relationship of retroperitoneal abscesses to surrounding structures is shown in Figure 43-15. Most retroperitoneal abscesses originate as inflammatory processes in the kidney and GI tract. Renal causes include infections related to renal lithiasis or previous urologic operative procedures. GI causes include appendicitis, diverticulitis, pancreatitis, and Crohn's disease. In one series from an urban center, tuberculosis of the spine was a common cause of retroperitoneal abscesses, with *Mycobacterium tuberculosis* being the second most common bacterial isolate after *E. coli.*[54]

The bacteriology of retroperitoneal abscesses is related to the cause. Infections originating from the kidney are often monomicrobial, involving gram-negative rods such as *Proteus mirabilis* and *E. coli.* Abscesses associated with diseases of the GI tract involve *E. coli, Enterobacter* spp., enterococci, and anaerobic species such as *Bacteroides.* These infections are multimicrobial and involve gram-negative bacilli, enterococci, and anaerobic species. Infections from hematogenous spread are usually monomicrobial and related to staphylococcal species. Tuberculosis of the spine is an important cause of retroperitoneal abscesses in immunocompromised individuals and in those immigrating from underdeveloped countries.

The most common symptoms of retroperitoneal abscesses include abdominal or flank pain (60% to 75%), fever and chills (30% to 90%), malaise (10% to 22%), and weight loss (12%). Patients with psoas abscesses may have referred pain to the hip, groin, or knee. The duration of symptoms is usually longer than 1 week. Patients with retroperitoneal abscesses often have concurrent, chronic illnesses, such as renal lithiasis, diabetes mellitus, HIV infection, or malignant neoplasms. CT demonstrates a low-density mass in the retroperitoneum, with surrounding inflammation. Gas may be present in as many as one third of these lesions.[54] CT provides important information about the location of the abscess and its relationship to contiguous organs and hence likely sources of the infection.

Treatment of retroperitoneal abscesses includes appropriate antibiotics and adequate drainage. Many reports have demonstrated the efficacy of CT-guided drainage in managing this aspect of treatment. Operative drainage through a retroperitoneal approach is indicated for lesions not amenable to percutaneous drainage or those that fail percutaneous drainage. The mortality rate for patients with retroperitoneal abscesses is related, in large part, to the presence of significant medical comorbidities.

Retroperitoneal Hematomas

Retroperitoneal hematomas usually occur after blunt or penetrating injuries, in the setting of abdominal aortic or visceral artery aneurysms, or after acute or chronic anticoagulation or fibrinolytic therapy. The diagnosis and management of retroperitoneal hematomas occurring in the setting of trauma or aneurysmal rupture are considered in detail in Chapters 16, 61, and 63.

TABLE 43-2 Cause and Relative Frequency of Retroperitoneal Abscesses*	
CAUSE	**FREQUENCY (%)**
Renal diseases	47
Gastrointestinal diseases, including diverticulitis, appendicitis, and Crohn's disease	16
Hematogenous spread from remote infections	11
Abscesses complicating operative procedures	8
Bone infections, including tuberculosis of the spine	7
Trauma	4.5
Malignant neoplasms	4
Miscellaneous causes	3

*Data are from three retrospective reviews[55-57] of 134 patients treated between 1971 and 2001.

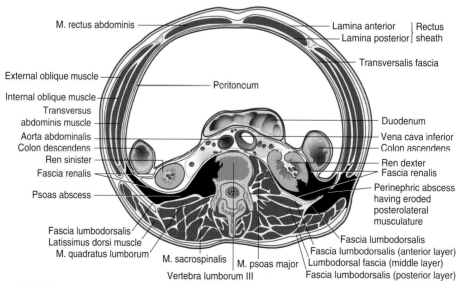

FIGURE 43-15 Anatomic relationships of retroperitoneal abscesses to surrounding structures. A psoas abscess *(left)* and perinephric abscess *(right)* are shown. (From McVay C: *Anson and McVay's surgical anatomy,* ed 6, Philadelphia, 1984, WB Saunders, p 735.)

Bleeding into the retroperitoneum may also complicate anticoagulant therapy for atrial fibrillation, deep venous thrombosis, or arterial catheterization during cardiac catheterization and endovascular procedures. Retroperitoneal hematomas have also been described in patients undergoing fibrinolytic therapy for peripheral or coronary arterial thrombosis and in patients with bleeding diatheses, such as hemophilia.

Patients present with abdominal or flank pain that may radiate into the groin, labia, or scrotum. Clinical evidence of acute blood loss may be present, depending on the volume of blood lost and the rapidity with which the patient bled. A palpable abdominal mass as well as physical evidence of ileus may be present. As many as 20% to 30% of patients will develop evidence of a femoral neuropathy.[55] The complete blood count may provide evidence of subacute or chronic blood loss or platelet deficiency. The prothrombin and partial thromboplastin times may demonstrate a coagulopathy. Microscopic hematuria is a common finding on urinalysis. CT establishes the diagnosis by demonstrating a high-density mass in the retroperitoneum, with surrounding stranding in the retroperitoneal tissue planes. These findings are readily distinguishable from the low-density mass characteristic of retroperitoneal abscesses.

Patients who develop retroperitoneal hematomas as a result of anticoagulation are best managed by the restoration of circulating blood volume and correction of the underlying coagulopathy. In rare circumstances, arteriography with embolization of a bleeding artery or operative exploration is required to stop the bleeding.

Retroperitoneal Fibrosis

Retroperitoneal fibrosis is characterized by chronic inflammation and fibrosis surrounding the abdominal aorta and iliac arteries that extend laterally to envelop surrounding structures, especially the ureters. Seventy percent of cases are idiopathic (Ormond disease), whereas 30% are associated with various drugs (most notably, ergot alkaloids or dopaminergic agonists), infections, trauma, retroperitoneal hemorrhage or retroperitoneal operations, radiation therapy, or primary or metastatic neoplasms. Many idiopathic cases are associated with inflammatory abdominal aortic aneurysms; thus, idiopathic retroperitoneal fibrosis might best be categorized with inflammatory abdominal aortic aneurysms and perianeurysmal retroperitoneal fibrosis as a form of chronic periaortitis.[56] The fibrosis is usually confined to the central and paravertebral spaces between the renal arteries and sacrum and tends to encase the aorta, inferior vena cava, and ureters. The process usually begins at the level of the aortic bifurcation and spreads cephalad. In 15% of cases, the fibrotic process extends outside the retroperitoneum to involve the peripancreatic and periduodenal spaces, pelvis, and mediastinum.

There is considerable evidence to suggest that idiopathic retroperitoneal fibrosis is a manifestation of a systemic autoimmune disease. A case-control study of 35 patients found that the disease is associated with HLA-DRB1*03, an allele linked to various autoimmune diseases, such as type 1 diabetes mellitus, myasthenia gravis, and systemic lupus erythematosus.[57] In some patients, disease will develop in the setting of a well-defined systemic autoimmune disorder (e.g., systemic lupus erythematosus) or so-called organ-specific autoimmune diseases (e.g., Hashimoto thyroiditis, sclerosing cholangitis). There are also histologic similarities between idiopathic retroperitoneal fibrosis and other systemic inflammatory conditions, such as large-vessel vasculitides.[56] Finally, systemic or constitutional symptoms are often present, such as fatigue, low-grade fever, weight loss, and myalgias.

Men are affected two to three times as often as women are. The mean age at presentation is 50 to 60 years, although the condition has also been reported in children and older adults. Patients may present with localized symptoms of side, back, or abdominal pain or lower extremity edema. Scrotal swelling is common, as is the occurrence of a varicocele or hydrocele. In most patients, localized symptoms are preceded by or coexist with systemic or constitutional symptoms (see earlier). Laboratory tests may demonstrate azotemia, and 80% to 100% of patients will have elevated concentrations of acute-phase reactants (e.g., erythrocyte sedimentation rate, C-reactive protein). The nonspecific nature of the clinical features of this disease contributes to the considerable delay between the onset of symptoms and the diagnosis. As such, ureteral involvement is present in 80% to 100% of cases.[56]

Evaluation of patients thought to have retroperitoneal fibrosis often starts with a CT scan. Without intravenous administration of contrast material, the CT scan will demonstrate a homogeneous fibrous plaque surrounding the lower abdominal aorta and the iliac arteries, which is usually isodense compared with surrounding muscle. MRI of early benign retroperitoneal fibrosis may show areas of high signal intensity on T2-weighted images as a result of the abundant fluid content and hypercellularity associated with the acute inflammation. In the mature and quiescent stages of benign retroperitoneal fibrosis, the low signal intensity on T1- and T2-weighted images is similar to that of psoas muscle.

The primary goals of treatment for patients with idiopathic retroperitoneal fibrosis are to stop the progression of retroperitoneal inflammation and fibrosis, to prevent or to relieve ureteral obstruction, to inhibit the systemic inflammatory response, and to improve the constitutional manifestations of the disease. The mainstay of treatment has been the administration of corticosteroids, which suppress the synthesis of proinflammatory cytokines and inhibit collagen synthesis and maturation. This will often result in a prompt improvement in symptoms, reduction in the size of the retroperitoneal mass, and relief of ureteral obstruction. Unfortunately, the optimal dose and duration of treatment have not been well established. Immunosuppressants such as mycophenolate mofetil, cyclophosphamide, azathioprine, methotrexate, cyclosporine, and tamoxifen have also been used to treat patients with idiopathic retroperitoneal fibrosis, particularly patients whose disease is unresponsive to steroids. Operative management of retroperitoneal fibrosis is generally performed to relieve ureteral obstruction by open ureterolysis, with intraperitoneal transposition and omental wrapping of the ureters. In most cases, when the clinical findings and imaging suggest the diagnosis of retroperitoneal fibrosis, the temporary placement of ureteral stents followed by medical therapy is the recommended course of action. Operative ureterolysis would be reserved for patients with refractory disease.

When retroperitoneal fibrosis is associated with an abdominal aortic aneurysm, repair of the aneurysm is warranted when the aortic diameter exceeds 4.5 to 5 cm. The effect of aneurysm repair of the periaortic fibrosis is unclear; some reports indicate resolution, and others report persistence or even progression of the inflammatory process.

Retroperitoneal Malignant Neoplasms

Malignant neoplasms in the retroperitoneum may result from the following:

- Extracapsular growth of a primary neoplasm of a retroperitoneal organ, such as the kidney, adrenal, colon, or pancreas

- Development of a primary germ cell neoplasm from embryonic rest cells
- Development of a primary malignant neoplasm of the retroperitoneal lymphatic system (e.g., lymphoma)
- Metastases from a remote primary malignant neoplasm into a retroperitoneal lymph node (e.g., testicular cancer)
- Development of a malignant neoplasm of the soft tissue of the retroperitoneum (e.g., sarcomas and desmoid tumors)

The most common primary malignant neoplasm of the retroperitoneum is a sarcoma.

Retroperitoneal sarcoma. Approximately 12,000 soft tissue sarcomas were diagnosed in the United States in 2014, of which 15% were retroperitoneal sarcomas.[58] The most common histologic subtypes are liposarcoma and leiomyosarcoma. Radiation is a known risk factor for the development of sarcomas, with radiation-associated sarcomas usually occurring approximately 10 years after exposure. Patients with von Recklinghausen disease (neurofibromatosis type 1) can develop malignant transformation of neurofibromas into malignant peripheral nerve sheath tumors; patients with Li-Fraumeni syndrome and hereditary retinoblastoma also have an increased incidence of sarcoma.

Most patients with a retroperitoneal sarcoma present with an asymptomatic abdominal mass, often after the primary tumor has reached a considerable size. Abdominal pain is present in 50% of patients; less common symptoms include GI hemorrhage, early satiety, nausea, vomiting, weight loss, and lower extremity swelling. Symptoms related to nerve compression by the tumor, such as lower extremity paresthesia and paresis, have also been associated with retroperitoneal sarcoma.

CT and MRI provide important information about the size and precise location of the primary tumor and its relationship to major vascular structures (Fig. 43-16). These studies will also document the presence or absence of metastatic disease in the lung or liver. These imaging modalities will also usually provide important diagnostic clues, thus obviating the need for image-guided biopsy in most cases.

Several findings can help distinguish retroperitoneal sarcomas from other retroperitoneal tumors. Lymphoma, especially with bulky retroperitoneal adenopathy, may appear as a mass arising from the retroperitoneum. The presence of constitutional symptoms, including fevers, night sweats, and weight loss, may suggest the diagnosis of lymphoma. A careful search for other evidence of lymphadenopathy is warranted in these patients. The spread of testicular cancer to the retroperitoneal lymph nodes may also be

manifested as a large retroperitoneal mass. Hence, workup of male patients should include a testicular examination and serologic testing for α-fetoprotein and human chorionic gonadotropin. Finally, the local extension of tumors arising in the adrenal gland or pancreas may also be considered in the differential diagnosis of patients with large retroperitoneal tumors.

Prognostic staging is difficult for sarcomas because there are many histologic types of sarcomas, with variables grades and locations. The latest edition of the American Joint Commission cancer staging system is notable in that it includes grade and depth to the fascia in addition to standard staging criteria, such as tumor size, nodal status, and distant metastasis.[59] Most retroperitoneal sarcomas are deep to the fascia and large, so grade is the main determinant of stage in nonmetastatic disease. Nodal disease had previously been classified as stage IV but is currently reassigned to stage III.

The goal of sarcoma treatment is complete en bloc resection of the tumor and any involved adjacent organs. As retroperitoneal sarcomas are rare tumors with several different histologic subtypes that may influence surgical treatment, a consensus approach from an international group of established experts was recently constructed to assist with management strategy.[60] Recommendations found within this consensus statement address preoperative assessment and biopsy, surgical approach, adjuvant and neoadjuvant therapy, and follow-up and may serve as a resource in addition to standard National Comprehensive Cancer Network guidelines. Lymph node metastases by sarcoma are rare (<5%); therefore, lymphadenectomy is not required unless there is evidence of lymph node involvement. The main prognostic factors for patients with retroperitoneal sarcomas are the size of the tumor, histologic grade, and resection status.[61] The difficulty of obtaining resection margins free of tumor is related to the juxtaposition or invasion of the tumor and retroperitoneal structures, such as the aorta, inferior vena cava, intra-abdominal viscera (colon, duodenum, kidney, pancreas, spleen), and adjacent muscles (psoas, rectus abdominis, diaphragm). The kidney is the most commonly resected organ; series have reported multiorgan resection in approximately 50% of cases.[62] A thoracoabdominal incision may be required for upper quadrant sarcomas, but this does not appear to increase morbidity greatly. It can be difficult pathologically to determine a negative margin resulting from the large surface area and anatomic constraints of the tumor. Most experts in treating this disease consider the goal of surgery to be complete resection, defined by removal of all gross disease (macroscopically negative

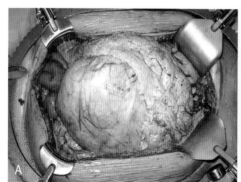 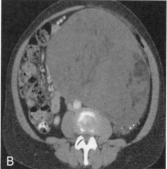

FIGURE 43-16 A, Intraoperative photograph of a large retroperitoneal sarcoma. **B,** CT scan of the same patient demonstrating the displacement of the aorta, inferior vena cava, and bowel to the right of the abdomen.

margin), with en bloc resection of adherent organs. Rates of resectability of the primary retroperitoneal sarcoma vary widely on the basis of the extent of disease at presentation, the surgeon's experience, and the institution's referral pattern. A review of several large series has reported complete resectability rates of 50% to 67%.[63]

There is no difference in survival for patients who undergo incomplete resection compared with those who are unresectable. Incomplete resection should be undertaken only for palliative purposes for all histologic types other than liposarcoma.[61] Incomplete resection of well-differentiated liposarcoma may prolong survival and has been shown to improve symptoms.[64] Local recurrence after surgery occurs in approximately 50% of patients, and distant metastases occur in 20% to 30%. The 5-year survival rate is approximately 50%.[64]

In patients with recurrent disease, complete resection of recurrent tumor is beneficial. In a report by Lewis and colleagues[61] at the Memorial Sloan Kettering Cancer Center, 35 of 61 patients with recurrent sarcoma underwent complete resection. This group of patients had a significantly higher survival rate than those undergoing incomplete resection (60% versus 18% 5-year disease-specific survival).

Unlike for extremity sarcoma, the role of external beam radiation for local control after surgical resection is limited by the low tolerance for radiation injury of the surrounding normal tissue. Postoperative radiotherapy and combined postoperative and intraoperative radiotherapy have been shown to improve recurrence rates but have not been clearly shown to have an effect on survival. Preoperative radiotherapy has some theoretical benefits, but there have been no prospective randomized trials of preoperative radiotherapy. Neoadjuvant or adjuvant chemotherapy is supported by limited and conflicting data, but unfortunately most agents used for sarcoma therapy have significant toxicity.

SELECTED REFERENCES

Chua TC, Moran BJ, Sugarbaker PH, et al: Early- and long-term outcome data of patients with pseudomyxoma peritonei from appendiceal origin treated by a strategy of cytoreductive surgery and hyperthermic intraperitoneal chemotherapy. *J Clin Oncol* 30:2449–2456, 2012.

This large multi-institutional retrospective study highlights the safety and improved outcomes using cytoreductive surgery with pseudomyxoma peritonei.

Fiore M, Rimareix F, Mariani L, et al: Desmoid-type fibromatosis: A front-line conservative approach to select patients for surgical treatment. *Ann Surg Oncol* 16:2587–2593, 2009.

This multi-institutional paper highlights the utility of a watch and wait approach for managing patients with desmoids.

Fleshman J, Sargent DJ, Green E, et al: Laparoscopic colectomy for cancer is not inferior to open surgery based on 5-year data from the COST Study Group trial. *Ann Surg* 246:655–662, 2007.

This important paper defined the incidence of port site recurrence after laparoscopic colectomy for colon cancer and established the equivalency of laparoscopic and open colectomy for the treatment of curable colon cancer.

Guillem JG, Wood WC, Moley JF, et al: ASCO/SSO review of current role of risk-reducing surgery in common hereditary cancer syndromes. *J Clin Oncol* 24:4642–4660, 2006.

This task force consensus statement outlines the current recommendations from the American Society of Clinical Oncology and Society of Surgical Oncology regarding surgery for desmoid tumors in patients with familial adenomatous polyposis.

Koulaouzidis A, Bhat S, Saeed AA: Spontaneous bacterial peritonitis. *World J Gastroenterol* 15:1042–1049, 2009.

This is a well-written and thorough review of the pathophysiology, bacteriology, and treatment of spontaneous bacterial peritonitis.

Martin LC, Merkle EM, Thompson WM: Review of internal hernias: Radiographic and clinical findings. *AJR Am J Roentgenol* 186:703–717, 2006.

This is a thorough and well-illustrated review of the types of congenital and acquired internal hernias.

Moller S, Henriksen JH, Bendtsen F: Ascites: Pathogenesis and therapeutic principles. *Scand J Gastroenterol* 44:902–911, 2009.

This is a well-written and thorough review of the pathophysiology of ascites formation in cirrhotics and the basic tenets of medical management.

Runyon BA, Montano AA, Akriviadis EA, et al: The serum-ascites albumin gradient is superior to the exudate-transudate concept in the differential diagnosis of ascites. *Ann Intern Med* 117:215–220, 1992.

This well-written paper established the use of serum-ascites albumin gradient in the elucidation of the pathophysiology of ascites formation.

Stewart JH, Shen P, Levine EA: Intraperitoneal hyperthermic chemotherapy for peritoneal surface malignancy: Current status and future directions. *Ann Surg Oncol* 12:765–777, 2005.

This review covers the rationale, technical aspects, and outcomes for intraperitoneal hyperthermic chemotherapy for several types of malignant neoplasms.

Trans-Atlantic RPS Working Group: Management of primary retroperitoneal sarcoma (RPS) in the adult: A consensus approach from the Trans-Atlantic RPS Working Group. *Ann Surg Oncol* 22:256–263, 2015.

This paper provides updated consensus statements on the management of retroperitoneal sarcoma.

Vaglio A, Salvarani C, Buzio C: Retroperitoneal fibrosis. *Lancet* 367:241–251, 2006.

This is a well-written and thorough review of the pathophysiology, immunology, and clinical features of retroperitoneal fibrosis.

REFERENCES

1. Cherry WB, Mueller PS: Rectus sheath hematoma: Review of 126 cases at a single institution. *Medicine (Baltimore)* 85:105–110, 2006.
2. Gurbuz AK, Giardiello FM, Petersen GM, et al: Desmoid tumors in familial adenomatous polyposis. *Gut* 35:377–381, 1994.
3. Kulaylat MN, Karakousis CP, Keaney CM, et al: Desmoid tumour: A pleomorphic lesion. *Eur J Surg Oncol* 25:487–497, 1999.
4. Stojadinovic A, Hoos A, Karpoff HM, et al: Soft tissue tumors of the abdominal wall: Analysis of disease patterns and treatment. *Arch Surg* 136:70–79, 2001.
5. Fiore M, Rimareix F, Mariani L, et al: Desmoid-type fibromatosis: A front-line conservative approach to select patients for surgical treatment. *Ann Surg Oncol* 16:2587–2593, 2009.
6. Lev D, Kotilingam D, Wei C, et al: Optimizing treatment of desmoid tumors. *J Clin Oncol* 25:1785–1791, 2007.
7. Gronchi A, Casali PG, Mariani L, et al: Quality of surgery and outcome in extra-abdominal aggressive fibromatosis: A series of patients surgically treated at a single institution. *J Clin Oncol* 21:1390–1397, 2003.
8. Bonvalot S, Ternes N, Fiore M, et al: Spontaneous regression of primary abdominal wall desmoid tumors: More common than previously thought. *Ann Surg Oncol* 20:4096–4102, 2013.
9. Bonvalot S, Eldweny H, Haddad V, et al: Extra-abdominal primary fibromatosis: Aggressive management could be avoided in a subgroup of patients. *Eur J Surg Oncol* 34:462–468, 2008.
10. Crago AM, Denton B, Salas S, et al: A prognostic nomogram for prediction of recurrence in desmoid fibromatosis. *Ann Surg* 258:347–353, 2013.
11. Salas S, Dufresne A, Bui B, et al: Prognostic factors influencing progression-free survival determined from a series of sporadic desmoid tumors: A wait-and-see policy according to tumor presentation. *J Clin Oncol* 29:3553–3558, 2011.
12. Nuyttens JJ, Rust PF, Thomas CR, Jr, et al: Surgery versus radiation therapy for patients with aggressive fibromatosis or desmoid tumors: A comparative review of 22 articles. *Cancer* 88:1517–1523, 2000.
13. Janinis J, Patriki M, Vini L, et al: The pharmacological treatment of aggressive fibromatosis: A systematic review. *Ann Oncol* 14:181–190, 2003.
14. Clark SK, Neale KF, Landgrebe JC, et al: Desmoid tumours complicating familial adenomatous polyposis. *Br J Surg* 86:1185–1189, 1999.
15. Hansmann A, Adolph C, Vogel T, et al: High-dose tamoxifen and sulindac as first-line treatment for desmoid tumors. *Cancer* 100:612–620, 2004.
16. Azzarelli A, Gronchi A, Bertulli R, et al: Low-dose chemotherapy with methotrexate and vinblastine for patients with advanced aggressive fibromatosis. *Cancer* 92:1259–1264, 2001.
17. Heinrich MC, McArthur GA, Demetri GD, et al: Clinical and molecular studies of the effect of imatinib on advanced aggressive fibromatosis (desmoid tumor). *J Clin Oncol* 24:1195–1203, 2006.
18. Fleshman J, Sargent DJ, Green E, et al: Laparoscopic colectomy for cancer is not inferior to open surgery based on 5-year data from the COST Study Group trial. *Ann Surg* 246:655–662, discussion 662–664, 2007.
19. Plaza JA, Perez-Montiel D, Mayerson J, et al: Metastases to soft tissue: A review of 118 cases over a 30-year period. *Cancer* 112:193–203, 2008.
20. Kashani A, Landaverde C, Medici V, et al: Fluid retention in cirrhosis: Pathophysiology and management. *QJM* 101:71–85, 2008.
21. Moller S, Henriksen JH, Bendtsen F: Ascites: Pathogenesis and therapeutic principles. *Scand J Gastroenterol* 44:902–911, 2009.
22. Runyon BA: Paracentesis of ascitic fluid. A safe procedure. *Arch Intern Med* 146:2259–2261, 1986.
23. Runyon BA, Montano AA, Akriviadis EA, et al: The serum-ascites albumin gradient is superior to the exudate-transudate concept in the differential diagnosis of ascites. *Ann Intern Med* 117:215–220, 1992.
24. Gines P, Cardenas A, Arroyo V, et al: Management of cirrhosis and ascites. *N Engl J Med* 350:1646–1654, 2004.
25. Kuiper JJ, de Man RA, van Buuren HR: Review article: Management of ascites and associated complications in patients with cirrhosis. *Aliment Pharmacol Ther* 26(Suppl 2):183–193, 2007.
26. Caruntu FA, Benea L: Spontaneous bacterial peritonitis: Pathogenesis, diagnosis, treatment. *J Gastrointestin Liver Dis* 15:51–56, 2006.
27. Berg RD: Bacterial translocation from the gastrointestinal tract. *Adv Exp Med Biol* 473:11–30, 1999.
28. Guarner C, Soriano G: Bacterial translocation and its consequences in patients with cirrhosis. *Eur J Gastroenterol Hepatol* 17:27–31, 2005.
29. Moore K: Spontaneous bacterial peritonitis (SBP). In Warrel DA, editor: *Oxford textbook of medicine* (vol 2), ed 4, New York, 2003, Oxford University Press, pp 739–741.
30. Levison ME, Bush LM: Peritonitis and intraperitoneal abscesses. In Mandell GL, Bennett JE, Dolin R, editors: *Principles and practice of infectious diseases* (vol 1), ed 6, Philadelphia, 2005, Elsevier Churchill Livingstone, pp 927–951.
31. Koulaouzidis A, Leontiadis GI, Abdullah M, et al: Leucocyte esterase reagent strips for the diagnosis of spontaneous bacterial peritonitis: A systematic review. *Eur J Gastroenterol Hepatol* 20:1055–1060, 2008.
32. Nguyen-Khac E, Cadranel JF, Thevenot T, et al: Review article: The utility of reagent strips in the diagnosis of infected ascites in cirrhotic patients. *Aliment Pharmacol Ther* 28:282–288, 2008.
33. Chavez-Tapia NC, Soares-Weiser K, Brezis M, et al: Antibiotics for spontaneous bacterial peritonitis in cirrhotic patients. *Cochrane Database Syst Rev* (1):CD002232, 2009.
34. Koulaouzidis A, Bhat S, Saeed AA: Spontaneous bacterial peritonitis. *World J Gastroenterol* 15:1042–1049, 2009.
35. Fernandez J, Navasa M, Garcia-Pagan JC, et al: Effect of intravenous albumin on systemic and hepatic hemodynamics and vasoactive neurohormonal systems in patients with cirrhosis and spontaneous bacterial peritonitis. *J Hepatol* 41:384–390, 2004.
36. Sanai FM, Bzeizi KI: Systematic review: Tuberculous peritonitis—presenting features, diagnostic strategies and treatment. *Aliment Pharmacol Ther* 22:685–700, 2005.
37. Kavanagh D, Prescott GJ, Mactier RA: Peritoneal dialysis–associated peritonitis in Scotland (1999-2002). *Nephrol Dial Transplant* 19:2584–2591, 2004.

38. Misdraji J, Yantiss RK, Graeme-Cook FM, et al: Appendiceal mucinous neoplasms: A clinicopathologic analysis of 107 cases. *Am J Surg Pathol* 27:1089–1103, 2003.
39. Ronnett BM, Yan H, Kurman RJ, et al: Patients with pseudomyxoma peritonei associated with disseminated peritoneal adenomucinosis have a significantly more favorable prognosis than patients with peritoneal mucinous carcinomatosis. *Cancer* 92:85–91, 2001.
40. Gonzalez-Moreno S, Sugarbaker PH: Right hemicolectomy does not confer a survival advantage in patients with mucinous carcinoma of the appendix and peritoneal seeding. *Br J Surg* 91:304–311, 2004.
41. Stewart JH, Shen P, Levine EA: Intraperitoneal hyperthermic chemotherapy for peritoneal surface malignancy: Current status and future directions. *Ann Surg Oncol* 12:765–777, 2005.
42. Chua TC, Moran BJ, Sugarbaker PH, et al: Early- and long-term outcome data of patients with pseudomyxoma peritonei from appendiceal origin treated by a strategy of cytoreductive surgery and hyperthermic intraperitoneal chemotherapy. *J Clin Oncol* 30:2449–2456, 2012.
43. Teta MJ, Mink PJ, Lau E, et al: US mesothelioma patterns 1973-2002: Indicators of change and insights into background rates. *Eur J Cancer Prev* 17:525–534, 2008.
44. Levy AD, Arnaiz J, Shaw JC, et al: From the archives of the AFIP: Primary peritoneal tumors: Imaging features with pathologic correlation. *Radiographics* 28:583–607, quiz 621–622, 2008.
45. Yan TD, Deraco M, Baratti D, et al: Cytoreductive surgery and hyperthermic intraperitoneal chemotherapy for malignant peritoneal mesothelioma: Multi-institutional experience. *J Clin Oncol* 27:6237–6242, 2009.
46. Levy AD, Rimola J, Mehrotra AK, et al: From the archives of the AFIP: Benign fibrous tumors and tumorlike lesions of the mesentery: Radiologic-pathologic correlation. *Radiographics* 26:245–264, 2006.
47. Horton KM, Lawler LP, Fishman EK: CT findings in sclerosing mesenteritis (panniculitis): Spectrum of disease. *Radiographics* 23:1561–1567, 2003.
48. Martin LC, Merkle EM, Thompson WM: Review of internal hernias: Radiographic and clinical findings. *AJR Am J Roentgenol* 186:703–717, 2006.
49. Cabot JC, Lee SA, Yoo J, et al: Long-term consequences of not closing the mesenteric defect after laparoscopic right colectomy. *Dis Colon Rectum* 53:289–292, 2010.
50. Nieuwenhuis MH, Mathus-Vliegen EM, Baeten CG, et al: Evaluation of management of desmoid tumours associated with familial adenomatous polyposis in Dutch patients. *Br J Cancer* 104:37–42, 2011.
51. Smith AJ, Lewis JJ, Merchant NB, et al: Surgical management of intra-abdominal desmoid tumours. *Br J Surg* 87:608–613, 2000.
52. Guillem JG, Wood WC, Moley JF, et al: ASCO/SSO review of current role of risk-reducing surgery in common hereditary cancer syndromes. *J Clin Oncol* 24:4642–4660, 2006.
53. Church J, Simmang C: Practice parameters for the treatment of patients with dominantly inherited colorectal cancer (familial adenomatous polyposis and hereditary nonpolyposis colorectal cancer). *Dis Colon Rectum* 46:1001–1012, 2003.
54. Paley M, Sidhu PS, Evans RA, et al: Retroperitoneal collections—a cause and radiological implications. *Clin Radiol* 52:290–294, 1997.
55. Loor G, Bassiouny H, Valentin C, et al: Local and systemic consequences of large retroperitoneal clot burdens. *World J Surg* 33:1618–1625, 2009.
56. Vaglio A, Salvarani C, Buzio C: Retroperitoneal fibrosis. *Lancet* 367:241–251, 2006.
57. Martorana D, Vaglio A, Greco P, et al: Chronic periaortitis and HLA-DRB1*03: Another clue to an autoimmune origin. *Arthritis Rheum* 55:126–130, 2006.
58. Siegel R, Ma J, Zou Z, et al: Cancer statistics, 2014. *CA Cancer J Clin* 64:9–29, 2014.
59. Soft tissue sarcoma. In Edge SB, Byrd DR, Compton CC, et al, editors: *AJCC cancer staging manual*, ed 7, New York, 2010, Springer, pp 291–298.
60. Trans-Atlantic RPS Working Group: Management of primary retroperitoneal sarcoma (RPS) in the adult: A consensus approach from the Trans-Atlantic RPS Working Group. *Ann Surg Oncol* 22:256–263, 2015.
61. Lewis JJ, Leung D, Woodruff JM, et al: Retroperitoneal soft-tissue sarcoma: Analysis of 500 patients treated and followed at a single institution. *Ann Surg* 228:355–365, 1998.
62. Russo P, Kim Y, Ravindran S, et al: Nephrectomy during operative management of retroperitoneal sarcoma. *Ann Surg Oncol* 4:421–424, 1997.
63. Mendenhall WM, Zlotecki RA, Hochwald SN, et al: Retroperitoneal soft tissue sarcoma. *Cancer* 104:669–675, 2005.
64. Shibata D, Lewis JJ, Leung DH, et al: Is there a role for incomplete resection in the management of retroperitoneal liposarcomas? *J Am Coll Surg* 193:373–379, 2001.

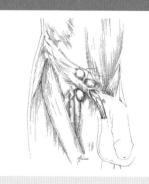

Hernias

Mark A. Malangoni, Michael J. Rosen

第四十四章　疝

OUTLINE

Inguinal Hernias
Femoral Hernias
Special Problems
Ventral Hernias
Unusual Hernias

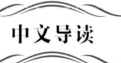

中文导读

　　本章共分为5节：①腹股沟疝；②股疝；③疝相关特殊问题；④腹壁疝；⑤少见类型疝。

　　第一节重点介绍了腹股沟疝的解剖、诊断和治疗方式。腹股沟疝是最常见的腹部疝。腹股沟区域的特殊解剖结构包括：腹外斜肌腱膜、腹内斜肌腱膜、腹横肌、腹横筋膜、Cooper韧带、腹股沟管、股管和腹膜前间隙等。腹股沟疝通常可分为斜疝和直疝，需注意分型和鉴别诊断，该部分详细介绍了各类型腹股沟疝的手术治疗方式，包括前入路组织修补、无张力补片修补、腹膜前间隙修补、腹腔镜修补（TAPP、TEP）等手术方式，并且对比了不同手术方式的治疗效果。

　　第二节简要地介绍了股疝的发生机制和治疗方式。同时指出：虽然股疝发生率远低于腹股沟疝，但是一旦发现应当及时接受手术治疗，以免发生严重的并发症——肠管嵌顿坏死。

　　第三节首先介绍了特殊类型的腹股沟疝，包括滑动性疝、复发性疝、绞窄性疝和双侧疝等。随后列举

了疝相关并发症，如手术部位感染、神经损伤和慢性疼痛综合征、缺血性睾丸炎和睾丸萎缩、输精管和内脏损伤、疝复发以及生活质量下降等。

　　第四节详细介绍了腹壁疝的定义、发病率、解剖、诊断和治疗方式。腹壁疝通常是由于前腹壁存在先天性或获得性缺损而发生的，可以分为：脐疝、上腹壁白线疝、切口疝等。腹壁疝，特别是切口疝，其修补手术中往往需要使用修补材料进行修补；修补材料可以分为合成补片、生物补片。腹壁疝修补手术过程中，补片放置的位置和方式非常重要，该部分详细介绍了相关理念和技巧。同时，组织分离技术也是腹壁疝修补手术的重要技巧。

　　第五节简要介绍少见类型的腹部疝，包括半月线疝、闭孔疝、腰疝、腹壁间疝、坐骨大孔疝、会阴疝、造口旁疝以及巨大腹壁疝等。

〔李兴睿〕

More than 600,000 hernias are repaired annually in the United States, making hernia repair one of the most common operations performed by general surgeons. Despite the frequency of this procedure, no surgeon has ideal results, and complications such as postoperative pain, nerve injury, surgical site infection, and recurrence remain.

Hernia is derived from the Latin word for rupture. A hernia is defined as an abnormal protrusion of an organ or tissue through a defect in its surrounding walls. Although a hernia can occur at various sites of the body, these defects most commonly involve the abdominal wall, particularly the inguinal region. Abdominal wall hernias occur only at sites at which the aponeurosis and fascia are not covered by striated muscle (Box 44-1). These sites most commonly include the inguinal, femoral, and umbilical areas; linea alba; lower portion of the semilunar line; and sites of prior incisions (Fig. 44-1). The so-called neck or orifice of a hernia is located at the innermost musculoaponeurotic layer, whereas the hernia sac is lined by peritoneum and protrudes from the neck. There is no consistent relationship between the area of a hernia defect and the size of a hernia sac.

A hernia is reducible when its contents can be replaced within the surrounding musculature, and it is irreducible or incarcerated when it cannot be reduced. A strangulated hernia has compromised blood supply to its contents, which is a serious and potentially fatal complication. Strangulation occurs more often in large hernias that have small orifices. In this situation, the small neck of the hernia obstructs arterial blood flow, venous drainage, or both to the contents of the hernia sac. Adhesions between the contents of the hernia and peritoneal lining of the sac can provide a tethering point that entraps the hernia contents and predisposes to intestinal obstruction and strangulation. A more unusual type of strangulation is a Richter hernia. In Richter hernia, a small portion of the antimesenteric wall of the intestine is trapped within the hernia, and strangulation can occur without the presence of intestinal obstruction.

BOX 44-1	Primary Abdominal Wall Hernias
Groin	**Pelvic**
Inguinal	Obturator
Indirect	Sciatic
Direct	Perineal
Combined	
Femoral	**Posterior**
	Lumbar
Anterior	Superior triangle
Umbilical	Inferior triangle
Epigastric	
Spigelian	

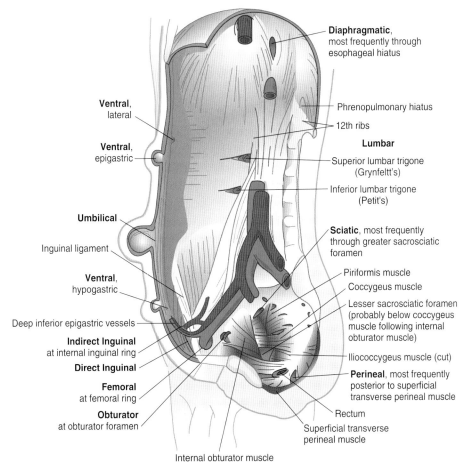

FIGURE 44-1 Types of abdominal wall hernias. (From *Dorland's illustrated medical dictionary*, ed 31, Philadelphia, 2007, WB Saunders, Plate 21.)

An external hernia protrudes through all layers of the abdominal wall, whereas an internal hernia is a protrusion of intestine through a defect in the peritoneal cavity. An interparietal hernia occurs when the hernia sac is contained within a musculoaponeurotic layer of the abdominal wall. In broad terms, most abdominal wall hernias can be separated into inguinal and ventral hernias. This chapter focuses on the specific aspects of each of these conditions individually.

INGUINAL HERNIAS

Inguinal hernias are classified as direct or indirect. The sac of an indirect inguinal hernia passes from the internal inguinal ring obliquely toward the external inguinal ring and ultimately into the scrotum. In contrast, the sac of a direct inguinal hernia protrudes outward and forward and is medial to the internal inguinal ring and inferior epigastric vessels. As indirect hernias enlarge, it sometimes can be difficult to distinguish between indirect and direct inguinal hernias. This distinction is of little importance because the operative repair of these types of hernias is similar. A pantaloon-type hernia occurs when there is both an indirect and direct hernia component.

Incidence

Hernias are a common problem; however, their true incidence is unknown. It is estimated that 5% of the population will develop an abdominal wall hernia, but the prevalence may be even higher. About 75% of all hernias occur in the inguinal region. Two thirds of these are indirect and the remainder are direct inguinal hernias. Femoral hernias represent only 3% of all groin hernias.

Men are 25 times more likely to have a groin hernia than women. An indirect inguinal hernia is the most common hernia, regardless of gender. In men, indirect hernias predominate over direct hernias at a ratio of 2 : 1. Indirect hernias are by far the most common type of hernia in women. The female-to-male ratio for femoral and umbilical hernias, however, is about 10 : 1 and 2 : 1, respectively. Although femoral hernias occur more frequently in women than in men, inguinal hernias remain the most common hernia in women. Femoral hernias are rare in men. Ten percent of women and 50% of men who have a femoral hernia have or will develop an inguinal hernia.

Indirect inguinal and femoral hernias occur more commonly on the right side. This is attributed to a delay in atrophy of the processus vaginalis after the normal slower descent of the right testis to the scrotum during fetal development. The predominance of right-sided femoral hernias is thought to be caused by the tamponading effect of the sigmoid colon on the left femoral canal.

The prevalence of hernias increases with age, particularly for inguinal, umbilical, and femoral hernias. The likelihood of strangulation and need for hospitalization also increase with aging. Strangulation, the most common serious complication of a hernia, occurs in only 1% to 3% of groin hernias and is more common at the extremes of life. Most strangulated hernias are indirect inguinal hernias; however, femoral hernias have the highest rate of strangulation (15% to 20%) of all hernias, and it is therefore recommended that all femoral hernias be repaired at the time of discovery.

Anatomy of the Groin

The surgeon must have a comprehensive understanding of the anatomy of the groin to select and to use various options for hernia repair properly. In addition, the relationships of muscles, aponeuroses, fascia, nerves, blood vessels, and spermatic cord structures in the inguinal region must be completely understood to obtain the lowest incidence of recurrence and to avoid complications. These anatomic considerations must be understood from the anterior and posterior approaches because both are useful in different situations (Figs. 44-2 and 44-3).

From anterior to posterior, the groin anatomy includes the skin and subcutaneous tissues, below which are the superficial circumflex iliac, superficial epigastric, and external pudendal arteries and accompanying veins. These vessels arise from and drain to the proximal femoral artery and vein, respectively, and are directed superiorly. If encountered during operation, these vessels can be retracted or even divided when necessary.

External Oblique Muscle and Aponeurosis

The external oblique muscle is the most superficial of the lateral abdominal wall muscles; its fibers are directed inferiorly and medially and lie deep to the subcutaneous tissues. The aponeurosis of the external oblique muscle is formed by a superficial and deep layer. This aponeurosis, along with the bilaminar aponeuroses of the internal oblique and transversus abdominis, forms the anterior rectus sheath and, finally, the linea alba by linear decussation. The external oblique aponeurosis serves as the superficial boundary of the inguinal canal. The inguinal ligament (Poupart ligament) is the inferior edge of the external oblique aponeurosis and extends from the anterior superior iliac spine to the pubic tubercle, turning posteriorly to form a shelving edge. The lacunar ligament is the fan-shaped medial expansion of the inguinal ligament, which inserts into the pubis and forms the medial border of the femoral space. The external (superficial) inguinal ring is an ovoid opening of the external oblique aponeurosis that is positioned superiorly and slightly laterally to the pubic tubercle. The spermatic cord exits the inguinal canal through the external inguinal ring.

Internal Oblique Muscle and Aponeurosis

The internal oblique muscle forms the middle layer of the lateral abdominal musculoaponeurotic complex. The fibers of the internal oblique are directed superiorly and laterally in the upper abdomen; however, they run in a slightly inferior direction in the inguinal region. The internal oblique muscle serves as the cephalad (or superior) border of the inguinal canal. The medial aspect of the internal oblique aponeurosis fuses with fibers from the transversus abdominis aponeurosis to form a conjoined tendon. This structure actually is present in only 5% to 10% of patients and is most evident at the insertion of these muscles on the pubic tubercle. The cremaster muscle fibers arise from the internal oblique, encompass the spermatic cord, and attach to the tunica vaginalis of the testis. These muscle fibers are essential to maintain the cremasteric reflex but have little relevance to the results of inguinal hernia repairs.

Transversus Abdominis Muscle and Aponeurosis and Transversalis Fascia

The transversus abdominis muscle layer is oriented horizontally throughout most of its area; in the inguinal region, these fibers course in a slightly oblique downward direction. The strength and continuity of this muscle and aponeurosis are important for the prevention and treatment of inguinal hernia.

The aponeurosis of the transversus abdominis covers anterior and posterior surfaces. The lower margin of the transversus abdominis arches along with the internal oblique muscle over the internal inguinal ring to form the transversus abdominis aponeu-

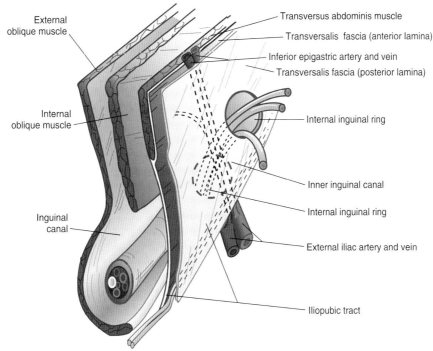

FIGURE 44-2 Nyhus's classic parasagittal diagram of the right midinguinal region illustrating the muscular aponeurotic layers separated into anterior and posterior walls. The posterior laminae of the transversalis fascia have been added, with the inferior epigastric vessels coursing through the abdominal wall medially to the inner inguinal canal. (From Read RC: The transversalis and preperitoneal fasciae: A re-evaluation. In Nyhus LM, Condon RE, editors: *Hernia*, ed 4, Philadelphia, 1995, JB Lippincott, pp 57-63.)

rotic arch. The transversalis fascia is the connective tissue layer that underlies the abdominal wall musculature. The transversalis fascia, sometimes referred to as the endoabdominal fascia, is a component of the inguinal floor. It tends to be denser in this area but still remains relatively thin.

The iliopubic tract is an aponeurotic band that is formed by the transversalis fascia and transversus abdominis aponeurosis and fascia. The iliopubic tract is located posterior to the inguinal ligament and crosses over the femoral vessels and inserts on the anterior superior iliac spine and inner lip of the wing of the ilium.

The inferior crus of the deep inguinal ring is composed of the iliopubic tract; the superior crus of the deep ring is formed by the transversus abdominis aponeurotic arch. The lateral border of the internal ring is connected to the transversus abdominis muscle, which forms a shutter mechanism to limit the development of an indirect hernia.

The iliopubic tract is an extremely important structure in the repair of hernias from the anterior and posterior approaches. It composes the inferior margin of most anterior repairs. The portion of the iliopubic tract lateral to the internal inguinal ring serves as the inferior border below which staples or tacks are not placed during a laparoscopic repair because the femoral, lateral femoral cutaneous, and genitofemoral nerves are located inferior to the iliopubic tract. Although it cannot always be visualized during posterior repairs, if the tacking device cannot be palpated on the anterior abdominal wall, one must assume it is below the iliopubic tract.

Pectineal (Cooper) Ligament

The pectineal (Cooper) ligament is formed by the periosteum and aponeurotic tissues along the superior ramus of the pubis. This structure is posterior to the iliopubic tract and forms the posterior border of the femoral canal. In approximately 75% of patients, there will be a vessel that crosses the lateral border of Cooper ligament that is a branch of the obturator artery. If this vessel is injured, troublesome bleeding can result. Cooper ligament is an important landmark for open and laparoscopic repairs and is a useful anchoring structure, particularly in laparoscopic repairs.

Inguinal Canal

The inguinal canal is about 4 cm in length and is located just cephalad to the inguinal ligament. The canal extends between the internal (deep) inguinal and external (superficial) inguinal rings. The inguinal canal contains the spermatic cord in men and the round ligament of the uterus in women.

The spermatic cord is composed of the cremaster muscle fibers, testicular artery and accompanying veins, genital branch of the genitofemoral nerve, vas deferens, cremasteric vessels, lymphatics, and processus vaginalis. These structures enter the cord at the internal inguinal ring, and vessels and vas deferens exit the external inguinal ring. The cremaster muscle arises from the lowermost fibers of the internal oblique muscle and encompasses the spermatic cord in the inguinal canal. The cremasteric vessels are branches of the inferior epigastric vessels and pass through the posterior wall of the inguinal canal through their own foramen.

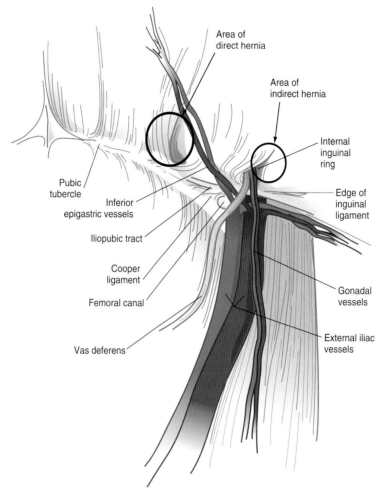

Area of
direct hernia

Area of
indirect hernia

Internal
inguinal
ring

Pubic
tubercle

Inferior
epigastric vessels

Edge of
inguinal
ligament

Iliopubic tract

Cooper
ligament

Gonadal
vessels

Femoral canal

External iliac
vessels

Vas deferens

FIGURE 44-3 Anatomy of the important preperitoneal structures in the right inguinal space. (From Talamini MA, Are C: Laparoscopic hernia repair. In Zuidema GD, Yeo CJ, editors: *Shackelford's surgery of the alimentary tract*, ed 5, vol 5, Philadelphia, 2002, WB Saunders, p 140.)

These vessels supply the cremaster muscle and can be divided to expose the floor of the inguinal canal during hernia repair without damaging the testis.

The inguinal canal is bounded superficially by the external oblique aponeurosis. The internal oblique and transversus abdominis musculoaponeuroses form the cephalad wall of the inguinal canal. The inferior wall of the inguinal canal is formed by the inguinal ligament and lacunar ligament. The posterior wall, or floor of the inguinal canal, is formed by the aponeurosis of the transversus abdominis muscle and transversalis fascia.

Hesselbach triangle refers to the margins of the floor of the inguinal canal. The inferior epigastric vessels serve as its superolateral border, the rectus sheath as the medial border, and the inguinal ligament and pectineal ligament as the inferior border. Direct hernias occur within Hesselbach triangle, whereas indirect inguinal hernias arise lateral to the triangle. It is not uncommon, however, for medium and large indirect inguinal hernias to involve the floor of the inguinal canal as they enlarge.

The iliohypogastric and ilioinguinal nerves and genital branch of the genitofemoral nerve are the important sensory nerves in the groin area (Fig. 44-4). The iliohypogastric and ilioinguinal nerves provide sensation to the skin of the groin, base of the penis,

and ipsilateral upper medial thigh. The iliohypogastric and ilioinguinal nerves lie beneath the internal oblique muscle to a point just medial and superior to the anterior superior iliac spine, where they penetrate the internal oblique muscle and course beneath the external oblique aponeurosis. The main trunk of the iliohypogastric nerve runs on the anterior surface of the internal oblique muscle and aponeurosis medial and superior to the internal ring. The iliohypogastric nerve may provide an inguinal branch that joins the ilioinguinal nerve. The ilioinguinal nerve runs anterior to the spermatic cord in the inguinal canal and branches at the superficial inguinal ring. The genital branch of the genitofemoral nerve innervates the cremaster muscle and skin on the lateral side of the scrotum and labia. This nerve lies on the iliopubic tract and accompanies the cremaster vessels to form a neurovascular bundle.

Preperitoneal Space

The preperitoneal space contains adipose tissue, lymphatics, blood vessels, and nerves. The nerves of the preperitoneal space of specific concern to the surgeon include the lateral femoral cutaneous nerve and genitofemoral nerve. The lateral femoral cutaneous nerve originates as a root of L2 and L3 and is occasionally a direct branch of the femoral nerve. This nerve courses along the anterior surface of the iliac muscle beneath the iliac fascia and passes under or through the lateral attachment of the inguinal ligament at the anterior superior iliac spine. This nerve runs beneath or occasionally through the iliopubic tract, lateral to the internal inguinal ring.

The genitofemoral nerve usually arises from the L2 or L1-L2 nerve roots. It divides into genital and femoral branches on the anterior surface of the psoas muscle. The genital branch enters the inguinal canal through the deep ring, whereas the femoral branch enters the femoral sheath lateral to the artery.

The inferior epigastric artery and vein are branches of the external iliac vessels and are important landmarks for laparoscopic hernia repair. These vessels course medial to the internal inguinal ring and eventually lie beneath the rectus abdominis muscle, immediately superficial to the transversalis fascia. The inferior epigastric vessels serve to define the types of inguinal hernia. Indirect inguinal hernias occur lateral to the inferior epigastric vessels, whereas direct hernias occur medial to these vessels.

The deep circumflex iliac artery and vein are located below the lateral portion of the iliopubic tract in the preperitoneal space. These vessels are branches of the inferior epigastric or external iliac

artery and vein. It is important to dissect only above the iliopubic tract during a laparoscopic hernia repair to avoid injury to these vessels.

The vas deferens courses through the preperitoneal space from caudad to cephalad and medial to lateral to join the spermatic cord at the deep inguinal ring.

Femoral Canal

The boundaries of the femoral canal are the iliopubic tract anteriorly, Cooper ligament posteriorly, and femoral vein laterally. The pubic tubercle forms the apex of the femoral canal triangle. This canal usually contains connective tissue and lymphatic tissue. A femoral hernia occurs through this space and is medial to the femoral vessels.

Diagnosis

A bulge in the inguinal region is the main diagnostic finding in most groin hernias. Most patients will have associated pain or vague discomfort in the region, but one third of patients will have no symptoms. Groin hernias are usually not extremely painful unless incarceration or strangulation has occurred. In the absence of physical findings, alternative causes for pain need to be consid-

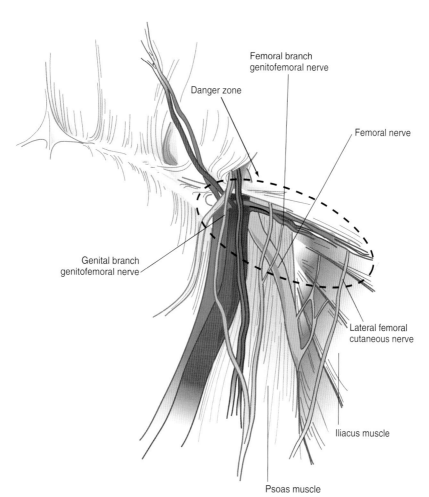

FIGURE 44-4 Important nerves and their relationship to inguinal structures (the right side is illustrated). (From Talamini MA, Are C: Laparoscopic hernia repair. In Zuidema GD, Yeo CJ, editors: *Shackelford's surgery of the alimentary tract*, ed 5, vol 5, Philadelphia, 2002, WB Saunders, p 140.)

ered. On occasion, patients may experience paresthesias related to compression or irritation of the inguinal nerves by the hernia. Masses other than hernias can occur in the groin region. Physical examination alone often differentiates between a groin hernia and these masses (Box 44-2).

The inguinal region is examined with the patient in the supine and standing positions. The examiner visually inspects and palpates the inguinal region, looking for asymmetry, bulges, or a mass. Having the patient cough or perform a Valsalva maneuver can facilitate identification of a hernia. The examiner places a fingertip over the inguinal canal and repeats the examination. Finally, a fingertip is placed into the external inguinal ring by invaginating the scrotum to detect a small hernia. A bulge moving lateral to medial in the inguinal canal suggests an indirect hernia. If a bulge progresses from deep to superficial through the inguinal floor, a direct hernia is suspected. This distinction is not critical because repair is approached the same way, regardless of the type of hernia. A bulge identified below the inguinal ligament is consistent with a femoral hernia.

A bulge of the groin described by the patient that is not demonstrated on examination presents a dilemma. Having the patient stand or ambulate for a time may allow an undiagnosed hernia to become visible or palpable. If a hernia is strongly suspected but undetectable, repeated examination at another time may be helpful.

Ultrasonography also can aid in the diagnosis. There is a high degree of sensitivity and specificity for ultrasound in the detection of occult direct, indirect, and femoral hernias.[1] Other imaging modalities are less useful. Computed tomography (CT) of the abdomen and pelvis may be useful for the diagnosis of obscure and unusual hernias as well as atypical groin masses.[2] On occasion, laparoscopy can be diagnostic and therapeutic for particularly challenging cases.

Classification

There are numerous classification systems for groin hernias. One simple and widely used system is the Nyhus classification (Box 44-3). Although their purpose is to promote a common language and understanding for communication of physicians and to allow appropriate comparisons of therapeutic options, these classifications are incomplete and contentious. Most surgeons continue to describe hernias by their type, location, and volume of the hernia sac.

Treatment
Nonoperative Management

Most surgeons recommend operation on discovery of a symptomatic inguinal hernia because the natural history of a groin hernia is that of progressive enlargement and weakening, with a small potential for incarceration and strangulation. However, in patients with minimal symptoms, the clinician is often faced with balancing the risk for hernia-related complications, such as incarceration and bowel strangulation, with the potential for complications in the short and long term. Fitzgibbons and colleagues[3] reported a prospective randomized trial of a watchful waiting strategy for men with asymptomatic or minimally symptomatic inguinal hernias. These investigators randomized more than 700 men to a watchful waiting or open tension-free hernia repair. At 2 years of follow-up, there were no deaths attributed to the study, and the risk for hernia incarceration in the watchful waiting group was extremely low, 0.3% of study participants or 1.8 events/1000 patient-years. Almost 25% of patients assigned to watchful waiting

---

BOX 44-2 **Differential Diagnosis of Groin and Scrotal Masses**
Inguinal hernia
Hydrocele
Varicocele
Ectopic testis
Epididymitis
Testicular torsion
Lipoma
Hematoma
Sebaceous cyst
Hidradenitis of inguinal apocrine glands
Inguinal lymphadenopathy
Lymphoma
Metastatic neoplasm
Femoral hernia
Femoral lymphadenopathy
Femoral artery aneurysm or pseudoaneurysm

---

crossed over to the surgical group, usually for pain related to the hernia that limited activity. In a later report, the crossover rate had increased to 68% at 10 years, with nearly 80% of men older than 65 years having an operation.[4] Patients who later had surgery did not have increased surgical site infections or higher recurrence rates than those who were initially assigned to early repair. A prospective randomized trial at a single institution in Great Britain had similar long-term results.[5] These studies provide conclusive evidence that a strategy of watchful waiting is safe for older patients with asymptomatic or minimally symptomatic inguinal hernias and that even though most patients eventually undergo repair, when they do, the operative risks and complication rates are no different from those of patients undergoing immediate repair. Watchful waiting can be a cost-effective management strategy for selected patients with no or minimal symptoms or who have suboptimal risk for operation. These results should not be applied to women, as women have not been included in these studies, or to patients with femoral hernias, which have a greater risk of strangulation than inguinal hernias.

Patients electing nonoperative management can occasionally have symptomatic improvement with the use of a truss. This approach is more commonly used in Europe. Spring trusses are more versatile than elastic ones, although most information on their use has been anecdotal. Correct measurement and fitting are important. Symptom control has been reported in about 30% of patients. Complications associated with the use of a truss include testicular atrophy, ilioinguinal or femoral neuritis, and hernia incarceration.

It is generally agreed that nonoperative management is not used for femoral hernias because of the high incidence of associated complications, particularly strangulation.

Operative Repair

Anterior repairs. Anterior repairs are the most common operative approach for inguinal hernias. Tension-free repairs are now standard, and there are a variety of different types. Older tissue types of repair are rarely indicated, except for patients with simultaneous contamination or concomitant bowel resection, when placement of a mesh prosthesis may be contraindicated.

BOX 44-3   **Nyhus Classification of Groin Hernia**

Type I
Indirect inguinal hernia: internal inguinal ring normal (e.g., pediatric hernia)

Type II
Indirect inguinal hernia: internal inguinal ring dilated but posterior inguinal wall intact; inferior deep epigastric vessels not displaced

Type III
Posterior wall defect
   A. Direct inguinal hernia
   B. Indirect inguinal hernia: internal inguinal ring dilated, medially encroaching on or destroying the transversalis fascia of Hesselbach triangle (e.g., scrotal, sliding, or pantaloon hernia)
   C. Femoral hernia

Type IV
Recurrent hernia
   A. Direct
   B. Indirect
   C. Femoral
   D. Combined

There are some technical aspects of the operation common to all anterior repairs. Open hernia repair is begun by making a transversely oriented linear or slightly curvilinear incision above the inguinal ligament and a fingerbreadth below the internal inguinal ring. The internal inguinal ring is located topographically at the midpoint between the anterior superior iliac spine and ipsilateral pubic tubercle. Dissection is continued through the subcutaneous tissues and Scarpa fascia. The external oblique fascia and external inguinal ring are identified. The external oblique fascia is incised through the superficial inguinal ring to expose the inguinal canal. The genital branch of the genitofemoral nerve and the ilioinguinal and iliohypogastric nerves are identified and avoided or mobilized to prevent transection and entrapment. The spermatic cord is mobilized at the pubic tubercle by a combination of blunt and sharp dissection. Improper mobilization of the spermatic cord too lateral to the pubic tubercle can cause confusion in the identification of tissue planes and essential structures and may result in injury to the spermatic cord structures or disruption of the floor of the inguinal canal.

The cremaster muscle of the mobilized spermatic cord is separated parallel to its fibers from the underlying cord structures. The cremaster artery and vein, which join the cremaster muscle near the inguinal ring, can usually be avoided but may need to be cauterized or ligated and divided. When an indirect hernia is present, the hernia sac is located deep to the cremaster muscle and anterior and superior to the spermatic cord structures. Incising the cremaster muscle in a longitudinal direction and dividing it circumferentially near the internal inguinal ring help expose the indirect hernia sac. The hernia sac is carefully separated from adjacent cord structures and dissected to the level of the internal inguinal ring. The sac is opened and examined for visceral contents if it is large; however, this step is unnecessary in small hernias. The sac can be mobilized and placed within the preperitoneal space, or the neck of the sac can be ligated at the level of the internal ring and any excess sac excised. If a large hernia sac is present, it can be divided with use of electrocautery to facilitate ligation. It is not necessary to excise the distal portion of the sac. If the sac is broad based, it may be easier to displace it into the peritoneal cavity rather than to ligate it. Direct hernia sacs protrude through the floor of the inguinal canal and can be reduced below the transversalis fascia before repair. A "lipoma" of the cord actually represents retroperitoneal fat that has herniated through the deep inguinal ring; this should be suture ligated and removed.

A sliding hernia presents a special challenge in handling the hernia sac. With a sliding hernia, a portion of the sac is composed of visceral peritoneum covering part of a retroperitoneal organ, usually the colon or bladder. In this situation, the grossly redundant portion of the sac (if present) is excised and the peritoneum reclosed. The organ and sac then can be reduced below the transversalis fascia, similar to the procedure for a direct hernia.

Tissue repairs. Although tissue repairs have largely been abandoned because of unacceptably high recurrence rates, they remain useful in certain situations. In strangulated hernias, for which bowel resection is necessary, mesh prostheses are contraindicated and a tissue repair is necessary. Available options for tissue repair include iliopubic tract, Shouldice, Bassini, and McVay repairs.

The iliopubic tract repair approximates the transversus abdominis aponeurotic arch to the iliopubic tract with the use of interrupted sutures (Fig. 44-5). The repair begins at the pubic tubercle and extends laterally past the internal inguinal ring. This repair was initially described using a relaxing incision (see later); however, many surgeons who use this repair do not perform a relaxing incision.

The Shouldice repair emphasizes a multilayer imbricated repair of the posterior wall of the inguinal canal with a continuous running suture technique. After completion of the dissection, the posterior wall of the inguinal canal is reconstructed by superimposing running suture lines progressing from deep to more superficial layers. The initial suture line secures the transversus abdominis aponeurotic arch to the iliopubic tract. Next, the internal oblique and transversus abdominis muscles and aponeuroses are sutured to the inguinal ligament. The Shouldice repair is associated with a very low recurrence rate and a high degree of patient satisfaction in highly selected patients.

The Bassini repair is performed by suturing the transversus abdominis and internal oblique musculoaponeurotic arches or conjoined tendon (when present) to the inguinal ligament. This once popular technique is the basic approach to nonanatomic hernia repairs and was the most popular type of repair done before the advent of tension-free repairs.

Cooper ligament repair, also known as the McVay repair, has traditionally been popular for the correction of direct inguinal hernias, large indirect hernias, recurrent hernias, and femoral hernias. Interrupted nonabsorbable sutures are used to approximate the edge of the transversus abdominis aponeurosis to Cooper ligament. When the medial aspect of the femoral canal is reached, a transition suture is placed to incorporate Cooper ligament and the iliopubic tract. Lateral to this transition stitch, the transversus abdominis aponeurosis is secured to the iliopubic tract. An important principle of this repair is the need for a relaxing incision. This incision is made by reflecting the external oblique aponeurosis cephalad and medial to expose the anterior rectus sheath. An incision is then made in a curvilinear direction, beginning 1 cm above the pubic tubercle throughout the extent of the anterior sheath to near its lateral border. This relieves tension on the suture line and results in decreased postoperative pain and hernia recurrence. The fascial defect is covered by the body of the rectus muscle, which prevents herniation at the relaxing incision site. The McVay repair is particularly suited for strangulated femoral hernias because it provides obliteration of the femoral space without the use of mesh.

Tension-free anterior inguinal hernia repair. The tension-free repair has become the dominant method of inguinal hernia repair (Fig. 44-6). Recognizing that tension in a repair is the principal cause of recurrence, current practices in hernia management use a synthetic mesh prosthesis to bridge the defect, a concept popularized by Lichtenstein. There are several options for placement of mesh during anterior inguinal herniorrhaphy, including the Lichtenstein approach, plug and patch technique, and sandwich technique, with both an anterior and preperitoneal piece of mesh.

In the Lichtenstein repair,[6] a piece of prosthetic nonabsorbable mesh is fashioned to fit the canal. A slit is cut into the distal lateral edge of the mesh to accommodate the spermatic cord. There are various preformed, commercially available prostheses available for use. Monofilament nonabsorbable suture is used to secure the mesh, beginning at the pubic tubercle and running a length of suture in both directions toward the superior aspect above the internal inguinal ring to the level of the tails of the mesh. The mesh is sutured to the aponeurotic tissue overlying the pubic tubercle medially, continuing superiorly along the transversus abdominis or conjoined tendon. The inferolateral edge of the mesh is sutured to the iliopubic tract or shelving edge of the inguinal ligament to a point lateral to the internal inguinal ring. At this point, the tails created by the slit are sutured together around the spermatic cord, snugly forming a new internal inguinal ring. It is important to protect the ilioinguinal nerve and

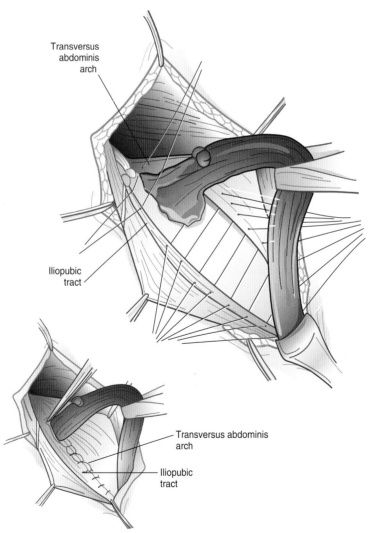

Transversus abdominis arch

Iliopubic tract

Transversus abdominis arch

Iliopubic tract

FIGURE 44-5 Iliopubic Tract Repair. *Top,* Sutures lateral to the cord complete reconstruction of the deep inguinal ring. These sutures encompass the transversus abdominis arch above and the cremaster origin and iliopubic tract below. *Bottom,* The complete repair is ready for wound closure. The reconstruction of the deep ring should be snug but also loose enough to admit the tip of a hemostat. (From Condon RE: Anterior iliopubic tract repair. In Nyhus LM, Condon RE, editors: *Hernia,* ed 2, Philadelphia, 1974, JB Lippincott, p 204.)

genital branch of the genitofemoral nerve from entrapment by placing them with the cord structures as they are passed through this newly fashioned internal inguinal ring or avoiding their enclosure in the repair.

Adapting the principles of tension-free repair, Gilbert[7] has reported using a cone-shaped plug of polypropylene mesh that when inserted into the internal inguinal ring would deploy like an upside-down umbrella and occlude the hernia. This plug is sewn to the surrounding tissues and held in place by an additional overlying mesh patch. This patch may not need to be secured by sutures; however, to do so requires dissection to create a sufficient space between the external and internal oblique muscles for the patch to lie flat over the inguinal canal. This so-called plug and

patch repair, an extension of Lichtenstein's original mesh repair, has now become the most commonly performed primary anterior inguinal hernia repair. Although this repair can be done without suture fixation by some experienced surgeons, most secure plug and patch with several monofilament nonabsorbable sutures, especially for very weak inguinal floors or large defects.

The sandwich technique involves a bilayered device, with three polypropylene components. An underlay patch provides a posterior repair similar to that of the laparoscopic approach, a connector functions similar to a plug, and an onlay patch covers the posterior inguinal floor. The use of interrupted fixating sutures is not mandatory, but most surgeons place three or four fixation sutures in this repair.

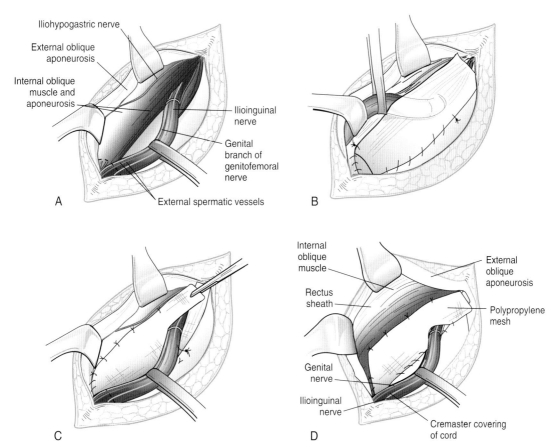

FIGURE 44-6 Lichtenstein Tension-Free Hernia Repair. **A,** This procedure is performed by careful dissection of the inguinal canal. High ligation of an indirect hernia sac is performed, and the spermatic cord structures are retracted inferiorly. The external oblique aponeurosis is separated from the underlying internal oblique muscle high enough to accommodate a 6- to 8-cm-wide mesh patch. Overlap of the internal oblique muscle edge by 2 to 3 cm is necessary. A sheet of polypropylene mesh is fashioned to fit the inguinal canal. A slit is made in the lateral aspect of the mesh, and the spermatic cord is placed between the two tails of the mesh. **B,** The spermatic cord is retracted in the cephalad direction. The medial aspect of the mesh overlaps the pubic bone by approximately 2 cm. The mesh is secured to the aponeurotic tissue overlying the pubic tubercle by a running suture of nonabsorbable monofilament material. The suture is continued laterally by suturing the inferior edge of the mesh to the shelving edge of the inguinal ligament to a point just lateral to the internal inguinal ring. **C,** A second monofilament suture is placed at the level of the pubic tubercle and continued laterally by suturing the mesh to the internal oblique aponeurosis or muscle approximately 2 cm from the aponeurotic edge. **D,** The lower edges of the two tails are sutured to the shelving edge of the inguinal ligament to create a new internal ring made of mesh. The spermatic cord structures are placed within the inguinal canal overlying the mesh. The external oblique aponeurosis is closed over the spermatic cord. (From Arregui ME, Nagan RD, editors: *Inguinal hernia: Advances or controversies?* Oxford, England, 1994, Radcliffe Medical.)

Another option for a tension-free mesh repair involves a pre-peritoneal approach using a self-expanding polypropylene patch.[8] A pocket is created in the preperitoneal space by blunt dissection, and then a preformed mesh patch is inserted into the hernia defect, which expands to cover the direct, indirect, and femoral spaces. The patch lies parallel to the inguinal ligament. It can remain without suture fixation, or a tacking suture can be placed.

The Stoppa-Rives repair uses a subumbilical midline incision to place a large mesh prosthesis into the preperitoneal space.[9] Blunt dissection is used to create an extraperitoneal space that extends into the prevesical space, beyond the obturator foramen, and posterolateral to the pelvic brim. This technique has the advantage of distributing the natural intra-abdominal pressure across a broad area to retain the mesh in a proper location. The Stoppa-Rives technique is particularly useful for large, recurrent, or bilateral hernias.

Preperitoneal repair. The open preperitoneal approach is useful for the repair of recurrent inguinal hernias, sliding hernias, femoral hernias, and some strangulated hernias.[10] A transverse skin incision is made 2 cm above the internal inguinal ring and is directed to the medial border of the rectus sheath. The muscles of the anterior abdominal wall are incised transversely, and the preperitoneal space is identified. If further exposure is needed, the anterior rectus sheath can be incised and the rectus muscle retracted medially. The preperitoneal tissues are retracted cephalad to visualize the posterior inguinal wall and the site of herniation. The inferior epigastric artery and veins are generally beneath the midportion of the posterior rectus sheath and usually do not need to be divided. This approach avoids mobilization of the spermatic cord and injury to the sensory nerves of the inguinal canal, which is particularly important for hernias previously repaired through an anterior approach. If the peritoneum is incised, it is sutured closed to avoid the evisceration of intraperitoneal contents into the operative field. The transversalis fascia and transversus abdominis aponeurosis are identified and sutured to the iliopubic tract with permanent sutures. Femoral hernias repaired by this approach require closure of the femoral canal by securing the repair to Cooper ligament. A mesh prosthesis is frequently used to obliterate the defect in the femoral canal, particularly with large hernias.

Laparoscopic repair. Laparoscopic inguinal hernia repair is another method of tension-free mesh repair based on a preperitoneal approach. The laparoscopic approach provides the mechanical advantage of placing a large piece of mesh behind the defect, covering the myopectineal orifice, and using the natural forces of the abdominal wall to disperse intra-abdominal pressure over a larger area to support the mesh in place. Proponents have touted quicker recovery, less pain, better visualization of anatomy, and usefulness for fixing all inguinal hernia defects. Critics have emphasized longer operative times, technical challenges, increased risk of recurrence, and increased cost. Laparoscopic repair is also associated with an approximately 0.3% risk of visceral or vascular injury.[11] Although controversy exists about the usefulness of laparoscopic repair for primary unilateral inguinal hernias, most agree that this approach has advantages for patients having bilateral or recurrent hernia repairs.[12] Adopting practice guidelines for the performance of laparoscopic hernia repairs could help control costs.

When considering the laparoscopic approach for repair of inguinal hernias, the surgeon has several options. The most popular techniques are totally extraperitoneal (TEP) and transab-

dominal preperitoneal (TAPP) approaches. The main difference between these two techniques is the sequence of gaining access to the preperitoneal space. In the TEP approach, the dissection begins in the preperitoneal space using a balloon dissector. With the TAPP repair, the preperitoneal space is accessed after initially entering the peritoneal cavity. Each approach has its merits. With the TEP approach, the preperitoneal dissection is quicker, and the potential risk for intraperitoneal visceral damage is minimized. However, the use of dissection balloons is costly, the working space is more limited, and it may not be possible to create a working space if the patient has had a prior preperitoneal operation. Also, if a large tear in the peritoneum is created during a TEP approach, the potential working space can become obliterated, necessitating conversion to a TAPP approach. For these reasons, knowledge of the transabdominal technique is essential in performing laparoscopic inguinal hernia repairs. The transabdominal approach allows identification of the groin anatomy before extensive dissection and disruption of natural tissue planes. The larger working space of the peritoneal cavity can make early experience with the laparoscopic approach easier.

There are no absolute contraindications to laparoscopic inguinal hernia repair other than the patient's inability to tolerate general anesthesia. Patients who have had extensive prior lower abdominal surgery can require significant adhesiolysis and may be best approached anteriorly. In particular, in patients who have had a radical retropubic prostatectomy with the preperitoneal space previously dissected, accurate and safe dissection can be challenging.

In the TEP approach, an infraumbilical incision is used. The anterior rectus sheath is incised, the ipsilateral rectus abdominis muscle is retracted laterally, and blunt dissection is used to create a space beneath the rectus. A dissecting balloon is inserted deep to the posterior rectus sheath, advanced to the pubic symphysis, and inflated under direct laparoscopic vision (Fig. 44-7). After it is opened, the space is insufflated, and additional trocars are placed. A 30-degree laparoscope provides the best visualization of the inguinal region (see Fig. 44-3). The inferior epigastric vessels are identified along the lower portion of the rectus muscle and serve as a useful landmark. Cooper ligament must be cleared from the pubic symphysis medially to the level of the external iliac vein. The iliopubic tract is also identified. Care must be taken to avoid injury to the femoral branch of the genitofemoral nerve and lateral femoral cutaneous nerve, which are located lateral to and below the iliopubic tract (see Fig. 44-4). Lateral dissection is carried out to the anterior superior iliac spine. Finally, the spermatic cord is skeletonized.

In the TAPP approach, an infraumbilical incision is used to gain access to the peritoneal cavity directly. Two 5-mm ports are placed lateral to the inferior epigastric vessels at the level of the umbilicus. A peritoneal flap is created high on the anterior abdominal wall, extending from the median umbilical fold to the anterior superior iliac spine. The remainder of the operation proceeds similar to a TEP procedure.

A direct hernia sac and associated preperitoneal fat are gently reduced by traction if not already reduced by balloon expansion of the peritoneal space. A small, indirect hernia sac is mobilized from the cord structures and reduced into the peritoneal cavity. A large sac may be difficult to reduce. In this case, the sac is divided with cautery near the internal inguinal ring, leaving the distal sac in situ. The proximal peritoneal sac is closed with a loop ligature to prevent pneumoperitoneum from occurring. After all hernias are reduced, a 12 × 14-cm piece of polypropylene mesh is inserted through a trocar and unfolded. It covers the direct, indirect, and femoral spaces and rests over the cord structures. It is imperative that the peritoneum be dissected at least 4 cm off the cord structures to prevent the peritoneum from encroaching beneath the mesh, which can lead to recurrence. The mesh is carefully secured with a tacking stapler to Cooper ligament from the pubic tubercle to the external iliac vein, anteriorly to the posterior rectus musculature and transversus abdominis aponeurotic arch at least 2 cm above the hernia defect, and laterally to the iliopubic tract. The mesh extends beyond the pubic symphysis and below the spermatic cord and peritoneum (Fig. 44-8). The mesh is not fixed in this area and tacks are not placed inferior to the iliopubic tract beyond the external iliac artery. Staples placed in this area may injure the femoral branch of the genitofemoral nerve or lateral femoral cutaneous nerve. Staples are also avoided in the so-called triangle of doom, bounded by the ductus deferens medially and spermatic vessels laterally, to avoid injury to the external iliac vessels and femoral nerve. As long as one can palpate the tip of the tacking device, these structures are not likely to be injured.

Results of Hernia Repair

The true measure of success for the various types of hernia repair is based on the results. The best information on the results of hernia repair is available from large prospective randomized trials, meta-analyses of clinical trials, and two large national registries, the Danish Hernia Database and the Swedish Hernia Register. The Danish Hernia Database includes more than 98% of inguinal hernia repairs; the capture rate of the Swedish Hernia Register is approximately 80%.[13,14] In spite of the randomized nature of some trials, caution must be used in interpreting the results. Many of these patients were highly selected, and most trials excluded recurrent hernias, obese individuals, and large inguinal hernias. Also, some follow-up results were completed by telephone interviews and not by physical examination. The national registries collect information only on operations, so the incidence of recurrence is lower than if all patients had been interviewed and examined.

The mortality of all types of repair is low, and there are no significant differences reported among the various techniques. There is a greater mortality associated with the repair of strangulated hernias. Otherwise, the risk of death is related to individual

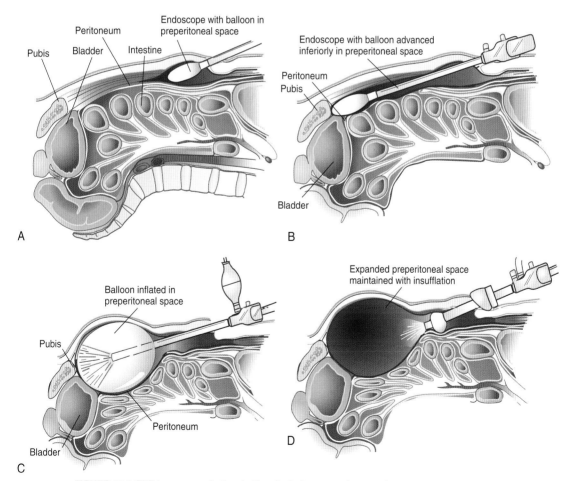

FIGURE 44-7 TEP Laparoscopic Hernia Repair. A, Access to the posterior rectus sheath is gained in the periumbilical region. A balloon dissector is placed on the anterior surface of the posterior rectus sheath. **B,** The balloon dissector is advanced to the posterior surface of the pubis in the preperitoneal space. **C,** The balloon is inflated, thereby creating an optical cavity. **D,** The optical cavity is insufflated by carbon dioxide, and the posterior surface of the inguinal floor is dissected.

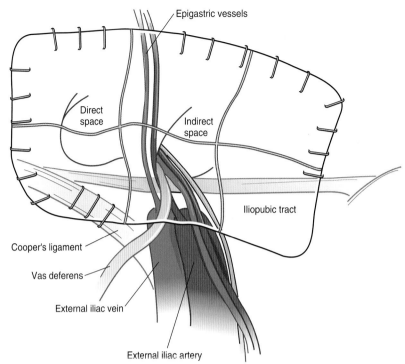

FIGURE 44-8 Prosthetic mesh placement for TEP hernia repair. (From Corbitt J: Laparoscopic transabdominal transperitoneal patch hernia repair. In Ballantyne GH, editor: *Atlas of laparoscopic surgery*, Philadelphia, 2000, WB Saunders, p 511.)

comorbid conditions and should be evaluated in each patient. The type of anesthetic does not affect the recurrence rate.[14] Open repairs can be performed under local anesthesia, which can be an advantage in operating on high-risk patients.

There are important differences in the results of primary hernia repair. Hernia recurrence is the primary outcome assessed by most studies. Large series, including multiple types of repairs, have suggested that recurrence ranges from 1.7% to 10%.[13-15]

The results of tissue repairs were often based on reports consisting of personal or single institutional series that were not prospective or randomized and had erratic follow-up periods. Not surprisingly, recurrence was variable.

Tension-free repairs have a lower rate of recurrence than tissue repairs.[14,16,17] Results from the Danish Hernia Database have demonstrated that hernia recurrence resulting in reoperation after the Lichtenstein repair is only 25% that of nonmesh repairs.[13] A Cochrane review reported that prosthetic mesh repairs have a 50% to 75% lower risk of hernia recurrence, a lower risk of chronic postherniorrhaphy groin pain, and an earlier return to work than open repairs.[16] The Shouldice repair has a higher recurrence rate than mesh repairs unless mesh is used.[17] A meta-analysis comparing the Lichtenstein, mesh plug, and bilayered repairs has reported no significant differences in the rate of recurrence, chronic groin pain, other complications, or time to return to work.[18] Approximately 50% of recurrences are found within 3 years after primary repair. Recurrence continues to occur after this time in nonmesh-based repairs but is uncommon with tension-free repairs. The bilayered repair was found to have a 20% hernia recurrence when used for large direct or recurrent hernias in one

study.[19] These results demonstrate the limitations of a fixed mesh size in these circumstances.

An extensive systematic review of randomized controlled trials was published in 2002 by the European Union Hernia Trialists Collaboration.[20] The authors reported a meta-analysis of 4165 patients in 25 studies. Based on the available data, the laparoscopic repair resulted in a more rapid return to normal activity and decreased persistent postoperative pain. The recurrence rate for the laparoscopic repair was lower compared with open nonmesh repairs; however, open and laparoscopic mesh repairs had similar recurrence rates.

A prospective trial sponsored by the Veterans Administration randomized 1983 patients to undergo an open Lichtenstein repair or laparoscopic repair, of which 90% were TEP repairs.[15] Most surgeons in this study may have had a suboptimal experience with the laparoscopic approach; only 25 prior repairs were necessary to be eligible to enroll patients, which is consistent with the seemingly high conversion rate of 5%. Despite these factors, the investigators found a twofold higher incidence of recurrence after laparoscopic repair (10%) than after open repair (5%). This difference in recurrence remained for primary hernias (10% laparoscopic versus 4% open); however, recurrent hernias repaired by the laparoscopic approach tended to have fewer re-recurrences (10% versus 14%). In another study by this group, surgeon inexperience with laparoscopy and surgeon age older than 45 years were both predictors of recurrence after laparoscopic repair.[18] A large cohort study and a recent meta-analysis have found a significantly higher risk of recurrence after laparoscopic repair that is nearly twice that of open repairs (4.1% versus 2.1%).[21,22] What can be concluded from these results? These results demonstrate that the laparoscopic repair of inguinal hernias has a definite learning curve to achieve an acceptably low recurrence rate.

In a Cochrane review of more than 1000 patients in eight nonrandomized trials, there was no difference in hernia recurrence between TAPP and TEP repairs.[23] TAPP procedures were associated with more port site hernias and vascular injuries, whereas the TEP approach had a greater conversion rate.

FEMORAL HERNIAS

A femoral hernia occurs through the femoral canal, which is bounded superiorly by the iliopubic tract, inferiorly by Cooper ligament, laterally by the femoral vein, and medially by the junction of the iliopubic tract and Cooper ligament (lacunar ligament). A femoral hernia produces a mass or bulge below the inguinal ligament. On occasion, some femoral hernias will present over the inguinal canal. In this case, the femoral hernia sac still exits inferior to the inguinal ligament through the femoral canal but ascends in a cephalad direction. Approximately 50% of men with a femoral hernia will have an associated direct inguinal hernia, whereas this relationship occurs in only 2% of women.

A femoral hernia can be repaired by the standard Cooper ligament repair, a preperitoneal approach, or a laparoscopic approach. The essential elements of femoral hernia repair include dissection and reduction of the hernia sac and obliteration of the defect in the femoral canal, either by approximation of the iliopubic tract to Cooper ligament or by placement of prosthetic mesh to obliterate the defect. The incidence of strangulation in femoral hernias is high; therefore, all femoral hernias should be repaired, and incarcerated femoral hernias should have the hernia sac contents examined for viability. In patients with a compromised bowel, the Cooper ligament approach is the preferred technique because mesh is contraindicated. When the incarcerated contents of a femoral hernia cannot be reduced, dividing the lacunar ligament can be helpful.

Femoral hernias were reported to occur in conjunction with inguinal hernias in 0.3% of patients in a large national hernia database of almost 35,000 patients.[24] The occurrence of a femoral hernia after repair of an inguinal hernia has been reported to be 15 times the normal expected rate. It is unclear whether this represents a femoral hernia overlooked at the prior operation or a propensity to development of a new hernia after inguinal hernia repair. Recurrence of femoral hernia after operation is only 2%. Recurrent femoral hernia repairs have a re-recurrence rate of about 10%.

SPECIAL PROBLEMS

Sliding Hernia

A sliding hernia occurs when an internal organ composes a portion of the wall of the hernia sac. The most common viscus involved is the colon or urinary bladder. Most sliding hernias are a variant of indirect inguinal hernias, although femoral and direct sliding hernias can occur. The primary danger associated with a sliding hernia is the failure to recognize the visceral component of the hernia sac before injury to the bowel or bladder. The sliding hernia contents are reduced into the peritoneal cavity, and any excess hernia sac is ligated and divided. After reduction of the hernia, one of the techniques described earlier can be used for repair of the inguinal hernia.

Recurrent Hernia

The repair of recurrent inguinal hernias is challenging, and results are associated with a higher incidence of secondary recurrence. Recurrent hernias almost always require placement of prosthetic mesh for successful repair. The exception is when infected mesh is associated with a recurrent hernia. Recurrences after anterior hernia repair using mesh are best managed by a laparoscopic or open posterior approach, with placement of a second prosthesis.

Strangulated Hernia

Repair of a suspected strangulated hernia is most easily done using a preperitoneal approach (see earlier). With this exposure, the hernia sac contents can be directly visualized and their viability assessed through a single incision. The constricting ring is identified and can be incised to reduce the entrapped viscus with minimal danger to the surrounding organs, blood vessels, and nerves. If it is necessary to resect strangulated intestine, the peritoneum can be opened and resection done without the need for a second incision.

Bilateral Hernias

The approach to repair of bilateral inguinal hernias is based on the extent of the hernia defect. Simultaneous repair of bilateral hernias has a similar recurrence rate to unilateral repair, regardless of whether the open or laparoscopic technique is used.[25] The use of a giant prosthetic reinforcement of the visceral sac (Stoppa repair)[9] or the laparoscopic repair is preferred for simultaneous repair of bilateral inguinal hernias.

Complications

There are myriad complications related to open and laparoscopic inguinal hernia repair (Table 44-1). Some are general complications that are related to underlying diseases and the effects of anesthesia. These vary by patient population and risk. In addition,

TABLE 44-1 Complications After Open and Laparoscopic Inguinal Hernia Repair (%)

COMPLICATION	OPEN REPAIR (N = 994)	LAPAROSCOPIC REPAIR (N = 989)
Intraoperative complications	1.9	4.8
Postoperative complications	19.4	24.6
Urinary retention	2.2	2.8
Urinary tract infection	0.4	1.0
Orchitis	1.1	1.4
Surgical site infection	1.4	1.0
Neuralgia, pain	3.6	4.2
Life-threatening complications	0.1	1.1
Long-term complications	17.4	18.0
Seroma	3.0	9.0
Orchitis	2.2	1.9
Infection	0.6	0.4
Chronic pain	14.3	9.8
Recurrence	4.9	10.1

From Neumayer L, Giobbie-Hurder A, Jonassen O, et al: Open mesh versus laparoscopic mesh repair of inguinal hernias. *N Engl J Med* 350:1819–1827, 2004.

there are technical complications that are directly related to the repair. Technical complications are affected by the experience of the surgeon and are more frequent during and after the repair of recurrent hernias. There is increased scarring and disturbed anatomy with hernia recurrence that can result in an inability to identify important structures at operation. This is the principal reason that we recommend using a different approach for recurrent hernias.

Although the overall complication rate from hernia repair has been estimated to be approximately 10%, many of these complications are transient and can be easily addressed. More serious complications from a large experience are listed in Table 44-1.

Surgical Site Infection

The risk for surgical site infection is estimated to be 1% to 2% after open inguinal hernia repair and slightly less with laparoscopic repairs. These are clean operations, and the risk for infection is primarily influenced by associated patient diseases. Most would agree that there is no need to use routine antimicrobial prophylaxis for hernia repair.[20] Prospective randomized clinical trials have not supported the routine use of perioperative antimicrobial prophylaxis for inguinal hernia repair for patients at low risk for infection.[26] Patients who have significant underlying disease, as reflected by an American Society of Anesthesiology score of 3 or more, receive perioperative antimicrobial prophylaxis with cefazolin, 1 to 2 g, given intravenously 30 to 60 minutes before the incision. Clindamycin, 600 mg intravenously, can be used for patients allergic to penicillin. Only a single dose of antibiotic is necessary. The placement of prosthetic mesh does not increase the risk for infection and does not affect the need for prophylaxis. Superficial surgical site infections are treated by opening the incision, local wound care, and healing by secondary intention. Some mesh infections will be manifested as a chronic draining sinus that tracks to the mesh or occur with extruded mesh. Deep surgical site infections usually involve the prosthetic mesh, which should be explanted.

The risk for infection can be decreased by using proper operative technique, preoperative antiseptic skin preparation, and appropriate hair removal. There is an increased risk for infection for patients who have had prior hernia incision infections, chronic skin infections, or infection at a distant site. These infections are treated before elective surgery.

Nerve Injuries and Chronic Pain Syndromes

Nerve injuries are an infrequent and underrecognized complication of inguinal hernia repair. Injury can occur from traction, electrocautery, transection, and entrapment. The use of prosthetic mesh can result in dysesthesias, which are usually temporary. The nerves most commonly affected during open hernia repair are the ilioinguinal, genital branch of the genitofemoral, and iliohypogastric nerves. During laparoscopic repair, the lateral femoral cutaneous and genitofemoral nerves are most often affected.[27] Rarely, the main trunk of the femoral nerve can be injured during open or laparoscopic inguinal hernia repair.

Transient neuralgias involving sensory nerves can occur and are usually self-limited and resolve within a few weeks after surgery. Persistent neuralgias usually result in pain and hyperesthesia in the area of distribution. Symptoms are often reproduced by palpation over the point of entrapment or hyperextension of the hip and may be relieved by flexion of the thigh. Transection of a sensory nerve usually results in an area of numbness corresponding to the distribution of the involved nerve.

With more attention to patient outcomes, chronic groin pain has replaced recurrence as the primary complication after open inguinal hernia repair. Approximately 10% of patients will have chronic postherniorrhaphy pain, defined as pain persisting more than 3 months after operation,[28] and pain has been reported to interfere with activities of daily living in 2% to 4%.[29] Strategies of routine nerve division in open surgery have not been associated with a reduction in chronic pain in mesh-based anterior repairs.[30] In contrast, routine ilioinguinal nerve division is associated with significantly more sensory disturbances. In laparoscopic repairs, by operating in a remote area to the commonly injured nerves and with judicious use of appropriately placed tacks, chronic groin pain intuitively is less common. Some reports comparing laparoscopic and open repairs have reported lower rates of chronic postoperative inguinal pain, but this observation remains controversial.

Various approaches to management of residual neuralgia have been described. Early symptoms are treated with anti-inflammatory agents, analgesics, and local anesthetic nerve blocks. Patients with nerve entrapment syndromes are best treated by repeated exploration with neurectomy and mesh removal through an anterior approach. Laparoscopic nerve injuries are minimized by not placing any tacks or staples below the lateral portion of the iliopubic tract. If nerve entrapment occurs, patients undergo reoperation to remove the offending tack or staple.

Ischemic Orchitis and Testicular Atrophy

Ischemic orchitis usually occurs from thrombosis of the small veins of the pampiniform plexus within the spermatic cord. This results in venous congestion of the testis, which becomes swollen and tender 2 to 5 days after surgery. The process may continue for an additional 6 to 12 weeks and usually results in testicular atrophy. Ischemic orchitis also can be caused by ligation of the testicular artery. It is treated with anti-inflammatory agents and analgesics. Orchiectomy is rarely necessary.

The incidence of ischemic orchitis can be minimized by avoiding unnecessary dissection within the spermatic cord. The incidence increases with dissection of the distal portion of a large hernia sac and in patients who have anterior operations for hernia recurrence or for spermatic cord disease. In these situations, the use of a posterior approach is preferred.

Testicular atrophy is a consequence of ischemic orchitis. It is more common after repair of recurrent hernias, particularly when an anterior approach is used. The incidence of ischemic orchitis increases by a factor of three or four with each subsequent hernia recurrence.

Injury to the Vas Deferens and Viscera

Injury to the vas deferens and intra-abdominal viscera is unusual. Most of these injuries occur in patients with sliding inguinal hernias when there is failure to recognize the presence of intra-abdominal viscera in the hernia sac. With large hernias, the vas deferens can be displaced in an enlarged inguinal ring before its entry into the spermatic cord. In this situation, the vas deferens is identified and protected.

Hernia Recurrence

Hernia recurrences are usually caused by technical factors, such as excessive tension on the repair, missed hernias, failure to include an adequate musculoaponeurotic margin in the repair, and improper mesh size and placement. Recurrence also can result from failure to close a patulous internal inguinal ring, the size of which is always assessed at the conclusion of the primary surgery. Other factors that can cause hernia recurrence are chronically elevated intra-abdominal pressure, a chronic cough, deep incisional infections, and poor collagen formation in the wound. Recurrences are more common in patients with direct hernias and usually involve the floor of the inguinal canal near the pubic tubercle, where suture line tension is greatest. The use of a relaxing incision when there is excessive tension at the time of primary hernia repair is helpful to reduce recurrence. A femoral hernia is found in approximately 5% to 10% of patients with an inguinal hernia recurrence and should always be investigated at surgery.[13]

Most recurrent hernias require the use of prosthetic mesh for successful repair.[30,31] Choosing a different approach (usually posterior) avoids dissection through scar tissue, improves visualization of the defect and reduction of the hernia, and decreases the incidence of complications, particularly ischemic orchitis and injury to the ilioinguinal nerve. Recurrences after initial prosthetic mesh repairs can be caused by displaced prostheses or the use of a prosthetic of inadequate size. Recurrences are best managed by placing a second prosthesis through a different approach.

A meta-analysis of 58 reports comparing synthetic mesh techniques with nonmesh repairs has demonstrated an almost 60% reduction in recurrence with the use of mesh.[20] This report concluded that there was no difference in the rate of hernia recurrence between laparoscopic and open approaches that used mesh. A recent meta-analysis of recurrent hernia repairs reported no difference between open and laparoscopic mesh repairs in re-recurrence or chronic groin pain.[32]

Recurrence is more common after repair of recurrent hernias and is directly related to the number of previous attempts at repair. Large population-based studies have reported a re-recurrence rate of 4% to 5% in the first 24 months, which increases to 7.5% at 5 years.[31,33] Tension-free and mesh-based repairs have the lowest rates of reoperation after recurrence and result in a reduction in recurrence of approximately 60% compared with more traditional repairs.[30]

There is a successive decrease in the time to hernia recurrence with each subsequent repair.[33] Re-recurrences are associated with increased operative times and a greater rate of complications.

Quality of Life

The major quality indicators that have been assessed for hernia repair are postoperative pain and return to work. Tension-free and laparoscopic mesh-based approaches have been demonstrated to be less painful than nonmesh repairs. Laparoscopic repairs have the least amount of postoperative pain and have been shown to provide a marginal advantage in reducing time off work.[12]

VENTRAL HERNIAS

A ventral hernia is defined by a protrusion through the anterior abdominal wall fascia. These defects can be categorized as spontaneous or acquired or by their location on the abdominal wall. Epigastric hernias occur from the xiphoid process to the umbilicus, umbilical hernias occur at the umbilicus, and hypogastric hernias are rare spontaneous hernias that occur below the umbilicus in the midline. Acquired hernias typically occur after surgical incisions and are therefore termed incisional hernias. Although not a true hernia, diastasis recti can present as a midline bulge. In this condition, the linea alba is stretched, resulting in bulging at the medial margins of the rectus muscles. Abdominal wall diastasis can occur at other sites in addition to the midline. There is no fascial ring or hernia sac, and unless it is significantly symptomatic, surgical correction is avoided.

Incidence

Based on national operative statistics, incisional hernias account for 15% to 20% of all abdominal wall hernias; umbilical and epigastric hernias constitute 10% of hernias. Incisional hernias are twice as common in women as in men. As a result of the almost 4 million laparotomies performed annually in the United States and the 2% to 30% incidence of incisional hernia, almost 150,000 ventral hernia repairs are performed each year. Several technical and patient-related factors have been linked to the occurrence of incisional hernias. There is no conclusive evidence demonstrating that the type of suture at the primary operation affects hernia formation.[34] Patient-related factors linked to ventral hernia formation include obesity, older age, male gender, sleep apnea, emphysema, and prostatism. It has been proposed that the same factors associated with destruction of the collagen in the lung result in poor wound healing, with increased hernia formation. Wound infection has been linked to hernia formation. Recent data suggest that the surgical technique used to close a midline laparotomy is highly associated with incisional hernia formation. The use of a suture to wound length ratio of 4:1 has been shown to significantly reduce incisional hernia formation compared with the 1-cm bites and 1-cm advancement suturing technique typically employed by most surgeons.[35]

Whether the type of initial abdominal incision influences the incisional hernia rate remains controversial. As noted, the incidence of ventral herniation after midline laparotomy ranges from 3% to 20% and doubles if the operation is associated with a surgical site infection. A meta-analysis of 11 studies examining the incidence of ventral hernia formation after various types of abdominal incisions has concluded that the risk is 10.5% for midline, 7.5% for transverse, and 2.5% for paramedian incisions.[36] A recently published prospective randomized trial has reported no difference in hernia formation in comparing midline versus transverse incisions after 1 year but noted a higher wound infection rate in the transverse incisions.[37] Given the likely similar rates of incisional hernia formation after transverse and midline incisions, the surgeon should plan the incision on the basis of the operative exposure desired to complete the procedure safely.

Few data are available about the natural history of untreated ventral hernias. As noted, asymptomatic or minimally symptomatic inguinal hernias purposely observed during 2 years have a low incidence of complications.[3] Whether this paradigm applies for asymptomatic ventral or incisional hernias is unclear. Because there is no prospective cohort available to determine the natural history of untreated ventral hernias, most surgeons recommend that these hernias be repaired when discovered.

Anatomy

The anatomy of the anterior abdominal wall is straightforward and considerably easier to grasp than the anatomy of the inguinal area. However, a clear understanding of the blood supply and innervation of the abdomen is important in performing advanced abdominal wall reconstruction. The lateral musculature is composed of three layers, with the fascicles of each directed obliquely at different angles to create a strong envelope for the abdominal contents. Each of these muscles forms an aponeurosis that inserts into the linea alba, a midline structure joining both sides of the abdominal wall. The external oblique is the most superficial muscle of the lateral abdominal wall. Deep to the external oblique lies the internal oblique muscle. The fibers of the external oblique course in an inferomedial direction (like hands in pockets), whereas those of the internal oblique muscle run deep to and opposite the external oblique. The deepest muscle layer of the abdominal wall is the transversus abdominis muscle. Its fibers course in a horizontal direction. These three lateral muscles give rise to aponeurotic layers lateral to the rectus, which contribute to the anterior and posterior layers of the rectus sheath.

The medial extension of the external oblique aponeurosis forms the anterior layer of the rectus sheath. At the midline, the two anterior rectus sheaths form the tendinous linea alba. On either side of the linea alba are the rectus abdominis muscles, whose fibers are directed longitudinally and run the length of the anterior abdominal wall. Below each rectus muscle lies the posterior layer of the rectus sheath, which also contributes to the linea alba.

Another important anatomic structure of the anterior abdominal wall is the arcuate line, which is located 3 to 6 cm below the umbilicus. The arcuate line delineates the point below which the posterior rectus sheath is absent. Above the arcuate line, the aponeurosis of the internal oblique muscle contributes to the anterior and posterior rectus sheaths, and the aponeurosis of the transversus abdominis muscle passes posterior to the rectus muscle to form the posterior rectus sheath. Below the arcuate line, the internal oblique and transversus abdominis aponeuroses pass completely anterior to the rectus muscle (Fig. 44-9). The posterior rectus sheath below the arcuate line is composed of the transversalis fascia and peritoneum only.

The abdominal wall receives most of its innervation from intercostal nerves 7 through 12 and the first and second lumbar nerves. These rami provide innervation to the lateral abdominal muscles and the rectus muscle and overlying skin. The nerves traverse through the lateral abdominal wall between the transversus abdominis and internal oblique muscles and penetrate the posterior rectus sheath just medial to the linea semilunaris.

The lateral abdominal muscles receive their blood supply from the lower three or four intercostal arteries, deep circumflex iliac artery, and lumbar arteries. The rectus abdominis has a more complex blood supply derived from the superior epigastric artery (a terminal branch of the internal mammary artery), inferior epigastric artery (a branch of the external iliac artery), and lower intercostal arteries. The superior and inferior epigastric arteries anastomose near the umbilicus. The periumbilical area provides critical perforator vessels that, if preserved, can decrease skin flap necrosis during extensive skin undermining (Fig. 44-10).

Diagnosis

The evaluation of abdominal wall hernias requires diligent physical examination. As with the inguinal region, the anterior abdominal wall is evaluated with the patient in standing and supine positions, and a Valsalva maneuver is also useful to demonstrate the site and size of a hernia. Imaging modalities may play a greater role in the diagnosis of more unusual hernias of the abdominal wall.

Classification
Umbilical Hernia

The umbilicus is formed by the umbilical ring of the linea alba. Intra-abdominally, the round ligament (ligamentum teres) and paraumbilical veins join into the umbilicus superiorly and the median umbilical ligament (obliterated urachus) enters inferiorly.

Umbilical hernias in infants are congenital and are common. They close spontaneously in most cases by the age of 2 years. Those that persist after the age of 5 years are frequently repaired surgically, although complications related to these hernias in children are unusual. There is a strong predisposition toward the development of these hernias in individuals of African descent. In the United States, the incidence of umbilical hernia is eight times higher in African American than in white infants.

Umbilical hernias in adults are largely acquired. These hernias are more common in women and in patients with conditions that result in increased intra-abdominal pressure, such as pregnancy, obesity, ascites, or chronic abdominal distention. Umbilical hernia is more common in those who have only a single midline aponeurotic decussation compared with the normal decussation of fibers from all three lateral abdominal muscles. Strangulation is unusual in most patients; however, strangulation or rupture can occur in chronic ascitic conditions. Small asymptomatic umbilical hernias barely detectable on examination need not be repaired. Adults who have symptoms, a large hernia, incarceration, thinning of the overlying skin, or uncontrollable ascites should have a hernia repair. Spontaneous rupture of umbilical hernias in patients with ascites can result in peritonitis and death.

Classically, repair was done using the vest over pants repair proposed by Mayo, which uses imbrication of the superior and inferior fascial edges. Because of increased tension on the repair and recurrence rates of almost 30% with long-term follow-up, however, the Mayo repair is rarely performed today. Instead, small defects are closed primarily after separation of the sac from the overlying umbilicus and surrounding fascia. Defects larger than 3 cm are closed using prosthetic mesh.[38] There are a number of techniques to place this mesh, and no prospective data have conclusively found clear advantages of one technique over another. Options for mesh implantation include bridging the defect, placing a preperitoneal underlay of mesh reinforced with suture repair, and placing it laparoscopically. The laparoscopic technique requires general anesthesia and is reserved for large defects or recurrent umbilical hernias.[39] There is no universal consensus on the most appropriate method of umbilical hernia repair.

Epigastric Hernia

Approximately 3% to 5% of the population has epigastric hernias. Epigastric hernias are two to three times more common in men. These hernias are located between the xiphoid process and umbilicus and are usually within 5 to 6 cm of the umbilicus. Like umbilical hernias, epigastric hernias are more common in individuals with a single aponeurotic decussation. The defects are small and often produce pain out of proportion to their size because of incarceration of preperitoneal fat. They are multiple in up to 20% of patients, and approximately 80% are in the midline. Repair usually consists of excision of the incarcerated preperitoneal tissue and simple closure of the fascial defect, similar to that for umbilical hernias. Small defects can be repaired under local anesthesia. Uncommonly, these defects can be sizable, can contain omentum or other intra-abdominal viscera, and may require mesh repairs. Epigastric hernias are better repaired anteriorly because the defect is small and fat that has herniated from within the peritoneal cavity is difficult to reduce.

Incisional Hernia

Of all hernias encountered, incisional hernias can be the most frustrating and difficult to treat. Incisional hernias occur as a result

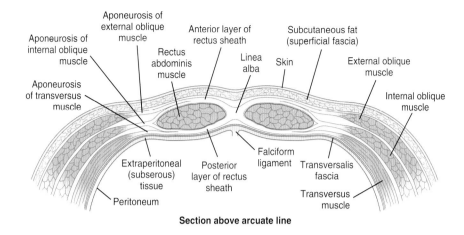

Section above arcuate line

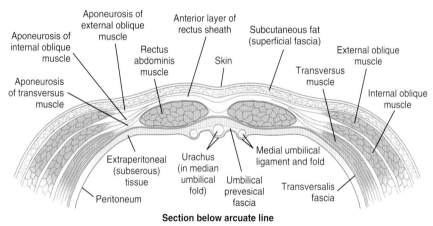

Section below arcuate line

FIGURE 44-9 Cross sections of the rectus abdominis muscle and aponeurosis above and below the arcuate line. (From Netter FT: *Atlas of human anatomy*, Summit, NJ, 1989, Ciba-Geigy, Plate 235.)

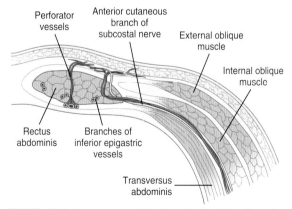

FIGURE 44-10 Cross section of the lateral abdominal wall detailing location of intercostal neurovascular bundle traveling between the transversus abdominis and internal oblique muscles.

of excessive tension and inadequate healing of a previous incision, which may be associated with surgical site infection. These hernias enlarge over time, leading to pain, bowel obstruction, incarceration, and strangulation. Obesity, advanced age, malnutrition, ascites, pregnancy, and conditions that increase intra-abdominal pressure are factors that predispose to the development of an incisional hernia. Obesity can cause an incisional hernia to occur because of increased tension on the abdominal wall from the excessive bulk of a thick pannus and large omental mass. Chronic pulmonary disease and diabetes mellitus have also been recognized as risk factors for the development of incisional hernia. Medications such as corticosteroids and chemotherapeutic agents and surgical site infection can contribute to poor wound healing and increase the risk for development of an incisional hernia.

Large hernias can result in loss of abdominal domain, which occurs when the abdominal contents no longer reside in the abdominal cavity. These large abdominal wall defects also can result from the inability to close the abdomen primarily because of bowel edema, abdominal packing, peritonitis, and repeated laparotomy. With loss of domain, the natural rigidity of the abdominal wall becomes compromised and the abdominal musculature is often retracted. Respiratory dysfunction can occur because these large ventral defects cause paradoxical respiratory abdominal motion. Loss of abdominal domain can also result in bowel edema, stasis of the splanchnic venous system, urinary retention, and constipation. Return of displaced viscera to the abdominal cavity during repair may lead to increased abdominal pressure, abdominal compartment syndrome, and acute respiratory failure.

There is no simple mechanism for communicating the complexity of a ventral incisional hernia. Defect size, location on the abdominal wall, loss of domain, patient comorbidities, presence of contamination, necessity for an ostomy, acuity of the presentation, and history of prior repairs with or without a prosthetic allow an infinite number of permutations. The absence of a universal classification system has hindered comparisons within the literature and at meetings, indirectly delaying meaningful conversations about repair techniques and prosthetic choice. The TNM model for cancer staging is an enviable model to strive for in hernia repair. As such, a recent group sought to stratify ventral hernias into stages using a limited number of preoperative variables to accurately predict the two most meaningful surgical outcomes: surgical site occurrence (SSO) and long-term hernia recurrence rates.

Two of the most popular ventral hernia classification tools to date have been generated from expert opinion: the Ventral Hernia Working Group grading scale and the European Hernia Society system. The Ventral Hernia Working Group grading scale uses patient comorbidities and wound class to predict SSO risk. The European Hernia Society system assesses hernia width and location; it was initially designed to gather data on recurrence risk.[40] Using data from 333 ventral hernia repairs with no filter for technique, investigators presented a multivariate analysis that identified hernia width (<10 cm, 10 to 20 cm, ≥20 cm) and the presence of contamination as the two variables associated with wound morbidity (SSO) and hernia recurrence. Hernia location and patient comorbidities were not significant in this model for either outcome measure. Hernias could be grouped into stages (I to III) using width and wound class alone (Table 44-2), with ordinal increments in both outcome measures. Stage I hernias are smaller than 10 cm/clean and associated with low SSO and recurrence risk. Stage II hernias are 10 to 20 cm/clean or smaller than 10 cm/contaminated and carry an intermediate risk of SSO and recurrence. Stage III hernias are either 10 cm and larger/contaminated or any hernia 20 cm or larger, and these are associated with high SSO and recurrence risk. Table 44-3 demonstrates the reported rates for SSO and recurrence using this system.

The staging system is simple but comprehensive in its ability to stratify patients by risk of wound morbidity and recurrence, the two chief outcome parameters of repair. Importantly, this system does not include intraoperative details, such as approach (open versus laparoscopic), mesh choice (biologic versus synthetic), or mesh position (onlay versus sublay). It is hoped that this platform can be the basis of future inclusion and exclusion criteria for studies regarding technique.

Treatment: Operative Repair

Primary repair of incisional hernias can be done when the defect is small (≤2 to 3 cm in diameter) and there is viable surrounding tissue or in cases in which the hernia was clearly a result of a technical error at the initial operation, such as a suture fracturing. Larger defects (>2 to 3 cm in diameter) have a high recurrence rate if closed primarily and are repaired with a prosthesis.[39] Recurrence rates vary between 10% and 50% and are typically reduced by more than 50% with the use of prosthetic mesh.[41] Prosthetic

material may be placed as an onlay patch to buttress a tissue repair, interposed between the fascial defect, sandwiched between tissue planes, or put in a sublay position. Depending on its location, several important properties of the mesh must be considered.

Prosthetic Materials for Ventral Hernia Repair

Synthetic materials. Various synthetic mesh products are available. Desirable characteristics of a synthetic mesh include its being chemically inert, resistant to mechanical stress while maintaining compliance, sterilizable, and noncarcinogenic; it should incite minimal inflammatory reaction and be hypoallergenic. The ideal mesh has yet to be defined. When selecting the appropriate mesh, the surgeon must consider the position of the mesh, whether it will be in direct contact with the viscera, and the presence or risk of infection. Mesh constructs can be classified on the basis of weight of the material, pore size, water angle (hydrophobic or hydrophilic), and whether an antiadhesive barrier present. In placing a mesh in the extraperitoneal position without the risk of bowel erosion, a macroporous unprotected mesh is appropriate. Both polypropylene and polyester mesh have been successfully placed in the extraperitoneal position. Polypropylene mesh is a hydrophobic macroporous mesh that allows the ingrowth of native fibroblasts and incorporation into the surrounding fascia. It is semirigid, somewhat flexible, and porous. Placing polypropylene mesh in an intraperitoneal position directly apposed to the bowel is avoided because of unacceptable rates of

TABLE 44-2 Incisional Hernia Staging System	
Stage I Risk: low recurrence, low SSO	<10 cm, clean
Stage II Risk: moderate recurrence, moderate SSO	<10 cm, contaminated 10-20 cm, clean
Stage III Risk: high recurrence, high SSO	≥10 cm, contaminated Any ≥20 cm

SSO, surgical site occurrence.

TABLE 44-3 Surgical Site Occurrence (SSO) and Recurrence Rates		
	SSO RATE	**RECURRENCE RATE**
Stage I Risk: low recurrence, low SSO <10 cm, clean	7/77 (10%)	7/77 (10%)
Stage II Risk: moderate recurrence, moderate SSO <10 cm, contaminated 10-20 cm, clean	30/151 (20%)	22/151 (15%)
Stage III Risk: high recurrence, high SSO ≥10 cm, contaminated Any ≥20 cm	44/105 (42%)	27/105 (26%)

enterocutaneous fistula formation.[42] Recently, lighter weight polypropylene mesh has been introduced to address some of the long-term complications of heavyweight polypropylene mesh. The definition of lightweight mesh was arbitrarily chosen at less than 50 g/m^2, with heavyweight mesh weighing more than 80 g/m^2. These lightweight mesh products often have an absorbable component of material that provides initial handling stability, typically composed of Vicryl (polyglactin 910) or Monocryl (poliglecaprone 25; Ethicon, Somerville, NJ).

Whether lightweight mesh results in improved patient outcomes is controversial. Two prospective randomized trials evaluating the incidence of postoperative pain after open inguinal hernia repair have shown mixed results.[43] In a randomized controlled trial evaluating lightweight versus heavyweight polypropylene mesh for ventral hernia repair, the recurrence rate in the lightweight group was more than twice that in the heavyweight group (17% for lightweight mesh versus 7% for heavyweight mesh), which approached statistical significance ($P = .052$).[44] Several investigators have reported concerning rates of central mesh failures with ultra-lightweight polypropylene mesh and lightweight polyester mesh.[45,46] Another recent finding with regard to large-pore lightweight mesh is its ability to resist bacterial contamination. Several animal studies have reported high rates of bacterial clearance with large-pore synthetic mesh when it is exposed to gastrointestinal flora and methicillin-resistant *Staphylococcus aureus*.[47,48] A large multicenter retrospective experience with 100 cases of large-pore polypropylene mesh used in clean contaminated and contaminated ventral hernia repairs was reported.[49] These authors noted excellent medium-term results with a 7% recurrence rate. Longer term data to verify the safety and durability of this approach are needed.

Polyester mesh is composed of polyethylene terephthalate and is a hydrophilic, heavyweight, macroporous mesh. This mesh has several different weaves that can yield a two-dimensional flat screen-like mesh and a three-dimensional multifilament weave. Unprotected polyester mesh should not be placed directly on the viscera because unacceptable rates of erosion and bowel obstruction have been reported.[42] When it is placed in the preperitoneal position in complex ventral hernia repairs, complication rates are low.[9,50]

When mesh is placed in an intraperitoneal position, several options are available. A single sheet of mesh with both sides constructed to reduce adhesions and a composite-type mesh with one side made to promote tissue ingrowth and the other to resist adhesion formation are available. Single-sheet mesh is composed of expanded polytetrafluoroethylene (ePTFE). This prosthetic has a visceral side that is microporous (3 μm) and an abdominal wall side that is macroporous (17 to 22 μm) and promotes tissue ingrowth. This product differs from other synthetic meshes in that it is flexible and smooth. Some fibroblast proliferation occurs through the pores, but PTFE is impermeable to fluid. Unlike polypropylene, PTFE is not incorporated into the native tissue. Encapsulation occurs slowly, and infection can occur during the encapsulation process. When it is infected, PTFE almost always must be removed.

To promote better tissue integration, composite mesh was developed. This product combines the attributes of polypropylene and PTFE by layering the two substances on top of one another. The PTFE surface serves as a permanent protective interface against the bowel and the polypropylene side faces superficially to be incorporated into the native fascial tissue. These materials have variable rates of contraction and, when placed together, can result in buckling of the mesh and visceral exposure to the polypropylene component. Other composite meshes recently have been developed that combine a macroporous mesh with a temporary, absorbable antiadhesive barrier. Basic constructs of these mesh materials include heavyweight or lightweight polypropylene or polyester. Absorbable barriers are typically composed of oxidized regenerated cellulose, omega-3 fatty acids, or collagen hydrogels. A number of small animal studies have validated the antiadhesive properties of these barriers, but currently no human trials exist evaluating the ability of these composite materials to resist adhesion formation.

Biologic materials. Biologic prostheses for ventral hernia repair are nonsynthetic, natural tissue mesh. There are numerous biologic grafts available for abdominal wall reconstruction (Table 44-4). These products can be categorized on the basis of the source material (e.g., human, porcine, bovine), postharvesting processing techniques (e.g., cross-linked, non–cross-linked), and sterilization techniques (e.g., gamma radiation, ethylene oxide gas sterilization, nonsterilized). These products are largely composed of acellular collagen and theoretically provide a matrix for neovascularization and native collagen deposition. These properties may provide advantages in infected or contaminated cases in which synthetic mesh is thought to be contraindicated. Ideal placement techniques are yet to be defined for these relatively new products; however, some general principles apply. These products function best when used as a fascial reinforcement rather than as a bridge or interposition repair.[51] The long-term durability of biologic mesh has recently been questioned in the largest series of biologic mesh use in a contaminated setting.[52] There are no prospective randomized data comparing the effectiveness of these natural tissue alternatives with that of synthetic mesh repairs in various settings of complex hernia repairs.

Operative Technique

Ventral hernias. It is generally agreed that all but the smallest incisional hernias can be repaired with mesh, and the surgeon has various options for placing the mesh. The onlay technique involves primary closure of the fascia defect and placement of a mesh over the anterior fascia. The major advantage of this approach is that the mesh is placed outside the abdominal cavity, avoiding direct interaction with the abdominal viscera. However, disadvantages include the large subcutaneous dissection, the increased likelihood of seroma formation, the superficial location of the mesh (which places it in jeopardy of contamination if the incision becomes infected), and the repair is usually under tension. Prospective analysis of this technique is not available, but a retrospective review has reported recurrence rates of 28%.[53] Interposition prosthetic repairs involve securing the mesh to the fascial edge without overlap. This results in a predictably high recurrence rate; the synthetic often pulls away from the fascial edge because of increased intra-abdominal pressure. A sublay or underlay technique involves placing the prosthetic below the fascial components. The mesh can be placed intraperitoneally, preperitoneally, or in the retrorectus (retromuscular) space. It is highly desirable to have the mesh placed beneath the fascia. With a wide overlap of mesh and fascia, the natural forces of the abdominal cavity act to hold the mesh in place and prevent migration. This can be accomplished by several techniques (Fig. 44-11).

Intraperitoneal mesh placement. After reopening of the prior incision and with the use of available dual-type mesh or composite mesh, the mesh can be placed in an intraperitoneal position at least 4 cm beyond the fascial margin and secured with

TABLE 44-4 **Biologic Mesh for Abdominal Wall Reconstruction and Postharvesting Processing Techniques**

PRODUCT	SOURCE	CROSS-LINKED	STERILIZATION METHOD
AlloDerm (LifeCell, Branchburg, NJ)	Human dermis	No	Ionic
AlloMax (Davol, Warwick, RI)	Human dermis	No	E beam
FlexHD (Ethicon, Sommerville, NJ)	Human dermis	No	Ethanol
Strattice (LifeCell, Branchburg, NJ)	Porcine dermis	No	Gamma irradiation
Permacol (Covidien, Norwalk, CT)	Porcine dermis	Yes	Ethanol
CollaMend (Davol, Warwick, RI)	Porcine dermis	Yes	Ethanol
XenMatrix (Davol, Warwick, RI)	Porcine dermis	No	Gamma irradiation
SurgiMend (TEI Biosciences, Boston, MA)	Bovine fetal dermis	No	Ethanol
Veritas (Synovis, St. Paul, MN)	Bovine	No	
Peri-Guard (Synovis, St. Paul, MN)	Bovine	Yes	
Surgisis (Cook, Bloomfield, IN)	Porcine intestine	No	Ethanol

interrupted mattress sutures. This technique requires raising sub-cutaneous flaps, and the mesh may be in direct contact with the abdominal contents.

The laparoscopic approach for ventral hernia repair relies on the same principles as the retrorectus repair; however, the mesh is placed within the peritoneal cavity. This repair is useful, particularly for large defects. Trocars are placed as far laterally as feasible based on the size and location of the hernia. The hernia contents are reduced, and adhesions are lysed. The surface area of the defect is measured, and a barrier-coated mesh is fashioned with at least 4 cm of overlap around the defect. The mesh is rolled, placed into the abdomen, and deployed. It is secured to the anterior abdominal wall with preplaced mattress sutures that are passed through separate incisions; tacking staples are placed between these sutures to secure the mesh 4 cm beyond the defect. There are fewer incisional complications with the laparoscopic approach because large incisions and subcutaneous undermining are avoided.

Myofascial releases. One of the underlying principles of abdominal wall reconstruction is to reestablish the linea alba. Restoring the linea alba to the midline provides the advantage of a functional abdominal wall, often protects the mesh from superficial wound issues, and might result in a more durable repair. In larger hernias, there are several options to provide the myofascial advancement necessary to reconstruct the midline and to restore contour to the abdominal wall. The basic tenets of these procedures are that the abdominal wall and rectus muscle are bounded by several different myofascial compartments, and by releasing one or more fascial bundles, advancement of the rectus muscle to the midline is possible. In essence, each of these procedures creates a local advancement flap of the rectus muscle. Great care should be taken to identify and to preserve the neurovascular structures to the rectus muscle to ensure a functional well-vascularized graft.

Posterior rectus sheath incision with retromuscular mesh placement. This technique involves placing prosthetic mesh in the extraperitoneal position in the preperitoneal space or retrorectus position. This technique was initially described by Stoppa.[9] A large piece of mesh is placed in the retromuscular space on top of the posterior rectus sheath or peritoneum. The compartment is accessed through an incision in the posterior rectus sheath approximately 1 cm from the medial edge of the rectus muscle. This space must be dissected laterally on both sides of the linea alba to a distance of 8 to 10 cm beyond the defect. Both leaflets of the posterior sheath are then sutured together to create an

Mesh placement options

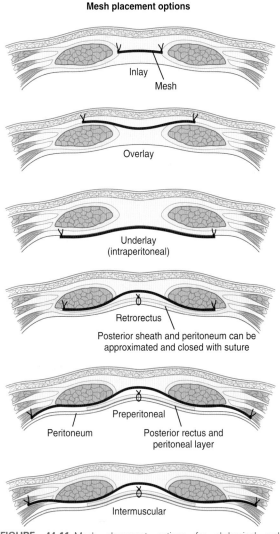

FIGURE 44-11 Mesh placement options for abdominal wall reconstruction.

extraperitoneal pocket in which to place the prosthetic material. The prosthetic mesh extends 5 to 6 cm beyond the superior and inferior borders of the defect. The use of transfascial sutures to secure the mesh remains controversial, and no definitive evidence exists supporting either approach. The authors selectively use transfascial sutures. With smaller defects, the mesh does not need to be sutured because it is held in place by intra-abdominal pressure (Pascal's principle), allowing eventual incorporation into the surrounding tissues. Alternatively, in larger defects, the mesh can be secured laterally with several sutures. This approach avoids contact between the mesh and abdominal viscera and has been shown in long-term studies to have a respectable recurrence rate (14%) in large incisional hernias.

Posterior component separation. The retrorectus space is bordered laterally by the linea semilunaris. In very large hernias or in those patients with atrophic narrowed rectus muscles, this might prevent adequate mesh overlap. Further advancement can be obtained by incising the posterior rectus sheath approximately 1 cm medial to the linea semilunaris. At this location, the posterior leaflet of the internal oblique and the transversus abdominis muscle are incised to gain access to the preperitoneum. This plane can be extended to the retroperitoneum and eventually to the psoas muscle if necessary.[54] Very large sheets of prosthetic mesh can be placed in this location with wide defect coverage.[55] A retrospective review from the Mayo Clinic, with a median follow-up of 5 years, has documented a 5% overall hernia recurrence rate in 254 patients who underwent complex ventral hernia repair during a 13-year period.[43] In one comparative analysis of posterior and anterior component separation, similar amount of fascial advancement was reported with a significant reduction in wound morbidity with use of the posterior approach.[55]

Anterior component separation. Another option for the repair of complex or large ventral defects is the anterior component separation technique (Fig. 44-12). This involves separating the lateral muscle layers of the abdominal wall to allow their advancement. Primary fascial closure at the midline is often possible. The procedure is performed by raising large subcutaneous flaps above the external oblique fascia. These flaps are carried laterally past the linea semilunaris. This lipocutaneous dissection itself can provide some advancement of the abdominal wall. Large perforating subcutaneous vessels can be preserved to prevent ischemic necrosis of the skin flaps. A relaxing incision is made 2 cm lateral to the linea semilunaris on the lateral external oblique aponeurosis from several centimeters above the costal margin to the pubis. The external oblique is then bluntly separated in the avascular plane, away from the internal oblique, allowing its advancement. Further relaxing incisions have been described to the aponeurotic layers of the internal oblique or transversus abdominis, but this can result in problematic lateral bulges or herniation at this site. Additional release can be safely achieved by incising the posterior rectus sheath. These techniques, when applied to both sides of the abdominal wall, can yield up to 20 cm of mobilization. Although this technique often allows tension-free closure of these large defects, recurrence rates as low as 20% have been reported with the use of prosthetic reinforcement in large hernias.[56] It is important that patients understand that a lateral bulge can occur after release of the external oblique aponeurosis. Recognizing the high recurrence rates with component separation alone, several authors have reported small series of biologic mesh reinforcement of these repairs.[51] To date, no randomized controlled trials have supported a lower recurrence rate with biologic prosthetic reinforcement. If a bioprosthetic is placed, it can be

secured with an underlay or onlay technique. No comparative data exist demonstrating the superiority of either repair technique.[57]

Endoscopic component separation. One of the major limitations of open component separation is that large skin flaps are necessary to access the lateral abdominal wall musculature. Recognizing these limitations, innovative, minimally invasive approaches to component separation have been described.[58] The basic principle of a minimally invasive component separation is to gain direct access to the lateral abdominal wall without creating a lipocutaneous flap. Typically, this is performed by a direct cutdown through a 1-cm incision off the tip of the 11th rib overlying the external oblique muscle (Fig. 44-13). The external oblique is split in the line of its fibers, and a standard bilateral inguinal hernia balloon dissector is placed in between the external and internal oblique muscles, toward the pubis. Three laparoscopic trocars are placed in the space created, and the dissection is carried from the pubis to several centimeters above the costal margin. The linea semilunaris is carefully identified, and the external oblique is incised from beneath the muscle, at least 2 cm lateral to the linea semilunaris. The muscle is released from the pubis to several centimeters above the costal margin. This procedure is performed bilaterally. Synthetic or biologic mesh can be used to reinforce the repair of the midline closure. These relatively new techniques are feasible, but long-term data demonstrating equivalency to open techniques are lacking.

Results of Incisional Hernia Repairs

Several prospective randomized trials have compared laparoscopic and open ventral hernia repairs (Table 44-5).[59-63] Although most of these studies were small, with fewer than 100 patients, the results tend to favor a laparoscopic approach for small to medium-sized defects. The incidences of postoperative complications and recurrence were less in hernias repaired laparoscopically. Several retrospective reports have demonstrated similar advantages for a laparoscopic approach. Based on the comparative trials listed in Table 44-5, laparoscopic incisional hernia repair results in fewer postoperative complications, lower infection rate, and decreased hernia recurrence.[54,56-60,64] Until an appropriately powered prospective randomized trial is performed, the ideal approach will largely be based on surgeon expertise and preference. In addition, these trials will need to provide guidance on the most appropriate hernia size to be repaired by either an open or a laparoscopic approach.

UNUSUAL HERNIAS

There are a number of hernias that occur infrequently, of various types.

Types
Spigelian Hernia
A spigelian hernia occurs through the spigelian fascia, which is composed of the aponeurotic layer between the rectus muscle medially and semilunar line laterally. Almost all spigelian hernias occur at or below the arcuate line. The absence of posterior rectus fascia may contribute to an inherent weakness in this area. These hernias are often interparietal, with the hernia sac dissecting posterior to the external oblique aponeurosis. Most spigelian hernias are small (1 to 2 cm in diameter) and develop during the fourth to seventh decades of life. Patients often present with localized

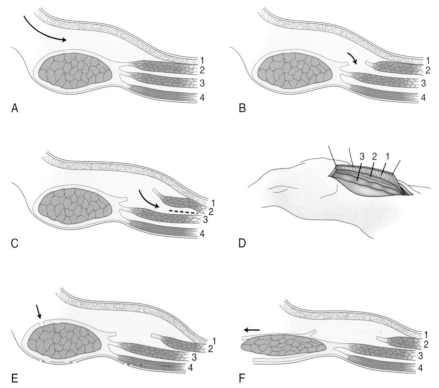

FIGURE 44-12 Component Separation Technique. A, The skin and subcutaneous fat are dissected free from the anterior sheath of the rectus abdominis muscle and the aponeurosis of the external abdominal oblique muscle. **B,** The external abdominal oblique is incised 1 to 2 cm lateral to the rectus abdominis muscle. **C,** The external abdominal oblique is separated from the internal abdominal oblique. **D,** The dissection is carried to the posterior axillary line. **E,** Additional length can be achieved by incising the posterior rectus sheath above the arcuate line. **F,** Care must be taken to avoid damaging the nerves and blood supply that enter the rectus abdominis posteriorly. (From de Vries Reilingh TS, van Goor H, Rosman C, et al: Components separation technique for the repair of large abdominal wall hernias. *J Am Coll Surg* 196:32–37, 2003.)

pain in the area without a bulge because the hernia lies beneath the intact external oblique aponeurosis. Ultrasound or CT of the abdomen can be useful to establish the diagnosis.

A spigelian hernia is repaired because of the risk for incarceration associated with its relatively narrow neck. The hernia site is marked before operation. A transverse incision is made over the defect and carried through the external oblique aponeurosis. The hernia sac is opened, dissected free of the neck of the hernia, and excised or inverted. The defect is closed transversely by simple suture repair of the transversus abdominis and internal oblique muscles, followed by closure of the external oblique aponeurosis. Larger defects are repaired with a mesh prosthesis. Recurrence is uncommon.

Obturator Hernia

The obturator canal is formed by the union of the pubic bone and ischium. This canal is covered by a membrane pierced at the medial and superior border by the obturator nerve and vessels. Weakening of the obturator membrane may result in enlargement of the canal and formation of a hernia sac, which can lead to intestinal incarceration and strangulation. The patient can present with evidence of compression of the obturator nerve, which causes pain in the anteromedial aspect of the thigh (Howship-Romberg sign) that is relieved by thigh flexion. Almost 50% of patients

with obturator hernia present with complete or partial bowel obstruction. An abdominal CT scan can establish the diagnosis, if necessary.

A posterior approach, open or laparoscopic, is preferred. This approach provides direct access to the hernia. After reduction of the hernia sac and contents, any preperitoneal fat within the obturator canal is reduced. If necessary, the obturator foramen is opened posterior to the nerve and vessels. The obturator nerve can be manipulated gently with a blunt nerve hook to facilitate reduction of the fat pad. The obturator foramen is repaired with prosthetic mesh, with care taken to avoid injury to the obturator nerve and vessels. Patients with compromised bowel usually require laparotomy.

Lumbar Hernia

Lumbar hernias can be congenital or acquired after an operation on the flank and occur in the lumbar region of the posterior abdominal wall. Hernias through the superior lumbar triangle (Grynfeltt triangle) are more common. The superior lumbar triangle is bounded by the 12th rib, paraspinal muscles, and internal oblique muscle. Less common are hernias through the inferior lumbar triangle (Petit triangle), which is bounded by the iliac crest, latissimus dorsi muscle, and external oblique muscle. Weakness of the lumbodorsal fascia through either of these areas results

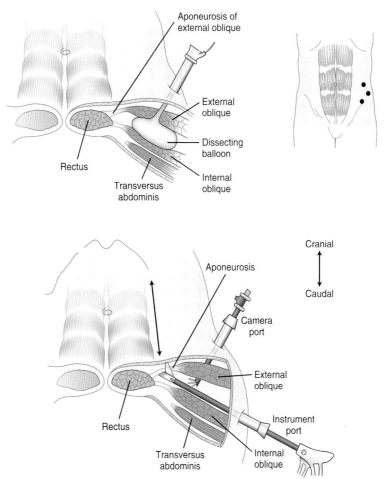

FIGURE 44-13 Endoscopic component separation: port placement and surgical technique.

TABLE 44-5 Comparative Randomized Studies Between Open and Laparoscopic Ventral Hernia Repair

STUDY	NO. OF PATIENTS		MESH USED		INTRAOPERATIVE COMPLICATIONS (%)		LOS (DAYS)		POSTOPERATIVE COMPLICATIONS (%)		FOLLOW-UP (MONTHS)		RECURRENCE (%)	
	LAP	OPEN	LAP	OPEN	LAP	OPEN	LAP	OPEN	LAP	OPEN	LAP	OPEN	LAP	OPEN
McGreevy et al,[60] 2003	65	71	ePTFE or polyester + collagen	PP	N/A	N/A	1.1	1.5	7.70	21.10	N/A	N/A	N/A	N/A
Lomanto et al,[61] 2006	50	50	Polyester + collagen	ePTFE	2	2	2.74	4.7	26	40	19.6	21	2	10
Bingener et al,[62] 2007	127	233	ePTFE, PP, or ePTFE	PP	N/A	N/A	N/A	N/A	33.10	43.30	36	36	13	9
Olmi et al,[59] 2007	85	85	Polyester + collagen	PP	N/A	N/A	2.7	9.9	16.50	29.40	24	24	2	4
Pring et al,[73] 2008	31	27	PTFE	PTFE	N/A	N/A	1	1	33	49	28	28	3.30	4.20
Asencio et al,[74] 2009	45	39	PTFE or PP	PP	6.70	0	3.46	3.33	5.20	33.30	12	12	9.70	7.90

ePTFE, expanded polytetrafluoroethylene; *LAP,* laparoscopic; *LOS,* length of stay; *N/A,* not available; *PP,* polypropylene.

in progressive protrusion of extraperitoneal fat and a hernia sac. Lumbar hernias are not prone to incarceration. Small lumbar hernias are frequently asymptomatic. Larger hernias may be associated with back pain. CT is useful for diagnosis.

Both open and laparoscopic repairs are useful. Satisfactory suture repair is difficult because of the immobile bone margins of these defects. Repair is best done by placement of prosthetic mesh, which is sutured beyond the margins of the hernia. There is usually sufficient fascia over the bone to anchor the mesh.

Interparietal Hernia

Interparietal hernias are rare and occur when the hernia sac lies between layers of the abdominal wall. These hernias most frequently occur in previous incisions. Spigelian hernias are almost always interparietal.

The correct preoperative diagnosis of interparietal hernia can be difficult. Many patients with complicated interparietal hernias present with intestinal obstruction. Abdominal CT can assist in the diagnosis. Large interparietal hernias usually require placement of prosthetic mesh for closure. When this cannot be done, the component separation technique may be useful to provide natural tissues to obliterate the defect.

Sciatic Hernia

The greater sciatic foramen can be a site of hernia formation. These hernias are extremely unusual and difficult to diagnose and frequently are asymptomatic until intestinal obstruction occurs. In the absence of intestinal obstruction, the most common symptom is the presence of an uncomfortable or slowly enlarging mass in the gluteal or intragluteal area. Sciatic nerve pain can occur, but sciatic hernia is a rare cause of sciatic neuralgia.

A transperitoneal approach is preferred if bowel obstruction or strangulation is suspected. Hernia contents can usually be reduced with gentle traction. Prosthetic mesh repair is usually preferred. A transgluteal approach can be used if the diagnosis is certain and the hernia is reducible, but most surgeons are not familiar with this approach. With the patient prone, an incision is made from the posterior edge of the greater trochanter across the hernia mass. The gluteus maximus muscle is opened, and the sac is visualized. The muscle edges of the defect are reapproximated with interrupted sutures, or the defect is obliterated with mesh.

Perineal Hernia

Perineal hernias are caused by congenital or acquired defects and are uncommon. These hernias may also occur after abdominoperineal resection or perineal prostatectomy. The hernia sac protrudes through the pelvic diaphragm. Primary perineal hernias are rare, occur most commonly in older multiparous women, and can be quite large. Symptoms are usually related to protrusion of a mass through the defect that is worsened by sitting or standing. A bulge is frequently detected on bimanual rectal-vaginal examination.

Perineal hernias are generally repaired through a transabdominal approach or combined transabdominal and perineal approaches. After the sac contents are reduced, small defects may be closed with nonabsorbable suture, whereas large defects are repaired with prosthetic mesh.

Loss of Domain Hernias

Loss of domain implies a massive hernia in which the herniated contents have resided for so long outside the abdominal cavity that they cannot simply be replaced into the peritoneal cavity. We typically classify loss of domain hernias into patients with and

without preoperative contamination. Each group is then subcategorized into two groups. Patients with a small hernia defect and a massive hernia sac (e.g., large inguinoscrotal hernias) require restoration of peritoneal cavity domain, whereas patients with a large defect and a massive hernia sac (open abdomen with skin graft) require restoration of peritoneal domain and complex reconstruction of the abdominal wall.

Before repair of these complex defects, the patient must undergo careful preoperative evaluation. A clear understanding of the morbidity and mortality associated with these reconstructive procedures is critical. Weight reduction, smoking cessation, optimization of nutrition, and glucose control are all important aspects of complex abdominal wall reconstruction. Previously, methods to stretch the abdominal wall gradually were used to allow the restoration of abdominal domain and closure. This was accomplished by insufflation of air into the abdominal cavity to create a progressive pneumoperitoneum. Repeated administrations of increasing volumes of air during 1 to 3 weeks allowed the muscles of the abdominal wall to become lax enough for primary closure of the defect. This technique is particularly suited for small defects and massive hernia sacs.[65] For large defects, some authors have also described a staged approach using ePTFE dual mesh for patients with loss of abdominal domain and lateral retraction of the abdominal wall musculature. The initial stage involves reduction of the hernia and placement of a large sheet of ePTFE dual mesh secured to the fascial edges with a running suture. Subsequent stages involve serial elliptical excision of the mesh until the fascia can be approximated in the midline without tension. Finally, the mesh is completely excised, and the fascia is reapproximated with component separation and a biologic underlay patch, if necessary.[66] This approach is technically feasible but does require multiple operations and long hospital stays, and it is associated with a fairly high morbidity rate.

Parastomal Hernia Repair

Parastomal hernia is a common complication of stoma creation. In fact, the creation of a stoma by strict definition is an abdominal wall hernia. The incidence of parastomal hernias is highest for colostomies and occurs in up to 50% of stomas. Fortunately, most patients remain asymptomatic, and life-threatening complications, such as bowel obstruction and strangulation, are rare. Unlike midline incisional hernia repair, routine repair of parastomal hernias is not recommended. Surgical repair should be reserved for patients experiencing symptoms of bowel obstruction, problems with pouch fit, or cosmetic issues.

Three general approaches are available for parastomal hernia repair. These techniques include primary fascial repair, stoma relocation, and prosthetic repair. Primary fascial repair involves hernia reduction and primary fascial reapproximation through a peristomal incision. This technique carries a predictably high recurrence rate. The advantage of this approach is that the abdomen often is not entered, making the operation less complex. Because of the high recurrence rate with this technique, it should be reserved for patients who will not tolerate a laparotomy. Stoma relocation improves results; however, it requires a laparotomy and predisposes to another parastomal hernia in the future. To reduce the rate of recurrent herniation, some surgeons reinforce the repair with biologic or synthetic mesh in a keyhole fashion around the new stoma site. Early results are promising, but long-term outcomes have not yet been reported.[67] Prosthetic repairs of parastomal hernias can provide excellent long-term results with a lower rate of hernia recurrence, but a higher rate of prosthetic complications must be accepted.

Regardless of the technique, a permanent foreign body placed in apposition to the bowel can result in erosion, obstruction, and disastrous complications. Several approaches to prosthetic mesh placement have been described. The mesh can be placed as an onlay patch, intra-abdominally, or in the retrorectus position. When the mesh is placed intraperitoneally, a keyhole is fashioned around the stoma site or placed as a flat sheet, lateralizing the stoma as it exits the abdomen, as described by Sugarbaker.[68] Several authors have described laparoscopic approaches to parastomal hernia repair, including keyhole and Sugarbaker-type repairs[69,70] (Fig. 44-14). A retromuscular repair that takes advantage of many of the advanced reconstructive techniques described in this chapter has recently been reported. In this approach, a laparotomy is performed, and the stoma is taken down and eventually resited to the contralateral side of the abdomen. A posterior component separation is then performed; a large mesh is deployed in the retromuscular space to cover the old stoma site and the entire midline incision, and it is used to prophylactically reinforce the new stoma site. The stoma is eventually brought out through a keyhole incision in the mesh and matured.[71] All these series are fairly small with fewer than 100 patients and have reported only short-term to medium-term follow-up, limiting our ability to make clear recommendations for this difficult problem.

Complications
Mesh Infection

Mesh infections are serious complications that can be difficult to treat. If ePTFE becomes infected, it requires removal with the resultant morbidity of another defect, which often must be closed under tension, leading to inevitable recurrence. In open ventral hernia repair, incisional and mesh infections are not infrequent. Use of the laparoscopic technique and placement of a large piece of mesh without undermining large subcutaneous tissue flaps avoid wound complications. In a series of almost 1000 patients who had laparoscopic ventral hernia repair, mesh infections occurred in less than 1% of cases.[72] Perhaps the greatest advantage of the laparoscopic approach for repairing ventral hernias is this reduction in infectious complications. Two randomized controlled trials have compared laparoscopic and open ventral hernia repair.[73,74]

Seromas

Seroma formation can occur after laparoscopic and open ventral hernia repair. In open ventral hernia repair, drains are often placed in an attempt to obliterate the dead space caused by the hernia and tissue dissection. These drains can cause mesh contamination, and seromas can form after drain removal. With laparoscopic repair, the hernia sac is not resected, and a seroma cavity will result. Most of these seromas will resolve over time as the mesh becomes incorporated on the hernia sac. Preoperative discussions with the patient describing the expectations of a temporary seroma are imperative before laparoscopic ventral hernia repair. We reserve aspiration for symptomatic or persistent seromas after 6 to 8 weeks.

Enterotomy

Intestinal injury during adhesiolysis can be catastrophic. Management of an enterotomy during a hernia repair is controversial and depends on the segment of intestine injured (small versus large bowel) and amount of spillage. Options include aborting the hernia repair, using a primary tissue or biologic tissue repair, and performing a delayed repair with prosthetic mesh in 3 to 4 days. When there is gross contamination, the use of synthetic mesh is contraindicated.

SELECTED REFERENCES

Anson BJ, McVay CB: Inguinal hernia: The anatomy of the region. *Surg Gynecol Obstet* 66:186–191, 1938.

Condon RE: Surgical anatomy of the transversus abdominis and transversalis fascia. *Ann Surg* 173:1–5, 1971.

Nyhus LM: An anatomic reappraisal of the posterior inguinal wall, with special consideration of the iliopubic tract and its relation to groin hernias. *Surg Clin North Am* 44:1305, 1960.

> These three references are classic descriptions of the anatomy of the groin. All are well illustrated.

Bisgaard T, Bay-Nielsen M, Kehlet H: Re-recurrence after operation for recurrent inguinal hernia. A nationwide 8-year follow-up study on the role of type of repair. *Ann Surg* 247:707–711, 2008.

> This long term population-based study provides useful information about the results of recurrent inguinal hernia repairs.

de Vries Reilingh TS, van Goor H, Charbon JA, et al: Repair of giant midline abdominal wall hernias: "Components separation technique" versus prosthetic repair: Interim analysis of a randomized controlled trial. *World J Surg* 31:756–763, 2007.

> This is a prospective randomized trial evaluating outcomes of open ventral hernia repair with synthetic mesh versus component separation without reinforcement.

Fitzgibbons RJ, Jr, Forse RA: Clinical practice. Groin hernias in adults. *N Engl J Med* 372:756–763, 2015.

> Recent review of the diagnosis and management of groin hernias in adults.

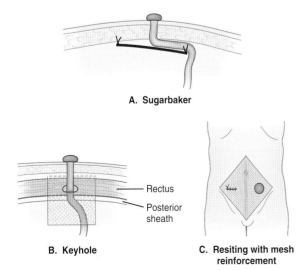

A. Sugarbaker

B. Keyhole

Rectus

Posterior sheath

C. Resiting with mesh reinforcement

FIGURE 44-14 Surgical approaches for parastomal hernia repair.

Forbes SS, Eskicioglu C, McLeod RS, et al: Meta-analysis of randomized controlled trials comparing open and laparoscopic ventral and incisional hernia repair with mesh. *Br J Surg* 96:851–858, 2009.

This is a meta-analysis evaluating eight prospective randomized trials comparing laparoscopic with open ventral hernia repair.

Itani KM, Hur K, Kim LT, et al: Veterans Affairs Ventral Incisional Hernia Investigators: Comparison of laparoscopic and open repair with mesh for the treatment of ventral incisional hernia: A randomized trial. *Arch Surg* 145:322–328, 2010.

This is a prospective randomized trial evaluating laparoscopic versus open ventral hernia repairs.

Neumayer L, Giobbie-Hurder A, Jonasson O, et al: Open mesh versus laparoscopic mesh repair of inguinal hernia. *N Engl J Med* 350:1819–1827, 2004.

Excellent prospective randomized trial comparing these two types of hernia repairs in Veterans Administration hospitals.

Zhao G, Gao P, Ma B, et al: Open mesh techniques for inguinal hernia repair: A meta-analysis of randomized controlled trials. *Ann Surg* 250:35–42, 2009.

Excellent meta-analysis of various techniques of tension-free repairs.

REFERENCES

1. Bradley M, Morgan D, Pentlow B, et al: The groin hernia—an ultrasound diagnosis? *Ann R Coll Surg Engl* 85:178–180, 2003.
2. Della Santa V, Groebli Y: [Diagnosis of non-hernia groin masses]. *Ann Chir* 125:179–183, 2000.
3. Fitzgibbons RJ, Jr, Giobbie-Hurder A, Gibbs JO, et al: Watchful waiting vs repair of inguinal hernia in minimally symptomatic men: a randomized clinical trial. *JAMA* 295:285–292, 2006.
4. Fitzgibbons RJ, Jr, Ramanan B, Arya S, et al: Long-term results of a randomized controlled trial of a nonoperative strategy (watchful waiting) for men with minimally symptomatic inguinal hernias. *Ann Surg* 258:508–515, 2013.
5. Chung L, Norrie J, O'Dwyer PJ: Long-term follow-up of patients with a painless inguinal hernia from a randomized clinical trial. *Br J Surg* 98:596–599, 2011.
6. Lichtenstein IL, Shulman AG, Amid PK, et al: The tension-free hernioplasty. *Am J Surg* 157:188–193, 1989.
7. Gilbert AI: Sutureless repair of inguinal hernia. *Am J Surg* 163:331–335, 1992.
8. Kugel RD: Minimally invasive, nonlaparoscopic, preperitoneal, and sutureless, inguinal herniorrhaphy. *Am J Surg* 178:298–302, 1999.
9. Stoppa RE: The treatment of complicated groin and incisional hernias. *World J Surg* 13:545–554, 1989.
10. Malangoni MA, Condon RE: Preperitoneal repair of acute incarcerated and strangulated hernias of the groin. *Surg Gynecol Obstet* 162:65–67, 1986.
11. Ahmad G, Duffy JM, Phillips K, et al: Laparoscopic entry techniques. *Cochrane Database Syst Rev* (2):CD006583, 2008.
12. Voyles CR, Hamilton BJ, Johnson WD, et al: Meta-analysis of laparoscopic inguinal hernia trials favors open hernia repair with preperitoneal mesh prosthesis. *Am J Surg* 184:6–10, 2002.
13. Bisgaard T, Bay-Nielsen M, Kehlet H: Re-recurrence after operation for recurrent inguinal hernia. A nationwide 8-year follow-up study on the role of type of repair. *Ann Surg* 247:707–711, 2008.
14. Nordin P, Haapaniemi S, van der Linden W, et al: Choice of anesthesia and risk of reoperation for recurrence in groin hernia repair. *Ann Surg* 240:187–192, 2004.
15. Neumayer L, Giobbie-Hurder A, Jonasson O, et al: Open mesh versus laparoscopic mesh repair of inguinal hernia. *N Engl J Med* 350:1819–1827, 2004.
16. McCormack K, Scott NW, Go PM, et al: Laparoscopic techniques versus open techniques for inguinal hernia repair. *Cochrane Database Syst Rev* (1):CD001785, 2003.
17. Amato B, Moja L, Panico S, et al: Shouldice technique versus other open techniques for inguinal hernia repair. *Cochrane Database Syst Rev* (4):CD001543, 2012.
18. Zhao G, Gao P, Ma B, et al: Open mesh techniques for inguinal hernia repair: A meta-analysis of randomized controlled trials. *Ann Surg* 250:35–42, 2009.
19. Schroder DM, Lloyd LR, Boccaccio JE, et al: Inguinal hernia recurrence following preperitoneal Kugel patch repair. *Am Surg* 70:132–136, discussion 136, 2004.
20. EU Hernia Trialists Collaboration: Repair of groin hernia with synthetic mesh: Meta-analysis of randomized controlled trials. *Ann Surg* 235:322–332, 2002.
21. El-Dhuwaib Y, Corless D, Emmett C, et al: Laparoscopic versus open repair of inguinal hernia: A longitudinal cohort study. *Surg Endosc* 27:936–945, 2013.
22. O'Reilly EA, Burke JP, O'Connell PR: A meta-analysis of surgical morbidity and recurrence after laparoscopic and open repair of primary unilateral inguinal hernia. *Ann Surg* 255:846–853, 2012.
23. Wake BL, McCormack K, Fraser C, et al: Transabdominal pre-peritoneal (TAPP) vs totally extraperitoneal (TEP) laparoscopic techniques for inguinal hernia repair. *Cochrane Database Syst Rev* (1):CD004703, 2005.
24. Mikkelsen T, Bay-Nielsen M, Kehlet H: Risk of femoral hernia after inguinal herniorrhaphy. *Br J Surg* 89:486–488, 2002.
25. Kald A, Fridsten S, Nordin P, et al: Outcome of repair of bilateral groin hernias: A prospective evaluation of 1,487 patients. *Eur J Surg* 168:150–153, 2002.
26. Aufenacker TJ, van Geldere D, van Mesdag T, et al: The role of antibiotic prophylaxis in prevention of wound infection after Lichtenstein open mesh repair of primary inguinal hernia: A multicenter double-blind randomized controlled trial. *Ann Surg* 240:955–960, discussion 960–961, 2004.
27. Grant AM, Scott NW, O'Dwyer PJ, et al: Five-year follow-up of a randomized trial to assess pain and numbness after laparoscopic or open repair of groin hernia. *Br J Surg* 91:1570–1574, 2004.
28. Fitzgibbons RJ, Jr, Forse RA: Clinical practice. Groin hernias in adults. *N Engl J Med* 372:756–763, 2015.
29. Simons MP, Aufenacker T, Bay-Nielsen M, et al: European

Hernia Society guidelines on the treatment of inguinal hernia in adult patients. *Hernia* 13:343–403, 2009.

30. Shulman AG, Amid PK, Lichtenstein IL: The 'plug' repair of 1402 recurrent inguinal hernias. 20-year experience. *Arch Surg* 125:265–267, 1990.

31. Haapaniemi S, Gunnarsson U, Nordin P, et al: Reoperation after recurrent groin hernia repair. *Ann Surg* 234:122–126, 2001.

32. Karthikesalingam A, Markar SR, Holt PJ, et al: Meta-analysis of randomized controlled trials comparing laparoscopic with open mesh repair of recurrent inguinal hernia. *Br J Surg* 97:4–11, 2010.

33. Sevonius D, Gunnarsson U, Nordin P, et al: Repeated groin hernia recurrences. *Ann Surg* 249:516–518, 2009.

34. Rucinski J, Margolis M, Panagopoulos G, et al: Closure of the abdominal midline fascia: Meta-analysis delineates the optimal technique. *Am Surg* 67:421–426, 2001.

35. Muysoms FE, Antoniou SA, Bury K, et al: European Hernia Society guidelines on the closure of abdominal wall incisions. *Hernia* 19:1–24, 2015.

36. Carlson MA, Ludwig KA, Condon RE: Ventral hernia and other complications of 1,000 midline incisions. *South Med J* 88:450–453, 1995.

37. Seiler CM, Deckert A, Diener MK, et al: Midline versus transverse incision in major abdominal surgery: A randomized, double-blind equivalence trial (POVATI: ISRCTN60734227). *Ann Surg* 249:913–920, 2009.

38. Luijendijk RW, Hop WC, van den Tol MP, et al: A comparison of suture repair with mesh repair for incisional hernia. *N Engl J Med* 343:392–398, 2000.

39. Wright BE, Beckerman J, Cohen M, et al: Is laparoscopic umbilical hernia repair with mesh a reasonable alternative to conventional repair? *Am J Surg* 184:505–508, discussion 508–509, 2002.

40. Petro CC, O'Rourke CP, Posielski NM, et al: Designing a ventral hernia staging system. *Hernia* 2015. [Epub ahead of print].

41. Anthony T, Bergen PC, Kim LT, et al: Factors affecting recurrence following incisional herniorrhaphy. *World J Surg* 24:95–100, discussion 101, 2000.

42. Leber GE, Garb JL, Alexander AI, et al: Long-term complications associated with prosthetic repair of incisional hernias. *Arch Surg* 133:378–382, 1998.

43. Koch A, Bringman S, Myrelid P, et al: Randomized clinical trial of groin hernia repair with titanium-coated lightweight mesh compared with standard polypropylene mesh. *Br J Surg* 95:1226–1231, 2008.

44. Conze J, Kingsnorth AN, Flament JB, et al: Randomized clinical trial comparing lightweight composite mesh with polyester or polypropylene mesh for incisional hernia repair. *Br J Surg* 92:1488–1493, 2005.

45. Petro CC, Nahabet EH, Criss CN, et al: Central failures of lightweight monofilament polyester mesh causing hernia recurrence: A cautionary note. *Hernia* 19:155–159, 2015.

46. Cobb WS, Warren JA, Ewing JA, et al: Open retromuscular mesh repair of complex incisional hernia: Predictors of wound events and recurrence. *J Am Coll Surg* 220:606–613, 2015.

47. Diaz-Godoy A, Garcia-Urena MA, Lopez-Monclus J, et al: Searching for the best polypropylene mesh to be used in bowel contamination. *Hernia* 15:173–179, 2011.

48. Harth KC, Blatnik JA, Anderson JM, et al: Effect of surgical wound classification on biologic graft performance in complex hernia repair: An experimental study. *Surgery* 153:481–492, 2013.

49. Carbonell AM, Criss CN, Cobb WS, et al: Outcomes of synthetic mesh in contaminated ventral hernia repairs. *J Am Coll Surg* 217:991–998, 2013.

50. Rosen MJ: Polyester-based mesh for ventral hernia repair: Is it safe? *Am J Surg* 197:353–359, 2009.

51. Jin J, Rosen MJ, Blatnik J, et al: Use of acellular dermal matrix for complicated ventral hernia repair: Does technique affect outcomes? *J Am Coll Surg* 205:654–660, 2007.

52. Rosen MJ, Krpata DM, Ermlich B, et al: A 5-year clinical experience with single-staged repairs of infected and contaminated abdominal wall defects utilizing biologic mesh. *Ann Surg* 257:991–996, 2013.

53. de Vries Reilingh TS, van Geldere D, Langenhorst B, et al: Repair of large midline incisional hernias with polypropylene mesh: Comparison of three operative techniques. *Hernia* 8:56–59, 2004.

54. Novitsky YW, Porter JR, Rucho ZC, et al: Open preperitoneal retrofascial mesh repair for multiply recurrent ventral incisional hernias. *J Am Coll Surg* 203:283–289, 2006.

55. Krpata DM, Blatnik JA, Novitsky YW, et al: Posterior and open anterior components separations: A comparative analysis. *Am J Surg* 203:318–322, discussion 322, 2012.

56. de Vries Reilingh TS, van Goor H, Charbon JA, et al: Repair of giant midline abdominal wall hernias: "Components separation technique" versus prosthetic repair : Interim analysis of a randomized controlled trial. *World J Surg* 31:756–763, 2007.

57. Ewart CJ, Lankford AB, Gamboa MG: Successful closure of abdominal wall hernias using the components separation technique. *Ann Plast Surg* 50:269–273, discussion 273–274, 2003.

58. Rosen MJ, Jin J, McGee MF, et al: Laparoscopic component separation in the single-stage treatment of infected abdominal wall prosthetic removal. *Hernia* 11:435–440, 2007.

59. Olmi S, Scaini A, Cesana GC, et al: Laparoscopic versus open incisional hernia repair: An open randomized controlled study. *Surg Endosc* 21:555–559, 2007.

60. McGreevy JM, Goodney PP, Birkmeyer CM, et al: A prospective study comparing the complication rates between laparoscopic and open ventral hernia repairs. *Surg Endosc* 17:1778–1780, 2003.

61. Lomanto D, Iyer SG, Shabbir A, et al: Laparoscopic versus open ventral hernia mesh repair: A prospective study. *Surg Endosc* 20:1030–1035, 2006.

62. Bingener J, Buck L, Richards M, et al: Long-term outcomes in laparoscopic vs open ventral hernia repair. *Arch Surg* 142:562–567, 2007.

63. DeMaria EJ, Moss JM, Sugerman HJ: Laparoscopic intraperitoneal polytetrafluoroethylene (PTFE) prosthetic patch repair of ventral hernia. Prospective comparison to open prefascial polypropylene mesh repair. *Surg Endosc* 14:326–329, 2000.

64. Iqbal CW, Pham TH, Joseph A, et al: Long-term outcome of 254 complex incisional hernia repairs using the modified Rives-Stoppa technique. *World J Surg* 31:2398–2404, 2007.

65. McAdory RS, Cobb WS, Carbonell AM: Progressive preoperative pneumoperitoneum for hernias with loss of domain. *Am Surg* 75:504–508, discussion 508–509, 2009.

66. Lipman J, Medalie D, Rosen MJ: Staged repair of massive incisional hernias with loss of abdominal domain: A novel approach. *Am J Surg* 195:84–88, 2008.

67. Taner T, Cima RR, Larson DW, et al: The use of human acellular dermal matrix for parastomal hernia repair in patients with inflammatory bowel disease: A novel technique to repair fascial defects. *Dis Colon Rectum* 52:349–354, 2009.

68. Sugarbaker PH: Peritoneal approach to prosthetic mesh repair of paraostomy hernias. *Ann Surg* 201:344–346, 1985.

69. Byers JM, Steinberg JB, Postier RG: Repair of parastomal hernias using polypropylene mesh. *Arch Surg* 127:1246–1247, 1992.

70. Janes A, Cengiz Y, Israelsson LA: Randomized clinical trial of the use of a prosthetic mesh to prevent parastomal hernia. *Br J Surg* 91:280–282, 2004.

71. Raigani S, Criss CN, Petro CC, et al: Single-center experience with parastomal hernia repair using retromuscular mesh placement. *J Gastrointest Surg* 18:1673–1677, 2014.

72. Heniford BT, Park A, Ramshaw BJ, et al: Laparoscopic repair of ventral hernias: Nine years' experience with 850 consecutive hernias. *Ann Surg* 238:391–399, discussion 399–400, 2003.

73. Pring CM, Tran V, O'Rourke N, et al: Laparoscopic versus open ventral hernia repair: A randomized controlled trial. *ANZ J Surg* 78:903–906, 2008.

74. Asencio F, Aguilo J, Peiro S, et al: Open randomized clinical trial of laparoscopic versus open incisional hernia repair. *Surg Endosc* 23:1441–1448, 2009.

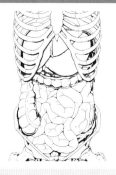

CHAPTER 45

Acute Abdomen

Ronald Squires, Steven N. Carter, Russell G. Postier

第四十五章 急腹症

中文导读

　　本章共分为12节：①解剖和生理；②病史；③体格检查；④实验室检查；⑤影像学检查；⑥腹腔内压力监测；⑦腹腔镜诊断；⑧鉴别诊断；⑨急诊手术术前准备；⑩特殊病人；⑪急腹症诊断流程；⑫总结。

　　第一节从解剖和生理方面介绍了内脏痛、腹壁痛和牵涉痛的成因、特点及鉴别要点。着重介绍了急腹症的常见病因，腹膜炎病理生理变化和分类，以及不同类型腹膜炎在常见病因、病原学特点、病理生理变化及临床表现方面的异同。

　　第二节介绍了病史采集的重要性和问诊技巧。病史采集需要注意的因素有：腹痛的起病缓急、疼痛程度、起始部位、放射痛范围、随时间的变化、加重因素；恶心、呕吐、腹泻、便秘、黑便等伴随症状；既往疾病、手术、药物使用史、月经史等，它们均对疾病诊断具有重要的指导意义。

　　第三节是关于体格检查，详细介绍了在急腹症诊断中，视诊、听诊、叩诊和触诊等体格检查的流程、内容、阳性体征的临床意义和操作时的注意事项。列举了具有重要诊断价值的典型征象：如Murphy征、腰大肌征等。

　　第四节主要讲述急腹症需要常规完善的实验室检查项目、临床意义。包括血红蛋白水平、白细胞分类计数、血清肌酐、尿素氮、淀粉酶和脂肪酶、尿HCG、大便常规等。

　　第五节主要讲述影像学检查方法在急腹症诊断中的作用及各种检查项目的优点和局限。CT不受肠气干扰，分辨率高，在急腹症的诊断方面有重要的价值。腹部平片适用于消化道穿孔、钙化病灶、肠梗阻的诊断。受肠气干扰的限制，腹部超声主要用于胆囊结石、胆管结石、泌尿系统和卵巢附件的检查，其价值逊于CT。

　　第六节主要介绍了腹腔压力的正常值，监测方法，升高的原因、以及在急腹症诊断治疗中的临床意义。重点讲述了腹腔内压力的分级及临床意义，特别是强调3～4级腹腔高压是剖腹探查的指征。

第七节主要讲述诊断性腹腔镜探查与传统超声、CT、腹腔灌洗相比具有更高的准确性（90%～100%）和敏感度，诊断的同时还可以进行相应治疗，由于可以避免开腹，尤其适用于重症病人。

第八节主要讲述急腹症的鉴别流程和注意事项。急腹症的鉴别诊断范围很大，通常根据病史、体格检查得到初步诊断并根据实验室检查和影像学检查进一步修正诊断。无法行CT等检查的重症病人可在床边行腹腔灌洗检查。如无法明确诊断而病情十分危重，应

果断行剖腹或腹腔镜探查。

第九节介绍了急腹症急诊手术术前常规处理，包括纠正水电解质酸碱平衡紊乱，抗生素的使用，留置胃管尿管，血型和交叉配血。同时把握手术时机，避免过分追求病人术前状况稳定而贻误最佳手术时机。

第十节主要介绍孕妇、儿童、合并重症疾病、免疫缺陷、病态肥胖等特殊人群急腹症的特点、诊断治疗面临的问题、解决方法和注意事项。

第十一节主要介绍了根据急腹症起病缓急，疼痛部位总结的诊断流程，对快速诊断和及时治疗具有一定的指导作用。

〔陈　琳〕

The term *acute abdomen* refers to signs and symptoms of abdominal pain and tenderness, a clinical presentation that often requires emergency surgical therapy. This challenging clinical scenario requires a thorough and expeditious workup to determine the need for operative intervention and to initiate appropriate therapy. Many diseases, some of which are not surgical or even intra-abdominal,[1] can produce acute abdominal pain and tenderness. Therefore, every attempt should be made to make a correct diagnosis so that the chosen therapy, often a laparoscopy or laparotomy, is appropriate. Despite improvements in laboratory and imaging studies, history and physical examination remain the mainstays of determining the correct diagnosis and initiating proper and timely therapy.

The diagnoses associated with an acute abdomen vary according to age and gender.[2] Appendicitis is more common in the young, whereas biliary disease, bowel obstruction, intestinal ischemia and infarction, and diverticulitis are more common in the elderly. Most of these diagnoses result from infection, obstruction, ischemia, or perforation.

Nonsurgical causes of an acute abdomen can be divided into three categories: endocrine and metabolic, hematologic, and toxins or drugs (Box 45-1).[3] Endocrine and metabolic causes include uremia, diabetic crisis, addisonian crisis, acute intermittent porphyria, acute hyperlipoproteinemia, and hereditary Mediterranean fever. Hematologic disorders are sickle cell crisis, acute leukemia, and other blood dyscrasias. Toxins and drugs causing an acute abdomen include lead and other heavy metal poisoning, narcotic withdrawal, and black widow spider poisoning. It is important to keep these possibilities in mind when evaluating a patient with acute abdominal pain (Box 45-1).

Because of the potential surgical nature of the acute abdomen, an expeditious workup is necessary (Box 45-2). The workup proceeds in the usual order of history, physical examination, and laboratory and imaging studies. Whereas imaging studies have increased the accuracy with which the correct diagnosis can be made, the most important part of the evaluation remains a thorough history and careful physical examination. Laboratory and imaging studies, although usually needed, are directed by the findings on history and physical examination.

ANATOMY AND PHYSIOLOGY

Abdominal pain is conveniently divided into visceral and parietal components. Visceral pain tends to be vague and poorly localized to the epigastrium, periumbilical region, or hypogastrium, depending on its origin from the primitive foregut, midgut, or hindgut (Fig. 45-1). It is usually the result of distention of a hollow viscus. Parietal pain corresponds to the segmental nerve roots innervating the peritoneum and tends to be sharper and better localized. Referred pain is pain perceived at a site distant from the source of stimulus. For example, irritation of the diaphragm may produce pain in the shoulder. Common referred pain sites and their accompanying sources are listed in Box 45-3. Determining whether the pain is visceral, parietal, or referred is important and can usually be done with a careful history.

Introduction of bacteria or irritating chemicals into the peritoneal cavity can cause an outpouring of fluid from the peritoneal membrane. The peritoneum responds to inflammation by increased blood flow, increased permeability, and the formation of a fibrinous exudate on its surface. The bowel also develops local or generalized paralysis. The fibrinous surface and decreased intestinal movement cause adherence between the bowel and omentum or abdominal wall and help to localize inflammation. As a result, an abscess may produce sharply localized pain with normal bowel sounds and gastrointestinal function, whereas a diffuse process, such as a perforated duodenal ulcer, produces generalized abdominal pain with a quiet abdomen. Peritonitis may affect the entire abdominal cavity or a portion of the visceral or parietal peritoneum.

Peritonitis is peritoneal inflammation from any cause. It is usually recognized on physical examination by severe tenderness to palpation, with or without rebound tenderness, and guarding. Peritonitis is usually secondary to an inflammatory insult, most

BOX 45-1 Nonsurgical Causes of the Acute Abdomen

Endocrine and Metabolic Causes
Uremia
Diabetic crisis
Addisonian crisis
Acute intermittent porphyria
Hereditary Mediterranean fever

Hematologic Causes
Sickle cell crisis
Acute leukemia
Other blood dyscrasias

Toxins and Drugs
Lead poisoning
Other heavy metal poisoning
Narcotic withdrawal
Black widow spider poisoning

BOX 45-2 Surgical Acute Abdominal Conditions

Hemorrhage
Solid organ trauma
Leaking or ruptured arterial aneurysm
Ruptured ectopic pregnancy
Bleeding gastrointestinal diverticulum
Arteriovenous malformation of gastrointestinal tract
Intestinal ulceration
Aortoduodenal fistula after aortic vascular graft
Hemorrhagic pancreatitis
Mallory-Weiss syndrome
Spontaneous rupture of spleen

Infection
Appendicitis
Cholecystitis
Meckel's diverticulitis
Hepatic abscess
Diverticular abscess
Psoas abscess

Perforation
Perforated gastrointestinal ulcer
Perforated gastrointestinal cancer
Boerhaave syndrome
Perforated diverticulum

Blockage
Adhesion induction small or large bowel obstruction
Sigmoid volvulus
Cecal volvulus
Incarcerated hernias
Inflammatory bowel disease
Gastrointestinal malignant neoplasm
Intussusception

Ischemia
Buerger disease
Mesenteric thrombosis or embolism
Ovarian torsion
Ischemic colitis
Testicular torsion
Strangulated hernias

often gram-negative infections with enteric organisms or anaerobes. It can result from noninfectious inflammation, a common example being pancreatitis. Primary peritonitis occurs more commonly in children and is most often due to pneumococcus or hemolytic streptococcus.[4] Adults with end-stage renal disease on peritoneal dialysis can develop infections of their peritoneal fluid, with the most common organisms being gram-positive cocci. Adults with ascites and cirrhosis can develop primary peritonitis, and in these cases the organisms are usually *Escherichia coli* and *Klebsiella*.

HISTORY

A detailed and organized history is essential to formulating an accurate differential diagnosis and subsequent treatment regimen. Modern advancements in imaging cannot and will never replace the need for a skilled clinician's careful history and bedside examination. The history must focus not only on the investigation of the pain complaints but also on past problems and associated symptoms as well. Questions should be open ended whenever possible and structured to disclose the onset, character, location, duration, radiation, and chronology of the pain experienced. It is tempting to ask a question such as, Is the pain sharp? or Does eating make it worse? This specific yes or no style can speed up the history taking by not allowing the patient to narrate, but it stands to miss vital details and potentially to skew the responses. A much better questioning style would be, How does the pain feel to you? or Does anything make the pain better or worse? Often, additional information can be gained by observing how the patient describes the pain that is experienced. Pain identified with one finger is often much more localized and typical of parietal innervation or peritoneal inflammation compared with an area of discomfort illustrated with the palm of the hand, which is more typical of the visceral discomfort of bowel or solid organ disease.

The intensity and severity of the pain are related to the underlying tissue damage. Sudden onset of excruciating pain suggests conditions such as intestinal perforation and arterial embolization with ischemia, although other conditions, such as biliary colic, can be manifested suddenly as well. Pain that develops and

worsens during several hours is typical of conditions of progressive inflammation or infection, such as cholecystitis, colitis, and bowel obstruction. The history of progressive worsening versus intermittent episodes of pain can help differentiate infectious processes that worsen with time compared with the spasmodic colicky pain associated with bowel obstruction, biliary colic from cystic duct obstruction, or genitourinary obstruction (Figs. 45-2 to 45-4). Equally important as the character of the pain is its location and radiation. Tissue injury or inflammation can trigger both visceral and somatic pain. Solid organ visceral pain in the abdomen is generalized in the quadrant of the involved organ, such as liver pain across the right upper quadrant of the abdomen. Small bowel pain is perceived as poorly localized periumbilical pain, whereas colon pain is centered between the umbilicus and the pubic symphysis. As inflammation expands to involve the peritoneal surface,

VISCUS	SEGMENTAL INNERVATIONS	NERVES	PLEXUSES

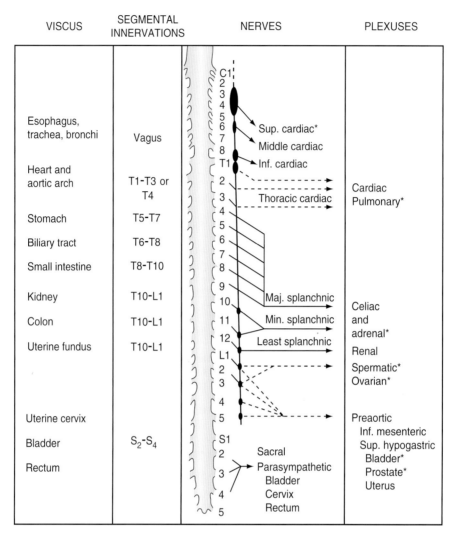

* No known sensory fibers in sympathetic rami.

FIGURE 45-1 Sensory innervation of the viscera. (From White JC, Sweet WH: *Pain and the neurosurgeon,* Springfield, Ill, 1969, Charles C Thomas, p 526.)

parietal nerve fibers from the spine allow focal and intense sensation. This combination of innervation is responsible for the classic diffuse periumbilical pain of early appendicitis that later shifts to become an intense focal pain in the right lower abdomen at McBurney point. If clinicians focus on the character of the current pain and do not thoroughly investigate its onset and progression, they will miss these strong historical clues (Figs. 45-5 and 45-6). Pain may also extend well beyond the diseased site. The liver shares some of its innervation with the diaphragm and may create referred pain to the right shoulder from the C3-C5 nerve roots. Genitourinary pain is another source of pain that commonly has a radiating pattern. Symptoms are primarily in the flank region originating from the splanchnic nerves of T11-L1, but pain often radiates to the scrotum or labia through the hypogastric plexus of S2-S4.

Activities that exacerbate or relieve the pain are also important. Eating will often worsen the pain of bowel obstruction, biliary colic, pancreatitis, diverticulitis, or bowel perforation. Food can provide relief from the pain of nonperforated peptic ulcer disease or gastritis. Clinicians will often recognize that they are evaluating

---

BOX 45-3   Locations of Referred Pain and Its Causes

Right Shoulder
Liver
Gallbladder
Right hemidiaphragm

Left Shoulder
Heart
Tail of pancreas
Spleen
Left hemidiaphragm

Scrotum and Testicles
Ureter

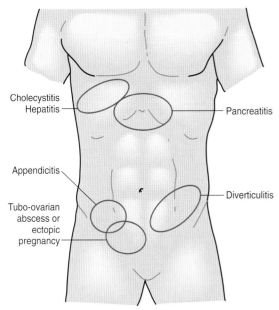

FIGURE 45-2 Character of pain: gradual, progressive pain.

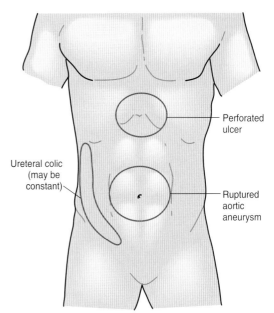

FIGURE 45-4 Character of pain: sudden, severe pain.

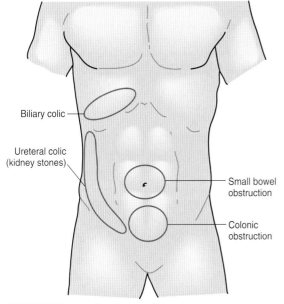

FIGURE 45-3 Character of pain: colicky, crampy, intermittent pain.

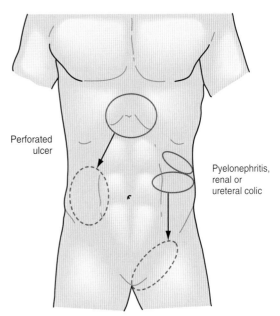

FIGURE 45-5 Referred pain. *Solid circles* are primary or most intense sites of pain.

peritonitis during the history. Patients with peritoneal inflammation will avoid any activity that stretches or jostles the abdomen. They describe worsening of the pain with any sudden body movement and will realize that there is less pain if their knees are flexed. The car ride to the hospital can be agonizing, with the patient feeling every bump along the way.

Associated symptoms can be important clues to the diagnosis. Nausea, vomiting, constipation, diarrhea, pruritus, melena, hematochezia, and hematuria can all be helpful symptoms if they are present and recognized. Vomiting may occur because of severe abdominal pain of any cause or as a result of mechanical bowel obstruction or ileus. Vomiting is more likely to precede the onset

of significant abdominal pain in many medical conditions, whereas the pain of an acute surgical abdomen is manifested first and stimulates vomiting through medullary efferent fibers that are triggered by the visceral afferent pain fibers. Constipation or obstipation can be a result of either mechanical obstruction or decreased peristalsis. It may represent the primary problem and require laxatives and prokinetic agents or merely be a symptom of an underlying condition. A careful history should include whether the patient is continuing to pass any gas or stool from the rectum. A complete obstruction is more likely to be associated with subsequent bowel ischemia or perforation related to either massive distention or a closed loop of small bowel that can occur. Diarrhea

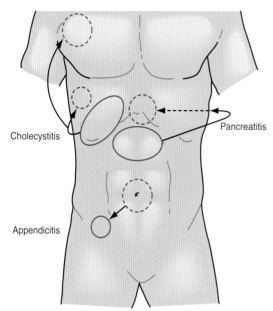

Cholecystitis

Pancreatitis

Appendicitis

FIGURE 45-6 Referred pain. *Solid circles* are primary or most intense sites of pain.

is associated with several medical causes of acute abdomen, including infectious enteritis, inflammatory bowel disease, and parasitic contamination. Bloody diarrhea can be seen in these conditions as well as in colonic ischemia.

The past medical history can potentially be more helpful than any other single part of the patient's evaluation. Previous illnesses or diagnoses can greatly increase or decrease the likelihood of certain conditions that would otherwise not be highly considered. Patients may, for example, report that the current pain is very similar to the kidney stone passage they experienced a decade prior. On the other hand, a prior history of appendectomy, pelvic inflammatory disease, or cholecystectomy can significantly shape the differential diagnosis. During the abdominal examination, all scars on the abdomen should be accounted for by the medical history obtained.

A history of medications as well as the gynecologic history of female patients is also important. Medications can both create acute abdominal conditions and mask their symptoms. Although a thorough discussion of the impact of all medications is beyond the scope of this chapter, several common drug classes deserve mention. High-dose narcotic use can interfere with bowel activity and lead to obstipation and obstruction. Narcotics also can contribute to spasm of the sphincter of Oddi and exacerbate biliary or pancreatic pain. Clearly, they also may suppress pain sensation and alter mental status, which can impair the ability to accurately diagnose the condition. Nonsteroidal anti-inflammatory agents are associated with an increased risk of upper gastrointestinal inflammation and perforation, whereas steroid medications can block protective gastric mucus production by chief cells and reduce the inflammatory reaction to infection, including advanced peritonitis. Immunosuppressant agents as a class both increase a patient's risk of acquiring a variety of bacterial or viral illnesses and also blunt the inflammatory response, diminishing the pain that is present and the overall physiologic response. Anticoagulants are much more prevalent in our emergency patients as the

population ages. These drugs may be the cause of gastrointestinal bleeds, retroperitoneal hemorrhages, or rectus sheath hematomas. They also can complicate the preoperative preparation of the patient and be the cause of substantial morbidity if their use goes unrecognized. Finally, recreational drugs can play a role in patients with an acute abdomen. Chronic alcoholism is strongly associated with coagulopathy and portal hypertension from liver impairment. Cocaine and methamphetamine can create an intense vasospastic reaction that can cause life-threatening hypertension as well as cardiac and intestinal ischemia.

The gynecologic health, and specifically the menstrual history, is crucial in evaluation of lower abdominal pain in a young woman. The likelihood of ectopic pregnancy, pelvic inflammatory disease, mittelschmerz, or severe endometriosis is heavily influenced by the details of the gynecologic history.

Very little has changed in the technique or goals of history taking since Zachary Cope first published his classic paper on the diagnosis of acute abdominal pain in 1921.[5] An exception is the application of computers to the "art" of history taking, which has been extensively studied in Europe.[6-10] Data were collected by physicians on detailed standardized forms during history and physical examinations and entered into computers programmed with a medical database of diseases and their associated signs and symptoms. The computer-generated diagnosis based on mathematical probabilities was as much as 20% more accurate than physicians left to their own methods. Statistically significant improvement was identified in timely laparotomy, shortened hospital stays, and reduced need for surgery and hospitalization.[6] However, statistically significant improvement in accuracy and efficiency has been realized without computer assistance if similar standardized forms are used for data collection. This has also been observed in the settings of trauma and critical care.

PHYSICAL EXAMINATION

An organized and thoughtful physical examination is critical to the development of an accurate differential diagnosis and the subsequent treatment algorithm. Despite newer technologies including high-resolution computed tomography (CT) scanning, ultrasound, and magnetic resonance imaging (MRI), the physical examination remains a key part of a patient's evaluation and must not be minimized. A skilled clinician will be able to develop a narrow and accurate differential diagnosis in most of his or her patients at the conclusion of the history and physical examination. Laboratory and imaging studies can then be used to further confirm the suspicions, to reorder the proposed differential diagnosis, or, less commonly, to suggest unusual possibilities not yet considered.

The physical examination should always begin with a general inspection of the patient to be followed by inspection of the abdomen itself. Patients with peritoneal irritation will experience worsened pain with any activity that moves or stretches the peritoneum. These patients will typically lie very still in the bed during the evaluation and often maintain flexion of their knees and hips to reduce tension on the anterior abdominal wall. Disease states that cause pain without peritoneal irritation, such as ischemic bowel or ureteral or biliary colic, typically cause patients to continually shift and fidget in bed while trying to find a position that lessens their discomfort (Fig. 45-7). Other important clues, such as pallor, cyanosis, and diaphoresis, may be observed during the general inspection as well.

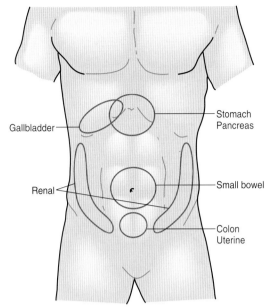

Gallbladder

Stomach
Pancreas

Renal

Small bowel

Colon
Uterine

FIGURE 45-7 Common locations for visceral pain.

Abdominal inspection should address the contour of the abdomen, including whether it appears distended or scaphoid and whether a localized mass effect is observed. Special attention should be paid to all scars present; if they are surgical in nature, they should correlate with the past surgical history provided. Fascial hernias may be suspected and can be confirmed during palpation of the abdominal wall. Evidence of erythema or edema of skin may suggest cellulitis of the abdominal wall; ecchymosis is sometimes observed with deeper necrotizing infections of the fascia or abdominal structures, such as the pancreas.

Auscultation can provide useful information about the gastrointestinal tract and the vascular system. Bowel sounds are typically evaluated for their quantity and quality. A quiet abdomen suggests an ileus, whereas hyperactive bowel sounds are found in enteritis and early ischemic intestine. The pitch and pattern of the sounds are also considered. Mechanical bowel obstruction is characterized by high-pitched tinkling sounds that tend to come in rushes and are associated with pain. Far-away echoing sounds are often present when significant luminal distention exists. Bruits heard within the abdomen reflect turbulent blood flow within the vascular system. These are most frequently encountered in the setting of high-grade arterial stenoses of 70% to 95% but can also be heard if an arteriovenous fistula is present. The clinician can also subtly test for the location and degree of pain during the auscultatory examination by varying the position and amount of pressure applied with the stethoscope. These data can then be compared with the findings during palpation and evaluated for consistency. Even though few patients will intentionally try to deceive the physician, some may exaggerate their pain complaints so as not to be disregarded or taken lightly.

Percussion is used to assess for gaseous distention of the bowel, free intra-abdominal air, degree of ascites, or presence of peritoneal inflammation. Hyperresonance, commonly referred to as tympany to percussion, is characteristic of underlying gas-filled loops of bowel. In the setting of bowel obstruction or ileus, this tympany is heard throughout all but the right upper quadrant where the liver lies beneath the abdominal wall. If localized dullness to percussion is identified anywhere other than the right

upper quadrant, an abdominal mass displacing the bowel should be considered. When liver dullness is lost and resonance is uniform throughout, free intra-abdominal air should be suspected. This air rises and collects beneath the anterior abdominal wall when the patient is in a supine position. Ascites is detected by looking for fluctuance of the abdominal cavity. A fluid wave or ripple can be generated by a quick firm compression of the lateral abdomen. The resulting wave should then travel across the abdominal wall. Movement of adipose tissue in the obese abdomen can be mistaken for a fluid wave. False-positive examinations can be reduced by first pressing the ulnar surface of the examiner's open palm into the midline soft tissue of the abdominal wall to minimize any movement of the fatty tissue while generating the wave with the opposite hand.

Peritonitis is also assessed by percussion. Older, traditional writings teach a technique of deep compression of the abdominal wall followed by abrupt release. This practice is excruciating in the setting of peritoneal inflammation and can create significant discomfort even in its absence. More sensitive and reliable methods can and should be used. Firmly tapping the iliac crest, the flank, or the heel of an extended leg will jar the abdominal viscera and elicit characteristic pain when peritonitis is present.

The final major step in the abdominal examination is palpation. Palpation typically provides more information than any other single component of the abdominal examination. In addition to revealing the severity and exact location of the abdominal pain, palpation can further confirm the presence of peritonitis as well as identify organomegaly or an abnormal mass lesion. Palpation should always begin gently and away from the reported area of pain. If considerable pain is induced at the outset of palpation, the patient is likely to voluntarily guard and continue to do so, limiting the information obtained. Involuntary guarding, or abdominal wall muscle spasm, is a sign of peritonitis and must be distinguished from voluntary guarding. To accomplish this, the examiner applies consistent pressure to the abdominal wall away from the point of maximal pain while asking the patient to take a slow, deep breath. In the setting of voluntary guarding, the abdominal muscles will relax during the act of inspiration; if guarding is involuntary, they remain spastic and tense.

Pain, when focal, suggests an early or well-localized disease process; diffuse pain on palpation is present with extensive inflammation or late presentations. If pain is diffuse, careful investigation should be carried out to determine where the pain is greatest. Even in the setting of extreme contamination from perforated peptic ulcers or colonic diverticula, the site of maximal tenderness often points to the underlying source.

Numerous unique physical findings have come to be associated with specific disease conditions and are well described as examination "signs" (Table 45-1). Murphy sign of acute cholecystitis results when inspiration during palpation of the right upper quadrant results in sudden worsening of pain because of descent of the liver and gallbladder toward the examiner's hand. Several signs help to localize the site of underlying peritonitis, including the obturator sign, the psoas sign, and Rovsing sign. Others, such as Fothergill sign and Carnett sign, help distinguish intra-abdominal disease from that of the abdominal wall.

Digital rectal examination needs to be performed in all patients with acute abdominal pain, checking for the presence of a mass, pelvic pain, or intraluminal blood. A pelvic examination should be included in all women in evaluating pain located below the umbilicus. Gynecologic and adnexal processes are best characterized by a thorough speculum and bimanual evaluation.

TABLE 45-1 **Abdominal Examination Signs**

Aaron sign	Pain or pressure in epigastrium or anterior chest with persistent firm pressure applied to McBurney point	Acute appendicitis
Bassler sign	Sharp pain created by compressing appendix between abdominal wall and iliacus	Chronic appendicitis
Blumberg sign	Transient abdominal wall rebound tenderness	Peritoneal inflammation
Carnett sign	Loss of abdominal tenderness when abdominal wall muscles are contracted	Intra-abdominal source of abdominal pain
Chandelier sign	Extreme lower abdominal and pelvic pain with movement of cervix	Pelvic inflammatory disease
Charcot sign	Intermittent right upper abdominal pain, jaundice, and fever	Choledocholithiasis
Claybrook sign	Accentuation of breath and cardiac sounds through abdominal wall	Ruptured abdominal viscus
Courvoisier sign	Palpable gallbladder in presence of jaundice	Periampullary tumor
Cruveilhier sign	Varicose veins at umbilicus (caput medusae)	Portal hypertension
Cullen sign	Periumbilical bruising	Hemoperitoneum
Danforth sign	Shoulder pain on inspiration	Hemoperitoneum
Fothergill sign	Abdominal wall mass that does not cross midline and remains palpable when rectus is contracted	Rectus muscle hematomas
Grey Turner sign	Local areas of discoloration around umbilicus and flanks	Acute hemorrhagic pancreatitis
Iliopsoas sign	Elevation and extension of leg against resistance create pain	Appendicitis with retrocecal abscess
Kehr sign	Left shoulder pain when supine and pressure placed on left upper abdomen	Hemoperitoneum (especially from splenic origin)
Mannkopf sign	Increased pulse when painful abdomen is palpated	Absent if malingering
Murphy sign	Pain caused by inspiration while applying pressure to right upper abdomen	Acute cholecystitis
Obturator sign	Flexion with external rotation of right thigh while supine creates hypogastric pain	Pelvic abscess or inflammatory mass in pelvis
Ransohoff sign	Yellow discoloration of umbilical region	Ruptured common bile duct
Rovsing sign	Pain at McBurney point when compressing the left lower abdomen	Acute appendicitis
ten Horn sign	Pain caused by gentle traction of right testicle	Acute appendicitis

LABORATORY STUDIES

A number of laboratory studies are considered routine in the evaluation of a patient with an acute abdomen (Box 45-4). They help confirm that inflammation or an infection is present and also aid in the elimination of some of the most common nonsurgical conditions. A complete blood count with differential is valuable as most but not all patients with an acute abdomen will have either a leukocytosis or bandemia. Serum electrolyte, blood urea nitrogen, and creatinine measurements will assist in evaluating the effect of such factors as vomiting and third space fluid losses. In addition, they may suggest an endocrine or metabolic diagnosis as the cause of the patient's problem. Serum amylase and lipase determinations may suggest pancreatitis as the cause of the abdominal pain, but levels can also be elevated in other disorders, such as small bowel infarction and duodenal ulcer perforation. Normal serum amylase and lipase levels do not exclude pancreatitis as a possible diagnosis because of the effects of chronic inflammation on enzyme production and timing factors. Liver function tests including total and direct bilirubin, serum aminotransferase, and alkaline phosphatase are helpful in evaluating potential biliary tract causes of acute abdominal pain. Lactate levels and arterial blood gas determinations can be helpful in diagnosis of intestinal ischemia or infarction. Urine testing, such as urinalysis, is helpful in the diagnosis of bacterial cystitis, pyelonephritis, and certain endocrine abnormalities, such as diabetes and renal parenchymal disease. Urine culture, although it can confirm a suspected urinary tract infection and direct antibiotic therapy, is not available in time to be helpful in the evaluation of an acute abdomen. Urinary measurements of human chorionic gonadotropin can either suggest pregnancy as a confounding factor in the patient's presentation or aid in decision making about therapy. The fetus of a pregnant patient with an acute abdomen is best protected by providing the best care to the mother,

BOX 45-4 **Helpful Laboratory Studies in the Acute Abdomen**

Hemoglobin
White blood cell count with differential
Electrolyte, blood urea nitrogen, and creatinine concentrations
Urinalysis
Urine human chorionic gonadotropin
Amylase and lipase levels
Total and direct bilirubin concentration
Alkaline phosphatase
Serum aminotransferase
Serum lactate levels
Stool for ova and parasites
C. difficile culture and toxin assay

including an operation if indicated.[11] Stool testing for occult blood can be helpful in the evaluation of these patients but is nonspecific. Stool for ova and parasite evaluation as well as culture and toxin assay for *Clostridium difficile* can be helpful if diarrhea is a component of the patient's presentation.

IMAGING STUDIES

Improvements in imaging techniques, especially multidetector CT scans, have revolutionized the diagnosis of the acute abdomen. The most difficult diagnostic dilemmas of the past, appendicitis in young women and ischemic bowel in the elderly, can now be diagnosed with much greater certainty and speed (Figs. 45-8 and 45-9).[12-14] This has resulted in more rapid operative correction of the problem with less morbidity and mortality. Despite its

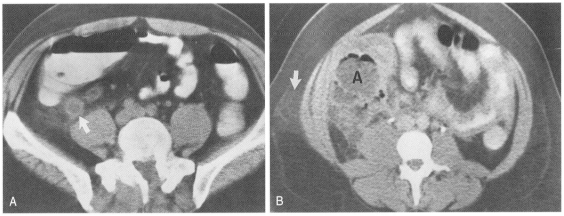

FIGURE 45-8 **Appendicitis.** **A,** CT scan of uncomplicated appendicitis. A thick-walled, distended, retrocecal appendix *(arrow)* is seen with inflammatory change in the surrounding fat. **B,** CT scan of complicated appendicitis. A retrocecal appendiceal abscess (A) with an associated phlegmon posteriorly found in a 3-week postpartum, obese woman. Inflammatory change extends through the flank musculature into the subcutaneous fat *(arrow)*.

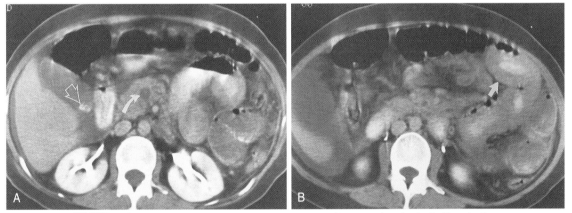

FIGURE 45-9 Small bowel infarction associated with mesenteric venous thrombosis. **A,** Note the low-density thrombosed superior mesenteric vein *(solid arrow)* and incidental gallstones *(open arrow)*. **B,** Thickening of proximal small bowel wall *(arrow)* coincided with several feet of infarcting small bowel at time of operation.

usefulness, CT is not the only imaging technique available and is also not the first step in imaging for most patients. In addition, none of the imaging techniques take the place of a careful history and physical examination.

Plain radiographs continue to play a role in imaging in patients with acute abdominal pain. Upright chest radiographs can detect as little as 1 mL of air injected into the peritoneal cavity. Lateral decubitus abdominal radiographs can also detect pneumoperitoneum effectively in patients who cannot stand. As little as 5 to 10 mL of gas may be detected with this technique.[15] These studies are particularly helpful in patients suspected of having a perforated duodenal ulcer as about 75% of these patients will have a large enough pneumoperitoneum to be visible (Fig. 45-10).[16] This obviates the need for further evaluation in most patients, allowing laparotomy with little delay.

Plain films also show abnormal calcifications. Approximately 5% of appendicoliths, 10% of gallstones, and 90% of renal stones contain sufficient amounts of calcium to be radiopaque. Pancreatic calcifications seen in many patients with chronic pancreatitis are visible on plain films, as are the calcifications in abdominal

aortic aneurysms, visceral artery aneurysm, and atherosclerosis in visceral vessels.

Upright and supine abdominal radiographs are helpful in identifying gastric outlet obstruction and obstruction of the proximal, mid, or distal small bowel. They can also aid in determining whether a small bowel obstruction is complete or partial by the presence or absence of gas in the colon. Colonic gas can be differentiated from small intestinal gas by the presence of haustral markings from the taeniae coli in the colonic wall. Obstructed colon appears as distended bowel with haustral markings (Fig. 45-11). Associated distention of small bowel may also be present, especially if the ileocecal valve is incompetent. Plain films can also suggest volvulus of either the cecum or sigmoid colon. Cecal volvulus is identified by a distended loop of colon in a comma shape with the concavity facing inferiorly and to the right. Sigmoid volvulus characteristically has the appearance of a bent inner tube with its apex in the right upper quadrant (Fig. 45-12).

Abdominal ultrasonography is extremely accurate in detecting gallstones and in assessing gallbladder wall thickness and the presence of fluid around the gallbladder.[17] It is also good at

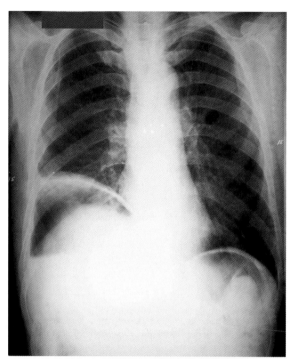

FIGURE 45-10 Upright chest radiograph depicting moderate-sized pneumoperitoneum consistent with perforation of abdominal viscus.

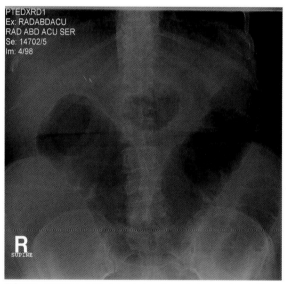

FIGURE 45-11 Upright abdominal radiograph in a patient with an obstructing sigmoid adenocarcinoma. Note the haustral markings on the dilated transverse colon that distinguished this from small intestine.

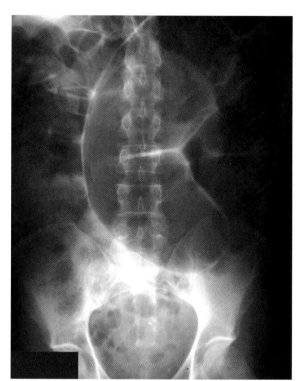

FIGURE 45-12 Upright abdominal radiograph in a patient with a sigmoid colon volvulus. Note the characteristic appearance of a bent inner tube with its apex in the right upper quadrant.

to the value of ultrasonography in the diagnosis of diseases that are manifested as an acute abdomen. Ultrasound has been found to be clinically inferior to CT scanning for the diagnosis of appendicitis.[18] In addition, ultrasound images are more difficult for most surgeons to interpret than are plain radiographs and CT images. Many hospitals have radiologic technologists available at all times to perform CT, but this is often not the case with ultrasonography. As CT has become more widely available and less likely to be hindered by abdominal air, it is becoming the secondary imaging modality of choice in the patient with an acute abdomen, following plain abdominal radiographs.

A number of studies have demonstrated the accuracy and utility of CT of the abdomen and pelvis in the evaluation of acute abdominal pain.[12-14] Many of the most common causes of the acute abdomen are readily identified by CT scanning, as are their complications. A notable example is appendicitis. Plain films and even barium enemas add little to the diagnosis of appendicitis; however, a well-performed CT scan is highly accurate in this disease. Prior experience suggested that optimal CT imaging for appendicitis should include intravenous, oral, and rectal contrast agents. Most recently, a large retrospective review of more than 9000 patients from 56 hospitals representing both urban and rural practices found no added diagnostic accuracy with the addition of enteral contrast material. Operative findings correlated with the CT observations 90% of the time whether or not enteral contrast material was used.[19]

It is equally important that an experienced radiologist, accustomed to reading abdominal CT scans, interpret the study to maximize the sensitivity and specificity of the examination. A prospective study from The Netherlands illustrated the variability

determining the diameter of the extrahepatic and intrahepatic bile ducts. Its usefulness in detecting common bile duct stones is limited. Abdominal and transvaginal ultrasonography can aid in the detection of abnormalities of the ovaries, adnexa, and uterus. Ultrasound can also detect intraperitoneal fluid. The presence of abnormal amounts of intestinal air in most patients with an acute abdomen limits the ability of ultrasonography to evaluate the pancreas or other abdominal organs. There are important limits of CT interpretation in the diagnosis of appendicitis. Three blinded groups of radiologists read CT scans of patients suspected of having appendicitis. All patients then underwent exploratory laparoscopy; 83% of patients were found to have appendicitis at surgery. Radiology group A was made up of radiology residents on call and trained in CT interpretation. Group B were on-call staff radiologists. Group C was represented by expert abdominal radiologists. For group A, B, and C radiologists, the sensitivity of CT scanning for the diagnosis of acute appendicitis was 81%, 88%, and 95%, respectively; the specificity was 94%, 94%, and 100%; and the negative predictive value was 50%, 68%, and 81%. Differences between groups A and C were statistically significant.[14] CT is also excellent in differentiating mechanical small bowel obstruction from paralytic ileus and can usually identify the transition point in mechanical obstruction (Fig. 45-13). Some of the most difficult diagnostic dilemmas, including acute intestinal ischemia and bowel injury after blunt abdominal trauma, can often be identified by this method.

Traumatic small bowel injuries can be a challenging clinical diagnosis. Associated abdominal wall, pelvic, or spinous injuries

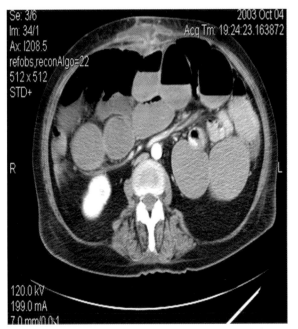

FIGURE 45-13 CT scan of a patient with a partial small bowel obstruction. Note the presence of dilated small bowel and decompressed small bowel. The decompressed bowel contains air, indicating a partial obstruction.

can be significant distracters that compromise an otherwise careful history and physical examination. In addition, many patients suffering a blunt abdominal trauma will have altered mental states from coexisting closed head injuries or from intoxicating substances. When a bowel injury is suspected, optimal CT scanning uses both oral and intravenous contrast agents. Zissin and colleagues[17] reported an overall sensitivity of 64%, specificity of 97%, and accuracy of 82% when diagnosing small bowel injury after blunt trauma using dual contrast CT scanning. Keys to the diagnosis include bowel wall thickening, any gas outside the lumen of the intestine, or a moderate to large amount of intraperitoneal fluid without visible solid abdominal organ injury.

INTRA-ABDOMINAL PRESSURE MONITORING

An elevated intra-abdominal pressure can be a symptom of an acute abdominal process or it can be the cause of the process. Abnormally increased intra-abdominal pressures diminish the blood flow to abdominal organs and decrease venous return to the heart while increasing venous stasis. Increased pressure in the abdomen can also press upward on the diaphragm, thereby increasing peak inspiratory pressures and decreasing ventilatory efficiency. Risk of esophageal reflux and pulmonary aspiration has also been associated with abdominal hypertension. It is important to consider the possibility of abdominal hypertension in any patient who presents with a rigid or significantly distended abdomen.

Normal intra-abdominal pressure is considered to be 5 to 7 mm Hg for a relaxed individual of average body build lying in a supine position. Obesity and elevation of the head of the bed can increase the normal resting abdominal pressure. Morbid obesity has been shown to increase "normal pressures" by 4 to 8 mm Hg; elevating the head of the bed to 30 degrees raises the pressure by 5 mm Hg on average.[20] Pressures are most commonly measured through the bladder by pressure transducer attached to a Foley catheter. Pressure readings are obtained at the end-expiration after instillation of 50 mL of saline into an otherwise empty bladder. Abnormally elevated pressures are those above 11 mm Hg and are graded 1 to 4 by severity (Table 45-2). Abdominal hypertension grades 1 and 2 can most always be treated adequately with medical interventions focusing on maintaining euvolemia, gut decompression with nasogastric tubes or laxatives and enemas, withholding of enteral feedings, catheter aspiration of ascitic fluid, abdominal wall relaxation, and judicious use of hypotonic intravenous fluids. Grades 3 and 4 often require surgical decompression by laparotomy with open packing of the abdomen if the severe hypertension and organ dysfunction do not respond promptly to aggressive medical intervention.

TABLE 45-2	**Abdominal Hypertension**						
	MESENTERIC PRESSURE	**CO**	**CVP**	**PIP**	**GFR**	**PERFUSION**	**TREATMENT**
Normal pressure	5-7 mm Hg	↔	↔	↔	↔	↔	None
Grade 1 hypertension	12-15 mm Hg	↔	↔ / ↑	↔ / ↑	↓	↓	Maintain euvolemia
Grade 2 hypertension	16-20 mm Hg	↓	↑ *	↑	↓	↓	Nonsurgical decompression
Grade 3 hypertension	21-25 mm Hg	↓ ↓	↑ ↑ *	↑ ↑	↓ ↓	↓ ↓	Surgical decompression
Grade 4 hypertension	>25 mm Hg	↓ ↓ ↓	↑ ↑ *	↑ ↑	↓ ↓ ↓	↓ ↓ ↓	Surgical decompression; reexplore

CO, cardiac output; *CVP*, central venous pressure; *GFR*, glomerular filtration rate; *PIP*, peak inspiratory pressure.
*Misleadingly elevated and not reflective of intravascular volume.

DIAGNOSTIC LAPAROSCOPY

A number of studies have confirmed the utility of diagnostic laparoscopy in patients with acute abdominal pain.[21-23] The purported advantages include high sensitivity and specificity, ability to treat a number of the conditions causing an acute abdomen laparoscopically, decreased morbidity and mortality, decreased length of stay, and decreased overall hospital costs. It may be particularly helpful in the critically ill, intensive care patient, especially if a laparotomy can be avoided.[24] Diagnostic accuracy is high, and reports show the accuracy ranges between 90% and 100%, with the primary limitation being recognition of retroperitoneal processes. This compares favorably with other diagnostic studies showing superiority to peritoneal lavage, CT scanning, or ultrasound of the abdomen.[25] Because of advances in equipment and increased availability, this technique is being used with greater frequency in these patients.

DIFFERENTIAL DIAGNOSIS

The differential diagnosis for acute abdominal pain is extensive. Conditions range from the mild and self-limited to the rapidly progressive and fatal. All patients must therefore be seen and evaluated immediately on presentation and reassessed at frequent intervals for changes in condition. Although many "acute abdomen" diagnoses will require surgical intervention for resolution, it is important to keep in mind that many causes of acute abdominal pain are medical in etiology (see Figs. 45-2 and 45-4).[26] Development of the differential diagnosis begins during the history and is further clarified during the physical examination. Refinements are then made with the assistance of laboratory analysis and imaging studies so that typically, one or two diagnoses rise above the rest. To be successful, this process requires a comprehensive knowledge of the medical and surgical conditions that create acute abdominal pain to allow individual disease features to be matched to patient demographics, symptoms, and signs.

Certain physical examination, laboratory, and radiographic findings are highly correlated with surgical disease (Box 45-5). At times, some patients will be too unstable to undergo comprehensive evaluations that require transportation to other departments, such as radiology. In this setting, peritoneal lavage can provide information suggesting pathologic processes requiring surgical intervention. The lavage can be performed under local anesthesia at the patient's bedside. A small incision is made in the midline adjacent to the umbilicus, and dissection is carried down to the peritoneal cavity. A small catheter or intravenous tubing is inserted, and 1000 mL of saline is infused. A sample of fluid is then allowed to siphon back out into the empty saline bag and is then analyzed for cellular or biochemical anomalies. This technique can provide sensitive evidence of hemorrhage or infection as well as of some types of solid or hollow organ injury.

Patients having emergency or life-threatening surgical disease are taken for immediate laparotomy; urgent diagnoses allow time for stabilization, hydration, and preoperative preparation as needed. The remaining acute abdominal patients are grouped as those with surgical conditions that sometimes require surgery, those with medical diseases, and those who as yet remain unclear. Hospitalized patients who do not go urgently to the operating room must be reassessed frequently and preferably by the same examiner to recognize potentially serious changes in condition that alter the diagnosis or suggest development of complications.

> ### BOX 45-5   Findings Associated With Surgical Disease in the Setting of Acute Abdominal Pain
>
> **Physical Examination and Laboratory Findings**
> Abdominal compartment pressures >30 mm Hg
> Worsening distention after gastric decompression
> Involuntary guarding or rebound tenderness
> Gastrointestinal hemorrhage requiring >4 units of blood without stabilization
> Unexplained systemic sepsis
> Signs of hypoperfusion (acidosis, pain out of proportion to examination findings, rising liver function test results)
>
> **Radiographic Findings**
> Massive dilation of intestine
> Progressive dilation of stationary loop of intestine (sentinel loop)
> Pneumoperitoneum
> Extravasation of contrast material from bowel lumen
> Vascular occlusion on angiography
> Fat stranding or thickened bowel wall with systemic sepsis
>
> **Diagnostic Peritoneal Lavage (1000 mL)**
> >250 white blood cells per milliliter of aspirate
> >300,000 red blood cells per milliliter of aspirate
> Bilirubin level higher than plasma level (bile leak) within aspirate
> Presence of particulate matter (stool)
> Creatinine level higher than plasma level in aspirate (urine leak)

Although the goal of every surgeon is to make the correct diagnosis preoperatively and to have planned the best possible surgical procedure before entering the operating suite, it must be emphasized that a clear diagnosis will not be able to be developed in every patient. Surgeons must always be willing to accept uncertainty and commit to abdominal exploration when examination findings warrant. Laboratory and imaging studies, although helpful, should never replace the bedside clinical judgment of an experienced surgeon. Patients are far more likely to be seriously or fatally harmed by delay of surgical treatment to perform confirmatory tests than by misdiagnoses discovered at operation. Laparoscopy has proved to be a valuable tool when the diagnosis is unclear. The presence of surgical disease can be confirmed in all but the most hostile abdominal environments, and as the surgeon's experience grows, more and more conditions are able to be treated laparoscopically as well. Even when conversion to open technique is required, laparoscopic evaluation facilitates more accurate positioning of the laparotomy incision, thereby reducing its length.

PREPARATION FOR EMERGENCY OPERATION

Patients with an acute abdomen vary greatly in their overall state of health at the time the decision to operate is made. Regardless of the patient's severity of illness, all patients require some degree of preoperative preparation. Intravenous access should be obtained and any fluid or electrolyte abnormalities corrected. Nearly all patients will require antibiotic infusions. The bacteria common in acute abdominal emergencies are gram-negative enteric organisms and anaerobes. Infusions of antibiotics to cover these organisms should be begun once a presumptive diagnosis is made. Patients with generalized paralytic ileus or vomiting benefit from nasogastric tube placement to decrease the likelihood of vomiting and aspiration. Foley catheter bladder drainage to assess urine output, a measure of adequacy of fluid resuscitation, is indicated in most patients. Preoperative urine output of 0.5 mL/kg/hr, systolic blood pressure of at least 100 mm Hg, and a pulse rate of 100 beats/min or less are indicative of an adequate intravascular volume. A common electrolyte abnormality requiring correction is hypokalemia. Preoperative acidosis may respond to fluid repletion and intravenous bicarbonate infusion. Acidosis due to intestinal ischemia or infarction may be refractory to preoperative therapy. Placement of a central venous catheter may facilitate resuscitation and allow accelerated correction of potassium concentration. Significant anemia is uncommon, and preoperative blood transfusions are usually unnecessary. However, most patients should have blood typed and crossmatched and available at operation. There is an inherent uncertainty in the operation that will be required in these patients, and having crossmatched blood available avoids transfusion delay if unexpected intraoperative events occur. The need for preoperative stabilization of patients must be weighed against the increased morbidity and mortality associated with a delay in the treatment of some of the surgical diseases that are manifested as an acute abdomen. The underlying nature of the disease process, such as infarcted bowel, may require surgical correction before stabilization of the patient's vital signs and restoration of acid-base balance can occur. Resuscitation should be viewed as an ongoing process and continued after the surgery is completed. Deciding when the maximum benefit of preoperative therapy in these patients has been achieved requires good surgical judgment.

ATYPICAL PATIENTS

Pregnancy

Acute abdominal pain in the pregnant patient creates several unique diagnostic and therapeutic challenges. Special emphasis must be placed on the possibility of gynecologic and surgical diseases when acute abdominal pain develops during pregnancy because of their frequency and morbidity if left unrecognized. Laparoscopy has had a major impact on the diagnosis and treatment of the gravid woman with acute abdominal pain and is now routinely employed for many clinical situations. Although case reports of fetal demise after laparoscopic surgery continue to be reported, its safety has been considered equal or superior to an open surgical approach in all trimesters of pregnancy.[27,28] A retrospective study and meta-analysis did call into question the safety of laparoscopic appendectomy compared with laparotomy, highlighting the need for more research into this area.[29,30] The greatest threat facing the pregnant patient with acute abdominal pain is the potential for delayed diagnosis. Delays in receiving surgical treatment have proved far more morbid than the operations themselves.[11,31] Delays occur for several reasons. Many times, symptoms are attributed to the underlying pregnancy, including abdominal pains, nausea, vomiting, and anorexia. Pregnancy can also alter the presentation of some disease processes and make the physical examination more challenging because of the enlarged uterus in the pelvis. The appendix rises out of the pelvis to within a few centimeters of the right anterolateral costal margin late in the third trimester (Fig. 45-14).[32] Laboratory studies such as white blood cell counts and other chemistries are also altered in pregnancy, making recognition of disease more difficult. In addition, physicians may hesitate to perform typical imaging studies, such as plain abdominal films or CT scans, because of concern over

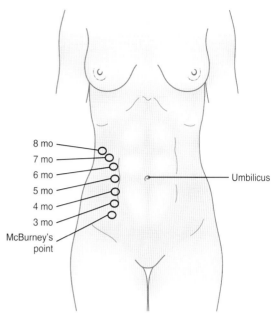

FIGURE 45-14 Location of maternal normal appendix during fetal gestation.

radiation exposure to the developing fetus. The lack of radiologic information can take a physician out of his or her diagnostic routine and cause extra emphasis to be placed on other modalities, such as vital signs and laboratory studies, which can confuse or underestimate the existing condition. Finally, physicians naturally tend to be more conservative in treating pregnant patients. First trimester miscarriage rates from nonobstetric surgeries have been reported to be as high as 38%, but most reports place the surgical miscarriage rate similar to spontaneous first trimester miscarriage rates of 8% to 16%.[27] Without controls, it is unclear if some of the increased miscarriage rates noted are secondary to the disease or the surgery itself. Surgery has not been associated with increased stillbirths and congenital abnormalities.[28] Abdominal surgery has been associated with an increased incidence of preterm labor in both the second and third trimesters of pregnancy, with the highest incidence in the third trimester. It is thought that preterm labor is less in the second trimester because of less uterine manipulation. Intraoperative care during pregnancy is focused on optimal care of the mother. If the fetus is previable, fetal heart tones should be measured before and after the surgery. If the fetus is viable, fetal heart sounds should be measured throughout the surgery with a provider capable of performing an emergent cesarean section readily available.[33]

Appendicitis is the most common nonobstetric disease requiring surgery, occurring in 1/1500 pregnancies.[29,33] Its symptoms typically consist of right lateral abdominal pain, nausea, and anorexia, yet "typical" presentations account for only 50% to 60% of cases.[34] Fever is uncommon unless the appendix is perforated with abdominal sepsis. Symptoms are sometimes attributed to the underlying pregnancy, and a high index of suspicion must be maintained. Laboratory studies can also be misleading. Leukocytosis as high as 16,000 cells/μL is common in pregnancy, and labor can increase the count to 21,000 cells/μL. Many authors have suggested that a neutrophil shift of more than 80% is suggestive of an acute inflammatory process such as appendicitis, yet others have observed that only 75% of patients with proven

TABLE 45-3   Modified Alvarado Scoring System for Appendicitis

FEATURE	SCORE
Symptoms	
Right iliac fossa pain	1
Nausea/vomiting	1
Anorexia	1
Signs	
Right iliac fossa tenderness	2
Fever	1
Rebound tenderness	1
Tests	
WBC ≥ 10,000	2
Left shift of neutrophils	1
Score ≥ 7	Surgery is recommended

From Brown MA, Birchard KR, Semelka RC: Magnetic resonance evaluation of pregnant patients with acute abdominal pain. *Semin Ultrasound CT MR* 26:206–211, 2005.

appendicitis had a shift, whereas as many as 50% of patients with a shift and pain were found to have a normal appendix.[11,30] Scoring systems have been advocated that assign numerical scores to certain symptoms, signs, and laboratory values to predict the likelihood of appendicitis. Although systems such as the Modified Alvarado Scoring System (Table 45-3) help predict the need for surgical intervention, they have not been validated in a model of pregnancy.[34] Ultrasound has been relied on as the first imaging tool in many centers. Graded compression ultrasound has been shown to have a sensitivity of 86% in the nonpregnant patient.[29] In a case series of 42 pregnant women with suspected appendicitis, graded compression ultrasound was found to be 100% sensitive, 96% specific, and 98% accurate.[35] Three women were excluded from the analysis because of a technically inadequate examination due to advanced gestational age (>35 weeks). Helical CT scanning has been established as a valuable tool for evaluation of the nonpregnant patient and shows promise as a second-line study in pregnancy. Compared with traditional CT scans, helical CT can provide a much faster study with radiation exposures of approximately 300 mrad to the fetus.[29] MRI now plays an important role in the diagnosis as well. MRI is not only capable of demonstrating the normal appendix, but it can also recognize an enlarged appendix, periappendiceal fluid, and inflammation.[36] The sensitivity and specificity reported in a retrospective review of 148 patients suspected of having acute appendicitis were 100% and 93%, respectively.[37]

The added difficulties in evaluating the pregnant patient with right lower quadrant abdominal pain have resulted in a significantly higher negative appendectomy rate compared with nonpregnant peers in the past. Although this diagnostic error rate would be unacceptable in a typical young healthy woman, it is widely accepted because of the fetal mortality suffered when appendicitis progresses to perforation before surgery. Perioperative fetal loss associated with appendectomy for early appendicitis is 3% to 5%, whereas it climbs to more than 20% in the setting of perforation.[31] With modern imaging, especially MRI, negative appendectomies have decreased without an associated increase in perforations.[36,37]

The second and third most common surgical diseases seen in pregnancy are biliary tract disorders and bowel obstructions. Surgery for biliary disease occurs in 1 to 6/10,000 pregnancies.[38] Symptoms of pain, nausea, and anorexia are the same as in nonpregnant patients. Even though the elevated estrogen levels should be more lithogenic, the incidence of disease is similar to that in nongravid women.[28] With few exceptions, the evaluation and treatment during pregnancy are similar to the evaluation and treatment of all patients with biliary disease. Ultrasound is the diagnostic test of choice. Alkaline phosphatase is elevated secondary to elevated estrogen, and normal values must be adjusted.

Laparoscopic cholecystectomy is the preferred technique for cholecystectomy.[28,38,39] Many studies have suggested laparoscopic cholecystectomy for all symptomatic disease secondary to high antepartum and postpartum recurrence and complications regardless of trimester.[28,38] Still, most surgeons try to treat simple biliary colic with conservative management in the first and third trimesters and plan elective laparoscopic cholecystectomy for the second trimester or the postpartum period to minimize fetal risk.[38] Gallstone pancreatitis and acute cholecystitis should be managed more carefully. Gallstone pancreatitis has been associated with fetal loss as high as 60%. If a woman does not respond quickly to conservative treatment with hydration, bowel rest, analgesia, and judicious use of antibiotics, further evaluation should be performed as surgery may be indicated.

Bowel obstructions are much less common, occurring in approximately 1 to 2/4000 pregnancies; the underlying cause is adhesions in two thirds of cases. Volvulus is the second most common cause, occurring in 25% of cases compared with only 4% of the nonpregnant population.[30] Signs and symptoms are typical but must not be attributed to "morning sickness." Colicky abdominal pain with rapid abdominal distention should key the clinician to the diagnosis. Three periods during gestation are associated with an increased risk of obstruction and correlate with rapid changes in uterine size.[30] The first is from 16 to 20 weeks when the uterus grows beyond the pelvis; the second is from 32 to 36 weeks when the fetal head descends; and the third is in the early postpartum period. The evaluation should be the same as for any patient, and there should be no hesitation to obtain abdominal radiographs if the situation warrants. As with other acute inflammatory processes in the abdomen, the maternal and fetal morbidity is most affected by delayed definitive treatment.

Pediatrics

Strategies for diagnosis of the acute abdomen in the pediatric population are the same as for adults. Appendicitis remains one of the primary causes of the acute abdomen in this age group. Although bowel obstructions and gallstone disease are seen, these entities are far less frequent than in adults. Intussusception should be maintained in the differential diagnosis, especially for those younger than 3 years. Gastroenteritis, perforations from foreign body ingestion, food poisoning, Meckel's diverticulitis, and *C. difficile* colitis are also potential causes. Presentations and examination findings are similar to those of adult patients. The primary challenge to making the correct diagnosis lies in obtaining an accurate history. Children will often be poor historians because of age, fear, or their general ability to describe their experience. A thorough history must therefore be also obtained from the child's parents as well. Diagnostic testing choices as well as treatments may be influenced by the age of the patient. Clinicians may be less inclined to perform studies that deliver ionizing radiation to young children. A retrospective study of 1228 children with suspected appendicitis evaluated the use of ultrasound as a first-line tool, with CT scanning used as an adjunct for equivocal studies.[40] This study showed that CT scanning was avoided in more than half of patients while maintaining a negative appendectomy rate of 8.1%. Finally, there is a growing experience in treating early appendicitis nonoperatively with antibiotics. A recent prospective nonrandomized study of 77 children with appendicitis found the immediate and 30-day success rates of nonoperative treatment to be 93% and 90%. Of the three patients who failed to respond to medical management, none progressed to perforated or complicated appendicitis. Children in the medically managed group were found to return to school 2 days sooner, had 14 fewer disability days, but incurred an 18-hour longer hospitalization on average.[41]

Acute Abdomen in the Critically Ill

The critically ill patient with a potential acute abdomen is a difficult challenge for intensivists and surgeons alike. Many of the underlying diseases and treatments encountered in the intensive care unit can predispose to acute abdominal disease. At the same time, unrecognized abdominal illness can be responsible for patients lingering in a critical state. Critically ill patients are often unable to appreciate symptoms to the same degree as healthy peers because of nutritional or immune compromise, narcotic analgesia, or antibiotic use. Many of these patients have an altered mental status or are intubated and cannot provide detailed information to their providers.

Cardiopulmonary bypass has been associated with several acute abdominal illnesses. Mesenteric ischemia, paralytic ileus, Ogilvie syndrome, stress peptic ulceration, acute acalculous cholecystitis, and acute pancreatitis have all been linked to the low-flow state of cardiopulmonary bypass, and incidence appears tied to the length of the cardiac procedure.[42,43] Vasoactive medications and ventilator support have also been linked to hypoperfusion and similar abdominal processes. When an acute abdominal complication occurs in an intensive care unit patient, it has a dramatic effect on outcome. Intensivists should maintain a high index of suspicion for the development of intra-abdominal disease and consult with surgeons early to maximize recovery potential. Surgeons must then work to exclude the possibility of abdominal disease using all of the methods described in this chapter as well as bedside ultrasound, paracentesis, or mini-laparoscopy so that early surgical intervention can be appropriately undertaken.[44]

Immunocompromised Patients With Acute Abdomen

Immunocompromised patients have variable presentations with acute abdominal diseases. The variability is highly correlated to the degree of immunosuppression. There is no reliable test for determining the degree of immunosuppression experienced by a given patient, so estimates are made by associations with certain disease states or medications. Mild to moderate compromise is experienced by the elderly, the malnourished, diabetics, transplant recipients on routine maintenance therapy, cancer patients, renal failure patients, and HIV patients with CD4 counts above 200/mm³. Although patients in this group have the same types of illnesses and infections as their immunocompetent peers, they still can present in an atypical fashion. Abdominal pain and systemic signs and symptoms are often tied to the development of inflammation. These patients may not be able to mount a full inflammatory response and therefore may experience less abdominal pain, have delayed development of fever, and have a blunted leukocytosis. Severely compromised patients typically include

transplant recipients having received high-dose therapy for rejection in the past 2 months, cancer patients on chemotherapy especially with neutropenia, and HIV patients with CD4 counts below 200/mm³. These patients present very late in their course, often with little or no pain, no fever, and vague constitutional symptoms followed by an overwhelming systemic collapse.

Pseudomembranous colitis has traditionally been associated with recent broad-spectrum antibiotic use, although it is increasingly seen in immunocompromised patients with diseases such as lymphoma, leukemia, and AIDS. Clinical manifestations commonly include diarrhea, dehydration, abdominal pain, fever, and leukocytosis, yet immunocompromised patients may fail to exhibit many of these findings because of their inability to mount a normal inflammatory response. Imaging studies such as CT of the abdomen become increasingly important in making early, accurate diagnoses when presentations are atypical. CT scans are useful in patients with complicated colitis without obvious operative indications. CT scans are useful to evaluate for megacolon, ileus, ascites, perforation, and colon wall thickening (Table 45-4).[45] These findings, when present, can greatly assist the clinician with forming the diagnosis of colitis. However, up to 14% of patients with proven pseudomembranous colitis will have had normal findings on CT examination, and therefore the diagnosis should not be ruled out solely on the basis of a negative scan. Early surgical consultation has been shown to decrease mortality.[46]

In addition, these patients may suffer from atypical infections, including peritoneal tuberculosis, fungal infections including aspergillus, endemic mycoses, and a variety of viral infections including cytomegalovirus and Epstein-Barr virus (Box 45-6). When an abdominal infection does occur, it is less likely to be walled off as a localized infection because of the lack of inflammatory reaction. All severely immunocompromised patients require prompt and thorough evaluation for any persistent abdominal complaints. All patients requiring hospitalization should receive a surgical consult to aid in timely diagnosis and treatment. High-resolution CT scanning can be of great benefit in these patients, but a low threshold for laparoscopy or laparotomy should be maintained for those with equivocal diagnostic test results and persistent symptoms that remain unexplained.

Acute Abdomen in the Morbidly Obese

Morbid obesity creates numerous challenges to the accurate diagnosis of acute abdominal processes. Many authors describe alterations in the signs and symptoms of peritonitis in the morbidly

TABLE 45-4 Frequency of Common CT Scan Observations in Pseudomembranous Colitis

CT FINDINGS	FREQUENCY (%)
Bowel wall thickening (>4 mm)	86
Pancolic distribution	46
Pericolic stranding	45
Ascites	38
Nodular or polypoid wall thickening	38
Mucosal enhancement	18
Bowel dilation	14
Accordion sign	14

From Tsiotos GG, Mullany CJ, Zietlow S, et al: Abdominal complications following cardiac surgery. *Am J Surg* 167:553–557, 1994.

obese.[47-49] Findings of overt peritonitis are often late and usually ominous, leading to sepsis, organ failure, and death.[47] Abdominal sepsis is a much more subtle diagnosis in this population and may be associated only with symptoms such as malaise, shoulder pain, hiccups, or shortness of breath.[48] Physical examination

findings can also be difficult to interpret. Severe abdominal pain is not common, and less specific findings, such as tachycardia, tachypnea, pleural effusion, and fever, may be the primary observation.[49] Appreciation of distention or intra-abdominal mass is also difficult because of the size and thickness of the abdominal wall.

Abdominal imaging is also adversely affected by obesity. Plain abdominal radiographs can require multiple images to view the entire abdomen, and clarity is reduced. CT and MRI scanning may be impossible to perform as a patient's girth or weight exceeds the size of the scanning aperture or the weight limit of the mechanized bed. In these settings, a high index of suspicion and low threshold for surgical exploration must be maintained. Laparoscopy is a valuable tool in these patients.

BOX 45-6   Causes of Acute Abdominal Pain in the Immunocompromised Patient

Opportunistic Infections

Endemic mycoses (coccidioidomycosis, blastomycosis, histoplasmosis)
Tuberculin peritonitis
Aspergillosis
Neutropenic colitis (typhlitis)
Pseudomembranous colitis
Cytomegalovirus colitis, gastritis, esophagitis, nephritis
Epstein-Barr virus
Hepatic abscesses (fungal or pyogenic)

Iatrogenic Conditions

Graft-versus-host disease with hepatitis or enteritis
Peptic ulcer or perforation from steroid use
Pancreatitis caused by steroids or azathioprine
Hepatic veno-occlusive disease (secondary to primary immunodeficiency or chemotherapy)
Nephrolithiasis caused by indinavir treatment of HIV

ALGORITHMS IN THE ACUTE ABDOMEN

Algorithms can aid in the diagnosis of the patient with an acute abdomen. As stated earlier, computer-assisted diagnosis has been shown to be more accurate than clinical judgment alone in a number of acute abdominal disease states. Algorithms are the basis for computer diagnosis and can be useful in making clinical decisions. The algorithms presented in Figures 45-15 to 45-20 are helpful in acute abdomen patients and can allow both a focused workup and expeditious therapy.

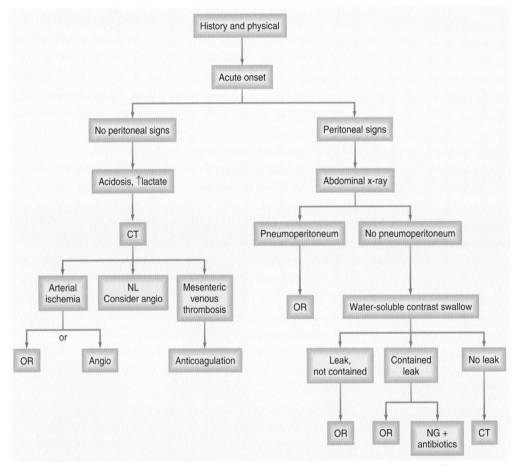

FIGURE 45-15 Algorithm for the treatment of acute-onset severe, generalized abdominal pain. *CT*, computed tomography; *NG*, nasogastric tube; *NL*, normal study; *OR*, operation.

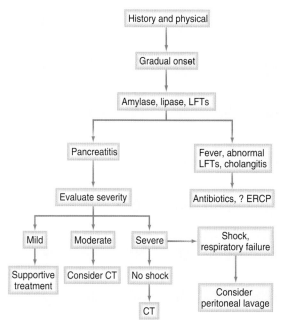

FIGURE 45-16 Algorithm for the treatment of gradual-onset severe, generalized abdominal pain. *CT*, computed tomography; *ERCP*, endoscopic retrograde cholangiopancreatography; *LFTs*, liver function tests.

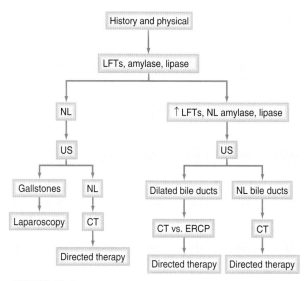

FIGURE 45-17 Algorithm for the treatment of right upper quadrant abdominal pain. *CT*, computed tomography; *ERCP*, endoscopic retrograde cholangiopancreatography; *LFTs*, liver function tests; *NL*, normal study; *US*, ultrasound.

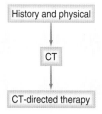

FIGURE 45-18 Algorithm for the treatment of left upper quadrant abdominal pain. *CT*, computed tomography.

SUMMARY

Evaluation and management of the patient with acute abdominal pain remain a challenging part of a surgeon's practice. Whereas advances in imaging techniques, use of algorithms, and computer assistance have improved the diagnostic accuracy for the conditions causing the acute abdomen, a careful history and physical examination remain the most important part of the evaluation. Even with these tools at hand, the surgeon must often make the decision to perform a laparoscopy or laparotomy with a good deal of uncertainty as to the expected findings. Increased morbidity and mortality associated with a delay in the treatment of many of the surgical causes of the acute abdomen argue for an aggressive and expeditious surgical approach.

Common Pitfalls

• Failure to thoroughly examine *and* document findings
• Failure to perform a rectal or vaginal examination when appropriate
• Failure to evaluate for hernias, including the scrotal region
• Failure to conduct a pregnancy test or to consider pregnancy in the diagnosis
• Failure to reassess the patient frequently while developing a differential diagnosis
• Failure to reconsider an established diagnosis when the clinical situation changes
• Failure to recognize immune compromise and to appreciate its masking effect on the historical and examination findings
• Allowing a normal laboratory value to dissuade a diagnosis when there is cause for clinical concern
• Failure to consult colleagues when appropriate
• Failure to take age- and situation-specific diagnoses into consideration
• Failure to make specific and concrete follow-up arrangements when monitoring a clinical situation on an outpatient basis
• Hesitancy to go to the operating room without a firm diagnosis when the clinical situation suggests surgical disease

SELECTED REFERENCES

Ahmad TA, Shelbaya E, Razek SA, et al: Experience of laparoscopic management in 100 patients with acute abdomen. *Hepatogastroenterology* 48:733–736, 2001.

A description of the usefulness of laparoscopy in a large series of patients with acute abdomen. A good review of this important diagnostic and therapeutic tool.

Cademartiri F, Raaijmaker RHJM, Kuiper JW, et al: Multidetector row CT angiography in patients with abdominal angina. *Radiographics* 24:969–984, 2004.

A good review of the computed tomographic characteristics of acute mesenteric ischemia. This outlines the radiographic findings that have greatly assisted in the diagnosis of this otherwise difficult condition.

Graff LG, Robinson D: Abdominal pain and emergency department evaluation. *Emerg Med Clin North Am* 19:123–136, 2001.

Good review of the spectrum of patients presenting with acute abdominal pain.

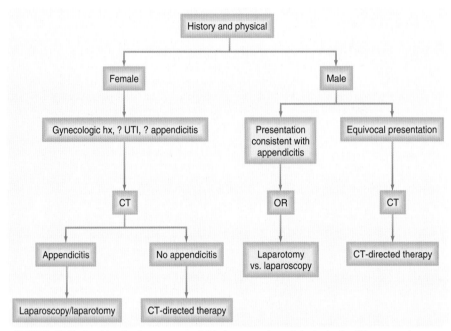

FIGURE 45-19 Algorithm for the treatment of right lower quadrant abdominal pain. *CT*, computed tomography; *hx*, history; *OR*, operation; *UTI*, urinary tract infection.

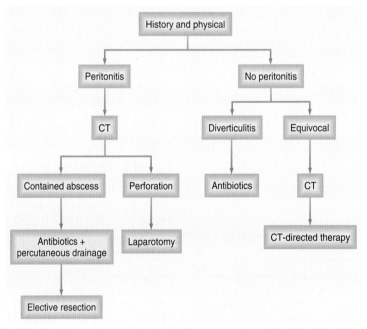

FIGURE 45-20 Algorithm for the treatment of left lower quadrant abdominal pain. *CT*, computed tomography.

Macari M, Balthazar EJ: The acute right lower quadrant: CT evaluation. *Radiol Clin North Am* 41:1117–1136, 2003.

A modern discussion of the role of computed tomography in the evaluation of patients with right lower quadrant abdominal pain.

Silen W: *Cope's early diagnosis of the acute abdomen*, ed 21, New York, 2005, Oxford University Press.

This is a classic monograph stressing the importance of history and physical examination in the diagnosis of the acute abdomen. Nearly all diseases manifesting as an acute abdomen are presented. A must read for the surgical resident.

Steinheber FU: Medical conditions mimicking the acute surgical abdomen. *Med Clin North Am* 57:1559–1567, 1973.

This classic article nicely reviews the various medical conditions that can be manifested as an acute abdomen. It is well written and remains pertinent to the evaluation of these patients.

REFERENCES

1. Sethuraman U, Siadat M, Lepak-Hitch CA, et al: Pulmonary embolism presenting as acute abdomen in a child and adult. *Am J Emerg Med* 27:514.e1–514.e5, 2009.
2. Graff LG, 4th, Robinson D: Abdominal pain and emergency department evaluation. *Emerg Med Clin North Am* 19:123–136, 2001.
3. Steinheber FU: Medical conditions mimicking the acute surgical abdomen. *Med Clin North Am* 57:1559–1567, 1973.
4. Gilbert JA, Kamath PS: Spontaneous bacterial peritonitis: An update. *Mayo Clin Proc* 70:365–370, 1995.
5. Silen W: *Cope's early diagnosis of the acute abdomen*, ed 21, New York, 2005, Oxford University Press.
6. Paterson-Brown S, Vipond MN: Modern aids to clinical decision-making in the acute abdomen. *Br J Surg* 77:13–18, 1990.
7. de Dombal FT: Computers, diagnoses and patients with acute abdominal pain. *Arch Emerg Med* 9:267–270, 1992.
8. Adams ID, Chan M, Clifford PC, et al: Computer aided diagnosis of acute abdominal pain: A multicentre study. *Br Med J (Clin Res Ed)* 293:800–804, 1986.
9. Wellwood J, Johannessen S, Spiegelhalter DJ: How does computer-aided diagnosis improve the management of acute abdominal pain? *Ann R Coll Surg Engl* 74:40–46, 1992.
10. McAdam WA, Brock BM, Armitage T, et al: Twelve years' experience of computer-aided diagnosis in a district general hospital. *Ann R Coll Surg Engl* 72:140–146, 1990.
11. Kort B, Katz VL, Watson WJ: The effect of nonobstetric operation during pregnancy. *Surg Gynecol Obstet* 177:371–376, 1993.
12. Macari M, Balthazar EJ: The acute right lower quadrant: CT evaluation. *Radiol Clin North Am* 41:1117–1136, 2003.
13. Cademartiri F, Raaijmakers RH, Kuiper JW, et al: Multidetector row CT angiography in patients with abdominal angina. *Radiographics* 24:969–984, 2004.
14. Lee R, Tung HK, Tung PH, et al: CT in acute mesenteric ischaemia. *Clin Radiol* 58:279–287, 2003.
15. Hof KH, Krestin GP, Steijerberg EW, et al: Interobserver variability in CT scan interpretation for suspected acute appendicitis. *Emerg Med J* 26:92–94, 2009.
16. Hanbidge AE, Buckler PM, O'Malley ME, et al: From the RSNA refresher courses: Imaging evaluation for acute pain in the right upper quadrant. *Radiographics* 24:1117–1135, 2004.
17. Zissin R, Osadchy A, Gayer G: Abdominal CT findings in small bowel perforation. *Br J Radiol* 82:162–171, 2009.
18. van Randen A, Bipat S, Zwinderman AH, et al: Acute appendicitis: Meta-analysis of diagnostic performance of CT and graded compression US related to prevalence of disease. *Radiology* 249:97–106, 2008.
19. Drake FT, Alfonso R, Bhargava P, et al: Enteral contrast in the computed tomography diagnosis of appendicitis: Comparative effectiveness in a prospective surgical cohort. *Ann Surg* 260:311–316, 2014.
20. De Keulenaer BL, De Waele JJ, Powell B, et al: What is normal intra-abdominal pressure and how is it affected by positioning, body mass and positive end-expiratory pressure? *Intensive Care Med* 35:969–976, 2009.
21. Ahmad TA, Shelbaya E, Razek SA, et al: Experience of laparoscopic management in 100 patients with acute abdomen. *Hepatogastroenterology* 48:733–736, 2001.
22. Perri SG, Altilia F, Pietrangeli F, et al: Laparoscopy in abdominal emergencies. Indications and limitations. *Chir Ital* 54:165–178, 2002.
23. Riemann JF: Diagnostic laparoscopy. *Endoscopy* 35:43–47, 2003.
24. Pecoraro AP, Cacchione RN, Sayad P, et al: The routine use of diagnostic laparoscopy in the intensive care unit. *Surg Endosc* 15:638–641, 2001.
25. Stefanidis D, Richardson WS, Chang L, et al: The role of diagnostic laparoscopy for acute abdominal conditions: An evidence-based review. *Surg Endosc* 23:16–23, 2009.
26. Hickey MS, Kiernan GJ, Weaver KE: Evaluation of abdominal pain. *Emerg Med Clin North Am* 7:437–452, 1989.
27. de Bakker JK, Dijksman LM, Donkervoort SC: Safety and outcome of general surgical open and laparoscopic procedures during pregnancy. *Surg Endosc* 25:1574–1578, 2011.
28. Pearl J, Price R, Richardson W, et al: Guidelines for diagnosis, treatment, and use of laparoscopy for surgical problems during pregnancy. *Surg Endosc* 25:3479–3492, 2011.
29. McGory ML, Zingmond DS, Tillou A, et al: Negative appendectomy in pregnant women is associated with a substantial risk of fetal loss. *J Am Coll Surg* 205:534–540, 2007.
30. Wilasrusmee C, Sukrat B, McEvoy M, et al: Systematic review and meta-analysis of safety of laparoscopic versus open appendicectomy for suspected appendicitis in pregnancy. *Br J Surg* 99:1470–1478, 2012.
31. Sadot E, Telem DA, Arora M, et al: Laparoscopy: A safe approach to appendicitis during pregnancy. *Surg Endosc* 24:383–389, 2009.
32. Hunt MG, Martin JN, Jr, Martin RW, et al: Perinatal aspects of abdominal surgery for nonobstetric disease. *Am J Perinatol* 6:412–417, 1989.
33. ACOG Committee on Obstetric Practice: ACOG Committee Opinion No. 474: Nonobstetric surgery during pregnancy. *Obstet Gynecol* 117:420–421, 2011.
34. Brown JJ, Wilson C, Coleman S, et al: Appendicitis in pregnancy: An ongoing diagnostic dilemma. *Colorectal Dis* 11:116–122, 2009.
35. Lim HK, Bae SH, Seo GS: Diagnosis of acute appendicitis in pregnant women: Value of sonography. *AJR Am J Roentgenol* 159:539–542, 1992.
36. Dewhurst C, Beddy P, Pedrosa I: MRI evaluation of acute appendicitis in pregnancy. *J Magn Reson Imaging* 37:566–575, 2013.
37. Pedrosa I, Lafornara M, Pandharipande PV, et al: Pregnant patients suspected of having acute appendicitis: Effect of MR imaging on negative laparotomy rate and appendiceal perforation rate. *Radiology* 250:749–757, 2009.
38. Veerappan A, Gawron AJ, Soper NJ, et al: Delaying cholecystectomy for complicated gallstone disease in pregnancy is associated with recurrent postpartum symptoms. *J Gastrointest Surg* 17:1953–1959, 2013.
39. Kuy S, Roman SA, Desai R, et al: Outcomes following cholecystectomy in pregnant and nonpregnant women. *Surgery* 146:358–366, 2009.

40. Krishnamoorthi R, Ramarajan N, Wang NE, et al: Effectiveness of a staged US and CT protocol for the diagnosis of pediatric appendicitis: Reducing radiation exposure in the age of ALARA. *Radiology* 259:231–239, 2011.

41. Minneci PC, Sulkowski JP, Nacion KM, et al: Feasibility of a nonoperative management strategy for uncomplicated acute appendicitis in children. *J Am Coll Surg* 219:272–279, 2014.

42. Guler M, Yamak B, Erdogan M, et al: Risk factors for gastrointestinal complications in patients undergoing coronary artery bypass graft surgery. *J Cardiothorac Vasc Anesth* 25:637–641, 2011.

43. Viana FF, Chen Y, Almeida AA, et al: Gastrointestinal complications after cardiac surgery: 10-year experience of a single Australian centre. *ANZ J Surg* 83:651–656, 2013.

44. Hecker A, Uhle F, Schwandner T, et al: Diagnostics, therapy and outcome prediction in abdominal sepsis: Current standards and future perspectives. *Langenbecks Arch Surg* 399:11–22, 2014.

45. Surawicz CM, Brandt LJ, Binion DG, et al: Guidelines for diagnosis, treatment, and prevention of *Clostridium difficile* infections. *Am J Gastroenterol* 108:478–498, quiz 499, 2013.

46. Sailhamer EA, Carson K, Chang Y, et al: Fulminant *Clostridium difficile* colitis: patterns of care and predictors of mortality. *Arch Surg* 144:433–439, 2009.

47. Mehran A, Liberman M, Rosenthal R, et al: Ruptured appendicitis after laparoscopic Roux-en-Y gastric bypass: Pitfalls in diagnosing a surgical abdomen in the morbidly obese. *Obes Surg* 13:938–940, 2003.

48. Byrne TK: Complications of surgery for obesity. *Surg Clin North Am* 81:1181–1193, 2001.

49. Hamilton EC, Sims TL, Hamilton TT, et al: Clinical predictors of leak after laparoscopic Roux-en-Y gastric bypass for morbid obesity. *Surg Endosc* 17:679–684, 2003.

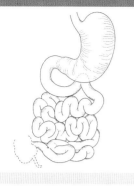

CHAPTER 46

Acute Gastrointestinal Hemorrhage

Ali Tavakkoli, Stanley W. Ashley

第四十六章　急性消化道出血

中文导读

　　本章共分为4节：①急性消化道出血病人的处理；②急性上消化道出血；③急性下消化道出血；④来源不明的急性消化道出血。

　　第一节介绍了急性消化道出血病人的处理，涵盖初步评估，复苏，病史和体格检查，出血点定位，危险分层。病人就诊时对其迅速的初步评估可以判断病情的紧急程度。出血越严重，越应该积极进行复苏。复苏应尽快稳定病人的血流动力学状态以及建立一种方法来监测正在进行的失血。仔细的病史采集和体格检查能为病因和出血来源提供线索，并能识别伴发的复杂情况，进一步的特异性检查可以明确诊断，对出血点进行定位。根据出血的来源，选择治疗性措施，控制出血并防止出血再发。当然，并非所有的消化道出血病人都需要住院或紧急评估，风险评分系统对危险程度进行分层方便病人的分诊。

　　第二节涵盖急性上消化道出血的定义，原因，诊断治疗方法。上消化道出血是指起源于屈氏韧带近端消化道的出血，其原因可以分为非静脉曲张性和门静脉高压相关性出血。内镜是诊断和治疗上消化道出血病人的基础，同时还有血管造影、药物干预、气囊压迫等诊断治疗方法。此外，必要时仍应行外科手术干预。在总述的基础上，该节又对诸如消化性溃疡、Mallory-Weiss撕裂、应激性胃炎以及门静脉高压相关性出血等导致急性上消化道出血的具体疾病进行了详细介绍。

　　第三节介绍了急性下消化道出血的特点，病因，诊断治疗原则。下消化道出血原因很多，可大到憩室病或血管病变引起的严重出血，亦可小到肛裂或痔引发的少量出血。以结肠出血为例，出血的具体病因包括憩室病、血管发育异常、肿瘤等。对下消化道出血进行评估时首先要评估肛门直肠出口出血，大出血时排除上消化道来源同样重要，后续评估取决于出血量，根据出血量选择下一步处理措施。血流动力学不稳定病人应送入手术室，迅速诊断并手术干预。

第四节介绍了来源不明的急性消化道出血。来源不明的（隐源性）消化道出血是一类经食管、胃、十二指肠及结肠镜检查均为阴性的消化道持续或复发性出血。其诊断仍依赖于内镜检查，重复上、下消化道内镜检查是发现遗漏病变的重要手段，另外，一些常规影像学检查手段如标记红细胞扫描、血管造影、小肠稀钡灌注等也被应用于出血的诊断。在一个含200例隐源性出血病人的研究中，小肠被发现是超过60%病例的出血来源，小肠出血的具体病因包括血管发育异常、肿瘤、克罗恩病等。隐源性显性出血的鉴别诊断繁杂多变，故其诊治需格外谨慎。

〔谢大兴〕

Acute gastrointestinal (GI) hemorrhage is a common clinical problem with diverse manifestations. Such bleeding may range from trivial to massive and can originate from virtually any region of the GI tract, including the pancreas, liver, and biliary tree. The site of bleeding is typically classified by the location relative to the ligament of Treitz. Upper GI hemorrhage from proximal to the ligament of Treitz is the most common site of acute GI bleeding. Peptic ulcer disease and variceal hemorrhage are the most common causes. Most of the lower GI bleeding is from the colon, with diverticula and angiodysplasias accounting for the majority of cases. In other cases, the small intestine is responsible. Obscure bleeding is defined as hemorrhage that persists or recurs after negative evaluation with endoscopy. Occult bleeding is not apparent to the patient until symptoms related to the anemia are manifested.

During the past 20 years, multiple factors have influenced the incidence of this disease. Increased use of certain medications (e.g., nonsteroidal anti-inflammatory drugs [NSAIDs] and selective serotonin reuptake inhibitors [SSRIs]) has increased prevalence of GI bleeding, whereas the use of proton pump inhibitors (PPIs) and agents that eradicate *Helicobacter pylori* has decreased the incidence of bleeding. The overall result is that the rate of hospitalization for GI bleeding has declined modestly by 4% between 1998 and 2006.[1] A national estimate of patient discharges with a primary diagnosis of GI bleeding in 2006 was 187 discharges per 100,000 capita. The incidence of GI bleeding increased with age, occurring in approximately 1% of those 85 years or older (1187 hospital discharges with primary diagnosis of GI bleeding per 100,000 capita).[1] Although the total economic burden of GI hemorrhage has not been formally assessed, cost of a hospital admission for upper GI bleeding has been estimated to be about $20,000 per admission with a direct in-hospital economic burden of $7.6 billion in 2009.[2] Importantly, patients who experience an upper GI bleed also have significantly higher health resource utilization and costs during the subsequent 12 months than patients without bleeding.[3]

Management of these patients is frequently multidisciplinary, involving emergency medicine, gastroenterology, intensive care, surgery, and interventional radiology. The importance of early surgical consultation in the care of these patients cannot be overemphasized. In addition to aiding in the resuscitation of the unstable patient, the surgical endoscopist in some settings establishes the diagnosis and initiates therapy. Even when the gastroenterologist assumes this role, early surgical consultation is recommended, especially in high-risk patients. Approximately 5% of patients, usually those who are often older and sicker, require surgical intervention.[4] Early consultation allows the establishment of treatment goals and limits for the initial nonoperative therapy and more time for preoperative preparation and evaluation as well as patient and family education should urgent surgical intervention become necessary.

Most patients with an acute GI hemorrhage stop bleeding spontaneously. This allows time for a more elective evaluation. However, in almost 15% of cases, major bleeding persists, requiring emergent resuscitation, evaluation, and treatment. Improvements in the management of such patients, primarily by means of endoscopy and directed therapy, have significantly reduced the length of hospitalization and overall mortality in the United States to 3%, with mortality rates of 10% reported by other groups, especially in the older patients.[4]

Determination of the site of bleeding is important for directing diagnostic interventions with minimal delay. However, attempts to localize the source should never precede appropriate resuscitative measures.

MANAGEMENT OF PATIENTS WITH ACUTE GASTROINTESTINAL HEMORRHAGE

In patients with GI bleeding, several fundamental principles of initial evaluation and management must be followed. A well-defined and logical approach to the patient with GI hemorrhage is outlined in Figure 46-1. On presentation, a rapid initial assessment permits a determination of the urgency of the situation. Resuscitation is initiated with stabilization of the patient's hemodynamic status and the establishment of a means for monitoring ongoing blood loss. A careful history and physical examination should provide clues to the cause and source of the bleeding and identify any complicating conditions or medications. Specific investigation should then proceed to refine the diagnosis. Therapeutic measures are then initiated, and bleeding is controlled and recurrent hemorrhage prevented.

Initial Assessment

The presentation of GI bleeding is variable, ranging from hemoccult-positive stool on rectal examination to exsanguinating hemorrhage; thus, a structured approach to the assessment is important. Adequacy of the patient's airway and breathing take

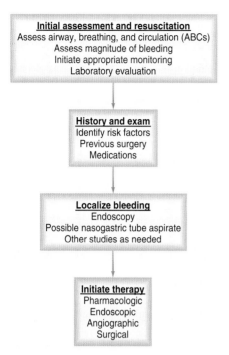

Initial assessment and resuscitation
Assess airway, breathing, and circulation (ABCs)
Assess magnitude of bleeding
Initiate appropriate monitoring
Laboratory evaluation

History and exam
Identify risk factors
Previous surgery
Medications

Localize bleeding
Endoscopy
Possible nasogastric tube aspirate
Other studies as needed

Initiate therapy
Pharmacologic
Endoscopic
Angiographic
Surgical

FIGURE 46-1 General approach to patients with acute GI hemorrhage.

first priority.[5] Once these are ensured, the patient's hemodynamic status becomes the dominant concern and forms the basis for further management. Initial evaluation should focus on rapid assessment of the magnitude of both the preexisting deficits and ongoing hemorrhage. Continuous reassessment of the patient's circulatory status determines the aggressiveness of subsequent evaluation and intervention. The history of the bleeding, both its magnitude and frequency, should also provide some guidance.

The severity of the hemorrhage can be generally determined on the basis of simple clinical parameters. Obtundation, agitation, and hypotension (systolic blood pressure <90 mm Hg in the supine position) associated with cool, clammy extremities are consistent with hemorrhagic shock and suggest a loss of more than 40% of the patient's blood volume. A resting heart rate above 100 beats/min with a decreased pulse pressure implies a 20% to 40% volume loss. In patients without shock, postural changes should be elicited by allowing the patient to sit up with the legs dangling for 5 minutes. A fall in blood pressure of more than 10 mm Hg or an elevation of the pulse of more than 20 beats/min again reflects at least a 20% blood loss. Patients with lesser degrees of bleeding may have no detectable alterations.

The hematocrit is not a useful parameter for assessing the degree of hemorrhage in the acute setting because the proportion of red blood cells (RBCs) and plasma initially lost is constant. The hematocrit does not fall until plasma is redistributed into the intravascular space and resuscitation with crystalloid solution is begun. Likewise, the absence of tachycardia may be misleading; some patients with severe blood loss may actually have bradycardia secondary to vagal slowing of the heart. Hemodynamic signs are less reliable in the elderly and patients taking beta blockers.

Resuscitation

The more severe the bleeding, the more aggressive the resuscitation. In fact, the single leading cause of morbidity and mortality

in these patients is multiorgan failure related to inadequate initial or subsequent resuscitation. Intubation and ventilation should be initiated early if there is any question of airway compromise. In patients with evidence of hemodynamic instability or those in whom ongoing bleeding is suspected, two large-bore intravenous lines should be placed, preferably in the antecubital fossae. Unstable patients should receive a 2-liter bolus of crystalloid solution, usually lactated Ringer solution , which most closely approximates the electrolyte composition of whole blood. The response to the fluid resuscitation should be noted. Blood should immediately be sent for type and crossmatch, hematocrit, platelet count, coagulation profile, routine chemistries, and liver function tests. A Foley catheter should also be inserted for assessment of end-organ perfusion. The oxygen-carrying capacity of the blood can be maximized by administering supplemental oxygen. Frequently, these patients benefit from early admission to and management in the intensive care unit (ICU).

The decision to transfuse blood depends on the response to the fluid challenge, the age of the patient, whether concomitant cardiopulmonary disease is present, and whether the bleeding continues. The initial effects of crystalloid infusion and the patient's ongoing hemodynamic parameters should be the primary criteria. Once again, this process requires an element of clinical judgment. For example, a young, healthy patient with an estimated blood loss of 20% who responds to the fluid challenge with a normalization of hemodynamics may not need any blood products, whereas an elderly patient with a significant cardiac history and the same blood loss probably requires a transfusion. In general, the hematocrit should be maintained above 30% in the elderly and above 20% in young, otherwise healthy patients. Likewise, the propensity of the suspected lesion to continue bleeding or to rebleed must play a role in this decision. For example, esophageal varices are very likely to continue to bleed and transfusion might be considered earlier than if a Mallory-Weiss tear, which has a low rebleeding rate, is considered the culprit. In general, packed RBCs are the preferred form of transfusion, although whole blood, preferably warmed, may be employed in circumstances of massive blood loss. Defects in coagulation and platelets should be replaced as they are detected, and patients who require high-volume transfusion should empirically receive both fresh-frozen plasma and platelets and calcium.

History and Physical Examination

Once the severity of the bleeding is assessed and resuscitation initiated, attention is directed to the history and physical examination. The history helps to make a preliminary assessment of the site and cause of bleeding and of significant medical conditions that may determine or alter the course of management.

Obviously, the characteristics of the bleeding provide important clues. The time at onset, volume, and frequency are important in estimating blood loss. Hematemesis, melena, and hematochezia are the most common manifestations of acute hemorrhage. Hematemesis is the vomiting of blood and is usually caused by bleeding from the upper GI tract, although rarely bleeding from the nose or pharynx can be responsible. It may be bright red or older and therefore take on the appearance of coffee grounds. Melena, the passage of black, tarry, and foul-smelling stool, generally suggests bleeding from the upper GI tract. Although the melanotic appearance typically results from gastric acid degradation, which converts hemoglobin to hematin, and from the actions of digestive enzymes and luminal bacteria in the small intestine, blood loss from the distal small bowel or right colon may have this appearance, particularly if transit is slow enough. Melena should not be confused with the greenish character of the stool in patients taking iron supplements. One way to distinguish these two is by performing a guaiac test, the result of which is negative in those receiving iron supplementation. Hematochezia refers to bright red blood from the rectum that may or may not be mixed with stool. Although this typically reflects a distal colonic source, if the magnitude is significant, even upper GI bleeds may produce hematochezia.

The medical history may provide a variety of clues to the diagnosis. Antecedent vomiting may suggest a Mallory-Weiss tear, whereas weight loss raises the specter of malignant disease. Even demographic data may prove useful; the elderly bleed from lesions such as angiodysplasias, diverticula, ischemic colitis, and cancer, whereas younger patients bleed from peptic ulcers, varices, and Meckel's diverticula. A past history of GI disease, bleeding, or operation should immediately begin to focus the differential diagnosis. Antecedent epigastric distress may point to a peptic ulcer, whereas previous aortic surgery suggests the possibility of an aortoenteric fistula. A history of liver disease prompts a consideration of variceal bleeding. Medication use may also be revealing. A history of ingestion of salicylates, NSAIDs, and SSRIs is common, particularly in the elderly.[6] These medications are associated with GI mucosal erosions that are typically seen in the upper GI tract but that occasionally can be seen in the small bowel and colon. GI bleeding in the setting of anticoagulation therapy, either warfarin or low-molecular-weight heparin, is still most commonly the result of GI disease and should not be ascribed to the anticoagulation alone.[7]

Physical examination may also be revealing. The oropharynx and nose can occasionally simulate symptoms of a more distal source and should always be examined. Abdominal examination is only occasionally helpful, but it is important to exclude masses, splenomegaly, and adenopathy. Epigastric tenderness is suggestive but not diagnostic of gastritis or peptic ulceration. The stigmata of liver disease, including jaundice, ascites, palmar erythema, and caput medusae, may suggest bleeding related to varices, although these patients commonly bleed from other sources as well. On occasion, the physical examination may reveal clues to more obscure diagnoses, such as the telangiectasias of Osler-Weber-Rendu syndrome or the pigmented lesions of the oral mucosa in Peutz-Jeghers syndrome. A rectal examination and anoscopy should be performed to exclude a low-lying rectal cancer or bleeding from hemorrhoids.

Localization

Subsequent management of the patient with acute GI hemorrhage depends on localization of the site of the bleeding. An algorithm for the diagnosis of acute GI hemorrhage is shown in Figure 46-2.

Although melena is usually from the upper GI tract, it can be the result of bleeding from the small bowel or colon. Likewise, hematochezia is sometimes the consequence of brisk upper GI bleeding. One approach to distinguishing these possibilities has been to insert a nasogastric (NG) tube and to perform a gastric lavage with examination of the aspirate. Increasing data, however, have shown that an NG tube is unreliable in localizing the bleeding site, and virtually all patients with significant bleeding should undergo upper endoscopy for direct visualization.

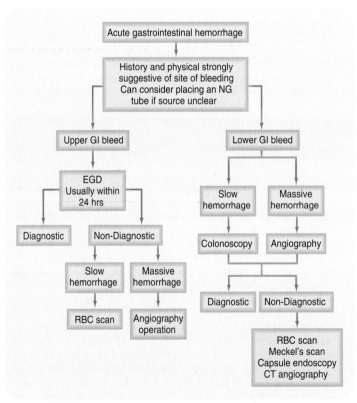

FIGURE 46-2 Algorithm for the diagnosis of acute GI hemorrhage.

Upper endoscopy under these circumstances is highly accurate both in identifying an upper GI lesion and, if evaluation is negative, in directing attention to a lower GI source. Early endoscopy with directed therapy has been shown to reduce resource utilization and transfusion requirements and to shorten hospital stay. The exact definition and timeline of an "early" endoscopy have been well studied and refined. There is little argument that in an unstable patient, an urgent endoscopy is often required; however, in those patients with overt signs of bleeding but who are otherwise stable, endoscopy within 6 or 12 hours has not been shown to be of any additional benefit compared with endoscopy performed within 24 hours.[8,9]

Clinicians should be aware that esophagogastroduodenoscopy (EGD) in the urgent or emergent setting is associated with reduced accuracy, often because of poor visualization, and a significant increase in the incidence of complications, including aspiration, respiratory depression, and GI perforation, compared with elective procedures. Airway protection is critical and may require endotracheal intubation if it has not been performed previously. Volume resuscitation should not be interrupted by the examination.

As shown in Figure 46-2, subsequent evaluation depends on the results of the upper endoscopy and the magnitude of the bleeding. Angiography or even surgery may prove necessary for massive hemorrhage, precluding endoscopy, from either the upper or lower GI tract. For slow or intermittent bleeding from the lower GI tract, colonoscopy is now the initial diagnostic maneuver of choice. When endoscopy is nondiagnostic, the tagged RBC scan is usually employed. For obscure bleeding, usually from the small bowel, capsule endoscopy is becoming the appropriate study. These diagnostic procedures are discussed subsequently in greater detail. Once the location of bleeding has been identified, appropriate therapy, as discussed in relevant sections later, can be initiated.

Risk Stratification

Not all patients with GI bleeding require hospital admission or emergent evaluation. For example, the patient with a small amount of rectal bleeding that has stopped can generally be evaluated on an outpatient basis. In many patients, however, the decision is less straightforward, and considerable recent effort has been devoted to the development of risk scoring tools to facilitate patient triage. These scoring systems have been used to predict the risk of rebleeding and mortality, to evaluate the need for ICU admission, and to determine the need for urgent endoscopy. Some scoring systems (e.g., APACHE II) are nonspecific to GI bleeding but can provide general information about the patient's condition and risk of adverse outcomes.

There have also been attempts to develop disease-specific scoring systems for upper GI bleeds. These scores help to identify those at higher risk of major bleeding or death and who warrant closer observation and more aggressive therapy. The commonly used scoring systems are the Rockall score, which takes into account endoscopic findings, and the Blatchford score, which does not require endoscopic data and can be used during initial assessment. Box 46-1 summarizes these scoring systems.

ACUTE UPPER GASTROINTESTINAL HEMORRHAGE

Upper GI bleeding refers to bleeding that arises from the GI tract proximal to the ligament of Treitz and accounts for nearly 80%

BOX 46-1 Commonly Used Risk Stratification Systems for Upper Gastrointestinal Bleeds

Blatchford Score
Blood urea nitrogen
Hemoglobin
Systolic blood pressure
Pulse
Presence of melena, syncope, hepatic or cardiac dysfunction

Rockall Score
Age (<60 years, 60-79 years, >80 years)
Comorbid disease (cardiac, hepatic, renal, or disseminated cancer)
Magnitude of the hemorrhage (systolic blood pressure <100 mm Hg, heart rate >100 beats/min) on presentation
Transfusion requirement
Endoscopic findings (Mallory-Weiss tears, nonmalignant lesions, or malignant lesions)
Stigmata of recent bleed

TABLE 46-1 Common Causes of Upper Gastrointestinal Hemorrhage

NONVARICEAL BLEEDING	80%	PORTAL HYPERTENSIVE BLEEDING	20%
Gastric and duodenal ulcers	30%-40%	Gastroesophageal varices	>90%
Gastritis or duodenitis	20%	Hypertensive portal gastropathy	<5%
Esophagitis	5%-10%	Isolated gastric varices	Rare
Mallory-Weiss tears	5%-10%		
Arteriovenous malformations	5%		
Tumors	2%		
Others	5%		

---

of significant GI hemorrhage. The causes of upper GI bleeding are best categorized as either nonvariceal sources or bleeding related to portal hypertension (Table 46-1). The nonvariceal causes account for approximately 80% of such bleeding, with peptic ulcer disease being the most common.[10] Although patients with cirrhosis are at high risk for development of variceal bleeding, nonvariceal sources can account for up to 50% of GI bleeds. However, because of greater morbidity and mortality of variceal bleeding, patients with cirrhosis should generally be assumed to have variceal bleeding and appropriate therapy initiated until an emergent endoscopy has demonstrated another cause for the hemorrhage.

The foundation for the diagnosis and management of patients with an upper GI bleed is an upper endoscopy. Multiple studies have demonstrated that early EGD, within 24 hours, results in reductions in blood transfusion requirements, a decrease in the need for surgery, and a shorter length of hospital stay. Endoscopic identification of the source of bleeding also permits an estimate of the risk of subsequent or persistent hemorrhage as well as facilitates operative planning should that prove necessary. It is somewhat surprising that studies have not shown any benefits in performing the endoscopies sooner (within 6 or 12 hours) than within 24 hours.[8,9] Although the best tool for localization of the bleeding source is EGD, this intervention is associated with increased risk and poor visualization in the acute setting, which may offset some of its benefits. In 1% to 2% of patients with upper GI hemorrhage, the source cannot be identified because of the excessive blood impairing the visualization of the mucosal surface.[11] Aggressive lavage of the stomach with room temperature normal saline solution before the procedure can be helpful. Use of promotility agents to enhance endoscopic visualization is not recommended.[12] If upper GI bleed is confirmed but identification of the actual source is still not possible, angiography may be appropriate in the reasonably stable patient, although operative intervention should be seriously considered if the blood loss is extreme or the patient is hemodynamically unstable. Tagged RBC scan is seldom necessary with a confirmed upper GI bleed, and contrast studies are usually contraindicated because they will interfere with subsequent maneuvers.

Specific Causes of Upper Gastrointestinal Hemorrhage
Nonvariceal Bleeding

Peptic ulcer disease. Peptic ulcer disease still represents the most frequent cause of upper GI hemorrhage, accounting for approximately 40% of all cases.[13] Approximately 10% to 15% of patients with peptic ulcer disease develop bleeding at some point in the course of their disease. Bleeding is the most frequent indication for operation and the principal cause for death in peptic ulcer disease.[14] Peptic ulcer disease is discussed in more detail in Chapter 48; this discussion focuses only on bleeding from ulcer disease.

The epidemiology of peptic ulcer has continued to change. The incidence of uncomplicated peptic ulcer disease has declined dramatically. This recent change has been attributed to better medical therapy, including the PPIs and regimens for eradication of *H. pylori*. Along with this decline, there has also been a decline in the number of hospitalizations for complicated peptic ulcer disease and number of surgical interventions, including suture repair of bleeding ulcers. When surgery for upper GI hemorrhage is undertaken, however, such operations are now typically performed in older patients with higher comorbidities.[14]

Bleeding develops as a consequence of acid-peptic erosion of the mucosal surface. Whereas chronic blood loss is common with any ulcer, significant bleeding typically results when there is involvement of an artery of the submucosa or, with penetration of the ulcer, of an even larger vessel. The most significant hemorrhage occurs when duodenal or gastric ulcers penetrate into branches of the gastroduodenal artery or left gastric arteries, respectively.

Management. Figure 46-3 outlines an approach to management. As stated previously, patients with clinical evidence of a GI bleed should receive an endoscopy within 24 hours, and while awaiting the EGD, they should be treated with a PPI. Although this approach has been shown to reduce the stigmata of a recent hemorrhage at index endoscopy, it had no impact on clinical outcomes such as transfusion requirements, mortality, or need for surgery; despite this, it is believed to be a cost-effective intervention for those suspected to have an upper GI bleed.[15]

After the index endoscopy, treatment strategies depend on the appearance of the lesion at endoscopy. Endoscopic therapy is instituted if bleeding is active or, when bleeding has already

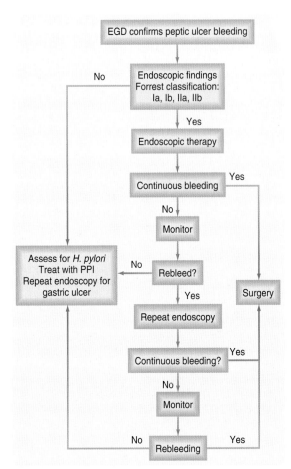

FIGURE 46-3 Algorithm for the diagnosis and management of nonvariceal upper GI bleeding.

TABLE 46-2 The Forrest Classification for Endoscopic Findings and Rebleeding Risks in Peptic Ulcer Disease

CLASSIFICATION		REBLEEDING RISK
Grade Ia	Active, pulsatile bleeding	High
Grade Ib	Active, nonpulsatile bleeding	High
Grade IIa	Nonbleeding visible vessel	High
Grade IIb	Adherent clot	Intermediate
Grade IIc	Ulcer with black spot	Low
Grade III	Clean, nonbleeding ulcer bed	Low

stopped, if there is a significant risk of rebleeding. The ability to predict the risk of rebleeding permits prophylactic therapy, closer monitoring, and earlier detection of hemorrhage in high-risk patients. The Forrest classification was developed in an attempt to assess this risk on the basis of endoscopic findings and to stratify the patients into low-, intermediate-, and high-risk groups (Table 46-2). Endoscopic therapy is recommended in cases of active bleeding as well as for a visible vessel (Forrest I-IIa). In cases of an adherent clot (Forrest IIb), the clot is removed and the underlying lesion evaluated. Ulcers with a clean base or a black spot, secondary to hematin deposition, are generally not treated endoscopically. Approximately 25% of patients undergoing EGD for upper GI bleed require an endoscopic intervention.[14]

Medical management. In cases of a confirmed peptic ulcer bleed, PPIs have been shown to reduce the risk of rebleeding and the need for surgical intervention. Therefore, patients with a suspected or confirmed bleeding ulcer should be started on a PPI.[12] Unlike perforated ulcers, which are commonly associated with *H. pylori* infection, the association between *H. pylori* infection and bleeding is less strong. Only 60% to 70% of patients with a bleeding ulcer are *H. pylori* positive.[16] This has generated some discussion as to the importance of *H. pylori* treatment in patients with a bleeding peptic ulcer. Several studies and a large meta-analysis, however, have shown that *H. pylori* treatment and eradication, in patients who test positive for the infection, result in decreased rebleeding.[17] Importantly, once the *H. pylori* infection has been eradicated, there is no need for long-term acid suppression, and there is no increased risk of further bleeding with this approach.[18] International consensus guidelines also recommend that patients treated for *H. pylori* should be tested to confirm eradication. Some guidelines also recommend that those who tested negative during the acute episode should be retested to confirm negative status. This is due to reports of high false-negative results of *H. pylori* testing during an acute bleed.[12]

In patients who are taking ulcerogenic medications such as NSAIDs or SSRIs and present with a bleeding GI lesion, these medications should be stopped. Patients should be started on a nonulcerogenic alternative, if possible, after their acute bleeding episode has resolved. In those taking NSAIDs, more specific cyclooxygenase 2 inhibitors had been a promising alternative. Concerns about the cardiotoxicity of these drugs have resulted in their withdrawal from the market, reducing the clinical use of these alternative medicines. Further affecting the popularity of these medications have been population-based studies showing that not all cyclooxygenase 2 inhibitors result in a decreased incidence of upper GI complications.[19] Therefore, an alternative approach has been to identify ways to reduce the adverse GI side effects of NSAIDs. To this end, studies have shown that *H. pylori* eradication in patients who are about to start these medications can reduce the incidence of adverse GI side effects, including bleeding.[20] These studies highlight the synergistic effect of *H. pylori* eradication and NSAID use. Although this approach can have a preventive role in regard to GI bleeding, NSAIDs cannot be recommended for those who present with a bleed, even after *H. pylori* eradication.[21]

Endoscopic management. Once the bleeding ulcer has been identified, effective local therapy can be delivered endoscopically to control the hemorrhage. The available endoscopic options include epinephrine injection, heater probes, and coagulation as well as the application of clips. Epinephrine injection (1:10,000) to all four quadrants of the lesion is successful in controlling the hemorrhage. It has been shown that large-volume injection (>13 mL) is associated with better hemostasis, suggesting that the endoscopic injection works, in part, by compressing the bleeding vessel and inducing tamponade. Epinephrine injection alone is associated with a high rebleeding rate; therefore, the standard practice as recommended by international consensus guidelines is to provide combination therapy. This usually means the addition of thermal therapy to the injection. The sources of thermal energy can be heater probes, monopolar or bipolar electrocoagulation, and laser or argon plasma coagulation (APC). The most commonly used energy sources are electrocoagulation for bleeding ulcers and APC for superficial lesions. A combination of injection

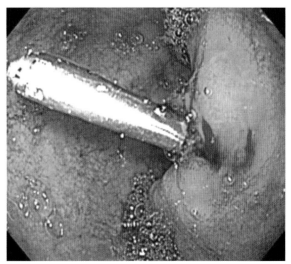

FIGURE 46-4 Hemoclip applied to a bleeding duodenal lesion. (Courtesy Linda S. Lee, MD, Brigham and Women's Hospital.)

with thermal therapy achieves hemostasis in 90% of bleeding peptic ulcer disease. Hemoclips (Fig. 46-4), which can be difficult to apply, may be particularly effective in dealing with a spurting vessel as they provide immediate control of hemorrhage.

Rebleeding of an ulcer is associated with a significant increase in mortality, and careful observation of patients at high risk of rebleeding using criteria previously described is important. In those who rebled, a second attempt at endoscopic control has been validated and is recommended. A second attempt at endoscopic hemostasis is successful in 75% of patients.[22] Although this will fail in 25% of patients who will then require emergent surgery, there does not appear to be any increase in morbidity or mortality with this treatment approach. Therefore, most clinicians would encourage a second attempt at endoscopic control before subjecting the patient to surgery.

Surgical management. Despite significant advances in endoscopic therapy, approximately 10% of patients with bleeding ulcers still require surgical intervention for effective hemostasis.[14] However, identifying patients who are likely to fail to respond to endoscopic therapy is difficult, and the timing of surgery is much debated. To assist in this decision making, several clinical and endoscopic parameters have been proposed that are thought to identify patients at high risk for failed endoscopic therapy. The clinical factors to consider are shock and a low hemoglobin level at presentation. At the time of endoscopy, although the Forrest classification is the most important indicator of rebleeding risk, the location and size of the ulcer are also significant. Ulcers larger than 2 cm, posterior duodenal ulcers, and gastric ulcers have significantly higher risk of rebleeding.[23,24] Patients with these characteristics need closer monitoring and possibly earlier surgical intervention. Clearly, clinical judgment and local expertise must play a critical role in this decision.

Indications for surgery have traditionally been based on the blood transfusion requirements. Increased blood transfusions have been clearly associated with increased mortality. Although a less definitive criterion than it was in the past, most surgeons still consider an ongoing blood transfusion requirement in excess of 6 units an indication for surgical intervention, particularly in the elderly, although an 8- to 10-unit loss may be more acceptable for

---

BOX 46-2 Indications for Surgery in Gastrointestinal Hemorrhage

Hemodynamic instability despite vigorous resuscitation (>6-unit transfusion)

Failure of endoscopic techniques to arrest hemorrhage

Recurrent hemorrhage after initial stabilization (with up to two attempts at obtaining endoscopic hemostasis)

Shock associated with recurrent hemorrhage

Continued slow bleeding with a transfusion requirement exceeding 3 units/day

---

the younger population. Current indications for surgery for peptic ulcer hemorrhage are summarized in Box 46-2. Secondary or relative indications include a rare blood type or difficult crossmatch, refusal of transfusion, shock on presentation, advanced age, severe comorbid disease, and a bleeding chronic gastric ulcer for which malignancy is a concern.

The first priority at operation should be control of the hemorrhage. Once this is accomplished, a decision must be made about the need for a definitive acid-reducing procedure. Each of these steps varies, depending on whether the lesion is a duodenal or gastric ulcer.

Duodenal ulcer. The first step in the operative management for a duodenal ulcer is exposure of the bleeding site. Because most of these lesions are in the duodenal bulb, longitudinal duodenotomy or duodenopyloromyotomy is performed. Hemorrhage can typically be controlled initially with pressure and then direct suture ligation with nonabsorbable suture. When ulcers are positioned anteriorly, four-quadrant suture ligation usually suffices. A posterior ulcer eroding into the pancreaticoduodenal or gastroduodenal artery may require suture ligature of the vessel proximal and distal to the ulcer as well as placement of a U-stitch underneath the ulcer to control the pancreatic branches.

Once the bleeding has been addressed, a definitive acid-reducing operation was traditionally considered. With the identification of the role of *H. pylori* infection in duodenal ulcer disease, the utility of such a procedure has been questioned on the basis of the argument that simple closure and subsequent treatment for *H. pylori* infection should be sufficient to prevent recurrence. This is reflected in current surgical practice, wherein rates of definitive ulcer therapy (gastrectomy or vagotomy) in patients hospitalized for peptic ulcer disease have declined significantly.

Historically, the choice between various operations has been based on the hemodynamic condition of the patient and on whether there is a long-standing history of refractory ulcer disease. The various operations for peptic ulcer disease are discussed in greater detail in Chapter 48. Because the pylorus has often been opened in a longitudinal fashion to control the bleeding, closure as a pyloroplasty combined with truncal vagotomy is the most frequently used operation for bleeding duodenal ulcer. There is some evidence to suggest that a parietal cell vagotomy may represent a better therapy for a bleeding duodenal ulcer in the stable patient, although some of this benefit may be abrogated if the pylorus has been divided. Today, inexperience of the surgeon with this procedure may be the determining factor. In a patient who has a known history of refractory duodenal ulcer disease or who has failed to respond to more conservative surgery, antrectomy with truncal vagotomy may be more appropriate. However, this procedure is more complex and should be undertaken rarely in a hemodynamically unstable patient.

Gastric ulcer. For bleeding gastric ulcers, control of bleeding is the immediate priority. Although this may initially require gastrotomy and suture ligation, this alone is associated with a high risk of rebleeding of almost 30%. In addition, because of a 10% incidence of malignancy, gastric ulcer resection is generally indicated. Simple excision alone is associated with rebleeding in as many as 20% of patients, so distal gastrectomy is generally preferred, although ulcer excision combined with vagotomy and pyloroplasty may be considered in the high-risk patient. Bleeding ulcers of the proximal stomach near the gastroesophageal junction are more difficult to manage. Proximal or near-total gastrectomies are associated with a particularly high mortality in the setting of acute hemorrhage. Options include distal gastrectomy combined with resection of a tongue of proximal stomach to include the ulcer or vagotomy and pyloroplasty combined with either wedge resection or simple oversewing of the ulcer.

Mallory-Weiss tears. Mallory-Weiss tears are mucosal and submucosal tears that occur near the gastroesophageal junction. Classically, these lesions develop in alcoholic patients after a period of intense retching and vomiting following binge drinking, but they can occur in any patient who has a history of repeated emesis. The mechanism, proposed by Mallory and Weiss in 1929, is forceful contraction of the abdominal wall against an unrelaxed cardia, resulting in mucosal laceration of the cardia as a result of the increased intragastric pressure.

Such lesions account for 5% to 10% of cases of upper GI bleeding. They are usually diagnosed on the basis of history. Endoscopy is frequently employed to confirm the diagnosis. To avoid missing the diagnosis, it is important to perform a retroflexion maneuver and to view the area just below the gastroesophageal junction. Most tears occur along the lesser curvature and less commonly on the greater curve. Supportive therapy is often all that is necessary because 90% of bleeding episodes are self-limited, and the mucosa often heals within 72 hours.

In rare cases of severe ongoing bleeding, local endoscopic therapy with injection or electrocoagulation may be effective. Angiographic embolization, usually with absorbable material such as a gelatin sponge, has been successfully employed in cases of failed endoscopic therapy. If these maneuvers fail, high gastrotomy and suturing of the mucosal tear are indicated. It is important to rule out the diagnosis of variceal bleeding in cases of failed endoscopic therapy by a thorough examination of the gastroesophageal junction. Recurrent bleeding from a Mallory-Weiss tear is uncommon.

Stress gastritis. Stress-related gastritis is characterized by the appearance of multiple superficial erosions of the entire stomach, most commonly in the body. It is thought to result from the combination of acid and pepsin injury in the context of ischemia from hypoperfusion states, although NSAIDs produce a similar appearance. In the 1960s and 1970s, it was a commonly encountered lesion in critically ill patients, with significant morbidity and mortality from bleeding. These lesions are different from the solitary ulcerations, related to acid hypersecretion, that occur in patients with severe head injury (Cushing ulcers). When stress ulceration is associated with major burns, these lesions are referred to as Curling ulcers. In contrast to NSAID-associated lesions, significant hemorrhage from stress ulceration was a common phenomenon. With improvements in the management of shock and sepsis as well as widespread use of acid suppressive therapy, significant bleeding from such lesions is rarely encountered.

In those who develop significant bleeding, acid suppressive therapy is often successful in controlling the hemorrhage. In rare cases when this fails, consideration should be given to administration of octreotide or vasopressin, endoscopic therapy, or even angiographic embolization. Historically, such cases were more commonly seen and, at times, dealt with surgically. The surgical choices included vagotomy and pyloroplasty with oversewing of the hemorrhage or near-total gastrectomy. These procedures carried mortality rates as high as 60%. Fortunately, they are seldom necessary today.

Esophagitis. The esophagus is infrequently the source for significant hemorrhage. When it does occur, it is most commonly the result of esophagitis. Esophageal inflammation secondary to repeated exposure of the esophageal mucosa to the acidic gastric secretions in gastroesophageal reflux disease leads to an inflammatory response that can result in chronic blood loss. Ulceration may accompany this, but the superficial mucosal ulcerations generally do not bleed acutely and are manifested as anemia or guaiac-positive stools. Various infectious agents may also cause esophagitis, particularly in the immunocompromised host (Fig. 46-5). With infection, hemorrhage can occasionally be massive. Other causes of esophageal bleeding include medications, Crohn's disease, and radiation.

Treatment typically includes acid suppressive therapy. Endoscopic control of the hemorrhage, usually with electrocoagulation or heater probe, is often successful. In patients with an infectious cause, targeted therapy is appropriate. Surgery is seldom necessary.

Dieulafoy lesion. Dieulafoy lesions are vascular malformations found primarily along the lesser curve of the stomach within 6 cm of the gastroesophageal junction, although they can occur elsewhere in the GI tract (Fig. 46-6). They represent rupture of unusually large vessels (1 to 3 mm) found in the gastric submucosa. Erosion of the gastric mucosa overlying these vessels leads to hemorrhage. The mucosal defect is usually small (2 to 5 mm) and may be difficult to identify.[25] Given the large size of the underlying artery, bleeding from a Dieulafoy lesion can be massive (Fig. 46-7).

Initial attempts at endoscopic control are often successful. Application of thermal or sclerosant therapy is effective in 80%

to 100% of cases. In cases that fail endoscopic therapy, angiographic coil embolization can be successful. If these approaches are unsuccessful, surgical intervention may be necessary; because of difficulties in visualization and palpation of these lesions, prior endoscopic tattooing can facilitate the procedure. A gastrostomy is performed, and attempts are made at identifying the bleeding source. The lesion can then be oversewn. In cases in which the bleeding point is not identified, a partial gastrectomy may be necessary.

Gastric antral vascular ectasia. Also known as watermelon stomach, gastric antral vascular ectasia (GAVE) is characterized by a collection of dilated venules appearing as linear red streaks converging on the antrum in longitudinal fashion, giving it the appearance of a watermelon. Acute severe hemorrhage is rare in GAVE, and most patients present with persistent, iron deficiency anemia from continued occult blood loss. Endoscopic therapy is indicated for persistent, transfusion-dependent bleeding and has been reportedly successful in up to 90% of patients. The preferred endoscopic therapy is APC (Fig. 46-8). Patients failing

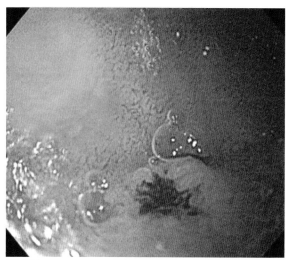

FIGURE 46-6 Dieulafoy lesion of the stomach. (Courtesy Linda S. Lee, MD, Brigham and Women's Hospital.)

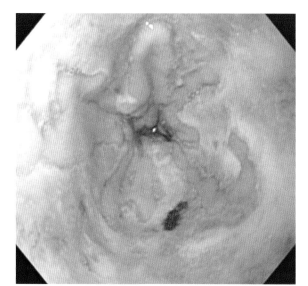

FIGURE 46-5 Bleeding esophageal ulcer secondary to herpes esophagitis. (Courtesy Scott A. Hande, MD, Brigham and Women's Hospital.)

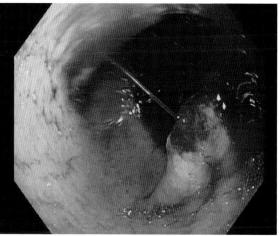

FIGURE 46-7 Bleeding Dieulafoy lesion with a spurting vessel. (Courtesy Marvin Ryou, MD, Brigham and Women's Hospital.)

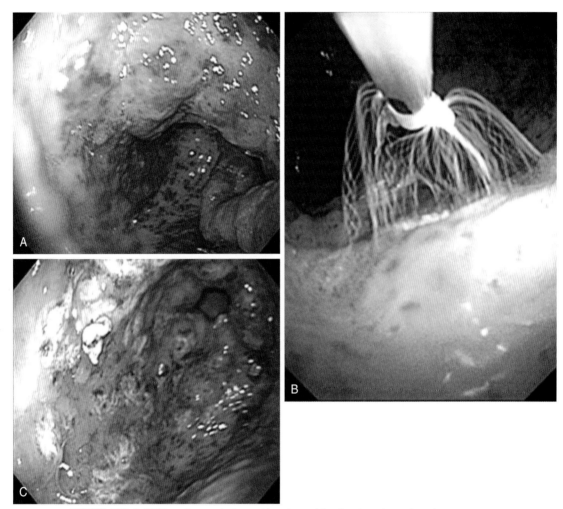

FIGURE 46-8 A, GAVE can be seen in the gastric antrum, giving the stomach a watermelon appearance. **B,** APC therapy of GAVE. **C,** Post-therapy appearance of GAVE. (Courtesy David L. Carr-Locke, MD, Brigham and Women's Hospital.)

to respond to endoscopic therapy should be considered for antrectomy.

Malignancy. Malignant neoplasms of the upper GI tract are usually associated with chronic anemia or hemoccult-positive stool rather than episodes of significant hemorrhage. On occasion, malignant neoplasms will be manifested as ulcerative lesions that bleed persistently. This is perhaps most characteristic of the GI stromal tumor (GIST), although it may occur with a variety of other lesions including leiomyomas and lymphomas. Although endoscopic therapy is often successful in controlling these bleeds, the rebleeding rate is high; therefore, when a malignant neoplasm is diagnosed, surgical resection is indicated. The extent of resection is dependent on the specific lesion and whether the resection is believed to be curative or palliative. Palliative resections for control of bleeding usually entail wedge resections. Standard cancer operations are indicated when possible, although this may depend on the hemodynamic stability of the patient.

Aortoenteric fistula. Primary aortoduodenal fistulas are rare lesions and likely to be fatal as they represent a rupture of the aorta to the bowel. The more common entity seen clinically is a graft-enteric erosion, which may develop in up to 1% of aortic

graft cases and can be manifested as a GI bleed (Fig. 46-9). Although the interval between surgery and hemorrhage can be days to years, the median interval is about 3 years. The sequence is thought to involve development of a pseudoaneurysm at the proximal anastomotic suture line in the setting of an infection, with subsequent fistulization into the overlying duodenum.

This diagnosis should be considered in all bleeding patients with a known abdominal aortic aneurysm or a previous prosthetic aneurysm repair. Hemorrhage in this situation is often massive and fatal unless immediate surgical intervention is undertaken. Typically, patients with bleeding from an aortoenteric fistula will present first with a "sentinel bleed." This is a self-limited episode that heralds the subsequent massive and often fatal hemorrhage. This should prompt urgent upper endoscopy because diagnosis at this stage can be lifesaving. Any evidence of bleeding in the distal duodenum (third or fourth portion) on EGD should be considered diagnostic. A computed tomography (CT) scan with intravenous administration of contrast material will demonstrate air around the graft (suggestive of an infection), possible pseudoaneurysm, and rarely intravenous contrast material in the duodenal lumen.

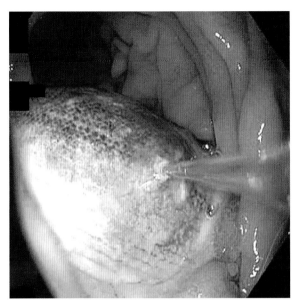

FIGURE 46-9 A vascular graft visualized during upper endoscopy for bleeding. (Courtesy Konrad Rajab, MD, Brigham and Women's Hospital.)

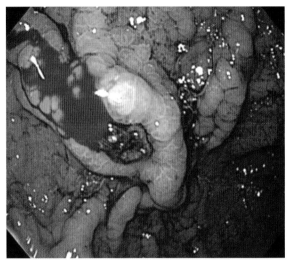

FIGURE 46-10 Bleeding from a percutaneous endoscopic gastrostomy site. (Courtesy David L. Carr-Locke, MD, Brigham and Women's Hospital.)

Therapy includes ligation of the aorta proximal to the graft, removal of the infected prosthesis, and extra-anatomic bypass. The defect in the duodenum is often small and can be repaired primarily. This is a complex and often morbid procedure.

Hemobilia. Hemobilia is often a difficult diagnosis to make. It is typically associated with trauma, recent instrumentation of the biliary tree, or hepatic neoplasms. This unusual cause of GI bleeding should be suspected in anyone who presents with hemorrhage, right upper quadrant pain, and jaundice. Unfortunately, this triad is seen in less than half of patients, and a high index of suspicion is required. Endoscopy can be helpful by demonstrating blood at the ampulla. Angiography is the diagnostic procedure of choice. If diagnosis is confirmed, angiographic embolization is the preferred treatment.

Hemosuccus pancreaticus. Another rare cause of upper GI bleeding is bleeding from the pancreatic duct. This is often caused by erosion of a pancreatic pseudocyst into the splenic artery. It is manifested with abdominal pain and hematochezia. As with hemobilia, it is a difficult diagnosis to make and requires a high index of suspicion in patients with abdominal pain, blood loss, and a past history of pancreatitis. Angiography is diagnostic and permits embolization, which is often therapeutic. In cases that are amenable to a distal pancreatectomy, the procedure often results in cure.

Iatrogenic bleeding. Upper GI bleeding may follow therapeutic or diagnostic procedures. As noted, hemobilia may be iatrogenic in nature, particularly after percutaneous transhepatic procedures. Endoscopic sphincterotomy represents another common cause for iatrogenic bleeding, which can occur in up to 2% of cases. It is often mild and self-limited. Late hemorrhage usually occurs within the first 48 hours and may require injection of the area with epinephrine. This is usually successful. Surgical intervention is rarely required.

Percutaneous endoscopic gastrostomy placement is an increasingly common procedure. Bleeding rates of up to 3% have been reported. Although the majority of these cases reflect bleeding from the incision site, some are due to bleeding from the gastric mucosa (Fig. 46-10). This can often be controlled endoscopically.

Upper GI bleeding can also be seen in patients who have recently undergone upper GI surgery. Any of the lesions previously mentioned could be responsible for postoperative hemorrhage, and these possibilities should be considered. In patients in whom a resection and anastomosis have been performed, the source of the bleeding may be the suture line or staple line. In patients in whom this is persistent and an intervention is needed, endoscopists are often concerned for the potential of suture or staple line disruption. However, it is safe to do this diagnostic or even therapeutic endoscopy, provided minimal insufflation is used and the procedure is done with care.[26]

Bleeding Related to Portal Hypertension

Upper GI bleeding is a serious complication of portal hypertension, most often in the setting of cirrhosis. Cirrhosis and portal hypertension are covered in more detail in Chapter 53; only bleeding related to portal hypertension is discussed here.

Hemorrhage related to portal hypertension is most commonly the result of bleeding from varices. These dilated submucosal veins develop in response to the portal hypertension, providing a collateral pathway for decompression of the portal system into the systemic venous circulation. They are most common in the distal esophagus and can reach sizes of 1 to 2 cm. As they enlarge, the overlying mucosa becomes increasingly tenuous, excoriating with minimal trauma (Fig. 46-11).

Although these varices are most commonly seen in the esophagus, they may also develop in the stomach and the hemorrhoidal plexus of the rectum. Portal hypertensive gastropathy, diffuse dilation of the mucosal and submucosal venous plexus of the stomach associated with overlying gastritis, is an incompletely understood entity in which the stomach acquires a snakeskin-like appearance with cherry-red spots. Unlike esophageal varices, it rarely causes major hemorrhage.

Gastroesophageal varices develop in approximately 30% of patients with cirrhosis and portal hypertension, and 30% in this group develop variceal bleeding. Compared with nonvariceal bleeding, variceal hemorrhage is associated with an increased risk of rebleeding, increased need for transfusions, longer hospital stays, and increased mortality. Hemorrhage is frequently massive, accompanied by hematemesis and hemodynamic instability. The hepatic functional reserve, estimated by Child criteria (see Chapter 53), correlates closely with outcomes in these patients. Recent advances in the field have resulted in a decrease in hospitalization rates for variceal bleeding.[27] Mortality rates have also improved but still remain high; the 6-week mortality rate after the first bleeding episode is almost 20%.[28] Treatment of variceal bleeding focuses on two aspects of care: control the acute hemorrhage and reduce the risk of rebleeding.

Management. Figure 46-12 provides an algorithm for management. As with other causes of GI bleeding, adequate resuscitation is imperative. Fluid resuscitation in patients with cirrhosis is

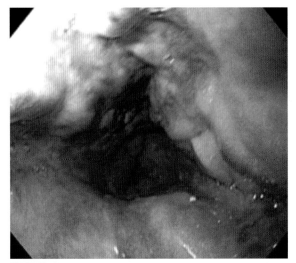

FIGURE 46-11 Nonbleeding esophageal varices secondary to cirrhosis. (Courtesy David L. Carr-Locke, MD, Brigham and Women's Hospital.)

a delicate balance. These patients frequently have hyperaldosteronism associated with fluid retention and ascites. For most of these patients, early admission to an ICU setting should be considered. A low threshold for intubation is appropriate. Defects in coagulation are common and should be aggressively corrected. A significant percentage of patients with variceal bleeding have underlying sepsis that may be associated with an aggravation in portal hypertension and lead to variceal bleeding. Studies have demonstrated that a 7-day empirical course of a broad-spectrum antibiotic (e.g., ceftriaxone) will lower the risk of rebleeding.[28]

Medical management. In patients with cirrhosis, pharmacologic therapy to reduce portal hypertension should be considered even while preparing for emergent upper endoscopy. Vasopressin produces splanchnic vasoconstriction and has been shown to significantly reduce bleeding compared with placebo. Unfortunately, this agent results in significant cardiac vasoconstriction, with resulting myocardial ischemia. Although vasopressin has been combined with nitroglycerin in clinical practice, somatostatin or its synthetic analogue, octreotide, is now the vasoactive agent of choice in the United States. Terlipressin is a newer vasopressin analogue with reduced side effects that does not need to be used as a continuous infusion. Terlipressin provides a 3% to 4% relative risk reduction in mortality in patients with acute variceal hemorrhage but is not currently available in the United States.[28]

Administration of these pharmacologic agents results in temporary control of bleeding and allows time for resuscitation and performance of the appropriate diagnostic and therapeutic maneuvers.

Endoscopic management. Early EGD is critical to evaluate the source of bleeding because more than half of bleeding is caused by nonvariceal sources, including peptic ulcer, gastritis, and Mallory-Weiss tears. In fact, studies have suggested that unlike in peptic ulcer bleeding, early endoscopy (within 15 hours of presentation) can affect survival in cases of variceal bleeding.[29]

Subsequent management is based on the endoscopic findings. If bleeding esophageal varices are identified, sclerotherapy and

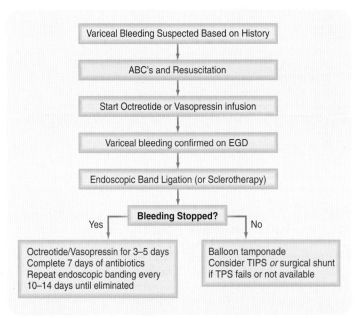

FIGURE 46-12 Algorithm for diagnosis and management of GI hemorrhage related to portal hypertension.

variceal banding have been shown to control hemorrhage effectively. Although sclerotherapy, which may use a variety of agents, is an easier procedure to perform, it is also associated with perforation, mediastinitis, and stricture. Banding seems to have a lower complication rate and, when expertise is available, should be the therapy of choice (Fig. 46-13). These endoscopic approaches, sometimes with up to three treatments during 24 hours, control the hemorrhage in up to 90% of patients with esophageal varices.

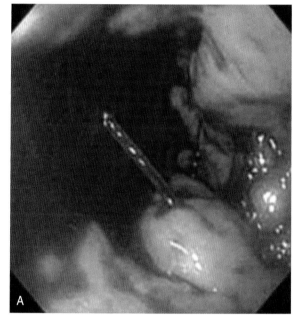

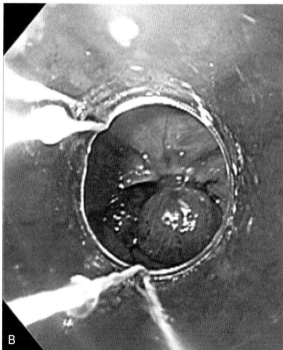

FIGURE 46-13 A, Actively bleeding varices. **B,** Effective control after variceal banding. (Courtesy David L. Carr-Locke, MD, Brigham and Women's Hospital.)

Unfortunately, gastric varices are not effectively managed by endoscopic techniques.

Other management. In cases in which pharmacologic or endoscopic therapies fail to control the hemorrhage, balloon tamponade can be successful in temporizing the hemorrhage. The Sengstaken-Blakemore tube consists of a gastric tube with esophageal and gastric balloons. The gastric balloon is inflated and tension is applied on the gastroesophageal junction. If this does not control the hemorrhage, the esophageal balloon is inflated as well, compressing the venous plexus between them. The Minnesota tube includes a proximal esophageal lumen for aspirating swallowed secretions. These tubes are associated with a high rate of complications related to both aspiration and inappropriate placement with esophageal perforation. Hemorrhage recurs on deflation in up to 50% of patients, and the balloon therapy itself has a 20% to 30% complication rate including aspiration pneumonia and esophageal tears. Currently, balloon tamponade is reserved for patients with massive hemorrhage to permit more definitive therapies. Recent trials using self-expanding esophageal stents to control massive variceal hemorrhage have also been encouraging, but their use remains experimental.[30]

In cases of refractory variceal bleeding that cannot be controlled endoscopically, emergent portal decompression is indicated. This is required in approximately 10% of patients with variceal bleeding.[31] Although randomized studies have shown equivalence between a transjugular intrahepatic portosystemic shunt (TIPS) and surgical shunting in these refractory cases,[32] this is most commonly achieved by means of a percutaneous TIPS, especially in an unstable patient. The TIPS procedure can be lifesaving in patients who are hemodynamically unstable from refractory variceal bleeding and is associated with significantly less morbidity and mortality than surgical decompression. Studies have shown that TIPS can control bleeding in 95% of cases. Rebleeding occurs in up to 20% within the first month, usually related to occlusion. Long-term patency rates are even lower, although many can be salvaged with careful surveillance and percutaneous techniques. In patients for whom TIPS is not available or fails, emergent surgical intervention is indicated, although this is seldom necessary today. Emergent surgical options are discussed in Chapter 53.

Unlike variceal hemorrhage, bleeding from portal hypertensive gastropathy is not amenable to endoscopic treatment because of the diffuse nature of the mucosal abnormalities. The underlying pathologic process involves elevated portal venous pressures, so pharmacologic therapies aimed at reducing portal venous pressure are indicated. If pharmacologic therapy fails to control acute bleeding, TIPS should be considered.[33]

Rarely, isolated gastric varices occur after splenic vein thrombosis. This is most commonly seen in the setting of pancreatitis. In these patients, central portal pressures are normal, but left-sided hypertension, decompressed from the spleen to the short gastric vessels, produces the varices. This is best treated by performing a splenectomy. Although the risk of variceal bleeding was thought to be high in this group and splenectomy was routinely recommended, recent data suggest that the incidence of variceal bleeding is in fact low (4% with a mean follow-up of 34 months), and splenectomy should not be routinely undertaken.[34]

Prevention of rebleeding. Once the initial bleeding has been controlled, prevention of recurrent hemorrhage should be a priority. If no further therapy is undertaken, approximately 70% of patients will have another bleed within 2 months. The risk of rebleeding is highest in the initial few hours to days after a first episode. Medical therapy to prevent recurrence includes a nonselective beta blocker, such as nadolol, and an antiulcer agent, such as a PPI or sucralfate. These are combined with endoscopic band ligation repeated every 10 to 14 days until all varices have been eradicated.

Although this aggressive approach results in a significant lowering of the rebleeding rate to less than 20%, it requires intensive medical follow-up and supervision.[35] In patients who are medically noncompliant or unable to tolerate such therapy, elective portal decompression should be considered if it has not already been performed. The choice between TIPS and operative decompression in the stable patient depends on the residual liver function. In general, patients with poor liver reserve who are on the liver transplant list should be considered for TIPS. This procedure provides a temporizing measure and avoids postoperative scarring of the porta hepatis, which could complicate the transplant procedure. Unfortunately, TIPS is associated with hepatic encephalopathy in up to 50% of patients within 1 year of the procedure.[36] Other shunt complications, such as thrombosis, can also occur in up to 30% of patients at 1 year. In those with good liver function who do not qualify for a transplant, surgical decompression is therefore preferred. This provides a more endurable long-term decompression, with a lower rate of hepatic encephalopathy. In those with good hepatic reserve, these advantages are thought to counterbalance the increased operative morbidity and mortality. The preferred elective shunt is a selective distal splenorenal shunt.

ACUTE LOWER GASTROINTESTINAL HEMORRHAGE

Compared with upper GI hemorrhage, lower GI bleeding is a less frequent reason for hospitalization; in fact, in looking at hospital discharge data in the United States, it is about half as common as bleeding from a location proximal to the ligament of Treitz.[1] The number of hospitalizations for this diagnosis, however, is slowly rising, increasing by 2% between 1998 and 2006. The mortality rate of lower GI bleeding is similar to that of upper GI bleeding at around 3%, but this rate increases with age to more than 5% in those 85 years or older. In more than 95% of patients with lower GI bleeding, the source of hemorrhage is the colon. The small intestine is only occasionally responsible, and because these lesions are not typically diagnosed with the combination of upper and lower endoscopy, they are considered in the section on obscure causes of GI bleeding. In general, the incidence of lower GI bleeding increases with age, and the cause is often age related (Table 46-3). Specifically, vascular lesions and diverticular disease affect all age groups but have an increasing incidence in middle-aged and elderly adults. In the pediatric population, intussusception is most commonly responsible, whereas Meckel's diverticulum must be considered in the differential in the young adult. The clinical presentation of lower GI bleeding ranges from severe hemorrhage with diverticular disease or vascular lesions to a minor inconvenience secondary to anal fissure or hemorrhoids.[37]

Diagnosis

Lower GI bleeding typically is manifested with hematochezia that can range from bright red blood to old clots. If the bleeding is slower or from a more proximal source, lower GI bleeding often is manifested as melena. Hemorrhage from the lower GI tract tends to be less severe and more intermittent and more commonly ceases spontaneously than upper GI bleeding. Compared with endoscopy in upper GI bleeding, no diagnostic modality is as

TABLE 46-3 Differential Diagnosis of Lower Gastrointestinal Hemorrhage

COLONIC BLEEDING	95%	SMALL BOWEL BLEEDING	5%
Diverticular disease	30%-40%	Angiodysplasias	
Anorectal disease	5%-15%	Erosions or ulcers (potassium, NSAIDs)	
Ischemia	5%-10%	Crohn's disease	
Neoplasia	5%-10%	Radiation	
Infectious colitis	3%-8%	Meckel's diverticulum	
Post-polypectomy	3%-7%	Neoplasia	
Inflammatory bowel disease	3%-4%	Aortoenteric fistula	
Angiodysplasia	3%		
Radiation colitis or proctitis	1%-3%		
Other	1%-5%		
Unknown	10%-25%		

sensitive or specific in making an accurate diagnosis in lower GI bleeding. Diagnostic evaluation is further complicated by the observation that in up to 40% of patients with lower GI bleeding, more than one potential source for bleeding is identified. If more than one source is identified, it is critical to confirm the responsible lesion before initiating aggressive therapy. This approach may occasionally require a period of observation with several episodes of bleeding before a definitive diagnosis can be made. In fact, in up to 25% of patients with lower GI hemorrhage, the bleeding source is never accurately identified.

An algorithm for the evaluation of lower GI hemorrhage is shown in Figure 46-14. Once resuscitation has been initiated, the first step in the workup is to rule out anorectal bleeding with a digital rectal examination and anoscopy or sigmoidoscopy. With significant bleeding, it is also important to eliminate an upper GI source. An NG aspirate that contains bile and no blood effectively rules out upper tract bleeding in most patients. However, when emergent surgery for life-threatening hemorrhage is being contemplated, preoperative or intraoperative EGD is usually appropriate.

Subsequent evaluation depends on the magnitude of the hemorrhage. With major or persistent bleeding, the workup should progress according to the patient's hemodynamic stability. The truly unstable patient who continues to bleed and requires ongoing aggressive resuscitation belongs in the operating room for expeditious diagnosis and surgical intervention. When hemorrhage is intermediate, resuscitation and hemodynamic stability permit a more directed evaluation and therapeutic intervention. Colonoscopy is the mainstay here because it allows both visualization of the pathologic process and therapeutic intervention in colonic, rectal, and distal ileal sources of bleeding. The usual adjuncts to colonoscopy include tagged RBC scan and angiography. If these modalities are not diagnostic, the source of the hemorrhage is considered obscure; such lesions and their evaluation are considered in the last section of this chapter.

Colonoscopy

Colonoscopy is most appropriate in the setting of minimal to moderate bleeding; major hemorrhage interferes significantly with visualization, and the diagnostic yield is low. In addition, in the unstable patient, sedation and manipulation may be associated with additional complications and can interfere with resuscitation. Although the blood is cathartic, gentle preparation with

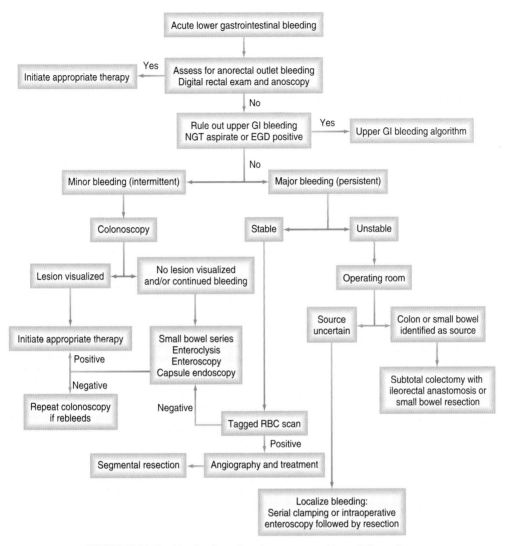

FIGURE 46-14 Algorithm for diagnosis and management of lower GI hemorrhage.

polyethylene glycol, either orally or through an NG tube, can improve visualization. Findings may include an actively bleeding site, clot adherent to a focus of mucosa or a diverticular orifice, or blood localized to a specific colonic segment, although this can be misleading because of retrograde peristalsis in the colon. Polyps, cancers, and inflammatory causes can frequently be seen. Unfortunately, angiodysplasias are often difficult to visualize, particularly in the unstable patient with mesenteric vascular constriction. Diverticula are identified in most patients, whether or not they are the source of the hemorrhage. Despite these limitations, the diagnostic yield of colonoscopy in experienced hands is reasonable. Because the majority of lower GI bleeds are self-limited, the timing of colonoscopy (within 24 hours) and experience of the colonoscopist are important in identifying the site of hemorrhage or stigmata of recent hemorrhage.[38]

Radionuclide Scanning

Radionuclide scanning with technetium Tc 99m (^{99m}Tc-labeled RBC) is the most sensitive but least accurate method for localization of GI bleeding. With this technique, the patient's own RBCs are labeled and reinjected. The labeled blood is extravasated into the GI tract lumen, creating a focus that can be detected scintigraphically. Initially, images are collected frequently and then at 4-hour intervals, for up to 24 hours. The RBC scan can detect bleeding as slow as 0.1 mL/min and is reported to be more than 90% sensitive (Fig. 46-15).[39] Unfortunately, the spatial resolution is low, and blood may move retrograde in the colon or distally in the small bowel. Reported accuracy of localization is in the range of only 40% to 60%, and it is particularly inaccurate in distinguishing right-sided from left-sided colonic bleeding. The RBC scan is not usually employed as a definitive study before surgery but instead as a guide to the utility of angiography; if the RBC scan is negative or only positive after several hours, angiography is unlikely to be revealing. Such an approach avoids the significant morbidity of angiography.

Computed Tomography Angiography

A study has shown that CT angiography may be better than scintigraphy at localizing the site of GI bleeding. Although sensitivity and specificity of the tests were similar, CT was better at localizing the site of bleeding, and the findings were more consistent to those at the time of subsequent therapeutic angiography.

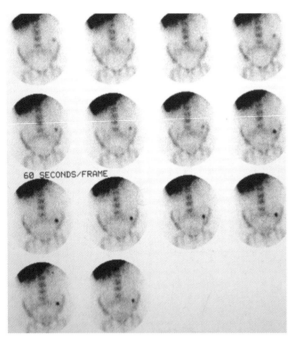

60 SECONDS/FRAME

FIGURE 46-15 A positive RBC scan localizing the bleeding to the left lower quadrant. (Courtesy Richard A. Baum, MD, Brigham and Women's Hospital.)

Although patients in this group received a greater amount of contrast dye, there was no adverse outcome on renal function.[40]

Mesenteric Angiography

Selective angiography, using either the superior or inferior mesenteric arteries, can detect hemorrhage in the range of 0.5 to 1.0 mL/min and is generally employed only in the diagnosis of ongoing hemorrhage. It can be particularly useful in identifying the vascular patterns of angiodysplasias. It may also be used for localizing actively bleeding diverticula. In addition, it has therapeutic capabilities. Catheter-directed vasopressin infusion can provide temporary control of bleeding, permitting hemodynamic stabilization, although as many as 50% of patients will rebleed when the medication is discontinued. It can also be used for embolization. Although the more limited collateral circulation of the colon has made this less appealing than in the upper GI tract, it has been suggested that such techniques can be applied safely in most patients. Typically, such therapy is reserved for patients whose underlying condition precludes surgical therapy. Unfortunately, angiography is associated with significant risk of complications, including hematomas, arterial thrombosis, contrast dye reactions, and acute renal failure.

Treatment

Therapeutic approaches with lower GI bleeding are clearly dependent on the lesion identified. The criteria for operation, shown in Box 46-2, are similar to those with upper GI hemorrhage, although there is a stronger tendency to delay until the site is clearly localized.

Specific Causes of Lower Gastrointestinal Tract Bleeding
Colonic Bleeding

Diverticular disease. In the United States, diverticula are the most common cause of significant lower GI bleeding. In the past,

diverticula were thought to be rare in patients younger than 40 years, but it is now an increasingly common diagnosis in this age group. Only 3% to 15% of individuals with diverticulosis experience any bleeding.[41] Bleeding generally occurs at the neck of the diverticulum and is believed to be secondary to bleeding from the vasa recti as they penetrate through the submucosa. Of those that bleed, more than 75% stop spontaneously, although approximately 10% will rebleed within a year and almost 50% within 10 years.[39] Although diverticular disease is much more common on the left side, right-sided disease is responsible for more than half the bleeding.

The best method of diagnosis and treatment is colonoscopy, although success is sometimes limited by the large amount of bleeding. If the bleeding diverticulum can be identified, epinephrine injection may control the bleeding. Electrocautery can also be used, and most recently, endoscopic clips have been successfully applied to control the hemorrhage. If bleeding ceases with these maneuvers or spontaneously, expectant management may be appropriate; however, this requires clinical judgment based on the magnitude of the hemorrhage and the patient's comorbidities, particularly cardiac disease.

If none of these maneuvers is successful or if hemorrhage recurs, angiography with embolization can be considered. Superselective embolization of the bleeding colonic vessel has gained popularity with high success rates (>90%), although the risk of ischemic complications continues to be of concern.[42] Under these circumstances, colonic resection is indicated. Certainty of the site of bleeding is critical. Blind hemicolectomy is associated with rebleeding in more than 50% of patients, and operation based on RBC scan localization alone can result in recurrent hemorrhage in up to one third of patients.[43] Subtotal colectomy does not eliminate the risk of recurrent hemorrhage and, compared with segmental resection, is accompanied by a significant increase in morbidity, particularly diarrhea in older patients, in whom the remaining rectum may never adapt.

Angiodysplasia. Angiodysplasias of the intestine, also referred to as arteriovenous malformations, are distinct from hemangiomas and true congenital arteriovenous malformations. They are thought to be acquired degenerative lesions secondary to progressive dilation of normal blood vessels within the submucosa of the intestine. Angiodysplasias have an equal gender distribution and are almost uniformly found in patients older than 50 years. These lesions are notably associated with aortic stenosis and renal failure, especially in the elderly. The hemorrhage tends to arise from the right side of the colon, with the cecum being the most common location, although they can occur in the rest of the colon and small bowel. Most patients present with chronic bleeding, but in up to 15%, hemorrhage may be massive. Bleeding stops spontaneously in most cases, but approximately 50% will rebleed within 5 years.

These lesions can be diagnosed by either colonoscopy or angiography. During colonoscopy, they appear as red stellate lesions with a surrounding rim of pale mucosa and can be treated with sclerotherapy or electrocautery. Angiography demonstrates dilated, slowly emptying veins and sometimes early venous filling. If these lesions are discovered incidentally, no further therapy is indicated. In acutely bleeding patients, they have been successfully treated with intra-arterial vasopressin, selective gel foam embolization, endoscopic electrocoagulation, or injection with sclerosing agents. If these measures fail or bleeding recurs and the lesion has been localized, segmental resection, most commonly right colectomy, is effective.

Neoplasia. Colorectal carcinoma is an uncommon cause of significant lower GI hemorrhage but is probably the most important one to rule out as more than 150,000 Americans are diagnosed each year with this cancer. The bleeding is usually painless, intermittent, and slow in nature. Frequently, it is associated with iron deficiency anemia. Polyps can also bleed, but more commonly the bleeding occurs after a polypectomy. Although bleeding in the pediatric population is discussed in Chapter 66, juvenile polyps are the second most common cause of bleeding in patients younger than 20 years. On occasion, other colonic neoplasms, most notably GISTs, can be associated with massive hemorrhage. The best diagnostic tool is colonoscopy. If the bleeding is attributable to a polyp, it can be treated with endoscopic therapy.

Anorectal disease. The major causes of anorectal outlet bleeding are internal hemorrhoids, anal fissures, and colorectal neoplasia. Although hemorrhoids are by far the most common of these entities, they account for only 5% to 10% of all acute lower GI bleeding. In general, anorectal hemorrhage is low-volume bleeding that is bright red blood per rectum seen in the toilet bowl and on the toilet paper. Most hemorrhoidal bleeding arises from internal hemorrhoids; these are painless and often accompanied by prolapsing tissue that reduces spontaneously or has to be manually reduced by the patient (Fig. 46-16). Anal fissure, on the other hand, produces painful bleeding after a bowel movement; bleeding is only occasionally the main symptom in these patients (Fig. 46-17).

Because anorectal disease is common, a careful investigation to rule out all other sources of bleeding, especially malignant neoplasia, is imperative before lower GI bleeding is attributed to such disease. Anal fissure can be treated medically with stool bulking agents (e.g., psyllium [Metamucil]), increased water intake, stool softeners, and topical nitroglycerin ointment or diltiazem to relieve sphincter spasm and to promote healing. Internal hemorrhoids should be treated with bulking agents, increased dietary fiber, and adequate hydration. A variety of office-based interventions, including rubber band ligation, injectable sclerosing agents, and infrared coagulation, have also been used. If these measures fail, surgical hemorrhoidectomy may be needed. Most anorectal bleeding is self-limited and responds to dietary and local measures.

Colitis. Inflammation of the colon is caused by a multitude of disease processes including inflammatory bowel disease (Crohn's disease, ulcerative colitis, and indeterminate colitis), infectious colitis (O157:H7 *Escherichia coli*, cytomegalovirus, *Salmonella*, *Shigella*, *Campylobacter* spp., and *Clostridium difficile*), radiation proctitis after treatment for pelvic malignant neoplasms, and ischemia.

Ulcerative colitis is much more likely than Crohn's disease to be manifested with GI bleeding. Ulcerative colitis is a mucosal disease that starts distally in the rectum and progresses proximally to occasionally involve the entire colon. Patients can present with up to 20 bloody bowel movements per day. These are usually accompanied by crampy abdominal pain and tenesmus. The diagnosis is secured by a careful history and flexible endoscopy with biopsy. Medical therapy with steroids, 5-aminosalicylic acid compounds, and immunomodulatory agents and supportive care are the mainstays of treatment. Surgical therapy is rarely indicated in the acute setting unless the patient develops a toxic megacolon or hemorrhage that is refractory to medical management.

In contrast, Crohn's disease typically is associated with guaiac-positive diarrhea and mucus-filled bowel movements but not with bright red blood. Crohn's disease can affect the entire GI tract. It is characterized by skip lesions, transmural thickening of the bowel wall, and granuloma formation. The diagnosis is made with endoscopy and contrast studies. Medical management consists of steroids, antibiotics, immunomodulators, and 5-aminosalicylic acid compounds. Because Crohn's disease is a relapsing and remitting disease, surgical therapy is used as a last resort. Massive colonic hemorrhage complicates ulcerative colitis in up to 15% of affected patients, whereas it occurs in only 1% of those with Crohn's colitis.[44]

Infectious colitis can cause bloody diarrhea. The diagnosis is usually established from the history and stool culture. *C. difficile* and cytomegalovirus colitis deserve special attention. *C. difficile* colitis usually is manifested with explosive, foul-smelling diarrhea in a patient with prior antibiotic use or hospitalization. Bloody bowel movements are not common but can be present, especially in severe cases in which there is associated mucosal sloughing. In

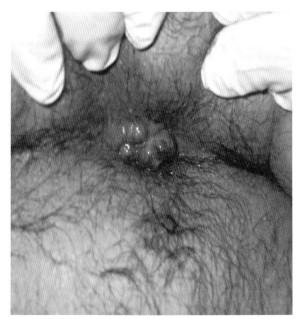

FIGURE 46-16 Bleeding and prolapsed hemorrhoids.

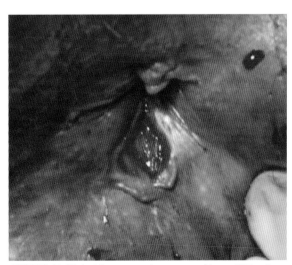

FIGURE 46-17 Anal fissures can be a source of lower GI bleeding.

North America, there has been an upsurge in the frequency and severity of *C. difficile*–associated colitis. Treatment consists of stopping antibiotics, supportive care, and oral or intravenous metronidazole or oral vancomycin. Cytomegalovirus colitis should be suspected in any immunocompromised patient who presents with bloody diarrhea. Endoscopy with biopsy confirms the diagnosis; treatment is intravenous ganciclovir.

Radiation proctitis has become much more common in the last several decades as the use of radiation to treat rectal cancer, prostate cancer, and gynecologic malignant neoplasms has increased. Patients present with bright red blood per rectum, diarrhea, tenesmus, and crampy pelvic pain. Flexible endoscopy reveals the characteristic bleeding telangiectasias (Fig. 46-18). Treatment consists of antidiarrheals, hydrocortisone enemas, and endoscopic APC. In cases of persistent bleeding, ablation with 4% formalin solution usually works well.

Mesenteric ischemia. Mesenteric ischemia can be secondary to either acute or chronic arterial or venous insufficiency. Predisposing factors include preexisting cardiovascular disease (atrial fibrillation, congestive heart failure, and acute myocardial infarction), recent abdominal vascular surgery, hypercoagulable states, medications (e.g., vasopressors and digoxin), and vasculitis. Acute colonic ischemia is the most common form of mesenteric ischemia. It tends to occur in the watershed areas of the splenic flexure and the rectosigmoid colon but can be right sided in up to 40% of patients. Patients present with abdominal pain and bloody diarrhea. CT will often show a thickened bowel wall. The diagnosis is generally confirmed with flexible endoscopy, which reveals edema, hemorrhage, and a demarcation between the normal and abnormal mucosa. Treatment focuses on supportive care consisting of bowel rest, intravenous antibiotics, cardiovascular support, and correction of the low-flow state. In 85% of cases, the ischemia is self-limited and resolves without incident, although some patients develop a colonic stricture. In the other 15% of cases, surgery is indicated because of progressive ischemia and gangrene. Marked leukocytosis, fever, a fluid requirement, tachycardia, acidosis, and peritonitis indicate a failure of the ischemia to resolve and the need for surgical intervention. During the surgery, resection of the ischemic intestine and creation of an end ostomy are indicated.[45]

ACUTE GASTROINTESTINAL HEMORRHAGE FROM AN OBSCURE SOURCE

Obscure GI hemorrhage is defined as bleeding that persists or recurs after an initial negative evaluation with EGD and colonoscopy. Obscure bleeding can be further subdivided into obscure-occult or obscure-overt bleeding. Obscure-occult bleeding is characterized by iron deficiency anemia or guaiac-positive stools without visible bleeding. If initial upper and lower endoscopy fails to identify a source for obscure-occult bleeding and the patient has no systemic signs of disease, these patients are often treated with iron therapy, and more than 80% resolve their symptoms in less than 2 years. Obscure-overt bleeding is characterized by recurrent or persistent visible bleeding.[46]

Obscure bleeding can be frustrating for both the patient and the clinician, particularly for obscure-overt bleeding, which cannot be localized despite obvious signs of bleeding that can be concerning to patients and necessitate aggressive diagnostic measures. Despite improved imaging technology including video capsule endoscopy, a source of bleeding may never be found in some patients. Those patients in whom a diagnosis is reached often have had multiple tests and several hospitalizations and have received blood transfusions. Further complicating the management of these patients is that obscure GI bleeds have a high rate of rebleeding; in one study evaluating patients with a negative capsule endoscopy, the rebleeding rates were 12.9%, 25.6%, and 31.5% at 1, 3, and 5 years, respectively.[47] Fortunately, obscure-overt bleeding is responsible for only about 1% of all GI bleeding. The differential diagnosis of obscure-overt bleeding is long and varied (Box 46-3) and includes a variety of small bowel lesions not previously described. In a series of 200 patients with obscure bleeding, the small bowel was identified as the source of bleeding in more than 60% of cases. In these patients, the most common cause was small bowel ulcers and erosions secondary to Crohn's disease, Meckel's diverticulum, or NSAIDs.[48]

Diagnosis
Repeated Endoscopy
The cause of obscure-overt bleeding is often a common lesion that is missed on initial evaluation. Repeated upper endoscopy and lower endoscopy are valuable tools in identifying missed lesions

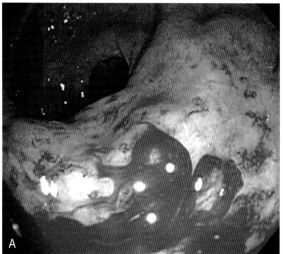

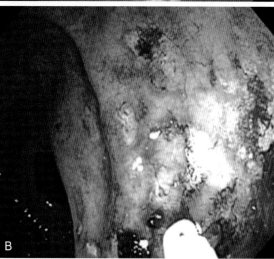

FIGURE 46-18 A, Rectal bleeding secondary to radiation damage. **B,** Effective control after application of APC treatment. (Courtesy David L. Carr-Locke, MD, Brigham and Women's Hospital.)

BOX 46-3 Differential Diagnosis of Obscure Gastrointestinal Bleeding

Upper Gastrointestinal Tract
Angiodysplasia
Peptic ulcer disease
Aortoenteric fistula
Neoplasia
HIV-related causes
Dieulafoy lesion
Lymphoma
Sarcoidosis
Hemobilia
Hemosuccus pancreaticus
GAVE
Metastatic cancer

Small Bowel
Crohn's disease
Meckel's diverticulum
Lymphoma
Radiation enteritis
Ischemia
HIV-related causes
Bacterial infection
Metastatic disease
Angiodysplasia
NSAID-induced erosions

Colon
Colitis
 Ulcerative colitis
 Crohn's colitis
 Ischemic colitis
 Radiation colitis
 Infective colitis
Solitary rectal ulcer
Amyloidosis
Lymphoma
Endometriosis
Angiodysplasia
Neoplasia
HIV-related causes
Hemorrhoids

as up to 35% of patients will have the bleeding source identified on second-look endoscopy. Most obscure GI hemorrhage is from a source distal to the ligament of Treitz. When repeated endoscopy fails to identify an obscure-overt bleeding source, investigation of the small bowel is warranted. This should proceed in an orderly fashion, depending on the degree of bleeding and the patient's hemodynamic status.

Conventional Imaging

The next step is probably a tagged RBC scan, although its utility in this setting has not been established, and as discussed previously, it may be misleading. Angiography may be more useful but usually requires significant ongoing hemorrhage. Provocative testing, which involves administration of anticoagulants, fibrinolytics, or vasodilators to increase hemorrhage during angiography, has been employed in small series with favorable results, but reluctance to induce uncontrolled hemorrhage has limited its use. Small bowel enteroclysis, which uses a tube to infuse barium, methylcellulose, and air directly into the small bowel, provides better imaging than simple small bowel follow-through. Because the yield has been reported to be very low and the test is poorly tolerated, it is now rarely used. An alternative to small bowel enteroclysis is CT enterography, which can identify gross lesions such as small bowel tumors and inflammatory conditions such as Crohn's disease. The limitation of small bowel radiography is that it cannot visualize angiodysplasias, the main cause of obscure small bowel hemorrhage.

In younger patients, usually younger than 30 years, part of the initial evaluation should be a Meckel's diverticulum scan. A Meckel's diverticulum with ectopic acid-secreting mucosa can ulcerate the small bowel and produce bleeding. This scan is performed by administration of ^{99m}Tc-pertechnetate that is taken up by the ectopic gastric mucosa in the diverticulum and localized with scintigraphy.

Small Bowel Endoscopy

The hemodynamically stable patient should undergo small bowel enteroscopy. Usually performed with a pediatric colonoscope, this is referred to as push endoscopy. It can reach about 50 to 70 cm past the ligament of Treitz in most cases and permits endoscopic management of some lesions. Overall, push enteroscopy is successful in 40% of patients. Sonde pull endoscopy uses an enteroscope that passes passively into the very distal small bowel. A balloon on the end of the scope permits normal small bowel peristalsis to carry the scope into the ileum; the mucosa is visualized as the scope is removed. This technique is cumbersome, does not permit intervention, and has largely been abandoned with the advent of capsule endoscopy.

Double-balloon endoscopy is another technique gaining in popularity. Although technically difficult, this approach is capable of providing a complete examination of the small bowel. In expert hands, double-balloon enteroscopy can identify a bleeding source in 77% of cases with occult bleeding, with the yield increasing to more than 85% if the endoscopy is performed within 1 month of an overt bleeding episode.[48] In cases of acute obscure-overt GI bleed, a study found that more bleeding lesions were identified by double-balloon endoscopy performed within 72 hours of admission than by video capsule endoscopy.[49] The advantage of double-balloon endoscopy is that as well as visualization, biopsies can be performed and therapeutic interventions undertaken.

Video Capsule Endoscopy

Capsule endoscopy uses a small capsule with a video camera, which is swallowed and acquires video images as it passes through the GI tract. This modality permits visualization of the entire GI tract but offers no interventional capability and is also time-consuming because someone has to watch the video to identify the bleeding source. This procedure is usually well tolerated, although it is contraindicated in patients with obstruction or a motility disorder. Capsule endoscopy is frequently used in the patient who is hemodynamically stable but continues to bleed. This technique has reported success rates as high as 90% in identifying small bowel disease. However, in a large national review of capsule endoscopy in obscure GI bleeding, the test failed to identify a source of bleeding in 30% to 40% of both obscure-occult and obscure-overt cases.[50]

Intraoperative Endoscopy

Intraoperative enteroscopy should be reserved for patients who have transfusion-dependent obscure-overt bleeding in whom an exhaustive search has failed to identify a bleeding source. This typically uses a pediatric colonoscope introduced through the mouth or through an enterotomy in the small bowel made by the surgeon. In the latter case, a sterile colonoscope is passed onto the field, introduced into the small bowel, and passed bidirectionally with the surgeon assisting to pass the bowel over the endoscope. Any suspicious areas are marked for possible resection or are dealt with endoscopically if feasible.

Treatment

Obscure GI hemorrhage requires a careful approach to diagnosis and management. Specific causes and their management are listed in the following section. Up to 25% of cases of obscure lower GI hemorrhage remain without a diagnosis, and 33% to 50% of patients will rebleed within 3 to 5 years.[46] Management strategies generally depend on the identification of a lesion. Iron replacement combined with intermittent transfusion is occasionally necessary, although this approach is not appealing. If possible, patients who are taking anticoagulants (e.g., warfarin, NSAIDs, aspirin, or clopidogrel) should be encouraged to stop these medications to lower rebleeding risks.[50]

Specific Causes of Small Bowel Bleeding
Angiodysplasias

Angiodysplasias are a common cause of small intestinal bleeding, accounting for 10% to 20%.[50] Most small intestinal vascular ectasias appear to occur in the jejunum, followed by the ileum and then the duodenum. The usual diagnostic tools are generally unsuccessful in identifying these lesions. Angiography is rarely positive. Instead, most small bowel vascular lesions require enteroscopy or capsule endoscopy for identification. In cases of severe hemorrhage requiring emergent operative intervention, intraoperative endoscopy may be helpful. These lesions have a high rebleeding rate, and segmental small bowel resection may be required. On occasion, these lesions may be diffuse; this may occur in heredity hemorrhagic telangiectasia (Osler-Weber-Rendu syndrome), acute renal failure, or von Willebrand disease. In this situation, there has been limited experience with estrogen and progesterone treatment, but it has been suggested that these agents may be of benefit.

Neoplasia

Small bowel tumors are not common but can be sources of occult or frank GI bleeding. Bleeding typically results from erosion of the mucosa overlying the tumor. GISTs have the greatest propensity for bleeding. Small bowel tumors are typically diagnosed by small bowel contrast series or spiral CT scan. Treatment involves surgical resection.

Crohn's Disease

Patients with Crohn's disease may also present with small bowel bleeding in association with terminal ileitis. Bleeding is not generally significant, nor is it usually the only presenting symptom. It is diagnosed by small bowel contrast series, and initial treatment is medical.

Meckel's Diverticulum

Meckel's diverticulum is a true diverticulum in that it contains all layers of the small bowel wall. It is a congenital remnant of the omphalomesenteric duct, occurring in approximately 2% of the general population. Often, heterotopic tissue is present at the base of the diverticulum. Bleeding from a Meckel's diverticulum is usually from an ulcerative lesion on the ileal wall opposite the diverticulum, resulting from acid production by ectopic gastric mucosa. If nuclear medicine imaging is negative and bleeding is relatively brisk, angiography may be helpful in the diagnosis. Surgical management usually requires a segmental resection to incorporate the opposing ileal mucosa, which is typically the site of bleeding.

Diverticula

Unlike a Meckel's diverticulum, small intestinal diverticula are false diverticula that do not involve all layers of the bowel. Bleeding from small bowel diverticula can present a diagnostic challenge. Capsule endoscopy or small intestinal contrast studies can confirm

the diagnosis of diverticula, and in the absence of other sources of bleeding, it may be assumed that the diverticula are the source of bleeding. In cases of profuse bleeding, angiography or intraoperative endoscopy may be used to identify the bleeding source.

SELECTED REFERENCES

Barkun AN, Bardou M, Kuipers EJ, et al: International consensus recommendations on the management of patients with nonvariceal upper gastrointestinal bleeding. *Ann Intern Med* 152:101–113, 2010.

> *An update on international consensus on management of upper GI bleeds.*

Gralnek IM: Obscure-overt gastrointestinal bleeding. *Gastroenterology* 128:1424–1430, 2005.

> *A concise discussion of the diagnostic approach to obscure bleeding, including the roles of small bowel fiberoptic and capsule endoscopy.*

Herrera JL: Management of acute variceal bleeding. *Clin Liver Dis* 18:347–357, 2014.

> *A review on current management of variceal bleeding.*

Rockey DC: Gastrointestinal bleeding. *Gastroenterol Clin North Am* 34:581–588, 2005.

> *A monograph covering all aspects of gastrointestinal hemorrhage.*

Sung JJ: Marshall and Warren Lecture 2009: Peptic ulcer bleeding: An expedition of 20 years from 1989–2009. *J Gastroenterol Hepatol* 25:229–233, 2010.

> *A review archiving the evolution of current endoscopic, pharmacologic, and surgical management of upper GI bleeding. There is also a discussion of some of the current controversies.*

REFERENCES

1. Zhao Y, Encinosa W: *Hospitalizations for gastrointestinal bleeding in 1998 and 2006: Statistical brief #65*, Rockville, Md, 2006, Healthcare Cost and Utilization Project (HCUP) Statistical Briefs.
2. Abougergi MS, Travis AC, Saltzman JR: The in-hospital mortality rate for upper GI hemorrhage has decreased over 2 decades in the United States: A nationwide analysis. *Gastrointest Endosc* 81:882–888, e1, 2015.
3. Cryer BL, Wilcox CM, Henk HJ, et al: The economics of upper gastrointestinal bleeding in a US managed-care setting: A retrospective, claims-based analysis. *J Med Econ* 13:70–77, 2010.
4. Quan S, Frolkis A, Milne K, et al: Upper-gastrointestinal bleeding secondary to peptic ulcer disease: Incidence and outcomes. *World J Gastroenterol* 20:17568–17577, 2014.

5. Meltzer AC, Klein JC: Upper gastrointestinal bleeding: Patient presentation, risk stratification, and early management. *Gastroenterol Clin North Am* 43:665–675, 2014.

6. Tata LJ, Fortun PJ, Hubbard RB, et al: Does concurrent prescription of selective serotonin reuptake inhibitors and non-steroidal anti-inflammatory drugs substantially increase the risk of upper gastrointestinal bleeding? *Aliment Pharmacol Ther* 22:175–181, 2005.

7. Rubin TA, Murdoch M, Nelson DB: Acute GI bleeding in the setting of supratherapeutic international normalized ratio in patients taking warfarin: Endoscopic diagnosis, clinical management, and outcomes. *Gastrointest Endosc* 58:369–373, 2003.

8. Tsoi KK, Ma TK, Sung JJ: Endoscopy for upper gastrointestinal bleeding: How urgent is it? *Nat Rev Gastroenterol Hepatol* 6:463–469, 2009.

9. Sarin N, Monga N, Adams PC: Time to endoscopy and outcomes in upper gastrointestinal bleeding. *Can J Gastroenterol* 23:489–493, 2009.

10. Enestvedt BK, Gralnek IM, Mattek N, et al: An evaluation of endoscopic indications and findings related to nonvariceal upper-GI hemorrhage in a large multicenter consortium. *Gastrointest Endosc* 67:422–429, 2008.

11. Cheng CL, Lee CS, Liu NJ, et al: Overlooked lesions at emergency endoscopy for acute nonvariceal upper gastrointestinal bleeding. *Endoscopy* 34:527–530, 2002.

12. Barkun AN, Bardou M, Kuipers EJ, et al: International consensus recommendations on the management of patients with nonvariceal upper gastrointestinal bleeding. *Ann Intern Med* 152:101–113, 2010.

13. Rockey DC: Gastrointestinal bleeding. *Gastroenterol Clin North Am* 34:581–588, 2005.

14. Wang YR, Richter JE, Dempsey DT: Trends and outcomes of hospitalizations for peptic ulcer disease in the United States, 1993 to 2006. *Ann Surg* 251:51–58, 2010.

15. Sung JJ: Marshall and Warren Lecture 2009: Peptic ulcer bleeding: An expedition of 20 years from 1989-2009. *J Gastroenterol Hepatol* 25:229–233, 2010.

16. Schilling D, Demel A, Nusse T, et al: *Helicobacter pylori* infection does not affect the early rebleeding rate in patients with peptic ulcer bleeding after successful endoscopic hemostasis: A prospective single-center trial. *Endoscopy* 35:393–396, 2003.

17. Gisbert JP, Khorrami S, Carballo F, et al: *H. pylori* eradication therapy vs. antisecretory non-eradication therapy (with or without long-term maintenance antisecretory therapy) for the prevention of recurrent bleeding from peptic ulcer. *Cochrane Database Syst Rev* (4):CD004062, 2003.

18. Liu CC, Lee CL, Chan CC, et al: Maintenance treatment is not necessary after *Helicobacter pylori* eradication and healing of bleeding peptic ulcer: A 5-year prospective, randomized, controlled study. *Arch Intern Med* 163:2020–2024, 2003.

19. Hippisley-Cox J, Coupland C, Logan R: Risk of adverse gastrointestinal outcomes in patients taking cyclo-oxygenase-2 inhibitors or conventional non-steroidal anti-inflammatory drugs: Population based nested case-control analysis. *BMJ* 331:1310–1316, 2005.

20. Chan FK, To KF, Wu JC, et al: Eradication of *Helicobacter pylori* and risk of peptic ulcers in patients starting long-term treatment with non-steroidal anti-inflammatory drugs: A randomised trial. *Lancet* 359:9–13, 2002.

21. Malfertheiner P, Megraud F, O'Morain C, et al: Current concepts in the management of *Helicobacter pylori* infection: The Maastricht III Consensus Report. *Gut* 56:772–781, 2007.

22. Lau JY, Sung JJ, Lam YH, et al: Endoscopic retreatment compared with surgery in patients with recurrent bleeding after initial endoscopic control of bleeding ulcers. *N Engl J Med* 340:751–756, 1999.

23. Guglielmi A, Ruzzenente A, Sandri M, et al: Risk assessment and prediction of rebleeding in bleeding gastroduodenal ulcer. *Endoscopy* 34:778–786, 2002.

24. Chung IK, Kim EJ, Lee MS, et al: Endoscopic factors predisposing to rebleeding following endoscopic hemostasis in bleeding peptic ulcers. *Endoscopy* 33:969–975, 2001.

25. Nguyen DC, Jackson CS: The Dieulafoy's lesion: An update on evaluation, diagnosis, and management. *J Clin Gastroenterol* 49:541–549, 2015.

26. Stiegmann GV: Endoscopic approaches to upper gastrointestinal bleeding. *Am Surg* 72:111–115, 2006.

27. Jamal MM, Samarasena JB, Hashemzadeh M, et al: Declining hospitalization rate of esophageal variceal bleeding in the United States. *Clin Gastroenterol Hepatol* 6:689–695, quiz 605, 2008.

28. Herrera JL: Management of acute variceal bleeding. *Clin Liver Dis* 18:347–357, 2014.

29. Hsu YC, Chung CS, Tseng CH, et al: Delayed endoscopy as a risk factor for in-hospital mortality in cirrhotic patients with acute variceal hemorrhage. *J Gastroenterol Hepatol* 24:1294–1299, 2009.

30. Dechene A, El Fouly AH, Bechmann LP, et al: Acute management of refractory variceal bleeding in liver cirrhosis by self-expanding metal stents. *Digestion* 85:185–191, 2012.

31. Chalasani N, Kahi C, Francois F, et al: Improved patient survival after acute variceal bleeding: A multicenter, cohort study. *Am J Gastroenterol* 98:653–659, 2003.

32. Henderson JM, Boyer TD, Kutner MH, et al: Distal splenorenal shunt versus transjugular intrahepatic portal systematic shunt for variceal bleeding: A randomized trial. *Gastroenterology* 130:1643–1651, 2006.

33. Lo GH, Liang HL, Chen WC, et al: A prospective, randomized controlled trial of transjugular intrahepatic portosystemic shunt versus cyanoacrylate injection in the prevention of gastric variceal rebleeding. *Endoscopy* 39:679–685, 2007.

34. Heider TR, Azeem S, Galanko JA, et al: The natural history of pancreatitis-induced splenic vein thrombosis. *Ann Surg* 239:876–880, discussion 880–882, 2004.

35. de la Pena J, Brullet E, Sanchez-Hernandez E, et al: Variceal ligation plus nadolol compared with ligation for prophylaxis of variceal rebleeding: A multicenter trial. *Hepatology* 41:572–578, 2005.

36. Riggio O, Angeloni S, Salvatori FM, et al: Incidence, natural history, and risk factors of hepatic encephalopathy after transjugular intrahepatic portosystemic shunt with polytetrafluoroethylene-covered stent grafts. *Am J Gastroenterol* 103:2738–2746, 2008.

37. Ghassemi KA, Jensen DM: Lower GI bleeding: Epidemiology and management. *Curr Gastroenterol Rep* 15:333, 2013.

38. Niikura R, Nagata N, Aoki T, et al: Predictors for identification of stigmata of recent hemorrhage on colonic diverticula in lower gastrointestinal bleeding. *J Clin Gastroenterol* 49:e24–e30, 2015.

39. Strate LL: Lower GI bleeding: Epidemiology and diagnosis. *Gastroenterol Clin North Am* 34:643–664, 2005.

40. Jacovides CL, Nadolski G, Allen SR, et al: Arteriography for lower gastrointestinal hemorrhage: Role of preceding abdominal computed tomographic angiogram in diagnosis and localization. *JAMA Surg* 150:650–656, 2015.

41. Niikura R, Nagata N, Shimbo T, et al: Natural history of bleeding risk in colonic diverticulosis patients: A long-term colonoscopy-based cohort study. *Aliment Pharmacol Ther* 41:888–894, 2015.

42. Lipof T, Sardella WV, Bartus CM, et al: The efficacy and durability of super-selective embolization in the treatment of lower gastrointestinal bleeding. *Dis Colon Rectum* 51:301–305, 2008.

43. Bender JS, Wiencek RG, Bouwman DL: Morbidity and mortality following total abdominal colectomy for massive lower gastrointestinal bleeding. *Am Surg* 57:536–540, discussion 540–541, 1991.

44. Pardi DS, Loftus EV, Jr, Tremaine WJ, et al: Acute major gastrointestinal hemorrhage in inflammatory bowel disease. *Gastrointest Endosc* 49:153–157, 1999.

45. Walker AM, Bohn RL, Cali C, et al: Risk factors for colon ischemia. *Am J Gastroenterol* 99:1333–1337, 2004.

46. Gralnek IM: Obscure-overt gastrointestinal bleeding. *Gastroenterology* 128:1424–1430, 2005.

47. Magalhaes-Costa P, Bispo M, Santos S, et al: Re-bleeding events in patients with obscure gastrointestinal bleeding after negative capsule endoscopy. *World J Gastrointest Endosc* 7:403–410, 2015.

48. Shinozaki S, Yamamoto H, Yano T, et al: Long-term outcome of patients with obscure gastrointestinal bleeding investigated by double-balloon endoscopy. *Clin Gastroenterol Hepatol* 8:151–158, 2010.

49. Aniwan S, Rerknimitr R, Kongkam P, et al: A combination of clinical risk stratification and fecal immunochemical test results to prioritize colonoscopy screening in asymptomatic participants. *Gastrointest Endosc* 81:719–727, 2015.

50. Min YW, Kim JS, Jeon SW, et al: Long-term outcome of capsule endoscopy in obscure gastrointestinal bleeding: A nationwide analysis. *Endoscopy* 46:59–65, 2014.

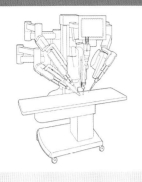

CHAPTER 47

Morbid Obesity

William O. Richards

第四十七章　病态肥胖

OUTLINE

中文导读

　　本章共分为14节：①肥胖问题的严重性；②病理生理学和相关的医学问题；③内科与外科治疗；④减肥外科的作用机制；⑤病人选择与术前评估；⑥特殊器材；⑦手术过程；⑧术后护理和随访；⑨转归；⑩并发症；⑪再次手术；⑫减肥外科中的争议；⑬探索性减肥手术方式；⑭结论。

　　第一节介绍了肥胖是美国可预防死亡的第二大原因，也是导致医疗费用增长的第二大可控因素。

　　第二节指出肥胖的病理生理尚不明确，疾病相关的遗传因素和环境因素仍有争议。而相关的代谢综合征不仅影响个体的健康，也导致一系列社会问题。

　　第三节介绍了减重手术与药物治疗的疗效对比，在减重效果、长期生存、心血管发病率等多方面，手术治疗都具有明显优势。

　　第四节探讨了各种减重手术的作用机制，包括限制性手术和吸收不良手术，以及代谢综合征的治疗机制。

　　第五节主要内容是减重手术的术前评估和病人选择，目前的标准是基于NIH和AHA/ACC/TOS指南。介绍了美国的相关医保政策及施行减重手术的资质和规则。

　　第六节介绍了为适应超胖病人所需要的诊所设施调整，以及手术室需要的特殊手术床、视频设备以及超长腹腔镜器械等。

　　第七节着重介绍了几种常见的减肥手术具体操作方法及其优缺点，如腹腔镜可调节胃束带手术（LAGB），Roux-en-Y胃旁路手术（RYGB），胆胰分流术（BPD），十二指肠转位术（DS）及腹腔镜袖状胃切除术（LSG）。

第八节着重讲述了术后几种严重并发症的诊断和处理：包括消化道漏和肺栓塞，同时强调了长期随访和监测的重要性。

第九节列举了几种主要减重术式的治疗效果，包括减重和合并症的改善。

第十节详细介绍了不同减重术式的各种并发症。

第十一节提出对先前减肥手术失败的病人再次施行减肥手术的适应证目前还未明确，而且手术失败的明确定义还不清楚。

第十二节主要讲减肥手术面临的一些争议，比如有研究者认为根据严格的BMI临界值无法识别出最有可能从手术中受益的目标人群，另外多年来减肥手术的标准一直是BMI，但有证据表明BMI并不能有效预测对心血管、糖尿病或癌症相关死亡率的影响。

第十三节临床探索性的减重术式。

总结：减重外科目前发展迅速，在治疗严重肥胖、2型糖尿病、高血压、血脂代谢异常等方面更为有效，但仍需要学界和社会的积极发展与推广。

〔吴剑宏〕

 Please access ExpertConsult.com to view the corresponding videos for this chapter.

The surgical treatment of morbid obesity is known as bariatric surgery. It has its origin in the 1950s, when malabsorptive operations were first performed for severe hyperlipidemia syndromes. Subsequently, jejunoileal bypass to produce weight loss began to be performed sporadically during the 1960s, then more frequently in the 1970s. This operation, however, produced unacceptable metabolic complications and has been completely abandoned while other effective, low-morbidity operations were developed.

This process has clearly pointed out two unique aspects of the field of bariatric surgery. The first is that this surgery involves the alteration of metabolic processes through fundamental changes in appetite, energy regulation, satiety, and metabolism, not just simply weight loss. The second is that long-term follow-up is essential to really gauge the effect of these operations on a patient's overall health. Long-term studies confirm that bariatric operations result in sustained long-term weight loss, alteration in the metabolic consequences of morbid obesity, and a substantial reduction in overall mortality from diabetes, cardiovascular complications, and cancer.[1-4] The accumulated weight of evidence that favors bariatric surgery and that has led to the most recent update in guidelines on the treatment of obesity is formulated and endorsed by the American College of Cardiology/American Heart Association Task Force on Practice Guidelines and The Obesity Society. The guidelines for obesity management are to "advise adults with a BMI ≥40 or BMI ≥35 with obesity-related comorbid conditions who are motivated to lose weight and who have not responded to behavioral treatment (with or without pharmacotherapy) with sufficient weight loss to achieve targeted health outcome goals that bariatric surgery may be an appropriate option to improve health and offer referral to an experienced bariatric surgeon for consultation and evaluation."[5]

OBESITY: THE MAGNITUDE OF THE PROBLEM

Until very recently, obesity was not recognized as a disease, which confounded the ability of physicians to be compensated for treatment they delivered and to treat the condition effectively. The American Medical Association officially recognized obesity as a disease in 2013 and in 2014 voted to approve the resolution "that our AMA, consistent with H-440.842 Recognition of Obesity as a Disease, work in concert with national specialty and state medical societies to advocate for patient access to the full continuum of care of evidence-based obesity treatment modalities (such as behavioral, pharmaceutical, psychosocial, nutritional, and surgical interventions)."

Morbid obesity is defined as being 100 pounds above ideal body weight, twice ideal body weight, or body mass index (BMI; measured as weight in kilograms divided by height in meters squared) of 40 kg/m². The last definition is more accepted internationally and has essentially replaced the former ones for all practical and scientific purposes. A consensus conference by the National Institutes of Health (NIH) in 1991 suggested that the term *severe obesity* is more appropriate for defining people of such size. This term is used interchangeably with *morbid obesity* in the remainder of this chapter.

It is estimated that more than one third of the U.S. adult population is obese, and prevalence of obesity in adolescents is 17%.[6] The percentage of obesity (BMI >30) in the United States increased 16 percentage points from 1980 to 2000, and the prevalence of morbidly obese adults (BMI >40) has increased to 6.3% of the adult U.S. population in 2010. If the current trend of linear increases in obesity prevalence continue unabated, 51% of the U.S. population will be obese in 2030. However, the most recent studies show that there has been no significant change in the prevalence of obesity in U.S. youth or adults from 2004 to the most recent survey in 2012, which suggests that the U.S. epidemic is slowing.[6]

Morbid obesity is the second leading cause of preventable death in the United States and is second only to smoking on the list of preventable factors responsible for increased health care costs. It is a sobering thought to realize that a 25-year-old morbidly obese man has a 22% reduction in life expectancy, or 12 years of life lost, compared with a normal-sized man. Moreover, the cost of care is staggering and may be as high as 9% of annual medical expenditures or $147 billion per year. There appears to be significant population heterogeneity between BMI and mortality that provides a survival advantage for class 1 obesity in older individuals (>70 years) but not in younger individuals.[7] Mortality also increases significantly for class 2/3 obesity (BMI >35/40), especially in those individuals who have at least a bachelor's degree education.[7] Thus, it appears that age, gender, education level, race, and income level all play a role in the effect of obesity and mortality.

PATHOPHYSIOLOGY AND ASSOCIATED MEDICAL PROBLEMS

The pathophysiology of severe obesity is poorly understood. Debate is ongoing about the relative genetic versus environmental components of the disease. There is a clear familial predisposition, and it is rare for a single family member to have severe obesity. There is increasing evidence that genes play a primary role in the development of obesity in certain individuals and populations. The genetic abnormality of leptin deficiency leads to severe childhood obesity in afflicted individuals but can be successfully treated with leptin. More recently, scientists have identified specific genes that are associated with obesity, including the *FTO* gene (fat mass and obesity related) that plays a role in controlling feeding behavior and energy expenditure; the *MC4R* deficiency gene (melanocortin 4 receptor), which is associated with obesity, increased fat mass, and insulin resistance; and the β_2-adrenergic receptor obesity genes that play a key role in regulation of lipolysis and thermogenesis.

Despite this solid evidence that genetics plays a significant role in obesity, the rapid increase in obesity from 1980 to the present day emphasizes the considerable environmental component of easily available, cheap, high-density, calorie-rich foods and physical inactivity that contributes to the problem as well.

Another theory suggests that bacteria within the gut, known as the microbiome, play an essential role in the metabolism and immune system. Simply giving low-dose penicillin (LDP) to newborn mice for 4 weeks increases obesity when the mice are later fed a high-fat diet. The predilection to obesity is transferrable to other mice when the LDP-selected gut bacteria are transferred to germ-free hosts, thus identifying that it is the action of the altered gut bacteria, not the antibiotics, that causes the obesity.[8] It is fascinating to hypothesize that the current epidemic of obesity relates to changes in the microbiome induced by the more frequent administration of antibiotics to children who reside in developed countries.

Although there is no definitive answer to the pathophysiology of severe obesity, it is clear that a severely obese individual has, in general, persistent hunger that is not satiated by amounts of food that satisfy the nonobese. This lack of satiety or maintenance of hunger with corresponding increases in calorie intake may be the single most important factor in the process. There appear to be fundamental differences in the satiety and appetite hormonal control of eating that have created the current epidemic.[9] This is hypothesized to occur when the brain's energy "set-point" rises to increase energy intake, through modulation of the individual's appetite.

We know that hormones, peptides, and vagal afferents to the brain have a major influence on satiety, appetite, and energy intake. Ghrelin, the only known orexigenic gut hormone, is also known as the hunger hormone and is secreted by P/D1 cells of the gastric fundus. Ghrelin stimulates release of various neuropeptides, such as neuropeptide Y and growth hormone, from the hypothalamus, which creates an orexigenic or increased appetite state.[9] Increased levels of ghrelin produce increased food intake, and increased levels develop in individuals after low-calorie diets, thus suggesting that one possible mechanism for the failure of most diets after 6 months is the increase in the appetite hormone ghrelin.

Morbid obesity is a metabolic disease associated with numerous medical problems, some of which are virtually unknown in the absence of obesity. Box 47-1 lists the most common. These problems must be carefully considered when one is contemplating offering a patient weight reduction surgery. The most frequent problem is the combination of arthritis and degenerative joint disease, present in at least 50% of patients seeking surgery for severe obesity. The incidence of sleep apnea is high. Asthma is present in more than 25%, hypertension in more than 30%, diabetes in more than 20%, and gastroesophageal reflux in 20% to 30% of patients. The incidence of these conditions increases with age and the severity and duration of severe obesity.

The *metabolic syndrome* includes type 2 diabetes mellitus caused by insulin resistance, dyslipidemia, and hypertension. Patients with this constellation of problems are obese, with central body obesity being the primary essential feature (waist circumference >35 inches in women or >40 inches in men). The syndrome is characterized by impaired hepatic uptake of insulin, systemic hyperinsulinemia, and tissue resistance to insulin. Patients with metabolic syndrome are at high risk for early cardiovascular death. Not listed in Box 47-1 are the associated societal discriminatory problems that severely obese individuals face. Public facilities in terms of seating, doorways, and restroom facilities often make access to events held in such settings unavailable to a severely obese person. Travel on public transportation is sometimes difficult if not impossible. Employment discrimination clearly exists for these individuals. Finally, the combination of low self-esteem, a frequent history of sexual or physical abuse, and these social difficulties coalesce to create a very high incidence of depression in the population of morbidly obese patients.

MEDICAL VERSUS SURGICAL THERAPY

Medical therapy for severe obesity has limited short-term success and almost nonexistent long-term success. Once severely obese, the likelihood that a person will lose enough weight by dietary means alone and remain at a BMI below 35 kg/m^2 is estimated at 3% or less. The NIH consensus conference recognized that for this population of patients, medical therapy has been largely unsuccessful in treating the problem. Review of the clinical trials of lifestyle interventions for prevention of obesity demonstrated that the majority of trials were completely ineffective, and the few that were marginally effective had an extremely small impact on BMI.[2,10]

The most striking evidence of efficacy comes from long-term follow-up trials comparing morbidly obese diabetics who underwent bariatric surgery with those who did not and were treated medically. The Swedish Obese Subjects (SOS) study is the first prospective controlled trial to provide long-term data on the

BOX 47-1   Medical Conditions Associated With Severe Obesity

Cardiovascular
Hypertension
Sudden cardiac death myocardial infarction
Cardiomyopathy
Venous stasis disease
Deep venous thrombosis
Pulmonary hypertension
Right-sided heart failure

Pulmonary
Obstructive sleep apnea
Hypoventilation syndrome of obesity
Asthma

Metabolic
Metabolic syndrome (abdominal obesity, hypertension, dyslipidemia, insulin resistance)
Type 2 diabetes
Hyperlipidemia
Hypercholesterolemia
Nonalcoholic steatotic hepatitis or nonalcoholic fatty liver disease

Gastrointestinal
Gastroesophageal reflux disease
Cholelithiasis

Musculoskeletal
Degenerative joint disease
Lumbar disk disease
Osteoarthritis
Ventral hernias

Genitourinary
Stress urinary incontinence
End-stage renal disease (secondary to diabetes and hypertension)

Gynecologic
Menstrual irregularities

Skin and Integumentary System
Fungal infections
Boils, abscesses

Oncologic
Cancer of the uterus, breast, colon, kidney, and prostate

Neurologic and Psychiatric
Pseudotumor cerebri
Depression
Low self-esteem
Stroke

Social and Societal
History of physical abuse
History of sexual abuse
Discrimination for employment
Social discrimination

effects of bariatric surgery on diabetes, cardiovascular events, cancer, and overall mortality. The study enrolled 2010 bariatric surgery subjects (gastric bypass, 13%; banding, 19%; vertical banded gastroplasty, 68%) and 2037 matched controls who received standard medical treatment and observed the subjects for 10 to 20 years. The SOS study was able to obtain follow-up on 98.9% of the subjects and found at 15 years after initiation that the surgery patients had lost 18% of their body weight, whereas the control group had only a 1% weight loss at 15 years as shown in Figure 47-1. The long-term sustained weight loss and reduction in comorbid conditions after bariatric surgery resulted in a 29% reduction in mortality in the bariatric surgery patients (adjusted hazard ratio, 0.71; 95% confidence interval, 0.54-0.92; $P = .01$) as shown in Figure 47-2. The most common cause of death in the

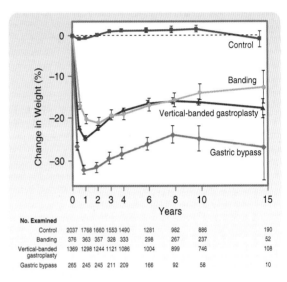

No. Examined										
Control	2037	1768	1660	1553	1490	1281	982	886		190
Banding	376	363	357	328	333	298	267	237		52
Vertical-banded gastroplasty	1369	1298	1244	1121	1086	1004	899	746		108
Gastric bypass	265	245	245	211	209	166	92	58		10

FIGURE 47-1 Weight loss during a 15-year period in the Swedish Obese Subjects study. (From Sjöström L, Narbro K, Sjöström CD, et al: Effects of bariatric surgery on mortality in Swedish obese subjects. *N Engl J Med* 357:741–752, 2007.)

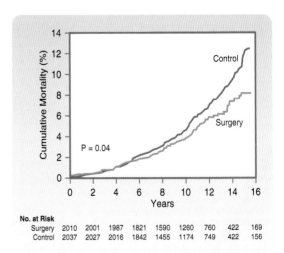

No. at Risk									
Surgery	2010	2001	1987	1821	1590	1260	760	422	169
Control	2037	2027	2016	1842	1455	1174	749	422	156

FIGURE 47-2 Swedish Obese Subjects study cumulative mortality. (From Sjöström L, Narbro K, Sjöström CD, et al: Effects of bariatric surgery on mortality in Swedish obese subjects. *N Engl J Med* 357:741–752, 2007.)

SOS study was cancer (47 in the control group and 29 in the surgery group). The incidence of myocardial infarction was significantly reduced in the surgery group compared with the control group (hazard ratio, 0.56), and the surgery group had a lower number of first-time cardiovascular events (hazard ratio, 0.67) compared with the control group. Most strikingly, the SOS trial showed an 80% decrease in the annual mortality of diabetic individuals in the surgical weight loss group versus the matched control patients (9% mortality in the surgery group versus 28% mortality in a control group).[3,4]

The SOS study also found higher rates of physical activity and improved quality of life compared with the matched control subjects at 10 years. Of note also is that it took 13 years of study to identify statistically improved survival compared with medical treatment in the SOS study, which points out the need for long-term follow-up.

Although the SOS trial is our best evidence of the profound salutary effects of bariatric surgery compared with medical therapy, other excellent long-term studies confirm the benefits of bariatric surgery. Several studies have compared patients undergoing laparoscopic adjustable gastric band (LAGB) with matched community control groups and have found consistently a sustained weight loss and survival advantage in the patients undergoing LAGB.[2] Adams[1] performed a retrospective cohort study of 7925 patients undergoing Roux-en-Y gastric bypass (RYGB) and compared their long-term outcomes with an equal number of matched controls who did not undergo surgery. After a mean follow-up of 7.1 years, the adjusted mortality from any cause was reduced 40% in the patients undergoing RYGB. The cause-specific mortality was reduced 60% for cancer, 56% for coronary artery disease, and 92% for diabetes in the surgery group.[1] After identifying such a positive effect for RYGB in the retrospective study, Adams conducted a different prospective trial of RYGB and compared outcomes after RYGB with a control group of obese patients who sought but did not undergo bariatric surgery (control group 1) and a matched control group of obese subjects who were not seeking bariatric surgery (control group 2). After 6 years, the patients undergoing RYGB had significantly higher rates of diabetes remission and weight loss as shown in Table 47-1. The patients who underwent RYGB had significant improvements in their cardiovascular and metabolic status compared with the two control groups, who generally worsened in all parameters measured during the 6-year period.[11]

There are multiple prospective, randomized clinical trials that compare bariatric surgery with medical therapy, and they all conclude that bariatric surgery is a significantly more effective treatment for weight loss, diabetes, and resolution of comorbidities than medical therapy. O'Brien[11] randomized obese adolescents to LAGB or to diet and lifestyle treatment. Patients randomized to LAGB lost 34.6 kg compared with the diet group, who lost only 3.0 kg at the end of the 2-year trial. In another randomized prospective trial of obese adults, the surgical LAGB group achieved a 21.6% initial body weight loss, whereas the medical group had only a 5.5% initial body weight loss.[12]

Level 1 evidence shown in Table 47-2 accumulated from randomized controlled trials shows that bariatric surgery (laparoscopic RYGB, LAGB, and laparoscopic sleeve gastrectomy [LSG]) is superior to medical therapy for treatment of type 2 diabetes.[13-16] Schauer and colleagues[16] randomized 150 obese patients with uncontrolled type 2 diabetes to one of three arms (i.e., intensive medical therapy, LSG, or laparoscopic RYGB); the primary end point was the proportion of patients 1 year after randomization who had glycated hemoglobin (HbA1c) level of 6.0% or less. Both surgery groups had significantly more patients who achieved glycemic control than in the medical group. Moreover, weight loss was much greater in the surgery groups compared with the medical group at 1 year after randomization. The use of medications to lower glucose, lipids, and blood pressure decreased sig-

TABLE 47-1 Results of the Prospective Clinical Trial of RYGB Matched to Two Medically Treated Control Groups

INCIDENCE (%)	RYGB	CONTROL GROUP 1	CONTROL GROUP 2
Initial weight loss	−27.7	+0.2	0
Diabetes	2	17	15
Hypertension	16	31	33
Low HDL-C	5	32	38
High LDL-C	4	25	30
High triglycerides	3	25	28

From Adams TD, Davidson LE, Litwin SE, et al: Health benefits of gastric bypass surgery after 6 years. *JAMA* 308:1122–1131, 2012. *HDL-C*, high-density lipoprotein cholesterol; *LDL-C*, low-density lipoprotein cholesterol.

TABLE 47-2 Randomized Prospective Trials of Bariatric Surgery versus Medical Therapy in Treatment of Obese Type 2 Diabetics

	SCHAUER[15] LAPAROSCOPIC RYGB	SCHAUER[15] LSG	IKRAMUDDIN[14] LAPAROSCOPIC RYGB	DIXON[13] LAGB
Hemoglobin A1c				
Medical therapy	5%*	5%*	9%*	13%†
Surgery	38%*	24%*	44%*	73%†
Percentage change in weight				
Medical therapy	−4.2	−4.2	−7.9	−1.7
Surgery	−24.5	−21.1	−26.1	−20.7
Triglycerides				
Medical therapy	−21.5%	−21.5%	−27%	−1.1%
Surgery	−45.9%	−31.5%	−59.2%	−37.7%

*Hemoglobin A1c <6.0%.
†Hemoglobin A1c <6.2%

nificantly in both surgery arms, whereas it increased for the patients randomized to medical treatment. Although four patients underwent reoperation, there were no deaths or life-threatening complications. In the most recent publication, Schauer[15] observed these patients for 3 years and found the beneficial effects of surgery to be sustained as shown in Table 47-2. This study also found at 3 years after randomization that both surgical groups (LSG, laparoscopic RYGB) had quality of life measures that were significantly better than in the medical therapy group.

Similar results have been demonstrated in a randomized trial comparing LAGB with intensive medical therapy in Australia. Dixon randomized 60 recently diagnosed diabetics who were also obese (BMI 30-40) patients to each group and identified that significantly more patients undergoing LAGB surgery achieved remission of diabetes at 2 years compared with the medically treated patients. Remission of diabetes was related to weight loss ($R^2 = 0.46$; $P < .001$).[13]

Another multinational multisite trial randomized 120 subjects with type 2 diabetes (HbA1c >8.0%) to laparoscopic RYGB or lifestyle and intensive medical management at four teaching hospitals in the United States and Taiwan. Ikrammuddin and colleagues[14] found at 1 year after induction of therapy that significantly more of the RYGB group achieved the primary end points (HbA1c <7.0%, low-density lipoprotein cholesterol <100 mg/dL, and systolic blood pressure <130 mm Hg) than did the patients randomized to lifestyle and intensive medical management (49% versus 19%). The number of cardiovascular and diabetes medications was significantly reduced in the patients undergoing surgery. They concluded that bariatric surgery results in substantial sustained weight loss and major improvements in diabetic control and lipids compared with intensive medical therapy.

The patients had significantly improved lipid levels after LAGB,[13] LSG,[15,16] and laparoscopic RYGB[14-16] compared with intensive medical treatment in the three randomized trials.

These studies and others have resulted in the increasing role of surgery. Moreover, consensus statements from organizations such as the International Diabetes Federation have concluded that bariatric surgery is a safe and effective treatment for obese type 2 diabetics who have not achieved recommended treatment targets with medical therapy.[17]

Despite this limited success with medical treatment, it is generally agreed that a severely obese patient needs to be given the chance to comply with an in-person, high-intensity comprehensive weight loss intervention.[5] A greater than 5% weight loss attained during a period of months at a rate of 0.5 to 2 lb/wk is the initial goal of medical therapy. Maintenance of the weight loss for 6 months defines the initial success with medical therapy, and further weight loss through a reduction in calories and an increase in physical activity is encouraged. Insurance funding for surgery has traditionally been linked to such an attempt or, for some insurance companies, a well-documented history of several such attempts. However, data showing any efficacy of a prolonged diet attempt as positively influencing outcomes after bariatric surgery are lacking.

Pharmacologic therapy has until recently focused on two medications, phentermine and orlistat. Phentermine has been available since 1959 and is the least expensive weight loss drug on the market. It works to decrease appetite and to increase resting energy expenditure. Orlistat inhibits pancreatic lipase and thereby reduces absorption of up to 30% of ingested dietary fat. Since 2012, two new medications, phentermine-topiramate

extended-release combination and lorcaserin, have been approved by the Food and Drug Administration. The phentermine-topiramate extended-release combination can achieve a 2-year sustained 5% body weight loss in 80% of patients. Lorcaserin has a low side-effect profile compared with other medications and was associated with 5.8% weight loss after 1 year of treatment. A maximum weight loss of up to 10% of body weight has been noted in unselected individuals taking either or both drugs; however, weight is regained within 12 to 18 months once the medications are stopped. For the severely obese individual, these drugs have not proved to be effective therapy alone.

MECHANISM OF ACTION OF BARIATRIC SURGERY

There are multiple theories on the mechanism of action of bariatric surgery. To a large degree, calorie restriction that induces long-term, sustained weight loss is responsible for much of the improvements in glucose metabolism, dyslipidemia, hypertension, and other metabolic effects associated with bariatric surgery. Our understanding of bariatric surgery can be categorized into restrictive (LAGB and LSG) and malabsorptive operations (RYGB, biliopancreatic diversion [BPD], and duodenal switch [DS]), which have profound effects on gastrointestinal peptides, hormones, and the enteroencephalic endocrine axis. The mechanism of action for the restrictive operations such as LSG and, in particular, LAGB is mediated through the decrease in appetite and early induction of satiety through the satiety center in the brain by vagal afferents that are triggered by enhancing the stretch receptors in the proximal stomach.[2,18] LAGB requires adjustment of the band diameter to induce satiety and weight loss; otherwise, the patients will not benefit from the procedure. To a large degree, the LSG affects weight loss through induction of satiety triggered by the same stretch receptors of the tubular stomach.

The RYGB is known as a malabsorptive procedure and has been highly effective in long-term sustained weight loss, with profound changes in glucose metabolism noted immediately after surgery and before significant weight loss. The small gastric pouch and early satiety induced by the gastric stretch fibers and the vagal feedback of the satiety center play some role in the weight loss after RYGB, but other mechanisms are thought to play a much larger role in the effectiveness of RYGB in weight loss. The brain-gut interaction known as the enteroencephalic endocrine axis has been recognized as the core physiologic control of eating, appetite, energy homeostasis, and metabolism. It is the complex interplay between the satiety/metabolism centers of the brain and the alimentary tract through nerves and hormones that exert control over the physiology of eating. Secretion of ghrelin, the only known orexigenic gut hormone, creates an orexigenic or increased appetite state. Conversely, when ghrelin levels fall after meals, the person achieves a sense of satiety. Most studies suggest that patients undergoing RYGB and LSG have suppressed postoperative levels of ghrelin, which is linked to the decreased appetite and calorie intake after surgery. Whereas this would explain the patients' loss of appetite and continued success with dieting, there are other studies that suggest no change or increased levels of ghrelin after RYGB.[9] Despite these conflicting studies, it is clear that RYGB induces a profound change in appetite and decreases calorie intake, in large part, through the changes in the enteroencephalic endocrine axis. RYGB is known to effect changes in glucagon-like peptide 1 (GLP-1), peptide YY, gastric inhibitory polypeptide, neuropeptide Y, leptin, and glucagon, just to name a few of the gastrointestinal hormones. The decrease in calorie intake and resulting profound loss of weight, particularly fat mass, results in twofold improvement in insulin muscle sensitivity and fourfold increase in hepatic insulin sensitivity at 1 year after RYGB, which has been largely attributed to the calorie restriction and loss of weight.[19]

Whereas weight loss after bariatric surgery does have substantial metabolic benefits, RYGB has an effect on beta cell function that is independent of weight loss. Cohen[20] demonstrated remission of diabetes in 88% of 66 patients with a BMI of 30 to 35 at a median of 5 years of follow-up. He demonstrated that weight loss after surgery did not correlate with improvements in glycemic control, whereas C-peptide response to glucose increased substantially, which suggests it was largely the improvement in beta cell function that improved the glycemic control after RYGB in the lower weight individual. Another experimental study in human subjects showed that RYGB alters the nutrient handling and results in greater disposal of glucose and amino acids than does calorie restriction in matched control subjects, which suggests that some of the salutary effects on glucose metabolism are independent of weight loss and directly attributable to RYGB.[21]

There are several mechanisms that can explain the weight-independent effects on glucose metabolism. The best explanation is the theory of incretin stimulation through bypass of the duodenum. The incretins are a family of peptides integral to the synthesis and regulation of insulin that are largely produced in the small and large intestine and are secreted in response to various nutrients. Bypass of the duodenum through RYGB increases nutrient exposure to incretin-secreting cells of the small and large intestine, which stimulates villus hyperplasia and also increases GLP-1 secretion, thereby improving glucose metabolism.[9,22,23] The improvement in beta cell function and glycemic control of RYGB could also occur because of the alteration of bile acid levels.[24]

Alterations in the gut microbiome induced by the bypass of the duodenum may also play a significant role in the long-lasting metabolic changes after bariatric surgery because we know that differences in the gut microbiome can fundamentally alter absorption of nutrients and therefore impart long-lasting increases in calorie intake and weight loss.[8] Increased numbers of H_2-oxidizing methanogen-producing bacteria were found in obese subjects compared with normal-weight or post-RYGB patients, suggesting that there is a large bacterial population shift after RYGB that alters food intake, digestion, and metabolism.[25] More work needs to be done on this intriguing subject.

Severe obesity is also related to the development of metabolic syndrome, a disorder of energy storage and utilization. Experimentally, multiple studies implicate the accumulation of inflammatory cells into adipose tissue (macrophages, T cells, B cells, and neutrophils) that serve as a driver of the insulin resistance and systemic inflammation. This is particularly true for the visceral adipose tissue (VAT), which has been identified as an important risk factor for development of insulin resistance in animal models, in which resection of VAT improves insulin sensitivity. The hypothesis that removal of omental fat would improve insulin sensitivity in human subjects was subjected to a randomized trial of gastric bypass surgery, with and without omentectomy, which demonstrated no added benefit to removal of VAT.[19] The study also showed that the markers of inflammation, such as C-reactive peptide, which are elevated before RYGB, are markedly reduced after RYGB, again demonstrating that the marked loss of fat mass has substantial benefits on metabolism and systemic inflammation.

PREOPERATIVE EVALUATION AND SELECTION

Eligibility

Selection of patients for bariatric surgery is based on currently accepted NIH and AHA/ACC/TOS guidelines.[5] Patients must have a BMI greater than 40 kg/m^2 without associated comorbid medical conditions or a BMI greater than 35 kg/m^2 with an associated comorbid medical problem. They must have also failed dietary and behavioral therapy. Several criteria must also be used as guidelines for indications for surgery, including psychiatric stability, motivated attitude, and ability to comprehend the nature of the operation and its resultant changes in eating behavior and lifestyle. Criteria for eligibility for bariatric surgery are given in Box 47-2. An inability to fulfill these criteria is a contraindication to bariatric surgery.

One criterion not listed in Box 47-2 that unfortunately is often a significant issue for a severely obese patient is insurance coverage for the operation. The Affordable Care Act (ACA) mandates that patients covered under the ACA Marketplace health plans must receive obesity screening and counseling without charging of copayment or coinsurance even if the patient has not met the yearly deductible. Remarkably, the ACA does not mandate coverage for bariatric surgery, and most Federal Marketplace insurance coverage does not cover bariatric surgery, despite that the writers of the ACA wanted to prevent bias against preexisting conditions and the overwhelming evidence that bariatric surgery is the only effective modality of long-term treatment in this population. Meanwhile, the medical societies recognize the need to refer severely obese individuals to bariatric surgeons.[5,17]

The Centers for Medicare and Medicaid Services (CMS), the federal agency that sets Medicare guidelines, established criteria for coverage of bariatric surgery in 2006. The ruling required that only surgeons in hospitals that are designated Centers of Excellence (COE) perform bariatric surgery. The unique requirements for Medicare beneficiaries were at least partly due to concern by policymakers that the morbidity and mortality associated with bariatric surgery were high and that the explosive growth in the number of hospitals and surgeons performing the operations did not match the hospital oversight of these procedures and the resulting complications. Flum and colleagues[26] evaluated the safety of bariatric surgery after the national coverage determination (NCD) and found a dramatic decrease in mortality (15% before NCD to 0.7% after NCD) that was largely explained by a shift in procedure type to lower risk procedures (e.g., LAGB) and a shift from high-risk patients to lower risk patients. They concluded that the majority of the decrease in mortality was not due to the NCD.

After the imposition of the CMS mandate, DeMaria[27] identified an operative mortality of 0.09% for COE participants and

---

BOX 47-2 Indications for Bariatric Surgery

Patients must meet the following criteria for consideration for bariatric surgery:

- BMI >40 kg/m^2 or BMI >35 kg/m^2 with an associated medical comorbidity worsened by obesity
- Failed dietary therapy
- Psychiatrically stable without alcohol dependence or illegal drug use
- Knowledgeable about the operation and its sequelae
- Motivated individual
- Medical problems not precluding probable survival from surgery

suggested that the imposition of the COE has been at least partially responsible for the decline in operative morbidity and mortality. Regardless, CMS removed the requirements for facility and surgeon certification to perform bariatric surgery in September 2013 partly on the basis of improvements in bariatric surgery outcomes since the 2006 ruling. After the ruling was made by CMS to forgo the requirement to undergo surgery at a certified COE, Morton and colleagues[28] published a paper that evaluated 117,478 bariatric patient discharges from 66 unaccredited and 79 accredited hospitals and found that the incidence of complications and mortality was significantly higher in the unaccredited centers. They also found that hospital accreditation was associated with safer outcomes, shorter length of stay, and lower total charges after bariatric surgery.[28]

Accreditation, improvement in communication, and structured quality programs have been important in the improvements in quality of care. The American Society for Metabolic and Bariatric Surgery (ASMBS) has published recommendations on credentialing of bariatric surgeons by hospitals recently that include the need for active participation within a structured bariatric surgery program and quality improvement program.[29] Although hospital-wide coordination of care, communication, and multidisciplinary teams must function well to achieve best results in bariatric surgery, a recent study showed that the technical skill of the individual surgeon was highly correlated with significantly fewer complications, readmissions, reoperations, and visits to the emergency department.[30] In summary, these studies show that the surgeon not only must achieve technical proficiency but also must engage the entire operative and hospital team to achieve excellent outcomes.

Medical contraindications to bariatric surgery are relative, and all patients with comorbid conditions are at greater risk. The surgeon must ensure that these risks are well understood by all patients before bariatric surgery, especially those at high risk. Ideally, several family members are included in these discussions. There are certain individuals who have end-stage organ dysfunction of the heart, lungs, or both. These patients are unlikely to gain the benefit of longevity and improved health.

Surgery is contraindicated in patients who are unable to ambulate because their level of debility precludes recovery during the rapid weight loss phase after surgery. Prader-Willi syndrome is another absolute contraindication because no surgical therapy affects the constant need to eat by these patients.

The U.S. Food and Drug Administration expanded the use of the LAP-BAND to include patients with BMI between 30 and 34 kg/m^2 who have an existing condition related to their obesity. Other contraindications to LAGB include cirrhosis, portal hypertension, autoimmune connective tissue disorders, chronic inflammatory conditions such as inflammatory bowel disease, and need for chronic administration of steroids.

Patients who weigh more than 500 pounds are at increased risk for mortality and have more complications. Many options for diagnostic testing, such as computed tomography (CT), are exceeded by this weight limit. At this weight, operating room tables, moving and lift equipment and teams, blood pressure cuffs, sequential compression device (SCD) boots, and any sort of invasive bedside procedures such as central venous catheters become extraordinarily difficult. It has been my practice to require patients weighing more than 500 pounds to lose weight down to that level by nonoperative methods.

Age is a controversial contraindication to bariatric surgery. For adolescents, most pediatric and bariatric surgeons recommend

that the operation be performed after the major growth spurt (mid to late teens), thus allowing increased maturity on the part of the patient. The Teen–Longitudinal Assessment of Bariatric Surgery (Teen-LABS) demonstrated that severely obese teens (<19 years) had multiple comorbid conditions and could undergo one of three commonly performed operations (laparoscopic RYGB, LSG, and LAGB) with no mortality and a favorable short-term complication profile.[31] Increasing experience will be required to determine which operation is most effective in adolescents.

Although in my practice I have generally set the age of 65 years as a rough cutoff for performing gastric bypass and 70 years for LAGB, patients older than 65 years have been individually evaluated. Such evaluations focus on the patient's relative physiologic age and potential for longevity rather than chronologic age. The duration and degree of obesity are the most important factors in evaluating an older patient. In general, the duration and the severity of obesity and the number of comorbid medical problems that exist lower the potential for such individuals to benefit from bariatric surgery.

General Bariatric Preoperative Evaluation and Preparation

Preoperative assessment of a bariatric surgical patient involves two distinct areas. One is a specific preoperative assessment of candidacy for bariatric surgery and evaluation for comorbid conditions. The second is a general assessment and preoperative preparation as for any major abdominal surgery, which is discussed in depth in Chapter 10. A team approach is required for optimal care of a morbidly obese patient as shown in Box 47-3, and Box 47-4 summarizes the steps and tests routinely performed for the preoperative evaluation of bariatric patients in the author's clinics. Proper preoperative patient education is essential, and attendance at educational sessions is mandatory. After preoperative testing is completed, a final counseling session with the surgeon and an education session with the nurse educator and nutritionist are held.

Data support the use of preoperative antibiotics and deep venous thrombosis (DVT) prophylaxis. A first-generation cephalosporin, in a dose appropriate for weight, is given preoperatively, and antibiotics are continued for less than 24 hours. Bariatric surgery patients are at moderate to high risk for venous thromboembolism (VTE), and they should receive mechanical prophylaxis such as early ambulation and use of SCDs. Most patients are at moderate or high risk for VTE, and the preponderance of data suggests that both chemoprophylaxis and mechanical measures be

---

BOX 47-3 **The Bariatric Multidisciplinary Team**

Surgeon
Assisting surgeon
Nutritionist
Anesthesiologist
Operating room nurse
Operating room scrub tech or nurse
Nurse care coordinator or educator
Secretary or administrator
Psychiatrist or psychologist
Primary care physician
Medical specialists for cardiac, pulmonary, gastrointestinal, endocrine, musculoskeletal, and neurologic conditions as indicated

BOX 47-4 Preoperative Evaluation and Postoperative Care

Before the Clinic Visit
Documented, medically supervised diet
Counseling and referral from the primary care physician
Reading a comprehensive written brochure or attendance at a seminar regarding operative procedures, expected results, and potential complications

Initial Clinic Visit
Group presentation on information in the booklet
Group presentation on preoperative and postoperative nutritional issues by the nutritionist
Individual assessment by the surgeon's team
Individual counseling session with the surgeon
Individual counseling session with the nutritionist
Screening blood tests

Subsequent Events and Evaluations
Full psychological assessment and evaluation as indicated
Medical specialist evaluations as indicated
Insurance approval for coverage of the procedure
Screening flexible upper endoscopy as indicated
Screening ultrasound of the gallbladder (if present)
Arterial blood gas analysis as indicated

Subsequent Clinic Visits
Counseling session with the surgeon (including selection of the date for surgery)
Education session with the nurse educator
Preoperative evaluation by the anesthesiologist
Final paperwork by the preadmissions center

used on the basis of individual assessment of clinical judgment and risk of bleeding. The Michigan Bariatric Surgery Collaborative (MBSC) identified that preoperative and postoperative use of low-molecular-weight heparin was associated with significantly lower rates of VTE compared with patients given unfractionated heparin.[32] High-risk patients (e.g., those with history of DVT, venous stasis ulcers, known or highly suspected pulmonary hypertension, hypoventilation syndrome of obesity, or need for reoperation during the initial hospitalization) are given low-molecular-weight heparin administered twice daily for a full 2-week course. The data are unclear about the use of prophylactic vena cava filters, and the ASMBS recommends their use only in combination with chemical and mechanical prophylaxis in extremely high risk individuals in whom the risks of VTE are greater than filter-related complications.

Evaluation of Specific Comorbid Conditions

Cardiovascular evaluation of a bariatric patient must include a history of recent chest pain and functional assessment of activity in relation to cardiac function. Patients with a history of recent chest pain or a change in exercise tolerance need to undergo a formal cardiology assessment, including stress testing as indicated. We almost never resort to invasive central monitoring with a Swan-Ganz catheter because central venous and pulmonary hypertension is routinely present and must not be interpreted as volume overload. The use of intraoperative transesophageal echocardiography is occasionally helpful in patients with cardiomyopathy.

Pulmonary assessment includes a search for obstructive sleep apnea because a significant number of patients undergoing bariatric surgery will have undiagnosed sleep apnea.[33] A history of falling asleep while driving or while at work or a history of feeling tired after a night's sleep coupled with a history of snoring or even witnessed apnea is strongly suggestive of the condition. Patients with suggestive histories of clinically significant sleep apnea need to undergo preoperative sleep study testing. If the patient is found to have the condition, use of a continuous or bilevel positive airway pressure apparatus postoperatively while sleeping can eliminate the stressful periods of hypoxia that would otherwise result. Although tolerated under normal circumstances, these hypoxic episodes in the immediate postoperative period are more dangerous because of the enhanced effect of narcotic pain medications and postoperative fluid shifts that affect hemodynamic stability.

Reactive asthma is another common problem of the severely obese and one that is underrecognized. It requires less preoperative preparation in terms of testing than sleep apnea does and is less dangerous.

Hypoventilation syndrome of obesity (pickwickian syndrome) is a diagnosis that should be suspected in the superobese (BMI >60) and by the patient's clinical appearance. Individuals with this diagnosis have plethoric faces, may appear clinically cyanotic, and clearly exhibit difficulty in normal respiratory efforts at baseline or with mild exertion. Arterial blood gas analysis reveals $PaCO_2$ higher than PaO_2 and an elevated hematocrit. Pulmonary artery pressure is greatly elevated. These patients have significantly increased high cardiopulmonary morbidity and mortality and require significant preoperative weight loss and optimization of the patient's cardiopulmonary physiology before the operative procedure. Prolonged ventilator support may be needed, and management of intravascular volume is based on the patient's baseline status.

Because there is an increased incidence of hypertension or diabetes in patients with concomitant renal disease, the serum creatinine value is an excellent preoperative screening test for baseline renal function.

Musculoskeletal conditions, especially arthritis and degenerative joint disease, are the most common group of comorbid diseases found in severely obese patients. More than half the patients have some form of these conditions, often to an advanced degree. Limited ambulation, joint replacement, severe back pain, and other sequelae are not uncommon. Before surgery, it is important for patients to understand that any preexisting structural damage cannot be reversed by weight loss. Fortunately, significant weight loss often alleviates or even reverses the chronic pain or disability from such conditions. Significant weight loss after bariatric surgery will make subsequent knee and hip replacement surgery more effective and safer.

Metabolic problems are common in severely obese patients, particularly hyperlipidemia, hypercholesterolemia, and type 2 diabetes mellitus. All are easily screened for by simple blood tests. Twenty percent to 30% of severely obese patients undergoing bariatric surgery have clinically significant type 2 diabetes. Diabetes needs to be controlled preoperatively to reduce the incidence of perioperative morbidity.

The skin must be examined for fungal infection and venous stasis changes, which are associated with a greatly increased incidence of postoperative DVT.

Umbilical or ventral hernias may be present. It has been my practice to postpone repair of ventral and incisional hernia until after significant weight loss. Repair of the hernias at the time of abdominoplasty enables the bariatric surgeon to complete physical reconstruction of the abdominal wall and to place prosthetic mesh to reinforce the abdominal wall, something that often cannot be accomplished during the initial bariatric procedure.

Cholelithiasis is the most prevalent of the several gastrointestinal conditions, and if gallstones are present, most surgeons agree that cholecystectomy needs to be performed simultaneously with the bariatric surgery. The incidence of gallstone or sludge formation after gastric bypass is approximately 30%. For patients undergoing malabsorptive operations, gallstone formation is so frequent that prophylactic cholecystectomy is a standard part of these procedures. However, for restrictive operations, screening ultrasound is recommended, particularly in patients undergoing RYGB, because endoscopic retrograde cholangiopancreatography is not possible. Ursodeoxycholic acid, 300 mg twice daily for 6 months postoperatively, reduces the incidence of gallstone formation to 3% in patients who follow this treatment plan. Our current recommendations for patients undergoing laparoscopic bariatric surgery are simultaneous cholecystectomy if gallstones are present and ursodiol therapy for 6 months after surgery if the gallbladder is normal.

Gastroesophageal reflux disease (GERD) is common in severely obese patients because of the increased abdominal pressure and shortened lower esophageal sphincter. Preoperative upper endoscopy is indicated in all patients who have GERD to detect Barrett esophagus and the presence of hiatal hernias and to evaluate the lower part of the stomach in patients undergoing RYGB.

A patient with nonalcoholic steatotic hepatitis (NASH) presents a potential problem. The size of the left lobe of the liver often inhibits the surgeon's ability to complete an operation laparoscopically. Patients with known enlarged fatty livers may benefit from calorie restriction, especially carbohydrate restriction, for a period of 5 to 10 days preoperatively. Bariatric surgery is beneficial for NASH; weight loss improves the prognosis. NASH is not a contraindication to bariatric surgery if there is no cirrhosis and portal hypertension or hepatocellular decompensation. Liver biopsy should be performed at the time of bariatric surgery in any patient whose liver appears abnormal.

SPECIAL EQUIPMENT

Clinic

The clinic for evaluating bariatric patients must be constructed with the needs of the patient in mind. The waiting area must contain comfortable benches with backs, not standard-size chairs. Doorways must be extra wide to accommodate wheelchairs. This is true for bathrooms as well, which must be equipped with toilets on the floor, not mounted on the wall. A scale that can weigh up to 800 pounds is necessary. Scales that use impedance to measure fat mass are useful in the evaluation and ongoing treatment of bariatric patients. The percentage of fat mass lost after surgery using the impedance scales is monitored to make sure that the patient is losing primarily fat mass and taking in enough protein to maintain muscle mass. Large-sized gowns, wide examining tables stable enough for large patients, and wide blood pressure cuffs are needed. A large room with appropriate seating is needed for the patient group education session.

Operating Room

The operating room needs to contain a hydraulically operated operating room table that can accommodate up to 800 pounds. Side attachments to widen the table as needed are required. Foam cushioning, extralarge SCD stockings, wide and secure padded straps for the abdomen and legs, and a footboard for the operating room table are all essential to safely secure the patient for placement in a steep reverse Trendelenburg position during surgery. Video telescopic equipment as used for any laparoscopic abdominal procedure is necessary. Two monitors, one near each shoulder, and high-flow insufflators able to maintain pneumoperitoneum are essential.

A 45-degree telescope, extralong staplers, atraumatic graspers, extralong trocars, and ultrasonic scalpel or other energy source instrument are essential for the laparoscopic operations. A fixed retractor device secured to the operating room table for clamping and holding the liver retractor is also essential. This can pose one of the most difficult technical challenges in patients with a large, thick liver. Sometimes, two retractors may be necessary for a large liver.

OPERATIVE PROCEDURES

Primary laparoscopic bariatric operations are preferred to the open procedures because of the overwhelming advantages of the laparoscopic approach, including reduced mortality, wound infections, pulmonary complications, thromboembolic complications, and rate of incisional hernias and decreased hospitalization.[33] Box 47-5 lists the major procedures to be described.

Vertical Banded Gastroplasty

This procedure has been abandoned in favor of other operations because of poor long-term weight loss, a high rate of late stenosis of the gastric outlet, and a tendency for patients to adopt a high-calorie liquid diet, thereby leading to regain of weight.

Laparoscopic Adjustable Gastric Banding

The LAGB procedure may be performed with any of multiple types of adjustable bands. The two bands approved for use by the Food and Drug Administration in the United States are the LAP-BAND (INAMED Health, Santa Barbara, CA) and the Realize band (Ethicon Endo-Surgery, Cincinnati, OH). The techniques of placement of the bands are similar; only the locking mechanisms, band shape and configuration, and adjustment schedules vary somewhat for the different types of bands. Their advantage over other bariatric procedures is individualized adjustability and a markedly lower initial operative morbidity and mortality.

Trocar placement for LAGB is shown in Figure 47-3. The surgeon stands to the patient's right; the assistant and the camera

---

> **BOX 47-5   Bariatric Operations: Mechanism of Action**
>
> **Restrictive**
> Vertical banded gastroplasty (historic purposes only)
> Laparoscopic adjustable gastric banding (LAGB)
> Laparoscopic sleeve gastrectomy (LSG)
>
> **Largely Restrictive, Moderately Malabsorptive**
> Roux-en-Y gastric bypass (RYGB)
>
> **Largely Malabsorptive, Mildly Restrictive**
> Biliopancreatic diversion (BPD)
> Duodenal switch (DS)

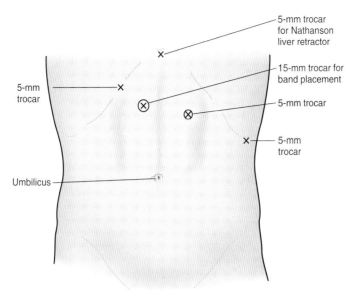

FIGURE 47-3 Trocar location for adjustable gastric banding.

operator are to the patient's left. Most surgeons place the patient in the supine position, but some prefer to have the patient's legs spread so that the surgeon can stand between the legs. The peritoneum at the angle of His is divided to create an opening in the peritoneum between the angle of His and the top of the spleen (Fig. 47-4A). The telescope is placed through the left upper quadrant port for this part of the operation to maximally view the angle of His area.

The pars flaccida technique has become the approach of choice for placing the adjustable band; it begins with dividing the gastrohepatic ligament in its thin area just over the caudate lobe of the liver. The anterior branch of the vagus nerve is spared, and any aberrant left hepatic artery is preserved. The base of the right crus of the diaphragm is identified. Care must be taken to clearly identify the crus because occasionally the vena cava can lie close to the caudate lobe. The surgeon gently follows the surface of the right crus posterior and inferior to the esophagus while aiming for the angle of His (Fig. 47-4B). A gentle spreading and pushing technique is used to create an avascular tunnel along this plane. Once the tip of the tunneling instrument is seen near the top of the spleen, it is gently pushed through any remaining peritoneal layers to complete the tunnel (Fig. 47-4C). The adjustable band has already been placed in the peritoneal cavity through the large 15-mm trocar located in the right upper quadrant before dissection of the pars flaccida. The narrow end of the band itself is grasped by the tunneling instrument and pulled through the tunnel from the greater to the lesser side of the stomach (Fig. 47-5). That end is then threaded through the locking mechanism of the band, after which the band is locked. Once the band has been locked in place, the buckle is adjusted to lie on the lesser curvature side of the stomach (Fig. 47-6). A 5-mm grasper inserted between the band and stomach ensures that the band is not too tight.

The anterior gastric wall is plicated over the band with three or four interrupted, nonabsorbable sutures (Fig. 47-7). There needs to be just enough stomach above the level of the band for incorporating that tissue into the suture. Suturing is carried as far posterolaterally as possible because this region has been the most frequent area of fundus herniation through the band. The band is thus ideally secured about 1 cm below the gastroesophageal junction with this technique.

The Silastic tubing leading from the band is pulled through the 15-mm trocar site in the right upper quadrant paramedian area to complete the laparoscopic portion of the operation. The trocar site incision is enlarged to reveal the anterior rectus fascia, which is exposed approximately 2 to 4 cm lateral to the existing fascial defect for the trocar, and the access port is connected to the inflation tubing. Four sutures inserted through the four holes on the access port are placed in the fascia, after which the port is tied to the fascia (Fig. 47-8). The redundant tubing is replaced in the abdominal cavity, with care taken to avoid kinking.

Roux-en-Y Gastric Bypass

The gastric bypass first described by Mason and Ito in 1969 incorporated a loop of jejunum anastomosed to a proximal gastric pouch. This operation proved unacceptable because of bile reflux, and RYGB, which eliminates bile reflux, has become one of the most commonly performed bariatric operations in the United States.

Described here is one technique that incorporates many of these modifications. There are certainly many variations of this technique, and many if not most will give excellent results. The essential principles of the operation are listed in Box 47-6.

The left subcostal region, near the midclavicular line, is an ideal location for the first trocar. Either a bladed trocar (United States Surgical Corporation, Norwalk, CT) or an optical trocar (Optiview, Ethicon Endo-Surgery) that dilates a tract under direct vision is placed. Subsequent trocars are placed under laparoscopic vision to achieve the configuration shown in Figure 47-9.

Once the omentum is mobilized, the ligament of Treitz is identified. A location approximately 30 to 40 cm distal to the ligament is chosen for division of the jejunum with an endoscopic stapler (Fig. 47-10). The mesentery is then further divided with staples or a harmonic scalpel.

The length of the Roux limb is influenced in our practices by the patient's weight. Patients with a BMI in the 40s will be well

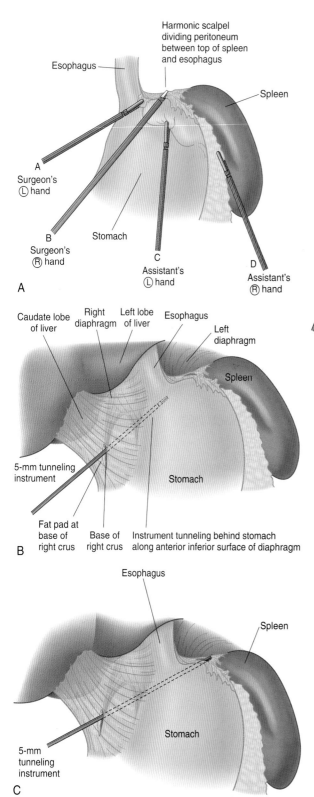

FIGURE 47-4 **A,** Dividing the peritoneum at the angle of His. **B,** Pars flaccida technique, in which the fat pad is divided at the base of the right crus. **C,** Tunnel posterior to the stomach completed.

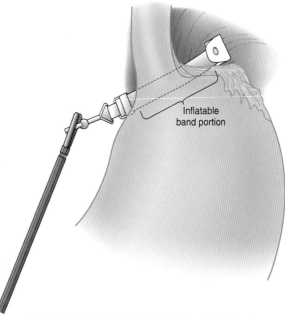

FIGURE 47-5 Pulling the LAP-BAND through the tunnel.

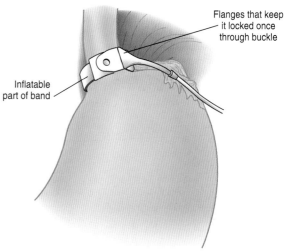

FIGURE 47-6 Locking the LAP-BAND.

served with a Roux limb of 80 to 120 cm, whereas a Roux limb of approximately 150 cm is constructed for patients with a BMI in excess of 50. The proximal jejunum is left to lay to the patient's right side, and the Roux limb is lifted cephalad and coiled in the curve of the transverse colon mesentery (Fig. 47-11). This technique allows the proximal jejunum to be aligned directly alongside the designated point on the Roux limb for the distal anastomosis. The stapler is placed through the surgeon's right-hand port because the bowel segments are easily aligned to facilitate placement of the stapler into enterotomies created in each segment of bowel at the desired location of the anastomosis (Fig. 47-12). Another firing of the stapler, this time from the left side of the patient, creates a large side-to-side anastomosis. Once the anastomosis is created, the stapler defect is closed with another fire of the stapler.

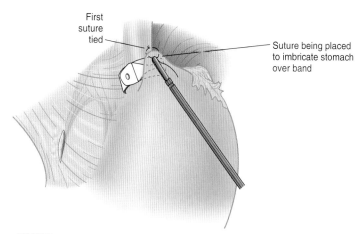

FIGURE 47-7 Imbricating the anterior aspect of the stomach over the LAP-BAND.

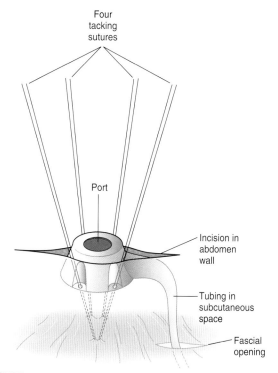

FIGURE 47-8 Passing the inflation tubing through the abdominal wall sufficiently far from the port site to prevent acute kinking of the tubing.

> ### BOX 47-6   Essential Components of Roux-en-Y Gastric Bypass
>
> Small proximal gastric pouch (15-20 mL)
> Gastric pouch constructed from the cardia of the stomach to prevent dilation and to minimize acid production
> Gastric pouch divided from the distal part of the stomach
> Roux limb at least 75 cm in length
> Enteroenterostomy constructed to avoid stenosis or obstruction
> Closure of all potential spaces for internal hernias using nonabsorbable sutures

The left lobe liver retractor is now placed, and the patient is placed in the reverse Trendelenburg position. Exposure of the angle of His allows division of the peritoneum between the top of the spleen and the gastroesophageal junction with the ultrasonic scalpel. The lesser sac is entered through the gastrohepatic ligament, 3 to 4 cm below the gastroesophageal junction. The blue load of the linear stapler is now fired multiple times to create a 10- to 15-mL proximal gastric pouch based on the upper lesser curvature of the stomach (Fig. 47-13). Once the gastric pouch is created, the Roux limb may be passed toward the proximal gastric pouch through a retrocolic or antecolic pathway. The antecolic, antegastric approach is preferred to prevent the risk of an internal hernia through the transverse mesocolon or a hernia formed by

the transverse mesocolon and the mesentery of the Roux limb in the retrocolic approach. The gastrojejunostomy may be performed with a circular stapler (Fig. 47-14) or a hand-sutured technique. The entire anastomosis is irrigated with saline, and a member of the operative team uses the endoscope to monitor occlusion of the Roux limb with an atraumatic 10-mm bowel clamp. Even the smallest leaks of air can be identified and closed with this technique. Studies have shown that use of this technique can dramatically reduce the incidence of postoperative leaks to very low levels. The mesenteric defect in the jejunojejunostomy is closed with a purse-string suture of 2-0 polypropylene that, combined with the antecolic Roux limb approach, has virtually eliminated a subsequent internal hernia (Fig. 47-15).

Biliopancreatic Diversion

BPD, like most bariatric operations that had been performed through an open approach, can be performed through a laparoscopic approach. BPD produces weight loss primarily on the basis of malabsorption, but it does have a restrictive component as well.

The anatomic configuration of BPD is shown in Figure 47-16. The intestinal tract is reconstructed to allow only a short, so-called common channel of the distal 50 cm of terminal ileum for absorption of fat and protein. The alimentary tract beyond the proximal part of the stomach is rearranged to include only the distal 200 cm of ileum, including the common channel. The proximal end of this ileum is anastomosed to the proximal end of the stomach after a distal hemigastrectomy is performed. The ileum proximal to the end that is anastomosed to the stomach is in turn anastomosed to the terminal ileum within the 50- to 100-cm distance from the ileocecal valve, depending on the surgeon's preference and the patient's size.

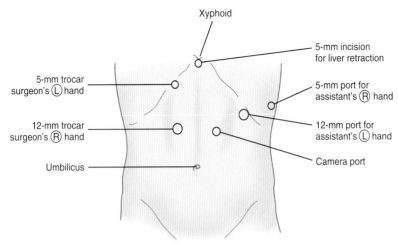

FIGURE 47-9 Trocar configuration for laparoscopic Roux-en-Y gastric bypass and for laparoscopic sleeve gastrectomy.

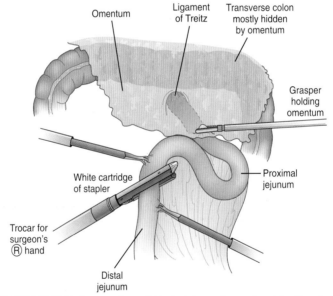

FIGURE 47-10 Placing a stapler to divide the jejunum for creation of the Roux limb.

Duodenal Switch

The DS configuration is shown in Figure 47-17. This modification was developed to help lessen the high incidence of marginal ulcers after BPD. The mechanism of weight loss is similar to that of BPD.

An appendectomy is followed by measurement of the terminal ileum. Notably in the DS procedure, the common channel is 100 cm and the entire alimentary tract is 250 cm. However, the major difference between DS and BPD is the gastrectomy and the proximal anatomy. Instead of a distal hemigastrectomy, a sleeve gastrectomy of the greater curvature of the stomach is performed. This procedure is done as the initial part of the operation because if the patient exhibits any intraoperative instability, the operation can be discontinued after the sleeve gastrectomy alone. A two-stage DS has been used in patients who have an extremely high BMI and are high operative risks. The sleeve gastrectomy alone usually produces enough weight loss to make the second stage of

the operation technically easier. This approach lowers the mortality rate despite the need to undergo two operative procedures. The first step of a laparoscopic DS is to perform the sleeve gastrectomy with a stapling technique that begins at the mid antrum, and a staple line is created parallel to the lesser curvature of the stomach with a 40 Fr to 60 Fr Maloney dilator placed along the lesser curve to prevent narrowing. The staple line is created with multiple firings of the stapler until the angle of His is reached. The goal is to produce a lesser curvature gastric sleeve with a volume of 150 to 200 mL.

After sleeve gastrectomy, the duodenum is divided with the stapler approximately 2 cm beyond the pylorus. The distal connections are performed as for BPD. The distal anastomosis is created at the 100-cm point proximal to the ileocecal valve. The proximal anastomosis is created between the proximal end of the 250 cm of terminal ileum and the first portion of the duodenum. The duodenoileostomy is an antecolic end-to-side anastomosis.

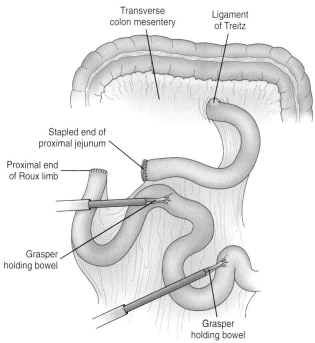

FIGURE 47-11 Measuring and laying out the jejunum to set up a distal anastomosis for the length of the Roux-en-Y gastric bypass.

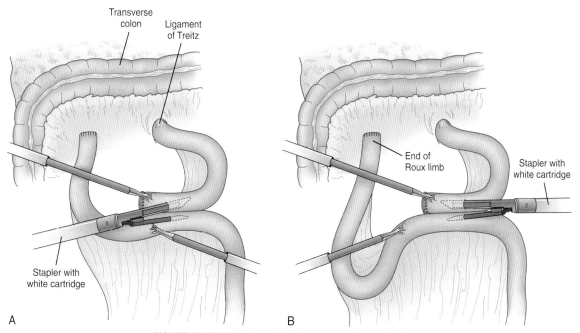

FIGURE 47-12 Placing the stapler to create an enteroenterostomy.

This anastomosis is one of the most critical parts of the operation and can be performed either with a circular stapler or using a hand-sewn technique. If the EEA stapler is used, the anvil is directly inserted through the staple line of the duodenal stump through a gastrotomy under suture guidance or through an oral approach with a nasogastric tube.

Laparoscopic Sleeve Gastrectomy

The LSG is now recognized as a primary procedure, and a *Current Procedural Terminology* code was assigned to the procedure in 2010. By 2012, there was a precipitous increase in the number of LSG procedures (0.9% to 36.3% of the total number of bariatric procedures) being performed in U.S. academic health centers from 2008 to 2012.[34] Advantages of the LSG are the technical simplicity of the procedure, preservation of the pylorus (avoidance of dumping), metabolic reduction of ghrelin levels,[9] no need for serial adjustments (as for the LAGB), reduction in internal hernias (seen after laparoscopic RYGB), reduction in malabsorption (seen with laparoscopic RYGB), and ability to later modify the gastric sleeve to either a laparoscopic RYGB or a DS configuration in a second stage of the operation.

The trocar placement is identical to that of laparoscopic RYGB (see Fig. 47-9). As a primary procedure, the surgeon takes down

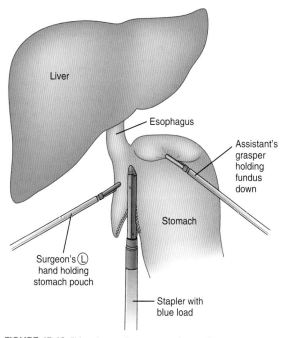

FIGURE 47-13 Firing the stapler to create the proximal gastric pouch.

the entire greater curvature, leaving intact the tissue within 3 cm of the pylorus and up to the angle of His and exposing the left crus of the diaphragm. Then, with use of a 32 Fr to 40 Fr bougie, the stomach is divided from the antrum to the angle of His by sequential firings of the stapler (Fig. 47-18). It is vitally important in this procedure to preserve the left gastric vessels and lesser curve blood supply and to prevent twisting or spiraling of the gastric tube. Most surgeons routinely suture the staple lines to reinforce the integrity and use some form of staple line reinforcement to prevent bleeding or leaks from the staple line.

Disadvantages of the procedure seem to focus on the Achilles heel of the operation, which is a leak along the long gastric staple line. Whereas a leak after gastric bypass is one of the most feared complications, leaks after LSG appear to be slightly more common than in laparoscopic RYGB and more difficult to treat.[35] The leaks are most likely to be located in the proximal third of the stomach. Management of the leak includes adequate drainage, by either CT-guided percutaneous catheter placement or operative approaches, with institution of total parenteral nutrition, no oral intake, antibiotics, and, in many cases, endoscopic stenting to prevent ongoing contamination of the peritoneal cavity.[35] The cause of leaks appears to be multifactorial, with early leaks (≤2 days postoperatively) related to stapler misfires or tissue trauma, whereas late leaks are related to ischemia and high intragastric pressure, particularly when there is distal stenosis, often at the incisura angularis. Diagnosis of leaks is best done with an oral contrast-enhanced CT scan of the abdomen if the patient has fever, tachycardia, and leukocytosis.

POSTOPERATIVE CARE AND FOLLOW-UP

Excellent surgical outcomes require the appropriate selection of patients, thorough preoperative preparation, technically well-performed operations, and attentive postoperative care. A bariatric patient requires particularly attentive and special postoperative

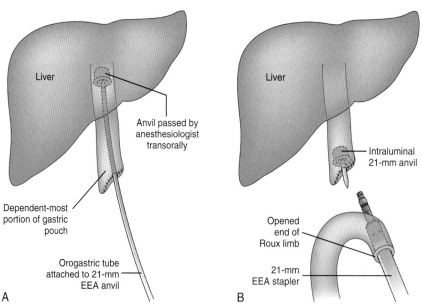

FIGURE 47-14 Creating the proximal anastomosis. **A,** Insertion of anvil transorally. **B,** Insertion of stapler through Roux limb and creation of stapled anastomosis.

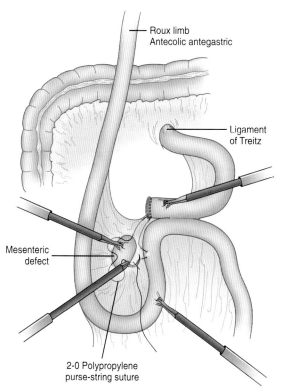

FIGURE 47-15 Closure of mesenteric defect using purse-string suture of 2-0 polypropylene.

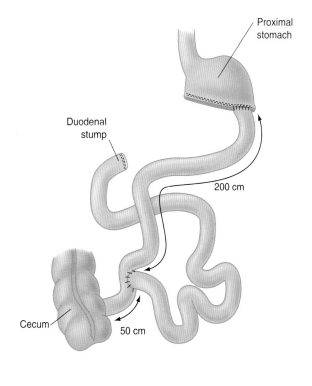

Alimentary channel = 250 (± 50) cm
Common channel = 50 cm

FIGURE 47-16 Anatomic configuration of biliopancreatic diversion.

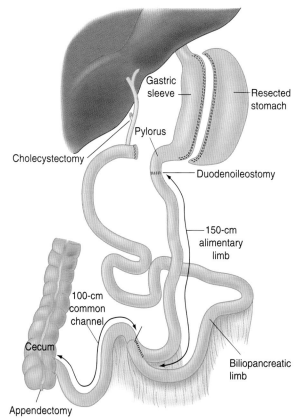

FIGURE 47-17 Anatomic configuration of the duodenal switch.

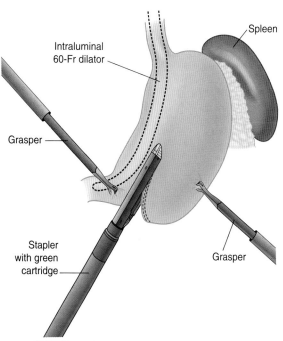

FIGURE 47-18 Creation of the sleeve gastrectomy.

care in several areas above and beyond that of the average surgical patient.

The most dreaded complication after bariatric surgery is a leak from the gastrointestinal tract. Tachycardia, at times accompanied by tachypnea or agitation, is often the only manifestation of this severe intra-abdominal problem. A severely obese patient may not be subject to the development of fever or signs of peritonitis, as would a patient with a normal body habitus. A high index of suspicion for leak must be present for the postoperative patients who demonstrate sustained tachycardia, fever, or increased pain. If a leak is suggested, a CT scan with oral administration of a contrast agent or possibly laparoscopy may be needed to establish the diagnosis before overwhelming sepsis occurs.

Appropriate fluid resuscitation is essential. A 200-kg patient who undergoes open gastric bypass can easily require 6 to 10 liters of fluid for replacement of maintenance, third-space, and operative fluid or blood losses. Our postoperative protocol after open surgery calls for 400 mL/hr of a balanced salt solution (usually lactated Ringer solution), with boluses given as needed for low urine output. A Foley catheter is used intraoperatively and urine output monitored carefully. Patients undergoing laparoscopic surgery usually have much less third-space and operative blood loss than do patients undergoing open surgery and can be managed with 125 mL/hr of intravenous fluids. Urine output intraoperatively is normally low because of the pneumoperitoneum and usually improves in the recovery room area. Some patients who have been taking diuretics chronically may not produce adequate urine output without diuretic use, but the surgeon must ensure that the patient is adequately volume resuscitated before giving diuretics. Higher than expected fluid requirements, oliguria, and tachycardia are a constellation of postoperative findings suggesting intra-abdominal problems.

Adequate pain control is essential. Narcotic requirements are decreased with a laparoscopic approach. A patient-controlled analgesia pump is appropriate and helpful. Non-narcotic intravenous pain medications have been extremely helpful in reducing postoperative pain, as have anesthetics injected locally in the incisions at the time of surgery.

DVT prophylaxis is important. Pulmonary embolism is one of the leading causes of death after open and laparoscopic bariatric surgery. We use a combination of early ambulation (the same day as surgery, generally within 4 to 6 hours), SCDs, and preoperative and postoperative subcutaneous administration of low-molecular-weight heparin (e.g., enoxaparin).[32]

Our standard practice is to obtain a CT scan of the gastrointestinal tract only if there are clinical signs of a leak, which include a temperature higher than 100° F or a sustained heart rate of more than 100 beats/min. If neither is present, a water trial is started with progression to bariatric clear liquids. Use of such an approach has led to excellent clinical results; however, the surgeon must investigate persistent tachycardia and fever, which can be the only signs of a clinically significant leak. Failure to diagnose and promptly to treat a leak after bariatric surgery often leads to catastrophic outcomes, whereas early intervention uniformly results in survival.

Discharge, regardless of the bariatric operation, occurs when the patient is mobile, is tolerating an oral liquid diet, has adequate pain control with oral analgesics, and exhibits no signs of problems (e.g., fever or wound cellulitis). The timing of discharge, once these criteria are met, is often influenced by cultural issues, patient expectation, or distance between home and the hospital. Thus, the duration of hospitalization is not always an accurate reflection of optimal outcomes in comparing published studies in the literature.

Although the schedule of postoperative visits varies, all patients must undergo long-term follow-up. This guarantees that the surgeon will obtain feedback on the operative results and helps ensure that any preventable long-term metabolic or other procedure-related complications will be avoided. The potential for such metabolic complications is inherently present for all of the malabsorptive procedures. The restrictive procedures have minimal health risks from metabolic complications but instead have their own set of potential problems, such as band slippage or erosion in patients undergoing LAGB. Moreover, improved weight loss occurs in patients who see their surgeon for adjustments to the band.

A typical regimen for monitoring a patient after LAGB would be to have the initial visit take place within the first month postoperatively to evaluate oral intake, food tolerance, and wound healing and to determine whether appropriate restriction has resulted from placement of the noninflated band. Subsequent visits, usually scheduled monthly to bimonthly in the beginning and then less frequently, involve counseling with a nutritionist and evaluation of weight loss and the need for band adjustment. A goal of 1 to 2 lb/wk of weight loss is adjusted for initial body weight. Inadequate weight loss is an indication for instillation of additional saline into the band system through the port. This is initially done under fluoroscopic control until the surgeon has sufficient experience and confidence to perform such adjustments in the office or clinic without fluoroscopic guidance. Blood tests are performed periodically throughout the patient's follow-up, depending on metabolic indications, the patient's underlying medical illnesses, and other indications for such tests.

After RYGB, a typical postoperative checkup regimen would include a visit within the first 2 weeks postoperatively to assess wound healing, to advance from a liquid diet to solid food, and to check overall recovery. Subsequent visits are scheduled at 6 weeks, 3 months, 6 months, and 1 year after surgery and then annually. Visits during the first year are for monitoring weight loss; those after the first year are for checking maintenance of weight loss and nutritional competence. The risk for iron, folate, vitamin A, vitamin D, or vitamin B_{12} deficiency exists for life.

Patients undergoing malabsorptive operations must understand the necessity of meticulous compliance with a strict follow-up plan. After BPD or DS, a patient is seen within the first 2 weeks to be certain that diarrhea is not too prolific and dehydration has not resulted. The patient must be taught the signs of dehydration and plans for its treatment. Replacement of fat-soluble vitamins is mandatory, and the patient's compliance must be documented. Initial visits after the first month take place monthly for the first several months until the risk of dehydration, poor protein intake, and significant metabolic consequences of rapid weight loss has decreased. The potential for protein-calorie malnutrition exists after these procedures, and it will usually be manifested during this time. Thereafter, as weight loss slows, periodic visits separated by 3-month intervals are indicated for the first year and then semiannually thereafter. Weight loss will taper after the first 12 to 18 months. Lifelong follow-up to assess fat-soluble vitamin deficiencies as well as protein levels, liver function, and metabolic stability is indicated after BPD or DS.

Most bariatric practices use patient support groups as a component of the postoperative support system. These groups are variously organized and managed but usually consist of patients who have undergone weight reduction surgery or are contemplating it; they meet to discuss personal experiences with respect to their surgery and recovery from it and the experience of losing weight and maintenance of lost weight. Groups that are vigorous and successful seem to provide an excellent forum for patients to exchange information as well as psychological and emotional support and encouragement to patients both before and after surgery.

RESULTS

Results of operations can be determined only after adequate long-term follow-up and with adequate numbers of operations performed by a variety of surgeons. The applicability of some operations may vary according to patient factors, such as size or previous abdominal surgery; however, there is considerable difference in utilization of bariatric surgery by race and gender that does not appear to be related to the prevalence of morbid obesity in that region.[36]

There are now considerable data demonstrating that bariatric procedures are effective in achieving long-term weight loss and improvement in comorbid diseases. The SOS trial[3,4] and the Utah studies[1,37] demonstrate superiority of bariatric surgery over medical treatment in weight loss, mortality, resolution of comorbidities, and patients' quality of life. These studies as well as multiple randomized trials comparing bariatric surgery with medical therapy demonstrate that bariatric surgery is much more effective than medical therapy for treatment of diabetes and obesity.[11,13-16] Resolution and improvement of comorbid conditions after all types of bariatric surgery have been confirmed in carefully performed prospective studies, such as the Longitudinal Assessment of Bariatric Surgery (LABS) Consortium, which was created and funded by the NIH to obtain long-term data of the safety and effectiveness of the bariatric surgical procedures currently performed in the United States. The consortium prospectively studied 2458 surgical cases (71% RYGB, 25% LAGB, and 5% other procedures) and found at 3 years of follow-up that RYGB and LAGB produced an initial weight loss of 32% and 16%, respectively. RYGB caused remission of diabetes in 68%, and LAGB induced remission in 29% of patients.[38] The results (weight loss, comorbidity resolution) of LSG fall in between those of the RYGB and the LAGB.[39] A comparison of the four major bariatric operations is shown in Table 47-3.

Laparoscopic Adjustable Gastric Banding

Patients undergoing LAGB experience an operation that may last as little as 1 hour in experienced hands. Discharge from the hospital after an overnight stay is the norm, with a few reports of same-day discharge but more frequent reports of longer hospital stays based on cultural norms and acceptance. Table 47-4 gives the results of LAGB in several large reported series in the literature with long-term follow-up.

The band is initially placed without adding any saline to distend it. Saline is added in 1.0- to 1.5-mL increments to produce a desired weight loss of 1 to 2 kg/wk. Excess weight loss (EWL) may lead to actual removal of a small amount of saline, whereas inadequate weight loss is an indication for the addition of more saline to the system to increase restriction of the band. The incidence of nutritional deficiencies is low after LAGB because there is no disruption of the normal gastrointestinal tract. One potential problem is esophageal dilation from chronic obstruction secondary to band slippage.

Weight loss after LAGB averaged 39.7 kg (61.2% EWL) and 34.8 kg in a meta-analysis of bariatric surgery (Table 47-4). The

TABLE 47-3 Results of the Four Major Bariatric Procedures

	BUCHWALD[40]	CARLIN[39]	HUTTER[45]
LAGB			
BMI weight loss	−10.4 kg/m²	NR	−7.1 kg/m²
EWL (%)	61.2	44	NR
Mortality (%)	0.1	0.07 (2949 patients)	0.05 (12,193 patients)
LSG			
BMI weight loss	NR	NR	−11.9 kg/m²
EWL (%)	NR	56	NR
Mortality (%)	NR	0.07 (2949 patients)	0.11 (944 patients)
RYGB			
BMI weight loss	−16.7 kg/m²	NR	−15.3 kg/m²
EWL (%)	61.6	67	NR
Mortality (%)	0.5 (5644 patients)	0.10 (2949 patients)	0.14 (14,491 patients)
BPD/DS			
BMI weight loss	−18.0 kg/m²	NR	NR
EWL (%)	70.1	NR	NR
Mortality (%)	1.1 (3030 patients)	NR	NR

BMI, body mass index; *BPD,* biliopancreatic diversion; *DS,* duodenal switch; *EWL,* excess weight loss; *LAGB,* laparoscopic adjustable gastric banding; *LSG,* laparoscopic sleeve gastrectomy; *NR,* not reported; *RYGB,* Roux-en-Y gastric bypass.

TABLE 47-4 Results of Laparoscopic Adjustable Gastric Banding Procedures

CRITERIA	O'BRIEN[12]	COURCOULAS[38]	HUTTER[45]	CARLIN[39]
No. of patients	714	588	12,193	2949
Age (years)	Mean = 47	18-78	Mean = 44	Mean = 46
Body mass index (kg/m²)	43.8	45.9	43.9	48
Follow-up (years)	10-15	3	1	3
Percentage of excess weight loss	47	NR	NR	44
Reduction in BMI (kg/m²)	NR	NR	−7.1	NR
Percentage of baseline weight loss	−21	−15.9	NR	−19
Resolution of type 2 diabetes (%)	NR	29.4	44	37

NR, not reported.

pattern of weight loss is such that weight loss continues after the first year, up to a maximal amount usually achieved by the third year. Studies with longer follow-up confirm that the weight loss may even improve slightly further after 3 years. Dixon collected 25 eligible studies with longer than 5-year follow-up; an EWL of approximately 50% to 55% occurs after 3 years and is maintained for up to 8 years after surgery.[2]

LAGB has been shown to resolve type 2 diabetes in 48% and to improve the condition in 81% of patients in the meta-analysis published.[40] LAGB was compared with medical treatment in a prospective randomized trial in Australia. This study demonstrated substantial weight loss in the surgical group associated with remission of type 2 diabetes in 73%; the medically treated patients had insignificant weight loss, and only 13% achieved remission of their diabetes.[13] Hypertension was resolved in 42% and improved in 71% of patients after this procedure.[40] Improvement in dyslipidemia associated with obesity (hypertriglyceridemia, low high-density lipoprotein cholesterol levels) was also noted after LAGB.[2] Another randomized trial compared weight loss after LAGB with medically treated patients and found that the LAGB group had significantly better weight loss than the medical group. Even in adolescents, the LAGB had much greater weight loss compared with the patients randomized to medical treatment.[11] Physical activity, self-esteem, and general health in adolescents have been shown to improve 2 years after LAGB compared with no improvement in the group randomized to medical therapy.[11] These randomized trials all support the use of the LAGB over medical therapy for weight loss, remission of diabetes, improvement in quality of life, and resolution of obesity-related comorbidities.[11,12]

Roux-en-Y Gastric Bypass

RYGB has an established track record that is longer than that of any other bariatric operation. Its performance has been modified over the years, and the results presented in Table 47-5 reflect data from studies in the era of its performance as a laparoscopic procedure. Resolution of comorbid conditions after open and laparoscopic RYGB has generally been excellent. Recovery after RYGB is improved after a laparoscopic approach.

Another important advantage of laparoscopic RYGB is a decrease in the incidence of wound complications and incisional hernia seen after open RYGB. Long-term follow-up of a prospective randomized trial comparing laparoscopic and open gastric bypass found a much higher rate of incisional hernias in the open surgery group. There was, however, no difference in the rate of resolution of comorbid conditions or weight loss between the two procedures. The duration of hospitalization has decreased in all patients undergoing RYGB. Patients undergoing laparoscopic RYGB are usually hospitalized for about 2 days.

Rubino has been a proponent of intestinal factors, particularly in the case of RYGB, of the effect of duodenal bypass on the improvement in diabetes unrelated to weight loss.[23] Long-term follow-up after RYGB shows that most patients who resolve their diabetes maintain good control of the diabetes unless they regain substantial amounts of weight.[41] Thus, whereas there may be a benefit to bypassing the duodenum, the sustained long-term weight loss appears to be an essential element of the salutary effects of RYGB on type 2 diabetes.

RYGB has also been shown to resolve the symptoms of pseudotumor cerebri as well as to cure the difficult problem of venous stasis ulcers. Immediate resolution of symptoms of GERD occurs in more than 90% of cases. The extremely small gastric pouch has a limited reservoir for holding gastric juice, and the cardia is a low acid-producing area of the stomach, so the Roux-en-Y reconstruction diverts gastric acid away from the esophagus immediately after surgery, thus accounting for its efficacy in alleviating heartburn.

Biliopancreatic Diversion and Duodenal Switch

Most malabsorptive procedures performed in the United States are the DS modification of BPD, so this section discusses the results of both operations. EWL (70%) after BPD/DS is the highest of the bariatric operations discussed in this chapter, with a mean weight loss of 46.4 and 53.1 kg found by meta-analysis (see Table 47-3).[40] Thus, some surgeons argue that superobese patients fare better and maintain weight loss better in the long term after undergoing DS than after other bariatric operations. Others point out that side effects, mortality, and morbidity are much higher with DS and therefore the incremental improvements in EWL are not justified.

BPD/DS has also been highly effective in treating comorbid conditions, including hypertension, diabetes, lipid disorders, and obstructive sleep apnea.[40]

After BPD, patients typically have between two and four bowel movements per day. Excessive flatulence and foul-smelling stools are the rule. Relatively selective malabsorption of starch and fat

TABLE 47-5	Results of Roux-en-Y Gastric Bypass			
CRITERIA	COURCOULAS[38]	HUTTER[45]	ADAMS[37]	CARLIN[39]
No. of patients	1691	14,491	418	2949
Age (years)	19-75	NR	18-72	Mean = 46
BMI (kg/m^2)	45.9	46.1	45.9	47
Follow-up (years)	3	1	6	1
Excess weight loss (%)	52	NR	NR	69
Reduction in BMI (kg/m^2)	NR	−15.3	NR	NR
Percentage of baseline weight loss	−31.5	NR	−27.7	−36
Resolution or improvement (%)				
Diabetes	67.5	83	62	80
Hypertension	38.2	79	42	45
Dyslipidemia	61.9	66	53-71*	63
Obstructive sleep apnea	NR	66	NR	66

NR, not reported.
*At 6 years after surgery for high triglyceride, low high-density lipoprotein cholesterol, and high low-density lipoprotein cholesterol levels.

provides the major mechanism of weight loss, although the partial gastric resection does contribute a restrictive component to the operation.

Surgeons caring for these patients must be alert to measure protein levels for confirmation of adequate absorption. When protein malnutrition does occur, the common channel may need to be lengthened with a reoperation. Patients must also be aware that their ability to absorb simple sugars, alcohol, and short-chain triglycerides is good and that overindulgence of sweets, milk products, soft drinks, alcohol, and fruit may produce excess weight gain.

Major considerations for achieving excellent results in patients offered BPD/DS include the ability to reliably monitor these patients and to confirm that they are being compliant with the recommendations to take appropriate vitamin supplements. Supplements include multivitamins as well as at least 2 g of oral calcium per day. Supplemental fat-soluble vitamins, including D, K, and A, are indicated monthly as well.

Laparoscopic Sleeve Gastrectomy

Because of a high incidence of morbidity and mortality (23% and 7%, respectively) in patients with a BMI greater than 60 kg/m^2 undergoing laparoscopic DS, surgeons developed the two-stage DS, with sleeve gastrectomy alone performed as the first stage to decrease morbidity in this population of superobese patients. The Clinical Issues Committee of the ASMBS performed a comprehensive review of the subject and found 13 studies in 821 high-risk patients undergoing a staged approach with LSG. On average, the preoperative BMI was 60 and, after 4 to 60 months of follow-up, the postoperative BMI was 45. The complications in this population of high-risk patients showed a leak rate of 1.2%, bleeding rate of 1.6%, and mortality of 0.24%. The ASMBS concluded that LSG has value as the initial stage of a bariatric surgery in a high-risk population (Table 47-6).

Currently, the LSG is accepted as a primary operation. The MBSC reported a 1-year follow-up on 2949 LSG patients matched in 23 baseline characteristics to an equal number of laparoscopic RYGB and LAGB cases shown in Table 47-3. This study found that the 1-year EWL was highest for the patients undergoing laparoscopic RYGB (69%), intermediate for LSG (60%), and lowest for LAGB (34%; $P < .0001$). Serious complications for LSG were lower than for laparoscopic RYGB (6.3% versus 10%;

$P < .0001$).[39] Longer term studies show a 48% EWL 6 to 8 years after LSG.[42] A randomized trial of LSG versus laparoscopic RYGB with 1-year follow-up demonstrates that LSG is associated with shorter operative time and a trend to fewer complications. Weight loss and improvement in comorbidities and quality of life were similar in LSG and laparoscopic RYGB 1 year after surgery.[43]

Advantages of the LSG are the technical ease of the procedure, induction of satiety through reduction in ghrelin levels, reduced need for postoperative adjustments as opposed to LAGB, preservation of the pylorus and avoidance of dumping, reduced risk of malabsorption, and apparent safety of the procedure in high-risk individuals. Use of the LSG is advantageous for some populations of patients as outlined in Table 47-7.

COMPLICATIONS

The various procedures are associated with complications that can occur with any intra-abdominal operation, such as pulmonary embolism. However, each operation has unique complications as well as different incidences of some of the shared common complications.

Multiple reports have shown laparoscopic procedures to be associated with fewer respiratory, surgical wound, and thrombotic complications.[33] The benefits touted for laparoscopic surgery go beyond the cosmetic and really do influence postoperative complication rates, which makes the laparoscopic technique our preferred approach in virtually every patient, including remedial operations. Analysis of the 30-day mortality after bariatric surgery was performed in the LABS, an NIH-supported 10-center observational cohort study of bariatric surgery outcomes performed between 2005 and 2009. Eighteen deaths (0.3%) in 6118 patients undergoing primary bariatric surgery were reported. The most common cause of death was sepsis (33%), followed by cardiac (28%) and pulmonary embolism (17%).

Laparoscopic Adjustable Gastric Banding

The mortality associated with LAGB (0.02% to 0.1%) has been significantly lower than that for RYGB (0.3% to 0.5%) or either of the malabsorptive operations (0.9% to 1.1%).[33] Complications for the procedure are described in this section and summarized in Table 47-8. A major complication of either RYGB or BPD/DS is

TABLE 47-6	Results of Laparoscopic Sleeve Gastrectomy				
CRITERIA	**EID**[42]	**SCHAUER**[15]	**BOZA**[48]	**HUTTER**[45]	**CARLIN**[39]
No. of patients	74	49	1000	944	2949
Age (years)	25-78	Mean = 48	14-77	Mean = 47	Mean = 46
BMI (kg/m^2)	66	36.1	37.4	46.2	48
Follow-up (years)	8	3	1	1	1
Excess weight loss (%)	46	NR	84.5	NR	60
Reduction in BMI (kg/m^2)	−20	−6.9	NR	−11.9	NR
Percentage of baseline weight loss	−30	−21.1	NR	NR	−30
Resolution or improvement (%)					
Diabetes	77	24 (achieved HbA1c <6.0%)	100*	55	66
Hypertension	74	NR	98*	68	40
Dyslipidemia	NR	NR	95*	35	40
Obstructive sleep apnea	NR	NR	NR	62	57

NR, not reported.
*Includes both resolution and improvement in condition at 1 year postop.

TABLE 47-7 Potential Role of Laparoscopic Sleeve Gastrectomy in Bariatric Surgery

CONDITION	PROCEDURES CONTRAINDICATED	POTENTIAL ADVANTAGE OF LSG
Iron deficiency anemia	RYGB, BPD	Preservation of duodenum
Crohn's small bowel disease	RYGB, DS, BPD, LAGB if taking steroids	Preservation of small bowel
Transplant patients taking immunosuppressive medications	LAGB if taking steroids; relative contraindication to RYGB, DS, and BPD	More stable absorption of antirejection medications
Cardiac failure patients	Malabsorption of medications by RYGB; DS and BPD a relative contraindication	More stable absorption of critically needed medications
Severe arthritis requiring nonsteroidal anti-inflammatory drugs	RYGB and BPD contraindicated because of ulcer risk	Preservation of stomach allows continued use of nonsteroidal anti-inflammatory drugs
Patients who may not be able to comply with frequent follow-up	LAGB, RYGB, DS, BPD	Less risk of malabsorption and reduced need for LAGB adjustments
Patients with preexisting vitamin deficiencies (e.g., vitamin D, iron)	RYGB, DS, BPD	Preservation of entire small bowel reduces risk of vitamin deficiencies
Autoimmune connective tissue disorder	LAGB	LSG may be a good option

BPD, biliopancreatic diversion; DS, duodenal switch; LAGB, laparoscopic adjustable gastric banding; LSG, laparoscopic sleeve gastrectomy; RYGB, Roux-en-Y gastric bypass.

TABLE 47-8 Complications After Laparoscopic Adjustable Gastric Banding

CRITERIA	FLUM[33]	O'BRIEN[12]	HUTTER[45]	BIRKMEYER[44]	INGE[31]	CARLIN[39]
No. of patients	1198	3227	12,193	5380	14	2949
Age (years)	18-78	Mean = 47	Mean = 44	Median = 47	13-19	Mean = 46
Mortality	0	0	0.05	0.4	0	0.07
Postoperative complications		NR	1.44		0	1.0
Venous thromboembolism	0.3	NR	0.05	0.11	0	0.2
Wound infection	NR	NR	0.6	1.3	0	0.7
Bleeding	NR	NR	1.1		0	0.2
Reoperations	NR	43	0.92	0.63	0	0.4
Erosions	NR	3.4	NR	NR	NR	NR
Slippage	NR	26	NR	NR	NR	NR
Explantation of band	NR	5.6	NR	NR	NR	NR

All numbers except number of patients and age represent percentages.
NR, not reported.

the risk of leakage from the anastomosis, which does not occur with LAGB; however, it appears that the need for reoperation and complications related to surgery occur in all types of bariatric procedures.

A common complication that plagued LAGB in the mid to late 1990s was the high incidence of band slippage because the band was placed around the proximal part of the stomach, with the posterior portion of the band free within the lesser sac, which allowed much more movement of the stomach and herniation of the fundus of the stomach through the band. O'Brien and colleagues[12] showed that the pars flaccida technique was associated with a much lower rate of slippage than the per gastric technique (4% versus 15%), and subsequently the pars flaccida technique has become the preferred approach.

Slippage is usually manifested as the sudden development of food intolerance or occasionally gastroesophageal reflux. The latter symptom is also indicative of any form of obstruction at the site of the band. Slippage is by far the most common cause of obstruction, but on occasion, erosion and fibrosis can also cause similar symptoms. A patient with obstructive symptoms or food intolerance should have a plain radiograph of the abdomen taken. In its appropriate position, the band is oriented in a diagonal direction, along the 2- to 8-o'clock axis in the epigastric region. A plain film showing the band in a horizontal or a 10- to 4-o'clock position

is diagnostic of slippage and altered band position. Slippage or any other obstructive process at the band site can cause acute life-threatening strangulation of the stomach or functional stenosis of the gastrointestinal tract at the proximal end of the stomach. As a result, esophageal dilation can occur if this situation is not fixed.

Erosion of the band into the lumen of the stomach is a far less frequent complication but requires reoperation. The incidence of erosion may increase with the passage of time. At this time, however, the incidence remains below 1% for many large series and up to 3% as noted earlier in the Australian collected experience. Erosion may be manifested as abdominal pain or as a port access site infection. In cases in which the band does erode into the stomach, it is presumed that the band is either too tight or the stomach was imbricated too close to the buckle of the band, which will cause erosion over time. Surprisingly, this complication is rarely life-threatening, and there are many reports in the literature describing removal of the eroded band, repair of the stomach, and replacement of a new band at the same operative setting.

Port access site problems are the most numerous of the complications that occur after LAGB. These problems also require reoperative therapy in most cases, but the procedure can often be performed under local anesthesia and does not involve the peritoneal cavity. Leakage of the access tubing is a common problem that occurs in up to 11% of cases. In addition, kinking of the tubing as it passes through the fascia is another relatively common reason for port access difficulties. Port site infection is the least common port access problem (<1%) but needs to be evaluated with upper endoscopy to be certain that band erosion has not occurred.

Roux-en-Y Gastric Bypass

The most recently reported mortality rates after laparoscopic RYGB have generally been in the 0.1% to 0.2% range for large series as shown in Table 47-9.[27,33,40] Compared with the open RYGB, the operative mortality and complication rates including splenectomy, wound infection, incisional hernia, respiratory complications, and VTE/pulmonary embolism are significantly lower for the laparoscopic approach. In contrast, the incidence of bowel obstruction, especially early bowel obstruction, appears to be higher in patients undergoing laparoscopic RYGB secondary to internal hernia.

Causes of mortality have varied but include pulmonary embolism, anastomotic leak, cardiac events, intra-abdominal abscess, and multiorgan failure. Mortality rates are obviously influenced heavily by patient selection. Male gender was associated with an increased risk for morbidity and mortality in older series but not in the most recent LABS experience.[33] The LABS study identified BMI and history of VTE as independent predictors of complications.[33] Complications specific to RYGB include anastomotic leaks from the proximal or distal anastomosis. Leaks from the gastrojejunostomy are more common and are generally the cause of a significant percentage of the life-threatening complications and deaths. Data suggest that a surgeon's operative skill significantly influences the leak rate, with the most experienced surgeons recording the lowest complication rates.[30] Whereas the older studies found a leak rate of 2.2% in open and laparoscopic RYGB, the more recent laparoscopic RYGB studies report anastomotic leak rates of 0.35% to 0.5%.[27,44,45]

Pulmonary embolism is one of the most feared complications after any form of bariatric surgery, and its incidence in large reported series of open RYGB sometimes exceeds 1%. Thrombotic complications such as DVT and pulmonary embolism appear to be less frequently associated with laparoscopic surgery than with open gastric bypass but still account for up to 30% of the major causes of death, and up to 80% of patients who die after bariatric surgery have evidence for VTE.

Although nausea and vomiting are not unusual in isolated circumstances after RYGB, especially in relation to a patient's adaptation to food restriction, if persistent, these symptoms can lead to the obvious problem of dehydration. This must be aggressively treated in the postoperative period or in association with a viral or other gastrointestinal illness compounding the problem and further limiting oral intake. Intravenous fluids are indicated when in doubt. This is the case for all bariatric operations, not just RYGB.

One specific problem that may arise with persistent vomiting after *any* of the bariatric operations and that is *imperative* for the surgeon to remember and to treat is Wernicke encephalopathy from prolonged vomiting. This neurologic deficit is preventable with appropriate administration of parenteral thiamine (vitamin B_1) when the patient has persistent and severe vomiting. If the neurologic symptoms become significant, they may often not be fully reversed despite thiamine therapy.

Because depression is so frequent in the population of patients undergoing bariatric surgery, severe postoperative depression may develop after any of the bariatric operations as well. When it does occur, the patient may completely stop eating, thereby producing what at first seems like a wonderful response, but if unrecognized, it can progress to loss of critical visceral and musculoskeletal protein mass, which can be life-threatening.

Another specific life-threatening complication that may result after RYGB is that of bowel obstruction. Patients who have a clinical or radiographic picture of small bowel obstruction after RYGB need a reoperation. The potential for internal hernias after this operation makes strangulation obstruction a frequent presentation. Patients with bowel obstruction are best diagnosed by an oral and intravenous contrast-enhanced CT scan of the abdomen to visualize the bypassed stomach and small bowel that may be obstructed or the mesenteric twist with volvulus of the Roux limb. These patients *must* be promptly treated before retrograde distention of the biliopancreatic limb and distal part of the stomach results in rupture of the distal gastric staple line with subsequent peritonitis.

Stenosis of the gastrojejunostomy may occur after RYGB and has been reported in 2% to 14% of patients in various series. The higher incidence seems to be associated with a circular stapler versus sutured anastomoses. Postoperative anastomotic stenosis is usually manifested at 4 to 6 weeks postoperatively as progressive intolerance to solids and then liquids. The problem is successfully treated with endoscopic balloon dilation. Unless a marginal ulcer is associated with the stenosis, the problem does not require a reoperation.

A marginal ulcer occurs after 2% to 10% of RYGB procedures. The incidence can be decreased by preoperative treatment of patients for *Helicobacter pylori* colonization of the stomach.

TABLE 47-9 Complications After Laparoscopic Roux-en-Y Gastric Bypass

CRITERIA	BIRKMEYER[44]	FLUM[33]	HUTTER[45]	INGE[31]	CARLIN[39]
No. of patients	9041	2975	14,491	161	2949
Age (years)	37-54	Mean = 44	Mean = 45	13-19	Mean = 46
Mortality	0.14	0.2	0.14	0	0.10
Leak/major wound complications	0.9	NR	0.8	1.8	0.6
Surgical site infection	8.7	NR	2.2	1.9	2.8
Pulmonary embolus/venous thromboembolism	0.5	0.4	0.17	0.6	0.3
Reoperation	2.5	NR	5.0	0.6	1.6
Bleeding	2.3	NR	1.1	0	2.3

All numbers except number of patients and age represent percentages.
NR, not reported.

Patients with a marginal ulcer typically have continuous boring epigastric pain. Treatment consists of medical therapy with proton pump inhibitors and avoidance of nonsteroidal anti-inflammatory drugs. Medical treatment resolves all marginal ulcers unless a fistula has formed to the lower part of the stomach and created an ongoing source of acid, thus exacerbating the ulcer. Surgery to divide the fistula is necessary to effect healing of the ulcer.

Iron and vitamin B_{12} deficiencies are the two most common long-term metabolic complications of RYGB. The incidence of iron insufficiency varies among reported series. Iron is preferentially absorbed in the duodenum and proximal jejunum. Hence, RYGB bypasses the area of maximal iron absorption in the gut. The iron deficiency, based on serum values, is between 15% and 40%, whereas actual iron deficiency anemia occurs in as many as 20% of patients after RYGB. This problem is easily treated in most cases with oral iron supplements. The gluconate form of iron is best absorbed in a nonacid environment.

The incidence of vitamin B_{12} deficiency after RYGB is reported as being 15% to 20%, although it rarely causes anemia. Vitamin B_{12} deficiency is due to inefficient absorption because of delayed mixing with intrinsic factor. Several preparations include intrinsic factor, which maximizes absorption in the terminal ileum. Other routes of vitamin B_{12} administration include sublingual medication, nasal spray, and parenteral injections.

Laparoscopic Sleeve Gastrectomy

The mortality rate after LSG (0.07% to 0.11%) is between that of the laparoscopic RYGB and the LAGB. The morbidity associated with LSG, including infections, reoperation, and VTE, is below that of laparoscopic RYGB but higher than that of LAGB as shown in Table 47-10. Malabsorption of vitamins and nutrients is much less for LSG compared with laparoscopic RYGB or the laparoscopic DS and makes the LSG ideally suited for patients with preexisting vitamin disorders or those who need full absorption of lifesaving medications as shown in Table 47-7.

However, the Achilles heel of the LSG is the occurrence of leaks, which are more common than in laparoscopic RYGB and more difficult to treat.[35] Despite the problem with leaks, many surgeons are opting to perform the LSG because of the advantages with the procedure. The advantages of the LSG are seen to be the technical simplicity, lower mortality, reduced malabsorption, effectiveness for weight loss, and resolution of comorbidities that is similar to that of laparoscopic RYGB.[34,39]

Biliopancreatic Diversion

Mortality rates after BPD/DS are 1.1%; surgical wound complications occur in 5.9% of patients, leaks develop in 1.8%, and reoperations occur 4.2% of the time.[40] The most significant and specific long-term complication seen after BPD is protein malnutrition, which occurs in 12% of patients. Treatment is hospitalization with 2 to 3 weeks of parenteral nutrition. This particular problem is usually manifested within the first few months after surgery, but it can occur sporadically, although less frequently, after surgery. In one series, 4% of patients eventually required a reoperation either to reverse the BPD completely or to lengthen the common channel. The revision rate was approximately 0.1% annually for the first 6 years, and the rehospitalization rate for malabsorption or diarrhea was 0.93% annually during that time. The percentage of patients averaging more than three bowel movements per day was 7%, and 34% of patients believed that the unpleasant odor of stools and flatus was a problem. Abdominal bloating was experienced in a third of patients more than once weekly. Bone pain was reported in 29% of patients. Metabolic complications and side effects included iron deficiency in 9%, low ferritin level in 25%, low calcium concentration in 8%, and low level of vitamin A in 5%. Elevated parathyroid hormone levels were present in 17%.

Malabsorption of fat-soluble vitamins is one of the major problems associated with BPD/DS. Two years after BPD, levels of vitamins D and A are significantly depressed, with vitamin D deficiency noted in 63% of patients and vitamin A deficiency in 69%. Lack of clinical correlation with these levels suggests that the problem may be more prevalent than originally reported or suspected from past series.

Although the complication of protein malnutrition and poor intake is theoretically most likely to occur soon after BPD/DS, the fact that late deaths occur from protein malnutrition and Wernicke encephalopathy suggests that these patients are always at risk for these problems. Marginal ulcers are a distinct problem of BPD, which has been addressed with the DS modification preserving the pylorus.

Perhaps it is the overall difficulty of the operation as well as the potential dangers of the operation that has relegated BPD to the least popular operation performed in the United States. Even the DS modification does not represent more than 2% of bariatric operations. Further studies are needed to evaluate the long-term consequences of BPD and DS to justify the performance of such operations as a primary procedure.

REOPERATIVE SURGERY

A controversial topic is the appropriateness of performing repeated bariatric operations for a failed procedure. The absolute definition

TABLE 47-10	Complications After Laparoscopic Sleeve Gastrectomy			
CRITERIA	**HUTTER[45]**	**BIRKMEYER[44]**	**CARLIN[39]**	**INGE[31]**
No. of patients	944	854	2949	67
Age (years)	Mean = 47	37-55	Mean = 46	13-19
Mortality	0.11	0	0.07	0
Leak perforation	0.74	0.35	0.9	1.5
Surgical site infection	2.0	2.2	2.2	3
Pulmonary embolus/venous thromboembolism	0.32	0.9	0.5	0
Reoperation	3.0	0.6	1.4	1.5
Bleeding	0.6	0.6	1.1	0

All numbers except number of patients and age represent percentages.

of a failed operation is unclear, but most surgeons would accept the criteria listed in Box 47-2 as appropriate when considering reoperation. If a patient has undergone an operation that has proved by experience to be ineffective, a repeated operation for failure of that procedure is appropriate. Complications of procedures, such as stenosis causing gastric outlet obstruction after vertical banded gastroplasty or metabolic complications after jejunoileal bypass, are obvious indications for revisional surgery. One mistake frequently made by a nonbariatric surgeon in correcting a complication of a bariatric operation is to simply perform a procedure that corrects the complication but does not provide for continued weight restriction. In these circumstances, a typical long-term course is for patients to slowly regain weight to their degree of obesity before the initial bariatric procedure and then to seek further surgical assistance.

In assessing a patient for the appropriateness of reoperative surgery, the surgeon must determine whether the original bariatric operation is intact and anatomically still appropriate for maintaining weight loss. If not, consideration for reoperation is appropriate. However, a patient who has failed an anatomically intact and well-constructed bariatric operation is, in our opinion, at high risk to fail a second or revisional bariatric operation. The incidence of infection, organ ischemia, anastomotic leakage, blood transfusion, and other severe intra-abdominal complications is increased in revisional surgery.

All bariatric operations have some incidence of failure, which includes inadequate weight loss, inadequate resolution of medical comorbid conditions, development of side effects negatively influencing lifestyle and satisfaction, development of complications requiring medical or surgical intervention, and complications requiring alteration or reversal of the operation. Analysis of the 449,753 bariatric operations logged into the Bariatric Outcomes Longitudinal Database (BOLD) shows that 4.4% were corrective operations (i.e., operations that addressed complications or incomplete treatment effect of the primary bariatric operation) and 1.9% were conversions (i.e., operations in which the primary bariatric procedure was converted to another bariatric procedure).[46] Only 6.3% of bariatric operations needed reoperation and even fewer needed conversion to another bariatric procedure, which points out the relative efficacy of the commonly performed bariatric procedures being performed currently. Moreover, the reoperations had a low mortality rate of 0.12% to 0.21% and a 1-year EWL of 36% to 39%. The data suggest that reoperations for failure are not that common, the clinical results are comparable to those of primary operations, and they are associated with comparable mortality rates.[46]

CONTROVERSIES IN BARIATRIC SURGERY

Some investigators have argued that guidelines for bariatric surgery, based on strict BMI cutoffs, fail to identify patients who would be most likely to benefit from surgery. For years, the criterion for bariatric surgery has been BMI, yet the evidence from the SOS trial shows that BMI did not predict the beneficial effect of surgery on cardiovascular, diabetic, or cancer-related mortality.[3] On the other hand, fasting hyperinsulinemia, which is reflective of insulin resistance, was predictive of the positive bariatric surgery results in overall mortality, cardiovascular events, and incidence of diabetes. If the aim of bariatric surgery is not just weight loss but to reduce mortality, to prevent diabetes, and to reduce cardiovascular events, Sjöström[3] suggests that preoperative insulin

and glucose levels are better criteria to select those patients who will benefit most from bariatric surgery.

Level 1 evidence also demonstrates the efficacy of bariatric surgery (RYGB, LSG, LAGB) over medical therapy in the treatment of type 2 diabetes patients with lower BMI.[13-16] The concept that bariatric surgery is better than medical management of type 2 diabetes is new and very controversial. Although more medical societies[5,17] are recognizing the benefits of bariatric surgery and even endorsing the referral to bariatric surgeons, it is unclear whether insurance guidelines for bariatric surgery will endorse the use of surgery as a primary treatment of diabetes or use metabolic variables rather than BMI as primary criteria for surgery.

INVESTIGATIONAL BARIATRIC PROCEDURES

A number of procedures have been investigated for weight loss surgery and either have been discredited or have not been accepted by the surgical community. Considerable evidence suggested that the visceral fat is an important risk factor in the development of metabolic syndrome X through the release of free fatty acids and adipokines directly into the portal vein. Animal studies demonstrated that surgical removal of the VAT improved insulin sensitivity. This was subjected to a randomized clinical trial that removed the greater omentum in obese subjects with type 2 diabetes and in obese subjects undergoing laparoscopic RYGB. Surgical removal of the omentum was not found to be a viable operation on the basis of measurement of liver and skeletal muscle insulin sensitivity using hyperinsulinemic-euglycemic clamp procedures that demonstrated omentectomy performed as either a primary or combination procedure with laparoscopic RYGB did not improve metabolic function.[19]

Considerable resources have been expended designing, creating, and then performing human trials of gastric stimulation. The original theory is that gastric stimulation can affect gastric electrical activity, which would induce gastric distention, impair emptying, and increase satiety. Another theory holds that gastric stimulation would affect the satiety hormones and the neuronal activity in the brain, which would induce weight loss. Numerous animal and short-term clinical trials in humans have shown that the most commonly used gastric stimulation devices induced a statistically significant weight loss during the first 12 months of implantation.[47] The Tantalus studies also targeted diabetics and demonstrated significant reductions in HbA1c at 3, 6, and 12 months after implantation. It appears that the weight loss in these early gastric stimulation trials is much less compared with currently used bariatric procedures but greater than the weight loss noted with diet and lifestyle treatments. For gastric stimulation to compete with current surgical therapies, there must be improvements in the treatment effect and an improvement in battery life to prevent the need for frequent battery replacement surgery.

Because the vagus nerve plays an important role in satiety, gastric emptying, and metabolism, surgeons have investigated the effects of blocking the vagus nerve through intermittent high-frequency electrical currents delivered by implantable electrodes placed laparoscopically around the abdominal vagal trunks. Early clinical trials of this technique were promising, and the randomized, double-blind, sham-controlled clinical trial of 239 human subjects showed a statistically significant difference in weight loss compared with the sham-treated group (9.2% versus 6.0%) at 12 months after surgery.[47] More studies are needed to compare the long-term effectiveness of vagal blockade with other obesity treatments and to determine the long-term safety of the procedure.

Endoscopic incisionless surgery has focused on the patients after RYGB who have either inadequate weight loss or significant weight regain and have a dilated gastrojejunostomy. The concept is that these patients lose restriction because of the dilated gastro-jejunostomy and thus overeat. Surgeons have tried endoscopic injection of sclerosing agents to create a scar and a smaller anas-tomosis with variable effects. Multiple ongoing studies are being performed to evaluate the effectiveness of various endoscopic suturing devices and injection therapies, all designed to reduce the size of the anastomosis and thus impose more restriction on the intake of food. These procedures have met with variable success and, in some circumstances, are not reimbursed by insur-ance companies, thus requiring the patients to pay out of pocket for the procedure.

There continues to be interest in endoscopic placement of a plastic sleeve to prevent nutrient exposure to the duodenum. Rubino[23] has been the major proponent of the theory that bypass of the duodenum improves glucose control in diabetics through reduction of the anti-incretin effect. Because the action of incre-tins in the distal small bowel is to increase beta cell proliferation, to increase insulin secretion, and to cause beta cell proliferation, increasing either the secretion or the effect of the incretins should improve the symptoms of diabetes.

Although recognized as standard bariatric procedures, laparo-scopic RYGB, LSG, and LAGB have been investigated as surgical treatment for diabetes in patients with a BMI (30 to 35) lower than commonly accepted as qualifying for bariatric surgery.[13-16] These studies, shown in Table 47-2, demonstrate that surgery had better outcomes than did medical therapy. In a 6-year prospective study of laparoscopic RYGB for diabetics with lower BMIs, Cohen[20] demonstrated a significant decrease in HbA1c from 9.7% to 5.9%. The investigators concluded that laparoscopic RYGB safely and effectively reduced cardiovascular risk and dia-betes in patients with BMIs of 30 to 35 kg/m².[20]

CONCLUSION

Surgical treatment of morbid obesity is no longer considered out of the mainstream of general surgery and is now a component of surgical residency training programs. It currently represents the fastest growing area of general surgery. Whereas patient demand for the procedure has vastly increased, at present, surgeons operate annually on less than 2% of the eligible patients who would benefit from bariatric surgery. This chapter has discussed all aspects of the performance of bariatric surgery in current surgical practice, including the most commonly performed procedures. Morbid obesity is unfortunately both incompletely understood and increasing in prevalence. Recent randomized clinical trials of bariatric surgery versus medical treatment in obese diabetics have shown that bariatric surgery is more effective in treatment of severe obesity, type 2 diabetes, hypertension, and dyslipidemia. With the positive results of bariatric surgery becoming more widely known, there has been movement by multiple medical societies to recognize the need for referral to a bariatric surgeon for evaluation. It is hoped that these data will also encourage the government and insurance companies to provide bariatric and metabolic surgery coverage.

SELECTED REFERENCES

Adams TD, Davidson LE, Litwin SE, et al: Health benefits of gastric bypass surgery after 6 years. *JAMA* 308:1122–1131, 2012.

Long-term follow-up of a prospective trial of 418 patients undergoing RYGB, a control group of 418 patients who sought but did not undergo bariatric surgery, and a second control group of 321 patients randomly selected from a population-based sample who were not seeking bariatric surgery. Patients undergoing RYGB lost significantly more weight than those in the two control groups (−27.7% versus 0.2% weight gain in control group 1 and 0% weight loss in control group 2). Diabetes remission was much greater in the surgery group compared with the two control groups (62%, 8%, and 6%, respectively). The authors concluded that RYGB was associated with much greater weight loss, diabetes remission, and lower risk of cardiovascular events 6 years after surgery.

Adams TD, Gress RE, Smith SC, et al: Long-term mortality after gastric bypass surgery. *N Engl J Med* 357:753–761, 2007.

A retrospective cohort study determined the long-term mor-tality among 7925 patients who underwent RYGB matched by age, sex, and BMI to 7925 severely obese persons who applied for driver's licenses. During a mean follow-up of 7.1 years, adjusted long-term mortality from any cause after RYGB decreased by 40% compared with that in the control group; cause-specific mortality in the surgery group decreased by 56% for coronary artery disease, by 92% for diabetes, and by 60% for cancer. They concluded that long-term total mortality after gastric bypass surgery was signifi-cantly reduced, particularly deaths from diabetes, heart disease, and cancer.

Birkmeyer JD, Finks JF, O'Reilly A, et al: Surgical skill and com-plication rates after bariatric surgery. *N Engl J Med* 369:1434–1442, 2013.

A study from the Michigan cooperative demonstrated that the surgeon's skill remains paramount in outcomes. The surgeons judged to be in the top quartile of technical skill on the basis of peer review of a video procedure showed sig-nificantly lower mortality (0.05% versus 0.26%; P = .01) and lower morbidity (5.2% versus 14.5%; P < .001) compared with the bottom quartile surgeons.

Buchwald H, Avidor Y, Braunwald E, et al: Bariatric surgery: A systematic review and meta-analysis. *JAMA* 292:1724–1737, 2004.

The authors reviewed the literature and selected 136 studies (22,094 patients) that they reviewed and subjected to meta-analysis. Bariatric surgery was found to be effective in weight loss and resulted in improvement or cure of serious comorbid conditions (diabetes, dyslipidemia, hypertension, and sleep apnea) in the majority of patients. This compre-hensive meta-analysis provides compelling data on the effectiveness and beneficial results of bariatric surgery in the literature.

Christou NV, Sampalis JS, Liberman M, et al: Surgery decreases long-term mortality, morbidity, and health care use in morbidly obese patients. *Ann Surg* 240:416–423, discussion 423-424, 2004.

> *In a study comparing matched control subjects with subjects who underwent bariatric surgery in Canada, Christou and coauthors demonstrated that weight loss surgery reduced the relative risk for mortality by 89% (95% confidence interval, 73% to 96%) 5 years after surgery. This is one of the substantial arguments for the effectiveness of bariatric surgery not only to reduce weight but also to ameliorate or to cure the comorbid conditions, which increases survival.*

Dixon JB, O'Brien PE, Playfair J, et al: Adjustable gastric banding and conventional therapy for type 2 diabetes: A randomized controlled trial. *JAMA* 299:316–323, 2008.

O'Brien PE, Dixon JB, Laurie C, et al: Treatment of mild to moderate obesity with laparoscopic adjustable gastric banding or an intensive medical program: A randomized trial. *Ann Intern Med* 144:625–633, 2006.

O'Brien PE, Sawyer SM, Laurie C, et al: Laparoscopic adjustable gastric banding in severely obese adolescents: A randomized trial. *JAMA* 303:519–526, 2010.

> *The Australian group has provided level I evidence of the superiority of bariatric surgery compared with medical treatment in three distinct scenarios. One study demonstrated that LAGB is superior in adolescents, whereas another showed that LAGB is superior in adult patients compared with medical therapy. Dixon's study showed a significantly improved weight loss and resolution of diabetes 2 years after LAGB surgery compared with a group of diabetics who were treated medically. Increasingly, the evidence is mounting that bariatric surgery provides better weight loss and resolution of comorbidities than does medical therapy in the severely obese patients.*

Hutter MM, Schirmer BD, Jones DB, et al: First report from the American College of Surgeons Bariatric Surgery Center Network: Laparoscopic sleeve gastrectomy has morbidity and effectiveness positioned between the band and the bypass. *Ann Surg* 254:410–420, discussion 420–422, 2011.

> *The first report from the American College of Surgeons Bariatric Surgery Center Network details the safety of LSG, LAGB, and laparoscopic RYGB. Overall mortality for the entire cohort of 28,616 patients was an extraordinarily low 0.12%. LSG had a 30-day operative mortality rate higher than LAGB but lower than laparoscopic RYGB. At 1 year, the LSG had a BMI reduction (11.9 kg/m^2) intermediate between LAGB (7.1 kg/m^2) and laparoscopic RYGB (15.3 kg/m^2). Improvement or resolution of the obesity comorbidities after LSG was in between the LAGB and laparoscopic RYGB.*

Ikramuddin S, Korner J, Lee WJ, et al: Roux-en-Y gastric bypass vs intensive medical management for the control of type 2 diabetes, hypertension, and hyperlipidemia: The Diabetes Surgery Study randomized clinical trial. *JAMA* 309:2240–2249, 2013.

> *A randomized prospective clinical trial comparing RYGB to intensive medical therapy in the control of type 2 diabetes, hypertension, and hyperlipidemia. At 12 months, 49% of the surgery group and only 11% of the intensive medical therapy group had achieved the primary end points (odds ratio, 4.8). They concluded that in mild to moderately obese diabetic subjects, the RYGB significantly improved the chances of achieving the composite end point. There were more serious adverse events in the group undergoing surgery, and they cautioned the readers that the potential benefits must be weighed against the risk of serious adverse events.*

Maggard MA, Shugarman LR, Suttorp M, et al: Meta-analysis: Surgical treatment of obesity. *Ann Intern Med* 142:547–559, 2005.

> *The authors assessed 147 studies on bariatric surgery to analyze weight loss, mortality, and complications. They found that laparoscopic gastric bypass resulted in fewer wound complications, incisional hernias, and respiratory complications than the open approach did. They concluded from the analysis of weight loss and resolution of comorbid conditions that bariatric surgery was more effective than medical treatment in patients with a BMI of 40 kg/m^2 or greater. This study amplifies the growing body of data supporting bariatric surgery as being safe and effective.*

Schauer PR, Bhatt DL, Kashyap SR: Bariatric surgery versus intensive medical therapy for diabetes. *N Engl J Med* 371:682, 2014.

Schauer PR, Kashyap SR, Wolski K, et al: Bariatric surgery versus intensive medical therapy in obese patients with diabetes. *N Engl J Med* 366:1567–1576, 2012.

> *The authors randomized 150 obese (BMI, 27-43) uncontrolled diabetics (HbA1c > 7.0%) to intensive medical therapy or to LSG or laparoscopic RYGB. Surgical groups had significant improvement in HbA1c, weight loss, and dyslipidemia and a reduction in the number of antihypertensive, lipid-lowering, and diabetic medications used at 1, 2, and 3 years after randomization. The surgical patients also had a significant improvement in quality of life, whereas there was no change in the quality of life for the medically treated patients. They concluded that " bariatric surgery represents a potentially useful strategy for the management of type 2 diabetes, allowing many patients to reach and maintain therapeutic targets of glycemic control that otherwise would not be achievable with intensive medical therapy alone." This study, now with 3-year follow-up showing sustained improvements for the surgical groups, adds to the strong evidence supporting bariatric surgery as safe and effective therapy for treatment of type 2 diabetes.*

Sjöström L: Review of the key results from the Swedish Obese Subjects (SOS) trial—a prospective controlled intervention study of bariatric surgery. *J Intern Med* 273:219–234, 2013.

> *An excellent review of the results of the Swedish Obese Subjects (SOS) trial. Bariatric surgery in 2010 obese subjects was associated with significant weight loss up to 20 years after surgery compared with a control group of 2037 who*

received standard medical care (18% versus 1%). Long-term mortality was reduced in the bariatric surgery patients (adjusted hazard ratio, 0.71). The bariatric surgery group also had decreased incidence of diabetes, myocardial infarction, stroke, and cancer. Their analysis also showed that high insulin or high glucose levels at baseline predicted success, whereas the level of BMI did not, which leads the authors to suggest that the selection based on BMI needs reevaluation and that use of insulin and glucose values would better predict outcomes with bariatric surgery and therefore would be a better selection criterion.

Sjöström L, Narbro K, Sjöström CD, et al: Effects of bariatric surgery on mortality in Swedish obese subjects. *N Engl J Med* 357:741–752, 2007.

This study compared a group of patients undergoing bariatric surgery with a group of matched control subjects and monitored them for 10.9 years. They had an unparalleled follow-up rate of 99.9% of the subjects in the study. They found a significant decrease in the weight and risk of death in individuals in the surgical weight loss group compared with control patients not undergoing surgery (unadjusted overall hazard ratio was 0.76 in the surgery group [P = .4] compared with the control group). This is the best long-term study indicating that bariatric surgery results in sustained weight loss, resolution of comorbid conditions, and increased survival in comparison to standard medical treatment.

REFERENCES

1. Adams TD, Gress RE, Smith SC, et al: Long-term mortality after gastric bypass surgery. *N Engl J Med* 357:753–761, 2007.
2. Dixon JB, Straznicky NE, Lambert EA, et al: Laparoscopic adjustable gastric banding and other devices for the management of obesity. *Circulation* 126:774–785, 2012.
3. Sjöström L: Review of the key results from the Swedish Obese Subjects (SOS) trial—a prospective controlled intervention study of bariatric surgery. *J Intern Med* 273:219–234, 2013.
4. Sjöström L, Narbro K, Sjöström CD, et al: Effects of bariatric surgery on mortality in Swedish obese subjects. *N Engl J Med* 357:741–752, 2007.
5. Jensen MD, Ryan DH, Apovian CM, et al: 2013 AHA/ACC/TOS guideline for the management of overweight and obesity in adults: A report of the American College of Cardiology/American Heart Association Task Force on Practice Guidelines and The Obesity Society. *Circulation* 129:S102–S138, 2014.
6. Ogden CL, Carroll MD, Kit BK, et al: Prevalence of childhood and adult obesity in the United States, 2011-2012. *JAMA* 311:806–814, 2014.
7. Zheng H, Yang Y: Population heterogeneity in the impact of body weight on mortality. *Soc Sci Med* 75:990–996, 2012.
8. Cox LM, Yamanishi S, Sohn J, et al: Altering the intestinal microbiota during a critical developmental window has lasting metabolic consequences. *Cell* 158:705–721, 2014.
9. Park CW, Torquati A: Physiology of weight loss surgery. *Surg Clin North Am* 91:1149–1161, vii, 2011.
10. Picot J, Jones J, Colquitt JL, et al: The clinical effectiveness and cost-effectiveness of bariatric (weight loss) surgery for obesity: A systematic review and economic evaluation. *Health Technol Assess* 13:1–190, 215-357, iii-iv, 2009.
11. O'Brien PE, Sawyer SM, Laurie C, et al: Laparoscopic adjustable gastric banding in severely obese adolescents: A randomized trial. *JAMA* 303:519–526, 2010.
12. O'Brien PE, MacDonald L, Anderson M, et al: Long-term outcomes after bariatric surgery: Fifteen-year follow-up of adjustable gastric banding and a systematic review of the bariatric surgical literature. *Ann Surg* 257:87–94, 2013.
13. Dixon JB, O'Brien PE, Playfair J, et al: Adjustable gastric banding and conventional therapy for type 2 diabetes: A randomized controlled trial. *JAMA* 299:316–323, 2008.
14. Ikramuddin S, Korner J, Lee WJ, et al: Roux-en-Y gastric bypass vs intensive medical management for the control of type 2 diabetes, hypertension, and hyperlipidemia: The Diabetes Surgery Study randomized clinical trial. *JAMA* 309:2240–2249, 2013.
15. Schauer PR, Bhatt DL, Kashyap SR: Bariatric surgery versus intensive medical therapy for diabetes. *N Engl J Med* 371:682, 2014.
16. Schauer PR, Kashyap SR, Wolski K, et al: Bariatric surgery versus intensive medical therapy in obese patients with diabetes. *N Engl J Med* 366:1567–1576, 2012.
17. Dixon JB, Zimmet P, Alberti KG, et al: Bariatric surgery: An IDF statement for obese type 2 diabetes. *Surg Obes Relat Dis* 7:433–447, 2011.
18. O'Brien PE: Bariatric surgery: Mechanisms, indications and outcomes. *J Gastroenterol Hepatol* 25:1358–1365, 2010.
19. Fabbrini E, Tamboli RA, Magkos F, et al: Surgical removal of omental fat does not improve insulin sensitivity and cardiovascular risk factors in obese adults. *Gastroenterology* 139:448–455, 2010.
20. Cohen RV, Pinheiro JC, Schiavon CA, et al: Effects of gastric bypass surgery in patients with type 2 diabetes and only mild obesity. *Diabetes Care* 35:1420–1428, 2012.
21. Khoo CM, Muehlbauer MJ, Stevens RD, et al: Postprandial metabolite profiles reveal differential nutrient handling after bariatric surgery compared with matched caloric restriction. *Ann Surg* 259:687–693, 2014.
22. Koshy AA, Bobe AM, Brady MJ: Potential mechanisms by which bariatric surgery improves systemic metabolism. *Transl Res* 161:63–72, 2013.
23. Rubino F, Schauer PR, Kaplan LM, et al: Metabolic surgery to treat type 2 diabetes: Clinical outcomes and mechanisms of action. *Annu Rev Med* 61:393–411, 2010.
24. Habegger KM, Al-Massadi O, Heppner KM, et al: Duodenal nutrient exclusion improves metabolic syndrome and stimulates villus hyperplasia. *Gut* 63:1238–1246, 2014.
25. Zhang H, DiBaise JK, Zuccolo A, et al: Human gut microbiota in obesity and after gastric bypass. *Proc Natl Acad Sci U S A* 106:2365–2370, 2009.
26. Flum DR, Kwon S, MacLeod K, et al: The use, safety and cost of bariatric surgery before and after Medicare's national coverage decision. *Ann Surg* 254:860–865, 2011.
27. DeMaria EJ, Pate V, Warthen M, et al: Baseline data from American Society for Metabolic and Bariatric Surgery–designated Bariatric Surgery Centers of Excellence using the Bariatric Outcomes Longitudinal Database. *Surg Obes Relat Dis* 6:347–355, 2010.
28. Morton JM, Garg T, Nguyen N: Does hospital accreditation impact bariatric surgery safety? *Ann Surg* 260:504–509, 2014.

29. Inabnet WB, 3rd, Bour E, Carlin AM, et al: Joint task force recommendations for credentialing of bariatric surgeons. *Surg Obes Relat Dis* 9:595–597, 2013.

30. Birkmeyer JD, Finks JF, O'Reilly A, et al: Surgical skill and complication rates after bariatric surgery. *N Engl J Med* 369:1434–1442, 2013.

31. Inge TH, Zeller MH, Jenkins TM, et al: Perioperative outcomes of adolescents undergoing bariatric surgery: The Teen-Longitudinal Assessment of Bariatric Surgery (Teen-LABS) study. *JAMA Pediatr* 168:47–53, 2014.

32. Birkmeyer NJ, Finks JF, Carlin AM, et al: Comparative effectiveness of unfractionated and low-molecular-weight heparin for prevention of venous thromboembolism following bariatric surgery. *Arch Surg* 147:994–998, 2012.

33. Flum DR, Belle SH, King WC, et al: Perioperative safety in the longitudinal assessment of bariatric surgery. *N Engl J Med* 361:445–454, 2009.

34. Nguyen NT, Nguyen B, Gebhart A, et al: Changes in the makeup of bariatric surgery: A national increase in use of laparoscopic sleeve gastrectomy. *J Am Coll Surg* 216:252–257, 2013.

35. Aurora AR, Khaitan L, Saber AA: Sleeve gastrectomy and the risk of leak: A systematic analysis of 4,888 patients. *Surg Endosc* 26:1509–1515, 2012.

36. Sudan R, Winegar D, Thomas S, et al: Influence of ethnicity on the efficacy and utilization of bariatric surgery in the USA. *J Gastrointest Surg* 18:130–136, 2014.

37. Adams TD, Davidson LE, Litwin SE, et al: Health benefits of gastric bypass surgery after 6 years. *JAMA* 308:1122–1131, 2012.

38. Courcoulas AP, Christian NJ, Belle SH, et al: Weight change and health outcomes at 3 years after bariatric surgery among individuals with severe obesity. *JAMA* 310:2416–2425, 2013.

39. Carlin AM, Zeni TM, English WJ, et al: The comparative effectiveness of sleeve gastrectomy, gastric bypass, and adjustable gastric banding procedures for the treatment of morbid obesity. *Ann Surg* 257:791–797, 2013.

40. Buchwald H, Avidor Y, Braunwald E, et al: Bariatric surgery: A systematic review and meta-analysis. *JAMA* 292:1724–1737, 2004.

41. Kim S, Richards W: Long-term follow-up of the metabolic profiles in obese patients with type 2 diabetes mellitus after Roux-en-Y gastric bypass. *Ann Surg* 251:1049–1055, 2010.

42. Eid GM, Brethauer S, Mattar SG, et al: Laparoscopic sleeve gastrectomy for super obese patients: Forty-eight percent excess weight loss after 6 to 8 years with 93% follow-up. *Ann Surg* 256:262–265, 2012.

43. Peterli R, Borbely Y, Kern B, et al: Early results of the Swiss Multicentre Bypass or Sleeve Study (SM-BOSS): A prospective randomized trial comparing laparoscopic sleeve gastrectomy and Roux-en-Y gastric bypass. *Ann Surg* 258:690–694, discussion 695, 2013.

44. Birkmeyer NJ, Dimick JB, Share D, et al: Hospital complication rates with bariatric surgery in Michigan. *JAMA* 304:435–442, 2010.

45. Hutter MM, Schirmer BD, Jones DB, et al: First report from the American College of Surgeons Bariatric Surgery Center Network: Laparoscopic sleeve gastrectomy has morbidity and effectiveness positioned between the band and the bypass. *Ann Surg* 254:410–420, discussion 420-422, 2011.

46. Sudan R, Nguyen NT, Hutter MM, et al: Morbidity, mortality, and weight loss outcomes after reoperative bariatric surgery in the USA. *J Gastrointest Surg* 19:171–178, 2015.

47. Ikramuddin S, Blackstone RP, Brancatisano A, et al: Effect of reversible intermittent intra-abdominal vagal nerve blockade on morbid obesity: The ReCharge randomized clinical trial. *JAMA* 312:915–922, 2014.

48. Boza C, Salinas J, Salgado N, et al: Laparoscopic sleeve gastrectomy as a stand-alone procedure for morbid obesity: Report of 1,000 cases and 3-year follow-up. *Obes Surg* 22:866–871, 2012.

48 CHAPTER

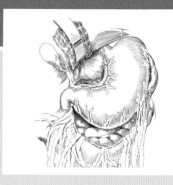

Stomach

Ezra N. Teitelbaum, Eric S. Hungness, David M. Mahvi

第四十八章　胃疾病

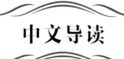

中文导读

　　本章共分为7节：①解剖学；②生理学；③消化性溃疡病；④应激性胃炎；⑤胃切除术后综合征；⑥胃癌；⑦其他胃部疾病。

　　第一节详细介绍了胃的大体解剖，包括胃的分区、血液供应、淋巴回流、神经支配，同时对于胃的形态以及胃显微解剖进行了相关阐述。

　　第二节详细介绍了胃功能的多肽调控，包括胃泌素、生长抑素、胃泌素释放肽、组胺、胃饥饿素的调控作用及原理。着重介绍了胃酸分泌中，刺激分泌的3个时相、壁细胞的激活及分泌、药物调控；胃的分泌功能中，对于胃液、内因子、胃蛋白酶原、黏液和碳酸氢盐也进行了阐述。胃动力学部分从生理、病理方面分别讲解了胃的运动及调节，介绍了胃排空的检查、评估方法，并列出了胃瘫的治疗方式及进展。最后还介绍了胃的屏障功能。

　　第三节介绍的是消化性溃疡病，在流行病学、发病机制等方面，特别强调了幽门螺杆菌感染在其中的作用；分别针对于十二指肠溃疡和胃溃疡做重点阐述，除了临床表现、诊断外，对于十二指肠溃疡出血、穿孔、出口梗阻的治疗方式也进行了描述，以及区别性地介绍了不同分型的胃溃疡和出血性、穿孔性、巨大胃溃疡治疗。文中提到虽然手术在治疗消化性溃疡中的作用降低，但是外科治疗在溃疡，特别是溃疡相关并发症上仍有着重要作用。

　　第四节是关于应激性胃炎方面，这也是临床常见的上消化道出血原因之一，该节将从发病机制、病理生理、临床表现和诊断以及治疗几个方面进行分类叙述。

　　第五节介绍的是胃切除术后综合征，指胃切除后引起的一些胃肠道及心血管症状，包括倾倒综合征、代谢紊乱、输入袢综合征、输出袢综合征、碱性反流性胃炎、胃瘫。

　　第六节是作者在本章中重点突出的部分，介绍了胃癌流行病学和危险因素，病理分型、分期，诊断治疗中的分期检查方法、分期工具，手术治疗方式和重建方式的选择，以及内镜治疗的方法和指征。同时对于微创治疗、辅助和新辅助治疗、姑息性和全身性治疗的进展也进行了介绍。同时在这一节里面作者也对

胃淋巴瘤、胃黏膜相关淋巴组织淋巴瘤、胃间质瘤、胃类癌、异位胰腺等疾病进行了分类叙述。

　　第七节是其他胃疾病的相关内容，包括肥厚性胃炎（Ménétrier Disease）、食管黏膜撕裂症、胃的杜氏病变、胃静脉曲张、胃扭转、胃石症，作者针对这些相对少见的胃疾病分别进行了介绍。

〔覃吉超〕

ANATOMY

Gross Anatomy

Divisions

The stomach begins as a dilation in the tubular embryonic foregut during the fifth week of gestation. By the seventh week, it descends, rotates, and further dilates with a disproportionate elongation of the greater curvature into its normal anatomic shape and position. Following birth, it is the most proximal abdominal organ of the alimentary tract. The most proximal region of the stomach is called the *cardia* and attaches to the esophagus. Immediately proximal to the cardia is a physiologically competent lower esophageal sphincter. Distally, the pylorus connects the distal stomach (antrum) to the proximal duodenum. Although the stomach is fixed at the gastroesophageal (GE) junction and pylorus, its large midportion is mobile. The fundus represents the superiormost part of the stomach and is floppy and distensible. The stomach is bounded superiorly by the diaphragm and laterally by the spleen. The body of the stomach represents the largest portion and is also referred to as the *corpus*. The body also contains most of the parietal cells and is bounded on the right by the relatively straight lesser curvature and on the left by the longer greater curvature. At the angularis incisura, the lesser curvature abruptly angles to the right. The body of the stomach ends here and the antrum begins. Another important anatomic angle (angle of His) is the angle formed by the fundus with the left margin of the esophagus (Fig. 48-1).

Most of the stomach resides within the upper abdomen. The left lateral segment of the liver covers a large portion of the stomach anteriorly. The diaphragm, chest, and abdominal wall bound the remainder of the stomach. Inferiorly, the stomach is attached to the transverse colon, spleen, caudate lobe of the liver, diaphragmatic crura, and retroperitoneal nerves and vessels. Superiorly, the GE junction is found approximately 2 to 3 cm below the diaphragmatic esophageal hiatus in the horizontal plane of the seventh chondrosternal articulation, a plane only slightly cephalad to the plane containing the pylorus. The gastrosplenic ligament attaches the proximal greater curvature to the spleen.

Blood Supply

The celiac artery provides most of the blood supply to the stomach (Fig. 48-2). There are four main arteries—the left and right gastric

arteries along the lesser curvature and the left and right gastroepiploic arteries along the greater curvature. In addition, a substantial quantity of blood may be supplied to the proximal stomach by the inferior phrenic arteries and by the short gastric arteries from the spleen. The largest artery to the stomach is the left gastric artery; it is not uncommon (15% to 20%) for an aberrant left hepatic artery to originate from it. Consequently, proximal ligation of the left gastric artery occasionally results in acute left-sided hepatic ischemia. The right gastric artery arises from the hepatic artery (or gastroduodenal artery). The left gastroepiploic artery originates from the splenic artery, and the right gastroepiploic artery originates from the gastroduodenal artery. The extensive anastomotic connection between these major vessels ensures that in most cases the stomach will survive if three out of four arteries are ligated, provided that the arcades along the greater and lesser curvatures are not disturbed. In general, the veins of the stomach parallel the arteries. The left gastric (coronary) and right gastric veins usually drain into the portal vein. The right gastroepiploic vein drains into the superior mesenteric vein, and the left gastroepiploic vein drains into the splenic vein.

Lymphatic Drainage

The lymphatic drainage of the stomach parallels the vasculature and drains into four zones of lymph nodes (Fig. 48-3). The

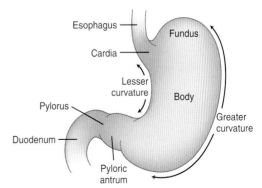

FIGURE 48-1 Divisions of the stomach. (From Yeo C, Dempsey DT, Klein AS, et al, editors: *Shackelford's surgery of the alimentary tract*, ed 6, Philadelphia, 2007, Saunders.)

superior gastric group drains lymph from the upper lesser curvature into the left gastric and paracardial nodes. The suprapyloric group of nodes drains the antral segment on the lesser curvature of the stomach into the right suprapancreatic nodes. The pancreaticolienal group of nodes drains lymph high on the greater curvature into the left gastroepiploic and splenic nodes. The inferior gastric and subpyloric group of nodes drains lymph along the right gastroepiploic vascular pedicle. All four zones of lymph nodes drain into the celiac group and into the thoracic duct. Although these lymph nodes drain different areas of the stomach, gastric cancers may metastasize to any of the four nodal groups, regardless of the cancer location. In addition, the extensive submucosal plexus of lymphatics accounts for the fact that there is frequently microscopic evidence of malignant cells several centimeters from gross disease.

Innervation

As shown in Figure 48-4, the extrinsic innervation of the stomach is parasympathetic (via the vagus) and sympathetic (via the celiac plexus). The vagus nerve originates in the vagal nucleus in the floor of the fourth ventricle and traverses the neck in the carotid sheath to enter the mediastinum, where it divides into several branches around the esophagus. These branches coalesce above the esophageal hiatus to form the left and right vagus nerves. It is not uncommon to find more than two vagal trunks at the distal esophagus. At the GE junction, the *left* vagus is *a*nterior, and the *right* vagus is *p*osterior (LARP).

The left vagus gives off the hepatic branch to the liver and continues along the lesser curvature as the anterior nerve of Latarjet. Although not shown, the so-called *criminal nerve of Grassi* is the first branch of the right or posterior vagus nerve; it is recognized as a potential cause of recurrent ulcers when left undivided. The right nerve gives a branch off to the celiac plexus and continues posteriorly along the lesser curvature. A truncal vagotomy is performed above the celiac and hepatic branches of the vagi, whereas a selective vagotomy is performed below. A highly selective vagotomy is performed by dividing the crow's feet to the proximal stomach while preserving the innervation of the antral and pyloric parts of the stomach. Most (90%) of the vagal fibers are afferent, carrying stimuli from the gut to the brain. Efferent vagal fibers originate in the dorsal nucleus of the medulla and synapse with neurons in the myenteric and submucosal plexuses. These neurons use acetylcholine as their neurotransmitter and influence gastric motor function and gastric secretion. In contrast, the sympathetic nerve supply comes from T5 to T10, traveling in the splanchnic nerve to the celiac ganglion. Postganglionic fibers travel with the arterial system to innervate the stomach.

The intrinsic or enteric nervous system of the stomach consists of neurons in Auerbach and Meissner autonomic plexuses. In these locations, cholinergic, serotoninergic, and peptidergic

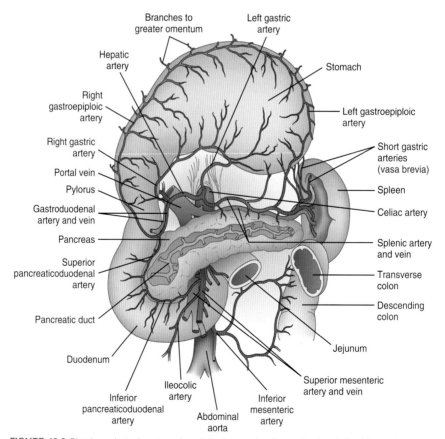

FIGURE 48-2 Blood supply to the stomach and duodenum showing anatomic relationships to the spleen and pancreas. The stomach is reflected cephalad. (From Yeo C, Dempsey DT, Klein AS, et al, editors: *Shackelford's surgery of the alimentary tract*, ed 6, Philadelphia, 2007, Saunders.)

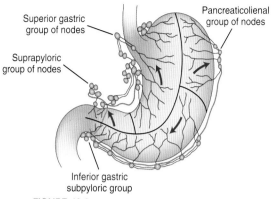

Superior gastric group of nodes

Suprapyloric group of nodes

Pancreaticolienal group of nodes

Inferior gastric subpyloric group

FIGURE 48-3 Lymphatic drainage of the stomach.

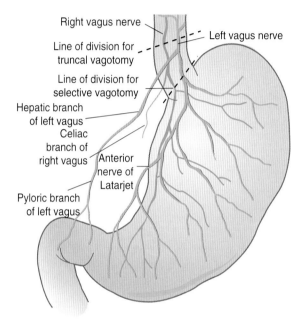

Right vagus nerve

Left vagus nerve

Line of division for truncal vagotomy

Line of division for selective vagotomy

Hepatic branch of left vagus

Celiac branch of right vagus

Anterior nerve of Latarjet

Pyloric branch of left vagus

FIGURE 48-4 Vagal innervation of the stomach. The line of division for truncal vagotomy is shown; it is above the hepatic and celiac branches of the left and right vagus nerves, respectively. The line of division for selective vagotomy is shown; this is below the hepatic and celiac branches. (From Mercer D, Liu T: Open truncal vagotomy. *Oper Tech Gen Surg* 5:8–85, 2003.)

TABLE 48-1	Gastric Cell Types, Location, and Function	
CELL TYPE	**LOCATION**	**FUNCTION**
Parietal	Body	Secretion of acid and intrinsic factor
Mucus	Body, antrum	Mucus
Chief	Body	Pepsin
Surface epithelial	Diffuse	Mucus, bicarbonate, prostaglandins (?)
Enterochromaffin-like	Body	Histamine
G	Antrum	Gastrin
D	Body, antrum	Somatostatin
Gastric mucosal interneurons	Body, antrum	Gastrin-releasing peptide
Enteric neurons	Diffuse	Calcitonin gene–related peptide, others
Endocrine	Body	Ghrelin

muscles. The middle layer of smooth muscle is circular and is the only complete muscle layer of the stomach wall. At the pylorus, this middle circular muscle layer becomes progressively thicker and functions as a true anatomic sphincter. The outer muscle layer is longitudinal and continuous with the outer layer of longitudinal esophageal smooth muscle. Within the layers of the muscularis externa is a rich plexus of autonomic nerves and ganglia, called *Auerbach myenteric plexus*. The submucosa lies between the muscularis externa and mucosa and is a collagen-rich layer of connective tissue that is the strongest layer of the gastric wall. In addition, it contains the rich anastomotic network of blood vessels and lymphatics and Meissner plexus of autonomic nerves. The mucosa consists of surface epithelium, lamina propria, and muscularis mucosae. The muscularis mucosae is on the luminal side of the submucosa and is probably responsible for the rugae that greatly increase epithelial surface area. It also marks the microscopic boundary for invasive and noninvasive gastric carcinoma. The lamina propria represents a small connective tissue layer and contains capillaries, vessels, lymphatics, and nerves necessary to support the surface epithelium.

Gastric Microscopic Anatomy

Gastric mucosa consists of columnar glandular epithelia. The cellular populations (and functions) of the cells forming this glandular epithelium vary based on their location in the stomach (Table 48-1). The glandular epithelium is divided into cells that secrete products into the gastric lumen for digestion (parietal cells, chief cells, mucus-secreting cells) and cells that control function (gastrin-secreting G cells, somatostatin-secreting D cells). In the cardia, the mucosa is arranged in branched glands, and the pits are short. In the fundus and body, the glands are more tubular, and the pits are longer. In the antrum, the glands are more branched. The luminal ends of the gastric glands and pits are lined with mucus-secreting surface epithelial cells, which extend down into the necks of the glands for variable distances. In the cardia, the glands are predominantly mucus-secreting. In the body, the glands are mostly lined from the neck to the base with parietal and chief cells (Fig. 48-5). There are a few parietal cells in the fundus and proximal antrum, but none in the cardia or prepyloric antrum. The endocrine G cells are present in greatest quantity in the antral glands.

neurons are present. However, the function of these neurons is poorly understood. Nevertheless, numerous neuropeptides have been localized to these neurons, including acetylcholine, serotonin, substance P, calcitonin gene–related peptide, bombesin, cholecystokinin (CCK), and somatostatin. Consequently, it is an oversimplification to think of the stomach as containing only parasympathetic (cholinergic input) and sympathetic (adrenergic input) supply. Moreover, the parasympathetic nervous system contains adrenergic neurons, and the sympathetic system contains cholinergic neurons.

Gastric Morphology

The stomach is covered by peritoneum, which forms the outer serosa of the stomach. Below it is the thicker muscularis propria, or muscularis externa, which is composed of three layers of smooth

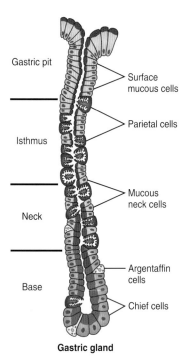

Gastric pit

Surface
mucous cells

Parietal cells

Isthmus

Mucous
neck cells

Neck

Argentaffin
cells

Base

Chief cells

Gastric gland

FIGURE 48-5 Cells residing within a gastric gland. (From Yeo C, Dempsey DT, Klein AS, et al, editors: *Shackelford's surgery of the alimentary tract*, ed 6, Philadelphia, 2007, Saunders.)

PHYSIOLOGY

The principal function of the stomach is to prepare ingested food for digestion and absorption as it is propulsed into the small intestine. The initial period of digestion requires that solid components of a meal be stored for several hours while they undergo a reduction in size and break down into their basic metabolic constituents.

Receptive relaxation of the proximal stomach enables the stomach to function as a storage organ. Receptive relaxation refers to the process whereby the proximal portion of the stomach relaxes in anticipation of food intake. This relaxation enables liquids to pass easily from the stomach along the lesser curvature, whereas the solid food settles along the greater curvature of the fundus. In contrast to liquids, emptying of solid food is facilitated by the antrum, which pumps solid food components into and through the pylorus. The antrum and pylorus function in a coordinated fashion, allowing entry of food components into the duodenum and returning material to the proximal stomach until it is suitable for delivery into the duodenum.

In addition to storing food, the stomach begins digestion of a meal. Starches undergo enzymatic breakdown through the activity of salivary amylase. Peptic digestion metabolizes a meal into fats, proteins, and carbohydrates by breaking down cell walls. Although the duodenum and proximal small intestine are primarily responsible for digestion of a meal, the stomach facilitates this process.

Regulation of Gastric Function

Gastric function is under neural (sympathetic and parasympathetic) and hormonal control (peptides or amines that interact with target cells in the stomach). An understanding of the roles of endocrine and neural regulation of digestion is critical to understanding gastric physiology. Abnormal secretion of gastrin and pepsin was thought to be the major causative factor in peptic ulcer disease (PUD). The discovery of *Helicobacter pylori* and the effect of this organism on ulcer disease have rendered moot many of the theoretical rationales for acid hypersecretion. However, a general understanding of gastric physiology and the specific impact of peptides on acid secretion is still critical to understanding the physiologic effects of gastric surgical procedures on digestion. We initially focus here on peptide regulation of gastric function and then describe the interactions of these peptides with neural inputs in regard to acid secretion and gastric function.

Gastric Peptides
Gastrin

Gastrin is produced by G cells located in the gastric antrum (see Table 48-1). It is synthesized as a prepropeptide and undergoes post-translational processing to produce biologically reactive gastrin peptides. Several molecular forms of gastrin exist. G-34 (big gastrin), G-17 (little gastrin), and G-14 (minigastrin) have been identified; 90% of antral gastrin is released as the 17–amino acid peptide, although G-34 predominates in the circulation because its metabolic half-life is longer than that of G-17. The pentapeptide sequence contained at the carboxyl terminus of gastrin is the biologically active component and is identical to that found on another gut peptide, CCK. CCK and gastrin differ by tyrosine sulfation sites. The release of gastrin is stimulated by food components in a meal, especially protein digestion products. Luminal acid inhibits the release of gastrin. In the antral location, somatostatin and gastrin release are functionally linked, and an inverse reciprocal relationship exists between these two peptides.

Gastrin is the major hormonal regulator of the gastric phase of acid secretion after a meal. Histamine, released from enterochromaffin-like (ECL) cells, is also a potent stimulant of acid release from the parietal cell. Gastrin also has considerable trophic effects on the parietal cells and gastric ECL cells. Prolonged hypergastrinemia from any cause leads to mucosal hyperplasia and an increase in the number of ECL cells and, under some circumstances, is associated with the development of gastric carcinoid tumors.

The detection of hypergastrinemia may suggest a pathologic state of acid hypersecretion but generally is the result of treatment with agents to reduce acid secretion, such as proton pump inhibitors (PPIs). Table 48-2 lists common causes of chronic hypergastrinemia. Hypergastrinemia that results from the administration of acid-reducing drugs is an appropriate response caused by loss of feedback inhibition of gastrin release by luminal acid. Lack of acid causes a reduction in somatostatin release, which causes increased release of gastrin from antral G cells. Hypergastrinemia can also occur in the setting of pernicious anemia or uremia or after surgical procedures such as vagotomy or retained gastric antrum after gastrectomy. In contrast, gastrin levels increase inappropriately in patients with gastrinoma (Zollinger-Ellison syndrome [ZES]). These gastrin-secreting tumors are not located in the antrum and secrete gastrin autonomously.

Gastrin initiates its biologic actions by activation of surface membrane receptors. These receptors are members of the classic G protein–coupled seven-transmembrane–spanning receptor family and are classified as type A or B CCK receptors. The gastrin or CCK-B receptor has high affinity for gastrin and CCK, whereas type A CCK receptors have an affinity for sulfated CCK analogues and a low affinity for gastrin. Binding of gastrin with the CCK-B

TABLE 48-2 Causes of Hypergastrinemia	
ULCEROGENIC CAUSES	**NONULCEROGENIC CAUSES**
Antral G cell hyperplasia or hyperfunction	Antisecretory agents (PPIs)
Retained excluded antrum	Atrophic gastritis
Zollinger-Ellison syndrome	Pernicious anemia
Gastric outlet obstruction	Acid-reducing procedure (vagotomy)
Short-gut syndrome	*Helicobacter pylori* infection
	Chronic renal failure

PPIs, Proton pump inhibitors.

receptor has been associated with elevated intracellular calcium levels.

Somatostatin

Somatostatin is produced by D cells and exists endogenously as the 14–amino acid peptide or 28–amino acid peptide. The predominant molecular form in the stomach is somatostatin-14. It is produced by diffuse neuroendocrine cells located in the fundus and antrum. In these locations, D cell cytoplasmic extensions have direct contact with the parietal cells and G cells, where somatostatin presumably exerts its actions through paracrine effects on acid secretion and gastrin release.[1] Somatostatin is able to inhibit parietal cell acid secretion directly but can also indirectly inhibit acid secretion through inhibition of gastrin release and downregulation of histamine release from ECL cells. The principal stimulus for somatostatin release is antral acidification, whereas acetylcholine from vagal fibers inhibits its release.

Somatostatin receptors are also seven-transmembrane–spanning receptors. Binding of somatostatin with its receptors is coupled to one or more inhibitory guanine nucleotide–binding proteins. Parietal cell somatostatin receptors appear to be a single subunit of glycoproteins with a molecular weight of 99 kDa, with equal affinity for somatostatin-14 and somatostatin-28. Somatostatin can inhibit parietal cell secretion through G protein–dependent and G protein–independent mechanisms. However, the ability of somatostatin to exert its inhibitory actions on cellular function is primarily thought to be mediated through the inhibition of adenylate cyclase, with a resultant reduction in cyclic adenosine monophosphate (cAMP) levels.

Gastrin-Releasing Peptide

Bombesin was discovered in 1970 in an extract prepared from skin of the amphibian *Bombina bombina* (European fire-bellied toad). Its mammalian counterpart is gastrin-releasing peptide (GRP). GRP is particularly prominent in nerves ending in the acid-secreting and gastrin-secreting portions of the stomach and is found in the circular muscular layer. In the antral mucosa, GRP stimulates gastrin and somatostatin release by binding to receptors located on the G and D cells, respectively. It is rapidly cleared from the circulation by a neutral endopeptidase and has a half-life of approximately 1.4 minutes. Peripheral administration of exogenous GRP stimulates gastric acid secretion, whereas central administration in the ventricles inhibits acid secretion. The inhibitory pathway activated is not mediated by a humoral factor, is unaffected by vagotomy, and appears to involve the sympathetic nervous system.

Histamine

Histamine plays a prominent role in parietal cell stimulation. Administration of histamine 2 (H_2) receptor antagonists almost completely abolishes gastric acid secretion in response to gastrin and acetylcholine. This suggests that histamine may be a necessary intermediary of gastrin-stimulated and acetylcholine-stimulated acid secretion. Histamine is stored in the acidic granules of ECL cells and in resident mast cells. Its release is stimulated by gastrin, acetylcholine, and epinephrine after receptor-ligand interactions on ECL cells. In contrast, somatostatin inhibits gastrin-stimulated histamine release through interactions with somatostatin receptors located on the ECL cell. The ECL cell plays an essential role in parietal cell activation possessing stimulatory and inhibitory feedback pathways that modulate the release of histamine and therefore acid secretion.

Ghrelin

Ghrelin is a 28–amino acid peptide predominantly produced by endocrine cells of the oxyntic mucosa of the stomach, with substantially lower amounts from the bowel, pancreas, and other organs. Removal of the acid-producing part of the stomach decreases circulating ghrelin by 80%. Ghrelin appears to be under endocrine and metabolic control, has a diurnal rhythm, likely plays a major role in the neuroendocrine and metabolic responses to changes in nutritional status, and may be a major anabolic hormone.

In human volunteers, ghrelin administration enhances appetite and increases food intake. In patients who have undergone a gastric bypass, ghrelin levels are 77% lower than levels in matched obese control subjects, a finding not seen after other forms of antiobesity surgery. Although the mechanism responsible for suppression of ghrelin levels after gastric bypass is unknown, it is suggested that ghrelin may be responsive to the normal flow of nutrients across the stomach. Other studies have suggested that ghrelin leads to a switch toward glycolysis and away from fatty acid oxidation, which would favor fat deposition. Ghrelin appears to be upregulated in times of negative energy balance and downregulated in times of positive energy balance, although the precise role of ghrelin in energy metabolism is unclear. Ghrelin may come to have a role in the treatment and prevention of obesity.

Gastric Acid Secretion

Gastric acid secretion by the parietal cell is regulated by three local stimuli—acetylcholine, gastrin, and histamine. These three stimuli account for basal and stimulated gastric acid secretion. Acetylcholine is the principal neurotransmitter modulating acid secretion and is released from the vagus and parasympathetic ganglion cells. Vagal fibers innervate not only parietal cells but also G cells and ECL cells to modulate release of their peptides. Gastrin has hormonal effects on the parietal cell and stimulates histamine release. Histamine has paracrine-like effects on the parietal cell and, as shown in Figure 48-6, plays a central role in the regulation of acid secretion by the parietal cell after its release from ECL cells. As depicted, somatostatin exerts inhibitory actions on gastric acid secretion. Release of somatostatin from antral D cells is stimulated in the presence of intraluminal acid to a pH of 3 or lower. After its release, somatostatin inhibits gastrin release through paracrine effects and modifies histamine release from ECL cells. In some patients with PUD, this negative feedback response is defective. Consequently, the precise state of acid secretion by the parietal cell depends on the overall influence of the positive and negative stimuli.

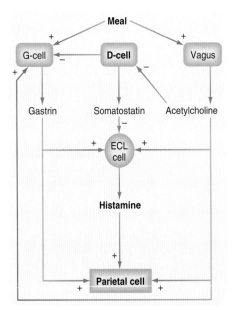

FIGURE 48-6 Central role of the enterochromaffin-like (ECL) cell in regulation of acid secretion by the parietal cell. As shown, ingestion of a meal stimulates vagal fibers to release acetylcholine (cephalic phase). Binding of acetylcholine to M_3 receptors located on the ECL cell, parietal cell, and G cell results in the release of histamine, hydrochloric acid, and gastrin. Binding of acetylcholine to M_3 receptors on D cells results in the inhibition of somatostatin release. After a meal, G cells are also stimulated to release gastrin, which interacts with receptors located on ECL cells and parietal cells to cause the release of histamine and hydrochloric acid (gastric phase). Release of somatostatin from D cells decreases histamine release and gastrin release from ECL cells and G cells. In addition, somatostatin inhibits parietal cell acid secretion (not shown). The principal stimulus for the activation of D cells is antral luminal acidification (not shown). (From Yeo C, Dempsey DT, Klein AS, et al, editors: *Shackelford's surgery of the alimentary tract*, ed 6, Philadelphia, 2007, Saunders.)

In the absence of food, there is always a basal level of acid secretion that is approximately 10% of maximal acid output. Under basal conditions, 1 to 5 mmol/hr of hydrochloric acid is secreted, and this is reduced after vagotomy or H_2 receptor blockade. Thus, it appears likely that basal acid secretion is caused by a combination of cholinergic and histaminergic input.

Stimulated Acid Secretion

Cephalic phase. Ingestion of food is the physiologic stimulus for acid secretion. Three phases of the acid secretory response to a meal have been described—cephalic, gastric, and intestinal. These three phases are interrelated and occur concurrently, not consecutively.

The cephalic phase originates with the sight, smell, thought, or taste of food, which stimulates neural centers in the cortex and hypothalamus. Although the exact mechanisms whereby senses stimulate acid secretion are not yet fully elucidated, it is hypothesized that several sites are stimulated in the brain. These higher centers transmit signals to the stomach by the vagus nerves, which release acetylcholine that activates muscarinic receptors located on target cells. Acetylcholine directly increases acid secretion by the parietal cells and can inhibit and stimulate gastrin release, the net effect being a slight increase in gastrin levels. Although the

intensity of the acid secretory response in the cephalic phase surpasses that of the other phases, it accounts for only 20% to 30% of the total volume of gastric acid produced in response to a meal because of the short duration of the cephalic phase.

Gastric phase. The gastric phase of acid secretion begins when food enters the gastric lumen. Digestion products of ingested food interact with microvilli of antral G cells to stimulate gastrin release. Food also stimulates acid secretion by causing mechanical distention of the stomach. Gastric distention activates stretch receptors in the stomach to elicit the long vagovagal reflex arc. It is abolished by proximal gastric vagotomy and is, at least in part, independent of changes in serum gastrin levels. However, antral distention also causes gastrin release in humans, a reflex that has been called the *pyloro-oxyntic reflex*. In humans, mechanical distention of the stomach accounts for approximately 30% to 40% of the maximal acid secretory response to a peptone meal, with the remainder caused by gastrin release. The entire gastric phase accounts for most (60% to 70%) of meal-stimulated acid output because it lasts until the stomach is empty.

Intestinal phase. The intestinal phase of gastric secretion is poorly understood but appears to be initiated by entry of chyme into the small intestine. It occurs after gastric emptying and lasts as long as partially digested food components remain in the proximal small bowel. It accounts for only 10% of the acid secretory response to a meal and does not appear to be mediated by serum gastrin levels. It has been hypothesized that a distinct acid stimulatory peptide hormone (entero-oxyntin) released from small bowel mucosa may mediate the intestinal phase of acid secretion.

Activation and Secretion by the Parietal Cell

The two second messengers principally involved in stimulation of acid secretion by parietal cells are intracellular cAMP and calcium. Synthesis of these two messengers activates protein kinases and phosphorylation cascades. The intracellular events following ligand binding to receptors on the parietal cell are shown in Figure 48-7. Histamine causes an increase in intracellular cAMP, which activates protein kinases to initiate a cascade of phosphorylation events that culminate in activation of H^+, K^+-ATPase. In contrast, acetylcholine and gastrin stimulate phospholipase C, which converts membrane-bound phospholipids into inositol triphosphate to mobilize calcium from intracellular stores. Increased intracellular calcium activates other protein kinases that ultimately activate H^+, K^+-ATPase in a similar fashion to initiate the secretion of hydrochloric acid.

H^+, K^+-ATPase is the final common pathway for gastric acid secretion by the parietal cell. It is composed of two subunits, a catalytic α-subunit (100 kDa) and a glycoprotein β-subunit (60 kDa). During the resting, or nonsecreting, state, gastric parietal cells store H^+, K^+-ATPase within intracellular tubulovesicular elements. Cellular relocation of the proton pump subunits through cytoskeletal rearrangements must occur for acid secretion to increase in response to stimulatory factors. The subsequent insertion and heterodimer assembly of the H^+, K^+-ATPase subunits into the microvilli of the secretory canaliculus causes an increase in gastric acid secretion. A KCl efflux pathway must exist to supply potassium to the extracytoplasmic side of the pump. Cytosolic hydrogen is secreted by H^+, K^+-ATPase in exchange for extracytoplasmic potassium (see Fig. 48-7), which is an electroneutral exchange and does not contribute to the transmembrane potential difference across the parietal cell. Secretion of chloride is accomplished through a chloride channel moving chloride from the parietal cell cytoplasm to the gastric lumen. However, the

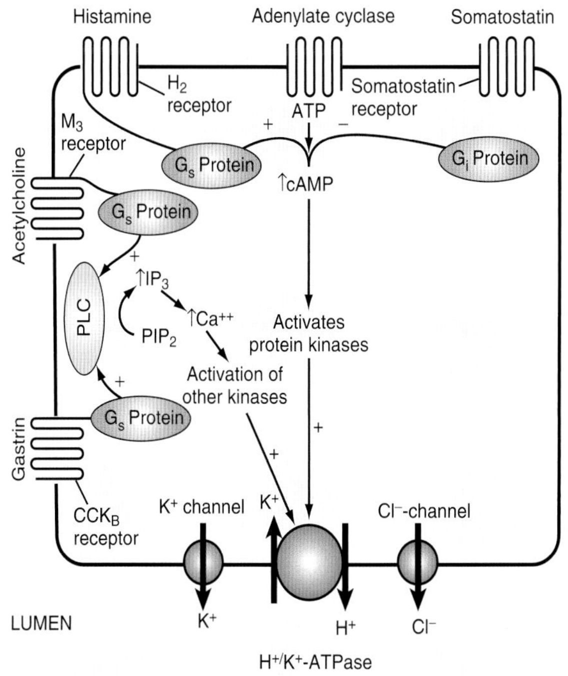

INTERSTITIUM

FIGURE 48-7 Intracellular signaling events in a parietal cell. As shown, histamine binds to H_2 receptors, stimulating adenylate cyclase through a G protein–linked mechanism. Adenylate cyclase activation causes an increase in intracellular cyclic adenosine monophosphate (cAMP) levels, which activates protein kinases. Activated protein kinases stimulate a phosphorylation cascade, with a resultant increase in levels of phosphoproteins that activate the proton pump. Activation of the proton pump leads to extrusion of cytosolic hydrogen in exchange for extracytoplasmic potassium. In addition, chloride is secreted through a chloride channel located on the luminal side of the membrane. Gastrin binds to type B cholecystokinin receptors, and acetylcholine binds to M_3 receptors. Following the interaction of gastrin and acetylcholine with their receptors, phospholipase C is stimulated through a G protein–linked mechanism to convert membrane-bound phospholipids into inositol triphosphate (IP_3). IP_3 stimulates the release of calcium from intracellular calcium stores, leading to an increase in intracellular calcium that activates protein kinases, which activate the H^+, K^+-ATPase. ATP, Adenosine triphosphate; ATPase, adenosine triphosphatase; G_i, inhibitory guanine nucleotide protein; G_s, stimulatory guanine nucleotide protein; PIP_2, phosphatidylinositol 4,5-diphosphate; PLC, phospholipase C. (From Yeo C, Dempsey DI, Klein AS, et al, editors: Shackelford's surgery of the alimentary tract, ed 6, Philadelphia, 2007, Saunders.)

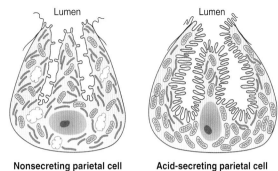

FIGURE 48-8 Diagrammatic representation of resting and stimulated parietal cells. Note the morphologic transformation between the nonsecreting parietal cell and stimulated parietal cell, with increases in secretory canalicular membrane surface area.

signal. The tyrosine-containing sequence is located on the cytoplasmic tail of the β-subunit and is highly homologous to the motif responsible for internalization of the transferrin receptor.

More than 1 billion parietal cells are found in the normal human stomach and are responsible for secreting approximately 20 mmol/hr of hydrochloric acid in response to a protein meal. Each individual parietal cell secretes 3.3 billion hydrogen ions/second, and there is a linear relationship between maximal acid output and parietal cell number. However, gastric acid secretory rates may be altered in patients with upper gastrointestinal (GI) disease. For example, gastric acid is often increased in patients with duodenal ulcer or gastrinoma, whereas it is decreased in patients with pernicious anemia, gastric atrophy, gastric ulcer, or gastric cancer. The lower secretory rates observed in patients with gastric ulcers are typically associated with proximal gastric ulcers, whereas distal, antral, or prepyloric ulcers are associated with acid secretory rates similar to rates in patients with duodenal ulcers.

Gastric acid plays a critical role in the digestion of a meal. It is required to convert pepsinogen into pepsin, elicits the release of secretin from the duodenum, and limits colonization of the upper GI tract with bacteria.

Pharmacologic Regulation

The diversity of mechanisms that stimulate acid secretion has resulted in the development of many site-specific drugs aimed at decreasing acid output by the parietal cell. The best-known site-specific antagonists are the group collectively known as the H_2 receptor antagonists. The most potent of the H_2 receptor antagonists is famotidine, followed by ranitidine, nizatidine, and cimetidine. The half-life for famotidine is 3 hours, and the half-life for the other H_2 receptor antagonists is approximately 1.5 hours. All H_2 receptor antagonists undergo hepatic metabolism, are excreted by the kidney, and do not differ much in bioavailability.

The PPIs represent the newest class of antisecretory agents. These substituted benzimidazoles, of which omeprazole is a prime example, inhibit acid secretion more completely because of their irreversible inhibition of the proton pump. PPIs are weak acids with a pK_a of 4 and become selectively localized in the secretory canaliculus of the parietal cell, which is the only structure in the body with a pH lower than 4. After oral administration, these agents are absorbed into the bloodstream as prodrugs and selectively concentrate in the secretory canaliculus. At low pH, they become ionized and activated, with the formation of an active

secretion or exchange of hydrogen for potassium requires energy in the form of adenosine triphosphate (ATP) because hydrogen is being secreted against a gradient of more than a million-fold. Because of this large energy requirement, the parietal cell also has the largest mitochondrial content of any mammalian cell, with a mitochondrial compartment representing 34% of its cell volume. In response to a secretagogue, the parietal cell undergoes a conformational change, and a several-fold increase in the canalicular surface area occurs (Fig. 48-8). In contrast to stimulated acid secretion, cessation of acid secretion requires endocytosis of H^+, K^+-ATPase, with regeneration of cytoplasmic tubulovesicles containing the subunits, and this occurs through a tyrosine-based sulfur group. Because the proton pump is located on the luminal surface, the transmembrane pump proteins are also exposed to acid or low pH. The cysteine residues on the α-subunit form a covalent disulfate bond with activated benzimidazoles, which irreversibly inhibits the proton pump. Because of the covalent nature of this bond, these PPIs have more prolonged inhibition of gastric acid secretion than H_2 blockers. For recovery of acid secretion to occur, new protein pumps need to be synthesized. As a result, these agents have a longer duration of action than their plasma half-life, with the intragastric pH being maintained higher than 3 for 18 hours or longer.

One notable side effect of all antisecretory agents is the elevation of serum gastrin levels. Serum gastrin levels are higher after treatment with PPIs than with H_2 receptor antagonists. This effect is accompanied by hyperplasia of G cells and ECL cells with long-term administration of these agents. Long-term administration of omeprazole has been found to cause ECL hyperplasia that could progress to carcinoid tumors in rats. However, this effect was not specific for omeprazole and was reproduced by other agents that caused prolonged inhibition of acid secretion and resultant hypergastrinemia.

Other Gastric Secretory Products

Gastric juice. Gastric juice is the result of secretion by the parietal cells, chief cells, and mucous cells, in addition to swallowed saliva and duodenal refluxate. The electrolyte composition of parietal and nonparietal gastric secretion varies with the rate of gastric secretion. Parietal cells secrete an electrolyte solution that is isotonic with plasma and contains 160 mmol/liter. The pH of this solution is 0.8. The lowest intraluminal pH commonly measured in the stomach is 2 because of dilution of the parietal cell secretion by other gastric secretions, which also contain sodium, potassium, and bicarbonate.

Intrinsic factor. Intrinsic factor is a 60-kDa mucoprotein secreted by the parietal cell that is essential for the absorption of vitamin B_{12} in the terminal ileum. It is secreted in amounts that far exceed the amounts necessary for vitamin B_{12} absorption. In general, secretion of intrinsic factor parallels gastric acid secretion, yet the secretory response is not linked to acid secretion. For example, PPIs do not block intrinsic factor secretion in humans, and they do not alter the absorption of labeled vitamin B_{12}. Intrinsic factor deficiency can develop in the patients with pernicious anemia or in patients undergoing total gastrectomy, and both groups of patients require vitamin B_{12} supplementation.

Pepsinogen. Pepsinogens are proteolytic proenzymes with a molecular weight of 42,500 that are secreted by the glands of the gastroduodenal mucosa. Two types of pepsinogens are secreted. Group 1 pepsinogens are secreted by chief cells and by mucous neck cells located in the glands of the acid-secreting portion of the stomach. Group 2 pepsinogens are produced by surface epithelial cells throughout the acid-secreting portion of the stomach, antrum, and proximal duodenum. Consequently, group 1 pepsinogens are secreted by the same glands that secrete acid, whereas group 2 pepsinogens are secreted by acid-secreting and gastrin-secreting mucosa. In the presence of acid, both forms of pepsinogen are converted to pepsin by removal of a short amino-terminal peptide. Pepsins become inactivated at a pH higher than 5, although group 2 pepsinogens are active over a wider range of pH values than group 1 pepsinogens. As a result, group 2 pepsinogens may be involved in peptic digestion in the presence of increased gastric pH, which commonly occurs in the setting of stress or in patients with gastric ulcer.

Mucus and bicarbonate. Mucus and bicarbonate combine to neutralize gastric acid at the gastric mucosal surface. They are secreted by the surface mucous cells and mucous neck cells located in the acid-secreting and antral portions of the stomach. Mucus is a viscoelastic gel that contains approximately 85% water and 15% glycoproteins. It provides a mechanical barrier to injury by contributing to the unstirred layer of water found at the luminal surface of the gastric mucosa. It also acts as an impediment to ion movement from the lumen to the apical cell membrane and is relatively impermeable to pepsins. Mucus is in a constant state of flux because it is secreted continuously by mucosal cells on one hand and solubilized by luminal pepsin on the other hand. Mucus production is stimulated by vagal stimulation, cholinergic agonists, prostaglandins, and some bacterial toxins. In contrast, anticholinergic drugs and nonsteroidal anti-inflammatory drugs (NSAIDs) inhibit mucus secretion. *H. pylori* secretes various proteases and lipases that break down mucin and impair the protective function of the mucous layer.

In the acid-secreting portion of the stomach, bicarbonate secretion is an active process, whereas in the antrum, active and passive secretion of bicarbonate occurs. However, the magnitude of bicarbonate secretion is considerably less than acid secretion. Although the luminal pH is 2, the pH observed at the surface epithelial cell is usually 7. The pH gradient found at the epithelial surface is a result of the unstirred layer of water in the mucous gel and of the continuous secretion of bicarbonate by the surface epithelial cells. Gastric cell surface pH remains higher than 5 until the luminal pH is less than 1.4. However, the luminal pH in patients with duodenal ulcers is frequently less than 1.4, so the cell surface is exposed to a lower pH in these patients. This reduction in pH may reflect a reduction in gastric bicarbonate secretion and decreased duodenal bicarbonate secretion and may explain why some patients with duodenal ulcers have a higher relapse rate after treatment.

Gastric Motility

Gastric motility is regulated by extrinsic and intrinsic neural mechanisms and by myogenic control. The extrinsic neural controls are mediated through parasympathetic (vagus) and sympathetic pathways, whereas the intrinsic controls involve the enteric nervous system (see "Anatomy"). In contrast, myogenic control resides in the excitatory membranes of the gastric smooth muscle cells.

Fasting Gastric Motility

The electrical basis of gastric motility begins with the depolarization of pacemaker cells located in the midbody of the stomach along the greater curvature. Once initiated, slow waves travel at 3 cycles/minute in a circumferential and antegrade fashion toward the pylorus. In addition to these slow waves, gastric smooth muscle cells are capable of producing action potentials, which are associated with larger changes in membrane potential than slow waves. Compared with slow waves, which are not associated with gastric contractions, action potentials are associated with actual muscle contractions. During fasting, the stomach goes through a cyclical pattern of electrical activity composed of slow waves and electrical spikes, which has been termed the *myoelectric migrating complex*. Each cycle of the myoelectric migrating complex lasts 90 to 120 minutes. The net effects of the myoelectric migrating complex are frequent clearance of gastric contents during periods of fasting. The exact regulatory mechanisms of myoelectric migrating complex activities are unknown, but these activities remain intact after vagal denervation.

Postprandial Gastric Motility

Ingestion of a meal results in a decrease in the resting tone of the proximal stomach and fundus, referred to as *receptive relaxation* and *gastric accommodation,* respectively. Because these reflexes are mediated by the vagus nerves, interruption of vagal innervation to the proximal stomach, such as by truncal vagotomy or proximal gastric vagotomy, can eliminate these reflexes, with resultant early satiety and rapid emptying of ingested liquids. In addition to its storage function, the stomach is responsible for the mixing and grinding of ingested solid food particles. This activity involves repetitive forceful contractions of the midportion and antral portion of the stomach, causing food particles to be propelled against a closed pylorus, with subsequent retropulsion of solids and liquids. The net effect is a thorough mixing of solids and liquids and sequential shearing of solid food particles to smaller than 1 mm.

The emptying of gastric contents is influenced by well-coordinated neural and hormonal mediators. Systemic factors, such as anxiety, fear, depression, and exercise, can affect the rate of gastric motility and emptying. Additionally, the chemical and mechanical properties and temperature of the intraluminal contents can influence the rate of gastric emptying. In general, liquids empty more rapidly than solids, and carbohydrates empty more readily than fats. An increase in the concentration or acidity of liquid meals causes a delay in gastric emptying. In addition, hot and cold liquids tend to empty at a slower rate than ambient temperature fluids. These responses to luminal stimuli are regulated by the enteric nervous system. Osmoreceptors and pH-sensitive receptors in the proximal small bowel have also been shown to be involved in the activation of feedback inhibition of gastric emptying. Inhibitory peptides proposed to be active in this setting include CCK, glucagon, vasoactive intestinal peptide, and gastric inhibitory polypeptide.

Abnormal Gastric Motility

Symptoms of abnormal gastric motility are nausea, fullness, early satiety, abdominal pain, and discomfort. Although mechanical obstruction can and should be ruled out with upper endoscopy or radiographic contrast studies, objective evaluation of a patient with a suspected motility disorder can be accomplished with gamma scintigraphy, real-time ultrasound, and magnetic resonance imaging (MRI). Gastric motility disorders usually encountered in clinical practice are gastric dysmotility after vagotomy, gastroparesis (secondary to diabetes, idiopathic, or medication related), and gastric motility dysfunction related to *H. pylori* infection. Vagotomy results in loss of receptive relaxation and gastric accommodation in response to meal ingestion, with resultant early satiety, postprandial bloating, accelerated emptying of liquids, and delay in emptying of solids. Clinical manifestations of diabetic gastropathy, which can occur in insulin-dependent or non–insulin-dependent patients, closely resemble the clinical picture of postvagotomy gastroparesis. Furthermore, structural changes have been identified in the vagus nerve of patients with diabetes, suggesting that a diabetic autonomic neuropathy may be responsible. However, the metabolic effects of diabetes have also been implicated. Specifically, hyperglycemia has been shown to cause a decrease in contractility of the gastric antrum, increase in pyloric contractility, and suppression of the migrating motor complex. Suppression of migrating motor complex activity is thought to be responsible for the accumulation of gastric bezoars seen in some

diabetic patients. In contrast, hyperinsulinemia, which is often associated with non–insulin-dependent diabetes, may play a role in the gastroparesis seen in non–insulin-dependent diabetes because it also leads to suppression of migrating motor complex activity.

Patients with *H. pylori* infection and nonulcer dyspepsia have also been demonstrated to have impaired gastric emptying accompanied by a reduction in gastric compliance. In rats, lipopolysaccharide derived from *H. pylori* causes a reduction in gastric emptying of a liquid meal for up to 12 hours by an unknown mechanism.

Gastric-Emptying Studies

There are numerous ways to assess gastric emptying. The saline load test is perhaps the simplest and is accomplished by instilling a known volume of saline into the stomach and aspirating the amount remaining at a certain time. Fluoroscopic procedures can also provide information on gastric emptying and may reveal mechanical causes that could contribute to a delay, such as gastric outlet obstruction. However, computerized radionucleotide scans are more commonly used to assess gastric emptying. This scintigraphy study is performed using a meal of radiolabeled egg whites. Scans are obtained immediately after ingestion of the meal, and at 1, 2, and 4 hours after the meal. Measurement of residual gastric contents at 4 hours provides the most sensitive means for diagnosing gastroparesis, as many patients with gastroparesis have equivocal results at 2 hours. Retention of greater than 60% of the meal at 2 hours or 10% at 4 hours indicates an abnormal study. At 4 hours, retention of 10% to 15% signifies mild gastroparesis; 15% to 35%, moderate; and greater than 35%, severe.

Treatment

Regardless of the cause of gastroparesis, initial treatment consists of modification of diet and environmental factors. Patients should be encouraged to eat multiple, small meals with little fat or fiber. Medications that affect gastric motility, such as opioids, calcium channel blockers, tricyclic antidepressants, and dopamine agonists, should be avoided and stopped when possible. Glycemic control should be optimized in diabetic patients. First-line medical therapy consisting of metoclopramide (Reglan), a dopamine antagonist that stimulates antral contractions, and erythromycin, a motilin agonist that acts by stimulating fundal contraction, has been shown to have some benefit, although the evidence is more compelling in diabetic patients.

Surgery for gastroparesis is rarely required, partly because poor improvement in symptoms was observed historically after traditional open operations including gastrojejunostomy and even gastrectomy. However, several less invasive and more effective options have been introduced more recently suggesting that surgery may play a larger role in the treatment of gastroparesis in the future. Pyloromyotomy and pyloroplasty are options for the surgical management of gastroparesis that function by lowering outflow resistance at the pylorus and enhancing any remaining gastric contractility. These operations can be performed laparoscopically, and a series of laparoscopic Heineke-Mikulicz pyloroplasties showed symptom improvement in 82% of patients with a reduction in gastric-emptying half-time from 180 minutes to 60 minutes, with few perioperative complications.[2] Surgical implantation of gastric electrostimulators has also been used as a treatment for refractory idiopathic and diabetic gastroparesis. In this technique, electrical leads are placed onto the antrum laparoscopically and connected to a subcutaneously positioned simulator that delivers high-frequency, low-energy current. In an initial crossover blinded study, patients had less vomiting when their simulator was activated compared with the off period of the study.[3] Although two subsequent trials, one involving patients with diabetes and the other patients with idiopathic gastroparesis, were unable to replicate these positive results during their blinded crossover periods, both showed an improvement in symptoms during a year-long unblinded stimulation period. Based on these data, the ultimate role and benefit of gastric simulation in the treatment of gastroparesis have yet to be conclusively determined.

Gastric Barrier Function

Gastric barrier function depends on physiologic and anatomic factors. Blood flow plays a critical role in gastric mucosal defense by providing nutrients and delivering oxygen to ensure that the intracellular processes that underlie mucosal resistance to injury can proceed unabated. Decreased gastric mucosal blood flow has minimal effects on ulcer formation until it approaches 50% of normal. When blood flow is reduced by more than 75%, marked mucosal injury results, which is exacerbated in the presence of luminal acid. After damage occurs, injured surface epithelial cells are replaced rapidly by the migration of surface mucous cells located along the basement membranes. This process is referred to as *restitution* or *reconstitution*. It occurs within minutes and does not require cell division.

Exposure of the stomach to noxious agents causes a reduction in the potential difference across the gastric mucosa. In normal gastric mucosa, the potential difference across the mucosa is −30 to −50 mV and results from the active transport of chloride into the lumen and sodium into the blood by the activity of Na^+, K^+-ATPase. Damage disrupts the tight junctions between mucosal cells, causing the epithelium to become leaky to ions (i.e., Na^+ and Cl^-) and a resultant loss of the high transepithelial electrical resistance normally found in gastric mucosa. In addition, damaging agents such as NSAIDs or aspirin possess carboxyl groups that are nonionized at a low intragastric pH because they are weak acids. Consequently, they readily enter the cell membranes of gastric mucosal cells because they are now lipid-soluble, whereas they will not penetrate the cell membranes at neutral pH because they are ionized. On entry into the neutral pH environment found in the cytosol, they become reionized, do not exit the cell membrane, and are toxic to the mucosal cells.

PEPTIC ULCER DISEASE

Epidemiology

Peptic ulcers are defined as erosions in the gastric or duodenal mucosa that extend through the muscularis mucosae. The incidence and prevalence of PUD in developed countries, including the United States, have been declining in recent years, as has the progression to complicated PUD, such as perforation and gastric outlet obstruction. This change is likely due to increases in the detection and eradication of *H. pylori* infection, the primary cause of PUD. A systematic review of epidemiologic studies of PUD reported a pooled annual incidence of 0.10% to 0.19% and an overall prevalence of 0.12% to 1.50%, with most studies showing a decline in rates of PUD over the last several decades. Although the incidence and hospitalization rates for PUD have been decreasing since the 1980s, it remains one of the most prevalent and costly GI diseases. Medical costs associated with PUD are an estimated $5.65 billion annually. An estimated 15,000 operations are performed each year in patients hospitalized with PUD.

Significant progress has been made over the past 2 decades, with total admissions for PUD decreasing by almost 30%. Admissions for complications of ulcer disease have also been decreasing, which has led to a significant decrease in ulcer-related mortality, from 3.9% in 1993 to 2.7% in 2006. Although overall mortality remains low, this still represents more than 4000 deaths caused by PUD each year.

The role of surgery in the treatment of ulcer disease has also decreased primarily as a result of a marked decline in elective surgical therapy for chronic disease, as the percentage of patients who require emergent surgery for complicated disease has remained constant, at 7% of hospitalized patients. This represents greater than 11,000 surgical procedures annually.

Much of this decline in ulcer incidence and the need for hospitalization has stemmed from increased knowledge of ulcer pathogenesis. Specifically, the role of *H. pylori* has been defined, and the risks of long-term NSAID use have been better elucidated. It is hoped that an increase in *H. pylori* eradication will result in not only a decrease of elective surgical procedures but also a decline in complications and mortality from emergent complications.

Pathogenesis

Peptic ulcers are caused by increased aggressive factors, decreased defensive factors, or both. Mucosal damage and subsequent ulceration result. Protective (or defensive) factors include mucosal bicarbonate secretion, mucus production, blood flow, growth factors, cell renewal, and endogenous prostaglandins. Damaging (or aggressive) factors include hydrochloric acid secretion, pepsins, ethanol ingestion, smoking, duodenal reflux of bile, ischemia, NSAIDs, hypoxia, and, most notably, *H. pylori* infection. Although it is now clear that most ulcers are caused by *H. pylori* infection or NSAID use, it is still important to understand all of the other protective and causative factors to optimize treatment and ulcer healing and prevent disease recurrence.

Helicobacter pylori Infection

It is now believed that 80% to 95% of duodenal ulcers and approximately 75% of gastric ulcers are associated with *H. pylori* infection. Infection with *H. pylori* has been shown to temporally precede ulcer formation, and when this organism is eradicated as part of ulcer treatment, ulcer recurrence is extremely rare. These observations have secured the place of *H. pylori* as the primary causative factor in the pathogenesis of PUD. *H. pylori* is a spiral or helical gram-negative rod with four to six flagella that resides in gastric-type epithelium within or beneath the mucous layer. This location protects the bacteria from acid and antibiotics. Its shape and flagella aid its movement through the mucous layer, and it produces enzymes that help it adapt to this hostile environment. Most notably, *H. pylori* is a potent producer of urease, which is capable of splitting urea into ammonia and bicarbonate, creating an alkaline microenvironment in the setting of an acidic gastric milieu. However, the secretion of this enzyme facilitates detection of the organism. *H. pylori* organisms are microaerophilic and can live only in gastric epithelium. Thus, *H. pylori* can also be found in heterotopic gastric mucosa in the proximal esophagus, in Barrett esophagus, in gastric metaplasia in the duodenum, within a Meckel's diverticulum, and in heterotopic gastric mucosa in the rectum.

The mechanisms responsible for *H. pylori*–induced GI injury are not fully elucidated, but the following four potential mechanisms have been proposed and likely interact to cause a derangement of normal gastric and duodenal physiology that leads to subsequent ulcer formation:

1. Production of toxic products that cause local tissue injury. Locally produced toxic mediators include breakdown products from urease activity (e.g., ammonia); cytotoxins; a mucinase that degrades mucus and glycoproteins; phospholipases that damage epithelial cells and mucous cells; and platelet-activating factor, which is known to cause mucosal injury and thrombosis in the microcirculation.
2. Induction of a local mucosal immune response. *H. pylori* can also cause a local inflammatory reaction in the gastric mucosa, attracting neutrophils and monocytes, which then produce numerous proinflammatory cytokines and reactive oxygen metabolites.
3. Increased gastrin levels with a resultant increase in acid secretion. In patients with *H. pylori* infection, basal and stimulated gastrin levels are significantly increased, presumably secondary to a reduction in antral D cells because of infection with *H. pylori*. However, the association of acid secretion with *H. pylori* is not as straightforward. Although *H. pylori*–positive healthy volunteers had a small increase or no increase in acid secretion compared with *H. pylori*–negative volunteers, *H. pylori*–infected patients with duodenal ulcers did have a marked increase in acid secretion. A decrease in serum levels of somatostatin as a result of *H. pylori* infection, which increases gastrin and acid secretion, could be the underlying causative mechanism behind the gastric hyperacidity.
4. Gastric metaplasia occurring in the duodenum. Metaplastic replacement of areas of duodenal mucosa with gastric epithelium likely occurs as a protective response to decreased duodenal pH, resulting from the above-described acid hypersecretion; this allows for *H. pylori* to colonize these areas of the duodenum, which causes duodenitis and likely predisposes to duodenal ulcer formation. The presence of *H. pylori* in the duodenum is more common in patients with ulcer formation compared with patients with asymptomatic infections isolated to the stomach.

Peptic ulcers are also strongly associated with antral gastritis. Studies performed before the *H. pylori* era demonstrated that almost all patients with peptic ulcers have histologic evidence of antral gastritis. It was later found that the only patients with gastric ulcers and no gastritis were those ingesting aspirin. It is now recognized that most cases of histologic gastritis are caused by *H. pylori* infection. Of patients with NSAID-associated ulcers, 25% have evidence of a histologic antral gastritis compared with 95% of patients with non–NSAID-associated ulcers. In most cases, the infection tends to be confined initially to the antrum and results in antral inflammation. The causative role of *H. pylori* infection in the pathogenesis of gastritis and PUD was first elucidated by Marshall and Warren in Australia in 1984. To prove this connection, Marshall himself ingested inocula of *H. pylori* after first confirming that he had normal gross and microscopic gastric mucosa. Within days, he developed abdominal pain, nausea, and halitosis as well as histologically confirmed presence of gastric *H. pylori* infection. Acute inflammation was observed histologically on days 5 and 10. By 2 weeks, acute inflammation had been replaced by chronic inflammation with evidence of a mononuclear cell infiltration. For their pioneering work, Marshall and Warren were jointly awarded the Nobel Prize in Medicine in 2005.

H. pylori infection usually occurs in childhood, and spontaneous remission is rare. There is an inverse relationship between infection and socioeconomic status. The reasons for this relationship are poorly understood, but it seems to be the result of factors such as sanitary conditions, familial clustering, and crowding. Such factors likely explain why developing countries have a comparatively higher rate of *H. pylori* infection, especially in children.

Numerous studies have demonstrated what appears to be a steady linear increase in the acquisition of *H. pylori* infection with age, especially in the United States and northern European nations. In the United States, *H. pylori* prevalence also varies among racial and ethnic groups.

H. pylori infection is associated with many common upper GI disorders, but most infected individuals are asymptomatic. Healthy U.S. blood donors have an overall prevalence of approximately 20% to 55%. *H. pylori* infection is almost always present in the setting of active chronic gastritis and is present in most patients with duodenal (80% to 95%) and gastric (60% to 90%) ulcers. Noninfected patients with gastric ulcers tend to be NSAID users. There is a weaker association with nonulcer dyspepsia. In addition, most patients with gastric cancer have current or past *H. pylori* infection. Although the association between *H. pylori* and cancer is strong, no causal relationship has been proven. However, *H. pylori*–induced chronic gastritis and intestinal metaplasia are thought to play a role. A meta-analysis of case-control studies comparing *H. pylori*–positive and *H. pylori*–negative individuals found that infection was associated with a twofold increased risk of developing gastric cancer. There is also a strong association between mucosa-associated lymphoid tissue (MALT) lymphoma and *H. pylori* infection. Regression of these lymphomas has been demonstrated after eradication of *H. pylori*.

Limited data are available to estimate the lifetime risk of PUD in patients with *H. pylori* infection. In a longitudinal study from Australia with a mean evaluation period of 18 years, 15% of *H. pylori*–positive subjects developed verified duodenal ulcer compared with 3% of seronegative individuals. In a 10-year study of patients with asymptomatic gastritis, 11% of patients with histologic gastritis developed PUD over a 10-year period compared with only 1% of patients without gastritis. Another factor implicating a causative role for *H. pylori* and ulcer formation is that eradication of *H. pylori* dramatically reduces ulcer recurrence. Many prospective trials showed that patients with *H. pylori* infection and non–NSAID-related ulcer disease who have documented eradication of the organism almost never (<2%) develop recurrent ulcers.

Nonsteroidal Anti-Inflammatory Drugs

Hospitalizations for bleeding upper GI lesions have increased together with the increased use of NSAIDs. The risk for bleeding and ulceration is proportional to the daily dosage of NSAIDs. The risk also increases with age older than 60 years, patients having a prior GI event, or concurrent use of steroids or anticoagulants. Consequently, the ingestion of NSAIDs is an important factor in ulcer pathogenesis, especially in regard to the development of complications and death.

NSAIDs are absorbed through the stomach and small intestine and function as systemic inhibitors of the cyclooxygenase enzymes. Cyclooxygenase enzymes form the rate-limiting step of prostaglandin synthesis in the GI tract. Prostaglandins promote gastric and duodenal mucosal protection via numerous mechanisms, including increasing mucin and bicarbonate secretion and increasing blood flow to the mucosal endothelium. The presence of NSAIDs disrupts these naturally protective mechanisms, increasing the risk of peptic ulcer formation in the stomach and the duodenum.

More than 3 million people in the United States use NSAIDs daily. Compared with the general population, NSAID users have a 2-fold to 10-fold increased risk for GI complications. The risk for mucosal injury or ulceration is roughly proportional to the anti-inflammatory effect associated with each NSAID. Compared with *H. pylori* ulcers, which are more frequently found in the duodenum, NSAID-induced ulcers are more often found in the stomach. *H. pylori* ulcers are also almost always associated with chronic active gastritis, whereas gastritis is not frequently found with NSAID-induced ulcers, occurring only approximately 25% of the time. When NSAID use is discontinued, the ulcers usually do not recur.

Acid

Acid plays an important but likely noncausative role in the formation of ulcers. In duodenal ulcers, there is a large overlap of acid levels between patients with ulcers and normal subjects. Almost 70% of patients with duodenal ulcers have an acid output within the normal range. Acid levels alone provide little information, and acid secretory testing is of little value in establishing a diagnosis of duodenal ulcer.

For types I and IV gastric ulcers, which are not associated with excessive acid secretion, acid acts as an important cofactor, exacerbating the underlying ulcer damage and attenuating the ability of the stomach to heal. For patients with type II or III gastric ulcers, gastric acid hypersecretion seems to be more common, and consequently these ulcers behave more like duodenal ulcers.

Duodenal Ulcer

Duodenal ulcer is a disease with numerous causes. The only requirements are acid and pepsin secretion in combination with infection by *H. pylori* or ingestion of NSAIDs.

Clinical Manifestations

Abdominal pain. Patients with duodenal ulcer disease can present in various ways. The most common symptom associated with duodenal ulcer disease is midepigastric abdominal pain that is usually well localized. The pain is generally tolerable and frequently relieved by food. The pain may be episodic, seasonal in the spring and fall, and worse during periods of emotional stress. Many patients do not seek medical attention until they have had the disease for many years. When the pain becomes constant, this suggests that there is deeper penetration of the ulcer. Referral of pain to the back is usually a sign of penetration into the pancreas. Diffuse peritoneal irritation is usually a sign of free perforation.

Diagnosis

History and physical examination are of limited value in distinguishing between gastric and duodenal ulceration. Routine laboratory studies include complete blood count; liver chemistries; and serum creatinine, serum amylase, and calcium levels. A serum gastrin level should also be obtained in patients with ulcers that are refractory to medical therapy or require surgery. An upright chest radiograph is usually performed when ruling out perforation. The two principal means of diagnosing duodenal ulcers are upper GI radiography and flexible upper endoscopy. Upper GI radiography is less expensive, and most (90%) ulcers can be diagnosed accurately by this means. However, approximately 5% of ulcers that appear radiographically benign are malignant. Because of the need to perform a biopsy to rule out malignancy, upper

endoscopy has replaced upper GI radiography as the primary test for the diagnosis and evaluation of PUD. Also, endoscopy has the advantage of being able to evaluate for other pathologies of the esophagus, stomach, and duodenum in addition to PUD that may be causing the patient's symptoms, such as esophagitis and gastritis. *H. pylori* testing should also be done in all patients with suspected PUD.

Upper gastrointestinal radiography. Diagnosis of duodenal ulcer by upper GI radiography requires the demonstration of barium within the ulcer crater, which is usually round or oval and may or may not be surrounded by edema. This study is useful to determine the location and depth of penetration of the ulcer and the extent of deformation from chronic fibrosis. A characteristic barium radiograph of a peptic ulcer is shown in Figure 48-9. The ability to detect ulcers on radiography requires the technical skills and abilities of the radiologist but also depends on the size and location of the ulcer. With single-contrast radiographic techniques, 50% of duodenal ulcers may be missed, whereas with double-contrast studies, 80% to 90% of ulcer craters can be detected. Despite this increased accuracy with double-contrast techniques, upper GI radiography has largely been replaced by flexible upper endoscopy as the method of choice for diagnosis and evaluation of gastric and duodenal ulcers.

Flexible upper endoscopy. Endoscopy is the most reliable method for diagnosing gastric and duodenal ulcers. In addition to providing a visual diagnosis, endoscopy provides the ability to sample tissue to evaluate for malignancy and *H. pylori* infection and may be used for therapeutic purposes in the setting of GI bleeding or obstruction.

Endoscopic evaluation of the stomach and duodenum has been shown to confirm a visual diagnosis of more than 90% of peptic ulcers, and this value is likely higher today with the use of high-definition endoscopes. When an ulcer has been detected endoscopically, biopsy is recommended in all cases to rule out malignancy. Larger ulcers and ulcers with irregular or heaped

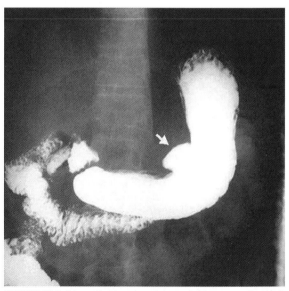

FIGURE 48-9 A large, benign-appearing gastric ulcer protrudes medially from the lesser curvature of the stomach *(arrow)*, just above the gastric incisura. (Courtesy Dr. Agnes Guthrie, Department of Radiology, University of Texas Medical School, Houston, TX.)

edges are more likely to harbor cancers. Multiple biopsy specimens should be taken of the ulcer for maximum diagnostic yield. An early study of the usefulness of endoscopic biopsy showed that the first biopsy sample taken of an ulcer had only a 70% sensitivity in detecting gastric cancer, whereas taking four biopsy specimens increased this yield to 95% and taking seven specimens increased it to 98%.

Helicobacter pylori *testing.* The gold standard for diagnosis of *H. pylori* is mucosal biopsy performed during upper endoscopy, but noninvasive tests offer an effective screening tool and do not require an endoscopic procedure. If endoscopy is to be performed, evaluation of biopsy samples with either a urease assay or histologic examination offers excellent diagnostic accuracy. Evaluation of serum antibodies is the test of choice for initial diagnosis when endoscopy is not required but has the drawback of remaining positive after treatment and eradication of infection. For monitoring treatment efficacy, stool antigen and urea breath testing are better choices.

Invasive Tests

Urease assay. Endoscopic biopsy specimens should be taken from the gastric body and the antrum and are then tested for urease. Sensitivity in diagnosing infection is greater than 90%, and specificity is 95% to 100%, meaning there are almost never false-positive results. However, the sensitivity of the test is lowered in patients who are taking PPIs, H_2 antagonists, or antibiotics. Rapid urease test kits are commercially available and can detect urease in gastric biopsy specimens within 1 hour with a similar level of diagnostic accuracy.

Histology. Endoscopy can also be performed with biopsy samples of gastric mucosa, followed by histologic visualization of *H. pylori* using routine hematoxylin-eosin stains or special stains (e.g., silver, Giemsa, Genta stains) for improved visibility. Sensitivity is approximately 95% and specificity is 99%, making histology slightly more accurate than the urease assay testing. Similar to urease assay, the sensitivity of histologic evaluation is lowered in patients taking PPIs or H_2 antagonists, but it remains the most accurate test available even in this setting. Histology additionally affords the physician the ability to assess the severity of gastritis and confirm the presence or absence of the organism; however, it is a more expensive option for evaluation of biopsy samples than the urease assay.

Culture. Culturing of gastric mucosa obtained at endoscopy can also be performed to diagnose *H. pylori*. The sensitivity is approximately 80%, and specificity is 100%. However, culture requires laboratory expertise, is not widely available, and is relatively expensive, and diagnosis requires 3 to 5 days. Nevertheless, it provides the opportunity to perform antibiotic sensitivity testing on isolates, if needed.

Noninvasive Tests

Serology. There are various enzyme-linked immunosorbent assay laboratory-based tests available and some rapid office-based immunoassays that are used to test for the presence of IgG antibodies to *H. pylori*. Serology has a 90% sensitivity but a more variable specificity rate between 76% and 96%, and tests need to be locally validated based on the prevalence of specific bacterial strains. Antibody titers can remain high for 1 year or longer; consequently, this test cannot be used to assess eradication after therapy. For these reasons, stool antigen and urea breath tests are the preferred modalities for diagnosis and evaluation of treatment efficacy in patients with PUD and suspected *H. pylori* infection.

Urea breath test. The carbon-labeled urea breath test is based on the ability of *H. pylori* to hydrolyze urea as a result of its production of urease. Both sensitivity and specificity are greater than 95%. As with other testing modalities, the sensitivity of the urea breath test is reduced in patients taking antisecretory medications and antibiotics. It is recommended that patients discontinue antibiotics for 4 weeks and PPIs for 2 weeks to ensure optimal test accuracy. The urea breath test is less expensive than endoscopy and samples the entire stomach. In evaluating treatment efficacy, false-negative results can occur if the test is performed too soon after treatment, so it is usually best to perform this test 4 weeks after therapy is completed.

Stool antigen. *H. pylori* bacteria are present in the stool of infected patients, and several assays have been developed that use monoclonal antibodies to *H. pylori* antigens to test fecal specimens. These tests have demonstrated sensitivities of greater than 90% and sensitivities of 86% to 92%.[1] Several studies demonstrated that stool antigen testing has an accuracy of greater than 90% in detecting eradication of infection after treatment, on par with invasive histology and noninvasive urea breath testing. Additionally, stool antigen testing is likely the most cost-effective method for assessing treatment efficacy.

Treatment

Medical management. Antiulcer drugs fall into three broad categories—drugs targeted against *H. pylori*, drugs that reduce acid levels by decreasing secretion or chemical neutralization, and drugs that increase the mucosal protective barrier. In patients with PUD and *H. pylori* infection, the focus of therapy is on eradication of the bacteria. In addition to medications, lifestyle changes, such as smoking cessation, discontinuing NSAIDs and aspirin, and avoiding coffee and alcohol, help promote ulcer healing.

Antacids. Antacids are the oldest form of therapy for PUD that reduce gastric acidity by reacting with hydrochloric acid, forming a salt and raising the gastric pH. Antacids differ greatly in their buffering ability, absorption, taste, and side effects. Magnesium antacids tend to be the best buffers but can cause significant diarrhea, whereas acids precipitated with phosphorus can occasionally result in hypophosphatemia and sometimes constipation. Antacids are most effective when ingested 1 hour after a meal because they can be retained in the stomach and exert their buffering action for longer periods. If taken on an empty stomach, antacids are emptied rapidly and have only a transient buffering effect. Because of this transient efficacy, the use of buffering antacids has largely been replaced by antisecretory therapy (either H_2 receptor antagonists or PPIs) for the treatment of PUD.

Sucralfate. Sucralfate is structurally related to heparin but does not have any anticoagulant effects. It has been shown to be effective in the treatment of ulcer disease, although its exact mechanism of action is not entirely understood. It is an aluminum salt of sulfated sucrose that dissociates under the acidic conditions in the stomach. It is hypothesized that the sucrose polymerizes and binds to protein in the ulcer crater to produce a protective coating that can last for 6 hours. It has also been suggested that it may bind and concentrate endogenous basic fibroblast growth factor, which appears to be important for mucosal healing. Treatment with sucralfate for 4 to 6 weeks results in duodenal ulcer healing that is superior to placebo and comparable to treatment with H_2 receptor antagonists such as cimetidine. However, the efficacy and role of sucralfate in healing gastric ulcers and ulcers caused by *H. pylori* infection has not been clearly established, and sucralfate is not included as part of initial treatment guidelines for PUD.

H₂ receptor antagonists. The H_2 receptor antagonists are structurally similar to histamine. Variations in ring structure and side chains cause differences in potency and side effects. Currently available H_2 receptor antagonists differ in their potency but only modestly in half-life and bioavailability. All undergo hepatic metabolism and are excreted by the kidney. Famotidine is the most potent, and cimetidine is the weakest. Continuous intravenous infusion of H_2 receptor antagonists has been shown to produce more uniform acid inhibition than intermittent administration. Many randomized controlled trials have indicated that all H_2 receptor antagonists result in duodenal ulcer healing rates of 70% to 80% after 4 weeks of therapy and 80% to 90% after 8 weeks.

Proton pump inhibitors. The most potent antisecretory agents are PPIs. These agents negate all types of acid secretion from all types of secretagogues. As a result, they provide a more complete and prolonged inhibition of acid secretion than H_2 receptor antagonists. H_2 receptor antagonists and PPIs are effective at night, but PPIs are more effective during the day. PPIs have a healing rate of 85% at 4 weeks and 96% at 8 weeks and produce more rapid healing of ulcers than standard H_2 receptor antagonists (14% advantage at 2 weeks and 9% advantage at 4 weeks). Because of this, PPIs have generally replaced H_2 receptor antagonists as primary therapy for PUD in the presence of and in the absence of *H. pylori* infection. PPIs require an acidic environment within the gastric lumen to become activated; thus, using antacids or H_2 receptor antagonists in combination with PPIs could have deleterious effects by promoting an alkaline environment and preventing activation of the PPIs. Consequently, antacids and H_2 receptor antagonists should not be used in combination with PPIs.

Treatment of helicobacter pylori *infection.* Before the discovery of *H. pylori* infection as the causative agent in greater than 95% of duodenal peptic ulcers, the primary form of treatment was the reduction of acid in the stomach, with or without increasing the protective barrier with drugs such as sucralfate. After it became clear that increased acid secretion was an effect of *H. pylori* infection, there was a paradigm shift that saw PUD as an infectious disease, rather than a consequence of pathologic acid secretion. Accordingly, treatment philosophy has shifted to focus on eradication of the infectious agent.

Current therapy is twofold in its approach, combining antibiotics against *H. pylori* with antacid medications. The primary goal of the antacids is to promote short-term healing by reducing pathologic acid levels and improve symptoms. *H. pylori* eradication helps with initial healing, but its primary efficacy is in preventing recurrence. There have been numerous trials comparing eradication therapy with ulcer-healing drugs alone or no treatment. Eradication of *H. pylori* has shown recurrence rates of 2%, with initial healing rates of 90%. Eradication rates after an initial course of therapy have been increasing, likely as a result of increased prevalence of antibiotic-resistant strains of *H. pylori;* at the present time, approximately 20% of patients fail initial therapy. For this reason, monitoring for infection eradication with a urea breath test, stool antigen, or repeat endoscopy with biopsy at 4 to 6 weeks after therapy is important, and many patients will require further treatment with alternative regimens.

The treatment of *H. pylori*–positive peptic duodenal ulcer disease is triple therapy aimed at the eradication of *H. pylori*, along with acid suppression (Box 48-1). This triple therapy includes a PPI and two antibiotics, usually amoxicillin (1 g BID) with clarithromycin (500 mg twice daily). In patients with penicillin allergies, metronidazole (500 mg twice daily) is substituted for

---

> **BOX 48-1   National Institutes of Health Consensus Panel Recommendations for *Helicobacter pylori* Treatment**
>
> Patients with active PUD who are *H. pylori*–positive
> - Use of NSAIDs should not alter treatment
> - Document eradication in patients with complications
>
> Ulcer patients in remission who are *H. pylori*–positive, including patients on maintenance H_2 receptor antagonist therapy
>
> *H. pylori*–positive patients with MALT lymphoma
>
> Controversial issues in *H. pylori*–positive patients
> - First-degree relatives of patients with gastric cancer
> - Immigrants from countries with high prevalence of gastric cancer
> - Individuals with gastric cancer precursor lesions (intestinal metaplasia)
> - Patients with dyspepsia not resulting from ulcer who insist on eradication (benefit versus risk)
> - Patients on long-term antisecretory therapy for reflux disease

---

> **BOX 48-2   Surgical Treatment Recommendations for Complications Related to Peptic Duodenal Ulcer Disease**
>
> Intractable: Parietal cell vagotomy ± antrectomy
> Bleeding: Oversewing of bleeding vessel with treatment of *H. pylori*
> Perforation: Patch closure with treatment of *H. pylori*
> Obstruction: Rule out malignancy and gastrojejunostomy with treatment of *H. pylori*

---

amoxicillin. In areas with high rates of clarithromycin resistance (>15% to 20%), it may be beneficial to substitute tetracycline, or another antibiotic, for initial therapy. Clinical guidelines generally recommend treatment with a 14-day course of triple therapy[4]; however, this is controversial, as a meta-analysis of randomized trials comparing treatment lengths found no significant increase in eradication rates when regimens of 7 days were compared with 10-day and 14-day schedules.[5] Side effects, which are generally mild and resolve with cessation of treatment, include diarrhea, nausea and vomiting, rash, and altered taste. For the 20% of patients with refractory disease, a treatment course with new antibiotics, such as metronidazole and tetracycline, is initiated, and quadruple therapy with the addition of bismuth is recommended.

Complicated Ulcer Disease

Ulcer disease was previously within the scope of the general surgeon, with ulcer surgery forming a major part of general surgery practice. With the shift in understanding of the disease from one primarily of aberrant acid physiology to one of infectious disease, this situation has changed significantly, with most patients with ulcers being treated and cured medically. The surgeon's role now is primarily to treat the approximately 20% of patients who have a complication from their disease, which includes hemorrhage, perforation, and obstruction (Box 48-2). Frequently included in discussions of complicated ulcer disease is an intractable ulcer. Although intractable disease no doubt exists, its definition is nebulous, and determining exactly when and what type of surgical intervention are required is primarily a matter of judgment. In the current era of excellent treatment options for *H.*

pylori infection and acid suppression, few patients who are truly compliant with medical therapy develop intractable ulcer disease in the absence of malignancy.

Hemorrhage. Upper GI bleeding is a relatively common problem, with an annual incidence of approximately 1 per 1000. Most nonvariceal bleeding (70%) is attributable to peptic ulcers. Most bleeding stops spontaneously and requires no intervention. However, persistent bleeding is associated with a 6% to 8% mortality. Several clinical scores have been created to risk-stratify patients presenting with upper GI bleeding to predict risk of rebleeding and overall morbidity and mortality. The most commonly used scores are the Blatchford and Rockall prediction scores.[6,7] The Blatchford score (Table 48-3) incorporates the patient's blood urea, hemoglobin, blood pressure, and other clinical parameters to predict the need for therapeutic intervention with transfusion, endoscopy, or surgery. A score of greater than zero has a sensitivity of 99% in predicting the need for such an intervention, and the score can serve as a useful screening tool for determining which patients are at risk for serious bleeding on initial presentation. The Rockall score (see Table 48-3) uses clinical variables and the findings of initial upper endoscopy to predict the risk of rebleeding and in-hospital mortality and is more helpful in determining whether a surgical intervention may be required after the patient has been initially resuscitated and evaluated.

The initial approach to an upper GI bleed is similar to the approach to a trauma patient. Large-bore intravenous access, rapid restoration of intravascular volume with fluid and blood products as the clinical situation dictates, and close monitoring for signs of rebleeding all are essential to effective management of these patients. The role of nasogastric (NG) lavage remains debatable; however, it can be useful as a predictor of high-risk patients and as an aid for later endoscopic intervention. Patients with bright red blood on NG lavage, as opposed to clear or coffee-ground lavage, are at much higher risk for persistent bleeding or rebleeding and warrant endoscopic intervention. If the NG lavage returns bilious fluid without blood, indicating the duodenal as well as gastric contents have been sampled, a lower GI source of bleeding (i.e., one distal to the ligament of Treitz) should be considered. In addition to its diagnostic usefulness, the NG tube can be used to lavage the stomach and duodenum before endoscopy, removing the clot and old blood that could obscure visualization of the source of bleeding. Given its relatively low risk and potential benefit, NG tube placement should be part of the treatment algorithm for these patients after appropriate intravascular access has been established and resuscitation begun.

Upper flexible endoscopy is the best initial procedure for diagnosis of the source of upper GI bleeding and for therapeutic intervention, especially in the setting of bleeding ulcers. Almost all patients with a potentially substantial acute upper GI bleed should undergo endoscopy within 24 hours. Although the data are inconclusive, early endoscopy has been shown to be a cost-effective strategy by triaging patients to more rapid intervention, if warranted, and by identifying low-risk patients without the need for prolonged observation (and therefore earlier hospital discharge). Additionally, more recent data from retrospective series using multivariate regression analysis to adjust for confounding variables suggest that early endoscopic intervention (within 12 hours from presentation) results in shorter hospital length of stay and possibly lower mortality in high-risk patients.[8]

Patients who are noted on endoscopy to have active bleeding, via an arterial jet or oozing, an adherent clot, or a visible vessel within the ulcer, are at high risk, and intervention is required. Patients without active bleeding, no visible vessel, and a clean

TABLE 48-3 Blatchford and Rockall Prediction Scores for Upper Gastrointestinal Bleeding

BLATCHFORD CLINICAL PREDICTION SCORE FOR UPPER GI BLEEDING[6]

VARIABLE	SCORE					
	0	1	2	3	4	6
Blood urea (mmol/liter)	<6.5		6.5-8	8-10	10-25	>25
Hemoglobin (g/dL) for men	>13	12-13		10-12		<10
Hemoglobin (g/dL) for women	>12	10-12				<10
Systolic BP (mmHg)	>109	100-109	90-99	<90		
Other factors		Pulse >100, presentation with melena	Presentation with syncope, hepatic disease, cardiac failure			

ROCKALL CLINICAL PREDICTION SCORE FOR UPPER GI BLEEDING[7]

VARIABLE	SCORE			
	0	1	2	3
Age	<60	60-79	>79	
Shock	Systolic BP ≥100 mm Hg and pulse <100	Systolic BP ≥100 mm Hg and pulse ≥100	Systolic BP <100 mm Hg	
Comorbidities	No major comorbidities		Heart failure, ischemic heart disease, other major comorbidity	Renal failure, liver failure, metastatic cancer
Diagnosis	Mallory-Weiss tear, no lesion identified, and no stigmata of recent bleeding	All other diagnoses	Upper GI malignancy	
Stigmata of recent hemorrhage	None or dark spot only		Blood in upper GI tract, adherent clot, visible or spurting vessel	

BP, Blood pressure.

TABLE 48-4 **Forrest Classification of Stigmata of Recent Hemorrhage on Endoscopic Examination of Peptic Ulcers and Relative Prevalence**

STIGMATA OF RECENT HEMORRHAGE	FORREST CLASSIFICATION	PREVALENCE (%) ON INPATIENT ENDOSCOPY PERFORMED FOR UPPER GI BLEEDING*
Active bleeding		10.7 (both spurting and oozing)
Active spurting	IA	
Active oozing	IB	
Recent hemorrhage		
Nonbleeding vessel	IIA	7.2
Adherent clot	IIB	7.1
Flat pigmented spot	IIC	14.3
No signs of hemorrhage		
Clean-based ulcer	III	48.6

From Enestvedt BK, Gralnek IM, Mattek N, et al: An evaluation of endoscopic indications and findings related to nonvariceal upper-GI hemorrhage in a large multicenter consortium. *Gastrointest Endosc* 67:422–429, 2008.
*The ulcer appearance was not described in 12.1% of patients.

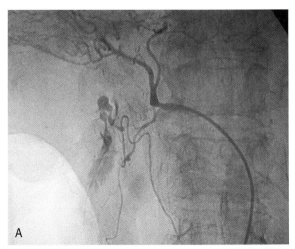

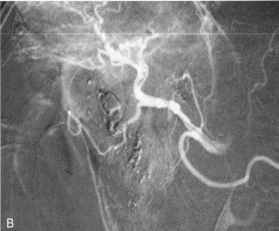

FIGURE 48-10 Endovascular control of a bleeding duodenal ulcer. **A,** An angiogram is obtained, which shows extravasation from a branch off of the gastroduodenal artery. **B,** A completion angiogram after glue embolization of the vessel shows resolution of the bleed with preservation of flow through the gastroduodenal artery. (From Loffroy R, Guiu B, Cercueil JP, et al: Refractory bleeding from gastroduodenal ulcers: Arterial embolization in high-operative-risk patients. *J Clin Gastroenterol* 42:361–367, 2008.)

ulcer base are low risk and do not require further intervention. The most commonly used system for classifying the endoscopic appearance of bleeding ulcers is the Forrest classification (Table 48-4), which stratifies the risk of rebleeding based on observed "stigmata of recent hemorrhage." Lower risk ulcers are much more frequently encountered than actively bleeding ones, even in the setting of inpatients undergoing endoscopy for diagnosis of upper GI bleeding. All patients undergoing endoscopic examination should be tested for *H. pylori* status. For high-risk patients requiring intervention, the best initial approach is endoscopic control, which results in primary hemostasis in approximately 90% of patients. The most common method of control is injection of a vasoconstrictor at the site of bleeding. With this method alone, primary hemostasis rates are high, but up to 30% of patients have rebleeding. This situation has led to the development of new techniques, including use of a second vasoconstrictor or sclerosing agent, thermocoagulation, and placement of clips at the site of bleeding. A 2009 meta-analysis compared the use of epinephrine alone with other forms of endoscopic monotherapy, most commonly thermal therapy or clips, and found these other approaches to be more effective in preventing rebleeding.[9] A dual approach, using epinephrine injection along with either thermal therapy or clips, showed an even better reduction in rebleeding rate, with a relative risk of 0.3 compared with epinephrine injection alone.

Guidelines for endoscopic control of bleeding published in 2010 advocate either the use of epinephrine plus an additional method or monotherapy with either thermocoagulation or clipping, but discourage the use of epinephrine alone. Although routine repeat endoscopy has not been shown to be beneficial, for patients who have rebleeding, repeat endoscopy does not increase their mortality and should be attempted before surgical intervention as long as the patient remains hemodynamically stable.

All high-risk patients should be placed in a monitored setting, preferably an intensive care unit, until all bleeding has stopped for 24 hours. As part of the 2010 consensus guidelines, all high-risk patients should be placed on a PPI administered intravenously, with an initial bolus followed by continuous infusion or intermittent dosing for up to 72 hours. Compared with a histamine blocker and placebo, intravenous PPI therapy showed lower rebleeding rates, a lower rate of emergency surgery, and decreased mortality. Additionally, high-dose intravenous PPIs were shown to be more effective than PPIs at standard dosing in preventing recurrent bleeding. Patients deemed high risk based on clinical factors who are awaiting endoscopy should begin therapy before endoscopy.

Although flexible upper endoscopy remains the standard first-line therapy for upper GI bleeding, another option for nonsurgical control of bleeding duodenal ulcers is catheter-directed angiography and endovascular embolization (Fig. 48-10). A meta-analysis of studies examining the use of arterial embolization of upper GI bleeding found a pooled technical success rate of 84% in stopping hemorrhage, with prevention of rebleeding in 67% of patients.[10] Another study retrospectively compared the effectiveness of arterial embolization and surgery for recurrent peptic ulcer bleeding after initial endoscopic therapy. Endovascular embolization was found to have higher rates of rebleeding (34% versus 13%, P = .01) but with fewer postintervention complications (41% versus 68%, P = .01). Mortality, transfusion requirements, and hospital length of stay were similar with the two approaches. Although it remains a relatively novel interventional modality, endovascular therapy for peptic ulcer bleeding offers an attractive approach in patients with recurrent bleeding after endoscopy who remain hemodynamically stable, especially patients who are poor surgical candidates based on other medical comorbidities.

Despite the use of PPIs and improved methods of endoscopic control, 5% to 10% of patients have persistent bleeding that requires surgical intervention. This group includes patients who become hemodynamically unstable and patients who continue to bleed and require ongoing blood transfusions (usually >6 U of packed red blood cells). The vessel most likely to be bleeding is the gastroduodenal artery because of erosion from a posterior ulcer. Although bleeding duodenal ulcers can be treated laparoscopically, the more typical approach is through an upper midline laparotomy, especially in patients who are hemodynamically unstable. A Kocher maneuver is performed to mobilize the duodenum. The anterior wall of the duodenal bulb is opened longitudinally, and the incision can be carried across the pylorus. The gastroduodenal artery is oversewn, with a three-point U stitch technique, which effectively ligates the main vessel (superior and inferior stitches) and prevents back-bleeding from any smaller branches (medial stitch), such as the transverse pancreatic artery, that head to the patient's left toward the body of the pancreas. One must be careful to avoid incorporating the common bile duct into the stitch. The course of the common bile duct can be identified by inserting a probe through the ampulla of Vater transduodenally or performing either a retrograde or an anterograde intraoperative cholangiogram. After the bleeding has been controlled, the duodenotomy is closed transversely to avoid narrowing (see Fig. 48-10).

Perforation. Patients with perforation typically complain of sudden-onset, frequently severe epigastric pain. For many, it is their first symptom of ulcer disease. Patients frequently have free air visible on the chest radiograph and have localized peritoneal signs on examination. Patients with more widespread spillage have diffuse peritonitis. For a small subset of patients, the perforation may seal spontaneously; however, operative intervention is required in almost all cases. Perforation has the highest mortality rate of any complication of ulcer disease, approaching 15%.

Perforation is a surgical disease, and conservative management means emergent surgical intervention. The perforation is usually in the first portion of the duodenum and can easily be accessed through an upper midline incision. Perforations smaller than 1 cm can generally be closed primarily and buttressed with a well-vascularized omentum. For larger perforations or ulcers with fibrotic edges that cannot be brought together without tension, a Graham patch repair with a tongue of healthy omentum is performed. Multiple stay sutures are placed that incorporate a bite of healthy tissue on the proximal and the distal side of the ulcer. The omentum is placed underneath these sutures, and they are tied to secure it in place and seal the perforation (Fig. 48-11). For very large perforations (>3 cm), control of the duodenal defect can be difficult. The defect should be closed by the application of

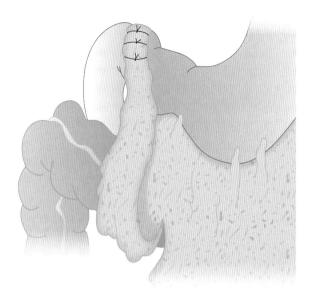

FIGURE 48-11 Graham patch repair of a perforated duodenal ulcer. A "tongue" of omentum is brought up to cover the ulcer defect and secured in position with a series of interrupted sutures. In Graham's original description, the ulcer defect is not closed, but if the tissue edges are healthy and come together without undue tension, a primary closure can be performed and reinforced with an omental patch. (From Baker RJ: Operation for acute perforated duodenal ulcer. In Nyhus LM, Baker RJ, Fischer JE, editors: *Mastery of surgery*, London, 1997, Little, Brown and Company.)

healthy tissue, such as omentum or jejunal serosa from a Roux-en-Y type limb. In such cases, a pyloric exclusion is typically performed by oversewing the pylorus using absorbable suture or stapling across it using a noncutting linear stapler. A gastrojejunostomy is created to bypass the duodenum in a Billroth II or Roux-en-Y fashion. Over several weeks, the pyloric exclusion stitches or staples give way, restoring normal GI anatomy after the perforation site has been given time to heal. Alternatively, a duodenostomy tube can be placed through the perforation with wide peritoneal drainage. Leakage of GI contents into the drain is likely, but in most cases sepsis will resolve. An alternative in this difficult situation is antrectomy and a Billroth II or Roux-en-Y reconstruction.

Perforations can also be treated laparoscopically. The results of two randomized controlled trials showed that patients undergoing laparoscopic repair have, as expected, less pain and parenteral narcotic use. They also have an earlier time to discharge. There was no difference in pulmonary complications or abdominal septic complications. A meta-analysis of studies comparing laparoscopic repair versus open repair, which included the randomized controlled trials along with prospective and retrospective cohort studies, showed overall similar outcomes, with longer operative times for laparoscopic repair.[11] However, these operating times have been decreasing in studies performed after 2001; in a recent randomized controlled trial, laparoscopic repair was faster than open repair. The conversion rate ranged from 10% to 15% in most reports. A case-matched analysis of the National Surgical Quality Improvement Program database comparing the two approaches found shorter hospital length of stay after laparoscopic repair with a trend toward decreased infectious complications postoperatively.[12] Based on these data, in experienced hands, laparoscopy appears to be the superior approach in patients with duodenal perforations who are hemodynamically stable.

For patients who are known to be negative for *H. pylori*, are taking long-term NSAIDs that they cannot discontinue, or have failed medical therapy in the past for their ulcer disease, an acid-reducing procedure can be added at the time of repair. These procedures are discussed later in the chapter and must be based on the clinical situation and comfort of the surgeon.

After repair, the stomach is decompressed until bowel activity returns. Drains should be kept in place until patients have eaten without a change in drain output or quality, which would suggest a leak. A routine contrast radiograph is not required before initiating eating but can be used to evaluate the security of the perforation closure should the patient exhibit symptoms or signs of enteric leak. All *H. pylori*–positive patients should undergo eradication with appropriate triple-therapy regimens.

Gastric outlet obstruction. Acute inflammation of the duodenum can lead to mechanical obstruction, with a functional gastric outlet obstruction manifested by delayed gastric emptying, anorexia, nausea, and vomiting. In cases of prolonged vomiting, patients may become dehydrated and develop a hypochloremic-hypokalemic metabolic alkalosis secondary to the loss of gastric juice rich in hydrogen and chloride. Chronic inflammation of the duodenum may lead to recurrent episodes of healing followed by repair and scarring, ultimately leading to fibrosis and stenosis of the duodenal lumen. In this situation, the obstruction is accompanied by painless vomiting of large volumes of gastric contents, with metabolic abnormalities similar to abnormalities seen in acute obstruction. The stomach can become massively dilated in this setting, and it rapidly loses its muscular tone. Marked weight loss and malnutrition are also common.

Gastric outlet obstruction from ulcer disease is now less common than obstruction from cancer. Cancer must be ruled out with endoscopy. Endoscopic dilation and *H. pylori* eradication are the mainstays of therapy. A study with an almost 5-year follow-up showed that patients who have an identifiable cause (e.g., *H. pylori* infection) that could be treated have good long-term results with endoscopic dilation, with a median of five dilations required, but no subsequent surgical therapy.[13] Patients with idiopathic duodenal ulcer disease causing gastric outlet obstruction who are treated with lifetime acid suppression also have good long-term results with endoscopic dilation. Patients with refractory obstruction are best managed with primary antrectomy and reconstruction along with vagotomy.

Intractable peptic ulcer disease. Intractability is defined as failure of an ulcer to heal after an initial trial of 8 to 12 weeks of therapy or if patients relapse after therapy has been discontinued. Intractable PUD is unusual for duodenal ulcer disease in the *H. pylori* era. Benign gastric ulcers that persist must be evaluated for malignancy. For any intractable ulcer, adequate duration of therapy, *H. pylori* eradication, and elimination of NSAID use must be confirmed. A serum gastrin level should also be determined in patients with ulcers refractory to medical therapy to rule out gastrinoma. Although rarely seen today, intractable duodenal ulcer should be treated with an acid-reducing operation. This can be a truncal vagotomy, selective vagotomy, or highly selective vagotomy, with or without an antrectomy.

Surgical procedures for peptic ulcers. Elective operative intervention has become rare as medical therapy has become more effective. The recognition of *H. pylori* and its eradication suggest that the intractability indication for surgery may apply only to

patients in whom the organism cannot be eradicated or who cannot be taken off NSAIDs. Patients who are noncompliant with acid suppression therapy may also fall into this category.

The goal of operative ulcer therapy is to reduce gastric acid secretion and this can be accomplished by removing vagal stimulation via vagotomy, gastrin-driven secretion by performing an antrectomy, or both. Vagotomy decreases peak acid output by approximately 50%, whereas vagotomy plus antrectomy decreases peak acid output by approximately 85%.

Truncal vagotomy. As shown in Figure 48-4, truncal vagotomy is performed by division of the left and right vagus nerves above the hepatic and celiac branches, just above the GE junction. Truncal vagotomy is probably the most common operation performed for duodenal ulcer disease. Most surgeons use some form of drainage procedure in association with truncal vagotomy. Pyloric relaxation is mediated by vagal stimulation, and a vagotomy without a drainage procedure can cause delayed gastric emptying. Classic truncal vagotomy, in combination with a Heineke-Mikulicz pyloroplasty, is shown in Figure 48-12. When the duodenal bulb is scarred, a Finney pyloroplasty or Jaboulay gastroduodenostomy may be a useful alternative. In general, there is little difference in the side effects associated with the type of drainage procedure performed, although bile reflux may be more common after gastroenterostomy, and diarrhea is more common after pyloroplasty. The incidence of dumping is the same for both.

Selective vagotomy. Selective vagotomy divides the main right and left vagus nerves just distal to the celiac and hepatic branches, and a pyloric drainage procedure is also performed. However,

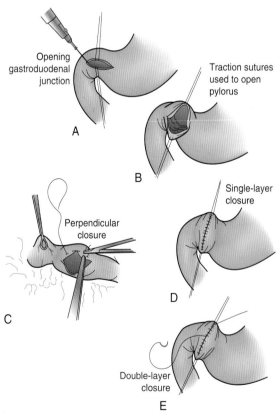

FIGURE 48-12 A-E, Heineke-Mikulicz pyloroplasty. (From Soreide JA, Soreide A: Pyloroplasty. *Oper Tech Gen Surg* 5:65–72, 2003.)

selective vagotomy results in higher ulcer recurrence rates than truncal vagotomy, with no advantage in terms of decreased post-gastrectomy symptoms. For these reasons, selective vagotomy has largely been abandoned as an option for acid-reducing surgery.

Highly selective vagotomy (parietal cell vagotomy). Highly selective vagotomy is also called *parietal cell vagotomy* or *proximal gastric vagotomy*. This procedure was developed after recognition that truncal vagotomy, in combination with a drainage procedure or gastric resection, adversely affects the pyloral antral pump function. A highly selective vagotomy divides only the vagus nerves supplying the acid-producing portion of the stomach within the corpus and fundus. This procedure preserves the vagal innervation of the gastric antrum and pylorus, so there is no need for routine drainage procedures. Consequently, the incidence of postoperative complications is lower. In general, the nerves of Latarjet are identified anteriorly and posteriorly, and the crow's feet innervating the fundus and body of the stomach are divided. These nerves are divided up until a point approximately 7 cm proximal to the pylorus or the area in the vicinity of the gastric antrum. Superiorly, division of these nerves is carried to a point at least 5 cm proximal to the GE junction on the esophagus (Fig. 48-13). Ideally, two or three branches to the antrum and pylorus should be preserved. The criminal nerve of Grassi represents a very proximal branch of the posterior trunk of the vagus, and great attention is needed to avoid missing this branch in the division process because it is frequently cited as a predisposition for ulcer recurrence if left intact.

The recurrence rates after highly selective vagotomy are variable and depend on the skill of the surgeon and duration of follow-up. Lengthy longitudinal follow-up is necessary to evaluate the results of this procedure because of the reported increase in recurrent ulceration with time. Recurrence rates of 10% to 15% have been reported for this procedure when performed by a skilled surgeon. These rates are slightly higher than the rates reported after truncal vagotomy in combination with pyloroplasty; however, selective vagotomy has lower rates of postvagotomy dumping syndrome and diarrhea.

Truncal vagotomy and antrectomy. Antrectomy is generally not performed for duodenal ulcers and is more commonly performed for gastric ulcers. Relative contraindications include cirrhosis; extensive scarring of the proximal duodenum that leaves a difficult or tenuous duodenal closure; and previous operations on the proximal duodenum, such as choledochoduodenostomy. When done in combination with truncal vagotomy, it is more effective at reducing acid secretion and recurrence than truncal vagotomy in combination with a drainage procedure or highly selective vagotomy. The recurrence rate for ulceration after truncal vagotomy and antrectomy is 0% to 2%. However, this low recurrence rate needs to be balanced against the 20% rate of postgastrectomy and postvagotomy syndromes in patients undergoing antrectomy, longer operative times, and increased postoperative morbidity.

Antrectomy requires reconstruction of GI continuity that can be accomplished by a gastroduodenostomy (Billroth I procedure [Fig. 48-14]) or gastrojejunostomy (either Billroth II procedure [Fig. 48-15] or Roux-en-Y reconstruction). For benign disease, gastroduodenostomy is generally favored because it avoids the problem of retained antrum syndrome, duodenal stump leak, and afferent loop obstruction associated with gastrojejunostomy after resection. If the duodenum is significantly scarred, gastroduodenostomy may be technically more difficult, necessitating gastrojejunostomy. If a gastrojejunostomy is performed, the loop of jejunum chosen for anastomosis is usually brought through the transverse mesocolon in a retrocolic fashion. The retrocolic anastomosis minimizes the length of the afferent limb and decreases the likelihood of twisting or kinking that could lead to afferent loop obstruction and predispose to the devastating complication of a duodenal stump leak. Although vagotomy and antrectomy are effective at managing ulcerations, they are used infrequently today in the treatment of patients with PUD. In general, operations of lesser magnitude are performed more frequently in the *H. pylori* era. The overall mortality rate for antrectomy is approximately 2% but is higher in patients with comorbid conditions, such as insulin-dependent diabetes or immunosuppression.

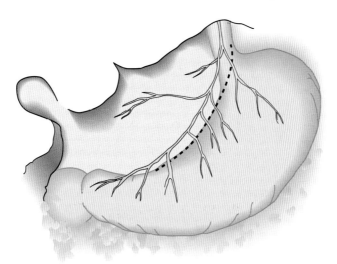

FIGURE 48-13 Anterior view of the stomach and anterior nerve of Latarjet. Note the line of dissection for parietal cell or highly selective vagotomy *(dashed line)*. The last major branches of the nerve are left intact, and the dissection begins 7 cm from the pylorus. At the gastroesophageal junction, the dissection is well away from the origin of the hepatic branches of the left vagus. (From Kelly KA, Teotia SS: Proximal gastric vagotomy. In Baker RJ, Fischer JE, editors: *Mastery of surgery*, Philadelphia, 2001, Lippincott Williams & Wilkins.)

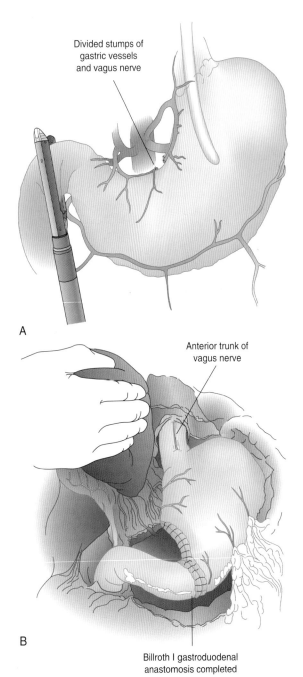

Divided stumps of
gastric vessels
and vagus nerve

A

Anterior trunk of
vagus nerve

B

Billroth I gastroduodenal
anastomosis completed

FIGURE 48-14 Hemigastrectomy with a Billroth I (gastroduodenal) anastomosis. (From Dempsey D, Pathak A: Antrectomy. *Oper Tech Gen Surg* 5:86–100, 2003.)

Approximately 20% of patients develop some form of postgastrectomy or postvagotomy complications (see later).

Gastric Ulcers

The modified Johnson anatomic classification system for gastric ulcers (i.e., types I through V, described in Table 48-5) was developed before the modern understanding that most ulcers are the consequence of *H. pylori* infection or NSAID usage. However, despite having an increased understanding of the mechanisms of how and why most ulcers develop, this historical classification

system is still relevant to surgical treatment because it dictates what operation should be performed in the setting of complications of such ulcers, most commonly perforation.

Gastric ulcers can occur at any location in the stomach, although they usually manifest on the lesser curvature, near the incisura. Approximately 60% of ulcers are in this location and are classified as type I gastric ulcers. These ulcers are generally not associated with excessive acid secretion and may occur with low to normal acid output. Most occur within 1.5 cm of the histologic transition zone between the fundic and antral mucosa and are not associated with duodenal, pyloric, or prepyloric mucosal abnormalities. In contrast, type II gastric ulcers (approximately 15%) are located in the body of the stomach in combination with a duodenal ulcer. These types of ulcers are usually associated with excess acid secretion. Type III gastric ulcers are prepyloric ulcers and account for approximately 20% of the lesions. They also behave similar to duodenal ulcers and are associated with hypersecretion of gastric acid. Type IV gastric ulcers occur high on the lesser curvature, near the GE junction. The incidence of type IV gastric ulcers is less than 10%, and they are not associated with excessive acid secretion. Type V gastric ulcers can occur at any location and are associated with long-term NSAID use. Finally, some ulcers may appear on the greater curvature of the stomach, but the incidence is less than 5%.

Gastric ulcers rarely develop before the age of 40 years, and the peak incidence occurs in individuals 55 to 65 years old. Gastric ulcers are more likely to occur in individuals in a lower socioeconomic class and are slightly more common in the non-white than white population. The exact pathogenesis of a benign gastric ulcer is less well understood than duodenal ulcers, but most are caused by *H. pylori* or NSAID use. Some clinical conditions that may predispose to gastric ulceration include chronic alcohol intake, smoking, long-term corticosteroid therapy, infection, and intra-arterial therapy. With regard to acid and pepsin secretion, the presence of acid appears to be essential to the production of a gastric ulcer; however, the total secretory output appears to be less important. In contrast to the acidification of the duodenum leading to ulcer formation, patients with gastric ulcers caused by *H. pylori* have normal or reduced gastric acid production. Ulcer formation is more likely due to an inflammatory response to the bacterial infection itself, which is most densely concentrated at the junction between the stomach body and antrum. Nevertheless, rapid healing follows antacid therapy, antisecretory therapy, or vagotomy even when the lesion-bearing portion of the stomach is left intact because in the presence of gastric mucosal damage, acid is ulcerogenic, even when present in normal or less than normal amounts.

Clinical Manifestations

The clinical challenge of gastric ulcer management is the differentiation between gastric carcinoma and benign ulcer. This is in contrast to duodenal ulcers, in which malignancy is extremely rare. Similar to duodenal ulcers, gastric ulcers are also characterized by recurrent episodes of quiescence and relapse. They also cause pain, bleeding, and obstruction and can perforate. Occasionally, benign ulcers have also been found to result in spontaneous gastrocolic fistulas. Surgical intervention is required in 8% to 20% of patients who develop complications from gastric ulcer disease. Hemorrhage occurs in approximately 35% to 40% of patients. Patients who develop significant bleeding from gastric ulcers usually are older, are less likely to stop bleeding spontaneously, and have higher morbidity and mortality rates than patients

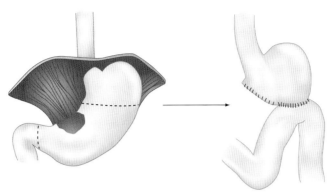

FIGURE 48-15 Subtotal gastrectomy with a Billroth II anastomosis.

TABLE 48-5	**Gastric Ulcer Types**	
TYPE	**LOCATION**	**ACID LEVEL**
I	Lesser curve at incisura	Low to normal
II	Gastric body with duodenal ulcer	Increased
III	Prepyloric	Increased
IV	High on lesser curve	Normal
V	Anywhere	Normal, NSAID-induced

NSAID, Nonsteroidal anti-inflammatory drug.

with bleeding from a duodenal ulcer. The most frequent complication of gastric ulceration is perforation. Most perforations occur along the anterior aspect of the lesser curvature. In general, older patients have increased rates of perforations, and larger ulcers are associated with higher morbidity and mortality. Similar to duodenal ulcers, gastric outlet obstruction can also occur in patients with type II or III gastric ulcers. However, one must carefully differentiate between benign obstruction and obstruction secondary to antral carcinoma.

Diagnosis and Treatment

The diagnosis and treatment of gastric ulceration generally mirror diagnosis and treatment of duodenal ulcer disease. The significant difference is the possibility of malignancy in a gastric ulcer. This critical difference demands that cancer be ruled out in acute and chronic presentations of gastric ulcer disease. Acid suppression and *H. pylori* eradication are important aspects of any treatment.

As with duodenal ulcers, intractable nonhealing ulcers are becoming increasingly less common. It is important to ensure that adequate time has elapsed and appropriate therapy has been administered to allow healing of the ulcer to occur; this includes confirmation that *H. pylori* has been eradicated and that NSAIDs have been eliminated as a potential cause. The presentation of a nonhealing gastric ulcer in the *H. pylori* era should raise serious concerns about the presence of an underlying malignancy. These patients should undergo a thorough evaluation with multiple biopsies to exclude malignancy before any surgical intervention (Fig. 48-16). The approach for a complicated gastric ulcer varies depending on the type of ulcer and its association with pathophysiologic acid levels. Types I and IV ulcers, which are not associated with increased acid levels, do not require acid-reducing vagotomy. Figure 48-17 is an algorithm for managing complicated gastric ulcers.

Type I gastric ulcers. For type I gastric ulcers, even with appropriate preoperative evaluation, malignancy is a major concern, and excision of a nonhealing ulcer is necessary. Excision can generally be accomplished by a wedge resection that includes the ulcer, although this depends on the exact anatomic location of the ulcer, its proximity to either the GE junction or the pylorus, and the length of the lesser curve of the stomach. A resection is generally curative and allows more intense pathologic examination of the specimen. Distal gastrectomy without vagotomy can also be performed but has a morbidity of 3% to 5%, with mortality ranging from 1% to 2%. Recurrence is less than 5%. There is no evidence that gastrectomy is superior to resection of the ulcer alone.

Type II and type III gastric ulcers. Because types II and III gastric ulcers are associated with increased gastric acid levels, surgery for intractable disease should focus on acid reduction. A distal gastrectomy in combination with truncal vagotomy should be performed. It has been shown that patients undergoing highly selective vagotomy for type II or III gastric ulcers have a poorer outcome than patients undergoing resection. However, some physicians advocate performing a laparoscopic parietal cell vagotomy and reserve resection for patients who develop ulcer recurrence.

Type IV gastric ulcers. Type IV gastric ulcers present a difficult management problem. Surgical treatment depends on ulcer size, distance from the GE junction, and degree of surrounding inflammation. Whenever possible, the ulcer should be excised. The preferred approach is to resect the ulcer without gastrectomy and the resultant morbidity of a small gastric remnant. Sometimes this approach is impossible, and a gastrectomy is necessary. The most aggressive approach is to perform a gastrectomy that includes a small portion of the esophageal wall and ulcer followed by a Roux-en-Y esophagojejunostomy to restore intestinal continuity. For type IV gastric ulcers that are located 2 to 5 cm from the GE junction, a distal gastrectomy with a vertical extension of the resection to include the lesser curvature with the ulcer can be performed (the Csendes procedure). After resection, bowel continuity is restored with an end-to-end gastroduodenostomy or gastrojejunostomy.

Bleeding gastric ulcers. Treatment of bleeding gastric ulcers depends on their cause and location; however, the initial approach is similar to duodenal ulcers. Patients require resuscitation, monitoring, and endoscopic investigation. Up to 70% of gastric ulcers are *H. pylori*–positive, so an attempt should be made to control the bleeding endoscopically, with multiple biopsy specimens of the ulcer obtained to rule out malignancy and concurrently obtained biopsy specimens of the body and antrum to test for *H.*

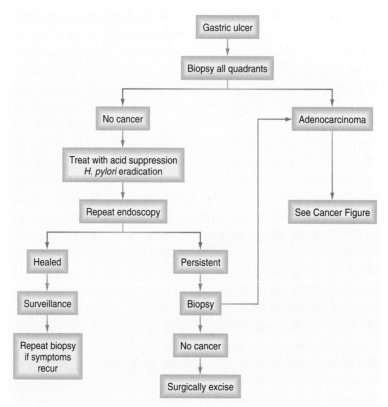

FIGURE 48-16 Algorithm for evaluation, treatment, and surveillance of a patient with a gastric ulcer.

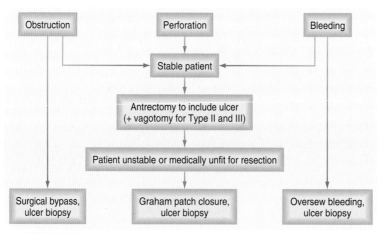

FIGURE 48-17 Algorithm for the management of complicated gastric ulcer disease.

pylori infection. Patients whose bleeding can be controlled and who are *H. pylori*–positive should undergo subsequent treatment for *H. pylori* infection. For bleeding that cannot be controlled, operative intervention again depends on the type of gastric ulcer. In all cases, the ulcer should ideally be excised with the addition of vagotomy depending on the cause of the ulcer (mostly for intractable ulcers that are not due to *H. pylori* infection or NSAID usage that can be stopped).

Perforated gastric ulcer. For perforated type I gastric ulcers that occur in patients in stable condition, distal gastrectomy with a Billroth I anastomosis is recommended. In unstable patients, simple patching of the gastric ulcer with biopsy and treatment for *H. pylori*, if positive, is recommended. However, even if the biopsy is negative, the risk for malignancy still needs to be ruled out; therefore, documentation of healing is required with repeat endoscopy and biopsy. Adding vagotomy for perforated type I gastric ulcers is unlikely to be of any value. Because they behave similar to duodenal ulcers, types II and III gastric ulcers can be simply treated with patch closure, with or without truncal vagotomy and pyloroplasty, depending on the medical condition, hemodynamic status, and extent of peritonitis, followed by treatment for *H. pylori* if positive.

Giant gastric ulcers. Giant gastric ulcers are defined as ulcers with a diameter of 2 cm or more. They are usually found on the lesser curvature and have a higher incidence of malignancy (10%) than smaller ulcers. These ulcers commonly penetrate into contiguous structures, such as the spleen, pancreas, liver, or transverse colon, and are falsely diagnosed as an unresectable malignancy, despite normal biopsy results. The incidence of malignancy ranges from 6% to 30% and increases with the size of the ulcer. Giant gastric ulcers have a high likelihood of developing complications (e.g., perforation or bleeding). Medical therapy heals 80% of these ulcers, although repeat endoscopy is indicated in 6 to 8 weeks. For complications or failure to heal, the operation of choice is gastrectomy including the ulcer bed, with vagotomy reserved for types II and III gastric ulcers. In a high-risk patient with significant underlying comorbid conditions, local excision combined with vagotomy and pyloroplasty may be considered; otherwise, resection has the highest chance for successful outcome.

Zollinger-ellison syndrome. ZES is a clinical triad consisting of gastric acid hypersecretion, severe PUD, and non–β-islet cell tumors of the pancreas. These tumors fall within the larger family of neuroendocrine tumors. The islet cell tumor produces gastrin and PUD. Hypergastrinemia associated with ZES accounts for most, if not all, clinical symptoms experienced by patients. Abdominal pain and PUD are the hallmarks of the syndrome and typically occur in more than 80% of patients. Patients may also exhibit diarrhea, weight loss, steatorrhea, and esophagitis. Endoscopy frequently demonstrates prominent gastric rugal folds, reflecting the trophic effect of hypergastrinemia on the gastric fundus in addition to evidence of PUD. Approximately one quarter of patients have ZES as part of multiple endocrine neoplasia type 1, an autosomal dominant syndrome.

Provocative tests are generally not required to establish the diagnosis of ZES because fasting plasma gastrin levels are usually elevated. Most patients with gastrinoma have elevated fasting serum gastrin levels (>200 pg/mL), and values higher than 1000 pg/mL are diagnostic. However, two thirds of patients with gastrinomas have fasting gastrin levels that are between 150 and 1000 pg/mL.[14] Diagnosing ZES in such patients is difficult because PPI use, *H. pylori* infection, and renal failure all can cause an elevation of fasting serum gastrin levels into this range. In patients with gastrin levels in this equivocal range, the most sensitive diagnostic test is the secretin-stimulated gastrin level. Serum gastrin samples are measured before and after intravenous secretin (2 U/kg) administration at 5-minute intervals for 30 minutes. An increase in the serum gastrin level of greater than 200 pg/mL above basal levels is specific for gastrinoma versus other causes of hypergastrinemia, which do not demonstrate this response.

After diagnosis of gastrinoma, acid suppression therapy is initiated, preferably with a high-dose PPI. Medical management is indicated preoperatively and for patients with metastatic or unresectable gastrinoma. The next step in management is localization and staging of the tumor. Most ZES gastrinomas are located in the duodenum or pancreas, within the "gastrinoma triangle"; the points of this triangle are made up of the cystic-common duct junction, the pancreas body-neck junction, and the junction between the second and third portions of the duodenum (Fig. 48-18). The best initial imaging study to localize the gastrin-secreting tumor is either computed tomography (CT) or MRI of the abdomen. However, these imaging modalities have a relatively low sensitivity in detecting tumors that are less than 1 cm in diameter as well as small liver metastases.[15] If initial imaging is nondiagnostic, localization can sometimes be achieved using

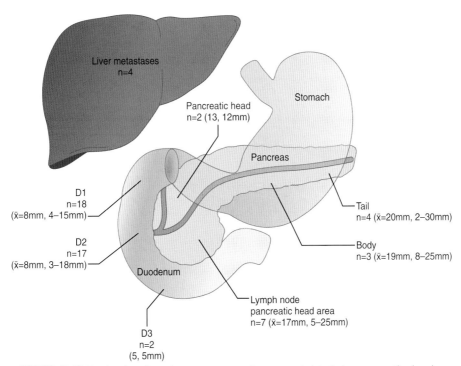

FIGURE 48-18 The location of gastrinomas at surgery that were not detected on preoperative imaging. Most tumors were located in the first and second portions of the duodenum and the head of the pancreas, within the so-called gastrinoma triangle. (From Norton JA, Fraker DL, Alexander HR, et al: Value of surgery in patients with negative imaging and sporadic Zollinger-Ellison syndrome. *Ann Surg* 256:509–517, 2012.)

somatostatin receptor scintigraphy or endoscopic ultrasound (EUS). Somatostatin receptor scintigraphy uses radionucleotide-labeled octreotide, which binds to the ZES tumor cells and can detect hepatic metastases in 85% to 95% of patients, as opposed to 70% to 80% using conventional cross-sectional imaging.

Localized gastrinoma should be resected; however, long-term cure rates are less than 40%. Although preoperative imaging is helpful in planning surgical resection, it is not necessary in all cases. In patients with ZES confirmed by gastrin levels but with negative imaging studies, the primary tumor can be localized on operative exploration in 98% of cases.[16] Once the tumor is located intraoperatively, a resection according to oncologic principles should be performed (rather than a tumor enucleation) because lymph node metastases are present in 43% to 82% of cases; however, this point is controversial. The role of surgery in patients with ZES and multiple endocrine neoplasia type 1 is also an area of debate, as these patients have higher recurrence rates and resection is rarely curative. Patients with tumor recurrence or metastatic disease are treated with chemotherapy (streptozotocin with 5-fluorouracil or doxorubicin or both), which results in clinical response rates of 20% to 45% but is never curative.

STRESS GASTRITIS

Stress gastritis, by definition, occurs after physical trauma, shock, sepsis, hemorrhage, or respiratory failure and may lead to life-threatening gastric bleeding. Stress gastritis is characterized by multiple superficial (nonulcerating) erosions that begin in the proximal or acid-secreting portion of the stomach and progress distally. They may also occur in the setting of central nervous system disease (Cushing ulcer) or as a result of thermal burn injury involving more than 30% of the body surface area (Curling ulcer).

Stress gastritis lesions typically change with time. They are considered early lesions if they appear within the first 24 hours. These early lesions are typically multiple and shallow, with discrete areas of erythema along with focal hemorrhage or an adherent clot. If the lesion erodes into the submucosa, which contains the blood supply, frank bleeding may result. On microscopy, these lesions appear as wedge-shaped mucosal hemorrhages with coagulation necrosis of the superficial mucosal cells. They are almost always seen in the fundus of the stomach and only rarely in the distal stomach. Acute stress gastritis can be classified as late if there is a tissue reaction or organization around a clot, or if an inflammatory exudate is present. This picture may be seen by microscopy 24 to 72 hours after injury. Late lesions appear identical to regenerating mucosa around a healing gastric ulcer. Both types of lesions can be seen endoscopically.

Pathophysiology

Although the precise mechanisms responsible for the development of stress gastritis remain to be fully elucidated, evidence suggests a multifactorial cause. Stress-induced gastric lesions appear to require the presence of acid. Other factors that may predispose to their development include impaired mucosal defense mechanisms against luminal acid, such as a reduction in blood flow, mucus, bicarbonate secretion by mucosal cells, or endogenous prostaglandins. All these factors render the stomach more susceptible to damage from luminal acid, with the resultant hemorrhagic gastritis. Stress is considered present when hypoxia, sepsis, or organ failure occurs. When stress is present, mucosal ischemia is thought to be the main factor responsible for the breakdown of these

normal defense mechanisms. There is little evidence to suggest that increased gastric acid secretion occurs in this situation. However, the presence of luminal acid appears to be a prerequisite for this form of gastritis to evolve. Moreover, complete neutralization of luminal acid or antisecretory therapy precludes the development of experimental stress gastritis.

Presentation and Diagnosis

Stress gastritis develops within 1 to 2 days after a traumatic event in more than 50% of patients. The only clinical sign may be painless upper GI bleeding that may be delayed at onset. The bleeding is usually slow and intermittent and may be detected by only a few flecks of blood in the NG tube or an unexplained decrease in hemoglobin level. Occasionally, there may be profound upper GI hemorrhage accompanied by hypotension and hematemesis. The stool is frequently guaiac-positive, although melena and hematochezia are rare. Endoscopy is required to confirm the diagnosis and differentiate stress gastritis from other sources of GI hemorrhage.

Prophylaxis

Because of the high mortality rate in patients with acute stress gastritis who develop massive upper GI hemorrhage, high-risk patients should be treated prophylactically. Because mucosal ischemia may alter many mucosal defense mechanisms that enable the stomach to withstand luminal irritants and protect itself from injury, every effort should be made to correct any perfusion deficits secondary to shock. The two strongest risk factors for developing clinically significant bleeding from gastric stress ulcers are coagulopathy and respiratory failure requiring prolonged mechanical ventilation (>48 hours). Patients in the intensive care unit without these risk factors are unlikely to develop significant bleeding (0.1% incidence). Additionally, prophylactically increasing the gastric pH may increase rates of ventilator-associated pneumonia and Clostridium difficile infection. For these reasons, only critically ill patients with coagulopathy or prolonged mechanical ventilation should receive prophylaxis.[17] Enteral nutrition reduces the risk of stress ulcer formation and should be initiated as soon as possible. Some experts advocate not administering prophylaxis to patients who are being fed enterally even if they have risk factors, although this is controversial. If prophylaxis is indicated, a PPI, rather than H_2 antagonists or sucralfate, should be used, although the evidence supporting this is weak, and further head-to-head comparisons are needed.

Treatment

Any patient with upper GI bleeding requires prompt and definitive fluid resuscitation with correction of any coagulation or platelet abnormalities. Treatment of the underlying sepsis plays a major role in treating the underlying gastric erosions. More than 80% of patients who present with upper GI hemorrhage stop bleeding with only supportive care. There is little evidence to suggest that endoscopy with electrocautery or heater probe coagulation has any benefit in the treatment of bleeding from acute stress gastritis. However, some studies suggested that acute bleeding can be effectively controlled by selective infusion of vasopressin into the splanchnic circulation through the left gastric artery. Vasopressin is administered by continuous infusion through the catheter at a rate of 0.2 to 0.4 IU/min for a maximum of 48 to 72 hours. If the patient has underlying cardiac or liver disease, vasopressin should not be used. Although vasopressin may decrease blood loss, it has not been shown to result in improved survival. Another angiographic technique that can be used is embolization of the left gastric artery if bleeding is identified on angiography. However, the extensive plexus of submucosal arterial vessels within the stomach makes this approach less appealing and not as successful.

Bleeding that recurs or persists, requiring more than 6 U of blood (3000 mL), is an indication for surgery. Because most lesions are in the proximal stomach or fundus, a long anterior gastrotomy should be made in this area. The gastric lumen is cleared of blood, and the mucosal surface is inspected for bleeding points. All bleeding areas are oversewn with figure-of-eight stitches taken deep within the gastric wall. Most superficial erosions are not actively bleeding and do not require ligation unless a blood vessel is seen at its base. The operation is completed by closing the anterior gastrotomy and performing a truncal vagotomy and pyloroplasty to reduce acid secretion. The incidence of rebleeding is less than 5% if bleeding points are carefully identified and secured. Less commonly, a partial gastrectomy combined with vagotomy is performed. Total gastrectomy should be performed rarely and only in patients with life-threatening hemorrhage refractory to other forms of therapy.

POSTGASTRECTOMY SYNDROMES

Gastric surgery results in numerous physiologic derangements caused by loss of reservoir function, interruption of the pyloric sphincter mechanism, and vagal nerve transection. These physiologic changes usually cause no long-term symptoms. The GI and cardiovascular symptoms may result in disorders collectively referred to as *postgastrectomy syndromes*. Approximately 25% of patients who undergo surgery for PUD subsequently develop some degree of postgastrectomy syndrome, although this frequency is much lower in patients who undergo highly selective vagotomy. The physiologic changes are not specific to PUD and can occur after gastrectomy for resection of neoplasm or Roux-en-Y gastric bypass for treatment of severe obesity. Only approximately 1% of patients become permanently disabled from their symptoms.

Dumping Syndrome

Dumping syndrome can be early (20 to 30 minutes after eating) or late (2 or 3 hours after a meal). Early dumping is more common, with more GI and fewer cardiovascular effects. GI symptoms include nausea and vomiting, a sense of epigastric fullness, cramping abdominal pain, and often explosive diarrhea. The cardiovascular symptoms include palpitations, tachycardia, diaphoresis, fainting, dizziness, flushing, and occasionally blurred vision. This symptom complex can develop after any operation on the stomach but is more common after partial gastrectomy with the Billroth II reconstruction. It is much less commonly observed after the Billroth I gastrectomy or after vagotomy and drainage procedures.

Early dumping occurs because of the rapid passage of food of high osmolarity from the stomach into the small intestine. This occurs because gastrectomy, or any interruption of the pyloric sphincteric mechanism, prevents the stomach from preparing its contents and delivering them to the proximal bowel in the form of small particles in isotonic solution. The resultant hypertonic food bolus passes into the small intestine, which induces a rapid shift of extracellular fluid into the intestinal lumen to achieve isotonicity. After this shift of extracellular fluid, luminal distention occurs and induces the autonomic responses listed earlier.

The basic defect of late dumping is also rapid gastric emptying; however, it is related specifically to carbohydrates being delivered rapidly into the proximal intestine. When carbohydrates are delivered to the small intestine, they are quickly absorbed, resulting in hyperglycemia, which triggers the release of large amounts of insulin to control the increasing blood sugar level. An overcompensation results so that profound hypoglycemia occurs in response to the insulin. This hypoglycemia activates the adrenal gland to release catecholamines, which results in diaphoresis, tremulousness, light-headedness, tachycardia, and confusion. The symptom complex is indistinguishable from insulin shock.

The symptoms associated with early dumping syndrome appear to be secondary to the release of several humoral agents, such as serotonin, bradykinin-like substances, neurotensin, and enteroglucagon. Dietary measures are usually sufficient to treat most patients. These include avoiding foods containing large amounts of sugar, frequent feeding of small meals rich in protein and fat, and separating liquids from solids during a meal.

In some patients without a response to dietary measures, long-acting octreotide agonists have ameliorated symptoms. These peptides not only inhibit gastric emptying but also affect small bowel motility so that intestinal transit of the ingested meal is prolonged. The side effects associated with administration of these synthetic peptides are relatively benign; however, the peptides are expensive. Many operative procedures have been advocated for the surgical treatment of these patients. The paucity of patients treated for PUD with gastrectomy or vagotomy has made remedial procedures for dumping exceedingly rare.

Metabolic Disturbances

The most common metabolic defect appearing after gastrectomy is anemia. Anemia is related to iron deficiency (more common) or impairment in vitamin B_{12} metabolism. More than 30% of patients undergoing gastrectomy have iron deficiency anemia. The exact cause is not fully understood but appears to be related to a combination of decreased iron intake, impaired iron absorption, and chronic blood loss. In general, the addition of iron supplements to the patient's diet corrects this metabolic problem.

Megaloblastic anemia from vitamin B_{12} deficiency only rarely develops after partial gastrectomy but is dependent on the amount of stomach removed. Vitamin deficiency occurs secondary to poor absorption of dietary vitamin B_{12} because of the lack of intrinsic factor. Patients undergoing subtotal gastrectomy should be placed on life-long vitamin B_{12} supplementation. If a patient develops a macrocytic anemia, serum vitamin B_{12} levels should be determined and, if abnormal, treated with long-term vitamin B_{12} therapy.

Osteoporosis and osteomalacia have also been observed after gastric resection and appear to be caused by deficiencies in calcium. If fat malabsorption is also present, the calcium malabsorption is aggravated further because fatty acids bind calcium. The incidence of this problem also increases with the extent of gastric resection and is usually associated with a Billroth II gastrectomy. Bone disease generally develops approximately 4 to 5 years after surgery. Treatment of this disorder usually requires calcium supplements (1 to 2 g/day) in conjunction with vitamin D (500 to 5000 U daily). Patients with Billroth II or Roux-en-Y reconstruction that bypasses the duodenum should also receive supplementation of the fat-soluble vitamins (vitamins A, D, E, and K).

Afferent Loop Syndrome

Afferent loop syndrome occurs as a result of partial obstruction of the afferent limb, which is unable to empty its contents. After obstruction of the afferent limb, pancreatic and hepatobiliary secretions accumulate within the limb, resulting in its distention, which causes epigastric discomfort and cramping. The intraluminal pressure eventually increases enough to empty the contents of the afferent loop forcefully into the stomach, resulting in bilious vomiting that offers immediate relief of symptoms. If the obstruction has been present for a long time, it can also be aggravated by the development of the blind loop syndrome. In this situation, bacterial overgrowth occurs in the static loop, and the bacteria bind with vitamin B_{12} and deconjugated bile acids; this results in a systemic deficiency of vitamin B_{12}, with the development of megaloblastic anemia.

In contrast to the diagnosis of an acute bowel obstruction, the diagnosis of chronic afferent loop obstruction may be problematic. Failure to visualize the afferent limb on upper endoscopy is suggestive of the diagnosis. Radionuclide studies imaging the hepatobiliary tree have also been used with some success in diagnosing this syndrome. Normally, the radionuclide should pass into the stomach or distal small bowel after being excreted into the afferent limb. If it does not, the possibility of an afferent loop obstruction should be considered.

Surgical correction is indicated for this mechanical problem. A long afferent limb is usually the underlying problem, so treatment involves the elimination of this loop. Remedies include conversion of the Billroth II construction into a Billroth I anastomosis, enteroenterostomy below the stoma, and creation of a Roux-en-Y procedure. The Roux-en-Y reconstruction is a good combination of efficacy and ease, especially in a patient with a previous vagotomy. Marginal ulceration from the diversion of duodenal contents from the gastroenteric stoma is a potential complication of the Roux-en-Y conversion.

Efferent Loop Obstruction

Obstruction of the efferent limb is rare. Efferent loop obstruction may occur at any time; however, more than 50% of cases do so within the first postoperative month. Establishing a diagnosis is difficult. Initial complaints may include left upper quadrant abdominal pain that is colicky in nature, bilious vomiting, and abdominal distention. The diagnosis is usually established by a GI contrast study of the stomach, with failure of barium to enter the efferent limb. Operative intervention is almost always necessary and consists of reducing the retroanastomotic hernia if this is the cause of the obstruction and closing the retroanastomotic space to prevent recurrence of this condition.

Alkaline Reflux Gastritis

After gastrectomy, reflux of bile is common. In a small percentage of patients, this reflux is associated with severe epigastric abdominal pain accompanied by bilious vomiting and weight loss. Although the diagnosis can be made by taking a careful history, hepatoiminodiacetic acid scans usually demonstrate biliary secretion into the stomach and sometimes into the esophagus. Upper endoscopy demonstrates friable, beefy red mucosa.

Most patients with alkaline reflux gastritis have had gastric resection performed with a Billroth II anastomosis. Although bile reflux appears to be the inciting event, numerous issues remain unanswered with respect to the role of bile in its pathogenesis. For example, many patients have reflux of bile into the stomach after gastrectomy without any symptoms. Moreover, there is no clear correlation between the volume or composition of bile and the subsequent development of alkaline reflux gastritis. Although the syndrome clearly exists, caution needs to be exercised to ensure that it is not overdiagnosed. After a diagnosis is made, therapy is directed at relief of symptoms. Most medical therapies that have been tried to treat alkaline reflux gastritis have not shown any consistent benefit. For patients with intractable symptoms, the surgical procedure of choice is conversion of the Billroth II anastomosis into a Roux-en-Y gastrojejunostomy, in which the Roux limb has been lengthened to more than 40 cm. In general, a Roux-en-Y procedure should be preferred over a Billroth II for reconstruction at the time of partial or subtotal distal gastrectomy to decrease the likelihood of alkaline reflux. A meta-analysis of randomized trials found that Roux-en-Y and Billroth II reconstructions resulted in the same rates of complications in the immediate postoperative period but that patients who underwent Roux-en-Y procedures had superior long-term quality of life because of lower rates of reflux esophagitis.

Gastric Atony

Gastric emptying is delayed after truncal and selective vagotomies but not after a highly selective or parietal cell vagotomy. With selective or truncal vagotomy, patients lose their antral pump function and have a reduction in the ability to empty solids. In contrast, emptying of liquids is accelerated because of loss of receptive relaxation in the proximal stomach, which regulates liquid emptying. Although most patients undergoing vagotomy and a drainage procedure manage to empty their stomach adequately, some patients have persistent gastric stasis that results in retention of food within the stomach for several hours. This condition may be accompanied by a feeling of fullness and occasionally abdominal pain. In still rarer cases, it may be associated with a functional gastric outlet obstruction.

The diagnosis of gastroparesis is confirmed by scintigraphic assessment of gastric emptying. However, other causes of delayed gastric emptying, such as diabetes mellitus, electrolyte imbalance, drug toxicity, and neuromuscular disorders, must also be excluded. In addition, a mechanical cause of gastric outlet obstruction, such as postoperative adhesions, afferent or efferent loop obstruction, and internal herniations, must be ruled out. Endoscopic examination of the stomach also needs to be performed to rule out any anastomotic obstructions.

In patients with a functional gastric outlet obstruction and documented gastroparesis, pharmacotherapy is generally used. The agents most commonly used are prokinetic agents such as metoclopramide and erythromycin. Metoclopramide exerts its prokinetic effects by acting as a dopamine antagonist and has cholinergic-enhancing effects because of facilitation of acetylcholine release from enteric cholinergic neurons. In contrast, erythromycin markedly accelerates gastric emptying by binding to motilin receptors on GI smooth muscle cells, where it acts as a motilin agonist. One of these two agents is usually sufficient to enhance gastric tone and improve gastric emptying. In rare cases of persistent gastric atony refractory to medical management, gastrectomy may be required.

GASTRIC CANCER

Epidemiology and Risk Factors

Incidence

Gastric cancer is the 14th most common cancer and cause of cancer death in the United States, with an estimated 22,000 new

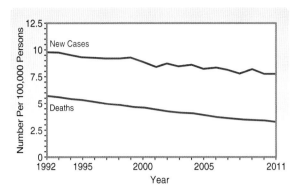

FIGURE 48-19 Age-adjusted incidence of gastric cancer, 1992-2011. (From National Cancer Institute, Surveillance Research Program: Fast Stats, 2009. <http://seer.cancer.gov/statfacts/html/stomach.html>, [Accessed October, 2014.])

cases/year and more than 10,000 deaths.[18] The disease affects men disproportionately, with more than 60% of new cases occurring in men. It is a disease of older individuals, with peak incidence in the seventh decade of life. Among racial groups, the disease is more common and has a higher mortality in African Americans, Asian Americans, and Hispanics compared with whites.

Worldwide, gastric cancer is the fourth most common cancer and the second leading cause of cancer death. It is especially prevalent in East Asia and South America and has been increasing in developing countries, which now have almost two thirds of all distal gastric cancer cases. In contrast, rates have been decreasing in the United States (Fig. 48-19). Among developed countries, Japan and Korea have the highest rates of the disease. Gastric cancer is the most common cancer in Japan. As a result, gastric cancer screening in Japan was started in the 1970s, and the mortality rate has decreased by 50% since that time. Although there has been an increase in proximal tumors in Japan, most are distal gastric cancers.

Risk Factors

The major risk factors for gastric cancer are discussed here; they include environmental and genetic factors (Box 48-3).

Helicobacter pylori Infection

In 1994, the International Agency for Research on Cancer labeled *H. pylori* a definite carcinogen. Numerous longitudinal prospective studies have demonstrated an association with the development of gastric cancer. In epidemiologic studies, *H. pylori* seropositivity has been associated with a relative risk of developing gastric cancer between 3.6 and 17. The primary mechanism is thought to be the presence of chronic inflammation. Long-term infection with the bacteria leads to gastritis, primarily within the gastric body, with ventral gastric atrophy. In some patients, gastritis progresses to intestinal metaplasia, dysplasia, and ultimately intestinal-type adenocarcinoma. A wide range of molecular alterations in intestinal metaplasia have been described and may affect the transformation into gastric cancer. These include overexpression of cyclooxygenase-2 and cyclin D2, *p53* mutations, microsatellite instability, decreased *p27* expression, and alterations in transcription factors such as CDX1 and CDX2. Intestinal metaplasia is a risk factor for the development of gastric carcinoma; however, not every patient with intestinal metaplasia develops invasive cancer. Host inflammatory responses play an important

BOX 48-3 Factors Associated With Increased Risk for Developing Stomach Cancer

Nutritional
Low fat or protein consumption
Salted meat or fish
High nitrate consumption
High complex carbohydrate consumption

Environmental
Poor food preparation (smoked, salted)
Lack of refrigeration
Poor drinking water (e.g., contaminated well water)
Smoking

Social
Low social class

Medical
Prior gastric surgery
H. pylori infection
Gastric atrophy and gastritis
Adenomatous polyps

Other
Male sex

role in this process. Specifically, individuals with high levels of interleukin-1 expression are at increased risk of gastric cancer development.

Some regional variances in the development of cancer may be attributed to the prevalence and virulence of *H. pylori*. It is more common in poor areas with less sanitation, and infection rates remain high in developing countries, with a concomitant increase in gastric cancer incidence. In contrast, the prevalence in more developed countries has been decreasing. The presence of the cytoxan-associated gene A *(cagA)* is associated with increased virulence and risk of gastric cancer. Countries with high levels of gastric cancer, such as Japan, have a much higher rate of *cagA*-positive *H. pylori* infection than countries with lower rates of gastric cancer, such as the United States.

Dietary Factors

High-salt foods, particularly foods with salted or smoked meats that contain high levels of nitrate, along with low intake of fruits and vegetables are linked to an increased risk of gastric cancer. The mechanism is thought to be the conversion of nitrates in the food to N-nitroso compounds by bacteria in the stomach. N-nitroso compounds are also found in tobacco smoke, another known risk factor for gastric cancer. Fresh fruits and vegetables contain ascorbic acid, which can remove the carcinogenic N-nitroso compounds and oxygen free radicals.

There is likely synergism between diet and *H. pylori* infection, with the bacteria increasing carcinogen production and inhibiting its removal. *H. pylori* has been shown to promote the growth of the bacteria that generate the carcinogenic N-nitroso compounds. At the same time, *H. pylori* can inhibit the secretion of ascorbic acid, preventing effective scavenging of oxygen free radicals and N-nitroso compounds. The increase in refrigeration over the past 70 years has likely contributed to the decrease in gastric cancer by reducing the amount of meat preserved by salting alone and allowing the increased storage and consumption of fresh fruits and vegetables.

Hereditary Risk Factors and Cancer Genetics

Gastric cancer is associated with several rare inherited disorders. Hereditary diffuse gastric cancer is an inherited form of gastric cancer. Patients with this disorder, resulting from a gene mutation for the cell adhesion molecule E-cadherin, have an 80% lifetime incidence of developing gastric cancer. Prophylactic total gastrectomy should be considered for patients with this mutation. In familial adenomatous polyposis, approximately 85% of patients have fundic gland polyps, with 40% of these having some type of dysplasia and more than 50% containing a somatic adenomatous polyposis coli mutation, which places these patients at risk of developing gastric cancer. These polyps, combined with the much higher frequency of potentially malignant duodenal polyps, warrant upper GI surveillance. Li-Fraumeni syndrome is an autosomal dominant disorder caused by a mutation in the tumor suppressor gene *p53*. These patients are at risk for numerous malignancies, including gastric cancer. Hereditary nonpolyposis colorectal cancer, or Lynch syndrome, which accounts for 2% to 3% of all colon and rectal cancers and is associated with microsatellite instability, is also associated with an increased risk of gastric and ovarian cancers.

Several genetic alterations have been identified that are associated with gastric adenocarcinoma. These changes can be classified as the activation of oncogenes, inactivation of tumor suppressor genes, reduction of cellular adhesion, reactivation of telomerase, and presence of microsatellite instability. The c-*met* protooncogene is the receptor for the hepatocyte growth factor and is frequently overexpressed in gastric cancer, as are the k-*sam* and c-*erbB2* oncogenes. Inactivation of the tumor suppressor genes *p53* and *p16* has been reported in diffuse and intestinal-type cancers, whereas adenomatous polyposis coli gene mutations tend to be more frequent in intestinal-type gastric cancers. Also, a reduction or loss in the cell adhesion molecule E-cadherin can be found in approximately 50% of diffuse-type gastric cancers. Microsatellite instability can be found in approximately 20% to 30% of intestinal-type gastric cancers. Microsatellites are lengths of DNA in which a short (one to five nucleotide) motif is repeated several times. Microsatellite instability reflects a gain or loss of repeat units in a germline microsatellite allele, indicating the clonal expansion that is typical of a neoplasm.

Other Risk Factors

Patients with pernicious anemia are at increased risk for developing gastric cancer. Achlorhydria is the defining feature of this condition; it occurs when chief and parietal cells are destroyed by an autoimmune reaction. The mucosa becomes very atrophic and develops antral and intestinal metaplasia. The relative risk for a patient with pernicious anemia developing gastric cancer is 2.1 to 5.6 of the general population.

Polyps. Adenomatous polyps carry a distinct risk for the development of malignancy in the polyp. Mucosal atypia is frequent, and progression from dysplasia to carcinoma in situ has been observed. The risk for the development of carcinoma is approximately 10% to 20% and increases with increasing size of the polyp. Endoscopic removal is indicated for pedunculated lesions and is sufficient if the polyp is completely removed and there are no foci of invasive cancer on histologic examination. If the polyp is larger than 2 cm, is sessile, or has a proven focus of invasive carcinoma, operative excision is warranted.

Fundic gland polyps (Fig. 48-20) are benign lesions that are thought to result from glandular hyperplasia and decreased luminal flow. They are strongly associated with PPI use and occur in one third of patients by 1 year. Dysplasia, although common in patients whose polyps result from familial adenomatous polyposis, has been described only as individual case reports for patients whose polyps result from PPI therapy. Such cases do not require excision, regular surveillance, or cessation of therapy.

Proton pump inhibitors. The use of PPIs has increased dramatically over the past 20 years because they have been proven to be an effective treatment for patients with GI reflux disease. They are often prescribed empirically as first-line treatment for dyspepsia. The impact of PPIs on the incidence of gastric cancer has not been elucidated.

Physiologically, PPIs, as their name suggests, block the hydrogen-potassium pump within the parietal cells, effectively blocking all acid secretion in the stomach. As a result, patients taking PPIs develop hypergastrinemia, which reverses with PPI withdrawal. The potential for cancer is at the intersection between *H. pylori*, already considered a carcinogen for gastric cancer, and the physiologic changes that are a consequence of PPI use. In patients with *H. pylori* taking long-term PPIs, the low-acid environment allows the bacteria to colonize the gastric body, leading to corpus gastritis. One third of these patients develop atrophic gastritis, which is significantly more common in patients with *H. pylori* who are taking PPIs. This atrophic gastritis quickly resolves

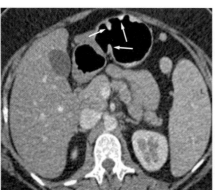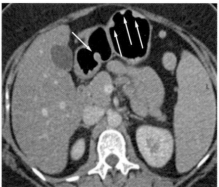

FIGURE 48-20 CT scan of fundic gland polyps. (Courtesy Dr. David Bentrem, Department of Surgery, Northwestern University Feinberg School of Medicine, Chicago, IL.)

after eradication of the *H. pylori*. At the present time, no study has shown the atrophic gastritis in this subset of patients to be associated with an increased cancer risk. However, in general, atrophic gastritis is considered a major risk factor for the development of gastric cancer. Additionally, several epidemiologic studies found an association with PPI therapy and the development of gastric cancer, although no evidence of causality has yet to be proven.[19] Therefore, PPIs are an effective first-line treatment for dyspepsia and remain an effective long-term therapy for patients with GE reflux disease. However, given the relationship between acid suppression, *H. pylori,* and the development of atrophic gastritis, a known risk factor for gastric cancer, in patients with persistent symptoms after initiation of therapy or who require long-term therapy, surveillance for and eradication of *H. pylori* is warranted.

Pathology

Numerous pathologic classification schemes of gastric cancer have been proposed. The Borrmann classification system was developed in 1926; it remains useful today for the description of endoscopic findings. This system divides gastric carcinoma into five types, depending on the lesion's macroscopic appearance (Fig. 48-21). One type, linitis plastica, describes a diffusely infiltrating lesion involving the entire stomach. Other classification systems have been proposed, but the most useful and widely used system is the one proposed by Lauren in 1965. This system separates gastric adenocarcinoma into intestinal or diffuse types based on histology, with both types having distinct pathology, epidemiology, and prognosis (Table 48-6).

The intestinal variant is more well differentiated and typically arises in the setting of a recognizable precancerous condition, such as gastric atrophy or intestinal metaplasia. Men are more commonly affected than women, and the incidence of intestinal-type gastric adenocarcinoma increases with age. These cancers are typically well differentiated, with a tendency to form glands. Metastatic spread is generally hematogenous to distant organs. The intestinal type is also the dominant histology in areas in which gastric cancer is epidemic, suggesting an environmental cause. Local rates of *H. pylori* prevalence likely play a large part in this increased environmental risk, as infection has been linked to the development of intestinal variant gastric cancer specifically.

The diffuse form of gastric adenocarcinoma consists of tiny clusters of small, uniform signet ring cells; is poorly differentiated; and lacks glands. It tends to spread submucosally, with less inflammatory infiltration than the intestinal type, with early metastatic spread via transmural extension and lymphatic invasion. It is generally not associated with chronic gastritis, is more common in women, and affects a slightly younger age group. The diffuse form also has an association with blood type A and familial occurrence, suggesting a genetic cause. Intraperitoneal metastases are frequent, and, in general, the prognosis is less favorable than for patients with intestinal-type cancers.

In 2010, the World Health Organization (WHO) revised their alternative classification system for gastric cancers based on morphologic features. In the WHO system, gastric cancer is divided into five main categories—adenocarcinoma, adenosquamous cell carcinoma, squamous cell carcinoma, undifferentiated carcinoma, and unclassified carcinoma. Adenocarcinomas are further subdivided into five types according to their growth pattern—papillary, tubular, mucinous, poorly cohesive (including signet ring cell carcinoma), and mixed adenocarcinoma. Although widely used, the WHO classification system offers little in terms of patient management, and there are a significant number of gastric cancers that do not fit into their categories. There is little evidence that any of the above-mentioned classification systems can add to the prognostic information provided by the American Joint Cancer Commission (AJCC) tumor, node, metastasis (TNM) staging system.

Diagnosis and Workup
Signs and Symptoms

The symptoms of gastric cancer are generally nonspecific and contribute to its frequently advanced stage at the time of diagnosis. Symptoms include epigastric pain, early satiety, and weight loss. These symptoms are frequently mistaken for more common benign causes of dyspepsia including PUD and gastritis. The pain associated with gastric cancer tends to be constant and nonradiating and is generally not relieved by eating. More advanced lesions may manifest with either obstruction or dysphagia depending on the location of the tumor. Some degree of GI bleeding is common, with 40% of patients having some form of anemia and 15% having frank hematemesis.

A complete history and physical examination should be performed, with special attention to any evidence of advanced disease, including metastatic nodal disease; supraclavicular (Virchow) or periumbilical (Sister Mary Joseph node); and evidence of

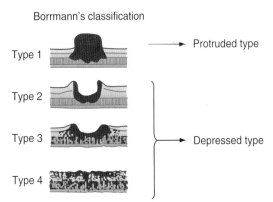

Borrmann's classification

Type 1 → Protruded type

Type 2

Type 3 → Depressed type

Type 4

FIGURE 48-21 Borrmann's pathologic classification of gastric cancer based on gross appearance. (From Iriyama K, Asakawa T, Koike H, et al: Is extensive lymphadenectomy necessary for surgical treatment of intramucosal carcinoma of the stomach? *Arch Surg* 124:309–311, 1989.)

TABLE 48-6	Lauren Classification System	
INTESTINAL	**DIFFUSE**
Environmental	Familial
Gastric atrophy, intestinal metaplasia	Blood type A
Men > women	Women > men
Increasing incidence with age	Younger age group
Gland formation	Poorly differentiated, signet ring cells
Hematogenous spread	Transmural, lymphatic spread
Microsatellite instability	Decreased E-cadherin
APC gene mutations	
p53, p16 inactivation	*p53, p16* inactivation

APC, Adenomatous polyposis coli.

intra-abdominal metastases such as hepatomegaly, jaundice, or ascites. Drop metastases to the ovaries (Krukenberg tumor) may be detectable on pelvic examination, and peritoneal metastases can be felt as a firm shelf (Blumer shelf) on rectal examination. Complete blood count, chemistry panel including liver function tests, and coagulation studies should be carried out.

Staging

The most widely used staging system at the present time is the AJCC TNM staging system. This system is based on the depth of tumor invasion (T), number of involved lymph nodes (N), and presence or absence of metastatic disease (M) (Table 48-7). Before 1997, N stage was determined by the anatomic location of the nodes with respect to the primary tumor, rather than the absolute number of nodes. This staging, based on anatomy, was intimately related to the D1 versus D2 anatomic lymphadenectomy debate (see later). The revised system does not differentiate among the locations of positive nodes. In the current staging system, a minimum of 15 nodes must be evaluated for accurate staging. Some experts have suggested that other factors be included in the T and N assessment, such as the location of the primary (cardia compared with distal tumors) because this may independently predict survival and emphasis on the percentage of positive nodes

(lymph node ratio) rather than the number of positive nodes. However, the current AJCC staging system does not reflect these factors.

The Siewert classification system is based on the anatomic location of adenocarcinomas (esophageal and gastric) that are in close proximity to the GE junction. This is an important distinction because such gastric cancers are more aggressive in nature and are treated in a similar manner to esophageal adenocarcinomas. There are three Siewert types: Type I tumors are tumors of the distal esophagus, within 1 to 5 cm above the GE junction; type II tumors have a tumor center located from 1 cm above the GE junction to 2 cm below it; type III tumors are termed subcardinal and are located between 2 and 5 cm caudad to the GE junction. In general, Siewert types I and II tumors are treated similar to esophageal adenocarcinoma, whereas type III tumors can be treated according to the guidelines for gastric adenocarcinoma described here, as long as the tumor does not extend into the GE junction.

Although not part of the formal AJCC staging system, the term *R status*, first described by Hermanek in 1994, is used to describe tumor status after resection and is important for determining the adequacy of surgery. R0 describes a microscopically margin-negative resection, in which no gross or microscopic tumor

TABLE 48-7 TNM Classification of Carcinoma of the Stomach

Primary Tumor (T)

TX	Primary tumor cannot be assessed
T0	No evidence of primary tumor
Tis	Carcinoma in situ; intraepithelial tumor without invasion of the lamina propria
T1	Tumor invades lamina propria, muscularis mucosae, or submucosa
T1a	Tumor invades lamina propria or muscularis mucosae
T1b	Tumor invades submucosa
T2	Tumor invades muscularis propria*
T3	Tumor penetrates subserosal connective tissue without invasion of visceral peritoneum or adjacent structures[†,‡]
T4	Tumor invades serosa (visceral peritoneum) or adjacent structures[†,‡]
T4a	Tumor invades serosa (visceral peritoneum)
T4b	Tumor invades adjacent structures

Regional Lymph Nodes (N)

NX	Regional lymph node(s) cannot be assessed
N0	No regional lymph node metastasis[§]
N1	Metastasis in 1-2 regional lymph nodes
N2	Metastasis in 3-6 regional lymph nodes
N3	Metastasis in 7 or more regional lymph nodes
N3a	Metastasis in 7-15 regional lymph nodes
N3b	Metastasis in 16 or more regional lymph nodes

Distant Metastasis (M)

M0	No distant metastasis
M1	Distant metastasis

ANATOMIC STAGE	PROGNOSTIC GROUP		
0	Tis	N0	M0
IA	T1	N0	M0
IB	T2	N0	M0
	T1	N1	M0
IIA	T3	N0	M0
	T2	N1	M0
	T1	N2	M0
IIB	T4a	N0	M0
	T3	N1	M0
	T2	N2	M0
	T1	N3	M0
IIIA	T4a	N1	M0
	T3	N2	M0
	T2	N3	M0
IIIB	T4b	N0	M0
	T4b	N1	M0
	T4a	N2	M0
	T3	N3	M0
IIIC	T4b	N2	M0
	T4b	N3	M0
	T4a	N3	M0
IV	Any T	Any N	M1

*A tumor may penetrate the muscularis propria with extension into the gastrocolic or gastrohepatic ligaments, or into the greater or

From Edge S, Byrd D, Compton C, et al, editors: *AJCC cancer staging manual*, ed 7, New York, 2010, Springer.
lesser omentum, without perforation of the visceral peritoneum covering these structures. In this case, the tumor is classified T3. If there is perforation of the visceral peritoneum covering the gastric ligaments or the omentum, the tumor should be classified T4.
[†]The adjacent structures of the stomach include the spleen, transverse colon, liver, diaphragm, pancreas, abdominal wall, adrenal gland, kidney, small intestine, and retroperitoneum.
[‡]Intramural extension to the duodenum or esophagus is classified by the depth of the greatest invasion in any of these sites, including the stomach.
[§]A designation of pN0 should be used if all examined lymph nodes are negative, regardless of the total number removed and examined.

remains in the tumor bed. R1 indicates removal of all macroscopic disease, but microscopic margins are positive for tumor. R2 indicates gross residual disease. Because the extent of resection can influence survival, some include this R designation to complement the TNM system. Long-term survival can be expected only after an R0 resection.

The AJCC system is not specific for nodal location, but the debate regarding lymphadenectomies for gastric cancer has continued. In the previous version of the Union Internationale Contre le Cancer (UICC) TNM system, N categories were defined by the location of lymph node metastases relative to the primary, with pN1 defined as positive nodes 3 cm or less from the primary and pN2 as positive nodes more than 3 cm from the primary or nodal metastases along named blood vessels. The Japanese Classification for Gastric Carcinoma (JCGC) staging system was designed to describe the anatomic locations of nodes removed during gastrectomy. There are 16 distinct anatomic locations of lymph nodes described, with the recommendation for nodal basin dissection dependent on the location of the primary (Fig. 48-22). The lymph node stations, or echelons, are numbered and further classified into groups of echelons corresponding to the location of the primary and reflect the likelihood of harboring metastases. The presence of metastasis to each lymph node group determines the N classification. For example, metastasis to any of the group 1 lymph nodes in the absence of disease in more distant lymph node groups is classified as N1. This grouping of regional lymph nodes is presented in Table 48-8. This system was not adopted by the AJCC. The AJCC pathologic staging system has been widely adopted in the United States.

Staging Workup

The goal of any preoperative staging is twofold. The first is to gain information on prognosis to counsel the patient and family effectively. The second is to determine the extent of disease to determine the most appropriate course of therapy. The three main treatment paths are resection (with or without subsequent adjuvant therapy), neoadjuvant therapy followed by resection, or treatment of systemic disease without resection (Fig. 48-23).

The main modalities for staging gastric adenocarcinoma and guiding therapy are endoscopy; EUS; cross-sectional imaging such as CT, MRI, or positron emission tomography (PET); and diagnostic laparoscopy. Their roles are discussed here.

Endoscopy and endoscopic ultrasound. Flexible endoscopy is the essential tool for the diagnosis of gastric cancer. It allows visualization of the tumor, provides tissue for pathologic diagnosis, and can serve as a treatment for patients with obstruction or bleeding (Fig. 48-24). On initial diagnostic endoscopy, if a suspicious mass or ulcer is encountered in the stomach, it is essential to obtain adequate tissue to confirm the correct diagnosis histologically. Multiple biopsy specimens (six to eight) should be taken of different areas of the lesion using endoscopic biopsy forceps. A single biopsy specimen results in a diagnostic sensitivity of 70%, whereas seven biopsy specimens increases this yield to 98%.[20] Small lesions (<2 cm in diameter) can be resected at the time of initial diagnostic endoscopy using endoscopic mucosal resection (EMR) or endoscopic submucosal dissection (ESD) techniques (described in further detail later). This resection can provide a more complete specimen to aid the pathologist in obtaining an accurate diagnosis and can potentially be curative for early-stage cancers, obviating the need for any further invasive surgical intervention.

Flexible upper endoscopy combined with ultrasound is now part of the standard workup for staging and risk-stratifying patients with gastric cancer properly. EUS provides the most accurate evaluation of the depth of tumor invasion (T category of TNM staging system) and possible nodal involvement (N

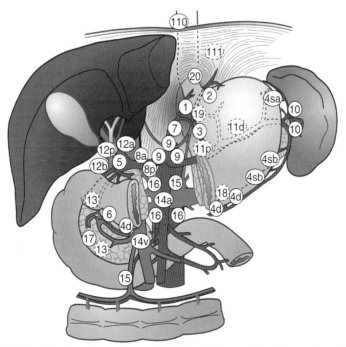

FIGURE 48-22 Lymph node station numbers as defined by the Japanese Gastric Cancer Association. (From Japanese Gastric Cancer Association: Japanese Classification of Gastric Carcinoma, 2nd English edition. *Gastric Cancer* 1:10–24, 1998.)

TABLE 48-8 **Grouping of Regional Lymph Nodes (Groups 1-3) by Location of Primary Tumor***

LYMPH NODE STATION (NO.)	DESCRIPTION	LOCATION OF PRIMARY TUMOR IN STOMACH		
		UPPER THIRD	MIDDLE THIRD	LOWER THIRD
1	Right paracardial	1	1	2
2	Left paracardial	1	3	M
3	Lesser curvature	1	1	1
4sa	Short gastric	1	3	M
4sb	Left gastroepiploic	1	1	3
4d	Right gastroepiploic	2	1	1
5	Suprapyloric	3	1	1
6	Infrapyloric	3	1	1
7	Left gastric artery	2	2	2
8a	Anterior common hepatic	2	2	2
8p	Posterior common hepatic	3	3	3
9	Celiac artery	2	2	2
10	Splenic hilum	2	3	M
11p	Proximal splenic	2	2	2
11d	Distal splenic	2	3	M
12a	Left hepatoduodenal	3	2	2
12b, p	Posterior hepatoduodenal	3	3	3
13	Retropancreatic	M	3	3
14v	Superior mesenteric vein	M	3	2
14a	Superior mesenteric artery	M	M	M
15	Middle colic	M	M	M
16al	Aortic hiatus	3	M	M
16a2, b1	Para-aortic, middle	M	3	3
16b2	Para-aortic, caudal	M	M	M

M, Lymph nodes regarded as distant metastasis.
*According to the Japanese Classification of gastric carcinoma (Japanese Gastric Cancer Association: Japanese Classification of Gastric Carcinoma—2nd English edition. *Gastric Cancer* 1:10–24, 1998).

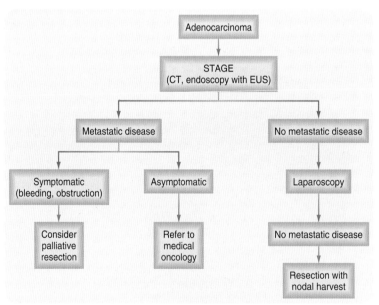

FIGURE 48-23 General staging and treatment strategy for gastric adenocarcinoma. *CT,* Computed tomography; *EUS,* endoscopic ultrasound.

category). EUS is performed using a flexible endoscope with a 7.5-MHz to 12-MHz ultrasound transducer. The stomach is filled with water to distend it and provide an acoustic window, and the stomach wall is visualized as five alternating hypoechoic and hyperechoic layers (Fig. 48-25*A*). The mucosa and submucosa

represent the first three layers (T1) (Fig. 48-25*B*). The fourth layer is the muscularis propria, invasion of which is a T2 tumor. Expansion of the tumor beyond the muscularis propria causing an irregular border correlates with expansion into the subserosa, or a T3 tumor. The serosa is the fifth layer, and loss of this bright

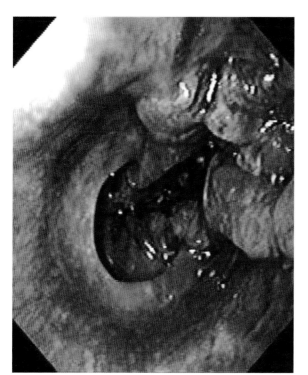

FIGURE 48-24 Endoscopic view of intestinal-type adenocarcinoma of the gastric cardia. (Courtesy Dr. David Bentrem, Department of Surgery, Northwestern University Feinberg School of Medicine, Chicago, IL.)

line correlates with penetration through it, indicating a T4a tumor. Direct invasion of surrounding structures, including named vessels, indicates a T4b tumor (Fig. 48-25C). Nodes are evaluated based on their size and ultrasound appearance and can additionally be sampled using fine-needle aspiration under EUS guidance.

The overall accuracy of EUS has been reported to be 85% for T stage and 80% for N stage; however, these studies considered accuracy retrospectively and not the predictive accuracy of EUS, and most were analyses of data obtained from single institutions. A larger, more recent study[21] showed lower accuracy of T and N stages. It considered the predictive accuracy of EUS for T and N stages and found them to be 57% and 50%, respectively. However, it showed improved accuracy when T and N stages were grouped together to differentiate high-risk versus low-risk disease, defined by the presence of any serosal (T3/T4) involvement or any nodal disease (>N0). When this classification system was used, the positive predictive value of EUS to identify advanced disease was 76%, and the negative predictive value to identify low-risk disease was 91% (Fig. 48-26).[21] From a prognostic and treatment standpoint, this classification may be more clinically relevant because an EUS finding indicative of advanced disease strongly correlates with decreased resectability and poorer disease-specific survival.

Another more recent study of 960 patients enrolled in a multi-institution gastric cancer database in the United States for the period 2000-2012[22] found that only 23% of patients underwent preoperative evaluation with EUS. Of patients who had preoperative EUS and then underwent resection without neoadjuvant chemotherapy or radiation therapy, the diagnostic accuracy of EUS in determining the exact T stage on pathologic examination was only 46.2% and was 66.7% for the N stage. Furthermore, the ability for EUS to differentiate between early-stage (T1/2) versus later stage (T3/4) tumors was only fair, with an area under

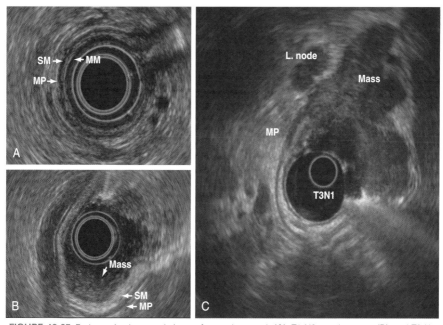

FIGURE 48-25 Endoscopic ultrasound views of normal stomach (A), T1 N0 gastric cancer (B), and T3 N1 gastric cancer (C). MM, Mucosa; MP, muscularis propria; SM, submucosa. (Courtesy Dr. Rajesh Keswani, Division of Gastroenterology, Department of Medicine, Northwestern University Feinberg School of Medicine, Chicago, IL.)

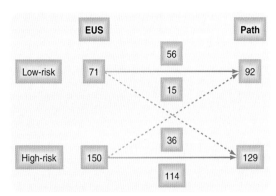

FIGURE 48-26 Predictive accuracy of endoscopic ultrasound (EUS) in gastric cancer. Of 71 patients identified as low risk (T1/2N0) on EUS, 56 were correctly staged, and 15 were understaged. Of 150 patients identified as high risk (T3/4, any N, or any T, N+) on EUS, 114 were correctly staged, and 36 were overstaged. (From Bentrem D, Gerdes H, Tang L, et al: Clinical correlation of endoscopic ultrasonography with pathologic stage and outcome in patients undergoing curative resection for gastric cancer. *Ann Surg Oncol* 14:1853–1859, 2007.)

the curve of 0.66; this is of vital importance because this distinction is often used to guide whether patients will receive neoadjuvant therapy before resection.

As the accuracy of EUS improves, it will likely play an increasing role in determining treatment algorithms in gastric cancer, much as it does in rectal cancer. At the present time, although individual T and N stage accuracy may be lacking, EUS has been shown to be a useful tool in differentiating between high-risk and low-risk patients, and this differentiation correlates with prognosis.

Computed tomography. CT of the chest, abdomen, and pelvis with oral and intravenous contrast agents is a mandatory component of the assessment of patients with gastric cancer and plays an important role in the evaluation of metastatic disease. CT is the primary method for detection of intra-abdominal metastatic disease, with an overall detection rate of approximately 85%. The sensitivity of CT for imaging peritoneal metastases is only 51%, with a high specificity of 96% if the study is positive.

CT has also been used in locoregional staging. The accuracy of T and N stages as determined by CT is less accurate than EUS. Although improved technology may increase the role for CT in locoregional evaluation and for neoadjuvant therapy, its primary role remains the evaluation of metastatic disease.

Positron emission tomography. The use of PET/CT for initial staging is limited because only 50% of gastric cancers are PET-avid. However, in patients with positive PET scans presumed to have advanced disease and patients considered for neoadjuvant therapy, there may be a role for PET. PET response to neoadjuvant therapy strongly correlates with survival, with a PET response seen within 14 days of treatment. PET may be an effective modality for monitoring response to these therapies, sparing unresponsive patients further toxic treatment. Additionally, in a study of patients with locally advanced tumors (T3/4) or N-positive on EUS, PET/CT was able to detect occult metastases that were missed on regular CT in 10% of patients.[23] Based on these data, the National Comprehensive Cancer Network guidelines now recommend PET/CT as part of routine staging for patients without evidence of metastatic disease on initial CT.

Laparoscopy. Staging laparoscopy is an integral part of the standard workup for gastric cancer. The high rate of occult metastatic disease makes laparoscopy an attractive staging modality. In the late 1990s, two large studies evaluated laparoscopy as a staging modality for patients with gastric cancer.[24,25] Both studies demonstrated high rates of occult metastatic disease (37% and 23%, respectively) in patients undergoing staging laparoscopy for gastric cancer who were previously thought to have no metastatic disease as assessed by CT. The overall sensitivity of laparoscopy for detecting metastatic disease was greater than 95%. For patients who had metastatic disease, fewer than 15% went on to require palliative gastrectomy. As a result of these studies, staging laparoscopy has been advocated as part of the workup for gastric cancer to avoid unnecessary laparotomy in patients without a clear need for laparotomy.

As CT technology has improved, the need for staging laparoscopy has been reexamined. However, a review of studies examining its usefulness showed that laparoscopy altered management in 9% to 60% of cases and specifically allowed patients to avoid an unnecessary laparotomy by detecting metastatic disease that was missed on preoperative staging in 9% to 44% of cases. Staging laparoscopy is a safe, low-risk procedure that can be planned as a single-stage procedure with resection; it can be done with minimal added risk in patients who undergo laparotomy and with no additional risk for patients who undergo an entirely laparoscopic resection. Meanwhile, there are many benefits of avoiding laparotomy, which include avoiding a delay in starting chemotherapy for patients with metastatic disease and limited life expectancy. Given the persistence of high rates of metastatic disease not detected by preoperative workup in many centers, even with improved imaging modalities, we believe that these benefits far outweigh the risk and that staging laparoscopy should be part of the workup for most patients with gastric cancer.

Treatment
Surgical Therapy

Complete resection of a gastric tumor with a wide margin of normal stomach remains the standard of care for resection with curative intent. All patients without metastatic disease or invasion of unresectable vascular structures such as the aorta, celiac trunk, proximal common hepatic, or proximal splenic arteries are candidates for curative resection. The extent of resection depends on the location of the tumor in the stomach and size of the tumor. For T4 tumors, any organ with invasion needs to be removed en bloc with the gastrectomy specimen to achieve a curative resection. The standard technique is via a laparotomy; however, minimally invasive techniques, including laparoscopy and completely endoscopic resection for very early tumors, have proven effective methods of treatment.

For cancers of the distal stomach, including the body and antrum, a distal gastrectomy is the appropriate operation. The proximal stomach is transected at the level of the incisura at a margin of at least 6 cm because studies have documented tumor spread as far as 5 cm laterally from the primary tumor, although some experts indicate that a 4-cm margin is adequate. Frozen section analysis should be performed before reconstruction. The distal margin is the proximal duodenum. The possibility of recurrence in the tumor bed (duodenal suture line and surface of the pancreas) suggests a Billroth II reconstruction rather than a Billroth I, which would result in less risk of gastric outlet obstruction secondary to tumor recurrence. If the patient is left with a small area of stomach proximal to the area of resection, a Roux-en-Y reconstruction should be performed to reduce the risk of alkaline reflux esophagitis.

For proximal lesions of the fundus or cardia, a total gastrectomy with a Roux-en-Y esophagojejunostomy or proximal gastrectomy is equivalent from an oncologic perspective. The postoperative anastomotic leak rate is higher for an esophagojejunostomy, but the margin is typically larger than for a gastrojejunostomy. When a negative margin can be achieved, a gastrojejunostomy is performed. However, to construct a tension-free anastomosis to the distal esophagus, a Roux-en-Y esophagojejunostomy is usually required. A hand-sewn or stapled technique may be used.

Minimally invasive techniques have been used for many GI tumors, and gastric cancer is no exception. Several studies have shown good short-term and long-term outcomes for the laparoscopic approach. A meta-analysis of trials comparing open and laparoscopic distal gastrectomy for treatment of gastric cancer found that a laparoscopic approach resulted in longer operative times but fewer complications and shorter hospital stays.[26] In this analysis, laparoscopy resulted in 3.9 fewer lymph nodes retrieved on average. However, a separate meta-analysis of eight trials in which D2 lymph node dissections (explained later) were specifically performed showed no difference in the number of lymph nodes resected between laparoscopic and open approaches.

Overall, laparoscopic gastrectomy has been shown to be a safe and effective treatment for gastric cancer. Although there appears to be a learning curve, when performed by an experienced surgeon, it has equivalent oncologic outcomes, with less postoperative pain, earlier initiation of oral feeding, and earlier discharge from the hospital.

Endoscopic Resection

For early gastric cancer with limited penetration of the gastric wall and no evidence of lymph node metastases, EMR can be carried out. EMR has been widely performed in Japan for decades and has been evaluated in the United States and Europe. There have been no randomized controlled trials comparing EMR with gastrectomy for early gastric cancer. Current practice is based on nonrandomized prospective studies and retrospective reviews. The most significant advantage of endoscopic resection is avoiding the need for gastrectomy, whether by laparotomy or laparoscopy. The major disadvantage is incomplete resection because of tumor size or unrecognized lymph node metastases. To avoid undertreating patients, several studies have sought to identify risk factors for harboring lymph node metastases. A Japanese study of 1196 patients with intramucosal gastric cancer without known lymph node disease who underwent resection found, in multivariate analysis, that lymphatic vessel invasion, histologic ulceration of the tumor, and larger size (≥30 mm) were independent risk factors for regional lymph node metastasis. Patients without any of these risk factors had only a 0.36% chance of having lymph node metastases.[27] Based on these data, the general guidelines for endoscopic resection of early gastric cancer are as follows: (1) tumor limited to the mucosa, (2) no lymphovascular invasion, (3) tumor smaller than 2 cm, (4) no ulceration, and (5) well or moderately well differentiated histopathology. Any of these listed findings on initial biopsy or during endoscopic resection is an indication for gastrectomy with lymph node dissection.

Endoscopic resection can be performed using one of two techniques: EMR or ESD. The basic principle for EMR involves elevating the tumor using a saline injection and then encircling the affected mucosa using a snare device to excise it with

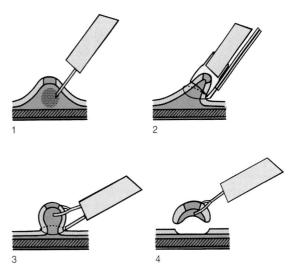

FIGURE 48-27 Endoscopic mucosal resection by strip biopsy: Saline is injected into the submucosal layer, and the area is elevated *(1)*. The top of the mound is pulled upward with forceps, and the snare is placed at the base of the lesion *(2 and 3)*. Electrosurgical current is applied through the snare to resect the mucosa, and the lesion is removed *(4)*. (From Tanabe S, Koizumi W, Kokutou M, et al: Usefulness of endoscopic aspiration mucosectomy as compared with strip biopsy for the treatment of gastric mucosal cancer. *Gastrointest Endosc* 50:819–822, 1999.)

electrocautery. Perforation rates are low, and bleeding rates are approximately 15%; these can generally be controlled without the need for further intervention (Fig. 48-27).

Long-term outcomes for properly selected patients are good. A 2007 multicenter retrospective review of 516 Korean patients showed complete resection in 77% of patients, 6% local recurrence rate for patients who had a complete resection, and no disease-specific mortality with 39-month median follow-up.[28] The data from the Japanese experience showed similar rates of complete resection and recurrence.

Some authors proposed expanding the eligibility criteria for endoscopic resection based on the results of several large studies of resected gastric cancer. A Japanese study of more than 5000 patients who underwent resection found that small tumors, regardless of ulcer status, and nonulcerated tumors, regardless of size, did not have associated lymph node disease.[29] It was also found that patients with submucosal invasion less than 500 μm behaved similarly to patients who had completely intramucosal tumors. Given these findings, the proposed extended criteria include all intramucosal tumors without ulceration, differentiated mucosal tumors smaller than 3 cm regardless of ulceration status, and tumors with limited (SM1) submucosal invasion that were smaller than 3 cm and without ulceration.

In treating these larger tumors or tumors with SM1 invasion, standard EMR techniques are generally ineffective. Given the size and depth, physicians treating patients under these extended criteria have used the ESD technique. This technique involves marking the borders of the lesion using electrocautery. A submucosal injection of epinephrine with indigo carmine hydrodissects the lesion, and an insulation-tipped knife is used to remove the lesion by dissecting a submucosal plane deep to the tumor and removing it en bloc. Any bleeding is controlled with electrocautery (Fig. 48-28).

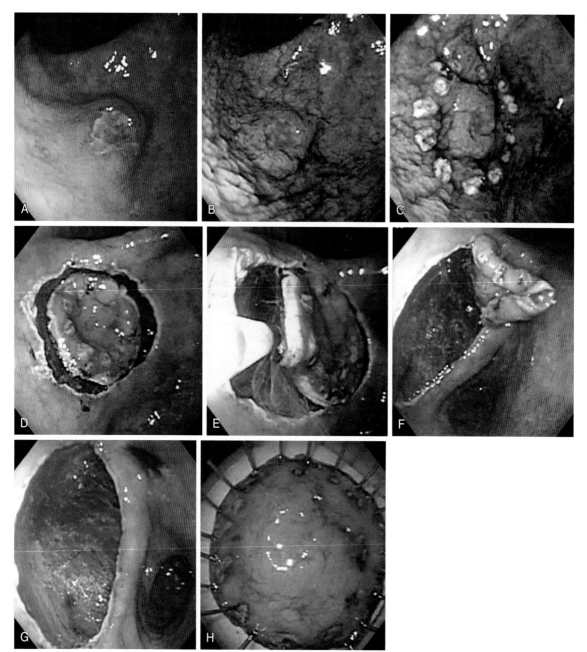

FIGURE 48-28 Procedure of endoscopic submucosal dissection. **A,** A type IIa+IIc early gastric cancer was located at the lesser curvature side of the antrum. **B,** Indigo carmine dye was sprayed around the lesion to define the margin accurately. **C,** Marking dots were made circumferentially at approximately 5 mm lateral to the margin of the lesion. **D,** After a submucosal injection of saline with epinephrine mixed with indigo carmine, a circumferential mucosal incision was performed outside the marking dots to separate the lesion from the surrounding non-neoplastic mucosa. **E** and **F,** After an additional submucosal injection, the submucosal connective tissue just beneath the lesion was directly dissected using an electrosurgical knife instead of using a snare. **G,** The lesion was completely resected, and the consequent artificial ulcer was seen. **H,** The resected specimen with a central early gastric cancer. (From Min B-H, Lee JH, Kim JJ, et al: Clinical outcomes of endoscopic submucosal dissection (ESD) for treating early gastric cancer: Comparison with endoscopic mucosal resection after circumferential precutting (EMR-P). *Dig Liver Dis* 41:201–209, 2009.)

There are limited data on the outcomes of patients undergoing EMR or endoscopic submucosal resection with extended criteria. A large series of 1627 patients who underwent resection using either EMR or ESD techniques found that patients with standard and extended criteria for endoscopic resection had similarly low local recurrence rates (0.9% and 1.1%) at median 32-month follow-up.[30] However, for patients undergoing extended criteria resection, ESD resulted in significantly higher rates of complete resection compared with EMR (83% versus 91%, P < .01). Based on these results, it seems reasonable to perform ESD for such extended criteria tumors. However, such procedures are technically challenging and surgeons should amass a large series of EMR resections for standard criteria tumors before attempting ESD procedures for oncologic indications, especially in the United States where fewer patients present with early-stage disease.

Clinical Decision Making

Endoscopic therapy for gastric cancer is well established in Eastern countries. Endoscopic resection is a safe and effective technique for patients who meet the criteria and will continue to play an increasing role in the treatment of this disease. Although several larger studies of patients who underwent gastrectomy with lymphadenectomy suggested that the eligibility could be safely expanded, two smaller studies of patients who underwent endoscopic resection under these criteria showed a higher rate of lymph node disease. Given that all these patients had early gastric cancer and were potentially curable with gastrectomy and lymphadenectomy, undertreatment in this group is especially concerning. As a matter of standard practice, patients with tumors larger than 2 cm, with ulceration or with any submucosal invasion, should be referred for gastrectomy with lymph node dissection if not part of a clinical trial.

Lymph node dissection. The extent of lymphadenectomy for gastric adenocarcinoma is an area of ongoing debate. Historically, lymphadenectomy for gastric adenocarcinoma was defined by, and is still often discussed in terms of, the location of the nodes relative to the primary tumor. The extent of dissection ranges from the more local D1 lymphadenectomy involving only perigastric nodes to clearance of the celiac axis, with or without splenectomy, in an extended D2 dissection to complete clearance of the celiac axis and periaortic nodes in a superextended D3 lymphadenectomy.

Several randomized trials compared the outcomes of patients undergoing D1 versus D2 dissection, with conflicting results. Whether these conflicting results are a result of different biology or of surgical technique is a matter of debate. The two large non-Japanese randomized trials (MRC and Dutch D1D2 trials) found that D2 lymphadenectomy resulted in higher rates of perioperative morbidity and increased mortality.[31,32] The MRC trial showed no difference in recurrence-free or overall survival outcomes at greater than 5-year follow-up.[33] Although the Dutch D1D2 trial showed lower recurrence rates and disease-free survival at 15-year follow-up in the D2 group, there was no difference in overall survival, possibly because of the increase in perioperative mortality for D2 patients. The results of both of these trials are confounded by the fact that patients undergoing concurrent splenectomy had much higher rates of perioperative morbidity and mortality, and the Dutch D1D2 trial group now advocates a D2 lymph node dissection with splenic preservation.

In contrast, the Japanese have shown increased survival in patients undergoing a D2 dissection, with no increased or minimal increase in morbidity. A meta-analysis of 12 randomized trials comparing lymph node dissections found that when the spleen was preserved, a D2 dissection resulted in superior recurrence-free survival, with a trend toward increased overall survival.[34] When taken together, these data illustrate that, in the absence of tumor invasion, the spleen should be spared during gastrectomy for gastric cancer and that a D2 lymph node dissection is likely oncologically superior but must be performed in a safe manner without added perioperative mortality to be of long-term benefit to the patient.

In 1997, the AJCC changed the TNM staging system so that N staging was defined not by the location of the nodes, but rather by the number of nodes. Along with this change was the recommendation that at least 15 lymph nodes be removed for adequate staging purposes. Several studies examined the impact of this change with respect to prognosis and outcomes. In multivariate analyses, only the number of nodes, not the location, was a significant predictor of mortality. When the number of nodes was used for staging, there was more consistency in survival rates, providing higher quality prognostic information for patients within a given stage (Table 48-9).

The improvement in survival rates may be caused by stage migration. Patients who were previously understaged are now classified as having node-positive disease status, improving the prognosis of both groups. Regardless, better stage homogeneity and reducing understaging are critical to clinical decisions on prognosis and potential treatments.

The number 15 nodes has become a marker for adequate lymphadenectomy. The number of nodes removed is related to hospital volume and whether the hospital is a National Comprehensive Cancer Network–National Cancer Institute institution (Table 48-10).[35] However, even at high-volume centers and National Comprehensive Cancer Network–National Cancer Institute centers, the percentage of patients who have more than 15 lymph nodes examined is less than 50%. Overall, only 23.8% of the more than 3000 patients studied had more than 15 lymph nodes examined. There is clearly room for improvement, regardless of the type of institution.

How does one achieve an adequate 15–lymph node resection? Some authors argue that the studies cited indicate evidence that a formal D2 resection should be the standard. This is also a systems issue in a given institution that depends not only on the surgeon but also on the pathology department. For the practicing surgeon, the focus should be on achieving a wide enough lymph node dissection to stage the patient adequately. Given the predominance of D1 resection in the United States and the overall failure to remove 15 lymph nodes consistently for analysis, simply clearing perigastric tissue is likely inadequate. There should be

TABLE 48-9 Median Survival According to Location of Positive Nodes Versus Number of Positive Nodes

SIZE	MEDIAN SURVIVAL (MONTHS)		
	1-6 PN	7-15 PN	>15 PN
<3 cm (n = 402)	38.8 (n = 311)	20.8 (n = 82)	9.5 (n = 9)
>3 cm (n = 233)	35.5 (n = 81)	19.7 (n = 96)	12.5 (n = 56)

Adapted from Karpeh MS, Leon L, Klimstra D, et al: Lymph node staging in gastric cancer: Is location more important than number? An analysis of 1038 patients. *Ann Surg* 232:362–371, 2000.
PN, Positive nodes.

TABLE 48-10   Lymph Node Resection Rates in Gastric Cancer*

VARIABLE	LYMPH NODES EXAMINED, MEDIAN NO. (INTERQUARTILE RANGE)	PATIENTS WITH AT LEAST 15 LYMPH NODES EXAMINED (%)
All hospitals	7 (3-14)	23.2
Hospital type		
NCCN-NCI	12 (6-20)	42.3
Other academic	8 (4-15)	25.5
Community	6 (3-12)	17.7
Hospital volume		
Highest	10 (5-18)	34.7
High	8 (4-14)	22.2
Moderate	6 (2-13)	17.8
Low	6 (3-12)	16.8

From Bilimoria KY, Talamonti MS, Wayne JD, et al: Effect of hospital type and volume on lymph node evaluation for gastric and pancreatic cancer. *Arch Surg* 143:671–678, 2008.
NCCN-NCI, National Comprehensive Cancer Network–National Cancer Institute.
*Stratified by hospital type and volume.

some attention to removing some fibrofatty tissue along named vessels. In a high-volume specialty center that can routinely perform a D2 resection without increased morbidity, wider resections are likely to be the more standard practice.

Adjuvant and Neoadjuvant Therapy

Gastric cancer remains a biologically aggressive cancer, with high recurrence and mortality rates. A review of more than 2000 patients who underwent R0 resection demonstrated recurrence rates of almost 30%, with most patients experiencing recurrence within the first 2 years (mean, 21.8 months).[36] For patients with recurrence, the prognosis was almost uniformly fatal, with a mortality rate of 94% and a mean survival time after recurrence of only 8.7 months. Other large series showed similar results.

Underlying these poor outcomes is the fact that the initial chemotherapy regimens for gastric cancer provide little benefit. Numerous primary studies and meta-analyses have shown inconclusive results. Overall, the survival for patients receiving adjuvant therapy was no better than surgery alone.

The Southwest Oncology Group (9008/INT-0116) reported a randomized controlled trial of 556 patients who had undergone curative gastrectomy alone or gastrectomy combined with adjuvant 5-fluorouracil and radiotherapy.[37] This study demonstrated a significant benefit for adjuvant therapy for overall survival (41% versus 50%) and recurrence-free survival (41% versus 64%). As a result, adjuvant chemoradiation has become the standard of care for patients undergoing curative gastrectomy in the United States. Several authors have criticized these results, noting a high rate of inadequate lymphadenectomy (54% of patients underwent a D0 resection). Given these findings, it is possible that some of the benefit from radiation was clearance of residual disease in the perigastric nodal basin. Furthermore, only 64% of patients randomly assigned to the treatment arm were able to complete therapy; 17% had to stop treatment because of toxic effects, and 5% progressed while on treatment.

Some of these study design deficiencies were addressed in the CLASSIC trial, which randomly assigned 1035 patients

undergoing gastrectomy with D2 lymph node dissection to either surgery alone or surgery followed by eight 3-week cycles of capecitabine plus oxaliplatin.[38] The trial was stopped early after patients in the adjuvant therapy group were found to have significantly higher rates of disease-free survival (74% versus 59%, $P < .0001$) and overall survival (83% versus 78%, $P < .05$) at median 3-year follow-up. In the chemotherapy group, 67% of patients received all eight cycles as planned per protocol. The ARTIST trial evaluated whether the addition of adjuvant radiotherapy would be beneficial to patients undergoing gastrectomy with D2 dissection and subsequent adjuvant chemotherapy with capecitabine and cisplatin.[39] There was no difference in outcomes found between the adjuvant chemotherapy and adjuvant chemotherapy plus radiotherapy groups, but radiotherapy improved disease-free survival in patients who had lymph node metastases on resection. A follow-up study with increased power is ongoing to examine the benefit of radiotherapy in this patient subgroup alone.

Given the relatively high rate of failure to complete adjuvant treatment in these trials, there has been increased focus on combined perioperative treatment for gastric cancer, rather than postoperative adjuvant therapy. The most significant results are those of the MAGIC trial, a randomized controlled study of 503 patients with stage II or higher gastric cancer that compared perioperative chemotherapy with surgery alone.[40] The treatment group received three 3-week cycles of epirubicin, cisplatin, and a continuous infusion of 5-fluorouracil preoperatively and three additional cycles postoperatively. More than 90% of patients who started the preoperative chemotherapy were able to complete it; however, only 65% of these patients went on to receive postoperative chemotherapy, and only 50% successfully completed both.

The treatment group had significantly better pathologic results and long-term outcomes. The chemotherapy group had a higher percentage of T1 and T2 tumors in the final specimens, along with a higher proportion of limited (N0 and N1) nodal disease compared with the surgery arm alone. The rates of local recurrence, distant metastases, and 5-year overall survival were significantly improved in the chemotherapy group compared with the surgery-only group (14.4% versus 20.6%, 24.4% versus 36.8%, and 36.3% versus 23%).

Similar to the Southwest Oncology Group (9008/INT-0116; SWOG Intergroup 0116) study, MAGIC has been criticized for inadequate staging (no laparoscopy) and inadequacy of lymph node dissection. However, in contrast to the Southwest Oncology Group trial, in which greater than 50% of patients had a D0 resection, most patients in the MAGIC trial had a D2 resection, with 15% undergoing a D1 resection. Given the ongoing debate over D1 versus D2 and the shifting focus toward lymph node count rather than anatomic location, the lymphadenectomy in the MAGIC trial is generalizable to the entire population of patients with gastric cancer who undergo curative gastrectomy. Further strengthening the case for perioperative chemotherapy are the results of the French trial FFCD 9703, which also studied combined neoadjuvant and adjuvant therapy.[41] The regimen in this trial was three preoperative cycles and three postoperative cycles of 5-fluorouracil and cisplatin, with a similar survival benefit for patients who received chemotherapy (5-year survival 38% versus 24%).

One limitation of both studies is the lack of stratification. Although only patients with clinically resectable advanced gastric cancer were included (penetration through the submucosa), they were not further stratified according to stage or other prognostic factors. Other investigators have shown that factors such as serosal involvement or nodal positivity are independent negative prognostic factors. Further studies examining which groups show the most benefit from these potentially toxic regimens will be essential. However, given the results of the MAGIC trial and FFCD 9703, patients with gastric cancer should be evaluated for preoperative systemic therapy.

Palliative Therapy and Systemic Therapy

Patients with unresectable or metastatic gastric cancer represent almost 50% of patients with the disease and have only a 3- to 5-month median survival with the best supportive therapy. Palliative therapy for gastric cancer involves attempts to improve survival and palliation of the symptoms of advanced disease. Many patients with advanced disease are asymptomatic, and palliation is focused on improvement in median survival. However, a significant subset of patients with unresectable gastric cancer have debilitating symptoms and should be considered for surgical therapy even in the setting of metastatic disease.

Chemotherapy improves survival in patients with unresectable tumors. A 2006 meta-analysis showed that triple therapy with 5-fluorouracil, cisplatin, and an anthracycline-based compound, generally epirubicin, was superior to single or double therapy (hazard ratio, 0.77 and 0.83 for triple therapy versus without epirubicin and without cisplatin, respectively).[42] Adverse reactions are common, with 50% of patients having severe neutropenia or GI complaints. Because of the high rate of chemotherapy side effects, single or dual agent therapy is recommended for older patients or patients with underlying medical comorbidities or poor functional status.

Although better than supportive care alone, results of systemic treatments remain relatively poor. Investigators continue to evaluate new treatment regimens with less toxicity. Thus, there has been increased interest in directed therapies that specifically target cancer cells at the molecular level. These include the epidermal growth factor receptor inhibitor cetuximab and the human epidermal growth factor receptor 2 (HER2) antagonist trastuzumab (Herceptin), which is approved for HER2-positive breast cancer. HER2 positivity has been reported in 6% to 35% of gastric cancers. Results of a phase III trial (ToGA trial) were first presented in 2009, evaluating 594 patients with HER2-overexpressing advanced gastric cancers. These patients were randomly assigned to receive capecitabine or 5-fluorouracil with cisplatin and Herceptin or cisplatin alone. The Herceptin group had a better median survival (13.8 months versus 11.1 months), and rates of severe complications did not differ between the groups.[43]

Cetuximab has been evaluated as monotherapy and in phase II trials as part of combination therapy with FOLFIRI (5-fluorouracil, levofolinic acid, and irinotecan; FOLCETUX study) or doxatel and cisplatin (DOCETUX study). In these limited efficacy trials, there was an increased overall response rate but no increase in overall survival. Phase III trials are required to determine the role of cetuximab in gastric cancer more accurately.

Complicated Gastric Cancer

Advanced gastric cancer represents a difficult challenge for the surgeon. Advanced disease is characterized by severe symptoms such as pain, obstruction, and bleeding. Determining the optimal treatment strategy for each patient can be complex and requires input and involvement of a multidisciplinary oncology team. The general approach for these problems is discussed here.

Locally advanced gastric cancer. Patients with advanced disease that is deemed unresectable because of adjacent organ involvement, generally the pancreas or spleen, or extensive nodal disease, including the para-aortic nodes, are particularly challenging. Data from two randomized controlled trials mentioned previously, the Dutch and British trials comparing D1 and D2 lymphadenectomy, including pancreaticosplenectomy as part of D2 resection, indicated that this multiorgan resection significantly increases morbidity and perioperative mortality. As a result, multiorgan resection has generally been abandoned in patients with gastric cancer. However, in both studies, multiorgan resection was performed regardless of tumor (T) status. In the British MRC study, no patients had pathologically confirmed T4 disease, suggesting that most, if not all, patients who had a multiorgan resection would have achieved an R0 resection even without pancreaticosplenectomy. This is in contrast to the data from several retrospective studies, including a review of 1133 patients who underwent R0 resection at Memorial Sloan Kettering Cancer Center. In that study, only male sex, depth of invasion, and nodal status were predictors of poor outcome on multivariate analysis.[44] Of the 268 patients who underwent an R0 multiorgan resection, the 5-year overall survival was 32%, with a median survival of 32 months.

Underlying all these studies, and the objective of performing multiorgan resection in general, is the desire to achieve an R0 resection. Patients with proven T4 disease who achieve an R0 resection have a clinically and statistically significant survival benefit over patients undergoing palliative resection only, with the palliative resection group having survival rates similar to rates for chemotherapy alone.

In an effort to increase the number of patients for whom an R0 resection can be achieved, several investigators explored the role of neoadjuvant therapy in otherwise unresectable disease. A 2009 phase II trial by Sym and colleagues[45] treated 49 patients with clinically unresectable gastric cancer with cisplatin, docetaxel, and capecitabine and found an overall R0 resection rate of 63% compared with historical rates of 30% to 60%. These patients were prospectively stratified according to which criteria made them unresectable—adjacent organ involvement, bulky para-aortic nodal disease, or limited peritoneal disease. For patients without peritoneal disease, the R0 resection rate was greater than 70%. Of all patients who achieved R0 resection, patients with adjacent organ involvement only had significantly better outcomes. At a median follow-up of 51 months, median progression-free and overall survival have yet to be reached, with a predicted 5-year overall survival of 54%. This small phase II trial demonstrated promising results, especially for patients with T4 disease, although these outcomes need to be further validated in phase III studies.

All these data suggest that multiorgan resection is beneficial in properly selected patients. The difficulty is how to select these patients properly. The percentage of patients with clinical T4 disease who have true T4 disease on final pathology ranges from 14% to 38.5%, with CT having only a 50% positive predictive value for true T4 disease. As preoperative staging modalities improve in accuracy, so will the ability to select patients properly for various treatment modalities, including multiorgan resection. In the meantime, for patients in whom an R0 resection can be performed, aggressive surgical therapy appears warranted. However, in patients who at the time of laparoscopy or laparotomy have clearly unresectable disease and who have no symptoms that would warrant resection, palliative resection should be avoided.

Complications

Patients with unresectable disease can develop complications such as bleeding, perforation, and obstruction. Treatment should be focused on maximum palliation and minimal morbidity. For patients with bleeding, endoscopic measures (e.g., cautery, clipping, injection) should be considered first-line therapy, and, similar to any acute GI hemorrhage, multiple attempts are reasonable in hemodynamically stable patients. If endoscopy is unsuccessful, angiography with coil embolization is a reasonable but generally unsuccessful option. If the patient is unstable and other methods are unsuccessful, surgical intervention is warranted. The resection should be tailored to the clinical situation. For patients with a short expected survival, limited resection to grossly negative margins is indicated. Patients with more localized disease can be treated with more aggressive gastric resection.

For patients with a gastric outlet obstruction, several options are available. Endoscopic dilation and stent placement can provide good short-term palliation; however, tumor progression and stent migration limit the long-term efficacy. Chemoradiotherapy has shown overall response rates of 50% and may alleviate outlet obstruction. For patients predicted to have a longer survival (e.g., patients without distant metastases or high-volume peritoneal disease), bypass with a gastrojejunostomy or palliative gastrectomy is a reasonable approach.

Perforation of gastric cancer requires surgical intervention. Primary closure of perforated, frequently necrotic, tumor is not generally possible. Given the relatively poor functional status and prognosis for many of these patients, closure with healthy omentum is a reasonable approach. If it can be done without excess morbidity, such as multiorgan resection, gastrectomy can also be performed.

Linitis plastica is a particularly aggressive form of the disease. These patients frequently have increased pain, obstruction, and poor gastric function. Symptom control and palliative chemoradiotherapy should be considered as the primary treatment. For patients with intractable symptoms not responding to other measures, a total gastrectomy can be performed.

Outcomes

The overall mortality rate for gastric cancer is 3.7 deaths/100,000 people, a decline of 35% since 1992. This incidence has been declining since 1930, likely because of changes in diet such as decreased sodium intake, changes in food storage and preparation, and decreased smoking. Nonetheless, the overall 5-year survival remains less than 25%. Many of these patients present at an advanced stage. For patients who undergo a potentially curative resection, overall 5-year survival rates range from of 24% to 57%; for the subset with early gastric cancer, cure rates are greater than 80%. For patients who present with distant disease, long-term survival is only 4% (Fig. 48-29). More than 63% of patients present with locally advanced or distant disease.

Recurrence

Recurrence rates after gastrectomy are high, from 40% to 80%, depending on the series. Most recurrences occur within the first 3 years. The locoregional failure rate ranges from 38% to 45%, whereas peritoneal dissemination as a component of failure occurs in 54% of patients in several series. Isolated distant metastases are uncommon because most patients with distant failure also have locoregional recurrence. The most common sites of locoregional recurrence are the gastric remnant at the anastomosis, in the

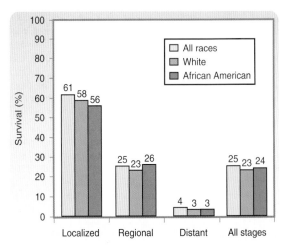

FIGURE 48-29 The 5-year relative survival rates in patients with selected cancers by race and stage at diagnosis, United States, 1996-2004. (From Jemal A, Siegel R, Ward E, et al: Cancer statistics. *CA Cancer J Clin* 59:225–249, 2009.)

gastric bed, and in the regional nodes. Hematogenous spread occurs to the liver, lung, and bone.

Surveillance. Although all patients should be followed systematically, the evidence for how this should occur is unclear. Because most recurrences occur within the first 3 years, surveillance examinations are more frequent in the first several years. Follow-up should include a complete history and physical examination every 4 months for 1 year, every 6 months for 2 years, and annually thereafter. Laboratory tests, including complete blood counts and liver function tests, should be performed as clinically indicated. Many physicians obtain chest x-rays and CT scans of the abdomen and pelvis routinely, whereas others obtain studies only when clinically suspicious of a recurrence. Annual endoscopy should be considered for patients who have undergone a subtotal gastrectomy.

Gastric Lymphoma
Epidemiology

The stomach is the most common site of lymphomas in the GI system. However, primary gastric lymphoma is still relatively uncommon, accounting for less than 15% of gastric malignancies and 2% of lymphomas. Patients often present with vague symptoms, such as epigastric pain, early satiety, and fatigue. Constitutional B symptoms are rare. Although overt bleeding is uncommon, more than 50% of patients present with anemia. Lymphomas occur in older patients, with the peak incidence in the sixth and seventh decades, and are more common in men (male-to-female ratio of 2:1). Gastric lymphomas, similar to carcinomas, usually occur in the gastric antrum but can arise from any part of the stomach. Patients are considered to have gastric lymphoma if the stomach is the exclusive or predominant site of disease.

Pathology

In the management of gastric lymphomas, as in the management of nodal lymphomas, it is important to determine not only the stage of disease but also the subtype of lymphoma. There are many classification systems for lymphomas (Table 48-11). The most common gastric lymphoma is diffuse large B cell lymphoma (55%), followed by gastric MALT lymphoma (40%), Burkitt

TABLE 48-11 Comparison of Gastrointestinal Lymphoma Classifications

WHO CLASSIFICATION	REAL	WORKING	LUKES-COLLINS	KLEL	RAPPAPORT
Extranodal marginal zone lymphoma (MALT lymphoma)	—	Small cleaved cell type	Small cleaved cell type	Immunocytoma	Well-differentiated lymphocytic
Follicular lymphoma	Follicular center lymphoma	Small cleaved cell type	Small cleaved cell type	Centroblastic-centrocytic, follicular and diffuse	Nodular, poorly differentiated lymphocytic
Mantle cell lymphoma	—	—	—	Centrocytic	Intermediately or poorly differentiated lymphocytic, diffuse or nodular
Diffuse large B cell lymphoma	Diffuse large B cell lymphoma	Large cleaved follicular center cell	Large cleaved follicular center cell	Centroblastic, B-immunoblastic	Diffuse mixed lymphocytic and histiocytic
Burkitt lymphoma	Burkitt lymphoma	Small noncleaved follicular center cell	Small noncleaved follicular center cell	Burkitt lymphoma with intracytoplasmic immunoglobulin	Undifferentiated lymphoma, Burkitt type

MALT, Mucosa-associated lymphoid tissue.

TABLE 48-12 Staging Systems for Primary Gastrointestinal Non-Hodgkin Lymphoma

STAGE				RELATIVE
ANN ARBOR*	RAO ET AL[†]	MUSSHOFF[‡]	DESCRIPTION	INCIDENCE (%)
IE	IE	IE	Tumor confined to GI tract	26
IIE	IIE	IIE	Tumor with spread to regional lymph nodes	26
IIE	IIIE	IIE	Tumor with nodal involvement beyond regional lymph nodes (para-aortic, iliac)	17
IIIE-IV	IVE	IIIE-IV	Tumor with spread to other intra-abdominal organs (liver, spleen) or beyond abdomen (chest, bone marrow)	31

*Carbone PP, Kaplan HS, Musshoff K, et al: Report of the Committee on Hodgkin's Disease Staging Classification. *Cancer Res* 31:1860–1861, 1971.
[†]Rao AR, Kagan AR, Kagan AR, et al: Management of gastrointestinal lymphoma. *Am J Clin Oncol* 7:213–219, 1984.
[‡]Musshoff K: [Clinical staging classification of non-Hodgkin's lymphomas (author's trans, German)]. *Strahlentherapie* 153:218–221, 1977.

lymphoma (3%), and mantle cell and follicular lymphomas (each <1%).

Diffuse large B cell lymphomas are generally primary lesions; however, they may also occur from progression of less aggressive lymphomas, such as chronic lymphocytic leukemia–small lymphocytic lymphoma, follicular lymphoma, and MALT lymphoma. Immunodeficiencies and *H. pylori* infection are risk factors for the development of primary diffuse large B cell lymphoma.

Burkitt lymphomas of the stomach are associated with Epstein-Barr virus infections, as they are in other sites. Burkitt lymphoma is very aggressive and tends to affect younger patients than other types of gastric lymphomas. Burkitt lymphoma is usually found in the cardia or body of the stomach as opposed to the antrum.

Evaluation

Endoscopy generally reveals nonspecific gastritis or gastric ulcerations. Occasionally, a submucosal growth pattern renders endoscopic biopsies nondiagnostic. EUS is useful to determine the depth of gastric wall invasion, specifically to identify patients at risk for perforation secondary to full-thickness involvement of the gastric wall. Evidence of distant disease should be sought through upper airway examination, bone marrow biopsy, and CT of the chest and abdomen to detect lymphadenopathy. Biopsies should be performed of any enlarged lymph nodes. Histologic *H. pylori*

testing should be performed and, if negative, confirmed by serology.

Staging

The best staging system is controversial. When possible, the TNM staging system should be used (using the criteria proposed for gastric carcinoma). Several other staging systems for primary gastric non-Hodgkin lymphoma are available (Table 48-12).

Treatment

Most centers use a multimodality treatment program for patients with gastric lymphoma. The role of resection in gastric lymphoma is controversial, and most patients are treated with chemotherapy alone. The risk for perforation in patients treated with chemotherapy has been overstated in the past and is now approximately 5%. The most common chemotherapeutic combination is CHOP (cyclophosphamide, hydroxydaunomycin [doxorubicin], Oncovin [vincristine], prednisone). A prospective randomized study evaluated several treatment strategies—surgical resection, resection plus radiation, resection plus chemotherapy, chemotherapy alone—in patients with early-stage (stage IE or IIE) disease.[43] The addition of chemotherapy was essential, with the surgery plus chemotherapy and chemotherapy-alone groups having significantly higher overall survival than the surgery-alone and surgery plus radiation groups. The addition of surgery to radiation therapy or chemotherapy did not improve outcomes. The primary role of surgery is for patients with limited gastric disease; patients with symptomatic recurrence of treatment failure; and patients who develop complications, such as bleeding, gastric outlet obstruction, or perforation.

The diagnosis of lymphoma discovered unexpectedly at surgery can be confirmed by frozen section. Also, fresh tissue should be sent for fluorescence-activated cell sorting, immunohistochemistry, and genetic analysis. Consideration should be given to bone marrow aspiration at the time of surgery. If isolated stage IE or IIE lymphoma is encountered, surgical removal of all gross disease is ideal. Patients with disseminated lymphoma cannot be cured surgically, and the operation should focus on obtaining enough tissue for diagnosis and the repair of perforations.

Mucosa-Associated Lymphoid Tissue Lymphomas

Numerous mucosal surfaces throughout the body have associated lymphoid tissue, including the lungs, small bowel, and stomach. In 1983, Isaacson and Wright noted that the histology of primary low-grade gastric B cell lymphoma resembled MALT. From that initial finding, it has been determined that in the setting of prolonged inflammation, these rests of lymphoid tissue can progress to low-grade lymphomas. The MALT lymphoma concept has been extended beyond the stomach to include other extranodal low-grade B cell lymphomas of the salivary gland, lung, and thyroid. These organs lack native lymphoid tissue; thus, the lymphomas at these sites arise from MALT acquired as a result of chronic inflammation.

Gastric MALT lymphoma is usually preceded by *H. pylori*–associated gastritis. Evidence of *H. pylori* infection can be found in almost every case of gastric MALT lymphoma. Epidemiologic studies have also linked *H. pylori* infection with gastric lymphomas. Genetically, MALT lymphoma is characterized by the translocations t(1;14)(p22;q32) and t(11;18)(q21;q21), both of which result in impaired responsiveness to apoptotic signaling and increased nuclear factor-κB activity. It has been suggested that t(11;18)(q21;q21) and *BCL-10* nuclear expression may predict for nonresponsiveness to treatment by *H. pylori* eradication and lymphoma regression.

Treatment

Given the strong association with *H. pylori* and the low-grade MALT lymphoma, there was interest in treating MALT lymphoma without chemotherapy. It has been suggested that early-stage MALT lymphomas and some cases of limited, diffuse large B cell lymphoma may be effectively treated by *H. pylori* eradication alone. Successful eradication resulted in remission in more than 75% of cases. However, careful follow-up is necessary, with repeat endoscopy in 2 months to document clearance of the infection and biannual endoscopy for 3 years to document regression. Some patients continued to demonstrate the lymphoma clone after *H. pylori* eradication, suggesting that the lymphoma became dormant rather than disappearing.

The presence of transmural tumor extension, nodal involvement, transformation into a large cell phenotype, t(11;18), and nuclear *BCL-10* expression all predict failure after *H. pylori* eradication alone. Additionally, a few patients with MALT lymphoma are *H. pylori*–negative. In these patients, consideration should be given to surgical resection, radiation, and chemotherapy. The 5-year disease-free survival rate with multimodality treatment is greater than 95% in stage IE disease and 75% in stage IIE disease.

Gastrointestinal Stromal Tumors

Gastrointestinal stromal tumors (GISTs) are the most common sarcomatous tumors of the GI tract. Originally thought to be a type of smooth muscle sarcoma, they are now known to be a distinct tumor derived from the interstitial cells of Cajal, an intestinal pacemaker cell. They can appear anywhere within the GI tract, although they are usually found in the stomach (40% to 60%), small intestine (30%), and colon (15%). GISTs vary considerably in their presentation and clinical course, ranging from small benign tumors to massive lesions with necrosis, hemorrhage, and wide metastases. Their pathology, presentation, and management as they relate to the stomach are discussed here.

Gastric GISTs can manifest at any age, although most typically they manifest in patients older than 50 years. They generally have an equal male-to-female ratio or a slight male predominance. They are rarely associated with familial syndromes such as GIST-paraganglioma syndrome (Carney triad), neurofibromatosis 1, and von Hippel-Lindau disease, but most develop de novo. Most GISTs manifest symptomatically, typically with bleeding or vague abdominal pain or discomfort. Bleeding is generally in the form of melena or, less frequently, frank hematemesis. Tumor rupture with intra-abdominal hemorrhage is uncommon, but when it occurs, it frequently requires emergent surgical intervention. Many patients remain asymptomatic, and their tumors are discovered incidentally at the time of other surgery or, increasingly, during imaging performed for other indications.

Patients are evaluated with upper endoscopy, on which a smooth-appearing, round, submucosal tumor can be identified, occasionally containing an area of central ulceration. Because of the submucosal nature of the tumor, obtaining tissue for histologic analysis via conventional endoscopic-forceps biopsy results in a low diagnostic yield. EUS-directed fine-needle aspiration results in superior diagnostic accuracy, with a sensitivity of 82% and specificity of 100% in diagnosing GIST.[46] Given the expense and specialized expertise involved in performing EUS-directed fine-needle aspiration, in addition to the fact that most submucosal GI tumors require surgical resection regardless of histology, some experts have argued that routine preoperative pathologic diagnosis is not needed for such tumors. CT of the abdomen and pelvis with an intravenous contrast agent is used to assess for metastatic disease. Pathologically, GISTs have smooth muscle and neuroendocrine features, consistent with their origin from the interstitial cells of Cajal. They are frequently identified by immunohistochemical staining for the c-*kit* proto-oncogene (CD117), which is overexpressed in 95% of these tumors, and for CD34, which is positive in 60% to 70% of GISTs.

The mainstay of treatment is complete surgical resection. Tumors greater than 2 cm in diameter should be resected, but the treatment for smaller tumors is controversial. Tumors that are less than 2 cm and have high-risk features on endoscopy and EUS, such as irregular borders, ulceration, and heterogeneity, should be resected, whereas tumors without such features can be observed with repeat endoscopy and EUS at 6- to 12-month intervals. Depending on tumor size, resection can include wide local excision, enucleation, sleeve gastrectomy, or total gastrectomy, with or without en bloc resection of adjacent organs. No specific surgical margin other than an R0 resection is required, and an anatomic resection according to lymph node basins is not required, as lymph node metastases are rare.

Recurrence rates are approximately 40%, and most patients who experience recurrence demonstrate metastasis to the liver, with one third having only isolated local recurrence. Recurrence can occur 20 years later, and long-term follow-up is warranted. Long-term disease-free survival is approximately 50%, with 20% to 80% of patients dying of their disease. Although there are no dichotomous criteria that are able to define benign versus malignant lesions histologically, the most important risk factors for malignancy are tumor size larger than 10 cm and more than five mitoses/50 high-power fields (HPF). Based on a long-term follow-up study of 1700 patients with gastric GISTs, guidelines for assessing malignant potential based on the combination of these two factors have been developed (Box 48-4).[47]

Adjuvant Therapy

Given the relatively high recurrence rates with increased disease-specific mortality for patients with larger lesions and increased mitotic rate, surgery alone for these patients appears inadequate.

BOX 48-4   Suggested Guidelines for Assessing Malignant Potential of Gastric Gastrointestinal Stromal Tumors of Different Sizes and Mitotic Activity

Benign (no tumor-related mortality)
- No larger than 2 cm, no more than 5 mitoses/50 HPF

Probably benign (<3% with progressive disease)
- >2 cm but ≤5 cm; no more than 5 mitoses/50 HPF

Uncertain or low malignant potential
- No larger than 2 cm; >5 mitoses/50 HPF

Low to moderate malignant potential (12%-15% tumor-related mortality)
- >10 cm; no more than 5 mitoses/50 HPF
- >2 cm but ≤5 cm; >5 mitoses/50 HPF

High malignant potential (49%-86% tumor-related mortality)
- >5 cm but ≤10 cm; >5 mitoses/50 HPF
- >10 cm; >5 mitoses/50 HPF

From Miettinen M, Sobin L, Lasota J: Gastrointestinal stromal tumors of the stomach: A clinicopathologic, immunohistochemical, and molecular genetic study of 1765 cases with long-term follow-up. *Am J Surg Pathol* 29:52–58, 2005.
HPF, High-power field.

However, adjuvant therapy was not effective until the discovery of the tyrosine kinase inhibitor imatinib (Gleevec). Originally designed to treat chronic myelogenous leukemia, it has proven in randomized controlled trials to be an effective treatment modality for patients with metastatic disease or disease that carries a high risk for recurrence. In patients with metastatic or unresectable disease, imatinib (400 mg daily) showed an overall 2-year survival of 70% compared with 25% for patients on traditional chemotherapy.[48] In the adjuvant setting, patients with c-*kit*–positive tumors 3 cm or larger who underwent complete resection and were treated with imatinib for 1 year had a recurrence rate of 8% compared with 20% for untreated patients.[49] This difference was even more pronounced for patients with larger tumors. The side effects were generally mild, with less than 1% of patients having any grade 3 or 4 toxicities.

The Scandinavian Sarcoma Group (SSG) XVIII trial compared an extended 36-month course of adjuvant imatinib versus a 12-month course after resection for high-risk GISTs (defined as >10 cm tumor, mitotic count >10/50 HPF, tumor >5 cm and mitotic count > per 50 HPF, or tumor rupture).[50] Patients in the extended treatment arm had higher recurrence-free survival (65.6% versus 47.9%) and overall survival (92.0% versus 81.7%) at 5 years after surgery. The results of this trial have established a 3-year course as the standard of care after surgical resection of high-risk GIST. Imatinib has also been reported to be successful in the neoadjuvant treatment of patients with nonmetastatic but unresectable disease, although this has not been evaluated in prospective randomized trials. However, as a result of current trials, for patients with metastatic disease and patients with resected primary disease at moderate risk of recurrence, indefinite treatment with imatinib has been approved by the U.S. Food and Drug Administration. Figure 48-30 is an algorithm for using imatinib in the treatment of GISTs in the neoadjuvant, adjuvant, and palliative settings.

Other Neoplasms
Gastric Carcinoid

Overall, carcinoid tumors (currently more appropriately classified as neuroendocrine tumors [NETs]) are a rare malignancy (0.49%

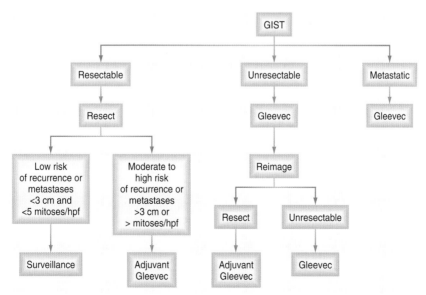

FIGURE 48-30 Algorithm for the workup and treatment of gastrointestinal stromal tumors (GISTs).

of all malignancies) that arise from neuroendocrine precursor cells and can manifest at any site in the body. The most common location is the GI tract, encompassing almost 68% of all NETs. The most common sites in the GI tract are the small intestine, rectum, and appendix.

The stomach has historically been a rare site for a GI NET; however, a marked increase has been noted over the past several decades. At the present time, the stomach is the location of almost 8% of GI NETs compared with 2% in 1950. They are also increasing as a percentage of all gastric tumors, increasing from 0.3% to 1.77% over the past 50 years. There are three types, two of which are associated with low acid and increased gastrin secretion and derive from gastric ECL cells. Type I, the most common, is associated with chronic atrophic gastritis and has a benign prognosis. These tumors are generally small and have an overall 5-year survival of greater than 95%. Type II is associated with ZES and multiple endocrine neoplasia type 1. The prognosis is still good, with long-term survival of 70% to 90% and slightly higher levels of metastases. Type III tumors are sporadic lesions with few ECL cells. They have a more than 50% rate of metastatic spread and a 5-year survival of less than 35%. The combined 5-year overall survival for all localized gastric NETs is 63%.

The treatment for localized NETs is complete removal. For small pedunculated lesions, complete removal can be accomplished endoscopically. Larger lesions may require wedge resection or partial gastrectomy. Patients with multiple gastric NETs may require total gastrectomy. For patients with recurrent or metastatic disease, somatostatin analogues can be used to decrease the burden of disease and treat carcinoid syndrome.

The incidence of gastric and small bowel NETs has increased eightfold over the past 5 to 10 years. Although more endoscopies for GI complaints account for some of the increase, there also appears to be growth in development of the disease. Given the relationship among hypergastrinemia, low-acid states, and NETs, some authors have asked whether the use of PPIs is responsible. The profound gastric acid suppression noted with PPIs has resulted in hypergastrinemia and gastric NET formation in in vivo animal studies. Although a direct causal link has not been shown in humans, database cohort studies have shown PPI use to be an independent risk factor for development of stomach and small bowel NETs. The clinical significance is unclear. With respect to small bowel NETs associated with PPI use, they tend to have a benign clinical course without any evidence of metastases, invasion of the muscle layer, or high mitotic rate. They can be treated successfully with local endoscopic excision with a low recurrence rate. Ongoing studies should define the long-term effects of PPIs and provide recommendations for surveillance of these patients.

Heterotopic Pancreas

Heterotopic pancreas (i.e., functioning pancreatic tissue is found in an abnormal anatomic location) is extremely rare, found in less than 0.2% of all autopsy specimens. Most occur in the proximal GI tract, with the stomach being the most common site. Symptomatic patients generally present with vague abdominal pain. There have been reports of pancreatitis, islet cell tumors, and pancreatic adenocarcinoma within these lesions. On endoscopy and CT, they are frequently small submucosal masses and may be confused with a GIST. The treatment is surgical excision, and the diagnosis is confirmed pathologically.

OTHER GASTRIC LESIONS

Hypertrophic Gastritis (Ménétrier Disease)

Ménétrier disease (hypoproteinemic hypertrophic gastropathy) is a rare, acquired premalignant disease characterized by massive gastric folds in the fundus and corpus of the stomach, giving the mucosa a cobblestone or cerebriform appearance. Histologic examination reveals foveolar hyperplasia (expansion of surface mucous cells), with absent parietal cells. The condition is associated with protein loss from the stomach, excessive mucus production, and hypochlorhydria or achlorhydria. The cause of Ménétrier disease is unknown, but it has been associated with cytomegalovirus infection in children and *H. pylori* infection in adults. Also, increased levels of transforming growth factor-α have been noted in the gastric mucosa of patients with the disease. Patients often present with epigastric pain, vomiting, weight loss, anorexia, and peripheral edema. Typical gastric mucosal changes can be detected by radiographic or endoscopic examination. Biopsy should be performed to rule out gastric carcinoma or lymphoma. A chromium-labeled albumin test reveals increased GI protein loss, and 24-hour pH monitoring reveals hypochlorhydria or achlorhydria. Medical treatment has yielded inconsistent results; however, some benefit has been shown with the use of anticholinergic drugs, acid suppression, octreotide, and *H. pylori* eradication. Total gastrectomy should be performed in patients who continue to have massive protein loss despite optimal medical therapy or if dysplasia or carcinoma develops.

Mallory-Weiss Tear

Mallory-Weiss tears are related to forceful vomiting, retching, coughing, or straining that results in disruption of the gastric mucosa high on the lesser curve at the GE junction. They account for 15% of acute upper GI hemorrhages and are rarely associated with massive bleeding. The overall mortality rate for the lesion is 3% to 4%, with the greatest risk for massive hemorrhage in alcoholic patients with preexisting portal hypertension. Most patients with active bleeding can be managed by endoscopic methods, such as multipolar electrocoagulation, epinephrine injection, endoscopic band ligation, or endoscopic hemoclipping. Angiographic intra-arterial infusion of vasopressin or transcatheter embolization may be useful in select high-risk cases. Operative intervention is rarely needed. If surgery is required, the lesion at the GE junction is approached through an anterior gastrotomy, and the bleeding site is oversewn with several deep 2-0 silk ligatures to reapproximate the gastric mucosa in an anatomic fashion.

Dieulafoy Gastric Lesion

Dieulafoy lesions account for 0.3% to 7% of nonvariceal upper GI hemorrhages. Bleeding from a gastric Dieulafoy lesion is caused by an abnormally large (1 to 3 mm), tortuous artery coursing through the submucosa. Erosion of the superficial mucosa overlying the artery occurs secondary to the pulsations of the large submucosal vessel. The artery is then exposed to the gastric contents, and further erosion and bleeding occur. Generally, the mucosal defect is 2 to 5 mm in size and is surrounded by normal-appearing gastric mucosa. The lesions generally occur 6 to 10 cm from the GE junction, generally in the fundus, near the cardia. In one series, 67% were located high in the body of the stomach, with 25% in the gastric fundus. Dieulafoy lesions are more common in men (2:1), with the peak incidence in the fifth decade. Most patients present with hematemesis. The classic presentation of a patient with a Dieulafoy lesion is sudden onset of massive, painless, recurrent hematemesis with hypotension.

Detection and identification of the Dieulafoy lesion can be difficult. The diagnostic modality of choice is esophagogastroduodenoscopy, which correctly identifies the lesion in 80% of patients. Because of the intermittent nature of the bleeding, repeated endoscopies may be needed to identify the lesion correctly. If the lesion can be identified endoscopically, attempts should be made to stop the bleeding using endoscopic modalities such as multipolar electrocoagulation, heater probe, noncontact laser photocoagulation, injection sclerotherapy, band ligation, or endoscopic hemoclipping. Angiography can be useful in cases in which endoscopy could not definitely identify the source. Angiographic findings may include a tortuous ectatic artery in the distribution of the left gastric artery, with accompanying contrast extravasation in the setting of acute bleeding. Embolization with absorbable gelatin sponge (Gelfoam) has been reported to control bleeding successfully in patients with Dieulafoy lesion, although the reported experience is limited.

Surgical therapy was once the only available treatment for Dieulafoy lesion, but it is now reserved for patients in whom other modalities have failed. Surgical management consists of gastric wedge resection to include the offending vessel. The difficulty at the time of exploration is locating the lesion, unless it is actively bleeding. The surgical procedure can be greatly facilitated by asking the endoscopist to tattoo the stomach when the lesion is identified. The traditional surgical approach has been through laparotomy with wide gastrotomy to identify the lesion with subsequent wide wedge resection. The lesion can also be approached laparoscopically, combined with intraoperative endoscopy. A wedge resection is performed with a linear stapling device using endoscopic transillumination to determine the resection margin.

Gastric Varices

Gastric varices are broadly classified into two types: GE varices and isolated gastric varices. Isolated gastric varices are subclassified into type 1 varices, located in the fundus of the stomach, and type 2, isolated ectopic varices located anywhere in the stomach.

Gastric varices can develop secondary to portal hypertension, in conjunction with esophageal varices, or secondary to sinistral hypertension from splenic vein thrombosis. In generalized portal hypertension, the increased portal pressure is transmitted by the left gastric vein to esophageal varices and by the short and posterior gastric veins to the fundic plexus and cardia veins. Isolated gastric varices tend to occur secondary to splenic vein thrombosis, which is usually the result of pancreatitis. Splenic blood flows retrograde through the short and posterior gastric veins into the varices and then hepatopetally through the coronary vein into the portal vein. Left-to-right retrograde flow through the gastroepiploic vein to the superior mesenteric vein can explain the development of ectopic varices in the stomach.

The incidence of bleeding from gastric varices has been reported to be between 3% and 30%, although it is less than 10% in most series. However, the incidence of bleeding can be as high as 78% in patients with splenic vein thrombosis and fundic varices. There are limited data on risk factors associated with hemorrhage in patients with gastric varices, although increasing size of the varices or a higher child status increases the risk for bleeding.

Gastric varices in the setting of splenic vein thrombosis are readily treated by splenectomy. Patients with bleeding gastric varices should have an imaging study to document splenic vein thrombosis before surgical intervention because gastric varices are more often associated with generalized portal hypertension.

Gastric varices in the setting of portal hypertension should be managed similarly to esophageal varices. The patient should be volume-resuscitated, with attention paid to the correction of abnormal coagulation profiles. Temporary tamponade can be attempted with a Sengstaken-Blakemore tube. Endoscopy serves as a diagnostic and therapeutic tool. Successful eradication of the esophageal varices through banding or sclerotherapy often results in obliteration of the gastric varices. Because gastric varices arise in the submucosa, a common complication associated with gastric variceal sclerotherapy is ulceration. A major problem with gastric varices is rebleeding, of which 50% is secondary to ulcers. Endoscopic variceal band ligation can achieve hemostasis in approximately 89% of patients; however, concerns about gastric perforations with this technique have tempered its use. Transjugular intrahepatic portosystemic shunting can be effective in controlling gastric variceal hemorrhage, with rebleeding rates of approximately 30%. A gastrorenal shunt between gastric varices and the left renal vein is present in 85% of patients with gastric varices. This spontaneous shunt decompresses the portal system and lessens the efficacy of transjugular intrahepatic portosystemic shunting. A balloon catheter can be inserted into the gastrorenal shunt through the left renal vein, and the shunt can be occluded by inflating the balloon. A sclerosant (e.g., ethanolamine oleate) is injected and left to remain until clots have formed in the varices. Balloon-occluded retrograde transvenous obliteration has been reported to have a high success rate (100%) with a low recurrence rate (0% to 5%). The major complication of this procedure is aggravation of esophageal varices secondary to an increase in portal pressure as a consequence of occluding the gastrorenal shunt. Also, ethanolamine oleate can cause hemolysis (treatable by haptoglobin administration), with subsequent renal damage.

Gastric Volvulus

Gastric volvulus is an uncommon condition. Torsion occurs along the stomach's longitudinal axis (organoaxial) in approximately two thirds of cases and along the vertical axis (mesenteroaxial) in one third (Fig. 48-31). Usually, organoaxial gastric volvulus occurs acutely and is associated with a diaphragmatic defect, whereas mesenteroaxial volvulus is partial (<180 degrees), recurrent, and not associated with a diaphragmatic defect. In adults, the diaphragmatic defects are usually traumatic or paraesophageal hernias, whereas in children, congenital defects such as the foramen of Bochdalek or eventration are involved. The major symptoms at presentation are abdominal pain that is acute in onset, distention, vomiting, and upper GI hemorrhage. The sudden onset of constant and severe upper abdominal pain, recurrent retching with production of little vomitus, and the inability to pass a NG tube constitute Borchardt triad. Plain films of the abdomen reveal a gas-filled viscus in the chest or upper abdomen. The diagnosis can be confirmed by barium contrast study or upper GI endoscopy. Acute volvulus is a surgical emergency. The stomach is reduced and uncoiled through a transabdominal approach. The diaphragmatic defect is repaired, with consideration given to a fundoplication in the setting of a paraesophageal hernia. In the unusual case in which strangulation has occurred (5% to 28%), the compromised segment of stomach is resected. Spontaneous volvulus, without an associated diaphragmatic defect, is treated by detorsion and fixation of the stomach by gastropexy or tube gastrostomy.

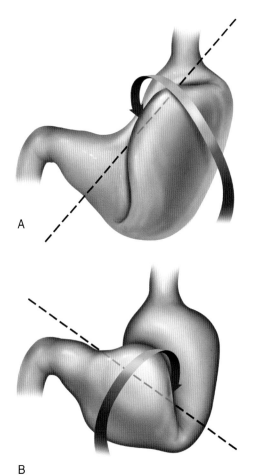

A

B

FIGURE 48-31 Torsion of the stomach along the longitudinal axis (organoaxial) **(A)** and along the vertical axis (mesoaxial) **(B)**. (From White RR, Jacobs DO: Volvulus of the stomach and small bowel. In Yeo CJ, Dempsey DT, Klein AS, et al, editors: *Shackelford's surgery of the alimentary tract*, ed 6, Philadelphia, 2007, Saunders.)

Bezoars

Bezoars are collections of nondigestible materials, usually of vegetable origin (phytobezoar) but also of hair (trichobezoar). Phytobezoars are most commonly found in patients who have undergone surgery of the stomach and have impaired gastric emptying. Diabetics with autonomic neuropathy are also at risk. The symptoms of gastric bezoars include early satiety, nausea, pain, vomiting, and weight loss. A large mass may be palpable on physical examination, and the diagnosis is confirmed by barium examination or endoscopy. In 1959, Dan and coworkers were the first to suggest enzymatic therapy to attempt dissolution of the bezoar. Papain, found in Adolph's Meat Tenderizer, is given in a dose of 1 tsp in 150 to 300 mL water several times daily. The sodium concentration in Adolph's Meat Tenderizer is high, so hypernatremia may result if large quantities are administered. Alternative enzymes such as cellulase have been used with some success. Generally, enzymatic débridement is followed by aggressive Ewald tube lavage or endoscopic fragmentation. Failure of these therapies necessitates surgical removal.

Trichobezoars are concretions of hair, generally found in long-haired girls or women who often deny eating their own hair (trichophagy). Symptoms include pain from gastric ulceration and fullness from gastric outlet obstruction, with occasional gastric perforation and small bowel obstruction. Trichobezoars tend to form a cast of the stomach, with strands of hair having been observed as far distally as the transverse colon. Small trichobezoars may respond to endoscopic fragmentation, vigorous lavage, or enzymatic therapy. However, these techniques are of limited usefulness, and larger trichobezoars require surgical removal. The small bowel should be examined to be ensure that additional bezoars are not present. Individuals with trichophagy require psychiatric care because recurrent bezoar formation is common.

SELECTED REFERENCES

Ahn JY, Jung HY, Choi KD, et al: Endoscopic and oncologic outcomes after endoscopic resection for early gastric cancer: 1370 cases of absolute and extended indications. *Gastrointest Endosc* 74:485–493, 2011.

> *This is a large retrospective series of patients undergoing endoscopic resection (either endoscopic mucosal resection or endoscopic submucosal dissection) for early-stage gastric cancers, generally those confined to the mucosa. This study found a very low local recurrence rate of approximately 1% at almost 3-year follow-up, suggesting these techniques are oncologically successful while obviating the need for gastrectomy in most patients. Most of the experience and data with these procedures come from East Asia, and further study is needed to determine the applicability of these procedures in Western populations, in which early-stage gastric cancer is much less frequent and endoscopic screening programs do not exist.*

Bang YJ, Kim YW, Yang HK, et al: Adjuvant capecitabine and oxaliplatin for gastric cancer after D2 gastrectomy (CLASSIC): A phase 3 open-label, randomised controlled trial. *Lancet* 379:315–321, 2012.

Lee J, Lim do H, Kim S, et al: Phase III trial comparing capecitabine plus cisplatin versus capecitabine plus cisplatin with concurrent capecitabine radiotherapy in completely resected gastric cancer with D2 lymph node dissection: The ARTIST trial. *J Clin Oncol* 30:268–273, 2012.

> *These two large randomized controlled trials examined the role of adjuvant therapy after surgical resection for localized gastric cancer. The CLASSIC trial found that adjuvant chemotherapy (capecitabine plus oxalaplatin) improved long-term disease-free and overall survival compared with surgery alone. The ARTIST trial evaluated the addition of adjuvant radiotherapy plus chemotherapy and showed no improvement compared with adjuvant chemotherapy alone. However, radiotherapy did result in an improvement in outcomes in patients who had lymph node metastases on surgical resection.*

Barkun AN, Bardou M, Kuipers EJ, et al: International consensus recommendations on the management of patients with nonvariceal upper gastrointestinal bleeding. *Ann Intern Med* 152:101–113, 2010.

This excellent overview of the prevalence of upper gastrointestinal hemorrhage includes an evidence-based assessment of various therapies. Recommendations are made regarding the role of endoscopy, methods of endoscopic control, pharmacologic interventions, proper monitoring and triaging, risk factors for rebleeding, and which patients have increased mortality.

Cunningham D, Allum WH, Stenning SP, et al: Perioperative chemotherapy versus surgery alone for resectable gastroesophageal cancer. *N Engl J Med* 355:11–20, 2006.

This major study showed a benefit to chemotherapy in gastric cancer. Patients underwent neoadjuvant treatment, and a much greater percentage were able to complete treatment compared with patients who completed the adjuvant trial. More patients had adequate lymphadenectomy than in the SWOG Intergroup 0116 trial.

Cuschieri A, Weeden S, Fielding J, et al: Patient survival after D1 and D2 resections for gastric cancer: Long-term results of the MRC randomized surgical trial. Surgical Co-operative Group. *Br J Cancer* 79:1522–1530, 1999.
Songun I, Putter H, Kranenbarg EM, et al: Surgical treatment of gastric cancer: 15-year follow-up results of the randomised nationwide Dutch D1D2 trial. *Lancet Oncol* 11:439–449, 2010.

These two randomized controlled trials were major challenges to the role of D2 lymphadenectomy in the non-Japanese population. Both studies showed increased perioperative morbidity and mortality with a D2 dissection without long-term survival benefit. They have been challenged on the grounds that patients in the D2 group were not stratified by whether they also underwent splenectomy, which later analysis showed as the major contributor to the increased operative morbidity. At 15-year follow-up in the Dutch trial, there was a benefit to D2 dissection in terms of cancer recurrence and disease-free survival, suggesting that if a spleen-sparing D2 dissection can be safely performed without adding perioperative morbidity, it will likely result in superior long-term oncologic outcomes.

DeMatteo RP, Ballman KV, Antonescu CR, et al: Adjuvant imatinib mesylate after resection of localised, primary gastrointestinal stromal tumour: A randomised, double-blind, placebo-controlled trial. *Lancet* 373:1097–1104, 2009.
Joensuu H, Eriksson M, Sundby Hall K, et al: One vs three years of adjuvant imatinib for operable gastrointestinal stromal tumor: A randomized trial. *JAMA* 307:1265–1272, 2012.

These two major randomized controlled trials established the role of adjuvant imatinib after surgical resection for the treatment of localized gastrointestinal stromal tumors (GISTs). The first study by DeMatteo and colleagues showed significantly less recurrence in patients who received imatinib compared with patients who did not; this was especially pronounced for patients at high risk of developing metastatic disease. The second trial by Joensuu and colleagues showed that a 36-month course of adjuvant imatinib was superior to a 12-month course in terms of disease-free and overall survival. These studies established long-term

adjuvant treatment with imatinib as the standard of care for patients with GISTs.

DeMatteo RP, Lewis JJ, Leung D, et al: Two hundred gastrointestinal stromal tumors: Recurrence patterns and prognostic factors for survival. *Ann Surg* 231:51–58, 2000.

The first major cohort study to characterize the natural progression of patients with gastrointestinal stromal tumors. This study demonstrated a relatively high rate of recurrence and subsequent metastases, which led to increased focus on the development of improved adjuvant therapies.

Fuccio L, Minardi ME, Zagari RM, et al: Meta-analysis: Duration of first-line proton-pump inhibitor based triple therapy for *Helicobacter pylori* eradication. *Ann Intern Med* 147:553–562, 2007.

The study by Fuccio and colleagues is a meta-analysis of trials comparing shorter durations of triple therapy for eradication of H. pylori (7 and 10 days) with the current standard of 14 days. This study found no difference in eradication rates, suggesting that shorter courses of therapy may be sufficient in the initial treatment of such patients.

Malfertheiner P, Megraud F, O'Morain CA, et al: Management of *Helicobacter pylori* infection—the Maastricht IV/Florence Consensus Report. *Gut* 61:646–664, 2012.

The Maastricht Consensus Report is a set of guidelines developed by an international panel of experts for the diagnosis and treatment of H. pylori. These guidelines summarize the most current evidence regarding the treatment of peptic ulcer disease caused by H. pylori infection.

REFERENCES

1. Vaira D, Malfertheiner P, Megraud F, et al: Diagnosis of *Helicobacter pylori* infection with a new non-invasive antigen-based assay. HpSA European study group. *Lancet* 354:30–33, 1999.
2. Toro JP, Lytle NW, Patel AD, et al: Efficacy of laparoscopic pyloroplasty for the treatment of gastroparesis. *J Am Coll Surg* 218:652–660, 2014.
3. Abell T, McCallum R, Hocking M, et al: Gastric electrical stimulation for medically refractory gastroparesis. *Gastroenterology* 125:421–428, 2003.
4. Malfertheiner P, Megraud F, O'Morain CA, et al: Management of *Helicobacter pylori* infection—the Maastricht IV/Florence Consensus Report. *Gut* 61:646–664, 2012.
5. Fuccio L, Minardi ME, Zagari RM, et al: Meta-analysis: Duration of first-line proton-pump inhibitor based triple therapy for *Helicobacter pylori* eradication. *Ann Intern Med* 147:553–562, 2007.
6. Blatchford O, Murray WR, Blatchford M: A risk score to predict need for treatment for upper-gastrointestinal haemorrhage. *Lancet* 356:1318–1321, 2000.
7. Rockall TA, Logan RF, Devlin HB, et al: Risk assessment after acute upper gastrointestinal haemorrhage. *Gut* 38:316–321, 1996.

8. Lim LG, Ho KY, Chan YH, et al: Urgent endoscopy is associated with lower mortality in high-risk but not low-risk nonvariceal upper gastrointestinal bleeding. *Endoscopy* 43:300–306, 2011.

9. Laine L, McQuaid KR: Endoscopic therapy for bleeding ulcers: An evidence-based approach based on meta-analyses of randomized controlled trials. *Clin Gastroenterol Hepatol* 7:33–47, quiz 31–32, 2009.

10. Mirsadraee S, Tirukonda P, Nicholson A, et al: Embolization for non-variceal upper gastrointestinal tract haemorrhage: A systematic review. *Clin Radiol* 66:500–509, 2011.

11. Lunevicius R, Morkevicius M: Systematic review comparing laparoscopic and open repair for perforated peptic ulcer. *Br J Surg* 92:1195–1207, 2005.

12. Byrge N, Barton RG, Enniss TM, et al: Laparoscopic versus open repair of perforated gastroduodenal ulcer: A National Surgical Quality Improvement Program analysis. *Am J Surg* 206:957–962, discussion 962–963, 2013.

13. Cherian PT, Cherian S, Singh P: Long-term follow-up of patients with gastric outlet obstruction related to peptic ulcer disease treated with endoscopic balloon dilation and drug therapy. *Gastrointest Endosc* 66:491–497, 2007.

14. Berna MJ, Hoffmann KM, Serrano J, et al: Serum gastrin in Zollinger-Ellison syndrome: I. Prospective study of fasting serum gastrin in 309 patients from the National Institutes of Health and comparison with 2229 cases from the literature. *Medicine (Baltimore)* 85:295–330, 2006.

15. Ito T, Igarashi H, Jensen RT: Zollinger-Ellison syndrome: Recent advances and controversies. *Curr Opin Gastroenterol* 29:650–661, 2013.

16. Norton JA, Fraker DL, Alexander HR, et al: Value of surgery in patients with negative imaging and sporadic Zollinger-Ellison syndrome. *Ann Surg* 256:509–517, 2012.

17. Dellinger RP, Levy MM, Rhodes A, et al: Surviving sepsis campaign: International guidelines for management of severe sepsis and septic shock: 2012. *Crit Care Med* 41:580–637, 2013.

18. Jemal A, Bray F, Center MM, et al: Global cancer statistics. *CA Cancer J Clin* 61:69–90, 2011.

19. Ahn JS, Eom CS, Jeon CY, et al: Acid suppressive drugs and gastric cancer: A meta-analysis of observational studies. *World J Gastroenterol* 19:2560–2568, 2013.

20. Graham DY, Schwartz JT, Cain GD, et al: Prospective evaluation of biopsy number in the diagnosis of esophageal and gastric carcinoma. *Gastroenterology* 82:228–231, 1982.

21. Bentrem D, Gerdes H, Tang L, et al: Clinical correlation of endoscopic ultrasonography with pathologic stage and outcome in patients undergoing curative resection for gastric cancer. *Ann Surg Oncol* 14:1853–1859, 2007.

22. Spolverato G, Ejaz A, Kim Y, et al: Use of endoscopic ultrasound in the preoperative staging of gastric cancer: A multi-institutional study of the US Gastric Cancer Collaborative. *J Am Coll Surg* 220:48–56, 2015.

23. Smyth E, Schoder H, Strong VE, et al: A prospective evaluation of the utility of 2-deoxy-2-[(18)F]fluoro-D-glucose positron emission tomography and computed tomography in staging locally advanced gastric cancer. *Cancer* 118:5481–5488, 2012.

24. Burke EC, Karpeh MS, Conlon KC, et al: Laparoscopy in the management of gastric adenocarcinoma. *Ann Surg* 225:262–267, 1997.

25. Lowy AM, Mansfield PF, Leach SD, et al: Laparoscopic staging for gastric cancer. *Surgery* 119:611–614, 1996.

26. Vinuela EF, Gonen M, Brennan MF, et al: Laparoscopic versus open distal gastrectomy for gastric cancer: A meta-analysis of randomized controlled trials and high-quality nonrandomized studies. *Ann Surg* 255:446–456, 2012.

27. Yamao T, Shirao K, Ono H, et al: Risk factors for lymph node metastasis from intramucosal gastric carcinoma. *Cancer* 77:602–606, 1996.

28. Kim JJ, Lee JH, Jung HY, et al: EMR for early gastric cancer in Korea: A multicenter retrospective study. *Gastrointest Endosc* 66:693–700, 2007.

29. Gotoda T, Yanagisawa A, Sasako M, et al: Incidence of lymph node metastasis from early gastric cancer: Estimation with a large number of cases at two large centers. *Gastric Cancer* 3:219–225, 2000.

30. Ahn JY, Jung HY, Choi KD, et al: Endoscopic and oncologic outcomes after endoscopic resection for early gastric cancer: 1370 cases of absolute and extended indications. *Gastrointest Endosc* 74:485–493, 2011.

31. Cuschieri A, Fayers P, Fielding J, et al: Postoperative morbidity and mortality after D1 and D2 resections for gastric cancer: Preliminary results of the MRC randomised controlled surgical trial. The Surgical Cooperative Group. *Lancet* 347:995–999, 1996.

32. Songun I, Putter H, Kranenbarg EM, et al: Surgical treatment of gastric cancer: 15-year follow-up results of the randomised nationwide Dutch D1D2 trial. *Lancet Oncol* 11:439–449, 2010.

33. Cuschieri A, Weeden S, Fielding J, et al: Patient survival after D1 and D2 resections for gastric cancer: Long-term results of the MRC randomized surgical trial. Surgical Co-operative Group. *Br J Cancer* 79:1522–1530, 1999.

34. Jiang L, Yang KH, Guan QL, et al: Survival and recurrence free benefits with different lymphadenectomy for resectable gastric cancer: A meta-analysis. *J Surg Oncol* 107:807–814, 2013.

35. Bilimoria KY, Talamonti MS, Wayne JD, et al: Effect of hospital type and volume on lymph node evaluation for gastric and pancreatic cancer. *Arch Surg* 143:671–678, discussion 678, 2008.

36. Yoo CH, Noh SH, Shin DW, et al: Recurrence following curative resection for gastric carcinoma. *Br J Surg* 87:236–242, 2000.

37. Macdonald JS, Smalley SR, Benedetti J, et al: Chemoradiotherapy after surgery compared with surgery alone for adenocarcinoma of the stomach or gastroesophageal junction. *N Engl J Med* 345:725–730, 2001.

38. Bang YJ, Kim YW, Yang HK, et al: Adjuvant capecitabine and oxaliplatin for gastric cancer after D2 gastrectomy (CLASSIC): A phase 3 open-label, randomised controlled trial. *Lancet* 379:315–321, 2012.

39. Lee J, Lim do H, Kim S, et al: Phase III trial comparing capecitabine plus cisplatin versus capecitabine plus cisplatin with concurrent capecitabine radiotherapy in completely resected gastric cancer with D2 lymph node dissection: The ARTIST trial. *J Clin Oncol* 30:268–273, 2012.

40. Cunningham D, Allum WH, Stenning SP, et al: Perioperative chemotherapy versus surgery alone for resectable gastroesophageal cancer. *N Engl J Med* 355:11–20, 2006.

41. Ychou M, Boige V, Pignon JP, et al: Perioperative chemotherapy compared with surgery alone for resectable

gastroesophageal adenocarcinoma: An FNCLCC and FFCD multicenter phase III trial. *J Clin Oncol* 29:1715–1721, 2011.

42. Wagner AD, Grothe W, Haerting J, et al: Chemotherapy in advanced gastric cancer: A systematic review and meta-analysis based on aggregate data. *J Clin Oncol* 24:2903–2909, 2006.

43. Bang YJ, Van Cutsem E, Feyereislova A, et al: Trastuzumab in combination with chemotherapy versus chemotherapy alone for treatment of HER2-positive advanced gastric or gastro-oesophageal junction cancer (ToGA): A phase 3, open-label, randomised controlled trial. *Lancet* 376:687–697, 2010.

44. Martin RC, 2nd, Jaques DP, Brennan MF, et al: Extended local resection for advanced gastric cancer: Increased survival versus increased morbidity. *Ann Surg* 236:159–165, 2002.

45. Sym SJ, Chang HM, Ryu MH, et al: Neoadjuvant docetaxel, capecitabine and cisplatin (DXP) in patients with unresect-able locally advanced or metastatic gastric cancer. *Ann Surg Oncol* 17:1024–1032, 2010.

46. Watson RR, Binmoeller KF, Hamerski CM, et al: Yield and performance characteristics of endoscopic ultrasound-guided fine needle aspiration for diagnosing upper GI tract stromal tumors. *Dig Dis Sci* 56:1757–1762, 2011.

47. Miettinen M, Sobin LH, Lasota J: Gastrointestinal stromal tumors of the stomach: A clinicopathologic, immunohisto-chemical, and molecular genetic study of 1765 cases with long-term follow-up. *Am J Surg Pathol* 29:52–68, 2005.

48. Blanke CD, Rankin C, Demetri GD, et al: Phase III random-ized, intergroup trial assessing imatinib mesylate at two dose levels in patients with unresectable or metastatic gastroin-testinal stromal tumors expressing the kit receptor tyrosine kinase: S0033. *J Clin Oncol* 26:626–632, 2008.

49. Dematteo RP, Ballman KV, Antonescu CR, et al: Adjuvant imatinib mesylate after resection of localised, primary gastro-intestinal stromal tumour: A randomised, double-blind, placebo-controlled trial. *Lancet* 373:1097–1104, 2009.

50. Joensuu H, Eriksson M, Sundby Hall K, et al: One vs three years of adjuvant imatinib for operable gastrointestinal stromal tumor: A randomized trial. *JAMA* 307:1265–1272, 2012.

49 | CHAPTER

Small Intestine

Jennifer W. Harris, B. Mark Evers

第四十九章 小肠疾病

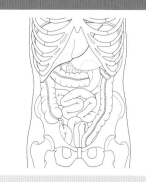

中文导读

本章共分为11节：①小肠的胚胎发育；②小肠解剖；③小肠生理；④小肠的运动；⑤小肠的内分泌功能；⑥小肠的免疫功能；⑦肠梗阻；⑧小肠炎性及感染性疾病；⑨小肠肿瘤；⑩小肠憩室疾病；⑪其他小肠疾病。

第一节阐述了小肠的发育过程及中肠与卵黄囊的关系。重点叙述了中肠发育过程中的旋转与卵黄囊的退化，以及与之相关的先天性疾病。同时介绍了小肠黏膜的形成，构成小肠黏膜隐窝的细胞及其功能。

第二节介绍了小肠的解剖，小肠动脉的来源、供应范围和侧支循环，小肠的静脉回流，小肠的神经支配，小肠的淋巴引流规律。阐述了小肠壁的显微结构。

第三节介绍了小肠的消化吸收功能。详细阐述了糖类、蛋白质、脂肪在小肠内的消化吸收过程，简要介绍了水、电解质和维生素的吸收。

第四节简要介绍了小肠平滑肌的收缩和小肠运动。概述了神经内分泌对小肠运动的影响。

第五节叙述小肠激素的分泌方式和作用类型，肠道激素受体的信号转导，并列表总结了各种主要肠道激素的刺激分泌条件、功能影响和临床意义。

第六节介绍了肠道相关的淋巴组织及各种免疫细胞在肠道中的作用。重点阐述了免疫系统在肠黏膜屏障中的作用，并图示说明了肠黏膜屏障的构成与作用机制。

第七节是本章的重点内容。简单介绍了肠梗阻诊治的历史、病因和病理生理，尤其是水电解质在肠腔内的聚集造成的影响。着重阐述了小肠梗阻的临床表现与诊断，包括：病史采集，体格检查，影像与实验室检查的方法和意义，并给出了典型病例的影像资料。强调了单纯梗阻和绞窄性梗阻的鉴别，尤其是病史采集和体格检查在诊断中的重要作用。治疗方面，不全性肠梗阻的主要治疗措施是液体复苏、抗感染、置管减压等。手术仍然是完全性肠梗阻的主要治疗手段，强调了手术时机的掌握。阐述了克罗恩病、放射性肠炎等特殊病因造成梗阻的手术指征。最后简述了一些特殊类型梗阻的诊治原则。

第八节简述了克罗恩病的历史、流行病学，详述了病因及病理。重点阐述了克罗恩病的肠道相关临床表现和肠外表现以及诊断，尤其是影像学、内镜以及血清指标在诊断中的应用。详细讲解了克罗恩病的非手术治疗、手术治疗（包括手术的指征、手术原则和术式选择）。另外，讲解了克罗恩病所致急性回肠炎、肠狭窄、肠壁穿透、消化道出血等特殊问题的处理。肠感染性疾病主要介绍了伤寒的病因和诊治及免疫缺陷所致各种类型肠炎的诊治。

第九节首先概述了小肠肿瘤的主要类型、发病率、临床表现和诊断。而后分述了小肠良性肿瘤和恶性肿瘤。良性肿瘤中简述了间质肿瘤、腺瘤、脂肪瘤、P-J综合征和血管瘤。恶性肿瘤中主要介绍了神经内分泌肿瘤、胃肠道间质瘤和腺癌的临床表现、诊断和治疗。

第十节简述了小肠憩室的分类及十二指肠憩室、空回肠憩室的临床表现和诊治。重点介绍了Meckel憩室的病因、临床表现、诊断和治疗。

第十一节简述了小肠溃疡、小肠异物。详细介绍了小肠瘘、肠气囊肿病、放射性肠炎、短肠综合征、十二指肠血管压迫症的诊治。

〔罗学来〕

The small intestine is a marvel of complexity and efficiency. The primary role of the small intestine is the digestion and absorption of dietary components after they leave the stomach. This process depends on a multitude of structural, physiologic, endocrine, and chemical factors. Exocrine secretions from the liver and pancreas enable complete digestion of the ingested dietary components. The enlarged surface area of the small intestinal mucosa then absorbs these nutrients. In addition to its role in digestion and absorption, the small bowel is the largest endocrine organ in the body and one of the most important organs of immune function. Given its essential role and complexity, it is amazing that diseases of the small bowel are not more frequent. This chapter describes the normal anatomy and physiology of the small intestine as well as disease processes involving the small bowel, which include obstruction, inflammatory and infectious diseases, neoplasms, diverticular disease, and miscellaneous disorders.

EMBRYOLOGY

The primitive gut is formed from the endodermal lining, the yolk sac, which is enveloped by the developing embryo as a result of cranial and caudal folding during the fourth week of fetal human gestation.[1] The endodermal layer gives rise to the epithelial lining of the digestive tract, and the splanchnic mesoderm surrounding the endoderm gives rise to the muscular connective tissue and all the other layers of the intestine. The splanchnic mesoderm wraps around the gut tube to form the mesenteries that suspend the gut within the body cavity; the mesoderm immediately adjacent to the endodermal tube also contributes to most of the wall of the gut tube. Nerves and neurons found in the wall are derived from the neural crest. Except for the duodenum, which is a primitive foregut structure, the small intestine is derived from the midgut. During the fifth week of fetal development, when the intestinal length is rapidly increasing, herniation of the midgut occurs through the umbilicus (Fig. 49-1). This midgut loop has a cranial and caudal limb, with the cranial limb developing into the distal duodenum, jejunum, and proximal ileum and the caudal limb becoming the distal ileum and proximal two thirds of the transverse colon. The juncture of the cranial and caudal limbs is where the vitelline duct joins to the yolk sac. This duct structure normally becomes obliterated before birth; however, it can persist as a Meckel's diverticulum in approximately 2% of the population. As the gut tube develops, the endoderm proliferates rapidly and temporarily occludes the lumen of the tube around the fifth week of gestation. Growth and expansion of mesoderm components in the wall, coupled with apoptosis of the endoderm during the seventh week, result in recanalization of the tube, and by the ninth week of gestation, the tube is again patent. This midgut herniation persists until about 10 weeks of fetal gestation, when the intestine returns to the abdominal cavity. After completing a 270-degree rotation from its initial starting point, the proximal jejunum reenters the abdomen and occupies the left side of the abdomen, with subsequent loops lying more to the right. The cecum enters last and is located temporarily in the right upper quadrant; however, with time, it descends to its normal position in the right lower quadrant.[1] Congenital anomalies of gut malrotation and fixation can occur during this process.

The primitive small bowel is lined by a sheet of cuboidal cells until about the ninth week of gestation, when villi begin to form in the proximal intestine and then proceed in a caudal fashion until the entire small bowel, and even the colon, for a time, are lined by these finger-like projections. Crypt formation begins in the tenth to twelfth weeks of gestation. The crypt layer of the small bowel is the site of continual cell renewal and proliferation. As the cells ascend the crypt-villous axis, proliferation ceases, and cells differentiate into one of the four main cell types: absorptive enterocytes, which compose about 95% of the intestinal cell

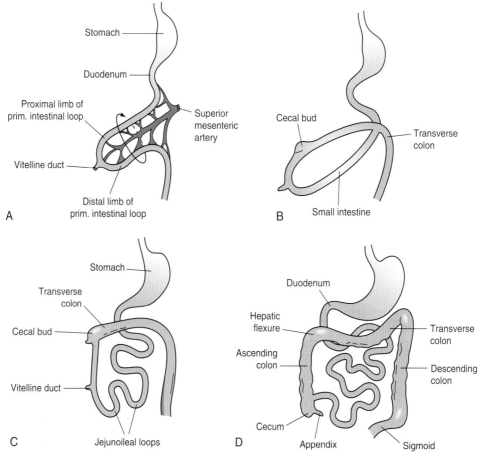

FIGURE 49-1 Rotation of the Intestine. **A,** The intestine after a 90-degree rotation around the axis of the superior mesenteric artery, the proximal loop on the right and the distal loop on the left. **B,** The intestinal loop after a further 180-degree rotation. The transverse colon passes in front of the duodenum. **C,** Position of the intestinal loops after reentry into the abdominal cavity. Note the elongation of the small intestine, with formation of the small intestine loops. **D,** Final position of the intestines after descent of the cecum into the right iliac fossa. (From Podolsky DK, Babyatshy MW: Growth and development of the gastrointestinal tract. In Yamada T, editor: *Textbook of gastroenterology* (vol 2). Philadelphia, 1995, JB Lippincott.)

population; goblet cells; Paneth cells; and enteroendocrine cells. An important distinction regarding Paneth cells is that they remain in the crypt bases, where they protect intestinal stem cells from damage by releasing signaling molecules that affect the host tissues and influence the microbial populations to maintain homeostasis in the intestine.[2] The other differentiating cells ascending the crypt-villous axis are eventually extruded into the intestinal lumen. Amazingly, with the exception of Paneth cells, epithelial cell turnover occurs rapidly, with a life span of 3 to 5 days in humans.

ANATOMY

Gross Anatomy

The entire small intestine, which extends from the pylorus to the cecum, measures 270 to 290 cm, with duodenal length estimated at approximately 20 cm, jejunal length at 100 to 110 cm, and ileal length at 150 to 160 cm. The jejunum begins at the duodenojejunal angle, which is supported by a peritoneal fold known as the *ligament of Treitz*. There is no obvious line of demarcation between the jejunum and the ileum; however, the jejunum is commonly considered to make up the proximal two fifths of the small intestine, and the ileum makes up the remaining three fifths. The jejunum has a somewhat larger circumference, is thicker than the ileum, and can be identified at surgery by examining mesenteric vessels (Fig. 49-2*A*). In the jejunum, only one or two arcades send out long, straight vasa recta to the mesenteric border, whereas the blood supply to the ileum may have four or five separate arcades with shorter vasa recta (Fig. 49-2*B*) The mucosa of the small bowel is characterized by transverse folds (plicae circulares), which are prominent in the distal duodenum and jejunum.

Neurovascular-Lymphatic Supply

The small intestine is served by rich vascular, neural, and lymphatic supplies, all traversing through the mesentery. The base of the mesentery attaches to the posterior abdominal wall to the left of the second lumbar vertebra and passes obliquely to the right and inferiorly to the right sacroiliac joint. The blood supply of the small bowel, except for the proximal duodenum, which is supplied by branches of the celiac axis, comes entirely from the superior mesenteric artery (Fig. 49-2*C*). The superior mesenteric artery courses anterior to the uncinate process of the pancreas and

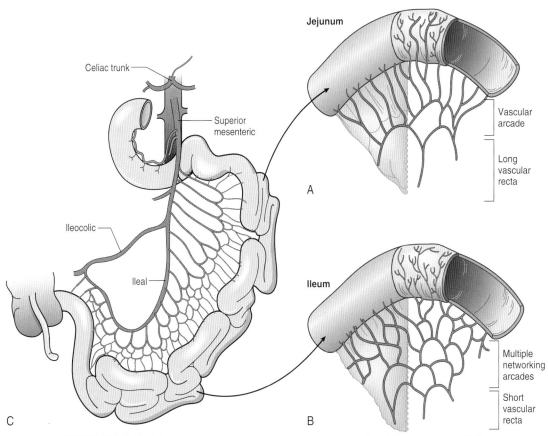

FIGURE 49-2 A, The jejunal mesenteric vessels form only one or two arcades with long vasa recta. **B,** The mesenteric vessels of the ileum form multiple vascular arcades with short vasa recta. **C,** The superior mesenteric artery, which courses anterior to the third portion of the duodenum, provides blood supply to the jejunoileum and distal duodenum. The celiac artery supplies the proximal duodenum. (Adapted from Keljo DJ, Gariepy CE: Anatomy, histology, embryology, and developmental anomalies of the small and large intestine. In Feldman M, Scharschmidt BF, Sleisenger MH, editors: *Sleisenger and Fordtran's gastrointestinal and liver disease: Pathology, diagnosis, management*, Philadelphia, 2002, WB Saunders, p 1646; illustration courtesy Matt Hazzard, University of Kentucky Medical Center, Lexington, KY.)

the third portion of the duodenum, where it divides to supply the pancreas, distal duodenum, entire small intestine, and ascending and transverse colons. There is an abundant collateral blood supply to the small bowel provided by vascular arcades coursing in the mesentery. Venous drainage of the small bowel parallels the arterial supply, with blood draining into the superior mesenteric vein, which joins the splenic vein behind the neck of the pancreas to form the portal vein.

The innervation of the small bowel is provided by parasympathetic and sympathetic divisions of the autonomic nervous system that, in turn, provide the efferent nerves to the small intestine. Parasympathetic fibers are derived from the vagus; they traverse the celiac ganglion and affect secretion, motility, and probably all phases of bowel activity. Vagal afferent fibers are present but apparently do not carry pain impulses. The sympathetic fibers come from three sets of splanchnic nerves and have their ganglion cells usually in a plexus around the base of the superior mesenteric artery. Motor impulses affect blood vessel motility and probably gut secretion and motility. Pain from the intestine is mediated through general visceral afferent fibers in the sympathetic system.

The lymphatics of the small intestine are noted in major deposits of lymphatic tissue, particularly in the Peyer's patches of the distal small bowel. Lymphatic drainage proceeds from the mucosa through the wall of the bowel to a set of nodes adjacent to the bowel in the mesentery. Drainage continues to a group of regional nodes adjacent to the mesenteric arterial arcades and then to a group at the base of the superior mesenteric vessels. From there, lymph flows into the cisterna chyli and then up the thoracic ducts, ultimately to empty into the venous system at the confluence of the left internal jugular and subclavian veins. The lymphatic drainage of the small intestine constitutes a major route for transport of absorbed lipid into the circulation and similarly plays a major role in immune defense and also in the spread of cells arising from cancers of the gut.

Microscopic Anatomy

The small bowel wall consists of four layers: serosa, muscularis propria, submucosa, and mucosa (Fig. 49-3).

The serosa is the outermost layer of the small intestine and consists of visceral peritoneum, a single layer of flattened mesoepithelial cells that encircles the jejunoileum, and the anterior surface of the duodenum.

The muscularis propria consists of two muscle layers, a thin outer longitudinal layer and a thicker inner circular layer of

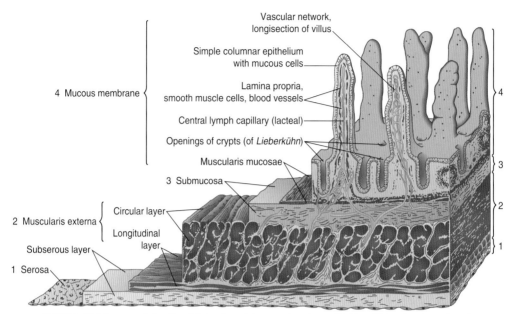

FIGURE 49-3 Layers of the Small Intestine. A large surface is provided by villi for the absorption of required nutriments. The solitary lymph follicles in the lamina propria of the mucous membrane are not labeled. In the stroma of both sectioned villi are shown the central chyle (lacteal) vessels or villous capillaries. (From Sobotta J, Figge FHJ, Hild WJ: *Atlas of human anatomy*, New York, 1974, Hafner.)

smooth muscle. Ganglion cells from the myenteric (Auerbach) plexus are interposed between the muscle layers and send neural fibers into both layers, thus providing electrical continuity between the smooth muscle cells and permitting conduction through the muscle layer.

The submucosa consists of a layer of fibroelastic connective tissue containing blood vessels and nerves. It is the strongest component of the intestinal wall and therefore must be included in anastomotic sutures. It contains elaborate networks of lymphatics, arterioles, and venules and an extensive plexus of nerve fibers and ganglion cells (Meissner plexus). The nerves from the mucosa and submucosa muscle layers are interconnected by small nerve fibers; cross connections between adrenergic and cholinergic elements have been described.

The mucosa can be divided into three layers: muscularis mucosae, lamina propria, and epithelial layers (Fig. 49-4). The muscularis mucosae is a thin layer of muscle that separates the mucosa from the submucosa. The lamina propria is a connective tissue layer between the epithelial cells and muscularis mucosae that contains a variety of cells, including plasma cells, lymphocytes, mast cells, eosinophils, macrophages, fibroblasts, smooth muscle cells, and noncellular connective tissue. The lamina propria, the base on which the epithelial cells lie, serves a protective role in the intestine to combat microorganisms that penetrate the overlying epithelium, secondary to a rich supply of immune cells. Plasma cells actively synthesize immunoglobulins and other immune cells in the lamina propria and release various mediators (e.g., cytokines, arachidonic acid metabolites, histamines) that can modulate various cellular functions of the overlying epithelium. The epithelial layer is a continual sheet of epithelial cells covering the villi and lining the crypts. The main functions of the crypt epithelium are cell renewal and exocrine, endocrine, water, and ion secretion; the main functions of the villous epithelium are digestion and absorption. Four main cell types are contained in the mucosal layer: absorptive enterocytes; goblet cells, which

secrete mucus; Paneth cells, which secrete lysozyme, tumor necrosis factor (TNF), and the cryptidins, which are homologues of leukocyte defensins thought to be related to the host mucosal defense system; and enteroendocrine cells, of which there are more than 15 distinct populations that produce the gastrointestinal hormones. The enteroendocrine cells also secrete a wide range of peptide hormones that, in a complex manner, control physiologic and homeostatic functions in the digestive tract, particularly postprandial secretion and motility.

The mucosa is designed for maximal absorptive surface area, with villi protruding into the lumen on microscopic examination. Villi are tallest in the distal duodenum and proximal jejunum and shortest in the distal ileum. Absorptive enterocytes represent the main cell type in the mucosa and are responsible for digestion and absorption. Their luminal surface is covered by microvilli that rest on a terminal web. The microvilli increase the absorptive capacity by 30-fold. To increase absorption further, the microvilli are covered by a fuzzy coat of glycoprotein, the glycocalyx.

PHYSIOLOGY

Digestion and Absorption

The complex process of digestion and eventual absorption of nutrients, water, electrolytes, and minerals is the main role of the small intestine. Liters of water and hundreds of grams of food are delivered to the small intestine daily, and with remarkable efficiency, almost all food is absorbed, except for indigestible cellulose. The stomach initiates the process of digestion with the breakdown of solids to particles 1 mm or smaller, which are then delivered to the duodenum, where pancreatic enzymes, bile, and brush border enzymes continue the process of digestion and eventual absorption through the small intestinal wall.[3] The small bowel is primarily responsible for the absorption of the dietary components (carbohydrates, proteins, and fats) as well as of ions, vitamins, and water.

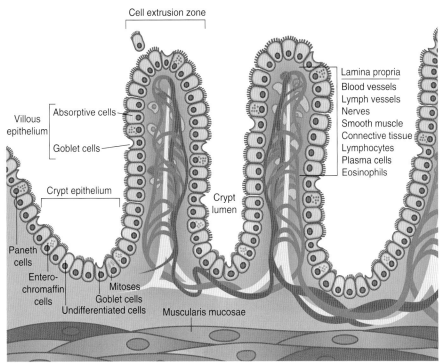

FIGURE 49-4 Schematic diagram of the histologic organization of the small intestinal mucosa. (Adapted from Keljo DJ, Gariepy CE: Anatomy, histology, embryology, and developmental anomalies of the small and large intestine. In Feldman M, Scharschmidt BF, Sleisenger MH, editors: *Sleisenger and Fordtran's gastrointestinal and liver disease: Pathology, diagnosis, management*, Philadelphia, 2002, WB Saunders, p 1646.)

Carbohydrates

An adult consuming a normal Western diet will ingest 300 to 350 g of carbohydrates a day, with about 50% consumed as starch, 30% as sucrose, 6% as lactose, and the remainder as maltose, trehalose, glucose, fructose, sorbitol, cellulose, and pectins.[3] Dietary starch is a polysaccharide consisting of long chains of glucose molecules. Amylose makes up about 20% of starch in the diet and is broken down at the α-1,4 bonds by salivary (i.e., ptyalin) and pancreatic amylases that convert amylose to maltotriose and maltose. Amylopectin, making up about 80% of dietary starch, has branching points every 25 molecules along the straight glucose chains; the α-1,6 glucose linkages in amylopectin produce the end products of amylase digestion—maltose, maltotriose, and the residual branch saccharides, the dextrins. In general, the starches are almost totally converted into maltose and other small glucose polymers before they have passed beyond the duodenum or upper jejunum. The remainder of carbohydrate digestion occurs as a result of brush border enzymes of the luminal surface.

The brush border of the small intestine contains the enzymes lactase, maltase, sucrase-isomaltase, and trehalase, which split the disaccharides as well as other small glucose polymers into their constituent monosaccharides (Table 49-1). Lactase hydrolyzes lactose into glucose and galactose. Maltase hydrolyzes maltose to produce glucose monomers. Sucrase-isomaltase is a complex of two subunits; sucrase hydrolyzes sucrose to yield glucose and fructose, and isomaltase hydrolyzes the α-1,6 bonds in α-limit dextrins to yield glucose. Glucose represents more than 80% of the final products of carbohydrate digestion, with galactose and

fructose usually representing no more than 10% of the products of carbohydrate digestion.

The carbohydrates are absorbed in the form of monosaccharides. Transport of the released hexoses (glucose, galactose, and fructose) is by specific mechanisms involved in active transport. The major routes of absorption are by three membrane carrier

TABLE 49-1   Characteristics of Brush Border Membrane Carbohydrases

ENZYME	SUBSTRATE	PRODUCTS
Lactase	Lactose	Glucose
	Galactose	
Maltase (glucoamylase)	α-1,4-linked oligosaccharides, up to nine residues	Glucose
Sucrase-isomaltase (sucrose-α-dextrinase)		
Sucrase	Sucrose	Glucose
		Fructose
Isomaltase	α-Limit dextrin	Glucose
Both enzymes	α-Limit dextrin	
	α-1,4-link at nonreducing end	Glucose
Trehalase	Trehalose	Glucose

From Marsh MN, Riley SA: Digestion and absorption of nutrients and vitamins. In Feldman M, Scharschmidt BF, Sleisenger MH, editors: *Sleisenger and Fordtran's gastrointestinal and liver disease: Pathophysiology, diagnosis, management* (vol 2). Philadelphia, 1998, WB Saunders, p 1480.

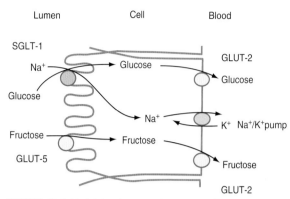

FIGURE 49-5 Model for glucose, galactose, and fructose transport across the intestinal epithelium. Glucose and galactose are transported into the enterocyte across the brush border membrane by the sodium-glucose cotransporter (SGLT-1) and then transported out across the basolateral membrane down their concentration gradients by GLUT-2. The low intracellular sodium concentration driving uphill sugar transport across the brush border is maintained by the Na+,K+ pump on the basolateral membrane. Glucose and galactose therefore stimulate sodium absorption across the epithelium. Fructose is transported across the cell down the concentration gradient across the brush border and basolateral membranes. GLUT-5 is the brush border fructose transporter, whereas GLUT-2 handles fructose transport across the basolateral membrane. (From Wright EM, Hirayama BA, Loo DDF, et al: Intestinal sugar transport. In Johnson LR, Alpers DH, Christensen J, et al, editors: *Physiology of the gastrointestinal tract*, ed 3, (vol 2). New York, 1994, Raven Press, p 1752.)

TABLE 49-2	**Principal Pancreatic Proteases**
ENZYME	**PRIMARY ACTION**
Endopeptidases	Hydrolyze interior peptide bonds of polypeptides and proteins
Trypsin	Attacks peptide bonds involving basic amino acids; yields products with basic amino acids at carboxyl-terminal end
Chymotrypsin	Attacks peptide bonds involving aromatic amino acids, leucine, glutamine, and methionine; yields peptide products with these amino acids at carboxyl-terminal end
Elastase	Attacks peptide bonds involving neutral aliphatic amino acids; yields products with neutral amino acids at carboxyl-terminal end
Exopeptidases	Hydrolyze external peptide bonds of polypeptides and protein
Carboxypeptidase A	Attacks peptides with aromatic and neutral aliphatic amino acids at carboxyl-terminal end
Carboxypeptidase B	Attacks peptides with basic amino acids at carboxyl-terminal end

From Castro GA: Digestion and absorption. In Johnson LR, editor: *Gastrointestinal physiology*, St. Louis, 1991, Mosby, pp 108–130.

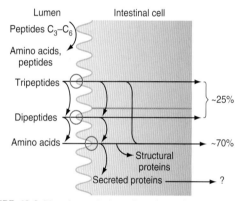

FIGURE 49-6 Digestion and absorption of proteins. (Adapted from Alpers DH: Digestion and absorption of carbohydrates and proteins. In Johnson LR, Alpers DH, Christensen J, et al, editors: *Physiology of the gastrointestinal tract*, ed 3, (vol 2). New York, 1994, Raven Press, p 1733.)

systems (Fig. 49-5): sodium-glucose transporter 1 (SGLT-1), glucose transporter 5 (GLUT-5), and glucose transporter 2 (GLUT-2).[3] Glucose and galactose are absorbed by a carrier-mediated active transport mechanism, which involves the cotransport of sodium (SGLT-1 transporter). As sodium diffuses into the inside of the cell, it pulls the glucose or galactose along with it, thus providing the energy for transport of the monosaccharide. The exit of glucose from the cytosol into the intracellular space is predominantly by a sodium-independent carrier (GLUT-2 transporter) located at the basolateral membrane. Fructose, the other significant monosaccharide, is absorbed from the intestinal lumen through a process of facilitated diffusion. The carrier involved in fructose absorption is GLUT-5, which is located in the apical membrane of the enterocyte. This transport process does not depend on sodium or energy. Fructose exits the basolateral membrane by another facilitated diffusion process involving the GLUT-2 transporter.

Protein

Protein digestion is initiated in the stomach, where gastric acid denatures proteins.[3] Digestion is continued in the small intestine, where the protein comes into contact with pancreatic proteases. Pancreatic trypsinogen is secreted in the intestine by the pancreas in an inactive form but becomes activated by the enzyme enterokinase, a brush border enzyme in the duodenum. Activated trypsin then activates the other pancreatic proteolytic enzyme precursors. The endopeptidases, which include trypsin, chymotrypsin, and elastase, act on peptide bonds at the interior of the protein molecule, producing peptides that are substrates for the exopeptidases (carboxypeptidases), which serially remove a single amino acid from the carboxyl end of the peptide (Table 49-2). This results in splitting of the complex proteins into dipeptides,

tripeptides, and some larger proteins, which are absorbed from the intestinal lumen by a sodium-mediated active transport mechanism and digested further by enzymes in the brush border and in the cytoplasm of the enterocytes (Fig. 49-6). These peptidase enzymes include aminopeptidases and several dipeptidases, which split the remaining larger polypeptides into tripeptides and dipeptides and some amino acids. The amino acids, dipeptides, and tripeptides are easily transported through the microvilli into the epithelial cells, where, in the cytosol, additional peptidases hydrolyze the dipeptides and tripeptides into single amino acids; these then pass through the epithelial cell membrane into the portal venous system. In normal humans, digestion and absorption of protein are usually 80% to 90% completed in the jejunum.

Fats

Emulsification. Most adults in North America consume 60 to 100 g/day of fat. Triglycerides, the most abundant fats, are composed of a glycerol nucleus and three fatty acids; small quantities of phospholipids, cholesterol, and cholesterol esters also are found in the normal diet. Essentially all fat digestion occurs in the small intestine, where the first step is the breakdown of fat globules into smaller sizes to facilitate further breakdown by water-soluble digestive enzymes, a process termed emulsification.[3] This process is facilitated by bile from the liver, which contains bile salts and the phospholipid lecithin. The polar parts of the bile salts and lecithin molecules are soluble in water, whereas the remaining portions are soluble in fat. Therefore, the fat-soluble portions dissolve in the surface layer of the fat globules, and the polar portions, projecting outward, are soluble in the surrounding aqueous fluids. This arrangement renders the fat globules more accessible to fragmentation by agitation in the small intestine. Therefore, a major function of bile salts, and especially lecithin in the bile, is to allow the fat globules to be readily fragmented by agitation in the intestinal lumen. With the increase in surface area of the fat globules resulting from the action of the bile salts and lecithin, the fats can now be readily attacked by pancreatic lipase, the most crucial enzyme in the digestion of triglycerides, which splits triglycerides into free fatty acids and 2-monoglycerides.

Micelle formation. Fat digestion is further accelerated by bile salts, which, secondary to their amphipathic nature, can form micelles. Micelles are small spherical globules composed of 20 to 40 molecules of bile salts with a sterol nucleus that is highly fat soluble and a hydrophilic polar group that projects outward. The mixed micelles thus formed are arrayed so that the insoluble lipid is surrounded by the bile salts oriented with their hydrophilic ends facing outward. Therefore, as quickly as the monoglycerides and free fatty acids are formed by lipolysis, they become dissolved in the central hydrophobic portion of the micelles, which then act to carry these products of fat hydrolysis to the brush borders of the epithelial cells, where absorption occurs.

Intracellular processing. The monoglycerides and free fatty acids, which are dissolved in the central lipid portion of the bile acid micelles, are absorbed through the brush border because of their highly lipid-soluble nature and simply diffuse into the interior of the cell.[3] After disaggregation of the micelle, bile salts remain within the intestinal lumen to enter into the formation of new micelles and act to carry more monoglycerides and fatty acids to the epithelial cells. The released fatty acids and monoglycerides in the cell re-form into new triglycerides. This re-formation of a triglyceride occurs in the cell through the interactions of intracellular enzymes that are associated with the endoplasmic reticulum.

The major pathway for resynthesis involves synthesis of triglycerides from 2-monoglycerides and coenzyme A (CoA)–activated fatty acids. Microsomal acyl-CoA lipase is necessary to synthesize acyl-CoA from the fatty acid before esterification. These reconstituted triglycerides then combine with cholesterol, phospholipids, and apoproteins to form chylomicrons, which consist of an inner core containing triglycerides and a membranous outer core of phospholipids and apoproteins. The chylomicrons pass from the epithelial cells into the lacteals, where they pass through the lymphatics into the venous system. From 80% to 90% of all fat absorbed from the gut is absorbed in this manner and transported to the blood by way of the thoracic lymph in the form of chylomicrons. Small quantities of short- to medium-chain fatty acids may be absorbed directly into the portal blood rather than being converted into triglycerides and absorbed into the lymphatics. These shorter chain fatty acids are more water soluble, which allows the direct diffusion into the bloodstream.

Enterohepatic circulation. The proximal intestine absorbs most of the dietary fat. Although the unconjugated bile acids are absorbed into the jejunum by passive diffusion, the conjugated bile acids that form micelles are absorbed in the ileum by active transport and are reabsorbed from the distal ileum. The bile acids then pass through the portal venous system to the liver for secretion as bile. The total bile acid pool (approximately 2 to 3 g) recirculates about six times every 24 hours through the enterohepatic circulation.[3] Almost all the bile salts are absorbed, with only about 0.5 g lost in the stool every day; this is replaced by resynthesis from cholesterol.

Water, Electrolytes, and Vitamins

Eight to 10 liters of water per day enter the small intestine. Much of this is absorbed, with only approximately 500 mL or less leaving the ileum and entering the colon[3] (Fig. 49-7). Water may be absorbed by the process of simple diffusion. In addition, water may be drawn in and out of the cell through a process of osmotic pressure, resulting from active transport of sodium, glucose, or amino acids into cells.

Electrolytes can be absorbed in the small bowel by active transport or by coupling to organic solute.[3] Na^+ is absorbed by active transport through the basolateral membranes. Cl^- is absorbed in the upper part of the small intestine by a process of passive diffusion. Large quantities of HCO_3^- must be reabsorbed, which is accomplished in an indirect fashion. As the Na^+ is absorbed, H^+ is secreted into the lumen of the intestine. It then combines with HCO_3^- to form carbonic acid, which then dissociates to form water and carbon dioxide. The water remains in the chyme, but the carbon dioxide is readily absorbed in the blood and is subsequently expired. Calcium is absorbed, particularly in the proximal intestine (duodenum and jejunum), by a process of active transport; absorption appears to be facilitated by an acid environment and is enhanced by vitamin D and parathyroid hormone. Iron is absorbed as a heme or nonheme component in the duodenum by an active process. Iron is then deposited within the cell as ferritin or transferred to the plasma bound to transferrin. The total absorption of iron is dependent on body stores of iron and the rate of erythropoiesis; any increase in erythropoiesis increases iron absorption. Potassium, magnesium, phosphate, and other ions also can be actively absorbed throughout the mucosa.

Vitamins are fat soluble (e.g., vitamins A, D, E, and K) or water soluble (e.g., ascorbic acid [vitamin C], biotin, nicotinic acid, folic acid, riboflavin [vitamin B_2], thiamine [vitamin B_1], pyridoxine [vitamin B_6], and cobalamin [vitamin B_{12}]).[3] The fat-soluble vitamins are carried in mixed micelles and transported in chylomicrons of lymph to the thoracic duct and into the venous system. The absorption of water-soluble vitamins appears to be more complex than originally thought. Vitamin C is absorbed by an active transport process that incorporates a sodium-coupled mechanism as well as a specific carrier system. Vitamin B_6 appears to be rapidly absorbed by simple diffusion into the proximal intestine. Vitamin B_1 is rapidly absorbed in the jejunum by an active process similar to the sodium-coupled transport system for vitamin C. Vitamin B_2 is absorbed in the upper intestine by facilitated transport. The absorption of vitamin B_{12} occurs primarily in the terminal ileum. Vitamin B_{12} is derived from cobalamin, which is freed in the duodenum by pancreatic proteases. The cobalamin binds to intrinsic factor, which is secreted by the stomach, and is protected from proteolytic digestion. Specific receptors in the terminal ileum take up the cobalamin–intrinsic factor complex, probably by translocation. In the ileal enterocyte,

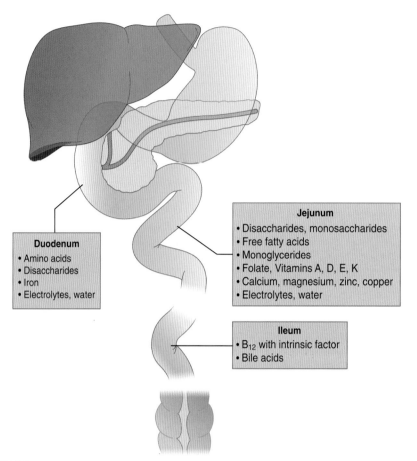

Duodenum
- Amino acids
- Disaccharides
- Iron
- Electrolytes, water

Jejunum
- Disaccharides, monosaccharides
- Free fatty acids
- Monoglycerides
- Folate, Vitamins A, D, E, K
- Calcium, magnesium, zinc, copper
- Electrolytes, water

Ileum
- B_{12} with intrinsic factor
- Bile acids

FIGURE 49-7 Absorption of water and electrolytes in the small bowel and colon. (Adapted from Westergaard H: Short bowel syndrome. In Feldman M, Scharschmidt BF, Sleisenger MH, editors: *Sleisenger and Fordtran's gastrointestinal and liver disease: Pathology, diagnosis, management*, Philadelphia, 2002, WB Saunders, p 1549.)

free vitamin B_{12} is bound to an ileal pool of transcobalamin II, which transports it into the portal circulation.

MOTILITY

Food particles are propelled through the small bowel by a complex series of muscle contractions.[3] Peristalsis consists of intestinal contractions passing aborally at a rate of 1 to 2 cm/sec. The major function of peristalsis is the movement of intestinal chyme through the intestine. Motility patterns in the small bowel vary greatly between the fed and fasted states. Pacesetter potentials, which are thought to originate in the duodenum, initiate a series of contractions in the fed state that propel food through the small bowel.

During the interdigestive (fasting) period between meals, the bowel is regularly swept by cyclical contractions that move aborally along the intestine every 75 to 90 minutes. These contractions are initiated by the migrating myoelectric complex, which is under the control of neural and humoral pathways. Extrinsic nerves to the small bowel are vagal and sympathetic. The vagal fibers have two functionally different effects; one is cholinergic and excitatory, and the other is peptidergic and probably inhibitory. Sympathetic activity inhibits motor function, whereas parasympathetic

activity stimulates it. Although intestinal hormones are known to affect small intestinal motility, the one peptide that has been clearly shown to function in this regard is motilin, which is found at its peak plasma level during phase III (intense bursts of myoelectrical activities resulting in regular, high-amplitude contractions) of migrating myoelectric complexes.

ENDOCRINE FUNCTION

Gastrointestinal Hormones

The gastrointestinal hormones are distributed along the length of the small bowel in a spatially specific pattern. In fact, the small bowel is the largest endocrine organ in the body. Although often classified as hormones, these agents do not always function in a truly endocrine fashion (i.e., discharged into the bloodstream, where an action is produced at some distant site; Fig. 49-8). Sometimes, these peptides are discharged and act locally in a paracrine or autocrine manner. In addition, these peptides may serve as neurotransmitters (e.g., vasoactive intestinal peptide). The gastrointestinal hormones play a major role in pancreaticobiliary and intestinal secretion and motility. In addition, certain gastrointestinal hormones exert a trophic effect on normal and neoplastic intestinal mucosa and pancreas. The location, major stimulants of release, and primary effects of the more important gastrointestinal

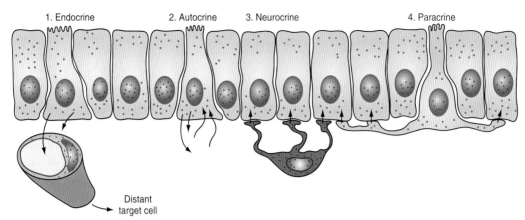

FIGURE 49-8 Actions of intestinal hormones may be through endocrine, autocrine, neurocrine, or paracrine effects. (Adapted from Miller LJ: Gastrointestinal hormones and receptors. In Yamada T, Alpers DH, Laine L, et al, editors: *Textbook of gastroenterology*, ed 3, (vol 1). Philadelphia, 1999, Lippincott Williams & Wilkins, p 37.)

hormones are summarized in Table 49-3. In addition, the diagnostic and therapeutic uses of gastrointestinal hormones are listed in Table 49-4. Field[4] presents a more in-depth discussion of the structure, molecular biology, and physiologic functions of these hormones and their impact on medical and surgical therapies.

Receptors

The gastrointestinal hormones interact with their cell surface receptors to initiate a cascade of signaling events that eventually culminate in their physiologic effects. These hormones primarily signal through G protein–coupled receptors that traverse the plasma membrane seven times and represent the largest group of receptors found in the body. The heterotrimeric G proteins, which are composed of α, β, and γ subunits, are the molecular switches for signal transduction. Agonist binding to the seven-transmembrane domain receptor is thought to cause a conformational change in the receptor that allows it to interact with the G proteins. Intracellular second messengers that can then be activated include cyclic adenosine monophosphate, Ca^{2+} cyclic guanosine monophosphate, and inositol phosphate.

In addition to the gastrointestinal hormones, receptors for a number of other peptides and growth factors are located in the gastrointestinal mucosa, including epidermal growth factor, transforming growth factor α and β, insulin-like growth factor, fibroblast growth factor, and platelet-derived growth factor. These peptides play a role in cell growth and differentiation and act through tyrosine kinase receptors, which have a single membrane-spanning domain.

A third class of surface receptors, the ion channel–linked receptors, are found most commonly in cells of neuronal lineage and usually bind specific neurotransmitters. Examples include receptors for excitatory (acetylcholine and serotonin) and inhibitory (γ-aminobutyric acid, glycine) neurotransmitters. These receptors undergo a conformational change on binding of the mediator that allows passage of ions across the cell membrane and results in changes in voltage potential.

IMMUNE FUNCTION

During the course of a normal day, we ingest a number of bacteria, parasites, and viruses. The large surface area of the small bowel mucosa represents a potential major portal of entry for these pathogens; the small intestine serves as a major immunologic barrier in addition to its important role in digestion and endocrine function. As a result of constant antigenic exposure, the intestine possesses abundant lymphoid cells (e.g., B and T lymphocytes) and myeloid cells (e.g., macrophages, neutrophils, eosinophils, mast cells). To deal with the constant barrage of potential toxins and antigens, the gut has evolved into a highly organized and efficient mechanism for antigen processing, humoral immunity, and cellular immunity. The gut-associated lymphoid tissue is localized in three areas—Peyer's patches, lamina propria lymphoid cells, and intraepithelial lymphocytes.

Peyer's patches are unencapsulated lymphoid nodules that constitute an afferent limb of the gut-associated lymphoid tissue, which recognizes antigens through the specialized sampling mechanism of the microfold (M) cells contained within the follicle-associated epithelium (Fig. 49-9). Antigens that gain access to the Peyer's patches activate and prime B and T cells in that site. The M cells cover the lymphoid follicles in the gastrointestinal tract and provide a site for the selective sampling of intraluminal antigens. Activated lymphocytes from intestinal lymphoid follicles then leave the intestinal tract and migrate into afferent lymphatics that drain into mesenteric lymph nodes. Furthermore, these cells migrate into the lamina propria. The B lymphocytes become surface immunoglobulin A (IgA). IgA-bearing lymphoblasts serve a critically important role in mucosal immunity.

B lymphocytes and plasma cells, T lymphocytes, macrophages, dendritic cells, eosinophils, and mast cells are scattered throughout the connective tissue of the lamina propria. Approximately 60% of the lymphoid cells are T cells. These T lymphocytes are a heterogeneous group of cells and can differentiate into one of several types of T effector cells. Cytotoxic T effector cells damage the target cells directly. Helper T cells are effector cells that help mediate induction of other T cells or the induction of B cells to produce humoral antibodies. T suppressor cells perform just the opposite function. Approximately 40% of the lymphoid cells in the lamina propria are B cells, which are primarily derived from precursors in Peyer's patches. These B cells and their progeny, plasma cells, are predominantly focused on IgA synthesis and, to a lesser extent, IgM, IgG, and IgE synthesis.

The intraepithelial lymphocytes are located in the space between the epithelial cells that line the mucosal surface and lie close to the basement membrane. It is thought that most of the

TABLE 49-3 Gastrointestinal Hormones

HORMONE	LOCATION	MAJOR STIMULANTS OF PEPTIDE SECRETION	PRIMARY EFFECTS
Gastrin	Antrum, duodenum (G cells)	Peptides, amino acids, antral distention, vagal and adrenergic stimulation, gastrin-releasing peptide (bombesin)	Stimulates gastric acid and pepsinogen secretion Stimulates gastric mucosal growth
Cholecystokinin	Duodenum, jejunum (I cells)	Fats, peptides, amino acids	Stimulates pancreatic enzyme secretion Stimulates gallbladder contraction Relaxes sphincter of Oddi Inhibits gastric emptying
Secretin	Duodenum, jejunum (S cells)	Fatty acids, luminal acidity, bile salts	Stimulates release of water and bicarbonate from pancreatic ductal cells Stimulates flow and alkalinity of bile Inhibits gastric acid secretion and motility and inhibits gastrin release
Somatostatin	Pancreatic islets (D cells), antrum, duodenum	Gut: fat, protein, acid, other hormones (e.g., gastrin, cholecystokinin) Pancreas: glucose, amino acids, cholecystokinin	Universal "off" switch Inhibits release of gastrointestinal hormones Inhibits gastric acid secretion Inhibits small bowel water and electrolyte secretion Inhibits secretion of pancreatic hormones
Gastrin-releasing peptide (mammalian equivalent of bombesin)	Small bowel	Vagal stimulation	Universal "on" switch Stimulates release of all gastrointestinal hormones (except secretin) Stimulates gastrointestinal secretion and motility Stimulates gastric acid secretion and release of antral gastrin Stimulates growth of intestinal mucosa and pancreas
Gastric inhibitory polypeptide	Duodenum, jejunum (K cells)	Glucose, fat, protein adrenergic stimulation	Inhibits gastric acid and pepsin secretion Stimulates pancreatic insulin release in response to hyperglycemia
Motilin	Duodenum, jejunum	Gastric distention, fat	Stimulates upper gastrointestinal tract motility May initiate the migrating motor complex
Vasoactive intestinal peptide	Neurons throughout the gastrointestinal tract	Vagal stimulation	Primarily functions as a neuropeptide Potent vasodilator Stimulates pancreatic and intestinal secretion Inhibits gastric acid secretion
Neurotensin	Small bowel (N cells)	Fat	Stimulates growth of small and large bowel mucosa Facilitates absorption of fats in the intestine Stimulates growth of cancer with neurotensin receptors

Enteroglucagon	Small bowel (L cells)	Glucose, fat	Glucagon-like peptide 1
			    Stimulates insulin release
			    Inhibits pancreatic glucagon release
			Glucagon-like peptide 2
			    Potent enterotrophic factor

Peptide YY	Distal small bowel, colon	Fatty acids, cholecystokinin	Inhibits gastric and pancreatic secretion Inhibits gallbladder contraction

TABLE 49-4 Diagnostic and Therapeutic Uses of Gastrointestinal Hormones

HORMONE	DIAGNOSTIC AND THERAPEUTIC USES
Gastrin	Pentagastrin (gastrin analogue) used to measure maximal gastric acid secretion
Cholecystokinin	Biliary imaging of gallbladder contraction
Secretin	Provocative test for gastrinoma Measurement of maximal pancreatic secretion
Glucagon	Suppresses bowel motility for endocrine spasm Relieves sphincter of Oddi spasm Provocative test for insulin, catecholamine, and growth hormone release
Somatostatin analogues	Treat carcinoid diarrhea and flushing Decrease secretion from pancreatic and intestinal fistulas Ameliorate symptoms associated with hormone-overproducing endocrine tumors Treat esophageal variceal bleeding

intraepithelial lymphocytes are T cells. On activation, the intraepithelial lymphocytes may acquire cytolytic functions that can contribute to epithelial cell death through apoptosis. These cells may be important in the immunosurveillance against abnormal epithelial cells.

As noted, one of the major protective immune mechanisms for the intestinal tract is the synthesis and secretion of IgA. The intestine contains more than 70% of the IgA-producing cells in the body. IgA is produced by plasma cells in the lamina propria and is secreted into the intestine, where it can bind antigens at the mucosal surface. The IgA antibody traverses the epithelial cell to the lumen by means of a protein carrier (the secretory component) that not only transports the IgA but also protects it against the intracellular lysosomes. IgA does not activate complement and does not enhance cell-mediated opsonization or destruction of infectious organisms or antigens, which is in sharp contrast to the role of other immunoglobulins. Secretory IgA inhibits the

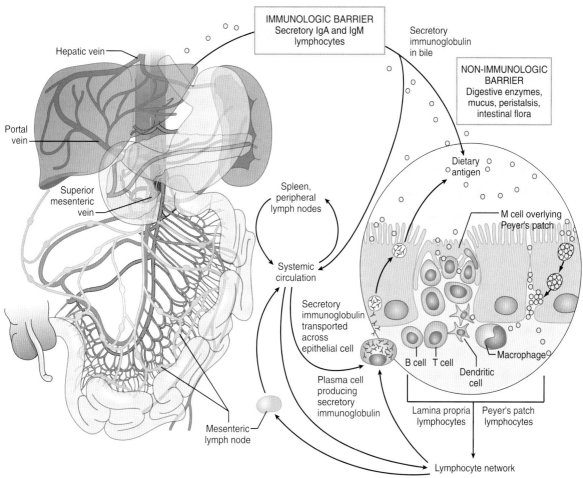

FIGURE 49-9 Mucosal Barrier of the Gut. Antigens contact specialized microfold (M) cells overlying Peyer's patches, which then process and present the antigen to the immune system. When B lymphocytes are stimulated by antigenic material, the cells develop into antibody-forming cells that secrete various types of immunoglobulins, the most important of which is IgA. (Adapted from Duerr RH, Shanahan F: Food allergy. In Targan SR, Shanahan F, editors: *Immunology and immunopathology of the liver and gastrointestinal tract*, New York, 1990, Igaku-Shoin, p 510; illustration courtesy Matt Hazzard, University of Kentucky Medical Center, Lexington, KY.)

adherence of bacteria to epithelial cells and prevents their colonization and multiplication. In addition, secretory IgA neutralizes bacterial toxins and viral activity and blocks the absorption of antigens from the gut.

OBSTRUCTION

The description of patients presenting with small bowel obstruction dates back to the third or fourth century BC, when Praxagoras created an enterocutaneous fistula to relieve a bowel obstruction. Despite this success with operative therapy, the nonoperative management of these patients with attempted reduction of hernias, laxatives, ingestion of heavy metals (e.g., lead, mercury), and leeches to remove toxic agents from the blood was the rule until the late 1800s, when antisepsis and aseptic surgical techniques made operative intervention safer and more acceptable. A better understanding of the pathophysiologic process of bowel obstruction, surgical advances, antibiotics, intestinal tube

decompression, and use of isotonic fluid resuscitation have greatly reduced the mortality rate for patients with a mechanical bowel obstruction. However, patients with a bowel obstruction still represent some of the most difficult and vexing problems that surgeons face with regard to correct diagnosis, optimal timing of therapy, and appropriate treatment. Ultimately, a clinical decision about the management of these patients dictates a thorough history and workup and heightened awareness of potential complications.

Causes

The causes of a small bowel obstruction can be divided into three major categories:
1. obstruction arising from extraluminal causes (e.g., adhesions, hernias, carcinomas, abscesses);
2. obstruction intrinsic to the bowel wall (e.g., primary tumors); and
3. intraluminal obturator obstruction (e.g., gallstones, enteroliths, foreign bodies, bezoars).

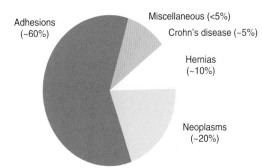

FIGURE 49-10 Common causes of small bowel obstruction in industrialized countries.

The cause of small bowel obstruction has changed dramatically since the 1900s.[5] At the turn of the 20th century, hernias accounted for more than 50% of mechanical intestinal obstructions. With the routine elective repair of hernias, this cause has dropped to the third most common cause of small bowel obstruction in industrialized countries. Adhesions secondary to previous surgery are now the most common cause of small bowel obstruction (Fig. 49-10).

Adhesions, particularly after pelvic operations (e.g., gynecologic procedures, appendectomy, colorectal resection), are responsible for more than 60% of all causes of bowel obstruction in the United States. This preponderance of lower abdominal procedures to produce adhesions that result in obstruction is thought to occur because the bowel is more mobile in the pelvis and more tethered in the upper abdomen (Box 49-1).

Malignant tumors account for approximately 20% of the cases of small bowel obstruction. Most of these tumors are metastatic lesions that obstruct the intestine secondary to peritoneal implants that have spread from an intra-abdominal primary tumor, such as ovarian, pancreatic, gastric, or colon cancer. Less often, malignant cells from distant sites, such as breast, lung, and melanoma, may metastasize hematogenously and account for peritoneal implants, resulting in an obstruction. Large intra-abdominal tumors may also cause small bowel obstruction through extrinsic compression of the bowel lumen. Primary colonic cancers, particularly those arising from the cecum and ascending colon, may be manifested as a small bowel obstruction. Primary small bowel tumors can cause obstruction but are exceedingly rare.

Hernias (typically ventral or inguinal hernias) represent the third leading cause of intestinal obstruction and account for approximately 10% of all cases. Internal hernias, generally related to prior abdominal surgery, can also result in small bowel obstruction. Less common hernias can also produce obstruction, such as femoral, obturator, lumbar, and sciatic hernias.

Crohn's disease is the fourth leading cause of small bowel obstruction and accounts for approximately 5% of all cases. Obstruction can result from acute inflammation and edema, which may resolve with conservative management. In patients with long-standing Crohn's disease, strictures can develop that may require resection and reanastomosis or strictureplasty.

An important cause of small bowel obstruction that is not routinely considered is obstruction associated with an intra-abdominal abscess, commonly from a ruptured appendix, diverticulum, or dehiscence of an intestinal anastomosis. The obstruction may be a result of a local ileus in the small bowel adjacent to the abscess. In addition, the small bowel can form a portion of the wall of the abscess cavity and become obstructed by kinking of the bowel at this point.

BOX 49-1 Causes of Mechanical Small Intestinal Obstruction in Adults

Lesions Extrinsic to the Intestinal Wall
Adhesions (usually postoperative)
Hernia
- External (e.g., inguinal, femoral, umbilical, or ventral hernias)
- Internal (e.g., congenital defects such as paraduodenal, foramen of Winslow, and diaphragmatic hernias or postoperative secondary to mesenteric defects)

Neoplastic
- Carcinomatosis
- Extraintestinal neoplasms

Intra-abdominal abscess

Lesions Intrinsic to the Intestinal Wall
Congenital
Malrotation
Duplications, cysts

Inflammatory
Crohn's disease
Infections
- Tuberculosis
- Actinomycosis
- Diverticulitis

Neoplastic
Primary neoplasms
Metastatic neoplasms

Traumatic
Hematoma
Ischemic stricture

Miscellaneous
Intussusception
Endometriosis
Radiation enteropathy/stricture

Intraluminal, Obturator Obstruction
Gallstone
Enterolith
Bezoar
Foreign body

Adapted from Tito WA, Sarr MG: Intestinal obstruction. In Zuidema GD, editor: *Surgery of the alimentary tract*, Philadelphia, 1996, WB Saunders, pp 375–416.

Miscellaneous causes of bowel obstruction account for 2% to 3% of all cases but should be considered in the differential diagnosis. These include intussusception of the bowel, which in the adult is usually secondary to a pathologic lead point, such as a polyp or tumor (Fig. 49-11); gallstones, which can enter the intestinal lumen by a cholecystenteric fistula and cause obstruction; enteroliths originating from jejunal diverticula; foreign bodies; and phytobezoars.

Pathophysiology

Early in the course of an obstruction, intestinal motility and contractile activity increase in an effort to propel luminal contents past the obstructing point. The increase in peristalsis that occurs

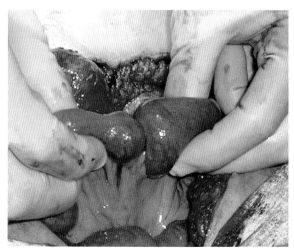

FIGURE 49-11 Jejunojenunal intussusception in an adult patient. (Courtesy Dr. Steven Williams, Nampa, ID.)

early in the course of bowel obstruction is present above and below the point of obstruction, thus accounting for the finding of diarrhea that may accompany partial or even complete small bowel obstruction in the early period. Later in the course of obstruction, the intestine becomes fatigued and dilates, with contractions becoming less frequent and less intense.

As the bowel dilates, water and electrolytes accumulate intraluminally and in the bowel wall itself. This massive third-space fluid loss accounts for the dehydration and hypovolemia. The metabolic effects of fluid loss depend on the site and duration of the obstruction. With a proximal obstruction, dehydration may be accompanied by hypochloremia, hypokalemia, and metabolic alkalosis associated with increased vomiting. Distal obstruction of the small bowel may result in large quantities of intestinal fluid into the bowel; however, abnormalities in serum electrolyte levels are usually less dramatic. Oliguria, azotemia, and hemoconcentration can accompany the dehydration. Hypotension and shock can ensue. Other consequences of bowel obstruction include increased intra-abdominal pressure, decreased venous return, and elevation of the diaphragm, compromising ventilation. These factors can serve to potentiate the effects of hypovolemia further.

As the intraluminal pressure increases in the bowel, a decrease in mucosal blood flow can occur. These alterations are particularly noted in patients with a closed loop obstruction, in which greater intraluminal pressures are attained. A closed loop obstruction, produced commonly by a twist of the bowel, can progress to arterial occlusion and ischemia if it is left untreated and may potentially lead to bowel perforation and peritonitis.

In the absence of intestinal obstruction, the jejunum and proximal ileum are almost sterile. With obstruction, however, the flora of the small intestine changes dramatically, in both the type of organism (most commonly *Escherichia coli*, *Streptococcus faecalis*, and *Klebsiella* spp.) and the quantity, with organisms reaching concentrations of 10^9 to 10^{10}/mL. Studies have shown an increase in the number of indigenous bacteria translocating to mesenteric lymph nodes and even systemic organs. Bacterial translocation amplifies the local inflammatory response in the gut, leading to intestinal leakage and subsequent increase in systemic inflammation. This inflammatory cascade may result in systemic sepsis and multiorgan failure if it is unrecognized and untreated.

Clinical Manifestations and Diagnosis

A thorough history and physical examination are critical to establishing the diagnosis and treatment of the patient with an intestinal obstruction. In most patients, a meticulous history and physical examination complemented by plain abdominal radiographs are all that is required to establish the diagnosis and to devise a treatment plan. More sophisticated radiographic studies may be necessary in certain patients in whom the diagnosis and cause are uncertain. However, a computed tomography (CT) scan of the abdomen should not be the starting point in the workup of a patient with intestinal obstruction.

History

The cardinal symptoms of intestinal obstruction include colicky abdominal pain, nausea, vomiting, abdominal distention, and obstipation. These symptoms may vary with the site and duration of obstruction. The typical crampy abdominal pain associated with intestinal obstruction occurs in paroxysms at 4- to 5-minute intervals and occurs less frequently with distal obstruction. Nausea and vomiting are more common with a higher obstruction and may be the only symptoms in patients with gastric outlet or high intestinal obstruction. An obstruction located distally is associated with less emesis; the initial and most prominent symptom is the cramping abdominal pain. Abdominal distention occurs as the obstruction progresses and the proximal intestine becomes increasingly dilated. Obstipation is a later development. It must be reiterated that patients, particularly in the early stages of bowel obstruction, may relate a history of diarrhea that is secondary to increased peristalsis. Therefore, the important point to remember is that a complete bowel obstruction cannot be ruled out on the basis of a history of loose bowel movements. The character of the vomitus is also important to obtain in the history. As the obstruction becomes more complete with bacterial overgrowth, the vomitus becomes more feculent, indicating a late and established intestinal obstruction.

Physical Examination

The patient with intestinal obstruction may present with tachycardia and hypotension, demonstrating the severe dehydration that is present. Fever suggests the possibility of strangulation. Abdominal examination demonstrates a distended abdomen, with the amount of distention somewhat dependent on the level of obstruction. Previous surgical scars should be noted. Early in the course of bowel obstruction, peristaltic waves can be observed, particularly in thin patients, and auscultation of the abdomen may demonstrate hyperactive bowel sounds with audible rushes associated with vigorous peristalsis (borborygmi). Late in the obstructive course, minimal or no bowel sounds are noted. Mild abdominal tenderness may be present, with or without a palpable mass; however, localized tenderness, rebound, and guarding suggest peritonitis and the likelihood of strangulation. A careful examination must be performed to rule out incarcerated hernias in the groin, femoral triangle, and obturator foramen. A rectal examination should *always* be performed to assess for intraluminal masses and to examine the stool for occult blood, which may be an indication of malignant disease, intussusception, or infarction.

Radiologic and Laboratory Studies

The diagnosis of intestinal obstruction is often immediately evident after a thorough history and physical examination. Therefore, plain radiographs usually confirm the clinical suspicion and define the site of obstruction more accurately. The accuracy of diagnosis of the small intestinal obstruction on plain abdominal radiographs is estimated to be approximately 60%, with an equivocal or a nonspecific diagnosis obtained in the remainder of cases. Characteristic findings on supine radiographs are dilated loops of small intestine, without evidence of colonic distention. Upright radiographs demonstrate multiple air-fluid levels, which often layer in a stepwise pattern (Fig. 49-12). Plain abdominal films

(Fig. 49-13*A*) may also demonstrate the cause of the obstruction (e.g., foreign bodies, gallstones [Fig. 49-13*B*]). In uncertain cases or when one is unable to differentiate partial from complete obstruction, further diagnostic evaluation may be required.

In the more complex patient in whom the diagnosis is not readily apparent, an abdominal CT scan can be helpful (Fig. 49-14). CT is particularly sensitive for diagnosing complete or high-grade obstruction of the small bowel and for determining

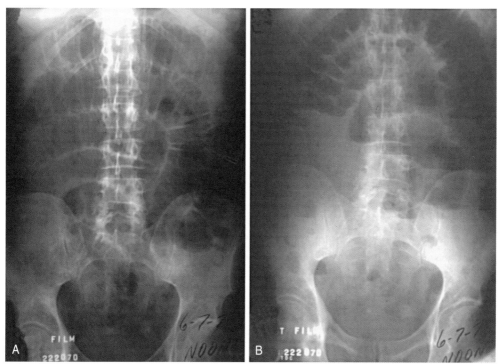

FIGURE 49-12 Plain abdominal radiographs of a patient with a complete small bowel obstruction. **A,** Supine film shows dilated loops of small bowel in an orderly arrangement, without evidence of colonic gas. **B,** Upright film shows multiple, short air-fluid levels arranged in a stepwise pattern. (Courtesy Dr. Melvyn H. Schreiber, The University of Texas Medical Branch, Galveston, TX.)

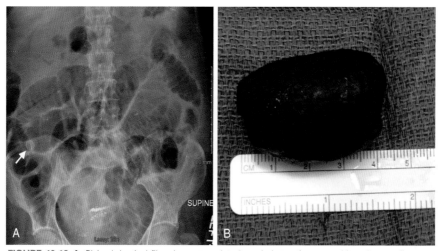

FIGURE 49-13 A, Plain abdominal film shows complete bowel obstruction caused by a large radiopaque gallstone *(arrow)* obstructing the distal ileum. **B,** The large gallstone responsible for the obstruction seen in the corresponding plain abdominal film. (Courtesy Dr. Kristin Long, University of Kentucky Medical Center, Lexington, KY.)

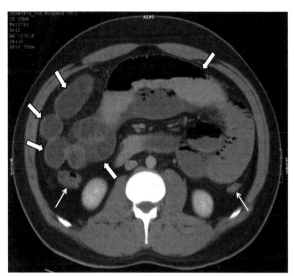

FIGURE 49-14 CT scan through the midabdomen shows dilated small bowel loops filled with fluid *(thick arrows)* and decompressed ascending and descending colon *(thin arrows)*. These are typical CT findings in small bowel obstruction. (Courtesy Dr. Eric Walser, The University of Texas Medical Branch, Galveston, TX.)

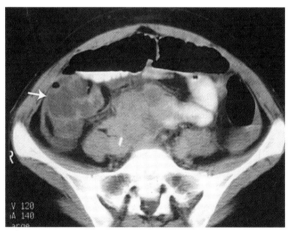

FIGURE 49-15 CT scan of the abdomen of a patient with a mechanical bowel obstruction secondary to an abscess in the right lower quadrant *(arrow)*. Multiple dilated and fluid-filled loops of small bowel are noted. (Courtesy Dr. Melvyn H. Schreiber, The University of Texas Medical Branch, Galveston, TX.)

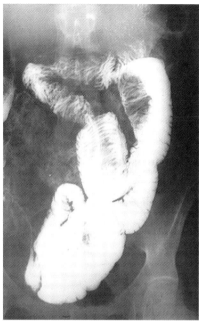

FIGURE 49-16 Barium study demonstrates jejunojejunal intussusception. (Courtesy Dr. Melvyn H. Schreiber, The University of Texas Medical Branch, Galveston, TX.)

the location and cause of obstruction. The CT examination is less sensitive, however, in patients with partial small bowel obstruction. In addition, CT is helpful if an extrinsic cause of bowel obstruction (e.g., abdominal tumors, inflammatory disease, or abscess) is suggested (Fig. 49-15). CT has also been described as useful for determining bowel strangulation, most commonly seen in the presence of hernia. Unfortunately, CT findings associated with strangulation are those of irreversible ischemia and necrosis. Importantly, the emergent surgical management of a toxic patient with a bowel obstruction identified by a thorough history and physical examination should not be delayed to perform further unnecessary and costly radiographic studies.

Barium studies, namely, enteroclysis, have been a useful adjunct in certain patients with a presumed obstruction.[6] This procedure involves the continued infusion of 500 to 1000 mL of thin barium sulfate and methylcellulose suspension into the intestine through a duodenal tube. The suspension is then viewed continuously with use of either fluoroscopy or standard radiographs taken at frequent intervals; therefore, this technique is a double-contrast procedure that allows detailed imaging of the entire small intestine. Enteroclysis has been advocated as the definitive study in patients for whom the diagnosis of low-grade, intermittent, small bowel obstruction is clinically uncertain. In addition, barium studies can precisely demonstrate the level of the obstruction as well as the cause of the obstruction in certain cases (Fig. 49-16). The main disadvantages of enteroclysis are the need for nasoenteric intubation, slow transit of contrast material in patients with a fluid-filled hypotonic small bowel, and enhanced expertise required by the radiologist to perform this procedure.

Ultrasound has been reported to be useful for pregnant patients because radiation exposure is a concern. Magnetic resonance imaging (MRI) has been described in patients with obstruction; however, it appears to be no better diagnostically than CT.

To summarize, plain abdominal radiographs are usually diagnostic of bowel obstruction in more than 60% of the cases, but further evaluation (possibly by CT or barium radiography) may be necessary in 20% to 30% of cases. CT examination is particularly useful in patients with a history of abdominal malignant disease, postsurgical patients, and patients who have no history of abdominal surgery and present with symptoms of bowel obstruction. Barium studies are recommended for patients with a history of recurring obstruction or low-grade mechanical obstruction to define the obstructed segment and degree of obstruction precisely.

Laboratory tests are usually not helpful in the actual diagnosis of patients with small bowel obstruction but are extremely important in assessing the degree of dehydration. Patients with a bowel obstruction should routinely have laboratory measurements of serum sodium, chloride, potassium, bicarbonate, and creatinine levels. The serial determination of serum electrolyte levels should be performed to assess the adequacy of fluid resuscitation. Dehydration may result in hemoconcentration, as noted by an elevated hematocrit value. This should be monitored because fluid resuscitation results in a decrease in the hematocrit, and some patients (e.g., those with intestinal malignant neoplasms) may require blood transfusions before surgery. In addition, the white blood cell count should be assessed. Leukocytosis may be found in patients with strangulation; however, an elevated white blood cell count does not necessarily denote strangulation. Conversely, the absence of leukocytosis does not eliminate strangulation as a possibility.

Simple Versus Strangulating Obstruction

Most patients with small bowel obstruction are classified as having simple obstructions that involve mechanical blockage of the flow of luminal contents without compromised viability of the intestinal wall. In contrast, a strangulated obstruction, which usually involves a closed loop obstruction in which the vascular supply to a segment of intestine is compromised, can lead to intestinal infarction. A strangulated obstruction is associated with an increased morbidity and mortality risk, and therefore recognition of early strangulation is important. In differentiating from simple intestinal obstruction, classic signs of strangulation have been described; these include tachycardia, fever, leukocytosis, and a constant, noncramping abdominal pain. However, a number of studies have convincingly shown that no clinical parameters or laboratory measurements can accurately detect or exclude the presence of strangulation in all cases. This reinforces the dictum that a careful history and physical examination are key for an accurate and timely diagnosis.

CT examination is useful only for detecting the late stages of irreversible ischemia (e.g., pneumatosis intestinalis, portal venous gas). Various serum determinations, including lactate dehydrogenase, amylase, alkaline phosphatase, and ammonia levels, have been assessed with no real benefit. Previous reports described limited success in discriminating strangulation by measuring serum D-lactate, creatine kinase isoenzyme (particularly the BB isoenzyme), or intestinal fatty acid–binding protein; however, these studies were ultimately abandoned as they showed no significant diagnostic benefits. Finally, noninvasive determinations of mesenteric ischemia have been described using a superconducting quantum interference device (SQUID) magnetometer to detect mesenteric ischemia noninvasively. Intestinal ischemia is associated with changes in the basic electrical rhythm of the small intestine. This technique remains investigational and is not in widespread clinical use.

Thus, it is important to remember that bowel ischemia and strangulation cannot be reliably diagnosed or excluded preoperatively in all cases by any known clinical parameter, combination of parameters, or current laboratory and radiographic examinations.

Treatment
Fluid Resuscitation and Antibiotics

Patients with intestinal obstruction are usually dehydrated and depleted of sodium, chloride, and potassium, requiring aggressive intravenous (IV) replacement with an isotonic saline solution such as lactated Ringer solution. Urine output should be monitored by the placement of a Foley catheter. After the patient has formed adequate urine, potassium chloride should be added to the infusion, if needed. Serial electrolyte level measurements as well as

hematocrit and white blood cell count are performed to assess the adequacy of fluid repletion. Because of large fluid requirements, some patients, particularly older patients, may require central venous assessment and, in select cases, the placement of a Swan-Ganz catheter. Broad-spectrum antibiotics are given prophylactically by some surgeons on the basis of the reported findings of bacterial translocation occurring even in simple mechanical obstructions; however, there is no substantial evidence to support the use of antimicrobial therapy in nontoxic-appearing patients or those without suspected bacterial overgrowth of the small intestine. Antibiotics are administered preoperatively in the event that the patient requires surgery.

Tube Decompression

In addition to IV fluid resuscitation, another important adjunct to the supportive care of patients with intestinal obstruction is nasogastric suction. Suction with a nasogastric tube empties the stomach, reducing the hazard of pulmonary aspiration of vomitus and minimizing further intestinal distention from preoperatively swallowed air. Nasogastric decompression in a patient with small bowel obstruction is still considered standard of care.

The use of long intestinal tubes (e.g., Cantor or Baker tube) has been advocated by some. However, prospective randomized trials have demonstrated no significant differences with regard to the decompression achieved, success of nonoperative treatment, or morbidity rate after surgical intervention compared with the use of nasogastric tubes. Furthermore, the use of these long tubes has been associated with a significantly longer hospital stay, duration of postoperative ileus, and postoperative complications in some series. Therefore, it appears that long intestinal tubes also offer no benefit in the preoperative setting over nasogastric tubes.

Patients with a partial intestinal obstruction may be treated conservatively with resuscitation and tube decompression alone. Resolution of symptoms and discharge without the need for surgery have been reported in up to 85% of patients with a partial obstruction.[5] Enteroclysis can assist in determining the degree of obstruction, with higher grade partial obstructions requiring earlier operative intervention. Although an initial trial of nonoperative management of most patients with partial small bowel obstruction is warranted, clinical deterioration of the patient or increasing small bowel distention on abdominal radiographs during tube decompression warrants prompt operative intervention. The decision to continue to treat a patient nonoperatively with a presumed bowel obstruction is based on clinical judgment and requires constant vigilance to ensure that the clinical course has not changed.

Operative Management

In general, the patient with a complete small bowel obstruction requires operative intervention. A nonoperative approach for selected patients with complete small intestinal obstruction has been proposed by some surgeons who argue that prolonged intubation is safe in these patients, provided no fever, tachycardia, tenderness, or leukocytosis is noted. Nevertheless, one must realize that nonoperative management of these patients is undertaken at a calculated risk of overlooking an underlying strangulated obstruction. This delay of definitive treatment often necessitates an urgent surgical intervention and can result in increased morbidity and mortality compared with patients who undergo a more prompt intervention. Retrospective studies have reported that a 12- to 24-hour delay of surgery in these patients is safe but that the incidence of strangulation and other complications increases significantly after this period.

The nature of the problem dictates the approach to management of the obstructed patient. Patients with intestinal obstruction secondary to an adhesive band may be treated with lysis of adhesions. Great care should be used in the gentle handling of the bowel to reduce serosal trauma and to avoid unnecessary dissection and inadvertent enterotomies. Incarcerated hernias can be managed by manual reduction of the herniated segment of bowel and closure of the defect.

The treatment of patients with an obstruction and history of malignant tumors can be particularly challenging. In the terminal patient with widespread metastasis, nonoperative management, if successful, is usually the best course; however, only a small percentage of cases of complete obstruction can be successfully managed nonoperatively. In this case, an intestinal bypass of the obstructing lesion, by whatever means, may offer the best option rather than a long and complicated operation that might entail bowel resection.

An obstruction secondary to Crohn's disease will often resolve with conservative management if the obstruction is acute. If a chronic fibrotic stricture is the cause of the obstruction, a bowel resection or strictureplasty may be required.

Patients with an intra-abdominal abscess can present in a manner indistinguishable from those with mechanical bowel obstruction. CT is particularly useful in diagnosing the cause of the obstruction in these patients; percutaneous drainage of the abscess may be sufficient to relieve the obstruction, but laparotomy and abdominal washout may be required for large and established abscesses. Laparoscopic drainage is also an option in cases not amenable to image-guided percutaneous drainage for patients who would not otherwise tolerate a laparotomy; it has reduced wound morbidity and is also useful in multiloculated collections and allows a washout of the peritoneal cavity at the same time.

Radiation enteropathy, as a complication of radiation therapy for pelvic malignant neoplasms, may cause bowel obstruction. Most cases can be treated nonoperatively with tube decompression and possibly corticosteroids, particularly during the acute setting. In the chronic setting, nonoperative management is rarely effective; it will require laparotomy, with possible resection of the irradiated bowel or bypass of the affected area.

At the time of exploration, it can sometimes be difficult to evaluate bowel viability after the release of a strangulation. If intestinal viability is questionable, the bowel segment should be completely released and placed in a warm, saline-moistened sponge for 15 to 20 minutes and then reexamined. If normal color has returned and peristalsis is evident, it is safe to retain the bowel. A prospective controlled trial comparing clinical judgment with the use of a Doppler probe or the administration of fluorescein for the intraoperative discrimination of viability has found that the Doppler flow probe added little to the conventional clinical judgment of the surgeon. In difficult borderline cases, fluorescein fluorescence may supplement clinical judgment. Intraoperative near-infrared angiography to determine the presence of ischemic bowel has shown promising results, but this technique is currently not in wide clinical use. Another approach to the assessment of bowel viability is the so-called second-look laparotomy 18 to 24 hours after the initial procedure. This decision should be made at the time of the initial operation. A second-look laparotomy is clearly indicated for a patient whose condition deteriorates after the initial operation.

Some studies have evaluated the efficacy of laparoscopic management of acute small bowel obstruction. The laparoscopic treatment of small bowel obstruction appears to be effective and leads to a shorter hospital stay and reduced overall complications in a highly selected group of patients.[7] Patients fitting the criteria for consideration of laparoscopic management include those with the following symptoms: mild abdominal distention allowing adequate visualization; proximal obstruction; partial obstruction; and anticipated single-band obstruction.

In particular, laparoscopic treatment has been found to be of greatest benefit in patients who have undergone fewer than three previous operations, were seen early after the onset of symptoms, and were thought to have adhesive bands as the cause. Currently, patients who have advanced, complete, or distal small bowel obstructions are not candidates for laparoscopic treatment. Similarly, patients with matted adhesions or carcinomatosis or those who remain distended after nasogastric intubation should be managed with conventional laparotomy. Therefore, the future role of laparoscopic procedures in the treatment of these patients remains to be completely defined. A multicenter, prospective, randomized trial comparing laparoscopic adhesiolysis to open surgery in patients with adhesive small bowel obstruction, diagnosed by CT scan, that fails to resolve with nonoperative management is currently accruing patients for evaluation.[7]

Management of Specific Problems
Recurrent Intestinal Obstruction

All surgeons can readily remember the complicated patient with multiple previous abdominal operations and a frozen abdomen who presents with yet another bowel obstruction. An initial nonoperative trial is usually desirable and often safe. In those patients who do not respond conservatively, reoperation is required. This can often be a long and arduous procedure, with great care taken to prevent enterotomies or adjacent organ injury. In these difficult patients, various surgical procedures and pharmacologic agents have been tried in an effort to prevent recurrent adhesions and obstruction.

External plication procedures have been described, in which the small intestine or its mesentery is sutured in large, gently curving loops. Common complications have included the development of fistulas, gross leakage, peritonitis, and death. Because of frequent complications and low overall success rate, these procedures have largely been abandoned. Several series have reported moderate success with internal fixation or stenting procedures using a long intestinal tube inserted through the nose, a gastrostomy, or even a jejunostomy and left in place for 2 weeks or longer. Complications associated with these tubes include prolonged drainage of bowel contents from the tube insertion site, intussusception, and difficult removal of the tube, which may require surgical reexploration.

Pharmacologic agents, including corticosteroids and other anti-inflammatory agents, cytotoxic drugs, and antihistamines, have been used with limited success. The use of anticoagulants, such as heparin, dextran solutions, dicumarol, and sodium citrate, has modified the extent of adhesion formation, but their side effects far outweigh their efficacy. Intraperitoneal instillation of various proteinases (e.g., trypsin, papain, pepsin), which cause enzymatic digestion of the extracellular protein matrix, has been unsuccessful. Hyaluronidase has been of questionable value, and conflicting results have been obtained with fibrinolytic agents such as streptokinase, urokinase, and fibrinolytic snake venoms. In a prospective multicenter trial, the use of a hyaluronate-based, bioresorbable membrane reduced the incidence and severity of postoperative adhesion formation.[8] Another study found that placement of this membrane reduced the severity but not the incidence of postoperative adhesion in patients undergoing a Hartmann procedure. Longer term, randomized studies will be required to determine the efficacy of this material in preventing adhesions and ultimately to prevent bowel obstructions.

To date, the most effective means of limiting the number of adhesions is a good surgical technique. This includes the gentle handling of the bowel to reduce serosal trauma, avoidance of unnecessary dissection, exclusion of foreign material from the peritoneal cavity (the use of absorbable suture material when possible, the avoidance of excessive use of gauze sponges, and the removal of starch from gloves), adequate irrigation and removal of infectious and ischemic debris, and preservation and use of the omentum around the site of surgery or in the denuded pelvis.

Acute Postoperative Obstruction

Small bowel obstruction that occurs in the immediate postoperative period presents a challenge in regard to diagnosis and treatment.[5] Diagnosis is often difficult because the primary symptoms of abdominal pain and nausea or emesis may be attributed to a postoperative ileus. Electrolyte deficiencies, particularly hypokalemia, can be a cause of ileus and should be corrected. Plain abdominal films are usually not helpful in distinguishing an ileus from obstruction. CT may be useful in this regard, and in particular, enteroclysis studies may be helpful in determining whether an obstruction exists and, if so, the level of the obstruction. More than 90% of early postoperative obstructions are partial and will resolve spontaneously, given ample time. Conservative management in the form of bowel rest, fluid resuscitation, electrolyte replacement, and parenteral nutrition, if necessary, is routinely successful. However, the development of complete obstruction or signs of strangulation mandates reoperative intervention. Postoperative bowel obstruction after laparoscopic surgery is more commonly associated with a definitive obstruction point, such as a port site hernia or an internal hernia, and should prompt a high index of suspicion for the need for operative intervention.

Ileus

An ileus is defined as intestinal distention and the slowing or absence of passage of luminal contents without a demonstrable mechanical obstruction. An ileus can result from a number of causes, including drug induced, metabolic, neurogenic, and infectious factors (Box 49-2).

BOX 49-2   Causes of Ileus

After laparotomy
Metabolic and electrolyte derangements (e.g., hypokalemia, hyponatremia,
    hypomagnesemia, uremia, diabetic coma)
Drugs (e.g., opiates, psychotropic agents, anticholinergic agents)
Intra-abdominal inflammation
Retroperitoneal hemorrhage or inflammation
Intestinal ischemia
Systemic sepsis

Adapted from Turnage RH, Bergen PC: Intestinal obstruction and ileus. In Feldman M, Scharschmidt FG, Sleisenger MH, editors: *Sleisenger and Fordtran's gastrointestinal and liver disease: Pathophysiology, diagnosis, management*, Philadelphia, 1998, WB Saunders, pp 1799–1810.

Pharmacologic agents that can produce an ileus include anticholinergic drugs, autonomic blockers, antihistamines, and various psychotropic agents, such as haloperidol and tricyclic antidepressants. One of the more common causes of drug-induced ileus in the operative patient is the use of opiates, such as morphine or meperidine. Metabolic causes of ileus are common and include hypokalemia, hyponatremia, and hypomagnesemia. Other metabolic causes include uremia, diabetic coma, and hypoparathyroidism. Neurogenic causes of an ileus include postoperative ileus, which occurs after abdominal operations. Spinal injury, retroperitoneal irritation, and orthopedic procedures on the spine or pelvis can result in an ileus. Finally, infections can result in an ileus; common infectious causes include pneumonia, peritonitis, and generalized sepsis from a nonabdominal source.

Patients often present in a manner similar to those with a mechanical small bowel obstruction. Abdominal distention, usually without the colicky abdominal pain, is the typical and most notable finding. Nausea and vomiting may occur but may also be absent. Patients with an ileus may continue to pass flatus and diarrhea, which may help distinguish these patients from those with a mechanical small bowel obstruction.

Radiologic studies may help distinguish ileus from small bowel obstruction. Plain abdominal radiographs may reveal distended small bowel as well as large bowel loops. In cases that are difficult to differentiate from obstruction, barium studies may be beneficial.

The treatment of an ileus is entirely supportive, with nasogastric decompression and IV fluids. The most effective treatment to correct the underlying condition may be aggressive treatment of the sepsis, correction of any metabolic or electrolyte abnormalities, and discontinuation of medications that may produce an ileus. Pharmacologic agents have been used but for the most part have been ineffective. Drugs that block sympathetic input (e.g., guanethidine) or stimulate parasympathetic activity (e.g., bethanechol, neostigmine) have been tried. Hormonal manipulation, using cholecystokinin or motilin, has been evaluated, but the results have been inconsistent. Erythromycin has been ineffective, and cisapride, although apparently beneficial in stimulating gastric motility, does not appear to alter intestinal ileus. Chewing gum has been suggested as an easy and inexpensive method to stimulate the cephalic phase of digestion (e.g., vagal cholinergic stimulation and the release of gastrointestinal hormones) and therefore a potential adjunct to prevent and to treat ileus. A more recent randomized trial demonstrated that chewing gum provides no benefit regarding return of bowel function or length of stay and even suggested that postoperative ileus may be further exacerbated by the use of sugared gum.

INFLAMMATORY AND INFECTIOUS DISEASES

Crohn's Disease

Crohn's disease is a chronic, transmural inflammatory disease of the gastrointestinal tract for which the definitive cause is unknown, although a combination of genetic and environmental factors has been implicated. Crohn's disease can involve any part of the alimentary tract from the mouth to the anus but most commonly affects the small intestine and colon. The most common clinical manifestations are abdominal pain, diarrhea, and weight loss. Crohn's disease can be complicated by intestinal obstruction or localized perforation with fistula formation. Medical and surgical treatments are palliative; however, operative therapy can provide effective symptomatic relief for patients with complications from Crohn's disease and produces a reasonable long-term benefit.

History

The first documented case of Crohn's disease was described by Morgagni in 1761. In 1913, the Scottish surgeon Dalziel described nine cases of intestinal inflammatory disease. However, it is the landmark paper by Crohn and colleagues in 1932 that provided, in eloquent detail, the pathologic and clinical findings of this inflammatory disease in young adults.[9] This classic paper crystallized the description of this inflammatory condition. Although many different (and sometimes misleading) terms have been used to describe this disease process, Crohn's disease has been universally accepted as its name.

Incidence and Epidemiology

Crohn's disease is the most common primary surgical disease of the small bowel. The incidence of Crohn's disease, which is rising in the United States for reasons that remain unclear, is estimated to be approximately 50 of 100,000 individuals in the general population.[10] The total direct and indirect costs for Crohn's disease in the United States have been estimated to be more than $800 million when factoring both inpatient hospital stays and outpatient visits. Crohn's disease primarily attacks young adults in the second and third decades of life. However, a bimodal distribution is apparent, with a second smaller peak occurring in the sixth decade of life. Crohn's disease is more common in urban dwellers, and although earlier reports suggested a somewhat higher female predominance, the two genders are affected equally. The risk for development of Crohn's disease is about twice as high in smokers as in nonsmokers. Several studies have indicated an increased incidence of Crohn's disease in women using oral contraceptives; however, more recent studies have shown no differences. Although Crohn's disease is uncommon in African blacks, blacks in the United States have rates similar to whites. Certain ethnic groups, particularly Jews, have a greater incidence of Crohn's disease than age- and gender-matched control subjects. Individuals born during the spring months (e.g., April to June) are more likely to develop Crohn's disease; there also appears to be a north-south gradient worldwide, and populations in higher latitudes have higher incidence rates than populations in lower latitudes. Of note, migrants moving from a low-risk region to a high-risk region have a risk for development of Crohn's disease that is similar to that in the high-risk region within one generation. There is a strong familial association, with the risk for development of Crohn's disease increased about 30-fold in siblings and 14- to 15-fold for all first-degree relatives. Other analyses supporting a genetic role for Crohn's disease have shown a concordance rate of only 3.7% in dizygotic twins but a 67% rate in monozygotic twins. More recent studies evaluating twins with and without Crohn's disease have used advanced genomic and proteomic techniques to show that intestinal microflora and epigenetic changes induced by environmental factors play an important role in disease development and progression in genetically susceptible individuals.[11]

Causes

The causes of Crohn's disease remain unknown. A number of potential causes have been proposed, with the most likely possibilities being infectious, immunologic, and genetic. Other possibilities that have met with various levels of enthusiasm include environmental and dietary factors, smoking, and psychosocial factors. Although these factors may contribute to the overall

disease process, it is unlikely that they represent the primary causative mechanism for Crohn's disease.

Infectious agents. Although a number of infectious agents have been proposed as potential causes of Crohn's disease, the two that have received the most attention are mycobacterial infections, particularly *Mycobacterium paratuberculosis* and enteroadherent *E. coli*. The existence of atypical mycobacteria as a cause for Crohn's disease was proposed by Dalziel in 1913. Subsequent studies using polymerase chain reaction (PCR) techniques have confirmed the presence of mycobacteria in intestinal samples of patients with Crohn's disease. Transplantation of tissue from patients with Crohn's disease has resulted in ileitis, but antimicrobial therapy directed against mycobacteria has not been effective in ameliorating the established disease process. Strains of enteroadherent *E. coli* are in higher abundance in patients with Crohn's disease compared with the general population based on PCR analysis. More recent studies have used fluorescent in situ hybridization to demonstrate increased numbers of *E. coli* in the lamina propria of patients with active Crohn's disease compared with those with inactive disease. Furthermore, an increased number of *E. coli* has been associated with a shorter time before relapse of the disease.

Immunologic factors. Immunologic abnormalities suggested as etiologic factors in patients with Crohn's disease have included humoral and cell-mediated immune reactions directed against intestinal cells, suggesting an autoimmune phenomenon. Attention has focused on the role of cytokines, such as interleukin (IL)-1, IL-2, IL-8, and TNF-α, as contributing factors in the intestinal inflammatory response. The role of the immune response remains controversial in Crohn's disease and may represent an effect of the disease process rather than an actual cause.

Genetic factors. Genetic factors play an important role in the pathogenesis of Crohn's disease because the single strongest risk factor for development of disease is having a first-degree relative with Crohn's disease. Several genome-wide association sequencing studies have been performed and have identified more than 70 genes associated with Crohn's disease (Table 49-5). The genes with the strongest and most frequently replicated associations with Crohn's disease are *NOD2*, *IL23R*, and *ATG16L1*. Putative inflammatory bowel disease loci have been identified on chromosomes 16q, 5q, 19p, 7q, and 3p. The *CARD15/NOD2* gene, which acts as a pattern recognition receptor, has been characterized on the *IBD1* locus of 16q12-13. *CARD15* leads to impaired activation of the transcription factor NF-κB and also specifically codes for a protein expressed in monocytes, macrophages, dendritic cells, epithelial cells, and Paneth cells; *NOD2* is associated with a decreased expression of antimicrobial peptides by Paneth cells. The *NOD2* gene has been associated with increased likelihood and earlier need for surgery in Crohn's disease; *CARD15* is also helpful in distinguishing Crohn's disease from ulcerative colitis as it is more strongly associated with Crohn's disease, especially in patients of northern European descent. The *FHIT* gene located on 3p14.2 has been identified as a tumor suppressor gene and is suggested to play a role in the pathogenesis of Crohn's disease as well as in the development and progression of Crohn's disease–related cancers. A complex cellular and molecular crosstalk occurs between these genes, namely, *NOD2/CARD15* and the autophagy gene *ATG16L1*, which is associated with a synergistic increase in earlier onset and disease severity, especially in smokers.[12] Genetic profiling may be helpful in selecting patients who will benefit from intensified treatment with immunomodulators and anti-TNF therapy, thus decreasing medical nonresponse.

TABLE 49-5   Genetic Polymorphisms Related to Crohn's Disease

Genes and the Diagnosis of Crohn's Disease

Genes related to innate pattern recognition receptors	NOD2/CARD15, OCTN, TLR
Genes related to epithelial barrier homeostasis	IBD5, DLG5
Genes related to molecular mimicry and autophagy	ATG16L1, IRGM, LRRK2
Genes related to lymphocyte differentiation	IL23R, STAT3
Genes related to secondary immune response and apoptosis	MHC, HLA

Genes and the Prognosis of Crohn's Disease

Genes related to age at Crohn's disease onset	TNFRSF6B, CXCL9, IL23R, NOD2, ATG16L1, CNR1, IL10, MDR1, DLG5, IRGM

Genes Related to Crohn's Disease Behavior

Stenotic/structuring behavior	NOD2, TLR4, IL12B, CX3CR1, IL10, IL6
Penetrating/fistulizing behavior	NOD2, IRGM, TNF, HLADRB1, CDKAL1
Inflammatory behavior	HLA
Granulomatous disease	TLR4/CARD15

Genes Related to Crohn's Disease Location

Upper gastrointestinal	NOD2, MIF
Ileal	IL10, CRP, NOD2, ZNF365, STAT3
Ileocolonic	ATG16L1, TCF4 (TCF7L2)
Colonic	HLA, TLR4, TLR1, TLR2, TLR6

Other Genes Related to Crohn's Disease

Genes related to Crohn's disease activity	HSP702, NOD2, PAI1, CNR1
Genes related to surgery	NOD2, HLAG
Genes related to dysplasia and cancer	FHIT
Genes related to extraintestinal manifestations	CARD15, FcRL3, HLADRB103, HLAB27, HLA-B44, HLA-B35, TNFa-308A, TNF-1031C, STAT3
Pharmacogenetics in Crohn's Disease	CARD15, NAT, TPMT, MDR1, MIF, DLG5, TNF, LTA

Adapted from Tsianos EV, Katsanos KH, Tsianos VE: Role of genetics in the diagnosis and prognosis of Crohn's disease. *World J Gastroenterol* 18:105–118, 2012.

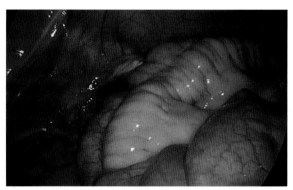

FIGURE 49-17 Laparoscopic evaluation of extensive fat wrapping caused by the circumferential growth of the mesenteric fat around the bowel wall. (Courtesy Dr. John Draus, University of Kentucky Medical Center, Lexington, KY.)

More recent genome-wide association sequencing studies in monozygotic twins have shown no reproducible differences within twin pairs in comparing whole genome sequences and tissue-specific variants in the intestinal mucosa directly affected by the inflammation of Crohn's disease.[11] These findings suggest that it is unlikely that somatic mutations have a substantial impact on the development of the disease, and simple mendelian inheritance cannot account for the pattern of occurrence. Therefore, it is likely that multiple causes (e.g., environmental factors) contribute to the cause and pathogenesis of this disease.

Pathology

The most common sites of occurrence of Crohn's disease are the small intestine and colon. Genetic variations may determine the involvement of varying locations throughout the intestine.[13] Ileal involvement has been shown with mutations of *IL10*, *CRP*, *NOD2*, *ZNF365*, and *STAT3*; ileocolonic involvement has been shown with mutations of *ATG16L1*, *TCF4*, and *TCF7L2*; and colonic involvement has been associated with mutations of *HLA*, *TLR4*, *TLR1*, *TLR2*, and *TLR6*. The involvement of the large and small intestine has been noted in about 55% of patients. Thirty percent of patients present with small bowel disease alone, and in 15%, the disease appears limited to the large intestine. The disease process is discontinuous and segmental. In patients with colonic disease, rectal sparing is characteristic of Crohn's disease and helps distinguish it from ulcerative colitis. Perirectal and perianal involvement occurs in about one third of patients with Crohn's disease, particularly those with colonic involvement. Crohn's disease can also involve the mouth, esophagus, stomach, duodenum, and appendix. Involvement of these sites can accompany disease in the small or large intestine, but in only rare cases have these locations been the only apparent sites of involvement.

Gross pathologic features. At exploration, thickened gray-pink or dull purple-red loops of bowel are noted, with areas of thick gray-white exudate or fibrosis of the serosa. Areas of diseased bowel separated by areas of grossly appearing normal bowel, called *skip areas*, are commonly encountered. A striking finding of Crohn's disease is extensive fat wrapping caused by the circumferential growth of the mesenteric fat around the bowel wall (Fig. 49-17). As the disease progresses, the bowel wall becomes increasingly thickened, firm, rubbery, and almost incompressible (Fig. 49-18). The uninvolved proximal bowel may be dilated secondary to obstruction of the diseased segment. Involved segments often are adherent to adjacent intestinal loops or other viscera, with internal fistulas common in these areas. The mesentery of the involved segment is usually thickened, with enlarged lymph nodes often noted.

On opening of the bowel, the earliest gross pathologic lesion is a superficial aphthous ulcer noted in the mucosa. With increasing disease progression, the ulceration becomes pronounced, and complete transmural inflammation results. The ulcers are characteristically linear and may coalesce to produce transverse sinuses with islands of normal mucosa in between, thus giving the characteristic cobblestone appearance.

Microscopic features. Mucosal and submucosal edema may be noted microscopically before any gross changes. A chronic inflammatory infiltrate appears in the mucosa and submucosa and extends transmurally. This inflammatory reaction is characterized

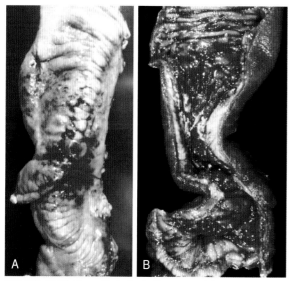

FIGURE 49-18 Gross Pathologic Features of Crohn's Disease. **A,** Serosal surface demonstrates extensive fat wrapping and inflammation. **B,** Resected specimen demonstrates marked fibrosis of the intestinal wall, stricture, and segmental mucosal inflammation. (Courtesy Dr. Mary R. Schwartz, Baylor College of Medicine, Houston, TX.)

by extensive edema, hyperemia, lymphangiectasia, intense infiltration of mononuclear cells, and lymphoid hyperplasia. Characteristic histologic lesions of Crohn's disease are noncaseating granulomas with Langerhans giant cells. Granulomas appear later in the course and are found in the wall of the bowel or in regional lymph nodes in 60% to 70% of patients (Fig. 49-19).

Clinical Manifestations

Crohn's disease can occur at any age, but the typical patient is a young adult in the second or third decade of life. The onset of disease is often insidious, with a slow and protracted course. Characteristically, there are symptomatic periods of abdominal pain and diarrhea interspersed with asymptomatic periods of varying lengths. With time, the symptomatic periods gradually become more frequent, more severe, and longer lasting. The most common symptom is intermittent and colicky abdominal pain, most commonly noted in the lower abdomen. The pain, however, may be more severe and localized and may mimic the signs and symptoms of acute appendicitis. Diarrhea is the next most frequent symptom and is present, at least intermittently, in about 85% of patients.[14] In contrast to ulcerative colitis, patients with Crohn's disease typically have fewer bowel movements, and the stools rarely contain mucus, pus, or blood. Systemic nonspecific symptoms include a low-grade fever present in about one third of the patients, weight loss, loss of strength, and malaise.

Clinically, Crohn's disease is often classified on the basis of age at onset, behavior, and site of origin. The Vienna Classification (Table 49-6) divides all patients into 24 distinct categories based on symptom onset (before or after the age of 40 years), disease behavior (nonstricturing/nonpenetrating, stricturing, or penetrating), and disease site (terminal ileum, colon, ileocolonic, upper gastrointestinal tract). This classification was developed to provide a reproducible staging of the disease, to help predict remission and relapse, and to direct therapy. The main intestinal complications of Crohn's disease include obstruction and perforation. Obstruction can occur as a manifestation of an acute exacerbation

of active disease or as the result of chronic fibrosing lesions, which eventually narrow the lumen of the bowel, producing partial or near-complete obstruction. Free perforations into the peritoneal cavity leading to a generalized peritonitis can occur in patients with Crohn's disease, but this presentation is rare. More commonly, fistulas occur between the sites of perforation and adjacent organs, such as loops of small and large intestine, urinary bladder, vagina, stomach, and sometimes the skin, usually at the site of a previous laparotomy. Localized abscesses can occur near the sites of perforation. Patients with Crohn's colitis may develop toxic megacolon and present with a marked colonic dilation, abdominal tenderness, fever, and leukocytosis. Bleeding is typically indolent and chronic, but massive gastrointestinal bleeding can occasionally occur, particularly in duodenal Crohn's disease associated with chronic ulcer formation.

Long-standing Crohn's disease predisposes to cancer of the small intestine and colon. These carcinomas typically arise at sites of chronic disease and more commonly occur in the ileum. Most are not detected until the advanced stages, and prognosis is poor. Although this relative risk for small bowel cancer in Crohn's disease is approximately 100-fold, the absolute risk is still small. Of greater concern is the development of colorectal cancer in patients with colonic involvement and a long duration of disease. Dysplasia is the putative precursor lesion for Crohn's disease–associated cancer. Patients with long-standing Crohn's disease should have an equally aggressive colonoscopic surveillance regimen as patients with extensive ulcerative colitis. Small bowel adenocarcinoma associated with Crohn's disease has an aggressive behavior and a strong predominance of extracellular mucin. In surgical specimens from patients with Crohn's disease, mucinous-appearing anal fistulas and ileal areas of adhesion/retraction should always be closely examined by a pathologist to evaluate for dysplasia or malignancy.[15]

Extraintestinal cancer, such as squamous cell carcinoma of the vulva and anal canal and Hodgkin and non-Hodgkin lymphomas, may be more frequent in patients with Crohn's disease, especially those treated with immunomodulators.

Perianal disease (fissure, fistula, stricture, or abscess) is common and occurs in 25% of patients with Crohn's disease limited to the small intestine, 41% of patients with ileocolitis, and 48% of patients with colonic involvement alone. Perianal disease may be the sole presenting feature in 5% of patients and may precede the onset of intestinal disease by months or even years. Crohn's disease should be suspected in any patient with multiple, chronic perianal fistulas.

Extraintestinal manifestations of Crohn's disease may be present in 30% of patients. The most common symptoms are skin lesions (Fig. 49-20), which include erythema nodosum and pyoderma gangrenosum, arthritis and arthralgias, uveitis and iritis, hepatitis and pericholangitis, and aphthous stomatitis. In addition, amyloidosis, pancreatitis, and nephrotic syndrome may occur in these patients. These symptoms may precede, accompany, or appear independently of the underlying bowel disease.

Diagnosis

A diagnosis of Crohn's disease should be considered in patients with chronic recurring episodes of abdominal pain, diarrhea, and weight loss. Typically, the diagnostic modalities most commonly used include barium contrast studies and endoscopy. Barium radiographic studies of the small bowel reveal a number of characteristic findings, including a cobblestone appearance of the mucosa composed of linear ulcers, transverse sinuses, and clefts.

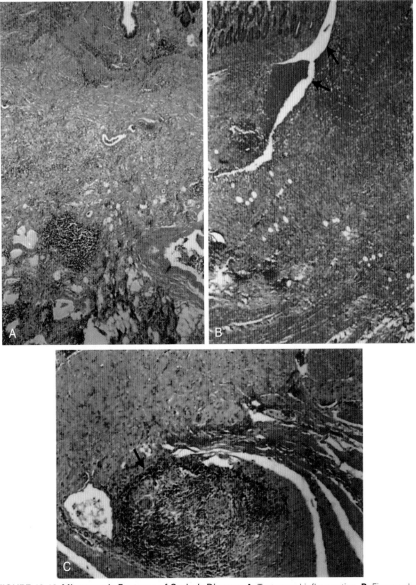

FIGURE 49-19 Microscopic Features of Crohn's Disease. **A,** Transmural inflammation. **B,** Fissure ulcer *(arrows).* **C,** Noncaseating granuloma located in the muscular layer of the small bowel *(arrow).* (Courtesy Dr. Mary R. Schwartz, Baylor College of Medicine, Houston, TX.)

TABLE 49-6 **Vienna Classification of Crohn's Disease**	
Age at diagnosis (years)	A1: <40
	A2: ≥40
Behavior	B1: Nonstricturing/nonpenetrating
	B2: Stricturing
	B3: Penetrating
Location	L1: Terminal ileum
	L2: Colon
	L3: Ileocolon
	L4: Upper gastrointestinal tract

Adapted from Gasche C, Scholmerich J, Brynskov J, et al. A simple classification of Crohn's disease: Report of the Working Party for the World Congresses of Gastroenterology, Vienna 1998. *Inflamm Bowel Dis* 6:8–15, 2000.

Long lengths of narrowed terminal ileum (Kantor string sign) may be present in long-standing disease (Fig. 49-21). Segmental and irregular patterns of bowel involvement may be noted. Fistulas between adjacent bowel loops and organs may be apparent (Fig. 49-22).

CT may be useful in demonstrating the marked transmural thickening; it can also greatly aid in diagnosing extramural complications of Crohn's disease, especially in the acute setting (Fig. 49-23). Both MRI and CT are equally accurate in assessing disease activity and bowel damage; however, MRI may be superior to CT in detecting intestinal strictures and ileal wall enhancement. More recent studies have suggested limiting the use of CT in patients with long-standing Crohn's disease because of its significant radiation exposure and need for numerous studies during the course of the disease. Other radiation-free modalities, such as

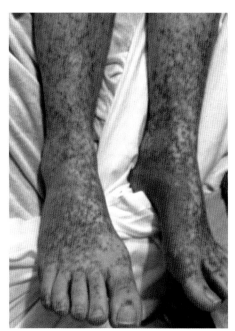

FIGURE 49-20 The most common extraintestinal presentations of Crohn's disease are skin lesions, which include erythema nodosum and pyoderma gangrenosum.

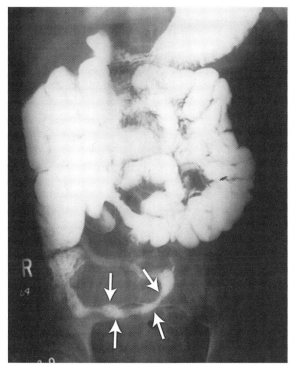

FIGURE 49-21 Small bowel series in a patient with Crohn's disease demonstrates a narrowed distal ileum (arrows) secondary to chronic inflammation and fibrosis. (Courtesy Dr. Melvyn H. Schreiber, The University of Texas Medical Branch, Galveston, TX.)

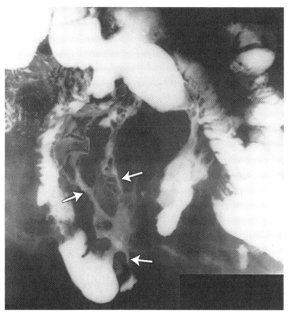

FIGURE 49-22 Crohn's disease with multiple short fistulous tracts communicating between the distal loops of ileum and the proximal colon (arrows). (Courtesy Dr. Melvyn H. Schreiber, The University of Texas Medical Branch, Galveston, TX. Adapted from Evers BM, Townsend CM Jr, Thompson JC: Small intestine. In Schwartz SI, editor: Principles of surgery, ed 7, New York, 1999, McGraw-Hill, p 1233.)

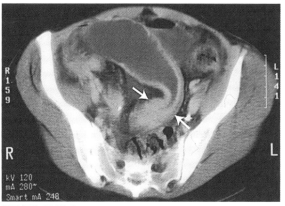

FIGURE 49-23 CT scan of a patient with Crohn's disease demonstrates marked thickening of the bowel (arrows) with a high-grade partial small bowel obstruction and dilated proximal intestine. (Courtesy Dr. Melvyn H. Schreiber, The University of Texas Medical Branch, Galveston, TX. Adapted from Evers BM, Townsend CM Jr, Thompson JC: Small intestine. In Schwartz SI, editor: Principles of surgery, ed 7, New York, 1999, McGraw-Hill, p 1233.)

MRI, ultrasound, and capsule endoscopy, should be considered in patients with long-standing Crohn's disease evaluated in an outpatient setting.[16] MRI enteroclysis is a useful adjunct to determine intestinal strictures as well as fistulas and sinus tracks; however, the relatively high cost, prolonged examination time, and limited availability may preclude many patients from receiving this procedure. Capsule endoscopy was approved by the Food and Drug Administration in 2001 and is helpful in the diagnosis of superficial mucosal abnormalities. The most commonly used criterion for an abnormal examination finding is the presence of three or more ulcers in the absence of nonsteroidal anti-inflammatory drug (NSAID) use.[17] The use of this modality is limited because of concern for capsule retention, which is defined as the presence of the capsule in the gastrointestinal tract for more than 2 weeks, which is of greater concern to patients with Crohn's disease, who have a significantly higher risk of retention (13%) compared with the general population (1% to 2.5%). Ultrasonography has limited value in the evaluation of patients with Crohn's disease and has an especially lower accuracy for detecting the disease proximal to the terminal ileum. One study determined that this modality failed to identify disease at this location in up to 67% of patients; however, ultrasound may be helpful in the assessment of undiagnosed right lower quadrant pain. When the colon is involved, sigmoidoscopy or colonoscopy may reveal characteristic aphthous ulcers with granularity and a normal-appearing surrounding mucosa. Intubation of the ileocecal valve during colonoscopy allows examination and biopsy of the terminal ileum but fails to evaluate other segments of the small intestine. With more progressive and severe disease, the ulcerations involve more and more of the bowel lumen and may be difficult to distinguish from ulcerative colitis. However, the presence of discrete ulcers and cobblestoning as well as the discontinuous segments of involved bowel favors a diagnosis of Crohn's disease. Endoscopic advances that allow better evaluation of the small intestine include single-balloon enteroscopy, double-balloon enteroscopy, and spiral enteroscopy; the most well established technique is double-balloon enteroscopy, which allows increased enteral intubation (240 to 360 cm) compared with push enteroscopy (90 to 150 cm) or ileocolonoscopy (50 to 80 cm). Limitations include specialized examiner skills and equipment, prolonged procedure times, and a 1% risk of complications (e.g., pancreatitis, perforation, or bleeding).

Serologic markers may also be useful in the diagnosis of Crohn's disease. In particular, perinuclear antineutrophil cytoplasmic antibody, anti–*Saccharomyces cerevisiae* antibody (ASCA), outer membrane porin of flagellin (anti-CBir1), and outer membrane porin of *E. coli* (OmpC-IgG) were able to predict the development of inflammatory bowel disease even in patients thought to be at low risk for development of disease.[18] ASCA has also been shown to be useful in differentiating Crohn's disease from ulcerative colitis as well as in determining patients who will require surgery in the future.

Noninvasive inflammatory markers, historically C-reactive protein and erythrocyte sedimentation rate, were used to aid in initial diagnosis, to rule out exacerbations, to monitor response to systemic therapy, and to predict relapse but were generally nonspecific and have largely been abandoned. Stool lactoferrin, an iron-binding protein in the secretory granules of neutrophils, and fecal calprotectin, a protein with antimicrobial properties released by squamous cells in response to inflammation, are inflammatory markers specific to the intestine that have shown promising results in the detection and surveillance of Crohn's disease. A prospective pilot study showed that both calprotectin and lactoferrin levels correlate well with endoscopic activity after ileocolonic resection for Crohn's disease.[19] Calprotectin had a sensitivity of 83% and a specificity of 93% to predict a risk of clinical recurrence, whereas lactoferrin had a sensitivity of 67% and a specificity of 71%. Despite being relatively inexpensive, these tests are still not widely available.

The differential diagnosis of Crohn's disease includes specific and nonspecific causes of intestinal inflammation. Bacterial inflammation (such as that caused by *Salmonella* and *Shigella*), intestinal tuberculosis, and protozoan infections (such as amebiasis) may be manifested as an ileitis. In the immunocompromised host, rare infections, particularly mycobacterial and cytomegalovirus (CMV) infections, have become more common and may cause ileitis. Acute distal ileitis may be a manifestation of early

TABLE 49-7 Diagnosis of Crohn's Colitis versus Ulcerative Colitis

PARAMETER	CROHN'S COLITIS	ULCERATIVE COLITIS
Symptoms and Signs		
Diarrhea	Common	Common
Rectal bleeding	Less common	Almost always
Abdominal pain (cramps)	Moderate to severe	Mild to moderate
Palpable mass	At times	No (unless large cancer)
Anal complaints	Frequent (>50%)	Infrequent (<20%)
Radiologic Findings		
Ileal disease	Common	Rare (backwash ileitis)
Nodularity, fuzziness	No	Yes
Distribution	Skip areas	Rectum extending upward and continuously
Ulcers	Linear, cobblestone, fissures	Collar-button
Toxic dilation	Rare	Uncommon
Proctoscopic Findings		
Anal fissure, fistula, abscess	Common	Rare
Rectal sparing	Common (50%)	Rare (5%)
Granular mucosa	No	Yes
Ulceration	Linear, deep, scattered	Superficial, universal

Crohn's disease, but it also may be unrelated, such as when it is caused by a bacteriologic agent (e.g., *Campylobacter*, *Yersinia*). Patients usually present in a similar fashion to those presenting with acute appendicitis, with a sudden onset of right lower quadrant pain, nausea, vomiting, and fever. These entities normally resolve spontaneously, and when they are noted during surgery, no biopsy or resection should be performed.

In most cases, Crohn's disease of the colon can be readily distinguished from ulcerative colitis; however, in 5% to 10% of patients, the delineation between Crohn's disease and ulcerative colitis may be difficult if not impossible to make (Table 49-7). Ulcerative colitis almost always involves the rectum most severely, with lessening inflammation from the rectum to the ileocolic area. In contrast, Crohn's disease may be worse on the right side of the colon than on the left side, and sometimes the rectum is spared. Ulcerative colitis also demonstrates continuous involvement from rectum to proximal segments, whereas Crohn's disease is segmental. Although ulcerative colitis involves the mucosa of the large intestine, it does not extend deep into the wall of the bowel, as does Crohn's disease. Bleeding is a more common symptom in ulcerative colitis. Perianal involvement and rectovaginal fistulas are unusual in ulcerative colitis but are more common in Crohn's disease. Other endoscopic features of Crohn's disease are skip lesions, asymmetrical involvement of bowel, and the cobblestone appearance that results from ulcerations interspersed with islands of edematous mucosa.

Management

Medical therapy. There is no cure for Crohn's disease. Therefore, medical therapies are directed toward inducing and maintaining remission as well as preventing acute exacerbations or complications of the disease.[20] Surgery is advocated for neoplastic and preneoplastic lesions, obstructing stenoses, suppurative complications, or medically intractable disease. Narcotic analgesia should be avoided except during the perioperative period because of the potential for tolerance and abuse in the setting of chronic disease.[10] Drugs that have demonstrated efficacy in the induction or maintenance of remission in Crohn's disease include corticosteroids; TNF antagonists, such as infliximab, adalimumab, and certolizumab; aminosalicylates, such as sulfasalazine and mesalamine; immunosuppressive agents, such as azathioprine (AZT), 6-mercaptopurine (6-MP), methotrexate (MTX), and tacrolimus (FK-506); and antibiotics. Other innovative therapies, such as leukocyte trafficking inhibitors, interleukin inhibitors, and probiotics, in addition to molecular targeted therapies are currently being investigated.

Aminosalicylates. Sulfasalazine (Azulfidine) is an aminosalicylate with 5-aminosalicylic acid as the active moiety. Although a clear benefit has been noted in patients with colonic involvement, the effectiveness of sulfasalazine alone in the treatment of Crohn's disease limited to the small bowel is controversial, and its use in maintenance therapy has fallen out of favor. Mesalamine, which is also an aminosalicylate, provides a slow release of 5-aminosalicylic acid with passage through the small bowel and colon. Clinical trials have demonstrated efficacy of mesalamine at a dosage of 4 g/day without an increase in side effects. Furthermore, although mesalamine has shown some efficacy as a postoperative maintenance strategy and is an acceptable first-line therapy, most patients, especially those with relapsing disease, are treated with immunosuppressive agents with or without TNF antagonist therapy.[21] Studies are currently being conducted to evaluate the efficacy of even higher dosages of mesalamine to determine its continued utility as an appropriate first-line therapy.

Corticosteroids. Corticosteroids, particularly prednisone, are beneficial in moderate to severe Crohn's disease. Prednisone is not ideal for maintenance therapy as more than 50% of patients, particularly smokers, treated with corticosteroids become "steroid dependent," and chronic treatment is associated with osteoporosis and increased relapse rates of Crohn's disease.[10] Patients with moderate to severe disease should be treated with high-dose (40 to 60 mg daily) prednisone until resolution of symptoms and resumption of weight gain. Parenteral corticosteroids are indicated for patients with severe disease once the presence of an abscess has been excluded. IV steroids should be tapered once the patient is experiencing clinical improvement. Currently, there are no standards for corticosteroid taper, but doses are generally tapered by 5 to 10 mg per week until 20 mg, and then by 2.5 to 5 mg weekly until cessation. Dual-energy x-ray absorptiometry scan, calcium and vitamin D supplementation, and consideration of bisphosphonate therapy are warranted once corticosteroid therapy is initiated to identify baseline bone density and to prevent steroid-induced loss of bone mineral density.

Budesonide is a glucocorticoid steroid with promising implications for the symptomatic treatment of Crohn's disease. It has a high first-pass hepatic metabolism, which allows targeted delivery to the intestine while mitigating the systemic effects of steroid therapy. Controlled ileal release budesonide (9 mg/day) is effective when active disease is confined to the ileum or right colon and has been shown to be more effective than either placebo or mesalamine.[10] Given a relatively good response and its relative safety, budesonide is recommended as the preferred primary treatment to mesalamine as first-line therapy for patients with mild to moderately active Crohn's disease with localized ileal disease.

Antibiotics. Certain antibiotics have also been found to be effective in the primary therapy for Crohn's disease. Promising results were initially reported for metronidazole, but later studies determined that it was no more effective than placebo for inducing remission. Other antibiotics that have been used with varying success include ciprofloxacin, rifaximin, clofazimine, ethambutol, isoniazid, and rifabutin. Antibiotic therapy has a clear role in the septic complications associated with Crohn's disease and is beneficial in perianal disease. The mechanism of action of antibiotics in Crohn's disease is unclear, and side effects of these antibiotics preclude their long-term use. Therefore, antibiotics may play an adjunctive role in the treatment of Crohn's disease and, in selected patients, may be useful in treating perianal disease, enterocutaneous fistulas, or active colonic disease but should not be used in maintenance therapy or to induce remission.

Immunosuppressive agents. The immunosuppressive agents AZT, MTX, and 6-MP are effective in maintenance therapy for and treatment of moderate to severe Crohn's disease. AZT and 6-MP are effective for maintaining steroid-induced remission, and weekly IV MTX is effective for steroid-dependent and refractory Crohn's disease.[10] Despite their potential toxicity, these drugs have proved to be relatively safe in these patients; the most common side effects are pancreatitis, hepatitis, fever, and rash. The more disconcerting complications of immunosuppressants include chronic liver disease, bone marrow suppression, and the potential for malignant transformation. No prospective controlled trial has evaluated dose escalation or initiation of therapy using these drugs. Genetic polymorphisms for thiopurine methyltransferase (TPMT), which is the primary enzyme that metabolizes AZT and 6-MP, have been identified and can potentially be used to regulate therapy according to the measurement of their metabolites (6-thioguanine nucleotides). Patients with decreased TPMT activity have a significantly increased risk of fatal bone marrow suppression, and previous studies have reported severe myelosuppression in patients who are wild-type or heterozygous carriers for TPMT variant alleles, suggesting that TPMT genotype testing may be a safe screening tool to determine which patients may have a genetic predisposition to adverse outcomes with AZT or 6-MP treatment.

Other immunosuppressive agents that have been used with some effectiveness include cyclosporine and FK-506. FK-506 inhibits the production of IL-2 by helper T cells and was found to be effective for fistula improvement, but not fistula remission, in patients with perianal Crohn's disease. Both of these agents have been used in patients with severe disease who do not respond to IV steroids. Low-dose cyclosporine was not found to be efficacious; however, in uncontrolled studies, FK-506 demonstrated some benefit in patients with steroid-refractory disease.

Anticytokine and cytokine therapies. The introduction of anti-TNF therapy for Crohn's disease was considered to be a breakthrough in medical management. The first anti-TNF agent introduced was infliximab, a chimeric monoclonal antibody to TNF-α, which is efficacious and safe in the treatment of moderate to severe Crohn's disease and effective as a monotherapy for maintenance therapy and steroid-induced remission. Multiple studies have shown that treatment with infliximab results in perineal fistula closure in approximately two thirds of patients. Although it is highly effective in certain Crohn's disease patients with penetrating disease and extraintestinal disease, not every patient responds to infliximab. Also, there is an increased risk for tuberculosis reactivation, invasive fungal and other opportunistic infections, demyelinating central nervous system lesions, activation of latent multiple sclerosis, and exacerbation of congestive heart disease. Other promising TNF antagonists include adalimumab (humanized IgG1 monoclonal antibody), which is an effective maintenance agent and can be self-administered, and certolizumab (humanized antibody fragment [Fab]), which is ideal in pregnant and nursing women as it is linked to a polyethylene glycol moiety and does not cross the placenta and is not excreted in breast milk.

Novel therapies. Other investigational therapeutic agents include leukocyte trafficking inhibitors, interleukin inhibitors, anti–adhesion molecule antibodies, and probiotics. Natalizumab, a recombinant humanized monoclonal antibody against α_4 integrin, showed effectiveness in the induction and maintenance of remission in patients with active Crohn's disease. It was removed from the market after several patients developed progressive multifocal leukoencephalopathy but was later reinstituted for refractory Crohn's disease and is currently available only in specialized centers worldwide. Vedolizumab is a humanized monoclonal antibody that specifically binds to $\alpha_4\beta_7$ integrin and blocks its interaction with mucosal addressin cell adhesion molecule 1 (MadCAM-1), thus inhibiting the translocation of memory T lymphocytes into inflamed gastrointestinal parenchymal tissues. Results from phase 3 trials appear promising regarding the use of vedolizumab in the treatment of both Crohn's disease and ulcerative colitis. Because MadCAM-1 is preferentially expressed on blood vessels in the gastrointestinal tract, vedolizumab is more gut specific and therefore a more targeted form of immunosuppression. Also, vedolizumab prevents the gastrointestinal mucosal or transmural inflammation without the nonspecific neurologic side effects seen in less selective α_4 integrin inhibitors, such as natalizumab.[22] Ustekinumab, a humanized IgG1 monoclonal antibody that inhibits IL-12/23 through targeting of a shared p40 subunit, has been shown in two large trials to be effective in severe Crohn's disease that is refractory to anti-TNF therapies, but it has yet to be approved and is only available through compassionate use measures at some centers. Compounds are also being evaluated that block certain signaling pathways (e.g., NF-κB, mitogen-activated protein kinases, and peroxisome proliferator-activated receptor-γ); in limited studies, some of these compounds have shown clinical improvement, but results have varied, and these agents are still under development.

Nutritional therapy. Nutritional therapy in patients with Crohn's disease has been used with varying success. The use of chemically defined elemental diets has been shown in some studies to reduce disease activity, particularly in patients with disease localized to the small bowel, and they have been shown to reduce corticosteroid-induced toxicities.[10] Liquid polymeric diets may be as effective as elemental feedings and are more acceptable to patients. With few exceptions, standard elemental diets have not been effective in the maintenance of remission in Crohn's disease. Total parenteral nutrition (TPN) has also been shown to be of use in patients with active Crohn's disease; however, complication rates exceed those for enteral nutrition. Although the primary role of nutritional therapy is questionable in patients with inflammatory bowel disease, there is definitely a secondary role for nutritional supplementation to replenish depleted nutrient stores, allowing intestinal protein synthesis and healing, and to prepare patients for operation.

Smoking cessation. Although the implication of tobacco abuse as a causative factor in the development of Crohn's disease has been difficult to prove, smoking clearly affects the disease course. Smoking is associated with the late bimodal onset of disease and has been shown to increase the incidence of relapse and failure of maintenance therapy. It also appears to be associated with the severity of disease in a linear dose-response relationship. Tobacco exposure is an independent predictor of need for maintenance treatment, specifically biologic therapy. Therefore, smoking cessation therapy is an important component of medical therapy.

Surgical treatment. Although medical management is indicated during acute exacerbations of disease, most patients with chronic Crohn's disease will require surgery at some time during the course of their illness. Approximately 70% of patients will require surgical resection within 15 years after diagnosis. Indications for surgery include failure of medical treatment, bowel obstruction, and fistula or abscess formation. Most patients can be treated with elective surgery, especially with the improvement of medical management in the past decade.[22] However, patients with intestinal perforation, peritonitis, excessive bleeding, or toxic megacolon require urgent surgery. Children with Crohn's disease and resulting systemic symptoms, such as growth retardation, may benefit from resection. The extraintestinal complications of Crohn's disease, although not primary indications for operation, often subside after resection of involved bowel, with the exception of ankylosing spondylitis and hepatic complications.

The aim of surgery for Crohn's disease has shifted from radical operation to achieve inflammation-free margins of resection to minimal surgery, intended to remove just grossly inflamed tissue or to increase the luminal diameter of the bowel (i.e., strictureplasty). Even if adjacent areas of bowel are clearly diseased, they should be ignored. Early in the history of surgical therapy for Crohn's disease, surgeons tended to perform wider resections with the hope of cure or significant remission. However, repeated wide resections resulted in no greater remissions or cure and led to the short bowel syndrome, which is a devastating surgical complication. Frozen sections to determine microscopic disease are unreliable and should be performed only in the event that malignant disease is suspected. It must be emphasized that operative treatment of a complication is limited to that segment of bowel involved with the complication, and no attempt should be made to resect more bowel, even though grossly evident disease may be apparent.

Laparoscopic surgery for patients with Crohn's disease has been determined to be safe and feasible in appropriately selected patients, for example, those with localized abscesses, simple intra-abdominal fistulas, perianastomotic recurrent disease, and disease limited to the distal ileum. A large comparative study evaluating laparoscopic colectomy for Crohn's colitis determined that the laparoscopic group had a significantly shorter median operative time, earlier return of bowel function, and shorter hospital stay.[23] Other investigators caution against a laparoscopic approach in morbidly obese patients as obesity is an independent risk factor for conversion to open surgery, and obesity was also shown to increase blood loss, operative times, and incidence of incisional hernia.[24] Multiple randomized clinical trials have verified that laparoscopic surgery is associated with a more rapid recovery of bowel function and shorter hospital stay; the rate of disease recurrence is similar compared with open procedures. Randomized controlled trials with long-term follow-up have demonstrated that patients undergoing laparoscopic ileocolonic resection for Crohn's disease had improved body image and satisfaction with cosmesis of surgery and less incidence of incisional hernia compared with the open surgery group. The potential for earlier recovery after laparoscopic resection has stimulated interest in extending the role of surgical resection in inducing remission; the LIR!C trial is a randomized multicenter trial currently under way to provide evidence as to whether infliximab treatment or surgery is the best treatment for recurrent distal ileitis in Crohn's disease.[25]

The decision to perform a primary anastomosis versus initial ostomy formation with delayed reconstruction can be a difficult one for those with Crohn's disease. Patients are often malnourished, are receiving intensive immunosuppressive therapy, or present with some element of intra-abdominal sepsis. In general, standard surgical principles should direct this decision. Patients with adequate nutrition and minimal intra-abdominal sepsis can safely undergo primary anastomosis at the initial operation, whereas malnourished and septic patients are best served by diversion, if possible. Although caution should be exercised in performing an anastomosis in the setting of high-dose immunosuppression, large series have confirmed that surgery is safe for patients with Crohn's disease while they are receiving perioperative infliximab or immunosuppressive therapy. Regarding anastomotic technique, several studies suggest that creating a wider anastomosis with a stapled functional end-to-end anastomosis may decrease fecal stasis and subsequent bacterial overgrowth, which are implicated in anastomotic recurrence in Crohn's disease. However, a randomized controlled trial comparing side-to-side anastomosis versus end-to-end anastomosis determined that there was no difference in overall complication rates, anastomotic leak rates, or rates of symptomatic recurrence, with only a slight increase in endoscopic recurrence in the end-to-end anastomosis group (43% versus 38%). Kono and associates[26] introduced a new antimesenteric functional end-to-end hand-sewn anastomosis designed to minimize anastomotic restenosis in Crohn's disease. Assessment after 5 years demonstrated that the surgical recurrence rate at the anastomosis was lower than in the conventional anastomosis group, but larger randomized controlled trials are required to definitively determine its overall benefit.

Specific Problems

Acute ileitis (nonstricturing, nonpenetrating). Patients can present with acute abdominal pain localized to the right lower quadrant and signs and symptoms consistent with a diagnosis of acute appendicitis. At exploration, the appendix is found to be normal, but the terminal ileum is edematous and beefy red, with a thickened mesentery and enlarged lymph nodes. This condition, known as *acute ileitis*, is a self-limited disease. Acute ileitis may be a manifestation of early Crohn's disease but is most often unrelated. Bacteriologic agents such as *Campylobacter* and *Yersinia* may cause acute ileitis. Intestinal resection should not be performed. Although in the past the management of the appendix was controversial, it is clear now that in the absence of acute inflammatory involvement of the appendix or the cecum, appendectomy should be performed. This eliminates the appendix as a source of abdominal pain in the future.

Stricturing disease. Intestinal obstruction is the most common indication for surgical therapy in patients with Crohn's disease. Obstruction in these patients is often partial, and nonoperative management is initially indicated. The success of nonoperative management can often be predicted on the basis of the chronicity of symptoms at the affected site. In patients for whom it is difficult to determine whether the site of obstruction is caused by an acute exacerbation or a chronically strictured segment, stool lactoferrin and calprotectin levels may help identify acute inflammation, whereas certain genetic markers (e.g., *NOD2*, *TLR4*, *CX3CR1*) may predict potential success of medical therapy. In case of a chronic strictured segment, medical therapy is rarely effective.

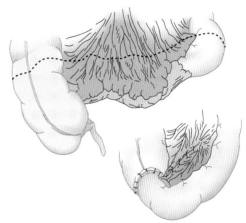

FIGURE 49-24 Resection of the ileum, ileocecal valve, cecum, and ascending colon for Crohn's disease of the ileum. Intestinal continuity is restored by end-to-end anastomosis.

Operative intervention is required for patients with complete obstruction and patients with partial obstruction whose condition does not resolve with nonoperative management. The treatment of choice for intestinal obstruction in patients with Crohn's disease is segmental resection of the involved segment with primary reanastomosis. This may involve segmental resection and primary anastomosis of a short segment of ileum if this is the site of the complication. More commonly, the cecum is involved contiguously with the terminal ileum, in which case resection of the involved terminal ileum and colon is required and the ileum is anastomosed to the ascending or transverse colon (Fig. 49-24).

In selected patients with obstruction caused by strictures (single or multiple), one option is to perform a strictureplasty that effectively widens the lumen but avoids intestinal resection. Strictureplasty is performed by making a longitudinal incision through the narrowed area of the intestine, followed by closure in a transverse fashion in a manner similar to that for a Heineke-Mikulicz pyloroplasty (Fig. 49-25A). For longer diseased segments (>10 cm), the strictureplasty can be performed similar to a Finney pyloroplasty (Fig. 49-25B) or a side-to-side isoperistaltic strictureplasty. Strictureplasty has the most application in patients in whom multiple short areas of narrowing are present over long segments of intestine, in those who have already had several previous resections of the small intestine, and when the areas of narrowing are caused by fibrous obstruction rather than by acute inflammation. This procedure preserves intestine and is associated with complication and recurrence rates comparable to those of resection and reanastomosis. Given the concerns for development of carcinoma at chronically strictured segments, full-thickness biopsy with frozen section of the stricture site has been advocated at the time of surgery to rule out malignant disease before strictureplasty is performed (Box 49-3).

In the past, bypass procedures were commonly used. There are two types of bypass operations: exclusion bypass and simple (continuity) bypass. For certain types of ileocecal disease associated with an abscess or phlegmon densely adherent to the retroperitoneum, the proximal transected end of the ileum is anastomosed to the transverse colon in an end-to-side fashion with or without construction of a mucous fistula using the distal transected end of the ileum (exclusion bypass), or an ileotransverse colonic anastomosis is made in a side-to-side fashion (continuity bypass).

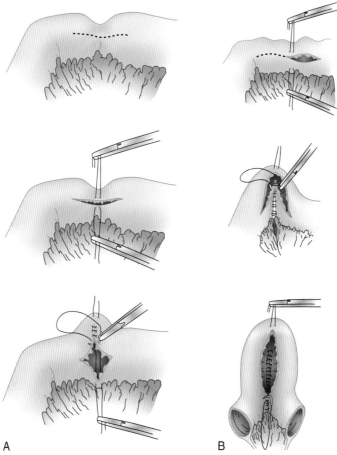

A   B

FIGURE 49-25 A, Technique of short strictureplasty in the manner of a Heineke-Mikulicz pyloroplasty. **B,** For longer diseased segments, strictureplasty may be performed in a manner similar to Finney pyloroplasty. (Adapted from Alexander-Williams J, Haynes IG: Up-to-date management of small-bowel Crohn's disease. In Mannick JA, editor: *Advances in surgery,* St. Louis, 1987, Mosby, pp 245–264.)

BOX 49-3   Contraindications to Strictureplasty

Excessive tension due to rigid and thickened bowel segments
Perforation of the intestine
Fistula or abscess formation at the intended strictureplasty site
Hemorrhagic strictures
Multiple strictures within a short segment
Malnutrition or hypoalbuminemia (<2.0 g/dL)
Suspicion of cancer at the intended strictureplasty site

Adapted from Yamamoto T, Watanabe T: Surgery for luminal Crohn's disease. *World J Gastroenterol* 20:78–90, 2014.

Currently, bypass with exclusion is used only in patients with severe gastroduodenal Crohn's disease not amenable to strictureplasty, older poor-risk patients, patients who have had several prior resections and cannot afford to lose any more bowel, and those in whom resection would necessitate entering an abscess or endangering a normal structure.

Penetrating disease. Fistula and abscess in patients with Crohn's disease are relatively common and usually involve the adjacent small bowel, colon, or other surrounding viscera (e.g.,

bladder). The presence of a radiographically demonstrable enteroenteral fistula without any signs of sepsis or other complications is not in itself an indication for surgery. Furthermore, penetrating disease is particularly sensitive to anticytokine therapy, and a conservative, surgical approach to Crohn's disease–related fistula is most appropriate. However, many of these patients will require eventual resection as the disease progresses and they have progressively worsening abdominal pain. Enterocutaneous fistulas may develop but are rarely spontaneous and are more likely to follow resection or drainage of intra-abdominal abscesses. Ideally, enterocutaneous fistulas should be managed by excising the fistula tract along with the diseased segment of intestine and performing a primary reanastomosis. If the fistula forms between two or more adjacent loops of diseased bowel, the involved segments should be excised. Alternatively, if the fistula involves an adjacent normal organ, such as the bladder or colon, only the segment of the diseased small bowel and fistulous tract should be resected, and the defect in the normal organ should simply be closed. Most patients with ileosigmoid fistulas do not necessarily require resection of the sigmoid because the disease is usually confined to the small bowel. However, if the segment of sigmoid is also found to have Crohn's disease, it should be resected along with the segment of diseased small bowel.

Perforation. Penetrating disease in the form of perforation into the free peritoneal cavity occurs occasionally but is not common in patients with Crohn's disease. Typically, penetration is manifested with a localized abscess densely adherent to the diseased segment of bowel. In cases of free perforation, the segment of involved bowel should be resected, and in the presence of minimal contamination, a primary anastomosis should be performed. If generalized peritonitis is present, a safer option may be to perform enterostomies until the intra-abdominal sepsis is controlled and then return for restoration of intestinal continuity. Abscesses can be treated with percutaneous drainage and antibiotics, although fistula or uncontrolled sepsis may ultimately develop, requiring resection with or without primary anastomosis.

Gastrointestinal bleeding. Although anemia from chronic blood loss is common in patients with Crohn's disease, life-threatening gastrointestinal hemorrhage is rare. The incidence of hemorrhage is more common in patients with Crohn's disease involving the colon rather than the small bowel. As with the other complications, the segment involved should be resected and intestinal continuity restored. Arteriography may be useful to localize the bleeding before surgery. In cases of bleeding associated with duodenal disease, endoscopic intervention is usually successful. However, in cases of failure, duodenotomy with oversewing of the bleeding ulcerative area is indicated.[22]

Urologic complications. Genitourinary complications occur in up to one third of patients with Crohn's disease. The most common urologic complication is ureteral obstruction, which is usually secondary to ileocolic disease with retroperitoneal abscess. Surgical treatment of the primary intestinal disease is adequate in most patients. In a few cases of long-standing inflammatory disease, periureteric fibrosis may be present and require ureterolysis with or without ureteral stenting.

Cancer. Patients with long-standing Crohn's disease of the small bowel and, in particular, the colon have an increased incidence of cancer. The management of these patients is the same as that for any patient—resection of the cancer with appropriate margins and regional lymph nodes. Patients with cancer associated with Crohn's disease commonly have a worse prognosis than those who do not have Crohn's disease, largely because the diagnosis in these patients is delayed. A strictureplasty should not be performed if malignant disease is suspected.

Colorectal disease. The same principle applies to patients with Crohn's disease limited to the colon as to those with disease to the small bowel, that is, surgical resection should be limited to the segment producing the complications. Indications for surgery include a lack of response to medical management and complications of Crohn's colitis, which include obstruction, hemorrhage, perforation, and toxic megacolon. Depending on the diseased segments, procedures commonly include segmental colectomy with colocolonic anastomosis, subtotal colectomy with ileoproctostomy, and, in patients with extensive perianal and rectal disease, total proctocolectomy with Brooke ileostomy. Laparoscopic colectomy for Crohn's colitis may be safely performed by experienced surgeons.[23] Patients with toxic megacolon should undergo colectomy, closure of the proximal rectum, and end ileostomy. Strictureplasty has limited usefulness in colonic Crohn's disease, and concerns of malignant transformation at an area of colonic obstruction should limit its application.

A particularly troubling problem after proctocolectomy in patients with Crohn's disease is delayed healing of the perineal wound. It has been found that more than half of perineal wounds are open 6 months after surgery in patients with Crohn's disease.

Persistent nonhealing wounds require excision with secondary closure. Large cavities or sinuses may be filled by using well-vascularized pedicles of muscle (e.g., gracilis, semimembranosus, rectus abdominis) or omentum or by using an inferior gluteal myocutaneous graft.

Although controversial, continence-preserving operations, such as ileal pouch–anal anastomosis or continent ileostomies (Kock pouch), may be considered in very carefully selected patients with Crohn's disease isolated to the colon who undergo thorough counseling about the increased risk of anastomotic failure and wound complication. However, they should never be considered in patients with evidence of terminal ileal or perianal disease as these patients have a significantly increased rate of recurrence of Crohn's disease in the pouch, fistulas to the anastomosis, and peripouch abscesses.[22]

Perianal disease. Diseases involving the perianal region include fissures and fistulas and are common in patients with Crohn's disease, particularly those with colonic involvement. The treatment of perianal disease should be nonoperative unless an abscess or complex fistula develops, and even in these cases, surgery should be approached cautiously and limited to addressing the specific problem with minimal tissue loss. Nonsuppurative, chronic fistulization or perianal fissuring is treated with antibiotics, immunosuppressive agents (e.g., AZT or 6-MP), and infliximab, which is the most widely supported therapy as it has shown the best results in fistula closure.[10] Several uncontrolled studies have shown some benefit with cyclosporine or FK-506 treatment.

Wide excision of abscesses or fistulas is not indicated, but more conservative interventions, including the liberal placement of drainage catheters and noncutting setons, are preferable. Definitive fistulotomy is indicated for most patients with superficial, low trans-sphincteric, and low intersphincteric fistulas, although one must recognize that some degree of anal stenosis may occur as a result of chronic inflammation. High trans-sphincteric, suprasphincteric, and extrasphincteric fistulas are usually treated with noncutting setons. Fissures are usually lateral, relatively painless, large, and indolent and often respond to conservative management. Abscesses should be drained, but large excisions of tissue *should not* be performed. Advancement flap closure of perineal fistulas may be required in certain cases. Selective construction of diverting stomas has good results in combination with optimal medical therapy to induce remission of inflammation. Proctectomy may be infrequently required in a subset of patients who have persistent and unremitting disease despite conservative medical and surgical therapy.

Duodenal disease. Crohn's disease of the duodenum occurs in approximately 1% to 5% of patients with Crohn's disease and occurs most commonly in the duodenal bulb.[22] Operative intervention is uncommon. The primary indication for surgery in these patients is duodenal obstruction that does not respond to medical therapy, with endoscopic balloon dilation and surgery being the mainstays of treatment. Gastrojejunostomy to bypass the disease rather than duodenal resection is the procedure of choice. Strictureplasties have been performed with success in selected patients and may avoid the marginal ulceration and diarrhea associated with gastrojejunostomy.

Prognosis

Crohn's disease is a chronic inflammatory disorder that is not medically or surgically curable; therefore, therapeutic approaches are required to induce and to maintain symptomatic control, to improve quality of life, and to minimize long-term complications.

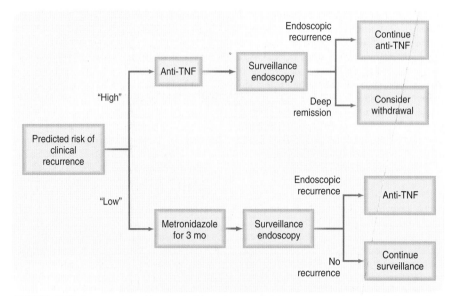

FIGURE 49-26 Suggested algorithm for deciding when to administer postoperative prophylaxis based on effectiveness of treatment. (Adapted from Vaughn BP, Moss AC: Prevention of post-operative recurrence of Crohn's disease. *World J Gastroenterol* 20:1147–1154, 2014.)

It is estimated that approximately 80% of patients will require surgery at some point in their lifetime.[27] Symptomatic recurrence varies from 40% to 80%, and endoscopic recurrence is much higher, with up to 90% of patients having visible lesions within 5 years. The only clearly modifiable risk factor is smoking cessation. Surgery is generally implicated in the event that the patient fails to respond to medical therapy or develops complications, but multiple studies have shown that patients report significant improvement in quality of life scores after surgical intervention. Although postsurgical recurrence is high, algorithms using careful endoscopic surveillance combined with biologic therapy play a role in the prevention of postoperative recurrence of Crohn's disease (Fig. 49-26). Although there is currently no cure for this disease, advances in medical and surgical therapies have clearly increased quality of life and disease-free progression.

Standardized mortality rates in patients with Crohn's disease are increased in those patients whose disease began before the age of 20 years and in those who have had disease present for longer than 13 years. Long-term survival studies have suggested that patients with Crohn's disease have a death rate approximately two to three times higher than that in the general population, which is most commonly related to chronic wound complications and sepsis. Gastrointestinal cancer remains the leading cause of disease-related death in patients with Crohn's disease; other causes of disease-related deaths include sepsis, thromboembolic complications, and electrolyte disorders.

Typhoid Enteritis

Typhoid fever remains a significant problem in developing countries, most commonly in areas with contaminated water supplies and inadequate waste disposal. It infects roughly 21.6 million people and kills an estimated 200,000 people every year worldwide. Children and young adults are most often affected. Improvements in sanitation have decreased the incidence of typhoid fever in industrialized countries. In the United States, most cases of typhoid fever arise in international travelers; however, unrecognized and untreated typhoid fever is a life-threatening illness of several weeks' duration with long-term morbidity.

Typhoid enteritis is an acute systemic infection caused primarily by *Salmonella typhi*. The pathologic events of typhoid fever are initiated in the intestinal tract after oral ingestion of the typhoid bacillus. These organisms penetrate the small bowel mucosa, making their way rapidly to the lymphatics and then systemically. Hyperplasia of the reticuloendothelial system, including lymph nodes, liver, and spleen, is characteristic of typhoid fever. Peyer's patches in the small bowel become hyperplastic and may subsequently ulcerate, with complications of hemorrhage or perforation.

The diagnosis of typhoid fever is confirmed by isolating the organism from blood (positive in 90% of the patients during the first week of the illness), bone marrow, and stool cultures. In addition, the finding of high titers of agglutinins against O and H antigens (Widal test) was used for decades but was found to be nonspecific and is no longer an acceptable clinical method. Assays for the diagnosis of *S. typhi* using PCR assay have had varying success. Combining assays of blood and urine achieved a sensitivity of 83% and reported specificity of 100%. Indirect hemagglutination, indirect fluorescent Vi antibody, and indirect enzyme-linked immunosorbent assay for IgM and IgG antibodies to *S. typhi* polysaccharide are promising, but the success rates of these assays vary greatly in the literature.

Typhoid fever and uncomplicated typhoid enteritis are treated by antibiotic administration. If a patient presents with clinical symptoms and has been in an endemic area, broad-spectrum empirical antibiotics should be started immediately. Treatment should not be delayed for confirmatory tests because prompt treatment drastically reduces the risk of complications and fatalities. Antibiotic therapy should be narrowed once more information is available. Chloramphenicol was initially the mainstay of treatment in the 1950s, but widespread antibiotic resistance occurred. Currently, the most widely used agents are fluoroquinolones and third-generation cephalosporins.

Complications requiring potential surgical intervention include hemorrhage and perforation. The incidence of hemorrhage was reported to be as high as 20% in some series, but with the availability of antibiotic treatment, this figure has decreased. When hemorrhage occurs, transfusion is indicated and usually suffices. Rarely, laparotomy must be performed for uncontrollable, life-threatening hemorrhage. Intestinal perforation through an ulcerated Peyer's patch occurs in approximately 2% of cases. Typically, it is a single perforation in the terminal ileum, and simple closure of the perforation is the treatment of choice. With multiple perforations, which occur in about 25% of patients, resection with primary anastomosis or exteriorization of the intestinal loops may be required.

Enteritis in the Immunocompromised Host

The acquired immunodeficiency syndrome (AIDS) epidemic as well as the widespread use of immunosuppressive agents after organ transplantation has resulted in a number of rare and exotic pathogens infecting the gastrointestinal tract. Almost all patients with AIDS have gastrointestinal symptoms during their illness, the most common of which is diarrhea. However, the surgeon may be asked to evaluate the immunocompromised patient with abdominal pain, an obvious acute abdomen, or gastrointestinal bleeding; a number of protozoal, bacterial, viral, and fungal organisms may be responsible.

Protozoa

Protozoa (e.g., *Cryptosporidium*, *Isospora*, and *Microsporidium*) are the most frequent class of pathogens causing diarrhea in patients with AIDS. The small bowel is the most common site of infection. Diagnosis may be established by acid-fast staining of the stool or duodenal secretions, but the introduction of specific antigen tests for stool examination has improved diagnostic capabilities. Immunochromatography cards for the rapid detection of protozoal proteins from a small sample of stool are available from several different commercial sources and are more sensitive and more specific (>90%) than the traditional microscopic examinations. Symptoms are most commonly related to diarrhea, which may be at times intractable. Current treatment regimens have not been entirely effective, but drugs such as cotrimoxazole and nitazoxanide appear to elicit a treatment response for cryptosporidiosis, and one study found no *Cryptosporidium* oocysts in the stools of patients receiving highly active antiretroviral therapy.[28]

Bacteria

Infections by enteric bacteria are more frequent and more virulent in individuals infected with human immunodeficiency virus (HIV) than in healthy hosts. *Salmonella*, *Shigella*, and *Campylobacter* are associated with higher rates of bacteremia and antibiotic resistance in the immunocompromised patient. The diagnosis of *Shigella* or *Salmonella* infection may be established by stool cultures. The diagnosis of *Campylobacter* infection is not as easily established because stool cultures are often negative, but PCR techniques evaluating stool and serum have shown promising diagnostic results in patients with negative cultures. These enteric infections are manifested clinically with high fever, abdominal pain, and diarrhea that may be bloody. Abdominal pain may mimic an acute abdomen. Bacteremia and serious infections should be treated by IV administration of imipenem antibiotics; ciprofloxacin is an attractive choice if the organisms are multiply resistant; the pregnant patient may be safely treated with erythromycin. The incidence of *Campylobacter* infection among patients

with AIDS who were treated with rifabutin prophylaxis was reported to be decreased compared with untreated controls.

Diarrhea caused by *Clostridium difficile* is more common in patients with AIDS because of the increased antibiotic use in this population compared with healthy hosts. Diagnosis is by standard assays of stool for *C. difficile* enterotoxin. Treatment with metronidazole or vancomycin is usually effective.

Mycobacteria

Mycobacterial infection is a frequent cause of intestinal disease in immunocompromised hosts. This can be secondary to *Mycobacterium tuberculosis* or *Mycobacterium avium complex* (MAC), which is an atypical mycobacterium related to the type that causes cervical adenitis (scrofula). The usual route of infection is by swallowed organisms that directly penetrate the intestinal mucosa. The luminal gastrointestinal tract is affected by MAC infection, with massive thickening of the proximal small intestine often noted (Fig. 49-27). Clinically, patients with MAC present with diarrhea, fever, anorexia, and progressive wasting.

The most frequent site of intestinal involvement of *M. tuberculosis* is the distal ileum and cecum, with approximately 90% of patients demonstrating disease at this site. The gross appearance can be ulcerative, hypertrophic, or ulcerohypertrophic. The bowel wall appears thickened, and an inflammatory mass often surrounds the ileocecal region. Acute inflammation is apparent, as are strictures and even fistula formation. The serosal surface is normally covered with multiple tubercles, and mesenteric lymph nodes are frequently enlarged and thickened; on sectioning, caseous necrosis is noted. The mucosa is hyperemic, edematous, and, in some cases, ulcerated. On histologic evaluation, the distinguishing lesion is a granuloma, with caseating granulomas found most commonly in the lymph nodes. Most patients com-

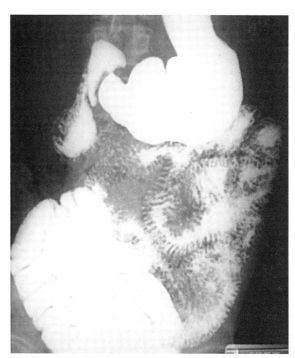

FIGURE 49-27 Barium radiograph of a patient with AIDS shows thickened intestinal folds consistent with enteritis secondary to atypical mycobacterium. (Courtesy Dr. Melvyn H. Schreiber, The University of Texas Medical Branch, Galveston, TX.)

plain of chronic abdominal pain that may be nonspecific, weight loss, fever, and diarrhea.

The diagnosis of mycobacterial infection is made by identification of the organism in tissue by direct visualization with an acid-fast stain, culture of the excised tissue, or PCR assay. Radiographic examinations usually reveal a thickened mucosa with distorted mucosal folds and ulcerations. CT may be useful and shows a thickening of the ileocecal valve and cecum.

The treatment of *M. tuberculosis* is similar in the immunocompromised or nonimmunocompromised host. The organism is usually responsive to multidrug antimicrobial therapy. The therapy for MAC infection is evolving; drugs that have been successfully used in vivo and in vitro include amikacin, ciprofloxacin, cycloserine, and ethionamide. Clarithromycin has also been successfully used in combination with other agents. Surgical intervention may be required for intestinal tuberculosis, particularly *M. tuberculosis*. Obstruction and fistula formation are the leading indications for surgery; however, with current treatment, most fistulas now respond to medical management. Surgery may be necessary for ulcerative complications when free perforation, perforation with abscess, or massive hemorrhage occurs. The treatment is usually resection with anastomosis.

Viruses

CMV is the most common viral cause of diarrhea in immunocompromised patients. Clinical manifestations include intermittent diarrhea accompanied by fever, weight loss, and abdominal pain. The manifestations of enteric CMV infection result from mucosal ischemic ulcerations, which account for the high rate of perforations noted with CMV. As a result of the diffuse ulcerating involvement of the intestine, patients may present with abdominal pain, peritonitis, or hematochezia. Diagnosis of CMV is made by demonstrating viral inclusions. The most characteristic form is an intranuclear inclusion, which is often surrounded by a halo, producing a so-called owl's eye appearance. There may also be cytoplasmic inclusions (Fig. 49-28). Cultures for CMV are usually positive when inclusion bodies are present, but these cultures are less sensitive and specific than histopathologic identification. Once CMV infection is diagnosed, treatment is usually effective with ganciclovir. An alternative to ganciclovir is foscarnet, a

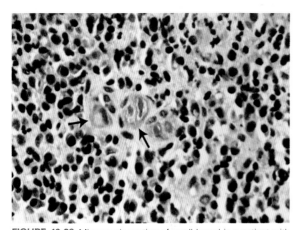

FIGURE 49-28 Microscopic section of small bowel in a patient with AIDS who has cytomegalovirus enteritis. Multiple large cells with intranuclear and intracytoplasmic inclusions typical of cytomegalovirus are demonstrated *(arrows)*. (Courtesy Dr. Mary R. Schwartz, Baylor College of Medicine, Houston, TX.)

pyrophosphate analogue that inhibits viral replication. Infections with other less common viruses, including adenovirus, rotavirus, and novel enteric viruses such as astrovirus and picornavirus, have been reported.

Fungi

Fungal infections of the intestinal tract have been recognized in patients with AIDS. Gastrointestinal histoplasmosis occurs in the setting of systemic infection, often in association with pulmonary and hepatic disease. Diagnosis is made by fungal smear and culture of infected tissue or blood. The infection is most commonly treated by the administration of amphotericin B. Coccidioidomycosis of the intestinal tract is rare and, like histoplasmosis, occurs in the context of systemic infection.

NEOPLASMS

General Considerations

Despite composing 75% of the length and 90% of the surface area of the gastrointestinal tract, the small bowel harbors relatively few primary neoplasms and less than 2% of gastrointestinal malignant neoplasms. Although uncommon, rates for new small intestine cancer cases have been increasing an average of approximately 2% each year during the last 10 years. In 2015, an estimated 9160 adults (4880 men and 4280 women) in the United States will be diagnosed with small bowel cancer, and approximately 1210 individuals (640 men and 570 women) will die of this disease. The 5-year survival for localized small bowel cancer is approximately 83%. Unfortunately, only 31% of patients are diagnosed with local disease; therefore, patients with regional and distant disease have 5-year survival rates of approximately 71% and 40%, respectively. This trend may be a reflection of the spread of AIDS and the increase in neoplasms, such as lymphomas, that occur in the immunocompromised host.

The mean age at presentation is 62 years in the setting of benign tumors and approximately 57 years for malignant lesions. The mean age at onset for both is approximately 59 years. Similar to other cancers, there appears to be a geographic distribution, with the highest cancer rates found among the Maori of New Zealand and ethnic Hawaiians. The incidence of small bowel cancer is particularly low in India, Romania, and other parts of eastern Europe. The incidence of small bowel neoplasia varies considerably, with benign lesions identified more often in autopsy series. In contrast, malignant neoplasms account for 75% of symptomatic lesions that lead to surgery. This reflects the fact that most benign neoplasms are asymptomatic and are most often identified as an incidental finding. Stromal tumors and adenomas are the most frequent of the benign tumors. Benign lesions appear to be more common in the distal small bowel, but these numbers may be somewhat misleading because of the relatively short length of the duodenum. Adenocarcinoma is the most common malignant neoplasm, accounting for 30% to 50% of malignant neoplasms of the small intestine; neuroendocrine tumors (NETs) account for 25% to 30% of small intestine malignant neoplasms. Adenocarcinomas are more numerous in the proximal small bowel, whereas the other malignant lesions are more common in the distal intestine.

Numerous risk factors and associated conditions related to neoplasia of the small bowel have been described. These include patients with familial adenomatous polyposis (FAP), hereditary nonpolyposis colorectal cancer, Peutz-Jeghers syndrome, Crohn's disease, gluten-sensitive enteropathy (i.e., celiac sprue), prior peptic ulcer disease, cystic fibrosis, and biliary diversion (e.g., previous cholecystectomy). Controversial factors that may contribute to small bowel cancers include smoking, heavy alcohol consumption (>80 g/day of ethanol), and consumption of red meat or salt-cured foods.

Although the molecular genetics of small bowel neoplasms have not been entirely characterized, similar to colorectal cancers, mutations of the *KRAS* gene are commonly found. Allelic losses, particularly involving tumor suppressor genes at chromosome locations 5q (the *APC* gene), 17q (the *p53* gene), and 18q (the *DCC* [*deleted in colon cancer*] and *DPC4* [*SMAD4*] genes), have been noted in some small bowel cancers. Recent findings demonstrate that approximately 15% of small intestinal adenocarcinomas have inactivation of DNA mismatch repair genes and display a high level of microsatellite instability (MSI-H). Interestingly, MSI-H is typical of small bowel carcinomas associated with celiac disease and indicates that aberrant CpG island methylation potentially links celiac disease and carcinogenesis. Furthermore, microarray analyses demonstrate a high percentage of small bowel tumors expressing both epidermal growth factor receptor and vascular endothelial growth factor (VEGF).

Clinical Manifestations

Symptoms associated with small bowel neoplasms are often vague and nonspecific and may include dyspepsia, anorexia, malaise, and dull abdominal pain, often intermittent and colicky. These symptoms may be present for months or years before surgery. Most patients with benign neoplasms remain asymptomatic, and the neoplasms are only discovered at autopsy or as incidental findings at laparotomy or upper gastrointestinal radiologic studies. Of the remainder, pain, most often related to obstruction, is the most frequent complaint. Usually, obstruction is the result of intussusception, and benign small tumors are the most common cause of this condition in adults. Hemorrhage is the next most common symptom. Bleeding is usually occult; hematochezia or hematemesis may occur, although life-threatening hemorrhage is uncommon.

Diagnosis

Because of the insidious nature of many of the small bowel neoplasms, a high index of suspicion must be present for these neoplasms to be diagnosed. In most series, a correct preoperative diagnosis is made in only 50% of symptomatic patients. An upper gastrointestinal tract series with small intestinal follow-through yields an accurate diagnosis in 53% to 83% of patients with malignant neoplasms of the small intestine (Fig. 49-29). CT enteroclysis appears to be an even more sensitive technique, with a diagnostic accuracy of approximately 95%, and MRI enteroclysis has a sensitivity and specificity of 98% and 97%, respectively.

Flexible endoscopy may be useful, particularly in diagnosing duodenal lesions, and the colonoscope can be advanced into the terminal ileum for visualization and biopsy of ileal neoplasms. Push enteroscopy has not been used routinely to evaluate lesions in the small bowel because this test may take up to 8 hours to perform and may not visualize the entire small bowel. Double-balloon enteroscopy can be a helpful adjunct; however, it should be reserved for cases in which biopsy or preoperative tattoo is required as it carries a risk of perforation, and other less invasive and highly accurate diagnostic tools are available. The sensitivity and specificity for diagnosis of a small bowel tumor by capsule endoscopy in the setting of obscure bleeding are between 89% and 95% and 75% and 95%, respectively.

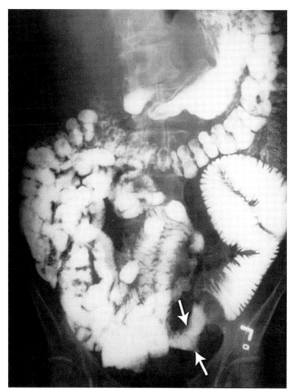

FIGURE 49-29 Barium radiograph demonstrates a typical apple core lesion *(arrows)* caused by adenocarcinoma of the small bowel, producing a partial obstruction with dilated proximal bowel. (Courtesy Dr. Melvyn H. Schreiber, The University of Texas Medical Branch, Galveston, TX.)

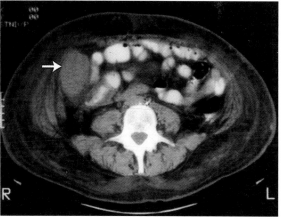

FIGURE 49-30 CT scan of abdomen demonstrates a small bowel neoplasm *(arrow)*. (Courtesy Dr. Melvyn H. Schreiber, The University of Texas Medical Branch, Galveston, TX.)

Plain films may confirm the presence of an obstruction; however, for the most part, they are useless in making a diagnosis of small bowel neoplasms. Angiography is of value in diagnosing and localizing tumors of vascular origin. CT of the abdomen can prove particularly useful in detecting extraluminal tumors, such as malignant gastrointestinal stromal tumors (GISTs), and can provide helpful information about the staging of malignant cancers (Fig. 49-30). Ultrasonography has not proved to be effective in making the preoperative diagnosis of small bowel neoplasm. Despite sophisticated imaging and diagnostic modalities, diagnosis of a small bowel tumor is often achieved only at the time of surgical exploration.

Benign Neoplasms

The most common benign neoplasms include benign stromal tumors, adenomas, and lipomas. Adenomas are the most common benign tumors reported in autopsy series, but stromal tumors are the most common benign small bowel lesions that produce symptoms. In general, when a benign tumor is identified at operation, resection is indicated because symptoms are likely to develop over time. At operation, a thorough search of the remainder of the small bowel is warranted because multiple tumors are not uncommon.

Stromal Tumors

Stromal tumors arise from the interstitial cell of Cajal, an intestinal pacemaker cell of mesodermal descent. Three histologic types of stromal tumors are noted on the basis of their cellular appearance; tumors may be fusiform (77%), epithelioid (8%), or mixed (15%).[29] Stromal tumors are three to four times more frequent than malignant GISTs and are most commonly found in the stomach (60%) and the jejunum and ileum (30%). They are rarely found in the duodenum (5%). More than 95% of stromal tumors express CD117, the c-*kit* proto-oncogene protein that is a transmembrane receptor for the stem cell growth factor, and 70% to 90% express CD34, the human progenitor cell antigen. These tumors infrequently stain positive for actin (20% to 30%), S100 (2% to 4%), and desmin (2% to 4%). The incidence is equal in men and women, and they are most frequently diagnosed in the fifth decade of life. In gross appearance, stromal tumors are firm, gray-white lesions with a whorled appearance noted on cut surface; microscopic examination demonstrates well-differentiated smooth muscle cells. These tumors may grow intramurally and cause obstruction. Alternatively, the tumors demonstrate intramural and extramural growth, sometimes achieving considerable size and eventually outgrowing their blood supply, resulting in bleeding manifestations, the most common indication for surgery in patients with benign stromal tumors. Surgical resection is necessary for appropriate treatment. The number of mitoses can vary substantially, between 0 and 150 mitoses per 50 high-power fields (hpf). Most benign tumors show a low mitotic index (<5 mitoses/50 hpf). The mitotic index is classified as low (<5 mitoses/50 hpf) or high (>5 mitoses/50 hpf); however, even mitotic counts higher than 2 mitoses/50 hpf imply an increased risk for local recurrence.

Adenomas. Adenomas account for approximately 15% of all benign small bowel tumors and are of three primary types: true adenomas, villous adenomas, and Brunner gland adenomas. Twenty percent of adenomas are found in the duodenum, 30% are found in the jejunum, and 50% are found in the ileum. Most of these lesions are asymptomatic; most occur singly and are found incidentally at autopsy. The most common presenting symptoms are bleeding and obstruction. Villous adenomas of the small bowel are rare but do occur, are most commonly found in the duodenum, and may be associated with the familial polyposis syndrome. Both true and villous adenomas are thought to proceed along a similar adenoma-carcinoma sequence as colorectal adenomas and should be considered premalignant. Villous adenomas have a particular propensity for malignant degeneration and may be of relatively large size (>5 cm) in diameter. They are usually noted

secondary to abdominal pain or bleeding; obstruction may also occur. The malignant potential of these lesions is reportedly between 35% and 55%. Treatment is determined by location and adenoma type. The options for treatment are endoscopic and surgical. In the jejunum and ileum, the treatment of choice is segmental resection. Although only 5% of adenomas occur in the duodenum, they cause symptoms more frequently, and decisions about surgical management must be carefully planned because of the potential morbidity (20% to 30%) associated with duodenal resection by pancreaticoduodenectomy or pancreas-preserving duodenectomy. Endoscopic ultrasound has recently emerged as a useful modality in the preintervention evaluation and may help guide management planning. Endoscopic resection of these neoplasms is a safe alternative and may delay a more aggressive and potentially morbid surgical procedure; however, some series showed that the lifelong risk of recurrence is approximately 50% after endoscopic treatment (i.e., snare excision, thermal ablation, argon plasma coagulation, or photodynamic therapy). Endoscopic mucosal resection is gaining acceptance as a useful technique for the treatment of duodenal adenomas and Brunner gland tumors. A single-center study found that endoscopic mucosal resection, even in the setting of large (>2 cm) sessile duodenal adenomas, had a high success rate for complete removal; however, the risk of delayed bleeding is significant. Other studies have shown that endoscopic mucosal resection is associated with an approximate 17% risk of other complications, including perforation, hemorrhage, and pancreatitis. Invasive changes or a recurrence after polypectomy necessitates a more definitive approach (e.g., pancreaticoduodenectomy).

Familial adenomas typically occur in the presence of FAP syndrome and require a different algorithm. Numerous studies have shown that adenomas in the duodenum can be found in 50% to 90% of cases, and increasing age was identified as an independent risk factor for adenoma development. Although these neoplasms grow slowly, FAP patients carry a 5% lifetime risk for development of duodenal adenocarcinoma, which represents the leading cause of cancer-related mortality in these patients; therefore, routine lifelong surveillance is a priority. To direct surveillance and treatment, patients are classified by the Spigelman classification (Table 49-8). Screening endoscopy with a forward- and side-viewing endoscope is performed at regular intervals with biopsy of all suspicious, villous, or large (>3 cm) adenomas in addition to random duodenal biopsy specimens. Frequency of endoscopic screening is 1 to 5 years, depending on the Spigelman classification (Box 49-4).[30] Endoscopic or surgical polypectomy

TABLE 49-8 Spigelman Classification for Duodenal Adenomatosis

PARAMETER	POINTS		
	1	2	3
No. of polyps	1-4	5-20	>20
Polyp size (mm)	1-4	5-10	>10
Histology	Tubular	Tubulovillous	Villous
Degree of dysplasia	Mild	Moderate	Severe

Stage 0, 0 points; stage I, 1-4 points; stage II, 5-6 points; stage III, 7-8 points; stage IV, 9-12 points.
From Johnson MD, Mackey R, Brown N, et al: Outcome based on management for duodenal adenomas: Sporadic versus familial disease. *J Gastrointest Surg* 14:229, 2010.

BOX 49-4   Recommended Surveillance Interval for Upper Gastrointestinal Endoscopic Examination in Relation to Spigelman Classification

Spigelman Classification (Surveillance Interval in Years)

0/I (5)

II (3)

III (1-2)

IV (consider surgery)

Adapted from Vasen HF, Möslein G, Alonso A, et al. Guidelines for the clinical management of familial adenomatous polyposis (FAP). *Gut* 57:704–713, 2008.

---

can be performed for large adenomas. Ablative therapy in the form of argon beam coagulation or photodynamic therapy has been attempted for these patients but with disappointing results. The presence of high-grade dysplasia, carcinoma in situ, or a Spigelman stage IV classification necessitates pancreaticoduodenectomy or pancreas-preserving duodenectomy. Adenomas of the remaining small bowel also occur more frequently in patients with FAP but are not as prevalent as duodenal disease in this population of patients.

Brunner gland adenomas represent benign hyperplastic lesions arising from the Brunner glands of the proximal duodenum. These adenomas may produce symptoms mimicking those of peptic ulcer disease. Diagnosis can usually be accomplished by endoscopy and biopsy, and symptomatic lesions in an accessible region can be resected by simple excision, either endoscopically or surgically. There is no malignant potential for Brunner gland adenomas, and a radical resection should not be used.

Lipomas. Lipomas, which are also included in the category of stromal tumors, are most common in the ileum and are manifested as single intramural lesions located in the submucosa. They usually occur in the sixth and seventh decades of life and are more frequent in men. Less than one third of these tumors are symptomatic, and of these, the most common manifestations are obstruction and bleeding from superficial ulcerations. The treatment of choice for symptomatic lesions is excision. Lipomas do not have malignant potential and therefore, when found incidentally, should be removed only if the resection is simple.

Peutz-Jeghers syndrome. Hamartomas of the small bowel occur as part of the Peutz-Jeghers syndrome, an inherited syndrome of mucocutaneous melanotic pigmentation and gastrointestinal polyps. The pattern of inheritance is autosomal dominant, with a high degree of penetrance. The classic pigmented lesions are small, 1- to 2-mm, brown or black spots located in the circumoral region of the face, buccal mucosa, forearms, palms, soles, digits, and perianal area. The entire jejunum and ileum are the most usual portions of the gastrointestinal tract involved with these hamartomas; however, 50% of patients may also have rectal and colonic lesions, and 25% of patients have gastric lesions. The most common symptom is recurrent colicky abdominal pain, usually as a result of intermittent intussusception. Lower abdominal pain associated with a palpable mass has been reported to occur in one third of patients. Hemorrhage as a result of autoamputation of the polyps occurs less frequently and is most commonly manifested by anemia. Acute life-threatening hemorrhage is uncommon but may occur. Although once considered a purely benign disease, adenomatous changes have been reported in 3% to 6% of hamartomas. Extracolonic cancers are common, occur-

ring in 50% to 90% of patients (small intestine, stomach, pancreas, ovary, lung, uterus, and breast). The small intestine represents the most frequent site for cancer compared with that of the general population. The treatment of complications of Peutz-Jeghers syndrome is directed mainly at the complication of obstruction or persistent bleeding. Resection should be limited to the segment of bowel that is producing complications and usually involves a limited resection. Because of the widespread nature of intestinal involvement, cure is not possible, and extensive resections are not indicated.

Hemangiomas. Hemangiomas are developmental malformations consisting of submucosal proliferation of blood vessels. They can occur at any level of the gastrointestinal tract; the jejunum is the most commonly affected small bowel segment. Hemangiomas account for 3% to 4% of all benign tumors of the small bowel and are multiple in 60% of patients. Hemangiomas of the small bowel may occur as part of an inherited disorder known as *Osler-Weber-Rendu disease.* In addition to the small bowel, hemangiomas may also be present in the lung, liver, and mucous membranes. Patients with Turner syndrome are likely also to have cavernous hemangiomas of the intestine. The most common symptom of small bowel hemangiomas is intestinal bleeding. Angiography and technetium Tc 99m red blood cell scanning are the most useful diagnostic studies. If a hemangioma is localized preoperatively, resection of the involved segment of intestine is warranted. If it is not identified, intraoperative transillumination and palpation can be helpful.

Malignant Neoplasms

Population-based analyses have shown that the incidence of malignant neoplasms of the small intestine has increased steadily during the past 3 decades. This increase has mirrored the increase in diagnosis of small bowel NETs, which have increased more than fourfold (from 2.1 to 9.3 new cases per million population) during the past 3 decades, whereas changes in the frequency of adenocarcinomas, stromal tumors, and lymphomas were less pronounced. Based on both the Surveillance, Epidemiology and End Results program and National Cancer Data Base, the distribution of typical malignant neoplasms of the small bowel from 1973 to 2004 is as follows: NETs, 37%; adenocarcinomas, 37%; lymphomas, 17%; and stromal tumors, 8%. Although the frequency of surgical intervention increased significantly for NETs (79% to 87%) and adjuvant chemotherapy increased for adenocarcinoma from 8% to 24%, the 5-year survival after resection remained unchanged over time for all histologic subtypes, even after adjustment for changes in patient demographics, tumor characteristics, and treatment approaches.[31] These findings highlight the need for more novel and effective treatment strategies.

In contrast to benign lesions, malignant neoplasms almost always produce symptoms, the most common of which are pain and weight loss. Obstruction develops in 15% to 35% of patients and, unlike the intussusception produced by benign lesions, is usually the result of tumor infiltration and adhesions. Diarrhea with tenesmus and passage of large amounts of mucus may occur. Gastrointestinal bleeding, manifested by anemia and guaiac-positive stools or occasionally by melena or hematochezia, occurs to varying degrees with malignant lesions and is more common with GISTs. A palpable mass may be felt in 10% to 20% of patients, and perforations develop in approximately 10%, usually secondary to lymphomas and sarcomas. Although presentation may be similar, each tumor type has a distinct biology that dictates management and prognosis.

Neuroendocrine Tumors

Intestinal NETs arise from enterochromaffin cells (Kulchitsky cells), which are considered neural crest cells and are situated at the base of the crypts of Lieberkühn. These cells are also known as argentaffin cells because of their staining by silver compounds. These tumors were first described by Lubarsch in 1888; in 1907, Oberndorfer coined the term *Karzinoide* to indicate the carcinoma-like appearance and the presumed lack of malignant potential. These tumors have been reported in a number of organs, including most commonly the lungs, bronchi, and gastrointestinal tract. Most patients with small bowel NETs are in their seventh decade of life. The median age for gastroenteric NET is 63 years. As noted in Chapter 38, a World Health Organization report updated the classification of NETs based on differentiation and grade of the tumor and not based on tumor site.[32] NETs are categorized as low grade (grade 1, G1), intermediate grade (grade 2, G2), or high grade (grade 3, G3) on the basis of appearance, mitotic rates, behavior (invasion of other organs, angioinvasion), and Ki-67 proliferative index. The distinction between well and poorly differentiated tumors is by far the most important; G1 and G2 tumors are considered well differentiated, and G3 tumors are poorly differentiated. The use of the word "carcinoid" to describe primary intestinal NETs is considered obsolete, although many clinicians continue to use this term. Certainly, it remains standard nomenclature to continue to refer to the syndrome as carcinoid syndrome.

NETs may be classified by the embryologic site of origin and secretory product. These tumors may be derived from the foregut (respiratory tract, thymus), midgut (jejunum, ileum and right colon, stomach, proximal duodenum), and hindgut (distal colon, rectum). Foregut NETs characteristically produce low levels of serotonin (5-hydroxytryptamine) but may secrete 5-hydroxytryptophan (5-HTP) or adrenocorticotropic hormone. Midgut NETs are characterized by having high serotonin production. Hindgut NETs rarely produce serotonin but may produce other hormones, such as somatostatin and peptide YY. The gastrointestinal tract is the most common site for NETs. After the appendix, the small intestine is the second most frequently affected site in the gastrointestinal tract. In the small intestine, NETs almost always occur within the last 2 feet of the ileum. NETs have a variable malignant potential and are composed of multipotential cells with the ability to secrete numerous humoral agents, the most prominent of which are serotonin and substance P (Table 49-9). In addition to these substances, NETs have been found to secrete corticotropin, histamine, dopamine, neurotensin, prostaglandins, kinins, gastrin, somatostatin, pancreatic polypeptide, calcitonin, and neuron-specific enolase.

The primary importance of NETs is the malignant potential of the tumors themselves. The carcinoid syndrome, which is characterized by episodic attacks of cutaneous flushing, bronchospasm, diarrhea, and vasomotor collapse, is present mostly in those patients with hepatic metastases. Primary sites that secrete directly into the venous system, bypassing the portal system (e.g., ovary, lung), give rise to the carcinoid syndrome without metastasis.

Pathology. Seventy percent to 80% of NETs are asymptomatic and found incidentally at the time of surgery. In the gastrointestinal tract, more than 90% of NETs are found in five typical sites: appendix (38%), small intestine (29%), colon (13%), stomach (12%), and rectum (8%). The changes in these distributions are associated with the increased incidence of NETs along with the changes of the World Health Organization classification of these tumors in 2010.[33] The malignant potential (ability to metastasize) is related to location, size, depth of invasion, and growth pattern. Only approximately 3% of appendiceal NETs metastasize, but about 35% of ileal NETs are associated with metastasis. Most (approximately 75%) gastrointestinal NETs are smaller than 1 cm in diameter, and about 2% of these are associated with metastasis. In contrast, NETs 1 to 2 cm in diameter and larger than 2 cm are associated with metastasis in 50% and 80% to 90% of cases, respectively.

In gross appearance, these tumors are small, firm submucosal nodules that are usually yellow on cut surface (Fig. 49-31A). They may be as subtle as a small whitish plaque seen on the antimesenteric border of the small intestine (Fig. 49-31B). Typically, they are associated with a larger mesenteric mass caused by nodal disease and desmoplastic invasion of the mesentery, which is often mistaken for the primary tumor. They tend to grow very slowly, but after invasion of the serosa, the intense desmoplastic reaction produces mesenteric fibrosis, intestinal kinking, and intermittent obstruction. Small bowel NETs are multicentric in 20% to 30% of patients. This tendency to multicentricity exceeds that of any other malignant neoplasm of the gastrointestinal tract. Another unusual observation is the frequent coexistence of a second primary malignant neoplasm of a different histologic type. This is usually a synchronous adenocarcinoma (most commonly in the large intestine) that can occur in 10% to 20% of patients with NETs. Multiple endocrine neoplasia type 1 is associated with NETs in approximately 10% of cases.

Clinical manifestations. In the absence of carcinoid syndrome, symptoms of patients with NETs of the small bowel are similar to those of patients with small bowel tumors of other histologic types. The most common symptom is abdominal pain, which is variably associated with partial or complete small intestinal obstruction. Obstructive symptoms can be caused by intussusception but usually occur secondary to a local desmoplastic reaction, apparently produced by humoral agents elaborated by the tumor. Diarrhea and weight loss may also occur. The diarrhea is a result of a partial bowel obstruction rather than the secretory diarrhea noted in patients with the malignant carcinoid syndrome. As mesenteric and nodal extension progresses, local venous engorgement and ultimately ischemia of the affected segment of intestine contribute to most symptoms and complications related to the tumor.

Malignant carcinoid syndrome. The malignant carcinoid syndrome is a relatively rare disease, occurring in less than 10%

TABLE 49-9 Secretory Products of Neuroendocrine Tumors*

AMINES	TACHYKININS	PEPTIDES	OTHER
5-HT	Kallikrein	Pancreatic polypeptide (40%)	Prostaglandins
5-HIAA (88%)	Substance P (32%)	Chromogranins (100%)	
5-HTP	Neuropeptide K (67%)	Neurotensin (19%)	
Histamine		HCG-α (28%)	
Dopamine		HCG-β	
		Motilin (14%)	

HCG, Human chorionic gonadotropin; *5-HIAA,* 5-hydroxyindoleacetic acid; *5-HT,* 5-hydroxytryptamine; *5-HTP,* 5-hydroxytryptophan.
*Values in parentheses represent percentage frequency.

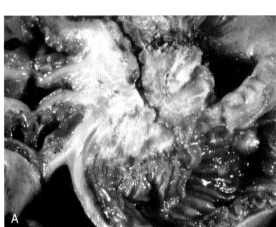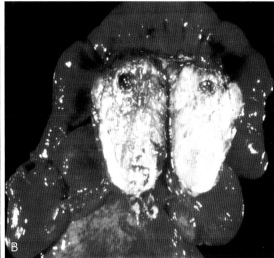

FIGURE 49-31 Gross pathologic characteristics of neuroendocrine tumor (NET). **A,** NET of the distal ileum demonstrates the intense desmoplastic reaction and fibrosis of the bowel wall. **B,** Mesenteric metastases from a NET of the small bowel. (Adapted from Evers BM, Townsend CM Jr, Thompson JC: Small intestine. In Schwartz SI, editor: *Principles of surgery,* ed 7, New York, 1999, McGraw-Hill, p 1245.)

of patients with NETs. The syndrome is usually associated with NETs of the gastrointestinal tract, particularly from the small bowel, but NETs in other locations, such as the bronchus, pancreas, ovary, and testes, have also been described in association with the syndrome. Because of the first-pass metabolism of the vasoactive peptides responsible for carcinoid syndrome, hepatic metastasis or extra-abdominal disease is necessary to elicit the syndrome. The classic description of the carcinoid syndrome typically includes vasomotor, cardiac, and gastrointestinal manifestations. A number of humoral factors are produced by NETs, but those considered to contribute to the carcinoid syndrome include serotonin, 5-HTP (a precursor of serotonin synthesis), histamine, dopamine, kallikrein, substance P, prostaglandin, and neuropeptide K. Most patients who exhibit malignant carcinoid syndrome have massive hepatic replacement by metastatic disease. However, tumors that bypass the liver, specifically ovarian and retroperitoneal NETs, may produce the syndrome in the absence of liver metastasis.

Common symptoms and signs include cutaneous flushing (80%); diarrhea (76%); hepatomegaly (71%); cardiac lesions, most commonly right-sided heart valvular disease (41% to 70%); and asthma (25%). Cutaneous flushing in the carcinoid syndrome may be of four varieties:

1. diffuse erythematous, which is short-lived and normally affects the face, neck, and upper chest;
2. violaceous, which is similar to a diffuse erythematous flush except that the attacks may be longer and patients may develop a permanent cyanotic flush, with watery eyes and injected conjunctivae;
3. prolonged flushes, which may last up to 2 or 3 days and involve the entire body and may be associated with profuse lacrimation, hypotension, and facial edema; and
4. bright-red patchy flushing, typically seen with gastric NETs.

The diarrhea associated with carcinoid syndrome is episodic (usually occurring after meals), watery, and often explosive. Increased circulating serotonin levels are thought to be the cause of the diarrhea because the serotonin antagonist methysergide effectively controls the symptom. Cardiac lesions usually involve

the right side of the heart, but left-sided lesions are present in 15% of patients and can lead to congestive heart disease and symptomatic left-sided heart failure. The three most common cardiac lesions are pulmonary stenosis (90%), tricuspid insufficiency (47%), and tricuspid stenosis (42%). Asthmatic attacks are usually observed during the flushing symptom, and serotonin and bradykinin have been implicated in this symptom. Malabsorption and pellagra (dementia, dermatitis, and diarrhea) are occasionally present and are thought to be caused by excessive diversion of dietary tryptophan.

Diagnosis. The elevation of various humoral factors forms the basis for diagnostic tests in patients with NETs and the carcinoid syndrome. NETs produce serotonin, which is then metabolized in the liver and the lung to the pharmacologically inactive 5-hydroxyindoleacetic acid (5-HIAA). Elevated urinary levels of 5-HIAA measured during 24 hours with high-performance liquid chromatography are highly specific although not sensitive. For the last decade, chromogranin A (CgA) has been a well-established marker for carcinoid disease; it is elevated in more than 80% of patients with NETs. CgA alone may be used for the diagnosis of NETs, given its specificity of 95%, but some investigators suggest that other tests should be used in conjunction with CgA for diagnostic purposes because its sensitivity is only 55%. A combination of serum CgA measurement with 24-hour urine 5-HIAA is an acceptable diagnostic combination with increased sensitivity. Studies have suggested that serum CgA and N-terminal pro-brain natriuretic peptide (NT-proBNP) may also be used in combination for both diagnosis and surveillance because patients with increased NT-proBNP and CgA levels showed worse overall survival than patients with elevated CgA alone. In terms of surveillance after resection or as a prognostic marker to monitor response to therapy, CgA levels have proven efficacy over urine 5-HIAA levels.

Plasma serotonin, substance P, neurotensin, neurokinin A, and neuropeptide K levels can be measured, but these peptides may not be elevated in all patients. Provocative tests using pentagastrin, calcium, or epinephrine may be used to reproduce the symptoms of NETs. More recently, pentagastrin has been used to differentiate between NETs and chronic atrophic gastritis but is generally not used for the diagnosis of NETs, given the diagnostic reliability of 5-HIAA, CgA, and NT-proBNP.

NETs of the small intestine are rarely diagnosed preoperatively. Barium radiographic studies of the small bowel may exhibit multiple filling defects as a result of kinking and fibrosis of the bowel (Fig. 49-32). A combination of anatomic and functional imaging techniques is routinely performed to optimize sensitivity and specificity.

Traditionally, CT scanning was the imaging modality of choice for identifying the site of disease and the presence of lymphatic or hematogenous metastases. CT scan findings depend on the size, the degree of mesenteric invasion and desmoplastic reaction, and the presence of regional lymph node invasion. If these entities are not well defined, CT has limited diagnostic capabilities in this disease. However, when CT scanning reveals a solid mass with spiculated borders and radiating surrounding strands that is associated with linear strands within the mesenteric fat and kinking of the bowel, a diagnosis of gastrointestinal NET can be made fairly confidently. CT angiography may be useful in cases associ-

ated with a large mesenteric process to identify encasement and pseudoaneurysm formation, typical of a malignant process in the mesentery. In general, MRI is not used in the diagnosis of gastrointestinal NETs but can be helpful in diagnosing metastatic disease, especially in the liver. Liver metastases are well demonstrated with MRI and usually have low signal intensity on T1-weighted images and high signal intensity on T2-weighted images. After the administration of a gadolinium-based contrast agent, liver metastases enhance peripherally in the hepatic arterial phase and appear as hypointense defects in the portal venous phase. Diffusion-weighted MRI and dynamic contrast-enhanced techniques represent promising advances in radiologic imaging, although these imaging techniques have not yet been validated for monitoring therapy of NETs.

Octreotide is a synthetic analogue of somatostatin, and indium In 111–labeled pentetreotide specifically binds to somatostatin receptor subtypes 2 and 5. Functional nuclear imaging studies capitalize on the concept of somatostatin receptor positivity as these imaging techniques are used to image many NETs, including those with somatostatin-binding sites. Scintigraphic localization has a higher sensitivity than CT for delineating and localizing NETs and is particularly useful in the identification of extra-abdominal metastatic disease or in cases in which the primary tumor cannot be identified by CT scan. An area of great interest is functional imaging by ^{18}F-fluorodeoxyglucose positron emission tomography ([18]FDG PET) scanning, although this imaging modality alone has limited capabilities because of the fact that [18]FDG is taken up only in high-grade NETs (e.g., high Ki-67 expression), whereas most NETs have low Ki-67 expression and are not apparent with this imaging modality. However, the addition of newer isotopes, such as ^{11}C-5-HTP and ^{18}F-L-dihydroxyphenylalanine (^{18}F-DOPA), has dramatically improved the sensitivity of PET for the diagnosis and surveillance of neuroendocrine malignant neoplasms.

Somatostatin receptor imaging with gadolinium Ga 68–DOTATATE PET/CT is increasingly used for managing patients with NETs. DOTATATE is an amide of 1,4,7,10-tetraazacyclododecane-1,4,7,10-tetraacetic acid (DOTA), which acts as a chelator for a radionuclide, and tyrosine-3-octreotate (TATE), a derivative of octreotide. The latter binds to somatostatin receptors and thus directs the radioactivity into the tumor. ^{68}Ga-DOTATATE PET/CT is a clinically useful imaging technique to localize primary tumors in patients with neuroendocrine metastases of unknown origin as well as to define the existence and extent of metastatic disease. Combining the two modalities may be even more helpful in diagnosing and managing NETs. In a study designed to investigate the relationship between PET/CT results and histopathologic findings in 27 patients with NETs, the sensitivity of ^{68}Ga-DOTATATE and [18]FDG PET/CT was 95% and 37%, respectively. The sensitivity in detecting liver, lymph node, and bone metastases and the primary lesion was 95%, 95%, 90%, and 93% for ^{68}Ga-DOTATATE and 40%, 28%, 28%, and 75% for [18]FDG, respectively. The peptide receptor radionuclide therapy agents yttrium-90 (^{90}Y) and lutetium-177 (^{177}Lu) are both diagnostic and therapeutic. The reason for developing compounds with high affinity for somatostatin receptors 2, 3, and 5 is to improve diagnostic sensitivity. These agents can also be used to adjust dosing of peptide receptor radionuclide therapy. A single-center study determined that the additional information provided by ^{68}Ga-DOTATATE PET/CT in the preoperative workup significantly influences surgical management in approximately 20% of patients treated for NET.[35] These findings are particularly

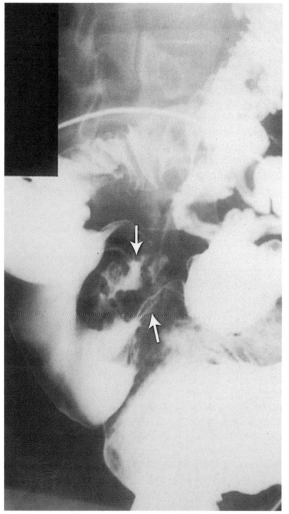

FIGURE 49-32 Barium radiograph of a NET of the terminal ileum demonstrates fibrosis with multiple filling defects and high-grade partial obstruction *(arrows)*. (Courtesy Dr. Melvyn H. Schreiber, The University of Texas Medical Branch, Galveston, TX.)

important because resection is the only curative treatment in patients with NETs of the small intestine, and accurate preoperative imaging is critical for surgical planning because findings of small and distant metastases may profoundly influence surgical management.

Treatment

Surgical therapy. The treatment of patients with small bowel NETs is based on tumor size and site and presence or absence of metastatic disease. For primary tumors smaller than 1 cm in diameter without evidence of regional lymph node metastasis, a segmental intestinal resection is adequate. For patients with lesions larger than 1 cm, with multiple tumors, or with regional lymph node metastasis, regardless of the size of the primary tumor, wide excision of bowel and mesentery is required. Lesions of the terminal ileum are best treated by right hemicolectomy. Small duodenal tumors can be excised locally; however, more extensive lesions may require pancreaticoduodenectomy.[36] A single-center, prospective, longitudinal study showed that a laparoscopic approach is safe and feasible in selected patients. Laparoscopy was associated with similar R0 (i.e., without residual microscopic tumor) resection and morbidity rates but a shorter hospital stay compared with laparotomy. Median follow-up was 39 months, and progression-free survival at 1, 3, and 5 years was as follows: 95%, 83%, and 75%, respectively, for R0 patients without liver metastasis; 92%, 83%, and 57%, respectively, for R0 patients with resected liver metastasis; and 82%, 58%, and 30%, respectively, for patients with R2 resection (i.e., evidence of residual tumor on visual examination). Overall survival and progression-free survival did not show any difference in comparing the laparoscopic and open groups.[37]

In addition to treatment of the primary tumor, it is important that the abdomen be thoroughly explored for multicentric lesions. In cases in which the mesenteric disease appears to involve a large portion of the mesentery, dissection of the tumor off the mesenteric vessels, with preservation of the blood supply to unaffected bowel, is appropriate, albeit technically demanding. Not only does removal of the mesenteric disease provide a significant survival advantage, but also mesenteric debulking ensures the most durable palliation for the patient.

Caution should be exerted in the anesthetic management of patients with NETs because anesthesia may precipitate a carcinoid crisis characterized by hypotension, bronchospasm, flushing, and tachycardia predisposing to arrhythmias. The treatment of carcinoid crisis is IV octreotide given as a bolus of 50 to 100 μg, which may be continued as an infusion at 50 μg/hr.

In patients with NETs and widespread metastatic disease, surgery is still indicated. In contrast to metastases from other tumors, there is a definite role for surgical debulking, which often provides beneficial symptomatic relief. In patients with limited hepatic involvement, metastasectomy has been shown to provide the most durable survival benefit compared with other treatment modalities.[36] Unfortunately, most patients are not candidates for liver resection because of extensive disease; recurrence after metastasectomy occurs in up to 75% of patients. In these cases, transarterial chemoembolization or radioembolization has been shown to provide liver-directed control of disease. Furthermore, resection of the primary tumor, with or without mesenteric resection, has been shown to improve survival and to slow progression of hepatic metastases in patients with unresectable disease. Although there have been some small series of hepatic transplantation for extensive liver metastases from NETs, unacceptably high recurrence rates limit this approach.

Medical therapy. Medical therapy for patients with malignant carcinoid syndrome is primarily directed toward the relief of symptoms caused by the excess production of humoral factors. Table 49-10 summarizes medical therapies for NET treatment. Somatostatin analogues are the standard of care for controlling symptoms of patients with functional gastrointestinal NETs, and they control symptoms in more than 70% of patients with carcinoid syndrome.[38] Somatostatin analogues such as octreotide (Sandostatin) and lanreotide and their depot formulations (Sandostatin LAR and Somatuline, respectively) relieve symptoms of the carcinoid syndrome (e.g., diarrhea, flushing) in most patients and delay progression. The results of a randomized phase 3 trial (PROMID) of 85 patients demonstrated that the median time to progression in patients with midgut NETs treated with octreotide LAR was more than twice as long compared with that of patients treated with placebo.[39] The landmark Controlled study of Lanreotide Antiproliferative Response In NeuroEndocrine Tumors (CLARINET) trial found that lanreotide, a somatostatin analogue, was associated with significantly prolonged progression-free survival among patients with metastatic enteropancreatic NETs of grade 1 or 2 (Ki-67 proliferative marker <10%).[40] Patients were randomly assigned to receive an extended-release aqueous-gel formulation of lanreotide or placebo once every 28 days for 96 weeks. The estimated rates of progression-free survival at 24 months were 65% in the lanreotide group and 33% in the placebo group.

Second-generation somatostatin analogues have been developed to address the limitations of the current regimens. Studies are ongoing using pan-receptor agonists (e.g., pasireotide) as well as chimeric dimers, which possess features of somatostatin and

TABLE 49-10 Medical Therapies for Neuroendocrine Tumor Treatment

Approved Therapeutics	
Somatostatin analogues	Octreotide (Sandostatin; Sandostatin LAR)
	Lanreotide (Somatuline depot)
Cytotoxic therapies	Streptozocin (pancreatic NET only)
mTOR inhibitor	Everolimus (Afinitor; pancreatic NET only)
Tyrosine kinase inhibitors	Sunitinib (Sutent; pancreatic NET only)
Used Off-Label	
Pan-receptor somatostatin agonists	Pasireotide (Signifor; approved indication for Cushing disease only)
Interferons	Interferon alfa
	Interferon alfa-2b
Cytotoxic therapies	5-Fluorouracil (5-FU)
	Cyclophosphamide (Cytoxan)
	Temozolomide (Temodar)
	Capecitabine (Xeloda)
Investigational	
Peptide receptor radionuclide therapy	^{90}Y conjugated with somatostatin analogues
	^{177}Lu isotopes conjugated with somatostatin analogues
Serotonin synthesis inhibitors	Telotristat etiprate (LX1032/LX1606)
VEGF inhibitors	Bevacizumab (Avastin)
Dopamine agonists	Dopastatins

Compiled with assistance of Lowell B. Anthony, MD, University of Kentucky.

dopamine agonists (dopastatins). These promising biologic therapies are thought to enhance symptom control by binding multiple receptors (somatostatin and dopamine receptors). Somatostatin receptor antagonists are also currently being developed for clinical use. Peptide receptor radionuclide therapy, ^{90}Y and ^{177}Lu isotopes conjugated with somatostatin analogues, appears to be efficacious in advanced NETs. These isotopes can be used for PET imaging as well as to determine the distribution of the agent and the dosimetry of the tumor. A study evaluating more than 1000 patients with metastatic NETs determined that tumor uptake is predictive for both survival after ^{90}Y-DOTA-TOC treatment and occurrence of renal toxicity as the kidney is the dose-limiting organ.[34] There is also an interest in targeting incretin receptor family members, particularly glucagon-like peptide 1 (GLP-1), which are overexpressed in NETs. The GLP-1 inhibitor Lys[40](Ahx-DTPA/DOTA[111]In)NH$_2$-exendin-4 is highly sensitive and can be detected up to 14 days after IV injection using a probe to facilitate surgical excision.

Interferon alfa was introduced as monotherapy for NET treatment in 1983. Interferon binds to two different receptors to elicit effects that include cell cycle inhibition at G$_1$/S, antiangiogenesis effects through downregulation of VEGF, and upregulation of somatostatin receptors, to name a few. Although some series showed tumor regression in 10% of patients and tumor stabilization in 65%, side effects, which included chronic fatigue, pancytopenia, thyroiditis, and systemic lupus erythematosus, were not tolerable. Pegylated interferon alfa-2b showed comparable survival rates to interferon alfa, but with more tolerable side effects. Some series have shown that given the upregulation of somatostatin receptors by interferon alfa, its combination with somatostatin analogues may be efficacious. Prospective randomized controlled trials demonstrated variable findings, but one retrospective study determined that combined treatment resulted in a longer progression-free survival (58 versus 55 months). Interferon is less expensive than somatostatin analogues, but the increased incidence of side effects and variable outcomes preclude the widespread use of this drug.[34]

In the past, the only available treatment for metastatic NETs was cytotoxic chemotherapy, most frequently combinations that included streptozotocin, 5-fluorouracil (5-FU), and cyclophosphamide. These treatments resulted in a median survival of around 2 years. Currently, the role of chemotherapy is confined predominantly to patients with metastatic disease who are symptomatic, are unresponsive to other therapies, or have high tumor proliferation rates. The duration of response, however, is short-lived. Temozolomide as monotherapy has acceptable toxicity and antitumoral effects in a small series of patients with advanced NETs, and in combination with capecitabine, it was shown to prolong survival in patients with well-differentiated, metastatic NETs who experienced progression with previous therapies. The use of cisplatin and etoposide has shown some promise, but only in patients with poorly differentiated NETs. Everolimus and sunitinib are approved for pancreatic NETs; lanreotide is approved for gastroenteropancreatic NETs without carcinoid syndrome.

Serotonin receptor antagonists have been used with limited success. Methysergide is no longer used because of the increased incidence of retroperitoneal fibrosis. Ketanserin and cyproheptadine have been shown to provide some control of symptoms, and other antagonists, such as ondansetron, may be even more effective. Serotonin synthesis inhibitors, such as telotristat etiprate (LX1032/LX1606), are effective in lowering serotonin levels and are in clinical development.

The treatment of metastatic NETs requires a multidisciplinary approach; combined modalities may be the best option, including surgical debulking, hepatic artery embolization, chemoembolization, or radioembolization and medical therapy. In addition, newer and more targeted therapies are being developed that may be useful in the future. Targeted therapy has progressed down four separate pathways. Given the hypervascular nature of NETs, antiangiogenesis therapy (e.g., bevacizumab) is being investigated in combination with cytotoxic and somatostatin therapy. Sunitinib, which is a multitargeted or selective tyrosine kinase inhibitor that is active against alpha-type and beta-type platelet-derived growth factor receptor (PDGFR) and vascular endothelial growth factor receptor (VEGFR), has been noted to decrease angiogenesis and to prolong progression-free survival in pancreatic NETs in multiple clinical trials, most notably those with mutations associated with exons 9 and 11.[34]

Tyrosine kinase inhibitors have been evaluated as systemic therapy and as a liver-directed chemoembolization strategy for NETs as well. The PI3K-AKT-mTOR pathway has also recently emerged as a potential target for systemic therapy. Agents such as everolimus, a mammalian target of rapamycin (mTOR) inhibitor, although initially developed as immunosuppressant therapy, have redefined themselves as potent antitumor agents and remain under active investigation for carcinoid disease. Everolimus is approved in the United States and Europe for the treatment of patients with advanced pancreatic NETs. The activity of everolimus remains under investigation in patients with intestinal NETs. In a randomized study of patients with advanced NETs associated with carcinoid syndrome, the addition of everolimus to octreotide therapy was associated with improved yet statistically insignificant progression-free survival. Further investigation is needed to determine whether primary tumor site or other clinical and molecular factors can affect response to mTOR inhibition. Although everolimus can slow tumor progression, significant tumor reduction is rarely obtained. Targeting of multiple signaling pathways is a treatment strategy that may provide better tumor control and overcome resistance mechanisms involved with targeting of a single pathway. Results of ongoing and future studies will provide important information about the added benefit of combining mTOR inhibitors with other targeted agents, such as VEGF pathway inhibitors, and cytotoxic chemotherapy in the treatment of advanced NETs.[41]

Prognosis. NETs have the best prognosis of all small bowel tumors, whether the disease is localized or metastatic. Resection of a NET localized to its primary site approaches a 100% survival rate. Five-year survival rates are approximately 65% in patients with regional disease and 25% to 35% in those with distant metastasis. Metastatic disease at the time of diagnosis is approximately 20% to 50%, and tumors recur in 40% to 60% of patients. When widespread metastatic disease precludes cure, extensive resection for palliation is indicated. In fact, long-term palliation often can be obtained because these tumors are relatively slow growing. A number of factors have been evaluated in an attempt to identify patients with NETs who have a poor prognosis. An elevated level of CgA, which is an independent predictor of an adverse prognosis, is probably the most useful factor identified.

Adenocarcinomas

Adenocarcinomas constitute approximately 50% of the malignant tumors of the small bowel. The peak incidence is in the seventh decade of life, and most series show a slight male predominance.

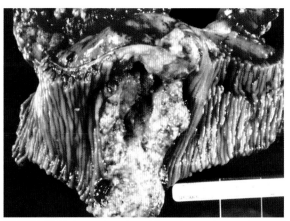

FIGURE 49-33 Large circumferential mucinous adenocarcinoma of the jejunum. (Courtesy Dr. Mary R. Schwartz, Baylor College of Medicine, Houston, TX.)

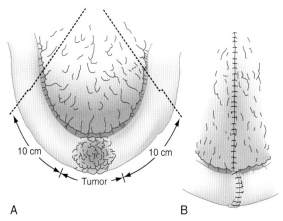

FIGURE 49-34 Surgical management of carcinoma of the small bowel. **A,** Malignant tumors should be resected with a wide margin of normal bowel and a wedge of mesentery to remove the immediate draining lymph nodes. **B,** End-to-end anastomosis of the small bowel and repair of the mesentery. (Adapted from Thompson JC: *Atlas of surgery of the stomach, duodenum, and small bowel,* St. Louis, 1992, Mosby–Year Book, p 299.)

Most of these tumors are located in the duodenum and proximal jejunum (Fig. 49-33). Those arising in association with Crohn's disease tend to occur at a somewhat younger age, and more than 70% arise in the ileum. Tumors of the duodenum tend to be manifested somewhat earlier than those in the most distal intestine because of the earlier presentation of symptoms, which are usually jaundice and chronic bleeding. Adenocarcinomas of the jejunum and ileum usually produce symptoms that may be more nonspecific and include vague abdominal pain and weight loss. Intestinal obstruction and chronic bleeding can also occur. Perforation is uncommon. As with adenocarcinomas in other organs, survival of patients with small bowel adenocarcinomas is related to the stage of disease at the time of diagnosis. Unfortunately, diagnosis is often delayed, and the disease is advanced at the time of surgery secondary to various factors (e.g., vagueness of symptoms, absence of physical findings, lack of clinical suspicion because of the rarity of these lesions).

Treatment of small bowel adenocarcinoma is determined by location and stage. Complete resection of the primary tumor with locoregional lymph node resection is mandatory. In an effort to downsize the tumor, neoadjuvant chemotherapy is appropriate to consider if there is tumor invasion into adjacent structures. Patients are then reevaluated for surgery after 2 to 3 months of treatment. Duodenal adenocarcinomas are treated with pancreaticoduodenectomy if the tumor is in the second portion of the duodenum or an infiltrating tumor in the proximal or distal duodenum. In addition, resection of the periduodenal, peripancreatic, and hepatic lymph nodes as well as resection of the involved vascular structures that originate from the celiac trunk and superior mesenteric arteries should be performed. Duodenal resection can be performed for a noninfiltrating tumor if it is located in the first, third, or fourth portion of the duodenum, but this is not recommended in the setting of residual microscopic tumor (R1 status) or grossly visible tumor after resection (R2 status) as these findings are associated with poor prognosis. An R0 resection with regional lymphadenectomy and jejunojejunal or ileoileal bypass should be performed in the setting of jejunal and ileal adenocarcinoma. If the terminal ileum is involved, an ileocecectomy with right colectomy should be performed with ligation of the ileocolic artery and subsequent regional lymphadenectomy (Fig. 49-34).

There is currently no standard adjuvant protocol for small bowel adenocarcinoma. Despite the previous lack of supporting evidence of traditional chemotherapy regimens, most guidelines suggest that patients with poorly differentiated cancers or those who had incomplete lymph node resections (<10 nodes identified) should at least be considered for adjuvant chemotherapy. Adjuvant regimens are often dictated by location, although studies have suggested that fluoropyrimidine and oxaliplatin may increase overall survival in patients with advanced disease. A prospective international phase 3 trial comparing observation versus adjuvant chemotherapy in patients with an R0 resection is currently accruing subjects. This trial proposes that in an adequately powered trial, adjuvant chemotherapy will result in an improvement in disease-free survival and overall survival compared with observation alone after potentially curative surgery for patients with stage I, II, and III small bowel adenocarcinoma. Studies have determined that FOLFOX (oxaliplatin, 5-FU, and leucovorin) and FOLFIRI (irinotecan, 5-FU, and leucovorin) significantly improve the performance status and progression-free survival in the treatment of metastatic small bowel adenocarcinoma. For metastatic small bowel adenocarcinoma, FOLFOX is considered first-line therapy, and FOLFIRI is an acceptable second-line strategy.

The prognosis of small bowel adenocarcinoma is poor, probably because of the delayed presentation and presence of advanced disease at diagnosis. Five-year survival rates are typically in the 14% to 33% range, although duodenal adenocarcinoma has a 5-year survival rate of 50%, probably because of the earlier symptom presentation and diagnosis. Lymph node invasion is the main prognostic factor for local small bowel adenocarcinoma; moreover, the number of lymph nodes assessed and the number of positive lymph nodes are of prognostic value. In stage III patients, more than three positive lymph nodes was associated with a worse 5-year disease-free survival rate than one or two positive lymph nodes (37% versus 57%, respectively). Multivariate analysis identified advanced age, advanced stage, ileal location, recovery of fewer than 10 lymph nodes, and number of positive nodes as significant predictors of poor overall survival. Thus, a curative resection at an early stage (stages I and II) should systematically include a regional lymphadenectomy.[42]

Lymphoma

Malignant lymphomas involve the small bowel primarily or as a manifestation of systemic disease. Approximately one third of gastrointestinal lymphomas occur in the small bowel, and these account for 5% of all lymphomas. Lymphomas constitute up to 25% of small bowel malignant tumors in the adult; in children younger than 10 years, they are the most common intestinal neoplasm. Lymphomas are most commonly found in the ileum, where there is the greatest concentration of gut-associated lymphoid tissue. Increased risk for development of primary small bowel lymphomas has been reported in patients with celiac disease and immunodeficiency states (e.g., AIDS). In gross appearance, small intestine lymphomas are usually large, with most larger than 5 cm; they may extend beneath the mucosa (Fig. 49-35). On microscopic examination, there is often diffuse infiltration of the intestinal wall. Symptoms of small bowel lymphoma include pain, weight loss, nausea, vomiting, and change in bowel habits. Perforation may occur in up to 25% of patients (Fig. 49-36). Fever is uncommon and suggests systemic involvement.

The treatment of small bowel lymphoma remains controversial. Traditionally, a combination of surgery, chemotherapy, and radiation therapy was used for all small bowel tumors. However, in the absence of symptoms, small bowel lymphomas are often chemoresponsive and do not require surgery. This can typically be predicted by cell type because B cell lymphomas are more chemosensitive than T cell lymphomas and have high remission rates with or without surgery. T cell lymphomas are traditionally more resistant to therapy and will progress to symptoms of obstruction or perforation if not resected. Regardless of cell type, resection is indicated at any onset of symptoms because progression to life-threatening hemorrhage or perforation portends a dismal prognosis. Five-year survival of 50% to 60% can be expected and is dictated by response to systemic therapy rather than by the success of surgical resection.

Gastrointestinal Stromal Tumors

Malignant GISTs arise from mesenchymal tissue and constitute about 20% of malignant neoplasms of the small bowel (Fig. 49-37). These tumors are more common in the jejunum and ileum, typically are diagnosed in the fifth and sixth decades of life, and occur with a slight male preponderance. Malignant GISTs are larger than 5 cm at the time of diagnosis in 80% of patients.

GISTs mostly arise from the muscularis propria and generally grow extramurally. Most common indications for surgery include bleeding and obstruction, although free perforation may occur as a result of hemorrhagic necrosis in large tumor masses. Typically, GISTs tend to invade locally and to spread by direct extension into adjacent tissues and hematogenously to the liver, lungs, and bone; lymphatic metastases are unusual. The most useful indicators of survival and the risk for metastasis include the size of the tumor at presentation, mitotic index, and evidence of tumor invasion into the lamina propria.

Treatment of GISTs continues to evolve and represents one of the first breakthroughs in signal transduction manipulation. Surgical management includes complete resection for localized GISTs, with extreme care to avoid rupture of the tumor capsule, which results in relapse in 100% of these patients. If capsule rupture occurs, these patients should receive adjuvant therapy regardless of the extent of the tumor before surgery. It is advisable to perform an en bloc resection, to include adjacent organs, for prevention of tumor capsule rupture. A laparoscopic approach in patients with large tumors is strongly discouraged. Radiologic criteria for unresectability include infiltration of the celiac trunk, superior mesenteric artery, or portal vein. Lymphadenectomy is

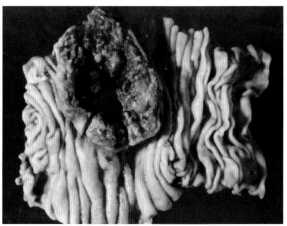

FIGURE 49-36 Small bowel lymphoma is manifested as perforation and peritonitis. (Courtesy Dr. Mary R. Schwartz, Baylor College of Medicine, Houston, TX.)

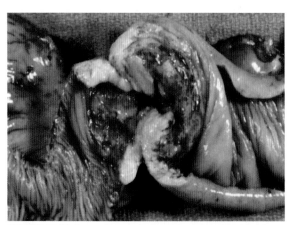

FIGURE 49-35 Gross photograph of primary lymphoma of the ileum shows replacement of all layers of the bowel wall with tumor. (Courtesy Dr. Mary R. Schwartz, Baylor College of Medicine, Houston, TX.)

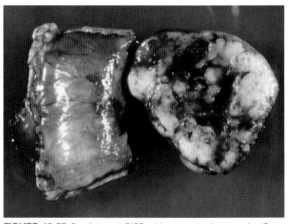

FIGURE 49-37 Small bowel GIST with hemorrhagic necrosis. (Courtesy Dr. Mary R. Schwartz, Baylor College of Medicine, Houston, TX.)

unnecessary, given the low frequency of lymph node metastasis.[29] Small GISTs (<2 cm) found incidentally in surgical specimens do not require further treatment. Before the development of tyrosine kinase inhibitors, adjuvant strategies for GISTs were lacking, and recurrence rates after resection were as high as 70%. However, the development of imatinib mesylate (Gleevec, formerly known as STI571) has significantly altered previous treatment strategies. Imatinib mesylate is a tyrosine kinase inhibitor that blocks the unregulated mutant c-*kit* tyrosine kinase and inhibits the BCR-ABL and PDGF tyrosine kinases. Multiple randomized trials have confirmed its efficacy as a first-line agent in the treatment of GIST (Fig. 49-38). Current guidelines suggest that patients with high-risk disease should receive 3 years of adjuvant

treatment with imatinib, but it is not recommended for low-risk patients after an R0 resection.

Relapse-risk assessment for primary GIST is critical as it provides prognostic information as well as estimates the potential benefits of imatinib. The current American Joint Committee on Cancer staging can be found in Table 49-11. This classification does not acknowledge recent evidence indicating that the type and location of the mutation have an effect on the risk of recurrence. For example, deletions affecting exon 11, codon 557/558 of the c-*kit* gene, and D842V PDGFRα mutations have a higher risk of recurrence within the first 3 to 4 years after surgery.[29] In fact, adjuvant imatinib therapy is not recommended in patients with D842V PDGFRα mutations, given its known resistance to this agent.

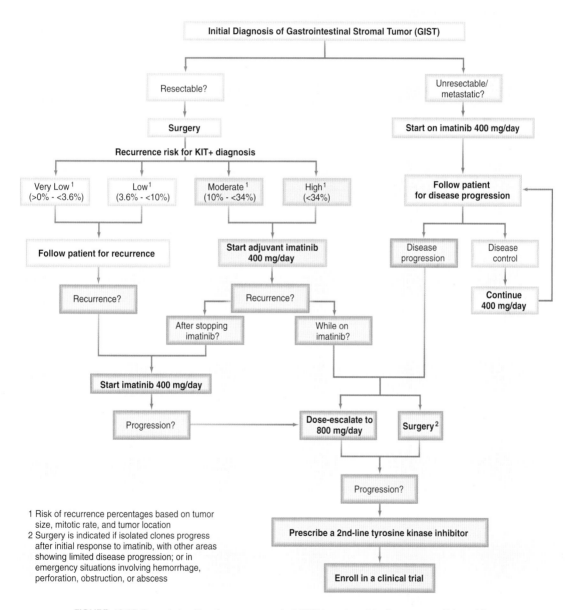

FIGURE 49-38 Current algorithm for management of GIST based on risk of recurrence. (Adapted from Pisters PW, Patel SR. Gastrointestinal stromal tumors: current management. J Surg Oncol. 2010 Jan 8. Gleevec® prescribing information. http://www.pharma.us.novartis.com/product/pi/pdf/gleevec_tabs.pdf. Accessed August 15, 2010.)

TABLE 49-11 Small Intestinal Gastrointestinal Tumor Classification

GROUP	PRIMARY TUMOR SIZE*	REGIONAL LYMPH NODE METASTASIS†	DISTANT METASTASIS‡	MITOTIC RATE
Stage I	T1 or T2	N0	M0	Low
Stage II	T3	N0	M0	Low
Stage IIIA	T1	N0	M0	High
	T4	N0	M0	Low
Stage IIIB	T2	N0	M0	High
	T3	N0	M0	High
	T4	N0	M0	High
Stage IV	Any T	N1	M0	Any rate
	Any T	Any N	M1	Any rate

*T1 Tumor ≤2 cm
T2 Tumor >2 cm but not >5 cm
T3 Tumor >5 cm but not >10 cm
T4 Tumor >10 cm in greatest dimension
†N0 No regional lymph node metastasis
N1 Regional lymph node metastasis
‡M0 No distant metastasis
M1 Distant metastasis
Adapted from Edge SB, Byrd DR, Compton CC, et al, editors: *AJCC cancer staging manual*, ed 7, New York, 2010, Springer, pp 181–189.

Imatinib is also a first-line treatment for unresectable and metastatic GISTs with characteristic tumor biology (Fig. 49-38). Genotyping is standard of care for patients with advanced or metastatic GIST. Standard-dose therapy (400 mg daily) is recommended as no survival advantage is offered by increasing the dose unless the patient has an exon 9 mutation. A European trial determined that patients with exon 9 mutations exhibited a dose-dependent decrease in risk of progression. Therefore, in this select group of patients, imatinib 400 mg twice per day should be given.

New molecular targeted therapies may provide better treatments for patients with genetic mutations and GISTs. In phase 3 clinical trials evaluating imatinib dosing in patients with metastatic GIST, there was no objective response in patients who carry the D842V PDGFRα mutation. A recent phase 2 trial evaluated dasatinib, an oral tyrosine kinase inhibitor of c-*kit*, PDGFR, ABL (Abelson murine leukemia viral oncogene homologue), and the proto-oncogene *Src* with a distinct binding affinity for c-*kit* and PDGFR, and showed that it has significant activity (as judged by CT response rates) in imatinib- and sunitinib-refractory GISTs; however, dasatinib did not meet the predefined 6-month progression-free survival rate of 30% in the population of patients. In vitro studies suggest that dasatinib may provide the best response in patients with a D842V PDGFRα mutation and could prove to be useful in this particular subset of patients.

Regorafenib is a second-generation tyrosine kinase inhibitor that targets c-*kit*, *RET*, *BRAF*, VEGFR, PDGFR, and fibroblast growth factor receptor. It is currently Food and Drug Administration approved and may be an effective treatment for advanced GISTs after failure of either imatinib or sunitinib. Nilotinib is a second-generation tyrosine kinase inhibitor active in chronic myeloid leukemia and has an inhibitory effect on c-*kit* and PDGF. Phase 3 trials have shown minimal differences between this drug and imatinib and sunitinib. Sorafenib is a VEGF, c-*kit*, PDGFR, and *BRAF* inhibitor and has been effective in imatinib- and sunitinib-resistant tumors. The combination of imatinib and doxorubicin has shown some benefit in patients with wild-type GISTs.

Metastatic Neoplasms

Metastatic tumors involving the small bowel are much more common than primary neoplasms. The most common metastases to the small intestine are those arising from other intra-abdominal organs, including the uterine cervix, ovaries, kidneys, stomach, colon, and pancreas. Small intestinal involvement is by direct extension or implantation of tumor cells. Metastases from extra-abdominal tumors are rare but may be found in patients with adenocarcinoma of the breast and carcinoma of the lung. Cutaneous melanoma is the most common extra-abdominal source to involve the small intestine, with involvement of the small intestine noted in more than 50% of patients dying of malignant melanoma (Fig. 49-39). Common symptoms include anorexia, weight loss, anemia, bleeding, and partial bowel obstruction. Treatment is palliative resection to relieve symptoms or, occasionally, bypass if the metastatic tumor is extensive and not amenable to resection. Interventional, nonoperative strategies for palliation of malignant bowel obstruction include endoscopic and radiologic placement of self-expandable metal stents, which are potential options to improve quality of life in patients with very poor performance status who may not tolerate a surgical procedure. Gastrostomy and jejunostomy tubes also may be placed to provide palliative decompression when other palliative methods are not possible.

DIVERTICULAR DISEASE

Diverticular disease of the small intestine is relatively common. It may be manifested as true or false diverticula. A true diverticulum contains all layers of the intestinal wall and is usually congenital. False diverticula consist of mucosa and submucosa protruding through a defect in the muscle coat and are usually acquired defects. Small bowel diverticula may occur in any portion of the small intestine. Duodenal diverticula are the most common acquired diverticula of the small bowel, and Meckel's diverticulum is the most common true congenital diverticulum of the small bowel.

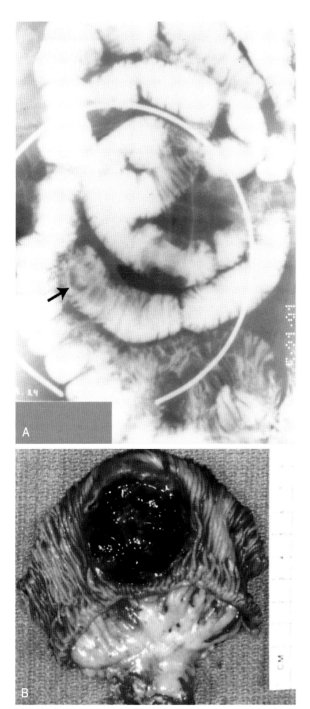

FIGURE 49-39 A, Barium radiograph shows target lesions consistent with metastatic melanoma of small bowel *(arrow).* **B,** Gross specimen demonstrating metastatic melanoma to the small bowel. (**A,** Courtesy Dr. Melvyn H. Schreiber, The University of Texas Medical Branch, Galveston, TX. **B,** Courtesy Dr. Mary R. Schwartz, Baylor College of Medicine, Houston, TX.)

Duodenal Diverticula
Incidence and Cause

First described by Chomel, a French pathologist, in 1710, diverticula of the duodenum are relatively common, representing the second most common site for diverticulum formation after the colon. The incidence of duodenal diverticula varies, depending on the age of the patient and method of diagnosis. Upper gastrointestinal radiographic studies identify duodenal diverticula in 1% to 5% of all studies, whereas endoscopic retrograde cholangiopancreatography identifies 9% to 23% of cases. Previous autopsy series report the incidence as being approximately 15% to 20%. Duodenal diverticula occur twice as often in women as in men and are rare in patients younger than 40 years. They have been classified as congenital or acquired, true or false, and intraluminal or extraluminal. Extraluminal duodenal diverticula are considerably more common than intraluminal diverticula, are acquired, and consist of mucosal or submucosal outpouchings herniated through a muscle defect in the bowel wall. Intraluminal duodenal diverticula (also known as windsock diverticula) are congenital and occur as a single saccular structure that is connected to the entire circumference or part of the wall of the duodenum to create a duodenal web. Incomplete recanalization of the duodenum during fetal development leads to intraluminal diverticula, which are exceedingly rare. In general, extraluminal diverticula usually occur within the second portion of the duodenum (62%) and less commonly in the third (30%) and fourth (8%) portions. They rarely occur in the first part of the duodenum (<1%). When they occur in the second portion, most (88%) are noted on the medial wall around the ampulla (i.e., periampullary), 8% are seen posteriorly, and 4% occur on the lateral wall.

Clinical Manifestations

The important thing to remember is that the overwhelming majority of duodenal diverticula are asymptomatic and are usually noted incidentally by an upper gastrointestinal series for an unrelated problem (Fig. 49-40). Upper gastrointestinal endoscopy identifies approximately 75% of duodenal diverticula, and the use of a side-viewing scope further increases the success rate. The diagnosis may be suggested by plain abdominal films showing an atypical gas bubble; CT can identify large diverticula by the presence of a mass-like structure interposed between the duodenum and pancreatic head containing air, air-fluid levels, fluid contrast material, or debris. Magnetic resonance cholangiopancreatography is particularly helpful to demonstrate the relationship of the diverticulum to the biliary and pancreatic ducts and associated pathologic changes in the biliary system and pancreas. Hemorrhage in diverticula is best diagnosed by a combination of angiography and scanning with ^{99m}Tc-labeled red blood cells; however, surgery should not be delayed to obtain imaging in the event of hemorrhage in a hemodynamically unstable patient. Less than 5% of duodenal diverticula will require surgery because of a complication of the diverticulum itself. Major complications of duodenal diverticula include obstruction of the biliary or pancreatic ducts that may contribute to cholangitis and pancreatitis, respectively, and hemorrhage, perforation, and, rarely, blind loop syndrome. Iatrogenic injuries, most commonly acquired during endoscopic instrumentation of an asymptomatic diverticulum, can lead to perforation or hemorrhage.

Only those diverticula associated with the ampulla of Vater are significantly related to complications of cholangitis and pancreatitis. In these patients, the ampulla usually enters the duodenum at the superior margin of the diverticulum rather than through the diverticulum itself. The mechanism proposed for the increased incidence of complications of the biliary tract is the location of the perivaterian diverticulum, which may produce mechanical distortion of the common bile duct as it enters the duodenum, resulting in partial obstruction and stasis. Hemorrhage can be

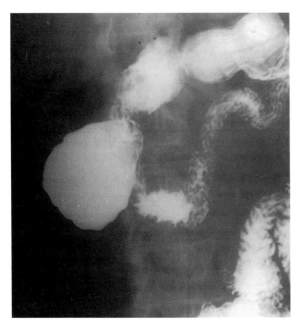

FIGURE 49-40 Large diverticulum arises from the second portion of the duodenum. (Courtesy Dr. Melvyn H. Schreiber, The University of Texas Medical Branch, Galveston, TX.)

caused by inflammation, leading to erosion of a branch of the superior mesenteric artery. Perforation of duodenal diverticula has been described but is rare. Finally, stasis of intestinal contents within a distended diverticulum can result in bacterial overgrowth, malabsorption, steatorrhea, and megaloblastic anemia (i.e., blind loop syndrome). Symptoms related to duodenal diverticula in the absence of any other demonstrable disease usually are nonspecific epigastric complaints that can be treated conservatively and may actually prove to be the result of another problem not related to the diverticulum itself.

Treatment

Most duodenal diverticula are asymptomatic and benign; when they are found incidentally, they should be left alone. For symptomatic duodenal diverticula, treatment consists of removal of the diverticulum, which can be accomplished endoscopically or surgically. Appropriate classification of these diverticula guides management. All intraluminal duodenal diverticula require treatment as recurrence of symptoms is certain. Curative treatment consists of removal of the intraluminal diverticulum by laparotomy and duodenotomy or by endoscopic resection. Large (>3 cm) or obstructing intraluminal duodenal diverticulum does not preclude endoscopic resection, but an endoscopic approach in the setting of massive hemorrhage or perforation with intra-abdominal contamination secondary to intestinal contents is discouraged. These entities are relatively rare and often require a multidisciplinary approach to determine the best treatment strategy.

Extraluminal duodenal diverticula should be resected in the setting of symptomatic disease or need for urgent surgery, such as free perforation or hemorrhage. Several operative procedures have been described for the treatment of the symptomatic extraluminal duodenal diverticula. The most common and effective treatment is diverticulectomy, which is most easily accomplished by performing a wide Kocher maneuver that exposes the duodenum. The diverticulum is then excised, and the duodenum is closed in

a transverse or longitudinal fashion, whichever produces the least amount of luminal obstruction. Because of the proximity of the ampulla, careful identification of the ampulla is essential to prevent injury to the common bile duct and pancreatic duct. For diverticula embedded deep within the head of the pancreas, a duodenotomy is performed, with invagination of the diverticulum into the lumen, which is then excised, and the wall is closed (Fig. 49-41*A-C*). Alternative methods that have been described for duodenal diverticula associated with the ampulla of Vater include an extended sphincteroplasty through the common wall of the ampulla in the diverticulum (Fig. 49-41*D-F*). Laparoscopic duodenal diverticulectomy has been determined to be safe and effective in patients with symptomatic and noncomplicated (i.e., not perforated or bleeding) diverticula. An endoscopic stapler is most commonly used to traverse and to resect the diverticulum at its base, and an omental patch reinforcement can be placed over the staple line.

The treatment of a perforated diverticulum may require procedures similar to those described for patients with massive trauma-related defects of the duodenal wall. The perforated diverticulum should be excised and the duodenum closed with a serosal patch from a jejunal loop. If the surrounding inflammation is severe, it may be necessary to divert the enteric flow away from the site of the perforation with a gastrojejunostomy or duodenojejunostomy. Interruption of duodenal continuity proximal to the perforated diverticulum may be accomplished by pyloric closure with suture or a row of staples. If the diverticulum is posterior and perforates into the substance of the pancreas, operative repair may be difficult and dangerous. Wide drainage with duodenal diversion may be all that is feasible in such cases. Great care should be taken if the perforation is adjacent to the papilla of Vater.

Jejunal and Ileal Diverticula
Incidence and Cause

Diverticula of the small bowel are much less common than duodenal diverticula, with an incidence ranging from 0.1% to 1.4% in autopsy series and 0.1% to 1.5% in upper gastrointestinal studies. Jejunal diverticula are more common and are larger than those in the ileum. These are false diverticula, occurring mainly in an older age group (after the sixth decade of life). These diverticula are multiple, usually protrude from the mesenteric border of the bowel, and may be overlooked at surgery because they are embedded within the small bowel mesentery (Fig. 49-42). The cause of jejunoileal diverticulosis is thought to be a motor dysfunction of the smooth muscle or the myenteric plexus, resulting in disordered contractions of the small bowel, generating increased intraluminal pressure and herniation of the mucosa and submucosa through the weakest portion of the bowel (i.e., the mesenteric side).

Clinical Manifestations

Jejunoileal diverticula are usually found incidentally at laparotomy or during an upper gastrointestinal study (Fig. 49-43); the great majority remain asymptomatic. Acute complications, such as intestinal obstruction, hemorrhage, and perforation, can occur but are rare. Chronic symptoms include vague chronic abdominal pain, malabsorption, functional pseudo-obstruction, and chronic low-grade gastrointestinal hemorrhage. Acute complications are diverticulitis with or without abscess or perforation, gastrointestinal hemorrhage, and intestinal obstruction. Stasis of intestinal flow with bacterial overgrowth (blind loop syndrome), caused by the jejunal dyskinesia, may lead to deconjugation of bile salts and

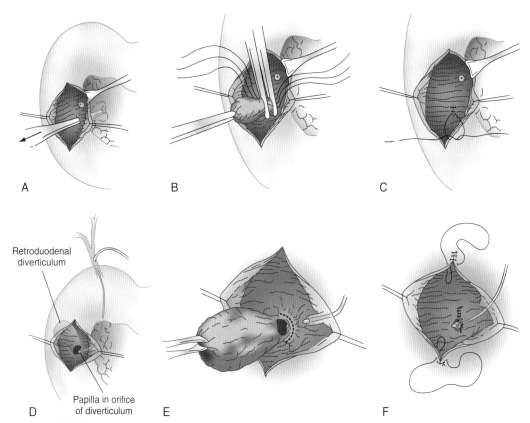

FIGURE 49-41 A-C, Treatment of a diverticulum protruding into the head of the pancreas. The duodenum is opened vertically. A clamp is used to invert the diverticulum into the lumen, where it is excised, and the posterior wall defect is closed. **D-F,** Management of the unusual duodenal diverticula that arise in the periampullary location. A tube stent should be placed into the common bile duct and passed distally into the duodenum to facilitate identification and later dissection of the sphincter of Oddi. The diverticulum is inverted into the lumen of the duodenum. The round opening in the wall of the base of the diverticulum is the site at which the ampullary structures were freed by a circumferential incision. **E,** Line of division of the base of the diverticulum *(heavy broken line),* which is accomplished by free-hand dissection. After the diverticulum has been removed, the stent and enveloping papilla are protruded into the defect left by the division of the base of the diverticulum. The mucosa and muscle wall of the papilla are then sewn circumferentially to the wall of the duodenum. (Adapted from Thompson JC: *Atlas of surgery of the stomach, duodenum, and small bowel,* St. Louis, 1992, Mosby–Year Book, pp 209–213.)

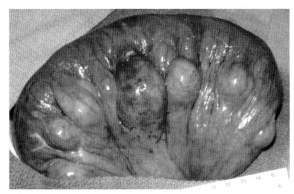

FIGURE 49-42 Multiple large jejunal diverticula located in the mesentery in an older patient presenting with obstruction secondary to an enterolith. (Adapted from Evers BM, Townsend CM Jr, Thompson JC: Small intestine. In Schwartz SI, editor: *Principles of surgery,* ed 7, New York, 1999, McGraw-Hill, p 1248.)

uptake of vitamin B_{12} by the bacterial flora, resulting in steatorrhea and megaloblastic anemia, with or without neuropathy.

Treatment

For incidentally noted, asymptomatic jejunoileal diverticula, no treatment is required. Treatment of complications of obstruction, bleeding, and perforation is usually by intestinal resection and end-to-end anastomosis. Patients presenting with malabsorption secondary to the blind loop syndrome and bacterial overgrowth in the diverticulum can usually be given antibiotics. Obstruction may be caused by enteroliths that form in a jejunal diverticulum and are subsequently dislodged and obstruct the distal intestine. This condition may be treated by enterotomy and removal of the enterolith, or sometimes the enterolith can be milked distally into the cecum. When the enterolith causes obstruction at the level of the diverticulum, bowel resection is necessary. When a perforation of a jejunoileal diverticulum is encountered, resection with reanastomosis is required because lesser procedures, such as simple closure, excision, and invagination, are associated with greater

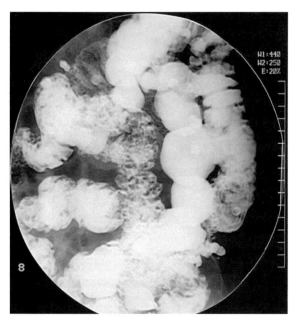

FIGURE 49-43 Multiple jejunal diverticula demonstrated by a barium contrast upper gastrointestinal study. (Courtesy Dr. Melvyn H. Schreiber, The University of Texas Medical Branch, Galveston, TX.)

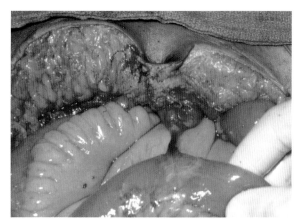

FIGURE 49-44 Omphalomesenteric remnant persisting as a fibrous cord from the ileum to the umbilicus.

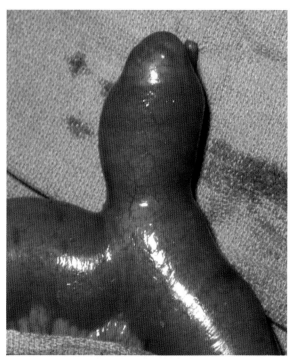

FIGURE 49-45 Common presentation of a Meckel's diverticulum projecting from the antimesenteric border of the ileum.

mortality and morbidity rates. Laparoscopic bowel resection with reanastomosis is a safe option in minimally contaminated surgical fields. In extreme cases, such as diffuse peritonitis, enterostomies may be required if judgment dictates that reanastomosis may be risky.

Meckel's Diverticulum

Incidence and Cause

Meckel's diverticulum is the most commonly encountered congenital anomaly of the small intestine, occurring in about 2% of the population. It was reported initially in 1598 by Hildanus and then described in detail by Johann Meckel in 1809. Meckel's diverticulum is located on the antimesenteric border of the ileum 45 to 60 cm proximal to the ileocecal valve and results from incomplete closure of the omphalomesenteric, or vitelline, duct. An equal incidence is found in men and women. Meckel's diverticulum may exist in different forms, ranging from a small bump that may be easily missed to a long projection that communicates with the umbilicus by a persistent fibrous cord (Fig. 49-44) or, much less commonly, a fistula. The usual manifestation is a relatively wide-mouthed diverticulum measuring about 5 cm in length, with a diameter of up to 2 cm (Fig. 49-45). Cells lining the vitelline duct are pluripotent; therefore, it is not uncommon to find heterotopic tissue within the Meckel's diverticulum, the most common of which is gastric mucosa (present in 50% of all Meckel's diverticula). Pancreatic mucosa is encountered in about 5% of diverticula; less commonly, these diverticula may harbor colonic mucosa.

Clinical Manifestations

Most Meckel's diverticula are benign and are incidentally discovered during autopsy, laparotomy, or barium studies (Fig. 49-46). The most common clinical presentation of Meckel's diverticulum is gastrointestinal bleeding, which occurs in 25% to 50% of patients who present with complications; hemorrhage is the most common symptomatic presentation in children 2 years of age or younger. This complication may be manifested as acute massive hemorrhage, anemia secondary to chronic bleeding, or a self-limited recurrent episodic event. The usual source of the bleeding is a chronic acid-induced ulcer in the ileum adjacent to a Meckel's diverticulum that contains gastric mucosa.

Another common presenting symptom of Meckel's diverticulum is intestinal obstruction, which may occur as a result of a volvulus of the small bowel around a diverticulum associated with a fibrotic band attached to the abdominal wall, intussusception, or, rarely, incarceration of the diverticulum in an inguinal hernia (Littre hernia). Volvulus is usually an acute event and, if allowed to progress, may result in strangulation of the involved bowel. In intussusception, a broad-based diverticulum invaginates and then is carried forward by peristalsis. This may be ileoileal or ileocolic

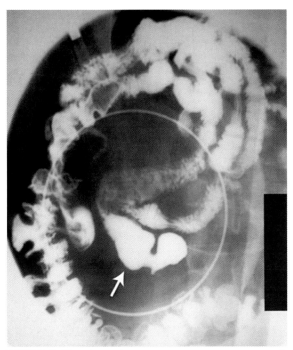

FIGURE 49-46 Barium radiograph demonstrates an asymptomatic Meckel's diverticulum *(arrow)*. (Courtesy Dr. Melvyn H. Schreiber, The University of Texas Medical Branch, Galveston, TX.)

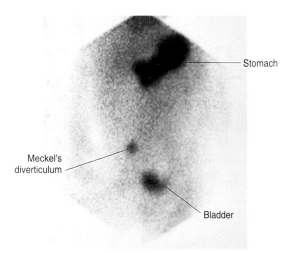

FIGURE 49-47 A ^{99m}Tc-pertechnetate scintigram from a child demonstrates a Meckel's diverticulum clearly differentiated from the stomach and bladder. (Courtesy Dr. Melvyn H. Schreiber, The University of Texas Medical Branch, Galveston, TX.)

and be manifested as acute obstruction associated with an urge to defecate, early vomiting, and occasionally the passage of the classic currant jelly stool. A palpable mass may be present. Although reduction of an intussusception secondary to Meckel's diverticulum can sometimes be performed by barium enema, the patient should still undergo resection of the diverticulum to negate subsequent recurrence of the condition.

Diverticulitis accounts for 10% to 20% of symptomatic presentations. This complication is more common in adult patients. Meckel's diverticulitis, which is clinically indistinguishable from appendicitis, should be considered in the differential diagnosis of a patient with right lower quadrant pain. Progression of the diverticulitis may lead to perforation and peritonitis. When the appendix is found to be normal during exploration for suspected appendicitis, the distal ileum should be inspected for the presence of an inflamed Meckel's diverticulum.

Neoplasms can also occur in a Meckel's diverticulum, with NET as the most common malignant neoplasm (77%). Other histologic types include adenocarcinoma (11%), which generally originates from the gastric mucosa, and GIST (10%) and lymphoma (1%).[43]

Diagnostic Studies

The diagnosis of Meckel's diverticulum may be difficult. Plain abdominal radiography, CT, and ultrasonography are rarely helpful. In children, the single most accurate diagnostic test for Meckel's diverticula is scintigraphy with sodium ^{99m}Tc-pertechnetate. The ^{99m}Tc-pertechnetate is preferentially taken up by the mucus-secreting cells of gastric mucosa and ectopic gastric tissue in the diverticulum (Fig. 49-47). The diagnostic sensitivity of this scan has been reported as high as 85%, with a specificity of 95% and an accuracy of 90% in the pediatric age group.

In adults, however, the sensitivity of ^{99m}Tc-pertechnetate scan falls to 63% because of the presence of less gastric mucosa in the diverticulum compared with that noted in the pediatric age group. The sensitivity and specificity can be improved by the use of pharmacologic agents. Cimetidine may be used to increase the sensitivity of scintigraphy by decreasing the peptic secretion, but not the radionuclide uptake, and retarding the release of pertechnetate from the diverticular lumen, thus resulting in higher radionuclide concentrations in the wall of the diverticulum. In adult patients, when nuclear medicine findings are normal, barium studies should be performed. False-negative results can occur because of inadequate gastric mucosal cells, inflammatory changes causing edema or necrosis, presence of outlet obstruction of the diverticulum, or low hemoglobin levels. In false-negative cases, mesenteric arteriography or double-balloon endoscopy can be helpful. In patients with acute hemorrhage, angiography is sometimes useful. Nevertheless, surgical intervention should not be delayed to obtain imaging for a patient with signs and symptoms of hemorrhage and hemodynamic instability.

Treatment

The treatment of a symptomatic Meckel's diverticulum should be prompt surgical intervention with resection of the diverticulum or resection of the segment of ileum bearing the diverticulum. Segmental intestinal resection is required for treatment of patients with bleeding because the bleeding site is usually in the ileum adjacent to the diverticulum. Resection of the diverticulum for nonbleeding Meckel's diverticula can be performed with a hand-sewn technique or stapling across the base of the diverticulum in a diagonal or transverse line to minimize the risk for subsequent stenosis. Reports have demonstrated the feasibility, effectiveness, and safety of laparoscopic diverticulectomy.

Although the treatment of complicated Meckel's diverticulum is straightforward, the optimal treatment of Meckel's diverticulum noted as an incidental finding is still debated. It is generally recommended that asymptomatic diverticula found in children during laparotomy be resected. The treatment of Meckel's diverticula encountered in the adult patient, however, remains controversial. A landmark paper by Soltero and Bill[44] formed the basis of the surgical management of asymptomatic Meckel's diverticula in adults for many years. In this study, the likelihood of a Meckel's diverticulum becoming symptomatic in the adult patient was estimated to be 2% or less, and given that the morbidity rates from incidental removal were 12% at the time, the recommendation was to not remove the incidental Meckel's diverticulum. This study was criticized, however, because it was not a population-based analysis. Further evidence supporting a conservative approach to the management of the incidental Meckel's diverticulum is provided in an analysis of 244 articles by Zani and colleagues[45] evaluating the incidence and outcomes of Meckel's diverticulum. In this study, a clear incidence of increased morbidity associated with incidental resection was noted; in fact, it was calculated that resection of an incidental Meckel's diverticulum would be required in more than 700 patients to avoid one death related to the diverticulum. However, other studies have challenged this more conservative approach to the adult patient with an incidental Meckel's diverticulum. For example, an epidemiologic population-based study by Cullen and associates[46] in 1994 initially challenged the practice of ignoring an incidentally found Meckel's diverticulum. A 6.4% rate of development of complications from the Meckel's diverticulum was calculated to occur over a lifetime. This incidence of complications did not appear to peak during childhood, as originally thought. Therefore, the recommendation from this study was that an incidentally found Meckel's diverticulum be removed at any age up to 80 years as long as no additional conditions (e.g., peritonitis) make removal hazardous. The rates of short- and long-term postoperative complications from prophylactic removal were low (~2%), and death was related to the primary operation or the general health of the patient and not to the diverticulectomy. Furthermore, in a recent population-based study evaluating patients from 1973 to 2006, the mean annual incidence of malignancy in a Meckel's diverticulum was noted to be approximately 1.44 per 10 million; therefore, the adjusted risk of cancer in the Meckel's diverticulum was at least 70 times higher than in any other ileal site, thus identifying a Meckel's diverticulum as a "hot spot" for malignant disease in the ileum.[43] Given the increased risk of malignant transformation over a lifetime, the authors advocated for removal of an incidental Meckel's diverticulum.

MISCELLANEOUS PROBLEMS

Small Bowel Ulcerations

Ulcerations of the small bowel are relatively uncommon and may be attributed to Crohn's disease, typhoid fever, tuberculosis, lymphoma, and ulcers associated with gastrinoma (Table 49-12). Drug-induced ulcerations can occur and were, in the past, attributed to enteric-coated potassium chloride tablets and corticosteroids. In addition, ulcerations of the small intestine in which no causative agent can be identified have been described. It has been suggested that small bowel complications from NSAIDs may be more common than originally considered. NSAID-induced ulcers occur more commonly in the ileum, with single or multiple ulcerations noted. Complications necessitating operative intervention include bleeding, perforation, and obstruction. In addition to ulcerations, NSAIDs are known to induce an enteropathy characterized by increased intestinal permeability leading to protein loss and hypoalbuminemia, malabsorption, and anemia. Treatment of complications from small bowel ulcerations is segmental resection and intestinal reanastomosis.

TABLE 49-12 Causes of Small Intestine Ulceration

CAUSE	EXAMPLES
Infections	Tuberculosis, syphilis, cytomegalovirus, typhoid, parasites, *Strongyloides* hyperinfection, *Campylobacter, Yersinia*
Inflammatory	Crohn's disease, systemic lupus erythematosus, celiac disease, ulcerative enteritis
Ischemia	Mesenteric insufficiency
Idiopathic	Primary ulcer, Behçet syndrome
Drug induced	Potassium, indomethacin, phenylbutazone, salicylates, antimetabolites
Radiation	Therapeutic, accidental
Vascular	Vasculitis, giant cell arteritis, amyloidosis (ischemic lesion), angiocentric lymphoma
Metabolic	Uremia
Hyperacidity	Zollinger-Ellison syndrome, Meckel's diverticulum, stomal ulceration
Neoplastic	Lymphoma, adenocarcinoma, melanoma
Toxic	Acute jejunitis (β-toxin–producing *Clostridium perfringens*), arsenic
Mucosal lesions	Lymphocytic enterocolitis

Adapted from Rai R, Bayless TM: Isolated and diffuse ulcers of the small intestine. In Feldman M, Scharschmidt BF, Sleisenger MH, editors: *Gastrointestinal and liver disease: Pathophysiology, diagnosis, management*, Philadelphia, 1998, WB Saunders, pp 1771–1778.

Ingested Foreign Bodies

Ingested foreign bodies, which can lead to subsequent perforation or obstruction of the gastrointestinal tract, are swallowed, usually accidentally, by children or adults. These include glass and metal fragments, pins, needles, toothpicks, fish bones, coins, whistles, toys, and broken razor blades (Fig. 49-48). Intentional ingestion of foreign bodies is sometimes seen in the prison population and those who are mentally unstable. For most patients, treatment is observation, which allows the safe passage of these objects through the intestinal tract. If the object is radiopaque, progress can be followed by serial abdominal films. Cathartic agents are contraindicated. Sharp pointed objects such as needles, razor blades, or fish bones may penetrate the bowel wall. If abdominal pain, tenderness, fever, or leukocytosis occurs, immediate laparotomy and surgical removal of the offending object are indicated. Laparotomy is also required for intestinal obstruction.

Small Bowel Fistulas

Despite improvements in surgical nutrition and critical care, mortality from enterocutaneous fistulas remains high, 10% in recent reports. Improvements in outcome are focused on prevention and, when fistulas occur, prompt recognition and intervention. Multidisciplinary care is critical to improve enterocutaneous fistula outcomes. Enterocutaneous fistulas are most commonly iatrogenic, as 75% to 85% occur during surgical intervention (e.g., anastomotic leakage, injury of the bowel or blood supply, erosion by suction catheters, laceration of the bowel by wire mesh or retention suture). The remaining 15% to 25% of fistula occurrences are associated with predisposing conditions such as Crohn's disease, malignant disease, radiation enteritis, diverticulitis, intra-abdominal sepsis, or trauma.

CLASSIFICATION	DESCRIPTION
Category	Low: <200 mL
	Intermediate: 200-500 mL
	High: >500 mL
Anatomy	Gastric, small bowel, colon, rectum
Etiology	Radiation, inflammatory bowel diseases,
	foreign body (e.g., mesh), iatrogenic injury

TABLE 49-13 **Fistula Classifications**

BOX 49-5 Factors Preventing Spontaneous Fistula Closure

High output (>500 mL/24 hr)
Severe disruption of intestinal continuity (>50% of bowel circumference)
Active inflammatory bowel disease of bowel segment
Cancer
Radiation enteritis
Distal obstruction
Undrained abscess cavity
Foreign body in the fistula tract
Fistula tract <2.5 cm long
Epithelialization of fistula tract

From Visschers RGJ, van Gemert WG, Winkens B, et al: Guided treatment improves outcome of patients with enterocutaneous fistulas. *World J Surg* 36:2341–2348, 2012.

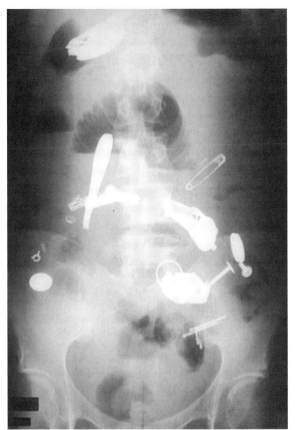

FIGURE 49-48 Plain abdominal film demonstrates a number of ingested foreign bodies in a patient presenting with a small bowel obstruction. (Courtesy Dr. Melvyn H. Schreiber, The University of Texas Medical Branch, Galveston, TX.)

Clinical Manifestations

Recognition of enterocutaneous fistulas is usually not difficult. The typical clinical presentation is that of a febrile postoperative patient with an erythematous wound. When a few skin sutures are removed, a purulent or bloody discharge is noted; leakage of enteric contents then occurs, sometimes immediately but often within 1 or 2 days. The diagnosis rarely eludes the surgeon for long. Small bowel fistulas can also be manifested with generalized peritonitis, although this is less common. Recently, the popularization of damage control laparotomy and staged management of the open abdomen has led to a more virulent form of small bowel fistula referred to as an *enteroatmospheric fistula*. These patients typically present with an open segment of intestine exposed through a large fascial defect, without a surrounding epidermal margin.

Enterocutaneous fistulas are classified according to their location and volume of daily output (Table 49-13). These factors dictate treatment and morbidity and mortality rates. Proximal fistulas are associated with higher output, greater fluid and electrolyte loss, and greater loss of digestive capacity. Distal fistulas tend to have lower output, making them easier to manage and more likely to close spontaneously. High-output fistulas are those that discharge 500 mL or more per 24 hours. Factors that prevent the spontaneous closure of fistulas are shown in Box 49-5. Once a fistula is identified, management should focus on prompt resus-

citation of the patient and consideration of potential factors that could prevent spontaneous closure. Successful management of patients with intestinal fistulas requires a coordinated staged approach that can be defined in three phases—stabilization, staging and supportive care, and definitive management.

Treatment

Stabilization. Historically, malnutrition and fluid losses were the leading causes of death in patients with small bowel fistula. However, with better nutritional supplementation and critical care support, sepsis has become the most common cause of death in affected patients. Nevertheless, the fluid losses and volume depletion associated with small bowel fistula cannot be marginalized. Visschers and coworkers[47] offer a guided treatment algorithm that prolongs periods of convalescence and improves spontaneous closure rates in patients with enterocutaneous fistulas (Box 49-6). Therefore, prompt fluid resuscitation and electrolyte replacement should occur on recognition of a fistula. Sepsis control is critical, and in the early period, CT scanning may be invaluable in identifying undrained abscesses, complete distal obstructions, or generalized intra-abdominal sepsis with peritonitis. All infections should be adequately drained percutaneously or operatively, if necessary, along with appropriate antibiotic administration. Once sepsis is controlled and the patient is resuscitated, effluent control with skin protection and adequate nutrition are necessary. Fistula output is best controlled by intubation of the fistula tract with a drain. Protection of the skin around the fistulous opening is important to prevent excoriation and destruction of the skin. This is most easily accomplished by using a Stomahesive product with applications of zinc oxide, aluminum paste ointment, or karaya powder. The suction catheter can be brought out through the end of the Stomahesive bag, which is cut to just fit the fistulous opening. This will allow collection and accurate measurement of

Adapted from Visschers RG, van Gemert WG, Winkens B, et al: Guided treatment improves outcome of patients with enterocutaneous fistulas. *World J Surg* 36:2341–2348, 2012. *ECF,* Enterocutaneous fistula.

the output. The use of TPN has been an important advance in the management of patients with high-output enterocutaneous fistulas and significantly prevents the problems of malnutrition. TPN is particularly valuable in the stabilization period to help minimize high-output fistula losses and for immediate nutritional repletion while the fistula is being delineated. However, if the patient can meet calorie goals without the use of TPN, especially when a high-output fistula is not present, enteral feeding is preferable and recommended.

Staging and supportive care. When sepsis has been controlled and nutritional therapy has been instituted, the fistula must be adequately staged. The combined use of fluoroscopic contrast studies, fistulography if necessary, and CT, along with the patient's clinical behavior, will characterize the anatomy and underlying pathology of the fistula. Some have advocated conservative man-

agement for up to 3 months to allow spontaneous closure. However, others have shown that after sepsis is controlled, more than 90% of small intestinal fistulas that closed did so within 1 month. Less than 10% of the fistulas closed after 2 months, and none closed spontaneously after 3 months. Therefore, a reasonable management plan would be to follow a 6-week period of convalescence, at which time, if closure has not been obtained, surgical management should be considered if the preoperative albumin level is above 25 g/liter. However, knowledge that spontaneous closure is unlikely should not prompt immediate reexploration at 8 weeks. In general, a period of 3 to 6 months is beneficial to allow the profound inflammatory response associated with intra-abdominal sepsis to subside completely and for the adhesion formation to stabilize. This period will provide a better opportunity for safe and successful operative intervention. Furthermore, as is the case with enteroatmospheric small bowel fistulas, it may take several months to stabilize the complex abdominal wound associated with the fistula.

Several adjuncts have been proposed to help assist in spontaneous fistula closure and management of the associated abdominal wound, although none are supported by vigorous level I data. Studies have suggested that bowel rest with TPN therapy improves fistula closure rates and time to closure in patients with high-output fistulas. Low-output fistulas can successfully be managed with enteral therapy while avoiding the known complications of parenteral therapy. Dysmotility agents such as loperamide and codeine can also assist with attempts at enteral therapy. Furthermore, newer techniques, such as fistuloclysis, in which the distal limb of a proximal fistula is intubated and enteral therapy is delivered to the distal bowel, have proved effective. Several randomized trials have evaluated the role of octreotide in the management of fistulas. Although octreotide has been shown to decrease fistula output, which can be useful in the presence of a high-output fistula, octreotide has not convincingly provided an improvement in spontaneous closure rates. Vacuum devices are valuable in the setting of enteroatmospheric fistulas to help contract the open abdominal wound around the associated fistula. Care should be given to avoid direct contact with visceral contents as this can cause new fistulas. Skin grafting up to the fistula has also been used in cases associated with an open abdomen, with a graft success rate of up to 80% in some series.

Definitive management. Once the patient's nutritional, fluid, and wound care needs have been addressed, reoperative intervention will ultimately be necessary for some patients. Surgery is most easily accomplished by entering the previous abdominal wound, with great care taken to avoid further damage to adherent bowel. The preferred operation is fistula tract excision and segmental resection of the involved segment of intestine and reanastomosis. Simple closure of the fistula after removal of the fistula tract almost always results in a recurrence of the fistula. If an unexpected abscess is encountered or if the bowel wall is rigid and distended over a long distance, thus making primary anastomosis unsafe, exteriorization of both ends of the intestine should be accomplished. Various bypass procedures have also been described as part of a staged approach in which exclusion of the segment containing the fistula is accomplished in the first reoperation, and then another operation is required for resection of the involved segment and fistula tract. Although this may be necessary in extreme circumstances, this is certainly not the preferred surgical management. Basic surgical considerations include attempting a one-stage procedure, careful adhesiolysis, addressing compromised tissues with wedge excision or intestinal resection, covering sutures with viable tissues, and avoiding friable areas that are not directly involved with the fistula.

In summary, enterocutaneous fistulas occur most commonly as a result of a previous operative procedure. Once identified, a three-phase approach of stabilization, staging and supportive care, and, in some cases, definitive surgical intervention is necessary. Most of these fistulas heal spontaneously within 6 weeks. If closure is not accomplished after this time, surgery is indicated.

Pneumatosis Intestinalis

Pneumatosis intestinalis is an uncommon condition manifesting as multiple gas-filled cysts of the gastrointestinal tract. The cysts may be located in the subserosa, submucosa, and, rarely, muscularis layer and vary in size from microscopic to several centimeters in diameter. They can occur anywhere along the gastrointestinal tract, from the esophagus to the rectum; however, they are most common in the jejunum, followed by the ileocecal region and colon. Extraintestinal structures such as mesentery, peritoneum, and falciform ligament may also be involved. There is an equal incidence in men and women, and the condition usually occurs in the fourth to seventh decades of life. Pneumatosis in neonates is usually associated with necrotizing enterocolitis. The cause of pneumatosis intestinalis has not been completely delineated. A number of theories have been proposed, of which the mechanical, mucosal damage, bacterial, and pulmonary hypotheses seem to be most promising.

Most cases of pneumatosis intestinalis are associated with chronic obstructive pulmonary disease or the immunocompromised state (e.g., in AIDS; after transplantation; in association with leukemia, lymphoma, vasculitis, or collagen vascular disease; and in patients undergoing chemotherapy or taking corticosteroids). Other associated conditions include inflammatory, obstructive, or infectious conditions of the intestine; iatrogenic conditions, such as endoscopy and jejunostomy placement; ischemia; and extraintestinal diseases, such as diabetes. Pneumatosis not associated with other lesions is referred to as *primary pneumatosis*.

In gross appearance, the cysts resemble cystic lymphangiomas or hydatid cysts. On histologic section, the involved portion has a honeycomb appearance. The cysts are thin walled and break easily. Spontaneous rupture gives rise to pneumoperitoneum. Symptoms are nonspecific, and in pneumatosis associated with other disorders, the symptoms may be those of the associated disease. Symptoms in primary pneumatosis intestinalis, when present, usually include diarrhea, abdominal pain, abdominal distention, nausea, vomiting, weight loss, and mucus in stools. Hematochezia and constipation have also been described. Complications associated with pneumatosis intestinalis occur in about 3% of cases and include volvulus, intestinal obstruction, hemorrhage, and intestinal perforation. Usually, pneumoperitoneum occurs in these patients, generally in association with small bowel rather than large bowel pneumatosis. Peritonitis is unusual. In fact, pneumatosis intestinalis represents one of the few cases of sterile pneumoperitoneum and should be considered in the patient with free abdominal air but no evidence of peritonitis.

The diagnosis is usually made radiographically by plain abdominal or barium studies. On plain films, pneumatosis intestinalis appears as radiolucent areas within the bowel wall, which must be differentiated from luminal intestinal gas (Fig. 49-49A). The radiolucency may be linear or curvilinear or appear as grape-like clusters or tiny bubbles. Alternatively, barium contrast or CT studies can be used to confirm the diagnosis (Fig. 49-49B). Visualization of intestinal cysts has also been described by ultrasound.

No treatment is necessary unless one of the very rare complications supervenes, such as rectal bleeding, cyst-induced volvulus, or tension pneumoperitoneum. Prognosis in most patients is that of the underlying disease. The important point is to recognize that pneumatosis intestinalis is a benign cause of pneumoperitoneum. Treatment should be directed at the underlying cause of the pneumatosis, and surgical intervention should be predicated on the clinical course of the patient.

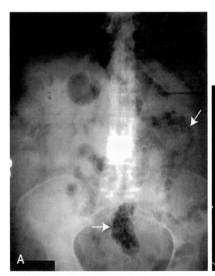 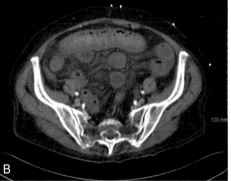

FIGURE 49-49 A, Plain abdominal film demonstrates pneumatosis intestinalis *(arrows).* **B,** CT findings consistent with curvilinear radiolucency appearing as tiny bubbles in the antimesenteric border of the bowel consistent with pneumatosis intestinalis. **(A,** Courtesy Dr. Melvyn H. Schreiber, The University of Texas Medical Branch, Galveston, TX. **B,** Courtesy Dr. Kristin Long, University of Kentucky Medical Center, Lexington, KY.)

Blind Loop Syndrome

Blind loop syndrome is a rare condition manifested by diarrhea, steatorrhea, megaloblastic anemia, weight loss, abdominal pain, and deficiencies of the fat-soluble vitamins as well as neurologic disorders. The underlying cause of this syndrome is bacterial overgrowth in stagnant areas of the small bowel produced by stricture, stenosis, fistulas, or diverticula (e.g., jejunoileal or Meckel's diverticulum). Under normal circumstances, the upper gastrointestinal tract contains fewer than 10^5 bacteria/mL, mostly gram-positive aerobes and facultative anaerobes. However, with stasis, the number of bacteria increases, with excessive proliferation of aerobic and anaerobic bacteria; bacteroides, anaerobic lactobacilli, coliforms, and enterococci are likely to be present in varying numbers. The bacteria compete for vitamin B_{12}, producing systemic deficiency of vitamin B_{12} and megaloblastic anemia.

The syndrome can be confirmed by a series of laboratory investigations. Bacterial overgrowth can be diagnosed with cultures obtained through an intestinal tube or by indirect tests such as the ^{14}C-xylose or ^{14}C-cholylglycine breath tests. Excessive bacterial use of ^{14}C substrate leads to an increase in ^{14}C-CO_2. After bacterial overgrowth and steatorrhea are confirmed, a Schilling test (^{57}Co-labeled vitamin B_{12} absorption) may be performed, which should reveal a pattern of urinary excretion of vitamin B_{12} resembling that of pernicious anemia (a urinary loss of 0% to 6% of vitamin B_{12} compared with the normal of 7% to 25%). In patients with blind loop syndrome, vitamin B_{12} excretion is not altered by the addition of intrinsic factor, but a course of a broad-spectrum antibiotic (e.g., tetracycline) should return vitamin B_{12} absorption to normal.

Treatment of patients with blind loop syndrome includes parenteral vitamin B_{12} therapy and broad-spectrum antibiotics. Tetracyclines have been the mainstay of treatment, but studies have shown that rifaximin and metronidazole demonstrate less resistance and are also effective. For most patients, a single course of therapy (7 to 10 days) is sufficient, and the patient may remain symptom free for months. Prokinetic agents have been used without real success. Surgical correction of the condition causing stagnation and blind loop syndrome produces a permanent cure and is indicated for patients who require multiple rounds of antibiotics or are receiving continuous therapy.

Radiation Enteritis

Radiation therapy is generally used as adjuvant therapy for various abdominal and pelvic cancers. In addition to tumor cells, however, other rapidly dividing cells in normal tissues may be affected by radiation. Surrounding normal tissue, such as the small intestinal epithelium, may sustain severe, acute, and chronic deleterious effects. Radiation injury to the small bowel can be subdivided into acute and chronic forms. Acute radiation-induced small bowel disease usually is manifested with colicky abdominal pain, bloating, loss of appetite, nausea, diarrhea, and fecal urgency during or shortly after a course of radiotherapy. Most patients notice symptoms during the second week of treatment, when tissue damage and inflammation are maximal, and symptoms peak by the fourth week when histologic changes are stable or improving.[48] Symptoms consistent with chronic radiation injury typically develop between 18 months and 6 years after a completed course of radiotherapy, but symptoms can be manifested up to 30 years after the treatment course.

The amount of radiation appears to correlate with the probability for development of radiation enteritis. Serious late complications are unusual if the total radiation dosage is less than 4000 cGy;

morbidity risk increases with dosages exceeding 5000 cGy. Other factors, including previous abdominal surgeries, preexisting vascular disease, hypertension, diabetes, and adjuvant treatment with certain chemotherapeutic agents (such as 5-FU, doxorubicin, dactinomycin, and MTX), contribute to the development of enteritis after radiation treatments. A previous history of laparotomy increases the risk for enteritis, presumably because of adhesions that fix portions of the small bowel into the irradiated field. Radiation damage leads to symptoms consisting mainly of diarrhea, abdominal pain, and malabsorption. The late effects of radiation injury are the result of damage to the small submucosal blood vessels, with a progressive obliterative arteritis and submucosal fibrosis, resulting eventually in thrombosis and vascular insufficiency. This injury may produce necrosis and perforation of the involved intestine but, more commonly, leads to stricture formation with symptoms of obstruction or small bowel fistulas.

Multiple strategies are used to reduce radiation injury to the small bowel (Box 49-7). Radiation enteritis may be minimized by adjusting ports and dosages of radiation to deliver optimal treatment specifically to the tumor and not to surrounding tissues. Placement of radiopaque markers, such as titanium clips, at the time of the original operation facilitates better targeting of the radiation treatment. A reduction in field size, multiple field arrangements, conformal radiotherapy techniques, and intensity-modulated radiotherapy can reduce toxicity related to radiotherapy. Methods designed to exclude the small bowel from the irradiated field include reperitonealization, omental transposition, and placement of absorbable mesh slings.

A number of pharmacologic interventions have also been described to reduce the side effects of radiation enteritis. Angiotensin-converting enzyme inhibitors and statins significantly reduce acute gastrointestinal symptoms during radical pelvic radiotherapy. Sucralfate, a highly sulfated polyanionic disaccharide thought to stimulate epithelial healing and to form a protective barrier over damaged mucosal surfaces, may help in the treatment of bleeding from radiation proctitis, but no evidence exists supporting its use in the prevention of radiation-induced small bowel disease. Superoxide dismutase, a free radical scavenger, has been used successfully to reduce complications. Other compounds that have been evaluated include glutathione, antioxidants (e.g., vitamin A, vitamin E, beta-carotene), histamine antagonists, and the combination of pentoxifylline and tocopherols, a class of chemical compounds with vitamin E activity. In addition, early studies have supported the use of probiotics as having a radioprotective effect in the gut; however, further studies are required before a final assessment can be made. The most effective radioprotectant agent appears to be amifostine (WR-2721), a sulfhydryl compound that is converted intracellularly to an active metabolite, WR-1065, which in turn binds to free radicals and protects the cell from radiation injury. A randomized controlled trial determined that glutamine offers little benefit, even when it is used before or during radiation therapy. Agents that may prove useful in the prevention of the acute symptoms of radiation enteritis include the hormones bombesin, growth hormone, glucagon-like peptide 2 (GLP-2), and insulin-like growth factor I (IGF-I), which have demonstrated effectiveness in experimental studies in preventing or reducing symptoms associated with radiation enteritis.

The treatment of acute radiation enteritis is directed at controlling symptoms. Antispasmodics and analgesics may alleviate abdominal pain and cramping, and diarrhea usually responds to opiates or other antidiarrheal agents. The use of corticosteroids for acute radiation enteritis is of uncertain value. Dietary manipulation, including oral elemental diets, has also been advocated to ameliorate the acute effects of radiation enteritis; however, results are conflicting. Antibiotics are frequently used in the setting of bacterial overgrowth. Bile acid malabsorption, thought to be responsible for diarrheal symptoms in 35% to 72% of patients with radiation-induced small bowel disease, responds well to cholestyramine, but it is not well-tolerated and many patients voluntarily discontinue use.

Operative intervention may be required for a subgroup of patients with the chronic effects of radiation enteritis. This subgroup of patients represents only a small percentage (1% to 2%) of the total number of patients who have received abdominal or pelvic irradiation. Indications for operation include obstruction, fistula formation, perforation, and bleeding, with obstruction being the most common presentation. Operative procedures include a bypass or resection with reanastomosis. Advocates for bypass procedures contend that this procedure is safer and controls the symptoms better than resection. Advocates of resection contend that the high morbidity and mortality rates previously reported with resection and reanastomosis reflect inadequate resection and anastomosis of diseased intestine. In patients presenting with obstruction, extensive lysis of adhesions should be avoided. Obstruction caused by rigid, fixed intestinal loops in the pelvis is best bypassed. If resection and reanastomosis are planned, at least one end of the anastomosis should be from intestine outside the irradiated field. Macroscopic findings may not be accurate in evaluating the full extent of radiation damage. Frozen section and laser Doppler flowmetry techniques have been used to assist resection and anastomosis. However, reports of their clinical usefulness are conflicting. Perforation of the intestine should be treated with resection and anastomosis. When reanastomosis is thought to be unsafe, the ends should be exteriorized.

Short Bowel Syndrome

The short bowel syndrome results from a total small bowel length that is inadequate to support nutrition. Of these cases of short bowel syndrome, 75% occur from massive intestinal resection. In the adult, mesenteric occlusion, midgut volvulus, and traumatic disruption of the superior mesenteric vessels are the most frequent causes. Multiple sequential resections, usually associated with recurrent Crohn's disease, account for 25% of patients. In neonates, the most common cause of short bowel syndrome is bowel resection secondary to necrotizing enterocolitis. The clinical hallmarks of short bowel syndrome include diarrhea, fluid and electrolyte deficiency, and malnutrition. Other complications include an increased incidence of gallstones caused by disruption of the enterohepatic circulation and of nephrolithiasis from hyperoxaluria. Specific nutrient deficiencies must be prevented, and levels must be monitored closely; these nutrients include iron, magnesium, zinc, copper, and vitamins. The likelihood that a patient with short bowel syndrome will be permanently dependent on TPN is thought to be primarily influenced by the length, location, and health of the remaining intestine. In patients with short bowel syndrome, postabsorptive levels of plasma citrulline, a nonprotein amino acid produced by intestinal mucosa, may provide an indicator to differentiate transient from permanent intestinal failure.

The bowel has a remarkable capacity to adapt after small bowel resection; in many cases, this process of intestinal adaptation, termed adaptive hyperplasia, effectively prevents severe complications resulting from the markedly decreased surface area available for absorption and digestion. However, any adaptive mechanism can be overwhelmed, and adaptation can be inadequate if too much small bowel is lost. Although there is considerable individual variation, resection of up to 70% of the small bowel usually can be tolerated if the terminal ileum and ileocecal valve are preserved. Length alone, however, is not the only determining factor of complications related to small bowel resection. For example, if the distal two thirds of the ileum, including the ileocecal valve, is resected, significant abnormalities of absorption of bile salts and vitamin B_{12} may occur, resulting in diarrhea and anemia, although only 25% of the total length of the small bowel has been removed. Proximal bowel resection is tolerated better than distal resection because the ileum can adapt and increase its absorptive capacity more efficiently than the jejunum.

Treatment

The most important issue to remember about short bowel syndrome is prevention. In patients with Crohn's disease, resections limited to the particular complication should be performed. In addition, during surgery for problems related to intestinal ischemia, the smallest possible resection should be performed, and if necessary, second-look operations should be carried out to allow the ischemic bowel to demarcate, thus potentially preventing unnecessary extensive resection of the bowel.

After massive small bowel resection, the treatment course may be divided into early and late phases. In its early phase, treatment is primarily directed at the control of diarrhea, replacement of fluid and electrolytes, and prompt institution of TPN in patients who cannot safely tolerate enteral feedings. Volume losses may exceed 5 liters/day, and vigorous monitoring of intake and output with adequate replacement must be carried out. Diarrhea in this early phase can be caused by a multitude of sources. For example, hypergastrinemia and gastric hypersecretion occur after massive small bowel resection and greatly contribute to diarrhea after a massive small bowel resection. Acid hypersecretion can be managed by H_2 receptor antagonists or proton pump blockers, such as omeprazole. Diarrhea may also be caused by ileal resection, resulting in disruption of the enterohepatic circulation and excessive amounts of bile salts entering the colon. Cholestyramine may be beneficial when diarrhea is related to the cathartic effects of unabsorbed bile salts in the colon. In addition, the judicious use of agents that inhibit gut motility (e.g., codeine, diphenoxylate) may be helpful. The long-acting somatostatin analogue octreotide also appears to reduce the amount of diarrhea during the early phase of short bowel syndrome. Some studies have suggested that octreotide may inhibit gut adaptation; other studies, however, have not confirmed this deleterious effect of octreotide.

As soon as the patient has recovered from the acute phase, enteral nutrition should be started. The most common types of enteral diets are elemental (e.g., Vivonex, Flexical) and polymeric (e.g., Isocal, Ensure). Controversy exists about the optimal diet for these patients. Initially, a high-carbohydrate, high-protein diet is appropriate to maximize absorption. Milk products should be avoided, and the diet should be begun at iso-osmolar concentrations and with small amounts. As the gut adapts, the osmolality, volume, and calorie content can be increased. The provision of nutrients in their simplest forms is an important part of the treatment. Simple sugars, dipeptides, and tripeptides are rapidly absorbed from the intestinal tract. Reduction in dietary fat has long been considered to be important in the treatment of patients with short bowel syndrome. Supplementation of the diet with 100 g or more of fat, however, should be carried out, often requiring the use of medium-chain triglycerides, which are absorbed in the proximal bowel. Vitamins, especially fat-soluble vitamins, as well as calcium, magnesium, and zinc supplementation should be provided. The roles of hormones administered systemically and glutamine administered enterally have been evaluated. The hormones neurotensin, bombesin, and GLP-2 have demonstrated marked mucosal growth in various experimental studies and have been shown to prevent the gut atrophy associated with TPN in experimental studies; combination therapy appears more efficacious than single-agent administration. Randomized controlled trials have shown that teduglutide, a GLP-2 analogue that is resistant to degradation by the proteolytic enzyme dipeptidyl peptidase 4 and therefore has a longer half-life than GLP-2, is well tolerated and has led to the restoration of intestinal functional and structural integrity through significant intestinotrophic and proabsorptive effects. It is the first targeted therapeutic agent to gain approval for use in adult short bowel syndrome with intestinal failure.[49]

Two other hormones not derived from the gut that have been evaluated extensively in various experimental and limited clinical trials include growth hormone and IGF-I. A meta-analysis of randomized controlled trials using growth hormone in short bowel syndrome suggests a possible short-term benefit in terms of body weight, lean body mass, and absorptive capacity; however, long-term efficacy was not noted. Somatropin, a recombinant human growth hormone that elicits anabolic and anticatabolic influence on various cells either as a direct effect or indirectly through IGF-I, is currently indicated to treat short bowel syndrome in conjunction with nutritional support. The combination of various trophic hormones with glutamine and a modified diet may prove more efficacious in the treatment of this difficult group of patients.

A number of surgical strategies have been attempted in patients who are chronically TPN dependent, with limited success; these include procedures to delay intestinal transit time, methods to increase absorptive area, and small bowel transplantation. Methods to delay intestinal transit time include the construction of various valves and sphincters, with inconsistent results reported. Antiperistaltic segments of small intestine have been constructed to slow the transit, thus allowing additional contact time for nutrient and fluid absorption. Moderate successes have been described with this technique. Other procedures, including colonic interposition, recirculating loops of small bowel, and retrograde electrical pacing, have been tried but were found to be unsuccessful in humans and

were largely abandoned. Surgical procedures to increase absorptive area include the intestinal tapering and lengthening procedure (e.g., Bianchi procedure), which improves intestinal function by correcting the dilation and ineffective peristalsis of the remaining intestine and by doubling the intestinal length while preserving the mucosal surface area.[50] Although beneficial in selected patients, potential complications can include necrosis of divided segments and anastomotic leaks.

Intestinal transplantation remains the standard of care for patients in whom intestinal rehabilitation attempts have failed and who are at risk of life-threatening complications of TPN. Patient survival after intestinal transplantation has significantly improved with the introduction of the immunosuppressive agent FK-506. The 1- and 5-year survival rates for isolated intestinal transplantation are 75% and 48%, respectively. Combined intestinal-liver transplants have comparable 1- and 5-year survival rates of approximately 66% and 54%, respectively. The challenges of small bowel transplantation continue to be the need for better immunosuppression and earlier detection of rejection.

Vascular Compression of the Duodenum

Vascular compression of the duodenum, also known as *superior mesenteric artery syndrome* or *Wilkie syndrome*, is a rare condition characterized by compression of the third portion of the duodenum by the superior mesenteric artery as it passes over this portion

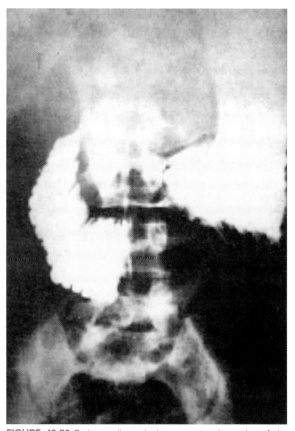

FIGURE 49-50 Barium radiograph demonstrates obstruction of the third portion of the duodenum secondary to superior mesenteric artery compression as a consequence of burn injury. (Adapted from Reckler JM, Bruck HM, Munster AM, et al: Superior mesenteric artery syndrome as a consequence of burn injury. *J Trauma* 12:979–985, 1972.)

of the duodenum. Symptoms include profound nausea and vomiting, abdominal distention, weight loss, and postprandial epigastric pain, which varies from intermittent to constant, depending on the severity of the duodenal obstruction. Weight loss usually occurs before the onset of symptoms and contributes to the syndrome.

This syndrome is most commonly seen in young asthenic individuals, with women being more commonly affected than men. Predisposing factors for vascular compression of the duodenum, aside from weight loss, include supine immobilization, scoliosis, and placement of a body cast, sometimes called the *cast syndrome*. An association between vascular compression of the duodenum and peptic ulcer has been observed. Vascular compression of the duodenum has been reported in association with anorexia nervosa and after proctocolectomy and J-pouch anal anastomosis, resection of an arteriovenous malformation of the cervical cord, abdominal aortic aneurysm repair, and orthopedic procedures, usually spinal surgery. One report in the literature described a family with a preponderance of vascular compression of the duodenum.

Diagnosis of this condition is made by a barium upper gastrointestinal series (Fig. 49-50) or hypotonic duodenography, which demonstrates abrupt or near-total cessation of flow of barium from the duodenum to the jejunum. CT has been useful in certain cases. Treatment of this syndrome varies. Conservative measures are tried initially and have been increasingly successful as definitive treatment. The operative treatment of choice for vascular compression of the duodenum is duodenojejunostomy.

SELECTED REFERENCES

Affronti A, Orlando A, Cottone M: An update on medical management on Crohn's disease. *Expert Opin Pharmacother* 16:63–78, 2015.

This represents a clear and concise review article highlighting critical issues in the management of Crohn's disease, new evidence from clinical trials, long-term prospective studies, and real-life experience, beyond the current guidelines.

Bilimoria KY, Bentrem DJ, Wayne JD, et al: Small bowel cancer in the United States: Changes in epidemiology, treatment, and survival over the last 20 years. *Ann Surg* 249:63–71, 2009.

This study represents a large, national database analysis of the overall increase of incidence of small intestine malignant neoplasms during the past two decades.

Caplin ME, Pavel M, Cwikla JB, et al: Lanreotide in metastatic enteropancreatic neuroendocrine tumors. *N Engl J Med* 371:224–233, 2014.

The landmark CLARINET trial (LanreotideAntiproliferativeResponse in patients with GEP-NET) is the largest phase 3, randomized, double-blind, placebo-controlled, multinational study that evaluated the antiproliferative effect of the somatostatin analogue lanreotide in patients with GEP-NETs. Lanreotide was associated with significantly prolonged progression-free survival among patients with grade 1 or 2 metastatic enteropancreatic neuroendocrine tumors.

Castano JP, Sundin A, Maecke HR, et al: Gastrointestinal neuroendocrine tumors (NETs): New diagnostic and therapeutic challenges. *Cancer Metastasis Rev* 33:353–359, 2014.

This paper summarizes the current understanding of the biology of somatostatin receptor, role of immunotherapy in neuroendocrine tumor (NET), new agents for peptide receptor radionuclide therapy, and methods to assess response and clinical benefit in NET.

Crohn BB, Ginzburg L, Oppenheimer GD: Regional ileitis: a pathologic and clinical entity. *JAMA* 99:1323–1329, 1932.

This landmark paper succinctly crystallizes the clinical course, differential diagnosis, and pathologic findings of regional ileitis in young adults. Although other terms have been applied to this disease process, based on the descriptions in this classic paper, Crohn's disease has been universally accepted as the name.

Thirunavukarasu P, Sathaiah M, Sukumar S, et al: Meckel's diverticulum—a high-risk region for malignancy in the ileum. Insights from a population-based epidemiological study and implications in surgical management. *Ann Surg* 253:223–230, 2011.

A national database study during 33 years that suggests Meckel's diverticulum is a high-risk area for ileal cancer and supports the resection of incidental Meckel's diverticulum.

Vasen HF, Moslein G, Alonso A, et al: Guidelines for the clinical management of familial adenomatous polyposis (FAP). *Gut* 57:704–713, 2008.

This article represents a thorough review of the literature and treatment guidelines for the clinical management of patients with FAP and their families.

REFERENCES

1. Moore KL, Persaud TVN: The digestive system. In Moore KL, Persaud TVN, editors: *The developing human: Clinically oriented embryology*, ed 9, Philadelphia, 2011, Elsevier, pp 255–286.
2. Bykov VL: Paneth cells: History of discovery, structural and functional characteristics and the role in the maintenance of homeostasis in the small intestine. *Morfologiia* 145:67–80, 2014.
3. Chung DH, Evers BM: The digestive system. In O'Leary JP, editor: *The physiologic basis of surgery*, ed 4, Philadelphia, 2007, Lippincott Williams & Wilkins, pp 475–507.
4. Field BC: Neuroendocrinology of obesity. *Br Med Bull* 109:73–82, 2014.
5. Zielinski MD, Bannon MP: Current management of small bowel obstruction. *Adv Surg* 45:1–29, 2011.
6. Maglinte DD: Fluoroscopic and CT enteroclysis: Evidence-based clinical update. *Radiol Clin North Am* 51:149–176, 2013.
7. Sallinen V, Wikstrom H, Victorzon M, et al: Laparoscopic versus open adhesiolysis for small bowel obstruction—a multicenter, prospective, randomized, controlled trial. *BMC Surg* 14:77, 2014.

8. Park CM, Lee WY, Cho YB, et al: Sodium hyaluronate–based bioresorbable membrane (Seprafilm) reduced early postoperative intestinal obstruction after lower abdominal surgery for colorectal cancer: The preliminary report. *Int J Colorectal Dis* 24:305–310, 2009.

9. Crohn BB, Ginzburg L, Oppenheimer GD: Regional ileitis: A pathologic and clinical entity. *JAMA* 99:1323–1329, 1932.

10. Lichtenstein GR: Current research in Crohn's disease and ulcerative colitis: Highlights from the 2010 ACG Meeting. *Gastroenterol Hepatol (N Y)* 6:3–14, 2010.

11. Petersen BS, Spehlmann ME, Raedler A, et al: Whole genome and exome sequencing of monozygotic twins discordant for Crohn's disease. *BMC Genomics* 15:564, 2014.

12. Vermeire S, Van Assche G, Rutgeerts P: Inflammatory bowel disease and colitis: New concepts from the bench and the clinic. *Curr Opin Gastroenterol* 27:32–37, 2011.

13. Tsianos EV, Katsanos KH, Tsianos VE: Role of genetics in the diagnosis and prognosis of Crohn's disease. *World J Gastroenterol* 18:105–118, 2012.

14. Spinelli A, Allocca M, Jovani M, et al: Review article: Optimal preparation for surgery in Crohn's disease. *Aliment Pharmacol Ther* 40:1009–1022, 2014.

15. Malvi D, Vasuri F, Mattioli B, et al: Adenocarcinoma in Crohn's disease: The pathologist's experience in a tertiary referral centre of inflammatory bowel disease. *Pathology* 46:439–443, 2014.

16. Fiorino G, Bonifacio C, Peyrin-Biroulet L, et al: Prospective comparison of computed tomography enterography and magnetic resonance enterography for assessment of disease activity and complications in ileocolonic Crohn's disease. *Inflamm Bowel Dis* 17:1073–1080, 2011.

17. Bourreille A, Ignjatovic A, Aabakken L, et al: Role of small-bowel endoscopy in the management of patients with inflammatory bowel disease: An international OMED-ECCO consensus. *Endoscopy* 41:618–637, 2009.

18. van Schaik FD, Oldenburg B, Hart AR, et al: Serological markers predict inflammatory bowel disease years before the diagnosis. *Gut* 62:683–688, 2013.

19. Yamamoto T, Shiraki M, Bamba T, et al: Faecal calprotectin and lactoferrin as markers for monitoring disease activity and predicting clinical recurrence in patients with Crohn's disease after ileocolonic resection: A prospective pilot study. *United European Gastroenterol J* 1:368–374, 2013.

20. Affronti A, Orlando A, Cottone M: An update on medical management on Crohn's disease. *Expert Opin Pharmacother* 16:63–78, 2015.

21. Terdiman JP, Gruss CB, Heidelbaugh JJ, et al: American Gastroenterological Association Institute guideline on the use of thiopurines, methotrexate, and anti-TNF-alpha biologic drugs for the induction and maintenance of remission in inflammatory Crohn's disease. *Gastroenterology* 145:1459–1463, 2013.

22. Yamamoto T, Watanabe T: Surgery for luminal Crohn's disease. *World J Gastroenterol* 20:78–90, 2014.

23. Umanskiy K, Malhotra G, Chase A, et al: Laparoscopic colectomy for Crohn's colitis. A large prospective comparative study. *J Gastrointest Surg* 14:658–663, 2010.

24. Krane MK, Allaix ME, Zoccali M, et al: Does morbid obesity change outcomes after laparoscopic surgery for inflammatory bowel disease? Review of 626 consecutive cases. *J Am Coll Surg* 216:986–996, 2013.

25. Eshuis EJ, Bemelman WA, van Bodegraven AA, et al: Laparoscopic ileocolic resection versus infliximab treatment of distal ileitis in Crohn's disease: A randomized multicenter trial (LIR!C-trial). *BMC Surg* 8:15, 2008.

26. Kono T, Ashida T, Ebisawa Y, et al: A new antimesenteric functional end-to-end handsewn anastomosis: Surgical prevention of anastomotic recurrence in Crohn's disease. *Dis Colon Rectum* 54:586–592, 2011.

27. Vaughn BP, Moss AC: Prevention of post-operative recurrence of Crohn's disease. *World J Gastroenterol* 20:1147–1154, 2014.

28. Wiwanitkit V, Srisupanant M: Cryptosporidiosis occurrence in anti-HIV-seropositive patients attending a sexually transmitted diseases clinic, Thailand. *Trop Doct* 36:64, 2006.

29. Poveda A, del Muro XG, Lopez-Guerrero JA, et al: GEIS 2013 guidelines for gastrointestinal sarcomas (GIST). *Cancer Chemother Pharmacol* 74:883–898, 2014.

30. Vasen HF, Moslein G, Alonso A, et al: Guidelines for the clinical management of familial adenomatous polyposis (FAP). *Gut* 57:704–713, 2008.

31. Bilimoria KY, Bentrem DJ, Wayne JD, et al: Small bowel cancer in the United States: Changes in epidemiology, treatment, and survival over the last 20 years. *Ann Surg* 249:63–71, 2009.

32. Reid MD, Balci S, Saka B, et al: Neuroendocrine tumors of the pancreas: Current concepts and controversies. *Endocr Pathol* 25:65–79, 2014.

33. Rindi G, Petrone G, Inzani F: The 2010 WHO classification of digestive neuroendocrine neoplasms: A critical appraisal four years after its introduction. *Endocr Pathol* 25:186–192, 2014.

34. Castano JP, Sundin A, Maecke HR, et al: Gastrointestinal neuroendocrine tumors (NETs): New diagnostic and therapeutic challenges. *Cancer Metastasis Rev* 33:353–359, 2014.

35. Ilhan H, Fendler WP, Cyran CC, et al: Impact of ^{68}Ga-DOTATATE PET/CT on the surgical management of primary neuroendocrine tumors of the pancreas or ileum. *Ann Surg Oncol* 22:164–171, 2015.

36. Coan KE, Gray RJ, Schlinkert RT, et al: Metastatic carcinoid tumors—are we making the cut? *Am J Surg* 205:642–646, 2013.

37. Figueiredo MN, Maggiori L, Gaujoux S, et al: Surgery for small-bowel neuroendocrine tumors: Is there any benefit of the laparoscopic approach? *Surg Endosc* 28:1720–1726, 2014.

38. Toumpanakis C, Caplin ME: Update on the role of somatostatin analogs for the treatment of patients with gastroenteropancreatic neuroendocrine tumors. *Semin Oncol* 40:56–68, 2013.

39. Anthony L, Freda PU: From somatostatin to octreotide LAR: Evolution of a somatostatin analogue. *Curr Med Res Opin* 25:2989–2999, 2009.

40. Caplin ME, Pavel M, Cwikla JB, et al: Lanreotide in metastatic enteropancreatic neuroendocrine tumors. *N Engl J Med* 371:224–233, 2014.

41. Chan J, Kulke M: Targeting the mTOR signaling pathway in neuroendocrine tumors. *Curr Treat Options Oncol* 15:365–379, 2014.

42. Aparicio T, Zaanan A, Svrcek M, et al: Small bowel adenocarcinoma: Epidemiology, risk factors, diagnosis and treatment. *Dig Liver Dis* 46:97–104, 2014.

43. Thirunavukarasu P, Sathaiah M, Sukumar S, et al: Meckel's diverticulum—a high-risk region for malignancy in the

ileum. Insights from a population-based epidemiological study and implications in surgical management. *Ann Surg* 253:223–230, 2011.

44. Soltero MJ, Bill AH: The natural history of Meckel's diverticulum and its relation to incidental removal. A study of 202 cases of diseased Meckel's diverticulum found in King County, Washington, over a fifteen year period. *Am J Surg* 132:168–173, 1976.

45. Zani A, Eaton S, Rees CM, et al: Incidentally detected Meckel diverticulum: To resect or not to resect? *Ann Surg* 247:276–281, 2008.

46. Cullen JJ, Kelly KA, Moir CR, et al: Surgical management of Meckel's diverticulum. An epidemiologic, population-based study. *Ann Surg* 220:564–568, discussion 568–569, 1994.

47. Visschers RG, van Gemert WG, Winkens B, et al: Guided treatment improves outcome of patients with enterocutaneous fistulas. *World J Surg* 36:2341–2348, 2012.

48. Stacey R, Green JT: Radiation-induced small bowel disease: Latest developments and clinical guidance. *Ther Adv Chronic Dis* 5:15–29, 2014.

49. Jeppesen PB: Pharmacologic options for intestinal rehabilitation in patients with short bowel syndrome. *JPEN J Parenter Enteral Nutr* 38:45S–52S, 2014.

50. Tappenden KA: Pathophysiology of short bowel syndrome: Considerations of resected and residual anatomy. *JPEN J Parenter Enteral Nutr* 38:14S–22S, 2014.

50 CHAPTER

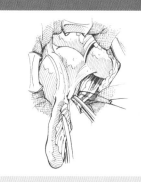

The Appendix

Bryan Richmond

第五十章　阑尾疾病

OUTLINE

Anatomy and Embryology
Appendicitis
Treatment of Appendicitis
Appendicitis in Special Populations
Neoplasms of the Appendix

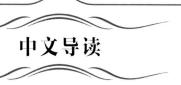

中文导读

本章共分5节：①解剖及胚胎学；②阑尾炎；③阑尾炎的治疗；④特殊人群阑尾炎；⑤阑尾肿瘤。

第一节主要讲述阑尾的解剖及胚胎发育相关基础知识，包括阑尾的胚胎发育起源、可能的免疫调节及肠道菌群调节功能、形态及解剖部位变异。特别介绍了阑尾解剖部位变异可能给阑尾炎带来不同的临床表现，给临床诊断及处理带来困扰。

第二节为本章的重点介绍内容。作者从医学史、病理生理学、病原学、鉴别诊断、临床表现、实验室检验、影像学检查等方面系统性介绍了阑尾炎这一临床常见疾病。"脐周向右下腹的转移性疼痛"为典型的阑尾炎主诉症状，体检阳性发现往往是"右下腹麦氏点压痛"。除了上述经典临床表现之外，阑尾炎还有各种不典型症状与体征。实验室检验及影像学检查也是确诊阑尾炎的重要工具，文中详细介绍了CT、彩超以及磁共振在阑尾炎诊断中的应用。

第三节作者首先以急性单纯性阑尾炎为例，介绍了阑尾切除的手术方式。然后，介绍了阑尾炎合并穿孔的处理原则；腹腔镜与开放式阑尾切除手术的优劣比较，认为腹腔镜手术优于开放式式。作者还对临床上较为难以处理的阑尾炎相关问题及争议话题进行了讨论及阐述，包括：阑尾炎的迟发症状及处理、术中阴性探查的处理原则、无并发症阑尾炎的非手术治疗、"慢性"阑尾炎、阑尾的"附带"切除（指在其他手术中顺带切除正常阑尾）等。

第四节主要介绍了特殊人群罹患阑尾炎时的临床特点及处理原则，包括妊娠合并阑尾炎、老年人阑尾炎及免疫缺陷合并阑尾炎。其中，重点介绍了妊娠合并阑尾炎的诊治。

第五节介绍阑尾肿瘤。阑尾肿瘤不多见，约有一半初诊为阑尾炎。最常见的阑尾肿瘤是阑尾类癌，阑尾腺癌相对少见。阑尾黏液性肿瘤是一种良性肿瘤，但是破裂之后处理棘手。

〔张　鹏〕

Please access ExpertConsult.com to view the corresponding videos for this chapter.

Appendicitis remains one of the most common diseases faced by the surgeon in practice. It is the most common urgent or emergent general surgical operation performed in the United States and is responsible for as many as 300,000 hospitalizations annually.[1] Although appendectomy is often the first "major" case performed by the young surgeon in training, few other operations will be learned that will have such a dramatic impact on the patient being treated.

It is estimated that as much as 6% to 7% of the general population will develop appendicitis during their lifetime, with the incidence peaking in the second decade of life.[2] Despite its high prevalence in Western countries, the diagnosis of acute appendicitis can be challenging and requires a high index of suspicion on the part of the examining surgeon to facilitate prompt treatment of this condition, thereby avoiding the substantial morbidity (and even mortality) associated with perforation. Appendicitis is much less common in underdeveloped countries, suggesting that elements of the Western diet, specifically a low-fiber, high-fat intake, may play a role in the development of the disease process.[3]

ANATOMY AND EMBRYOLOGY

The appendix is a midgut organ and is first identified at 8 weeks of gestation as a small outpouching of the cecum. As gestation progresses, the appendix becomes more elongated and tubular as the cecum rotates medially and becomes fixed in the right lower quadrant of the abdomen. The appendiceal mucosa is of the colonic type, with columnar epithelium, neuroendocrine cells, and mucin-producing goblet cells lining its tubular structure.[3] Lymphoid tissue is found in the submucosa of the appendix, leading some to hypothesize that the appendix may play a role in the immune system. In addition, evidence suggests that the appendix may serve as a reservoir of "good" intestinal bacteria and may aid in recolonization and maintenance of the normal colonic flora.[4] Consensus about this has not been achieved, however. Successful removal of the appendix has not been definitively demonstrated to have any known adverse sequelae.

As a midgut organ, the blood supply of the appendix is derived from the superior mesenteric artery. The ileocolic artery, one of the major named branches of the superior mesenteric artery, gives rise to the appendiceal artery, which courses through the *mesoappendix*. The mesoappendix also contains lymphatics of the appendix, which drain to the ileocecal nodes, along the blood supply from the superior mesenteric artery.[3,5]

The appendix is of variable size (5 to 35 cm in length) but averages 9 cm in length in adults. Its base can be reliably identified by defining the area of convergence of the taeniae at the tip of the cecum and then elevating the appendiceal base to define the course and position of the tip of the appendix, which is variable in location. The appendiceal tip may be found in a variety of locations, with the most common being retrocecal (but intraperitoneal) in approximately 60% of individuals, pelvic in 30%, and retroperitoneal in 7% to 10%. Agenesis of the appendix has been reported, as has duplication and even triplication.[3,5] Knowledge of these anatomic variations is important to the surgeon because the variable position of the appendiceal tip may account for differences in clinical presentation and in the location of the associated abdominal discomfort. For example, patients with a retroperitoneal appendix may present with back or flank pain, just as patients with the appendiceal tip in the midline pelvis may present with suprapubic pain. Both of these presentations may result in a delayed diagnosis as the symptoms are distinctly different from the classically described anterior right lower quadrant abdominal pain associated with appendiceal disease.

APPENDICITIS

History

The first appendectomy was reported in 1735 by a French Surgeon, Claudius Amyand, who identified and successfully removed the appendix of an 11-year-old boy that was found within an inguinal hernia sac and that had been perforated by a pin. Although autopsy findings consistent with perforated appendicitis appeared sporadically thereafter in the literature, the first formal description of the disease process, including the common clinical features and a recommendation for prompt surgical removal, was in 1886 by Reginald Heber Fitz of Harvard University.[3]

Notable advances in surgery for appendicitis include McBurney's description of his classic muscle-splitting incision and technique for removal of the appendix in 1894 and the description of the first laparoscopic appendectomy by Kurt Semm in 1982.[3] Laparoscopic appendectomy has become the preferred method for management of acute appendicitis among surgeons in the United States and may be accomplished using several (typically three) trocar sites or through single-incision laparoscopic surgical techniques. Finally, but of no less significance, was the development of broad-spectrum antibiotics, interventional radiologic techniques, and better surgical critical care strategies, all of which have resulted in substantial improvements in the care of patients with appendiceal perforation and its subsequent complications.

Pathophysiology and Bacteriology

Appendicitis is caused by luminal obstruction.[3] The appendix is vulnerable to this phenomenon because of its small luminal diameter in relation to its length. Obstruction of the proximal lumen of the appendix leads to elevated pressure in the distal portion because of ongoing mucus secretion and production of gas by bacteria within the lumen. With progressive distention of the appendix, the venous drainage becomes impaired, resulting in mucosal ischemia. With continued obstruction, full-thickness ischemia ensues, which ultimately leads to perforation. Bacterial overgrowth within the appendix results from bacterial stasis distal to the obstruction.[3] This is significant because this overgrowth results in the release of a larger bacterial inoculum in cases of perforated appendicitis (Table 50-1). The time from onset of obstruction to perforation is variable and may range anywhere from a few hours to a few days. The presentation after perforation is also variable. The most common sequela is the formation of an abscess in the periappendiceal region or pelvis. On occasion, however, free perforation occurs that results in diffuse peritonitis.[3]

Because the appendix is an outpouching of the cecum, the flora within the appendix is similar to that found within the colon. Infections associated with appendicitis should be considered polymicrobial, and antibiotic coverage should include agents that address the presence of both gram-negative bacteria and anaerobes. Common isolates include *Escherichia coli*, *Bacteroides fragilis*, enterococci, *Pseudomonas aeruginosa*, and others.[6] The choice and duration of antibiotic coverage and the controversies surrounding the need for cultures are discussed later in the chapter.

The causes of the luminal obstruction are many and varied. These most commonly include fecal stasis and fecaliths but may also include lymphoid hyperplasia, neoplasms, fruit and vegetable material, ingested barium, and parasites such as ascarids. Pain of appendicitis has both visceral and somatic components. Distention of the appendix is responsible for the initial vague abdominal pain (visceral) often experienced by the affected patient. The pain typically does not localize to the right lower quadrant until the tip becomes inflamed and irritates the adjacent parietal peritoneum (somatic) or perforation occurs, resulting in localized peritonitis.[3]

Differential Diagnosis

Appendicitis must be considered in every patient (who has not had an appendectomy) who presents with acute abdominal pain.[7] Knowledge of disease processes that may have similar presenting symptoms and signs is essential to avoid an unnecessary or incorrect operation. Consideration of the patient's age and gender may help narrow the list of possible diagnoses. In children, other

considerations include but are not limited to mesenteric adenitis (often seen after a recent viral illness), acute gastroenteritis, intussusception, Meckel's diverticulitis, inflammatory bowel disease, and (in males) testicular torsion. Nephrolithiasis and urinary tract infection may be manifested with right lower quadrant pain in either gender.[3]

In women of childbearing age, the differential diagnosis is expanded even further. Gynecologic problems may be mistaken for appendicitis and result in a higher negative appendectomy rate than in male patients of comparable age. These include ruptured ovarian cysts, *mittelschmerz* (midcycle pain occurring with ovulation), endometriosis, ovarian torsion, ectopic pregnancy, and pelvic inflammatory disease.[3,7]

Two other patient populations deserve mention. In the elderly, consideration must be given to acute diverticulitis and malignant disease as possible causes of lower abdominal pain. In the neutropenic patient, *typhlitis* (also known as neutropenic enterocolitis) should also be considered within the differential diagnosis. Appendicitis in these special populations is discussed later in the chapter.

Presentation
History

Patients presenting with acute appendicitis typically complain of vague abdominal pain that is most commonly periumbilical in origin and reflects the stimulation of visceral afferent pathways through the progressive distention of the appendix. Anorexia is often present, as is nausea with or without associated vomiting. Either diarrhea or constipation may be present as well. As the condition progresses and the appendiceal tip becomes inflamed, resulting in peritoneal irritation, the pain localizes to its classic location in the right lower quadrant. This phenomenon remains a reliable symptom of appendicitis[3,7] and should serve to further increase the clinician's index of suspicion for appendicitis (Fig. 50-1).

Whereas these symptoms represent the "classic" presentation of appendicitis, the clinician must be aware that the disease may be manifested in an atypical fashion. For example, patients with a retroperitoneal appendix may present in a more subacute manner, with flank or back pain, whereas patients with an appendiceal tip in the pelvis may have suprapubic pain suggestive of urinary tract infection.[3,7] We have on occasion encountered patients presenting with symptoms of small bowel obstruction who were found to be obstructed by multiple interloop abscesses as a consequence of unrecognized appendiceal perforation. Although cases such as these are less common than the typical presentation, knowledge of these variations is essential to maintain the necessary index of suspicion to permit a prompt and accurate diagnosis.

Physical Examination

Patients with appendicitis typically appear ill. They frequently lie still because of the presence of localized peritonitis, which makes any movement painful. Tachycardia and mild dehydration are often present to varying degrees. Fever is frequently present, ranging from low-grade temperature elevations ($<38.5°$ C) to more impressive elevations of body temperature, depending on the status of the disease process and the severity of the patient's inflammatory response. Absence of fever does not exclude a diagnosis of appendicitis.[1,3,7]

Abdominal examination typically reveals a quiet abdomen with tenderness and guarding on palpation of the right lower quadrant. The location of the tenderness is classically over McBurney point, which is located one-third the distance between the anterior supe-

TABLE 50-1 Bacteria Commonly Isolated in Perforated Appendicitis

TYPE OF BACTERIA	PATIENTS (%)
Anaerobic	
Bacteroides fragilis	80
Bacteroides thetaiotaomicron	61
Bilophila wadsworthia	55
Peptostreptococcus spp.	46
Aerobic	
Escherichia coli	77
Viridans streptococcus	43
Group D streptococcus	27
Pseudomonas aeruginosa	18

Adapted from Bennion RS, Thompson JE: Appendicitis. In Fry DE, editor: *Surgical infections*, Boston, 1995, Little, Brown, pp 241–250.

GENERAL APPROACH TO THE PATIENT WITH SUSPECTED APPENDICITIS

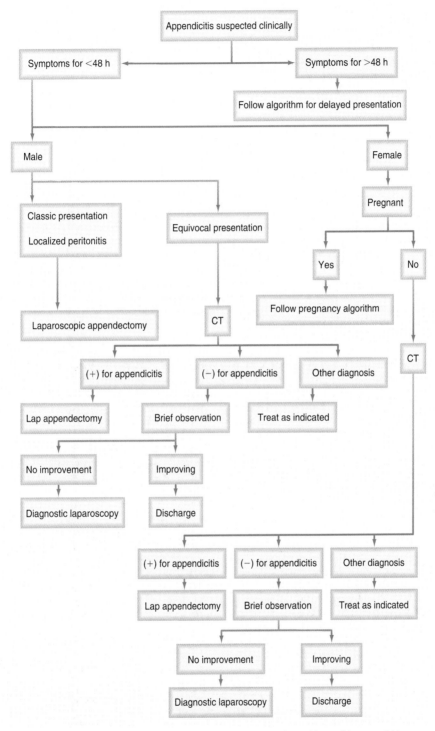

FIGURE 50-1 Suggested algorithm for the approach to the patient with possible appendicitis.

rior iliac spine and the umbilicus. The pain and tenderness are typically accompanied by localized peritonitis as evidenced by the presence of rebound tenderness. Diffuse peritonitis or abdominal wall rigidity due to involuntary spasm of the overlying abdominal wall musculature is strongly suggestive of perforation.[1,3]

A number of signs have been described to aid in the diagnosis of appendicitis. These include the Rovsing sign (the presence of right lower quadrant pain on palpation of the left lower quadrant), the obturator sign (right lower quadrant pain on internal rotation of the hip), and the psoas sign (pain with extension of the ipsilateral hip), among others.[1] Although these are of historical interest, it is important to realize that they are simply indicators of localized peritonitis rather than a diagnostic of a specific disease process. Still, they are useful maneuvers to perform in examining a patient with suspected appendicitis and are supportive of the diagnosis if it is suspected clinically.

Rectal examination findings are typically normal. However, a palpable mass or tenderness may be present if the appendiceal tip is located within the pelvis or if a pelvic abscess is present. In female patients, pelvic examination is important to exclude pelvic disease. However, cervical motion tenderness, a finding typically associated with pelvic inflammatory disease, may be present in appendicitis because of irritation of the pelvic organs from the adjacent inflammatory process.[3]

Laboratory Studies

Laboratory studies should be interpreted with caution in cases of suspected appendicitis and should be used to support the clinical picture rather than definitively to prove or to exclude the diagnosis. A leukocytosis, often with a "left shift" (a predominance of neutrophils and sometimes an increase in bands), is present in 90% of cases. A normal white blood cell count is found in 10% of cases, however, and it should not be used as an isolated test to exclude the presence of appendicitis.[8] Urinalysis is typically normal as well, although the finding of trace leukocyte esterase or pyuria is not unusual and is presumably due to the proximity of the inflamed appendix to the bladder or ureter. If the presentation is strongly suggestive of appendicitis, a "positive" urinalysis should not be used as an isolated test to refute the diagnosis. Pregnancy testing is mandatory in women of childbearing age. C-reactive protein has been demonstrated to be neither sensitive nor specific in diagnosing (or excluding) appendicitis.[1,8]

No symptom or sign has been demonstrated to be discriminatory and predictive of appendicitis.[1,8] The same may be said of laboratory tests, which are also weakly predictive when considered in isolation. Rather, it is the assessment of the collective body of information that allows more precise diagnosis.[1,8]

Imaging Studies

A variety of radiographic studies may be used to diagnose appendicitis. These consist of plain radiographs, computed tomography (CT) scanning, ultrasound (US), and magnetic resonance imaging (MRI).

Plain radiographs are frequently obtained in the emergency department setting for the evaluation of acute abdominal pain but lack both sensitivity and specificity for the diagnosis of appendicitis and are rarely helpful. Findings that may support the diagnosis include the presence of a calcified fecalith in the right lower quadrant, although this finding must be placed into the appropriate clinical context and is typically present in only 5% of cases.[9] Pneumoperitoneum, if present, should alert the clinician to other causes of a perforated viscus (such as a perforated ulcer or diverticulitis), as this is not typically observed in cases of appendicitis, even with perforation.

CT scanning is the most common imaging study to diagnose appendicitis and is highly effective and accurate.[9] Modern helical CT scans have the advantage of being operator independent and easy to interpret. CT has been shown to have a sensitivity of 90% to 100%, a specificity of 91% to 99%, a positive predictive value of 92% to 98%, and a negative predictive value of 95% to

100%.[9,10] The recommended imaging protocol from the Infectious Diseases Society of America (IDSA) and the Surgical Infection Society includes the intravenous administration of contrast material only. Oral and rectal administration of contrast material is not recommended.[11]

The diagnosis of appendicitis on CT is based on the appearance of a thickened, inflamed appendix with surrounding "stranding" indicative of inflammation. The appendix is typically more than 7 mm in diameter with a thickened, inflamed wall and mural enhancement or "target sign" (Fig. 50-2). Periappendiceal fluid or air is also highly suggestive of appendicitis and suggests perforation. In cases in which the appendix is not visualized, the absence of inflammatory findings on CT suggests that appendicitis is not present.[12] Although we do not recommend CT in cases in which appendicitis is strongly suspected on clinical grounds based on supportive history and physical and laboratory findings, published data do suggest that use of CT in equivocal cases does indeed reduce the negative appendectomy rate.[13]

US has been used for diagnosis of appendicitis since the 1980s. As US technology has become more advanced, so has its ability to visualize the appendix. The US probe is applied to the area of pain in the right lower quadrant, and graded compression is used to collapse normal surrounding bowel and to diminish the interference encountered with overlying bowel gas. The inflamed appendix is typically enlarged, immobile, and noncompressible (Fig. 50-3). If the appendix cannot be visualized, the study is inconclusive and cannot be relied on to guide treatment. Although US provides the advantage of avoiding ionizing radiation, the technology is highly operator dependent. The sensitivity is reported to range from 78% to 83%, whereas the specificity ranges from 83% to 93%. Its greatest utility appears to be in the evaluation of the pediatric or pregnant patient, in whom the associated radiation exposure from CT is undesirable.[9]

MRI is typically reserved for use in the pregnant patient; the study is performed without contrast agents. If it is obtained in a pregnant woman, the study should be noncontrasted. MRI offers excellent resolution and is accurate in diagnosing appendicitis. Criteria for MRI diagnosis include appendiceal enlargement (>7 mm), thickening (>2 mm), and the presence of inflammation.[9] The sensitivity of MRI is reported to be 100%, the specificity 98%, the positive predictive value 98%, and the negative predictive value 100%. MRI is also operator independent and offers highly reproducible results. Drawbacks associated with the use of MRI include its higher cost, motion artifact, greater difficulty in interpretation by nonradiologists who may have limited experience with the technology, and limited availability (especially in the after-hours emergency setting).[9]

TREATMENT OF APPENDICITIS

Acute Uncomplicated Appendicitis

The appropriate treatment of acute uncomplicated appendicitis is prompt appendectomy. The patient should undergo fluid resuscitation as indicated, and the intravenous administration of broad-spectrum antibiotics directed against gram-negative and anaerobic organisms should be initiated immediately.[11] Operation should proceed without undue delay.

For open appendectomy, the patient is placed in the supine position. The choice of incision is a matter of the surgeon's preference, whether it is an oblique muscle-splitting incision (McArthur-McBurney; Fig. 50-4), a transverse incision (Rockey-Davis), or a conservative midline incision. The cecum is grasped

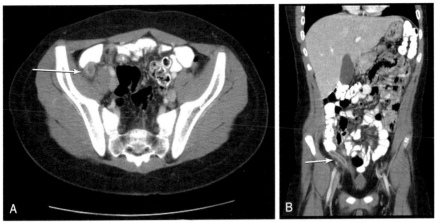

FIGURE 50-2 CT scan of the abdomen demonstrating classic findings of acute appendicitis. **A,** Sagittal view with *arrow* demonstrating a thickened, inflamed, and fluid-filled appendix (target sign). **B,** Coronal view of same patient. The *arrow* points to the thickened, elongated appendix with periappendiceal fat stranding and fluid around the appendiceal tip.

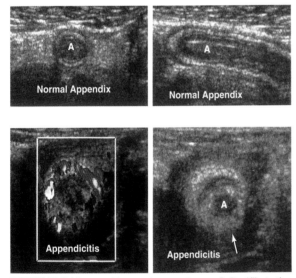

FIGURE 50-3 Ultrasound image of a normal appendix *(top)* illustrating the thin wall in coronal *(left)* and longitudinal *(right)* planes. In appendicitis, there is distention and wall thickening *(bottom, right),* and blood flow is increased, leading to the so-called ring of fire appearance. *A,* Appendix.

working ports are then placed, typically in the left lower quadrant and in either the suprapubic area or supraumbilical midline, based on the surgeon's preference. We have found it to be advantageous for both the surgeon and assistant to stand to the left side of the patient with the left arm tucked. This allows optimum triangulation of the camera and working instruments. Atraumatic graspers are used to elevate the appendix, and the mesoappendix is carefully divided using the harmonic scalpel. The base is then secured with endoloops and the appendix divided. Alternatively, the appendix may be divided with an endoscopic stapler. We prefer this technique in cases in which the entire appendix is friable because it allows the staple line to be placed slightly more proximally, on the edge of the healthy cecum, thereby reducing the risk of leakage from breakdown of a tenuous appendiceal stump. Retrieval of the appendix is accomplished by the use of a plastic retrieval bag. The pelvis is irrigated, the trocars are removed, and the wounds are closed. Laparoscopic appendectomy may also be performed with single-site laparoscopic surgical techniques as well, although this technique remains less commonly performed than the traditional multitrocar approach.

Antibiotic administration is not continued beyond a single preoperative dose.[11] Oral alimentation is begun immediately and advanced as tolerated. Discharge is usually possible the day after operation.

Perforated Appendicitis

The operative strategy for perforated appendicitis is similar to that for uncomplicated appendicitis with a few notable exceptions. First of all, the patient may require a more aggressive resuscitation before proceeding to the operating theater. As with uncomplicated appendicitis, antibiotic therapy should be initiated immediately on diagnosis.[11]

Both the open and laparoscopic approaches are acceptable for the treatment of perforated appendicitis. Although the technique of appendectomy for perforation is the same as for simple appendicitis, the level of difficulty encountered in removing a friable, gangrenous, perforated appendix can be a challenge to the most experienced surgeon and requires gentle meticulous handling of the friable appendix and inflamed periappendiceal tissues to avoid

by the taeniae and delivered into the wound, allowing visualization of the base of the appendix and delivery of the appendiceal tip. The mesoappendix is divided, and the appendix is crushed just above the base, ligated with an absorbable ligature, and divided. The stump is then either cauterized or inverted by a purse-string or Z suture technique. Finally, the abdomen is thoroughly irrigated and the wound closed in layers.

For laparoscopic appendectomy, the patient is placed in the supine position. The bladder is emptied by a straight catheter or by having the patient void immediately before the procedure. The abdomen is entered at the umbilicus, and the diagnosis is confirmed by inserting the laparoscope (Fig. 50-5). Two additional

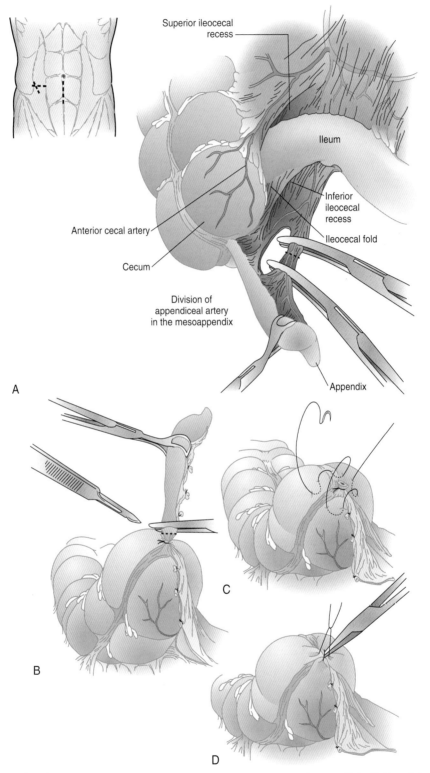

FIGURE 50-4 A, *Left,* Location of possible incisions for an open appendectomy. *Right,* Division of the mesoappendix. **B,** Ligation of the base and division of the appendix. **C,** Placement of purse-string suture or Z stitch. **D,** Inversion of the appendiceal stump. (From Ortega JM, Ricardo AE: Surgery of the appendix and colon. In Moody FG, editor: *Atlas of ambulatory surgery*, Philadelphia, 1999, WB Saunders.)

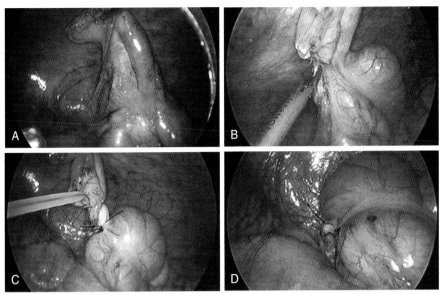

FIGURE 50-5 Laparoscopic appendectomy. **A,** Visualization and upward retraction of appendix. **B,** Division of mesoappendix using harmonic scalpel. **C,** Application of endoloops to appendix. Two loops are used to secure the base; a third loop is applied distally to avoid spillage of the luminal contents. The specimen is then divided between the endoloops. **D,** View of completed appendectomy after removal of the specimen. (*Note:* Depending on the surgeon's preference, an endoscopic stapling device may be used to divide the mesoappendix and appendix instead of the harmonic scalpel and endoloops.)

tissue injury. Cultures are not mandatory unless the patient has had exposure to a health care environment or has had recent exposure to antibiotic therapy because these factors increase the likelihood of encountering resistant bacteria. However, we routinely obtain them because they sometimes yield resistant bacteria and are helpful in tailoring the switch to oral therapy on discharge.[11] Once the appendix is successfully removed, careful attention should be given to the clearance of infectious material, including spilled fecal material or fecaliths, from the abdomen. This task may be accomplished by large-volume irrigation, with special attention given to the right lower quadrant and pelvis. Drains are not routinely placed unless a discrete abscess cavity is present. If an abscess cavity is present, a single closed suction Jackson-Pratt drain is placed within its base and left for several days. If an open technique was used, the skin and subcutaneous tissues are left open for 3 or 4 days to prevent development of wound infection, at which time the wound may be closed at the bedside with sutures, clips, or Steri-Strips, depending on the surgeon's preference.

Postoperatively, broad-spectrum antibiotics are continued for 4 to 7 days in accordance with IDSA guidelines.[11] If culture specimens were obtained, antibiotic therapy should be modified in accordance with the results. Nasogastric suction is not employed routinely but may be necessary if postoperative ileus develops. Oral alimentation is begun after return of bowel sounds and passage of flatus and advanced as tolerated. Once the patient is tolerating a diet, is afebrile, and has a normal white blood cell count, the patient may be discharged home.

If the patient develops fever, leukocytosis, pain, and delayed return of bowel function, the possibility of a postoperative abscess must be entertained. Abscess complicates perforated appendicitis in 10% to 20% of cases and represents the major source of morbidity related to perforation.[1,3] A CT scan with intravenous administration of a contrast agent is diagnostic and also allows simultaneous placement of a percutaneous drain within the abscess cavity.[9] If CT drainage is not technically possible because of the location of the abscess, laparoscopic, transrectal, or transvaginal drainage is an alternative.

Laparoscopic versus Open Appendectomy

The debate about the choice of open versus laparoscopic appendectomy for the treatment of appendicitis remains a major point of controversy among surgeons. Although no level I data exist to support one approach over another, a study published in 2010 examined this issue in detail. Ingraham and colleagues[14] analyzed results from 222 hospitals comparing laparoscopic versus open appendectomy using the American College of Surgeons National Surgical Quality Improvement Program. In all, 24,969 laparoscopic and 7714 open procedures were included in the analysis. Although the data were limited by the retrospective nature, the investigators observed that laparoscopic appendectomy was associated with lower risk of wound complications and deep surgical site infection in uncomplicated appendicitis. In complicated appendicitis, laparoscopic appendectomy was associated with fewer wound complications but a slightly higher incidence of intra-abdominal abscess. The overall conclusion, however, was that the laparoscopic approach was associated with an overall lower incidence of complications than the open procedure. The conclusions evident from a number of studies indicate that both approaches are acceptable and that the advantages with laparoscopy, although small, were a lower overall morbidity, reduced wound complications, reduced postoperative pain, and perhaps a slightly shorter recovery time. The slightly higher risk of intra-abdominal abscess formation after laparoscopic appendectomy in cases of complicated appendicitis was a negative aspect of laparoscopic appendectomy, although the authors acknowledged that this has not been observed in all studies.[15]

We prefer the laparoscopic approach for several reasons. Laparoscopy allows examination of the entire peritoneal space, making it exceptionally useful to exclude other intra-abdominal disease that may be manifested in a similar fashion, such as diverticulitis or tubo-ovarian abscess, whereas visualization of these structures would not be possible through a right lower quadrant incision. We find it to be technically simpler in most patients, particularly the obese, and have been impressed with our ability to discharge patients within several hours of the operation.

The debate about the superiority of laparoscopic versus open appendectomy will likely continue as a clearly superior choice has not been conclusively demonstrated. What does appear clear, however, is that regardless of the surgeon's preferred approach, the most important aspect of appendectomy is that it be done promptly and safely.

Delayed Presentation of Appendicitis

Patients may occasionally present several days to even weeks after the onset of appendicitis. In these cases, the treatment should be individualized on the basis of the nature of the presentation (Fig. 50-6). Although rare, a patient may present with diffuse peritonitis. More commonly, however, patients present with localized right lower quadrant pain and fever, with a history that is compatible with appendicitis. A mass may be palpable in children or thin patients. Immediate exploration and attempted appendectomy in these patients may result in substantial morbidity, including failure to identify the appendix, postoperative abscess or fistula, and unnecessary extension of the operation to include ileocecectomy, all due to the extreme induration and friability of the involved tissues. For this reason, in general, treatment for these patients is initially accomplished nonoperatively.[16-20] Fluid resuscitation is initiated, and broad-spectrum antibiotic therapy is initiated. A CT scan is obtained, and perforated appendicitis with a localized abscess or phlegmon is confirmed (Fig. 50-7). If a localized abscess is identified, CT-guided percutaneous drainage is performed for source control. The drainage catheter is typically left in place for 4 to 7 days, during which the patient is treated with antibiotic therapy and after which time it is removed. If CT-guided drainage is not technically feasible, operative drainage may be accomplished through transrectal or transvaginal approaches. Laparoscopic drainage is another option that we have found to be exceptionally useful. This technique is performed by visualizing the inflammatory mass with the laparoscope and then entering the abscess with a laparoscopic suction tip, evacuating the purulent material, and placing a drain within the residual abscess cavity. Postoperative management is identical to that of patients who are successfully drained percutaneously. If a periappendiceal phlegmon is present or if the amount of fluid present is not sufficient to drain, the patient may be treated with antibiotics alone, typically for 4 to 7 days also, as recommended by IDSA guidelines for treatment of intra-abdominal infection.[11]

Traditionally, after successful nonoperative treatment of complicated appendicitis, patients were advised to undergo removal of the appendix, a procedure known as interval appendectomy, several weeks to months later. This practice has been reexamined. The rationale for interval appendectomy is based on the potential for development of recurrent appendicitis and the subsequent risks associated with emergent removal or reperforation of the appendix. However, the actual risk of recurrent appendicitis appears to be small, 8% at 8 years in one study of 6400 pediatric patients.[21] The findings in this study as well as similar results reported by others have led them to conclude that interval appendectomy should be reserved only for patients who present with symptoms of recurrent appendicitis.[21,22] In addition, the presence of an appendicolith on CT has also been shown to be predictive of a higher risk of recurrent appendicitis and has been used as a justification to proceed with interval appendectomy in that subgroup of patients. This selective approach to interval appendectomy has also been demonstrated to be more cost-effective than its routine performance in all affected patients.[22]

A systematic review published by Hall and colleagues[23] examining the role of interval appendectomy found that the overall risk of recurrent appendicitis was 20.5%. All recurrences were seen within 3 years, and 80% of these occurred within 6 months. In addition, the morbidity of interval appendectomy was significant, with complications reported in 23 of the studies, for an overall rate of 3.4%. Other authors have reported significant associated morbidity with interval appendectomy as well, with rates as high as 18%.[24]

One argument favoring interval appendectomy in adults has been the observation by some investigators of a higher incidence of appendiceal neoplasms found in interval appendectomy specimens.[8,25-27] Also, perforated tumors of the cecum may be manifested in a similar fashion as perforated appendicitis.[28] For this reason, colonoscopy is recommended in all adult patients as routine follow-up after nonoperative management of complicated appendicitis.[29] To date, no large-scale randomized controlled trials examining the outcomes of patients who do or do not undergo interval appendectomy after successful nonoperative treatment have been conducted. For this reason, this issue is likely to remain controversial for some time.

The Normal-Appearing Appendix at Operation

In cases of "negative appendectomy," in which a normal appendix is identified at operation, there is controversy as to whether the appendix should be removed.[30,31] Before that particular issue is examined, it is important to emphasize the need to thoroughly evaluate the abdomen for other causes of pain severe enough to warrant an operation. The abdominal and pelvic organs should be assessed for any abnormalities. In our experience, this is most easily done through the laparoscopic approach, which we think is a major advantage of laparoscopy over an open approach. Note should be made of any free fluid as such a finding may suggest perforation. The terminal 60 cm of ileum should be examined for a Meckel's diverticulum and the serosa of the small bowel for any stigmata of Crohn's disease, such as inflammation, stricture formation, or the characteristic "creeping fat" appearance of the mesentery. Inspection of the ileal mesentery may reveal enlarged lymph nodes suggestive of mesenteric adenitis. The uterine adnexa should be examined for any evidence of tubo-ovarian or salpingeal disease, such as ovarian torsion, tubo-ovarian abscess, endometriosis, or ruptured ovarian cysts. The sigmoid colon should be examined for evidence of acute diverticulitis, especially in cases in which a redundant sigmoid colon is found in the right lower quadrant. If these are all normal, attention should be turned to the upper abdomen for examination of the gallbladder and duodenum. Inability to perform an adequate evaluation of the intra-abdominal organs or demonstration of disease of other organs requiring intervention may require conversion to a midline laparotomy if necessary.

We routinely remove the normal appendix for several reasons. First, many causes of right lower quadrant pain discussed before may be recurrent, such as pain from ruptured ovarian cysts or

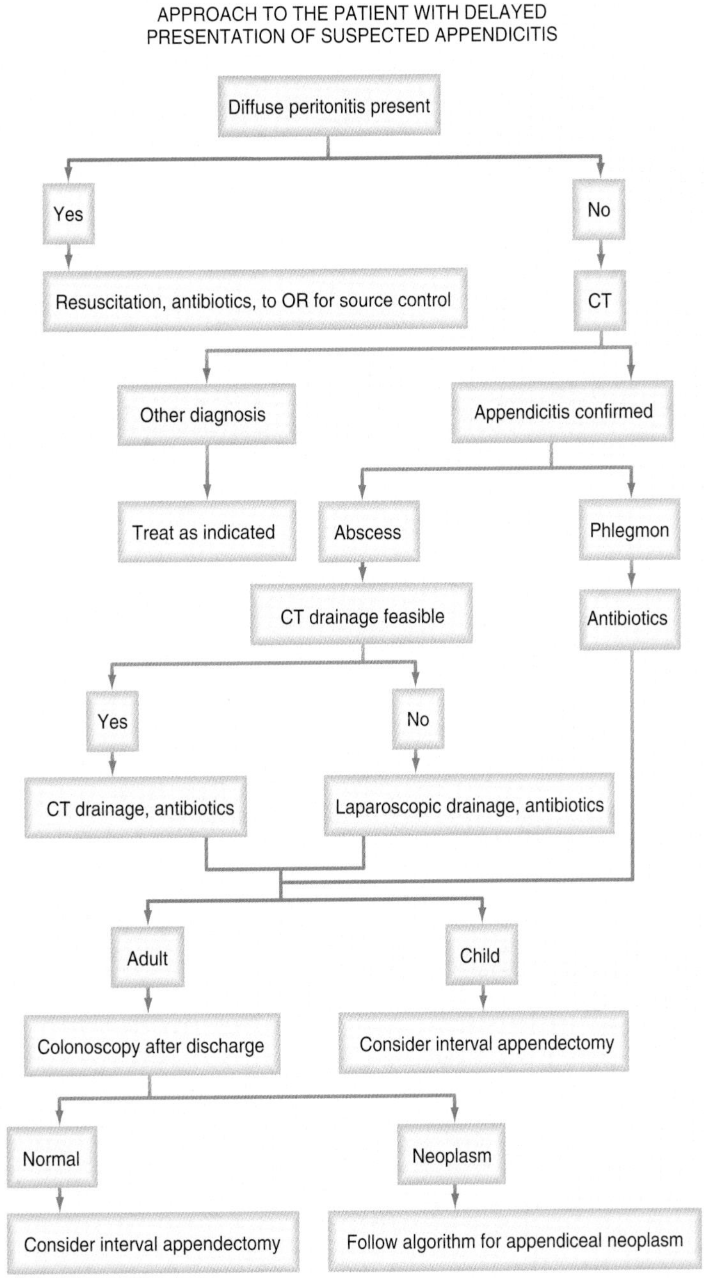

APPROACH TO THE PATIENT WITH DELAYED
PRESENTATION OF SUSPECTED APPENDICITIS

FIGURE 50-6 Suggested algorithm for managing the patient with delayed presentation of appendicitis.

mesenteric adenitis. Appendectomy is also advisable in cases of Crohn's disease when suggested by findings at operation, unless the base of the appendix and cecum are involved. In this scenario, appendectomy is deferred to avoid breakdown of the inflamed stump and subsequent fistula formation. In these clinical circumstances, appendectomy is advisable because it removes appendicitis from the differential diagnosis when the patient presents with recurrent right lower quadrant pain. In addition, abnormalities of the appendix not apparent on gross inspection at the time of operation are sometimes identified on pathologic examination.[30,31]

Nonoperative Treatment of Uncomplicated Appendicitis

Although prompt appendectomy is the standard of care, a number of studies have challenged this concept and have supported antibiotic therapy alone as a definitive treatment for acute uncomplicated appendicitis. Two meta-analyses analyzing the results of randomized controlled trials examining this issue concluded that nonoperative treatment was associated with a lower risk of complications (12% in the nonoperative group versus 18% in the appendectomy group; $P = .001$).[32,33] Appendectomy, however, outperformed the nonoperative group in overall treatment failure

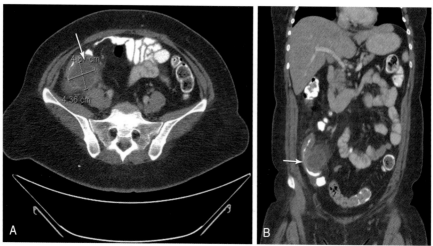

FIGURE 50-7 Sagittal **(A)** and coronal **(B)** CT images demonstrate an appendiceal abscess in a patient who presented with a 2-week history of abdominal pain and was found to have a palpable mass on examination. The *arrows* point to a periappendiceal abscess cavity. She was successfully managed with percutaneous drainage and antibiotic therapy.

rate (40% nonoperative versus 9% in the appendectomy group; $P < .001$). The authors concluded that antibiotic therapy was safe as a treatment for uncomplicated appendicitis but was associated with a significantly, perhaps prohibitively high failure rate compared with appendectomy.[32,33] For this reason, our practice is to reserve nonoperative therapy only for acute uncomplicated appendicitis for those patients in whom the operative risk is prohibitive. Failures of nonoperative therapy in these high-risk patients are then managed with adjunctive treatment measures, such as CT-guided drainage of periappendiceal abscesses.

"Chronic" Appendicitis as a Cause of Abdominal Pain

On occasion, patients will present with a history of recurrent right lower quadrant pain, and a surgical opinion will be sought as to the benefit of elective appendectomy for treatment of this condition. Modest epidemiologic data exist to suggest that appendicitis may spontaneously resolve, so it is conceivable that appendicitis may wax and wane in some patients.[1] In addition, some patients with pain are found to have a thickened appendix or an appendicolith on CT but have no evidence of a systemic illness or acute periappendiceal inflammation. In some cases, appendectomy will produce relief of symptoms, and in these cases, examination of the appendix will sometimes reveal findings consistent with chronic inflammation.[31,34] We will consider, on a case by case basis, elective appendectomy in cases in which the history is consistent with appendiceal disease and there is radiographic (CT) evidence of appendiceal disease.

More troubling, however, is the patient with pain in the absence of radiographic evidence of appendiceal disease. We typically pursue a multidisciplinary workup in these patients involving input from specialists in gastroenterology and gynecology as well as surgery. Appendectomy is typically not offered unless disease is demonstrated radiographically; however, if diagnostic laparoscopy is performed to investigate or to exclude other disease (typically by a gynecologist), we will typically perform appendectomy, an approach advocated by others.[35] We have found that as with the management of any chronic pain syndrome, manage-

ment of expectations is critical in caring for this very difficult group of patients.

Incidental Appendectomy

Incidental appendectomy is the term applied when a grossly normal appendix is removed at the time of an unrelated procedure, such as a hysterectomy, cholecystectomy, or sigmoid colectomy. Once commonly performed, incidental appendectomy has become a controversial procedure. The theoretical benefit is that of eliminating the patient's risk for development of appendicitis in the future, a concept that is thought to be most beneficial in patients younger than 35 years because of their greater lifetime risk for development of the disease compared with older patients.[16] Data suggesting that incidental appendectomy may be performed with no additional morbidity have been criticized for not having been properly risk adjusted. When these data were scrutinized further, Wen and coworkers actually demonstrated that incidental appendectomy was associated with an increase in both morbidity and mortality.[36] Other investigators have demonstrated that incidental appendectomy does not appear to be cost-effective as a preventive measure.[37] Finally, the recent finding that the appendix may actually have a role in the maintenance of healthy colonic flora makes the practice of incidental appendectomy even more controversial.[4] For these reasons, we advocate careful inspection of the appendix for abnormalities during abdominal operations as part of a thorough exploration but do not advocate appendectomy unless an abnormality is detected.

APPENDICITIS IN SPECIAL POPULATIONS

Appendicitis in the Pregnant Patient

Appendicitis remains the most common nonobstetric emergency in pregnancy and is consequently the most frequent reason for general surgical intervention in this group of patients.[38] The diagnosis of appendicitis in pregnancy presents a special challenge to the surgeon. As with all conditions in pregnancy, the surgeon must consider the welfare of two patients, the mother and fetus, when considering possible diagnoses, workup, and treatment (Fig. 50-8).

In pregnancy, appendicitis has a typical clinical presentation in only 50% to 60% of cases.[38] The common symptoms of early appendicitis, such as nausea and vomiting, are nonspecific and are also often associated with normal pregnancy. The normal febrile response to illness may be blunted in pregnancy. Also, the physical examination of the pregnant patient is difficult and is altered because of the effect of the gravid uterus and its displacement of the appendix to a more cephalad location within the abdomen. Lower quadrant pain in the second trimester produced by traction on the suspensory ligaments of the uterus, a phenomenon known as round ligament pain, is a common occurrence and further complicates the clinical picture further because 50% of cases of appendicitis occur in the second trimester. Finally, biochemical and laboratory indicators used to support the diagnosis of appendicitis in the nonpregnant patient are unreliable in pregnancy. For example, a mild physiologic leukocytosis of pregnancy is a normal finding. C-reactive protein levels may also be physiologically elevated in pregnancy. In addition, the surgeon must be concerned about the possibility of obstetric emergencies as a cause of abdominal pain, such as preterm labor, placental

abruption, or uterine rupture.[38-40] All of these factors have contributed to the high rate of negative appendectomy in pregnant patients, as high as 25% to 50%, when it is based on clinical presentation alone.[38]

The impact of appendicitis on the pregnant patient is severe. The risk of preterm labor has been shown to be 11% and fetal loss 6% with complicated appendicitis.[41] These data would appear to favor an aggressive, early approach to appendicitis in the pregnant patient. Complicating this approach, however, was the finding in the same series that negative appendectomy was also associated with preterm labor and fetal loss (10% and 4%, respectively). The lowest rates of preterm labor and fetal loss (6% and 2%, respectively) were seen in cases of uncomplicated appendicitis.[41] For these reasons, preoperative accuracy of diagnosis is crucial in the pregnant patient with suspected appendicitis.

Routine imaging is recommended in pregnant patients. The initial study of choice is US with graded compression.[42] It has the advantage of being safe, inexpensive, and readily available. In addition, US may provide information as to fetal well-being and obstetric causes of abdominal pain, such as placental abruption. Scanning patients in a left posterior oblique or left lateral decubitus position rather than in the traditional supine position has

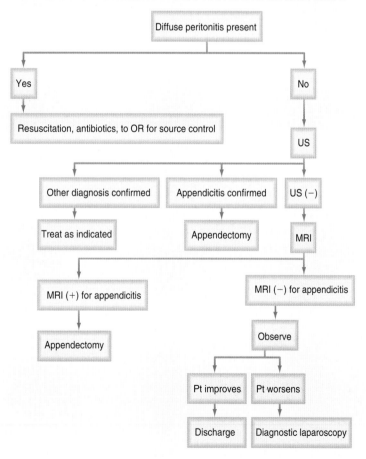

APPROACH TO THE PREGNANT PATIENT WITH SUSPECTED APPENDICITIS

FIGURE 50-8 Suggested algorithm for managing the pregnant patient with possible appendicitis.

been advocated to increase the chances of visualizing the appendix. The criteria for US diagnosis are the same as in the nonpregnant patient and have been discussed previously. Unfortunately, the sensitivity (78%) and specificity (83%) of US appear to be reduced in pregnancy because of the presence of the gravid uterus.[42]

If US examination findings are equivocal, MRI without gadolinium contrast, with its excellent soft tissue contrast resolution and lack of ionizing radiation, remains a safe alternative for confirmation or exclusion of appendicitis in the pregnant patient. In addition, the excellent sensitivity and specificity are preserved in the pregnant patient (Fig. 50-9). A patient in whom MRI findings are normal likely does not require appendectomy. Routine use of MRI in pregnant patients has been demonstrated to reduce the negative appendectomy rate by 47% without a significant increase in the perforation rate, and it has been shown to be a cost-effective study.[42] For these reasons, we encourage liberal use of MRI in pregnant patients suspected to have acute appendicitis without frank peritonitis. However, MRI may not be available in some institutions and may be available only on a limited basis or during limited times in other institutions. The decision about any delay in appendectomy to obtain an MRI study is a complex one and should be made using all available clinical and imaging data available because there are potentially severe consequences associated with both negative appendectomy and appendiceal perforation.

If US is inconclusive and MRI scanning is not immediately available, CT scanning for diagnosis of appendicitis in pregnancy has been reported. A study published in 2008 demonstrated that the use of CT was associated with an 8% negative appendectomy rate, compared with 54% by clinical assessment alone and 32% by clinical assessment combined with US. The authors concluded that CT should be used if US examination findings are equivocal and argued that the amount of radiation delivered during a limited CT examination is below the threshold required to induce fetal malformations and that most cases of appendicitis in pregnancy occur in the second or third trimester, when organogenesis in already complete.[42] Although protocols vary, if CT is used during pregnancy for equivocal cases, care should be taken to perform as limited a study as possible with avoidance of intravenous admin-

istration of contrast material. Further study is required before the routine use of CT can be accepted in this clinical scenario.

The choice of laparoscopic versus open technique for appendectomy in pregnancy also merits discussion. Current Society of American Gastrointestinal and Endoscopic Surgeons guidelines state that laparoscopic appendectomy is safe in pregnancy and is the standard of care in pregnant patients.[43] Two studies, both small and retrospective, have shown no increased fetal loss with laparoscopic appendectomy compared with open appendectomy. Another study reported higher preterm labor and overall complication rates in the open group compared with the laparoscopic group.[40] Others have reported higher fetal loss rates with laparoscopic appendectomy (5.6% versus 3.1%) compared with open appendectomy.[44] It is apparent that this debate would be best resolved through randomized controlled trials, which to date have not been performed.

Our institutional experience with laparoscopic appendectomy in pregnancy has been positive, making it our preferred approach to the pregnant patient. In our hands, we believe it allows an easier identification of the highly variable location of the appendix, a more expeditious removal, and an opportunity for more thorough evaluation of the abdomen for any associated pathologic process. We do routinely use an open access approach (Hasson technique) for initial trocar placement to avoid any chance of injury to the gravid uterus.

Appendicitis in the Elderly

Although it is not the peak age for its occurrence, appendicitis is not infrequently seen in elderly patients and should remain in the differential diagnoses of any elderly patient presenting with acute abdominal pain who has not had an appendectomy. The most important aspect is to realize the expanded differential diagnosis that must be considered in the elderly. Other possible diagnoses include but are not limited to acute diverticulitis (uncomplicated or complicated), malignant disease, intestinal ischemia, ischemic colitis, complicated urinary tract infection, and perforated ulcer. Appendicitis may also be manifested in an atypical manner, so a high index of suspicion must be maintained. A careful history and physical examination may aid in diagnosis, but this may have little value in certain circumstances, such as in patients with dementia or an altered mental status. The higher perforation rate in the elderly population, as high as 40% to 70%, combined with the frequent coexistence of comorbidities resulting in higher morbidity makes the diagnosis and treatment of appendicitis in the elderly a challenge, to say the least.[3]

When faced with an elderly patient with diffuse peritonitis, immediate laparotomy should be performed without unnecessary delay. When the pain is localized and peritonitis is absent, CT scanning of the abdomen should be performed to confirm the diagnosis and to evaluate for other pathologic changes. Laparoscopic appendectomy is safe in the elderly and is our procedure of choice in this group of patients. Exceptions include patients with severe cardiomyopathy, in whom we prefer the open approach to avoid the deleterious effects of pneumoperitoneum in patients with marginal cardiac function.[45] We have also successfully performed open appendectomy under spinal anesthesia in patients who are "pulmonary cripples" and in whom the risk of general surgery is prohibitive and likely to result in ventilator dependence.

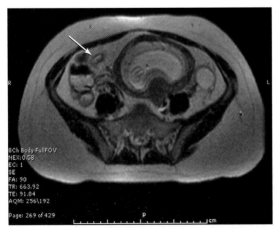

FIGURE 50-9 MRI scan with T1-weighted axial image of the abdomen in a gravid woman. The *arrow* highlights the thickened appendix. (From Parks NA, Schroeppel TJ: Update on imaging for acute appendicitis. *Surg Clin North Am* 91:141–154, 2011.)

Appendicitis in the Immunocompromised Patient

Appendicitis in the immunocompromised patient is managed in

the same manner as in the immunocompetent patient, with prompt appendectomy. The key in the evaluation of this population lies in maintenance of a high index of suspicion because the lack of the ability to mount an immune response may result in absence of fever, leukocytosis, and peritonitis. For this reason, early use of CT imaging is advisable. This allows confirmation of the diagnosis of appendicitis as well as the exclusion of diagnoses, such as neutropenic enterocolitis (typhlitis), that may be amenable to nonoperative treatment.[46]

NEOPLASMS OF THE APPENDIX

Neoplasms of the appendix, although rare, require appropriate treatment. An unanticipated appendiceal neoplasm may be encountered at any elective or emergency operation. It is estimated that 50% of appendiceal neoplasms present as appendicitis and are diagnosed on pathologic examination of the surgical specimen, but variable presentations have been reported. It is reported that appendiceal neoplasms are identified in 0.7% to 1.7% of pathology specimens. In addition, an appendiceal mass is sometimes noted as an incidental finding on abdominal CT (Fig. 50-10). The pathologic classification and biologic behavior of appendiceal neoplasms are diverse, which serves to make the classification, terminology, and treatment recommendations even more confusing.[1] Overall, appendiceal neoplasms are thought to account for 0.4% to 1% of all gastrointestinal malignant neoplasms.[1]

After appendectomy for presumed appendicitis, the incidence of unexpected findings in the surgical specimen is low. Still, if identified, appropriate counseling and treatment are essential. Carcinoid tumors are the most common tumor primary identified in the appendix.[16] These neoplasms arise from neuroendocrine cells from within the appendix and are detected in 0.3% to 0.9% of appendectomy specimens.[1] These are typically small, well-circumscribed lesions that are located within the more distal aspect of the appendix.

The biologic behavior of carcinoid tumors is highly variable. Size appears to be the best predictor of malignant behavior and metastatic potential, more so than histologic features, including lymphovascular invasion. Carcinoids smaller than 1 cm are typically thought to behave in a benign manner and are cured with appendectomy. Carcinoids larger than 2 cm are treated more aggressively, however. Other considerations include whether the carcinoid involves the base of the appendix or extends into the mesoappendix. Patients with carcinoids larger than 2 cm, with involvement of the base, or with extension to the mesoappendix should undergo right hemicolectomy with regional lymphadenectomy. For lesions between 1 and 2 cm in size, recommendations should be made after careful consideration of the individual tumor characteristics as metastases have been reported.[1,47]

Adenocarcinoma of the appendix is rare and occurs at a frequency of 0.08% to 0.1% of all appendectomies.[1] Treatment is identical to that of cecal adenocarcinoma and consists of right hemicolectomy with regional lymphadenectomy. Chemotherapy is also identical to that of adenocarcinoma of the colon, with adjuvant administration of 5-fluorouracil, leucovorin, and oxaliplatin (FOLFOX) to selected patients. FOLFOX has also been used in the neoadjuvant setting in patients with mucinous adenocarcinoma before cytoreductive (debulking) surgery.[48]

Mucinous tumors of the appendix are appendiceal tumors that are not frankly malignant but, if ruptured, can result in intraperitoneal spread and the development of pseudomyxoma peritonei (PMP). Classification and nomenclature of these lesions are confusing and not universally agreed on.[1] Because PMP results as a consequence of perforation and direct peritoneal seeding from the appendiceal contents, the surgeon should use great caution to avoid rupturing an intact appendix if mucocele or mucinous neoplasm is suspected on preoperative imaging or diagnosed intraoperatively. If PMP occurs, treatment by extensive cytoreductive surgery involving removal of any involved organs combined with heated intraperitoneal chemotherapy is typically employed[49] and is associated with long-term survival.

Although many appendiceal neoplasms are diagnosed on final pathologic examination, the mass will occasionally be visible at the time of appendectomy. An excellent algorithm for the management of the incidentally identified appendiceal mass was proposed by Wray and colleagues, and a modified version is provided for review (Fig. 50-11).[1] This algorithm is useful both in cases of appendicitis and in cases in which an appendiceal tumor is identified incidentally. The availability of frozen-section diagnosis may provide additional help with intraoperative decision making.

SELECTED REFERENCES

Ingraham AM, Cohen ME, Bilimoria KY, et al: Comparison of outcomes after laparoscopic versus open appendectomy for acute appendicitis at 222 ACS NSQIP hospitals. *Surgery* 148:625–635, discussion 635–637, 2010.

> *The authors provide one of the largest series to date, nearly 32,000 patients, comparing outcomes of laparoscopic versus open appendectomy using the ACS NSQIP database.*

McGory ML, Zingmond DS, Tillou A, et al: Negative appendectomy in pregnant women is associated with a substantial risk of fetal loss. *J Am Coll Surg* 205:534–540, 2007.

> *This article, which demonstrates that fetal loss is not only highest with appendiceal rupture but also increased with negative appendectomy, highlights the need for accurate diagnosis in the pregnant patient.*

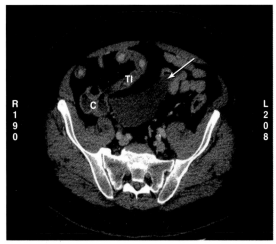

FIGURE 50-10 CT scan of the abdomen in a patient with a benign 10-cm mucocele. The axial image shows a distended fluid-filled mass medial to the appendix *(arrow)*, without associated inflammation. *C*, Cecum; *TI*, terminal ileum.

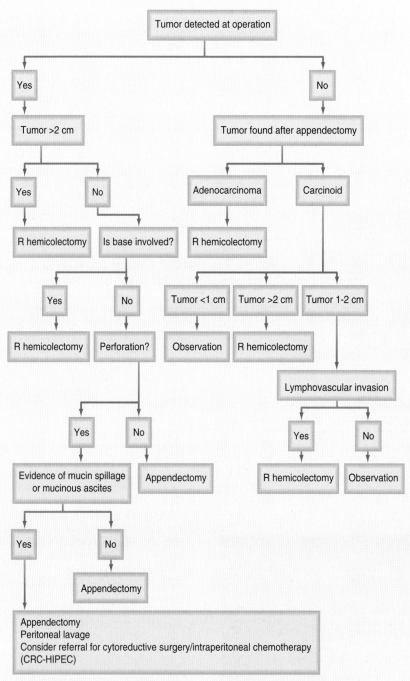

FIGURE 50-11 Suggested algorithm for managing the patient with an appendiceal neoplasm.

Parks NA, Schroeppel TJ: Update on imaging for acute appendicitis. *Surg Clin North Am* 91:141–154, 2011.

> The authors present a thorough, evidence-based review of the current available imaging studies used to diagnose appendiceal disease along with the clinical circumstances in which they are most useful.

Silen W: *Cope's early diagnosis of the acute abdomen*, ed 22, New York, 2010, Oxford University Press.

> This classic text, now in its 22nd edition, provides a masterful overview of the differential diagnoses and subtle historical findings of appendicitis and related disease. It is a timeless source of wisdom and is considered a "must read" by many surgeons.

Solomkin JS, Mazuski JE, Bradley JS, et al: Diagnosis and management of complicated intra-abdominal infection in adults and children: Guidelines by the Surgical Infection Society and the Infectious Diseases Society of America. *Clin Infect Dis* 50:133–164, 2010.

> This consensus statement from the IDSA and SIS provides evidence-based guidelines for the treatment of complicated intra-abdominal infections, including appendicitis.

Wray CJ, Kao LS, Millas SG, et al: Acute appendicitis: Controversies in diagnosis and management. *Curr Probl Surg* 50:54–86, 2013.

> This timely and well-written review article details some of the controversial issues relating to surgery of the appendix and includes an excellent overview of the treatment of appendiceal neoplasms.

REFERENCES

1. Wray CJ, Kao LS, Millas SG, et al: Acute appendicitis: Controversies in diagnosis and management. *Curr Probl Surg* 50:54–86, 2013.
2. Addiss DG, Shaffer N, Fowler BS, et al: The epidemiology of appendicitis and appendectomy in the United States. *Am J Epidemiol* 132:910–925, 1990.
3. Prystowsky JB, Pugh CM, Nagle AP: Current problems in surgery. Appendicitis. *Curr Probl Surg* 42:688–742, 2005.
4. Randal Bollinger R, Barbas AS, Bush EL, et al: Biofilms in the large bowel suggest an apparent function of the human vermiform appendix. *J Theor Biol* 249:826–831, 2007.
5. Deshmukh S, Verde F, Johnson PT, et al: Anatomical variants and pathologies of the vermix. *Emerg Radiol* 21:543–552, 2014.
6. Chen CY, Chen YC, Pu HN, et al: Bacteriology of acute appendicitis and its implication for the use of prophylactic antibiotics. *Surg Infect (Larchmt)* 13:383–390, 2012.
7. Silen W: *Cope's early diagnosis of the acute abdomen*, ed 22, New York, 2010, Oxford University Press.
8. Andersson RE: Meta-analysis of the clinical and laboratory diagnosis of appendicitis. *Br J Surg* 91:28–37, 2004.
9. Parks NA, Schroeppel TJ: Update on imaging for acute appendicitis. *Surg Clin North Am* 91:141–154, 2011.
10. Birnbaum BA, Wilson SR: Appendicitis at the millennium. *Radiology* 215:337–348, 2000.
11. Solomkin JS, Mazuski JE, Bradley JS, et al: Diagnosis and management of complicated intra-abdominal infection in adults and children: Guidelines by the Surgical Infection Society and the Infectious Diseases Society of America. *Clin Infect Dis* 50:133–164, 2010.
12. Brown MA: Imaging acute appendicitis. *Semin Ultrasound CT MR* 29:293–307, 2008.
13. Drake FT, Florence MG, Johnson MG, et al: Progress in the diagnosis of appendicitis: A report from Washington State's Surgical Care and Outcomes Assessment Program. *Ann Surg* 256:586–594, 2012.
14. Ingraham AM, Cohen ME, Bilimoria KY, et al: Comparison of outcomes after laparoscopic versus open appendectomy for acute appendicitis at 222 ACS NSQIP hospitals. *Surgery* 148:625–635, discussion 635-637, 2010.
15. Fleming FJ, Kim MJ, Messing S, et al: Balancing the risk of postoperative surgical infections: A multivariate analysis of factors associated with laparoscopic appendectomy from the NSQIP database. *Ann Surg* 252:895–900, 2010.
16. Teixeira PG, Demetriades D: Appendicitis: Changing perspectives. *Adv Surg* 47:119–140, 2013.
17. Deelder JD, Richir MC, Schoorl T, et al: How to treat an appendiceal inflammatory mass: Operatively or nonoperatively? *J Gastrointest Surg* 18:641–645, 2014.
18. Lugo JZ, Avgerinos DV, Lefkowitz AJ, et al: Can interval appendectomy be justified following conservative treatment of perforated acute appendicitis? *J Surg Res* 164:91–94, 2010.
19. Fawley J, Gollin G: Expanded utilization of nonoperative management for complicated appendicitis in children. *Langenbecks Arch Surg* 398:463–466, 2013.
20. Zhang HL, Bai YZ, Zhou X, et al: Nonoperative management of appendiceal phlegmon or abscess with an appendicolith in children. *J Gastrointest Surg* 17:766–770, 2013.
21. Puapong D, Lee SL, Haigh PI, et al: Routine interval appendectomy in children is not indicated. *J Pediatr Surg* 42:1500–1503, 2007.
22. Raval MV, Lautz T, Reynolds M, et al: Dollars and sense of interval appendectomy in children: A cost analysis. *J Pediatr Surg* 45:1817–1825, 2010.
23. Hall NJ, Jones CE, Eaton S, et al: Is interval appendicectomy justified after successful nonoperative treatment of an appendix mass in children? A systematic review. *J Pediatr Surg* 46:767–771, 2011.
24. Iqbal CW, Knott EM, Mortellaro VE, et al: Interval appendectomy after perforated appendicitis: What are the operative risks and luminal patency rates? *J Surg Res* 177:127–130, 2012.
25. Willemsen PJ, Hoorntje LE, Eddes EH, et al: The need for interval appendectomy after resolution of an appendiceal mass questioned. *Dig Surg* 19:216–220, discussion 221, 2002.
26. Carpenter SG, Chapital AB, Merritt MV, et al: Increased risk of neoplasm in appendicitis treated with interval appendectomy: Single-institution experience and literature review. *Am Surg* 78:339–343, 2012.

27. Furman MJ, Cahan M, Cohen P, et al: Increased risk of mucinous neoplasm of the appendix in adults undergoing interval appendectomy. *JAMA Surg* 148:703–706, 2013.

28. Gaetke-Udager K, Maturen KE, Hammer SG: Beyond acute appendicitis: Imaging and pathologic spectrum of appendiceal pathology. *Emerg Radiol* 21:535–542, 2014.

29. Lai HW, Loong CC, Chiu JH, et al: Interval appendectomy after conservative treatment of an appendiceal mass. *World J Surg* 30:352–357, 2006.

30. Garlipp B, Arlt G: [Laparoscopy for suspected appendicitis. Should an appendix that appears normal be removed?]. *Chirurg* 80:615–621, 2009.

31. Chiarugi M, Buccianti P, Decanini L, et al: "What you see is not what you get." A plea to remove a 'normal' appendix during diagnostic laparoscopy. *Acta Chir Belg* 101:243–245, 2001.

32. Varadhan KK, Neal KR, Lobo DN: Safety and efficacy of antibiotics compared with appendicectomy for treatment of uncomplicated acute appendicitis: Meta-analysis of randomised controlled trials. *BMJ* 344:e2156, 2012.

33. Mason RJ, Moazzez A, Sohn H, et al: Meta-analysis of randomized trials comparing antibiotic therapy with appendectomy for acute uncomplicated (no abscess or phlegmon) appendicitis. *Surg Infect (Larchmt)* 13:74–84, 2012.

34. Giuliano V, Giuliano C, Pinto F, et al: Chronic appendicitis "syndrome" manifested by an appendicolith and thickened appendix presenting as chronic right lower abdominal pain in adults. *Emerg Radiol* 12:96–98, 2006.

35. Teli B, Ravishankar N, Harish S, et al: Role of elective laparoscopic appendicectomy for chronic right lower quadrant pain. *Indian J Surg* 75:352–355, 2013.

36. Wen SW, Hernandez R, Naylor CD: Pitfalls in nonrandomized outcomes studies. The case of incidental appendectomy with open cholecystectomy. *JAMA* 274:1687–1691, 1995.

37. Wang HT, Sax HC: Incidental appendectomy in the era of managed care and laparoscopy. *J Am Coll Surg* 192:182–188, 2001.

38. Brown JJ, Wilson C, Coleman S, et al: Appendicitis in pregnancy: An ongoing diagnostic dilemma. *Colorectal Dis* 11:116–122, 2009.

39. Flexer SM, Tabib N, Peter MB: Suspected appendicitis in pregnancy. *Surgeon* 12:82–86, 2014.

40. Peled Y, Hiersch L, Khalpari O, et al: Appendectomy during pregnancy—is pregnancy outcome depending by operation technique? *J Matern Fetal Neonatal Med* 27:365–367, 2014.

41. McGory ML, Zingmond DS, Tillou A, et al: Negative appendectomy in pregnant women is associated with a substantial risk of fetal loss. *J Am Coll Surg* 205:534–540, 2007.

42. Khandelwal A, Fasih N, Kielar A: Imaging of acute abdomen in pregnancy. *Radiol Clin North Am* 51:1005–1022, 2013.

43. Korndorffer JR, Jr, Fellinger E, Reed W: SAGES guideline for laparoscopic appendectomy. *Surg Endosc* 24:757–761, 2010.

44. Walsh CA, Tang T, Walsh SR: Laparoscopic versus open appendicectomy in pregnancy: A systematic review. *Int J Surg* 6:339–344, 2008.

45. Richmond BK, Thalheimer L: Laparoscopy associated mesenteric vascular complications. *Am Surg* 76:1177–1184, 2010.

46. Hernandez-Ocasio F, Palermo-Garofalo CA, Colon M, et al: Right lower quadrant abdominal pain in an immunocompromised patient: Importance for an urgent diagnosis and treatment. *Bol Asoc Med P R* 103:51–53, 2011.

47. Boudreaux JP, Klimstra DS, Hassan MM, et al: The NANETS consensus guideline for the diagnosis and management of neuroendocrine tumors: Well-differentiated neuroendocrine tumors of the jejunum, ileum, appendix, and cecum. *Pancreas* 39:753–766, 2010.

48. Sugarbaker PH, Bijelic L, Chang D, et al: Neoadjuvant FOLFOX chemotherapy in 34 consecutive patients with mucinous peritoneal carcinomatosis of appendiceal origin. *J Surg Oncol* 102:576–581, 2010.

49. Wagner PL, Austin F, Maduekwe U, et al: Extensive cytoreductive surgery for appendiceal carcinomatosis: Morbidity, mortality, and survival. *Ann Surg Oncol* 20:1056–1062, 2013.

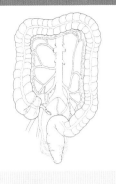

CHAPTER 51

Colon and Rectum

Najjia N. Mahmoud, Joshua I.S. Bleier, Cary B. Aarons,
E. Carter Paulson, Skandan Shanmugan, Robert D. Fry

第五十一章 结直肠疾病

中文导读

本章共分12节：①结肠、直肠的胚胎学；②结肠、直肠和盆底解剖；③结肠生理学；④术前肠道准备；⑤憩室性疾病；⑥结肠扭转；⑦大肠梗阻和假性肠梗阻；⑧炎症性肠病；⑨感染性结肠炎；⑩结肠缺血性疾病；⑪结直肠肿瘤；⑫盆底疾病和便秘。

第一节描述了结肠及直肠在胚胎形成过程中的起源及发育过程。

第二节分别介绍了结肠、直肠、直肠旁筋膜、盆底的相关解剖，同时对于相关的动脉血供、静脉和淋巴回流，以及神经支配进行阐述。

第三节从营养物质的再循环，结肠的吸收、分泌、运动、粪便形成、排泄这几个方面进行介绍。

第四节分别对肠道准备的意义、机械性肠道准备的方式、肠道抗生素的使用等方面进行阐述。

第五节介绍了憩室的发病机制，针对非复杂性憩室炎以及复杂性憩室炎进行了详细讲述。

第六节是结肠扭转的内容，从发病机制、检查、治疗选择上进行了讲解。

第七节是关于大肠梗阻和假性肠梗阻的内容，将梗阻划分为动力性（机械性）和非动力性（假性梗阻），并从这两个方面进行了介绍。

第八节是炎症性肠病，这是本章的重点内容之一，分别从溃疡性结肠炎和克罗恩结肠炎两大块进行介绍，从各自的流行病学、病因学、组织学、病理学特征、临床表现、诊断、药物治疗、手术指征以及手术方式选择上进行详细阐述。

第九节介绍了感染性结肠炎不同致病菌的特点、

诊断要点及治疗方案。

　　第十节重点介绍结肠缺血的病因、诊断方式以及手术适应证。

　　第十一节是结直肠肿瘤，这是本章的重点，首先从遗传学上分类描述相关癌基因及抑癌基因，阐述了结直肠癌的起源及发生发展，区分了遗传性癌综合征和散发性结直肠癌；从病因、诊断方法、分期方法、手术方式、手术范围、术后治疗以及随访等方面进行

了系统描述，特别针对直肠肿瘤的局部切除、经肛门手术方式以及选择指征进行了介绍。最后阐述的还包括了结直肠癌的预防和筛查的内容。

　　第十二节从诊断、检查、评估开始，介绍了盆底疾病和便秘等内容，重点介绍了直肠脱垂、内脱垂、孤立性直肠溃疡综合征、直肠前膨出、便秘等疾病的特点以及治疗方法。

〔曹志新〕

EMBRYOLOGY OF THE COLON AND RECTUM

No comprehensive discussion of colorectal anatomy is complete without a thorough understanding of the genesis of the gastrointestinal (GI) tract. Knowledge of the developmental anatomy of the foregut, midgut, and hindgut establishes a context in which to consider mature structural and functional anatomic relationships.

The endodermal roof of the yolk sac gives rise to the primitive gut tube. At the beginning of the third week of development, the gut tube is divided into three regions; the midgut, which opens ventrally, is positioned between the foregut in the head fold and the hindgut in the tail fold. Development progresses through the stages of physiologic herniation, return to the abdomen, and fixation. The acquisition of length and the formation of dedicated blood and lymphatic supplies take place during this time (Fig. 51-1).

Foregut-derived structures end at the second portion of the duodenum and rely on the celiac artery for blood supply. The midgut, extending from the duodenal ampulla to the distal transverse colon, is based on the superior mesenteric artery (SMA). The distal third of the transverse colon, descending colon, and rectum evolve from the hindgut fold and are supplied by the inferior mesenteric artery (IMA). Venous and lymphatic channels mirror their arterial counterparts and follow the same embryologic divisions. At the dentate line, endoderm-derived tissues fuse with the ectoderm-derived proctodeum, or ingrowth from the anal pit.

Distal rectal development is complex. The cloaca is a specialized area of the primitive distal rectum composed of endoderm- and ectoderm-derived tissues. This area is incorporated into the anal transition zone, which surrounds the dentate line in the adult. The cloaca exists in a continuum with the hindgut, but at approximately the sixth week, it begins to divide and to differentiate into anterior urogenital and posterior anal and sphincter elements. Simultaneously, the urogenital and GI tracts are separated by caudal migration of the urogenital septum. During the tenth week of development, the external anal sphincter is formed from the posterior cloaca as the descent of the urogenital septum becomes complete. The internal anal sphincter is formed by the twelfth week from enlarged circular muscle layers of the rectum.

ANATOMY OF THE COLON, RECTUM, AND PELVIC FLOOR

The colon and rectum constitute a tube of variable diameter approximately 150 cm in length. The terminal ileum empties into the cecum through a thickened, nipple-shaped invagination, the ileocecal valve. The cecum is a capacious sac-like segment of the proximal colon, with an average diameter of 7.5 cm and length of 10 cm. Although it is distensible, acute dilation of the cecum to a diameter of more than 12 cm, which can be measured by a plain abdominal radiograph, can result in ischemic necrosis and perforation of the bowel wall. Surgical intervention may be required when this degree of cecal distention is caused by obstruction or pseudo-obstruction (Fig. 51-2).

The appendix extends from the cecum approximately 3 cm below the ileocecal valve as a blind-ending elongated tube, 8 to 10 cm in length. The proximal appendix is fairly constant in location, whereas the end can be located in a wide variety of positions relative to the cecum and terminal ileum. Most commonly, it is retrocecal (65%), followed by pelvic (31%), subcecal (2.3%), preileal (1.0%), and retroileal (0.4%). Clinically, the appendix is found at the convergence of the taeniae coli. Another clinical aid useful for detecting the location of the appendix through a small abdominal incision is the identification of the fold of Treves, the only antimesenteric epiploic appendage normally found on the small intestine, marking the junction of the ileum and cecum.

The ascending colon, approximately 15 cm in length, runs upward toward the liver on the right side; like the descending colon, the posterior surface is fixed against the retroperitoneum, whereas the lateral and anterior surfaces are true intraperitoneal structures. The white line of Toldt represents the fusion of the mesentery with the posterior peritoneum. This subtle peritoneal landmark serves as a guide for the surgeon for mobilizing the colon and mesentery from the retroperitoneum.

The transverse colon is approximately 45 cm in length. Hanging between fixed positions at the hepatic and splenic flexures, it is completely invested in visceral peritoneum. The nephrocolic ligament secures the hepatic flexure and directly overlies the right kidney, duodenum, and porta hepatis. The phrenocolic ligament lies ventral to the spleen and fixes the splenic flexure in the left upper quadrant. The angle of the splenic flexure is higher,

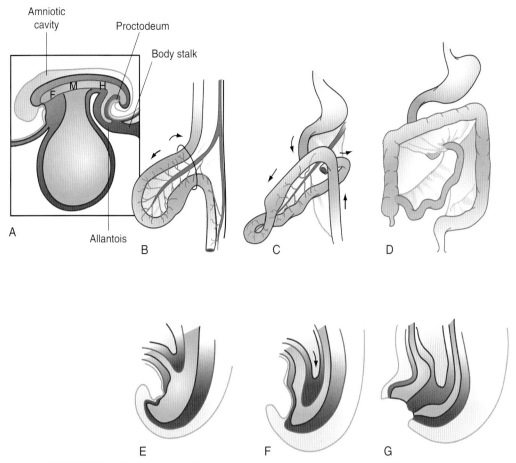

FIGURE 51-1 At the third week of development, the primitive tube can be divided into three regions **(A)**: the foregut (F) in the head fold, the hindgut (H) with its ventral allantoic outgrowth in the smaller tail fold, and the midgut (M) between these two portions. Stages of development of the midgut are physiologic herniation **(B),** return to the abdomen **(C),** and fixation **(D).** At the sixth week, the urogenital septum migrates caudally **(E)** and separates the intestinal and urogenital tracts **(F, G).** (From Corman ML, editor: *Colon and rectal surgery,* ed 4, Philadelphia, 1998, Lippincott-Raven, p 2.)

more acute, and more deeply situated than that of the hepatic flexure. The splenic flexure is typically approached by dissecting the descending colon along the line of Toldt from below and then entering the lesser sac by reflecting the omentum from the transverse colon. This maneuver allows mobilization of the flexure to be achieved, with minimal traction required for exposure. Attached to the superior aspect of the transverse colon is the greater omentum, a fused double layer of visceral and parietal peritoneum (four total layers) that contains variable amounts of stored fat. Clinically, it is useful in preventing adhesions between surgical abdominal wounds and underlying bowel and is often used to cover intraperitoneal contents as incisions are closed. The omentum can be mobilized and placed between the rectum and vagina after repair of a high rectovaginal fistula or used to fill the pelvic and perineal space left after excision of the rectum. The living tissue of the greater omentum makes a good patch in difficult situations, such as treatment of a perforated duodenum, when closure of inflamed and friable tissues is impossible or ill-advised.

The descending colon lies ventral to the left kidney and extends downward from the splenic flexure for approximately 25 cm. It is smaller in diameter than the ascending colon. At the level of the pelvic brim, there is a transition between the relatively thin-walled, fixed, descending colon and the thicker, mobile sigmoid colon. The sigmoid colon varies in length from 15 to 50 cm (average, 38 cm) and is very mobile. It is a small-diameter, muscular tube on a long floppy mesentery that often forms an omega loop in the pelvis. The mesosigmoid is frequently attached to the left pelvic sidewall, producing a small recess in the mesentery known as the intersigmoid fossa. This mesenteric fold is a surgical landmark for the underlying left ureter.

The rectum, along with the sigmoid colon, serves as a fecal reservoir. There is some controversy about the definition of the proximal and distal extent of the rectum. Some consider the rectosigmoid junction to be at the level of the sacral promontory; others consider it to be the point at which the taeniae converge. Anatomists consider the dentate line the distal extent of the rectum, whereas surgeons typically view this union of columnar

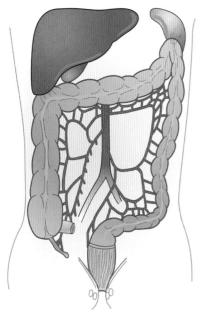

FIGURE 51-2 Anatomy of the colon and rectum, coronal view. The diameter of the right colon is larger than the diameter of the left side. Note the higher location of the splenic flexure compared with the hepatic flexure and the extraperitoneal location of the rectum.

and squamous epithelium as existing within the anal canal and consider the end of the rectum to be the proximal border of the anal sphincter complex. The rectum is 12 to 15 cm in length and lacks taeniae coli or epiploic appendices. It occupies the curve of the sacrum in the true pelvis, and the posterior surface is almost completely extraperitoneal in that it is adherent to presacral soft tissues and thus is outside the peritoneal cavity. The anterior surface of the proximal third of the rectum is covered by visceral peritoneum. The peritoneal reflection is 7 to 9 cm from the anal verge in men and 5 to 7.5 cm in women. This anterior peritoneal-ized space is called the pouch of Douglas, pelvic cul-de-sac, or rectouterine pouch and may serve as the site of so-called drop metastases from visceral tumors. These peritoneal metastases can form a mass in the cul-de-sac (called Blumer's shelf) that can be detected by a digital rectal examination.

The rectum possesses three involutions or curves known as the valves of Houston. The middle valve folds to the left, and the proximal and distal valves fold to the right. These valves are more properly called folds because they have no specific function as impediments to flow. They are lost after full surgical mobilization of the rectum, a maneuver that may provide approximately 5 cm of additional length to the rectum, greatly facilitating the surgeon's ability to fashion an anastomosis deep in the pelvis.

The posterior aspect of the rectum is invested with a thick, closely applied mesorectum. A thin layer of investing fascia (fascia propria) coats the mesorectum and represents a distinct layer from the presacral fascia against which it lies. During proctectomy for rectal cancer, mobilization and dissection of the rectum proceed between the presacral fascia and fascia propria. Total mesorectal excision is a well-described oncologic maneuver that makes good use of the tissue planes investing the rectum to achieve a relatively bloodless rectal and mesorectal dissection. The lymphatics are contained within the mesorectum, and total mesorectal excision adheres to the basic surgical oncologic principle of removal of the

cancer in continuity with its blood and lymphatic supplies. Resection of the rectum by this technique, and based on a thorough understanding of anatomy, has been shown to reduce markedly the incidence of subsequent local recurrence of rectal cancer.

Pararectal Fascia

The endopelvic fascia is a thick layer of parietal peritoneum that lines the walls and floor of the pelvis. The portion that is closely applied to the periosteum of the anterior sacrum is the presacral fascia. The fascia propria of the rectum is a thin condensation of the endopelvic fascia that forms an envelope around the mesorectum and continues distally to help form the lateral rectal stalks. The lateral rectal stalks or ligaments are actually anterolateral structures containing the middle rectal artery. The stalks reside close to the mixed autonomic nerves, containing sympathetic and parasympathetic nerves, and division of these structures close to the pelvic sidewall may injure these nerves, resulting in impotence and bladder dysfunction (Fig. 51-3).

The rectosacral fascia, or Waldeyer fascia, is a thick condensation of endopelvic fascia connecting the presacral fascia to the fascia propria at the level of S4 that extends to the anorectal ring. Waldeyer fascia is an important surgical landmark, and its division during dissection from an abdominal approach provides entry to the deep retrorectal pelvis. Dissection between the fascia propria and presacral fascia follows the principles of surgical oncology and minimizes the risk for vascular or neural injuries. Disruption of the presacral fascia may lead to injury of the basivertebral venous plexus, resulting in massive hemorrhage. Disruption of the fascia propria during an operation for rectal cancer may significantly increase the incidence of subsequent recurrence of cancer in the pelvis if mesorectum is then left behind.

Pelvic Floor

The muscles of the pelvic floor, like those of the anal sphincter mechanism, arise from the primitive cloaca. The pelvic floor, or diaphragm, consists of the pubococcygeus, iliococcygeus, and puborectalis, a group of muscles that together form the levator ani. The pelvic diaphragm resides between the sacrum, obturator fascia, ischial spines, and pubis. It forms a strong floor that supports the pelvic organs and, with the external anal sphincter, regulates defecation. The levator hiatus is an opening between the decussating fibers of the pubococcygeus that allows egress of the anal canal, urethra, and dorsal vein in men and the anal canal, urethra, and vagina in women. The puborectalis is a strong, U-shaped sling of striated muscle coursing around the rectum just above the level of the anal sphincters. Relaxation of the puborectalis straightens the anorectal angle and permits descent of feces; contraction produces the opposite effect. The puborectalis is in a state of continual contraction, a factor vital to the maintenance of continence. Puborectalis dysfunction is an important cause of defecation disorders. The pubococcygeus and iliococcygeus most likely participate in continence by applying lateral pressure to narrow the levator hiatus (Figs. 51-4 and 51-5).

Arterial Supply and Venous and Lymphatic Drainage

Knowledge of the embryologic development of the intestinal tract provides an excellent foundation for understanding the anatomic blood supply. The foregut is supplied by the celiac artery, the midgut by the SMA, and the hindgut by the IMA (Figs. 51-6 and 51-7). Anatomic redundancy confers survival advantages, and in the intestinal tract, this feature is provided by extensive communication between the major arteries and collateral blood supply

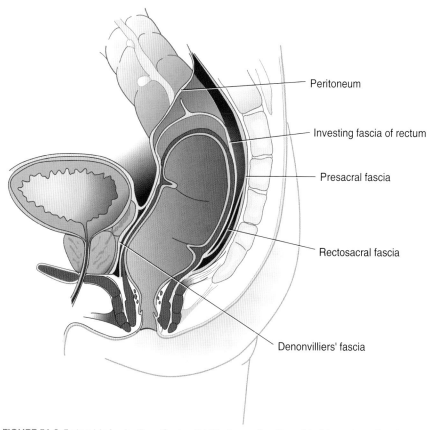

FIGURE 51-3 Endopelvic fascia. (From Gordon PH, Nivatvongs S, editors: *Principles and practice of surgery for the colon, rectum and anus*, ed 2, St. Louis, 1999, Quality Medical Publishing, p 10.)

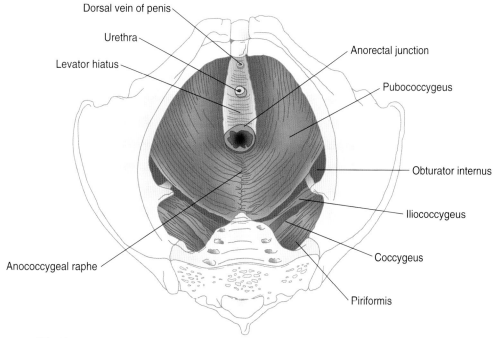

FIGURE 51-4 Levator muscles. (From Gordon PH, Nivatvongs S, editors: *Principles and practice of surgery for the colon, rectum and anus*, ed 2, St. Louis, 1999, Quality Medical Publishing, p 18.)

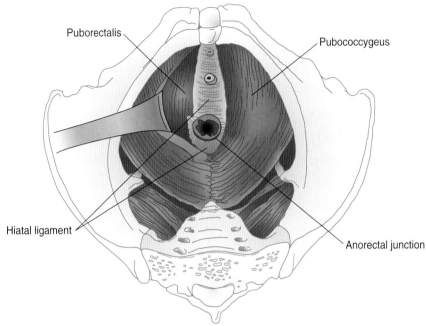

Puborectalis

Pubococcygeus

Hiatal ligament

Anorectal junction

FIGURE 51-5 Hiatal ligament. (From Gordon PH, Nivatvongs S, editors: *Principles and practice of surgery for the colon, rectum and anus*, ed 2, St. Louis, 1999, Quality Medical Publishing, p 18.)

(Fig. 51-8). The territory of the SMA ends at the distal portion of the transverse colon, and that of the IMA begins in the region of the splenic flexure. A large collateral vessel, the marginal artery, connects these two circulations and forms a continuous arcade along the mesenteric border of the colon. Vasa recta from this artery branch off at short intervals and supply the bowel wall directly (Fig. 51-9). The SMA supplies the entire small bowel, giving off 12 to 20 jejunal and ileal branches to the left and up to three main colonic branches to the right. The ileocolic artery is the most constant of these branches; it supplies the terminal ileum, cecum, and appendix. The right colic artery is absent in 2% to 18% of specimens; when present, it may arise directly from the SMA or as a branch of the ileocolic or middle colic artery. It supplies the ascending colon and hepatic flexure and communicates with the middle colic artery through collateral marginal artery arcades. The middle colic artery is a proximal branch of the SMA. It generally divides into right and left branches, which supply the proximal and distal transverse colon, respectively. Anatomic variations of the middle colic artery include complete absence in 4% to 20% and the presence of an accessory middle colic artery in 10% of specimens. The left branch of the middle colic artery may supply territory also supplied by the left colic artery through the collateral channel of the marginal artery. This collateral circulation in the area of the splenic flexure is the most inconsistent of the entire colon and has been referred to as a watershed area, vulnerable to ischemia in the presence of hypotension. In some studies, up to 50% of specimens were found to lack clearly identified arteries in a small segment of colon at the confluence of the blood supplies of the midgut and hindgut. These individuals rely on adjacent vasa recta in this area for arterial supply to the bowel wall. In practice, surgeons avoid making anastomoses in the region of the splenic flexure, fearing that the blood supply will not be sufficient to permit healing of the

anastomosis, a situation that could lead to anastomotic leak and sepsis.

The IMA originates from the aorta at the level of L2 to L3, approximately 3 cm above the aortic bifurcation. The left colic artery is the most proximal branch, supplying the distal transverse colon, splenic flexure, and descending colon. Two to six sigmoid branches collateralize with the left colic artery and form arcades that supply the sigmoid colon and contribute to the marginal artery.

The arc of Riolan is a collateral artery, first described by Jean Riolan (1580-1657), that directly connects the proximal SMA with the proximal IMA and may serve as a vital conduit when one or the other of these arteries is occluded. It is also known as the meandering mesenteric artery and is highly variable in size. Flow can be forward (IMA stenosis) or retrograde (SMA stenosis), depending on the site of obstruction. Such obstruction results in increased size and tortuosity of this meandering artery, which may be detected by arteriography; the presence of a large arc of Riolan thus suggests occlusion of one of the major mesenteric arteries (Fig. 51-10).

The IMA terminates in the superior rectal (superior hemorrhoidal) artery, which courses behind the rectum in the mesorectum, branching and then entering the rectal submucosa. Here, the capillaries form a submucosal plexus in the distal rectum at the level of the anal columns. The anal canal also receives arterial blood from the middle rectal (hemorrhoidal) and inferior rectal (hemorrhoidal) arteries. The middle rectal artery is a branch of the internal iliac artery. It is variable in size and enters the rectum anterolaterally, passing alongside and slightly anterior to the lateral rectal stalks. It has been reported to be absent in 40% to 80% of specimens studied. The inferior rectal artery is a branch of the pudendal artery, which itself is a more distal branch of the internal iliac. From the obturator canal, it traverses the obturator

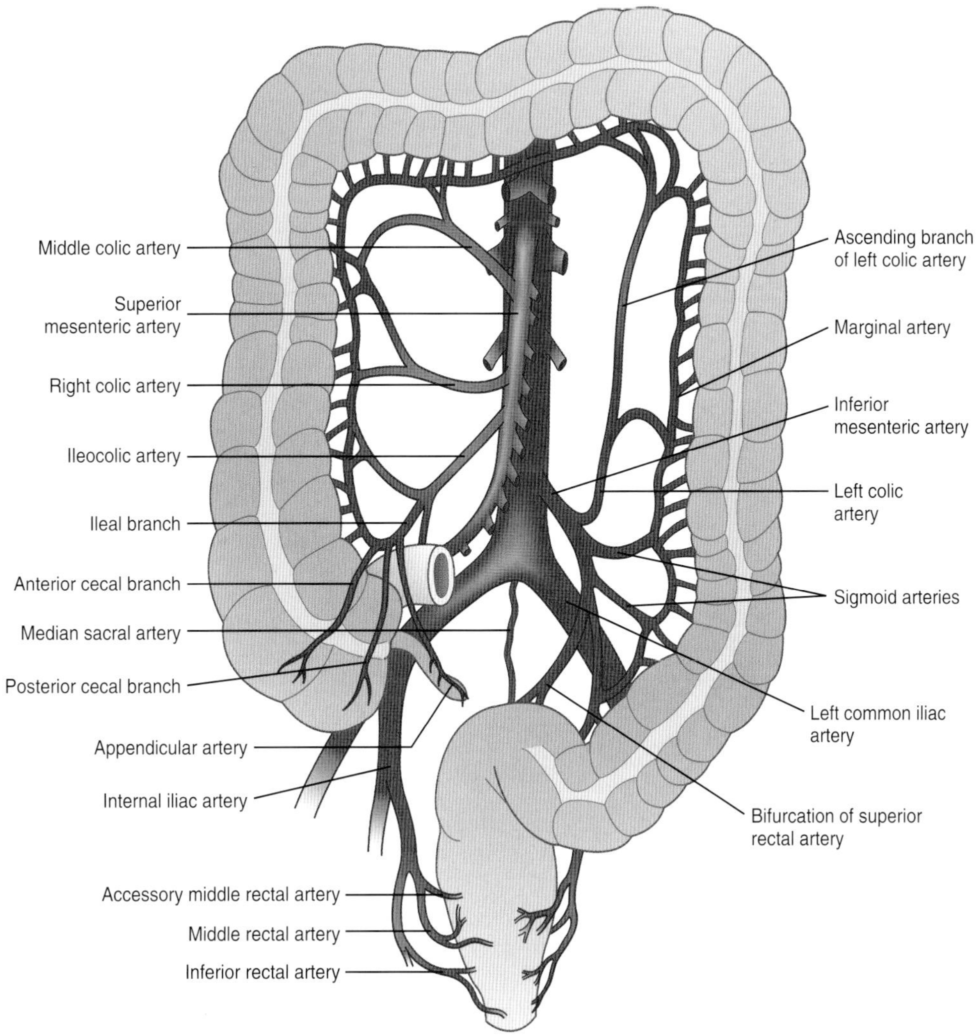
Middle colic artery
Superior mesenteric artery
Right colic artery
Ileocolic artery
Ileal branch
Anterior cecal branch
Median sacral artery
Posterior cecal branch
Appendicular artery
Internal iliac artery
Accessory middle rectal artery
Middle rectal artery
Inferior rectal artery
Ascending branch of left colic artery
Marginal artery
Inferior mesenteric artery
Left colic artery
Sigmoid arteries
Left common iliac artery
Bifurcation of superior rectal artery

FIGURE 51-6 Arterial supply of the colon. (From Gordon PH, Nivatvongs S, editors: *Principles and practice of surgery for the colon, rectum and anus*, ed 2, St. Louis, 1999, Quality Medical Publishing, p 23.)

fascia, ischiorectal fossa, and external anal sphincter to reach the anal canal. This vessel is encountered during the perineal dissection of an abdominoperineal resection.

The venous drainage of the colon and rectum mirrors the arterial blood supply. Venous drainage from the right and proximal transverse colon empties into the superior mesenteric vein, which coalesces with the splenic vein to become the portal vein. The distal transverse colon, descending colon, sigmoid, and most of the rectum drain into the inferior mesenteric vein, which empties into the splenic vein to the left of the aorta. The anal canal is drained by the middle and inferior rectal veins into the internal iliac vein and subsequently the inferior vena cava. The bidirectional venous drainage of the anal canal accounts for differences in patterns of metastasis from tumors arising in this region (Fig. 51-11).

Lymphatic drainage also follows the arterial anatomy. The wall of the large bowel is supplied with a rich network of lymphatic capillaries that drain to extramural channels paralleling the arterial supply. Lymphatics from the colon and proximal two thirds of the rectum ultimately drain into the para-aortic nodal chain, which empties into the cisterna chyli. Lymphatics draining the distal rectum and anal canal may drain to the para-aortic nodes or laterally, through the internal iliac system, to the superficial inguinal nodal basin. Although the dentate line roughly marks the level where lymphatic drainage diverges, classic studies by Block and Enquist using dye injection demonstrated that spread through lymphatic channels occurs to adjacent pelvic organs, such as the vagina and broad ligament, when injections are administered as high as 10 cm proximal to the dentate line (Figs. 51-12 and 51-13).

Lymph nodes are commonly grouped into levels according to their location. Epicolic nodes are located along the bowel wall and in the epiploic appendices. Nodes adjacent to the marginal artery are paracolic. Intermediate nodes are located along the main branches of the large blood vessels; primary nodes are located on the SMA or IMA. Lymph node invasion by metastatic cancer is an important prognostic factor for patients with colorectal cancer. Accurate pathologic assessment of lymph nodes is essential for accurate staging, which serves as a determinant for treatment of patients with colorectal cancer.

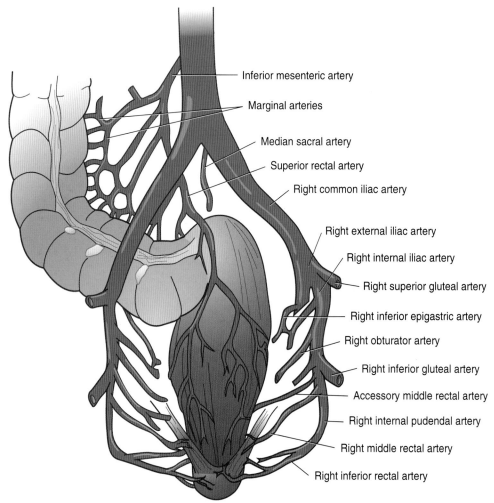

Inferior mesenteric artery

Marginal arteries

Median sacral artery

Superior rectal artery

Right common iliac artery

Right external iliac artery

Right internal iliac artery

Right superior gluteal artery

Right inferior epigastric artery

Right obturator artery

Right inferior gluteal artery

Accessory middle rectal artery

Right internal pudendal artery

Right middle rectal artery

Right inferior rectal artery

FIGURE 51-7 Arterial supply of the rectum. (From Gordon PH, Nivatvongs S, editors: *Principles and practice of surgery for the colon, rectum and anus*, ed 2, St. Louis, 1999, Quality Medical Publishing, p 24.)

Nerves

Preganglionic sympathetic nerves from T6 to T12 synapse in preaortic ganglia. Postsympathetic fibers then course along blood vessels to reach the right and transverse colon. The right and transverse colon parasympathetic supply comes from the right vagus nerve. Parasympathetic fibers follow branches of the SMA to synapse in the wall of the bowel. The left colon and rectum receive sympathetic supply from the preganglionic lumbar splanchnics of L1 to L3. These synapse in the preaortic plexus located above the aortic bifurcation, and the postganglionic elements follow the branches of the IMA and superior rectal artery to the left colon, sigmoid, and rectum. The lower rectum, pelvic floor, and anal canal receive postganglionic sympathetics from the pelvic plexus. The pelvic plexus is adherent to the pelvic sidewalls and is adjacent to the lateral stalks. It receives sympathetic branches from the presacral plexus that condense at the sacral promontory into the left and right hypogastric nerves. These sympathetic nerves, which descend into the pelvis dorsal to the superior rectal artery, are responsible for delivery of semen to the posterior

prostatic urethra. Failure to preserve at least one of the hypogastric nerves during rectal dissection results in ejaculatory dysfunction in men.

The pelvic parasympathetic nerves, or nervi erigentes, arise from S2 to S4. Preganglionic parasympathetic nerves merge with postganglionic sympathetics after the latter emerge from the sacral foramina. These nerve fibers, through the pelvic plexus, surround and innervate the prostate, urethra, seminal vesicles, urinary bladder, and muscles of the pelvic floor. Rectal dissection may disrupt the pelvic plexus and its subdivisions, resulting in neurogenic bladder and sexual dysfunction. Rates of bladder and erectile dysfunction after rectal surgery are as high as 45%. The degree and type of dysfunction are affected by the level of the neurologic injury. A high IMA ligation severing the hypogastric nerves near the sacral promontory results in sympathetic dysfunction characterized by retrograde ejaculation and bladder dysfunction. Injury to the mixed parasympathetic and sympathetic periprostatic plexus results in impotence and an atonic bladder.

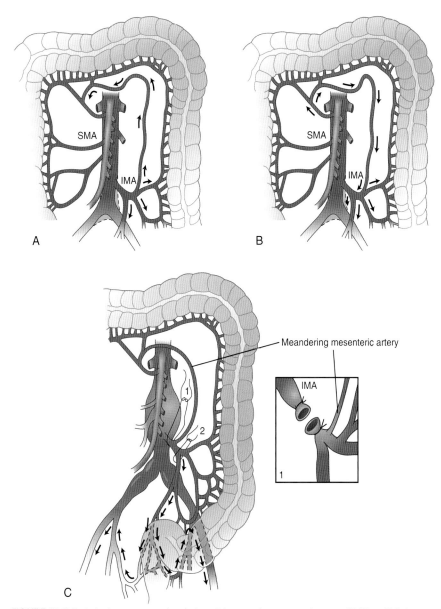

FIGURE 51-8 Pathologic anatomy and occlusion of the superior mesenteric artery (SMA) and inferior mesenteric artery (IMA). **A,** Occlusion of the SMA. **B,** Occlusion of the IMA. **C,** Ligating the IMA: *1,* correct location of ligation *(inset)*; *2,* incorrect location of ligation. (From Gordon PH, Nivatvongs S, editors: *Principles and practice of surgery for the colon, rectum and anus,* ed 2, St. Louis, 1999, Quality Medical Publishing, p 28.)

PHYSIOLOGY OF THE COLON

Generally speaking, the function of the colon is the recycling of nutrients, whereas the function of the rectum is the elimination of stool. The recycling of nutrients depends on the metabolic activity of the colonic flora, colonic motility, and mucosal absorption and secretion. Stool elimination involves dehydration of colonic contents and defecation.

Recycling of Nutrients

During the digestive process, ingested nutrients are diluted within the intestinal lumen by biliopancreatic and GI secretions. The small intestine absorbs most ingested nutrients and some of the fluid and bile salts secreted into the lumen. However, the ileal effluent is still rich in water, electrolytes, and nutrients that resist digestion. The colon has the functional ability to recover these substances to avoid unnecessary losses of fluids, electrolytes, nitrogen, and energy. To accomplish this, the colon depends highly on its bacterial flora.

Colonic Flora

Nutrients are digested within the intestinal lumen with the aid of biliopancreatic and GI secretions. By the time the chyme reaches the terminal ileum, most of the nutrients have been absorbed,

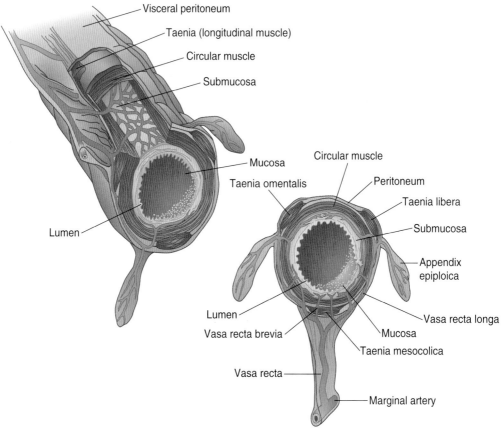

FIGURE 51-9 Cross-sectional anatomy of the colon, with vasa brevia and vasa recta. (From Gordon PH, Nivatvongs S, editors: *Principles and practice of surgery for the colon, rectum and anus*, ed 2, St. Louis, 1999, Quality Medical Publishing, p 26.)

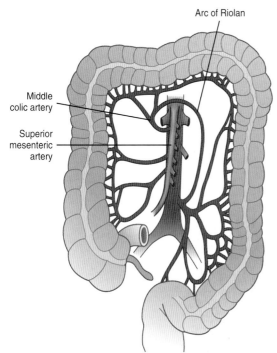

FIGURE 51-10 Arc of Riolan. (From Gordon PH, Nivatvongs S, editors: *Principles and practice of surgery for the colon, rectum and anus*, ed 2, St. Louis, 1999, Quality Medical Publishing, p 27.)

leaving a succus entericus composed of electrolyte-rich fluid, bile salts, and some proteins and starches that have resisted digestion. An enormous quantity of autochthonous flora, consisting of more than 400 bacterial species, resides in the large intestine. Large bowel contents may contain as many as 10^{11} to 10^{12} bacterial cells per gram, contributing approximately 50% of fecal mass. Most of these colonic species are anaerobes. These bacteria feed on proteins sloughed from the bowel wall and undigested complex carbohydrates.

Colonic microflora provide several important functions to the host, including barrier functions that help maintain epithelial integrity, nutritive functions that use plant polysaccharides, developmental functions that stimulate epithelial cell differentiation and angiogenesis, and, finally, immune functions through the gut. Gut-associated lymphoid tissue contributes to both innate and adaptive immunity.[1] Short-chain fatty acids (SCFAs) are produced by microbial breakdown and fermentation of dietary starches. These fatty acids are the principal source of nutrition for the colonocyte. *Bacteroides* species predominate throughout the colon, composing two thirds of the total counts of the proximal colon and almost 70% of the bacteria in the rectum. *Escherichia, Klebsiella, Proteus, Lactobacillus,* and enterococci are the predominant species of facultative anaerobes.

Prebiotics and Probiotics

Probiotics can be defined as dietary supplements that contain live cultures of bacteria and yeast that are beneficial to colonic and

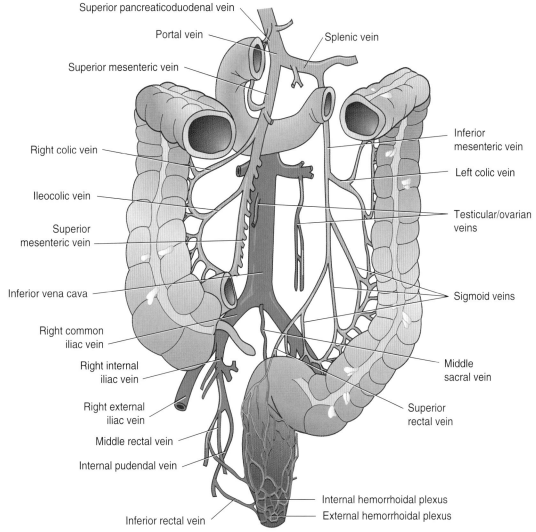

FIGURE 51-11 Venous drainage of the colon and rectum. (From Gordon PH, Nivatvongs S, editors: *Principles and practice of surgery for the colon, rectum and anus*, ed 2, St. Louis, 1999, Quality Medical Publishing, p 30.)

host function. The two most widely used agents are *Lactobacillus* and *Bifidobacterium*. Studies have indicated that probiotics may have widespread health benefits, including stimulation of immune function, anti-inflammatory effects, and suppression of entero-pathogenic colonization.[2] In addition, they may increase the digestibility of dietary proteins, enhance absorption of amino acids, and play a protective or therapeutic role against *Clostridium difficile*–associated diarrhea.[3] The ultimate role of probiotics has not yet been determined. There are conflicting data in regard to whether they work more effectively as primary therapy or as prophylaxis against recurrent *C. difficile*–associated diarrhea. Indications for their use are evolving but may include necrotizing enterocolitis in neonates, patients with HIV-AIDS, and neutropenic patients undergoing chemotherapy. Further research is needed, but the evidence for probiotic use in various settings is encouraging.

Prebiotics are nondigestible oligosaccharides (e.g., inulin) that help the host by stimulating the growth of certain species of beneficial intestinal bacteria. There is a growing body of data

suggesting health benefits; however, there is currently little evidence to guide recommendations for their use.

Fermentation

Unlike most of the mucosal lining of the proximal GI tract, colonic mucosa does not receive its primary nutrition from the bloodstream. Instead, nutrient requirements are fulfilled from the colonic luminal contents. The primary energy source for the colonocyte is the SCFA butyrate. The manner in which this interaction occurs illustrates the essential symbiotic interaction between the colon and its resident bacterial flora.

The main source of energy for intestinal bacteria is dietary fiber, composed of complex carbohydrates (starches and nonstarch polysaccharides [NSPs]). This fiber is metabolized by the process of fermentation. Not all complex carbohydrates are fermented in the same manner, which underlies many of the dietary recommendations for bulking agents. Lignin and psyllium are components of plants that are not fermented by human colonic flora; they are hydrophilic, thus leading to water resorption and stool

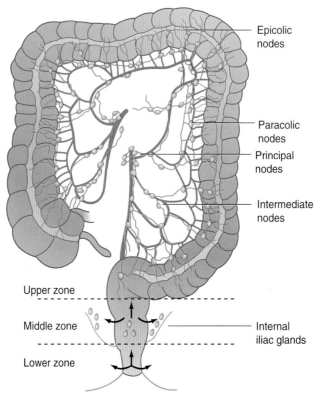

FIGURE 51-12 Lymphatic drainage of the colon. (From Corman ML, editor: *Colon and rectal surgery*, ed 4, Philadelphia,1998, Lippincott-Raven, p 21.)

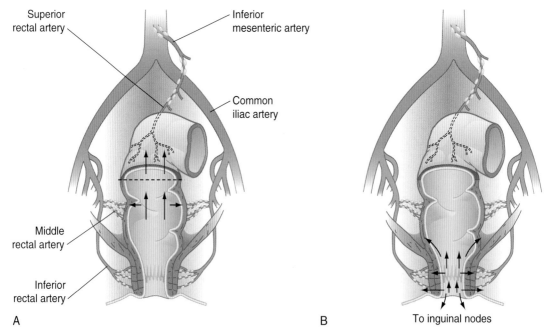

FIGURE 51-13 Lymphatic drainage of the rectum **(A)** and anal canal **(B)**. (From Gordon PH, Nivatvongs S, editors: *Principles and practice of surgery for the colon, rectum and anus*, ed 2, St. Louis, 1999, Quality Medical Publishing, p 32.)

bulking. Celluloses are partially fermented, whereas fruit pectins are completely metabolized by colonic bacteria. Diets high in nonfermentable NSPs contribute to stool bulk and increased transit time; highly fermentable NSPs provide minimal bulk but enhanced colonocyte nutrition.

The end products of fermentation are SCFAs and gas—carbon dioxide, methane, and hydrogen. In addition to NSPs, colonic bacteria ferment poorly absorbed starches and proteins from the upper GI tract, known as resistant starches. Although highly variable from person to person, with daily variability dependent on diet, the gases produced by bacterial fermentation compose approximately 50% to 75% of flatus, with the remainder consisting of swallowed air.[4]

Protein fermentation, otherwise known as putrefaction, results in the formation of potentially toxic metabolites, including phenols, indoles, and amines. The production of these toxins is inhibited in many intestinal bacteria by the presence of alternative carbohydrate energy sources. This process becomes accentuated more distally in the colon as carbohydrate sources become scarcer. These deleterious end products of bacterial metabolism can lead to mucosal injury and reactive hyperproliferation, which have been hypothesized to promote carcinogenesis. Also, the presence of bulking agents decreases intracolonic pressures and may serve to prevent the formation of colonic diverticula. It can be seen, then, how providing adequate sources of various forms of dietary carbohydrates can serve positive roles in colonic health. These principles underlie the recommendations for dietary fiber, as do the evolving data on the helpful nature of probiotics and prebiotics.

Short-Chain Fatty Acids

The primary end products of bacterial fermentation are SCFAs. Absorption of SCFAs in the large intestine is efficient; only 5% to 10% is lost in the feces. The three primary fatty acids produced are acetate, propionate, and butyrate in a ratio of 3 : 1 : 1. SCFAs have key roles in colonic and also overall human metabolism. They are metabolized in three main sites: (1) colonocytes use butyrate as their primary energy source; (2) hepatocytes metabolize all three SCFAs to various degrees for use in gluconeogenesis; and (3) muscle cells oxidize acetate to generate energy. Metabolism of the SCFAs can provide up to 70% of colonocyte energy needs, reduce glucose oxidation, and spare other essential amino acids for metabolism. SCFAs also influence GI motility through the ileocolonic brake mechanism, which is defined as the inhibition of gastric emptying and nutrients reaching the ileocolonic junction.

Acetate, the principal SCFA in the colon, is primarily absorbed and transported to the liver, where it is the primary substrate for cholesterol synthesis. Nonabsorbable, nonfermentable dietary fiber, such as psyllium, may decrease the production of acetate and may have a beneficial effect on cholesterol levels. Similarly, propionate, which has a glycolytic role in the liver, may also lower serum lipid levels by inhibiting cholesterol synthesis. Butyrate is the primary energy source for colonic epithelial cells and may also play an important role in maintaining cellular health by arresting the proliferation of neoplastic colonocytes while paradoxically being trophic for normal colonocytes. In addition, butyrate serves to regulate and to stabilize cell adhesion molecules.

Urea Recycling

It was long believed that urea is the end product of nitrogen metabolism in humans. This is true in the sense that humans, and mammals in general, do not produce urease. However, colonic bacteria are rich in urease. When urea is labeled with a tracer (e.g.,

radioisotope, heavy isotope) and injected intravenously, 10% of the urea nitrogen is not recovered in urine but is incorporated into body protein. Bacteria firmly adherent to the colonic epithelium mediate this process of urea recycling, which produces urease. A low-protein and high-fiber diet, such as that of the Papua New Guinea highlanders, further increases urea recycling. These individuals ingest only 10 mg of protein per kilogram per day and have normal health, with normal muscle mass and serum proteins. Adaptation to this low-protein diet has made the colon efficient in recycling nitrogen to the point that it may even absorb some essential amino acids (e.g., lysine). Urea recycling has been exploited as a therapy for renal failure by excluding nonessential amino acids from the diet to promote maximal urea recycling and to diminish the need for dialysis.

However, one pathologic condition in which urea recycling is not beneficial is liver failure. When the liver cannot reuse the urea nitrogen absorbed by the colon, ammonia crosses the blood-brain barrier and produces false neurotransmitters, which results in hepatic coma.

Absorption

The total absorptive area of the colon is estimated at approximately 900 cm^2. Between 1000 and 1500 mL of fluid is poured into the cecum by the daily ileal effluent. The total volume of water in stool is only 100 to 150 mL/day. This 10-fold reduction in water across the colon represents the most efficient site of absorption in the GI tract per surface area. The net absorption of sodium is even higher. Although the ileal effluent contains 200 mEq/liter of sodium, stool contains only 25 to 50 mEq/liter. One major difference between sodium and water absorption in the colon is that although water is absorbed passively, sodium requires active transport. Sodium is transported against chemical and electrical gradients at the expense of energy consumption.

The colonic epithelium can use various fuels; however, n-butyrate is oxidized in preference to glutamine, glucose, or ketone bodies. Because mammalian cells do not produce n-butyrate, the colonic epithelium relies on luminal bacteria to produce it through the fermentation of dietary fiber. The lack of n-butyrate, such as that resulting from the inhibition of fermentation by broad-spectrum antibiotics, leads to less sodium and water absorption and thus diarrhea. Conversely, the perfusion of the colonic lumen with n-butyrate stimulates sodium and water absorption. n-Butyrate, acetate, and propionate are SCFAs produced through bacterial fermentation; these constitute the main anions in stool. Other physiologic effects of SCFAs on the colon include stimulation of blood flow, mucosal cell renewal, and regulation of intraluminal pH for homeostasis of the bacterial flora.

In addition to recovering sodium and water, the colonic mucosa absorbs bile acids. The colon absorbs bile acids that escape absorption by the terminal ileum, thus making the colon part of the enterohepatic circulation. Bile acids are passively transported across the colonic epithelium by nonionic diffusion. When the colonic absorptive capacity is exceeded, colonic bacteria deconjugate bile acids. Deconjugated bile acids can then interfere with sodium and water absorption, leading to secretory, or choleretic, diarrhea. Choleretic diarrhea is seen early after right hemicolectomy as a transient phenomenon and more permanently after extensive ileal resection.

Secretion

The physiologic role of colon secretion is demonstrated in patients with chronic renal failure. Uremic patients can remain normokalemic while ingesting a normal amount of potassium before requiring dialysis. This phenomenon is associated with a compensatory increase in colonic secretion and fecal excretion of potassium. This effect is blocked by spironolactone, which illustrates the effect of aldosterone on colonic potassium secretion. Potassium secretion requires both Na^+,K^+-ATPase and Na^+-K^+-$2Cl^-$ cotransport on the basolateral membrane and an apical potassium channel.

Many forms of colitis are associated with increased potassium secretion, such as inflammatory bowel disease (IBD), cholera, and shigellosis. In addition, some forms of colitis impair colonic absorption or produce secretion of chloride, such as collagenous and microscopic colitis and congenital chloridorrhea. Chloride is secreted by colonic epithelium at a basal rate, which is increased in pathologic conditions such as cystic fibrosis and secretory diarrhea. Secretion of chloride also requires the coupling of Na^+,K^+-ATPase and Na^+-K^+-$2Cl^-$ cotransport to exit passively through the apical membrane. Calcium and cyclic adenosine monophosphate both stimulate chloride secretion, whereas bicarbonate and SCFAs inhibit chloride secretion.

Colonic secretion of H^+ and bicarbonate is coupled to the absorption of Na^+ and Cl^-, respectively. It is through these exchangers that the colon is linked to systemic acid-base metabolism. The supply of H^+ and bicarbonate for these exchangers is maintained by the hydration of CO_2, catalyzed by colonic carbonic anhydrase. Changes in systemic pH induce changes in the activity of carbonic anhydrase, eliciting elimination of H^+ or bicarbonate as needed to bring the systemic pH back to normal.

Motility

Colonic motility is a highly complex process, made difficult to investigate by a lack of standardized terminology and measurements. In addition, movement through the colon is relatively slow compared with the proximal GI tract, and studies require prolonged observation.

Colonic motility patterns may be more simply divided into two primary patterns, segmental activity and propagated activity. Segmental activity consists of single contractions or rhythmic bursts of contractions. The purpose of these segmental contractions is to propel fecal matter distally through a directed pressure gradient toward the rectum in discrete distances and to allow mixing, which promotes optimal absorption. The second pattern is propagated activity, commonly classified on the basis of amplitude as low-amplitude or high-amplitude propagated contractions. High-amplitude propagated contractions have been historically referred to as mass movements, or migrating motor complexes, whose role is shifting large quantities of contents through the colon. These have an important role in defecation, with mass movements propelling larger volumes of fecal matter to the distal colon and emptying of the descending colon into the sigmoid colon and rectum. Little is known about low-amplitude propagated contractions, but they are associated with distention of the viscus and passage of flatus.[5]

There seems to be a circadian rhythm to colonic motility, with maximum peaks of activity immediately after waking and after meals. Sleep is associated with a decrease in colonic motility.

Not surprisingly, food ingestion results in an increase of overall colonic motility for approximately 2 hours. This reflex is stimulated not only by gastric distention but also by the central nervous system, initiated by visualization of food. In addition, meal composition affects colonic responses. Increased activity in response to carbohydrate meals is fairly short-lived, whereas fatty meals elicit longer term responses.

Ultimately, transit in the colon is controlled by the autonomic nervous system. Parasympathetic innervation reaches the colon through the vagus and pelvic nerves. The enteric nervous system in the colon is arranged in several plexuses—subserosal, myenteric (Auerbach), submucosal (Meissner), and mucosal plexuses. Sympathetic innervation originates in the superior and inferior mesenteric ganglia and reaches the colon through perivascular plexuses.

Formation of Stool

The frequency of defecation is just as variable among individuals as is their perception of abnormal stool frequency. An individual who passes more than three loose stools daily is considered to have diarrhea, whereas fewer than three weekly stools is considered constipation. Any frequency within that range is considered normal, although many individuals will still seek medical attention for what they perceive as diarrhea or constipation. Many factors influence colonic transit rate. Colonic transit is longer in women than in men and longer in premenopausal than in postmenopausal women. Conversely, colonic transit time is shortened in smokers. In normal subjects, supplementation with NSPs does not shorten colonic transit time, although it does increase fecal weight. In patients with idiopathic constipation, however, NSPs, in the form of psyllium seeds, shorten colonic transit time and increase stool weight.

Defecation

Normal defecation requires adequate colonic transit time, stool consistency, and fecal continence. Fecal continence implies deferment of stool elimination; discrimination among gas, liquid, and solid stool; and selective elimination of gas without stool. There is some controversy about the actual role of the rectum under resting conditions. Some have proposed that the rectum is simply a conduit, which under resting conditions should be empty. If stool arrives at the rectum, the anorectal inhibitory reflex is triggered, forcing the subject to hold defecation by voluntary contraction of the external sphincter. However, any surgeon who performs routine rigid proctosigmoidoscopies in the office is well aware that a patient can have a rectum full of stool without any awareness. This leads to the opposing view, which regards the rectum as a reservoir. Just as stool triggers the anorectal inhibitory reflex, it also triggers a rectocolic reflex. This reflex allows continuous filling of the rectum with fecal material until the colon is emptied.

The mechanisms involved in fecal continence are not fully understood. A certain reservoir capacity is needed to achieve fecal continence. A stiff nondistensible rectum, such as in radiation proctitis, may produce incontinence, even when the sphincter muscles are competent. Some of the internal and external sphincter muscle fibers are necessary for adequate continence, although many patients have part of the sphincter severed during a fistulotomy and are still continent. Probably the only factor needed for fecal continence is innervation of the sphincter. The motor nerve fibers, which produce contraction of the sphincter fibers, and also all the sensory innervation are important to empty the rectum adequately.

PREOPERATIVE WORKUP AND STOMA PLANNING

Today, routine preoperative testing guidelines exist to streamline the process to elective surgery. They are dependent on the planned procedure, the patient's comorbidities, and the American Society of Anesthesiologists class of the patient. Detailed description of preoperative management and workup for surgical patients is discussed elsewhere. However, additional preoperative evaluation specific to major colon and rectal procedures may also include the following considerations:

- Evaluation of nutritional status
- Use of a preoperative mechanical bowel preparation (MBP) or oral antibiotics
- Preoperative counseling for stoma care, education, and marking
- Colonoscopy to exclude synchronous lesions
- Postoperative fluid and pain management

Nutritional Assessment

Preoperative malnutrition is an important predictor of poor clinical outcomes in patients undergoing major colorectal operations. The additional stress of a major abdominal surgery further induces a catabolic response and insulin resistance. Therefore, nutritional parameters for chronically ill patients and especially those with IBD should be assessed before consideration for elective surgery. Serum albumin is an indicator of long-term nutrition (21 days), whereas serum prealbumin can gauge short-term nutritional status (3 to 5 days). Low preoperative albumin (<3.5 g/dL) has been further shown to be a risk factor for anastomotic leak after colorectal surgery. These two indices may also identify patients who may benefit from preoperative supplemental nutrition, such as total parenteral nutrition. The decision to initiate total parenteral nutrition should also be judicious because of its known albeit low association with infectious complications. Nonetheless, elective operations should be delayed if possible until the patient is nutritionally replete.

Preoperative Bowel Preparation

Purging the feces and reducing the concentration of colonic intraluminal bacteria before operations on the colon is a practice that has been challenged in recent years. The normal, or autochthonous, microbial organisms in the colon compose up to 90% of the dry weight of feces, reaching concentrations of up to 10^9 organisms/mL of feces. The anaerobic *Bacteroides* is the most common colonic microbe, whereas *Escherichia coli* is the most common aerobe. *Pseudomonas, Enterococcus, Proteus, Klebsiella,* and *Streptococcus* spp. are also present in large numbers.

The process of preparing the colon for an elective operation has traditionally involved two factors, purging of the fecal contents (mechanical preparation) and administration of antibiotics effective against colonic bacteria. Tradition has held that an unprepared colon (i.e., one that contains intraluminal feces) poses an unacceptably high rate of failure of the anastomosis to heal. However, experience with primary repair of traumatic colonic injuries, along with reports from Europe describing elective operations conducted safely without the use of preoperative purging, has led to reconsideration of the true value of purging the colon before colonic surgery. Because the colonocytes receive nutrition from intraluminal free fatty acids produced by fermentation from colonic bacteria, there are concerns that purging may actually be detrimental to healing of a colonic anastomosis. In the United States at present, the addition of a preoperative MBP with or without oral antibiotics is controversial and is left to the surgeon's discretion. Nonetheless, a variety of MBP regimens and antibiotic combinations are in current use. A clear superiority of one over another has not been found; however, for some patients, certain bowel preparations may have adverse physiologic consequences.

Knowledge of the history of bowel preparation practices, current controversies, and data is useful.

Complete bowel obstruction and free perforation are absolute contraindications to bowel preparation. For colonoscopy, properties of preparations are judged by safety, tolerance of the patient, and efficacy or preparation quality. In the past, 4 to 5 days of clear liquids along with laxatives (such as senna, castor oil, and bisacodyl), whole bowel nasogastric irrigation, mannitol irrigation, and repeated enemas were among the regimens used. Tolerance of patients of these methods is poor; they are associated with dehydration, electrolyte abnormalities, and severe abdominal cramping and are generally not well tolerated by older or infirm patients.

In the 1980s, polyethylene glycol–electrolyte solution, a nonabsorbed, sodium sulfate–based liquid, was developed as an oral MBP. Patients are required to drink at least 2 to 4 liters of the solution, along with additional fluids. Abdominal cramping, nausea, and vomiting are common side effects of the preparation, and prophylactic antiemetics are often administered routinely. In the 1990s, oral sodium phosphate solutions and pills were developed in response to dissatisfaction of patients with the large fluid volume required for polyethylene glycol preparation, and these preparations have been found in most trials to be more tolerable, with higher rates of satisfaction and compliance of patients. Sodium phosphate, in liquid or pill form, has been linked more frequently than polyethylene glycol to rare but serious electrolyte imbalances. In patients with impaired renal function, hyperphosphatemia, hypernatremia, hypokalemia, and hypocalcemia can occur. In response to concerns about toxicity, the Food and Drug Administration removed oral sodium phosphate bowel preparations from the market in 2008; however, they are still available as over-the-counter medications in other countries. Thus, polyethylene glycol–electrolyte solution is the recommended bowel preparation in patients with renal insufficiency, cirrhosis, ascites, or congestive heart failure as well as physiologically in normal patients. Ultimately, comfort of the patient and economic factors may determine MBP practices if the efficacy is similar. Patients favor preparations that are low in volume, are palatable, have easy to complete regimens, and are either reimbursed by health insurance or are inexpensive. Physicians are advised to select a preparation that is safe to administer in light of existing comorbid conditions and those preparations that will not interact with previously prescribed medications. The ideal bowel preparation has to balance the intraoperative expectations of the surgeon with the safety profile and comfort of the patient.

For patients undergoing colonoscopy, the quality of the bowel preparation is essential for performing an accurate examination. However, for patients undergoing surgical resection, the necessity of mechanical bowel preparation has been questioned. In a 2011 update to the initial Cochrane review from 2005, Guenaga and colleagues evaluated 13 randomized controlled studies that compared MBP versus no preparation during elective colorectal surgery while looking at the primary outcome of anastomotic leakage.[6] The overall anastomotic leakage rate was 4.4% in the group with MBP (101 of 2275 participants) compared with 4.5% in the group without MBP (103 of 2258 participants) and was not statistically significant. Before conclusions are drawn, it is important to note that although the goals of many of these studies appear the same, there is significant heterogeneity in their methodology. There is significant variability among the populations of patients, and more pertinent prognostic factors for anastomotic leakage may include the indications for surgery, the patient's comorbidities and acuity, the surgeon's experience, the surgical technique, and the location of intestinal anastomosis.

Antibiotic use in colorectal surgery is a well-established practice that reduces infectious complications. Elective colorectal cases are classified as clean contaminated and, as such, benefit from routine single-dose administration of parenteral antibiotics 30 minutes before an incision to reduce rates of superficial and deep wound infection. It has been shown that when operative times are prolonged, additional doses at 4-hour intervals are required. When the operation is completed, postoperative administration of antibiotics for a clean contaminated case, such as a routine segmental resection, does not reduce infectious complications further and may promote *C. difficile* colitis, *Candida* infection, and the emergence of bacterial antibiotic resistance. Polk and Lopez-Mayer showed a reduction in postoperative infection rates from 30% to 8% with the routine use of preoperative parenteral antibiotics. Gomez-Alonzo and colleagues repeated these results, showing a decrease from 39% to 9%. Antibiotics active against both aerobes and anaerobes are ideal; a second- or third-generation cephalosporin alone or a combination of a fluoroquinolone plus metronidazole or clindamycin is typical.

The efforts to reduce surgical site infections (SSIs) have recently included the implementation of the Surgical Care Improvement Project guidelines and the push to incorporate standardized prophylactic parenteral antibiotic measures. The correct and timely administration of antibiotics has now become a performance measure for quality improvement projects nationwide. The role of appropriate parenteral antibiotics before incision is well established in reducing SSI. However, the role of oral antibiotics in conjunction with preoperative mechanical bowel preparation has been recently questioned. Despite the current trends among surgeons to omit oral nonabsorbable antibiotics, the data suggest that this omission may be premature. The use of additional oral antibiotics, theoretically to reduce the bacterial load further, is widely accepted but not as well validated. In a survey of colon and rectal surgeons, 87% indicated that both oral and parenteral antibiotic use is part of their routine preparation for elective colon operations. A typical preparation consists of erythromycin base (1 g) and neomycin (1 g) given in three preoperative doses the day before surgery. However, this regimen is associated with a high incidence of nausea and abdominal cramps, and some surgeons prefer to prescribe oral ciprofloxacin or metronidazole.

In a 2002 meta-analysis by Lewis (N = 215), the study showed a significant reduction in SSIs for patients with MBP plus oral antibiotics (from 17% to 5%); all patients received a standard preoperative parenteral antibiotic regimen.[7] Similarly, a 2012 retrospective study conducted by Cannon and colleagues showed a 57% decrease in SSIs when MBP and oral antibiotics were used in elective colon resections (N = 9940).[8] These results were echoed by Bellows and colleagues, who showed in their 2011 meta-analysis that the combination of oral antibiotics and MBP reduced the incidence of SSI after colorectal surgery by 43% compared with parenteral antibiotics alone. In 2011, the Michigan Surgical Quality Collaborative evaluated 2011 elective colectomies performed during 16 months; MBP without oral antibiotics was administered to 49.6% of patients, whereas 36.4% received MBP and oral antibiotics. In this large, well-designed study, patients receiving oral antibiotics were significantly less likely to have any SSI (4.5% versus 11.8%; P = .0001), to have an organ space infection (1.8% versus 4.2%; P = .044), or to have a superficial SSI (2.6% versus 7.6%; P = .001). Interestingly, they also found that patients receiving bowel preparation with oral antibiotics

were also less likely to have a prolonged ileus (3.9% versus 8.6%; P = .011) and had similar rates of *C. difficile* colitis (1.3% versus 1.8%; P = .58).[5] Thus, it seems there are reliable data supporting the use of oral antibiotics as an adjunct to a preoperative MBP as a means of reducing postoperative SSI.

Planning Intestinal Stomas

The techniques of fashioning a stoma have been developed to provide diversion of waste until conditions are attained that permit the restoration of normal intestinal continuity. If it is anticipated that the creation of a stoma will be part of an operation, appropriate preparations should be made to optimize the outcome of the procedure. Preoperative consultation with an enterostomal therapist is helpful in most circumstances. This consultation provides the opportunity for education, counseling, and appropriate stoma site selection and marking. Such preparation significantly increases the patient's satisfaction and quality of life scores of patients who require permanent or temporary stomas.[9]

The preferred location of a stoma should be in an area of the anterior abdominal wall where there are no creases that could prohibit the satisfactory seal of the appliance to the peristomal skin. The stoma should be visible to the patient—not on the underside of a large pannus in an obese individual—and easily accessible. Most surgeons think that it is desirable to bring the stoma through the rectus muscle, traversing an appropriately sized aperture (2 cm) that does not constrict the blood supply to the stoma but does not result in a peristomal hernia. In a normal-sized patient, the preferred site for stoma location is through the rectus muscle, slightly inferior to the umbilicus at the apex of the naturally occurring tissue mound of the abdomen (Fig. 51-14).

Stoma Types

A colostomy is an anastomosis fashioned between the colon and skin of the abdominal wall. Colostomies may be temporary or permanent, depending on the disease and conditions for which they are created. However, appropriate planning and careful

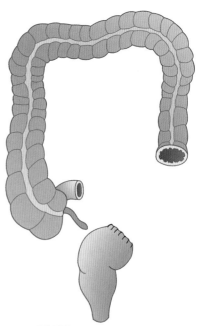

FIGURE 51-14 Selecting a site.

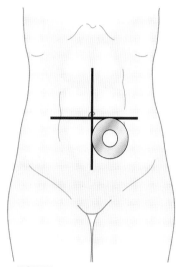

FIGURE 51-15 Hartmann operation.

technical considerations should be given to the creation of any colostomy because history has shown that even colostomies intended to be temporary may prove to be permanent in a significant number of patients.[10]

A colostomy may be indicated to divert colonic contents temporarily from a pathologic process in the distal colon or rectum, such as an obstructing rectal cancer or phlegmon of the sigmoid colon associated with diverticulitis. A loop colostomy using the sigmoid or the transverse colon can be useful for this, expedient, and able to be completed laparoscopically. Other circumstances are more appropriately treated by an end colostomy, in which the end of the sigmoid or, more commonly, descending colon is brought out the abdominal wall. An end colostomy is an essential component of an abdominal perineal proctectomy performed for rectal cancer. Resection of the sigmoid colon with closure of the rectal stump and fashioning of a descending colon is usually referred to as a Hartmann operation (Fig. 51-15). An ileostomy is the union of the terminal ileum to the skin of the abdominal wall. As described for colostomy, an ileostomy may also be fashioned as a loop or an end stoma. A temporary loop ileostomy may be fashioned to protect a distal anastomosis, such as a coloanal anastomosis in a patient who has received preoperative chemoradiation for rectal cancer, or to protect an ileal pouch–anal anastomosis (IPAA) in a patient treated with restorative proctocolectomy for ulcerative colitis. An end ileostomy is required if the colon and rectum must be removed and the anal sphincter cannot be preserved.

Physiologic Considerations and Practical Implications
Colostomy

For practical purposes, the dominant physiologic properties of the proximal colon are the completion of digestion of complex carbohydrates by fermentation, retention of electrolytes, and absorption of water. The more distal colon participates to less of an extent in these processes and serves as a reservoir for the waste products of digestion pending elimination. In some cases, the collateral communication through the marginal artery is not sufficient to sustain the sigmoid colon, so it is generally preferred to fashion a distal colostomy from the descending colon, which has

a more reliable blood supply than the sigmoid colon (especially if the IMA has been divided). In addition, the sigmoid colon is often afflicted with diverticulosis and the thickening of the colonic wall associated with that disease process, so the more pliable and capacious descending colon is the preferred choice for a left-sided colostomy.

The more proximal the site of the colon that is selected to fashion a colostomy, the more likely it is that the effluent will be liquid and foul-smelling. Descending colostomies that pass formed feces are relatively easy to care for with a well-fitting enterostomal appliance, whereas transverse colostomies that expel significant amounts of feculent liquid are difficult to care for and frequently leak and prolapse. Colostomies from the right colon are particularly troublesome because there is a copious amount of liquid foul-smelling effluent that is difficult to contain with an appliance. In addition, the motility characteristics of the colon are such that the more proximal the site of the colon selected to fashion a colostomy, the higher is the likelihood of prolapse through the stoma. This is distressing to the patient and makes maintenance of the stoma exceedingly difficult. As a general rule, with modern enterostomal techniques, it is much easier to care for an ileostomy than to care for a wet colostomy or a colostomy fashioned from the proximal colon.

Transverse colostomies, although at times useful to protect a distal anastomosis or to divert colonic contents from a distal obstruction, should almost always be considered a temporary diversion to a transient problem. A transverse loop colostomy fashioned at skin level will completely divert the fecal stream for a period of at least 6 weeks, but with the passage of time and the natural maturation of the colostomy, the spur, or posterior wall of the colostomy, will retract and the stoma will no longer divert completely. In addition, the incidence of significant prolapse from a transverse loop colostomy is high and increases over time. It is usually (but not always) the distal limb of the loop colostomy that prolapses through the stoma site.

Ileostomy

The terminal ileum normally delivers up to 2 liters of succus entericus to the cecum during a 24-hour period. There is a remarkable adaptation following the construction of a stoma from the very distal ileum in that after several weeks, the absorptive capacity of the ileum increases to the extent that approximately 900 mL of effluent will be expected to be produced by the ileum during a 24-hour period. However, the intestinal adaptation cannot completely compensate for the loss of the absorptive capacity of the colon, and ileostomy patients need to recognize the need to increase their intake of fluid. Supplemental sodium chloride may often be necessary for ileostomates, although liberal addition of salt to the daily diet usually will suffice.

The ileal chyme is liquid and contains digestive substances that are normally inactivated in the colon. If the skin adjacent to the ileostomy is exposed to the effluent, significant erosion of the peristomal skin can occur. Therefore, the ileostomy is fashioned to protrude above the skin surface as a spigot that pours the ileal contents into an enterostomal appliance fitted to the abdominal skin at the base of the ileostomy to protect the skin from the corrosive properties of the ileal effluent.

Technical Considerations
End Descending Colostomy

As noted, it is generally preferable to use the descending colon, rather than the sigmoid colon, for the creation of a colostomy.

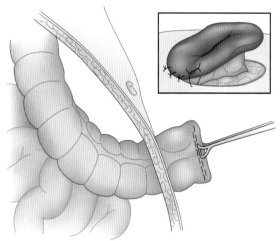

FIGURE 51-16 End colostomy.

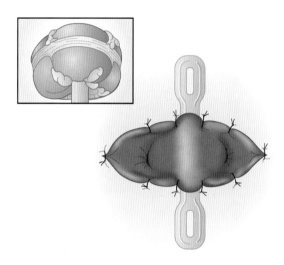

FIGURE 51-17 Loop colostomy.

The most common indication for an end descending colostomy is abdominal perineal resection for rectal cancer. In this case, we recommend dividing the IMA close to the aorta (for oncologic and anatomic reasons; see later). The sigmoid colon should be resected with the rectum, with care taken to preserve the mesentery to the descending colon. The blood supply to the descending colon will be maintained through the collateral circulation from the marginal artery, and this collateral circulation is better maintained by dividing the IMA close to its origin. The colon is then mobilized from the posterior abdominal wall and the prerenal (Gerota) fascia in such a manner that the entire descending colon and its mesentery lie anterior to the small bowel (Fig. 51-16). With use of this technique, there is no remaining lateral attachment of the colonic mesentery for the small intestine to twist around, and it is not necessary to approximate the mesentery of the descending colon to the lateral peritoneum to prevent an internal hernia.

The closed end of the descending colon is brought through an abdominal wall aperture created through the left rectus muscle at the site selected and marked before the operation. The colostomy is matured by approximating the wall of the colon to the skin with interrupted absorbable sutures. Some surgeons place the sutures in such a fashion to elevate the colostomy above skin level slightly, but this is not necessary with a descending colon because the effluent is formed and noncorrosive, and maintaining an appliance does not require eversion of the stoma.

Loop Colostomy

A loop colostomy may provide diversion from a distal obstruction (e.g., rectal cancer, diverticulitis) while simultaneously decompressing the limb of the colon leading to the obstruction. The most commonly performed type of loop colostomy is the transverse loop colostomy, but as noted, this stoma has the disadvantages of liquid effluent, eventual prolapse, and only temporary complete diversion. Although a loop transverse colostomy is certainly indicated in certain circumstances, consideration should be given to a loop ileostomy or loop descending colostomy. The loop ileostomy is easier to care for and to maintain an appliance, and the effluent of the loop descending colostomy is thicker, with less fluid loss and less chance of prolapse of the more distally placed colostomy. The technique of fashioning the descending loop

colostomy is essentially the same as for the transverse loop colostomy; the transverse loop is often technically easier because it is mobile and more easily accessible in the midabdomen.

The transverse colon is brought through an abdominal wall aperture, usually selected in the midline well cephalad to the umbilicus and well above a midline incision if the operation is conducted through such an incision. The exteriorized loop of colon is supported over a plastic stoma rod (Fig. 51-17). The antimesenteric surface of the colon is incised in a longitudinal incision, and the edges of the resulting colostomy are sutured to the skin of the abdominal wall with absorbable sutures. The supporting rod is removed after the fifth postoperative day. This stoma will provide complete diversion of the feces and gas from the proximal colon while simultaneously venting the distal colon. However, after a period of approximately 6 weeks, the posterior wall of the stoma (spur) will retract, and feces from the proximal colon can spill over into the distal limb.

Ileostomy

In forming an ileostomy, the ileum is brought through the abdominal wall at a site selected before the operation to ensure that the location is ideal for maintaining the seal of an appliance (i.e., away from natural abdominal wall creases, scars, hernias). A disc of skin is excised, the dissection is carried longitudinally through the center of the rectus muscle, and the posterior fascia is divided (Fig. 51-18). The abdominal wall aperture should be approximately 2.5 cm in diameter, thus admitting two fingers (Fig. 51-19). Sufficient length of well-vascularized ileum is brought through the abdominal wall to permit creation of a spigot that will protrude well above skin level (Brooke configuration), allowing the ileal contents to pour into an appliance sealed to the adjacent skin (Fig. 51-20). The ileostomy is completed by approximating the full thickness of the divided wall of the ileum to the subcuticular tissue of the abdominal skin of the stoma site, placing sutures in so as to maintain the everted configuration of the stoma (Figs. 51-21 and 51-22).

By use of these same principles, a loop ileostomy may be fashioned (Figs. 51-23 and 51-24). The loop ileostomy can be fashioned over an ileostomy rod, but a rod is not necessary to maintain the configuration of the stoma. Some surgeons prefer not to use a supporting rod because it may interfere with maintaining the

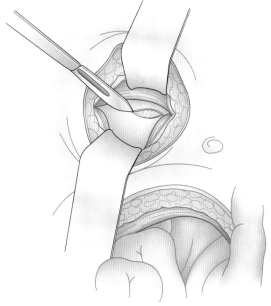

FIGURE 51-18 Dividing fascia for ileostomy.

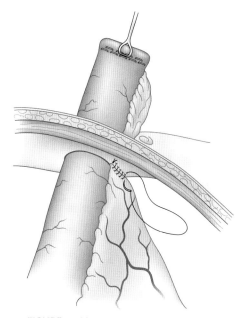

FIGURE 51-20 Ileum brought through aperture.

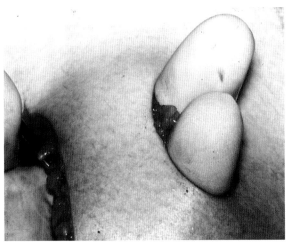

FIGURE 51-19 Aperture for ileostomy.

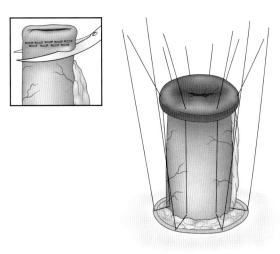

FIGURE 51-21 Maturing ileostomy.

seal of the appliance. If an ileostomy rod is used, it can be removed on the fifth postoperative day.

Postoperative Management Protocols

Major colon and rectal procedures are commonly performed in the United States, and therefore the postoperative management of these patients has come under scrutiny with the focus on decreasing morbidity, mortality, and health care cost. Evidence-based studies have now generated standardized fast-track protocols or enhanced recovery pathways to streamline the postoperative management of these patients, to limit complications, and to limit length of stay by enhancing early recovery of bowel function. These protocols include several of the following key elements:

- Appropriate selection of patients
- Minimally invasive surgery
- Perioperative fluid management
- Early enteric feeding

- Early ambulation
- Multimodality postoperative analgesia

Patients selected for inclusion in enhanced recovery pathways should understand the goals of the protocol and be able to physiologically tolerate reduced fluids and narcotics. Even so, participation in some but not all of the elements of an enhanced recovery pathway may still confer benefit. The cornerstones of the concept include intraoperative and postoperative fluid restriction as well as limitation of opiates and use of alternative pain control strategies. Acetaminophen, nonsteroidal anti-inflammatory drugs, gabapentin, and use of epidurals and cutaneous analgesic approaches have all been incorporated into various enhanced recovery protocols.

In a comprehensive meta-analysis, 13 randomized controlled studies (1910 patients) were analyzed, and in comparison with traditional care, enhanced recovery after surgery programs were associated with significantly decreased primary hospital stay

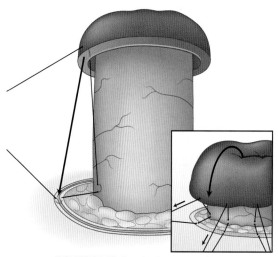

FIGURE 51-22 Creating ileostomy spigot.

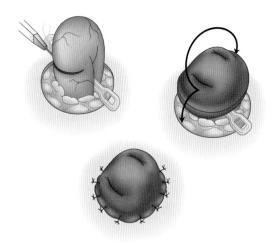

FIGURE 51-23 Completing loop ileostomy.

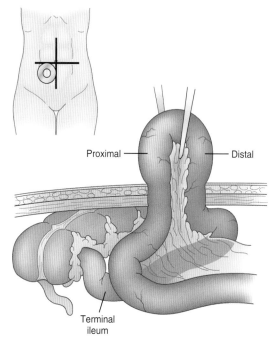

Proximal — — Distal

Terminal
ileum

FIGURE 51-24 Loop ileostomy in continuity.

(weighted mean difference, −2.44 days; 95% confidence interval [CI], −3.06 to −1.83 days; P < .00001), total hospital stay (weighted mean difference, −2.39 days; 95% CI, −3.70 to −1.09 days; P = .0003), total complications (relative risk, 0.71; 95% CI, 0.58-0.86; P = .0006), and general complications (relative risk, 0.68; 95% CI, 0.56-0.82; P < .0001).[11] No significant differences were found for readmission rates, surgical complications, and mortality. However, despite these favorable initial results, protocols for enhanced recovery after surgery have not been widely implemented. This is not unexpected as most protocols incorporate 8 to 20 elements and require the persistence and involvement of a multidisciplinary team of surgeons, anesthesiologist, nurses, stoma therapist, and hospital administration.

More recent adjuncts to the postoperative management in major colon and rectal surgery include the abandonment of nasogastric tubes and administration of early enteral feeding. A Cochrane review in 2007 revealed that patients without a nasogastric tube after undergoing lower GI surgery experience early return of bowel function, fewer primary complications, and decreased length of stay. In addition, randomized controlled trials have shown that early postoperative enteral feeding in patients undergoing elective colorectal surgery is safe and effective

and decreases both postoperative complications and hospital length of stay with no differences to the risk of anesthetic anastomotic dehiscence, pneumonia, wound infection, vomiting, and mortality.

Clearly, the implementation of enhanced recovery after surgery protocols and the contemporary evolution of postoperative management for elective colorectal surgery have significant benefits to the patient and health care costs.

DIVERTICULAR DISEASE

Background

Diverticular disease encompasses a range of signs and symptoms directly related to the presence of diverticula in the colon wall. These include infection, perforation, bleeding, fistula, and occasionally obstruction due to chronic inflammation. Diverticulosis was first described in the mid-19th century and appears to be an unfortunate product of the Industrial Revolution, which brought with it marked changes in diet. The incidence has been noted to increase with age and has been largely on the rise in the United States and other Western societies. Approximately 30% of those older than 60 years and roughly 60% to 80% of those older than 80 years may be affected. Only 10% to 20% of people with diverticula develop symptoms, which in the United States accounts for roughly 300,000 hospitalizations annually and 1.5 million outpatient visits, all of which comes at a considerable annual cost estimated to exceed $2 billion.[12]

Pathophysiology

Diverticula are abnormal outpouchings or sacs of the colon wall that occur most commonly because of interactions of high intraluminal pressures, disordered motility, alterations in colonic structure, and diets low in fiber. Diverticula are formed on the mesenteric side of the antimesenteric taeniae coli in areas of relative weakness in the bowel where small arterioles (vasa recta)

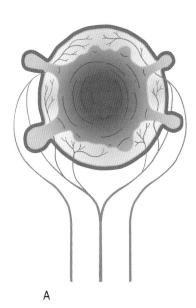
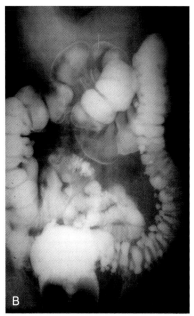

A

B

FIGURE 51-25 A, Pathogenesis of diverticular disease. Diverticula are herniations of the mucosa through the points of entry of blood vessels across the muscular wall. Because the diverticula are formed only by the mucosa rather than by the entire wall of the intestine, they are called false diverticula. Note that the diverticula form only between the mesenteric taenia and each of the two lateral taeniae. Because there are no perforating vessels, diverticula do not form on the antimesenteric side of the colon. **B,** Radiograph of barium enema with extensive sigmoid diverticulosis.

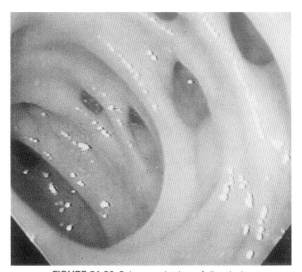

FIGURE 51-26 Colonoscopic view of diverticula.

penetrate the muscular layers as they traverse the colon wall. This results in the protrusion of the mucosa and submucosa through the layers of muscle, termed a pseudodiverticulum or false diverticulum (Fig. 51-25). A true diverticulum involves all of the layers of the intestinal wall.

The sigmoid and descending colon are the most commonly affected areas and in this disease process are characterized by hypertrophy of the muscular layers and associated decreased luminal diameter (Fig. 51-26). The resulting disordered motility in these segments and increase in luminal pressure facilitate the herniation of diverticula through the muscular coat. Deficiency

in dietary fiber further aids in the overall pathogenesis of diverticulosis because there is less bulking of stool within the colon. This resulting decrease in colonic luminal content requires the generation of increased colonic pressures to propel the feces forward.

Evaluation

Diverticulitis results from the perforation of a colonic diverticulum, which leads to pericolonic inflammation as there is extravasation of feculent fluid through the ruptured diverticulum. Patients will typically present with localized abdominal pain in the left lower quadrant because the sigmoid colon is the most commonly affected site. Other symptoms may include change in bowel habits, anorexia, nausea, fever, and urinary urgency if there is associated inflammation of the bladder. Physical examination often reveals abdominal distention and localized tenderness due to focal peritonitis in the left lower quadrant if the perforation is contained. A tender mass may also be appreciated if there is a large associated phlegmon. Diffuse peritonitis with rebound and guarding is indicative of a free intra-abdominal perforation with widespread contamination. Leukocytosis is a common laboratory finding.

The diagnosis of diverticulitis can often be made by eliciting these findings on a thorough history and physical examination; however, several radiologic studies can be used to confirm the diagnosis. Barium enema studies were primarily used before the advent of computed tomography (CT) scans and have largely been abandoned as a primary tool as they provide information only about the luminal surface of the colon and cannot be performed if perforation is suspected. If a contrast enema is performed, the contrast agent should be water soluble (Fig. 51-27). CT scan of the abdomen and pelvis is now considered by most to be the standard

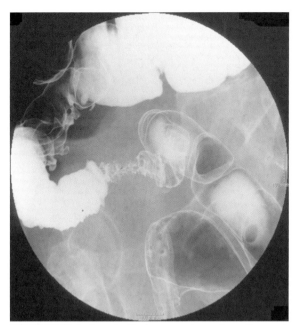

FIGURE 51-27 Radiograph of barium enema in a patient with a previous attack of diverticulitis. Note stricture in sigmoid colon. Colonoscopy was necessary to exclude cancer.

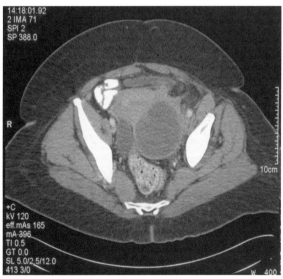

FIGURE 51-28 CT scan of pelvis showing diverticulitis with abscess.

for the evaluation of acute diverticulitis. CT scan provides useful information on the location, extent, and severity of disease as well as pathologic changes outside of the colon, such as an abscess or colovesical fistula. These findings are immensely useful in operative planning. If an abscess is detected by CT scan, it can also be a useful modality for guidance for percutaneous drainage (Fig. 51-28). Ultrasound and magnetic resonance imaging (MRI) have also been used to establish the diagnosis; however, their use varies by institution, and these procedures are not as reliable or expedient as CT scans. Sigmoidoscopy should be approached with caution in the acute setting because distention of the colon could result in worsening perforation.

Management

The management of acute diverticulitis primarily depends on the severity of disease at presentation, and subsequently the approach to care should be individualized. Acute diverticulitis is often broadly clinically divided into uncomplicated and complicated disease on the basis of the findings on initial presentation. Patients with complicated diverticulitis are characterized by the presence of an abscess, fistula, obstruction, or free perforation. The majority of these patients will require surgery. Those with uncomplicated disease are found to have pericolonic inflammation in the presence of diverticula without any of these complications.[13]

Uncomplicated Diverticulitis

The majority of patients with uncomplicated diverticulitis can be managed in the outpatient setting with a regimen of antibiotics and short-term diet modification as their symptoms resolve. This can be accomplished successfully and safely if the patient is afebrile with stable vital signs, is able to tolerate an oral diet, and is without evidence of immunosuppression or significant comorbid conditions. Antibiotics should be tailored to gram-negative rods and anaerobes. Those patients who do not meet these criteria or who have significant concerning peritonitis on physical examination should be admitted to the hospital for bowel rest, intravenous (IV) antibiotics, and judicious analgesia. Patients with uncomplicated diverticulitis usually respond promptly with marked improvement in symptoms within 48 hours; therefore, failure to improve in this interval should prompt further evaluation to ensure that there has been no progression in the severity of the disease. After the resolution of symptoms, colonoscopy should be performed in 4 to 6 weeks to confirm the presence of diverticula and to exclude any neoplasm or other colonic disease, such as IBD or other colitides, that could mimic the symptoms of diverticulitis. Contrast enema can be helpful in delineating the extent of colonic diverticula but is limited in definitely excluding neoplasms.

After the resolution of the initial episode of acute uncomplicated diverticulitis, approximately 33% of patients will have recurrent attacks or continue to have symptoms; however, only a small percentage of those who are hospitalized and roughly 1% of patients with diverticulosis will ultimately require surgery. Historically, the recommendation for elective surgery was based on the number of recurrences, as providers feared the progression to complicated disease with subsequent exacerbations of diverticulitis.[14-16] Current recommendations suggest that the decision for surgery should be individualized, taking into consideration the frequency and severity of recurrences. The patient's overall medical condition and comorbidities should also be included in the analysis.[17,18]

The goal of elective colectomy is to remove the affected segment of colon (usually the sigmoid colon) and to perform a primary anastomosis of the healthy remaining bowel. An important technical consideration after sigmoid colectomy is that the anastomosis should be made to the upper rectum to minimize the risk of recurrent disease. There is a large body of evidence to support that this can be achieved with either a laparoscopic or open approach with similar morbidity and mortality. The short-term benefits of laparoscopy, including less pain, quicker recovery of bowel function, and shorter hospital stays, can be achieved with minimally invasive sigmoid colectomy for diverticulitis. A hand-assisted laparoscopic approach has been advocated by some surgeons who believe that this technique facilitates the division of fused tissue planes while maintaining the benefits of laparoscopy.

Complicated Diverticulitis

Abscess. Diverticulitis complicated by a pelvic or pericolonic abscess is a challenging clinical entity. Patients often present with abdominal pain, fever, leukocytosis, and an ileus due to the associated inflammation of the small bowel. The management of these abscesses depends primarily on the radiographic appearance, size, and location with respect to the other intra-abdominal organs. Large (≥4 cm) pericolonic abscesses can often be managed successfully with percutaneous drainage with CT or ultrasound guidance to reduce the inflammation and to avoid a transabdominal approach by laparotomy. Smaller abscesses, which are typically not amenable to percutaneous drainage, can be managed by combining antibiotics and observation with interval imaging to ensure complete resolution. Failure of percutaneous drainage or antibiotic therapy should mandate more urgent surgical management.

The Hinchey classification is commonly used to describe the severity of diverticular disease complicated by perforation and is an additional tool that may be used to guide overall management:

Stage I: Small, confined pericolonic or mesenteric abscess
Stage II: Larger, walled-off pelvic abscess
Stage III: Generalized purulent peritonitis
Stage IV: Generalized fecal peritonitis

Hinchey stages I and II can often be managed with administration of antibiotics and percutaneous drainage, if technically feasible. If this is successful and the inflammation is allowed to subside, an urgent problem can be converted to an elective one whereby colectomy can be performed and a primary anastomosis can be achieved. Preoperative evaluation with colonoscopy is critical. Current guidelines support the recommendation of elective resection after a single episode of complicated diverticulitis.[17] Hinchey stage III and stage IV generally constitute surgical emergencies that require immediate surgical exploration as patients will present with generalized peritonitis and potentially signs of overwhelming sepsis (fever, tachycardia, hypotension). Abdominal radiographs or CT scans may reveal intraperitoneal free air in addition to inflammation associated with the perforated segment of colon. After resuscitation, operative goals should include washout of the abdominal contamination and resection of the diseased colon. In the setting of a grossly contaminated field, primary anastomosis is not a safe option; therefore, the appropriate strategy should be the Hartmann procedure: segmental resection, a proximal end colostomy, and closure of the rectal stump. Primary anastomosis with or without proximal diversion has been studied extensively in retrospective series in the setting of acute diverticulitis with peritonitis. Although it is feasible if the intra-abdominal contamination is minimal, its application should be individualized on the basis of patient and intraoperative factors.

Given the high morbidity associated with emergent colectomy for perforated diverticulitis, laparoscopic lavage has emerged as an attractive alternative therapeutic approach for patients with Hinchey stage III classification. The procedure entails a diagnostic laparoscopy followed by irrigation with warmed saline to clear the intra-abdominal contamination as well as placement of drains near the perforated segment. Neither colectomy nor colostomy is performed, and patients are treated with perioperative antibiotics. They are also monitored closely postoperatively to ensure that the peritonitis resolves. Patients who fail to improve are considered for colectomy. This has been fertile ground for study in the past decade; several studies show low morbidity and mortality rates as well as short length of hospital stay. Importantly, successful

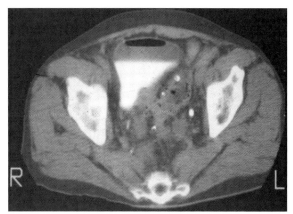

FIGURE 51-29 CT scan of pelvis. The patient has diverticulitis, and air in the bladder indicates a fistula between the sigmoid and the bladder.

laparoscopic lavage may obviate the need for elective resection in many patients. Two large reviews showed elective resection rates of 38% and 51%, with low reported rates of recurrent diverticulitis in those who did not have elective surgery. The safety and efficacy of laparoscopic lavage have yet to be proven in a prospective, randomized fashion.

Fistula. Fistulas to adjacent organs are a relatively common complication of diverticulitis as the associated inflammation of the sigmoid colon causes local attachments and ultimately communication with the bowel. The dome of the bladder is the most common site of fistulas, but the vagina and small bowel are also notable sites. On occasion, colocutaneous fistulas may be formed at the site of prior percutaneous drainage. Patients with colovesical fistulas will frequently present with recurrent urinary tract infections but may also report pneumaturia or fecaluria. Evidence on CT scan of air in the bladder that has not been instrumented is pathognomonic for a colovesical fistula (Fig. 51-29). Sigmoidvesicular fistulas are more common in men than in women because the uterus prevents the sigmoid from adhering to the bladder. A barium enema may reveal a colovesical fistula up to 50% of the time, and cystoscopy usually reveals cystitis and bullous edema at the site of the fistula.

Initial treatment includes broad-spectrum antibiotics to ensure resolution of the inflammation. A colonoscopy to examine the affected colon and to exclude colon cancer or Crohn's disease as the cause of the fistula is important for preoperative planning. Elective resection of the involved colon and fistula tract should then be performed with subsequent primary anastomosis. If a small defect is encountered in the bladder, it may not be necessary to close this primarily, as healing will occur spontaneously if the bladder is drained with a Foley catheter for 7 days after the operation. Larger defects will require primary closure with absorbable sutures combined with Foley drainage. Fistulas to the small bowel will typically require resection and primary anastomosis.

Obstruction. Obstruction due to stricture formation is rarely associated with acute diverticulitis. However, this may occur because of chronic inflammation resulting in narrowing of the lumen. Most often, the obstruction is partial and insidious, but patients can occasionally have significant obstructive symptoms. Preoperative colonoscopy to exclude carcinoma is critical before elective resection; however, if this is not feasible because of luminal narrowing, a retrograde contrast study or CT enterography may be helpful in evaluating the remainder of the proximal colon.

Small bowel obstruction is possible in the setting of acute diverticulitis if the bowel becomes adherent to the phlegmon or abscess. In such circumstances, the appropriate treatment is to pass a nasogastric tube for decompression while addressing the obstruction by treating the infection with antibiotics or percutaneous drainage of the abscess.

Special Considerations
The Immunocompromised Patient
Diverticulitis in the immunocompromised or transplant patient represents a unique challenge for the surgeon. Whereas diverticulitis is not more prevalent in this cohort, studies indicate that they are at greater risk of presenting with recurrent and complicated disease. As a result, there should be a lower threshold for sigmoid colectomy after a single attack of diverticulitis in these patients because of their diminished ability to combat an infectious insult. Prophylactic colectomy in pretransplant patients remains controversial.

Right-Sided Diverticulitis
Diverticulitis of the right colon is relatively rare. Patients with cecal diverticulitis are typically younger by comparison to those with sigmoid diverticulitis and will present with right-sided abdominal pain. This can be a challenging clinical entity as the differential diagnosis can be broad, including acute appendicitis, Meckel's diverticulitis, cholecystitis, pelvic inflammatory disease, pyelonephritis, mesenteric adenitis, and ischemic colitis. A thorough history and evaluation with CT scan are instrumental in making the proper diagnosis. Similar to sigmoid diverticulitis, the CT scan for cecal diverticulitis will show fat stranding or associated abscess or phlegmon. Patients who have recurrent episodes or complicated disease should be considered for resection with a right colectomy.

Diverticulitis in Young Patients
Historically, diverticulitis in younger patients (<50 years) was considered more virulent and associated with worse clinical outcomes and higher recurrence rates. Therefore, elective resection was recommended after one episode even with uncomplicated disease. Further study has shown that initial reports were plagued by selection bias and missed or delayed diagnoses, making a true comparison between younger and older cohorts difficult. Current guidelines do not recommend routine elective resection on the basis of young age (<50 years).[17]

COLONIC VOLVULUS

Volvulus describes the condition in which the bowel becomes twisted on its mesenteric axis, a situation that results in partial or complete obstruction of the bowel lumen and a variable degree of impairment of its blood supply. The condition usually affects the colon. Although colonic volvulus is relatively rare in the United States, ranking behind cancer and diverticulitis, it is responsible for approximately 4% of cases of large bowel obstruction. However, in the region known as the volvulus belt, an area extending along South America, Africa, the Middle East, India, and Russia, colonic volvulus is more common and accounts for approximately 50% of all cases of colonic obstruction.

Any portion of the large bowel can twist if that segment is attached to a long and floppy mesentery that is fixed to the retroperitoneum by a narrow base of origin. However, the mesenteric anatomy is such that volvulus is most common in the sigmoid colon, with less frequent occurrences involving the right colon and terminal ileum (usually referred to as cecal volvulus), the cecum alone (the condition permitted by a highly mobile cecum, called a cecal bascule, that is mobile in a caudad to cephalad direction), and, most rarely, the transverse colon.

Sigmoid volvulus accounts for two thirds of all cases of colonic volvulus. The condition is permitted by an elongated segment of bowel accompanied by a lengthy mesentery with a narrow parietal attachment, a situation that allows the two ends of the mobile segment to come close together and to twist around the narrow mesenteric base. Associated factors include chronic constipation and aging, with the average age at presentation being in the seventh to eighth decade of life. There is an increased incidence of the condition in institutionalized patients afflicted with neuropsychiatric conditions and treated with psychotropic drugs. These medications may predispose to volvulus by affecting intestinal motility. The increased incidence of volvulus in the so-called volvulus belt countries has been attributed to a diet high in fiber and vegetables.

Patients with sigmoid volvulus may present as acute or subacute intestinal obstruction, with signs and symptoms indistinguishable from those caused by cancer of the distal colon. There is usually a sudden onset of severe abdominal pain, vomiting, and obstipation. The abdomen is generally markedly distended and tympanitic, with the distention often more dramatic than would be associated with other causes of obstruction. There is always the possibility that the condition is associated with ischemia caused by mural ischemia resulting from the increased tension of the distended bowel wall or by arterial occlusion caused by torsion of the mesenteric arterial supply. Therefore, severe abdominal pain, rebound tenderness, and tachycardia are ominous signs.

There may be a history of previous episodes of acute volvulus that spontaneously resolved. In this case, marked abdominal distention may occur with minimal tenderness.

Radiographic findings are often dramatic and enable prompt diagnosis and treatment (Fig. 51-30). Abdominal radiographs

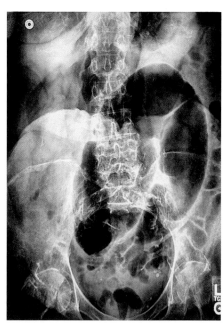

FIGURE 51-30 Plain film of sigmoid volvulus. Note bent inner tube appearance.

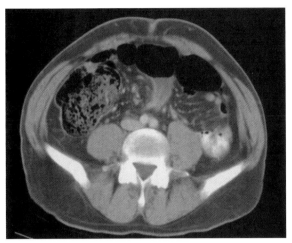

FIGURE 51-31 CT scan of abdomen in patient with sigmoid volvulus. Note characteristic whorl in mesentery.

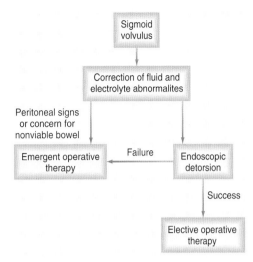

FIGURE 51-33 Algorithm for the management of volvulus.

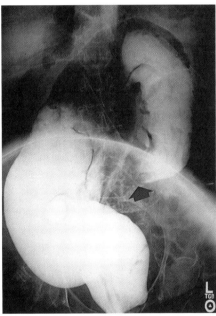

FIGURE 51-32 Radiograph of barium enema with sigmoid volvulus. Contrast material and air fill the rectum and distal sigmoid colon. The contrast material stops abruptly at the point of torsion.

reveal a markedly dilated sigmoid colon that resembles a bent inner tube, with its apex in the right upper quadrant. An air-fluid level may be seen in the dilated loop of colon, and gas is usually absent from the rectum. CT, although not necessary to establish the diagnosis, will typically reveal a characteristic mesenteric whorl (Fig. 51-31). A contrast enema typically demonstrates the point of obstruction with the pathognomonic bird's beak deformity revealing the twist that obstructs the sigmoid lumen (Fig. 51-32).

Treatment of the sigmoid volvulus begins with appropriate resuscitation and, in most cases, involves nonoperative decompression. Decompression relieves the acute problem and allows resection as an elective procedure, which can be accomplished with reduced morbidity and mortality. Patients with signs of colonic necrosis are not eligible for nonoperative decompression.

Decompression can be achieved by placement of a rectal tube through a rigid proctoscope, but more often a flexible sigmoidoscope is used. Decompression results in a sudden gush of gas and fluid, with a decrease in the abdominal distention. The reduction should be confirmed with an abdominal radiograph. The rectal tube should be taped to the thigh and left in place for 1 or 2 days to allow continued decompression and to prevent immediate recurrence of the volvulus. The bowel can then be cleansed with cathartics and a complete colonoscopic examination performed. If detorsion of the volvulus cannot be accomplished with a rectal tube or flexible sigmoidoscope, laparotomy with resection of the sigmoid colon (Hartmann operation) is required (Fig. 51-33).

Even if detorsion of the sigmoid is successful, elective sigmoid resection is indicated in most cases because of the extremely high recurrence rate, which approaches 70%. Colonoscopy should be performed before elective resection to exclude an associated neoplasm. The operation can be conducted through a small left lower quadrant incision or by a laparoscopic approach. Because the elongated colon and mesentery require almost no mobilization, resection with primary anastomosis is easily accomplished.

For patients with signs of colonic necrosis or in whom endoscopic detorsion has failed, the traditional treatment has been a sigmoid colectomy with closure of the rectum and end colostomy (Hartmann procedure). Some surgeons have recently demonstrated, however, that resection with primary anastomosis, with or without protection from a proximal ostomy (transverse colostomy or ileostomy), may be accomplished in the acute setting. For patients who have had successful endoscopic detorsion but have significant comorbidities, endoscopic colopexy may also be an option.

Although the term *cecal volvulus* is ingrained in the literature, true volvulus of the cecum probably never occurs. There is a well-recognized condition, a cecal bascule, in which the cecum folds in a cephalad direction anteriorly over a fixed ascending colon. Although gangrene may develop, this is exceedingly rare because there is no major vessel obstruction. The cecal bascule commonly causes intermittent bouts of abdominal pain because the mobile cecum permits intermittent episodes of isolated cecal obstruction that are spontaneously relieved as the cecum falls back into its normal position.

The condition commonly referred to as cecal volvulus is actually a cecocolic volvulus. It consists of an axial rotation of the terminal ileum, cecum, and ascending colon, with concomitant twisting of the associated mesentery. This is a relatively rare condition, accounting for less than 2% of all cases of adult intestinal obstruction and approximately 25% of all cases of colonic volvulus in the United States. Cecocolic volvulus is possible because of a lack of fixation of the cecum to the retroperitoneum. Studies on cadavers have shown that between 11% and 22% of people have a right colon that is sufficiently mobile to allow a volvulus to occur. Factors that have been implicated in causing a cecal volvulus include previous surgery, pregnancy, malrotation, and obstructing lesions of the left colon. Cecocolic volvulus is somewhat more common in women, whereas sigmoid volvulus occurs with equal frequency in men and women. Cecocolic volvulus affects a younger age group (most common in the late 50s) than sigmoid volvulus.

The typical presentation of patients with cecocolic volvulus is the sudden onset of abdominal pain and distention. In the early phases of a cecocolic volvulus, the pain is mild or moderate in intensity. If the condition is not relieved and ischemia occurs, the pain increases significantly. Physical examination may reveal asymmetrical distention of the abdomen, with a tympanitic mass palpable in the left upper quadrant or midabdomen. Plain radiographs of the abdomen reveal a dilated cecum that is usually displaced to the left side of the abdomen. The distended cecum generally assumes a gas-filled comma shape, the concavity of which faces inferiorly and to the right. On occasion, the distended cecum appears as a circular shape with a narrow, triangular density pointing superiorly and to the right. Haustral markings in the distended loop indicate that the dilated bowel is colon. The torsion results in obstruction of the small bowel, and the radiographic pattern of dilated small intestine can cause diagnostic difficulty.

Although there have been reports of detorsion of cecocolic volvulus with a colonoscope, most cases require surgery to correct the volvulus and to prevent ischemia. If ischemia has already occurred, an immediate operation is obviously required. Contrast enema can sometimes be helpful to confirm the diagnosis and to exclude a carcinoma of the distal bowel as a precipitating cause of the volvulus (Fig. 51-34). Although there have been reports of endoscopic detorsion of cecal volvulus, the success rate is significantly lower than in sigmoid volvulus, and the procedure is associated with the risks of increasing distention because of insufflation of air during the procedure. Surgical intervention is therefore warranted in almost all cases of cecocolic volvulus.

Right colectomy is the procedure of choice. Primary anastomosis is usually preferred unless the volvulus has resulted in frankly gangrenous bowel, in which case resection of the gangrenous bowel with ileostomy is a safer approach. There have been many reports of correcting cecocolic volvulus with cecopexy, which should avoid the complication associated with an anastomosis. However, the procedure to provide fixation of the cecum is extensive and entails elevating and attaching a flap of peritoneum over the surface of the cecum and ascending colon. The recurrence rates are high with cecopexy, and right colectomy remains the procedure of choice for most surgeons.

Volvulus of the transverse colon is extremely rare and tends to be associated with other abnormalities, such as congenital bands and distal obstructing lesions, and pregnancy. Clinical features are indistinguishable from other causes of large bowel obstruction. Radiologic examination is not particularly useful because many

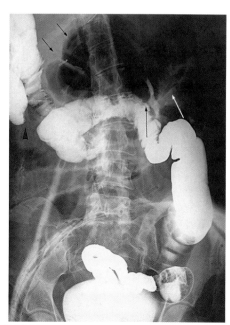

FIGURE 51-34 Radiograph of barium enema in a patient with cecal volvulus. The contrast material stops abruptly at the proximal end of the hepatic flexure *(arrowhead)*. The dilated air-filled cecum crosses the midline of the abdomen toward the left upper quadrant *(arrows)*. (Courtesy Dr. Dina F. Caroline, Temple University Hospital, Philadelphia.)

cases are misdiagnosed as sigmoid volvulus. A contrast study may show a bird's beak deformity, indicating a volvulus. In such cases, colonoscopic reduction may result in detorsion and relief of obstruction. Elective resection should follow to prevent recurrence.

LARGE BOWEL OBSTRUCTION AND PSEUDO-OBSTRUCTION

Large bowel obstruction can be classified as dynamic (mechanical obstruction) or adynamic (pseudo-obstruction). Mechanical obstruction is characterized by blockage of the large bowel (luminal, mural, or extramural), resulting in increased intestinal contractility as a physiologic response to relieve the obstruction. Pseudo-obstruction is characterized by the absence of intestinal contractility, often associated with decreased or absent motility of the small bowel and stomach.

Colorectal cancer is the single most common cause of large intestinal obstruction in the United States, whereas colonic volvulus is the more common cause in Russia, eastern Europe, and Africa. Approximately 2% to 5% of patients with colorectal cancer in the United States present with complete obstruction. Intraluminal causes of colorectal obstruction include fecal impaction, inspissated barium, and foreign bodies. Intramural causes, in addition to carcinoma, include inflammation (e.g., diverticulitis, Crohn's disease, lymphogranuloma venereum, tuberculosis, schistosomiasis), Hirschsprung's disease (aganglionosis), ischemia, radiation, intussusception, and anastomotic stricture. Extraluminal causes include adhesions (the most common cause of small bowel obstruction but rarely a cause of colonic obstruction), hernias, tumors in adjacent organs, abscesses, and volvulus.

The signs and symptoms of large bowel obstruction depend on the cause and location of the obstruction. Cancers arising in the rectum or left colon are more likely to obstruct than those arising in the more capacious proximal colon. Regardless of the cause of the blockage, the clinical manifestations of large bowel obstruction include the failure to pass stool and flatus associated with increasing abdominal distention and cramping abdominal pain.

The colon becomes distended as gas (approximately two thirds is swallowed air, and the remainder includes the products of bacterial fermentation), stool, and liquid accumulate proximal to the site of blockage. If the obstruction is the result of a segment of colon trapped by a hernia or by a volvulus, the blood supply can become compromised, or strangulated. The venous return is blocked initially, causing localized swelling that can in turn occlude the arterial supply with resultant ischemia that, if uncorrected, can progress to necrosis or gangrene. The strangulation at first involves only the entrapped, or incarcerated, segment of bowel, but the colon proximal to that segment becomes progressively dilated because of the obstruction.

Another route to vascular compromise of the obstructed colon occurs if the bowel proximal to the point of obstruction distends to the extent that the intramural pressure within the intestinal wall exceeds the capillary pressure, depriving the bowel of adequate oxygenation. This route to ischemic necrosis can occur with mechanical obstruction and pseudo-obstruction.

A closed loop obstruction occurs when the proximal and distal parts of the bowel are occluded. A strangulated hernia or volvulus almost always leads to this condition. The more common form of closed loop obstruction, however, is seen when a cancer occludes the lumen of the colon in the presence of a competent ileocecal valve. In this situation, increasing colonic distention causes the pressure in the cecum to become so high that the vessels in the bowel wall are occluded, and necrosis and perforation can occur.

The treatment of large bowel obstruction obviously depends on the cause of the obstruction, and specific treatments are covered in the discussion of those entities (see later). However, some principles of diagnosis and treatment can be generalized. The obstruction needs to be relieved with some expediency before compromise of the blood supply results in ischemia and gangrene. The diagnosis should be established to guide appropriate treatment. History and physical examination provide important clues. The abdomen should be palpated for masses, the groins inspected for hernias, and a digital rectal examination performed to exclude rectal cancer. Plain films of the abdomen provide considerable information concerning the location of the obstruction and, in some situations, may be diagnostic of a volvulus. A CT scan is helpful in revealing an inflammatory process, such as an abscess associated with diverticulitis, and identifying the site of the obstruction. If a volvulus or distal sigmoid cancer is suspected, a water-soluble contrast enema may establish the diagnosis. Treatment options vary considerably, depending on the diagnosis, the condition of the bowel, and the status of the patient. It is helpful to establish the diagnosis before an operation to guide therapy properly. If the cause of the obstruction is a cancer of the distal or mid rectum, the preferred treatment is to relieve the obstruction with a loop sigmoid colostomy and then to treat the cancer with neoadjuvant chemoradiation, with a plan to resect the primary lesion at a later time after treatment. On the other hand, if the obstructing cancer is in the sigmoid colon, the surgical options include Hartmann operation (sigmoidectomy with descending colostomy and closure of the rectal stump or mucous fistula) and sigmoidectomy with primary colorectal anastomosis

(with or without intraoperative colonic lavage if the colon is in good condition and the patient is stable).

Right-sided colonic obstruction, whether caused by cancer or the result of volvulus, is generally treated by resection and primary anastomosis of the ileum and transverse colon if the bowel is well perfused and relatively nonedematous and the patient is hemodynamically stable. If any one of those conditions is not met, temporary end ileostomy and mucous fistula or long Hartmann is indicated. In general, a stable patient with an early obstruction and well-perfused, nonedematous bowel can be considered for primary anastomosis. A safe choice and acceptable choice in emergency bowel surgery and obstruction in general is a temporary diverting stoma.

Pseudo-obstruction of the colon, also called Ogilvie syndrome, after its description by Sir William Heneage Ogilvie in 1948, describes the condition of distention of the colon, with signs and symptoms of colonic obstruction, in the absence of an actual physical cause of the obstruction. Ogilvie described two patients with clinical features of colonic obstruction despite normal findings on a barium enema study. Both patients underwent laparotomy for the condition; neither had mechanical obstruction, but both had unsuspected malignant disease involving the area of the celiac axis and semilunar ganglion. The cause of the dilation was attributed to the malignant infiltration of the sympathetic ganglia. Subsequently, there have been numerous descriptions of cases of colonic distention in the absence of mechanical obstruction and without malignant involvement of the visceral autonomic nerves. Very few cases of pseudo-obstruction have malignant infiltration of the autonomic nerves as the cause; in fact, the exact pathogenesis of the syndrome remains unknown, and it has been associated with a heterogeneous group of conditions.

Primary pseudo-obstruction is a motility disorder that is a familial visceral myopathy (hollow visceral myopathy syndrome) or a diffuse motility disorder involving the autonomic innervation of the intestinal wall. The latter may be modified by a disturbance of intestinal hormones or may be principally caused by disordered autonomic innervation.

Secondary pseudo-obstruction is more common and has been associated with neuroleptic medications, opiates, severe metabolic illness, myxedema, diabetes mellitus, uremia, hyperparathyroidism, lupus, scleroderma, Parkinson disease, and traumatic retroperitoneal hematomas. One mechanism thought to play a role in the pathogenesis is sympathetic overactivity overriding the parasympathetic system. Indirect support for this theory has been derived from the success in treating the syndrome with neostigmine, a parasympathomimetic agent. Further support comes from reports of immediate resolution of the syndrome after administration of an epidural anesthetic that provides sympathetic blockade.

Pseudo-obstruction may be manifested in an acute or chronic form. The acute variety usually affects patients with chronic renal, respiratory, cerebral, or cardiovascular disease. It generally involves only the colon, whereas the chronic form affects other parts of the GI tract, usually is manifested as bouts of subacute and partial intestinal obstruction, and tends to recur periodically.

Acute colonic pseudo-obstruction should be suspected when a medically ill patient suddenly develops abdominal distention. The abdomen is tympanitic and usually nontender, and bowel sounds are generally present. Plain abdominal radiographs reveal a distended colon, with the right and transverse segments tending to be most dramatically affected. The radiologic appearance is one of large bowel obstruction.

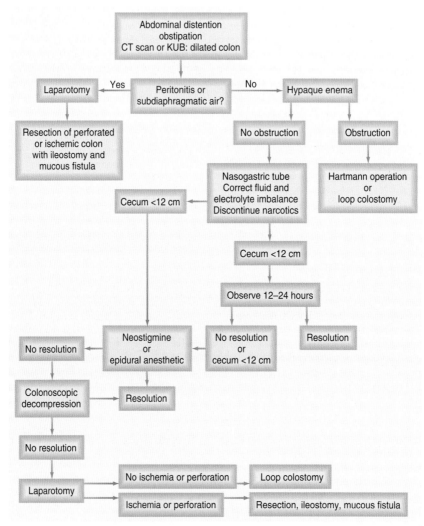

FIGURE 51-35 Algorithm for Ogilvie syndrome management.

The most useful investigation is a water-soluble contrast enema, which should be performed in all patients in whom the diagnosis is suspected, provided they are stable enough to tolerate the procedure (Fig. 51-35). The contrast enema can reliably differentiate between mechanical obstruction and pseudo-obstruction, a differentiation that is essential to guide appropriate therapy.

Colonoscopy is an alternative diagnostic investigation for pseudo-obstruction and has the attractive advantage that it can be used for treatment. However, colonoscopy runs the risk of distending the proximal colon even more, with insufflation of more air, and at present, the water-soluble contrast enema is generally the preferred initial test.

When the diagnosis of acute pseudo-obstruction is suspected, treatment should accompany the diagnostic evaluation. Initial treatment includes nasogastric decompression, replacement of extracellular fluid deficits, and correction of electrolyte abnormalities. All medications that inhibit bowel motility, such as opiates and antihistamines, should be discontinued. Ambulation, if possible, is encouraged. The patient's response is monitored by serial abdominal examinations and radiography. Most patients improve with this regimen. Until the mid-1990s, the treatment

generally used when the colonic distention failed to resolve with supportive measures was colonoscopic decompression. Although this approach was usually successful, it required skilled personnel and equipment and carried the risk for colonic perforation from instrument trauma and insufflation. In addition, the procedure often had to be repeated because of recurrence of the colonic distention.

Sympathetic blockade by epidural anesthesia has been shown to relieve colonic pseudo-obstruction successfully. However, at present, the trend has been to treat this condition with neostigmine, a parasympathomimetic agent. It is obviously imperative that mechanical obstruction be excluded by water-soluble contrast enema or colonoscopy before the administration of neostigmine because the subsequent high pressures generated in the colon against a distal obstruction could cause colonic perforation.

Neostigmine enhances parasympathetic activity by competing with acetylcholine for acetylcholinesterase binding sites. In the treatment of colonic pseudo-obstruction, 2.5 mg of neostigmine is given intravenously over 3 minutes. The resolution of the condition is indicated within less than 10 minutes of administration of the drug by the passage of stool and flatus by the patient. The recurrence rates after the administration of neostigmine appear to be far lower than those associated with colonoscopic decompression, with satisfactory decompression being achieved in approximately 90% of patients after a single administration of the medication.

A significant side effect of neostigmine is bradycardia, and all patients must be monitored by telemetry during administration of the drug. Atropine must be immediately available; patients with significant cardiac disease or asthma are not candidates for this treatment.

If treatment with neostigmine, an epidural anesthetic, or colonoscopic decompression is not successful, or if signs of peritonitis or intestinal perforation occur, laparotomy is required. In the absence of perforation or ischemia, a loop colostomy is indicated to vent the proximal and distal colon. Any areas of perforation or ischemia must be resected.

INFLAMMATORY BOWEL DISEASE

The term *inflammatory bowel disease* is generally used to describe two diseases of unknown cause with similar general characteristics, ulcerative colitis and Crohn's disease. The distinction between the two entities can usually be established on the basis of clinical and pathologic criteria, including history and physical examination, radiologic and endoscopic studies, gross appearance, and histology. However, in approximately 10% to 15% of patients with inflammatory disease confined to the colon, a clear distinction cannot be made, and the disease is labeled indeterminate colitis. The medical treatment and surgical management of ulcerative colitis and Crohn's disease often differ significantly, so each entity is discussed separately here. A comparison of the characteristics of ulcerative colitis and Crohn's disease is presented in Table 51-1.

Ulcerative Colitis
Epidemiology and Cause
Ulcerative colitis occurs more commonly in developed countries and is relatively unusual in Asia, Africa, and South America. There appears to be a seasonal variation in the activity of the disease, with onset and relapse occurring statistically more often between August and January. The incidence of the disease has remained relatively stable during the past 25 years, with new cases reported as 4 to 6 cases/100,000 white adults per year, with a prevalence ranging from 40 to 100 cases/100,000. All ages are susceptible, but it more commonly affects patients younger than 30 years. A small secondary peak in the incidence occurs in the sixth decade. Both genders are equally affected, but the condition is more common in whites, Ashkenazi Jews, and persons of northern European ancestry.

Although the cause of ulcerative colitis is unknown, its prevalence in industrialized countries and the increased incidence in individuals who migrate from low-risk to high-risk areas suggest an environmental influence. Speculation on the influence of dietary factors has included inadequate fiber intake, chemical food additives, refined sugars, and cow's milk. However, none of these have been demonstrated to play a definitive role. Infectious agents, including *C. difficile* and *Campylobacter jejuni,* have been implicated as playing a causative role in the pathogenesis, but such a role has not been confirmed.

Smoking appears to confer a protective effect against the development of ulcerative colitis as well as providing a therapeutic influence; nicotine has been reported to induce remission in some

TABLE 51-1 Comparisons of Ulcerative Colitis and Crohn's Colitis

	ULCERATIVE COLITIS	CROHN'S COLITIS
Gross Appearance		
Thickened wall	0	4+
Thickened mesentery	0	3+
Serosal fat wrapping	0	4+
Segmental disease	0	4+
Microscopic Appearance		
Transmural	0	4+
Lymphoid aggregates	0	4+
Granulomas	0	3+
Clinical Features		
Bleeding per rectum	3+	1+
Diarrhea	3+	3+
Obstructive symptoms	1+	3+
Anal or perianal disease	Rare	4+
Risk for cancer	2+	3+
Small bowel disease	0	4+
Colonoscopic Features		
Distribution	Continuous	Discontinuous
Rectal disease	4+	1+
Friability	4+	1+
Aphthous ulcers	0	4+
Deep longitudinal ulcers	0	4+
Cobblestoning	0	4+
Pseudopolyps	2+	2+
Operative Treatment		
Total proctocolectomy	Curative	Combined disease: colon and rectum
Segmental resection	Rare	Absence of anorectal disease
Ileal pouch	Preferred by most patients	Contraindicated
Complications		
Postoperative recurrence	0	4+
Fistulas	Rare	4+
Sclerosing cholangitis	1+	Rare
Cholelithiasis	0	2+
Nephrolithiasis	0	2+

cases. This is in contrast to Crohn's disease, which is more common in smokers and appears to be aggravated by the habit. Both ulcerative colitis and Crohn's disease are more common in women who use oral contraceptives compared with those who do not. Patients who have had an appendectomy appear to be at decreased risk for development of ulcerative colitis.

A family history of IBD is a significant risk factor. Several studies have demonstrated the existence of family aggregates with ulcerative colitis and a high degree of concordance in monozygotic twins. The genetic predisposition for ulcerative colitis is not inherited in a classic mendelian pattern, suggesting the influence of environmental factors on an individual's susceptibility. Genetic abnormalities found to be associated with ulcerative colitis are variations in DNA repair genes and class II major histocompatibility complex genes. Patients with ulcerative colitis display specific alleles of group HLA and DR2 (HLA-DRB1), with an association between certain alleles and expression of the disease. The DR1501 allele is associated with a more benign course, whereas the DR1502 allele is associated with a more virulent form of the disease.

Another theory of the cause of IBD concerns an altered immunologic response to external and host antigens. Although anticolon antibodies have been identified in blood and tissue of patients with IBD, there is little evidence that these play a pathogenic role. Other studies have shown that defective cell-mediated immunity, leukocyte chemotactic impairment, and abnormalities of antigen-specific helper and suppressor T cells may be involved in the pathogenesis.

Pathologic Features

Gross appearance. Ulcerative colitis is a disease in which the major pathologic process involves the mucosa and submucosa of the colon, with sparing of the muscularis. Despite the name, ulceration of the mucosa is not invariably present. In fact, the typical gross appearance of ulcerative colitis is hyperemic mucosa. Friable and granular mucosa is common in more severe cases, and ulceration may not be readily evident, especially early in the course of the disease. However, ulceration may appear and vary widely, from small superficial erosions to patchy ulceration of the full thickness of the mucosa (Fig. 51-36). The rectum is invariably involved with the inflammatory process. In fact, rectal involvement (proctitis) is the hallmark of the disease, and the diagnosis should be questioned if the rectal mucosa is not affected. The mucosal inflammation extends in a continuous fashion for a variable distance into the more proximal colon. Pseudopolyps, or inflammatory polyps, represent regeneration of inflamed mucosa and are composed of a variable mixture of non-neoplastic colonic mucosa and inflamed lamina propria (Fig. 51-37).

As implied earlier, a diagnostic characteristic of ulcerative colitis is continuous uninterrupted inflammation of the colonic mucosa, beginning in the distal rectum and extending proximally to a variable distance. This is in contrast to Crohn's disease, in which normal segments of colon (skipped areas) may be interspersed between distinct segments of colonic inflammation. The entire colon, including the cecum and appendix, may be involved in ulcerative colitis. In contrast to Crohn's disease, ulcerative colitis does not involve the terminal ileum, except in cases of backwash ileitis, when the ileal mucosa may appear inflamed in the presence of extensive proximal colonic involvement. However, in such cases, contrast studies usually reveal the inflamed ileum to be dilated, in contrast to the frequently narrowed and contracted ileum characteristic of Crohn's disease.

Colonic strictures can occur in 5% to 12% of patients with chronic ulcerative colitis. Although these strictures are most often benign, caused by hypertrophy of the muscularis, cancer must be excluded as the cause of any colonic stricture occurring in the setting of ulcerative colitis. Three important features are suggestive of malignant strictures: appearance later in the course of ulcerative colitis (60% after 20 years versus 0% before 10 years); location proximal to the splenic flexure (86% malignant); and large bowel obstruction caused by the stricture (Fig. 51-38).

Histologic appearance. The typical microscopic finding in ulcerative colitis is inflammation of the mucosa and submucosa. The most characteristic lesion is the crypt abscess, in which collections of neutrophils fill and expand the lumina of individual crypts of Lieberkühn (Fig. 51-39). Crypt abscesses, however, are not specific for ulcerative colitis and can be seen in Crohn's disease and infectious colitis. Hematochezia often results from the marked vascular congestion. Crypt branching may be seen in chronic ulcerative colitis and is an important characteristic. The number of goblet cells in the crypts is diminished, as is mucus production.

It has been stressed that the inflammatory process in ulcerative colitis spares the muscular layer of the colon, a characteristic that differentiates it from Crohn's disease, which is characterized by transmural inflammation or involvement of all layers of the

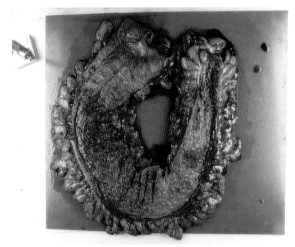

FIGURE 51-36 Ulcerative colitis: macroscopic appearance of colitis extending continuously from the rectum *(upper right)* to the mid–ascending colon *(upper left)*. The proximal colon appears spared, with normal colonic folds. Most of the colon exhibits erythema and granularity of the mucosal surface. (Courtesy Dr. Jeffrey P. Baliff, Thomas Jefferson University, Philadelphia.)

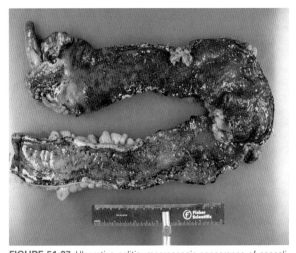

FIGURE 51-37 Ulcerative colitis: macroscopic appearance of pancolitis. The entire length of the colonic mucosa exhibits prominent flattening, erythema, and friability, with focal areas of green-yellow exudate. There is a suggestion of linear ulcerations along the bowel axis. Overall, the colon is narrowed and shortened. The terminal ileum *(upper left)* is spared. (Courtesy Dr. Jeffrey P. Baliff, Thomas Jefferson University, Philadelphia.)

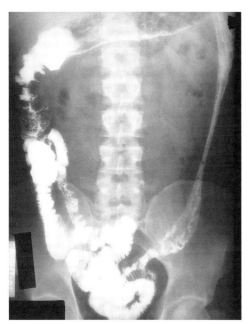

FIGURE 51-38 Radiograph of stricture in chronic ulcerative colitis. Colonoscopy revealed chronic inflammation but no dysplasia or cancer.

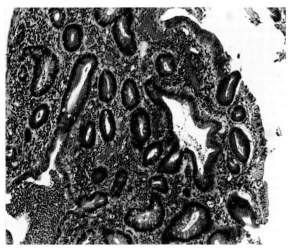

FIGURE 51-39 Histologic section of active ulcerative colitis. There is glandular architectural distortion manifested by irregular branching and orientation of glands relative to the surface. The lamina propria is expanded with inflammatory cells, and intraepithelial neutrophils are present. A crypt abscess is noted *(lower left)*. (Courtesy Dr. Jeffrey P. Baliff, Thomas Jefferson University, Philadelphia.)

intestinal wall. However, in rare cases of severe inflammation, all layers of the colon may be involved, and perforation may occur if treatment is delayed. However, the inflammatory process in such cases (toxic megacolon) is atypical and may be related to factors such as prolonged colonic distention with vascular compromise.

Numerous studies have demonstrated that antineutrophil cytoplasmic antibodies with a perinuclear staining pattern are seen in up to 86% of patients with mucosal ulcerative colitis. The presence of perinuclear antineutrophil cytoplasmic antibodies has

been used as a diagnostic test to help differentiate ulcerative colitis from Crohn's disease.

Clinical Presentation

Ulcerative colitis and colonic Crohn's disease often have similar clinical presentations. Both may be manifested with diarrhea and the passage of mucus. Patients with ulcerative colitis tend to have more urgency than those with Crohn's disease, likely because ulcerative colitis is invariably associated with distal proctitis. Rectal bleeding is also common in ulcerative colitis; although it may be present in patients with Crohn's disease, it is typically not as severe. Patients with acute-onset ulcerative colitis often complain of abdominal discomfort, but the pain is seldom as severe as that found in patients with Crohn's disease. A tender abdominal mass suggestive of a phlegmon or abscess is more commonly associated with Crohn's disease.

Perianal disease is an uncommon finding in patients with ulcerative disease, whereas it may be the only presenting symptom of Crohn's disease. It is interesting and seemingly paradoxical that rectal involvement is present in almost 100% of patients with ulcerative colitis, whereas anal involvement is rare. In contrast, patients with Crohn's disease may have normal rectal mucosa (so-called rectal sparing), although anal disease (e.g., fissures, fistulas, abscesses) is common.

Extraintestinal Manifestations

Extraintestinal manifestations of ulcerative colitis include arthritis, ankylosing spondylitis, erythema nodosum, pyoderma gangrenosum, and primary sclerosing cholangitis (PSC). Arthritis, particularly of the knees, ankles, hips, and shoulders, occurs in approximately 20% of patients, typically in association with increased activity of intestinal disease. Ankylosing spondylitis occurs in 3% to 5% of patients and is most prevalent in patients who are HLA-B27 positive or have a family history of ankylosing spondylitis. Erythema nodosum arises in 10% to 15% of patients with ulcerative colitis and often occurs in conjunction with peripheral arthropathy. Pyoderma gangrenosum typically is manifested on the pretibial region as an erythematous plaque that progresses into an ulcerated painful wound. Most patients who develop this condition have underlying active IBD. Arthritis, ankylosing spondylitis, erythema nodosum, and pyoderma gangrenosum typically improve or completely resolve after colectomy.

PSC occurs in 5% to 8% of patients with ulcerative colitis. Most patients with IBD who develop PSC are younger than 40 years, and most are men. Genetics likely play a role because patients with ulcerative colitis who have the HLA-B8 or HLA-DR3 haplotype are 10 times more likely to develop PSC. Patients with PSC and ulcerative colitis typically have a more quiescent disease course; however, the risk for colon cancer in these patients is up to five times greater than in patients with ulcerative colitis alone. These tumors are more likely to arise proximal to the splenic flexure. PSC may be asymptomatic and diagnosed only by abnormal laboratory test results, or it may be manifested with symptoms of obstructive jaundice and abdominal pain. The disease is progressive and ultimately fatal unless liver transplantation is undertaken. Colectomy has no effect on the course of PSC.

Diagnosis

Endoscopic examination of the colon and rectum is essential in the diagnosis of IBD. In the acute phase of the disease, proctosigmoidoscopy is often sufficient because the rectum is invariably inflamed in patients with ulcerative colitis. Complete colonoscopy offers little additional information in the acute setting and increases the risk for colonic perforation. The presence of diffuse, confluent, symmetrical disease from the dentate line proximally is consistent with ulcerative colitis; the mucosal appearance can vary from loss of the normal vessel pattern secondary to edema in the early stages of the disease to frank ulceration in more advanced disease. If the inflammation extends beyond the level of the sigmoidoscope, a full colonoscopy should be carried out after the disease is more quiescent.[19,20]

Conditions other than ulcerative colitis can be manifested with similar symptoms of diarrhea and bleeding; it is important to identify these conditions because their treatment may be considerably different. Crohn's disease has features similar to those of ulcerative colitis; however, the rectum is spared in 40% of patients with Crohn's colitis, even in the presence of perianal disease. An upper GI radiograph with a small bowel follow-through should be obtained to rule out the possibility of small bowel involvement, a finding that would suggest Crohn's disease. Collagenous colitis is a condition that generally occurs in women older than 50 years. It typically is manifested with profuse watery diarrhea and is characterized histologically by marked thickening of the colonic subepithelial basement membrane. On endoscopic evaluation, the mucosa appears normal in most patients, and the diagnosis is made by endoscopic biopsy. Treatment of collagenous colitis is typically medical.

In addition to multiple mucosal biopsy specimens from serial sites, stool samples should be sent to the laboratory to look for bacteria, ova, and parasites. Infectious conditions that mimic ulcerative colitis include colitis caused by *C. difficile,* cytomegalovirus, *Entamoeba histolytica, C. jejuni,* and *Salmonella enteritidis.*

Risk for Carcinoma

One of the most serious sequelae of ulcerative colitis is the development of colorectal carcinoma.[21] The most important risk factors include prolonged duration of the disease, pancolonic disease, continuously active disease, and severity of inflammation. The cumulative risk for cancer increases with the duration of the disease, reaching 25% at 25 years, 35% at 30 years, 45% at 35 years, and 65% at 40 years. Patients with disease confined to the left side of the colon have a lower risk for development of carcinoma than patients with disease involving the entire colon. Carcinomas arising in ulcerative colitis tend to be poorly differentiated and highly aggressive tumors.[22] As noted, a colonic stricture in a patient with ulcerative colitis must be presumed to be carcinoma until proved otherwise. If malignant disease cannot be ruled out by endoscopy, the presence of a stricture is an indication for operative intervention (Figs. 51-40 to 51-42).

There is considerable debate about the optimal method of surveillance colonoscopy in patients with ulcerative colitis. The American Cancer Society guidelines recommend surveillance colonoscopy every 1 to 2 years, beginning 8 years after the onset of pancolitis and 12 to 15 years after the onset of left-sided colitis. This strategy is based on the premise that a dysplastic lesion can be detected endoscopically before invasive carcinoma has developed (Fig. 51-43). Traditionally, 10 random biopsy specimens were recommended; however, it has been suggested that at least 30 specimens be obtained.

The risk for cancer varies with the degree of dysplasia; carcinoma is found in 10% of those displaying low-grade dysplasia, in 30% to 40% with high-grade dysplasia, and in more than 50% of colons with dysplasia associated with a lesion or mass. Neoplastic lesions can develop in dysplasia associated with a lesion or mass

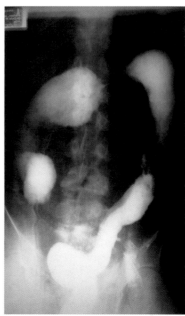

FIGURE 51-40 Radiograph of barium enema demonstrating stricture in transverse colon of patient with ulcerative colitis of 15 years' duration.

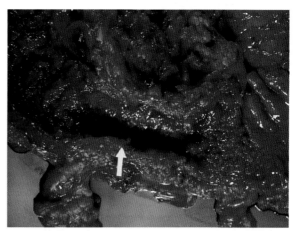

FIGURE 51-41 Resected colon from patient in Figure 51-40, revealing the stricture *(arrow)* to be invasive cancer. The patient had liver metastases.

or in a coincidental adenoma, and approximately 25% of carcinomas in patients with ulcerative colitis are not associated with dysplasia elsewhere in the colon.

A meta-analysis of 10 prospective studies was performed to determine whether colonoscopic surveillance of dysplasia was a reasonable alternative to prophylactic colectomy. Less than 3% of patients who had no dysplasia during the initial evaluation went on to develop evidence of dysplasia. In patients with high-grade dysplasia, however, 32% were found to have invasive carcinoma at the time of colectomy. These tumors tended of earlier stage compared with tumors in patients in whom the diagnosis of cancer was made before colectomy. When high-grade dysplasia is found and has been confirmed by a second independent pathologist, proctocolectomy should be recommended. This is also true for patients who have dysplasia associated with a lesion or mass.

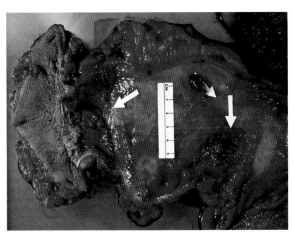

FIGURE 51-42 Resected rectum from patient in Figure 51-40, showing invasive cancers in the rectum *(arrows)*.

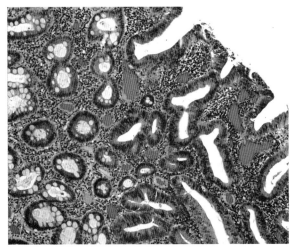

FIGURE 51-43 Flat high-grade dysplasia arising in ulcerative colitis. Compared with the normal crypt epithelium *(left)*, high-grade epithelial dysplasia exhibits an increased nuclear-to-cytoplasmic ratio, hyperchromaticity, and loss of polarity *(right)*. (Courtesy Dr. Jeffrey P. Baliff, Thomas Jefferson University, Philadelphia.)

If low-grade dysplasia is confirmed, strong consideration should also be given to proctocolectomy. Multiple areas of dysplasia, either high or low grade, are an indication for proctocolectomy.

Flow cytometry of colonoscopic biopsy specimens may also be useful for detecting dysplasia. A strong correlation between DNA aneuploidy and polyploidy and the presence of dysplasia has been found. Although the presence of these abnormalities should not serve as an indication for colectomy, they may indicate a need for more frequent colonoscopic surveillance.

Treatment
Medical therapy. Medical management of ulcerative colitis has undergone a significant evolution. The combination of steroids, antimetabolites, immunomodulators, and biologics has significantly advanced the efficacy of the management of acute colitis flares as well as chronic maintenance. Treatment groups can be broadly classified into aminosalicylates, corticosteroids, immunomodulators, and biologics.

In overview, current guidelines of the European consensus conference on management of ulcerative colitis state that patients with steroid-dependent ulcerative colitis should be maintained with thiopurines; the use of methotrexate in ulcerative colitis is no longer supported; and in patients with steroid-resistant, severely active ulcerative colitis, use of cyclosporine or infliximab is recommended.

Aminosalicylates. Aminosalicylates, including 5-aminosalicylic acid formulations and mesalamine, are first-line medications used to induce and to maintain remission in patients with mild to moderately active ulcerative colitis. A Cochrane analysis confirmed that 5-aminosalicylic acid is superior to placebo in maintaining clinical or endoscopic remission with a dose-dependent effect. Common adverse events include abdominal pain, nausea, diarrhea, and dyspepsia.

Corticosteroids. Steroid treatment is considered to be the most effective therapy in inducing remission in patients who do not have adequate response to 5-aminosalicylic acid formulations. Most patients see an effect within 7 to 14 days. Oral steroid doses of prednisone are generally 40 to 60 mg, followed by a taper of 5 to 10 mg per week after remission is achieved. In general, therapy then transitions to thiopurine or aminosalicylate therapy.

In hospitalized patients, treatment of severe ulcerative colitis flares requires the use of IV steroids, such as methylprednisolone or hydrocortisone. This generally results in greater than 50% remission, with response rates as high as 80%. Long-term side effects of systemic corticosteroids include infections, weight gain, hyperglycemia, hirsutism, and hypertension. Bone loss will occur within 6 months of continuous treatment. Systemic steroids are not indicated as long-term therapy, and inability to transition to a long-term treatment denotes steroid-refractory disease. Because of the side-effect profile, oral budesonide, a corticosteroid with high topical activity and low systemic absorption, may be used. However, budesonide was found to have lower efficacy than oral mesalamine after 8 weeks of treatment. Formulations of budesonide designed to be released in the colon show significant improvement over placebo.

Immunomodulators
Thiopurines. Thiopurines are the most commonly used immunomodulators in patients with moderate to severe ulcerative colitis requiring long-term treatment. These medications are not sufficient to be used in treating severe acute flares; rather, they are used chronically, in the transition from initial steroid control to maintenance therapy. The efficacy of azathioprine was evaluated in two randomized controlled trials. A meta-analysis showed a trend toward a benefit of azathioprine compared with placebo for the treatment of active colitis, but this did not reach statistical significance. In quiescent disease, however, there was a statistically significant benefit in the use of azathioprine compared with placebo in preventing relapse. In comparing the efficacy of azathioprine with the use of mesalamine in steroid-dependent ulcerative colitis, after a 6-month follow-up, azathioprine was significantly more effective than mesalamine at achieving clinical and endoscopic remission. More recently, a study was conducted in patients with steroid-dependent ulcerative colitis treated with azathioprine during a 3-year period. This showed sustained efficacy for maintenance of clinical remission off steroids.

Methotrexate. There are few data to support the use of methotrexate in ulcerative colitis. Oren and colleagues conducted a placebo-controlled trial showing no benefit of oral methotrexate in ulcerative colitis patients. In comparing the use of methotrexate with 6-mercaptopurine and mesalamine, there is a significantly higher remission rate observed in patients with ulcerative colitis treated with 6-mercaptopurine compared with mesalamine but not with methotrexate compared with mesalamine.

Tacrolimus. Tacrolimus is appropriate as second-line therapy in patients with severely active ulcerative colitis unresponsive to steroids. In a placebo-controlled trial evaluating the use of tacrolimus in 60 patients with moderate to severe ulcerative colitis, high-dose tacrolimus achieved a nearly 70% clinical improvement compared with 10% of patients treated with placebo. Clinical remission was seen in 20%. This comes at the price of a significant side-effect profile. A more recent randomized controlled trial of 60 patients with steroid-refractory ulcerative colitis showed a response rate of 50% with oral tacrolimus compared with 13% with placebo (*P* = .003) after 2 weeks of treatment.

Cyclosporine. Cyclosporine is another immunomodulator indicated for second-line therapy in the case of severe, steroid-refractory ulcerative colitis. Treatment is usually initiated after 3 to 5 days of failed steroid response. If treatment by cyclosporine fails, surgery is typically indicated within 4 to 7 days. In a placebo-controlled trial, 20 patients who were nonresponsive to IV corticosteroids were randomized to cyclosporine or placebo. In the cyclosporine group, 9 of 11 patients (82%) had a response within a mean of 7 days compared with 0 of 9 patients who received placebo. Cyclosporine use is associated with significant, dose-dependent side effects, including nephrotoxicity, hepatotoxicity, seizures, and lymphoproliferative disorders. As a result, current recommendations are for low-dose (2 mg/kg daily) treatment when appropriate. A study looking at the long-term colectomy-sparing results with the use of cyclosporine showed that transitioning to oral 6-mercaptopurine therapy rather than to oral cyclosporine is associated with a significantly decreased risk of colectomy at 5 years.

Biologics. The use of various anti–tumor necrosis factor-α (TNF-α) monoclonal antibodies is well supported in the case of severe ulcerative colitis refractory to steroids. Typically, before the use of these drugs, the coexistence of cytomegalovirus infection, *C. difficile* infection, and purified protein derivative reactivity as well as any active infection must be ruled out.

The best studied of this group is infliximab. Infliximab was the first anti–TNF-α antibody that was approved by the Food and Drug Administration for the treatment of moderate to severe ulcerative colitis. It is a chimeric (human and murine) monoclonal antibody to TNF-α that is administered by infusion at 6-week intervals. A Cochrane review on the use of infliximab in moderate to severe steroid-refractory ulcerative colitis showed that infliximab was more effective than placebo in inducing clinical remission. Because of the murine component, acute infusion reactions have been observed in 8% to 12% of patients.[23]

Adalimumab is a humanized monoclonal antibody that works in a similar fashion and is effective in patients who cannot tolerate infliximab. Like infliximab, it can induce clinical remission in patients with steroid-refractory moderate to severe ulcerative colitis and in one study rescued 40% of patients who had been previously treated with infliximab. It is also effective as first-line therapy. Golimumab and certolizumab pegol are additional fully human anti–TNF-α monoclonal antibodies that have shown significant efficacy in the treatment of moderate to severe ulcerative colitis.

Current guidelines support the use of either anti–TNF-α medications or thiopurines for maintenance therapy in ulcerative colitis. In addition, anti–TNF-α medications are second-line therapy for severe, steroid-refractory ulcerative colitis and can be effective in avoiding colectomy.[23]

BOX 51-1   **Ulcerative Colitis: Indications for Surgery**
Intractability
Dysplasia, carcinoma
Massive colonic bleeding
Toxic megacolon

The impact of preoperative biologics on the rate of postoperative complications has been a subject of considerable debate. Initial data seemed to suggest a possible increase in postoperative complications with the use of preoperative infliximab; however, a systematic review of data showed that there was no significant difference in the complication rate between infliximab and control groups.

Indications for surgery. Indications for the surgical management of ulcerative colitis include fulminant colitis with toxic megacolon, massive bleeding, intractable disease, and dysplasia or carcinoma (Box 51-1). Malnutrition and growth retardation may necessitate resection in pediatric and adolescent patients.

Fulminant colitis and toxic megacolon. Patients with fulminant colitis typically present with high fever, severe abdominal pain, tenderness, tachycardia, and leukocytosis. These patients require hospitalization with IV hydration, nasogastric decompression, high-dose IV steroids if the patient is steroid dependent, and broad-spectrum antibiotics. IV hyperalimentation may be useful, depending on the patient's nutritional status and length of illness before the fulminant episode. Patients should be closely monitored with serial abdominal examinations and leukocyte counts. Deterioration or lack of improvement within 48 to 72 hours of the initiation of medical treatment warrants an urgent procedure because the mortality rate is increased fourfold in patients with colonic perforation.

Toxic megacolon is a serious life-threatening condition that can occur in patients with ulcerative colitis, Crohn's colitis, and infectious colitides such as pseudomembranous colitis, in which the bacterial infiltration of the walls of the colon creates a dilation of the colon that progresses to the point of imminent perforation. This decompensation results in a necrotic thin-walled bowel in which pneumatosis can often be seen radiographically. Although some patients with toxic megacolon have been successfully treated medically, a high rate of recurrence with subsequent urgent operation has been reported. Aggressive preoperative stabilization is required, using volume resuscitation with crystalloid solutions to prevent dehydration secondary to third-space fluid losses, stress-dose steroids for patients previously receiving steroid therapy, and broad-spectrum antibiotics.

Although a restorative proctocolectomy with IPAA as a single-stage procedure has been reported for toxic megacolon, proctectomy and anastomosis are generally ill-advised in the acutely ill patient with an unprepared bowel. Total proctocolectomy in the urgent setting carries a prohibitively high mortality rate, and the leak rate from a primary anastomosis is unacceptably high. Whereas the goal in elective surgery is to remove all the colonic or dysplastic mucosa, the aim in emergent surgery is to rescue the patient from a life-threatening situation. A total abdominal colectomy with ileostomy and preservation of the rectum is therefore the preferred operation for this condition. This procedure can be expeditiously performed with relatively low morbidity and mortality, and it serves the main purpose of removing the diseased colon and avoiding a difficult and morbid pelvic dissection.

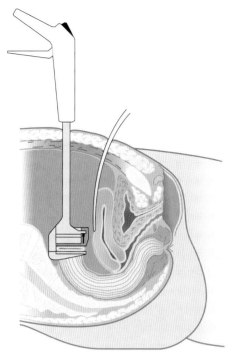

FIGURE 51-44 Closure of rectal stump after resection of abdominal colon.

Preserving the rectum leaves the option of fashioning an ileorectal anastomosis in the future (Fig. 51-44). This is particularly important for patients in whom the diagnosis is unclear and a subsequent ileoanal pouch might be contraindicated (e.g., in Crohn's disease). Some controversy exists about management of the distal segment of bowel. The remaining rectum or rectosigmoid can be delivered as a mucous fistula placed subcutaneously or closed as a Hartmann pouch. Each management strategy has its proponents, but no randomized prospective trial has been performed to date that has shown superiority of any of these options. In general, if the tissue of the rectal stump appears necrotic and fragile, a mucous fistula will prevent stump blowout and sepsis.

The blow-hole procedure was advocated in the past for treatment of patients with severe toxic megacolon in whom the distended colonic wall was so thin and fragile that any handling during the conduct of an operation would risk perforation of the colon, with massive peritoneal contamination. Currently, it is distinctly unusual that operative intervention is delayed to such a degree, but the operation may be advantageous in such dire circumstances. The technique consists of performing a skin-level (blow-hole) transverse colostomy; sometimes the left colon is decompressed with a simultaneous, second, sigmoid skin-level colostomy. Fashioning a loop ileostomy is an essential component of this operation. The operation was often rewarded with dramatic improvement in the patient's condition. After recovery from the acute illness, usually during a period of several months, the patient could then be treated with restorative proctocolectomy with IPAA or total proctocolectomy, depending on the circumstances.

Massive bleeding. Massive hemorrhage from ulcerative colitis is an uncommon event, occurring in less than 5% of patients requiring operation. Patients obviously require resuscitation and stabilization before surgery, with replenishment of extracellular volume and transfusions, as needed. Subtotal colectomy is the procedure of choice and will usually suffice. However, if bleeding continues from the remaining rectal mucosa, emergency proctectomy may be required.

Intractability. Colitis with debilitating symptoms refractory to medical therapy is the most common indication for operative therapy. Patients with intractable disease have persistent symptoms such as crampy abdominal pain, frequent bowel movements, stool urgency, and anemia. It has been demonstrated that patients' quality of life after surgery for ulcerative colitis is improved, regardless of the procedure performed. Complications of long-term steroid therapy, such as diabetes mellitus, avascular necrosis of the femoral head, cataracts, psychiatric problems, osteoporosis, and weight gain, are a frequent indication for surgical resection, even though the patient's symptoms may be controlled while receiving steroids. Indeed, steroid dependence is considered failure of medical management. Elective surgery should also be considered for patients with significant extracolonic manifestations refractory to nonoperative measures.

Dysplasia or carcinoma. The finding of dysplastic changes in the colon or carcinoma is an indication for surgical intervention (see earlier). The presence of cancer may influence the procedure selected or the sequence of staged procedures. It does not exclude the possibility of performing an ileoanal pouch, but the location and stage of the cancer must also be taken into consideration.

Surgical procedures. Elective surgical options for ulcerative colitis include total proctocolectomy with ileostomy, restorative proctocolectomy with IPAA, and total proctocolectomy with a continent ileal reservoir (Kock pouch). Segmental colectomy for ulcerative colitis, in contrast to Crohn's disease, has been shown to be an inadequate procedure for controlling disease. For example, in the case of colitis confined to the left side, a proctosigmoidectomy with an end descending colostomy or coloanal anastomosis invariably results in the recurrence of disease in the remaining colon within a short time and is contraindicated.

In the past, abdominal colectomy with ileorectal anastomosis was advocated for patients with ulcerative colitis and rectal sparing. However, these patients are exceedingly rare. The inflammatory process typical of ulcerative colitis almost always involves the rectum, and an anastomosis of the ileum to the inflamed rectum invariably results in intractable diarrhea. Patients with true rectal sparing and left colitis most likely have Crohn's disease. In that situation, a segmental colectomy or subtotal colectomy with rectal anastomosis is an appropriate procedure.

Total proctocolectomy with end ileostomy. Total proctocolectomy has the advantage of removing all diseased mucosa, thereby preventing further inflammation and the potential for progression to dysplasia or carcinoma. The major disadvantage of this procedure is the need for a permanent ileostomy. In addition, despite improvements in bowel preparation, antibiotics, and surgical technique, a total proctocolectomy still has a fairly high morbidity rate. Most of the morbidity is related to perineal wound healing, adhesions, the ileostomy, and complications of pelvic dissection. Perineal wound problems may be reduced if an intersphincteric proctectomy is performed. This approach involves a dissection between the internal and external sphincters, preserving the external sphincter and levator ani for a more secure perineal wound closure.

Total proctocolectomy with end ileostomy was one of the earliest operations performed for ulcerative colitis and, despite advances in sphincter-saving procedures, continues to have a role. Older patients, those with poor sphincter function, and patients with carcinomas in the distal rectum may be candidates for this procedure.

Total proctocolectomy with continent ileostomy. The continent ileostomy was introduced by Kock in 1969 and became popular in the 1970s because it offered control of evacuations for patients with an ileostomy. A single-chambered reservoir is fashioned by suturing several limbs of ileum together after the antimesenteric border has been divided. The outflow tract is intussuscepted into the reservoir to create a valve that provides obstruction to the pouch contents (continence). As the pouch distends, pressure over the valve causes it to close and to retain stool, permitting patients to wear a simple bandage over a skin-level stoma. Between two and four times daily, the patient introduces a tube through the valve to evacuate the pouch.

The major problem with the Kock pouch is the high complication rate necessitating reoperation in up to 50% of patients. The most common problem is a slipped valve, which occurs when the intussuscepted limb everts and the continent nipple is lost. This leads to the inability of the pouch to remain continent or the inability to intubate the pouch, leading to spontaneous emptying of the pouch as it overflows. Revision of the nipple valve corrects this problem. Other complications include inflammation of the ileal pouch mucosa (so-called pouchitis) in 15% to 30% of cases, fistula formation (10%), and stoma stricture (10%).

Since the introduction of restorative proctocolectomy and IPAA, the popularity of the continent ileostomy has declined, and it is now seldom used. High complication and reoperation rates have dampened enthusiasm among surgeons for the technique. Although ulcerative colitis patients in whom IPAA is contraindicated may be candidates, realistically, only a few centers presently offer the operation. The most common surgery related to continent ileostomies is revisional surgery. The Kock procedure should not be performed in obese patients, debilitated patients, or any patient with a physical or mental handicap that would prohibit safe catheterization of the reservoir. The procedure is contraindicated in patients with Crohn's disease because of the high incidence of its recurrence, causing failure of the pouch.

Total proctocolectomy with ileal pouch–anal anastomosis. Restorative proctocolectomy with IPAA has become the most common definitive operation for the surgical treatment of ulcerative colitis. The procedure involves a near-total proctocolectomy, with preservation of the anal sphincter complex. A single-chambered pouch is fashioned from the distal 30 cm of the ileum (Fig. 51-45) and sutured to the anus using a double-stapled technique (Fig. 51-46). Alternatively, a hand-sewn anastomosis may be fashioned between the pouch and anus after stripping the distal rectal mucosa from the internal anal sphincter (mucosectomy; Fig. 51-47).

A critical consideration in restorative proctocolectomy is fashioning a tension-free anastomosis between the ileal reservoir and anal dentate line. Usually, there is sufficient mesenteric length for an ileal pouch, fashioned from the distal 30 cm of ileum, to reach the anus without unacceptable tension. However, occasionally, the anatomy will be such that specific maneuvers are required to allow the pouch to reach that level. It should be routine to mobilize the

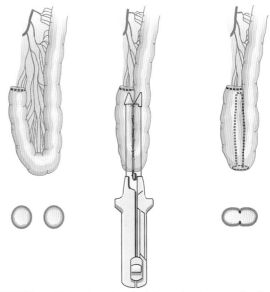

FIGURE 51-45 Creation of an ileal J pouch using a cutting linear stapler. For replacement of the rectum, a reservoir is created from the distal ileum. The stapler joins two limbs of intestine with staples while dividing the intervening wall. The diameter of the pouch so created is twice as large as the original diameter of the ileum.

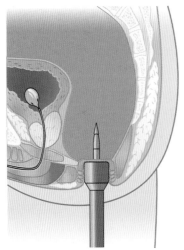
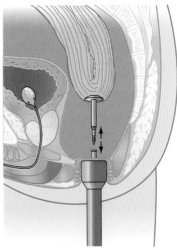

FIGURE 51-46 Fashioning of stapled ileal pouch–anal anastomosis.

posterior attachment of the entire small bowel mesentery to the third portion of the duodenum, exposing the inferior portion of the head of the pancreas. An estimate of the ease of the pouch reaching the anus can be made by drawing the selected apex of the anticipated pouch over the symphysis pubis, with the expectation that it should extend 6 cm beyond the pubis to reach the anal canal easily (Fig. 51-48). This length may occasionally be obtained without further maneuvers, but an additional 2 to 5 cm

of length will generally be necessary. To achieve this length, we usually divide the remnant of the ileocolic artery close to its origin from the SMA (Fig. 51-49). This is aided by transilluminating the mesentery to visualize the mesenteric arteries. The SMA will sustain the viability of the pouch after excision of the ileocolic artery. The apex of the pouch can be moved a few centimeters in either direction to determine the point that will reach the farthest. The peritoneum of the mesentery may be serially incised on its anterior and posterior surfaces; these relaxing incisions can confer an additional 1 or 2 cm of length and are especially beneficial if the mesentery has been thickened by adhesions from previous surgery (Fig. 51-50). These maneuvers will almost always suffice to provide adequate mesenteric length to fashion an anastomosis between the apex of the ileal pouch and anus.[24] In rare cases, the anatomy may be such that the ileal pouch will not extend to reach the anus. An alternative to be considered if the ileal pouch will not reach the anus, despite the maneuvers described, is to close the ileal enterotomy at the apex of the pouch, leave the pouch residing in the pelvis above the anus, and fashion a loop ileostomy proximal to the pouch. There have been several reports of successful IPAAs achieved several months later, when postoperative mesenteric lengthening permits adequate length for the pouch to reach the anus.

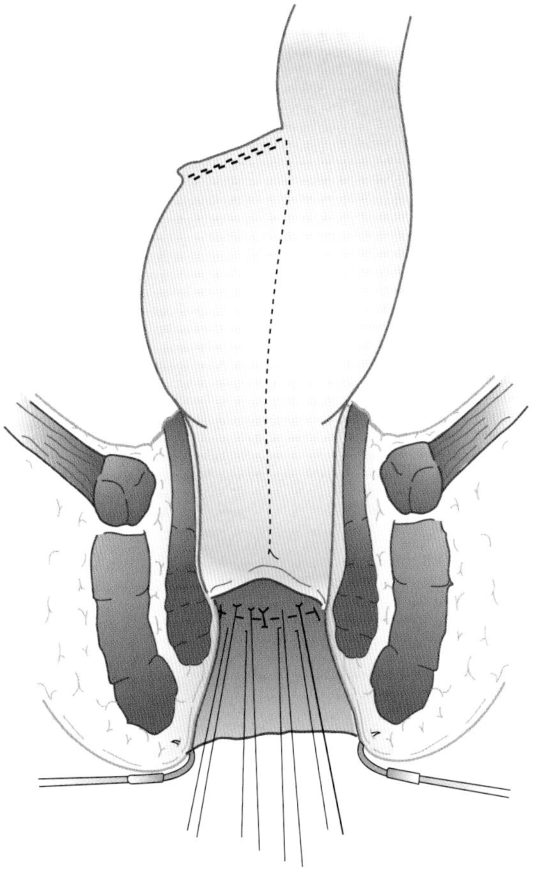

FIGURE 51-47 Hand-sewn ileal pouch–anal anastomosis after anorectal mucosectomy.

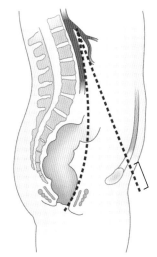

FIGURE 51-48 Estimation of J pouch length.

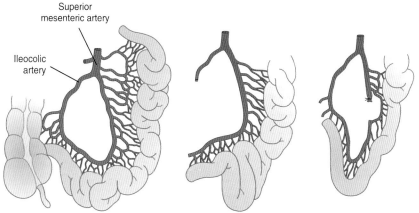

Superior mesenteric artery

Ileocolic artery

FIGURE 51-49 Division of IMA close to SMA.

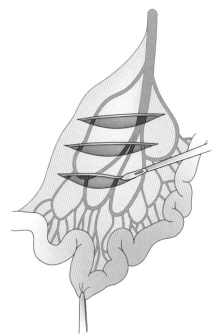

FIGURE 51-50 Peritoneal relaxing incisions create 1 to 2 cm of length.

Some controversy exists concerning the advantages of performing a mucosectomy as a routine component of the procedure. The double-stapling technique may leave a small remnant of rectal mucosa at the anastomosis, which may be at risk for development of dysplasia and cancer. Large retrospective long-term analyses of outcomes of this technique have failed to bear this out. Mucosectomy has, however, been complicated by cancer arising at the anastomosis and extraluminally in the pelvis, from islands of glands that remain after the mucosa is incompletely removed. Although cancer is exceedingly rare, the mucosectomy technique may conceal retained rectal mucosa in more than 20% of patients. The double-stapling technique permits surveillance and biopsy of the remaining mucosa. Avoiding the mucosectomy preserves the anal transition zone, which contains nerve endings involved in differentiating liquid and solid stool from gas, and is thus thought to provide superior postoperative continence.

Controversy also exists about temporary fecal diversion. The pouch and anastomosis were traditionally protected with a diverting loop ileostomy; however, there are some proponents of the single-stage procedure without diversion. This approach has the advantage of a single operation that avoids the complications accompanying an ileostomy. Disadvantages, however, include an increased risk for pelvic sepsis, usually caused by anastomotic leak of a pouch suture line or the anal anastomosis. Most surgeons routinely perform a two-stage operation in high-risk patients, particularly those taking steroids preoperatively.[25]

Patients who undergo total proctocolectomy and IPAA typically have between five and seven bowel movements in a 24-hour period. Function continues to improve with time, with numerous studies demonstrating a decrease in the number of daily bowel movements during the ensuing 3 to 24 months after reestablishment of continuity.

Restorative proctocolectomy and IPAA are associated with early and late complications. A common complication is small bowel obstruction, occurring in up to 27% of patients. Another significant complication is pelvic sepsis. Anastomotic and pouch suture line leaks are devastating complications that can lead to pelvic abscess and seriously threaten the integrity and functionality of the pouch. Treatment of pelvic sepsis secondary to pouch leaks usually requires a diverting ileostomy and drainage of the abscesses. Delayed ileostomy closure after resolution of IPAA complications has no deleterious functional effects. A pouch-vaginal fistula is a specific form of pelvic sepsis that is difficult to manage but fairly rare, occurring in less than 10% of cases. Persistence of the fistula after surgical closure (and often temporary diversion) usually signifies underlying Crohn's disease and may result in the loss of the pouch in a significant number of patients.

Inflammation of the mucosa of the ileal pouch, or pouchitis, occurs in 7% to 33% of patients with ulcerative colitis treated by IPAA. Pouchitis typically is manifested with increased stool frequency, fever, bleeding, cramps, and dehydration. The cause is unknown but may be related to bacterial overgrowth, mucosal ischemia, or other local factors. Episodes usually respond to rehydration and oral antibiotics, usually metronidazole or ciprofloxacin. Probiotics have been reported to provide dramatic resolution in some cases of pouchitis resistant to antibiotic therapy. The diagnosis of Crohn's disease must also be entertained in patients with significant pouchitis that does not respond to medical treatment.[26]

In some cases, the preoperative distinction between Crohn's disease and ulcerative colitis can be difficult, and the pathologist may label the disease indeterminate colitis. Patients with Crohn's disease are not candidates for IPAA because the high incidence of recurrent inflammation in the pouch can cause abscesses, fistulas, and loss of the reservoir. Patients with indeterminate colitis who undergo restorative proctocolectomy and IPAA who do not develop Crohn's disease have results that are more encouraging; patients with indeterminate colitis are generally considered candidates for IPAA if they understand that they are at increased risk for pouch complications related to underlying Crohn's disease.

Summary of elective operations. A suggested algorithm for elective operations for patients with intractable ulcerative colitis is presented in Figure 51-51. Older patients or those with fecal incontinence should undergo a total proctocolectomy with an end ileostomy. Younger patients with no evidence of rectal dysplasia should be offered restorative proctocolectomy and IPAA with a double-stapled anastomosis and diverting loop ileostomy. Patients with confirmed rectal dysplasia should be treated with mucosectomy and a hand-sewn IPAA. Patients with significant debility who are poor operative candidates should undergo a total abdominal colectomy with a very low Hartmann closure and an end ileostomy.

Postoperative care. Postoperative care after restorative proctocolectomy with IPAA is similar to that for other major colorectal procedures. Nasogastric tubes are usually removed at the completion of the procedure, and liquid diets are offered to patients in the early recovery period. Diet is advanced with return of bowel function, as evidenced by ileostomy function. If a pelvic drain is used, it is typically removed after 48 to 72 hours. Bladder catheters are typically left in place for 3 to 4 days, depending on the difficulty of pelvic dissection. A contrast enema is performed approximately 10 weeks postoperatively to ensure an intact IPAA. If the enema shows a leak, the contrast examination is repeated in 6 weeks; almost 95% of anastomotic leaks heal in the absence of pelvic sepsis. If the radiograph shows no leak, the diverting ileostomy is closed.

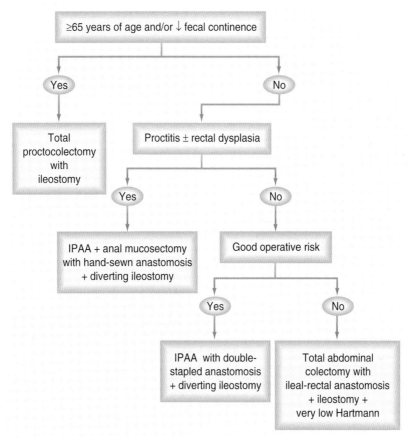

FIGURE 51-51 Elective operations for ulcerative colitis.

Laparoscopic Approaches for Ulcerative Colitis

As with all surgical approaches for colon and rectal surgery, minimally invasive options have fast become standard of care. Despite the complexity of the surgical approaches for ulcerative colitis, laparoscopy and other minimally invasive approaches have been shown to be safe and efficacious in the application for all aspects of surgery for ulcerative colitis. A large retrospective review of the National Surgical Quality Improvement Program database from 2005 to 2008 for all patients undergoing surgery for ulcerative colitis showed that a laparoscopic approach was used in more than 29% of patients with rates increasing each year, starting at 18.5% in 2005 and reaching 41% in 2008. A laparoscopic approach was associated with a lower complication rate in total abdominal colectomy (18.8% versus 41.7%; $P < .0001$) and IPAA (18.2% versus 29.9%; $P = .005$) as well as an overall lower mortality rate (0.2% versus 1.7%; $P = .046$). Laparoscopic abdominal colectomy for severe ulcerative colitis in a hemodynamically stable patient is safe and associated with decreased ileus and shorter length of stay. In addition, patients are able to undergo subsequent restorative proctectomy sooner than patients who have open abdominal colectomy. Although undoubtedly some of these data reflect selection bias, they do validate the proof of principle that the laparoscopic approach in surgery for ulcerative colitis is safe and feasible in experienced hands.

Crohn's Colitis

Originally described as regional ileitis, Crohn's disease is a nonspecific IBD that may affect any segment of the GI tract. Of patients with Crohn's disease, 15% have disease limited to the colon. The inflammatory process may affect the entire colon and mimic ulcerative colitis, or it may affect only segments of the colon (Fig. 51-52). This section discusses Crohn's colitis; additional discussions of Crohn's disease are found elsewhere in this text.

Epidemiology and Cause

A rapid increase in the incidence of Crohn's disease occurred between 1965 and 1980, and since then, the incidence has increased at a slow pace. This is in contrast to the incidence of ulcerative colitis, which has been relatively constant during the same time. The incidence of Crohn's disease varies between 1 and 10/100,000, depending on the geographic location, with the highest incidence in Scandinavian countries and Scotland, followed by England and North America. Similar to ulcerative colitis, there is a bimodal age distribution, with peaks between the ages of 15 and 30 years and a second smaller peak between 55 and 80 years of age. Crohn's disease is more common among patients of Jewish descent and occurs more frequently in urban residents.

The cause of Crohn's disease has not yet been determined. Three prevalent theories include response to a specific infectious agent, a defective mucosal barrier allowing an increased exposure to antigens, and an abnormal host response to dietary antigens. One infectious agent that has generated some interest is *Mycobacterium paratuberculosis,* which has been isolated in up to 65% of tissue samples from Crohn's disease patients. A statistically significant association between the onset of Crohn's disease and prior

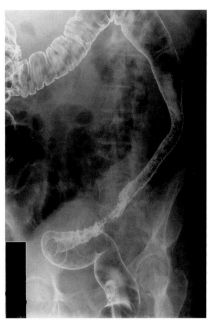

FIGURE 51-52 Crohn's colitis. This barium enema radiograph demonstrates segmental inflammation of the left colon, characteristic of Crohn's disease. The rectum is spared, a clinical finding that is useful in distinguishing Crohn's colitis from ulcerative colitis. The rectal mucosa is almost always affected in patients with ulcerative colitis, whereas the pattern of colonic inflammation is variable in Crohn's colitis.

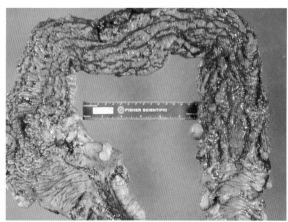

FIGURE 51-53 Crohn's colitis. Linear ulceration of the mucosa, giving the appearance of a railroad track or bear claw ulcers.

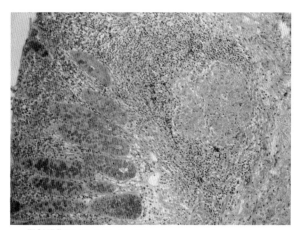

FIGURE 51-54 Crohn's colitis with noncaseating granuloma.

use of antibiotics has also been observed. Smoking appears to be a risk factor for Crohn's disease, and after intestinal resection, the risk of recurrence is greatly increased in smokers. Several studies have also shown an increased risk in patients taking oral contraceptives.

Advances in molecular biology have intensified the search for genetic factors and pathogenetic mechanisms in Crohn's disease. The *NOD2/CARD15* gene, located on chromosome 16, has been shown to be involved in the activation of nuclear factor κB, a transcription factor that plays a significant role in Crohn's disease. Specific genotypes may also determine susceptibility, location, and behavior of Crohn's disease.

Pathologic Features

Gross appearance. Crohn's disease is a transmural, predominantly submucosal inflammation characterized by a thickened colonic wall. The affected mucosa observed by endoscopy is often described as having a cobblestone appearance. In severe disease, the bowel wall may be entirely encased by creeping fat of the mesentery, and strictures may develop in the small and large intestines. The mucosa may demonstrate long, deep linear ulcers that resemble railroad tracks or bear claws (Fig. 51-53). Normal mucosa may intervene between areas of inflammation, causing skip areas characteristic of the disease.

Histologic appearance. Crohn's disease is characterized microscopically by transmural inflammation, submucosal edema, lymphoid aggregation, and, ultimately, fibrosis. The pathognomonic histologic feature of Crohn's disease is the noncaseating granuloma, a localized, well-formed aggregate of epithelioid histiocytes surrounded by lymphocytes and giant cells (Fig. 51-54). Granulomas are found in 50% of specimens resected in Crohn's disease; however, the number identified by endoscopic biopsy is far smaller.

Clinical Presentation

Patients with Crohn's disease may present with a wide spectrum of severity, from subtle symptoms to overwhelming fulminant disease. The characteristic triad of symptoms—abdominal pain, diarrhea, and weight loss—mimics that of viral gastroenteritis or irritable bowel syndrome. Other symptoms may include anorexia, fever, and recurrent oral aphthous ulcers. Patients with a family history of Crohn's disease tend to present with more extensive disease. In contrast to ulcerative colitis, in which the rectum is invariably involved, only 60% of patients with Crohn's colitis have rectal disease. Two thirds of patients with Crohn's colitis have involvement of the entire colon.

Anal disease, including anal fistulas, fissures, strictures, edematous skin tags, and erosion of the anoderm, occurs in up to 30% of patients with Crohn's disease of the terminal ileum and in more than 50% of patients with colonic disease. Anal disease in a patient with colitis suggests a diagnosis of Crohn's disease.

Diagnosis

The differential diagnosis of Crohn's colitis includes ulcerative colitis and various infectious agents. As for patients with ulcerative colitis, stool should be sent for culture and examined for ova and parasites. The diagnosis of Crohn's colitis is made by a combination of clinical, endoscopic, and radiologic features. Barium

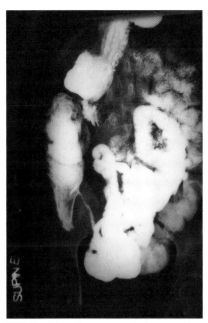

FIGURE 51-55 Small bowel contrast study demonstrating string sign caused by inflammation and narrowing of the terminal ileum.

enema may not demonstrate any abnormalities in mild and early disease; colonoscopy is the more sensitive diagnostic modality. The disease is often patchy in distribution; however, some patients may have granular and friable mucosa in a continuous pattern involving the entire colon and rectum. Edema of the mucosa and aphthous ulcers are present in early Crohn's disease, with deep linear ulcers present in more severe disease and strictures more prevalent in chronic disease. It is at times difficult to distinguish Crohn's disease from ulcerative colitis, particularly if the rectum is involved. Biopsy samples should be obtained. However, unless a granuloma is identified, distinguishing between the two diseases may still be difficult.

An air-contrast enema may provide useful information in making the diagnosis and determining the extent of the disease. Characteristic radiologic findings in Crohn's colitis are skip lesions, contour defects, longitudinal and transverse ulcers, a cobblestone-like mucosal pattern, strictures, thickening of the haustral margin, and irregular nodular defects. A small bowel series, CT enterography, or magnetic resonance enterography should be performed in all patients with suspected Crohn's disease or ulcerative colitis to study the small bowel. Involvement of the small intestine strongly favors the diagnosis of Crohn's disease (Fig. 51-55).

Treatment

Medical therapy. Because surgery for Crohn's disease is not curative, and it is reserved only for specific indications, the medical management of Crohn's colitis takes a more prominent role. As with ulcerative colitis, the categories of medications fall into similar groups (i.e., aminosalicylates, corticosteroids, immunomodulators, and biologic therapies). Treatment is divided into management of acute disease according to severity and maintenance.

In contrast to ulcerative colitis, the isolated use of thiopurines (azathioprine, 6-mercaptopurine) as single agents is not thought to be adequate for maintenance of remission in Crohn's disease; however, they have been shown to reduce cutaneous fistulous

disease by 50%. A notable risk with the chronic use of thiopurines (either alone or in combination with anti–TNF-α medications) is the risk of lymphoma, particularly in young men. Methotrexate may be a useful alternative in the case of thiopurine failure or intolerance.

In particular, the use of the anti–TNF-α biologics has revolutionized management of acute and chronic Crohn's disease. Infliximab and adalimumab are both approved for use and are effective in inducing and maintaining remission in moderate to severe or steroid-refractory disease. They have also shown remarkable activity in active perianal disease, significantly decreasing the number of fistulas. One of the other advantages of the biologics is rapidity of clinical efficacy, measured in weeks compared with months for thiopurines.

As with ulcerative colitis, debate arose as to the risks that biologic therapy posed in increasing postoperative complications after surgery for refractory Crohn's disease in patients who were being treated preoperatively. A systematic review reported on all relevant data through 2012, including more than 1100 patients. The investigators concluded that there was no significant increase in major or minor complications, reoperation rate, or mortality in patients who were undergoing preoperative infliximab therapy versus alternative regimens.

Indications for surgery. The indications for surgery in patients with Crohn's colitis are presented in Box 51-2. Operative treatment in Crohn's disease is intended to relieve symptoms when medical management has failed, to correct complications, and to prevent the development of cancer.

Intractability. Patients who fail to respond to optimal medical therapy for Crohn's disease and remain symptomatic are referred for surgical consultation. As with ulcerative colitis, this represents the most common indication for operative treatment of Crohn's disease.

Intestinal obstruction. Intestinal obstruction in Crohn's disease may be caused by active inflammation, a fibrotic (fibrostenosis) stricture from chronic disease, or an abscess or phlegmon causing a mass effect. Adhesions from previous abdominal operations must also be considered. Obstruction typically involves the small intestine, although large bowel obstruction from strictures may occur. Initial treatment includes bowel rest, nasogastric decompression, IV fluids, and anti-inflammatory medications (usually steroids). Resection with diversion is typically the appropriate operation if the obstruction involves the colon or terminal ileum. Primary anastomosis is generally done in proximal small bowel obstructions.

Intra-abdominal abscess. An intra-abdominal abscess in Crohn's disease is the result of intestinal perforation caused by transmural inflammation. An abscess is usually diagnosed by CT and can often be managed nonoperatively with CT-guided percutaneous drainage and antibiotics. If percutaneous drainage is not feasible or the patient does not respond to this therapy, laparotomy, drainage of the abscess, and resection of the involved bowel are indicated.

Fistulas. Fistulas may develop between the intestine and any other intra-abdominal organ, including the bladder, bowel, uterus, vagina, and stomach. Up to 35% of patients with Crohn's disease develop fistulas, most of which involve the small intestine. Asymptomatic enteroenteric or enterocolic fistulas may not require operative therapy. A common fistula associated with Crohn's disease is an ileosigmoid fistula, which usually is caused by ileal disease with secondary involvement of the sigmoid. Symptomatic patients should undergo resection of the terminal ileum. When the inflammation in the sigmoid colon is minimal, the sigmoid defect can be primarily closed. Extensive inflammation in the sigmoid, however, also requires resection of the sigmoid colon. Colovesical and colovaginal fistulas require resection of the diseased bowel and closure of the bladder or vagina, with interposition of omentum between the bowel and contiguous organ.

Enterocutaneous fistulas in Crohn's disease may develop spontaneously, typically with ileal disease, or as the result of an early postoperative anastomotic breakdown. Patients are initially treated with bowel rest and drainage of any intra-abdominal abscess. Parenteral nutrition and medical treatment of the disease may result in spontaneous closure of the fistula; however, operative treatment is often necessary.

Fulminant colitis and toxic megacolon. Patients with Crohn's disease may present with fulminant colitis in a fashion similar to patients with ulcerative colitis presenting with toxic megacolon. Fulminant colitis typically is manifested with high fever, severe abdominal pain, tenderness, tachycardia, and leukocytosis. Patients should be monitored in an intensive care unit and given IV fluids, bowel rest, antibiotics, and steroids. If there is evidence of clinical deterioration or if there is no significant improvement within 48 to 72 hours, subtotal colectomy with an end ileostomy is indicated. Because the pathologic process in Crohn's disease involves inflammation of the entire bowel wall, the colonic dilation characteristic of toxic megacolon may not occur in patients with Crohn's disease, but the toxicity of the colitis may be no less severe.

Massive bleeding. Massive bleeding, although less common in Crohn's disease than in ulcerative colitis, occurs in 13% of patients in some reviews. The terminal ileum represents the most common site of bleeding. If the disease involves the colon and spares the ileum and the bleeding does not respond to medical therapy, flexible sigmoidoscopy or proctoscopy should be performed to rule out a rectal source. Appropriate operative treatment in rare cases of colonic bleeding for Crohn's colitis is abdominal colectomy and ileostomy or ileorectal anastomosis if the rectum is not inflamed.

Cancer. The risk for development of carcinoma of the colon is not as high as the risk in long-standing, chronic ulcerative colitis, but it is present; therefore, patients with chronic active disease require periodic colonoscopic surveillance and biopsy. The presence of high-grade dysplasia is an indication for colectomy. Patients who have undergone intestinal bypass for Crohn's disease have an increased risk for development of carcinoma; therefore, bypassed segments of Crohn's disease should be resected, if possible.

Extracolonic manifestations. Extraintestinal manifestations of Crohn's disease are similar to those associated with ulcerative colitis. With the exception of PSC, cirrhosis, and ankylosing spondylitis, most extracolonic manifestations of Crohn's disease improve after resection of the diseased bowel.

Growth retardation. Young patients with Crohn's disease and ulcerative colitis may have impaired growth and mental development. Growth failure is often the result of prolonged inadequate calorie intake; therefore, nutritional support is an important component of care in these patients. Resection of severely diseased segments of bowel before puberty may help eliminate growth retardation and premature closure of bone epiphyses.

Surgical procedures. Because surgical intervention is not curative, medical therapy is the mainstay of treatment for Crohn's disease. Recurrence rates after surgery are high, and the risk continues with the passage of time. Therefore, an important principle in the surgical treatment of Crohn's disease is to resect only enough bowel to improve symptoms or to correct complications. Intestine should be resected with the aim of obtaining margins free of disease by gross inspection. Frozen sections of the margins of resection are unnecessary because positive microscopic margins are not predictive of postoperative recurrence. Resection of grossly normal-appearing intestine may eventually lead to short bowel syndrome, with insufficient absorptive surface to maintain nutrition. A suggested algorithm for elective operations for patients with intractable Crohn's disease is presented in Figure 51-56.

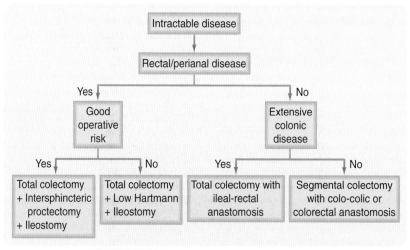

FIGURE 51-56 Elective operations for Crohn's colitis.

Ileocecal resection. Ileocecal resection is indicated for patients with severe disease of the terminal ileum resulting in obstruction or perforation. It typically involves resection of approximately 6 to 12 inches of the terminal ileum and cecum, with an anastomosis created between the ileum and ascending colon. The terminal ileum is transected 2 cm proximal to grossly apparent Crohn's disease. Strictureplasty is not indicated for disease of the terminal ileum. In most series, the recurrence rate of Crohn's disease requiring re-resection in patients who have undergone ileocolic resection is approximately 50% in 10 years.

On occasion, patients presenting with acute distal ileal disease (fever, right lower quadrant abdominal pain, leukocytosis) are misdiagnosed as having appendicitis. Traditional therapy for patients with terminal ileitis found at the time of surgery for appendicitis has been to perform an appendectomy when the cecum is normal, to leave the ileum in place, and to treat with medical therapy after surgery. However, it is reported that more than 90% of patients found to have terminal ileitis at the time of appendectomy sparing the terminal ileum require ileocolic resection for complications of Crohn's disease within 12 years. Terminal ileitis may also be caused by *Yersinia enterocolitica* and *Campylobacter* spp., and distinguishing these processes from Crohn's disease intraoperatively may be difficult.

Total proctocolectomy with end ileostomy. Total proctocolectomy with end ileostomy involves removing all the abdominal colon, rectum, and anus and is indicated for patients with Crohn's disease involving the entire colon and rectum or when fecal incontinence is too severe to warrant preserving the rectum. Disadvantages of this procedure include delayed healing of the perineal wound and problems with malabsorption. Intersphincteric proctectomy decreases the incidence of perineal wound complications, as does placement of a tissue flap. Rapid small bowel transit and malabsorption of nutrients may occur more frequently after this procedure in patients with Crohn's disease compared with patients with ulcerative colitis because variable amounts of terminal ileum may be involved in the disease process.

Total abdominal colectomy with ileorectal anastomosis. Total abdominal colectomy with ileorectal anastomosis is indicated for patients with Crohn's colitis with sparing of the rectum and anus and offers the best functional result in patients who wish to maintain intestinal continuity. After this procedure, patients may expect to have between four and six bowel movements daily. The major disadvantage of the operation is the high likelihood of recurrence requiring completion proctectomy and ileostomy. Numerous studies have shown that approximately 50% of patients require proctectomy within 10 years.

Segmental colon resection. Between 10% and 20% of patients with Crohn's colitis have disease limited to a segment of colon. Segmental colon resection may therefore be an option for patients with limited colonic disease associated with stricture or obstruction. It is contraindicated for patients with severe rectal or anal disease. As with total abdominal colectomy and ileorectal anastomosis, the major disadvantage of segmental colon resection is the high rate of recurrence requiring subsequent operations. Within 5 years, recurrence rates range between 30% and 50%, with 60% of patients requiring reoperation by 10 years. Despite these high recurrence rates, segmental colectomy may be a good option for patients with limited disease who wish to avoid an ostomy.

Postoperative recurrence. A number of risk factors have been identified for recurrence of Crohn's disease after resection, including duration and severity of Crohn's disease before initial resection, smoking, and the presence of granulomas in the resected specimen. Longer disease-free resection margins and various types of anastomoses (i.e., end to side or side to side) have not been shown to affect recurrence rates. The reoperative rate for patients with Crohn's disease is 4% to 5% per year. In patients with Crohn's disease limited to the colon, total proctocolectomy has the lowest recurrence, with rates varying between 10% and 25%, depending on the length of follow-up.

Minimally Invasive Approaches to Surgical Management of Crohn's Disease

The benefits enjoyed by minimally invasive colon and rectal surgery have been successfully applied and validated for use in Crohn's disease. Compared with open surgery, a laparoscopic approach offers the same benefits, such as decreased pain, and has lower wound complication rates, decreased ileus, better cosmesis, and shorter hospital stays. Although it is technically more difficult, there have been numerous reports in the literature validating its use. A recent meta-analysis by Tan looked at almost 900 patients undergoing laparoscopic and open surgery for Crohn's disease. Ileocolic resection was the most common operation performed. This study confirmed an improvement in recovery of bowel function and decreased length of stay at the cost of slightly longer operative times. In addition, overall morbidity was significantly lower in the laparoscopic group (12.8% versus 20%). With respect to laparoscopic colectomy, short-term outcomes of 125 consecutive patients undergoing colectomy during a 7-year period were examined. In this series, the laparoscopic cohort had a significantly higher body mass index and a similar duration of disease. Again, the laparoscopic group showed decreased ileus and shorter hospital stays. The minimally invasive group was also associated with shorter operative times, decreased blood loss, and decreased complications, which probably reflects increasing proficiency with laparoscopy. The conversion rate from laparoscopy to open surgery was approximately 10%.

INFECTIOUS COLITIS

Various forms of infectious enteritis are brought to the attention of the surgeon because they may present as an acute abdomen, masquerade as IBD, or progress to the point that surgical treatment is required. *C. difficile* infection is one of most common infectious colitides requiring surgical attention in the United States. It is discussed in detail in this section. Other infectious colitides that may, more rarely, require surgical evaluation or treatment are discussed briefly at the end of this section.

Clostridium difficile Infection

C. difficile is a gram-positive, spore-forming anaerobic microorganism related to the bacteria that cause tetanus and botulism. It is almost always a health care–associated infection, and it is the pathogen most commonly associated with nosocomial infectious diarrhea. Prior treatment with antibiotics, particularly clindamycin, cephalosporins, and some penicillins and fluoroquinolones, is the most significant risk factor for development of *C. difficile* infection. In general, pathologic growth of *C. difficile* is suppressed by the normal (autochthonous) bacteria of the colon, but antibiotics that suppress the colonic flora permit overgrowth of *C. difficile,* which releases toxins that cause diarrhea.

C. difficile produces two toxins (A and B), both of which are important in the pathogenesis of pseudomembranous colitis. Toxin

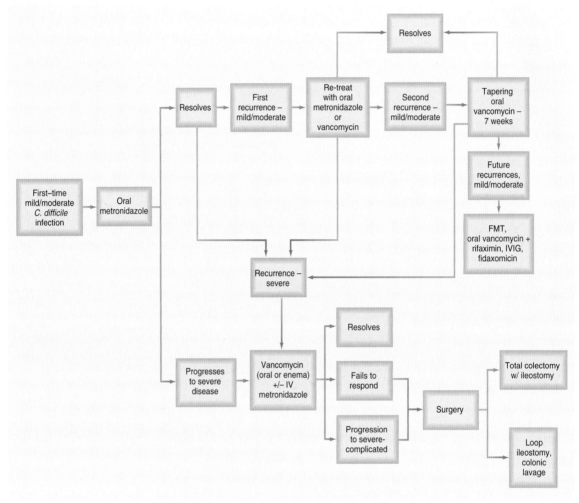

FIGURE 51-57 Algorithm for the management of *C. difficile* colitis.

A, the toxin that directly leads to the development of colitis, is released by the bacterium and binds to a colonocyte glycoprotein receptor. This leads to the destruction of the colonocyte and the release of inflammatory mediators. Toxin A is also a chemoattractant for neutrophils and activates macrophages and mast cells, resulting in further inflammation and systemic symptoms of sepsis. Toxin B is also a potent cytotoxin and has the potential to cause colitis, even in strains of *C. difficile* that do not produce toxin A.

C. difficile colitis typically begins within 4 to 9 days after the initiation of antibiotics, although 25% of patients may not become symptomatic until up to 10 weeks after a course of antibiotics. The clinical presentation generally includes watery diarrhea with or without abdominal pain, fever, or ileus. Laboratory diagnosis can be made by demonstrating the toxins in the stool with an enzyme-linked immunosorbent assay (ELISA). These tests can be performed within hours; however, in the past, they were limited by a relatively low sensitivity. Often, multiple tests were required to confirm a negative result. More recently, however, the sensitivity of the ELISA test has reached greater than 90%, making it the initial test of choice in patients with suspected *C. difficile* infection. Alternatively, polymerase chain reaction testing can be used to identify DNA from the *C. difficile* toxins in the stool. This is more expensive than the ELISA assay but may eventually become the test of choice. If the diagnosis remains unclear, proctoscopy or flexible sigmoidoscopy may reveal inflamed mucosa covered by yellowish plaque-like membranes or pseudomembranes. These are pathognomonic for *C. difficile* infection and are seen in approximately 25% of patients with mild disease and 87% of patients with fulminant colitis.

Infection can range from mild diarrhea to fulminant infection with toxic megacolon, colonic perforation, and systemic sepsis (Fig. 51-57). Treatment should be tailored to the severity of the disease. Surgical therapy is generally required only for fulminant cases recalcitrant to medical management. There is some evidence that early surgical intervention reduces morbidity and mortality, so early surgical consultation is warranted.

For patients with diagnosed *C. difficile* infection, initial management includes cessation of concomitant antibiotic treatment, when possible, and judicious fluid and electrolyte management (Fig. 51-57). For patients with a first-time episode of mild to moderate *C. difficile* infection, the Infectious Diseases Society of America recommends treatment with oral metronidazole (250 to 500 mg three or four times a day for 14 days).[27] In patients who fail to respond to metronidazole treatment within 3 to 4 days but remain clinically stable, oral vancomycin (125 mg four times a day for 10 days) should be started.

There are patients who will respond to initial treatment but have recurrent episodes of mild to moderate *C. difficile* infection. In these cases, oral metronidazole or oral vancomycin can be repeated. If a patient has a second recurrence, a tapering multi-week (often 7-week) course of oral vancomycin is currently the recommended therapy.

Some patients develop refractory or recurrent *C. difficile* colitis; the pathologic bacteria cannot be eradicated with repeated and prolonged treatment by vancomycin or metronidazole. In these patients, diarrhea and hematochezia recur or persist but do not progress to a state of severe toxicity.

Fidaxomicin is a macrolide antibiotic that has been shown to be as effective as oral vancomycin, particularly in patients who require continuation of their concomitant antibiotics. It is much more costly than either metronidazole or vancomycin. It currently should be considered in patients with recurrent *C. difficile* infection after oral metronidazole and vancomycin therapy, in patients who cannot tolerate metronidazole or vancomycin, and possibly in patients who require continuation of other antibiotics during treatment for first-time *C. difficile* infection. Other studies have shown that rifaximin, a broad-spectrum antibiotic selective for the GI tract, can be beneficial for recurrent infection when it is used in combination with oral vancomycin.

Intravenous immune globulin (IVIG) has been used to treat recalcitrant and recurrent *C. difficile* colitis, but evidence is limited as to its true efficacy. Monoclonal antibodies directed specifically against the *C. difficile* toxins A and B have shown some promise, but this is a new treatment and not widely available. Studies are under way to better assess the safety and efficacy of monoclonal antibody treatment.

Perhaps the most promising treatment emerging for recurrent and recalcitrant *C. difficile* infection is fecal microbiota transplantation (FMT). Using FMT, donor stool is administered to the patient through one of a variety of described routes (nasogastric tube, colonoscopic lavage, upper endoscopy). Although it has long been recognized that the restoration of the bowel flora by FMT is successful at treatment of recalcitrant and recurrent *C. difficile* infection, FMT has not been popular, given obvious logistical disadvantages. In the past several years, however, multiple randomized trials and reviews have reported success rates for recurrent *C. difficile* infection of greater than 80% with FMT. A review of the literature, including more than 500 patients treated, suggests that FMT is safe and effective in recurrent *C. difficile* infections. FMT is currently recognized as perhaps the most successful treatment for recurrent *C. difficile* infection and is being used more frequently at many centers.[28]

Unfortunately, some patients develop severe and severe-complicated infection. In patients diagnosed with severe *C. difficile* infection, oral vancomycin is the initial treatment of choice. Patients with severe-complicated infection, as manifested by an ileus, peritonitis, or sepsis, for example, should be treated with IV metronidazole in combination with high-dose oral vancomycin, if tolerated. The administration of vancomycin by enema or orally through a nasogastric tube is recommended in patients who cannot tolerate oral medication. These patients require intensive care to manage their complicated volume status and hemodynamic instability that result from hypovolemia, sepsis, and shock.

In rare instances, severe cases of *C. difficile* colitis may require surgical intervention. Deciding when to surgically intervene in these cases remains difficult. On occasion, the disease progresses to overwhelming sepsis, toxic megacolon, and colonic perforation. In these cases, operative intervention is mandatory. In other cases,

however, the decision is not so clear. Patients with severe disease who fail to progress with optimal medical management may require surgery. Unfortunately, there are no trials or guidelines that define failure of medical management, so the decision to operate requires considerable surgical judgment. There is evidence that earlier surgical intervention reduces morbidity and mortality. Most advocate continuing medical treatment for severe *C. difficile* colitis for 3 to 5 days before surgical intervention in a clinically stable patient.

When surgery is indicated, abdominal colectomy with ileostomy and rectal preservation has traditionally been the procedure of choice. Segmental colectomy, colostomy, and ileostomy have not been shown to be effective treatment for this pancolonic disease. The colon should be divided at the distal sigmoid or the rectosigmoid junction, which allows control of the disease while providing the possibility for future ostomy reversal. If there is concern for the integrity of the distal staple line, the rectal stump can and should be externalized as a mucous fistula. Some surgeons advocate drainage of the rectal stump transanally with a drain, whereas others discuss irrigation of the stump with vancomycin enemas. There are few data to support the efficacy of these practices. Unfortunately, the mortality rate associated with colectomy for severe *C. difficile* colitis remains higher than 50%.[28]

Because of the high mortality of abdominal colectomy with ileostomy, other surgical techniques have been explored. The most promising is laparoscopic creation of a loop ileostomy with intra-operative, antegrade colonic lavage using polyethylene glycol. Neal and colleagues have reported the largest series of patients treated in this manner (N = 42).[29] All patients were given a loop ileostomy and intraoperative colonic lavage with polyethylene glycol and were subsequently treated with 10 days of vancomycin enemas and IV metronidazole. In this series, 3 of 42 patients subsequently required colectomy, whereas the mortality was only 19%. No other reported studies have duplicated these results, but the procedure is becoming more widespread. If evidence continues to support the efficacy of this procedure in treating severe-complicated *C. difficile* infection, it may supplant initial abdominal colectomy as the surgical treatment of choice.

Based on a review of the current literature, Figure 51-57 demonstrates one possible treatment algorithm for patients diagnosed with *C. difficile* colitis. As evidence mounts to support newer medical treatments, such as monoclonal antibodies and FMT, and less invasive surgical therapies, this algorithm is likely to evolve, leading, it is hoped, to higher success rates and lower morbidity and mortality for patients with this infection.

Other Colonic Infections

Other infectious pathogens can cause diarrhea and colitis but only rarely require surgical intervention. Some of the more common are reviewed here. Bacterial colitis can be caused by a variety of pathogens. *Campylobacter jejuni,* a spiral, microaerophilic, gram-positive rod, is a leading cause of infectious colitis worldwide and has become one of the major causes of infectious diarrhea in the United States. Symptoms most often include fever, watery diarrhea, and abdominal pain, often 2 to 4 days after exposure to improperly prepared chicken or beef. This infection can mimic appendicitis or Crohn's disease as it has a predilection for involvement of the cecum and terminal ileum. Endoscopic evaluation usually shows an edematous, inflamed mucosa, and histologic examination is usually nonspecific; definitive diagnosis is by stool culture. Treatment of mild *Campylobacter* enteritis is supportive only; severe cases have traditionally been treated with ciprofloxacin, but in recent years, fluoroquinolone resistance has been reported in up to 80% of *C. jejuni* isolates. Macrolides should be regarded as the treatment of choice when necessary. Rarely, surgical intervention is necessary when toxic megacolon, with hemorrhage or perforation, develops.

Yersinia enterocolitica, a gram-negative coccobacillus, also causes enteric infections after exposure to contaminated water or food, most commonly in children and young adults. Patients infected with *Yersinia* typically present with bloody diarrhea and abdominal pain. Similar to *C. jejuni* infection, *Yersinia* infection often mimics appendicitis or Crohn's disease. Diagnosis is made by isolation of the bacteria from the stool. *Yersinia* enteritis often resolves with supportive care alone; however, in more severe cases, patients should be treated with trimethoprim-sulfamethoxazole or a fluoroquinolone. As for other infectious colitides, surgery is reserved for complications of the infection, including ulcerative ileitis, toxic megacolon, perforation, and intussusception.

Salmonella typhi and *S. enteritidis* are the most commonly identified pathogens in patients with gastroenteritis but differ widely in their worldwide distribution. *S. typhi* causes enteric fever in underdeveloped countries, whereas *S. enteritidis* is a common cause of food-borne gastroenteritis in the United States. Symptoms include abdominal pain and cramping, diarrhea, and vomiting. Severe septicemia may also occur if the organism enters the bloodstream. Diagnosis is based on culture of the organism from the stool or blood. Medical management includes treatment with fluoroquinolones or third-generation cephalosporins. Surgical intervention is warranted in cases of perforation, obstruction, and hemorrhage.

Shigella is a leading cause of dysentery in developing countries. Like other enteric infections, *Shigella* infection is often manifested with fever, abdominal pain, and watery diarrhea but often progresses to bloody diarrhea. Elevated fecal leukocytes and stool culture are used for diagnosis. Trimethoprim-sulfamethoxazole and ciprofloxacin can be used to treat severe cases. *Shigella* often affects the rectum and sigmoid most significantly, and endoscopy can reveal focal ulcerations with mucosal edema and bleeding. In children, this infection can lead to rectal prolapse. In adults, perforation and obstruction may develop, requiring surgical intervention.

Cytomegalovirus is a viral cause of colitis most often seen in immunocompromised hosts, such as patients with advanced HIV infection or transplant patients. The presentation varies but usually includes fevers, often bloody diarrhea, and abdominal pain. Diagnosis is made by endoscopic findings of patchy erythema and biopsy specimens showing pathognomonic inclusion bodies. Infection, especially in the immunocompromised host, can progress to sepsis, toxic megacolon, and colon perforation. Primary treatment is ganciclovir. As with other infectious colitides, surgery is reserved only for complication. Of note, in patients presenting with fulminant diarrhea and colitis believed to be due to IBD, cytomegalovirus infection should be ruled out (along with *C. difficile* infection) before definitive surgical intervention for IBD.

ISCHEMIC COLITIS

It has long been recognized that ligation of a major colonic artery can result in segmental colonic gangrene. It was not until the 1960s, however, that Boyle identified five patients with "reversible vascular occlusion of the colon." Soon after that, Marston coined the term *ischemic colitis.* Today, ischemic colitis accounts for more

than 50% of all GI ischemic episodes, making it the most common form of GI ischemia. As with infectious colitis, its spectrum of presentation, including abdominal pain, bloody diarrhea, fever, and sepsis, often brings it to the attention of surgeons. Although most cases, when identified and treated promptly, do not require surgical intervention, delay in diagnosis can result in the need for emergency colectomy and poor patient outcome.

Anatomy

Understanding the vascular anatomy of the colon is important in understanding the distribution and presentation of ischemic colitis. As mentioned earlier, the colon is supplied by three major arterial sources: the SMA, the IMA, and the bilateral iliac arteries. The SMA supplies the cecum, right colon, and proximal transverse colon through its ileocolic, right colic, and middle colic branches. The IMA supplies the distal transverse colon and left colon through its left colic branch. There is a variable branch, originating either from the left colic or the IMA itself, that supplies the distal left colon and sigmoid colon. Finally, the terminal IMA forms the superior hemorrhoidal artery that supplies blood to the rectum. The iliac arteries also supply the rectum through the inferior and middle hemorrhoidal branches. Of note, the colon has multiple vascular collaterals connecting the major arterial vessels that are important in understanding ischemic colitis. The marginal artery of Drummond runs parallel to the colon, connecting the SMA and IMA circulation. In patients with vascular disease who experience gradual occlusion of the IMA, this marginal artery can provide the majority of blood flow to the left and sigmoid colon. In addition, the arc of Riolan is a variable collateral vessel that connects the SMA, through the middle colic vessel, to the IMA, through the left colic. Watershed areas describe regions of the colon at the border of territory supplied by the two main arteries, the SMA and the IMA, areas often dependent on the collateral vessels for blood supply. Griffith point is the region of the splenic flexure where the circulations of the IMA and SMA meet. Sudeck point describes an area in the sigmoid colon at the junction of the sigmoid and superior hemorrhoidal vessels. These watershed areas are particularly susceptible to ischemia during periods of low blood flow. The rectum, on the other hand, has a robust dual blood supply, from both the IMA and the iliac circulation, and is rarely the victim of ischemic injury.

Causes

Ischemic colitis results from occlusive and nonocclusive causes. Occlusive causes include events that acutely cut off the blood supply to a major arterial branch to the colon. This is most often due to a thromboembolism from the left side of the heart, particularly as a result of atrial fibrillation. In addition, colonic ischemia is a well-known risk of aortic reconstructive surgery that results in occlusion of the IMA, such as during an abdominal aortic aneurysm repair. In these patients, if collateral circulation is not sufficient, acute occlusion of the IMA can result in sigmoid and left colon ischemia.

Nonocclusive causes of colonic ischemia are wide ranging, and the risk factors are multifactorial. Known risk factors for ischemic colitis include age older than 65 years, cardiac arrhythmias, irritable bowel syndrome, constipation, and chronic obstructive pulmonary disease. In younger patients, risk factors include vasculitis, medication, long-distance running, and sickle cell disease. In addition, any systemic condition, such as profound shock, resulting in hypotension and low blood flow can result in colonic ischemia.

Classification

Marston and colleagues first described three categories of ischemic colitis: gangrenous, stricturing, and transient. Today, in the acute phase, the clinical management is dependent on two classifications: partial thickness (which can be transient or stricturing) and full thickness with gangrene. In partial-thickness ischemia, the vascular insult is limited to the mucosa and sometimes the submucosa. When treated appropriately, this is generally transient and resolves without the need for acute surgical intervention. On occasion, as discussed later, partial-thickness ischemic colitis can resolve but result in scarring and stricturing of the involved colon, a condition that may eventually require segmental colectomy if symptomatic. Partial-thickness ischemia can also progress into a chronic, segmental ischemia with recurrent sepsis and colonic ulceration. In full-thickness ischemia, the entire thickness of the bowel wall is compromised, colonic perforation is common, and urgent surgical intervention is necessary. Identifying partial-thickness versus full-thickness ischemia in the acute setting is of paramount importance in determining the appropriate treatment, including the need for timely surgical intervention.

Presentation and Diagnosis

Regardless of cause, the majority of ischemic colitis initially is manifested as abdominal pain and cramping, fever, and the development of often bloody diarrhea. These symptoms can vary considerably, depending on the length and thickness of the colon that is affected. Partial-thickness ischemia of a short segment of colon may result in only mild abdominal pain and passage of a small amount of bloody diarrhea. Full-thickness ischemia can result in peritonitis, high fever, leukocytosis, and acidosis. As mentioned, rapid and accurate diagnosis is critical in the treatment of ischemic colitis and is obviously facilitated by a high suspicion for ischemic colitis in the setting of mild to moderate abdominal pain, fever, and bloody diarrhea.

Abdominal radiography is often the first study performed in the workup of ischemic colitis, but the results, including ileus or a dilated segment of colon, are generally nonspecific. Thumbprinting, a sign caused by intestinal wall edema, is more specific for ischemia but is not diagnostic. The presence of free intraperitoneal air on plain abdominal radiography suggests bowel perforation and can direct immediate operative management.

The use of barium enema in the diagnosis of acute ischemic colitis has become obsolete. The risk for perforation and barium peritonitis in this circumstance is unacceptable. Water-soluble contrast studies also carry a risk for perforation of the compromised colon and are avoided in the acute setting. Contrast enemas, however, are useful for the evaluation of chronic ischemic strictures that can develop after an episode of transient partial-thickness ischemia (Fig. 51-58).

Abdominal CT is useful in the assessment of patients with abdominal pain and suspected colonic ischemia. It allows examination of the entire abdomen and pelvis to rule out other sources of pain. Findings suggestive of colonic ischemia on CT scan include colonic wall thickening or pneumatosis, pericolonic stranding, and portal venous air. Endoscopy provides the advantage of direct visualization of the colonic mucosa. It also allows biopsy samples to be taken and culture specimens to be obtained to rule out other possible causes of the patient's symptoms. Whereas all segments of the colon may be involved, it is rarely necessary to visualize the colon beyond the level of the splenic flexure to establish a diagnosis. If right-sided ischemia is suspected, full colonoscopy may be required. The finding of hemorrhagic, pale mucosa with patches of inflammation interspersed between healthy mucosa is typical of partial-thickness ischemic injury. The major disadvantage of endoscopy is its inability, except in severe cases, to distinguish between partial-thickness and full-thickness ischemia.

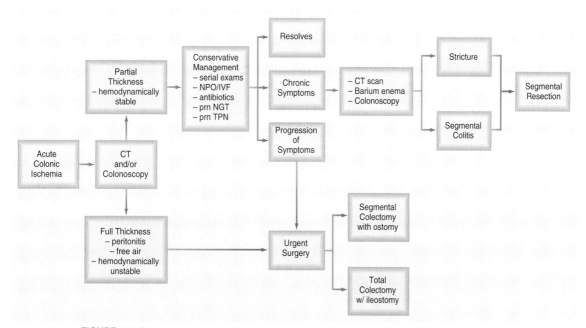

FIGURE 51-58 Treatment algorithm for ischemic colitis. *IVF*, intravenous fluids; *NGT*, nasogastric tube; *NPO*, nothing by mouth; *TPN*, total parenteral nutrition.

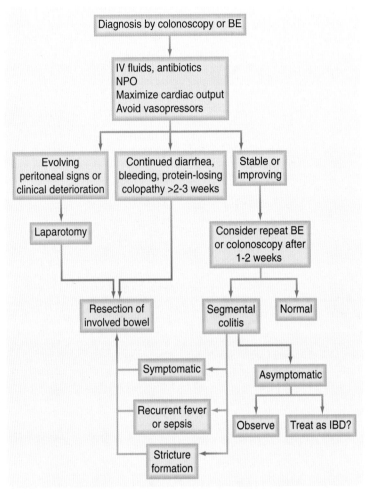

FIGURE 51-59 Management of colonic ischemia. *BE,* Barium enema.

Treatment

The majority of patients with ischemic colitis do not require urgent surgical intervention (Fig. 51-59). In one review, only 21% of patients admitted to the hospital with a diagnosis of ischemic colitis required surgery during that admission. For stable patients without evidence of full-thickness ischemia or bowel perforation, conservative management consists of bowel rest, nasogastric tube if ileus is present, IV fluids, and serial abdominal examinations. Efforts should be made to ensure optimal blood flow, including treatment of hypotension and hydration. There is evidence that colonic ischemia can result in bacterial translocation and sepsis; therefore, broad-spectrum antibiotics to cover both aerobic and anaerobic organisms are recommended. Patients should be closely monitored for the resolution of abdominal pain, return of normal bowel function, and normalization of any acidosis or leukocytosis. The majority of these patients will recover without long-term consequences. Failure to improve or worsening of symptoms, however, during the first 24 to 28 hours raises the concern for the development of full-thickness ischemia. Repeated imaging with either endoscopy or CT scanning is recommended at that time, assuming the patient remains stable, to help guide management. Hemodynamic instability, peritonitis, or concern for perforation dictates that the patient undergo surgical exploration and colonic resection.

On occasion, partial-thickness colonic ischemia will resolve initially, but a chronic stricture at the site of the ischemia develops. In patients with symptoms suggestive of a postischemic stricture, including constipation, abdominal pain, and narrow stools, evaluation with a contrast enema or a colonoscopy can confirm the diagnosis. Indications for surgical resection of a stricture include obstructive symptoms, inability to rule out malignant disease, and inability to survey the colon proximal to the stricture. In these cases, as the acute ischemic episode is long resolved, segmental colonic resection with primary anastomosis is reasonable.

Still other patients with acute, partial-thickness ischemia will go on to develop a chronic, segmental ischemia. This can be manifested as recurrent bouts of sepsis, bloody diarrhea, and abdominal pain. On endoscopy, these areas appear as areas of inflammation and ulceration consistent with segmental colitis. These patients may require elective segmental colectomy. Assuming the bowel on either side of the involved segment is healthy and well perfused, primary anastomosis is acceptable.

Finally, there are patients who require emergency exploration for colonic ischemia. These are patients who develop or present with peritonitis, sepsis, and concern for full-thickness ischemia with perforation. Unlike for mesenteric ischemia involving the small bowel, revascularization procedures to establish blood flow to the colon are not indicated. The resection required depends on

---

BOX 51-3 Colonic Ischemia: Indications for Surgery

Acute Indications
Peritoneal signs
Massive bleeding
Universal fulminant colitis, with or without toxic megacolon

Subacute Indications
Failure of an acute segmental ischemic colitis to respond within 2 to 3 weeks, with continued symptoms or a protein-losing colopathy
Apparent healing but with recurrent bouts of sepsis

Chronic Indications
Symptomatic colon stricture
Symptomatic segmental ischemic colitis

TABLE 51-2 Familial Risk and Colon Cancer

FAMILIAL SETTING*	APPROXIMATE LIFETIME RISK OF COLON CANCER
General U.S. population	6%
One first-degree relative with colon cancer	2- to 3-fold increased
Two first-degree relatives with colon cancer	3- to 4-fold increased
First-degree relative with colon cancer diagnosed at ≤50 years	3- to 4-fold increased
One second- or third-degree relative with colon cancer	1.5-fold increased
Two second- or third-degree relatives with colon cancer	2- to 3-fold increased
One first-degree relative with adenomatous polyp	2-fold increased

From Burt RW: Colon cancer screening. *Gastroenterology* 119:837–853, 2000.
*First-degree relatives include parents, siblings, and children. Second-degree relatives include grandparents, aunts, and uncles. Third-degree relatives include great-grandparents and cousins.

---

the operative findings. Ischemia involving the entire colon is rare, but such cases require total colectomy with ileostomy. More often, the ischemia involves a recognizable segment of colon. In these cases, segmental resection is appropriate. If there is concern for evolving ischemia, leaving the bowel in discontinuity and the abdomen open in preparation for a planned second-look laparotomy is prudent. If there is little concern for ongoing ischemia, a one-stage operation is reasonable, but deciding between primary anastomosis and ostomy can be difficult. In general, if emergent colon resection is required for colonic ischemia, the safest approach is to fashion an end ostomy with either a mucous fistula, if possible, or Hartmann closure of the distal colon or rectum. A summary of the indications for surgery is presented in Box 51-3.

NEOPLASIA

Adenocarcinoma of the colon and rectum is the third most common site of new cancer cases and deaths in men (following prostate and lung or bronchus cancer) and women (following breast and lung or bronchus cancer) in the United States. It was estimated that in 2015, there were 106,100 new cases of colon cancer (552,010 men and 54,090 women) and 40,870 new cases of rectal cancer (23,580 men and 17,290 women) diagnosed. In 2015, 49,920 Americans (25,240 men and 24,680 women) were predicted to die of colorectal cancer. It remains the second leading cause of cancer death in the United States. The lifetime risk for development of colorectal cancer in the United States is 5.51% (1 in 18) for men and 5.10% (1 in 20) for women. The risk for development of invasive colorectal cancer increases with age, with more than 90% of new cases being diagnosed in patients older than 50 years. The incidence of colorectal cancer from 1998 to 2005 decreased at a rate of 2.8%/year for men and 2.2%/year for women. The death rate for men and women decreased 4.3% annually during the period from 2002 to 2005. There has been a significant increase in 5-year survival rates during the last 30 years. The 5-year survival for colon cancer was 52% from 1975 to 1977, 59% from 1984 to 1986, and 65% from 1996 to 2004. The 5-year survival for Americans with rectal cancer was 49% from 1975 to 1977, 57% from 1984 to 1986, and 67% from 1996 to 2004.[30]

Colorectal cancer occurs in hereditary, sporadic, and familial forms. Hereditary colorectal cancer has been extensively described and is characterized by family history, young age at onset, and the presence of other specific tumors and defects. Familial adenomatous polyposis (FAP) and hereditary nonpolyposis colorectal cancer (HNPCC) are the subject of many studies that have provided significant insights into the pathogenesis of colorectal cancer.

Sporadic colorectal cancer occurs in the absence of family history, generally affects an older population (60 to 80 years of age), and usually is manifested as an isolated colon or rectal lesion. Genetic mutations associated with the cancer are limited to the tumor itself, unlike in hereditary disease, in which the specific mutation is present in all cells of the affected individual. Nevertheless, the genetics of colorectal cancer initiation and progression can, in some circumstances, proceed along similar pathways in the hereditary and sporadic forms of the disease. Studies of the relatively rare inherited models of the disease have greatly enhanced the understanding of the genetics of the far more common sporadic form.

The concept of familial colorectal cancer is relatively recent. Lifetime risk for colorectal cancer increases for members in families in which the index case is young (<50 years) and the relative is close (first-degree relative). The risk increases as the number of family members with colorectal cancer rises (Table 51-2). An individual who is a first-degree relative of a patient diagnosed with colorectal cancer before the age of 50 years is twice as likely as an individual in the general population to develop the cancer. This more subtle form of inheritance has been the subject of much investigation. Genetic polymorphisms, gene modifiers, and defects in tyrosine kinases have all been implicated in various forms of familial colorectal cancer.

Colorectal Cancer Genetics
The field of colorectal cancer genetics was revolutionized in 1988 by the description of the genetic changes involved in the progression of a benign adenomatous polyp to invasive carcinoma. Since then, there has been an explosion of additional information about the molecular and genetic pathways that result in colorectal cancer. Tumor suppressor genes, DNA mismatch repair (MMR)

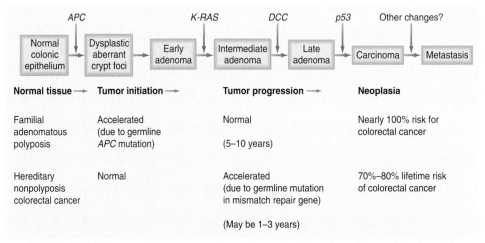

FIGURE 51-60 Adenoma-carcinoma sequence in sporadic and hereditary colorectal cancer. (From Ivanovich JL, Read TE, Ciske DJ, et al: A practical approach to familial and hereditary colorectal cancer. *Am J Med* 107:68–77, 1999.)

genes, proto-oncogenes, and promoter hypermethylation events all contribute to colorectal neoplasia in the sporadic and inherited forms. The Fearon-Vogelstein adenoma-carcinoma multistep model of colorectal neoplasia represents one of the best-known models of carcinogenesis (Fig. 51-60). This sequence of tumor progression involves damage to proto-oncogenes and tumor suppressor genes. The multistep carcinogenesis model can serve as a template to illustrate how certain early mutations produce accumulated defects resulting in neoplasia. The specific contributing mutations in genes such as adenomatous polyposis coli *(APC)* have been intensely studied. It is important to view this model and others as progressive and in flux while interconnected cell cycle control pathways and new functions for well-known genes are becoming apparent (Table 51-3).

Specific Genes and Mutations
Tumor Suppressor Genes

Tumor suppressor genes produce proteins that inhibit tumor formation by regulating mitotic activity and providing inhibitory cell cycle control. Tumor formation occurs when these inhibitory controls are deregulated by mutation. Point mutations, loss of heterozygosity, frame-shift mutations, and promoter hypermethylation are all types of genetic and epigenetic changes that can cause failure of a tumor suppressor gene. The first genes mutated in the sequence are often referred to as gatekeeper genes because they provide cell cycle inhibition and regulatory control at specific checkpoints in cell division. The failure of regulation of normal cellular function by tumor suppressor genes is appropriately described by the term *loss of function*. Both alleles of the gene must be nonfunctional to initiate tumor formation.

The *APC* gene is a tumor suppressor gene located on chromosome 5q21. Its product is 2843 amino acids in length and forms a cytoplasmic complex with GSK-3β (a serine-threonine kinase), β-catenin, and axin. β-Catenin, a multifunctional protein, is a structural component of the epithelial cell adherens junctions and the actin cytoskeleton; it also binds in the cytoplasm to Tcf/LEF and is then transported into the nucleus, where it activates transcription of genes such as c-*myc* and others that regulate cellular growth and proliferation. *APC* therefore participates in cell cycle control by regulating the intracytoplasmic pool of β-catenin.

TABLE 51-3	Gene Mutations That Promote Colorectal Cancer	
MUTATION TYPE	**GENES INVOLVED**	**TYPE OF DISEASE CAUSED**
Germline	*APC*	Familial adenomatous polyposis
	MMR	HNPCC (Lynch syndrome)
Somatic	Oncogenes: *myc, ras, src, erbB*	Sporadic disease
	Tumor suppressor genes: *TP53, DCC, APC*	
	MMR genes: *bMSH2, bMLH1, bPMS1, bPMS2, bMSH6, bMSH3*	
Genetic polymorphism	*APC*	Familial colon cancer in Ashkenazi Jews

DCC, Deleted in colorectal carcinoma.

The Wnt signaling proteins are closely associated with the *APC*–β-catenin pathway. *APC* also influences cell cycle proliferation by regulating Wnt expression. Wnt gene products are extracellular signaling molecules that help regulate tissue development throughout the organism. The Wnt signaling proteins are closely associated with the *APC*–β-catenin pathway. Under normal conditions, reduced intracytoplasmic β-catenin levels inhibit Wnt expression. When *APC* is mutated, however, β-catenin levels rise and Wnt is activated. Overexpression of Wnt leads to activation of Wnt target genes, such as cyclin D1 and *MYC,* which drive cell proliferation and tumor formation.

The earliest mutations in the adenoma-carcinoma sequence occur in the *APC* gene. The earliest phenotypic change present is known as aberrant crypt formation, and the most consistent genetic aberrations within these cells are abnormally short proteins known as *APC* truncations. Most clinically relevant derangements in *APC* are truncation mutations created by inappropriate transcription of premature termination codons.

A germline *APC* truncation mutation is responsible for the autosomal dominant inherited disease FAP. Thirty percent of cases of FAP are de novo germline mutations, presenting without a family history of the disease. FAP is rare, with an estimated incidence of 1 in 10,000 live births in the United States, occurring without gender predilection. It is typically characterized by more than 100 adenomatous polyps present in the colon and rectum. These polyps often number in the thousands and are almost always manifested by the late second or early third decade of life (Fig. 51-61). Because some of these polyps proceed through the adenoma-carcinoma sequence, most patients with FAP die of colon cancer by their fifth decade of life in the absence of surgical intervention. FAP is of great interest to those studying sporadic colorectal cancer because *APC* truncation mutations similar to those found in *APC* patients occur in 85% of sporadic colorectal cancers.

Most *APC* truncation mutations occur in the mutational cluster region of the gene, an area responsible for β-catenin binding. However, genotype-phenotype correlations exist with mutations in other regions of the gene. For example, mutations close to the 5′ end of the gene produce a short truncated protein that causes the syndrome known as attenuated FAP or (AFAP). These patients usually have far less than the hundreds of polyps usually associated with FAP, and the disease has a tendency to spare the rectum.

Classic FAP is characterized by truncation mutations occurring in the gene from codon 1250 to codon 1464. Mutations occurring farther along the gene toward the 3′ end are rare and most likely result in a much attenuated phenotype or no detectable abnormality (Fig. 51-62).

The variability of the FAP phenotype is also demonstrated by the presence or absence of extraintestinal manifestations of disease. In the past, the term *Gardner syndrome* was used to describe the coexpression of profuse colonic adenomatous polyps along with osteomas of the mandible and skull, desmoid tumors of the mesentery, and periampullary neoplasms.

Many other associated disorders have been subsequently described, including thyroid papillary tumors, medulloblastomas, hypertrophic gastric fundic polyps, and congenital hypertrophy of the retinal pigmented epithelium of the iris (CHRPE). The expression of extraintestinal manifestations of FAP is dependent on mutation location, with most of these signs seen only when the truncation occurs in a very small area of the mutational cluster region.

Another *APC* mutation implicated in approximately 25% of colorectal cancers afflicting Ashkenazi Jews is the I1307 point mutation caused by the substitution of a lysine for isoleucine at codon 1307. This was initially believed to be a genetic polymorphism, a substitution that does not affect the protein structure. However, it is now recognized as probably the most important cause of familial colorectal cancer in this population.

MYH Mutations and *MYH*-Associated Polyposis

A number of families have been characterized with a phenotype resembling that of FAP or AFAP but without a discoverable *APC* gene defect. In 2002, a report of a Welsh family (family N) with apparent recessive inheritance of multiple colorectal polyps and a cancer was published. On analysis of tumor *APC*, frequent somatic mutations were found characterized by G : C to T : A substitutions typically caused by oxidative DNA damage. The authors found that those family members affected had two distinct mutations in the *MYH* gene, a gene responsible for base excision-repair and used to repair oxidative DNA damage, thereby indicating that unlike FAP, its inheritance pattern is recessive in nature. From

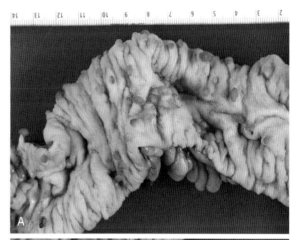
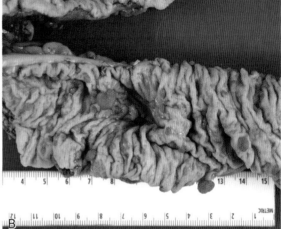
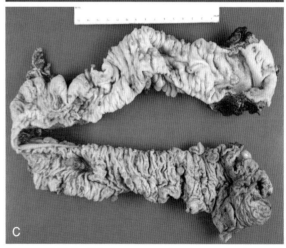

FIGURE 51-61 Familial adenomatous polyposis, macroscopic appearance. The colonic mucosa exhibits numerous small polyps, both pedunculated and sessile. The entire colon contained hundreds of polyps. (Courtesy Dr. Jeffrey P. Baliff, Thomas Jefferson University, Philadelphia.)

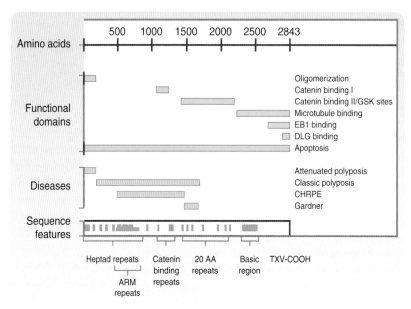

FIGURE 51-62 Functional and pathogenic properties of *APC*. The product of *APC* is a protein heterodimer 2843 amino acids in length. The figure depicts the functional domains of *APC* schematically as *blue bars* where regional mutations result in loss of protein binding, as described in the column on the right side of the figure. Mutations in these regions result in truncations that may affect cellular structure and cell signaling, such as the inability to bind catenins and interference with microtubule binding. Cellular processes such as apoptosis are affected by mutations occurring at many sites along the gene. Some mutational effects are unknown, such as those preventing EB1 and DLG binding (proteins with unclear functions). Diseases are similarly represented by *tan bars*. Mutations within the regions depicted result in the disease phenotypes described in the right column, including attenuated polyposis, classic polyposis, CHRPE, and Gardner syndrome (extraintestinal manifestations of FAP). (From Kinzler KW, Vogelstein B: Lessons from hereditary colorectal cancer. *Cell* 87:159–170, 1996.)

several subsequent surveys of kindreds with familial colorectal cancer or polyp inheritance patterns, it has become clear that a number of *MYH* mutations exist and may coexist in the same patient. The mutation has been characterized in northern European, Indian, and Pakistani populations; it appears to affect the production of polyps and tumors by promoting *APC* defects and is called *MYH*-associated polyposis (MAP). Although the proportion of colorectal cancers attributable to germline *MYH* mutations is unknown, all patients with biallelic *MYH* mutations are at increased risk for colorectal cancer. Greater numbers of polyps (100 to 1000) and even extracolonic manifestations, such as duodenal adenomas, are associated with the presence of more than one germline *MYH* mutation in a single patient.[31]

It is evident that the MAP phenotype is highly variable and that clinical management, for now, should follow guidelines previously established for FAP and AFAP. Surgery in carriers who have polyps is IPAA or ileorectal anastomosis, depending on the status of the rectum. Colonoscopic and duodenal surveillance every 1 or 2 years for those with biallelic mutations is warranted, given the uncertainty of the natural history of the disease.

It remains unclear whether heterozygotes are at increased risk for colorectal cancer; all offspring of those with the disease can be reasonably assured that they are heterozygotes unless they too have multiple polyps, an extremely unlikely event. However, it is certain that patients with MAP need to be distinguished from those with FAP or AFAP because it implies increased risk in siblings rather than in offspring. For those with biallelic mutations, spouses can also be tested in the unlikely event that both spouses possess a recessive *MYH* allele at the same locus.

The most frequently mutated tumor suppressor gene in human neoplasia is *p53 (TP53)*, located on chromosome 17p. Mutations in *p53* are present in 75% of colorectal cancers and occur rather late in the adenoma-carcinoma sequence. Under normal conditions, *p53* acts by inducing apoptosis in response to cellular damage or by causing G_1 cell cycle arrest, allowing DNA repair mechanisms to occur. One of the features of mutated *p53* is that it is unable to activate the *BAX* gene to induce apoptosis. For its role in regulating apoptosis, *p53* is known as the guardian of the genome. The minority of colon cancer patients who have intact *p53* in their tumors may possess a survival advantage. Studies have indicated that prognostic significance may be related to tumor *p53* status.

A number of genes on chromosome 18q are implicated in colorectal cancer, including *SMAD2, SMAD4*, and *DCC*. SMAD proteins are involved in the transforming growth factor-β signal transduction pathway. *SMAD2* and *SMAD4* are mutated in 5% to 10% of sporadic colorectal cancers. *DCC* is a large gene involved in cell-cell or cell-matrix interactions. It is not clear how *DCC* is directly involved in colorectal neoplasia. *DPC4* is a gene adjacent to *DCC* and may be the tumor suppressor gene deleted in 18q mutations.

Mismatch Repair Genes

MMR genes are called caretaker genes because of their important role in policing the integrity of the genome and correcting DNA replication errors. MMR genes that undergo a loss of function contribute to carcinogenesis by accelerating tumor progression. Mutations in MMR genes (including *hMLH1, hMSH2, hMSH3, hPMS1, hPMS2,* and *hMSH6*) result in the HNPCC syndrome. Approximately 3% of colorectal cancers in the United States are caused by HNPCC. Mutations in MMR genes produce microsatellite instability. Microsatellites are repetitive sequences of DNA that appear to be randomly distributed throughout the genome. Stability of these sequences is a good measure of the general integrity of the genome. MMR gene mutations result in errors in S phase when DNA is newly synthesized and copied. Microsatellite instability exists in 10% to 15% of sporadic tumors and in 95% of tumors in patients with HNPCC.

Oncogenes

Proto-oncogenes are genes that produce proteins that promote cellular growth and proliferation. Mutations in proto-oncogenes typically produce a gain of function and can be caused by mutation in only one of the two alleles. After mutation, the gene is called an oncogene. Overexpression of these growth-oriented genes contributes to the uncontrolled proliferation of cells associated with cancer. The products of oncogenes can be divided into categories. For example, growth factors (e.g., transforming growth factor-β, epidermal growth factor, insulin-like growth factor), growth factor receptors (e.g., erbB2), signal transducers (e.g., src, abl, ras), and nuclear proto-oncogenes and transcription factors (myc) are all oncogene products that appear to have a role in the development of colorectal neoplasia. The *ras* proto-oncogene is located on chromosome 12, and mutations are believed to occur early in the adenoma-carcinoma sequence. Mutated *ras* has been found to be present in aberrant crypt foci and adenomatous polyps. Activated *ras* leads to constitutive activity of the protein, which stimulates cellular growth.

Adenoma-Carcinoma Sequence

The adenoma-carcinoma sequence is recognized as the process through which most colorectal carcinomas develop. Clinical and epidemiologic observations have long been cited to support the hypothesis that colorectal carcinomas evolve through a progression of benign polyps to invasive carcinoma, and the elucidation of the genetic pathways to cancer described earlier has confirmed the validity of this hypothesis. However, before the molecular genesis of colorectal cancer was appreciated, there was considerable controversy about whether colorectal cancer arises de novo or evolves from a polyp that was initially a benign precursor. Although there have been a few documented cases of small colon cancers arising de novo from normal mucosa, these are rare, and the validity of the adenoma-carcinoma sequence is now accepted by almost all authorities. The historical observations that led to the hypothesis are of interest because of the therapeutic implications implicit in an understanding of the adenoma-carcinoma sequence. Observations that provided support for the hypothesis include the following:

- Larger adenomas are found to harbor cancers more often than smaller ones, and the larger the polyp, the higher the risk for cancer. Although the cellular characteristics of the polyp are important, with villous adenomas carrying a higher risk than tubular adenomas, the size of the polyp is also important. The risk for cancer in a tubular adenoma smaller than 1 cm in diameter is less than 5%, whereas the risk for cancer in a tubular adenoma larger than 2 cm is 35%. A villous adenoma larger than 2 cm carries a 50% chance of containing a cancer.
- Residual benign adenomatous tissue is found in most invasive colorectal cancers, suggesting progression of the cancer from the remaining benign cells to the predominant malignant ones.

- Benign polyps have been observed to develop into cancers. There have been reports of the direct observation of benign polyps that were not removed progressing over time into malignant neoplasms.
- Colonic adenomas occur more frequently in patients who have colorectal cancer. Almost one third of all patients with colorectal cancer will also have a benign colorectal polyp.
- Patients who develop adenomas have an increased lifetime risk for development of colorectal cancer.
- Removal of polyps decreases the incidence of cancer. Patients with small adenomas have a 2.3 times increased risk for cancer after the polyp is removed, compared with an eightfold increased incidence of colorectal cancer in patients with polyps who do not undergo polypectomy.
- Populations with a high risk for colorectal cancer also have a high prevalence of colorectal polyps.
- Patients with FAP will develop colorectal cancer in almost 100% of cases in the absence of surgical intervention. The adenomas that characterize this syndrome are histologically the same as sporadic adenomas.
- The peak incidence for the discovery of benign colorectal polyps is 50 years of age. The peak incidence for the development of colorectal cancer is 60 years of age. This suggests a 10-year time span for the progression of an adenomatous polyp to a cancer. It has been estimated that a polyp larger than 1 cm in diameter has a cancer risk of 2.5% in 5 years, 8% in 10 years, and 24% in 20 years.

These observations and studies by molecular biologists have documented that colonic mucosa progresses through stages to the eventual development of an invasive cancer. Colonic epithelial cells lose the normal progression to maturity and cell death and begin proliferating in an increasingly uncontrolled manner. With this uncontrolled proliferation, the cells accumulate on the surface of the bowel lumen as a polyp. With more proliferation and increasing cellular disorganization, the cells extend through the muscularis mucosae to become invasive carcinoma. Even at this advanced stage, the process of colorectal carcinogenesis generally follows an orderly sequence of invasion of the muscularis mucosae, pericolic tissue, and lymph nodes and, finally, distant metastasis (Figs. 51-63 and 51-64).

Colorectal Polyps

A colorectal polyp is any mass projecting into the lumen of the bowel above the surface of the intestinal epithelium. Polyps arising from the intestinal mucosa are generally classified by their gross appearance as pedunculated (with a stalk; Fig. 51-65) or sessile (flat, without a stalk; Fig. 51-66). They are further classified by their histologic appearance as tubular adenoma (with branched tubular glands), villous adenoma (with long finger-like projections of the surface epithelium; Fig. 51-67), or tubulovillous adenoma (with elements of both cellular patterns). The most common benign polyp is the tubular adenoma, constituting approximately 65% to 80% of all polyps removed. Approximately 10% to 25% of polyps are tubulovillous, and 5% to 10% are villous adenomas. Tubular adenomas are most often pedunculated; villous adenomas are more commonly sessile. The degree of cellular atypia is variable across the span of polyps, but there is generally less atypia in tubular adenomas, and severe atypia or dysplasia (precancerous cellular change) is found more often in villous adenomas. The incidence of invasive carcinoma being found in a polyp is dependent on the size and histologic type of the polyp. As noted, there is less than a 5% incidence of carcinoma

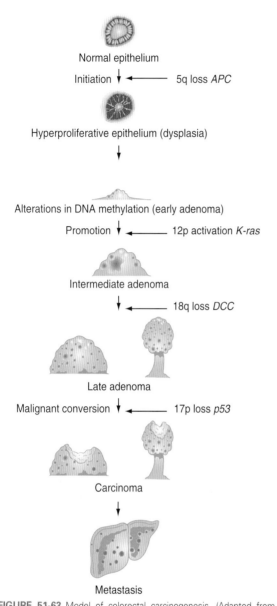

Normal epithelium

Initiation ↓ ←——— 5q loss *APC*

Hyperproliferative epithelium (dysplasia)

↓

Alterations in DNA methylation (early adenoma)

Promotion ↓ ←——— 12p activation *K-ras*

Intermediate adenoma

↓ ←——— 18q loss *DCC*

Late adenoma

Malignant conversion ↓ ←——— 17p loss *p53*

Carcinoma

↓

Metastasis

FIGURE 51-63 Model of colorectal carcinogenesis. (Adapted from Corman ML, editor: *Colon and rectal surgery*, ed 4, Philadelphia,1998, Lippincott-Raven, p 593.)

in an adenomatous polyp smaller than 1 cm in diameter, whereas there is a 50% chance that a villous adenoma larger than 2 cm in diameter will contain a cancer.

The treatment of an adenomatous or villous polyp is removal, usually by colonoscopy. The presence of any polypoid lesion is an indication for a complete colonoscopy and polypectomy, if feasible. Polyps on a stalk are often removed by a snare passed through the colonoscope, whereas sessile (flat) polyps present technical problems with this method because of the danger of perforation associated with the snare technique. Although it is often feasible to elevate the sessile polyp from the underlying muscularis with saline injection, permitting subsequent endoscopic excision, sessile lesions that are large or have a central depression or cannot be "lifted" with saline may be perforation

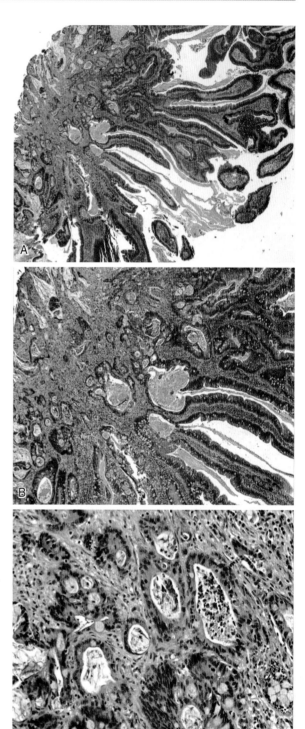

FIGURE 51-64 Colon adenocarcinoma arising in an adenoma, microscopic appearance. **A,** Tubulovillous adenoma with finger-like projections *(right)* reveals a deeper area of infiltrating glands *(left).* **B,** Glands have penetrated the muscularis mucosae. **C,** On high power, neoplastic angulated glands with central dirty necrosis present within a desmoplastic stroma. (Courtesy Dr. Jeffrey P. Baliff, Thomas Jefferson University, Philadelphia.)

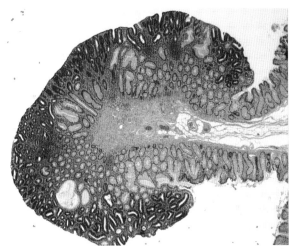

FIGURE 51-65 Pedunculated adenomatous polyp, microscopic appearance. The head of the polyp is lined with dysplastic epithelium, whereas the stalk is lined with nondysplastic epithelium. (Courtesy Dr. Jeffrey P. Baliff, Thomas Jefferson University, Philadelphia.)

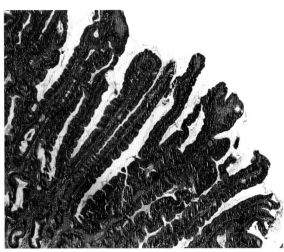

FIGURE 51-67 Villous adenoma. This photomicrograph reveals the finger-like projections that give the appearance of villi. (Courtesy Dr. Jeffrey P. Baliff, Thomas Jefferson University, Philadelphia.)

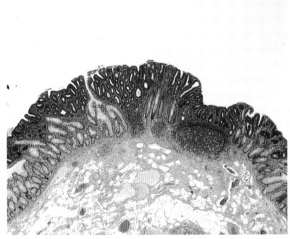

FIGURE 51-66 Sessile adenomatous polyp, microscopic appearance. This tubular adenoma is called *sessile* because of its broad base, the preservation of the muscularis mucosae underneath, and the absence of a stalk. (Courtesy Dr. Jeffrey P. Baliff, Thomas Jefferson University, Philadelphia.)

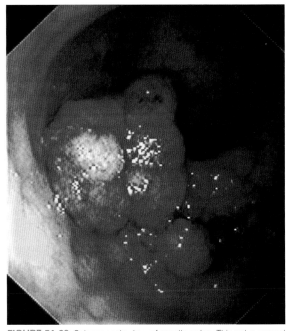

FIGURE 51-68 Colonoscopic view of sessile polyp. This polyp proved to be a carcinoma after it was removed by segmental resection.

risks and should be surgically excised by segmental colectomy for complete removal and lymph node examination (Fig. 51-68).

Adenomatous polyps should be considered precursors of cancer, and when cancer arises in a polyp, careful consideration needs to be given to ensure the adequacy of treatment. Invasive carcinoma describes the situation in which malignant cells have extended through the muscularis mucosae of the polyp, whether it is on a stalk or a sessile lesion. Cellular changes confined to the muscularis mucosae above the lamina propria do not metastasize, and the cellular abnormalities should be described as atypia or dysplasia. Complete endoscopic excision of this type of polyp is adequate treatment.

If invasive carcinoma penetrates the muscularis mucosae, the risk for lymph node metastasis and local recurrence must be considered to determine whether a more extensive resection is required. Haggitt and colleagues have proposed a classification for polyps containing cancer according to the depth of invasion, as follows (Fig. 51-69):

Level 0: Carcinoma does not invade the muscularis mucosae (carcinoma in situ or intramucosal carcinoma)

Level 1: Carcinoma invades through the muscularis mucosae into the submucosa but is limited to the head of the polyp

Level 2: Carcinoma invades the level of the neck of the polyp (junction between the head and stalk)

Level 3: Carcinoma invades any part of the stalk

Level 4: Carcinoma invades into the submucosa of the bowel wall below the stalk of the polyp but above the muscularis propria

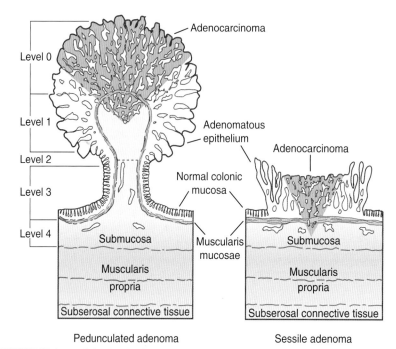

FIGURE 51-69 Anatomic landmarks of pedunculated and sessile adenomas. (From Haggitt RC, Glotzbach RE, Soffer EE, et al: Prognostic factors in colorectal carcinoma arising in adenomas: Implications for lesions removed by endoscopic polypectomy. *Gastroenterology* 89:328–336, 1985.)

By definition, all sessile polyps with invasive carcinoma are level 4 by Haggitt's criteria.

If a polyp contains a histologically poorly differentiated invasive carcinoma or if there are cancer cells observed in the lymphovascular spaces, there is a more than 10% chance of metastases, and these lesions should be treated aggressively. A pedunculated polyp with invasion to levels 1, 2, and 3 has a low risk for lymph node metastasis or local recurrence, and complete excision of the polyp is adequate if the poor prognostic factors mentioned earlier are absent and margins are negative. A sessile polyp containing invasive cancer has at least a 10% chance of metastasis to regional lymph nodes, but if the lesion is well or moderately differentiated, there is no lymphovascular invasion noted, and the lesion can be completely excised, the depth of invasion by the cancer may provide useful prognostic information. There is a high risk for lymph node and distant metastases associated with sessile cancers in the rectum, and these lesions should be treated aggressively.

Hyperplastic polyps are the most common colonic polyps but are usually small and composed of cells showing dysmaturation and hyperplasia. The small diminutive polyps have been regarded as benign in nature, with no neoplastic potential. The histologic appearance of these polyps is serrated (saw-toothed; Figs. 51-70 and 51-71). Of these polyps, 90% are smaller than 3 mm in diameter, and these diminutive lesions are generally considered to have no malignant potential. However, adenomatous changes can be found in hyperplastic polyps, and therefore the polyps should be excised for histologic examination. These serrated adenomas have been observed to be associated with the development of cancers that predominate in the right side of the colon, more frequently in older women and smokers. They appear to be associated with the microsatellite instability characteristic of defects in DNA repair mechanisms.

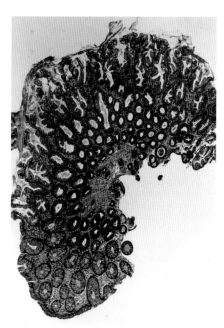

FIGURE 51-70 Hyperplastic polyp. Elongated crypts reveal a serrated (saw-toothed) or star-shaped appearance. There is no epithelial dysplasia. (Courtesy Dr. Jeffrey P. Baliff, Thomas Jefferson University, Philadelphia.)

Hereditary Cancer Syndromes (Table 51-4)
Familial Adenomatous Polyposis

FAP is the prototypical hereditary polyposis syndrome. The discovery of the gene responsible for the transmission of the disease, the *APC* gene, located on chromosome 5q21, lagged behind the

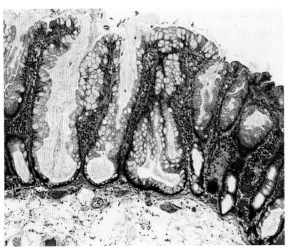

FIGURE 51-71 Sessile serrated adenoma. This view shows basilar crypt dilation, epithelium proliferating in a serrated (saw-toothed) manner, and so-called crypt architectural dysplasia in the form of mal-oriented crypts, with one crypt extending horizontally. There is no cytologic dysplasia of the epithelium. (Courtesy Dr. Jeffrey P. Baliff, Thomas Jefferson University, Philadelphia.)

first descriptions of cases of FAP by an entire century. In 1863, Virchow reported a 15-year-old boy with multiple colonic polyps. In 1882, Cripps described the occurrence of numerous colonic polyps in multiple family members. In 1927, Cockayne demonstrated that FAP was genetically transmitted in an autosomal dominant fashion. Dukes was the first to establish some form of a familial tumor registry, which he reported with Lockhart-Mummery in 1930. Throughout the 20th century, many reports described various extraintestinal manifestations associated with FAP. In 1986, Lemuel Herrera demonstrated that the underlying genetic abnormality was a mutation in the *APC* gene.

The common expression of the syndrome is the invariable presence of multiple colonic polyps; frequent occurrence of gastric, duodenal, and periampullary polyps; and occasional association of extraintestinal manifestations, including epidermoid cysts, desmoid tumors in the abdomen, osteomas, and brain tumors. Gastric and duodenal polyps occur in approximately 50% of affected individuals. Most of the gastric polyps represent fundic gland hyperplasia, rather than adenomatous polyps, and have limited malignant potential. However, duodenal polyps are adenomatous in nature and should be considered premalignant. Patients with FAP have an increased risk for ampullary cancer. Adenomatous polyps and cancer have also been found in the jejunum and ileum of patients with FAP. Rare extraintestinal malignant neoplasms in FAP patients include cancers of the extra-hepatic bile ducts, gallbladder, pancreas, adrenals, thyroid, and liver. An interesting marker for FAP is CHRPE, which can be detected by indirect ophthalmoscopy in approximately 75% of affected individuals.

The gene is expressed in 100% of patients with the mutation. Autosomal dominance results in expression in 50% of offspring. There is a negative family history in 10% to 20% of affected individuals, who apparently acquire the syndrome as the result of a spontaneous germline mutation. All patients with the defective gene will develop cancer of the colon if left untreated. The average age at discovery of a new patient with FAP is 29 years. The average age of a patient who is newly discovered to have colorectal cancer

related to FAP is 39 years. Eponymous polyposis syndromes now recognized to belong to the general disorder of FAP include Gardner syndrome (colonic polyps, epidermal inclusion cysts, osteomas) and Turcot syndrome (colonic polyps, brain tumors).

Osteomas usually present as visible and palpable prominences in the skull, mandible, and tibia of individuals with FAP. They are almost always benign. Radiographs of the maxilla and mandible may reveal bone cysts, supernumerary and impacted molars, or congenitally absent teeth. Desmoid tumors can present in the retroperitoneum and abdominal wall of affected patients, usually after surgery. These tumors seldom metastasize but are often locally invasive; direct invasion of the mesenteric vessels, ureters, or walls of the small intestine can result in death.

Surgical treatment of patients with FAP is directed at removal of all affected colonic and rectal mucosa. Restorative proctocolectomy with IPAA has become the most commonly recommended operation. The procedure is usually accompanied by a distal rectal mucosectomy to ensure that all premalignant colonic mucosa is removed, and the IPAA is fashioned between the ileal pouch and dentate line of the anal canal. Patients who undergo this procedure for FAP have a better functional result than patients similarly treated for ulcerative colitis. The incidence of inflammation in the ileal pouch (pouchitis) is much lower in patients with FAP than in patients with ulcerative colitis.

An alternative approach, total abdominal colectomy with ileorectal anastomosis, was used extensively before the development of the technique of IPAA and has certain advantages. If an FAP patient has relatively few polyps in the rectum, consideration may be given to this option. The abdominal colon is resected and an anastomosis fashioned between the ileum and rectum. It is technically a simpler operation to perform, and the pelvic dissection is avoided. This eliminates the potential complication of injury to the autonomic nerves that could result in impotence. In addition, there is theoretically less risk for anastomotic leak from the relatively simple ileorectal anastomosis fashioned in the peritoneal cavity compared with the long suture (or staple) lines required to form the ileal pouch and then to fashion the anastomosis between the ileal pouch and anus.

An additional argument in favor of abdominal colectomy and ileorectal anastomosis is the observation that sulindac and celecoxib have caused the regression of adenomatous polyps in some patients with FAP. The disadvantages are that the rectum remains at high risk for the formation of new precancerous polyps, a proctoscopic examination is required every 6 to 12 months to detect and to destroy any new polyps, and there is a definite increased risk for cancer arising in the rectum with the passage of time.

It has been suggested that genetic testing may help make the decision between restorative proctocolectomy with IPAA and abdominal colectomy with ileorectal anastomosis. It has been observed that the risk for rectal cancer is almost three times higher in FAP patients with a mutation after codon 1250 than in patients with mutations before this codon. This may influence the decision to offer abdominal colectomy with ileorectal anastomosis to those whose mutation occurs proximal to codon 1250 if proctoscopic examination reveals no or few polyps in the rectum.

Patients who choose to be treated by abdominal colectomy with ileorectal anastomosis should realize that the risk for development of rectal cancer is real and has been shown to be 4%, 5.6%, 7.9%, and 25% at 5, 10, 15, and 20 years after the operation, respectively. Even though sulindac and celecoxib can produce partial regression of polyps, semiannual surveillance of the rectal

TABLE 51-4 Hereditary Cancer Syndromes

	HEREDITARY NONPOLYPOSIS COLON CANCER	HEREDITARY ADENOMATOUS POLYPOSIS SYNDROMES		HEREDITARY HAMARTOMATOUS POLYPOSIS SYNDROMES			
		FAMILIAL ADENOMATOUS POLYPOSIS (FAP)/GARDNER SYNDROME	TURCOT SYNDROME	COWDEN DISEASE	FAMILIAL JUVENILE POLYPOSIS	PEUTZ-JEGHERS SYNDROME	RUVALCABA-MYHRE-SMITH SYNDROME (BANNAYAN-ZONANA SYNDROME)
GI Features	Small number of colorectal polyps	Hundreds to thousands of colorectal polyps; duodenal adenomas and gastric polyps, usually fundic gland	Colorectal polyps, which may be few or resemble classic FAP	Polyps most commonly of colon and stomach	Juvenile polyps mostly in colon but throughout GI tract; defined by ≥10 juvenile polyps	Small number of polyps throughout GI tract but most common in small intestine	Hamartomatous GI polyps, usually lipomas, hemangiomas, or lymphangiomas
Other Clinical Features	Muir-Torre variant: sebaceous adenomas, keratoacanthomas, sebaceous epitheliomas, and basal cell epitheliomas	Osteomas, desmoid tumors, epidermoid cysts, and congenital hypertrophy of retinal epithelium	Brain tumors, including cerebellar medulloblastoma and glioblastomas	Mucocutaneous lesions, thyroid adenomas and goiter, fibroadenomas and fibrocystic disease of the breast, uterine leiomyomas, macrocephaly	Congenital abnormalities in at least 20%, including malrotation, hydrocephalus, cardiac lesions, Meckel's diverticulum, mesenteric lymphangioma	Pigmented lesions of skin; benign and malignant genital tumors	Dysmorphic facial features, macrocephaly, seizures, intellectual impairment, pigmented macules of shaft and glans of penis
Malignancy Risk	70%-80% lifetime risk for colorectal cancer; 30%-60% lifetime risk for endometrial cancer; ↑ risk for ovarian cancer, gastric carcinoma, transitional cell carcinoma of the ureters and renal pelvis, small bowel cancer, and sebaceous carcinomas	Colorectal cancer risk approaches 100%; ↑ risk for periampullary malignant disease, thyroid carcinoma, central nervous system tumors, hepatoblastoma	Colorectal carcinoma and brain tumors	10% risk for thyroid cancer and up to 50% risk for adenocarcinoma of breast in affected women	9% to 25% risk for colorectal cancer; ↑ risk for gastric, duodenal, and pancreatic cancer	↑ Risk for GI malignant disease and pancreatic cancer and adenoma malignum of cervix; unknown risk for breast cancer	Malignant GI tumors identified but lifetime risk for malignant disease unknown

Screening Recommendations

Colonoscopy at age 20-25 years; repeat every 1-3 years; transvaginal ultrasound or endometrial aspiration at age 20-25 years; repeat annually (expert opinion only)	Flexible proctosigmoidoscopy at age 10-12 years; repeat every 1-2 years until age of 35 years; after the age of 35 years, repeat every 3 years; upper GI endoscopy every 1-3 years starting when polyps first identified	Same as for FAP; also consider imaging of the brain	Annual physical examination with special attention to thyroid; mammography at age 30 years or 5 years before earliest breast cancer case in the family; routine colon cancer surveillance (expert opinion only)	Screening by age 12 years if symptoms have not yet arisen; colonoscopy with multiple random biopsy specimens every several years (expert opinion only)	Upper GI endoscopy, small bowel radiography, colonoscopy every 2 years; pancreatic ultrasound and hemoglobin levels annually; gynecologic examination, cervical smear, pelvic ultrasound annually; clinical breast examination and mammography at age 25 years; clinical testicular examination and testicular ultrasound in males with feminizing features (expert opinion only)	No known published recommendations

Genetic Basis

AD	AD	AD	AD	AD	AD	AD
MLH1 (chromosome 3p) MSH2 (chromosome 2p) MSH6/GTMP (chromosome 2p) PMS1 (chromosome 2q) PMS2 (chromosome 7q)	APC (chromosome 5q)	APC mutations identified predominantly in families with cerebellar medulloblastoma; MLH1, PMS2 mutations identified in families with predominance of glioblastomas	PTEN (chromosome 10q)	AD inheritance in some families; Subset of families with mutation in SMAD4 (DRC4) (chromosome 10q)	STK11 (chromosome 19p)	PTEN (chromosome 10q) in some

Genetic Testing

Clinical testing of MLH1 and MSH2 genes available	Clinical testing of APC gene available	Clinical testing of APC and MLH1 genes available	Research testing of PTEN gene available	Families being collected for research studies only	Research testing of STK11 gene available	Research testing of PTEN gene available

AD, Autosomal dominant; GI, gastrointestinal; ↑, increased.

mucosa is required, and approximately one third of patients treated by abdominal colectomy and ileorectal anastomosis develop florid polyposis of the rectum that will require proctectomy (and ileostomy or IPAA) within 20 years.

Polyps of the stomach and duodenum are not uncommon in patients with FAP. The gastric polyps are usually hyperplastic and do not require surgical removal. However, the duodenal and ampullary polyps are generally neoplastic and require attention. A reasonable surveillance program is for upper GI surveillance every 2 years after the age of 30 years and endoscopic polypectomy, if possible, to remove all large adenomas from the duodenum. If numerous polyps are identified, the endoscopy obviously should be repeated with greater frequency. If an ampullary cancer is discovered at an early stage, pancreatoduodenectomy (Whipple procedure) is indicated.

The abdominal desmoid tumor can be an especially vexing and difficult extraintestinal manifestation of FAP. After surgical procedures, dense fibrous tissue forms in the mesentery of the small intestine or within the abdominal wall in some patients with FAP. If the mesentery is involved, the intestine can be tethered or invaded directly by the tumor. The locally invasive tumor can also encroach on the vascular supply to the intestine. Small desmoid tumors confined to the abdominal wall are appropriately treated by resection, but the surgical treatment of mesenteric desmoids is dangerous and generally futile. There have been sporadic reports of regression of desmoid tumors after treatment with sulindac, tamoxifen, low-dose methotrexate, radiation, and various types of chemotherapy. The initial treatment is usually with sulindac or tamoxifen.

The ability to identify the genetic mutation in most patients with FAP—although the mutation may not be identified in as many as 20% of patients with a well-documented, transmissible FAP syndrome—permits a method of screening family members at risk for inheriting the mutation. It is imperative that the *APC* mutation be clearly identified in the DNA of a family member known to have the disease. The DNA of other family members can then be analyzed directly, requiring only a venipuncture. If the analysis demonstrates noninheritance of a mutated *APC* gene, the individual can avoid annual endoscopic screening and should require only an occasional colonoscopy.

Lynch Syndrome

Lynch syndrome (also called hereditary nonpolyposis colon cancer or HNPCC) is the most frequently occurring hereditary colorectal cancer syndrome in the United States and western Europe. It accounts for approximately 3% of all cases of colorectal cancer and for approximately 15% of these cancers in patients with a family history of colorectal cancer. Alder S. Warthin, Chairman of Pathology at the University of Michigan, initially recognized this hereditary syndrome in 1885. Dr. Warthin's seamstress prophesied that she would die of cancer because of her strong family history of endometrial, gastric, and colon cancer. Dr. Warthin's investigations of her family's medical records revealed a pattern of autosomal dominant transmission of the cancer risk. This family (family G) has been further studied and characterized by Henry Lynch, who described the prominent features of the syndrome, including onset of cancer at a relatively young age (mean, 44 years), proximal distribution (70% of cancers located in the right colon), predominance of mucinous or poorly differentiated (signet cell) adenocarcinoma, increased number of synchronous and metachronous cancers, and, despite all these poor prognostic indicators, a relatively good outcome after surgery. Originally, two

hereditary syndromes were initially described. Lynch I syndrome is characterized by cancer of the proximal colon occurring at a relatively young age; Lynch II syndrome is characterized by families at risk for both colorectal and extracolonic cancers, including cancers of endometrial, ovarian, gastric, small intestinal, pancreatic, and ureteral and renal pelvic origin. Currently, the term *Lynch syndrome* refers to both patterns, and it is understood that there is overlap between the two described variants.

Before the genetic mechanisms underlying the Lynch syndrome were understood, is was defined by the Amsterdam criteria, which required three criteria for the diagnosis:
1. Colorectal cancer in three family members (first-degree relatives)
2. Involvement of at least two generations
3. At least one affected individual being younger than 50 years at the time of diagnosis

These requirements were recognized as being too restrictive, and the modified Amsterdam criteria expanded the cancers to be included to not only colorectal but also endometrial, ovarian, gastric, pancreatic, small intestinal, ureteral, and renal pelvic cancers. Further liberalization for identifying patients with HNPCC occurred with the introduction of the Bethesda criteria (Box 51-4).

Molecular biologists have demonstrated that the increased cancer risk in these syndromes is caused by malfunction of the DNA repair mechanism. Specific genes that have been shown to be responsible for the syndrome include *hMSH2* (located on chromosome 2p21), *hMLH1* (3p21), *hMSH6* (2p16-21), and *hPMS2* (7p21). A mutation in *hMSH2* has been shown to be responsible for the cancer prevalence in cancer family G. Mutations in *hMSH2* or *hMLH1* account for more than 90% of identifiable mutations in patients with Lynch syndrome. The

---

BOX 51-4 Clinical Criteria for Hereditary Nonpolyposis Colorectal Cancer

Amsterdam Criteria
At least three relatives with colon cancer and all of the following:
- One affected person is a first-degree relative of the other two affected persons
- Two successive generations affected
- At least one case of colon cancer diagnosed before the age of 50 years
- FAP excluded

Modified Amsterdam Criteria
Same as the Amsterdam criteria, except that cancer must be associated with HNPCC (colon, endometrium, small bowel, ureter, renal pelvis) instead of specifically colon cancer

Bethesda Criteria
The Amsterdam criteria or one of the following:
- Two cases of HNPCC-associated cancer in one patient, including synchronous or metachronous cancer
- Colon cancer and a first-degree relative with HNPCC-associated cancer and/or colonic adenoma (one case of cancer diagnosed before age 45 years and adenoma diagnosed before age 40 years)
- Colon or endometrial cancer diagnosed before age 45 years
- Right-sided colon cancer that has an undifferentiated pattern (solid, cribriform) or signet cell histopathologic characteristics diagnosed before age 45 years
- Adenomas diagnosed before age 40 years

initially reported difference in the types of cancers in Lynch I and II syndromes cannot be accounted for by mutations in specific MMR genes. The cancer family syndrome involving *hMSH6* is characterized by an increased incidence of endometrial carcinoma.

The mainstay of the diagnosis of Lynch syndrome is a detailed family history. Still, as many as 20% of newly discovered cases of HNPCC are caused by spontaneous germline mutations, so a family history may not accurately reflect the genetic nature of the syndrome. Colorectal cancer, or a Lynch syndrome–related cancer, arising in a person younger than 50 years should raise suspicion for this syndrome. Genetic counseling and testing should be offered. If the individual proves to have Lynch syndrome by identification of a mutation in one of the known MMR genes, other family members can be tested after obtaining genetic counseling. However, failure to identify a causative MMR gene mutation in a patient with a suggestive history does not exclude the diagnosis of Lynch syndrome. In as many as 50% of patients with a family history that clearly demonstrates Lynch syndrome–type transmission of cancer susceptibility, DNA testing will fail to identify the causative gene.

The management of patients with Lynch syndrome is somewhat controversial, but the need for close surveillance in patients known to carry the mutation is obvious. It is usually recommended that a program of surveillance colonoscopy begin at the age of 20 years. Colonoscopy is repeated every 2 years until the age of 35 years and then annually thereafter. In women, periodic vacuum curettage is begun at age 25 years, as are pelvic ultrasound and determination of CA-125 levels. Annual tests for occult blood

in the urine should also be carried out because of the risk for ureteral and renal pelvic cancer.

It has been shown that annual colonoscopy and removal of polyps, when found, will decrease the incidence of colon cancer in patients with HNPCC. However, there have been well-documented cases of invasive colon cancers occurring 1 year after a negative colonoscopy. It is obvious that the slow evolution from benign polyp to invasive cancer is not a feature of the pathogenesis in HNPCC patients, and this phenomenon of accelerated carcinogenesis mandates frequent (annual) colonoscopic examinations. Even with annual colonoscopic examinations, there is a documented risk for colon cancer, but when a cancer arises while the patient is under a vigorous surveillance program, the cancer stage is usually favorable (Fig. 51-72).

When colon cancer is detected in a patient with Lynch syndrome, an abdominal colectomy–ileorectal anastomosis is the procedure of choice. If the patient is a woman with no further plans for childbearing, a prophylactic total abdominal hysterectomy and bilateral salpingo-oophorectomy are recommended. The rectum remains at risk for the development of cancer, and annual proctoscopic examinations are mandatory after abdominal colectomy. Other forms of cancer associated with Lynch syndrome are treated according to the same criteria as for nonhereditary cases. The role of prophylactic colectomy for patients with Lynch syndrome has been considered in some cases, but this has not received universal acceptance. It is an interesting but well-documented fact that the prognosis is better for cancer patients with Lynch syndrome than for non–Lynch syndrome patients with cancer of the same stage.

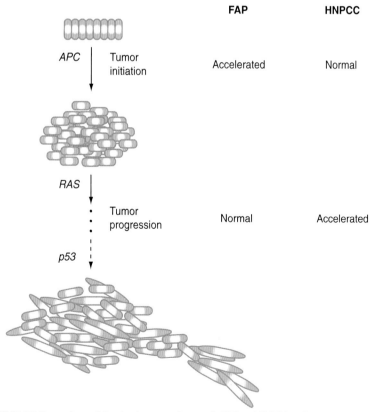

	FAP	HNPCC
APC ↓ Tumor initiation	Accelerated	Normal
RAS ... *p53* ↓ Tumor progression	Normal	Accelerated

FIGURE 51-72 Comparison of the development of cancer in FAP and HNPCC patients. (From Kinzler KW, Vogelstein B: Lessons from hereditary colorectal cancer. *Cell* 87:159–170, 1996.)

Peutz-Jeghers Syndrome

Peutz-Jeghers syndrome is an autosomal dominant syndrome characterized by the combination of hamartomatous polyps of the intestinal tract and hyperpigmentation of the buccal mucosa, lips, and digits. Germline defects in the tumor suppressor serine-threonine kinase 11 *(STK11)* gene are implicated in this rare autosomal dominant inherited disease. Although the syndrome was first described by Hutchinson in 1896, later separate descriptions by Peutz and then Jeghers in the 1940s brought recognition to the condition. The syndrome is associated with an increased (2% to 10%) risk for cancer of the intestinal tract, with cancers reported throughout the intestinal tract, from the stomach to the rectum. There is also an increased risk for extraintestinal malignant neoplasms, including cancer of the breast, ovary, cervix, fallopian tubes, thyroid, lung, gallbladder, bile ducts, pancreas, and testicles.

The polyps may cause bleeding or intestinal obstruction (from intussusception). If surgery is required for these symptoms, an attempt should be made to remove as many polyps as possible with the aid of intraoperative endoscopy and polypectomy. Any polyp that is larger than 1.5 cm should be removed if possible. It is reasonable to survey the colon endoscopically every 2 years, and patients should be screened periodically for malignant neoplasms of the breast, cervix, ovary, testicle, stomach, and pancreas.

Juvenile Polyposis Syndrome

Juvenile polyposis is an autosomal dominant syndrome with high penetrance that carries an increased risk for both GI and extraintestinal cancer. The syndrome is usually discovered because of GI bleeding, intussusception, or hypoalbuminemia associated with protein loss through the intestine. The juvenile polyps in this syndrome are predominantly hamartomas, but the hamartomas may contain adenomatous elements, and adenomatous polyps also are common. There is an increased cancer risk in afflicted individuals, with a malignant potential of at least 10% in patients with multiple juvenile polyps. Mutations in the tumor suppressor gene *SMAD4* are believed to cause up to 50% of reported cases.

In patients with relatively few juvenile polyps, endoscopic polypectomy should be carried out. However, patients with numerous polyps should be treated with abdominal colectomy, ileorectal anastomosis, and frequent endoscopic surveillance of the rectum. If the diffuse form of polyposis involves the rectal mucosa, consideration should be given to restorative proctocolectomy with IPAA. Sporadic juvenile polyps can occur as well and can be a lead point for intussusception. Juvenile polyps are benign polyps composed of cystic dilations of glandular structures within the fibroblastic stroma of the lamina propria. They are relatively uncommon yet may cause bleeding or intussusception. Therefore, the polyps should be treated by endoscopic removal.

Sporadic Colon Cancer

It is important to recognize the increased risk for cancer in patients with hereditary cancer syndromes, but the most common form of colorectal cancer is sporadic in nature, without an associated strong family history. Although the cause and pathogenesis of adenocarcinoma are similar throughout the large bowel, significant differences in the use of diagnostic and therapeutic modalities separate colonic from rectal cancers. This distinction is largely because of the confinement of the rectum by the bony pelvis and possible biologic differences that may mandate more aggressive treatment and surveillance, stage per stage, for rectal cancer. The limited mobility of the rectum allows MRI to generate better

images and increases its sensitivity. In addition, the proximity of the rectum to the anus permits easy access of ultrasound probes for more accurate assessment of the extent of penetration of the bowel wall and the involvement of adjacent lymph nodes. The limited accessibility of the rectum, proximity to the anal sphincter, and close association with the autonomic nerves supplying the bladder and genitalia require special and unique consideration in planning of treatment for cancer of the rectum. Therefore, colon and rectal adenocarcinomas are discussed separately.

The signs and symptoms of colon cancer are varied, nonspecific, and somewhat dependent on the location of the tumor in the colon as well as the extent of constriction of the lumen caused by the cancer. In the past 4 decades, the incidence of cancer in the right colon has increased in comparison to cancer arising in the left colon and rectum. This is an important consideration in that about 40% of all colon cancers are located proximal to the area that can be visualized by the flexible sigmoidoscope. Colorectal cancers can bleed, causing red blood to appear in the stool (hematochezia). Bleeding from right-sided colon tumors can produce dark tarry stools (melena). Often, the bleeding is asymptomatic and detected only by anemia discovered by a routine hemoglobin determination. Iron deficiency anemia in any man or nonmenstruating woman should lead to a search for a source of bleeding from the GI tract. Bleeding is often associated with colon cancer, but in approximately one third of patients with a proven colon cancer, the hemoglobin level is normal and the stool test results are negative for occult blood.

Cancers located in the left colon are often constrictive in nature. Patients with left-sided colon cancers may notice a change in bowel habit, most often reported as increasing constipation. Sigmoid cancers can mimic diverticulitis, presenting with pain, fever, and obstructive symptoms. At least 20% of patients with sigmoid cancer also have diverticular disease, making the correct diagnosis difficult at times. Sigmoid cancers can also cause colovesical or colovaginal fistulas. Such fistulas are more commonly caused by diverticulitis, but it is imperative that the correct diagnosis be established because the treatment of colon cancer is substantially different from treatment of diverticulitis.

Cancers in the right colon more often are manifested with melena, fatigue associated with anemia, or, if the tumor is advanced, abdominal pain. Although obstructive symptoms are usually associated with cancers of the left colon, any advanced colorectal cancer can cause a change in bowel habits and intestinal obstruction (Figs. 51-73 and 51-74).

Colonoscopy is the "gold standard" for establishing the diagnosis of colon cancer. It permits biopsy of the tumor to verify the diagnosis while allowing inspection of the entire colon to exclude metachronous polyps or cancers; the incidence of a synchronous cancer is approximately 3%. Colonoscopy is generally performed even after a cancer is detected by barium enema to obtain a biopsy specimen and to detect (and remove) small polyps that may be missed by the contrast study (Fig. 51-75).

Staging

Staging may be defined as the process whereby objective data are assembled to define the state of progression of disease. Data are summated to provide a designated stage for an individual's disease, from which inferences may be drawn about the likelihood of residual disease and hence the chance of cure with or without further treatment.

At present, the stage of the tumor is assessed by indicating the depth of penetration of the tumor into the bowel wall (T stage),

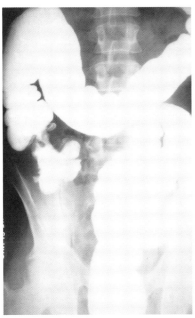

FIGURE 51-73 Radiograph of barium enema demonstrating apple core or napkin ring lesion caused by a constricting carcinoma.

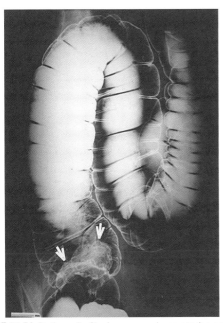

FIGURE 51-74 Radiograph of barium enema demonstrating a polypoid carcinoma arising in the cecum of a 35-year-old woman (arrows). (Courtesy Dr. Dina F. Caroline, Temple University Hospital, Philadelphia.)

the extent of lymph node involvement (N stage), and the presence or absence of distant metastases (M stage). The standard staging system was based on a system developed in 1932 by Cuthbert Dukes, a pathologist at St. Mark's Hospital in London, that was later modified. The classification was developed for rectal cancer, but it was generally also used to describe the stage of colon cancer. The Dukes classification is simple to remember but has rapidly been replaced by the American Joint Committee on Cancer (AJCC) staging system. This classification is in use by most

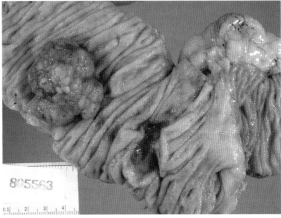

FIGURE 51-75 Resected right colon containing large benign sessile polyp adjacent to an ulcerated carcinoma.

hospitals in the United States and was developed by the AJCC and approved by the International Union Against Cancer. This classification, known as the TNM (tumor, node, metastasis) system, combines clinical information obtained preoperatively with data obtained during surgery and after histologic examination of the specimen. There have been numerous and significant modifications in the system since its introduction in 1987; the seventh edition of the *AJCC Cancer Staging Manual* has taken into account survival and relapse data that refine the prognostic value of accurate staging of colorectal cancer (Table 51-5).[22]

Rules for Classification

Clinical staging. A clinical assessment of the stage of disease (cTNM) is based on evidence obtained by medical history, physical examination, and endoscopy. Examinations designed to detect metastatic disease include chest radiographs, CT (including pelvis, abdomen, and chest), MRI, and positron emission tomography (PET) or fused PET/CT scans. Clinical staging in patients with rectal cancer often determines whether preoperative adjuvant treatment is indicated. Modalities to assess the preoperative stage of rectal cancer include endorectal ultrasound, pelvic CT, and pelvic MRI, with or without an endorectal coil.

Pathologic staging. The pathologic examination of the resected specimen (pTNM) provides a basis for prognosis and consideration of the need for further (adjuvant) treatment. Patients who were given a clinical stage (cTNM) before the initiation of preoperative adjuvant treatment, usually combined radiation therapy and chemotherapy, will have a modified pathologic stage assessed after examination of the surgically resected specimen; that stage is indicated by the y prescript (ypTNM).

Cancer cells confined within the glandular basement membrane (intraepithelial) or lamina propria (intramucosal) with no extension through the muscularis mucosae are not associated with a risk of metastasis and are defined as in situ carcinoma, pTis.

Accumulated survival data reviewed by the AJCC have allowed the provision of more accurate prognostic data with further stratification based on accuracy of staging. For example, it is now recognized that outcomes are different for tumors within the pT4 category based on extent of disease. T4 cancers that penetrate to the surface of the visceral peritoneum (pT4a) have a better prognosis than tumors that directly invade or adhere to other organs (pT4b), and the staging classification has been refined to reflect this. In addition, it is recognized that increasing numbers of

TABLE 51-5 American Joint Committee on Cancer TNM Staging System for Colorectal Cancer

STAGE	FEATURES
Primary Tumor (T)	
TX	Primary tumor cannot be assessed
T0	No evidence of primary tumor
Tis	Carcinoma in situ—intraepithelial or invasion of lamina propria*
T1	Tumor invades submucosa
T2	Tumor invades muscularis propria
T3	Tumor invades through the muscularis propria into pericolorectal tissues
T4a	Tumor penetrates to the surface of the visceral peritoneum[†]
T4b	Tumor directly invades or is adherent to other organs or structures[†,‡]
Regional Lymph Nodes (N)	
NX	Regional lymph nodes cannot be assessed
N0	No regional lymph node metastasis
N1	Metastasis in one to three regional lymph nodes
N1a	Metastasis in one regional lymph node
N1b	Metastasis in two or three regional lymph nodes
N1c	Tumor deposit(s) in the subserosa, mesentery, or nonperitonealized pericolic or perirectal tissues without regional nodal metastasis
N2	Metastasis in four or more regional lymph nodes
N2a	Metastasis in four to six regional lymph nodes
N2b	Metastasis in seven or more regional lymph nodes
Distant Metastasis (M)	
M0	No distant metastasis
M1	Distant metastasis
M1a	Metastasis confined to one organ or site (e.g., liver, lung, ovary, nonregional node)
M1b	Metastases in more than one organ/site or the peritoneum

STAGE GROUPING

STAGE	T	N	M	DUKES[§]	MAC[§]
0	Tis	N0	M0	—	—
I	T1	N0	M0	A	A
	T2	N0	M0	A	B1
IIA	T3	N0	M0	B	B2
IIB	T4a	N0	M0	B	B2
IIC	T4b	N0	M0	B	B3
IIIA	T1-T2	N1/N1c	M0	C	C1
	T1	N2a	M0	C	C1
IIIB	T3-T4a	N1/N1c	M0	C	C2
	T2-T3	N2a	M0	C	C1/C2
	T1-T2	N2b	M0	C	C1
IIIC	T4a	N2a	M0	C	C2
	T3-T4a	N2b	M0	C	C2
	T4b	N1-N2	M0	C	C3
IVA	Any T	Any N	M1a	—	—
IVB	Any T	Any N	M1b	—	—

STAGE	FEATURES
Histologic Grade (G)	
GX	Grade cannot be assessed
G1	Well differentiated
G2	Moderately differentiated
G3	Poorly differentiated
G4	Undifferentiated
Residual Tumor (R)	
R0	Complete resection, margins histologically negative, no residual tumor left after resection (e.g., primary tumor, regional nodes)

TABLE 51-5	American Joint Committee on Cancer TNM Staging System for Colorectal Cancer—cont'd	
STAGE	**FEATURES**
R1	Incomplete resection, margins histologically involved, microscopic tumor remains after resection of gross disease (primary tumor, regional nodes)
R2	Incomplete resection, margins macroscopically involved or gross disease remains after resection (e.g., primary tumor, regional nodes, or liver metastasis)

From Edge S, Byrd D, Compton C, et al, editors: *AJCC cancer staging manual*, ed 7, New York, 2010, Springer.

*This includes cancer cells confined within the glandular basement membrane (intraepithelial) or mucosal lamina propria (intramucosal), with no extension through the muscularis mucosae into the submucosa.

†Direct invasion in T4 includes invasion of other organs or other segments of the colorectum as a result of direct examination (e.g., invasion of the sigmoid colon by a carcinoma of the cecum) or, for cancers in a retroperitoneal or subperitoneal location, direct invasion of other organs or structures by extension beyond the muscularis propria (i.e., respectively, a tumor on the posterior wall of the descending colon invading the left kidney or lateral abdominal wall, or a mid or distal rectal cancer with invasion of prostate, seminal vesicles, cervix, or vagina).

‡Tumor that is adherent to other organs or structures, grossly, is classified as cT4b. However, if no tumor is present in the adhesion, microscopically, the classification should be pT1-4a, depending on the anatomic depth of wall invasion. The V and L classifications should be used to identify the presence or absence of vascular or lymphatic invasion, whereas the PN site-specific factor should be used for perineural invasion.

§Dukes B is a composite of better (T3 N0 M0) and worse (T4 N0 M0) prognostic groups, as is Dukes C (any T N1 M0 and any T N2 M0). MAC is the modified Astler-Coller classification.

involved lymph nodes are associated with a worsening prognosis, and the most recent classification system takes this into account.

The recent AJCC manual also recognizes prognostic factors in addition to serum carcinoembryonic antigen (CEA) levels that should be ascertained. These include the following: tumor deposits, the number of satellite tumor deposits discontinuous from the edge of the cancer that are not associated with a residual lymph node; a tumor regression grade that permits the pathologic response to neoadjuvant therapy to be graded; the circumferential resection margin, the distance from the edge of tumor to the nearest dissected margin of the surgical resection; microsatellite instability; perineural invasion, histologic cancerous invasion of the regional nerves; and *KRAS* mutation status. The *KRAS* mutation has been shown to be associated with lack of response to treatment with monoclonal antibodies directed against the epidermal growth factor receptor (EGFR) in patients with metastatic colorectal cancer.

Tumor regression grade. Although the data are not definitive, it appears that a significant pathologic response to preoperative adjuvant treatment is associated with a better prognosis. Patients with minimal or no residual disease after therapy may have a better prognosis than patients with extensive residual cancer. A four-point regression grade has been developed to assess the response to neoadjuvant therapy (Table 51-5).

Obstructing Colon Cancers

In patients with tumors causing complete obstruction, the diagnosis is best established by resection of the tumor without the benefit of preoperative colonoscopy and often without benefit of good staging. A water-soluble contrast enema is often useful in such circumstances to establish the anatomic level of the obstruction. Primary anastomosis between the proximal colon and the colon distal to the tumor has been avoided in the past in the presence of obstruction because of a high risk for anastomotic leak associated with this approach. Thus, such patients were usually treated by resection of the segment of colon containing the obstructing cancer, suture closure of the distal sigmoid or rectum,

and construction of a colostomy (Hartmann operation). Intestinal continuity could be reestablished later by taking down the colostomy and fashioning a colorectal anastomosis.

Alternatives to this approach have been to resect the segment of left colon containing the cancer and then to cleanse the remaining colon with saline lavage by inserting a catheter through the appendix or ileum into the cecum and irrigating the contents from the colon. A primary anastomosis between the prepared colon and rectum can then be fashioned without the need for a temporary colostomy. This can be done only in patients who are hemodynamically stable and have pliable, nonedematous, well-vascularized bowel. More recently, endoscopic techniques have been developed that permit the placement of a stent introduced with the aid of a colonoscope that traverses the obstructed tumor and expands, re-creating a lumen, relieving the obstruction, and permitting a bowel preparation and elective operation with primary colorectal anastomosis. This can be of temporary benefit, allowing the edema to resolve and the patient's bowel to be prepared. Stents can, however, be complicated by perforation and erosion and are used either in the palliative setting or as a short bridge to surgery. Complete obstruction of the right colon or cecum by cancer occurs less frequently because the stool is more liquid. These patients present with signs and symptoms of a small bowel obstruction. If an obstruction of the proximal colon is suspected, a water-soluble contrast study is useful to verify the diagnosis and to evaluate the distal colon for the presence of a synchronous lesion. Obstructing cancer of the proximal colon is treated by right colectomy, with primary anastomosis between the ileum and transverse colon, as long as the terminal ileum is viable, the patient is stable, and the bowel is minimally edematous. Otherwise, end ileostomy with long Hartmann or mucous fistula is required.

Patients with nonobstructing tumors should undergo a thorough evaluation for metastatic disease. This includes a thorough physical examination, chest radiograph, and measurement of the CEA level. CT or MRI to inspect the intra-abdominal cavity for metastases and to search for other intra-abdominal disease is an important aspect of preoperative staging. If possible, a colonoscopy should be done to evaluate the remainder of the colon and rectum, and additional disease should be ruled out. CT colonography (virtual colonoscopy) or contrast enema can be helpful if there are technical difficulties that precluded colonoscopy. Liver function tests are no longer required as they are neither sensitive nor specific for liver metastases. Complete blood count and electrolyte panels with blood urea nitrogen and creatinine measurement are required as well.

The objective of surgery for colon adenocarcinoma is the removal of the primary cancer with adequate margins, regional lymphadenectomy, and restoration of the continuity of the GI tract by anastomosis. The extent of resection is determined by the location of the cancer, its blood supply and draining lymphatic system, and the presence or absence of direct extension into adjacent organs. It is important to resect the lymphatics, which parallel the arterial supply, to the greatest extent possible in an attempt to render the abdomen free of lymphatic metastases. If hepatic metastases are subsequently detected, they may still be resected for cure in some cases if the abdominal disease has been completely eradicated.

To restore the continuity of the GI tract, an anastomosis is fashioned with sutures or staples, joining the ends of the intestine (small or large). It is important that both segments of the intestine used for the anastomosis have an excellent blood supply and that there is no tension on the anastomosis. For lesions involving the cecum, ascending colon, and hepatic flexure, a right hemicolectomy is the procedure of choice. This involves removal of the bowel from 4 to 6 cm proximal to the ileocecal valve to the portion of the transverse colon supplied by the right branch of the middle colic artery (Fig. 51-76). An anastomosis is fashioned

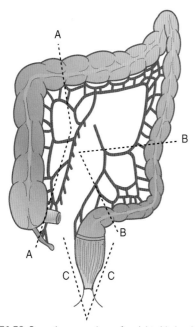

FIGURE 51-76 Operative procedures for right-sided colon cancer, sigmoid diverticulitis, and low-lying rectal cancer. Right hemicolectomy involves resection of a few centimeters of terminal ileum and colon up to the division of the middle colic vessels into right and left segments *(A)*. Sigmoidectomy consists of removal of the colon between the partially retroperitoneal descending colon and the rectum *(B)*. Abdominoperineal resection of the rectum is performed in a combined approach through the abdomen and through the perineum for the resection of the entire rectum and anus *(C)*.

between the terminal ileum and transverse colon. An extended right hemicolectomy is the procedure of choice for most transverse colon lesions; this involves division of the right and middle colic arteries at their origin, with removal of the right and transverse colon supplied by these vessels. The anastomosis is fashioned between the terminal ileum and proximal left colon. A left hemicolectomy (resection from the splenic flexure to the rectosigmoid junction) is the procedure of choice for tumors of the descending colon, whereas a sigmoidectomy is appropriate for tumors of the sigmoid colon. Most surgeons prefer to avoid incorporating the proximal sigmoid colon into an anastomosis because of the often tenuous blood supply from the IMA and frequent involvement of the sigmoid colon with diverticular disease.

Abdominal colectomy (sometimes called subtotal colectomy or total colectomy) entails removal of the entire colon from the ileum to the rectum, with continuity restored by an ileorectal anastomosis. Because of loss of the absorptive and storage capacity of the colon, this procedure causes an increase in stool frequency. Patients younger than 60 years generally tolerate this well, with gradual adaptation of the small bowel mucosa, increased water absorption, and an acceptable stool frequency of one to three movements daily. In older individuals, however, abdominal colectomy may result in significant chronic diarrhea. Abdominal colectomy is indicated for patients with multiple primary tumors, for individuals with HNPCC, and occasionally for those with completely obstructing sigmoid cancers.

Treatment and Follow-up

Although the prognosis can be refined by careful and accurate pathologic staging, patients treated with appropriate resection for stage I colon cancer generally have a 5-year survival rate of approximately 90%. The 5-year survival rate for patients with stage II colon cancer treated surgically is approximately 75%. The survival of patients with stage III disease, with lymph node metastasis, is approximately 50%; and patients with stage IV disease (distant metastases) have a poor prognosis, with a 5-year survival of less than 5%.

Further treatment and follow-up of patients treated by segmental colectomy for colon cancer is directed by the stage of the disease. Approximately 85% of recurrences are detected within 2 years of the time of resection, so the follow-up strategy should be especially intensive during that period.

A reasonable strategy to observe patients with stage I colon cancer is a colonoscopic examination 1 year after the operation to inspect the anastomosis but also to detect any new or missed polyps. The colonoscopy should be repeated annually if any polyps are detected and removed, until an examination reveals the absence of polyps. Then, a colonoscopy should be offered every 5 years unless a strong family history or other genetic risk factor is present, in which case more frequent endoscopic examinations are obviously indicated. A CEA level should be determined every 3 months during the first 2 years, even if the preoperative CEA level was normal. A rising CEA level requires further tests to search for metastatic disease, including a CT scan (or MRI) of the abdomen and chest and possibly a PET scan. The goal of close follow-up testing is to detect early recurrence that is amenable to treatment. Isolated hepatic or pulmonary metastases are amenable to resection, with a 5-year survival rate of 20%. Multiple or unresectable metastases may respond to current chemotherapeutic agents.

Postoperative treatment of patients with stage II colon cancer is somewhat controversial. To date, no large randomized trial has shown a benefit from adjuvant chemotherapy for this heterogeneous group of patients. An attempt to stratify patients may identify a subset that would benefit from chemotherapy. The 5-year survival rate of patients with stage IIA disease is 85%, compared with 72% for stage IIB disease, which is actually worse than for patients with node-positive stage IIIA disease. The American Society of Clinical Oncology suggests a course of 5-fluorouracil (5-FU)–based adjuvant chemotherapy for stage II patients with at least one poor prognostic indicator, including insufficient lymph node sampling (<12 nodes resected with the specimen), T4 lesions, poorly differentiated histology, or bowel perforation. Whether oxaliplatin-based regimens should be used in stage II disease in addition to 5-FU–leucovorin is controversial, but current practice in most areas appears to favor the addition of oxaliplatin in early-stage disease. Further follow-up of stage II patients includes a CEA level every 3 months for 2 years, then every 6 months for a total of 5 years, and annual CT scans of the abdomen and chest for at least the first 3 years.

Patients with stage III disease clearly benefit from adjuvant chemotherapy. The addition of oxaliplatin to the 5-FU–leucovorin regimen (FOLFOX) has resulted in an improvement of disease-free survival rates at 3 years to 78% (compared with 73% with 5-FU–leucovorin alone). Irinotecan (Camptosar) has been investigated as an addition to 5-FU–based therapy in the adjuvant setting on the basis of its benefit against metastatic disease. Unfortunately, irinotecan has not demonstrated efficacy in the adjuvant setting and is not currently used for the treatment of patients with stage III disease.

The method of delivery of chemotherapeutic agents is evolving. Continuous infusion of 5-FU is now generally considered to be superior to bolus infusions, with less toxicity. An oral fluoropyrimidine, capecitabine (Xeloda), has been shown to be at least equivalent to 5-FU.

The treatment of patients with stage IV disease depends on the location and extent of the metastases. In general, for asymptomatic patients with stage IV disease, a chemotherapy first approach is often used. It allows the patient to benefit immediately from systemic therapy without a waiting period for healing after surgery. Most patients with asymptomatic stage IV disease do not benefit from removal of the primary lesion. Removal is not associated with long-term benefits. However, there are many situations in which metastasectomy is associated with reasonable long-term survival, with approximately 15% to 24% of patients surviving at 5 years. Hepatic or pulmonary lesions may be amenable to resection, typically after three to six cycles of chemotherapy and then reimaging to determine response. Good responders with resectable disease may have survival rates approaching 25% at 5 years. Agents complementing the 5-FU regimens that remain the keystone of therapy are effective for metastatic disease and are being studied in the adjuvant setting. These are the monoclonal antibodies bevacizumab (Avastin), cetuximab (Erbitux), and panitumumab (Vectibix). Cetuximab is a chimeric (mouse-human) monoclonal antibody; panitumumab, a fully human monoclonal antibody, binds to and inhibits the EGFR, which is overexpressed in 60% to 80% of colorectal cancers and is associated with a shorter survival time. Cetuximab and panitumumab are effective only on tumors that do not have a mutation of the *KRAS* gene.[32] Accordingly, genetic testing is now recommended to confirm the absence of *KRAS* mutations (indicating the presence of the *KRAS* wild-type gene) before the use of these EGFR inhibitors is recommended. These agents have shown clinical efficacy in patients with metastatic colorectal cancer, both as monotherapy and in combination with irinotecan and FOLFOX. Bevacizumab, a vascular endothelial growth factor inhibitor, has also improved survival when added to regimens that include irinotecan, 5-FU–leucovorin, or oxaliplatin.

Rectal Cancer

Cancers arising in the distal 15 cm of the large bowel share many of the genetic, biologic, and morphologic characteristics of colon cancers. However, the unique anatomy of the rectum, with its retroperitoneal location in the narrow pelvis and proximity to the urogenital organs, autonomic nerves, and anal sphincters, makes surgical access relatively difficult. In addition, precise dissection in appropriate anatomic planes is essential because dissection medial to the endopelvic fascia investing the mesorectum may doom the patient to local recurrence of the disease, and dissection laterally to the avascular anatomic space risks injury to the mixed autonomic nerves, causing impotence in men and bladder dysfunction in men and women.

Furthermore, the biologic properties of the rectum, combined with its anatomic distance from the small intestine afforded by its retroperitoneal pelvic location, provide an opportunity for treatment by radiation therapy that is not feasible for colon tumors. The large bowel can tolerate properly delivered radiation doses up to 6000 cGy, whereas such levels of radiation targeted at colon tumors would include small bowel in the treatment field. The small bowel cannot withstand radiation doses of this level without complications of radiation enteritis, including stricture, hemorrhage, and perforation.

The treatment of rectal cancer has changed significantly during the past 25 years; there is considerable controversy concerning the precise role of surgery, radiation therapy, and chemotherapy and the ideal timing of each modality with relation to the others. Although information from clinical trials has provided data supporting the multimodality treatment of rectal cancer, the criteria for selection of patients remains controversial. However, some generalities can be made:

- Radiation therapy offers significant benefit to many patients with rectal cancer, and preoperative radiation is superior to postoperative radiation. Preoperative radiation (combined with chemotherapy) is used for locally advanced distal rectal cancers (within 10 to 15 cm of the anal verge, stage II or higher).
- Chemotherapy that has shown efficacy in the adjuvant setting in the treatment of colon cancer is also beneficial in the adjuvant setting for patients with rectal cancer. The combination of neoadjuvant (preoperative) radiation (usually 4500 to 5040 cGy) with infusional 5-FU–leucovorin, 5-FU alone, or capecitabine often results in dramatic reduction in tumor size (downstaging) and may result in apparently complete eradication of the tumor in up to 20% of cases.[33,34] Although interest has grown in use of chemoradiation as the sole treatment for patients who have demonstrated a complete clinical response to chemoradiation, the ability to predict which patients actually have a complete response has been shown to be difficult. At least one series has shown that a complete clinical response occurs in only 10% of patients treated with neoadjuvant chemoradiation. There is considerable interest in elucidating factors associated with complete eradication of rectal cancer by nonoperative treatment, and strategies and methods for predicting a complete clinical response have been attracting international interest.[33,35,36]
- The best course of neoadjuvant treatment is not clear, but there are regional preferences that may offer equivalent oncologic

outcomes. In Europe, the short course of radiation (25 Gy), followed by extirpative surgery (low anterior resection or abdominal perineal resection), is the most common approach.[37] In the United States, stage II or higher rectal cancers are more commonly treated with preoperative chemoradiation consisting of 4500 to 5040 cGy of radiation in conjunction with infusional 5-FU–based chemotherapy or oral capecitabine. The radiation is delivered during a period of 5 to 6 weeks, and surgery (low anterior resection or abdominal perineal resection, laparoscopic or open) is done 6 to 10 weeks after completion of the radiation therapy. A diverting stoma (ileostomy) is usually fashioned to protect the anastomosis, and the stoma is then closed 10 weeks later, when studies show satisfactory healing of the anastomosis.

- Neoadjuvant therapy is not a substitute for a properly performed surgical procedure. As discussed later, dissection in the proper plane is essential to achieve adequate margins and to remove the rectal lymphatics that may harbor metastases. A total mesorectal resection is appropriate for cancer of the mid and distal rectum, but the mesorectum can be divided below a cancer of the proximal rectum (>10 cm above the anus) to allow preservation of the distal rectum for the anastomosis. If a total mesorectal excision is performed and the anal sphincters are preserved, the anastomosis to establish continence will need to join the colon to the top of the anal canal.

The most common symptom of rectal cancer is hematochezia. Unfortunately, this is often attributed to benign anorectal disease, and the correct diagnosis is consequently delayed until the cancer has reached an advanced stage. Other symptoms include mucus discharge, tenesmus, and change in bowel habit.

The differential diagnosis of rectal cancer includes ulcerative colitis, Crohn's proctocolitis, radiation proctitis, and procidentia. On occasion, so-called hidden rectal prolapse or internal intussusception of the sigmoid into the rectum can produce a solitary rectal ulcer that mimics an ulcerating cancer. It is thought that the chronic trauma from the recurrent intussusception results in ulceration of the rectal mucosa. The mucosal trauma from intussusception can also form a polypoid lesion characterized by the presence of benign columnar epithelium and mucous cysts residing deep to the muscularis mucosae. This histologic pattern (colitis cystica profunda) can be confused with invasive adenocarcinoma, and it is obviously important to recognize this as a benign process.

The preoperative assessment of patients with rectal cancer is similar to that described for patients with colon cancer, with some significant differences—the requirement for precise characterization of the cancer with respect to the anal sphincters and the extent of invasion, as determined by depth of penetration into the bowel wall and spread to adjacent lymph nodes. A complete colonoscopic examination should be done to exclude synchronous tumors in the colon, but the precise location of the rectal tumor is best determined by examination with a rigid proctosigmoidoscope or flexible sigmoidoscopy. The depth of penetration can be estimated by digital rectal examination (superficially invasive tumors are mobile, whereas the lesions become tethered and fixed with increasing depth of penetration), and endorectal ultrasound or MRI can provide an accurate assessment of the extent of invasion of the bowel wall (Fig. 51-77).

Local Excision

Local excision of a rectal cancer may be appropriate for a small cancer in the distal rectum that has not penetrated into the

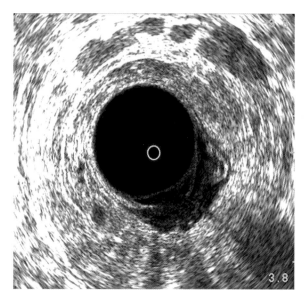

FIGURE 51-77 Endorectal ultrasound of patient with T3N1 rectal cancer. The cancer penetrates through all layers of the rectal wall, and an enlarged lymph node is clearly visible.

muscularis mucosa (T1N0). This is accomplished through a transanal approach and involves excision of the full thickness of the rectal wall underlying the tumor. Tumors located in the distal 3 to 5 cm of the rectum present the greatest challenge for the surgeon. Thorough and adequate assessment of tumors in this location is mandatory to select the proper treatment. If the tumor is confined to the submucosa (T1N0), excision by a transanal approach is an attractive option. In such circumstances, the incidence of lymphatic metastases is less than 8%, a factor that should be considered in contemplating the morbidity and functional loss that would be associated with an abdominal perineal resection.[38,39] Cancers in this location that invade or penetrate the muscular wall of the rectum have a high incidence of local recurrence after transanal excision (>20%), and consideration should be given to treatment that is more aggressive than local excision. The preferred course of treatment requires consideration of many factors, including the patient's overall health and preferences. However, T2N0 rectal cancers mandate a more aggressive approach than full-thickness local excision alone. Proctectomy with total mesorectal excision (abdominoperineal resection or low anterior resection) is the only strategy that ensures examination of the local lymph nodes and is associated with 5-year survival rates in excess of 95% for stage I T2N0 rectal cancers. This high cure rate needs to be balanced with the functional issues that arise postoperatively and the morbidity of the procedure. It is also acceptable to discuss and to offer full-thickness local excision with chemoradiation for small, good-risk T2N0 lesions. Recent evidence has suggested that this strategy offers results comparable to radical excision. Lesions that meet criteria for this option should be small (<3 cm), distal, and accessible and harbor no poor histopathologic features (poor differentiation, lymphoneural or perineural invasion).[40]

Local excision does not allow complete removal of lymph nodes in the mesorectum, so operative staging is limited. In addition, definitive treatment of early-stage rectal cancers by local excision has been shown to be associated with a threefold to fivefold higher recurrence rate compared with similar stage cancers treated by radical surgical resection before guidelines for specific selection criteria. Over time, the selection criteria have been refined to select only patients for this procedure who will have acceptable long-term outcomes. The operation is indicated for mobile tumors smaller than 3 cm in diameter that involve less than 30% of the rectal wall circumference and that are located in the distal rectum. These tumors should be stage T1 (limited to the submucosa), be well or moderately differentiated histologically, and have no vascular or lymphatic invasion. There should be no evidence of nodal disease on preoperative ultrasound or MRI. Adherence to these principles results in acceptable local recurrence rates compared with treatment by abdominal perineal resection. Local excision is also used for palliation of more advanced cancer in patients with severe comorbid disease, in whom extensive surgery carries a high risk for morbidity or mortality. Various technical approaches have been described to achieve transanal local excision, including use of a proctoscope equipped with a magnifying camera (transanal endoscopic microsurgery), but all approaches require complete excision of the cancer, with adequate margins of normal tissue. Although many surgeons suture the rectal defect closed after the local excision, this is not mandatory because the operative site is below the peritoneal reflection. Unfortunately, as experience has accumulated with this approach, it has become clear that close follow-up is mandatory in that approximately 8% of T1 lesions recur, and the recurrence rate for T2 lesions has been shown in some series to exceed 20%. As noted, most clinicians believe that local excision is not adequate treatment for a T2 rectal cancer and further treatment is required, adjuvant radiation plus chemotherapy or radical excision (low anterior resection or abdominal perineal resection; see earlier).

Transanal Endoscopic Microsurgery

Transanal endoscopic microsurgery is an approach for the local excision of favorable rectal tumors (T1 cancers and sessile polyps) through a device designed to provide access to the mid and proximal rectum. The endosurgical device is a large (4-cm-diameter) proctoscope through which four functions—carbon dioxide insufflation, water irrigation, suction, and monitoring of intrarectal pressure—are simultaneously regulated. The transanal microsurgery endoscope itself is closed and sealed, so that the rectum distends when carbon dioxide is insufflated into the system. This distention facilitates visualization afforded by binocular lenses attached to the system.

The endoscope is inserted through the anus and positioned to provide optimum visualization of and access to the tumor. Positioning of the endoscope is critical for success of the operation, and the patient must be placed in the proper position on the operating table to permit it to be adequately secured in a stable position. Long operating instruments are then inserted through ports in the system and used to excise the tumor under direct vision. The advantages of the technique include excellent exposure to tumors in a difficult area of access. The complications associated with the technique are the same as for standard transanal local excision—bleeding, urinary retention, perforation into the peritoneal cavity, and fecal soilage. The dilation of the anal sphincters by the large endoscope may be associated with subsequent fecal incontinence, but this appears to be a transient problem in most circumstances.

Fulguration

The technique of fulguration, which eradicates the cancer by using an electrocautery device that destroys the tumor by creating a full-thickness eschar at the tumor site, requires extension of the

eschar into the perirectal fat, thus destroying both the tumor and rectal wall. The procedure can be used only for lesions below the peritoneal reflection. Complications associated with this approach are postoperative fever and significant bleeding, which can occur as late as 10 days after the operation. Obviously, this technique cannot provide a specimen to assess the pathologic stage because the tumor and margins are disintegrated by fulguration. The procedure is reserved for patients with a prohibitive operative risk and limited life expectancy; it has largely been replaced by transanal excision, which provides the advantage of examination and more adequate staging of the specimen. Better anesthesia techniques and supportive patient care have rendered this technique virtually obsolete.

Abdominal Perineal Resection

Complete excision of the rectum and anus, by concomitant dissection through the abdomen and perineum, with suture closure of the perineum and creation of a permanent colostomy, was first described by Ernest Miles and is thus sometimes referred to as the Miles procedure. The rectum and sigmoid colon are mobilized through an abdominal incision. The pelvic dissection, done through the abdominal incision, mobilizes the mesorectum in continuity with the tumor-bearing rectum. The pelvic dissection is carried to the level of the levator ani muscles. The perineal portion of the operation excises the anus, anal sphincters, and distal rectum. Although there are different approaches to performing this operation, recent experience has shown that positioning the patient in the prone position for the perineal excision permits a more cylindrical specimen (wider margins of normal tissue) to be obtained, with a reduction in positive circumferential margins, which should reduce the incidence of local recurrence.[41] An abdominal perineal resection is indicated when the tumor involves the anal sphincters or is too close to the sphincters for adequate margins to be obtained and in patients in whom sphincter-preserving surgery is not possible because of unfavorable body habitus or poor preoperative sphincter control. A well-fashioned colostomy will often provide a superior quality of life to coloanal anastomosis in an older patient or in a patient who is preoperatively fecally incontinent.

Low Anterior Resection

Resection of the rectum through an abdominal approach offers the advantage of removing the portion of bowel containing the cancer and the mesorectum completely, which contains the lymphatic channels that drain the tumor bed. The term *anterior resection* (an abbreviation for the more correct term, *anterior proctosigmoidectomy with colorectal anastomosis*) indicates resection of the proximal rectum or rectosigmoid above the peritoneal reflection. The term *low anterior resection* indicates that the operation entails resection of the rectum below the peritoneal reflection through an abdominal approach. The sigmoid colon is almost always included with the resected specimen because diverticulosis often involves the sigmoid, and the blood supply to the sigmoid is often not adequate to sustain an anastomosis if the IMA is transected. For cancers involving the lower half of the rectum, the entire mesorectum, which contains the lymph channels draining the tumor bed, should be excised in continuity with the rectum. This technique, total mesorectal excision, produces the complete resection of an intact package of the rectum and its adjacent mesorectum, enveloped within the visceral pelvic fascia with uninvolved circumferential margins. The use of the technique of total mesorectal excision has resulted in a significant increase in 5-year survival rates (50% to 75%), a decrease in local recurrence rates (30% to 5%), and a decrease in the incidence of impotence and bladder dysfunction (85% to <15%).[42]

Intestinal continuity is reestablished by fashioning an anastomosis between the descending colon and rectum, which has been greatly facilitated by the introduction of the circular stapling device. After the colorectal anastomosis has been completed, it should be inspected with a proctoscope inserted through the anus. If there is concern about the integrity of the anastomosis or if the patient has received high-dose preoperative chemoradiation, a temporary proximal ileostomy should be made to permit complete healing of the anastomosis.[43] The stoma can be closed in approximately 10 weeks if proctoscopy and contrast studies verify the integrity of the anastomosis.

An end-to-end anastomosis between the descending colon and distal rectum or anus may result in significant alteration of bowel habits attributed to the loss of the normal rectal capacity (Fig. 51-78). Patients treated with this operation often experience frequent small bowel movements (low anterior resection syndrome or clustering). This problem can be partially addressed by fashioning a colonic J pouch as the proximal component of the anastomosis (Fig. 51-79). As experience has accumulated with this approach, it appears that improvement in bowel function is significant for cancers located in the distal rectum, but if the anastomosis is created above 9 cm from the anal verge, there is little benefit of a J pouch compared with an end-to-end anastomosis. The limbs of the J pouch should be relatively short (6 cm) because patients with larger pouches have a significant incidence of difficulty with evacuation. It is generally thought to be preferable to avoid using the sigmoid colon as the proximal component of a

colorectal anastomosis because the blood supply to the sigmoid from the IMA may be tenuous, and the presence of diverticular disease, common in the sigmoid colon, is often considered to be a risk factor for anastomotic leak. In obese patients and in patients with a narrow pelvis, it may not be technically feasible to fashion a J pouch as the proximal component of the low pelvic anastomosis because the bulk of the pouch simply will not fit into the narrow pelvis. In such cases, a reservoir can be devised with a coloplasty.[44,45] This technique provides a rectal reservoir by making an 8- to 10-cm colotomy 4 to 6 cm from the divided end of the colon. The colotomy is closed transversely to provide increased rectal space and capacitance (Figs. 51-80 and 51-81).

Sphincter-Sparing Abdominal Perineal Resection With Coloanal Anastomosis

Abdominal perineal resection is required when a cancer in the distal rectum cannot be resected with adequate margins while preserving the anal sphincter. However, the use of preoperative radiation and chemotherapy has been shown, in some cases, to shrink the tumor to an extent that acceptable margins can be achieved.[46] If the anal sphincters do not need to be sacrificed to achieve adequate margins based on oncologic principles, a permanent stoma may be avoided with a sphincter-sparing abdominal perineal resection, with an anastomosis between the colon and anal canal. This procedure has particular application for young patients with rectal tumors who have a favorable body habitus and good preoperative sphincter function. The operation can be conducted in a variety of ways, but all methods involve mobilizing the sigmoid colon and pelvic rectum through an abdominal approach, dissecting the rectal mucosa from the anal sphincters

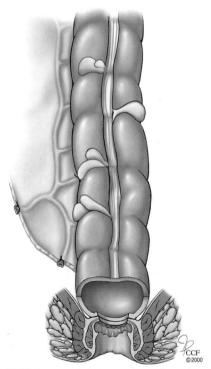

FIGURE 51-78 Anastomosis between descending colon and anus, following complete resection of the rectum. The absence of the rectum often results in frequent small bowel movements, a phenomenon known as clustering or low anterior resection syndrome. (Courtesy Cleveland Clinic Foundation, Cleveland, 2000.)

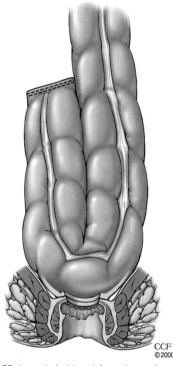

FIGURE 51-79 J pouch fashioned from descending colon to form proximal portion of coloanal anastomosis. This increases its capacitance to decrease the frequency of bowel movements. (Courtesy Cleveland Clinic Foundation, Cleveland, 2000.)

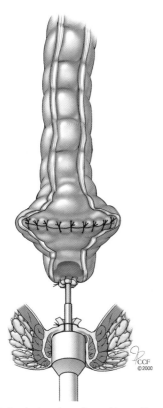

FIGURE 51-80 A coloplasty is performed by making an 8- to 10-cm colotomy 4 to 6 cm from the cut end of the colon. The longitudinal colotomy is made between the taeniae on the antimesenteric side. It is closed transversely with absorbable sutures. An end-to-end stapled anastomosis then joins the colon to the distal rectum or anus. (Courtesy Cleveland Clinic Foundation, Cleveland, 2000.)

at the level of the dentate line, and completing the resection of the most distal rectum through the anal approach. An anastomosis is then fashioned between the descending colon and anus, often using a J pouch or coloplasty procedure described earlier for the low colorectal anastomosis. The anastomosis is made with sutures placed through a transanal approach by the surgeon in the perineal field. Low anterior resection syndrome describes a functional disorder created by removal of the rectum and fashioning of a coloanal anastomosis. It can occur no matter how the anastomosis is constructed, and a patient facing rectal cancer surgery with a consideration for sphincter preservation must be made aware of this as it can seriously and adversely affect quality of life.[42,47]

PELVIC FLOOR DISORDERS AND CONSTIPATION

Disorders of the pelvic floor can be classified as primarily colorectal, urologic, or gynecologic. Often, problems requiring the attention of multiple specialists present in a synchronous fashion, a condition known as complex prolapse. Rectal prolapse (procidentia), enterocele, rectocele, and functional disorders of the muscles of the pelvic floor (anismus, levator spasm) are among the pelvic floor disorders treated by surgeons. A functional disorder is defined by the concurrent presence of normal anatomy and abnormal function. Surgeons are often consulted concerning functional disorders of the large bowel or pelvic floor. These problems do not

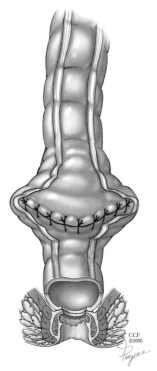

FIGURE 51-81 The completed stapled coloplasty with anastomosis. (Courtesy Cleveland Clinic Foundation, Cleveland, 2000.)

usually require operative intervention; in fact, the surgical literature is replete with examples of failed operations to correct these problems. However, the signs and symptoms of these disorders mimic surgical diseases and require proper recognition and treatment. Although chronic constipation is often considered an example of a functional problem, surgery is a consideration for some patients who fail to respond to medical management. The surgical evaluation and management of these disorders is discussed in this section.

Diagnosis: Testing and Evaluation
Anorectal Physiology Laboratory Testing
Anorectal physiology testing refers to the systematic evaluation of anal canal resting and squeeze pressures, anal reflexes, pudendal nerve conduction velocities, and electromyographic muscle fiber recruitment. Measurement of anal canal pressures (manometry) involves the use of water-filled balloons attached to catheters and transducers placed in the anal canal. The measurement of resting and squeeze pressures at various points in the anal canal reflects the strength, tone, and function of the internal and external sphincter. Normal resting and squeeze values are 40 to 80 mm Hg. Resting pressure reflects the function of the internal sphincter, whereas squeeze pressure measures external sphincter (voluntary muscle) contributions. Measurement of anal canal pressures is useful in the evaluation of conditions ranging from incontinence to obstructive defecation. Electromyographic recruitment refers to the motor unit potential of the puborectalis muscle and is compared for rest, squeeze, and push (simulated defecation). An increase in the recruitment of fibers during straining is pathognomonic for the syndrome of paradoxical puborectalis, or inappropriate puborectalis contraction. Pudendal nerve terminal motor latency times are measured with a special transducer attached to

a glove-like apparatus designed to be worn on the finger and hand. A digital rectal examination is required, with application of the finger electrode to the right and left levator ani complex. Values between 1.8 and 2.2 milliseconds are normal. Prolonged values are seen in traumatic injuries of the vagina or anal canal (obstetric in cause), sacral nerve root damage, or chronic diseases such as diabetes.

Defecography

Defecography is an extremely useful modality for determining the precise nature of various pelvic floor abnormalities. Barium paste is placed in the vagina and rectum after the patient ingests a water-soluble contrast agent to opacify the small bowel. As the patient evacuates the rectal barium paste, abnormalities occurring during the act of defecation can be recorded with fluoroscopic videotaping. A vast amount of functional and anatomic information can be gathered from this test. The presence of multiple anatomic abnormalities, such as rectocele, enterocele, and vaginal vault prolapse, can be efficiently evaluated. Functional problems such as paradoxical puborectalis syndrome have characteristic defecographic patterns and can be evaluated in this way. Many contributing anatomic problems can be readily identified.

Rectal Prolapse (Procidentia)
Causes and Symptoms

Most information about how patients develop rectal prolapse is based on observation of the clinical characteristics of those suffering from this problem. The condition was documented in the Hippocratic Corpus, and since then, descriptions of causes and rectifying procedures have been numerous. However, two competing theories of rectal prolapse did evolve. In 1912, Alexis Moschcowitz proposed that a rectal prolapse was caused by a sliding herniation of the pouch of Douglas through the pelvic floor fascia into the anterior aspect of the rectum. His theory was based on the fact that the pelvic floor of prolapse patients is mobile and unsupported and on the observation that other adjacent structures can occasionally be seen alongside the rectal component of the prolapse. With the advent of defecography in 1968, however, Broden and Snellman were able to show convincingly that procidentia is basically a full-thickness rectal intussusception starting approximately 3 inches above the dentate line and extending beyond the anal verge. Both explanations take into consideration the weakness of the pelvic floor in rectal prolapse cases, the concept of herniation, and the observation that there are abnormal anatomic features that characterize this condition.

Women aged 50 years and older are six times as likely as men to present with rectal prolapse. The peak age of incidence is the seventh decade in women, whereas the relatively few men afflicted with the syndrome may develop prolapse at the age of 40 years or younger. One striking characteristic of young male patients is their tendency to have psychiatric disorders, and many are institutionalized. Young male patients with procidentia also tend to take constipating medications and report significant symptoms related to bowel function.

Anatomy and Pathophysiology

Patients with prolapse are frequently found to have specific anatomic characteristics. Diastasis of the levator ani, abnormally deep cul-de-sac, redundant sigmoid colon, patulous anal sphincter, and loss of the rectal sacral attachments are commonly described.

Large case reviews aimed at elucidating other predisposing factors have supported several observations. Chronic or lifelong

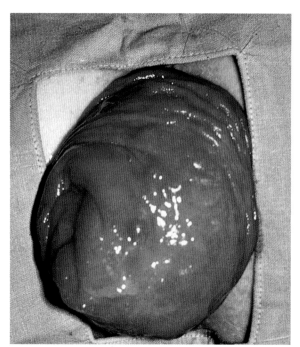

FIGURE 51-82 Procidentia, or rectal prolapse. The entire rectum has protruded through the anal canal.

constipation with a component of straining is present in more than 50% of patients, and 15% experience diarrhea. Contrary to the common assumption that rectal prolapse is a consequence of multiparity, 35% of patients with rectal prolapse are nulliparous. Once a prolapse is apparent, fecal incontinence becomes a predominant symptomatic feature, occurring in 50% to 75% of cases. Proximal bilateral pudendal neuropathy is present in incontinent prolapse patients and is responsible for denervation atrophy of the external sphincter musculature. This finding is absent in normal controls. It is speculated that pudendal nerve damage is responsible for pelvic floor and anal sphincter weakening and may be the underlying cause of a spectrum of pelvic floor disorders. Pudendal nerve damage can result from direct trauma (e.g., obstetric injury), chronic diseases (e.g., diabetes), and neoplastic processes causing sacral nerve root damage.

Symptoms of prolapse progress as the prolapse develops. Often, the prolapse initially comes down with defecation or straining, only to reduce spontaneously afterward. Patients describe a mass or large lump that they may have to push back in after defecation (Fig. 51-82). The presenting complaint may be the concurrent fecal incontinence that results from the prolapse or a sensation of chronic moisture and mucous drainage in the perineal area. Minimal or spontaneously reducible prolapses may progress to a chronically prolapsed rectum, requiring digital reduction. Chronically prolapsed rectal mucosa may become thickened or ulcerated and cause significant bleeding. On occasion, the presentation of rectal prolapse can be dramatic when the prolapsed segment becomes incarcerated below the level of the anal sphincter. Emergent operative therapy is indicated in this situation.

Differential Diagnosis and Investigation

A common pitfall in the diagnosis of rectal prolapse is the potential for confusion with prolapsed incarcerated internal hemorrhoids. These conditions may be distinguished by close inspection of the direction of the prolapsed tissue folds. In the case of rectal prolapse, the folds are always concentric, whereas hemorrhoidal tissue develops radial invaginations defining the hemorrhoidal cushions. Prolapsed incarcerated hemorrhoids produce extreme pain and can be accompanied by fever and urinary retention. Unless it is incarcerated, rectal prolapse is easily reducible and painless.

Before operative intervention, a careful history, physical examination, and colonoscopy should be performed. Of patients with rectal prolapse, 35% complain of urinary incontinence and another 15% have a significant vaginal vault prolapse. These symptoms will require evaluation and potential multidisciplinary surgical intervention.

If the diagnosis is suspected from the history but not detected on physical examination, confirmation can be obtained by asking the patient to produce the prolapse by straining while on a toilet. Inspection of the perineum with the patient in the sitting or squatting position is helpful for this purpose. In the event that the prolapse is still elusive, defecography (see earlier) may reveal the problem.

Although uncommon, a neoplasm may form the lead point for a rectal intussusception. For this reason, and because this age group has the highest incidence of colorectal neoplasia, colonoscopy or barium enema should precede an operation. A significant finding on colonoscopic inspection may change the operative approach.

Anal manometry and pudendal nerve terminal motor latency tests can be ordered preoperatively to evaluate symptoms of incontinence further. However, these test results rarely change the operative strategy. A finding of increased nerve conduction periods (nerve damage) may have postoperative prognostic significance for continence, although more studies are required to confirm this. Patients with evidence of nerve damage may have a higher rate of incontinence after surgical correction of the prolapse. Decreased anal squeeze or resting pressures are expected with this condition and may predate the actual development of the prolapse. Routine manometric studies for obvious prolapse are usually not done.

Operative Repair

The number of procedures described in the literature, historically and in recent times, is breathtaking. More than 50 types of repair have been documented, most of historical interest only. Approaches have generally included anal encirclement, mucosal resection, perineal proctosigmoidectomy, anterior resection with or without rectopexy, rectopexy alone, and a host of procedures involving the use of synthetic mesh affixed to the presacral fascia. The apparent enthusiasm and ingenuity of surgeons in their quest to define the ideal prolapse operation serve only to highlight its elusiveness. Two predominant approaches, abdominal and perineal, are considered in the operative repair of rectal prolapse. The surgical approach is dictated by the comorbidities of the patient, the surgeon's preference and experience, and the patient's age. It is generally believed that the perineal approach results in less perioperative morbidity and pain and a reduced length of hospital stay. These advantages have, until relatively recently, been considered to be offset by a higher recurrence rate, but data are unclear on this point, however, and a properly executed perineal operation may yield the same good long-term results as an abdominal procedure. This point will be clarified by ongoing long-term studies. All of the abdominal operations for prolapse can be performed laparoscopically. Data suggest that the surgical approach (laparoscopic versus open) does not influence the recurrence rates in experienced hands.

Abdominal approaches

Ripstein repair and anterior mesh repairs. The Ripstein repair involves placement of a prosthetic mesh around the mobilized rectum, with attachment of the mesh to the presacral fascia below the sacral promontory. Recurrence rates for this procedure range from 2.3% to 5%. The bowel is mechanically prepared for this procedure with a polyethylene glycol or sodium phosphate solution. The procedure involves mobilizing the rectum on both sides and posteriorly down to the levator ani muscle plate. Recent data suggest that mobilizing anteriorly down to the levators as well helps reduce rates of anterior prolapse even further. Division of the upper portion of the lateral rectal ligaments has been described, but some advocate leaving them wholly intact because the rates of postoperative constipation are 50% higher in patients with divided lateral stalks. After mobilization of the rectum, a 5-cm band of rectangular mesh is placed around its anterior aspect at the level of the peritoneal reflection, and both sides of the mesh are sutured with nonabsorbable suture to the presacral fascia, approximately 1 cm from the midline. Sutures are used to secure the mesh to the rectum anteriorly, and the rectum is pulled upward and posteriorly. Various materials have been recommended to secure the rectum, including autologous fascia lata, synthetic nonabsorbable products such as Marlex (Chevron Phillips Chemical, The Woodlands, Tex), Teflon (DuPont, Wilmington, Del), and absorbable prosthetics such as polyglycolic acid. The recurrence rates for all these materials are less than 10%, although follow-up times and evaluation criteria among studies have varied and strict comparisons cannot be made. Complications include large bowel obstruction, erosion of the mesh through the bowel, ureteric injury or fibrosis, small bowel obstruction, rectovaginal fistula, and fecal impaction. Postoperative morbidity rates are 20%, but most of these complications are minor. Although mesh rectopexy results in significant improvement in fecal incontinence (50%), no rectal prolapse operation should be advocated as a procedure to restore continence, and patients, especially those with prolapse for longer than 2 years, should be warned of the possibility that incontinence could persist.

A significant complication of this operation is the incidence of new-onset or worsened constipation. Fifteen percent of patients experience constipation for the first time after Ripstein rectopexy, and at least 50% of those who are constipated preoperatively are made worse. Although some of these difficulties are attributed to complications of the procedure, such as mesh stricture, obstruction at the level of the repair, or rectal dysfunction after lateral stalk division, a subset of patients will be found to have slow-transit constipation characterizing a global motility disorder. Some advocate routine preoperative transit studies to select these patients out, but a good bowel habit history will usually suffice. The cause of any severe, unremitting postoperative defecation or obstruction problem should be investigated with a barium enema and perhaps with a small bowel study. Strictures, obstructions, adhesions, and fistulas may be identified by radiography.

Fiber, fluids, and stool softeners are useful in the management of functional constipation after rectal prolapse repairs of any type. On occasion, mild laxatives such as milk of magnesia, magnesium citrate, or polyethylene glycol–based therapies may be necessary for short periods. Newer treatments for constipation involve oral administration of 5-HT$_4$ receptor agonists (e.g., tegaserod maleate) and may prove invaluable in the short-term treatment of this problem.

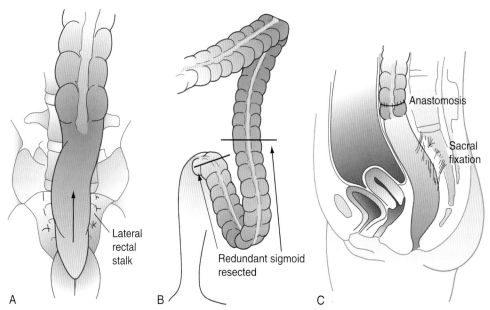

FIGURE 51-83 Anterior resection with rectopexy, or the Frykman-Goldberg procedure, for rectal prolapse. **A,** After full mobilization by sharp dissection, the tissues lateral to the rectal wall are swept away laterally. **B,** Resection of the redundant sigmoid colon. **C,** Anastomosis is completed, and rectopexy sutures are placed. (From Gordon PH, Nivatvongs S, editors: *Principles and practice of surgery for the colon, rectum and anus,* ed 2, St Louis, 1999, Quality Medical Publishing.)

Resection rectopexy. Resection rectopexy is a technique first described by Frykman and Goldberg in 1969 and popularized in the United States in the past 35 years (Fig. 51-83). Lack of artificial mesh, ease of operation, and reduction of redundant sigmoid colon are the principle advantages of the procedure. Recurrence rates are low, ranging from 2% to 5%, and major complication rates range from 0% to 20% and relate to obstruction or anastomotic leak. Basically, the sigmoid colon and rectum are mobilized to the level of the levators. The lateral ligaments are divided, elevated from the deep pelvis, and sutured to the presacral fascia. Again, as in anterior mesh repairs, anterior mobilization has gotten renewed interest because of the observed lower incidence of recurrence with this technique. The mesentery of the sigmoid colon is then divided, with preservation of the IMA, and a tension-free anastomosis is created. A revised version of this procedure involves preservation of the lateral stalks and unilateral fastening of the rectal mesentery to the sacrum at the level of the sacral promontory. Sigmoid resection is a unique feature of this procedure. It appears to reduce constipation by 50% in those who complain preoperatively of this symptom in some studies. Interestingly, in patients who complain of incontinence before surgery, this symptom consistently improves in approximately 35%, even with the sigmoid resection. A variant of this procedure involves forgoing the sigmoid resection in those who report no history of constipation and whose predominant complaint is fecal incontinence and doing the mobilization and rectopexy alone.

Perineal approaches

Perineal proctosigmoidectomy and the Altemeier procedure. Perineal proctosigmoidectomy was first introduced by Mikulicz in 1899 and remained the favored treatment for prolapse in Europe for many years. Miles advocated this procedure in the United Kingdom, and it was promoted in the United States by Altemeier at the University of Cincinnati. As the abdominal approaches gained favor, principally because of the reduced recurrence rates, the perineal approach was increasingly reserved only for those with the highest operative risk. However, renewed interest in the technique has accompanied studies showing reduced recurrence rates, and a number of surgeons believe that strong consideration should be given to this technique in repairing prolapse in young men who have an increased risk for autonomic nerve injury resulting in impotence.

The Altemeier procedure combines a perineal proctosigmoidectomy with an anterior levatorplasty (Fig. 51-84). The latter procedure is performed to correct the levator diastasis commonly associated with this condition. Theoretically, restoration of fecal continence is enhanced by this additional maneuver. As always, the large bowel is mechanically cleansed. The patient is placed in the prone jackknife position, and a Foley catheter is placed. The rectal mucosa is serially grasped with Babcock or Allis clamps until a full-thickness prolapse is demonstrated. A full-thickness circumferential incision is made 1.5 cm proximal to the dentate line. The low peritoneal reflection can usually be incised anteriorly and the peritoneal cavity entered. The mesentery of the rectum and sigmoid colon is sequentially clamped and tied until no redundant bowel remains. The colon is transected at this point, and an anastomosis is fashioned between the colon and anal canal with sutures or staples.

Patients undergoing perineal proctosigmoidectomy are generally older and have significantly more comorbidities than those who are considered for abdominal repair. Complication rates are less than 10%, and recurrence rates have been reported as high as 16%, although, as mentioned, some series have demonstrated significantly lower recurrence rates. Complications include bleeding from the staple or suture line, pelvic abscess, and, rarely, dehiscence of the suture line, with perineal evisceration. Lack of an abdominal incision, reduced pain, and reduced length of hospitalization make this procedure an attractive option.

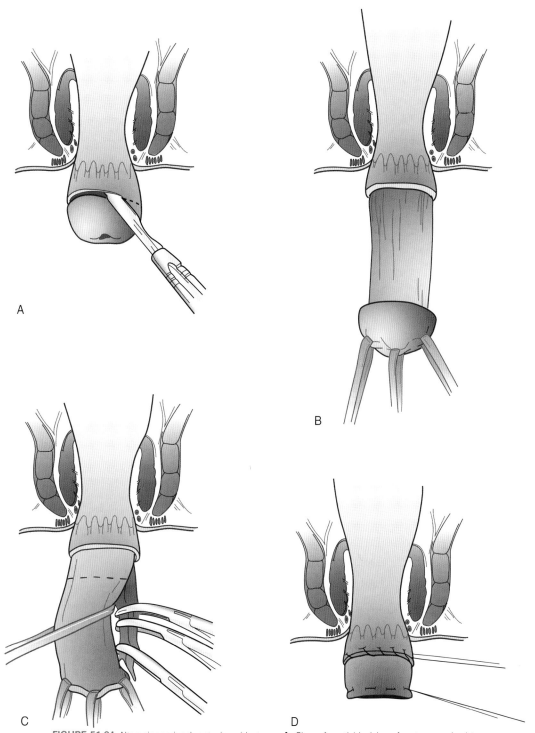

A

B

C

D

FIGURE 51-84 Altemeier perineal rectosigmoidectomy. **A,** Circumferential incision of rectum proximal to dentate line. **B,** Delivery of redundant rectum and sigmoid colon. **C,** Ligation of blood supply to rectum. **D,** Placement of purse-string suture on proximal bowels and excision of redundant colon and rectum; whip stitch placed on rectal stump. *Continued*

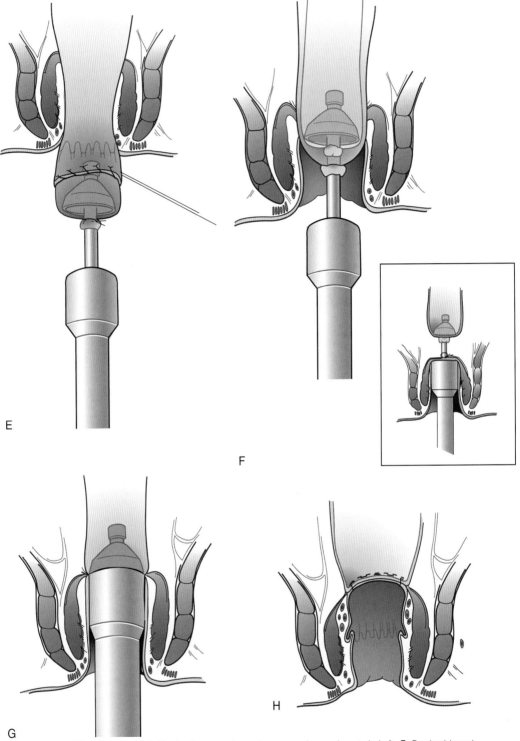

E

F

G

H

FIGURE 51-84, cont'd **E,** Proximal purse-string suture secured around central shaft. **F,** Proximal bowel advanced through anus and distal purse-string tied. **G,** Approximation of anvil to cartridge and activation of stapler. **H,** Completed anastomosis. (From Gordon PH, Nivatvongs S, editors: *Principles and practice of surgery for the colon, rectum and anus*, ed 2, St Louis, 1999, Quality Medical Publishing.)

Anal encirclement. Anal encirclement is one of the oldest surgical techniques for rectal prolapse described. Thiersch described silver wire anal encirclement in 1891. Since then, it has been tried with a wide variety of materials, including stainless steel wire, nonabsorbable mesh, small Silastic bands, nylon suture, and polypropylene. Anal encirclement does not correct the fecal incontinence associated with prolapse, and the recurrence rate is high (>30%), as is the morbidity. Erosion of the wire into the sphincter, anovaginal fistula formation, rectal prolapse incarceration, fecal impaction, and infection can occur. Reoperative rates of 7% to 59% have been reported. The safety of current anesthetic techniques and the low morbidity and relative functional success of perineal proctectomy have made anal encirclement, for the most part, a procedure of the past.

Internal Prolapse and Solitary Rectal Ulcer Syndrome

Two areas of controversy related to rectal prolapse involve the treatment of solitary rectal ulcer syndrome (SRUS) and internal intussusception of the rectal mucosa. Although identified as an ulcer, the gross pathologic features of SRUS can range from a typical crater-like ulcer with a fibrinous central depression to a polypoid lesion. It is always located on the anterior aspect of the rectum, 4 to 12 cm from the anal verge, and is thought to correspond to the location of the puborectalis sling. It is frequently although not exclusively associated with internal intussusception or full-thickness rectal prolapse. Patients are typically young and female, however, with an average age of 25 years and a history of straining and difficult evacuation.

The rectal ulcer is usually found on proctoscopy or flexible sigmoidoscopy and commonly is manifested with rectal bleeding in the setting of straining or constipation. The cause of SRUS remains somewhat unclear, but speculation centers on chronic ischemia. The fold with the ulcer is thought to form the lead point of an intussusception into the anal canal. Chronic, repeated straining or prolapse of this lead point produces ischemia, tissue

breakdown, and ulceration. Possible digital self-disimpaction may also be a contributing factor. Histology reveals a thick layer of fibrosis obliterating the lamina propria and a central fibrinous exudate. Other common pathologic findings include the presence of mucus-filled glands misplaced in the submucosa and lined with normal colonic epithelium (colitis cystica profunda). Differentiating SRUS from malignant disease, infection, or Crohn's disease is important but not difficult. The anterior location in the context of classic symptoms and pathologic findings is conclusive.

Defecography is the radiologic procedure of choice for diagnostic evaluation and usually reveals the underlying disorder. Full-thickness rectal prolapse, internal prolapse, paradoxical puborectalis syndrome (failure of relaxation of the pelvic floor musculature on straining), and thickened rectal folds are common findings.

Data regarding the treatment of this unusual disorder are retrospective, and studies have been small, but several common observations have been made. In general, one third of patients with SRUS also suffer from full-thickness rectal prolapse. Abdominal prolapse repairs have resulted in a cure rate of 80% in patients with SRUS and full-thickness rectal prolapse. In the same study, patients treated with the same procedure for mucosal prolapse and SRUS fared far worse; only 25% of patients responded to operative intervention. In most studies, dietary management, pelvic floor retraining (biofeedback), and short-term use of topical anti-inflammatory medications containing mesalamine result in remission for those with internal prolapse or pelvic muscle dysfunction. Prompt diagnosis of the underlying problem and appropriate treatment can be difficult but are the keys to cure. Local excision usually results in a larger nonhealing wound and has no role in management. Rarely, symptoms of severe bleeding, pain, and spasm may require a temporary diverting sigmoid colostomy.

Internal intussusception was first described in the late 1960s, when defecography was first developed and came into widespread use. The condition is also called internal or hidden prolapse and is confined to the rectal mucosa and submucosa, which separates

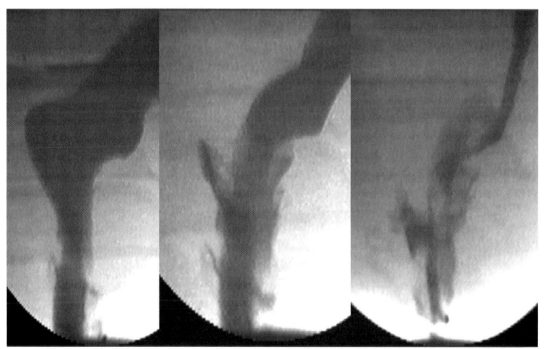

FIGURE 51-85 Defecogram showing progression of internal intussusception.

from the muscularis mucosae layer and slides down the anal canal (Fig. 51-85). Internal intussusception can be identified in a significant proportion of the asymptomatic population and appears to represent a normal variant. However, there are advocates of internal prolapse repair when it is found in patients who complain of dysfunctional defecation. The transanal Delorme mucosal resection procedure involves circumferential removal of redundant anal canal and distal rectal mucosa and imbrication of the muscularis layer with serial vertical sutures. Although satisfactory results were reported for this procedure in the 1990s, experience has been discouraging, and enthusiasm for the procedure has waned.

Abdominal repairs such as the Ripstein procedure have also been advocated as an alternative for symptomatic patients. Unfortunately, the results of these studies are not conclusive. Of patients who underwent repair by an abdominal approach, only 24% to 38% reported improvement, whereas a significant number experienced worsening. As for patients with SRUS, the treatment of patients with incomplete or obstructed defecation should be initially evaluated with defecography. Studies have not supported operative intervention for these disorders when internal intussusception alone is present.

Rectocele

A rectocele is an abnormal sac-like projection of the anterior rectum that extends from the distal rectum to the distal anal canal. It usually begins just above the sphincter complex (Figs. 51-86 and 51-87). The cause of rectoceles is multifactorial. Stretching of the endopelvic fascia from antecedent pelvic floor injury, followed by chronic increased intra-abdominal pressure, causes an anterior full-thickness herniation of the rectum into the vagina. Rectal pressures are higher than those in the vagina; therefore, pressure tends to push the rectum anteriorly and stretch and shift the rectovaginal septum as well. The major symptom of rectocele is stool trapping, a form of obstructed defecation. Women commonly describe requiring vaginal pressure to reduce the bulge, effectively stenting the anterior rectum and enabling defecation.

Criteria for operative intervention include symptomatic stool trapping requiring digital evacuation or vaginal support and the presence of large protruding rectoceles that push vaginal mucosa beyond the introitus, producing dryness, ulceration, and discomfort. Although small rectoceles are common, it is rare that a rectocele smaller than 2 cm is symptomatic.

There are two major operative approaches to rectoceles, transanal and transvaginal. Although the transvaginal approach has been criticized by surgeons because the repair is done on the low-pressure side of the rectovaginal septum, it does have certain distinct advantages. The bowel is fully prepared and the patient is placed in the lithotomy position. After the submucosal injection of lidocaine with 1% epinephrine, a swath of vagina is excised, starting at the vaginal introitus and carried to the apex of the vagina. The size of this segment is determined by the depth of the rectocele. The goal is to excise a full-thickness segment of vagina, to dissect out and to reduce an enterocele if one is found in the rectovaginal septum, and then to obliterate the deep cul-de-sac by suturing the cut edges of the vagina closed, allowing the space to contract by fibrosis.

Alternatively, several approaches for the transanal correction of rectocele have been described. This technique was probably best described by Sullivan, who expected 80% of patients to have good to excellent results. An incision is made longitudinally in the rectum over the bulge above the sphincters. The incision's length varies with the size of the rectocele. The underlying vagina is exposed and imbricated to obliterate the sac, and the rectum is separately imbricated and closed over that with absorbable sutures. Unfortunately, direct comparisons in the literature between these techniques are absent. However, the largely unsubstantiated argument has been made by surgeons that a repair based in the high-pressure or rectal side of the bulge may reduce recurrence. No matter the technique, patient selection and follow-up are crucial. In one study, only 54% of patients who underwent rectocele repair obtained relief from their symptoms of obstructive defecation. Paradoxical puborectalis syndrome was not ruled out and

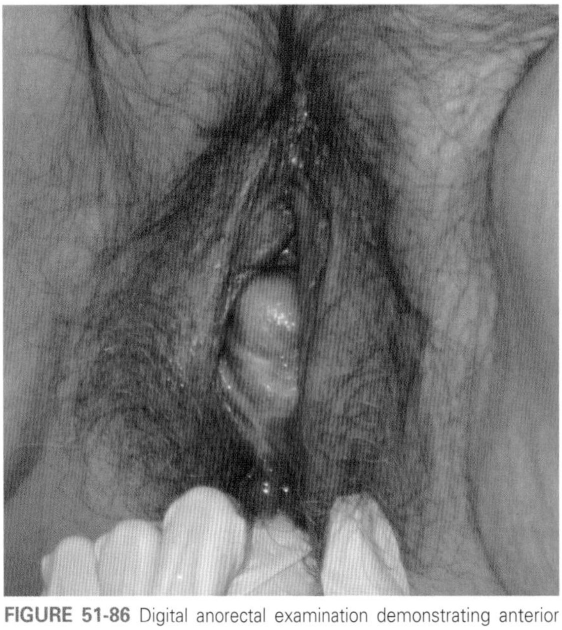

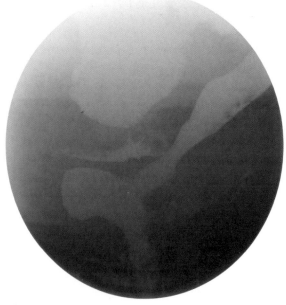

FIGURE 51-86 Digital anorectal examination demonstrating anterior rectocele protruding from the vaginal introitus.

FIGURE 51-87 Triple-contrast radiograph demonstrates large anterior rectocele. Contrast material is also in the vagina and small intestine.

was responsible for continued problems. Postoperative biofeed-back therapy is appropriate in these cases. Defecography evaluation is helpful to distinguish these problems before surgery.

Constipation

Constipation is a symptom, and it is often used by patients to describe different problems. It occurs frequently in older populations; in one survey, 50% of women and 30% of men older than 65 years were affected. Although functional constipation appears to occur most often in older patients, a small subset of patients present at a young age with severe unremitting symptoms. These patients are evaluated differently (see later). Although most individuals describe constipation in terms of reduced stool frequency, up to 25% use the term to indicate straining, excessive pushing, or a feeling of incomplete defecation. Normal stool frequencies range from three times weekly to three times daily. The causes of constipation are numerous, but the evaluation of constipation is relatively straightforward and the indications for surgery are few

(Fig. 51-88). The initial evaluation of constipation should elicit information about acuteness of symptoms, stool frequency, changes in stool form, presence or absence of blood in the stool, new medications, and any newly diagnosed illnesses. The physical examination should always include a rectal examination and proctoscopy. New-onset constipation can be divided into categories for further diagnostic consideration. These categories are depression or debilitation, new medications, endocrine conditions such as hypothyroidism, and obstructed defecation. For our purposes, we focus on surgically correctable causes while recognizing that most constipation is chronic and functional and is rectified simply by the addition of fluid and fiber to the diet.

A patient whose symptoms include straining and incomplete defecation with a normal stool frequency should be evaluated for obstructive defecation. The best way to obtain the most information is through the physical examination and defecography. Symptomatic rectoceles are those that fail to empty completely on defecography. Associated anatomic abnormalities (e.g., vaginal

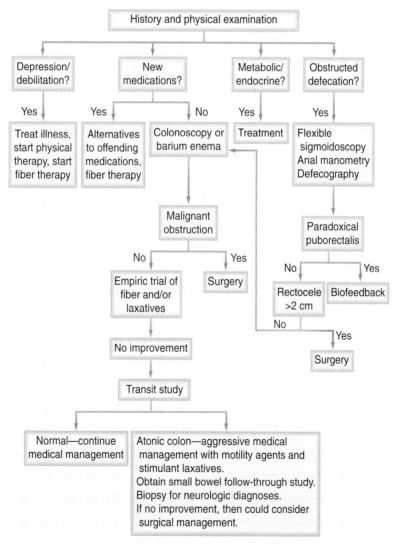

FIGURE 51-88 Algorithm for management of patients with constipation.

vault prolapse, enterocele) can be concurrently corrected. Anal manometry with electromyographic recruitment is an invaluable investigatory tool for the patient with normal anatomy and suspected paradoxical puborectalis syndrome. Biofeedback therapy is indicated in these cases. On occasion, surgically correctable rectocele and functional defecatory disorders coexist. In this situation, biofeedback is usually initiated and rectocele repair is done subsequently.

The primary concern for the physician evaluating new-onset constipation is to rule out large bowel malignant disease. A patient who presents with complaints of an acute change in bowel habits should be evaluated by colonoscopy in the absence of obvious causes, such as narcotic use. Suspect medications should be immediately stopped, and reevaluation should take place shortly thereafter. No improvement or a guaiac-positive stool should lead to a colonoscopic examination. Barium enema is acceptable as well, but flexible sigmoidoscopy, even combined with stool guaiac testing, fails to detect 25% of right-sided malignant neoplasms. A normal finding on colonoscopic examination is reassuring and should lead to trials of dietary therapy. Fluid intake should be increased to 2 liters/day at a minimum, and fiber therapy should be instituted. Caffeinated beverages should be avoided. There are many other laxative-based strategies for the short-term treatment of functional constipation. Long-term failure to respond to these strategies necessitates further investigation.

Transit Studies

Measurement of the colonic transit time is a valuable aid in the establishment of a diagnosis of slow-transit constipation, or colonic inertia. Although many different techniques exist to assess colonic transit times, the main goal of testing is to establish whole gut and segmental transit values. A common and simple test has been devised by Martelli. The patient is asked to refrain from the use of laxatives or constipating medications such as iron supplements for 3 to 4 days before the test. The patient ingests a capsule containing 20 radiopaque markers, and an abdominal radiograph is obtained on each subsequent day for a total of 7 days or until the markers are expelled. The capsules are quantified in three areas of the colon—right, left, and rectosigmoid. Normal subjects expel 80% of markers within 5 days after ingestion. Slow-transit constipation is diagnosed in patients who fail to meet these criteria.

Slow-transit constipation: colonic inertia. It has been estimated that 2% of the population suffers from chronic, unremitting functional constipation. The cause of this syndrome is not well understood, but it has been suggested that most of the motility alterations in slow-transit constipation might be of neuropathic origin, and there is some evidence suggesting that subtle alterations of the enteric nervous system, not evident on conventional histologic examination, may be present in these patients. Most patients are female, with a mean age younger than 30 years. Most of them will report that they were constipated as children and that the constipation worsened during adolescence and early adulthood. Bowel movement frequency is widely variable and ranges from once or twice weekly to once every 2 to 3 weeks. Abdominal pain, bloating, and nausea accompany the constipation and make these patients miserable. Frequent use of over-the-counter laxatives and enemas characterizes this group, and concurrent psychiatric conditions such as depression are common. Although malignant disease in this group is exceedingly rare, it should be ruled out. A barium enema is a useful initial examination; not only does it screen for large obvious lesions, but the

morphology of the colon and presence of dilation can also be evaluated. A transit study is the next diagnostic step. Biopsies are usually not indicated unless a strong suspicion of neuropathic constipation is harbored. A loss of the argyrophil plexus, with a marked increase in Schwann cells indicating extrinsic damage to the myenteric plexus, may be found. This damage is thought to result from chronic laxative abuse. A delay in gastric emptying and small bowel follow-through has been noted in some patients, implying a global motility problem. This motility problem may be responsible for the mixed surgical outcomes reported.

An aggressive bowel regimen is always the first course of action after the diagnosis of slow-transit constipation. A combination of laxatives, fiber, and polyethylene glycol–based solutions can be helpful. A new class of laxative approved for short-term use is 5-HT$_4$ receptor agonists. These may prove beneficial and merit investigation.

Surgery for idiopathic colonic inertia is controversial. The most commonly described procedure is subtotal colectomy with ileorectal anastomosis. Traditionally, only patients with symptoms in the setting of megacolon or megarectum were considered for operative intervention, but now more patients with a normal-caliber colon and severe refractory constipation are being referred for surgery. The costs and inconvenience associated with medical therapy for severe chronic constipation are not inconsiderable. Intuitively, surgery may seem like an attractive option. However, the data concerning lasting cure are unclear. In most series that included more than 20 patients and had longer than 2-year follow-up, results ranged from 33% to 94% success rates (regular defecation without the use of laxatives). The wide range of results is concerning. It has been noted that often the symptoms of nausea, bloating, and abdominal pain can persist and be accompanied by incapacitating diarrhea. In effect, many patients trade one symptom complex for another. There have been only a few small prospective studies exercising strict selection criteria for surgery that include normal defecography results and diffuse delay on transit study. These patients appear to fare best in follow-up, enjoying a 94% success rate as defined by good or excellent patient satisfaction scores. Subtotal colectomy with ileorectal anastomosis is an option for patients with normal-caliber colonic inertia but should not be advocated as a perfect solution. Careful selection criteria applied to motivated, psychologically well-adjusted individuals result in the best long-term surgical results.

Slow-transit constipation: colonic inertia with megacolon. A small but important subset of constipation is neurologic in origin. In contrast to colonic inertia with a normal colon, as a group, 50% of these patients are male. Surgical intervention is usually indicated in these cases because medical therapy eventually fails. Among these entities, Chagas disease, adult Hirschsprung's disease, and neuronal intestinal dysplasia are considered. Commonly, all these causes are manifested with slow-transit constipation in the presence of a dilated colon. A dilated rectum is a variable finding and is typically absent in Hirschsprung's disease.

Hirschsprung's disease is occasionally diagnosed in adulthood. These patients are typically young men in their 20s with lifelong evacuation complaints. Commonly, in these cases, a short, distal segment of rectum is involved. The remainder of the colon is dilated from chronic distal partial obstruction. Stool is characteristically absent from the distal rectum, similar to the physical finding in children. Barium enema characteristically demonstrates a narrow distal rectum with proximal dilated colon. Anal manometric findings reveal an absent rectoanal inhibitory reflex, indicating that the rectum has lost its neurologically mediated ability to relax in response to the presence of a fecal load. Histologic diagnosis is made on biopsy of the distal rectal mucosa at least 3 cm above the dentate line to avoid the normal aganglionic segment in this area. Suction mucosal and superficial punch biopsies are both diagnostic and can be done in the office setting. Acetylcholinesterase staining of the submucosa and lamina propria reveals an increased number of large brown-stained nerve fibers and is considered 99% accurate in establishing the diagnosis. A discussion of surgical interventions for this problem is found elsewhere in this text (see Chapter 66).

Megacolon is the most common complication of intestinal trypanosomiasis. The organism involved is *Trypanosoma cruzi,* a parasite endemic to South America. Nerve damage resulting from trypanosomiasis causes megacolon and megarectum. Fecal impaction and sigmoid volvulus are the most common complications. Subtotal colectomy for this problem results in a residual dyskinetic rectum; therefore, pull-through procedures with excision of the colon and rectum and creation of an ileal reservoir (ileal J pouch or Park pouch) are preferable.

Neuronal intestinal dysplasia describes two distinct congenital defects of the intestinal mural ganglia. Type A is seen predominantly in children and consists of hypoplasia of the sympathetic innervation. Type B is present in children and adults and is characterized by dysplasia of the submucosal plexus, resulting in weak forward propulsion of stool. On histologic evaluation, hyperplasia and giant ganglia with 7 to 10 nerve cells are present. Acetylcholinesterase staining shows a dense plexus of parasympathetic fibers with increased activity. Laxative therapy in these individuals is usually a short-term strategy, and most patients fail to respond to treatment. Surgical resection with ileorectal anastomosis is the treatment of choice.

SELECTED REFERENCES

Clinical Outcomes of Surgical Therapy Study Group: A comparison of laparoscopically assisted and open colectomy for colon cancer. *N Engl J Med* 350:2050–2059, 2004.

A multi-institutional study demonstrating similar results for laparoscopically assisted colectomy and open colectomy performed for colon cancer.

Corman ML, editor: *Colon and rectal surgery,* ed 5, Philadelphia, 2005, Lippincott Williams & Wilkins.

A surgeon's view of the entire spectrum of colon and rectal surgery. Scattered throughout the text are 139 thumbnail biographical sketches of historical surgeons filled with fun factoids.

Feingold D, Steele SR, Lee S, et al: Practice parameters for the treatment of sigmoid diverticulitis. *Dis Colon Rectum* 57:284–294, 2014.

A comprehensive overview of evidence-based practices related to the surgical management of diverticulitis sponsored by the American Society of Colon and Rectal Surgeons.

Gordon PL, Nivatvongs S, editors: *Principles and practice of surgery for the colon, rectum, and anus,* ed 3, London, 2007, Informa Healthcare.

This text provides excellent anatomic illustrations and detailed descriptions of all aspects of diseases of the colon, rectum, and anus. The discussion of anorectal abscesses and fistula-in-ano is particularly helpful.

Haggitt RC, Glotzbach RE, Soffer EE, et al: Prognostic factors in colorectal carcinomas arising in adenomas: Implications for lesions removed by endoscopic polypectomy. *Gastroenterology* 89:328–336, 1985.

Description of Haggitt's criteria, a classification for polyps with adenocarcinoma that assesses malignant potential according to the depth of invasion.

Miles WE: Pathology of spread of cancer of rectum and its bearing on surgery of cancerous rectum. *Surg Gynecol Obstet* 52:350–359, 1931.

Classic article describing the lymphatic pathways whereby rectal cancer spreads, providing the rationale for abdominal perineal resection as a superior operation to perineal proctectomy.

Sauer R, Becker H, Hohenberger W, et al: Preoperative versus postoperative chemoradiotherapy for rectal cancer. *N Engl J Med* 351:1731–1740, 2004.

The only randomized controlled trial of preoperative versus postoperative chemoradiation that has been done, which demonstrated superiority of the neoadjuvant technique.

Vogelstein B, Fearon ER, Hamilton SR, et al: Genetic alterations during colorectal-tumor development. *N Engl J Med* 319:525–532, 1988.

An excellent description of the most common molecular pathways in the development of colorectal adenocarcinoma.

Wolff BG, Fleshman JW, Beck DE, editors: *The ASCRS textbook of colon and rectal surgery,* New York, 2016, Springer.

This text is sponsored by the American Society of Colon and Rectal Surgeons, with chapters written by recognized authorities in their field.

REFERENCES

1. Pai R, Kang G: Microbes in the gut: A digestable account of host-symbiont interactions. *Indian J Med Res* 128:587–594, 2008.
2. Parkes GC, Sanderson JD, Whelan K: The mechanisms and efficacy of probiotics in the prevention of *Clostridium difficile–*associated diarrhoea. *Lancet Infect Dis* 9:237–244, 2009.
3. McFarland LV: Evidence-based review of probiotics for antibiotic-associated diarrhea and *Clostridium difficile* infections. *Anaerobe* 15:274–280, 2009.
4. Wong JM, de Souza R, Kendall CW, et al: Colonic health: Fermentation and short chain fatty acids. *J Clin Gastroenterol* 40:235–243, 2006.
5. Englesbe MJ, Brooks L, Kubus J, et al: A statewide assessment of surgical site infection following colectomy: The role

of oral antibiotics. *Ann Surg* 252:514–519, discussion 519–520, 2010.

6. Guenaga KF, Matos D, Wille-Jorgensen P: Mechanical bowel preparation for elective colorectal surgery. *Cochrane Database Syst Rev* (9):CD001544, 2011.

7. Lewis RT: Oral versus systemic antibiotic prophylaxis in elective colon surgery: A randomized study and meta-analysis send a message from the 1990s. *Can J Surg* 45:173–180, 2002.

8. Cannon JA, Altom LK, Deierhoi RJ, et al: Preoperative oral antibiotics reduce surgical site infection following elective colorectal resections. *Dis Colon Rectum* 55:1160–1166, 2012.

9. American Society of Colon and Rectal Surgeons Committee Members, Wound Ostomy Continence Nurses Society Committee Members: ASCRS and WOCN joint position statement on the value of preoperative stoma marking for patients undergoing fecal ostomy surgery. *J Wound Ostomy Continence Nurs* 34:627–628, 2007.

10. Francone TD, Saleem A, Read TA, et al: Ultimate fate of the leaking intestinal anastomosis: Does leak mean permanent stoma? *J Gastrointest Surg* 14:987–992, 2010.

11. Zhuang CL, Ye XZ, Zhang XD, et al: Enhanced recovery after surgery programs versus traditional care for colorectal surgery: A meta-analysis of randomized controlled trials. *Dis Colon Rectum* 56:667–678, 2013.

12. Sheth AA, Longo W, Floch MH: Diverticular disease and diverticulitis. *Am J Gastroenterol* 103:1550–1556, 2008.

13. Janes SE, Meagher A, Frizelle FA: Management of diverticulitis. *BMJ* 332:271–275, 2006.

14. Anaya DA, Flum DR: Risk of emergency colectomy and colostomy in patients with diverticular disease. *Arch Surg* 140:681–685, 2005.

15. Strate LL, Liu YL, Syngal S, et al: Nut, corn, and popcorn consumption and the incidence of diverticular disease. *JAMA* 300:907–914, 2008.

16. Chapman JR, Dozois EJ, Wolff BG, et al: Diverticulitis: A progressive disease? Do multiple recurrences predict less favorable outcomes? *Ann Surg* 243:876–883, discussion 880–883, 2006.

17. Rafferty J, Shellito P, Hyman NH, et al: Practice parameters for sigmoid diverticulitis. *Dis Colon Rectum* 49:939–944, 2006.

18. Rocco A, Compare D, Caruso F, et al: Treatment options for uncomplicated diverticular disease of the colon. *J Clin Gastroenterol* 43:803–808, 2009.

19. Dignass A, Lindsay JO, Sturm A, et al: Second European evidence-based consensus on the diagnosis and management of ulcerative colitis part 2: Current management. *J Crohns Colitis* 6:991–1030, 2012.

20. Blonski W, Buchner AM, Lichtenstein GR: Treatment of ulcerative colitis. *Curr Opin Gastroenterol* 30:84–96, 2014.

21. Kiran RP, Khoury W, Church JM, et al: Colorectal cancer complicating inflammatory bowel disease: Similarities and differences between Crohn's and ulcerative colitis based on three decades of experience. *Ann Surg* 252:330–335, 2010.

22. Edge SB, Byrd DR, Compton CC, et al: *AJCC cancer staging manual*, ed 7, New York, 2010, Springer-Verlag.

23. Khan KJ, Dubinsky MC, Ford AC, et al: Efficacy of immunosuppressive therapy for inflammatory bowel disease: A systematic review and meta-analysis. *Am J Gastroenterol* 106:630–642, 2011.

24. Metcalf DR, Nivatvongs S, Sullivan TM, et al: A technique of extending small-bowel mesentery for ileal pouch–anal anastomosis: Report of a case. *Dis Colon Rectum* 51:363–364, 2008.

25. Remzi FH, Fazio VW, Gorgun E, et al: The outcome after restorative proctocolectomy with or without defunctioning ileostomy. *Dis Colon Rectum* 49:470–477, 2006.

26. Shen B, Fazio VW, Remzi FH, et al: Clinical approach to diseases of ileal pouch–anal anastomosis. *Am J Gastroenterol* 100:2796–2807, 2005.

27. Cohen SH, Gerding DN, Johnson S, et al: Clinical practice guidelines for *Clostridium difficile* infection in adults: 2010 update by the Society for Healthcare Epidemiology of America (SHEA) and the Infectious Diseases Society of America (IDSA). *Infect Control Hosp Epidemiol* 31:431–455, 2010.

28. Eaton SR, Mazuski JE: Overview of severe *Clostridium difficile* infection. *Crit Care Clin* 29:827–839, 2013.

29. Neal MD, Alverdy JC, Hall DE, et al: Diverting loop ileostomy and colonic lavage: An alternative to total abdominal colectomy for the treatment of severe, complicated *Clostridium difficile* associated disease. *Ann Surg* 254:423–427, discussion 427–429, 2011.

30. Jemal A, Siegel R, Xu J, et al: Cancer statistics, 2010. *CA Cancer J Clin* 60:277–300, 2010.

31. Sampson JR, Jones S, Dolwani S, et al: MutYH (MYH) and colorectal cancer. *Biochem Soc Trans* 33:679–683, 2005.

32. Karapetis CS, Khambata-Ford S, Jonker DJ, et al: K-ras mutations and benefit from cetuximab in advanced colorectal cancer. *N Engl J Med* 359:1757–1765, 2008.

33. Habr-Gama A, Perez RO, Nadalin W, et al: Long-term results of preoperative chemoradiation for distal rectal cancer correlation between final stage and survival. *J Gastrointest Surg* 9:90–99, discussion 99-101, 2005.

34. O'Neill BD, Brown G, Heald RJ, et al: Non-operative treatment after neoadjuvant chemoradiotherapy for rectal cancer. *Lancet Oncol* 8:625–633, 2007.

35. Guillem JG, Diaz-Gonzalez JA, Minsky BD, et al: cT3N0 rectal cancer: Potential overtreatment with preoperative chemoradiotherapy is warranted. *J Clin Oncol* 26:368–373, 2008.

36. Nyasavajjala SM, Shaw AG, Khan AQ, et al: Neoadjuvant chemo-radiotherapy and rectal cancer: Can the UK watch and wait with Brazil? *Colorectal Dis* 12:33–36, 2010.

37. Stephens RJ, Thompson LC, Quirke P, et al: Impact of short-course preoperative radiotherapy for rectal cancer on patients' quality of life: Data from the Medical Research Council CR07/National Cancer Institute of Canada Clinical Trials Group C016 randomized clinical trial. *J Clin Oncol* 28:4233–4239, 2010.

38. Okabe S, Shia J, Nash G, et al: Lymph node metastasis in T1 adenocarcinoma of the colon and rectum. *J Gastrointest Surg* 8:1032–1039, discussion 1039–1040, 2004.

39. Bentrem DJ, Okabe S, Wong WD, et al: T1 adenocarcinoma of the rectum: Transanal excision or radical surgery? *Ann Surg* 242:472–477, discussion 477-479, 2005.

40. Kesisoglou I, Sapalidis K: Treatment of early rectal cancer. *Tech Coloproctol* 14(Suppl 1):S33–S34, 2010.

41. West NP, Finan PJ, Anderin C, et al: Evidence of the oncologic superiority of cylindrical abdominoperineal excision for low rectal cancer. *J Clin Oncol* 26:3517–3522, 2008.

42. Schmidt CE, Bestmann B, Kuchler T, et al: Ten-year historic cohort of quality of life and sexuality in patients with rectal cancer. *Dis Colon Rectum* 48:483–492, 2005.

43. Matthiessen P, Hallbook O, Rutegard J, et al: Defunctioning stoma reduces symptomatic anastomotic leakage after low anterior resection of the rectum for cancer: A randomized multicenter trial. *Ann Surg* 246:207–214, 2007.

44. Ho YH: Techniques for restoring bowel continuity and function after rectal cancer surgery. *World J Gastroenterol* 12:6252–6260, 2006.

45. Remzi FH, Fazio VW, Gorgun E, et al: Quality of life, functional outcome, and complications of coloplasty pouch after low anterior resection. *Dis Colon Rectum* 48:735–743, 2005.

46. Rullier E, Laurent C, Bretagnol F, et al: Sphincter-saving resection for all rectal carcinomas: The end of the 2-cm distal rule. *Ann Surg* 241:465–469, 2005.

47. Cornish JA, Tilney HS, Heriot AG, et al: A meta-analysis of quality of life for abdominoperineal excision of rectum versus anterior resection for rectal cancer. *Ann Surg Oncol* 14:2056–2068, 2007.

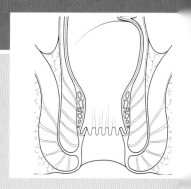

52 CHAPTER

Anus

Amit Merchea, David W. Larson

第五十二章　肛门疾病

OUTLINE

Disorders of the Anal Canal
Pelvic Floor Disorders
Common Benign Anal Disorders
Less Common Benign Anal Disorders
Neoplastic Disorders

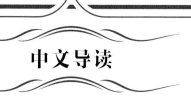

中文导读

　　本章共分为5节：①肛管疾病；②盆底疾病；③肛门常见良性病变；④肛门罕见良性病变；⑤肛门肿瘤。

　　第一节从肛管的解剖、生理学特征、症状及体征、常见的检查手段等几个方面对肛管疾病进行了系统性的阐述，概述肛管的正常解剖学和生理学特征，结合疼痛、出血、分泌物及排便习惯改变等常见肛管疾病的临床表现，介绍了体格检查、内镜检查及影像学检查的基本情况。

　　第二节重点介绍了大便失禁、直肠脱垂、直肠膨出等三种常见的盆底疾病。从临床特征、克利夫兰评分及常见的内外科治疗方式对大便失禁进行概述；从病理生理学特征、术前评估及常见的手术方式对直肠脱垂进行概述；从临床表现和治疗手段两方面对直肠膨出进行了介绍。

　　第三节涵盖痔疮、肛裂、肛周脓肿、肛瘘、藏毛窦等几种肛门常见良性病变，阐明其病因、临床表现及诊治原则。其中着重阐述了内痔和外痔的临床特

征和鉴别诊断要点，介绍了痔疮的分度及包括痔切除术、套扎术、吻合器痔上黏膜环切术等常见的手术方式。介绍了肛裂的常见病因、临床表现和内外科治疗手段。介绍了肛周脓肿的分类及治疗方式。重点介绍了肛瘘的Park分类及预测肛瘘内口的Goodsall规律，及肛瘘的治疗原则和手术方式。简述了藏毛窦的病因和治疗原则。

　　第四节肛门罕见良性病变，包括：直肠阴道瘘，肛周性传播疾病，肛周化脓性汗腺炎及肛周克罗恩病的临床特征及诊治原则。简述了直肠阴道瘘的外科手术原则和方式，简单介绍了常见的肛周性传播疾病的临床表现。概述了肛周化脓性汗腺炎的临床特征及治疗手段。重点介绍肛周克罗恩病的活动指数评分、临床表现和治疗方案。

　　第五节主要阐述了肛门常见良、恶性肿瘤的临床

表现和诊治原则。概述了尖锐湿疣、肛门上皮内瘤变（AIN）、瘤状癌、肛周佩吉特病（Paget's Disease）等常见良性射治疗、化学治疗瘤的临床特征和治疗原则，重点介绍了肛门鳞状细胞癌的TNM分期，放射治疗、

化学治疗及手术指征。对于肛门黑色素瘤，腺癌及基底细胞癌等恶性肿瘤的临床特征及治疗方式做了简要介绍。

〔高　纯〕

DISORDERS OF THE ANAL CANAL

The anal canal remains an area of medicine and surgery plagued by obscurity and limited provider knowledge. Many conditions are in fact common and benign, but some lead to incapacitating interference with the patient's daily life. Provider limitations in both experience and traditional knowledge often lead to misdiagnosis or maltreatment. Therefore, attempts to improve our fund of knowledge of the anatomy and function of the anal canal and the basic physiology of the pelvic floor should facilitate accurate diagnosis and management of both common and rare conditions.

Anatomy

The anal canal extends from the anorectal ring at the most distal aspect of the rectum to the skin of the anal verge and is approximately 4 cm in length. The internal and external sphincter muscles along with the pelvic floor structures contribute significantly to the regulation of defecation and continence. The anus is bounded by the coccyx posteriorly, the ischiorectal fossa bilaterally, and the perineal body and either vagina or urethra anteriorly.

The sphincter apparatus of the anal canal consists of the internal and external sphincters and can be considered as two tubular structures overlying each other. The circular muscle layer of the rectum continues distally to form the thickened and rounded internal sphincter, which terminates approximately 1.5 cm below the dentate line, just cephalad to the external sphincter (intersphincteric groove). The external sphincter is elliptical and surrounds the internal sphincter superiorly and is continuous with the puborectalis and levator ani muscles (Fig. 52-1). The perineal body is formed by the constitution of the external sphincter, bulbospongiosus, and transverse perineal muscles anteriorly. The paired levator ani muscles form the bulk of the pelvic floor, and their fibers decussate medially with the contralateral side to fuse with the perineal body around the prostate or vagina.

The internal sphincter is tonically contracted independent of voluntary control. It receives innervation by the autonomic nervous system. The external sphincter, under voluntary control, is innervated by the inferior rectal branch of the internal pudendal nerve and perineal branch of the fourth sacral nerve. Thus, the loss of bilateral S3 nerve roots (either surgically or otherwise) will result in incontinence. If all sacral nerve roots on either side are sacrificed, normal function is preserved. Similarly, if S1-S3 remains intact on only one side, the patient would maintain anorectal control.

Distal to the anal verge, the perianal skin becomes anoderm, which is a modified squamous lining without hair. At the dentate line, the squamous epithelium transitions to columnar epithelium; this region is referred to as the anal transition zone. Proximal to this area, the lining becomes exclusively gastrointestinal columnar epithelium.

Physiology

The process of defecation and maintenance of continence constitute the principal function of the anus. Various factors affect our ability to effectively achieve these functions—the coordinated sensory and muscular activities of the anus and pelvic floor, the compliance of the rectum, and the consistency, volume, and timing of the fecal movements are all critical to avoidance of fecal incontinence or defecatory disorders.

As the external sphincter contracts, the anal canal lengthens. With straining, it shortens. The internal anal sphincter imparts the resting pressure ($\sim$90 cm H_2O). Squeeze pressure, generated by external sphincter contraction, more than doubles resting pressure. The pressure differential between the rectum and anal canal (low to high) is the principal mechanism that provides continence. The anorectal angle is the angle between the anal canal and the rectum. This angle is approximately 75 to 90 degrees at rest and becomes more obtuse, straightening with straining and evacuation. The ability of the puborectalis to relax and to allow this straightening of the angle facilitates defecation.

Diagnostic Evaluation of the Anus

Anorectal disorders are common. Therefore, basic principles including careful history and physical examination should occur before elaborate testing.

History

It is important to elicit symptoms of pain, bleeding, discharge (purulent or fecal), and any alteration of bowel habits (frequency, consistency). Other past medical, social (including sexual), and family history may be relevant in diagnosing anorectal disease.

Bleeding is among the most common presenting symptoms of diseases of the anus and large bowel. Specific details about the nature of the bleeding can help localize the source in the alimentary tract. Blood that drips, is separate from stools, and is bright red is usually seen with rectal outlet bleeding, as from internal hemorrhoids. Blood on toilet tissue may be associated with minor hemorrhoidal disease but also with anal fissure, although anal fissure is typically accompanied by severe pain at defecation. Passage of clots or melena may indicate a more proximal source of bleeding. One must always give consideration to evaluation of the more proximal bowel to exclude serious conditions, such as cancer. This should be of prime importance when initial

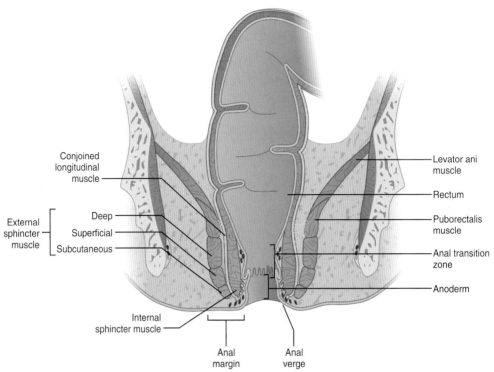

FIGURE 52-1 The anal canal musculature and pelvic floor muscles are depicted.

anorectal examination cannot confirm a bleeding source, when the patient has greater than average risk of cancer, or when bleeding does not resolve promptly after initiation of appropriate treatment.

Anal or rectal pain occurring during or immediately after stooling is another common presenting complaint. Severe pain during defecation, often described by patients as passing glass, is usually associated with anal fissure. Pain, either with or without defecation, that is throbbing in nature is most often seen with an abscess or poorly draining fistula. Patients may also complain of purulent, mucoid, or feculent discharge. A deep-seated rectal pain unrelated to defecation often characterizes proctalgia fugax or levator ani syndrome. This is characterized by painful episodes of short duration (<20 to 30 minutes) that are often relieved by walking, warm baths, or other maneuvers.

Physical Examination

Adequate visualization of the external anal anatomy and the anal canal by anoscopy requires appropriate positioning of the patient (either left lateral or, more commonly, prone jackknife) and good lighting. Skin tags, excoriations, scars, and any changes in color or appearance of perianal skin should be easily recognized. A patulous anus may indicate incontinence and possibly prolapse. Inspection while straining (even with the patient on the commode) may help differentiate the presence of hemorrhoids from rectal prolapse. A careful and systematic digital examination allows the identification of any palpable abnormalities of the anal canal. Finally, the resting tone and strength of the squeeze pressure of the anal sphincter can be assessed.

Anoscopy or proctosigmoidoscopy (flexible or rigid) after enema preparation enables visualization of the anus, rectum, and left colon. Mucosal inflammation is identified by loss of the

normal vascular pattern with erythema, granularity, friability, and even ulcerations. Gross lesions (polyps or carcinoma) should be readily identifiable. Biopsy specimens of any suspicious findings should be obtained for histologic diagnosis.

Other investigations, such as stool culture, specialized imaging (ultrasound, magnetic resonance imaging [MRI], defecography), and specialized physiologic testing, may be helpful adjuncts and should be obtained as clinically appropriate.

PELVIC FLOOR DISORDERS

Incontinence

Fecal incontinence is defined as the recurrent uncontrolled passage of fecal material for at least 1 month in an individual with a developmental age older than 4 years. The reported prevalence of fecal incontinence varies considerably. It has been estimated to occur in 2% to 15% of noninstitutionalized adults.[1] Fecal incontinence can have a significant impact on people's lives, causing physical discomfort, embarrassment, and social isolation. Furthermore, the financial costs and caregiver burden are substantial with real risk of underreporting.

Clinical Evaluation

Obtaining a complete medical history and thorough physical examination is imperative in determining the cause of the fecal incontinence, which will ultimately guide therapy. Defining the extent of the incontinence can be accomplished by a simple history—major incontinence represented by complete loss of solid stool, and minor incontinence by occasional staining or seepage. Mucus seepage from prolapsing hemorrhoids or large secretory villous polyp, urgency from colitis or proctitis, and overflow incontinence from fecal impaction may be inappropriately confused with true incontinence. The severity of the incontinence should be established by assessing the patient's control of flatus and liquid and solid stool and by the impact of symptoms on quality of life. Numerous scoring systems for fecal incontinence exist and can help quantify the problem objectively (Table 52-1).

The cause of fecal incontinence is often multifactorial with combinations of both anatomic and physiologic dysfunctions. Anatomic defects in the sphincter may be the result of trauma from previous surgical procedures, impalement, or obstetric injuries. Moreover, physiologic changes may occur from these anatomic changes, over time or directly, that may lead to sphincter dysfunction, decreased rectal compliance, or decreased sensation. All of these issues may contribute to or have an impact on the degree of incontinence even years after the inciting events.

The most common nonanatomic causes of fecal incontinence should include associated gastrointestinal disorders, such as diarrhea, which can aggravate continence.[2] A physical examination may reveal anatomic abnormalities that account for the incontinence, such as the presence of prolapse, hemorrhoids, or abscess/fistula. A proper digital rectal examination can highlight a weak resting tone and squeeze pressure or a patulous anus and the presence of scars, defects, deformities, or keyhole abnormalities. Endoscopy remains critical to exclude proctitis, impaction, neoplasia, or other rectal mucosal abnormalities that may be contributing factors.

To confirm physical examination findings, the use of focused diagnostic tests may be required. Anorectal manometry confirms the extent of impairment of the internal and external sphincters. Manometry may identify asymmetry, suggesting anatomic defects amenable to repair. Balloon expulsion testing during manometry may demonstrate impairments in rectal sensation. Endoanal ultrasound or MRI may also be employed to detect structural defects of the anal sphincters, rectal wall, and puborectalis muscle.

Treatment

Medical management. Medical management is the initial option for patients with mild incontinence that may not significantly affect quality of life in patients without a reparable anatomic abnormality. Medications to slow transit, to decrease frequency, and to increase stool consistency can be used. Biofeedback training uses noninvasive methods to strengthen the anal musculature and to improve sensation. Nearly 90% of patients note improvement in quality of life.[3] A bowel management program, including antidiarrheal medications (loperamide), bulking agents (methylcellulose), and anticholinergic agents (hyoscyamine), has been successful for some patients.[4] Medical management can also be complementary to surgical therapy and may be carried out before or after surgery to optimize surgical results.

Surgical repair. Surgical options range from the traditional anatomic approaches, such as sphincter repair, to newer techniques like sacral nerve stimulation and the artificial bowel sphincter. For patients with intractable symptoms or failure of other therapeutic measures, colostomy remains a definitive cure. For defined anatomic defects, the most common surgical approach is the sphincteroplasty, in which the separated muscle ends are dissected, reapproximated, and sutured. This can be done in an overlapping fashion or by simply reapproximating the sphincter (Fig. 52-2).[5] The overlapping sphincteroplasty is associated with low rates of morbidity and mortality and reasonable rates of short-term success, with good to excellent results achieved in 55% to 68% of patients.[6] Long-term results of sphincteroplasty have demonstrated a deterioration of continence over time, with only 40% having good to excellent control at a median follow-up of 10 years.[7]

The use of injectable materials for the treatment of fecal incontinence has recently gained attention. In this procedure, a bulking agent (silicone, collagen, carbon microbeads, or dextranomer–hyaluronic acid) is injected into the intersphincteric space to augment the internal anal sphincter. There are limited data for these approaches; however, a single randomized controlled trial did demonstrate short-term improvement in 50% of patients undergoing injection with dextranomer–hyaluronic acid (Solesta; Salix Pharmaceuticals, Raleigh, NC).[8]

More complex approaches to treatment of fecal incontinence include the dynamic graciloplasty, sacral nerve stimulator, and artificial bowel sphincter. The use of the gracilis muscle as a flap encircling the anal canal is reserved for patients in whom the bulk of the anal sphincter is missing and requires complete reconstruction. Results of graciloplasty have been favorable, with the majority of patients maintaining continence and the ability to defer defecation at 5 years.[9] Sacral nerve stimulation has been traditionally used in patients in whom the anal sphincter is intact but there is an associated neurologic injury or poor innervation. A prospective multicenter trial demonstrated success rates of up to 85% at 2 years with a decrease in the number of incontinent episodes per week by approximately 70%.[10] More recent investigation has been conducted to determine its effectiveness in the setting of a defined anal sphincter defect (<180 degrees); many patients have noted significant improvement in these settings.[11] With increasing use of sacral nerve stimulation, the use of an artificial bowel sphincter has been limited. Complications associated with its use are erosion, infection, and obstruction. A review had demonstrated little change in the rate of device explantation or infection in spite of novel surgical techniques and approaches to placement.[12] An algorithm for the treatment of fecal incontinence is presented (Fig. 52-3).

TABLE 52-1 Cleveland Clinic Fecal Incontinence Score					
TYPE	NEVER	RARELY	SOMETIMES	USUALLY	ALWAYS
Solid	0	1	2	3	4
Liquid	0	1	2	3	4
Gas	0	1	2	3	4
Pad use	0	1	2	3	4
Quality of life impact	0	1	2	3	4

From Jorge JM, Wexner SD: Etiology and management of fecal incontinence. *Dis Colon Rectum* 36:77–97, 1993.
Responses are scored and summed. A score of 0 indicates perfect continence, 20 is complete incontinence; rarely, <1/month; sometimes, >1/month; usually, >1/week; always, >1/day.

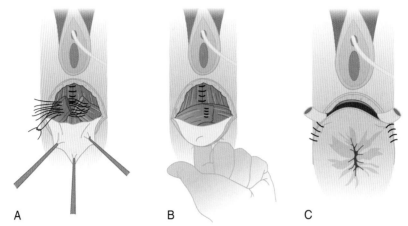

A   B   C

FIGURE 52-2 Overlapping Sphincteroplasty. **A,** An anterior curvilinear incision is made on the perineum between the anus and vagina. The disrupted ends of the external sphincter are dissected free, and the muscle ends are overlapped and reapproximated with suture. A levatorplasty is also concurrently performed. **B,** Digital rectal examination can judge for appropriate tightness of the repair. **C,** The incision is then reapproximated. Some surgeons may leave drains or a small gap in the closure to allow drainage.

Prolapse of the Rectum
Pathogenesis and Clinical Presentation

Prolapse of the rectum, or procidentia, is an uncommon problem (incidence of 0.25% to 0.4%) characterized by eversion of the rectum through the anus.[13] The prolapse may be complete, characterized by protrusion of all layers of the rectal wall, or partial, characterized by a mucosal prolapse only. Risk factors that increase the risk of prolapse include female sex, age older than 40 years, multiparity, vaginal delivery, prior pelvic surgery, chronic straining, dementia, and pelvic floor anatomic defects.

The symptoms of early prolapse may be vague, including discomfort or a sensation of incomplete evacuation during defecation, bleeding, and seepage. Many patients have a long history of constipation and straining. When prolapse is complete, protrusion of the rectum is generally obvious. In patients with occult prolapse, a feeling of pressure and sensation of incomplete evacuation may be the only symptoms.

Preoperative Evaluation

The preoperative assessment should focus on defining the extent of the prolapse; the presence of associated conditions, such as constipation and pelvic floor dysfunction; and other potentially related complications, such as incontinence. Any of these factors may influence management. Nearly 50% of patients have constipation, and the majority have fecal incontinence.[14] If the presence and extent of the prolapse are not readily apparent, examination while straining on the commode may make it more evident. Complete prolapse demonstrates full-thickness rectal protrusion with concentric rings (Fig. 52-4); this should be differentiated from prolapsed hemorrhoids, which demonstrate radial folds. Associated complex pelvic floor abnormalities (cystocele, enterocele, rectocele, vaginal vault prolapse) can be assessed by dynamic pelvic floor MRI; identification of these additional pathologic processes may alter the surgical approach.

Complete lower gastrointestinal tract evaluations should be performed as indicated. On endoscopy, a solitary rectal ulcer 6 to 8 cm anteriorly may be evidenced by redness or ulceration of the anterior rectal wall. Additional tests can be ordered but have limited value and are not typically required. Manometry identifies the presence of sphincter damage but does not predict recovery. Despite the ability of pudendal nerve terminal motor latency to predict a high risk for postoperative anal incontinence, it rarely influences the management. In patients with severe constipation, colonic transit studies may be valuable; although it is exceedingly rare, these patients may respond better to a more extensive colonic resection.

Surgical Correction

Surgical repair of rectal prolapse may be conducted through a perineal approach (Delorme or Altemeier procedure) or an abdominal approach (rectopexy with or without resection and mesh fixation). Insufficient data exist to definitely demonstrate which surgical approach is superior.[15,16] The perineal approach is less morbid for the patient but has a higher recurrence rate; thus, it is best suited for patients with high operative risk and limited life expectancy. Abdominal approaches (laparoscopic, robotic, or open) are preferred for younger patients, particularly those with constipation or associated pelvic floor disorders.

Perineal procedures. For patients with a short (3 to 4 cm) prolapse, a mucosal sleeve resection with muscularis plication (Delorme procedure) is ideal (Fig. 52-5). Recurrence rates associated with this procedure range from 10% to 15%. Mortality and major morbidity are low, approximately 1% and 14%, respectively.[17] Improvement in incontinence is observed in as many as 69% of patients. Prolapse recurrence is common and is likely underestimated because this procedure is performed in patients with limited life expectancies and therefore short follow-up.

The Altemeier procedure (perineal rectosigmoidectomy) involves a full-thickness rectal resection, starting just above the dentate line. The bowel and associated mesentery are resected. Because the pelvic cavity is entered, care must be taken to avoid injury to the small bowel. A full-thickness anastomosis is completed once the prolapsed bowel is resected. For patients with incontinence, a levatorplasty may be added to the resection.

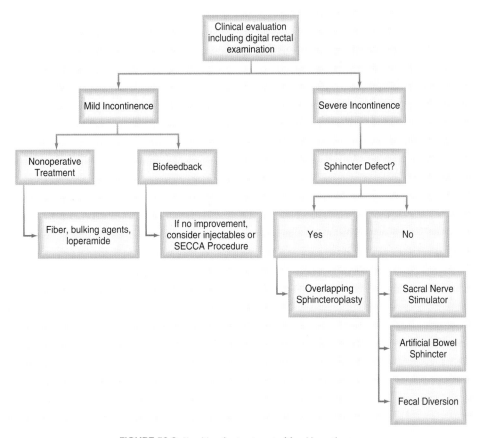

FIGURE 52-3 Algorithm for treatment of fecal incontinence.

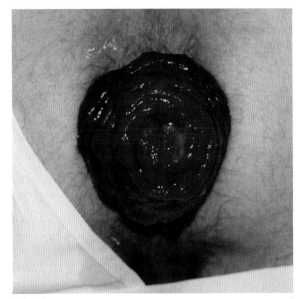

FIGURE 52-4 Full-thickness rectal prolapse. The prolapsed rectal wall appears as concentric folds circumferentially. With prolapsed hemorrhoids, these concentric rings are not seen. (Courtesy Mayo Foundation for Medical Education and Research, Rochester, Minn.)

Long-term results are similar to those described for the Delorme procedure.[18]

Abdominal procedures. The abdominal approaches include rectal mobilization to the pelvic floor, with or without anterior resection (dependent on the presence of constipation), followed by rectopexy of the rectum to the sacral promontory, with or without mesh. Preservation of the lateral stalks is believed to improve function but results in a greater risk for recurrence. If resection and anastomosis are being performed, they should be performed high rather than low in the rectum; this decreases the risk of anastomotic leak. Once it is completely mobilized, the rectum is retracted cephalad out of the pelvis and secured with sutures at the level of the sacral promontory. Resection with rectopexy is generally completed in those patients with symptoms of constipation and is associated with low recurrence rates (0% to 9%). Constipation has been shown to improve in up to 50% of patients. Minimally invasive (laparoscopic or robotic assisted) techniques have been described; however, meta-analyses have yet to identify a significant improvement in function or recurrence rates with this approach compared with more traditional open techniques.[16,19] The universal benefits of minimally invasive approaches (reduced pain, shorter return of bowel function, decreased length of stay) are still evident.

Rectopexy with mesh fixation, and no resection, avoids the risks for resection and anastomosis with low recurrence rates. The mesh can be placed anteriorly or posteriorly. Complications can result, however, from the presence of a foreign body, and symptoms

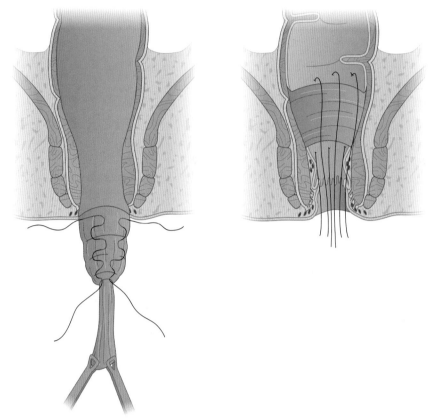

FIGURE 52-5 Delorme Repair. Mucosal sleeve resection is performed and followed by muscle plication, anastomosing the proximal mucosal resection site to the distal mucosa, proximal to the dentate. (Courtesy Mayo Foundation for Medical Education and Research, Rochester, Minn.)

of constipation are often aggravated. In one described technique of anterior mesh fixation, the rectum is minimally mobilized in an effort to avoid autonomic nerve injury and to decrease the risk of increased constipation and poor function postoperatively.[20] In this technique, the right lateral peritoneum is incised overlying the sacral promontory and extended along the rectum toward the pouch of Douglas. Denonvilliers fascia is incised, opening the rectovaginal septum. No rectal mobilization or lateral dissection is performed. A piece of permanent mesh is fixed to the ventral distal rectum and to the sacral promontory using nonabsorbable sutures. Care is taken to not place the rectum on traction. The incised peritoneum can be closed over the mesh, protecting it from the abdominal viscera. Reviews of this technique have demonstrated a low morbidity with less than 5% risk of recurrence.[21]

Incontinence and Biofeedback

Incontinence secondary to pudendal nerve damage from chronic stretching may improve after prolapse repair, except in those patients in whom the lateral stalks are divided. Although the majority of patients report excellent satisfaction with results, the most common reasons for dissatisfaction include persistent constipation or incontinence. The role of biofeedback for treating persistent postoperative incontinence or for preventing recurrent prolapse in patients with pelvic floor dysfunction has not been well established. However, it can be beneficial to some patients, and it is noninvasive.

Rectocele
Clinical Evaluation

Rectocele, like sigmoidocele and enterocele, is associated with a posterior vaginal defect. Symptoms include a vaginal bulge or prolapse of the anterior rectal wall into the vagina, obstructed defecation, and, in many cases, the need to digitally compress the vagina or to digitize the rectum or perineum to evacuate. The cause of rectocele is likely to be multifactorial as it is often associated with a number of other pelvic floor disorders, including constipation, paradoxical muscle contraction, and neuropathies or anatomic disorders from vaginal childbirth.[22] A careful rectovaginal examination will reveal the size of the defect where the rectum prolapse extends to the vagina.

Defecography (fluoroscopic or magnetic resonance) can demonstrate dynamic information on rectal emptying. A rectocele is diagnosed if the distance between the line of the anterior border of the anal canal and the maximal point of bulge of the anterior rectal wall into the posterior vaginal wall is more than 2 cm. It is the most useful test for understanding the relevance of the rectocele in the defecation process and for identification of additional pelvic floor abnormalities.

Treatment

Treatment, when the rectocele is symptomatic, initially involves the optimization of bowel function through diet, fiber supplementation, and good bowel habits. Nonsurgical therapies include the use of pessaries and biofeedback. A pessary has been associated with resolution of prolapse symptoms, but many of these patients are older and have less severe prolapse. Biofeedback has met with limited success, providing only partial relief in most patients.[23]

Surgical treatment. Patients should be considered for surgical correction if the rectocele is larger than 2 cm or the patient has to digitize the vagina or rectum to assist with defecation. Approach to surgical repair is through a transvaginal, transperineal, or transanal technique. All repairs can be completed with or without mesh and may include a levatorplasty. Symptomatic improvement has been observed in 73% to 79% of properly selected patients. A newer technique, the stapled transanal rectal resection, has been investigated for treatment of rectocele associated with internal rectal prolapse causing obstructed defecation. This procedure uses two circular staplers, one anteriorly to resect the rectocele and a second posteriorly to resect the mucosal prolapse. Whereas many patients note improvement in their symptoms, this has been associated with a high rate of fecal urgency and potential for anal stenosis.[24]

COMMON BENIGN ANAL DISORDERS

Hemorrhoids

Presentation and Evaluation

Hemorrhoids are normal, vascular tissue within the submucosa located in the anal canal. They are thought to aid in anal continence by providing bulk to the anal canal. They are typically located in the left lateral, right anterior, and right posterior quadrants of the canal. Hemorrhoids can be external or internal; the differentiation is based on physical examination. External hemorrhoids are distal to the dentate line and are covered with anoderm; these may periodically engorge, causing pain and difficulty with hygiene. Thrombosis of these external hemorrhoids results in severe pain. Internal hemorrhoids are characterized by bright red, painless bleeding or prolapse. Internal hemorrhoids are stratified into four grades that summarize their severity and influence treatment options (Table 52-2). The patient may report dripping or squirting of blood in the toilet. Occult blood loss resulting in anemia is rare, and other causes of anemia, such as a more proximal colorectal lesion, should be investigated. Prolapse of hemorrhoidal tissue may occur, extending below the dentate line; many of these patients complain of mucus and fecal leakage and pruritus.

The physical examination should include inspection of the anus, digital rectal examination, and anoscopy. Examination during straining may make prolapse more evident (Fig. 52-6). Digital examination should focus on anal canal tone and exclusion of other palpable lesions, especially low rectal or anal canal neoplasms. Given that most patients confuse numerous other anorectal symptoms for hemorrhoidal disease, it is imperative that other anorectal diseases be considered and excluded. Anoscopy is generally sufficient to arrive at the correct diagnosis, but complete endoscopic evaluation of the proximal bowel should always be considered to exclude proximal mucosal disease, particularly neoplasia, if the extent of hemorrhoidal disease is incongruent with the patient's symptoms, the patient is due for colonoscopic surveillance, or the patient has risk factors for colon cancer, such as a family history. Depending on the extent of the hemorrhoidal disease and the patient's symptoms, treatment can either be nonsurgical or involve formal hemorrhoidectomy.

Treatment

Nonoperative management. Dietary modifications including fiber supplementation and increasing fluid intake may improve symptoms of prolapse and bleeding. Bulking of the stool permits a soft, formed stool for avoidance of excessive straining and promotion of better bowel habits. Bleeding symptoms are generally reduced during a period of weeks with the use of fiber supplementation alone. Patients with prolapse of internal plus external hemorrhoids will generally benefit from additional interventions.

First-, second-, and some third-degree internal hemorrhoids can usually be treated with office procedures. Results are typically more favorable for lower degree hemorrhoids. Rubber band ligation remains one of the simplest and widely used office-based procedures for treatment of hemorrhoids. Sedation is not required, and ligation is carried out through an anoscope, using a ligator (Fig. 52-7). Although rare, severe perineal sepsis has been reported after rubber band ligation; thus, patients should be instructed to be aware of delayed or increasing pain, inability to void, or fever. Patients with larger hemorrhoids are likely to be better served by a surgical approach, which is more durable and effective. In patients undergoing one or more bandings, relief of symptoms was noted in 80%, with failure predicted in patients who required four or more bandings.[25] Relative contraindications to banding include immunocompromised patients (chemotherapy, HIV/AIDS), presence of coagulopathy, and patients taking anticoagulation or antiplatelet medications (excluding aspirin products).

Sclerotherapy involves the injection of a low volume (3 to 5 mL) of a sclerosant (e.g., 3% normal saline) into the internal hemorrhoid. This technique has good short-term success, but the hemorrhoidal disease tends to recur in longer follow-up. The benefit to this technique is its application in patients with bleeding tendency or who are taking anticoagulants that cannot be stopped. Infrared and laser coagulation involves the use of light energy to cause coagulation and necrosis, causing fibrosis of the submucosa in the region of the hemorrhoid.

Surgical treatment. Hemorrhoidectomy is a durable option and has the best long-term results. It should be considered whenever patients fail to respond to more conservative repeated attempts to treat the disease. Hemorrhoidectomy should be considered in patients who continue to present with severe prolapse and require manual reduction (grade III) or cannot be reduced (grade IV); for those hemorrhoids complicated by strangulation, ulceration, fissure, or fistula; and for those patients who have symptomatic external hemorrhoids. Patients with thrombosed external hemorrhoids may ideally undergo excision in the office, during the period of maximum pain (generally the first 72 hours). In this case, the thrombosed external hemorrhoid should be excised, not incised, as this may increase the risk of rethrombosis (Fig. 52-8). Those patients presenting after the period of maximum pain are best served by supportive measures. In patients presenting

TABLE 52-2	Internal Hemorrhoids Grading
GRADE	**SYMPTOMS AND SIGNS**
First degree	Bleeding; no prolapse
Second degree	Prolapse with spontaneous reduction
Third degree	Prolapse requiring manual reduction
Fourth degree	Prolapsed, cannot be reduced

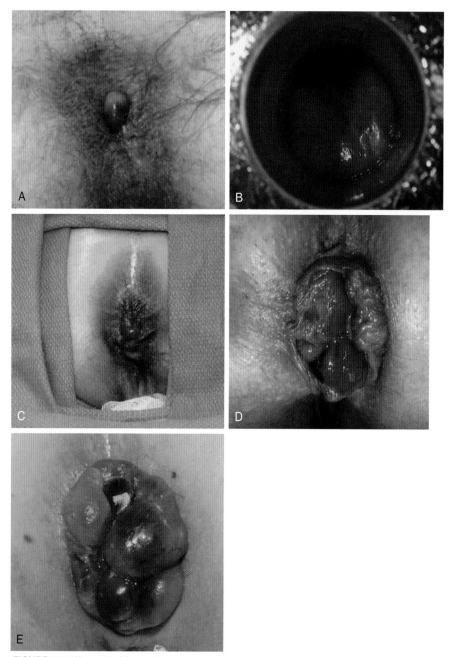

FIGURE 52-6 Hemorrhoids. A, Thrombosed external. **B,** Internal, first-degree internal as seen through anoscope. **C,** Internal prolapsed and reduced spontaneously, second degree. **D,** Internal prolapsed, requiring manual reduction, third degree. **E,** Inability to be reduced, strangulated, fourth degree. (Courtesy Mayo Foundation for Medical Education and Research, Rochester, Minn.)

with complex internal or external hemorrhoids, operative hemorrhoidectomy can be performed as an outpatient procedure.

Closed (Ferguson) hemorrhoidectomy consists of simultaneous excision of internal and external hemorrhoids (Fig. 52-9). With use of a large anoscopic retractor, such as the Fansler, an elliptical incision is made encompassing the complete hemorrhoidal column. Care must be taken to not excise excessive amounts of tissue and to ensure that sufficient anoderm is preserved to avoid the complication of anal stenosis. The excision site

is then closed with a continuous absorbable suture. The open (Milligan-Morgan) hemorrhoidectomy differs in that the excision site is not closed and left open. Postoperative complications include urinary retention (in up to 30% of patients), fecal incontinence (2%), infection (1%), delayed hemorrhage (1%), and stricture (1%). Patients typically recover quickly and are able to return to work within 1 to 2 weeks.

Other techniques involving the application of ultrasonic (Harmonic Scalpel; Soma, Bloomfield, CT) or electrical energy

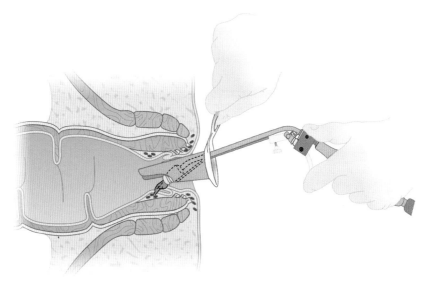

FIGURE 52-7 Rubber Band Ligation. The internal hemorrhoid is identified proximal to the dentate line; the area of proposed banding should be pinched to test for sensation before banding. The hemorrhoid is drawn into the ligator by use of either forceps or the suction device of a suction ligator. The band is then placed. (Courtesy Mayo Foundation for Medical Education and Research, Rochester, Minn.)

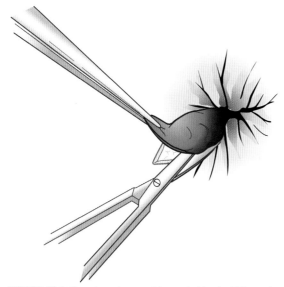

FIGURE 52-8 Thrombosed external hemorrhoids should be excised, not incised, after the area has been infiltrated with local anesthetic. There is no need to close the excision site. (Courtesy Mayo Foundation for Medical Education and Research, Rochester, Minn.)

(LigaSure; Covidien, Boulder, CO) devices have been applied to the operative treatment of hemorrhoids. Both methods remove the excess hemorrhoidal tissue, with minimal lateral thermal injury in the hope of decreasing postoperative pain and edema. Various studies have investigated their efficacy and have demonstrated decreased postoperative pain and analgesic use in these groups compared with traditional techniques, with similar short-term success rates.[26,27]

Stapled hemorrhoidopexy is a technique that results in excision of a circumferential portion of the lower rectal and upper anal canal mucosa and submucosa with a circular stapling device (Fig. 52-10). The procedure is completed by first reducing the hemorrhoidal tissue into the anal canal. A purse-string suture is placed 3 to 4 cm above the dentate line, ensuring that all the redundant tissue is incorporated circumferentially. Overly aggressive placement of the sutures may inadvertently incorporate the vaginal wall anteriorly, resulting in a rectovaginal fistula. In addition, if the suture is placed too close to the dentate line, it could result in severe and intractable pain.

Results of stapled hemorrhoidopexy are varied. A meta-analysis of randomized controlled trials comparing this with conventional hemorrhoidectomy found that the stapled procedure was safe but on long-term follow-up was associated with a higher rate of recurrence and reoperation (Fig. 52-11).[28]

Anal Fissures
Presentation and Evaluation
An anal fissure is a linear ulcer usually found in the midline, distal to the dentate line (Fig. 52-12). These lesions are typically easily seen by visual inspection of the anal verge with gentle spreading of the buttocks. Location may vary; most fissures are identified in the posterior midline, and anterior midline fissures are still more common that lateral fissures. Other associated findings include a sentinel tag at the distal portion of the fissure and a hypertrophied anal papilla proximal to the fissure. Fissures occurring in the lateral positions should raise the possibility of other associated diseases, such as Crohn's disease, tuberculosis, syphilis, HIV/AIDS, or carcinoma. Anal fissure most often is manifested with excruciating anal pain (because of its location extending onto the very sensitive anoderm) with defecation and bleeding.

Patients typically describe a preceding episode of constipation. Digital and anoscopic examination may result in severe pain and is not necessary if the fissure can be visualized. Examination under anesthesia, with or without biopsy of the fissure, or endoscopic examination should be performed if it is refractory to medical management.

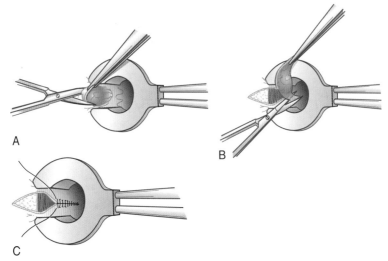

FIGURE 52-9 Closed Hemorrhoidectomy. **A,** An elliptical incision is made surrounding the hemorrhoidal tissues, and these are excised from distal to proximal. **B,** Care is taken to preserve the sphincter muscle. **C,** The feeding vascular pedicle at the proximal point is sutured and the defect closed with a running absorbable suture. In the open technique, this excision site is not closed with suture. (Courtesy Mayo Foundation for Medical Education and Research, Rochester, Minn.)

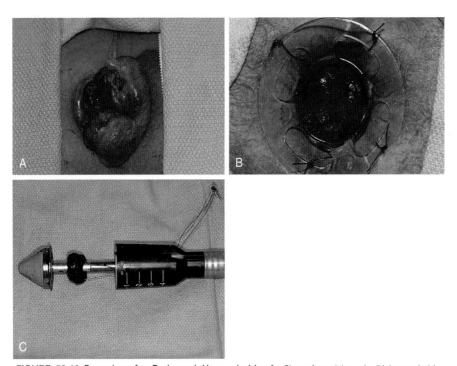

FIGURE 52-10 Procedure for Prolapsed Hemorrhoids. **A,** Circumferential grade IV hemorrhoids. **B,** The stapling device has an obturator that is placed in the internal canal to aid in reduction of tissue and placement of purse-string suture in the mucosa above the dentate line. **C,** Stapling device demonstrating circumferential excision of anal canal and hemorrhoid mucosa.

Pathogenesis

The cause of anal fissure is likely to be multifactorial. The passage of large and hard stools, low-fiber diet, previous anal surgery, trauma, and infection may be contributing factors. Increased resting anal canal pressures and reduced anal blood flow in the posterior midline have also been postulated as causes. These possibilities have led to the introduction of several medical approaches.

Treatment

Given that a hypertonic sphincter and large, hard stools may contribute to anal fissures, most medical therapies are directed to

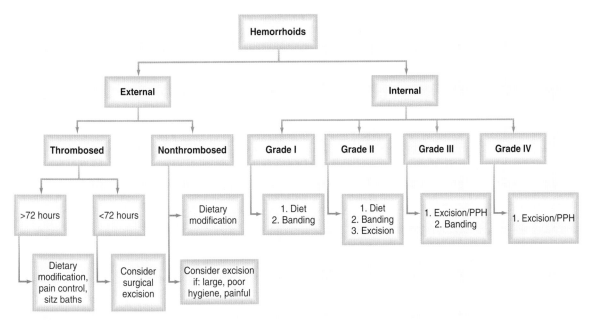

FIGURE 52-11 Algorithm for the treatment of hemorrhoids. *PPH,* procedure for prolapse and hemorrhoids.

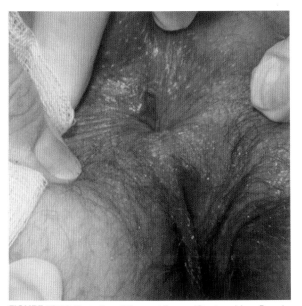

FIGURE 52-12 Posterior midline anal fissure. (Courtesy Mayo Foundation for Medical Education and Research, Rochester, Minn.)

achieve the goals of relaxation of the anal sphincter without causing fecal incontinence, passage of soft and formed stools, and relief of pain. Many pharmacologic agents have been considered, including topical nitric oxide (e.g., nitroglycerin), calcium channel blockers (e.g., diltiazem, nifedipine), and botulinum toxin injections.

Nonsurgical therapy is safe and often effective, with limited side effects, and should be the first-line therapy for anal fissure. However, a subset of patients may benefit from upfront surgical intervention, and the treatment should generally be individualized (Fig. 52-13).

Medical management. Medical therapies for acute anal fissures (those presenting within 6 weeks of symptom onset) are effective. Medical management includes topical and oral pharmacotherapy in addition to diet modification and bulking agents.[29] Topical therapy is popular, given its fewer side effects compared with oral therapies.

Topical nitrates (0.2% to 0.4% nitroglycerin) or calcium channel blockers (0.2% nifedipine or 2% diltiazem) are commonly prescribed. A meta-analysis compared nonsurgical treatments and found that nitroglycerin was significantly better than placebo (49% versus 36%; $P < .0009$) in healing anal fissures, but there was a 50% late recurrence rate. Calcium channel blockers were equally effective but exhibited fewer side effects.[29]

Temporary chemodenervation of the internal anal sphincter can be achieved by injection of botulinum toxin (Botox). This results in relaxation of the internal anal sphincter and is believed to promote increased blood flow to the affected anoderm, allowing the fissure to heal. Success is variable, with reported rates of 60% to 80% being achieved. Up to 10% of patients may develop temporary incontinence to flatus, with rare temporary fecal incontinence. Presently, there is no agreed on standard dose, site of injection, or number or timing of injections in the administration of botulinum toxin. Our practice is to inject 20 units of botulinum toxin into the internal anal sphincter on each side of the fissure. In patients who are nonresponders to diet modification and topical pharmacotherapy, such as topical nitroglycerin or calcium channel blockers, and who wish to avoid surgery, botulinum injection may be a reasonable alternative treatment.

Surgical management. Patients with severe or chronic fissures and those who have failed to respond to medical therapy may benefit from surgery. Lateral internal sphincterotomy remains the operation of choice and has been shown to be superior to all other medical therapies, anal dilation, or fissurectomy.[30] Lateral internal sphincterotomy can be carried out by the closed or open (Fig. 52-14) technique, depending on the surgeon's preference. There is no significant difference between these techniques for rate of

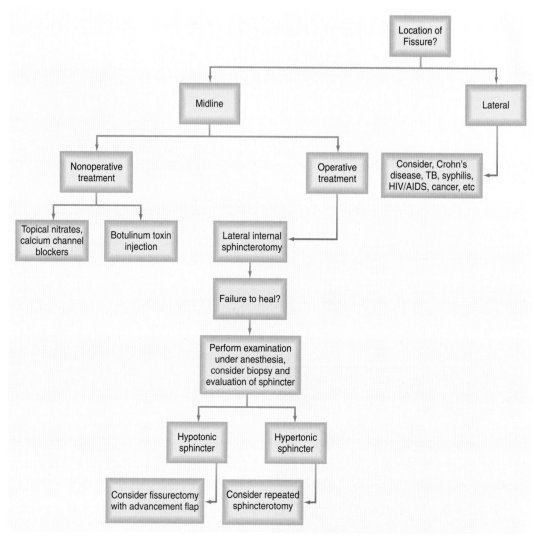

FIGURE 52-13 Algorithm for the treatment of anal fissure.

healing or rate of incontinence. In terms of the extent of sphincterotomy, studies have investigated whether sphincterotomy to the level of the dentate line is superior to sphincterotomy to the fissure apex. Those with sphincterotomy to the level of the dentate had a higher rate of fissure healing, with no statistical difference in rate of incontinence.[30] The risk of incontinence with sphincterotomy is not negligible. A meta-analysis demonstrated an overall rate of incontinence of 14%. Incontinence of flatus occurred in 9% of patients. Incontinence of liquid or solid stool occurred in 2% of all patients.[31] It is important to evaluate for any preexisting incontinence before undertaking surgical intervention so as not to further compromise sphincter function.

In patients with chronic or recurrent fissure with hypotensive anal sphincter, fissurectomy with endoanal advancement flap is an alternative surgical approach.

Anorectal Suppuration

The most common cause of anorectal suppuration is nonspecific cryptoglandular infection. Other less common although not necessarily rare causes include Crohn's disease and hidradenitis

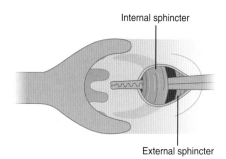

FIGURE 52-14 Lateral Internal Sphincterotomy. A large operating anoscope is placed into the anal canal. A small incision is made along the intersphincteric groove. The mucosa is elevated from the sphincter, and the underlying internal sphincter is elevated off the external sphincter. This is divided either to the level of the dentate line or to the proximal extent of the fissure. (Courtesy Mayo Foundation for Medical Education and Research, Rochester, Minn.)

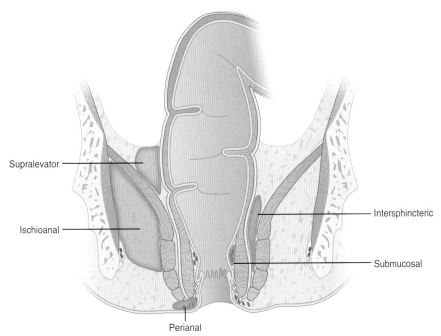

Supralevator

Ischioanal

Intersphincteric

Submucosal

Perianal

FIGURE 52-15 Anatomic locations and classification of perianal/perirectal abscesses.

suppurativa. The abscess represents the acute manifestation and the fistula the chronic sequela.[32]

Anorectal abscesses generally originate in the intersphincteric space. The infectious process may remain isolated within the intersphincteric space, or it may extend vertically upward or downward, horizontally, or circumferentially. Abscesses are generally classified into perianal, ischiorectal, intersphincteric, and supralevator (Fig. 52-15).

Clinical Presentations of Various Types of Abscesses

An intersphincteric abscess is limited to the primary site of origin. These abscesses may be asymptomatic; however, classically, the patient will present with pain out of proportion to physical examination findings. Downward extension results in a perianal abscess, exhibited by a tender swelling at the anal margin.

Upward extension may result in a supralevator abscess. These abscesses may be difficult to diagnose because the patient may complain of vague pelvic or anorectal discomfort, and there is a lack of external manifestations. Supralevator abscesses may also result from pelvic infectious processes, such as diverticulitis. In rare instances, these may extend downward into the ischiorectal or intersphincteric space.

Horizontal spread may traverse the internal sphincter internally into the anal canal or externally across the external sphincter into the ischiorectal fossa, forming an ischiorectal abscess. These abscesses may become large as external physical examination findings may be subtle, and the infection may initially or insufficiently be treated with only antibiotics, allowing expansion to the roof of the fossa or through the pelvic floor into the supralevator space. Patients may complain of pain and fever before an obvious fluctuant mass is detected. A complex horseshoe abscess may result if the infectious process spreads circumferentially from one side to the other of the intersphincteric space, supralevator space, or ischiorectal fossa.

Treatment

Acute anorectal abscesses should be incised and drained at the time of diagnosis. If the abscess is superficial and simple, this can most often be done under local anesthesia in the office setting. In the presence of immunosuppression (AIDS, diabetes mellitus, chemotherapy), systemic symptoms (fever), or more complicated large abscesses, definitive treatment should be undertaken in the operating room under anesthesia. The location and method of drainage are determined by the location of the abscess.

For a perianal abscess, a simple skin incision is adequate. The incision should be kept as close as possible to the anal verge, without injury to the underlying sphincter muscle, to minimize the length of any potential fistula that may form. Intersphincteric abscesses are drained into the anal canal by dividing the internal anal sphincter at the level of the abscess. The cause of a supralevator abscess must be determined before drainage; supralevator abscesses, if not the result of upward extension of an ischiorectal abscess, should be drained into the lower rectum and upper anal canal or transabdominally if the result of an abdominal source. Ischiorectal abscesses should be drained through an appropriate incision through the skin and subcutaneous tissue overlying the infected space (Fig. 52-16). If the abscess is deep within the fossa, needle localization of the purulent material may help guide the surgeon for the optimal location of the skin incision. Care should be taken to avoid vigorous débridement of the abscess cavity as there exists a low risk of injury to the inferior rectal branch of the internal pudendal nerve. Abscesses that are not adequately treated may result in a devastating and sometimes lethal necrotizing infection of the perineum. In these situations, wide débridement of infectious and necrotic tissue is necessary, often combined with broad-spectrum antibiotics.

Recurrent abscesses may result if there has been inadequate drainage, presence of a fistula, or underlying immunosuppression. In this setting, examination under anesthesia may be warranted

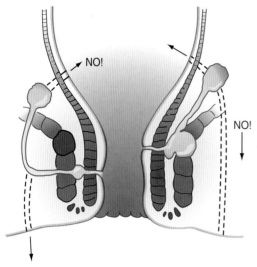

FIGURE 52-16 Sites of Drainage for Abscesses. It is important that the location of the incision is appropriate to avoid creation of extrasphincteric or suprasphincteric fistulas. (From Parks AG, Gordon PH, Hardcastle JD: A classification of fistula-in-ano. *Br J Surg* 63:1–12, 1976.)

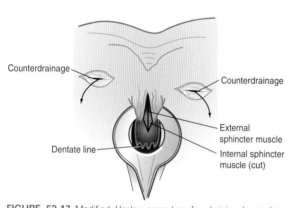

FIGURE 52-17 Modified Hanley procedure for draining horseshoe abscesses. (From Gordon PH: Anorectal abscesses and fistula-in-ano. In Gordon PH, Nivatvongs S, editors: *Principles and practice of surgery for the colon, rectum, and anus*, ed 2, St Louis, 1992, Quality Medical, p 232.)

> ### BOX 52-1   Parks Classification of Fistula in Ano
>
> Intersphincteric: The fistula is confined to the intersphincteric plane.
> Trans-sphincteric: The fistula traverses the external sphincter, communicating with the ischiorectal fossa.
> Suprasphincteric: The fistula extends cephalad over the external sphincter and perforates the levator ani.
> Extrasphincteric: The fistula extends from the rectum to the perianal skin, external to the sphincter apparatus.

From Parks AG, Gordon PH, Hardcastle JD: A classification of fistula-in-ano. *Br J Surg* 63:1–12, 1976.

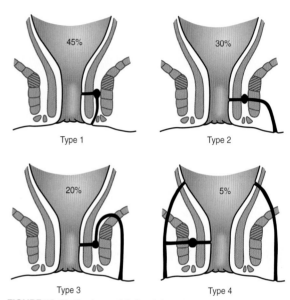

FIGURE 52-18 Fistulas and their relationship to the sphincter apparatus: type 1, intersphincteric; type 2, trans-sphincteric; type 3, suprasphincteric; type 4, extrasphincteric. (From Parks AG, Gordon PH, Hardcastle JD: A classification of fistula-in-ano. *Br J Surg* 63:1–12, 1976.)

after imaging studies of the abdomen or pelvis (e.g., MRI or computed tomography [CT]) have been obtained. Horseshoe abscesses result from circumferential spread of the infectious process. A modified Hanley procedure that drains the deep postanal space and lateral extensions of the abscess should be performed. A posterior midline incision is made extending from the subcutaneous portion of the external sphincter over the abscess to the tip of the coccyx, separating the superficial external sphincter and unroofing the deep postanal space and its lateral extension (Fig. 52-17). Lateral incisions can be made and setons placed to drain any anterior extensions of the abscess.

Antibiotics and abscess culture have a limited role in the treatment of uncomplicated anal suppuration but should be considered in patients with immunosuppression, systemic illness, or a history of prolonged and frequent antibiotic use.

Ancillary imaging studies (CT scan, MRI, endoanal ultrasound, fistulography) may have some utility in select cases, but treatment is generally based on clinical findings. These studies may be helpful to guide management in patients with complex or recurrent disease.

Fistula in Ano

Fistula in ano can develop in approximately 40% of patients during the acute phase of sepsis or even be discovered within 6 months of initial therapy. Fistulas are categorized by the Parks classification (Box 52-1 and Fig. 52-18).

Clinical Presentations

The most common anal fistula is an intersphincteric fistula. Most frequently, the fistula traverses directly downward to the anal margin. In some cases, however, the track may travel upward in the rectal wall (high blind track), with or without a perineal opening.

In trans-sphincteric fistulas, the track travels across the external sphincter and into the ischiorectal fossa, terminating at the perineal skin. If it passes through the muscle at a low level, it is uncomplicated and treatment is relatively simple; however, if it involves the upper two thirds of the sphincter, repair is more complicated. Care must be taken in probing these fistulas to avoid inadvertent puncture of the lower rectum, creating an iatrogenic extrasphincteric fistula. Suprasphincteric fistulas are rare and can be difficult to treat. With these fistulas, the trajectory is above all the muscles of importance to continence. Furthermore, the fistula may have an additional extension into the pelvis, parallel to the rectum (high blind track).

Finally, an extrasphincteric fistula is also rare and often results from iatrogenic injury. It travels from the perineal skin to the rectal wall above the levator ani. The track is completely outside the sphincter apparatus. Treatment often involves the need for a colostomy.

Treatment

Adequate and appropriate treatment is dependent on correct classification of the fistula and identification of the internal and external openings, the course of the track, and the amount of sphincter muscle involved. Surgical treatment remains the primary modality of treatment for noninflammatory bowel disease–related fistulas. Examination under anesthesia allows a complete anorectal examination and appropriate classification of the disease. Digital examination may reveal a palpable nodule in the wall of the anal canal, an indication of the primary opening. A probe can be placed gently from the external skin opening to the internal anal canal opening.

Management of simple fistulas (those with minimal involvement of the sphincter complex—low trans-sphincteric fistulas, intersphincteric fistulas) is often done by laying the track open by fistulotomy. Depending on the length or depth of the track, it may be marsupialized to promote healing. Recurrence and incontinence rates are generally low but heavily dependent on operator judgment and experience. Goodsall's rule (Fig. 52-19) is useful for predicting the anatomy of simple fistulas. If direct probing cannot identify the internal opening, injection of a mixture of methylene blue and hydrogen peroxide may help identify it.

Complex fistulas often require more than simple fistulotomy to resolve. A variety of techniques exist for their treatment, which again is dependent on the classification and accurate identification of the internal opening. For fistulas that involve more than 30% of the sphincter, those distal to the dentate line, or high trans-sphincteric fistulas, a draining seton (suture or elastic) is placed loosely through the track to facilitate drainage of any sepsis and to preserve the sphincter. This may be converted to a cutting seton, which is periodically tightened at regular intervals to slowly cut through the involved sphincter muscle and to promote fibrosis to avoid disruption of the sphincter and the resulting incontinence. Success rates are variable and have ranged from 60% to 100%; many patients ultimately experience some level of incontinence, more often to flatus than to liquid or solids.

Other methods of fistula closure in the setting of complex disease include the use of biologic material to promote the closure of fistulas without division of any sphincter muscle (fibrin glue or porcine-derived fistula plug). Both products promote healing of the track by providing an extracellular matrix that serves as a scaffolding, allowing ingrowth of host tissue for incorporation and remodeling. Fibrin glue contains human pooled plasma fibrinogen and thrombin. The fibrin glue is injected into the anal fistula track starting from the internal opening and filling the track from internal to external. A comprehensive review of the literature has

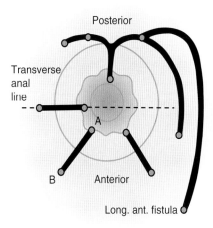

FIGURE 52-19 Goodsall's Rule. The predicted relationship of internal and external fistula orifices is depicted. The internal opening is marked *A*. The long anterior fistula is often an exception to the rule. (From Schrock TR: Benign and malignant disease of the anorectum. In Fromm O, editor: *Gastrointestinal surgery*, New York, 1985, Churchill Livingstone, p 612.)

reported that successful fibrin glue injection results are varied and range from 14% to 60%.[32]

A bioprosthetic fistula plug is also available to serve as a matrix for tissue ingrowth and to obliterate the fistula track. It is inserted into the fistula and then secured at the internal opening. The external opening is widened and left open to allow drainage. Over time, tissue will grow into the plug and replace the matrix, obliterating the fistula track. There are limited data about the success of this approach, but its low morbidity and low risk make it an attractive option in patients with complex fistulas.

High fistulas or other persistent fistulas may be treated by a sliding advancement flap made of mucosa, submucosa, and circular muscle to cover the internal opening. Success rates are again variable, ranging from 13% to 56%, and some patients still report changes in continence, even though the sphincter is not violated.[32]

Finally, a newer technique, ligation of the intersphincteric fistula track, has been developed (Fig. 52-20). This involves dissection in the intersphincteric plane for identification of the fistula track and ligation of it to obliterate the communication with the anal canal. This approach limits risk to the sphincter mechanism and has shown promise with success rates of 60% to 94%.[32]

Pilonidal Disease

Pilonidal infections and chronic pilonidal sinuses are usually found in the midline of the sacrococcygeal region of young hirsute men. The incidence of disease is approximately 26 per 100,000 population. The presence of hair in the gluteal cleft seems to play a central role in the pathogenesis of this disease. This is consistent with the observation that pilonidal disease rarely occurs in those with less body hair. Other risk factors include obesity, local trauma, sedentary lifestyle, deep natal cleft, and family history. Diagnosis is generally a clinical one; patients may present with a

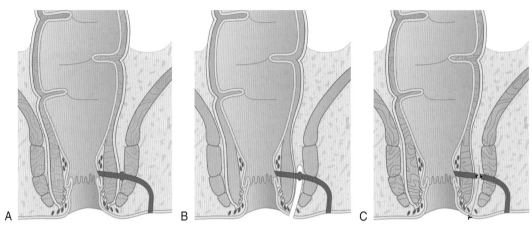

A   B   C

FIGURE 52-20 Ligation of intersphincteric fistula track. This procedure preserves the sphincter and minimizes any risk of incontinence.

chronic inflammation or a sinus with persistent drainage. Acutely, there may be an abscess or multiple complex subcutaneous tracks.

Treatment

Acute management. Acute presentation often involves a painful fluctuant abscess or a draining infected sinus. Both are generally managed in the office with simple treatments; more definitive surgical procedures are reserved for patients who develop a recurrence. Abscesses can be drained with use of local anesthesia. The abscess extends to either side of the midline cleft, and incision and drainage should be performed down to the subcutaneous tissues, off the midline to allow complete drainage and to lower wound complications. The surrounding skin should be shaved weekly to prevent the reintroduction of hair. Laser hair removal can also be considered to accomplish effective, long-lasting hair removal.[33] Recurrent or chronic disease develops in 10% to 15% of patients and may eventually require more extensive surgical management.

Surgical management. The simplest approach for chronic pilonidal disease is midline excision and primary closure. An alternative approach involves marsupialization, whereby the areas of midline pits and sinuses are excised and the wound is reduced in size by suturing the wound edges to the fibrous base of the wound. This has been shown to decrease time for complete wound healing but requires meticulous wound care until the incision has healed. A systematic review compared healing by primary versus secondary intention and found that recurrence rates were the lowest with healing by secondary intention but faster with primary closure. There was no difference in surgical site infections. In addition, when closure was performed, those who underwent off-midline closure had better outcomes than those closed in the midline.[34]

In patients with recurrent disease who have undergone multiple prior surgical interventions, flap-based procedures, such as a V-Y advancement flap, rhomboid flap, Z-plasty, Bascom cleft lip repair, or Karydakis flap, may be beneficial.

Limited comparative studies of the various flap-based procedures exist. A rhomboid fasciocutaneous flap that serves to flatten the gluteal cleft has been shown to have lower recurrence rates compared with a V-Y advancement flap. A Karydakis flap and rhomboid flap are essentially equivalent in published series. In most practices, the complex flap closures are reserved for patients with refractory disease for whom previous simple measures have failed.

LESS COMMON BENIGN ANAL DISORDERS

Rectovaginal Fistula

A rectovaginal or anovaginal fistula is a communication between the rectum or anus and vagina. Rectovaginal fistulas may be congenital or acquired through trauma, inflammatory bowel disease, irradiation, neoplasia, infection, or other rare causes. The most common cause is obstetric-related trauma from unsuccessful repair of third- or fourth-degree perineal laceration or pressure necrosis secondary to prolonged labor. Patients complain of passage of gas, feces, mucus, or blood through the vagina. In the setting of traumatic injuries, anal manometry and endoanal ultrasound may demonstrate the severity of the underlying sphincter defect and help guide the surgical approach.

Surgical Repair

Before embarking on surgical repair of rectovaginal fistulas, it is important to consider the underlying disease, size of the fistula, presence of active inflammation, and severity of symptoms. Small, low-output fistulas may close spontaneously. However, those associated with inflammatory bowel disease, radiation therapy, or underlying infection may resolve only with medical or surgical therapy. High rectovaginal fistulas (upper third of the vagina) generally require a transabdominal approach, whereas low rectovaginal fistulas can be repaired transvaginally, transrectally, or transperineally.

An endorectal advancement flap, sphincteroplasty, and transperineal procedures can all be employed for the repair of a truly low-lying fistula (anovaginal fistula).[35] An endorectal advancement flap consists of a flap of rectal mucosa, submucosa, and underlying internal anal sphincter muscle that is advanced to cover the primary opening in the rectum or anus. The flap is best suited for the initial repair or for patients without an underlying sphincter defect. The transperineal approach (perineoproctotomy) converts the rectovaginal fistula into a fourth-degree tear. The tissues are then reapproximated in a normal anatomic fashion with the internal, external, and levator muscles in discrete layers. This should be reserved for patients with preexisting sphincter defects for whom other more conservative approaches have failed.[35]

For high rectovaginal fistulas, a transabdominal approach is often required. This approach requires mobilization of the rectovaginal septum, division of the fistula, and subsequent closure of the rectal and vaginal defects. Placement of a viable pedicle of tissue between the two structures may help augment the repair and promote healing. In some cases, no rectal resection is necessary. In the setting of severe prior radiation exposure, inflammatory bowel disease, or neoplasia, rectal excision is required. A low anterior resection or coloanal anastomosis may be possible, preserving the sphincters and allowing normal evacuation.[35]

Sexually Transmitted Diseases and Acquired Immunodeficiency Syndrome

Multiple partners and anal receptive intercourse increase the risk for transmission of sexually transmitted disease (STD), which can be bacterial, viral, or parasitic in origin (Box 52-2). The site and manner of infection dictate the symptoms of presentation.

Clinical Presentation

Patients with STDs may present with varied but often overlapping symptoms that may include pruritus, bloody or purulent rectal discharge, tenesmus, diarrhea, and fever. Proctoscopic examination may demonstrate proctitis, mucopurulent discharge, ulceration, and abscesses. Diagnosis is aided by clinical findings based on physical examination, endoscopy, and cultures.

Patients infected with molluscum contagiosum develop painless flattened, round, and umbilicated dermal lesions. Endoscopy often demonstrates vesicles, ulcers, and friability. Similar endoscopic findings may be seen in herpes or anal warts. The diagnosis is obtained by cultures, scrapings, or biopsy. Treatment for herpes infection is with the antiviral acyclovir. Other viral lesions are generally treated by destruction or excision.[36]

Parasitic STDs have a greater incidence of systemic symptoms, such as fever, abdominal cramping, and bloody diarrhea. *Entamoeba histolytica* characteristically causes hourglass-shaped ulcerations. More diffuse ulceration is seen with *Giardia lamblia*. Diagnosis is based on biopsy specimens or scrapings and specific stains.

AIDS. Anorectal disease affects approximately one third of patients with HIV infection and can cause significant morbidity. Pain and bleeding are the most frequent presenting complaints. The most common findings in this population of patients include abscesses, fistulas, infectious proctitis, condyloma, anal intraepithelial neoplasia (AIN), and cancer. Herpes, cytomegalovirus, and *Chlamydia* spp. are the most typical infectious agents. Examination should include inspection of the perianal skin, palpation of the lymph nodes (may be enlarged in syphilis or herpes simplex infection), and visualization of the anal canal. Mucopurulent anal discharge that is associated with pain may be secondary to gonorrhea, chlamydia, or herpes. One should also consider obtaining a Gram stain or culture as indicated.

Neoplastic disorders are more prevalent in men who have sex with men, and this is even greater in those who are HIV positive. These disorders include condyloma, AIN, epidermoid carcinoma, and Kaposi sarcoma.[37] Treatment of anal condyloma is not different on the basis of HIV positivity status; however, the recurrence rates and conversion to malignancy are higher for those who are HIV positive. In those patients with squamous cell carcinoma, whether invasive or in situ disease, CD4 count and treatment with antiretroviral therapy are key adjuncts to success with local excision or chemoradiotherapy.

Anal condyloma and human papillomavirus (HPV) infections are considered STDs. However, these infections are discussed later, with other neoplastic disorders.

Hidradenitis Suppurativa

Hidradenitis suppurativa primarily involves the intertriginous skin regions of the axilla, inframammary, groin, perianal, and perineal areas. Hidradenitis has traditionally been considered the result of occlusion of apocrine glands by keratotic debris. This occlusion leads to bacterial proliferation, suppuration, and spread of inflammation to surrounding subcutaneous tissues. Subcutaneous tracks and pits develop; the infected tissues ultimately become fibrotic and thickened. Many bacterial organisms have been identified, including *Streptococcus milleri, Staphylococcus aureus, Staphylococcus epidermidis,* and *Staphylococcus hominis.*

Clinical Presentation

Perianal hidradenitis can be manifested as early acute or late chronic, severe form; the condition most commonly is first manifested with an inflammatory, painful nodule. The nodules may spontaneously regress and then recur or rupture and drain. Fistulas or sinus tracks may ultimately develop that intermittently release purulent debris. After repeated interventions, dense scarring and fibrosis may develop. The appearance is classic (Fig. 52-21). In rare cases, squamous malignant neoplasms may also be

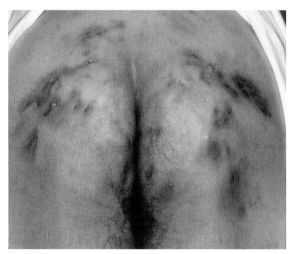

FIGURE 52-21 Hidradenitis suppurativa. (Courtesy Mayo Foundation for Medical Education and Research, Rochester, Minn.)

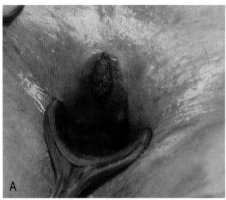
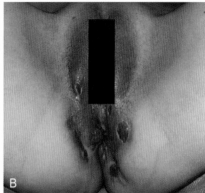

FIGURE 52-22 Perineal Crohn's disease. **A,** Crohn's disease fissures demonstrate deep and shaggy edges, significant ulceration, and abundant granulation tissue. **B,** Perianal Crohn's disease can be complicated by multiple fistulas and abscesses, complicating treatment and requiring combination surgical and medical therapy. (Courtesy Mayo Foundation for Medical Education and Research, Rochester, Minn.)

present. To ensure appropriate treatment, hidradenitis must be differentiated from Crohn's disease–related fistulas or cryptoglandular infection. Hidradenitis fistulas arise distal to the dentate line in the anal skin, differentiating them from cryptoglandular fistulas, which communicate with the dentate line, and Crohn's disease, which may have tracks to the anorectum proximal to the dentate line.

Treatment

The general goals in treatment are to reduce the extent of disease, to remove chronic infection/sinuses, and to limit scar formation. To exclude the possibility of malignancy, liberal biopsies should be performed. For acute disease, the mainstay of therapy remains incision and drainage. In an effort to reduce the risk of recurrence, medical management includes the use of topical clindamycin, which may have additional benefit in treating secondary infections. Oral antibiotic treatment, with clindamycin, minocycline, doxycycline, or amoxicillin–clavulanic acid (Augmentin), may also have some benefit in acute flares of mild disease.

Sinus tracks that are chronic and superficial can be unroofed or laid open. Avoiding curettage of the epithelized track may facilitate rapid healing and minimize scarring. Extensive, deep and fibrotic disease may require wide excision, although this is associated with recurrence rates of approximately 50%. Wide excision may lead to large wounds, which can be managed with delayed healing and dressing changes, flaps, or skin grafts. Involvement of a plastic surgeon to assist with closure or wound management is sometimes necessary. Healing by secondary intention requires significant wound care, and it can often take weeks to months for complete healing to be accomplished.

Crohn's Disease of the Anorectum
Clinical Presentation

Perianal complications of Crohn's disease can affect approximately 40% of patients. In these patients, the presence of perianal disease is often predicted by the location and activity of more proximal gastrointestinal disease. The majority (>90%) of patients with rectal disease will have perianal disease. This is compared with approximately 40% of patients with isolated colonic disease, whereas up to 5% of patients with perianal disease will have no disease in the proximal gastrointestinal tract.[38] Those patients younger than 40 years and nonwhites are also more likely to

present with perianal disease. Perianal Crohn's disease may include fissures, fistulas, and abscesses. Patients may have a varied presentation including pain, swelling, drainage, incontinence, fever, and bleeding (Fig. 52-22).

Evaluation and Treatment

In evaluating patients with Crohn's disease, one must determine if the anal pathologic change is secondary to Crohn's disease or, especially in the setting of quiescent disease, a common anorectal problem unrelated to the underlying disease. It is important that the examination be complete (including endoscopy). Obtaining a thorough examination may require anesthesia for diagnostic and therapeutic purposes, particularly in the patient experiencing pain that limits an office examination. In the absence of rectal or anal Crohn's disease, common anorectal conditions (fissure, fistula, or abscess) may be treated by standard approaches. The surgeon must be cautious when treating a Crohn's disease patient with anorectal problems; however, undertreatment of symptomatic conditions should also be avoided. The disease activity can be objectively measured by the Perianal Crohn's Disease Activity Index, a scoring system that evaluates the fistulizing disease in five categories: discharge, pain, restriction of sexual activity, type of perianal disease, and degree of induration (Table 52-3).[39]

Crohn's disease fissures often are multiple, off-midline lesions. Although conservative measures, such as sitz baths, stool softeners, oral analgesics, and nifedipine ointment, may be tried, patients will often require medical treatment to control the disease. Sphincterotomy and fissurectomy should be avoided when Crohn's disease is present. In the case of anorectal suppuration caused by Crohn's disease, a combination of surgical and medical therapy is advised.[40,41] Abscesses should be drained, and the anus and rectum should be completely evaluated for fistulas or other inflammation. For fistulas, treatment should be based on the symptoms and relationship of the fistula to the sphincter complex. Simple, low to mid fistulas may be treated with fistulotomy or staged with seton placement. In addition, antibiotics may complement the treatment. Complex fistulizing disease or fistulizing disease with extensive proctitis requires drainage with setons and initiation of immunomodulator therapy, such as infliximab or azathioprine and mercaptopurine. In severe cases, diversion or even proctectomy is sometimes required. In patients treated with azathioprine and mercaptopurine, a complete response is seen in nearly 40%

TABLE 52-3 Perianal Crohn's Disease Activity Index

ELEMENTS	SCORE
Discharge	
None	0
Minimal mucous	1
Moderate mucous or purulent	2
Substantial	3
Gross fecal soiling	4
Pain or Restriction of Activity	
None	0
Mild discomfort, no restriction	1
Moderate discomfort, some limitation	2
Marked discomfort, marked limitation	3
Severe pain, severe limitation	4
Restriction of Sexual Activity	
None	0
Slight restriction	1
Moderate restriction	2
Marked restriction	3
Unable to engage in sexual activity	4
Type of Perianal Disease	
None	0
Anal fissure or mucosal tear	1
<3 Perianal fistulas	2
>3 Perianal fistulas	3
Sphincter ulceration	4
Degree of Induration	
None	0
Minimal	1
Moderate	2
Substantial	3
Gross fluctuance/abscess	4

From Irvine EJ: Usual therapy improves perianal Crohn's disease as measured by a new disease activity index. McMaster IBD Study Group. *J Clin Gastroenterol* 20:27–32, 1995.

of patients. The use of maintenance infliximab has been associated with decreased rate of recurrence, fewer hospitalizations, and fewer procedures performed for fistulizing disease.

NEOPLASTIC DISORDERS

There is a wide spectrum of benign and malignant neoplastic lesions of the anus. Defining the anatomy of the anal canal is important in differentiating the appropriate treatment modalities for various lesions.

The American Joint Commission on Cancer (AJCC) has defined three anatomic regions in which anal or perianal squamous cell cancer may be manifested: anal canal, perianal, or skin. Anal canal lesions are defined as those lesions that cannot be visualized or are incompletely visualized by gentle traction of the buttocks. Perianal lesions are completely visible and arise within 5 cm of the anal opening when the buttocks are gently spread. Skin lesions are outside of the 5-cm radius.[42]

Clinical Evaluation

Initial assessment should begin with a complete history and physical examination. The extent and duration of the symptoms, such as bleeding, pain, changes in continence, and weight loss, should be documented. The perianal area should be closely examined for changes in the normal skin. Digital rectal examination establishes tumor location, fixation, and function of the sphincter muscles. Anoscopy or rigid proctosigmoidoscopy can help determine the size and relation of the tumor to the dentate line, anal verge, or anorectal ring. One should also examine for any pathologic lymphadenopathy. Staging studies investigating for distant disease include chest, abdominal, and pelvic CT. Pelvic MRI for staging purposes is encouraged to determine exact tumor size and nodal involvement. A positron emission tomography scan should be considered in those with T2 or greater tumors or those with positive nodal involvement.

Anal Margin (Perianal) Tumors

Neoplastic lesions that exclusively involve the skin of the anal margin are treated like skin lesions at any other skin site unless treatment would compromise the sphincter mechanism.

Condyloma Acuminatum

Condyloma acuminatum (anogenital wart) is caused by HPV. It remains the most common virally transmitted STD in the United States. Viral subtypes, such as HPV-6 and HPV-11, are found more commonly in benign warts, whereas HPV-16 and HPV-18 tend to be aggressive and are associated with dysplasia and progression to cancer. Acquiring condyloma is directly related to sexual activity and is more common in immunocompromised individuals.

Clinical presentation. Patients may complain of pruritus, bleeding, pain, discharge, or a palpable mass. Examination typically reveals pinkish warts of varying sizes that may coalesce to form a mass (Fig. 52-23A). Anoscopy may reveal disease within the anal canal. The diagnosis is generally made by direct inspection of the perineum and genitals; anoscopy and proctosigmoidoscopy must be performed as the disease often extends intra-anally, and some patients have disease limited to the anal canal. Histology confirms the diagnosis. High-resolution anoscopy with or without 5% acetic acid may improve detection of disease.

Diagnostic evaluation. The most important factors contributing to the successful management of condylomata acuminata are the extent of disease, presence of underlying contributing conditions, and risk of malignancy. Condylomas are often found in other sites around the perineum or genitals, and these areas should be thoroughly evaluated; concurrent treatment of nonanal sites helps limit the risk of relapse. In addition, sexual partners are at risk for contracting the disease and should also undergo evaluation and treatment.

Patients with condylomata acuminata should be screened for any immunologic compromise. This may be secondary to HIV infection, medication related (transplant patients), or oncologic related. Immunosuppression increases the risk of malignancy in patients with condyloma or undergoing treatment for condyloma, and these patients should be closely observed. HIV testing should be considered if it has not previously been conducted, and tissue samples should be obtained for HPV and AIN evaluation. High-resolution anoscopy can help locate sites of high-risk lesions.[43]

Treatment. Treatment approaches involve physical or chemical destruction, immunologic therapies, and surgery. Despite the various multimodal therapies, recurrence rates of 30% to 70% have been reported. Chemical agents include podophyllin,

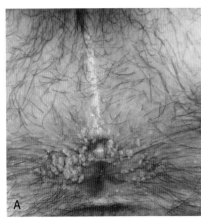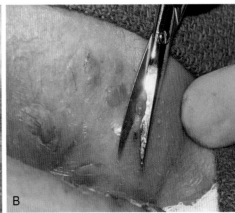

FIGURE 52-23 A, Perianal condyloma acuminatum. **B,** Sharp excision of condyloma. (Courtesy Mayo Foundation for Medical Education and Research, Rochester, Minn.)

trichloroacetic acid, and 5-fluorouracil (5-FU). Podophyllin is cytotoxic and can be irritating to normal skin. Its use should be limited to those patients with minimal extra-anal disease. Care must be taken to avoid systemic toxicity. Although it is simple and inexpensive, the results are often disappointing, with high recurrence rates reported. Trichloroacetic acid can be used perianally and intra-anally and is less irritating than podophyllin. The recurrence rate with both agents is much higher than with surgical excision. Another topical immune therapy is imiquimod, which creates an inflammatory response that destroys the condyloma. Current recommendations are for the topical application of imiquimod 5% cream three times weekly (for 6 to 10 hours). This can be used as a primary treatment or as an adjunct after initial resection or destruction of disease. Although it is not currently approved for intra-anal use, some centers have applied this medication in this manner with similar results.

Destruction of the condyloma by electrocauterization with a needle tip cautery is effective and used extensively, and it is often combined with excision of larger lesions. Carbon dioxide laser is also an effective tool, but the cost is higher without evidence of increased efficacy. Excision at the base with small scissors can also be performed; it is precise, minimizes destruction of the skin, and can be used on larger lesions (Fig. 52-23*B*). General or regional anesthesia is often necessary. All options, however, are associated with a significant chance of recurrence. Thus, close follow-up of patients is recommended.

Anal Intraepithelial Neoplasia

There exists variability and confusion in regard to the terminology describing anal squamous intraepithelial lesions. The AJCC classifies these lesions as low-grade anal intraepithelial lesions (LSIL) to include AIN I (low grade) and high-grade anal intraepithelial lesions (HSIL) to include AIN II-III (moderate or high grade). The term *Bowen disease*, which has been ascribed variably to anal squamous cell carcinoma in situ, AIN II, and AIN III, further complicates the discussion as there is little if any biologic difference between these entities. The term *Bowen disease* should be abandoned for the more universal term HSIL.

Treatment. Treatment should be individualized to the patient and disease process. Historically, the recommendation has been for anal mapping and treatment according to the extent and location of the disease. In situ lesions that are unifocal can be managed with local excision to achieve negative margins. In some cases,

wounds can be of sufficient size to require wound closure with more complex means other than primary approximation; various flap techniques have been previously described. Whereas this would provide excellent local control, recurrence rates remained high.[44] More frequently and in a less morbid approach, high-resolution anoscopy with acetic acid to aid in lesion visualization has allowed directed destruction. Perianal disease can be treated with topical application of imiquimod, as described earlier, which has been associated with complete clinical and histologic clearance of AIN in some reports. Multifocal anal canal disease is usually focally ablated. All patients should be closely observed for recurrence and for invasive disease. Interval of follow-up should be determined on the basis of grade of dysplasia, extent of disease, and presence of immunosuppression. Patients who are immunocompromised may have an increased risk for development of invasive disease.

Verrucous Carcinoma

Verrucous carcinoma is also referred to as giant condyloma acuminatum or Buschke-Löwenstein tumor. These large lesions are slow growing and may be complicated by fistulization, infection, or malignant transformation. Wide local excision is recommended; in rare cases when all disease cannot be removed, abdominal perineal resection (APR) is necessary. Those tumors that progress to invasive squamous cell carcinoma are associated with a poor prognosis. However, some may respond favorably to combined chemoradiotherapy.

Squamous Cell Carcinoma

Squamous cell carcinoma of the anal canal is five times more common than perianal squamous cell carcinoma. Cancers of the anal margin (those occurring within 5 cm of the squamous mucocutaneous junction) that are small (T1) and well differentiated may be treated by wide local excision. Any anal margin lesions that are greater than T1 or node positive should be treated like primary squamous cell cancers of the anal canal with definitive chemoradiation (see later). Patients with stage IV metastatic disease may benefit from cisplatin-based chemotherapy with or without radiation therapy.

Paget Disease

Extramammary Paget disease of the anus is a rare intraepithelial adenocarcinoma. Paget disease more commonly is manifested in

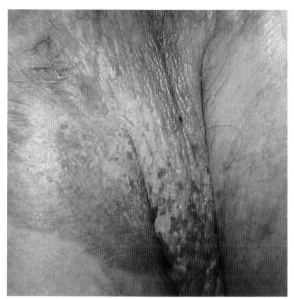

FIGURE 52-24 Perianal Paget disease. (Courtesy Mayo Foundation for Medical Education and Research, Rochester, Minn.)

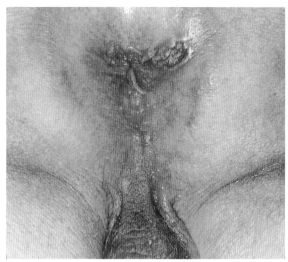

FIGURE 52-25 Basal cell carcinoma of anal margin. (Courtesy Mayo Foundation for Medical Education and Research, Rochester, Minn.)

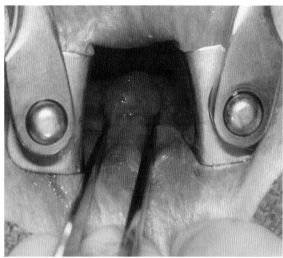

FIGURE 52-26 Squamous cell carcinoma of anal canal. (Courtesy Mayo Foundation for Medical Education and Research, Rochester, Minn.)

older patients (usually in the seventh decade of life) and is often seen in areas of high density of apocrine sweat glands.[45] Over time, these can develop into an invasive cancer of the underlying apocrine glands. The most common presenting symptom is intractable itching, and some patients with long-standing symptoms are misdiagnosed with pruritus ani. The typical appearance is an eczematous, well-demarcated plaque with occasional ulceration and scaling (Fig. 52-24). Histology demonstrates the presence of periodic acid–Schiff–positive (because of significant mucin) Paget cells (large, vacuolated cytoplasm with eccentric nuclei), confirming the diagnosis. Extramammary Paget disease is associated with an underlying invasive carcinoma in 30% to 45% of patients. However, visceral malignant neoplasms may be seen in up to 50% of patients.

Treatment is based on the local extent of the disease and presence or absence of invasion. Limited, noninvasive disease is best managed by wide local excision and closure of the defect primarily or with V-Y advancement flaps. Recurrences can generally be treated with re-excision as long as disease remains noninvasive. In patients medically unfit for surgery and with noninvasive disease, other techniques can be used, such as topical 5-FU, imiquimod, cryotherapy, or argon beam laser therapy. Close observation in these cases is advised, and biopsies for symptoms are recommended.[45] For patients with an invasive component, consideration should be given to radical resection with APR. Five-year disease-specific survival ranges from 50% to 70% of all patients with extramammary Paget disease.

Basal Cell Carcinoma

Basal cell carcinoma is a rare type of anal tumor. In gross appearance, these lesions are characteristic for pearly borders, with central depression (Fig. 52-25). In most cases, these tumors can be treated by wide local excision, reserving APR for extensive lesions or those involving the sphincter mechanism.

Malignant Anal Canal Neoplasms
Squamous Cell Carcinoma

Squamous cell carcinoma of the anal canal typically is manifested as a mass, sometimes with bleeding and pruritus (Fig. 52-26).

Many patients are initially misdiagnosed and ultimately present late. Some have reported only 10% of patients being diagnosed with tumors confined to the epithelium and subepithelial tissues.

AJCC staging for anal canal cancers is based on the size of the tumor and local invasion of adjacent organs or structures (Table 52-4).[42] A tumor that is 2 cm or smaller is designated T1, larger than 2 cm but not more than 5 cm is T2, and larger than 5 cm is T3. Any size tumor that invades a local structure is designated T4. Staging of disease includes CT of the chest, abdomen, and pelvis and pelvic MRI. Positron emission tomography scanning should be considered for larger (T2 or greater) tumors or any node-positive disease. HIV testing and checking a CD4 count should also be considered if indicated.

Historically, treatment consisted of surgery alone or radiation therapy alone. Epithelial or subepithelial tumors were locally excised, and more advanced lesions underwent APR. The introduction of multimodality therapy combining chemotherapy and

TABLE 52-4 TNM Staging Classifications for Anal Malignant Neoplasms

Primary Tumor (T)

TX	Primary tumor cannot be assessed
T0	No evidence of primary tumor
Tis	Carcinoma in situ (Bowen disease, high-grade squamous intraepithelial lesion [HSIL], anal intraepithelial neoplasia II-III [AIN II-III])
T1	Tumor 2 cm or less in greatest dimension
T2	Tumor more than 2 cm but not more than 5 cm in greatest dimension
T3	Tumor more than 5 cm in greatest dimension
T4	Tumor of any size that invades adjacent organ(s) (e.g., vagina, urethra, bladder*)

Regional Lymph Nodes (N)

NX	Regional lymph nodes cannot be assessed
N0	No regional lymph node metastasis
N1	Metastasis in perirectal lymph node(s)
N2	Metastasis in unilateral internal iliac and/or inguinal lymph node(s)
N3	Metastasis in perirectal and inguinal lymph nodes and/or bilateral internal iliac and/or inguinal lymph nodes

Distant Metastasis (M)

M0	No distant metastasis
M1	Distant metastasis

Stage Grouping

0	Tis	N0	M0
I	T1	N0	M0
II	T2	N0	M0
	T3	N0	M0
IIIA	T1	N1	M0
	T2	N1	M0
	T3	N1	M0
	T4	N0	M0
IIIB	T4	N1	M0
	Any T	N2	M0
	Any T	N3	M0
IV	Any T	Any N	M1

From Edge S, Byrd D, Compton C, et al, editors: *AJCC cancer staging manual,* ed 7, New York, 2010, Springer.
*Invasion of the rectal wall, perirectal skin, subcutaneous tissue, or sphincter muscles is not classified as T4.

radiation therapy promised to preserve continence, to avoid colostomy, and to offer similar or improved survival.

Nigro was the first to promote radiation therapy with chemotherapy as definitive treatment for squamous cell cancers of the anal canal. The current protocol includes infusional 5-FU with mitomycin C and external beam radiation to the pelvis with a minimum dose of 45 Gy. The inguinal nodes, pelvis, anus, and perineum should be included in the radiation fields. Patients with T2 lesions and residual disease after 45 Gy, T3 or T4 tumors, or node-positive disease are usually treated with an additional 9 to 14 Gy for a total dose of 54 to 59 Gy. In patients treated with APR for persistent or locally recurrent disease, 5-year actuarial survival is reported at 57%.[46]

Despite high success rates with definitive chemoradiotherapy, 15% to 30% of patients will have recurrence or fail to respond completely.[47] Patients with persistent disease up to 6 months after treatment generally require APR. Those who have local recurrence are also recommended for APR. In the setting of isolated inguinal node recurrence, groin dissection is generally required with consideration for radiation therapy to the inguinal node basins if no prior radiotherapy was given. Up to 50% of patients treated with salvage APR can expect a 5-year cure. This is compared with approximately 27% of patients treated with salvage radiation and concurrent cisplatin-based chemotherapy who can expect cure.

In those patients presenting with anal squamous cell carcinoma in the setting of HIV infection, disease severity (CD4 count and use of antiretroviral therapy) has a significant impact on success of standard chemoradiation. The current consensus is that standard protocols for chemoradiotherapy should be attempted, regardless of HIV status, and that medical management of the patient's HIV infection be optimized. The 2-year survival rates for HIV-positive patients have been reported to be the same as for HIV-negative patients, 77% and 75%, respectively.[48]

Melanoma

Melanoma of the anal canal is a rare tumor that can be manifested as a mass, pain, or bleeding. Tumors can be amelanotic and are sometimes incidentally found during histopathologic examination of tissue obtained from an unrelated procedure, for example, a hemorrhoidectomy specimen. Outcomes for patients with anal melanoma are poor, with 5-year survival rates dependent on the extent of disease: 32%, 17%, and 0% for local, regional, and distant disease, respectively.[49] Extent of surgery has not been shown to correlate with long-term outcomes. It remains controversial whether the optimal surgical approach involves wide local excision or APR. Whichever approach is chosen, obtaining R0 resection remains a significant predictor for the best survival rates: 19% 5-year survival for R0 cases and 6% 5-year survival for cases with involved margins.

Adenocarcinoma

Adenocarcinoma of the anal canal is rare and thought to arise from the columnar epithelium of canal ducts. Differentiating distal rectal cancer from true anal canal cancer may be difficult, and it is not necessary as the treatment for both is the same. These patients should be treated with multimodality therapy consisting of chemoradiotherapy and APR. This approach is superior to local excision[50] and radiation therapy alone.

SELECTED REFERENCES

Madoff RD, Mellgren A: One hundred years of rectal prolapse surgery. *Dis Colon Rectum* 42:441–450, 1999.

A historical perspective of surgery to repair rectal prolapse, summarizing much of the relevant data.

Nelson RL, Chattopadhyay A, Brooks W, et al: Operative procedures for fissure in ano. *Cochrane Database Syst Rev* (11):CD002199, 2011.

An evidence-based review of the data on different surgical approaches to chronic anal fissure.

Nelson RL, Thomas K, Morgan J, et al: Nonsurgical therapy for anal fissure. *Cochrane Database Syst Rev* (2):CD003431, 2012.

An evidence-based review of the data on nonsurgical approaches to chronic anal fissure.

Parks AG, Gordon PH, Hardcastle JD: A classification of fistula-in-ano. *Br J Surg* 63:1–12, 1976.

A classic description of the anatomy, data, and classification of anorectal suppurative disease, including abscesses and fistulas.

Steele SR, Kumar R, Feingold DL, et al: Practice parameters for the management of perianal abscess and fistula-in-ano. *Dis Colon Rectum* 54:1465–1474, 2011.

A well-referenced summary of the current standards in the diagnosis and treatment of perianal suppurative disease.

Steele SR, Varma MG, Melton GB, et al: Practice parameters for anal squamous neoplasms. *Dis Colon Rectum* 55:735–749, 2012.

A comprehensive review of diagnostic and treatment issues pertinent to anal squamous neoplasms.

Tou S, Brown SR, Malik AI, et al: Surgery for complete rectal prolapse in adults. *Cochrane Database Syst Rev* (4):CD001758, 2008.

A comprehensive review of the varying techniques for rectal prolapse repair.

REFERENCES

1. Whitehead WE, Borrud L, Goode PS, et al: Fecal incontinence in US adults: Epidemiology and risk factors. *Gastroenterology* 137:512–517, 517.e1–517.e2, 2009.
2. Whitehead WE, Bharucha AE: Diagnosis and treatment of pelvic floor disorders: What's new and what to do. *Gastroenterology* 138:1231–1235, 1235.e1–1235.e4, 2010.
3. Heymen S, Scarlett Y, Jones K, et al: Randomized controlled trial shows biofeedback to be superior to pelvic floor exercises for fecal incontinence. *Dis Colon Rectum* 52:1730–1737, 2009.
4. Omar MI, Alexander CE: Drug treatment for faecal incontinence in adults. *Cochrane Database Syst Rev* (6):CD002116, 2013.
5. Galandiuk S, Roth LA, Greene QJ: Anal incontinence–sphincter ani repair: Indications, techniques, outcome. *Langenbecks Arch Surg* 394:425–433, 2009.
6. Malouf AJ, Norton CS, Engel AF, et al: Long-term results of overlapping anterior anal-sphincter repair for obstetric trauma. *Lancet* 355:260–265, 2000.
7. Oom DM, Gosselink MP, Schouten WR: Anterior sphincteroplasty for fecal incontinence: A single center experience in the era of sacral neuromodulation. *Dis Colon Rectum* 52:1681–1687, 2009.
8. Maeda Y, Laurberg S, Norton C: Perianal injectable bulking agents as treatment for faecal incontinence in adults. *Cochrane Database Syst Rev* (2):CD007959, 2013.
9. Murphy J, Chan CL, Scott SM, et al: Rectal augmentation: Short- and mid-term evaluation of a novel procedure for severe fecal urgency with associated incontinence. *Ann Surg* 247:421–427, 2008.
10. Wexner SD, Coller JA, Devroede G, et al: Sacral nerve stimulation for fecal incontinence: Results of a 120-patient prospective multicenter study. *Ann Surg* 251:441–449, 2010.
11. Ratto C, Litta F, Parello A, et al: Sacral nerve stimulation in faecal incontinence associated with an anal sphincter lesion: A systematic review. *Colorectal Dis* 14:e297–e304, 2012.
12. Hong KD, Dasilva G, Kalaskar SN, et al: Long-term outcomes of artificial bowel sphincter for fecal incontinence: A systematic review and meta-analysis. *J Am Coll Surg* 217:718–725, 2013.
13. Stein EA, Stein DE: Rectal procidentia: Diagnosis and management. *Gastrointest Endosc Clin N Am* 16:189–201, 2006.
14. Madoff RD, Mellgren A: One hundred years of rectal prolapse surgery. *Dis Colon Rectum* 42:441–450, 1999.
15. Tou S, Brown SR, Malik AI, et al: Surgery for complete rectal prolapse in adults. *Cochrane Database Syst Rev* (4):CD001758, 2008.
16. Sajid MS, Siddiqui MR, Baig MK: Open vs laparoscopic repair of full-thickness rectal prolapse: A re-meta-analysis. *Colorectal Dis* 12:515–525, 2010.
17. Lieberth M, Kondylis LA, Reilly JC, et al: The Delorme repair for full-thickness rectal prolapse: A retrospective review. *Am J Surg* 197:418–423, 2009.
18. Altomare DF, Binda G, Ganio E, et al: Long-term outcome of Altemeier's procedure for rectal prolapse. *Dis Colon Rectum* 52:698–703, 2009.
19. Purkayastha S, Tekkis P, Athanasiou T, et al: A comparison of open vs. laparoscopic abdominal rectopexy for full-thickness rectal prolapse: A meta-analysis. *Dis Colon Rectum* 48:1930–1940, 2005.
20. D'Hoore A, Cadoni R, Penninckx F: Long-term outcome of laparoscopic ventral rectopexy for total rectal prolapse. *Br J Surg* 91:1500–1505, 2004.
21. D'Hoore A, Penninckx F: Laparoscopic ventral recto(colpo)pexy for rectal prolapse: Surgical technique and outcome for 109 patients. *Surg Endosc* 20:1919–1923, 2006.
22. Lukacz ES, Lawrence JM, Contreras R, et al: Parity, mode of delivery, and pelvic floor disorders. *Obstet Gynecol* 107:1253–1260, 2006.
23. Mimura T, Roy AJ, Storrie JB, et al: Treatment of impaired defecation associated with rectocele by behavioral retraining (biofeedback). *Dis Colon Rectum* 43:1267–1272, 2000.
24. Boccasanta P, Venturi M, Stuto A, et al: Stapled transanal rectal resection for outlet obstruction: A prospective, multicenter trial. *Dis Colon Rectum* 47:1285–1296, discussion 1296–1297, 2004.
25. Iyer VS, Shrier I, Gordon PH: Long-term outcome of rubber band ligation for symptomatic primary and recurrent internal hemorrhoids. *Dis Colon Rectum* 47:1364–1370, 2004.
26. Chen CW, Lai CW, Chang YJ, et al: Results of 666 consecutive patients treated with LigaSure hemorrhoidectomy for symptomatic prolapsed hemorrhoids with a minimum follow-up of 2 years. *Surgery* 153:211–218, 2013.
27. Tsunoda A, Sada H, Sugimoto T, et al: Randomized controlled trial of bipolar diathermy vs ultrasonic scalpel for closed hemorrhoidectomy. *World J Gastrointest Surg* 3:147–152, 2011.

28. Giordano P, Gravante G, Sorge R, et al: Long-term outcomes of stapled hemorrhoidopexy vs conventional hemorrhoidectomy: A meta-analysis of randomized controlled trials. *Arch Surg* 144:266–272, 2009.

29. Nelson RL, Thomas K, Morgan J, et al: Nonsurgical therapy for anal fissure. *Cochrane Database Syst Rev* (2):CD003431, 2012.

30. Nelson RL, Chattopadhyay A, Brooks W, et al: Operative procedures for fissure in ano. *Cochrane Database Syst Rev* (11):CD002199, 2011.

31. Garg P, Garg M, Menon GR: Long-term continence disturbance after lateral internal sphincterotomy for chronic anal fissure: A systematic review and meta-analysis. *Colorectal Dis* 15:e104–e117, 2013.

32. Steele SR, Kumar R, Feingold DL, et al: Practice parameters for the management of perianal abscess and fistula-in-ano. *Dis Colon Rectum* 54:1465–1474, 2011.

33. Steele SR, Perry WB, Mills S, et al: Practice parameters for the management of pilonidal disease. *Dis Colon Rectum* 56:1021–1027, 2013.

34. Al-Khamis A, McCallum I, King PM, et al: Healing by primary versus secondary intention after surgical treatment for pilonidal sinus. *Cochrane Database Syst Rev* (1):CD006213, 2010.

35. Saclarides TJ: Rectovaginal fistula. *Surg Clin North Am* 82:1261–1272, 2002.

36. El-Attar SM, Evans DV: Anal warts, sexually transmitted diseases, and anorectal conditions associated with human immunodeficiency virus. *Prim Care* 26:81–100, 1999.

37. Simard EP, Pfeiffer RM, Engels EA: Cumulative incidence of cancer among individuals with acquired immunodeficiency syndrome in the United States. *Cancer* 117:1089–1096, 2011.

38. Fry RD, Shemesh EI, Kodner IJ, et al: Techniques and results in the management of anal and perianal Crohn's disease. *Surg Gynecol Obstet* 168:42–48, 1989.

39. Irvine EJ: Usual therapy improves perianal Crohn's disease as measured by a new disease activity index. McMaster IBD Study Group. *J Clin Gastroenterol* 20:27–32, 1995.

40. Poupardin C, Lemann M, Gendre JP, et al: Efficacy of infliximab in Crohn's disease. Results of a retrospective multicenter study with a 15-month follow-up. *Gastroenterol Clin Biol* 30:247–252, 2006.

41. Schwartz DA, Pemberton JH, Sandborn WJ: Diagnosis and treatment of perianal fistulas in Crohn disease. *Ann Intern Med* 135:906–918, 2001.

42. Edge SB, Compton CC: The American Joint Committee on Cancer: The 7th edition of the AJCC cancer staging manual and the future of TNM. *Ann Surg Oncol* 17:1471–1474, 2010.

43. Steele SR, Varma MG, Melton GB, et al: Practice parameters for anal squamous neoplasms. *Dis Colon Rectum* 55:735–749, 2012.

44. Margenthaler JA, Dietz DW, Mutch MG, et al: Outcomes, risk of other malignancies, and need for formal mapping procedures in patients with perianal Bowen's disease. *Dis Colon Rectum* 47:1655–1660, discussion 1660–1661, 2004.

45. McCarter MD, Quan SH, Busam K, et al: Long-term outcome of perianal Paget's disease. *Dis Colon Rectum* 46:612–616, 2003.

46. Mariani P, Ghanneme A, De la Rochefordiere A, et al: Abdominoperineal resection for anal cancer. *Dis Colon Rectum* 51:1495–1501, 2008.

47. Gunderson LL, Winter KA, Ajani JA, et al: Long-term update of US GI intergroup RTOG 98-11 phase III trial for anal carcinoma: Survival, relapse, and colostomy failure with concurrent chemoradiation involving fluorouracil/mitomycin versus fluorouracil/cisplatin. *J Clin Oncol* 30:4344–4351, 2012.

48. Gervaz P, Buchs N, Morel P: Diagnosis and management of anal cancer. *Curr Gastroenterol Rep* 10:502–506, 2008.

49. Podnos YD, Tsai NC, Smith D, et al: Factors affecting survival in patients with anal melanoma. *Am Surg* 72:917–920, 2006.

50. Chang GJ, Gonzalez RJ, Skibber JM, et al: A twenty-year experience with adenocarcinoma of the anal canal. *Dis Colon Rectum* 52:1375–1380, 2009.

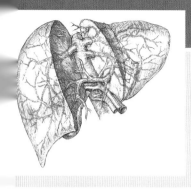

The Liver

Vikas Dudeja, Yuman Fong

第五十三章 肝疾病

中文导读

本章共分为7节：①肝脏外科发展历史；②肝脏解剖与生理；③肝硬化门静脉高压症；④肝脏感染性疾病；⑤肝脏肿瘤；⑥胆道出血；⑦病毒性肝炎。

第一节从古巴比伦人描述肝脏解剖开始，详细阐述了肝脏解剖和肝脏手术发展历程。随着麻醉、重症管理、抗生素和放射介入技术的进步，肝脏手术的安全性得到大幅提升，全肝移植甚至活体供肝切取都渐渐成为常规手术，而且肝脏手术微创化进展很快，腹腔镜肝切除以及机器人肝切除都得到了快速发展。

第二节详细介绍了肝脏大体解剖、胚胎发育及功能解剖，对于门静脉、肝动脉、肝静脉、胆管和肝内神经淋巴系统进行了分类阐述，着重突出了胆汁排泄系统、胆汁形成和肝肠循环等内容。作为人体最重要的代谢器官，本章节也对肝脏参与胆红素、糖类、脂质、蛋白质和维生素代谢等内容进行了详细阐述，同

时作者也介绍了肝脏是如何参与机体凝血和解毒的，并对肝脏再生领域进行了展望。

第三节作者从门静脉高压症的定义出发，对于其病理生理、慢性肝病和门静脉高压症的评估等方面详细加以阐述，重点介绍了食管胃底静脉曲张破裂出血的治疗，涉及内镜、药物、介入、手术等方面，当然也包括门静脉高压症预防出血治疗等问题。

第四节作者重点介绍了两种非寄生虫性感染性疾病（细菌性肝脓肿和阿米巴肝脓肿）和一种寄生虫性感染性疾病（肝包虫病），分别从疾病的流行病学、病理生理、临床表现、鉴别诊断、治疗和结局等方面进行了详细叙述。

第五节也是作者在本章内突出介绍的部分，代表

性疾病有肝脏良性实质性肿瘤（肝细胞腺瘤、局灶性结节增生、血管瘤等）、原发性肝脏恶性肿瘤（肝细胞癌和肝内胆管癌）、转移性肝脏肿瘤（结直肠癌肝转移、神经内分泌肿瘤肝移植、其他恶性肿瘤肝转移等）。对于上述瘤种，作者都从临床表现、诊断与鉴别诊断、治疗预后等方面分别详细介绍，力求对于读者的临床实践有所帮助。

第六节是胆道出血，这也是临床常见的上消化道出血原因之一，作者也对其常见原因、临床表现和诊断治疗进行了分类叙述。

第七节是病毒性肝炎的相关内容。病毒性肝炎作为临床上肝硬化和肝癌的重要病因之一，一直是临床医生关注的焦点问题之一。因此最后部分，作者也对于病毒性肝炎分类、流行病学与传播、发病机制与临床表现，以及如何预防和治疗等临床医生比较感兴趣的部分进行了重点阐述。

〔陈孝平　朱　鹏〕

HISTORICAL PERSPECTIVE

The surface anatomy of the liver was described as early as 2000 BC by the ancient Babylonians. Even Hippocrates understood and described the seriousness of liver injury. In 1654, Francis Glisson was the first physician to describe the essential anatomy of the blood vessels of the liver accurately. The beginnings of liver surgery are described as rudimentary excisions of eviscerated liver from penetrating trauma. The first documented case of a partial hepatectomy is credited to Berta, who amputated a portion of protruding liver in a patient with a self-inflicted stab wound in 1716.

In the late 1800s, the first gastrectomies and cholecystectomies were being performed in Europe. At that time, surgery on the liver was regarded as dangerous if not impossible. In 1897, Elliot, in his report on liver surgery for trauma, said that the liver was so "friable, so full of gaping vessels and so evidently incapable of being sutured that it had always seemed impossible to successfully manage large wounds of its substance." European surgeons began to experiment with techniques of elective liver surgery on animals in the late 1800s. The credit for the first elective liver resection is a matter of debate and many surgeons have been given credit, but it certainly occurred during this period.

The early 1900s saw some small but significant advances in liver surgery. Techniques for suturing major hepatic vessels and the use of cautery for small vessels were applied and reported. The most significant advance of that time was probably that of J. Hogarth Pringle. In 1908, he described digital compression of the hilar vessels to control hepatic bleeding from traumatic injuries. The modern era of hepatic surgery was ushered in by the development of a better understanding of liver anatomy and formal anatomic liver resection. Credit for the first anatomic liver resection is usually given to Lortat-Jacob, who performed a right hepatectomy in 1952 in France. Pack from New York and Quattelbaum from Georgia performed similar operations within the next year and were unlikely to have had any knowledge of Lortat-Jacob's report. Descriptions of the segmental nature of liver anatomy by Couinaud, Goldsmith, and Woodburne in 1957 opened the door even wider and introduced the modern era of liver surgery.

Despite these improvements, hepatic surgery was plagued by tremendous operative morbidity and mortality from the 1950s into the 1980s. Operative mortality rates in excess of 20% were common and usually related to massive hemorrhage. Many surgeons were reluctant to perform hepatic surgery because of these results, and understandably, many physicians were reluctant to refer patients for hepatectomy. With the courage of patients and their families as well as the persistence of surgeons, safe hepatic surgery has now been realized. A complete list is not possible here, but courageous hepatic surgeons such as Blumgart, Bismuth, Longmire, Fortner, Schwartz, Starzl, and Ton deserve mention.

Advances in anesthesia, intensive care, antibiotics, and interventional radiologic techniques have also contributed tremendously to the safety of major hepatic surgery. Total hepatectomy with liver transplantation and live donor partial hepatectomy for transplantation are now performed routinely in specialized transplantation centers. Partial hepatectomy for a large number of indications is now performed throughout the world in specialized centers, with mortality rates of 5% or less. Partial hepatectomy on normal livers is now consistently performed, with mortality rates of 1% to 2%.

Safely performed open hepatic surgery with its liberal use in the management of a wide variety of diseases is now a reality. Moreover, minimally invasive approaches to liver surgery have been developed and are now being used in significant numbers. However, the learning curve remains steep, and the indications for this technique are still being carefully defined. Use of robotics in liver surgery may help in addressing the issues with learning curve with laparoscopy. The addition of robotics offers advanced suturing and articulation that closely approximate the open surgery. This allows a greater proportion of cases to be performed in total minimally invasive fashion.[1] The role of robotics in liver surgery is rapidly evolving. Thermal ablative techniques to treat hepatic tumors, including radiofrequency and microwave ablation, have exploded in popularity. Finally, techniques to improve the safety of liver resection further, such as portal vein embolization to induce preoperative hypertrophy of the future liver remnant (FLR), have been developed and are now being used.

ANATOMY AND PHYSIOLOGY

Anatomy

Gross Anatomy

A precise knowledge of the anatomy of the liver is an absolute prerequisite to performing surgery on the liver or biliary tree. During the last several decades, a greater appreciation for the complex anatomy beyond the misleading minimal external markings has been realized. The anatomic contributions of Couinaud (see later) and the description of the segmental nature of the liver should be embraced and studied by students of hepatic surgery.

General description and topography. The liver is a solid gastrointestinal organ whose mass (1.2 to 1.6 kg) largely occupies the right upper quadrant of the abdomen. The costal margin coincides with the lower margin of the liver, and the diaphragm drapes over the superior surface of the liver. The large majority of the right liver and most of the left liver are covered by the thoracic cage. The posterior surface straddles the inferior vena cava (IVC). A wedge of liver extends to the left side of the abdomen. The liver is invested in peritoneum except for the gallbladder fossa, porta hepatis, and posterior aspect of the liver on either side of the IVC in two wedge-shaped areas. The region of liver to the right of the IVC is called the bare area of the liver. The peritoneal duplications on the liver surface are referred to as ligaments. The diaphragmatic peritoneal duplications are referred to as the coronary ligaments, whose lateral margins on either side are the right and left triangular ligaments. From the center of the coronary ligament emerges the falciform ligament, which extends anteriorly as a thin membrane connecting the liver surface to the diaphragm, abdominal wall, and umbilicus.

The ligamentum teres (the obliterated umbilical vein) runs along the inferior edge of the falciform ligament from the umbilicus to the umbilical fissure. The umbilical fissure is on the inferior surface of the left liver and contains the left portal pedicle. In early descriptions of hepatic anatomy, the falciform ligament, the most obvious surface marker of the liver, was used as the division of the right and left lobes of the liver. However, this description is inaccurate and of minimal usefulness to the hepatobiliary surgeon (see later for detailed segmental anatomy). On the posterior surface of the left liver, running from the left portal vein in the porta hepatis toward the left hepatic vein and the IVC is the ligamentum venosum (obliterated sinus venosus) that also runs in a fissure (Fig. 53-1). Hepatic arterial blood and portal venous blood enter the liver at the hilum and branch throughout the liver as a single portal pedicle unit, which also includes a bile duct. These portal triads are invested in a peritoneal sheath that invaginates at the hepatic hilum. Venous drainage is through the right, middle, and left hepatic veins that empty directly into the suprahepatic IVC.

Normal development and embryology. The developing liver shares a common progenitor with the biliary tree and pancreas. During embryogenesis, signals are transmitted from the cardiac mesenchyme and septum transversum. The molecules regulating this (e.g., fibroblast growth factor, bone morphogenetic protein, Wnt) have begun to be elucidated. The liver primordium begins to form in the third week of development as an outgrowth of endodermal epithelium, known as the hepatic diverticulum or liver bud. The connection between the hepatic diverticulum and the future duodenum narrows to form the bile duct, and an outpouching of the bile duct forms into the gallbladder and cystic duct. Hepatic cells develop cords and intermingle with the vitelline and umbilical veins to form hepatic sinusoids.

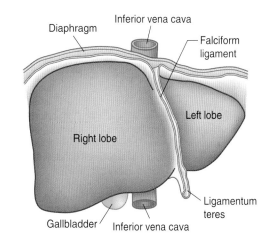

A

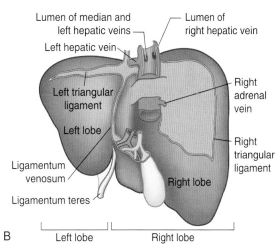

B

FIGURE 53-1 A, Historically, the liver was divided into right and left lobes by the external marking of the falciform ligament. On the inferior surface of the falciform ligament, the ligamentum teres can be seen entering the umbilical fissure. **B,** The posterior and inferior surface of the liver is shown. The liver embraces the IVC posteriorly in a groove. The lumens of the three major hepatic veins and right adrenal vein can be seen directly entering the IVC. The bare area, bounded by the right and left triangular ligaments, is illustrated. To the left of the IVC is the caudate lobe, which is bounded on its left side by a fissure containing the ligamentum venosum. The lesser omentum terminates along the edge of the ligamentum venosum, and thus the caudate lobe lies within the lesser sac and the rest of the liver lies in the supracolic compartment. A layer of fibrous tissue can be seen bridging the right lobe to the caudate lobe posterior to the IVC, thus encircling it. This ligament of tissue must be divided on the right side in mobilizing the right liver off the IVC. (From Blumgart LH, Hann LE: Surgical and radiologic anatomy of the liver and biliary tract. In Blumgart LH, Fong Y, editors: *Surgery of the liver and biliary tract*, London, 2000, WB Saunders, pp 3–34.)

Simultaneously, hematopoietic cells, Kupffer cells, and connective tissue form from the mesoderm of the septum transversum. The mesoderm of the septum transversum connects the liver to the ventral abdominal wall and foregut. As the liver protrudes into the abdominal cavity, these structures are stretched into thin membranes, ultimately forming the falciform ligament and lesser omentum. The mesoderm on the surface of the developing liver differentiates into visceral peritoneum, except superiorly, where contact between the liver and mesoderm (future diaphragm) is maintained, forming a bare area devoid of visceral peritoneum (Fig. 53-2).

The primitive liver plays a central role in the fetal circulation. The vitelline veins carry blood from the yolk sac to the sinus venosus and ultimately form a network of veins around the foregut (future duodenum) that drain into the developing hepatic sinusoids. These vitelline veins eventually fuse to form the portal, superior mesenteric, and splenic veins. The sinus venosus, which empties into the fetal heart, becomes the hepatocardiac channel and then the hepatic veins and retrohepatic IVC. The umbilical veins, which are paired early on, carry oxygenated blood to the fetus. Initially, the umbilical veins drain into the sinus venosus, but at week 5 of development, they begin to drain into the hepatic sinusoids. The right umbilical vein ultimately disappears, and the left umbilical vein later drains directly into the hepatocardiac channel, bypassing the hepatic sinusoids through the ductus venosus. In the adult liver, the remnant of the left umbilical vein becomes the ligamentum teres, which runs in the falciform ligament into the umbilical fissure, and the remnant of the ductus venosus becomes the ligamentum venosum at the termination of the lesser omentum under the left liver (Fig. 53-3).

The adult liver is a complex system of numerous cell types, including hepatocytes, cholangiocytes, neuroendocrine cells, hepatic progenitors (known as oval cells), myofibroblastic

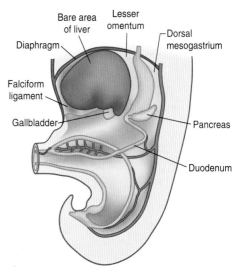

FIGURE 53-2 An approximately 36-day-old embryo is shown. The extensions of the septum transversum can be seen developing as the liver protrudes into the abdominal cavity, stretching out and forming the lesser omentum and the falciform ligament. The liver is completely invested in visceral peritoneum, except for a portion next to the diaphragm known as the bare area. (From Sadler TW: *Langman's medical embryology*, ed 5, Baltimore, 1985, Williams & Wilkins.)

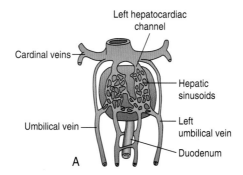

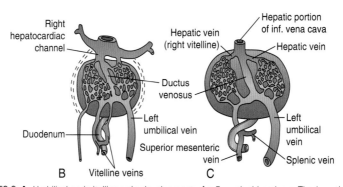

FIGURE 53-3 A, Umbilical and vitelline vein development of a 5-week-old embryo. The hepatic sinusoids have developed, and although there are channels that bypass these sinusoids, the vitelline and umbilical veins are beginning to drain into them. **B,** In the second month, the vitelline veins drain directly into the hepatic sinusoids. The ductus venosus has formed and accepts oxygenated blood from the left umbilical vein, bypasses the hepatic sinusoids, and directly enters the hepatocardiac channel. **C,** By the third month, the vitelline veins have formed into the portal system (splenic, superior mesenteric, and portal veins). The right umbilical vein has disappeared, and the left umbilical vein (future ligamentum teres) drains into the sinus venosus, bypassing the hepatic sinusoids. Note the development of the IVC and hepatic veins. (From Sadler TW: *Langman's medical embryology*, ed 5, Baltimore, 1985, Williams & Wilkins.)

mesenchymal cells (known as hepatic stellate cells and portal myofibroblasts), resident macrophages (known as Kupffer cells), and vascular endothelial cells.

Functional Anatomy

Historically, the liver was divided into left and right lobes by the obvious external landmark of the falciform ligament. Not only was this description oversimplified, but it was anatomically incorrect in relation to the blood supply to the liver. Our understanding of functional liver anatomy has become more sophisticated.

The functional anatomy of the liver (Figs. 53-4 and 53-5) is composed of eight segments, each supplied by a single portal triad

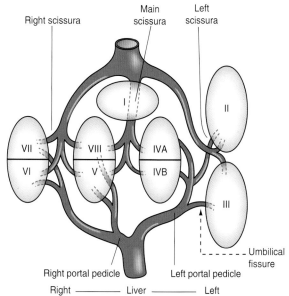

FIGURE 53-4 Schematic Depiction of the Segmental Anatomy of the Liver. Each segment receives its own portal pedicle (triad of portal vein, hepatic artery, and bile duct). The eight segments are illustrated, and the four sectors, divided by the three main hepatic veins running in scissurae, are shown. The umbilical fissure (not a scissura) is shown to contain the left portal pedicle. (From Blumgart LH, Hann LE: Surgical and radiologic anatomy of the liver and biliary tract. In Blumgart LH, Fong Y, editors: *Surgery of the liver and biliary tract*, London, 2000, WB Saunders, pp 3–34.)

(also called a pedicle) composed of a portal vein, hepatic artery, and bile duct. These segments are further organized into four sectors separated by scissurae containing the three main hepatic veins. The four sectors are even further organized into the right and left liver. The terms *right liver* and *left liver* are preferable to the terms *right lobe* and *left lobe* because there is no external mark that allows the identification of the right and left liver. This system was originally described in 1957 by Goldsmith and Woodburne and by Couinaud. It defines hepatic anatomy because it is most relevant to surgery of the liver. The functional anatomy is more often seen as cross-sectional imaging (Fig. 53-6).

The main scissura contains the middle hepatic vein, which runs in an anteroposterior direction from the gallbladder fossa to the left side of the vena cava. It divides the liver into right and left hemilivers. The line of the main scissura is also known as Cantlie line. The right liver is divided into anterior (segments V and VIII) and posterior (segments VI and VII) sectors by the right scissura, which contains the right hepatic vein. The right portal pedicle is composed of the right hepatic artery, portal vein, and bile duct. It splits into right anterior and right posterior pedicles, which supply the segments of the anterior and posterior sectors.

The left liver has a visible fissure along its inferior surface called the umbilical fissure. The ligamentum teres, containing the remnant of the umbilical vein, runs into this fissure. The falciform ligament is contiguous with the umbilical fissure and ligamentum teres. The umbilical fissure is not a scissura and does not contain a hepatic vein; it contains the left portal pedicle, which contains the left portal vein, hepatic artery, and bile duct. This pedicle runs in this fissure and branches to feed the left liver. The left liver is split into anterior (segments III and IV) and posterior (segment II, the only sector composed of a single segment) sectors by the left scissura. The left scissura runs posterior to the ligamentum teres and contains the left hepatic vein.

At the hilum of the liver, the right portal triad has a short extrahepatic course of approximately 1 to 1.5 cm before entering the substance of the liver and branching into anterior and posterior sectoral branches. The left portal triad, however, has a long extrahepatic course of up to 3 to 4 cm and runs transversely along the base of segment IV in a peritoneal sheath, which is the upper end of the lesser omentum. This connective tissue is known as the hilar plate (Fig. 53-7). The continuation of the left portal triad runs anteriorly and caudally in the umbilical fissure and gives branches to segments II and III and recurrent branches to segment IV.

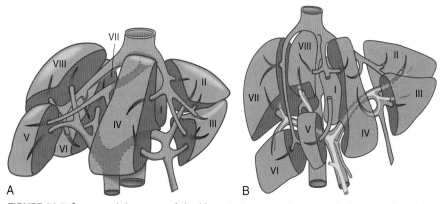

FIGURE 53-5 Segmental Anatomy of the Liver. **A,** As seen at laparotomy in the anatomic position. **B,** In the ex vivo position. (From Blumgart LH, Hann LE: Surgical and radiologic anatomy of the liver and biliary tract. In Blumgart LH, Fong Y, editors: *Surgery of the liver and biliary tract*, London, 2000, WB Saunders, pp 3–34.)

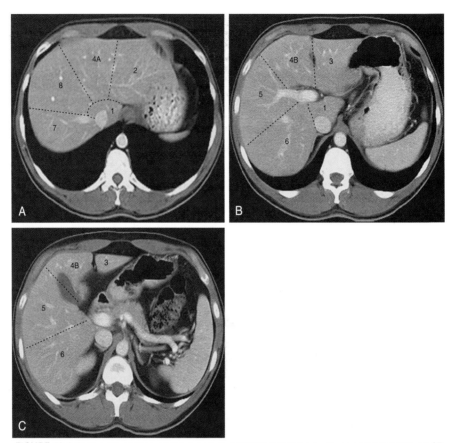

FIGURE 53-6 Segmental anatomy of the liver is demonstrated at three levels on contrast-enhanced CT images. **A,** At the level of the hepatic veins, the caudate lobe (segment 1) is seen posteriorly embracing the vena cava. Segment 2 is separated from segment 4A by the left hepatic vein. Segment 4A is separated from segment 8 by the middle hepatic vein, and segment 8 is separated from segment 7 by the right hepatic vein. **B,** At the level of the portal vein bifurcation, segment 3 is visible as it hangs inferiorly in its anatomic position and is separated from segment 4B by the umbilical fissure. Note that segment 2 is not visible at this level. Terminal branches of the middle hepatic vein separate segment 4B from segment 5, and terminal branches of the right hepatic vein separate segment 5 from segment 6. Note that segments 4A, 8, and 7 are not visible at this level. Segment 1 is seen posterior to the portal vein and embracing the vena cava. **C,** Below the portal bifurcation, one can see the inferior tips of segments 3 and 4B. The terminal branches of the middle hepatic vein and the gallbladder mark the separation of segment 4B from segment 5. Segments 5 and 6 are separated by the distal branches of the right hepatic vein. Note how the right liver hangs well inferior to the left liver.

The caudate lobe (segment I) is the dorsal portion of the liver. It embraces the IVC on its posterior surface and lies posterior to the left portal triad inferiorly and the left and middle hepatic veins superiorly. The main bulk of the caudate lobe is to the left of the IVC, but inferiorly it traverses between the IVC and left portal triad, where it fuses to the right liver (segments VI and VII). This part of the caudate lobe is known as the right portion or the caudate process. The left portion of the caudate lobe lies in the lesser omental bursa and is covered anteriorly by the gastrohepatic ligament (lesser omentum) that separates it from segments II and III anteriorly. The gastrohepatic ligament attaches to the ligamentum venosum (sinus venosus remnant) along the left side of the left portal triad (Fig. 53-8).

The vascular inflow and biliary drainage to the caudate lobe come from both the right and left pedicles. The right side of the caudate, the caudate process, largely derives its portal venous supply from the right portal vein or the bifurcation of the main portal vein. The left portion of the caudate derives its portal

venous inflow from the left main portal vein. The arterial supply and biliary drainage are generally through the right posterior pedicle system for the right portion and through the left main pedicle for the left portion. The hepatic venous drainage of the caudate is unique because a number of posterior small veins drain directly into the IVC.

The posterior edge of the left side of the caudate terminates as a fibrous component that attaches to the crura of the diaphragm and also runs posteriorly, wrapping behind the IVC and attaching to segment VII of the right liver. In up to 50% of people, this fibrous component is composed partially or completely of liver parenchyma. Thus, liver tissue may completely encircle the IVC. This structure is known as the caval ligament and is important to recognize in mobilizing the right liver or the caudate lobe off the vena cava.

Anomalous development of the liver is uncommonly encountered. Complete absence of the left liver has been reported. A tongue of tissue extending inferiorly off the right liver has been

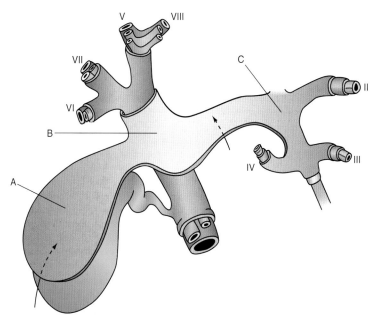

FIGURE 53-7 The plate system: the cystic plate between the gallbladder and liver (A); the hilar plate at the biliary confluence at the base of segment IV (B); and the umbilical plate above the umbilical portion of the portal vein (C). Shown are the plane of dissection of the cystic plate for cholecystectomy and the hilar plate for exposure of the hepatic duct confluence and main left hepatic duct *(arrows)*. (From Blumgart LH, Hann LE: Surgical and radiologic anatomy of the liver and biliary tract. In Blumgart LH, Fong Y, editors: *Surgery of the liver and biliary tract*, London, 2000, WB Saunders, pp 3–34.)

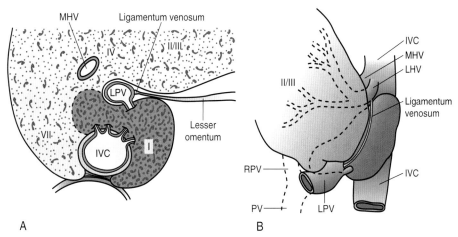

A   B

FIGURE 53-8 **Anatomy of the Caudate Lobe (Segment I). A,** Seen in cross section, most of the caudate is to the left of the IVC and lies posterior to the lesser omentum, which separates the caudate from segments II and III. The termination of the lesser omentum at the ligamentum venosum is demonstrated. The caudate lobe traverses to the right, insinuating itself between the IVC and the left portal vein (LPV), where it attaches to the right liver. Note the proximity of the middle hepatic vein (MHV) to these structures. **B,** Segments II and III have been rotated to the patient's right, exposing the left side of the caudate. (From Blumgart LH, Hann LE: Surgical and radiologic anatomy of the liver and biliary tract. In Blumgart LH, Fong Y, editors: *Surgery of the liver and biliary tract*, London, 2000, WB Saunders, pp 3–34.)

described (Riedel lobe). Rare cases of supradiaphragmatic liver in the absence of a hernia sac have been noted.

Portal vein. The portal vein provides approximately 75% of the hepatic blood inflow. Despite being postcapillary and largely deoxygenated, its high flow rate provides 50% to 70% of the liver's oxygen requirement. The lack of valves in the portal venous system provides a system that can accommodate high flow at low pressure. This also allows the measurement of portal venous pressure at any point along the system.

The portal vein forms behind the neck of the pancreas at the confluence of the superior mesenteric vein and the splenic vein. The length of the main portal vein ranges from 5.5 to 8 cm, and its diameter is usually approximately 1 cm. Cephalad to its formation behind the neck of the pancreas, the portal vein runs behind the first portion of the duodenum and into the hepatoduodenal ligament, where it runs along the right border of the lesser omentum, usually posterior to the common bile duct and proper hepatic artery.

The portal vein divides into main right and left branches at the hilum of the liver. The left branch of the portal vein runs transversely along the base of segment IV and into the umbilical fissure, where it gives off branches to segments II and III and feedback branches to segment IV. The left portal vein also gives off posterior branches to the left side of the caudate lobe. The right portal vein has a short extrahepatic course; it usually enters the substance of the liver, where it splits into anterior and posterior sectoral branches. These sectoral branches can occasionally be seen extrahepatically and can come off the main portal vein before its bifurcation. There is usually a small caudate process branch off the main right portal vein or at the right portal vein bifurcation that comes off posteriorly to supply this portion of liver (Fig. 53-9).

There are a number of connections between the portal and systemic venous systems. Under conditions of high portal venous pressure, these portosystemic connections may enlarge secondarily to collateral flow. This concept is reviewed in more detail later in the chapter, but the most significant portosystemic collateral locations are the following: the submucosal veins of the proximal stomach and distal esophagus receive portal flow from the short gastric veins and the left gastric vein and can result in varices, with the potential for hemorrhage; the umbilical and abdominal wall veins recanalize from flow through the umbilical vein in the ligamentum teres, resulting in caput medusae; the superior hemorrhoidal plexus receives portal flow from inferior mesenteric vein tributaries and can form large hemorrhoids; and other retroperitoneal communications yield collaterals that can make abdominal surgery hazardous.

The anatomy of the portal vein and its branches is relatively constant and has much less variation than the biliary ductal and hepatic arterial systems. The portal vein is rarely found anterior to the neck of the pancreas and duodenum. Entrance of the portal vein directly into the vena cava has also been described. Very rarely, a pulmonary vein may enter the portal vein. Finally, there may be a congenital absence of the left branch of the portal vein. In this situation, the right branch courses through the right liver and curves around peripherally to supply the left liver, or the right anterior sectoral vein can arise from the left portal vein.

Hepatic artery. The hepatic artery, representing high-volume oxygenated systemic arterial flow, provides approximately 25% of the hepatic blood flow and 30% to 50% of its oxygenation. The common description of the arterial supply to the liver and biliary tree is present only approximately 60% of the time (Fig. 53-10). The celiac trunk originates directly off the aorta, just below the aortic diaphragmatic hiatus, and gives off three branches—splenic artery, left gastric artery, and common hepatic artery. The common hepatic artery passes forward and to the right along the superior

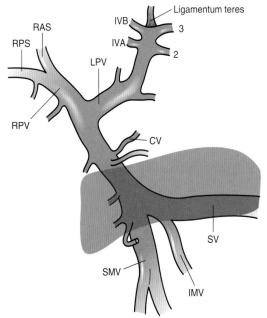

FIGURE 53-9 **Anatomy of the Portal Vein.** The superior mesenteric vein (SMV) joins the splenic vein (SV) posterior to the neck of the pancreas *(shaded area)* to form the portal vein. Note the entrance of the inferior mesenteric vein (IMV) into the splenic vein, the most common anatomic arrangement. In its course superiorly in the edge of the lesser omentum posterior to the common bile duct and hepatic artery, the portal vein receives venous effluent from the coronary vein (CV). At the hepatic hilum, the portal vein bifurcates into a larger right portal vein (RPV) and a smaller left portal vein (LPV). The LPV runs transversely at the base of segment IV and enters the umbilical fissure to supply the segments of the left liver. Just before the umbilical fissure, the LPV usually gives off a sizable branch to the caudate lobe. The RPV enters the substance of the liver and splits into right anterior sectoral (RAS) and right posterior sectoral (RPS) branches. It also gives off a posterior branch to the right side of the caudate lobe–caudate process. (From Blumgart LH, Hann LE: Surgical and radiologic anatomy of the liver and biliary tract. In Blumgart LH, Fong Y, editors: *Surgery of the liver and biliary tract*, London, 2000, WB Saunders, pp 3–34.)

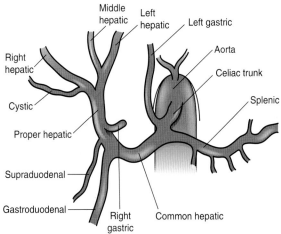

FIGURE 53-10 **Most Common Anatomy of the Celiac Axis and Hepatic Arterial System.** The celiac axis, just below the diaphragmatic hiatus, trifurcates into the splenic, left gastric, and common hepatic arteries. The common hepatic artery heads to the right and turns superiorly toward the hilum. At the point of this turn, the gastroduodenal artery is given off, and the proper hepatic artery is formed. The common hepatic artery gives off right and left hepatic arteries in the hilum. Note the middle hepatic artery off the proximal left hepatic artery, which goes on to supply segment IV. The cystic artery usually comes off the right hepatic artery within the triangle of Calot. (From Blumgart LH, Hann LE: Surgical and radiologic anatomy of the liver and biliary tract. In Blumgart LH, Fong Y, editors: *Surgery of the liver and biliary tract*, London, 2000, WB Saunders, pp 3–34.)

border of the pancreas and runs along the right side of the lesser omentum, where it ascends toward the hepatic hilum, lying anterior to the portal vein and to the left of the bile duct. At the point where the common hepatic artery begins to head superiorly toward the hepatic hilum, it gives off the gastroduodenal artery, followed by the supraduodenal artery and right gastric artery. The common hepatic artery beyond the takeoff of the gastroduodenal is called the proper hepatic artery; it divides into right and left hepatic arteries at the hilum. The left hepatic artery heads vertically toward the umbilical fissure to supply segments II, III, and IV. The left hepatic artery usually also gives off a middle hepatic artery branch that heads toward the right side of the umbilical fissure and supplies segment IV. The right hepatic artery usually runs posterior to the common hepatic bile duct and enters Calot triangle, bordered by the cystic duct, common hepatic duct, and liver edge, where it gives off the cystic artery to supply the gallbladder and then continues into the substance of the right liver.

Unlike portal vein anatomy, hepatic arterial anatomy is extraordinarily variable (Fig. 53-11). An accessory vessel is described as an aberrant origin of a branch that is in addition to the normal branching pattern. A replaced vessel is described as an aberrant origin of a branch that substitutes for the lack of the normal branch. The hepatic artery usually originates off the celiac trunk. However, branches or the entire hepatic arterial system can originate off the superior mesenteric artery (SMA). The right and left hepatic arteries can also arise separately off the celiac axis. Replaced or accessory right hepatic arteries come off the SMA and are present approximately 11% to 21% of the time. Hepatic vessels replaced to the SMA run behind the head of the pancreas, posterior to the portal vein in the portacaval space. The right hepatic artery, in its usual branching pattern, can also course anterior to the common hepatic duct. A replaced or accessory left hepatic artery is present approximately 3.8% to 10% of the time, originates from the left gastric artery, and courses within the lesser omentum, heading toward the umbilical fissure. Other important variations include the origin of the gastroduodenal artery, which has been found to originate from the right hepatic artery and is occasionally duplicated. The anatomy of the cystic artery is also variable; knowledge of these variations is of particular importance in the performance of cholecystectomy (Fig. 53-12). An accessory cystic artery can originate from the proper hepatic artery or gastroduodenal artery, where it runs anterior to the bile duct. A single cystic artery can originate anywhere off the proper hepatic artery or gastroduodenal artery or directly from the celiac axis. These variant cystic arteries can run anterior to the bile duct and are not necessarily present in the triangle of Calot. All these variations in hepatic arterial anatomy are of obvious importance during hepatic resection, hepatic arterial pump placement, cholecystectomy, and hepatic interventional radiologic procedures.

Hepatic veins. The three major hepatic veins drain from the superior-posterior surface of the liver directly into the IVC (see Figs. 53-4 to 53-6). The right hepatic vein runs in the right scissura between the anterior and posterior sectors of the right liver and drains most of the right liver after a short (1-cm) extrahepatic course into the right side of the IVC. The left and middle hepatic veins usually join intrahepatically and enter the left side of the IVC as a single vessel, although they may drain separately. The left hepatic vein runs in the left scissura between segments II and III and drains segments II and III; the middle hepatic vein runs in the portal scissura between segment IV and the anterior sector of the right liver, composed of segments V and VIII, and drains segment IV and some of the anterior sector of the right liver. The

umbilical vein is an additional vein that runs under the falciform ligament, between the left and middle veins, and usually empties into the left hepatic vein. A number of small posterior venous branches from the right posterior sector and caudate lobe drain directly into the IVC. A substantial inferiorly located accessory right hepatic vein is commonly encountered. There is also often a venous tributary from the caudate lobe that drains superiorly into the left hepatic vein.

Biliary system. The intrahepatic bile ducts are the terminal branches of the right and left hepatic ductal branches that invaginate Glisson capsule at the hilum, along with their corresponding portal vein and hepatic artery branches, forming the peritoneal covered portal triads also known as portal pedicles. Along these intrahepatic portal pedicles, the bile duct branches are usually superior to the portal vein, whereas the hepatic artery branches run inferiorly. The left hepatic bile duct drains segments II, III, and IV, which constitute the left liver. The intrahepatic ductal branches of the left liver join to form the main left duct at the base of the umbilical fissure, where the left hepatic duct courses transversely across the base of segment IV to join the right hepatic duct at the hilum. In its transverse portion, the left hepatic duct drains one to three small branches from segment IV. The right hepatic duct drains the right liver and is formed by the joining of the anterior sectoral duct (draining segments V and VIII) and the posterior sectoral duct (draining segments VI and VII). The posterior sectoral duct runs in a horizontal and posterior direction; the anterior sectoral duct runs vertically. The main right hepatic duct bifurcates just above the right portal vein. The short right hepatic duct meets the longer left hepatic duct to form the confluence anterior to the right portal vein, constituting the common hepatic duct. The caudate lobe (segment I) has its own biliary drainage, which is usually through right and left systems. However, in up to 15% of individuals, drainage is through the left system only, and in 5%, it is through the right system only.

The common hepatic duct drains inferiorly. Below the takeoff of the cystic duct, it is referred to as the common bile duct. The common bile duct usually measures 10 to 15 cm in length and is typically 6 mm in diameter. The common hepatic (bile) duct runs along the right side of the hepatoduodenal ligament (free edge of the lesser omentum) to the right of the hepatic artery and anterior to the portal vein. The common bile duct continues inferiorly behind the first portion of the duodenum and into the head of the pancreas in an inferior and slightly rightward direction. The intrapancreatic distal common bile duct then joins with the main pancreatic duct (of Wirsung), with or without a common channel, and enters the second portion of the duodenum through the major papilla of Vater. At the choledochoduodenal junction, a complex muscular complex known as the sphincter of Oddi regulates bile flow and prevents reflux of duodenal contents into the biliary tree. There are three major parts to this sphincter: (1) the sphincter choledochus, which is a circular muscle that regulates bile flow and the filling of the gallbladder; (2) the pancreatic sphincter, present to variable degrees, which surrounds the intraduodenal pancreatic duct; and (3) the sphincter ampullae, made up of longitudinal muscle, which prevents duodenal reflux.

The gallbladder is a biliary reservoir that lies against the inferior surface of segments IV and V of the liver, usually making an impression against the liver. A peritoneal layer covers most of the gallbladder, except for the portion adherent to the liver. Here, the gallbladder adheres to the liver by a layer of fibroconnective tissue known as the cystic plate, an extension of the hilar plate (see Fig. 53-7). Variable in size but usually about 10 cm long and 3 to

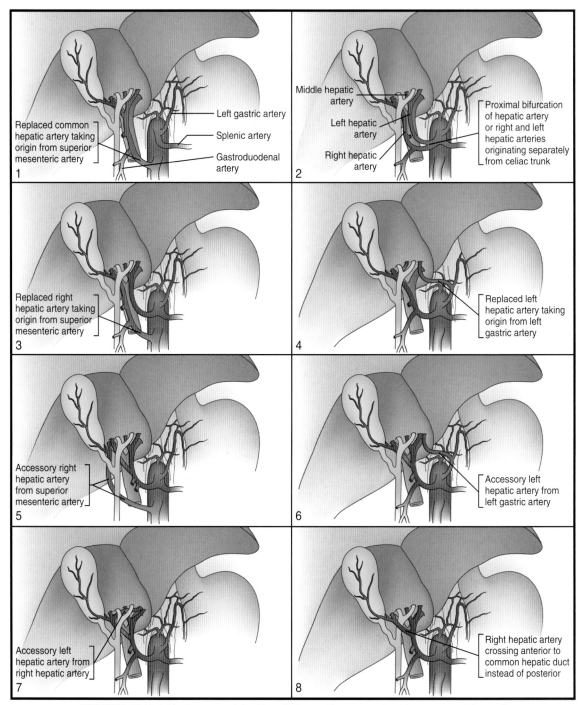

1 Replaced common hepatic artery taking origin from superior mesenteric artery

Left gastric artery

Splenic artery

Gastroduodenal artery

2 Middle hepatic artery

Left hepatic artery

Right hepatic artery

Proximal bifurcation of hepatic artery or right and left hepatic arteries originating separately from celiac trunk

3 Replaced right hepatic artery taking origin from superior mesenteric artery

4 Replaced left hepatic artery taking origin from left gastric artery

5 Accessory right hepatic artery from superior mesenteric artery

6 Accessory left hepatic artery from left gastric artery

7 Accessory left hepatic artery from right hepatic artery

8 Right hepatic artery crossing anterior to common hepatic duct instead of posterior

FIGURE 53-11 **Variable Anatomy of the Hepatic Artery.** The common hepatic artery can originate off the SMA instead of the celiac axis. A replaced or accessory right hepatic artery comes off the SMA and runs posterior to the head of the pancreas, to the right of the portal vein, and behind the common bile duct into the hilum. A replaced or accessory left hepatic artery originates off the left gastric artery and runs through the lesser omentum into the umbilical fissure. (From Netter FH: Netter anatomy collection. *www.netterimages.com.* © Elsevier Inc. All rights reserved.)

5 cm wide, the gallbladder is composed of a fundus, body, infundibulum, and neck, which ultimately empty into the cystic duct. The fundus usually projects just slightly beyond the liver edge anteriorly; when it is folded on itself, it is described as a phrygian cap. Continuing toward the bile duct, the body of the gallbladder is usually close to the second portion of the duodenum and transverse colon. The infundibulum (or Hartmann pouch) hangs forward along the free edge of the lesser omentum and can fold in front of the cystic duct. The portion of gallbladder between the infundibulum and cystic duct is referred to as the neck. The cystic

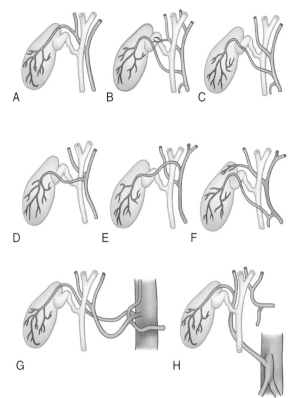

FIGURE 53-12 Variations in the Anatomy of the Cystic Artery. A, Most common anatomy. B, Double cystic artery, one off the proper hepatic artery. C, Origin off the proper hepatic artery and coursing anterior to the bile duct. D, Originating off the right hepatic artery and coursing anterior to the bile duct. E, Originating from the left hepatic artery and coursing anterior to the bile duct. F, Originating off the gastroduodenal artery. G, Originating off the celiac axis. H, Originating from a replaced right hepatic artery. (From Blumgart LH, Hann LE: Surgical and radiologic anatomy of the liver and biliary tract. In Blumgart LH, Fong Y, editors: *Surgery of the liver and biliary tract*, London, 2000, WB Saunders, pp 3–34.)

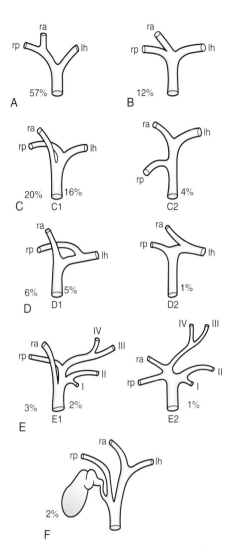

FIGURE 53-13 Variations of the Hepatic Duct Confluence. A, Most common anatomy. B, Trifurcation at the confluence. C, Either of the right sectoral ducts drains into the common hepatic duct. D, Either of the right sectoral ducts drains into the left hepatic duct. E, Absence of a hepatic duct confluence. F, Absence of right hepatic duct and drainage of right posterior sectoral duct into the cystic duct. (From Blumgart LH, Hann LE: Surgical and radiologic anatomy of the liver and biliary tract. In Blumgart LH, Fong Y, editors: *Surgery of the liver and biliary tract*, London, 2000, WB Saunders, pp 3–34.)

duct is variable in its length, course, and insertion into the main biliary tree. The first portion of the cystic duct is usually tortuous and contains mucosal duplications, referred to as the folds of Heister, which regulate the filling and emptying of the gallbladder. The cystic duct usually joins the common hepatic duct to form the common bile duct.

Knowledge of the multiple and frequent variations in the anatomy of the biliary tree is absolutely essential for performing hepatobiliary procedures. Anomalies of the hepatic ductal confluence are common and are present approximately one third of the time. The most common anomalies of the biliary confluence involve variations in the insertion of the right sectoral ducts. Usually, this is the posterior sectoral duct. The confluence can be a trifurcation of the right anterior sectoral, right posterior sectoral, and left hepatic ducts. Either of the right sectoral ducts can drain into the left hepatic duct, the common hepatic duct, the cystic duct, or, rarely, the gallbladder (Fig. 53-13).

Anomalies of the gallbladder itself are rare. Agenesis of the gallbladder, bilobar gallbladder with two ducts or a single duct, septations, and congenital diverticulum of the gallbladder have been described. Anomalies of the position of the gallbladder are more common; these include an intrahepatic position and, rarely,

location on the left side of the liver. The gallbladder can also have a long mesentery, which can predispose it to torsion.

The position and entry of the cystic duct into the main ductal system are also variable. Double cystic ducts draining a unilocular gallbladder and drainage into hepatic duct branches have been reported. The cystic duct usually joins the common hepatic duct at an angle; but it can run parallel and enter it more distally, and in this situation, the cystic duct can be fused to the hepatic duct along its parallel course by connective tissue. The cystic duct can also run a spiral course anteriorly or posteriorly and enter the left side of the common hepatic duct. Finally, the cystic duct can be very short or even absent (Fig. 53-14).

The supraduodenal and infrahilar bile ducts are predominantly supplied by two axial vessels that run at 3- and 9-o'clock positions.

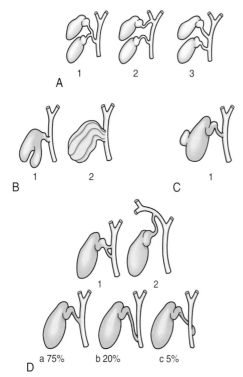

FIGURE 53-14 Variations in the Anatomy of the Gallbladder and Cystic Duct. **A,** Bilobar gallbladder. **B,** Septations of the gallbladder. **C,** Diverticulum of the gallbladder. **D,** Variations in cystic duct anatomy. The three types of union of the cystic duct and common hepatic duct are illustrated. (From Blumgart LH, Hann LE: Surgical and radiologic anatomy of the liver and biliary tract. In Blumgart LH, Fong Y, editors: *Surgery of the liver and biliary tract*, London, 2000, WB Saunders, pp 3–34.)

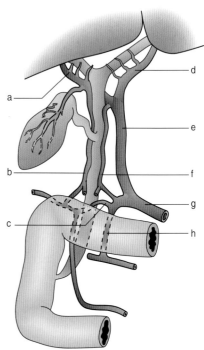

FIGURE 53-15 The blood supply to the common bile duct and common hepatic duct is illustrated: right hepatic artery (a); 9:00 artery (b); retroduodenal artery (c); left hepatic artery (d); proper hepatic artery (e); 3:00 artery (f); common hepatic artery (g); gastroduodenal artery (h). (From Blumgart LH, Hann LE: Surgical and radiologic anatomy of the liver and biliary tract. In Blumgart LH, Fong Y, editors: *Surgery of the liver and biliary tract*, London, 2000, WB Saunders, pp 3–34.)

These vessels are derived from the superior pancreaticoduodenal, right hepatic, cystic, gastroduodenal, and retroduodenal arteries. It has been estimated that only 2% of the arterial supply to this portion of the bile duct is segmental, arising directly off the proper hepatic artery. The bile duct and its bifurcation in the hilum derive their arterial blood supply from a rich network of multiple small branches from surrounding vessels. Similarly, the retropancreatic bile duct derives its arterial supply from the retroduodenal artery, which provides a rich network of multiple small branches (Fig. 53-15). Venous drainage of the bile duct parallels the arterial supply and drains into the portal venous system. The venous drainage of the gallbladder empties into the veins that drain the bile duct and does not flow directly into the portal vein.

Nerves. The innervation of the liver and biliary tract is through sympathetic fibers originating from T7 through T10 as well as parasympathetic fibers from both vagal nerves. The sympathetic fibers pass through celiac ganglia before giving off postganglionic fibers to the liver and bile ducts. The right-sided celiac ganglia and right vagal nerve form an anterior hepatic plexus of nerves that runs along the hepatic artery. The left-sided celiac ganglia and left vagal nerve form a posterior hepatic plexus that runs posterior to the bile duct and portal vein. The hepatic arteries are supplied by sympathetic fibers, whereas the gallbladder and extrahepatic bile ducts receive innervation from sympathetic and parasympathetic fibers. The clinical significance of these nerves is still not well understood. Acute distention of the liver, and thus the liver

capsule, can result in right upper quadrant pain, which may be referred to the right shoulder through phrenic nerve innervation of the diaphragmatic peritoneum.

Lymphatics. Most lymph node drainage from the liver is to the hepatoduodenal ligament. From here, lymphatic drainage usually continues along the hepatic artery to the celiac lymph nodes and then to the cisterna chyli. Lymphatic drainage can also follow the hepatic veins to lymph nodes in the area of the suprahepatic IVC and through the diaphragmatic hiatus. The lymphatic drainage of the gallbladder and most of the extrahepatic biliary tract is generally into the lymph nodes of the hepatoduodenal ligament. This drainage may follow along the hepatic artery to the celiac lymph nodes, but it can also flow into lymph nodes behind the head of the pancreas or within the aortocaval groove.

Microscopic Anatomy

Functional unit of the liver. The organization of hepatic parenchyma into microscopic functional units has been described in a number of ways, referred to as an acinus or a lobule (Fig. 53-16). This was originally described by Rappaport and then modified by Matsumoto and Kawakami. A lobule is made up of a central terminal hepatic venule surrounded by four to six terminal portal triads that form a polygonal unit. This unit is lined on its periphery between each terminal portal triad by terminal portal triad branches. In between the terminal portal triads and the central hepatic venule, hepatocytes are arranged in one-cell-thick plates, surrounded on each side by endothelium-lined and blood-filled sinusoids. Blood flows from the terminal portal triad through the

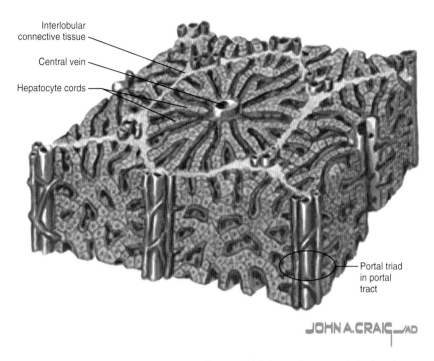

Interlobular connective tissue

Central vein

Hepatocyte cords

Portal triad in portal tract

JOHN A.CRAIG—AD

Hepatic Lobule. Liver arranged as series of hexagonal lobules, each composed of series of hepatocyte cords (plates) interspersed with sinusoids. Each lobule surrounds a central vein and is bounded by 6 peripheral portal triads (low magnification).

FIGURE 53-16 Schematic illustration of a hepatic lobule seen as a three-dimensional polyhedral unit. The terminal portal triads (hepatic artery, portal vein, and bile duct) are at each corner and give off branches along the sides of the lobule. Hepatocytes are in single-cell sheets with sinusoids on either end aligned radially toward a central hepatic venule. (From Netter FH: Netter anatomy collection. *www.netterimages.com.* © Elsevier Inc. All rights reserved.)

sinusoids into the terminal hepatic venule. Bile is formed within the hepatocytes and empties into terminal canaliculi, which form on the lateral walls of the intercellular hepatocyte. These ultimately coalesce into bile ducts and flow toward the portal triads. This functional hepatic unit provides a structural basis for the many metabolic and secretory functions of the liver.

Between the terminal portal triad and central hepatic venule are three zones that differ in their enzymatic makeup as well as exposure to nutrients and oxygenated blood. There is debate about the shape of these zones and their relationship to the basic lobular unit, but in general, zones 1 through 3 splay out from the terminal portal triad toward the central hepatic venule. Zone 1 (periportal zone) is an environment rich in nutrients and oxygen. Zone 2 (intermediate zone) and zone 3 (perivenular zone) are exposed to environments that are poorer in oxygen and nutrients. The cells of the different zones differ enzymatically and respond differently to toxin exposure and hypoxia. This anatomic arrangement also explains the phenomenon of centrilobular necrosis from hypotension because zone 3 is the most susceptible to decreases in oxygen delivery.

Hepatic microcirculation. Terminal portal venous and hepatic arterial branches directly supply the hepatic sinusoids with blood. The portal branches provide a constant but minimal flow into this low-volume system; the arterial branches provide the sinusoids with pulsatile but low-volume flow that enhances flow in the sinusoids. Hepatic arterial branches terminate in a plexus around the terminal bile ductules and provide nutrients. Arterial and portal vein flow varies inversely in the sinusoids and can be

compensatory. Local control of blood flow in the sinusoids likely depends on arteriolar sphincters and contraction of the sinusoidal lining by endothelial cells and hepatic stellate cells or portal myofibroblasts. Blood within the sinusoids empties directly into terminal hepatic venules at the center of a functional lobule. This process results in the unidirectional flow of blood in the liver from zone 1 to zone 3.

The endothelium-lined sinusoids of the hepatic lobule represent the functional unit of the liver, where afferent blood flow is exposed to functional hepatic parenchyma before being drained into hepatic venules (Fig. 53-17). The hepatic sinusoids are 7 to 15 μm wide but can increase in size by up to 10-fold. This yields a low-resistance and low-pressure (generally 2 to 3 mm Hg) system. The sinusoidal endothelial cells account for 15% to 20% of the total hepatic cell mass.

Sinusoidal endothelial cells are separated from hepatocytes by the space of Disse (perisinusoidal space). This is an extravascular fluid compartment into which hepatocytes project microvilli, which allows proteins and other plasma components from the sinusoids to be taken up by the hepatocytes. Within this space, the endothelial cells are specialized in that they lack intercellular junctions and a basement membrane but contain multiple large fenestrations. This arrangement provides for the maximal contact of hepatocyte membranes with this extravascular fluid compartment and blood in the sinusoidal space. Thus, this system permits bidirectional movement of solutes (high- and low-molecular-weight substances) into and out of hepatocytes, providing tremendous filtration potential. On the other hand, the fenestrations of

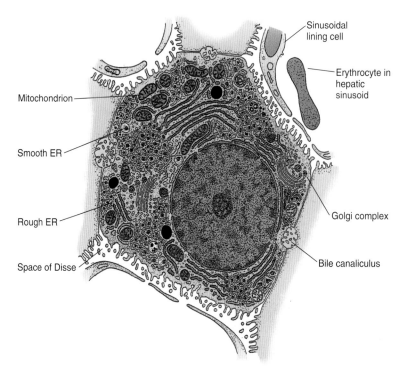

FIGURE 53-17 A hepatocyte and its sinusoidal and lateral domains. *ER*, endoplasmic reticulum. (From Ross MH, Reith EJ, Romrell LJ. The liver. In Ross RH, Reith EJ, Romrell LJ: *Histology: A text and atlas*, Baltimore, 1989, Williams & Wilkins, pp 471–478.)

the endothelial cells restrict movement of molecules between the sinusoids and hepatocytes and vary in response to exogenous and endogenous mediators.

Other cell types are found along the sinusoidal lining. Kupffer cells, derived from the macrophage-monocyte system, are irregularly shaped cells that also line the sinusoids insinuating between endothelial cells. Kupffer cells are phagocytic, can migrate along sinusoids to areas of injury, and play a major role in the trapping of foreign substances and initiating inflammatory responses. Major histocompatibility complex II antigens are expressed on Kupffer cells but do not confer efficient antigen presentation compared with macrophages elsewhere in the body. Other lymphoid cells also exist in hepatic parenchyma, such as natural killer, natural killer T, CD4 T, and CD8 T cells. These provide the liver with an innate immune system. Hepatic stellate cells, previously known as Ito cells, are cells high in retinoid content (accounting for their phenotypic identification) found in the space of Disse. They have dendritic processes that contact hepatocyte microvilli and also wrap around endothelial cells. The major functions of these stellate cells include vitamin A storage and the synthesis of extracellular collagen and other extracellular matrix proteins. In acute and chronic hepatic liver injuries, hepatic stellate cells are activated to a myofibroblastic state associated with morphologic changes, cellular contractility, decreases in intracellular vitamin A, and production of extracellular matrix. Ultimately, stellate cells play a central role in the development and progression of hepatic fibrosis to cirrhosis and are the target for the development of antifibrotic treatments.

Hepatocytes. Hepatocytes are complex multifunctional cells that make up 60% of the hepatic cellular mass and 80% of the cytoplasmic mass of the liver (Fig. 53-17). The hepatocyte is a

polyhedral cell with a central spherical nucleus. As noted, hepatocytes are arranged in single-cell-layer plates lined on either side by blood-filled sinusoids. Every hepatocyte has contact with adjacent hepatocytes, the biliary space (bile canaliculus), and the perisinusoidal space, enabling these cells to perform their broad range of functions. Among the many essential functions of the hepatocyte are the following: uptake, storage, and release of nutrients; synthesis of glucose, fatty acids, lipids, and numerous plasma proteins (including C-reactive protein and albumin); production and secretion of bile for digestion of dietary fats; and degradation and detoxification of toxins.

To carry out these functions, the plasma membrane of the hepatocyte is organized in a specific manner into three specific domains. The sinusoidal membrane is exposed to the space of Disse and has multiple microvilli that provide a surface specialized in the active transport of substances between the blood and hepatocytes. The lateral domain exists between neighboring hepatocytes and contains gap junctions that provide for intercellular communication. The canalicular membrane is a tube containing microvilli formed by two apposed hepatocytes. These bile canaliculi are sealed by zonula occludens (tight junctions), which prevent the escape of bile. The bile canaliculi form a ring around the hepatocyte that drains into small bile ducts known as canals of Hering, which empty into a bile duct at a portal triad. The canalicular membrane contains adenosine triphosphate (ATP)–dependent active transport systems that enable solutes to be secreted into the canalicular membrane against large concentration gradients.

The hepatocyte is one of the most diverse and metabolically active cells in the body, as reflected by its abundance of organelles. There are 1000 mitochondria/hepatocyte, occupying approximately 20% of the cell volume. Mitochondria generate energy

(ATP) through oxidative phosphorylation and provide the energy for the metabolic demands of the hepatocyte. The hepatocyte mitochondria are also essential for fatty acid oxidation. The monoclonal antibody HepPar1 (hepatocyte paraffin 1) identifies a unique antigen on hepatocyte mitochondria and is widely used to identify hepatocytes or hepatocellular neoplasms on immunohistochemical examination.

An extensive system of interconnected membrane complexes made up of smooth and rough endoplasmic reticulum and the Golgi apparatus compose what is known as the hepatocyte microsomal fraction. These complexes have a diverse range of functions, including the following: synthesis of structural and secreted proteins; metabolism of lipids and glucose; production and metabolism of cholesterol; glycosylation of secretory proteins; bile formation and secretion; and drug metabolism. Finally, hepatocytes also contain lysosomes, which are intracellular single-membrane vesicles that contain a number of enzymes. These vesicles store and degrade exogenous and endogenous substances. Coordination of these numerous organelles in the hepatocyte allows these cells to accomplish a large variety of functions.

Functions

The unique anatomic arrangement of the liver provides a remarkable landscape on which the multiple central and critical functions of this organ can be carried out. The liver is the center of metabolic homeostasis; it serves as the regulatory site for energy metabolism by coordinating the uptake, processing, and distribution of nutrients and their subsequent energy products. The liver also synthesizes a large number of proteins, enzymes, and vitamins that participate in a tremendously broad range of body functions. Finally, the liver detoxifies and eliminates many exogenous and endogenous substances, serving as the major filter of the human body. The following sections summarize this broad range of functions.

Energy

The liver is the critical intermediary between dietary sources of energy and the extrahepatic tissues that require this energy. The liver receives dietary byproducts through the portal circulation and sorts, metabolizes, and distributes them into the systemic circulation. The liver also plays a major role in regulating endogenous sources of energy, such as fatty acids and glycerol from adipose tissues and lactate, pyruvate, and certain amino acids from skeletal muscle. The two major sources of energy that the liver releases into the extrahepatic circulation are glucose and acetoacetate. Glucose is derived from the glycogenolysis of stored glycogen and from gluconeogenesis from lactate, pyruvate, glycerol, propionate, and alanine. Acetoacetate is derived from the β-oxidation of fatty acids. Also, storage lipids such as triacylglycerols and phospholipids are synthesized and stored as lipoproteins by the liver. These can be circulated systemically for uptake by peripheral tissues. These complex and essential functions are regulated by hormones, overall nutritional state of the organism, and requirements of obligate glucose-requiring tissues.

Functional Heterogeneity

To add to the metabolic complexity of the liver, hepatocytes vary in their function, depending on their location within the lobule. This functional heterogeneity of hepatocytes is anatomically related to their location in the three zones of the lobule and is specifically related to the distance from the incoming portal triad. For example, cells located in the periportal zone (zone 1)

are exposed to a high concentration of substrates. Thus, uptake of oxygen and solutes is greater here. A critically important function of hepatocytes, however, is their ability to change their metabolic functionality and to be recruited to perform specific functions under varying physiologic conditions, regardless of anatomic location. Sinusoids in the periportal zone are narrower and more tortuous, facilitating increased uptake of substrate by the hepatocytes in this area. In contrast, sinusoids in zone 3 (perivenous) have larger fenestrations, allowing uptake of larger molecules. Thus, sinusoids are also variable in form and function.

Enzymatic makeup, plasma membrane proteins, and ultrastructure are also heterogeneous among the hepatocyte population. This cellular protein variability can also be distinguished on the basis of the hepatocyte location within the lobule. Glucose uptake and release, bile formation, and synthesis of albumin and fibrinogen take place in the periportal zone, whereas glucose catabolism, xenobiotic metabolism, and synthesis of α_1-antitrypsin and α-fetoprotein (AFP) occur in the perivenous zone. Another example of enzymatic heterogeneity according to lobular zones is the location of the urea cycle enzymes in zone 3, adjacent to the terminal hepatic veins. The functional hepatocyte heterogeneity and its anatomic relationship to the lobular unit account for patterns of damage from metabolic or physiologic insults to the liver.

Blood Flow

There is a dual blood supply to the liver that comes from the portal vein and hepatic artery. The portal vein provides approximately 75% of the blood flow to the liver, which is oxygen poor but rich in nutrients. The hepatic artery provides the other 25% of the blood flow, which is oxygen rich and represents systemic arterial blood flow. The large flow rate of the portal vein is still able to provide 50% to 70% of the afferent oxygenation to the liver. Overall, hepatic blood flow represents about 25% of the cardiac output, demonstrating its central role in whole body metabolism. Hepatic blood flow is decreased during exercise and increased after ingestion of food. Carbohydrates have the most profound effect on hepatic blood flow. Hepatic arterial pressure is representative of systemic arterial pressure. Portal pressure is generally 6 to 10 mm Hg, and sinusoidal pressure is usually 2 to 4 mm Hg.

Hepatic blood flow is regulated by various factors. Differences in afferent and efferent vessel pressures as well as muscular sphincters located at the inlet and outlet of the sinusoids play a major role. Muscular sphincter tone is regulated by the autonomic nervous system, circulating hormones, bile salts, and metabolites. Specific endogenous factors known to affect hepatic blood flow include glucagon, histamine, bradykinin, prostaglandins, nitric oxide, and many gut hormones, including gastrin, secretin, and cholecystokinin. The sinusoids are also the primary regulators of hepatic blood flow through contraction and expansion of their endothelial cells, Kupffer cells, and hepatic stellate cells.

A one-way reciprocal relationship between hepatic artery and portal vein flow has been demonstrated. Increases in hepatic arterial flow accompany decreases in portal vein flow, but the opposite does not occur. Hepatic arterial compensation, however, cannot provide complete compensation to support hepatic parenchyma in total portal vein occlusion, which is likely the cause of ipsilateral atrophy in this case. Experimental evidence has suggested that the buildup of adenosine in the liver plays an important role in this hepatic arterial compensatory response.

Bile Formation

One of the major functions of the liver is bile production and secretion. The physiologic role of bile is twofold. The first is to dispose of substances secreted into bile; the second is to provide enteric bile salts to aid in the digestion of fats. Bile is a substance containing organic and inorganic solutes produced by an active process of secretion and subsequent concentration of these solutes. The concentration of inorganic solutes in bile in the main biliary tree resembles that of plasma (Table 53-1). In the case of bile loss (e.g., from an external biliary fistula), the high concentrations of protein and electrolytes must be considered in replacing the losses. The osmolality of bile is approximately 300 mOsmol/kg and is accounted for by the inorganic solutes. The major organic solutes in bile are bile acids, bile pigments, cholesterol, and phospholipids.

The contents of bile are generally absorbed from the bloodstream through sinusoids into the hepatocyte through the sinusoidal membrane. Bile is initially secreted by hepatocytes into the canaliculi through specialized microvilli containing lateral membranes of the hepatocytes that form the canaliculi. Tight junctions along the canalicular membranes prevent leakage of bile in the normal state. This also provides a route for paracellular secretion of solutes and water into bile. The canaliculi coalesce into larger bile ductules containing biliary epithelium, which then form the intrahepatic and extrahepatic biliary tree. Thus, the liver, in part, serves as an epithelial structure that moves solutes from the blood to the bile and provides a route of secretion for bile into the intestines.

Approximately 1500 mL of bile is secreted daily, and much of this (≈80%) is secreted by hepatocytes into canaliculi. Such canalicular bile flow is largely the result of water flow in response to active solute transport. Bile acids are transported from the sinusoidal blood into the hepatocyte by ATP-requiring active transport. Intracellular transport to the canalicular membrane is through bile acid–binding proteins that are transported by a vesicular system derived from the Golgi apparatus. The bile acids are then actively pumped into the canaliculus through an ATP-requiring active transport system. It is well recognized that bile flow has a linear association with bile acid secretion, known as bile acid–dependent flow. Because bile acids form micelles in the bile and do not provide osmotic potential, it is likely that flow related to bile acid secretion is secondary to ions that accompany the bile acids (counterions). Bile flow can also occur in the near-absence of bile acid secretion, known as bile acid–independent flow. Experimental evidence has suggested that bile acid–independent flow is at least partially the result of biliary glutathione secretion.

Once bile has passed from the canaliculi to the biliary ductules and then to main bile ducts, bile undergoes further reabsorption and secretion. The epithelial cells of the biliary tract actively reabsorb and secrete water and electrolytes. Secretion is generally through a chloride channel activated by secretin, its most powerful activator, and its subsequent activation of cyclic adenosine monophosphate production. There is usually a net secretion of water and electrolytes, accounting for the other 20% of biliary secretion. Ultimately, bile becomes highly enriched in bicarbonate ions. Many organic substances, such as glutathione, are degraded in the biliary tree. Many drugs can be secreted into the biliary tree in a highly concentrated form (e.g., ceftriaxone). The gallbladder acts as the reservoir of the biliary tree; its function is to store bile in the fasting state. The gallbladder reabsorbs water, concentrating stored bile, and secretes mucin. Contraction of the gallbladder is mediated hormonally, largely through cholecystokinin, in response to a meal, with the simultaneous relaxation of the sphincter of Oddi and release of bile into the duodenum.

Enterohepatic Circulation

Bile salts are primarily produced in the liver and secreted to be used in the biliary tree and intestine. The primary bile salts cholic acid and chenodeoxycholic acid are produced in the liver from cholesterol and subsequently conjugated with glycine or taurine in the hepatocyte. Once secreted in the gut, the primary bile acids are modified by intestinal bacteria to form the secondary bile acids deoxycholic acid and lithocholic acid. Bile acids are reabsorbed passively into the jejunum and actively into the ileum. Thus, the bile acids reenter the portal venous system, and up to 90% of the bile acids are extracted by hepatocytes. Only a small fraction spills over into the systemic circulation because of efficient hepatic extraction, which accounts for low levels of plasma bile acids. After hepatic extraction, bile acids are recirculated into the canaliculi and back into the biliary tree, completing the circuit. A small amount of intestinal bile acids is not absorbed by the portal system and is excreted in the stool. Thus, the active secretion of bile salts from hepatocytes into bile and from ileal enterocytes into the portal vein is the engine behind the enterohepatic circulation.

The enterohepatic circulation is more than a unique mechanism for reusing physiologically valuable bile acids. This circulation of bile constitutes the major mechanism for eliminating excess cholesterol because cholesterol is consumed during the production of bile salts and is excreted in the feces by mixed micelles formed by organic biliary solutes. Bile salts also play a critical role in the absorption of dietary fats, fat-soluble vitamins (i.e., vitamins A, D, E, and K), and lipophilic drugs. Water movement from hepatocytes into bile and water absorption through the small bowel are also regulated by bile salts. The enterohepatic circulation is therefore central to a number of solubilization, transport, and regulatory functions.

Bilirubin Metabolism

Bilirubin is the result of heme breakdown. An early phase of heme breakdown, accounting for 20% of bilirubin, is from hemoproteins (heme-containing enzymes) and occurs within 3 days of labeling with radioactive heme. A late phase of heme breakdown, accounting for 80% of bilirubin, is from senescent red blood cells. This occurs approximately 110 days after administration of radioactive labeled heme and is consistent with the life span of red

TABLE 53-1	Solute Concentrations of Hepatic Bile		
SOLUTE	**CONCENTRATION**
Na^+	132-165 mEq/L
K^+	4.2-5.6 mEq/L
Ca^{2+}	1.2-4.8 mEq/L
Mg^{2+}	1.4-3.0 mEq/L
Cl^-	96-126 mEq/L
HCO_3^-	17-55 mEq/L
Bile acids	3-45 mM
Phospholipid	25-810 mg/dL
Cholesterol	60-320 mg/dL
Protein	300-3000 mg/L

blood cells. Heme is initially broken down into a green biliverdin by heme oxygenase, which is then broken down into the orange bilirubin by biliverdin reductase.

Circulating bilirubin is bound to albumin, which protects many organs from the potentially toxic effects of this compound. The bilirubin-albumin complex enters hepatic sinusoidal blood, where it enters the space of Disse through the large sinusoidal fenestrations. The bilirubin-albumin complex is disassociated in this space. Free bilirubin is internalized into the hepatocyte, where it is conjugated to glucuronic acid. Conjugated bilirubin is then secreted in an energy-dependent fashion into canalicular bile against a large concentration gradient. Bilirubin is secreted with bile into the gastrointestinal tract. Within the gastrointestinal tract, bilirubin is deconjugated by intestinal bacteria to a group of compounds known as urobilinogens. These urobilinogens are further oxidized and reabsorbed into the enterohepatic circulation and secreted into bile. A small percentage of the reabsorbed urobilinogens is excreted into urine. These oxidized urobilinogens account for the colored compounds that contribute to the yellow color of urine and the brown color of stool.

Bilirubin has long been known to be a toxic compound and is the agent responsible for neonatal encephalopathy and cochlear damage secondary to severe unconjugated hyperbilirubinemia (kernicterus). The binding of serum bilirubin to albumin protects the tissues from exposure to bilirubin. However, binding sites can be overwhelmed by increasing amounts of bilirubin or displaced by other binding agents (e.g., various drugs). The mechanism of bilirubin toxicity appears to be related to a number of its effects. Free bilirubin can uncouple oxidative phosphorylation, inhibit ATPases, decrease glucose metabolism, and inhibit a broad spectrum of protein kinase activities.

Portosystemic shunts, such as those seen with cirrhosis and portal hypertension, decrease the first-pass hepatic clearance of bilirubin, resulting in a mildly increased serum unconjugated hyperbilirubinemia. A number of disorders can result in an unconjugated serum hyperbilirubinemia, including neonatal hyperbilirubinemia, an increased bilirubin load caused by hemolytic syndromes, and inherited enzymatic deficiencies such as Crigler-Najjar and Gilbert syndromes. Disorders presenting with serum conjugated hyperbilirubinemia include cholestasis, Dubin-Johnson, and Rotor syndromes.

Carbohydrate Metabolism

The liver is the center of carbohydrate metabolism because it is the major regulator of storage and distribution of glucose to the peripheral tissues and, in particular, to glucose-dependent tissues such as the brain and erythrocytes. Both liver and muscle are capable of storing glucose in the form of glycogen, but only the liver can break down glycogen to provide glucose for systemic circulation. Glycogen that is broken down can be used only in muscle and is therefore not a source of systemically circulated glucose.

In the fed state, carbohydrate absorbed through the intestines (mostly glucose) is circulated systemically. Carbohydrates reaching the liver are rapidly converted to glycogen for storage. The liver contains up to 65 g of glycogen per kilogram of liver tissue. Excess carbohydrate is mostly converted to fatty acids and stored in adipose tissue. In the postabsorptive state (between meals, nonfasting), there is no further systemic glucose coming directly from the gut, and the liver becomes the primary source of circulating glucose by the breakdown of glycogen. This is crucial for the brain and erythrocytes, which rely on glucose for their

metabolism. In the postabsorptive state, most other tissues begin to rely on fatty acids derived from adipose tissue as their primary fuel. Highly active muscle may deplete its own glycogen and depend on liver-derived glucose for its substrate in the postabsorptive state. After 48 hours of fasting, hepatic glycogen is depleted and the liver shifts from glycogenolysis to gluconeogenesis. The substrate for hepatic gluconeogenesis is mostly from amino acids (mainly alanine) derived from muscle breakdown, but they also come from glycerol derived from adipose breakdown. During a prolonged fast, fatty acids from adipose breakdown are β-oxidized in the liver, which releases ketone bodies that then become the primary fuel for the brain.

Transition in and out of these various metabolic states and regulation of carbohydrate metabolism are mostly influenced by glucose concentration in sinusoidal blood and hormonal influences (e.g., insulin, catecholamines, glucagon). In the fasting state, during anaerobic metabolism, lactate is produced, largely from muscle. The liver uses this lactate, which is converted to pyruvate that enters into the gluconeogenic pathways to produce glucose. This cycle is known as the Cori cycle.

Derangements of carbohydrate metabolism are common in liver disease. Cirrhotics often demonstrate abnormal glucose tolerance. Its mechanism is not completely clear but is probably related to associated insulin resistance. This phenomenon is not caused by shunting of glucose-containing blood away from the liver. Hypoglycemia is a distinctly uncommon entity in chronic liver disease because of the remarkable resilience of the liver and its metabolic function. Only with massive hepatocyte loss in fulminant hepatic failure does gluconeogenesis fail and hypoglycemia ensue.

Lipid Metabolism

Fatty acids are synthesized in the liver during states of glucose excess, when the liver's ability to store glycogen has been exceeded. Adipocytes have a limited ability to synthesize fatty acids. Therefore, the liver is the predominant source of synthesized fatty acids, although they are largely stored in adipose tissue. During lipolysis, free fatty acids are transported to the liver, where they are metabolized. Fatty acids in the liver undergo esterification with glycerol to form triglycerides for storage or transportation, or they undergo β-oxidation, yielding energy in the form of ATP and ketone bodies. In general, this process is regulated by the nutritional state; starvation favors oxidation, and the fed state favors esterification.

There is a constant cycling of fatty acids between the liver and adipose tissue that is under a delicate balance, which can easily be offset, resulting in fatty infiltration of the liver. A few factors influence this balance; for example, hepatic uptake of fatty acids is a function of plasma concentrations. Although there is no limit to the liver's ability to esterify fatty acids, its ability to dispose of or to break down fatty acids is limited, as is its ability to secrete triglycerides in the form of lipoproteins. Therefore, conditions of increased circulating fatty acids can easily override the liver's ability to handle them, resulting in fatty accumulation in the liver. This is known as steatosis or, when it is associated with chronic inflammation in more advanced cases, steatohepatitis. A number of conditions have been associated with hepatic steatosis, such as diabetes, steroid use, starvation, obesity, and extensive administration of cytotoxic chemotherapeutic agents. Fatty liver associated with alcohol intake has a number of causes; it is related to increased lipolysis, reduced oxygenation, and augmented esterification of hepatic fatty acids and may also be related to relative starvation in the chronic alcoholic.

Protein Metabolism

The liver is also a central site for the metabolism of proteins and is involved in synthesis of protein, catabolism of proteins into energy or storage forms, and management of excess amino acids and nitrogen waste. Ingested protein is broken down into amino acids that are circulated throughout the body, where they are used as the building blocks for proteins, enzymes, and hormones. Excess amino acids not used in peripheral tissues are generally handled by the liver, in which they are oxidized for energy—providing 50% of the liver's energy needs—or converted into glucose, ketone bodies, or fats. When amino acids are catabolized for energy production throughout the body, ammonia, glutamine, glutamate, and aspartate are produced. These products are largely processed in the liver, where the waste nitrogen is converted to urea through the urea cycle, and the urea is generally excreted in the urine. Thus, the liver is central and critical to the body's nitrogen balance and amino acid metabolism.

Although the liver can catabolize most amino acids, yielding energy or other storable energy forms such as glucose and fats, notable exceptions are the branched-chain amino acids. Branched-chain amino acids cannot be catabolized in the liver and are mostly dealt with by muscle. It has been postulated that this may act as a so-called safety net that helps spare the liver some of the demands of protein and amino acid metabolism.

The liver also is the main site of synthesis for many proteins involved in such wide-ranging and critical functions as coagulation, transport, copper and iron binding, and protease inhibition. These proteins include ceruloplasmin, iron storage and binding proteins, and α_1-antitrypsin. Albumin is made exclusively in the liver and is the predominant serum binding protein. Hepatic insufficiency or specific genetic abnormalities can result in altered amounts and functions of these proteins, with wide-ranging pathologic effects.

The liver is also responsible for the so-called acute-phase response, a synthetic response by protein to trauma or infection. Its purpose is to restrict organ damage, to maintain vital hepatic function, and to control defense mechanisms. The response is incited by proinflammatory cytokines such as interleukin-1 (IL-1), IL-6, and tumor necrosis factor, which induce acute-phase protein gene expression in the liver. Some of the well-known hepatic acute-phase proteins are α_1-, α_2-, and β-globulin as well as C-reactive protein and serum amyloid A. An equally important part of this response is its termination. Anti-inflammatory cytokines such as IL-1 receptor antagonist, IL-4, and IL-10 appear to play important roles. The acute-phase response is usually completed in 24 to 48 hours but, in the context of ongoing injury, can be prolonged.

Vitamin Metabolism

Along with the intestine, the liver is responsible for the metabolism of the fat-soluble vitamins A, D, E, and K. These vitamins are obtained exogenously and absorbed in the intestine. Their adequate intestinal absorption is critically dependent on adequate fatty acid micellization, which requires bile acids.

Vitamin A is from the retinoid family and is involved in normal vision, embryonic development, and adult gene regulation. Storage of vitamin A is solely in the liver and occurs in the hepatic stellate cells. Overingestion of vitamin A can result in hepatic toxicity. Vitamin D is involved in calcium and phosphorus homeostasis. One of vitamin D's activation steps (25-hydroxylation) occurs in the liver. Vitamin E is a potent antioxidant and protects membranes from lipid peroxidation and free radical formation. Finally, vitamin K is a critical cofactor in the post-translational γ-carboxylation of the hepatically synthesized coagulation factors II, VII, IX, and X as well as of protein C and protein S, the so-called vitamin K–dependent cofactors. Cholestasis syndromes can result in the inadequate absorption of these vitamins secondary to poor micellization in the intestine. The associated vitamin deficiency syndromes, such as metabolic bone disease (vitamin D deficiency), neurologic disorders (vitamin E deficiency), and coagulopathy (vitamin K deficiency), can subsequently occur.

The liver is also involved in the uptake, storage, and metabolism of a number of water-soluble vitamins, including thiamine, riboflavin, vitamin B_6, vitamin B_{12}, folate, biotin, and pantothenic acid. The liver is responsible for converting some of these water-soluble vitamins to active coenzymes, transforming some to storage metabolites, and using some for enterohepatic circulation (e.g., vitamin B_{12}).

Coagulation

The liver is responsible for synthesizing almost all the identified coagulation factors as well as many of the fibrinolytic system components and several plasma regulatory proteins of coagulation and fibrinolysis. As noted, the liver is critical for the absorption of vitamin K, synthesizes the vitamin K–dependent coagulation factors, and contains the enzyme that activates these factors. Also, the reticuloendothelial system of the liver clears activated clotting factors, activated complexes of the coagulation and fibrinolytic systems, and end products of fibrin degradation. Diseases of the liver are often associated with thrombocytopenia, qualitative platelet abnormalities, vitamin K deficiency with impaired modulation of vitamin K–dependent coagulation factors, and disseminated intravascular coagulation. It is no surprise that liver disease is firmly associated with coagulation disorders that are often challenging to deal with.

Warfarin, one of the most commonly dispensed anticoagulants, acts in the liver by blocking vitamin K–dependent activation of factors II, VII, IX, and X. Factor VII has the shortest half-life of the coagulation factors; its deficiency is manifested clinically as abnormalities of the measured prothrombin time (PT) or international normalized ratio (INR). Patients with hepatic synthetic dysfunction similarly have an abnormal PT.

Metabolism of Drugs and Toxins (Xenobiotics)

The human body is exposed to an inordinate amount of foreign chemicals during a lifetime. This poses a challenge to our ability to detoxify and to eliminate these potentially harmful chemicals. Many of these chemicals are not incorporated into cellular metabolism and are referred to as xenobiotics. The liver plays a central role in handling them through an enormously complex and numerous set of enzymes and reaction pathways, which are increasingly recognized as new chemicals are discovered.

Hepatic-based reactions to xenobiotics are broadly classified into phase I and phase II reactions. Phase I reactions, through oxidation, reduction, and hydrolysis, increase the polarity and thus water solubility of compounds. This in turn allows easier excretion. Phase I reactions do not necessarily detoxify chemicals and may, in fact, create toxic metabolites. Phase I reactions occur in the cytochrome P450 (CYP) system. Phase II reactions generally act to create a less toxic or less active byproduct. This is generally accomplished through transferase reactions, in which a compound is usually coupled to a conjugate, rendering the xenobiotic more innocuous.

Regeneration

The liver possesses the unique quality of adjusting its volume to the needs of the body. This is observed clinically in its regeneration after partial hepatectomy or after toxic liver injury. It is also seen in liver transplantation, in that donor liver size mismatches adjust to the new host. This quality is highly conserved evolutionarily because of the critical functions of the liver and the fact that the liver is the first line of exposure to ingested toxic agents.

Liver regeneration is a hyperplastic response of all cell types of the liver, in which the microscopic anatomy of the functional liver is maintained. Much information that we have about the regenerative response of the liver is based on experimental evidence in rodents. Normally quiescent hepatocytes rapidly enter the cell cycle after partial hepatectomy. Maximal hepatocyte DNA synthesis occurs 24 to 36 hours after partial hepatectomy, and maximal DNA synthesis occurs in the other cell types by 48 to 72 hours later. Most of the increase in hepatic mass in rodents is seen by 3 days after partial hepatectomy, and it is usually almost complete after 7 days.

In the late 1960s, it was recognized that circulating factors were responsible, in part, for the regenerative response, and much research has focused on the humoral and genetic control of hepatic regeneration. The major circulating factors that have been identified, largely from rodent studies, are hepatocyte growth factor, epidermal growth factor, transforming growth factors, insulin, and glucagon and the cytokines tumor necrosis factor-α, IL-1, and IL-6. These factors, when infused into a normal host, do not result in hepatic growth, indicating that hepatocytes must be primed in some way before responding to these growth factors. Remarkable progress in the understanding of liver regeneration has been made because of the development of improved genetic and molecular biologic techniques. Hundreds of genes involved at all stages of regeneration have been identified by RNA microarray techniques. Also, numerous cytokine-dependent and growth factor–independent pathways have been further defined. A complete description is beyond the scope of this chapter, however, and many questions still remain.

Future Developments

The study of the liver and its physiology continues to be a remarkable and exciting field. As the fields of molecular biology and genetic manipulation have exploded, so has the field of hepatology. Given the lack of alternative options to transplantation for patients with end-stage liver failure, tissue engineering and attempts to provide exogenous hepatic functional support continue to be studied. Liver repopulation with transplanted cells—hepatocytes or hepatic progenitor and stem cells—may also provide future options for patients with liver failure. Although the identification of specific and reliable markers for hepatic stem cells has been elusive, the concepts of liver progenitors and stem cells and their potential usefulness for hepatic repopulation have gained acceptance, making this an exciting area of research. Ongoing genetic comparisons of normal and diseased liver using new molecular biology and cell biology techniques will provide clues about the genetic regulation of liver diseases. Great strides have been made in the effectiveness of gene therapy, and many groups continue to study liver-directed gene therapy strategies to treat acquired and inherited disorders. Ongoing molecular biology studies are researching hepatic cell cycle regulation, with implications for hepatocarcinogenesis. Research studies about the pathogenesis of hepatic fibrosis and, perhaps more exciting, reversal of this process are ongoing and likely to result in significant advances in the future.

Assessment of Liver Function

A wide variety of tests are available to evaluate hepatic diseases. Screening for hepatic disease, assessing hepatic function, diagnosing specific disorders, and prognosticating are critical in the management of hepatic disease. For the surgeon, assessment of hepatic function and estimation of the ability of a hepatic remnant to be sufficient after liver resection are also of obvious importance. Unfortunately, most measures of hepatic disease are gross indicators and lack sensitivity, specificity, and accuracy. We have divided these hepatic function tests into three categories—routine screening, specific diagnostic, and quantitative tests.

Routine Screening Tests

Screening blood tests are often used to determine whether there is disease in the hepatobiliary system. Standard liver function tests (LFTs) are generally not tests of function and are not always specific to hepatic disease. Nonetheless, they are valuable as a general screening tool that can provide basic indications to recognize the presence of hepatic disease and to yield clues about the cause of that disease. Total bilirubin, direct bilirubin (conjugated), and indirect bilirubin (unconjugated) levels can be affected by a number of processes related to bilirubin metabolism. Unconjugated hyperbilirubinemia can be a reflection of increased bilirubin production (e.g., hemolysis), drug effects, inherited enzymatic disorders, or physiologic jaundice of the newborn. Conjugated hyperbilirubinemia is generally a result of cholestasis or mechanical biliary obstruction but can also be seen in some inherited disorders or hepatocellular disease.

The transaminases alanine aminotransferase (ALT) and aspartate aminotransferase (AST) are the most common serum markers of hepatocellular necrosis, with subsequent leak of these intracellular enzymes into the circulation. AST is found in other organs, such as the heart, muscle, and kidney, but ALT is liver specific. However, the degree of elevation of these enzyme levels has never been shown to be of prognostic value. Alkaline phosphatase (ALP) is expressed in liver, bile ducts, bone, intestine, placenta, kidney, and leukocytes. Isoenzyme determinations can sometimes be helpful for distinguishing the source of an elevated ALP level. Elevations of ALP levels in hepatobiliary diseases are generally secondary to cholestasis or biliary obstruction. Such elevations are caused by increased production of this enzyme. The ALP level can also be increased in malignant disease of the liver. Gamma-glutamyl transpeptidase (GGT) is an enzyme in many organs in addition to the liver, such as the kidneys, seminal vesicles, spleen, pancreas, heart, and brain. Its level can be elevated in diseases affecting any of these tissues. It is also induced by alcohol intake and is elevated in biliary obstruction. Thus, it is also a nonspecific marker of liver disease but can be helpful in determining whether an elevated ALP level is from hepatic disease. 5′-Nucleotidase is also found in a wide variety of organs in addition to the liver, but increased levels are fairly specific to hepatic disease. Like GGT, it can be helpful in determining whether an elevated ALP level is secondary to hepatic disease.

Albumin is synthesized exclusively in the liver and can be used as a general measure of hepatic synthetic function. Because chronic malnutrition and acute injury or inflammation can decrease albumin synthesis, these factors must be taken into account in evaluating a low serum albumin level. Because of the remarkable protein synthetic capacity of the liver, hypoalbuminemia is a marker of severe liver disease. However, it lacks sensitivity, and large decreases in hepatic function are required to be reflected in albumin levels. In general, it is most helpful in chronic liver disease.

Clotting factors are largely synthesized in the liver; abnormalities of coagulation can be a marker of hepatic synthetic dysfunction. Measurement of specific clotting factors, such as factors V and VII, has been used to evaluate hepatic function in the transplantation population. PT or INR is the best test to measure the effects of hepatic disease on clotting, and prolonged PT or elevated INR is usually a marker of advanced chronic liver disease. Hepatic disease can also affect clotting through intravascular coagulation and vitamin K malabsorption.

Specific Diagnostic Tests

Once screening tests, along with clinical findings, have suggested liver disease, specific tests can be used to help elucidate the cause and to guide treatment, if necessary. Hepatitis serologies are important to determine the presence of viral hepatitis. Autoimmune antibodies are used to diagnose primary biliary cirrhosis (e.g., antimitochondrial), primary sclerosing cholangitis (e.g., antineutrophil), and autoimmune hepatitis. α_1-Antitrypsin and ceruloplasmin levels assist in the diagnosis of α_1-antitrypsin deficiency and Wilson disease, respectively. Tumor markers such as AFP and carcinoembryonic antigen (CEA) can be helpful in the diagnosis and management of primary and metastatic tumors of the liver.

In general, the LFTs discussed in this section are gross, nonspecific, and of little if any prognostic value. Many attempts have been made to formulate dynamic and quantitative tests of hepatic function based on the liver's ability to clear various exogenously administered substances. Despite many years of research, it still remains unclear whether these tests of hepatic function are any better than scoring systems derived from simple blood tests and clinical observations. For example, the aminopyrine breath test is based on CYP clearance of radiolabeled aminopyrine. A breath test measuring radiolabeled CO_2 as a breakdown product of aminopyrine is performed after administration at a specified time. The results largely depend on the functional hepatic mass, which is generally not depleted until end-stage liver disease has developed. There are varying results of studies comparing the aminopyrine breath test with standard LFTs and scoring systems; its main value appears to be prognosis in chronic liver disease, but it is clearly not an effective test to detect subclinical hepatic dysfunction.

Substances such as antipyrine and caffeine can evaluate liver function in a similar way, with similar results. The lidocaine clearance test yields similar information to the aminopyrine test because it is based on its clearance by the hepatic CYP test. Lidocaine clearance is dependent on blood flow and a complex distribution process, but measurement of one of its metabolites, monoethylglycinexylidide, has greatly simplified the test. It has been shown to have some prognostic value in the transplantation population. The galactose elimination test is based on the liver's role in phosphorylating galactose and converting it to glucose. The rate at which galactose is eliminated from the bloodstream can be used as a measure of hepatic function. Problems related to this test are that the enzymes involved are genetically heterogeneous, and considerable extrahepatic metabolism occurs. Also, multiple blood draws are necessary, which makes the test cumbersome. The value of this test is probably in assessing the prognosis of patients with chronic liver disease rather than in screening. Indocyanine green is a dye removed by the liver by a carrier-mediated process and excreted into bile. This dye is rapidly cleared from the bloodstream and is not metabolized. This is the only test that has been shown to have some prognostic ability in cirrhotic

TABLE 53-2	**Child-Pugh Classification**		
	NO. OF POINTS		
FACTOR	**1**	**2**	**3**
Bilirubin (mg/dL)	<2	2-3	>3
Albumin (g/dL)	>3.5	2.8-3.5	<2.8
Prothrombin time (increased seconds)	1-3	4-6	>6
Ascites	None	Slight	Moderate
Encephalopathy	None	Minimal	Advanced

Class A, 5-6 points; class B, 7-9 points; class C, 10-15 points.

patients undergoing liver resection, although this is not universally demonstrated in studies, nor is it universally accepted.

Quantitative Tests

A large number of scoring systems based on clinical observation and standard blood tests have been proposed. The most commonly used system is Pugh's modification of the Child score (Table 53-2). Although all these systems are less than perfect and not universally accepted, the Child-Pugh score is commonly used for cirrhotic patients who require liver surgery. Mortality and survival rates after hepatectomy have been shown to correlate with this score but are not always related to liver failure. Child-Pugh class B and C patients have higher perioperative mortality after any partial hepatectomy than Child-Pugh class A patients, who can generally withstand a major hepatectomy.[1,2] The presence of portal hypertension has been shown to predict poor outcome after partial hepatectomy. Portal hypertension in cirrhotic patients is usually manifested as thrombocytopenia, splenomegaly, and presence of intra-abdominal varices on imaging or at endoscopy. The best evidence for portal hypertension is a hepatic vein wedge pressure higher than 10 mm Hg, which has been shown to correlate strongly with postoperative liver failure.

PORTAL HYPERTENSION

Cirrhosis is the end result of a healing response initiated by chronic liver injury. Cirrhosis is characterized by development of fibrous septa surrounding regenerating hepatocellular nodules. Besides development of synthetic deficiencies, cirrhosis is associated with development of portal hypertension. At present, effective treatments for cirrhosis are nonexistent. As a result, its treatment has largely been focused on the treatment of resultant portal hypertension and its complications. The major challenge for the hepatologist or surgeon who is treating patients with cirrhosis and end-stage liver disease is determining when definitive treatment (e.g., liver transplantation) rather than palliative treatment (e.g., interventions to prevent recurrent variceal hemorrhage) should be applied.

Definition

Portal hypertension is defined by a portal pressure higher than 5 mm Hg. However, higher pressures (8 to 10 mm Hg) are typically required to begin stimulating the development of portosystemic collateralization. Collateral vessels usually develop where the portal and systemic venous circulations are in close apposition (Fig. 53-18). The collateral network through the coronary and short gastric veins to the azygos vein is clinically the most important because it results in formation of esophagogastric varices.

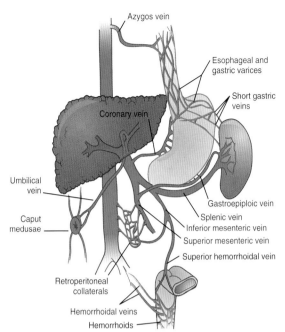

Azygos vein

Esophageal and
gastric varices

Short gastric
veins

Coronary vein

Umbilical
vein

Gastroepiploic vein
Splenic vein
Inferior mesenteric vein
Superior mesenteric vein

Caput
medusae

Superior hemorrhoidal vein

Retroperitoneal
collaterals

Hemorrhoidal veins
Hemorrhoids

FIGURE 53-18 Portosystemic collateral pathways develop where the portal venous and systemic venous systems are in close apposition. (From Rikkers LF: Portal hypertension. In Miller TA, editor: *Physiologic basis of modern surgical care,* St Louis, 1988, Mosby, pp 417–428.)

However, other sites include a recanalized umbilical vein from the left portal vein to the epigastric venous system (caput medusae), retroperitoneal collateral vessels, and the hemorrhoidal venous plexus. In addition to extrahepatic collateral vessels, a significant fraction of portal venous flow passes through anatomic and physiologic (e.g., capillarization of hepatic sinusoids) intrahepatic shunts. As hepatic portal perfusion decreases, hepatic arterial flow generally increases (buffer response).[2]

Pathophysiology

Portal hypertension usually occurs because of increased portal venous resistance that is prehepatic, intrahepatic, or posthepatic in location. Several factors may contribute to this, including the following: increased passive resistance secondary to fibrosis and regenerative nodules; increased hepatic vascular resistance caused by active vasoconstriction by norepinephrine, endothelin, and other humoral vasoconstrictors; and increased portal venous inflow secondary to a hyperdynamic systemic circulation and splanchnic hyperemia. The last one is a major contributor to the maintenance of portal hypertension as portal systemic collaterals develop. Unfortunately, the exact causes remain unknown, but splanchnic hormones, decreased sensitivity of the splanchnic vasculature to catecholamines, and increased production of nitrous oxide and prostacyclin may be involved. Understanding the pathophysiology of portal hypertension may have therapeutic implications because these factors may represent targets for treatment.

The most common cause of prehepatic portal hypertension is portal vein thrombosis. This accounts for approximately 50% of cases of portal hypertension in children. When the portal vein is thrombosed in the absence of liver disease, hepatopetal (to the liver) portal collateral vessels develop to restore portal perfusion.

This combination is termed cavernomatous transformation of the portal vein. Isolated splenic vein thrombosis (left-sided portal hypertension) is usually secondary to pancreatic inflammation or neoplasm. The result is gastrosplenic venous hypertension, with superior mesenteric and portal venous pressures remaining normal. The left gastroepiploic vein becomes a major collateral vessel, and gastric rather than esophageal varices develop. This variant of portal hypertension is important to recognize because it is easily reversed by splenectomy alone.

The site of increased resistance in intrahepatic portal hypertension may be at the presinusoidal, sinusoidal, or postsinusoidal level. Frequently, more than one level may be involved. The most common cause of intrahepatic presinusoidal hypertension is schistosomiasis. In addition, many causes of nonalcoholic cirrhosis result in presinusoidal portal hypertension. In contrast, alcoholic cirrhosis, the most common cause of portal hypertension in the United States, usually causes increased resistance to portal flow at the sinusoidal (secondary to deposition of collagen in the space of Disse) and postsinusoidal (secondary to regenerating nodules distorting small hepatic veins) levels.

Posthepatic or postsinusoidal causes of portal hypertension are rare; they include Budd-Chiari syndrome (hepatic vein thrombosis), constrictive pericarditis, and heart failure. Rarely, increased portal venous flow alone, secondary to massive splenomegaly (e.g., idiopathic portal hypertension) or a splanchnic arteriovenous fistula, causes portal hypertension.

Assessment of Chronic Liver Disease and Portal Hypertension

The key aspects of assessing a patient with suspected chronic liver disease or complications of portal hypertension are the following: diagnosis of the underlying liver disease; estimation of functional hepatic reserve; definition of portal venous anatomy and hepatic hemodynamic evaluation; and identification of the site of upper gastrointestinal hemorrhage, if present. These diagnostic categories take on varying degrees of importance, depending on the clinical situation. For example, estimation of functional hepatic reserve is useful in determining the risk associated with therapeutic intervention and whether definitive (e.g., hepatic transplantation) or palliative (e.g., endoscopic variceal ligation or a shunt procedure) treatment is indicated.

Variceal Hemorrhage

Bleeding from esophagogastric varices is the single most life-threatening complication of portal hypertension. It is responsible for approximately one third of all deaths in patients with cirrhosis. Approximately 50% of these deaths are caused by uncontrolled bleeding. The risk for death from bleeding is mainly related to the underlying hepatic functional reserve. Patients with extrahepatic portal venous obstruction and normal hepatic function rarely die of bleeding varices, whereas those with decompensated cirrhosis (e.g., Child-Pugh class C) may face a mortality rate in excess of 50%. Once bleeding is controlled, the greatest risk for rebleeding from varices is within the first few days after the onset of hemorrhage; the risk declines rapidly between that point and 6 weeks. Subsequently, the risk returns to the prehemorrhage rate.

Treatment

In a patient with upper gastrointestinal bleeding, general measures are instituted; these include securing the airway (especially in an encephalopathic patient), ensuring adequate access (two large-bore intravenous lines), fluid infusion, type and crossmatch of blood, and judicious blood and products transfusion. Therapy for portal hypertension and variceal bleeding has evolved over time and now encompasses a spectrum of treatment modalities, in which sequential therapies are often necessary.[3,4] For acutely bleeding patients with portal hypertension, nonoperative treatments are generally used as a first-line approach as these patients are high operative risks because of decompensated hepatic function. Endoscopic treatment (e.g., sclerosis or ligation) has become the mainstay of nonoperative treatment of acute hemorrhage because bleeding can be controlled in more than 85% of patients. This allows an interval of medical management for improvement of hepatic function, resolution of ascites and encephalopathy, and enhancement of nutrition before definitive treatment for prevention of recurrent bleeding is instituted. Pharmacotherapy can also be initiated, and trials have suggested that it may be as effective as endoscopic treatment. Balloon tamponade, which is infrequently used, can be lifesaving in patients with exsanguinating hemorrhage when other nonoperative methods are not successful. A transjugular intrahepatic portosystemic shunt (TIPS) is another treatment option whereby a percutaneous connection is created within the liver, between the portal and systemic circulations, to reduce portal pressure in patients with complications related to portal hypertension. TIPS has replaced operative shunts for managing acute variceal bleeding when pharmacotherapy and endoscopic treatment fail to control bleeding. As a result, emergency surgical intervention in most centers is reserved for select patients who are not TIPS candidates.

Endoscopy. About 80% to 90% of acute variceal bleeding episodes are successfully controlled by endoscopic measures. Sclerotherapy and band ligation of varices are the two main options available for control of acute variceal bleeding. Data suggest that band ligation is better than sclerotherapy in the initial control of bleeding and is associated with fewer complications. The literature also suggests that sclerotherapy, but not band ligation, may increase portal pressures. Thus, at this time, band ligation is the modality of choice for initial control of variceal bleeding. Endoscopic sclerotherapy may be used if technology for band ligation is not available. Early endoscopy, preferably within 12 hours of admission, with an attempt at control of bleeding is recommended. Patients should be started on vasoactive drugs early, and endoscopy with band ligation is performed after initial resuscitation.

Pharmacotherapy. Pharmacotherapy works by reducing variceal blood flow, which in turn reduces variceal pressure. Medical therapy should be initiated at the onset of variceal bleeding. Because infections are common in patients with variceal bleeding, antibiotic prophylaxis should be initiated. This has been shown to decrease the infection rate by more than 50%, to decrease rebleeding, and to improve survival. Randomized trials have also shown that somatostatin and its longer acting analogue octreotide are as efficacious as endoscopic treatment for control of acute variceal bleeding. Because of the minimal adverse effects and ease of administration, octreotide is now commonly used as an adjunct to endoscopic therapy. In fact, the combination of octreotide and endoscopic therapy is more effective than octreotide alone in controlling bleeding and is the preferred treatment for most patients. In severe cases of hemorrhage, vasopressin can be used to diminish splanchnic blood flow. However, because of the adverse systemic effects of vasopressin, nitroglycerin should be simultaneously infused and then titrated to achieve blood pressure control.

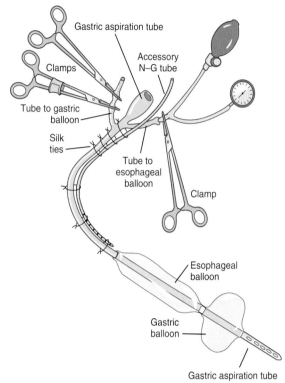

FIGURE 53-19 Modified Sengstaken-Blakemore tube. Note the accessory nasogastric tube for suctioning of secretions above the esophageal balloon and the two clamps, one secured with tape, to prevent inadvertent decompression of the gastric balloon. (From Rikkers LF: Portal hypertension. In Goldsmith H, editor: *Practice of surgery*, Philadelphia, 1981, Harper & Row, pp 1–37.)

Variceal tamponade. Controlled trials have demonstrated that balloon tamponade is as effective as pharmacotherapy and endoscopic therapy in controlling acute variceal bleeding. The major advantages of variceal tamponade using the Sengstaken-Blakemore tube are immediate cessation of bleeding in more than 85% of patients and the widespread availability of this device (Fig. 53-19). However, there are also significant disadvantages of balloon tamponade, including frequent recurrent hemorrhage in up to 50% of patients after balloon deflation, considerable discomfort for the patient, and a high incidence of serious complications when it is used incorrectly by an inexperienced health care provider.

Interventional approaches. In most institutions, TIPS has become the preferred treatment for acute variceal bleeding when pharmacotherapy and endoscopic treatment fail. With TIPS, a functional portacaval side-to-side shunt is established. TIPS is able to control bleeding in almost all patients. However, TIPS is associated with risk of encephalopathy. Furthermore, in the case of shunt dysfunction, there is risk of recurrent bleeding. Use of polytetrafluoroethylene (PTFE) covered stents has been a major step forward. PTFE stents have higher patency rates over time and reduced mortality rates.[5] Use of TIPS in patients with multiorgan failure or in patients with decompensated liver disease is associated with high 30-day mortality. In such patients, early use of TIPS, rather than after failure of other therapies, may be associated with better outcomes.

Operative approaches. Operative procedures are typically reserved for those situations in which TIPS is not indicated or is not available. Selection of the appropriate emergency operation should mainly be guided by the experience of the surgeon. Although nonoperative therapies are effective in most patients with acute variceal bleeding, an emergency operation should be promptly carried out when less invasive measures fail to control hemorrhage or are not indicated. The most common situations requiring urgent or emergency surgery are failure of acute endoscopic treatment, failure of long-term endoscopic therapy, hemorrhage from gastric varices or portal hypertensive gastropathy, and failure of TIPS placement.

Esophageal transection with a stapling device is rapid and relatively simple, but rebleeding rates after this procedure are high. Moreover, there is little evidence that operative mortality rates are lower than after surgical portal decompression.

A commonly performed shunt operation in the emergency setting is the portacaval shunt because it rapidly and effectively decompresses the portal venous circulation. Impressive results have been achieved by Orloff and colleagues,[6] but not by others, when an emergency portacaval shunt is used as routine therapy for acute variceal bleeding. In patients who are not actively bleeding at the time of surgery and in those in whom bleeding is temporarily controlled by pharmacotherapy or balloon tamponade, a more complex operation, such as the distal splenorenal shunt, may be appropriate. The major disadvantage of emergency surgery is that operative mortality rates exceed 25% in most reported series. Early postoperative mortality is usually related to the status of hepatic functional reserve rather than to the type of emergency operation selected.

Prevention of Recurrent Variceal Hemorrhage

After a patient has bled from varices, the likelihood of a repeated episode exceeds 70%. Because most patients with variceal hemorrhage have chronic liver disease, the challenge of long-term management is prevention of recurrent bleeding and maintenance of satisfactory hepatic function. Options available for definitive treatment include pharmacotherapy, chronic endoscopic treatment, TIPS, shunt operations (e.g., nonselective, selective, partial), various nonshunt procedures, and liver transplantation. The most effective treatment regimen usually requires two or more of these therapies in sequence. In most centers, initial treatment consists of pharmacotherapy or endoscopic therapy, with portal decompression by means of TIPS or an operative shunt reserved for failures of first-line treatment. Hepatic transplantation is used for patients with end-stage liver disease.

Pharmacotherapy. A meta-analysis of controlled trials of nonselective β-adrenergic blockade has shown that this treatment significantly decreases the likelihood of recurrent hemorrhage and demonstrates a trend toward decreased mortality.[7] The combination of a beta blocker and long-acting nitrate (e.g., isosorbide 5-mononitrate) has been shown to be more effective than variceal ligation.[8] Combination therapy is also more effective than beta blockade alone. Long-term pharmacotherapy should be used only in compliant patients who are observed closely by their physician.

Endoscopic therapy. Several controlled trials and a meta-analysis comparing endoscopic sclerotherapy with variceal ligation have shown a significant advantage to variceal ligation. Complications are less frequent after variceal ligation, and fewer treatment sessions are required to eradicate varices (Fig. 53-20). Rebleeding and mortality rates also appear to be lower after variceal ligation. The combination of variceal ligation and pharmacotherapy with nonselective beta blockade is more effective than variceal ligation alone.[9] This result has been confirmed in a meta-analysis that

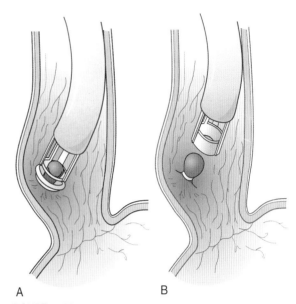

FIGURE 53-20 Endoscopic ligation of esophageal varices. **A,** The varix is drawn into the ligator by suction. **B,** An O ring is applied. (From Turcotte JG, Roger SE, Eckhauser FE: Portal hypertension. In Greenfield LJ, Mulholland MW, Oldham KT, editors: *Surgery: Scientific principles and practice,* Philadelphia, 1993, JB Lippincott, p 899.)

included the data from 17 randomized controlled trials.[10] In this trial, combination of beta blocker and endoscopic treatment significantly reduced rebleeding rates at 6, 12, and 24 months. Furthermore, mortality at 24 months was significantly lower for the combined treatment group. Thus, at this time, combination therapy should be recommended as the first line of treatment for secondary prophylaxis of variceal bleeding.

Several controlled trials comparing chronic endoscopic therapy with conventional medical management have been completed. Although fewer patients receiving endoscopic treatment than medical treatment experienced rebleeding in all the investigations, recurrent bleeding still occurred in approximately 50% of endoscopic therapy patients. Rebleeding is most frequent during the initial year. Rebleeding rate decreases by about 15% annually thereafter. Although a single episode of recurrent hemorrhage does not signify failure of therapy, uncontrolled hemorrhage, multiple major episodes of rebleeding, and hemorrhage from gastric varices and hypertensive gastropathy all require that endoscopic therapy be abandoned and another treatment modality substituted. Endoscopic treatment failure secondary to rebleeding occurs in as many as one third of patients. Thus, chronic endoscopic therapy is a rational initial treatment for many patients who bleed from esophageal varices, but subsequent treatment with TIPS, a shunt procedure, a nonshunt operation, or liver transplantation should be anticipated for a significant percentage of patients. Because of its relatively high failure rate, a course of chronic endoscopic therapy should not be undertaken for noncompliant patients and those living a long distance from advanced medical care.

Interventional therapy. TIPS is being increasingly used for definitive treatment of patients who bleed from portal hypertension (Fig. 53-21). A major limitation of TIPS, however, is a high incidence (up to 50%) of shunt stenosis or shunt thrombosis within the first year. Shunt stenosis, which is usually secondary to neointimal hyperplasia, is more common than thrombosis and

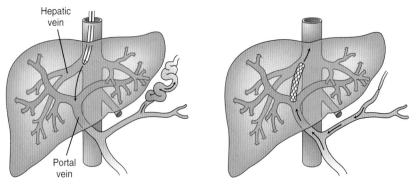

Hepatic
vein

Portal
vein

FIGURE 53-21 Transjugular Intrahepatic Portosystemic Shunt Placement. The IVC is accessed through right internal jugular vein. If the right internal jugular vein is unsuitable, left internal jugular vein may also be used. Through this access, a 5F catheter is placed into the right hepatic vein and wedged into a peripheral branch. Wedged hepatic venography is then performed with CO_2 gas to opacify the portal venous system. Using the wedged hepatic venogram image as a guide, a needle is advanced through the wall of the right hepatic vein and directed in an antero-inferior direction to access the right PV. Once the portal vein is cannulated CO_2 is injected into the parenchymal tract to exclude transgression of the bile duct or hepatic artery. Once proper placement is confirmed TIPS endoprosthesis is deployed which creates a shunt between the portal vein and the hepatic vein, thus decreasing resistance and decompressing varices.

can often be resolved by balloon dilation of the TIPS or, in some cases, by placement of a second shunt. Total shunt occlusion occurs in 10% to 15% of patients. Shunt stenosis and shunt thrombosis are often followed by recurrent portal hypertensive bleeding. TIPS stenosis and occlusion have become less frequent with use of PTFE covered stents.

TIPS has been compared with chronic endoscopic therapy in 11 randomized controlled trials. Fewer patients rebled after TIPS (19%) than after endoscopic treatment (47%), but encephalopathy was significantly more common in TIPS patients (34%). TIPS dysfunction developed in 50% of patients. The major advantage of TIPS is that it is a nonoperative approach. Thus, it would appear to be the ideal therapy when only short-term portal decompression is required. Liver transplantation candidates who fail to respond to endoscopic therapy or pharmacotherapy are therefore well suited for TIPS followed by transplantation when a donor organ becomes available. As a result, the patient is protected from bleeding in the interim, and the transplantation procedure may be facilitated by the lower portal pressure. Another group of patients in whom TIPS may be advantageous includes those with advanced hepatic functional decompensation who are unlikely to survive long enough for the TIPS to malfunction. Because it functions as a side-to-side portosystemic shunt, TIPS is also effective for the treatment of medically intractable ascites.

Surgical therapy. Portosystemic shunts are clearly the most effective means of preventing recurrent hemorrhage in patients with portal hypertension. These procedures are effective because they all decompress the portal venous system to varying degrees by shunting portal flow into the lower pressure systemic venous system. However, diversion of portal blood, which contains hepatotropic hormones, nutrients, and cerebral toxins, is also responsible for the adverse consequences of shunt operations, namely, portosystemic encephalopathy and accelerated hepatic failure. Depending on whether they completely decompress, compartmentalize, or partially decompress the portal venous circulation, portosystemic shunts can be classified as nonselective, selective, or partial. In addition to variceal decompression, selective and partial portosystemic shunts also aim to preserve hepatic portal perfusion and therefore to prevent or to minimize the adverse consequences of these procedures.

Nonselective shunts. Commonly used nonselective shunts, all of which completely divert portal flow, include the end-to-side portacaval shunt (Eck fistula), side-to-side portacaval shunt, large-diameter interposition shunts, and conventional splenorenal shunt (Fig. 53-22). The end-to-side portacaval shunt is the prototype of nonselective shunts and is the only shunt procedure that has been compared with conventional medical treatment in randomized controlled trials. Figure 53-23 combines survival data from four controlled investigations of the therapeutic portacaval shunt, performed in patients with prior variceal hemorrhage. The most common causes of death in medically treated and shunted patients were rebleeding and accelerated hepatic failure, respectively. Although no survival advantage could be demonstrated for shunt patients, all these studies had a crossover bias in favor of medically treated patients, several of whom received a shunt when they developed intractable recurrent variceal hemorrhage. In addition, almost all the trial patients had alcoholic cirrhosis; therefore, these results do not necessarily apply to other causes of portal hypertension. Other important findings of these randomized trials included reliable control of bleeding in shunted patients, variceal rebleeding in more than 70% of medically treated patients, and spontaneous, often severe encephalopathy in 20% to 40% of shunted patients.

All the other nonselective shunts in Figure 53-22 maintain continuity of the portal vein, thereby connecting the portal and systemic venous systems in a side-to-side fashion. Therefore, these procedures decompress the splanchnic venous circulation and intrahepatic sinusoidal network. Because the liver and intestines are both important contributors to ascites formation, side-to-side portosystemic shunts are the most effective shunt procedures for relieving ascites as well as for preventing recurrent variceal bleeding. Because they completely divert portal flow, like the end-to-side portacaval shunt, however, side-to-side shunts also accelerate hepatic failure and lead to frequent postshunt encephalopathy.

The conventional splenorenal shunt consists of anastomosis of the proximal splenic vein to the renal vein. Splenectomy is also performed. Because the smaller proximal rather than the larger distal end of the splenic vein is used, shunt thrombosis is more common after this procedure than after the distal splenorenal shunt. Although early series noted that postshunt encephalopathy

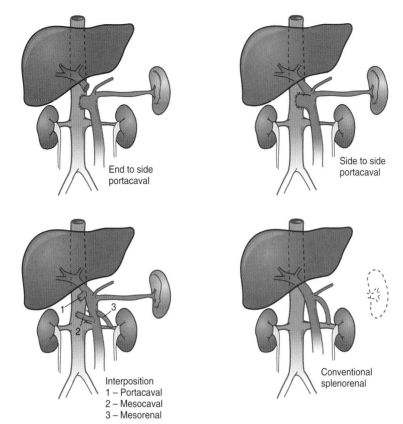

FIGURE 53-22 Nonselective shunts completely divert portal blood flow away from the liver. (From Rikkers LF: Portal hypertension. In Moody FG, Carey LC, Scott Jones RS, et al, editors: *Surgical treatment of digestive disease*, Chicago, 1986, Year Book Medical, pp 409–424.)

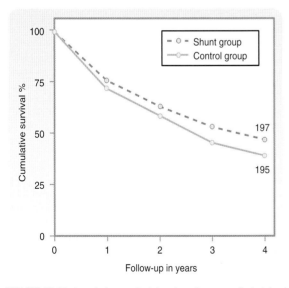

FIGURE 53-23 Cumulative survival data from four controlled trials of the portacaval shunt versus conventional medical management. (From Boyer TD: Portal hypertension and its complications: Bleeding esophageal varices, ascites, and spontaneous bacterial peritonitis. In Zakim D, Boyer TD, editors: *Hepatology: A textbook of liver disease*, Philadelphia, 1982, WB Saunders, pp 464–499.)

was less common after the conventional splenorenal shunt than after the portacaval shunt, subsequent analyses have suggested that this low frequency of encephalopathy was probably a result of restoration of hepatic portal perfusion after shunt thrombosis developed in many patients. A conventional splenorenal shunt that is of sufficient caliber to remain patent gradually dilates and eventually causes complete portal decompression and portal flow diversion. A purported advantage of the procedure is that hypersplenism is eliminated by splenectomy. The thrombocytopenia and leukopenia that accompany portal hypertension, however, are rarely of clinical significance, making splenectomy an unnecessary procedure in most patients.

In summary, nonselective shunts effectively decompress varices. Because of complete portal flow diversion, however, they are complicated by frequent postoperative encephalopathy and accelerated hepatic failure. Side-to-side nonselective shunts effectively relieve ascites and prevent variceal hemorrhage. Presently, nonselective shunts are only rarely indicated. TIPS, also a nonselective shunt, is the preferred therapy for most situations in which nonselective shunts were previously used (e.g., patients with both variceal bleeding and medically intractable ascites). In general, a nonselective shunt is constructed only when a TIPS cannot be performed or when a TIPS fails.

Selective shunts. The hemodynamic and clinical shortcomings of nonselective shunts stimulated development of the concept of selective variceal decompression. In 1967, Warren and colleagues introduced the distal splenorenal shunt. In the following year, Inokuchi and associates reported their initial results with the

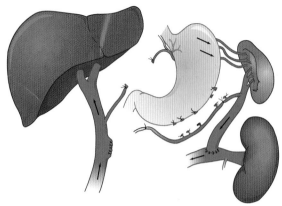

FIGURE 53-24 The distal splenorenal shunt provides selective variceal decompression through the short gastric veins, spleen, and splenic vein to the left renal vein. Hepatic portal perfusion is maintained by interrupting the umbilical vein, coronary vein, gastroepiploic vein, and any other prominent collaterals. (From Salam AA: Distal splenorenal shunts: Hemodynamics of total versus selective shunting. In Baker RJ, Fischer JE, editors: *Mastery of surgery*, ed 4, Philadelphia, 2001, Lippincott Williams & Wilkins, pp 1357–1366.)

left gastric–venacaval shunt, which consists of interposition of a vein graft between the left gastric (coronary) vein and IVC. Therefore, it directly and selectively decompresses esophagogastric varices. However, only a minority of patients with portal hypertension have appropriate anatomy for this operation; experience with it has been limited to Japan, and no controlled trials have been conducted.

The distal splenorenal shunt consists of anastomosis of the distal end of the splenic vein to the left renal vein and interruption of all collateral vessels (e.g., coronary vein and gastroepiploic veins) that connect the superior mesenteric vein and gastrosplenic components of the splanchnic venous circulation (Fig. 53-24). This results in separation of the portal venous circulation into a decompressed gastrosplenic venous circuit and high-pressure superior mesenteric venous system that continues to perfuse the liver. Although the procedure is technically demanding, it can be mastered by most well-trained surgeons who are knowledgeable in the principles of vascular surgery.

Not all patients are candidates for the distal splenorenal shunt. Because sinusoidal and mesenteric hypertension is maintained and important lymphatic pathways are transected during dissection of the left renal vein, the distal splenorenal shunt tends to aggravate rather than to relieve ascites. Thus, patients with medically intractable ascites should not undergo this procedure. However, the larger population of patients who develop transient ascites after resuscitation from a variceal hemorrhage are candidates for a selective shunt. Another contraindication to a distal splenorenal shunt is prior splenectomy. A splenic vein diameter less than 7 mm is a relative contraindication to the procedure because the incidence of shunt thrombosis is high when a small-diameter vein is used. Although selective variceal decompression is a sound physiologic concept, the distal splenorenal shunt remains controversial after an extensive clinical experience spanning almost 40 years.

Although the distal splenorenal shunt results in portal flow preservation in more than 85% of patients during the early postoperative interval, the high-pressure mesenteric venous system gradually collateralizes to the low-pressure shunt, resulting in loss

of portal flow in approximately 50% of patients by 1 year. The degree and duration of portal flow preservation depend on the cause of portal hypertension and the technical details of the operation (the extent to which mesenteric and gastrosplenic venous circulations are separated). Although portal flow is maintained in most patients with nonalcoholic cirrhosis and noncirrhotic portal hypertension (e.g., portal vein thrombosis), portal flow rapidly collateralizes to the shunt in patients with alcoholic cirrhosis.

Modification of the distal splenorenal shunt by purposeful or inadvertent omission of coronary vein ligation results in early loss of portal flow. Even when all major collateral vessels are interrupted, portal flow may be gradually diverted through a pancreatic collateral network (pancreatic siphon). This pathway can be discouraged by dissecting the full length of the splenic vein from the pancreas, splenopancreatic disconnection, which results in better preservation of hepatic portal perfusion, especially in patients with alcoholic cirrhosis. However, this extension of the procedure makes it technically more challenging and a significant disadvantage in an era when fewer shunts are being placed because of increased use of endoscopic therapy, TIPS, and liver transplantation.

Six of the seven controlled comparisons of the distal splenorenal shunt and nonselective shunts have included predominantly alcoholic cirrhotic patients. None of these trials has demonstrated an advantage to either procedure with respect to long-term survival. Three of the studies found a lower frequency of encephalopathy after the distal splenorenal shunt, whereas the other trials showed no difference in the incidence of this postoperative complication. In contrast to survival, encephalopathy is a subjective end point that was assessed with various methods in the trials. Another important end point in comparing treatments for variceal hemorrhage was the effectiveness with which recurrent bleeding was prevented. In almost all uncontrolled and controlled series of the distal splenorenal shunt, this procedure was equivalent to nonselective shunts in preventing recurrent hemorrhage. Mainly because of these inconsistent results of the controlled trials, there is no consensus as to which shunting procedure is superior in patients with alcoholic cirrhosis. Because the quality of life (e.g., lower encephalopathy rate) was significantly better in the distal splenorenal shunt group in three of the trials, there appears to be an advantage to selective variceal decompression, even in this population.

Considerably fewer data are available regarding selective shunting in nonalcoholic cirrhosis and noncirrhotic portal hypertension. Because hepatic portal perfusion after the distal splenorenal shunt is better preserved in these disease categories, one might expect improved results. A single controlled trial in patients with schistosomiasis (presinusoidal portal hypertension) has demonstrated a lower frequency of encephalopathy after the distal splenorenal shunt than after a conventional splenorenal shunt (nonselective). Another large series from Emory University has shown that distal splenorenal shunt is associated with better survival in patients with nonalcoholic cirrhosis than in those with alcoholic cirrhosis. However, this has not been a consistent finding in all centers in which the distal splenorenal shunts have been performed.

Several controlled trials have also compared the distal splenorenal shunt with chronic endoscopic therapy. In these investigations, recurrent hemorrhage was more effectively prevented by selective shunting than by sclerotherapy. However, hepatic portal perfusion was maintained in a significantly higher fraction of patients undergoing sclerotherapy. Despite this hemodynamic advantage, encephalopathy rates were similar after both therapies.

The two North American trials were dissimilar with respect to the effect of these treatments on long-term survival. Sclerotherapy with surgical rescue for the one third of sclerotherapy failures resulted in significantly better survival than selective shunt alone, whereas 85% of sclerotherapy failures could be salvaged by surgery. In contrast, a similar investigation conducted in a sparsely populated area (Intermountain West and Plains) showed superior survival after the distal splenorenal shunt. Only 31% of sclerotherapy failures could be salvaged by surgery in this trial. The survival results of these two studies suggest that endoscopic therapy is a rational initial treatment for patients who bleed from varices if sclerotherapy failure is recognized and these patients promptly undergo surgery or TIPS. However, patients living in remote areas are less likely to be salvaged by shunt surgery when endoscopic treatment fails, and therefore a selective shunt may be preferable initial treatment for such patients.

In one nonrandomized comparison to TIPS, the distal splenorenal shunt had lower rates of recurrent bleeding, encephalopathy, and shunt thrombosis. Ascites was less prevalent after TIPS. A multicenter randomized trial comparing TIPS and the distal splenorenal shunt for the elective treatment of variceal bleeding in good-risk cirrhotic patients has shown generally equivalent results for these two procedures. Rebleeding rates were not significantly different between the distal splenorenal shunt (6%) and TIPS (11%), but this represents the lowest reported rate of rebleeding after TIPS. This was likely secondary to meticulous surveillance of TIPS patency by duplex ultrasound and angiography. Frequent reintervention in TIPS patients (82% compared with 11% for distal splenorenal shunt patients) was necessary to achieve these results. In this trial, postshunt encephalopathy and survival were similar after the two procedures.

Partial shunts. The objectives of partial and selective shunts are the same: effective decompression of varices, preservation of hepatic portal perfusion, and maintenance of some residual portal hypertension. Initial attempts at partial shunting consisted of small-diameter vein-to-vein anastomoses. In general, these thrombosed or dilated with time and thereby became nonselective shunts.

More recently, a small-diameter interposition portacaval shunt using a PTFE graft, combined with ligation of the coronary vein and other collateral vessels, was described (Fig. 53-25). When the prosthetic graft is 10 mm or less in diameter, hepatic portal perfusion is preserved in most patients, at least during the early postoperative interval. Early experience with this small-diameter prosthetic shunt is that less than 15% of shunts have thrombosed, and most of these have been successfully opened by interventional radiologic techniques. A small prospective randomized trial of partial (8 mm in diameter) and nonselective (16 mm in diameter) interposition portacaval shunts has shown a lower frequency of encephalopathy after the partial shunt but similar survival after both types of shunts. In another controlled trial, the small-diameter interposition shunt was discovered to have a lower overall failure rate than TIPS.

Hepatic transplantation. Liver transplantation is not a treatment for variceal bleeding but rather needs to be considered for all patients who present with end-stage hepatic failure, whether or not it is accompanied by bleeding. Transplantation in patients who have bled secondary to portal hypertension is the only therapy that addresses the underlying liver disease in addition to providing reliable portal decompression. Because of economic

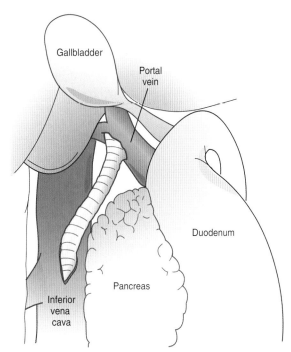

FIGURE 53-25 A small-diameter (8 to 10 mm) interposition portacaval shunt partially decompresses the portal venous system and may preserve hepatic portal perfusion. (From Sarfeh IJ, Rypins EB, Mason GR: A systematic appraisal of portacaval H-graft diameters: Clinical and hemodynamic perspectives. *Ann Surg* 204:356–363, 1986.)

factors and a limited supply of donor organs, liver transplantation is not available to all patients. Also, transplantation is not indicated for some of the more common causes of variceal bleeding, such as schistosomiasis (normal liver function) and active alcoholism (noncompliance).

There is accumulating evidence that variceal bleeders with well-compensated hepatic functional reserve (Child-Pugh class A and B+) are initially better served by nontransplantation strategies. The first-line treatment for such patients should be pharmacologic and endoscopic therapy. For those who fail to respond to first-line therapy, an operative shunt or TIPS can be performed. These can also be applied under circumstances in which pharmacologic or endoscopic treatment would be risky, such as patients with gastric varices and those geographically separated from tertiary medical care.

Patients with variceal bleeding who are transplantation candidates include nonalcoholic cirrhotic patients and abstinent alcoholic cirrhotic patients with limited hepatic functional reserve (Child-Pugh class B and C) or a poor quality of life secondary to the disease (e.g., encephalopathy, fatigue, bone pain). In these patients, the acute hemorrhage should be treated with endoscopic therapy and pharmacotherapy and the patient's transplantation candidacy immediately activated. If endoscopic treatment and pharmacotherapy are ineffective, a TIPS should be inserted as a short-term bridge to transplantation.

If a nontransplantation procedure (e.g., operative shunt or TIPS) is performed initially, these patients should be carefully assessed at regular intervals of 6 to 12 months. Hepatic transplantation should be considered when other complications of cirrhosis develop or hepatic functional decompensation is evident clinically or by careful assessment with quantitative LFTs.

Algorithm for Management of Variceal Hemorrhage

An algorithm for definitive management of variceal hemorrhage is shown in Figure 53-26. Patients are first grouped according to their transplantation candidacy. This decision is based on a number of factors, including cause of portal hypertension, abstinence for alcoholic cirrhotic patients, presence or absence of other diseases, and physiologic rather than chronologic age.

Transplantation candidates with decompensated hepatic function or a poor quality of life secondary to their liver disease should undergo transplantation as soon as possible.

Most future transplantation and nontransplantation candidates should undergo initial endoscopic treatment or pharmacotherapy unless they bleed from gastric varices or portal hypertensive gastropathy or live in a remote geographic location and have

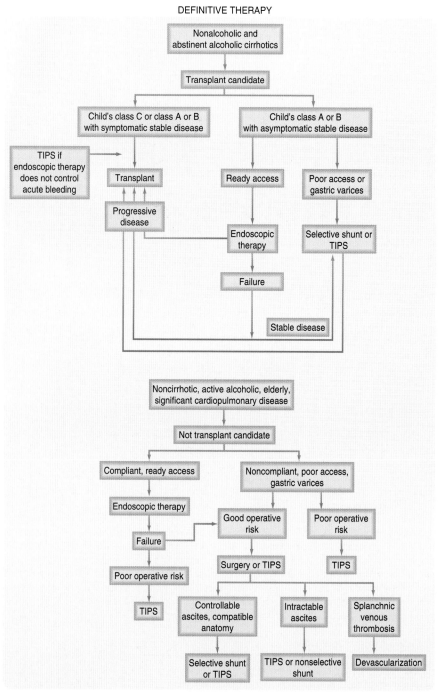

FIGURE 53-26 Algorithm for definitive therapy of variceal hemorrhage (see text for details). (Adapted from Rikkers LF: Portal hypertension. In Levine BA, Copeland E, Howard R, et al, editors: *Current practice of surgery* (vol 3), New York, 1995, Churchill Livingstone.)

limited access to emergency tertiary care. Patients who live in remote locations and those who fail to respond to endoscopic and drug therapy should receive a selective shunt or TIPS. A controlled trial has shown that if careful surveillance of TIPS patency and frequent TIPS reinterventions are done, these procedures are equally efficacious.

Until improvements in TIPS technology are fully realized, the distal splenorenal shunt is likely to remain a more durable long-term solution and a reasonable alternative for TIPS failure. However, a TIPS is more commonly done, and few surgeons who are experienced in shunt surgery remain. Therefore, it is likely that operative shunts will play an even smaller role in the management of variceal bleeding in the future than they do now. Patients with medically intractable ascites in addition to variceal bleeding are best treated with TIPS when less invasive measures fail to control bleeding. If the TIPS eventually fails, an open side-to-side shunt can then be constructed if the patient has reasonable hepatic function and is not a transplantation candidate. On the other hand, TIPS is clearly indicated for patients with endoscopic treatment failure who may require transplantation in the near future and for nontransplantation candidates with advanced hepatic functional deterioration. Future transplantation candidates should be carefully monitored so that they undergo transplantation at the appropriate time before they become poor operative risks.

The treatment algorithm for variceal bleeding has changed considerably since the 1970s, during which time endoscopic therapy, liver transplantation, and TIPS have become available to these patients. Nontransplantation operations are now less frequently necessary, the survival results are better because patients at high operative risk are managed by other means, and emergency surgery has almost been eliminated.

INFECTIOUS DISEASES

Pyogenic Abscess

Epidemiology

Ochsner and DeBakey, in their classic paper on pyogenic liver abscess in 1938, described 47 cases and reviewed the world literature. This was the largest experience at that time and the first serious attempt to study this disease. In that era, pyogenic liver abscess was largely a disease of people in their 20s and 30s, mostly the result of acute appendicitis. With the marked changes in medical care since then, notably effective antibiotics and prompt effective treatments for acute inflammatory disorders, and an aging population, the spectrum of this disease has changed. Pyogenic liver abscess is now mostly seen in patients in their 50s to 60s and is more often related to biliary tract disease or is cryptogenic in nature.

However, the incidence of pyogenic liver abscess has remained similar. In 1938, Ochsner and DeBakey reported an incidence of 8/100,000 hospital admissions, whereas in 1975, Pitt and Zuidema reported 13/100,000 hospital admissions. Two large autopsy studies, one from 1901 and another from 1960, have reported similar incidences of pyogenic liver abscess, 0.45% and 0.59%, respectively. More recent studies from the 1980s through the 2000s have suggested small but significant increases in the incidence of pyogenic liver abscess as high as 22/100,000 hospital admissions.[11] These figures may be declining on the basis of more recent data. This may reflect better, more available, and more frequently used high-quality imaging techniques. Hospital admission practices also affect these numbers. A recent population-based study from North America calculated an annual incidence of 3.6 cases/100,000 population.[12] There is no significant gender, ethnic, or geographic differences in disease frequency; the male-to-female ratio is approximately 1.5:1. Comorbid conditions associated with pyogenic abscess are cirrhosis, diabetes, chronic renal failure, and a history of malignant disease.

Pathogenesis

The liver is probably exposed to portal venous bacterial loads on a regular basis and usually clears this bacterial load without problems. The development of a hepatic abscess occurs when an inoculum of bacteria, regardless of the route of exposure, exceeds the liver's ability to clear it. This results in tissue invasion, neutrophil infiltration, and formation of an organized abscess. The potential routes of hepatic exposure to bacteria are the biliary tree, portal vein, hepatic artery, direct extension of a nearby nidus of infection, and trauma. The relative contribution of these routes to the formation of hepatic abscess is summarized in Table 53-3.

Along with cryptogenic infections, infections from the biliary tree are the most common identifiable cause of hepatic abscess. Biliary obstruction results in bile stasis with the potential for subsequent bacterial colonization, infection, and ascension into the liver. This process is known as ascending suppurative cholangitis. The nature of biliary obstruction is mostly related to stone disease or malignant disease. In Asia, intrahepatic stones and cholangitis (recurrent pyogenic cholangitis; see later) are common causes, whereas in the West, malignant obstruction has become a more predominant cause. Other factors associated with increased risk include Caroli disease, biliary ascariasis, and biliary tract surgery. The common link between all causes of hepatic abscesses from the biliary tree is obstruction and bacteria in the biliary tract. Prior biliary-enteric anastomosis has also been associated with hepatic abscess formation, likely because of unimpeded exposure of the biliary tree to enteric organisms.

The portal venous system drains the gastrointestinal tract; therefore, any infectious disorder of the gastrointestinal tract can

TABLE 53-3   Pyogenic Abscesses Attributable to Specific Cause

YEAR OF REPORT	NO. OF PATIENTS	CAUSE (%)					
		PORTAL VEIN	HEPATIC ARTERY	BILIARY TREE	DIRECT EXTENSION	TRAUMA	CRYPTOGENIC
1927-1938 (one study*)	622	42	—	—	17	4	20
1945-1982 (eight studies)	521	17	9	38	10	4	16
1970-1999 (eight studies)	1264	5	3	38	1	2	43

*Ochsner A, DeBakey M, Murray S: Pyogenic abscess of the liver. *Am J Surg* 40:292–319, 1938. This is the classic study of Ochsner and DeBakey that reviewed 286 previously reported cases and 47 new cases.

result in an ascending portal vein infection (pyelophlebitis), with exposure of the liver to large amounts of bacteria. Historically, untreated appendicitis was considered the most common cause of hepatic abscess, but with the advent of antibiotics and the development of prompt and effective treatment of acute intra-abdominal infections, portal venous infections of the liver have become less frequent. The most common causes of pyelophlebitis are diverticulitis, appendicitis, pancreatitis, inflammatory bowel disease, pelvic inflammatory disease, perforated viscus, and omphalitis in the newborn. Hepatic abscess has also been associated with colorectal malignant disease. In a case-control study from Taiwan, the incidence of gastrointestinal cancers was increased fourfold among patients with pyogenic liver abscess compared with controls.[13]

Any systemic infection (e.g., endocarditis, pneumonia, osteomyelitis) can result in bacteremia and infection of the liver through the hepatic artery. Microabscess formation is a relatively common finding at autopsy in patients dying of sepsis, but these patients are generally not included in analyses of pyogenic liver abscess. Hepatic abscess from systemic infections may also reflect an altered immune response, such as in patients with malignant disease, AIDS, or disorders of granulocyte function. Children with chronic granulomatous disease are particularly susceptible.

Hepatic abscess can be the result of direct extension of an infectious process. Common examples include suppurative cholecystitis, subphrenic abscess, perinephric abscess, and even perforation of the bowel directly into the liver.

Penetrating and blunt trauma can also result in an intrahepatic hematoma or an area of necrotic liver, which can subsequently develop into an abscess. Bacteria may have been introduced from the trauma, or the affected area may be seeded from systemic bacteremia. Hepatic abscesses associated with trauma can be manifested in a delayed fashion up to several weeks after injury. Other mechanisms of iatrogenic hepatic necrosis, such as hepatic artery embolization or, more recently, thermal ablative procedures, can be complicated by abscess. This is an uncommon complication of these procedures but is seen more often when there has been a previous biliary-enteric anastomosis.

Usually, no cause for a hepatic abscess is found. Cryptogenic abscesses predominate in many series and are more common in some case reports. Possible explanations for cryptogenic hepatic abscess are undiagnosed abdominal disease, resolved infectious process at the time of presentation, and host factors such as diabetes or malignant disease rendering the liver more susceptible to transient hepatic artery or portal vein bacteremia. In patients with cryptogenic hepatic abscess who have undergone computed tomography (CT) and ultrasonography, it has been argued whether a diligent search for a cause should ensue. In series evaluating colonoscopy and endoscopic retrograde cholangiopancreatography (ERCP) in patients with cryptogenic abscess, the yield has been low and often is only fruitful in patients with some objective finding that might have suggested a subclinical abnormality (e.g., mildly elevated bilirubin level). In general, these patients should undergo a thorough history, physical examination, and laboratory workup in search of abnormalities in the intestinal tract or biliary tree. Further invasive procedures or imaging studies should be based on clinical suspicions raised by this workup.

Pathology and Microbiology

Most hepatic abscesses involve the right hemiliver, accounting for about 75% of cases. The explanation for this is not known, but preferential laminar blood flow to the right side has been postulated. The left liver is involved in approximately 20% of the cases; the caudate lobe is rarely involved (5%). Bilobar involvement with multiple abscesses is uncommon. Approximately 50% of hepatic abscesses are solitary. Hepatic abscesses can vary in size from less than 1 mm to 3 or 4 cm in diameter and can be multiloculated or a single cavity. At abdominal exploration, hepatic abscesses appear tan and are fluctuant to palpation, although deeper abscesses may not be visible and can be difficult to palpate. Surrounding inflammation can cause adhesions to local structures.

Studies of the microbiology of hepatic abscesses have had variable results, for a number of reasons. In early series, sterile abscesses were commonly reported but probably reflected inadequate culture techniques, whereas in modern series, few abscesses are sampled before the administration of antibiotics. Also, the heterogeneity of the routes of infection makes the microbiology variable. Abscesses from pyelophlebitis or cholangitis tend to be polymicrobial, with a high preponderance of gram-negative bacilli. Systemic infections, on the other hand, usually cause infection with a single organism.

Although the rate of sterility reported by Ochsner's review in 1938 was approximately 50%, series in the 1990s reported sterile abscess rates in approximately 10% to 20% of cases. Many hepatic abscesses are polymicrobial in nature and account for approximately 40% of cases. Some have suggested that solitary abscesses are more likely to be polymicrobial. Anaerobic organisms are involved approximately 40% to 60% of the time. The most common organisms cultured are *Escherichia coli* and *Klebsiella pneumoniae*. Other commonly encountered organisms are *Staphylococcus aureus*, *Enterococcus* sp., viridans streptococci, and *Bacteroides* spp. *Klebsiella* is frequently associated with gas-forming abscesses. Enterococci and viridans streptococci are generally found in polymicrobial abscesses, whereas staphylococcal infections are typically caused by a single organism. Uncommonly encountered organisms (<10% of cultures) include species of *Pseudomonas*, *Proteus*, *Enterobacter*, *Citrobacter*, *Serratia*, beta-hemolytic streptococci, microaerophilic streptococci, *Fusobacterium*, *Clostridium*, and other rare anaerobes. Blood cultures are positive in approximately 50% to 60% of cases. Of note, highly resistant organisms in patients with indwelling biliary catheters, multiple episodes of cholangitis, and repeated use of antibiotics are being encountered as the use of these catheters becomes more common. Fungal and mycobacterial hepatic abscesses are rare and are almost always associated with immunosuppression, usually from chemotherapy.

Clinical Features

The classic description of the presenting symptoms of hepatic abscess is fever, jaundice, and right upper quadrant pain, with tenderness to palpation. Unfortunately, this presentation is present in only 10% of cases. Fever, chills, and abdominal pain are the most common presenting symptoms, but a broad array of nonspecific symptoms can be present (Table 53-4). A study from Taiwan of 133 patients found fever in 96% of patients, chills in 80%, abdominal pain in 53%, and jaundice in 20%. Many of the symptoms, such as malaise and vomiting, were constitutional in nature. Involvement of the diaphragm may result in symptoms of cough or dyspnea. Rarely, patients can present with peritonitis secondary to rupture. Cases of rupture into the pleural space or pericardium have been reported but are distinctly uncommon. The duration of presenting symptoms is variable, ranging from an acute illness to a chronic presentation lasting months. It has been

TABLE 53-4	Pyogenic Abscesses With Noted Symptoms									
		SYMPTOM (%)								
YEAR OF REPORT	NO. OF PATIENTS	FEVER, CHILLS	NIGHT SWEATS	MALAISE	ANOREXIA, WEIGHT LOSS	NAUSEA, VOMITING	DIARRHEA	ABDOMINAL PAIN	CHEST PAIN	COUGH
1927-1938 (one study*)	333	94	—	—	—	33	—	92	—	—
1945-1982 (eight studies)	494	88	8	58	62	40	17	66	14	13
1970-1995 (ten studies)	1314	72	9	25	33	30	14	59	16	6

*Ochsner A, DeBakey M, Murray S: Pyogenic abscess of the liver. *Am J Surg* 40:292–319, 1938. This is the classic study of Ochsner and DeBakey that reviewed 286 previously reported cases and 47 new cases.

suggested that acute presentation is associated with identifiable abdominal disease, whereas a chronic presentation is often associated with a cryptogenic abscess. A rare complication specific to *Klebsiella* hepatic abscesses is endogenous endophthalmitis, occurring in approximately 3% of cases. This serious complication is more common in diabetics. The best chance to preserve visual function is with early diagnosis and treatment.

On physical examination, fever and right upper quadrant tenderness are the most common findings. Tenderness is present in 40% to 70% of patients. Jaundice is also found in approximately 25% of cases and is often secondary to underlying biliary disease. Chest findings are often found in approximately 25% of patients, and hepatomegaly is also commonly noted in approximately 50%. Ascites, splenomegaly, and severe sepsis are uncommon signs of hepatic abscesses.

Nonspecific abnormalities of blood tests are common in pyogenic abscesses. Leukocytosis is present in 70% to 90% of patients, and anemia is commonly encountered. Abnormalities of LFT results are generally present. The ALP level is mildly elevated in 80% of patients, whereas total bilirubin concentration is elevated 20% to 50% of the time. Transaminases are mildly elevated in approximately 60% of patients. Severe abnormalities of liver function are almost always associated with underlying biliary disease. Hypoalbuminemia or mild elevations of the PT and INR can be present and reflect a degree of chronicity. None of these blood tests specifically help diagnose a hepatic abscess. However, together they may suggest a liver abnormality that often leads to imaging studies.

The most essential element to establishing the diagnosis of hepatic abscess is radiographic imaging. Chest radiographs are abnormal approximately 50% of the time, and findings generally reflect subdiaphragmatic disease, such as an elevated right hemidiaphragm, right pleural effusion, or atelectasis. On occasion, these can be left-sided findings in the case of an abscess involving the left liver. Plain abdominal radiographs, in rare cases, can be helpful. They can show air-fluid levels or portal venous gas (Fig. 53-27).

Ultrasound and CT are the mainstays of diagnostic modalities for hepatic abscess. Ultrasound usually demonstrates a round or oval area that is less echogenic than the surrounding liver. Ultrasound can reliably distinguish solid from cystic lesions. The limitations of ultrasound are in its ability to visualize lesions high up in the dome of the liver and that it is a user-dependent modality.

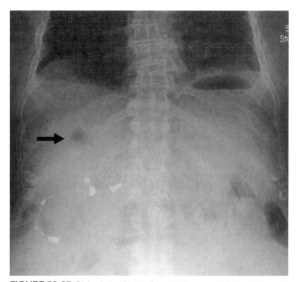

FIGURE 53-27 Plain abdominal radiograph demonstrating an abnormal collection of air in the right upper quadrant consistent with a pyogenic hepatic abscess *(arrow)*.

The sensitivity of ultrasound in diagnosing hepatic abscess is 80% to 95%. CT demonstrates similar findings to ultrasound, and lesions are of lower attenuation than surrounding hepatic parenchyma. High-quality CT scans can demonstrate very small abscesses and can more easily identify multiple small abscesses. The abscess wall usually has an intense enhancement on contrast-enhanced CT. The sensitivity of CT in diagnosing hepatic abscess is 95% to 100%. Both CT and ultrasound are useful in diagnosing other intra-abdominal pathologic processes, such as biliary disease (ultrasound) and inflammatory disorders such as appendicitis and diverticulitis (CT). Magnetic resonance imaging (MRI) can be helpful in distinguishing the cause of many hepatic masses and evaluating the biliary tree for pathologic changes, but it does not appear to have any distinct advantage over CT in diagnosing hepatic abscess.

Differential Diagnosis

Differentiating pyogenic abscess from other cystic infective diseases of the liver, such as amebic abscess or echinococcal cyst, is

TABLE 53-5 Features of Amebic versus Pyogenic Liver Abscess

CLINICAL FEATURES	AMEBIC ABSCESS	PYOGENIC ABSCESS
Age	20-40 years	>50 years
Male-to-female ratio	≥10:1	1.5:1
Solitary versus multiple	Solitary 80%*	Solitary 50%
Location	Usually right liver	Usually right liver
Travel in endemic area	Yes	No
Diabetes	Uncommon (≈2%)	More common (≈27%)
Alcohol use	Common	Common
Jaundice	Uncommon	Common
Elevated bilirubin	Uncommon	Common
Elevated alkaline phosphatase	Common	Common
Positive blood culture	No	Common
Positive amebic serology	Yes	No

*In acute amebic abscess, 50% are solitary.

important because of differences in treatment. Pyogenic abscess (see later) is largely treated by antibiotics and drainage. Amebic abscess is mainly treated by antibiotics, whereas echinococcal cysts often require surgical management. Fortunately, echinococcal cysts can usually be diagnosed by history and characteristic radiologic findings (see later). The presentations of amebic and pyogenic abscess, however, are more similar, with some notable exceptions that are critical in distinguishing the two (Table 53-5). Amebic abscesses generally occur in young Hispanic men, whereas pyogenic abscess tends to occur in patients 50 to 60 years of age, with no predominant gender or race. Fever is common in both, but chills and symptoms of a severe acute bacteremia are more common in pyogenic abscess. On serologic testing, *Entamoeba histolytica* antibodies are almost always present in amebic abscesses but are uncommon in patients with pyogenic abscess. A study comparing 471 patients with amebic abscess to 106 patients with pyogenic abscess found age older than 50 years, pulmonary findings on physical examination, multiple abscesses, and low amebic serology titers to be independently predictive of pyogenic abscess. On occasion, differentiating the two is not possible, and diagnostic aspiration or a trial of antiamebic antibiotics may be necessary. Unfortunately, aspiration is diagnostic in amebic abscess only approximately 10% to 20% of the time.[14]

Treatment

Before the availability of antibiotics and the routine use of drainage procedures, untreated hepatic pyogenic abscess was almost uniformly fatal. It was not until the classic review by Ochsner and DeBakey in 1938 (see earlier) that routine surgical drainage was used and dramatic reductions in mortality were noted. Open surgical drainage of pyogenic abscesses was the sole treatment (with the addition of antibiotics eventually) for hepatic abscess until the 1980s. Since then, less invasive percutaneous drainage techniques and intravenous (IV) antibiotics have been used. Laparotomy is generally reserved for failures of percutaneous drainage.

Once the diagnosis of pyogenic hepatic abscess is suspected, broad-spectrum IV antibiotics should be started immediately to control ongoing bacteremia and its associated complications. Blood samples and specimens of the abscess from aspiration should be sent for aerobic and anaerobic cultures. In immunosuppressed patients, mycobacterial and fungal cultures of the aspirate should be considered. Patients who are at risk for amebic infections should have blood samples drawn for amebic serology. Until cultures have specifically identified the offending organisms, broad-spectrum antibiotics covering gram-negative, gram-positive, and anaerobic organisms should be used. Combinations such as ampicillin, an aminoglycoside, and metronidazole or a third-generation cephalosporin with metronidazole are appropriate. The optimal duration of antibiotic treatment is not well defined and must be individualized, depending on the success of the drainage procedure. Antibiotics should certainly be continued while there is evidence of ongoing infection, such as fever, chills, or leukocytosis. Beyond this, it is unclear how long to continue antibiotics, but recommendations are usually for 2 weeks or more.

Percutaneous drainage for pyogenic hepatic abscesses was first reported in 1953 but did not gain widespread acceptance until the 1980s with the development of high-quality imaging and expertise in interventional radiologic techniques. During the last 25 years, percutaneous catheter drainage has become the treatment of choice for most patients (Fig. 53-28). Success rates range from 66% to 90%.[11,13] The obvious advantages are the simplicity of treatment (usually at the time of radiologic diagnosis) and avoidance of general anesthesia and a laparotomy. Relative contraindications to percutaneous catheter drainage include the presence of ascites, coagulopathy, and proximity to vital structures. Percutaneous drainage of multiple abscesses is usually met with a higher failure rate, but reports have demonstrated a high enough success rate that percutaneous approaches should be made first, reserving surgery for failures. A retrospective study comparing surgical with percutaneous drainage for large abscesses (>5 cm) has shown a better success rate with surgical drainage. Despite this, two thirds of percutaneous treatments were successful, and the overall morbidity and mortality rates were similar. There has never been a randomized prospective comparison between percutaneous and surgical therapy for hepatic abscess. However, case series have suggested that for most cases, there are similar success and mortality rates. Modern series attempting to compare these two techniques retrospectively must be read with caution because most patients treated surgically have failed to respond to other less invasive techniques. In general, surgery should be reserved for patients who require surgical treatment of the primary pathologic process (e.g., appendicitis) or for those who have failed to respond to percutaneous techniques. Laparoscopic drainage procedures have been reported with some success, and this can be considered a reasonable option to pursue in select cases.[11]

Percutaneous aspiration without the placement of an indwelling drain has been investigated by a number of groups. Success rates are generally 60% to 90% and are somewhat similar to those for percutaneous catheter drainage.[15] Most patients, however, require more than one aspiration, and 25% of patients require three or more aspirations. One randomized trial has evaluated percutaneous aspiration versus percutaneous catheter drainage. Success rates were 60% in the aspiration group and 100% in the catheter group. All but one patient in the aspiration group had a single aspiration. Another randomized trial of 64 patients has compared aspiration alone with catheter drainage. There were similar outcomes in terms of treatment success rate, hospital stay, antibiotic duration, and mortality. In the aspiration-only group, 40% required two aspirations and 20% required three aspirations. In general, catheter drainage remains the treatment of choice, although a trial of a single aspiration is reasonable to consider.

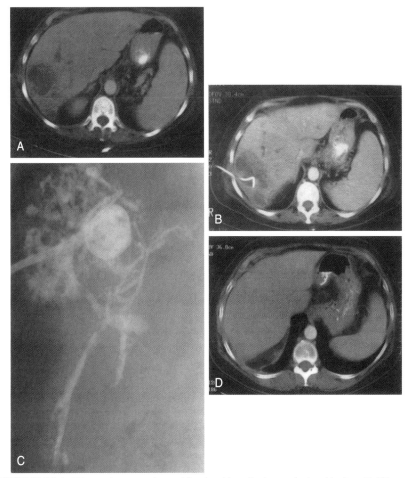

FIGURE 53-28 **A,** CT scan demonstrating multiloculated hepatic abscess in the right liver. **B,** CT scan at the time of percutaneous drainage. **C,** Contrast study through the drainage catheter demonstrating typical irregular loculated appearance as well as communication with biliary tree. **D,** Follow-up CT scan 3 months after treatment demonstrating complete resolution of abscess. (From Brown KT, Getrajdman GI: Interventional radiologic techniques in the liver and biliary tract. In Blumgart LH, Fong Y, editors: *Surgery of the liver and biliary tract,* London, 2000, WB Saunders, pp 575–594.)

Some investigators have reported success with antibiotics alone. Most of these patients, however, have had a diagnostic aspiration and thus at least a partial drainage. Also, other series have reported that antibiotic treatment without drainage carries a prohibitively high mortality (59% to 100%). In patients who are not surgical candidates or who refuse any invasive procedure, an attempt at antibiotic treatment is reasonable. However, this is not recommended in other situations.

Liver resection is occasionally required for hepatic abscess. This may be required for an infected hepatic malignant neoplasm, hepatolithiasis, or intrahepatic biliary stricture. If hepatic destruction from infection is severe, some patients may benefit from resection.

Outcomes

Mortality from pyogenic hepatic abscess has dramatically improved during the last 70 years. Before the routine use of surgical drainage, pyogenic abscess was uniformly fatal. With the routine use of surgical drainage and the use of IV antibiotics, mortality was reduced to approximately 50%, a figure that stayed relatively constant from 1945 until the early 1980s. Since then, the mortality has been reported from 10% to 20%, and series from the 1990s have demonstrated a mortality rate below 10%.[15] The most recent series from Memorial Sloan Kettering Cancer Center (MSKCC) has reported a 3% mortality. A number of studies have analyzed factors predictive of a poor outcome in patients with hepatic pyogenic abscess. The presence of malignant disease, factors associated with malignant disease (e.g., jaundice, markedly elevated LFT results), and signs of sepsis appear to be consistent markers of poor prognosis. Signs of chronic disease, such as hypoalbuminemia, are also often associated with a poor outcome. Finally, signs of severe infection, such as marked leukocytosis, APACHE II (Acute Physiology and Chronic Health Evaluation II) scores, abscess rupture, bacteremia, and shock, are also associated with mortality.

Amebic Abscess

Epidemiology

Amebiasis is largely a disease of tropical and developing countries but is also a significant problem in developed countries because of immigration and travel between countries. *E. histolytica* is endemic in Mexico, India, Africa, and parts of Central and South America. In 1995, the World Health Organization estimated that 40 to 50 million people suffer from amebic colitis or amebic liver abscess worldwide, resulting in 40,000 to 100,000 deaths each year.[14] Before this, estimates of amebiasis were unreliable because *E. histolytica* (the pathogenic form) was not differentiated from *Entamoeba dispar* (the nonpathogenic form). Male homosexuals with diarrhea, previously thought to harbor *E. histolytica,* were actually found to be infected with *E. dispar,* which requires no treatment. Epidemiologic studies specifically addressing *E. histolytica* infections have estimated that as many as 55% of those in endemic regions are infected, although less than 50% are symptomatic.

In contrast to pyogenic hepatic abscesses, patients with amebic liver abscesses tend to be Hispanic men, 20 to 40 years of age, with a history of travel to (or origination from) an endemic area. Poverty and cramped living conditions are associated with higher rates of infection. A male preponderance of more than 10:1 has been reported in almost all studies. For unclear reasons, menstruating women have a low incidence of invasive amebiasis, and pregnancy appears to abrogate this resistance. Heavy alcohol consumption is commonly reported and may render the liver more susceptible to amebic infection. Patients with impaired host immunity also appear to be at higher risk of infection and have higher mortality rates. Patients with amebic liver abscess without a history of travel to an endemic area often have associated immunosuppression, such as HIV infection, malnutrition, chronic infection, or chronic steroid use.[16]

Pathogenesis

E. histolytica is a protozoan and exists as a trophozoite or a cyst. All other species in the genus *Entamoeba* are considered nonpathogenic, and not all strains of *E. histolytica* are considered virulent. Ingestion of *E. histolytica* cysts through a fecal-oral route is the cause of amebiasis. Humans are the principal host, and the main source of infection is human contact with a cyst-passing carrier. Contaminated water and vegetables are also routes of human infection. Once ingested, the cysts are not degraded in the stomach and pass to the intestines, where the trophozoite is released and passed on to the colon. In the colon, the trophozoite can invade mucosa, resulting in disease.

It is thought that the trophozoites reach the liver through the portal venous system. There is no evidence for trophozoites passing through lymphatics. As implied by its name, *E. histolytica* trophozoites can lyse tissues through a complex set of events, including cell adherence, cell activation, and subsequent release of enzymes, resulting in necrosis. The principal mechanism is probably enzymatic cellular hydrolysis. Amebic liver abscesses are formed by progressing, localized hepatic necrosis producing a cavity containing acellular proteinaceous debris surrounded by a rim of invasive amebic trophozoites. Early development of an amebic liver abscess is associated with an accumulation of polymorphonuclear leukocytes, which are then lysed by the trophozoites.

Antiamebic antibodies develop rapidly in patients with invasive disease or an amebic hepatic abscess. Secretory immunoglobulin A (IgA) antibodies have been shown to inhibit adherence to colonic epithelium in vitro. However, the development of these antibodies does not halt the progression of disease. Interestingly, children who lack antiamebic IgG have innate resistance to invasive infection, suggesting an alternative immune-mediated response. There is now evidence that a cell-mediated helper T cell response is probably the major mechanism of resistance.

Pathology

Hepatic amebic abscess is essentially the result of liquefaction necrosis of the liver producing a cavity full of blood and liquefied liver tissue. The appearance of this fluid is typically described as resembling anchovy sauce; the fluid is odorless unless secondary bacterial infection has taken place. The progressive hepatic necrosis continues until Glisson capsule is reached because the capsule is resistant to hydrolysis by the amebae. Thus, amebic abscesses tend to abut the liver capsule. Because of the resistance of Glisson capsule, the cavity is typically crisscrossed by portal triads protected by this peritoneal sheath. Early on, the formed cavity is ill-defined, with no real fibrous response around the edges. However, a chronic abscess can ultimately develop a fibrous capsule and may even calcify. Like pyogenic abscesses, amebic abscesses tend to occur mainly in the right liver.

Clinical Features

Approximately 80% of patients with amebic liver abscess present with symptoms lasting from a few days to 4 weeks. The duration of symptoms has been found to be typically less than 10 days. The presenting clinical signs and symptoms are summarized in Table 53-6. The typical clinical picture is a patient 20 to 40 years of age who has recently traveled to an endemic area, with fever, chills, anorexia, right upper quadrant pain and tenderness, and hepatomegaly. The abdominal pain is typically constant, dull, and localized to the right upper quadrant. Although some studies report higher numbers, approximately 25% of patients have diarrhea despite an obligatory colonic infection. Synchronous hepatic abscess is found in one third of patients with active amebic colitis.

TABLE 53-6 Signs, Symptoms, and Laboratory Findings in Amebic Liver Abscess*

PARAMETER	AVERAGE	RANGE	NO. OF CASES REVIEWED
Symptoms and Signs			
Abdominal pain (%)	92	73-100	1701
Fever (%)	90	72-100	2192
Abdominal tenderness (%)	78	40-100	1424
Hepatomegaly (%)	62	20-100	1539
Anorexia (%)	47	28-89	499
Weight loss (%)	39	11-83	871
Diarrhea (%)	23	12-40	1426
Jaundice (%)	22	5-50	1630
Laboratory Tests			
Stool cysts, trophozoites (%)	12	4-30	4908
Amebae in cyst aspirate (%)	42	30-76	1402
Hemoglobin (g/dL)	12.1	10.2-12.8	229
Alkaline phosphatase (% >120 U/liter)	76	65-91	589
Total bilirubin (g/dL)	1.4	0.8-2.4	509
Albumin (g/dL)	2.8	2.3-3.4	404
AST (× upper limit normal)	1.7	1.0-2.5	459

*In an extensive literature review.

Jaundice, as a result of a large abscess compressing the biliary tree, is not as rare as was once thought, with an average 22% of patients presenting with this feature worldwide. Weight loss and myalgias may occur when symptoms have been present for weeks. Pleuritic or right shoulder pain can occur if there is irritation of the right hemidiaphragm. Symptoms and tenderness may be epigastric or left sided if the abscess is located in the left liver. Rupture into the peritoneum with peritonitis occurs infrequently; when it does occur, it is more often with left-sided abscesses. Rare cases of rupture into the pleural space, pericardium, and other intraabdominal organs have also been reported.

Patients presenting acutely (symptoms <10 days) versus those with a chronic presentation (>2 weeks) differ clinically. Acute presentations are typically more dramatic, with high fevers, chills, and significant abdominal tenderness. In the acute presentation, 50% of patients have multiple lesions, whereas with the chronic presentation, more than 80% of patients have a single right-sided lesion. A more complicated course tends to ensue in the acute presentation, but response to therapy is similar in both groups.

Laboratory abnormalities are common in amebic abscess (Table 53-6). Patients typically have a mild to moderate leukocytosis, without eosinophilia. Anemia is common. Mild abnormalities of LFT results, including albumin, PT-INR, ALP, AST, and bilirubin levels, are typical. The most common LFT abnormality is an elevated PT-INR. Because more than 70% of patients with amebic liver abscess do not have detectable amebae in their stool, the most useful laboratory evaluation is the measurement of circulating antiamebic antibodies, which are present in 90% to 95% of patients. A number of serologic tests have been devised over the years. An indirect hemagglutinin test was used extensively in the past and has a sensitivity of 90%. This test has largely been replaced by enzyme immunoassays, which detect presence of antibodies against the parasite and are simple, rapidly performed, and inexpensive. An enzyme immunoassay has a reported sensitivity of 99% and specificity higher than 90% in patients with hepatic abscess. Unfortunately, the presence of antibodies may reflect prior infection, and interpretation can be difficult in endemic areas. Ongoing studies are focusing on identifying specific *E. histolytica* antigens in an attempt to identify acute infection. The antigen detection kits have been evaluated in endemic areas. These kits can detect the *E. histolytica* lectin antigen in the serum and liver abscess pus and in small studies have been shown to have high sensitivity. However, the sensitivity may decrease if the test is performed after treatment with metronidazole.[17]

Radiologic studies are a critical element in the diagnosis of amebic liver abscess. Plain chest radiographs are abnormal in approximately 50% of cases, usually demonstrating an elevated right diaphragm, pleural effusion, or atelectasis. Abdominal ultrasound has a reported accuracy of approximately 90% when it is combined with a typical history and clinical presentation. Typical findings on abdominal ultrasound are a rounded lesion abutting the liver capsule (see earlier) without significant rim echoes, interpreted as an abscess wall. The contents of the cavity are usually hypoechoic and nonhomogeneous (Fig. 53-29). These findings on ultrasound are found in 40% to 70% of cases. Abdominal CT scanning is probably more sensitive than ultrasound and is helpful in differentiating amebic from pyogenic abscess, with rim enhancement noted in the pyogenic abscess (Fig. 53-30). CT can also be helpful in identifying simple cysts and necrotic tumors. MRI of the liver has no distinct advantages over CT or ultrasound in typical cases but may be helpful in differentiating atypical lesions. Nuclear medicine studies, such as gallium scanning or technetium

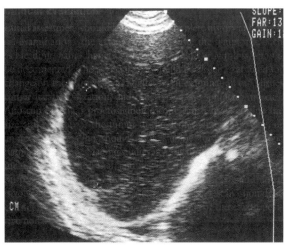

FIGURE 53-29 Typical ultrasound image of an amebic hepatic abscess. Note the peripheral location, rounded shape with poor rim, and internal echoes. (From Thomas PG, Ravindra KV: Amebiasis and biliary infection. In Blumgart LH, Fong Y, editors: *Surgery of the liver and biliary tract*, London, 2000, WB Saunders, pp 1147–1166.)

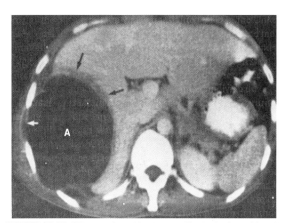

FIGURE 53-30 CT scan of amebic abscess. The lesion is peripherally located and round. The rim is nonenhancing but shows peripheral edema *(black arrows)*. Note the extension into the intercostal space *(white arrow)*.

Tc 99m liver scans, can be helpful in differentiating pyogenic from amebic abscesses because the amebic abscesses typically do not contain leukocytes and therefore do not light up on these scans.[18]

When this workup is still not definitive and diagnostic uncertainty persists, two options should be considered. First, a therapeutic trial of antiamebic drugs can be used. If a rapid improvement occurs, this supports the diagnosis. In situations in which amebic serology is inconclusive and a therapeutic trial of antibiotics is deemed inappropriate or has failed to improve symptoms, the second option, a diagnostic aspiration, should be considered. A pyogenic abscess would have bacteria and leukocytes, whereas an amebic abscess would contain the typical so-called anchovy sauce. Cultures of amebic abscess are usually negative and do not contain leukocytes. In patients for whom neoplasm or hydatid disease is in the differential diagnosis, aspiration should not be performed.

Differential Diagnosis

The differential diagnosis of an amebic liver abscess can be broad and include diseases such as viral hepatitis, echinococcal disease, cholangitis, cholecystitis, and even other inflammatory abdominal disorders, such as appendicitis. Malignant lesions of the liver can also have similar presentations in atypical situations. On occasion, primary pulmonary disorders must be considered. Usually, the most important distinction to be made is between pyogenic and amebic abscess. The essential elements of this distinction are summarized in Table 53-5 and in the earlier section on pyogenic abscess.

Treatment

The mainstay of treatment for amebic abscesses is metronidazole (750 mg orally, three times daily for 10 days), which is curative in more than 90% of patients. Clinical improvement is usually seen within 3 days. Other nitroimidazoles (e.g., secnidazole, tinidazole) are also as effective and are commonly used outside the United States. If response to metronidazole is poor or the drug is not tolerated, other agents can be used. Emetine hydrochloride is effective against invasive amebiasis, particularly in the liver, but requires intramuscular injections and has serious cardiac side effects. A more attractive option is chloroquine, but this is a less effective agent. After treatment of the liver abscess, it is recommended that luminal agents such as iodoquinol, paromomycin, and diloxanide furoate be administered to treat the carrier state.

Therapeutic needle aspiration of amebic abscesses has been proposed. However, a Cochrane systematic review did not support any benefit of therapeutic aspiration in addition to metronidazole treatment over metronidazole treatment alone to hasten clinical or radiologic resolution of amebic liver abscesses.[19] In general, aspiration is recommended for diagnostic uncertainty (see earlier), with failure to respond to metronidazole therapy in 3 to 5 days, or in abscesses thought to be at high risk for rupture. Abscesses larger than 5 cm in diameter and in the left liver are thought to carry a higher risk of rupture, and aspiration should be considered.

Outcomes

Although amebic liver abscesses usually respond rapidly to treatment, there are uncommon complications of which one must be aware. The most frequent complication of amebic abscess is rupture into the peritoneum, pleural cavity, or pericardium. The size of the abscess appears to be the most important risk factor for rupture, and the overall incidence of rupture ranges from 3% to 17%. Most peritoneal ruptures tend to be contained by the diaphragm, abdominal wall, or omentum, but rupture can fistulize into a hollow viscus. A peritoneal rupture usually is manifested as abdominal pain, peritonitis, and a mass or generalized distention. Laparotomy was advocated in the past for this complication, but now many patients are treated successfully with percutaneous drainage. Laparotomy is indicated in cases of doubtful diagnosis, hollow viscus perforation, fistulization resulting in hemorrhage or sepsis, and failure of conservative therapy. Rupture into the pleural space usually results in a large and rapidly accumulated effusion that collapses the involved lung. Treatment consists of thoracentesis, but if secondary bacterial infection ensues, more aggressive surgical approaches may be necessary. Rupture can occur into the bronchi and is usually self-limited with postural drainage and bronchodilators. Rarely, a left-sided abscess may rupture into the pericardium and can be manifested as an asymptomatic pericardial effusion or even tamponade. This must be treated with aspiration or drainage through a pericardial window. Other complications include compression of the biliary tree or IVC from a very large abscess and the development of a brain abscess.

The mortality for all patients with amebic liver abscess is approximately 5% and does not appear to be affected by the addition of aspiration to metronidazole therapy or by chronicity of symptoms. When an abscess ruptures, mortality ranges from 6% to as high as 50%. Factors independently associated with poor outcome are elevated serum bilirubin level (>3.5 mg/dL), encephalopathy, hypoalbuminemia (<2.0 g/dL), multiple abscess cavities, abscess volume larger than 500 mL, anemia, and diabetes. Although clinical improvement after adequate treatment with antiamebic agents is the rule, radiologic resolution of the abscess cavity is usually delayed. The average time to radiologic resolution is 3 to 9 months, and in some patients, it can take years. Studies have shown that more than 90% of the visible lesions disappear radiologically, but a small percentage of patients are left with a clinically irrelevant residual lesion.

Hydatid Cyst

Hydatid disease or echinococcosis is a zoonosis that occurs primarily in sheep-grazing areas of the world but is common worldwide because the dog is a definitive host. Echinococcosis is endemic in Mediterranean countries, the Middle East, Far East, South America, Australia, New Zealand, and east Africa.[20] Humans contract the disease from dogs, but there is no human-to-human transmission.[21,22]

There are three species that cause hydatid disease. *Echinococcus granulosus* is the most common, and *Echinococcus multilocularis* and *Echinococcus ligartus* account for a small number of cases.[20] Dogs are the definitive host of *E. granulosus;* the adult tapeworm is attached to the villi of the ileum. Up to thousands of ova are passed daily and deposited in the dog's feces. Sheep are the usual intermediate host, but humans are an accidental intermediate host. Humans are an end stage to the parasite. In the human duodenum, the parasitic embryo releases an oncosphere containing hooklets that penetrate the mucosa, allowing access to the bloodstream. In the blood, the oncosphere reaches the liver (most commonly) or lungs, where the parasite develops its larval stage—the hydatid cyst.

Three weeks after infection, a visible hydatid cyst develops, which then slowly grows in a spherical manner. A pericyst or fibrous capsule derived from host tissues develops around the hydatid cyst. The cyst wall itself has two layers, an outer gelatinous membrane (ectocyst) and an inner germinal membrane (endocyst). Brood capsules are small, intracystic cellular masses in which future worm heads develop into scoleces. In a definitive host, the scoleces develop into an adult tapeworm; but in the intermediate host, they can differentiate only into a new hydatid cyst. Freed brood capsules and scoleces are found in the hydatid fluid and form the so-called hydatid sand. Daughter cysts are true replicas of the mother cyst. Hydatid cysts can die with degeneration of the membranes, development of cystic vacuoles, and calcification of the wall. Calcification of a hydatid cyst, however, does not always imply that the cyst is dead.

Hydatid cysts are diagnosed in equal numbers of men and women at an average age of about 45 years. Approximately 75% of hydatid cysts are located in the right liver and are solitary. The clinical presentation of a hydatid cyst is largely asymptomatic until complications occur. The most common presenting symptoms are abdominal pain, dyspepsia, and vomiting. The most frequent sign is hepatomegaly. Jaundice and fever are each present in approximately 8% of patients. Bacterial superinfection of a hydatid cyst can occur and be manifested like a pyogenic abscess. Rupture of the cyst into the biliary tree or bronchial tree or free rupture into the peritoneal, pleural, or pericardial cavities can occur. Free ruptures can result in disseminated echinococcosis or a potentially fatal anaphylactic reaction. In cases of diagnostic uncertainty, a battery of serologic tests are available to evaluate antibody response, but all are plagued by low sensitivity and specificity.

Ultrasound is most commonly used worldwide for the diagnosis of echinococcosis because of its availability, affordability, and accuracy. A number of findings on ultrasound can be diagnostic but depend on the stage of the cyst at the time of the examination. A simple hydatid cyst is well circumscribed with budding signs on the cyst membrane and may contain free-floating hyperechogenic hydatid sand. A rosette appearance is seen when daughter cysts are present. The cyst can be filled with an amorphous mass, which can be diagnostically misleading. Calcifications in the wall of the cyst are highly suggestive of hydatid disease and can be helpful in the diagnosis (Fig. 53-31). Similar findings are seen on CT or MRI scans. These cross-sectional imaging studies can also evaluate extrahepatic disease and demonstrate detailed hepatic anatomic relationships to the cyst. In patients with suspected biliary involvement, ERCP or percutaneous transhepatic cholangiography may be necessary.

Although the treatment of hepatic hydatid cysts is primarily surgical, alternative options are in evolution.[23] In general, most cysts should be treated; but in older patients with small, asymptomatic, densely calcified cysts, conservative management is appropriate. In preparation for an operation, preoperative steroids have been recommended but are not universally used. The anesthesiologist should have epinephrine and steroids available in case of an anaphylactic reaction. A number of operations have been used, but in general, the abdomen is completely explored, the liver mobilized, and the cyst exposed. Packing off the abdomen is important because rupture can result in anaphylaxis and diffuse seeding. The cyst is usually then aspirated through a closed suction system and flushed with a scolicidal agent, such as hypertonic saline. The cyst is then unroofed, which can then be followed by a number of possibilities, including excision (or pericystectomy), marsupialization procedures, leaving the cyst open, drainage of the cyst, omentoplasty, and partial hepatectomy to encompass the cyst. Total pericystectomy or formal partial hepatectomy can also be performed without entering the cyst (Fig. 53-32). Both radical (resection) and conservative (drainage and evacuation) surgical approaches appear to be equally effective at controlling disease, although a prospective comparison has never been performed. When bile duct communication is diagnosed preoperatively or at operation, it must be meticulously sought after. Simple suture repair is often sufficient, but major biliary repairs, approaches through the common bile duct, or postoperative ERCP may be necessary. Laparoscopic techniques for drainage and unroofing of cysts have been reported in a number of series, with encouraging results. Recurrence rates after surgical treatment range from 1% to 20% but are generally 5% or less in experienced centers.

In the past, percutaneous aspiration of hydatid cysts was contraindicated because of the risk of rupture and uncontrolled spillage. However, percutaneous aspiration with injection of scolicidal agents has been reported with high success rates in highly selected

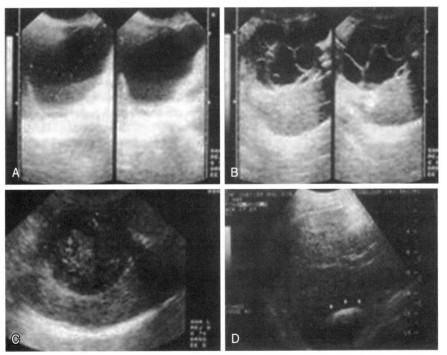

FIGURE 53-31 Ultrasound image demonstrating typical characteristics of a hydatid cyst at varying stages. **A,** Simple hydatid cyst with hydatid sand. **B,** Daughter and granddaughter cysts and typical rosette appearance. **C,** Hydatid cyst filled with amorphous mass, giving a solid or semisolid appearance. **D,** Calcified cyst with eggshell appearance. (From Thomas PG, Ravindra KV: Amebiasis and biliary infection. In Blumgart LH, Fong Y, editors: *Surgery of the liver and biliary tract,* London, 2000, WB Saunders, pp 1147–1166.)

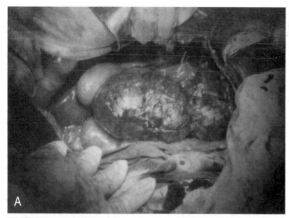

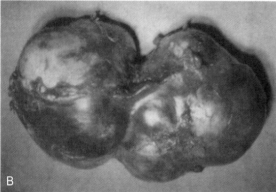

FIGURE 53-32 A, Peripheral hydatid cyst of the left liver. **B,** Intact specimen after pericystectomy. Note that the entire pericyst has been removed. (From Milicevic MN: Hydatid disease. In Blumgart LH, Fong Y, editors: *Surgery of the liver and biliary tract,* London, 2000, WB Saunders, pp 1167–1204.)

patients.[24] This technique is known as PAIR (puncture, aspiration, injection, and reaspiration) and has become more accepted in some centers. Two randomized trials, one comparing PAIR with surgery (*N* = 50) and one comparing PAIR with medical therapy, have shown similar success rates. These trials were small and had significant methodologic problems, limiting the ability to draw firm conclusions.[25] Although surgery remains the treatment of choice, further prospective trials are clearly indicated to address this interesting and potentially useful technique. Treatment of echinococcosis with albendazole or mebendazole is effective at shrinking cysts in many patients with *E. granulosus* infection, but cyst disappearance occurs in well below 50% of patients. Preoperative treatment may decrease the risk of spillage and is a reasonable and safe practice.[15] Medical therapy without definitive resection or drainage should be considered only for widely disseminated disease or poor surgical candidates.

Recurrent Pyogenic Cholangitis

Recurrent pyogenic cholangitis (RPC) is a syndrome of repeated attacks of cholangitis secondary to biliary stones and strictures that involve the extrahepatic and intrahepatic ducts. The condition has many names but is often referred to as Oriental cholangiohepatitis or hepatolithiasis. The disease is almost exclusively found in Asians and Asian medical centers. However, it is also seen in Asian immigrants throughout the world. Men and women are equally affected, and historically, the disease strikes at an early age (20 to 40 years) in patients from lower socioeconomic classes.[26]

The cause of RPC is unknown but is related to recurrent infection of biliary radicals with gut bacteria. Ultimately, stones and strictures develop in the biliary tree, but it is not known which occurs first. The stones are bilirubinate stones; in some patients, no stones are found and only biliary sludge is demonstrated. An association between RPC and *Clonorchis sinensis* and *Ascaris lumbricoides* infection has been noted, but a true causal relationship has never been proven.[27]

Strictures can be found anywhere in the biliary tree but usually involve the intrahepatic main hepatic ducts, most often the left hepatic duct. The gallbladder is involved only in approximately 20% of cases. Cirrhosis and liver failure are seen only in long-standing disease, usually after multiple operations. Other complications include choledochoduodenal fistulas and acute pancreatitis from common bile duct stones. An increased incidence of cholangiocarcinoma has been noted, but a causal relationship is difficult to prove.

The typical patient with RPC is a young Asian of a lower socioeconomic background who presents with repeated bouts of cholangitis. The symptoms and presentation are those of cholangitis. These include fever, right upper quadrant abdominal pain, and jaundice. Biliary obstruction is usually incomplete, and therefore marked jaundice and pruritus are not common. There is usually leukocytosis and abnormal LFT results consistent with biliary obstruction. Evaluation of the anatomic distribution of disease is critical to formulation of a sound therapeutic plan. A combination of ultrasound, CT, and direct cholangiography is often necessary to evaluate these patients. Direct cholangiography is performed endoscopically or transhepatically and is considered an important study complementing the cross-sectional imaging. Magnetic resonance cholangiopancreatography can combine cross-sectional imaging and cholangiography in one noninvasive test and may ultimately replace direct cholangiography.

In an acute presentation, most patients improve with conservative management, allowing time for radiologic studies and planning of a definitive operation, which is the treatment of choice. If intervention is necessary during the acute phase, it must focus on adequate decompression of the biliary tree through open common bile duct exploration or endoscopic papillotomy with stenting. Although nonoperative approaches, such as percutaneous transhepatic cholangioscopic lithotomy, have been developed, surgical treatment remains the treatment of choice. Percutaneous transhepatic cholangioscopic lithotomy is generally used for poor-risk surgical patients and those who have failed to respond to surgical treatment. Stone clearance rates are high (>80%) and necessary for a successful long-term outcome. Unfortunately, stone recurrence is common and is mostly related to the presence of biliary strictures.[28]

The goal of operative approaches is to clear the biliary tree of stones and to bypass, resect, or enlarge strictures.[29] Many cases require only exploration of the common bile duct, with or without hepaticojejunostomy. In complicated cases, providing permanent access to the biliary tree for interventional radiologic procedures by extending the end of the Roux-en-Y hepaticojejunostomy to the skin or subcutaneous space has been a successful approach (Fig. 53-33). Other potentially necessary procedures include stricturoplasty and partial hepatectomy. Partial hepatectomy is advocated for patients with intrahepatic strictures, hepatic atrophy, liver abscess, or suspicion of cholangiocarcinoma.[30]

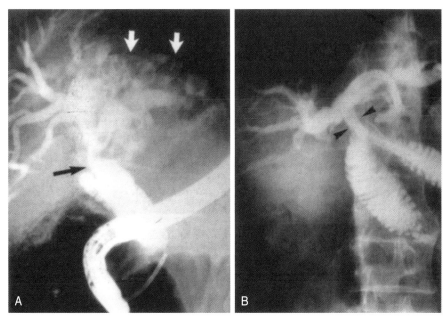

FIGURE 53-33 A, Cholangiogram of a patient with recurrent pyogenic cholangitis and a common hepatic duct stricture *(black arrow)*. There are numerous stones inside dilated left ducts *(white arrows)*. **B,** A hepaticojejunostomy to the segment III duct *(arrowheads)* has been performed, and a flexible choledochoscope is shown passing through the anastomosis into the peripheral left ducts. All stones have been cleared. (From Fan ST, Wong J: Recurrent pyogenic cholangitis. In Blumgart LH, Fong Y, editors: *Surgery of the liver and biliary tract*, London, 2000, WB Saunders, pp 1205–1225.)

In a large series from Asia, where surgery and hepatectomy are liberally applied, surgical mortality rates are 1%. Moreover, with aggressive treatment, there is almost a 100% stone clearance rate. Long-term outcome is excellent, with a less than 5% stone recurrence rate. Long-term survival is mostly related to the presence of cholangiocarcinoma, which is found in approximately 10% of patients. Particularly complicated cases can have a higher rate of recurrent symptoms.

NEOPLASMS

Solid Benign Neoplasms

It is estimated that benign focal liver masses are present in approximately 10% to 20% of the population in developed countries. With the increasing use of rapidly improving radiologic examinations, these entities have been encountered more frequently. Familiarity with the clinical characteristics, natural history, imaging characteristics, and indications for surgery in these tumors is essential. Many benign lesions can be adequately characterized by modern imaging studies, such as CT, ultrasound, and MRI. In unclear cases, serum tumor markers (e.g., AFP, CEA) and a search for a primary tumor in the case of suspected metastases should be carried out. A resection might be necessary to make a definitive diagnosis. Laparoscopy for assessment, biopsy, or resection has become an important diagnostic technique as well.[31,32]

Liver Cell Adenoma

Liver cell adenoma (LCA) is a relatively rare benign proliferation of hepatocytes in the context of a normal liver. It is predominantly found in young women (aged 20 to 40 years) and is often associated with steroid hormone use, such as long-term oral contraceptive pill (OCP) use. Male anabolic hormone use can also predispose to development of LCA. The female-to-male ratio is approximately 11:1. LCAs are usually singular, but multiple lesions have been reported in 12% to 30% of cases. Interestingly, cases with multiple adenomas are not associated with OCP use and do not have as dramatic a female preponderance. On histologic evaluation, LCAs are composed of cords of benign hepatocytes containing increased glycogen and fat. Bile ductules are not observed histologically, and the normal architecture of the liver is absent in these lesions. Hemorrhage and necrosis are commonly seen.[33] On the basis of detailed molecular pathology correlation studies, a French collaborative group has recently proposed a molecular-pathologic classification whereby the adenomas are classified as β-catenin mutated adenoma, *HNF1A* mutated adenoma, inflammatory adenoma, and not otherwise specified adenoma.[34,35] Molecular studies have also identified genetic signatures associated with a higher risk of malignant transformation. Specifically, highest risk of malignant transformation is observed in LCA with β-catenin activation.[35,36] Patients with LCA present with symptoms approximately 50% to 75% of the time. Upper abdominal pain is common and may be related to hemorrhage into the tumor or local compressive symptoms. The physical examination is usually unrevealing, and tumor markers are normal. Dramatic presentations with free intraperitoneal rupture and bleeding can occur. Imaging tends to be characteristic and obviates the need for tissue diagnosis most of the time.[37-39] Because of intratumoral hemorrhage, the necrosis and fat component of LCA tends to be heterogeneous on CT. On contrast-enhanced CT, LCA tends to have peripheral enhancement with centripetal progression. MRI scans of LCA also have specific imaging characteristics, including a well-demarcated heterogeneous mass containing fat or hemorrhage. Despite high-quality imaging, resection may sometimes be necessary to secure a diagnosis in difficult cases. Intriguingly, studies are elucidating a correlation between the molecular subtypes described and imaging characteristics.[40]

The two major risks of LCA are rupture, with potentially life-threatening intraperitoneal hemorrhage, and malignant transformation. Quantifying the risk of rupture is difficult, but it has been estimated to be as high as 30% to 50%, with all instances of spontaneous rupture occurring in lesions 5 cm and larger.[39] Although there are numerous reports of transformation of LCA into hepatocellular carcinoma (HCC), the true risk of transformation is probably low. Hepatic adenomas with β-catenin activation should be considered for early surgical intervention as malignant transformation most commonly occurs in this subtype.[36,41]

Patients who present with acute hemorrhage need emergent attention. If possible, hepatic artery embolization is a helpful and usually effective temporizing maneuver. Once the patient is stabilized and appropriately resuscitated, a laparotomy and resection of the mass are required. Symptomatic masses should be similarly resected. Patients with asymptomatic LCAs taking OCPs can be watched for regression after stopping of the OCPs, although progression and rupture have been observed in this setting. Behavior of LCAs during pregnancy has been unpredictable, and resection before a planned pregnancy is usually recommended. Overall, the surgeon must compare the risks of expectant management with serial imaging studies and AFP measurements against those of resection. Resection is usually recommended because of low mortality in experienced hands and the risks of observation. Margin status is not important in these resections, and limited resections can be performed. The management of adenomatosis is controversial, but large lesions should probably be resected because of the risk of rupture, whereas the risk of malignancy is low in lesions smaller than 5 cm.[42] On occasion, liver transplantation is necessary for aggressive forms of adenomatosis.[43,44]

Focal Nodular Hyperplasia

Focal nodular hyperplasia (FNH) is the second most common benign tumor of the liver after hemangioma and is predominantly discovered in young women.[39] FNH is characterized by a central fibrous scar with radiating septa, although no central scar is seen in approximately 15% of cases (Fig. 53-34). On microscopic examination, FNH contains cords of benign-appearing hepatocytes divided by multiple fibrous septa originating from a central scar. Typical hepatic vascularity is not seen, but atypical biliary epithelium is found scattered throughout the lesion. The central scar often contains a large artery that branches out into multiple smaller arteries in a spoke wheel pattern. The cause of FNH is not known, but the most common theory is that FNH is related to a developmental vascular malformation. Female hormones and OCPs have been implicated in the development and growth of FNH, but the association is weak and difficult to prove.

In most patients, FNH is an incidental finding at laparotomy or, more commonly, on imaging studies. If symptoms are noted, vague abdominal pain is most often present, but a variety of nonspecific symptoms have been described. It is often difficult to ascribe these reported symptoms to the presence of FNH, and therefore other possible causes must be sought. Physical examination is usually unrevealing, and mild abnormalities of liver function may be found. Serum AFP levels are normal.

With advances in hepatobiliary imaging, most cases of FNH can be diagnosed radiologically with reasonable certainty. Contrast-enhanced CT and MRI have become accurate methods of diagnosing FNH.[45] FNH typically shows strong hypervascularity in the

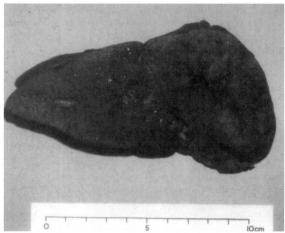

FIGURE 53-34 Cross section of resected focal nodular hyperplasia. Note the well-defined central scar. (From Hugh TJ, Poston GJ: Benign liver tumors and masses. In Blumgart LH, Fong Y, editors: *Surgery of the liver and biliary tract*, London, 2000, WB Saunders, pp 1397–1422.)

arterial phase of CT or MRI with central nonenhancing scar. The enhancement fades over time, and the lesion becomes isointense to the liver parenchyma in the portal and delayed phases. When no central scar is seen, however, radiologic diagnosis is difficult, and differentiation from LCA or a malignant mass, especially fibrolamellar HCC, can sometimes be impossible. On occasion, histologic confirmation is necessary, and resection is recommended for definitive diagnosis. Fine-needle aspiration for the diagnosis of FNH has been recommended but is often unrevealing.

Most FNH tumors are benign and indolent. Rupture, bleeding, and infarction are exceedingly rare, and malignant degeneration of FNH has never been reported. The treatment of FNH therefore depends on diagnostic certainty and symptoms. Asymptomatic patients with typical radiologic features do not require treatment.[39] If diagnostic uncertainty exists, resection may be necessary for histologic confirmation. Symptomatic patients should be thoroughly investigated to look for other pathologic processes to explain the symptoms. Careful observation of symptomatic FNH with serial imaging is reasonable because symptoms may resolve in a significant number of cases. Patients with persistent symptomatic FNH or an enlarging mass should be considered for resection. Because FNH is a benign diagnosis, resection must be performed, with minimal morbidity and mortality.[46]

Hemangioma

Hemangioma is the most common benign tumor of the liver.[39] It occurs in women more than in men (3:1 ratio) and at a mean age of approximately 45 years. Small capillary hemangiomas are of no clinical significance, whereas larger cavernous hemangiomas more often come to the attention of the liver surgeon (Fig. 53-35). Cavernous hemangiomas have been associated with FNH and are also theorized to be congenital vascular malformations. The enlargement of hemangiomas is by ectasia rather than by neoplasia. They are usually solitary and less than 5 cm in diameter, and they occur with equal incidence in the right and left hemilivers. Lesions larger than 5 cm are arbitrarily called giant hemangiomas. Involution or thrombosis of hemangiomas can result in dense fibrotic masses that may be difficult to differentiate from malignant tumors. On microscopic examination, they are

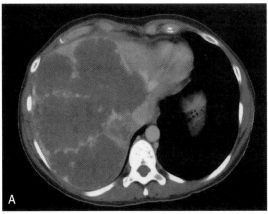

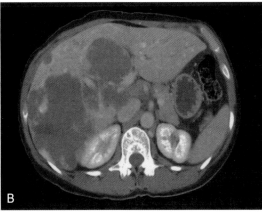

FIGURE 53-35 **A** and **B**, CT scans of a large cavernous hemangioma showing displacement of left and middle hepatic veins and abutment of the left portal vein. The mass was symptomatic and required an extended right hepatectomy for removal.

endothelium-lined, blood-filled spaces separated by thin fibrous septa.[47,48]

Hemangiomas are usually asymptomatic and found incidentally on imaging studies. Large compressive masses may cause vague upper abdominal symptoms. Symptoms ascribed to a liver hemangioma, however, mandate a search for other disease because an alternative cause of symptoms will be found in approximately 50% of cases. Rapid expansion or acute thrombosis can occasionally cause symptoms. Spontaneous rupture of liver hemangiomas is exceedingly rare. An associated syndrome of thrombocytopenia and consumptive coagulopathy known as Kasabach-Merritt syndrome is rare but well described.

LFT results and tumor markers are usually normal in liver hemangiomas. Radiologic investigation can make the diagnosis reliably in most cases. CT and MRI are usually sufficient if a typical peripheral nodular enhancement pattern is seen.[45,47] Isotope-labeled red blood cell scans are an accurate test but are rarely necessary if high-quality CT and MRI are available. Percutaneous biopsy of a suspected hemangioma is potentially dangerous and inaccurate. Therefore, biopsy is not recommended.

The natural history of liver hemangioma is generally benign; it appears that most remain stable for a long time, with a low risk of rupture or hemorrhage.[39] Growth and development of symptoms do occur, however, occasionally requiring resection. There has never been a report of malignant degeneration of a liver

hemangioma. An asymptomatic patient with a secure diagnosis can therefore be simply observed.[39] Symptomatic patients should undergo a thorough evaluation looking for alternative explanations for the symptoms but are candidates for resection if no other cause is found. Rupture, significant change in size, and development of the Kasabach-Merritt syndrome are indications for resection. In rare cases of diagnostic uncertainty, resection may be necessary for a definitive diagnosis to be made. Resection of liver hemangiomas should be performed, with minimal morbidity and mortality. The preferred approach to resection is enucleation with arterial inflow control, but anatomic resections may be necessary in some cases. Surgery on large central hemangiomas can be associated with significant morbidity.

Liver hemangiomas in children are common, accounting for approximately 12% of all childhood hepatic tumors.[49] They are usually multifocal and can involve other organs. Large hemangiomas in children can result in congestive heart failure secondary to arteriovenous shunting. Untreated symptomatic childhood hemangiomas are associated with high mortality. On the other hand, almost all small capillary hemangiomas resolve. Symptomatic childhood hemangiomas may be treated with therapeutic embolization; medical therapy should be initiated for congestive heart failure. Radiation and chemotherapeutic agents have been used, but experience has been limited. Resection may be necessary for symptomatic lesions or rupture.

Other Benign Tumors

Most benign solid liver tumors are LCAs, FNHs, or hemangiomas, but there are other benign hepatic tumors. However, these are rare and can be difficult to differentiate from malignant neoplasms. Macroregenerative nodules, previously known as adenomatous hyperplasia, are single or multiple, well-circumscribed, bile-stained, bulging surface nodules that occur primarily in cirrhotics and result from the hyperplastic response to chronic liver injury. These lesions have malignant potential and can be difficult to distinguish from HCC. Nodular regenerative hyperplasia is a benign diffuse micronodular (usually <2 cm) process associated with lymphoproliferative disorders, collagen vascular diseases, and the use of steroids or chemotherapy. Nodular regenerative hyperplasia has no malignant potential and is not associated with cirrhosis. Biopsy may be necessary to distinguish these focal nodules from malignant neoplasms.

Mesenchymal hamartomas are rare solitary tumors of childhood that account for 5% of pediatric liver tumors. They are usually large cystic masses found in the right liver that present as progressive, painless, abdominal distention. Resection of mesenchymal hamartomas may be necessary in the case of large lesions causing a mass effect.

Fatty tumors of the liver are rarely encountered but can usually be distinguished by typical characteristics on CT or MRI scans. Fatty tumors of the liver include primary lipomas, myelolipomas (which contain hematopoietic tissue), angiolipomas (which contain blood vessels), and angiomyolipomas (which contain smooth muscle). Focal fatty change in the liver can be confused with a neoplastic process and is becoming more common with improved imaging and the increasing incidence of hepatic steatosis.

Benign fibrous tumors of the liver can become large and symptomatic, requiring resection. Inflammatory pseudotumors of the liver are localized masses of inflammatory cells that can mimic a neoplasm. The cause of these inflammatory lesions is unknown but may be related to thrombosed vessels or old abscesses. Other extremely rare benign hepatic tumors include leiomyomas, myxomas, schwannomas, lymphangiomas, and teratomas.

Intrahepatic biliary cystadenomas or bile duct adenomas are rare but can cause biliary symptoms. Biliary hamartomas and biliary hyperplasia are common and are often seen as small white surface lesions that can mimic small metastatic tumors at abdominal exploration. Adrenal and pancreatic rests have also been found in the liver.

Primary Solid Malignant Neoplasms
Hepatocellular Carcinoma

Epidemiology. HCC is the most common primary malignant neoplasm of the liver and one of the most common malignant neoplasms worldwide, accounting for more than 1 million deaths annually. The geographic distribution of HCC is clearly related to the incidence of hepatitis B virus (HBV) infection. The highest incidence of disease (>10 to 20 cases/100,000) is found in Southeast Asia and tropical Africa. The lowest incidence (1 to 3 cases/100,000) is found in Australia, North America, and Europe. In high-incidence areas, rates are variable. For example, Taiwan has an incidence of 150 cases/100,000, and Singapore has an incidence of 28 cases/100,000. Epidemiologic evidence strongly suggests that HCC is largely related to environmental factors; the incidence of HCC in immigrants eventually approaches that of the local population after several generations. An exception to this is that whites living in high-prevalence areas tend to have a low incidence of HCC. This is likely related to the continuation of the lifestyle and environment of their home country. It is probable that the variation in incidence rates among immigrants is related to HBV carrier rates. A significant rise in the incidence of HCC in the United States and other Western countries has been noted during the last 35 years. However, recent data suggest that at least in the United States, the epidemic may have peaked as the incidence rates have stabilized in the last few years.[50,51] The explanation for the observed increase during the last few decades is not understood, but the emergence of hepatitis C virus (HCV) infection and immigration patterns have been suggested.[52-54] Risk of HCC is further increased in obese patients and in those with nonalcoholic fatty liver disease and nonalcoholic steatohepatitis.[55] Given that obesity and its ensuing complications are increasing at epidemic proportion in the Western world, obesity as the cause of HCC is becoming more important. Recent data also suggest that addressing the environmental factors can lead to reduction in incidence of HCC. In Taiwan, treatment of chronic hepatitis B and C under the auspices of a national viral hepatitis therapy program has met with a reduction in incidence and mortality due to HCC.[56]

HCC is two to eight times more common in men than in women in low- and high-incidence areas. Although sex hormones may play a minor role in the development of HCC, the higher incidence in men is probably related to higher rates of associated risk factors, such as HBV infection, cirrhosis, smoking, alcohol abuse, and higher hepatic DNA synthesis in cirrhosis. In general, the incidence of HCC increases with age, but a tendency to development of HCC earlier in high-incidence areas has been noted. For example, in Mozambique, 50% of patients with HCC were found to be younger than 30 years. This may be related to differing ages at infection and the natural histories of hepatitis B and C.

Causative factors. A large number of associations between hepatic viral infections, environmental exposure, alcohol use, smoking, genetic metabolic diseases, cirrhosis, and OCP use and the development of HCC have been recognized. Overall, 75% to 80% of HCC cases are related to HBV (50% to 55%) or HCV (25% to 30%) infections. It is also clear from research that the development of HCC is a complex and multistep process that involves any number of these risk factors.[54,57]

Many years of research have documented a clear association between persistent HBV infection and the development of HCC.[58] Studies have estimated relative risks of 5 to 100 for the development of HCC in HBV-infected individuals compared with noninfected individuals. Other evidence includes the following observations: geographic areas high in HBV infection have high rates of HCC; HBV infection precedes the development of HCC; the sequence of HBV infection to cirrhosis to HCC is well documented; and the HBV genome is found in the HCC genome. The HBV has no known oncogenes, but insertional mutagenesis into hepatocytes may be a contributing factor to the development of HCC. Another proposed mechanism is related to cirrhosis and chronic hepatic inflammation, which is present in 60% to 90% of patients with HBV infection and HCC. Cirrhosis, however, is not a prerequisite for the development of HBV-related HCC. The risk of HCC is not simply related to HBV exposure but requires chronic infection (i.e., chronically positive HBV surface antigen). There is a higher risk of persistent infection (carrier state) when the infection is acquired at birth or during early childhood. Familial clustering of HCC is probably related to early vertical transmission of the virus and establishment of the chronic carrier state.

Hepatitis C has been discovered to be a major cause of chronic liver disease in Japan, Europe, and the United States, where there is a relatively low rate of HBV infection. Antibodies to the HCV are found in 76% of patients with HCC in Japan and Europe and in 36% of patients in the United States. HBV and HCV infections are both independent risk factors for the development of HCC but probably act synergistically when an individual is infected with both viruses. Although the natural history of HCV infection is not completely understood, it appears to be one of chronic infection, with a benign early course. However, the ultimate development of cirrhosis and HCC may ensue. Studies on the rates of progression to cirrhosis estimate a median time of 30 years, but differing progression rates yield a range of less than 20 years to more than 50 years. Factors associated with a more rapid progression include male gender, chronic alcohol use, and older age at the time of infection. HCV is an RNA virus that does not integrate into the host genome, and therefore the pathogenesis of HCV-related HCC may be related more to chronic inflammation and cirrhosis than to direct carcinogenesis.[59,60]

The true relationship of cirrhosis and HCC is difficult to ascertain, and suggestions of causation remain speculative. Cirrhosis is not required for the development of HCC, and hepatocarcinogenesis is not an inevitable result of cirrhosis. The relationship of cirrhosis and HCC is further complicated by the fact that they share common associations. Furthermore, some associations (e.g., HBV infection, hemochromatosis) are associated with higher risk of HCC, whereas others (e.g., alcohol, primary biliary cirrhosis) are associated with a lower risk of HCC. Research has demonstrated that cirrhotic livers with higher DNA replication rates are associated with the development of HCC.

Chronic alcohol abuse has been associated with an increased risk of HCC, and there may be a synergistic effect with HBV and HCV infection. Alcohol causes cirrhosis but has never been shown to be directly carcinogenic in hepatocytes. Thus, alcohol likely acts as a cocarcinogen. Cigarette smoking has been linked to the development of HCC, but the evidence is not consistent, and the contributing risk independent of viral hepatitis is likely to be small. Aflatoxin, produced by *Aspergillus* spp., is a powerful hepatotoxin. With chronic exposure, aflatoxin acts as a carcinogen and increases the risk of HCC. The offending fungi grow on grains, peanuts, and food products in tropical and subtropical regions. Ingestion of contaminated foods results in aflatoxin exposure. Levels of aflatoxin in these implicated foods are regulated in the United States.

Other chemicals have also been implicated as carcinogens related to HCC. These include nitrites, hydrocarbons, solvents, pesticide, and vinyl chloride. Thorotrast (colloidal thorium dioxide) is an angiographic medium that was used in the 1930s. It emits high levels of long-lasting radiation and has been associated with hepatic fibrosis, angiosarcoma, cholangiosarcoma, and HCC. Associations with inherited metabolic liver diseases, such as hereditary hemochromatosis, α_1-antitrypsin deficiency, and Wilson disease, have also been implicated as risk factors for HCC. Associations with hormonal manipulations, such as the use of OCPs and anabolic steroids, have been suggested but are weak and are probably better linked specifically to adenoma and well-differentiated HCC. Research has been focusing on relationships of HCC with diabetes, obesity, and metabolic syndrome.[55,61-63]

Clinical presentation. Most commonly, patients presenting with HCC are men 50 to 60 years of age who complain of right upper quadrant abdominal pain and weight loss and have a palpable mass. In countries endemic for HBV, presentation at a younger age is common and probably related to childhood infection. Unfortunately, in unscreened populations, HCC tends to be manifested at a later stage because of the lack of symptoms in early stages. Presentation at an advanced stage is often with vague right upper quadrant abdominal pain that sometimes radiates to the right shoulder. Nonspecific symptoms of advanced malignant disease, such as anorexia, nausea, lethargy, and weight loss, are also common. Another common presentation of HCC is hepatic decompensation in a patient with known mild cirrhosis or even in patients with unrecognized cirrhosis.

HCC can rarely be manifested as a rupture, with the sudden onset of abdominal pain followed by hypovolemic shock secondary to intraperitoneal bleeding. Other rare presentations include hepatic vein occlusion (Budd-Chiari syndrome), obstructive jaundice, hemobilia, and fever of unknown origin. Less than 1% of cases of HCC are manifested with a paraneoplastic syndrome, usually hypercalcemia, hypoglycemia, and erythrocytosis. Small, incidentally noted tumors have become a more common presentation because of the knowledge of specific risk factors, screening programs for diagnosed HBV or HCV infection, and increasing use of high-quality abdominal imaging.

Diagnosis. Radiologic investigation is a critical part of the diagnosis of HCC. In the past, liver radioisotope scans and angiography were common methods of diagnosis, but ultrasound, CT, and MRI have replaced these studies. Ultrasound plays a significant role in screening and early detection of HCC, but definitive diagnosis and treatment planning rely on CT or MRI. Contrast-enhanced CT and MRI protocols aimed at diagnosing HCC take advantage of the hypervascularity of these tumors, and arterial-phase images are critical to assess the extent of disease adequately.[64,65] CT and MRI also evaluate the extent of disease in terms of peritoneal metastases, nodal metastases, and extent of vascular and biliary involvement. Detection of bland or tumor thrombus in the portal or hepatic venous system is also important and can be diagnosed with any of these modalities (Fig. 53-36).

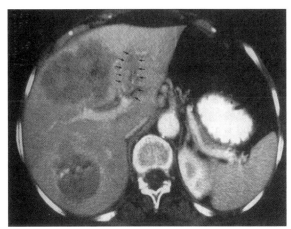

FIGURE 53-36 Contrast-enhanced CT scan demonstrating multifocal hepatocellular carcinoma. The left portal vein is invaded and expanded by tumor. (From Roddie ME, Adam A: Computed tomography of the liver and biliary tree. In Blumgart LH, Fong Y, editors: *Surgery of the liver and biliary tract*, London, 2000, WB Saunders, pp 309–340.)

AFP measurements can be helpful in the diagnosis of HCC. However, AFP measurement is associated with multiple problems. First, AFP measurements have low sensitivity and specificity. The specificity and positive predictive values of AFP improve with higher cutoff levels (e.g., 400 ng/mL) but at the cost of sensitivity. False-positive elevations of serum AFP levels can be seen in inflammatory disorders of the liver, such as chronic active viral hepatitis. Furthermore, AFP is not specific to HCC and can be elevated with intrahepatic cholangiocarcinoma and colorectal metastases. With improvements in imaging technology and the ability to detect smaller tumors, AFP is largely used as an adjunctive test in patients with liver masses. AFP levels are particularly useful in monitoring treated patients for recurrence after normalization of levels.

Since the proposal of guidelines for the diagnosis of HCC by the Barcelona-2000 European Association for the Study of the Liver conference[66] and the American Association for the Study of Liver Disease,[67] new data have accumulated and the recommendations have evolved.[68,69] AFP used to play a major role in the diagnosis of HCC larger than 2 cm.[67] However, given the excellent performance of contrast-enhanced imaging modalities, AFP does not play a critical role in the diagnosis of HCC anymore.[68,69] For hepatic nodules 1 to 2 cm in size on a background of cirrhosis, a contrast-enhanced triple-phase CT and MRI scan is now recommended.[68,69] If typical features of HCC on imaging (arterially enhancing mass with washout of contrast material in delayed phases) are observed, diagnosis of HCC is presumed. For lesions larger than 2 cm, a single study may suffice. However, for lesions 1 to 2 cm in size, contrast-enhanced CT and MRI have a sensitivity of 53% to 62%, specificity of approximately 100%, positive predictive value of 95% to 100%, and negative predictive value of 80% to 84%.[70] Performance of both MRI and CT in a sequential fashion can increase the sensitivity and may be required for difficult cases.[70]

Patients with appropriate risk factors and suggestive radiologic features, with or without an elevated AFP level, who are candidates for potentially curative surgical therapy do not require preoperative biopsy unless the diagnosis is in question. Percutaneous fine-needle aspiration of HCC does run a small risk of tumor cell spillage (estimated to be ≈1%) and rupture or bleeding, especially in cirrhotic livers and subcapsular tumors. Once the diagnosis of HCC has been made, the disease must be staged to develop an appropriate treatment plan. Most patients with HCC have two diseases, and survival is as much related to the tumor as it is to cirrhosis. Staging includes an extent of disease and extent of cirrhosis workup.

In assessing the extent of disease, the common sites of metastases must be considered. HCC largely metastasizes to the lung, bone, and peritoneum. Preoperative history should focus on symptoms referable to these areas. Extent of disease in the liver, including macrovascular invasion and the presence of multiple liver masses, must also be considered. Cross-sectional abdominal imaging, including arterial-phase images (see earlier), yields information on the extent of disease in the liver as well as peritoneal disease. Preoperative chest CT is mandatory because lung metastases are usually asymptomatic. Routine bone scans are not performed unless there are suggestive symptoms or signs.

Assessment of liver function is absolutely critical in considering treatment options for a patient with HCC. Liver resection is considered the treatment of choice for HCC, and the risk of postoperative liver failure and death must be considered. This risk is related to the degree of cirrhosis, portal hypertension, amount of liver resected (functional liver reserve), and regenerative potential response. Other successful treatments are available for HCC, such as ablative techniques, embolization techniques, and liver transplantation. Therefore, a complete assessment of tumor and liver function must be carried out. A number of tests of liver function are available, generally divided into clinical assessment and functional tests, and there are many clinical assessment schemes (see earlier). However, Child-Pugh status is used most often. Child-Pugh class C patients are not candidates for resectional therapy, whereas Child-Pugh class A patients can usually tolerate some extent of liver resection. Many consider Child-Pugh class B patients to be candidates for operation, but they are generally borderline, and therapy must be individualized.

Outside of scoring systems, it has been demonstrated that significant portal hypertension, regardless of biochemical assessments, is highly predictive of postoperative liver failure and death. Portal hypertension can be assessed directly through hepatic vein wedge pressures, but it is usually obvious on high-quality imaging in the form of splenomegaly, a cirrhotic-appearing liver, and intra-abdominal varices. Blood work usually demonstrates marked cytopenias. Most typically, patients have thrombocytopenia. Functional tests of liver function have been well described but are not routinely used in most Western centers because the results of studies evaluating their predictive value have been mixed.

Staging laparoscopy has been used as a staging tool in HCC and spares about one in five patients a nontherapeutic laparotomy. Laparoscopy yields additional information about the extent of disease in the liver, extrahepatic disease, and cirrhosis. The yield of laparoscopy is dictated by the extent of disease and is only selectively used. The presence of clinically apparent cirrhosis, radiologic evidence of vascular invasion, or bilobar tumors increases the yield to 30%, whereas without these factors, the yield is 5%.[71]

There are a number of staging systems for HCC, but none have been shown to be particularly superior; they probably depend on the specific population in which the disease is being staged as well as the cause of HCC in that particular population of patients. The TNM staging system is not routinely used for HCC because it does not accurately predict survival; it does not take liver function into account. Moreover, the TNM staging system relies on pathology that is frequently unavailable preoperatively. The Okuda staging system is an older but simple and effective system that takes liver function and tumor-related factors into account. It adds up a single point for the presence of tumor involving more than 50% of the liver, presence of ascites, albumin level less than 3 g/dL, and bilirubin level higher than 3 mg/dL. The Okuda staging system reliably distinguishes patients with a prohibitively poor prognosis from those with potential for long-term survival. The most well validated staging system is the Cancer of the Liver Italian Program (CLIP), which was rigorously developed and has been prospectively validated (Table 53-7). An example of a scoring system that is probably population specific is the Chinese University Prognostic Index (CUPI), which takes into account TNM stage, symptoms, and ascites and the levels of AFP, bilirubin, and ALP; it appears to apply mainly to HBV-related HCC in China.

Pathology. On histologic evaluation, HCC is graded as well, moderately, or poorly differentiated. The grade of HCC, however, has never been shown to predict outcome accurately. In gross appearance, the growth patterns of HCC have been classified in a number of ways. The most useful scheme divides HCC into three distinct growth patterns that have distinct relationships to outcome. The hanging type of HCC is connected to the liver by a small vascular stalk and is easily resected without sacrifice of a significant amount of adjacent non-neoplastic liver tissue. This type can grow to substantial size without involving much normal liver tissue. The pushing type of HCC is well demarcated and often contains a fibrous capsule. It is characterized by growth that displaces vascular structures rather than invading them. This type is usually resectable. The last type is called the infiltrative type of HCC, which tends to invade vascular structures, even at a small size. Resection of the infiltrative type is often possible, but positive histologic margins are common. Small tumors (<5 cm) usually do not fall into any of these groups and are often discussed as a separate entity.

Finally, HCC can be manifested in a multifocal manner. Most HCC probably starts as a single tumor, but ultimately multiple satellite lesions can develop secondary to portal vein invasion and metastases. Multifocal tumors throughout the liver probably represent the end stage of HCC, with multiple metastases and multiple primary tumors.

TABLE 53-7	**Cancer of the Liver Italian Program Score***		
CLINICAL PARAMETERS		**CUTOFF VALUES**	**POINTS**
Child-Pugh class		A	0
		B	1
		C	2
Tumor morphology		Uninodular, <50% extension	0
		Multinodular, <50% extension	1
		Massive or extension >50%	2
AFP level		<400 ng/dL	0
		>400 ng/dL	1
Portal vein thrombosis		No	0
		Yes	1

*Score ranges from 0 to 6; a score of 4 to 6 is generally considered advanced disease, whereas a score of 0 to 3 has the potential for long-term survival.

BOX 53-1 Treatment Options for Hepatocellular Carcinoma

Surgical
Resection
Orthotopic liver transplantation

Ablative
Ethanol injection
Acetic acid injection
Thermal ablation (cryotherapy, radiofrequency ablation, microwave)

Transarterial
Embolization
Chemoembolization

Radiotherapy
Combination transarterial and ablative: external beam radiation

Systemic
Chemotherapy
Hormonal
Immunotherapy

Treatment. There are a large number of treatment options for patients with HCC, reflecting the heterogeneity of this disease and the lack of a proven superior treatment, except complete resection (Box 53-1). Deciding on a treatment regimen for any one patient must take into consideration the stage of malignancy, condition of the patient and of the liver, and experience of the treating physician.

Complete excision of HCC by partial hepatectomy or by total hepatectomy and liver transplantation is the treatment of choice, when possible, because it has the highest chance of long-term survival. In general, however, only 10% to 20% of patients are considered to have resectable disease. Historically, mortality rates for partial hepatectomy have ranged from 1% to 20%, but if it is performed in healthy patients without advanced cirrhosis, most series have a mortality rate of less than 5%. Advances in surgical technique have also allowed the development of limited segmental resections when appropriate, which preserves liver function and improves early postoperative recovery. Selection of the appropriate patient for resection is critical and must take into account the condition of the liver and extent of disease. Patients with Child-Pugh class B or C cirrhosis or portal hypertension do not tolerate resection. The volume of the FLR is also an important consideration and is associated with postoperative complications and mortality. Preoperative portal vein embolization is an effective strategy to increase the volume and function of the FLR and should be used liberally in patients with Child-Pugh class A cirrhosis with a small FLR (i.e., <30% to 40% of the total liver volume) who are being considered for a major resection. The overall postresection survival rates for HCC are 58% to 100% at 1 year, 28% to 88% at 3 years, 11% to 75% at 5 years, and 19% to 26% at 10 years. These results obviously depend on the stage of the tumor and degree of cirrhosis in each particular series. Together, they give a sense of the possibilities.

A variety of prognostic factors predictive of survival after resection have been identified, but none are universally agreed on. The most commonly cited negative prognostic factors are tumor size, cirrhosis, infiltrative growth pattern, vascular invasion, intrahepatic metastases, multifocal tumors, lymph node metastases,

margin less than 1 cm, and lack of a capsule. The best outcomes are found in patients with single small tumors, but size alone should not contraindicate resection. Especially for patients with large tumors that are outside the criteria for transplantation, not many therapeutic options are available. In such patients with adequate liver function, adequate functional liver remnant, and resectable tumors, surgical resection may offer the best possible outcomes. Multifocal tumors and major vascular invasion are generally associated with a poor outcome, but some groups advocate resection in highly select patients.[72,73] A randomized controlled trial corroborated these findings. In this study, patients with multifocal HCC outside Milan criteria were randomized to resection or transarterial chemoembolization.[74] In this study, resection provided better overall survival for patients with multifocal HCC compared with transarterial chemoembolization, suggesting that resection may be an option for these patients.

Theoretically, orthotopic liver transplantation is the ideal treatment for HCC because it addresses the liver dysfunction and cirrhosis and the HCC. The limitations of transplantation are the need for chronic immunosuppression and the lack of organ donors. There has been growing interest in the use of partial hepatectomy from live donors, which addresses the lack of organ donors but remains a somewhat controversial approach. Early series of transplantation for HCC had high recurrence rates and relatively poor long-term survival, largely attributed to the fact that most of these patients were undergoing transplantation for advanced disease. Refinements in patient selection—namely, patients with single tumors smaller than 5 cm or no more than three tumors 3 cm in size—have resulted in improved outcomes.[75,76] Long-term survival rates with more stringent selection criteria have ranged from 50% to 85%. Studies have begun to expand the indications for orthotopic liver transplantation without a major effect on long-term survival but likely an increase in overall recurrence rates. Comparison of results of resection with transplantation is difficult, and the two should be viewed as complementary rather than competitive.[77] Patients with advanced cirrhosis (Child class B and C) and early-stage HCC should be considered for transplantation, whereas those with Child class A cirrhosis have similar results with transplantation and resection and should probably be resected.[78-80]

A number of other nonsurgical local ablative therapies are available for the treatment of small tumors. Percutaneous ethanol injection (PEI) is a useful technique for ablating small tumors. The tumor is killed by a combination of cellular dehydration, coagulative necrosis, and vascular thrombosis. Most tumors smaller than 2 cm can be ablated with a single application of PEI, but larger tumors may require multiple injections. Long-term survival after PEI for tumors smaller than 5 cm has been reported to range from 24% to 40%, but no randomized trials have compared PEI with resection. Percutaneous injection of acetic acid is a technique similar to PEI but has stronger necrotizing abilities, making it more useful in septated tumors.

Thermal ablative techniques that freeze or heat tumors to destroy them have become popular. Cryotherapy uses a specialized cryoprobe to freeze and thaw tumor and surrounding liver tissue, with resulting necrosis. Cryotherapy is usually performed at laparotomy or laparoscopically, but it has been performed with percutaneous techniques. One advantage is that the ice ball formed is easily monitored with ultrasound. Disadvantages include a heat sink effect limiting the usefulness of freezing near major blood vessels and a relatively high complication rate of 8% to 41%. Reported 2-year survival rates for cryoablation of HCC range from 30% to 60%, but no comparative studies to resection have been carried out. Radiofrequency ablation (RFA) uses high-frequency alternating current to create heat around an inserted probe, resulting in temperatures higher than 60° C (140° F) and immediate cell death. Although initially limited to smaller tumors, improvements in technology have created RFA probes reportedly able to ablate tumors as large as 7 cm. Nonetheless, the efficacy of RFA for HCCs larger than 3 cm is limited because of increased local recurrence rates. RFA is also limited by the protective effect of blood vessels and does not ablate well in these areas. The procedure can easily be performed percutaneously, with low complication rates, and optimal guidance systems are being developed. Recent data suggest that resection may be superior to RFA for small HCCs in terms of both disease-free and overall survival.[81]

Transarterial therapy for HCC is based on the fact that most of the tumor's blood supply is from the hepatic artery. Today, the transarterial therapy is applied in a percutaneous fashion, thus avoiding morbidity and mortality of laparotomy. Percutaneous transarterial embolization can induce ischemic necrosis in HCC, resulting in response rates as high as 50% (Fig. 53-37). Attempts to improve the efficacy of arterial embolization have included adding chemotherapeutic agents (chemoembolization) to the bland embolization particles and oils, such as ethiodized oil (Ethiodol), that are selectively taken up by HCCs.[82] Although chemoembolization has not been shown to be superior to bland embolization with regard to survival, a trial suggested an improvement in local control with chemoembolization.[83] Seven randomized trials have compared embolization or chemoembolization with conservative management. Two of these trials and a meta-analysis have confirmed an overall survival advantage from the embolization strategies.[84-86] The selection of appropriate candidates for embolization is important, and treatment should generally be limited to patients with preserved liver function and asymptomatic multinodular tumors without vascular invasion. Poor selection will result in a higher incidence of treatment-induced liver failure, offsetting the potential benefits.

External beam radiation therapy (EBRT) has a limited role in the treatment of HCC, although occasional dramatic responses are seen. EBRT is limited by damage to normal liver parenchyma and to surrounding organs, but newer methods of conformal radiotherapy and breath-gated techniques are improving the usefulness of this treatment modality. Intra-arterial injections of iodine-131 with Ethiodol or yttrium-90 in glass microspheres have also been used to deliver localized radiation to HCCs, with reports of dramatic response rates. Transarterial radiotherapy is a potentially promising therapy for HCC as a primary or adjuvant therapy.[82]

Systemic chemotherapy with a variety of agents (e.g., cisplatin, doxorubicin, etoposide, 5-fluorouracil [5-FU], mitomycin C, amsacrine, mitoxantrone, picibanil, tamoxifen, uracil, VM-26) has been ineffective and has had a minimal role in the treatment of HCC. Response rates are generally below 20% and of short duration. Systemic immunotherapy and hormonal therapy have been used in small numbers of patients with HCC, with some early promising results, but have not yet demonstrated superiority to standard regimens.

Most recently, sorafenib, a molecular targeted therapy that inhibits the serine-threonine kinases Raf-1 and B-Raf and the receptor tyrosine kinase activity of vascular endothelial growth factor receptors 1, 2, and 3 and platelet-derived growth factor β, was evaluated. Llovet and colleagues[87] randomized 599 patients with advanced-stage HCC and Child-Pugh level A cirrhosis to oral sorafenib or placebo. The median overall survival was 10.7 months in the sorafenib group and 7.9 months in the placebo group ($P < .001$), a difference of 2.8 months. The median time to radiologic progression was 5.5 months in the sorafenib group and 2.8 months in the placebo group ($P < .001$), a difference of 2.7 months. Neither group demonstrated any complete responses by radiologic criteria. Although the adverse event profile of sorafenib was similar to the placebo group, this and earlier studies have shown that sorafenib is best tolerated in patients with Child-Pugh class A cirrhosis. With better understanding of the molecular pathogenesis, there is hope that novel therapeutics will be increasingly evaluated in this disease.[87]

In summary, a plethora of treatment options are available for treatment of HCC. Selection of the appropriate treatment modality is based on disease extent, presence or absence of portal hypertension, and liver reserve. Patients with resectable disease with maintained liver reserve and absence of portal hypertension are best treated with resection. Patients with advanced underlying liver disease and with portal hypertension are best treated with liver transplantation. Liver transplantation is applicable only if the tumor is 5 cm or smaller or there are two or three tumors, the largest of which is 3 cm or smaller. Expanded criteria for transplantation are being increasingly used. In patients with very small tumors and with multiple comorbidities, percutaneous ablative techniques may be applied. The efficacy of ablation decreases with increasing size of the tumor. For multifocal disease in the absence of macrovascular invasion and extrahepatic disease, neither resection nor transplantation is applicable, and trans-arterial therapies offer the best results. For symptomatic patients with advanced disease, with macrovascular involvement, and in the presence of extrahepatic disease, sorafenib is an option. For patients with extensive disease who are symptomatic with deterioration of their performance status and who have severe deterioration of their liver function, any treatment modality is unlikely to provide significant benefit, and these patients should be offered supportive treatment only.

Distinct variants of HCC. Fibrolamellar HCC[88] is a variant of HCC with remarkably different clinical features, summarized in Table 53-8. This tumor generally occurs in younger patients without a history of cirrhosis. The tumor is usually well demarcated and encapsulated and may have a central fibrotic area. The central scar can make distinguishing this tumor from FNH difficult. On histologic evaluation, fibrolamellar HCC is composed of large polygonal tumor cells embedded in a fibrous stroma, forming lamellar structures (Fig. 53-38). Fibrolamellar HCC does not produce AFP but is associated with elevated neurotensin levels. In general, fibrolamellar HCC has a better prognosis than

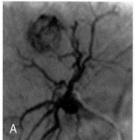
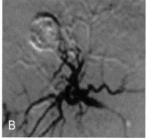

FIGURE 53-37 Angiograms demonstrating hypervascular hepatocellular carcinoma before **(A)** and after **(B)** embolization.

TABLE 53-8 **Comparison of Standard Hepatocellular Carcinoma and Fibrolamellar Hepatocellular Carcinoma**		
PARAMETER	HCC	FIBROLAMELLAR HCC
Male-to-female ratio	2:1-8:1	1:1
Median age	55 years	25 years
Tumor	Invasive	Well circumscribed
Resectability	<25%	50%-75%
Cirrhosis	90%	5%
AFP positive	80%	5%
Hepatitis B positive	65%	5%

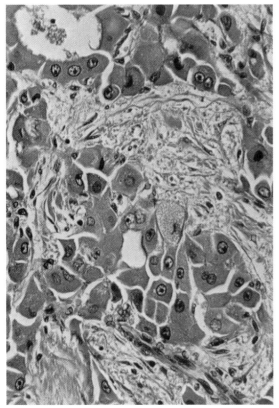

FIGURE 53-38 Fibrolamellar HCC. Abundant collagen is evident interconnecting clusters of cells. The cells are often in single-layer sheets. An acinus is present in the left upper field.

HCC, probably related to high resectability rates, lack of chronic liver disease, and a more indolent course. Long-term survival can be expected in approximately 50% to 75% of patients after complete resection, but recurrence is common and occurs in at least 80% of patients. The presence of lymph node metastases predicts a worse outcome. Resection of lymph node metastases and recurrent disease has been advocated because of a lack of alternative therapy and the possibility of long-term survival. A study identified a chimeric transcript that is expressed in fibrolamellar HCC but not in the adjacent normal liver.[89] The study also suggested that this transcript codes for a chimeric protein containing the catalytic domain of protein kinase A, thus suggesting that this gain of kinase activity may have a role in the pathogenesis of fibrolamellar HCC. Elucidation of such novel processes can lead to development of novel targeted therapies against this disease, which typically strikes young, healthy people.

Rarely, HCC can be manifested as a mixed hepatocellular-cholangiocellular tumor, with cellular differentiation of both types present. Whether this is two separate tumors growing into each other or mixed differentiation of the same tumor is not known. These mixed tumors tend to have a prognosis that is worse than for standard HCC but better than expected for intrahepatic cholangiocarcinoma.

A clear cell variant of HCC also exists, in which the cells contain a clear cytoplasm. These tumors can resemble renal cell neoplasms. The clear cell variant may have a better prognosis than standard HCC, but this is a subject of debate. A pleomorphic or giant cell variant of HCC has also been reported. Cells in this type are multinucleated, pleomorphic, and large and likely to originate from primary hepatic cells. Some HCCs show evidence of sarcomatoid differentiation and are referred to as a sarcomatoid variant or carcinosarcoma. These tumors tend not to produce AFP and have a higher incidence of metastases at presentation.

Childhood HCC is a distinct entity that represents almost 25% of pediatric liver tumors but rarely occurs in infancy. Viral hepatitis is associated with childhood HCC in Asia but less so in the United States. Other inherited metabolic liver diseases (see earlier) are often associated with childhood HCC. As in adult HCC, complete resection is the only potentially curative treatment. There is a high incidence of multifocality, vascular invasion, and extrahepatic metastases, resulting in relatively poor long-term survival rates of 10% to 20%.

Intrahepatic Cholangiocarcinoma

Cholangiocarcinoma is an uncommon neoplasm, with an incidence of 1 to 2/100,000 in the United States, and can develop anywhere along the biliary tree, from the ampulla of Vater to the peripheral intrahepatic bile ducts. Most of these tumors (40% to 60%) involve the biliary confluence (Klatskin tumor), but approximately 10% emanate from intrahepatic ducts and are known as intrahepatic cholangiocarcinoma (IHC). IHC is the second most common primary hepatic neoplasm. Studies on the incidence and natural history of IHC have been confused by the fact that in the past, many of these tumors were mistaken for metastatic adenocarcinoma because biopsy is unable to differentiate the two.

Historically, the most common risk factors for the development of cholangiocarcinoma (all types) were primary sclerosing cholangitis, choledochal cyst disease, hepatolithiasis,[90] and RPC. Recent epidemiologic evidence has now linked IHC to HBV infection,[91] HCV infection,[53] cirrhosis, nonalcoholic steatohepatitis,[92] and diabetes.[93] Increases in the diagnosis of IHC in the United States are likely related to better recognition of the disease, changed classification, and perhaps the rise in HCV infections in the 1960s and 1970s.[94,95]

The clinical presentation of IHC is similar to that of HCC. These tumors are asymptomatic in early stages. When present, the most common symptoms are right upper abdominal pain and weight loss. Jaundice occurs less commonly as these tumors tend to arise in the periphery of the liver. More commonly, patients present with incidentally found liver masses on cross-sectional imaging. Unlike in HCC, the AFP levels are normal, although CEA or CA 19-9 levels can be elevated in some cases. Because metastatic adenocarcinoma to liver is more common, IHC is a diagnosis of exclusion, and a search for a primary tumor with upper and lower gastrointestinal endoscopy and cross-sectional imaging of the chest, abdomen, and pelvis should be carried out. If a biopsy has been performed, it is often read as adenocarcinoma. Although special stains may suggest diagnosis of IHC, they are not conclusive. On CT and MRI, IHC is seen as a focal hepatic mass that may be associated with peripheral biliary dilation. The mass typically has peripheral or central enhancement on contrast-enhanced scans. Intrahepatic metastases, lymph node metastases, and growth along the biliary tree are often encountered.

Complete resection is the treatment of choice for IHC. Resectability rates generally range up to 60%, and long-term survival in unresected patients is rare. If it is completely resected, 3-year survival rates range from 16% to 61%, and 5-year survival rates range from 24% to 44%. Factors associated with a poor outcome include multifocality, lymph node metastases, vascular invasion, and positive margins. Because of the rarity of IHC, little is known about the effectiveness of radiation therapy and chemotherapy for IHC in the adjuvant setting. Thus, their application is not routine. Chemotherapy is largely considered ineffective for IHC, but it is hoped that improvements in chemotherapy for other gastrointestinal tumors will translate into improved outcomes. Regional hepatic artery chemotherapy has been under study and may be a promising approach.

Other Primary Malignant Neoplasms

Hepatoblastoma is the most common primary hepatic tumor of childhood. There are approximately 50 to 70 new cases per year in the United States. Rare cases of adult hepatoblastoma have been reported, but overall, the median age at presentation is 18 months, and almost all cases occur before the age of 3 years. Hepatoblastoma has been associated with the familial polyposis syndrome. There are a number of histologic subtypes, but in general, the tumor is derived from fetal or embryonic hepatocytic progenitors, and mesenchymal elements are often present. This tumor generally is manifested as an asymptomatic mass. Mild anemia and thrombocytosis are commonly found at presentation. Serum AFP levels are elevated in 85% to 90% of patients and can serve as a useful marker for therapeutic response. Most studies have supported the use of chemotherapy followed by resection, and survival appears to be dependent on complete resection. Chemotherapy can serve to downstage tumors, which facilitates resection. In patients without metastatic disease or the anaplastic variant, long-term survival rates of 60% to 70% can be expected with complete resection. Interestingly, 50% of patients with pulmonary metastases can be cured with resection of the hepatic tumor and chemotherapy or resection of the pulmonary metastases.

A variety of sarcomas can rarely be manifested as primary liver tumors, but they must always be considered metastatic lesions until proven otherwise. Angiosarcoma is probably the best-described primary hepatic sarcoma because of its well-known association with vinyl chloride or Thorotrast exposure. Angiosarcoma typically is manifested as multiple hepatic masses and can appear in childhood. Long-term survival is uncommon with primary hepatic angiosarcoma. Other sarcomas, including leiomyosarcoma, malignant fibrous histiocytoma, embryonic sarcoma, and primary hepatic rhabdoid tumors, have been described but are rare. The last two lesions are typically seen in the pediatric population.

Non-Hodgkin lymphoma can be manifested primarily in the liver, with or without extrahepatic disease. Primary hepatic lymphoma should be treated in the same manner as lymphoma elsewhere in the body if the diagnosis can be made before a liver resection.

Primary hepatic neuroendocrine tumors or carcinoid tumors have been described but are probably extremely rare. Distinguishing the rare primary hepatic neuroendocrine tumor from a metastatic lesion can be difficult because the extrahepatic primary tumor can be radiologically occult for many years, and the liver is the most common site of metastases.

Malignant germ cell tumors of the liver including teratomas, choriocarcinomas, and yolk sac tumors are very rare and are principally described in the pediatric population.

Epithelioid hemangioendothelioma of the liver is a rare malignant vascular tumor that is manifested with multiple bilateral hepatic masses. Extrahepatic metastases occur in approximately 25% of patients and clinical behavior is unpredictable, with some patients having a prolonged indolent course. Most patients ultimately die of liver failure, but cases of successful transplantation have been reported.

Metastatic Tumors

The most common malignant tumors of the liver are metastatic lesions. The liver is a common site of metastases from gastrointestinal tumors, presumably because of dissemination through the portal venous system. The most relevant metastatic tumor of the liver to the surgeon is colorectal cancer because of the well-documented potential for long-term survival after complete resection. However, a large number of other tumors commonly metastasize to the liver, including cancers of the upper gastrointestinal system (stomach, pancreas, biliary), genitourinary system (renal, prostate), neuroendocrine system, breast, eye (melanoma), skin (melanoma), soft tissue (retroperitoneal sarcoma), and gynecologic system (ovarian, endometrial, cervical). The large majority of metastatic liver tumors that present with concomitant extrahepatic disease will have unresectable liver disease or are not curable with resection, limiting the role of the surgeon to highly select cases. Metastatic adenocarcinoma to the liver of unknown primary is often a primary IHC, and this diagnosis must always be kept in mind.

Traditionally, cancer spread to a distant site was considered a systemic disease in which locoregional therapies (i.e., surgery) were not effective. Some metastatic tumors to the liver and, in particular, metastatic colorectal cancer have been shown to be an exception to this rule. More than 35 years of clinical research has documented that metastatic colorectal cancer isolated in the liver can be resected, with the potential for long-term survival and cure.[96-98] Advances in systemic and regional chemotherapy have also broadened the number of patients eligible for surgical therapy and probably have improved long-term survival after resection.[99] Selection of patients is the most important aspect of surgical therapy for metastatic disease in the liver, and clinical follow-up of resected patients has identified those most and least likely to benefit. Although long-term survival is common and occurs in up to 50% to 60% of patients in current series, recurrence and chronic multimodal therapy are common, occurring in approximately 75% of patients. Therefore, an important aspect of treatment is realistic expectations and honest patient education. Tumors other than colorectal cancer manifested as isolated or limited hepatic metastases can also be resected for potential long-term survival, but data on these other tumors are sparse and less compelling than for colorectal cancer.

Colorectal Metastases

There are more than 50,000 cases of colorectal liver metastases a year in the United States. Most of these cases are associated with widespread disease or unresectable hepatic disease. It is estimated that approximately 5% to 10% of these patients are candidates for a potentially curative liver resection. With improved response rates to modern chemotherapy and advances in hepatic surgery, however, more patients are now candidates for hepatectomy than in the past; at present, up to 20% of patients may be candidates. In the distant past, patients with hepatic colorectal metastases generally presented with symptoms and signs of advanced malignant disease, such as pain, ascites, jaundice, weight loss, and a palpable mass. Presentation with these symptoms is a poor prognostic sign; few of these patients are candidates for therapy aside from chemotherapy or supportive care. This has led most physicians to observe patients with resected primary colorectal cancer carefully who are potential candidates for aggressive therapy with serial physical examinations, cross-sectional imaging studies, LFTs, and determination of CEA levels. Although not supported by randomized trials, clinical observations have indicated that patients who are carefully observed with serial physical examinations, cross-sectional imaging studies, LFTs, and determination of CEA levels are those often found to have resectable metachronous disease and the greatest potential for long-term survival. In addition to these patients, some are found to have synchronous metastatic disease at the time of diagnosis of the primary colorectal cancer on preoperative imaging or at laparotomy.[100]

Although an elevated CEA level is not specific for recurrent colorectal cancer, a rising CEA level on serial examinations and a new solid mass on imaging studies are diagnostic of metastatic disease. Mild elevations in LFT results are common in metastatic colorectal cancer to the liver but are not effective as a screening tool. The levels most commonly elevated are those of ALP, GGT, and lactate dehydrogenase. Imaging of hepatic metastases with high-quality CT or MRI is important for determining resectability and operative planning. Most physicians use thin-cut (5 mm), high-resolution, dynamic, contrast-enhanced helical scanning techniques. Timing with IV administration of a contrast agent should correspond to the portal venous phase to maximize hepatic parenchymal enhancement, which improves the disparity between parenchyma and tumor.

Once a patient with colorectal liver metastases is considered a candidate for surgical therapy, a complete extent of disease workup must be performed. Colonoscopy should be performed if it has been longer than 1 year since the last examination to rule out local recurrence or metachronous colorectal lesions. Complete abdominal and pelvic cross-sectional imaging must also be performed. Chest CT is often performed but is of low yield. Many studies have evaluated the added benefit of positron emission tomography (PET) scans to detect occult extrahepatic disease. Approximately 25% of patients have a change in management based on PET scan findings, but this is highly variable, depending on the quality of cross-sectional imaging, radiologic interpretation, and patient selection (Fig. 53-39). A randomized trial of PET/CT versus CT in patients with potentially resectable colorectal liver metastases has been published.[101] In this trial, the use of PET/CT did not result in significant changes in surgical management, and there was no difference in resectability or long-term outcomes between the two groups. This trial provides definitive evidence that routine use of PET does not significantly affect outcomes among patients with potentially resectable colorectal cancer liver metastasis. With use of staging laparoscopy, 10% of patients are spared a nontherapeutic laparotomy, and the yield of laparoscopy correlates with the number of poor prognostic factors present, allowing it to be used on a selective basis.

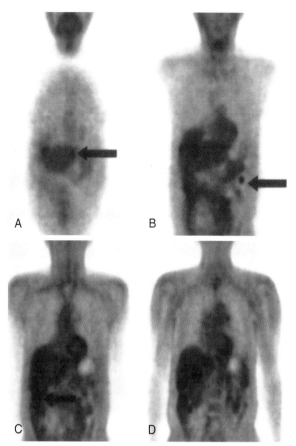

FIGURE 53-39 PET scan in a patient diagnosed with colorectal cancer synchronously metastatic to the liver after resection of the colonic tumor. The scan demonstrates hypermetabolic activity throughout the liver but also shows two areas in the left upper quadrant consistent with an omental lesion as well as an anastomotic recurrence. A recent CT scan demonstrated liver disease only. (From Akhurst T, Larson SM: The role of nuclear medicine in the diagnosis and management of hepatobiliary diseases. In Blumgart LH, Fong Y, editors: *Surgery of the liver and biliary tract,* London, 2000, WB Saunders, pp 271–308.)

To date, a prospective trial comparing surgery with no treatment or chemotherapy alone has not been performed, nor is this likely ever to be done. Therefore, the rationale for liver resection comes from retrospective comparisons of these treatment strategies. The surgeon must understand the natural history of colorectal liver metastases left untreated or treated with systemic chemotherapy to interpret survival data associated with hepatectomy appropriately. Before the 1980s, most hepatic metastases were left untreated. Two key studies retrospectively identified patients with isolated single hepatic metastases or multiple but resectable tumors who received no therapy. One study documented a 10% 3-year survival and the other a 2% 5-year survival for patients with limited and potentially resectable disease. It was clear from these studies that long-term survival is extremely rare without treatment and that survival is closely related to the extent of disease. In the past, 5-FU–based systemic chemotherapy was ineffective as sole therapy for hepatic colorectal metastases, with median survivals of approximately 12 months and response rates of 20% to 30%. Tremendous advances in systemic chemotherapy for metastatic colorectal cancer have now been achieved.

Combination chemotherapy, including 5-FU with irinotecan or oxaliplatin combined with targeted antiangiogenic antibodies such as bevacizumab (anti–vascular endothelial growth factor antibody) or cetuximab (anti–epidermal growth factor antibody), has now resulted in response rates of more than 50% and median survivals of 20 months and longer for patients with advanced disease.[97] Although response rates and survival have improved, durable complete response and 5-year survival are rare with the administration of chemotherapy alone.

The sporadic partial hepatectomies performed for metastatic colorectal cancer before the 1980s were appropriately viewed with great skepticism. The high morbidity and mortality for liver surgery at that time and the questionable rationale of resecting bloodborne metastases were the major issues. During the last 30 years, however, large series have demonstrated that liver surgery can now be practiced with acceptable safety and that patients with isolated and resectable hepatic metastases have the potential for long-term survival. Five-year survival rates range from 25% to 58%. There is also a clear trend toward longer survival in more recent series (Table 53-9). Perioperative mortality in experienced centers is consistently less than 5% and in many series has been less than 2%. Almost all demonstrate that almost 50% of patients

undergoing a liver resection for metastatic colorectal cancer will survive 3 years and 20% will survive 10 years. Despite the low operative mortality, liver surgery is still associated with significant morbidity rates of 30% to 50%.[102] Complications are most commonly bleeding, bile leak, abscess, and other generalized cardiorespiratory complications. With improvements in chemotherapy, a higher proportion of patients undergoing hepatectomy have been treated preoperatively. However, some studies have shown that preoperative chemotherapy is associated with hepatic toxicity (steatohepatitis and sinusoidal obstructive syndrome) and higher rates of postoperative liver failure.

From these large series, we have learned much about prognostic factors as well as which patients are most likely to benefit from a liver resection for hepatic colorectal metastases. Although not all studies agree, it has been found that poor prognostic factors include extrahepatic metastases, involved lymph nodes with the primary colorectal tumor, synchronous presentation (or shorter disease-free interval), larger number of tumors, bilobar involvement, CEA level elevation more than 200 ng/mL, size of largest hepatic tumor more than 5 cm, and involved histologic margins. In a series of 1001 liver resections from MSKCC, a multivariate analysis[103] identified five preoperative factors as the

TABLE 53-9 Results of Hepatic Resection for Hepatic Colorectal Metastases*

| STUDY | NO. OF PATIENTS | OPERATIVE MORTALITY RATE (%) | SURVIVAL RATE (%) | | | MEDIAN SURVIVAL (MONTHS) |
			1-YEAR	5-YEAR	10-YEAR	
Adson, 1984	141	2	82	25	—	24
Hughes, 1986	607	—	—	33	—	—
Schlag, 1990	122	4	85	30	—	32
Doci, 1991	100	5	—	30	—	28
Gayowski, 1994	204	0	91	32	—	33
Scheele, 1995	469	4	83	33	20	40
Fong, 1995	577	4	85	35	—	40
Jenkins, 1997	131	4	81	25	—	33
Rees, 1997	150	1	94	37	—	
Jamison, 1997	280	4	84	27	20	33
Fong, 1999	1001	3	89	37	22	42
Minagawa, 2000	235	0	—	35	26	37
Scheele, 2000	597	—	—	36	—	35
Choti, 2002	226	1	—	40[†]	26	46
Abdalla, 2004	190	—	—	58	—	Not reached
Nicoli, 2004	228	0.9		16	9	
Andres, 2008	210	0.5	95	40	—	—
de Jong, 2009	243	—	—	47	—	36
House, 2010	1600					
1985-1998	1037	2.5	—	35	16	43
1999-2004	563	0.5	—	43	—	64
Faitot, 2014[‡]	272					
One stage	155	3	85	35		37.2
Two stage	117	4	82	49		34.5
Saxena, 2014	701	2	86	33	20	35
Marques, 2012[§]	676					
Preoperative chemotherapy[‖]	334	3.9	91	43		
No preoperative chemotherapy	342	3.4	93	55		

*In selected series with more than 100 patients.
[†]The 5-year survival rate in the patients operated on in the most current time period in this study was 58%.
[‡]Long-term results of two-stage hepatectomy versus one-stage hepatectomy used in combination with ablation approaches.
[§]Combined data from two hepatobiliary centers, data analyzed with respect to receipt of preoperative chemotherapy or not.
[‖]Number of tumors higher in the preoperative chemotherapy group (2.8 ± 2.2) compared with those with no preoperative therapy (1.8 ± 1.6).

TABLE 53-10 Clinical Risk Score and Survival in 1001 Patients Undergoing Liver Resection for Metastatic Colorectal Cancer*

SCORE	SURVIVAL RATE (%)			MEDIAN SURVIVAL (MONTHS)
	1-YEAR	3-YEAR	5-YEAR	
0	93	72	60	74
1	91	66	44	51
2	89	60	40	47
3	86	42	20	33
4	70	38	25	20
5	71	27	14	22

Adapted from Fong Y, Fortner J, Sun RL, et al: Clinical score for predicting recurrence after hepatic resection for metastatic colorectal cancer: Analysis of 1001 consecutive cases. *Ann Surg* 230:309–318, 1999.
*Each of the following five risk factors equals 1 point: node-positive primary, disease-free interval <12 months, >1 tumor, size >5 cm, carcinoembryonic antigen level >200 ng/mL. Score is total number of points in an individual patient.

most influential on outcome: size larger than 5 cm, disease-free interval less than 1 year, more than one tumor, lymph node–positive primary, and CEA level higher than 200 ng/mL. Using these five factors, we have developed a risk score predictive of recurrence after liver resection (Table 53-10).

Traditionally, the presence of extrahepatic disease, four or more hepatic metastases, close margins, and inability to resect all disease in the liver have been considered contraindications to hepatectomy. The only one of these historic contraindications that holds true today is the inability to resect all disease. Recent reports have shown that hepatectomy for four or more metastases is associated with an approximate 5-year survival of 33%, despite a high recurrence rate. Although the width of the closest margin has been shown to be associated with outcome, it is often confounded by its relationship to an overall poor prognostic tumor (i.e., multiple synchronous tumors).[104] However, close or involved margins do not appear to preclude the possibility of long-term survival, but patients with positive margins tend to fair poorly. Nonetheless, attempts at wide margins more than 1 cm are appropriate, when possible.[105] Resection of extrahepatic metastases that present simultaneously with liver metastases has been shown to be associated with long-term survival in highly select cases.[106] The sites that appear to be associated with the best outcomes in this situation are limited lung metastases, locoregional recurrences of the primary tumor, and portal lymph nodes. These results have been further confirmed in a meta-analysis of 50 studies including 3481 patients with colorectal liver metastases with extrahepatic disease.[107] Selection of patients is critical for this aggressive approach and generally requires preoperative chemotherapy to exclude progression and consideration of the overall bulk of metastatic disease.

Although long-term survival after liver resection for hepatic colorectal metastases is clearly possible, recurrence of disease is common. Overall, approximately 75% of patients have recurrence, but in high-risk situations (e.g., four or more tumors, extrahepatic disease), recurrence rates approach 100%. Approximately 50% of recurrences are isolated to the liver, and a small number of these patients (≈5% of all patients undergoing liver resection) are candidates for a second liver resection. These highly select patients who undergo a second liver resection with complete removal of all disease can expect further 5-year survival rates of 30% to 40%. Limited and isolated lung recurrences can also be resected, with the potential for further long-term survival. Furthermore, multiple lines of effective chemotherapy are now available, associated with prolongation of survival. Because of the potential for further effective therapeutic interventions after liver resection, patients eligible for such treatment should be observed with serial CEA level determinations and imaging studies to detect recurrences at an early, potentially treatable phase.

Adjuvant chemotherapy has been used in an attempt to reduce recurrence and to improve long-term survival. Prospective randomized clinical trials have shown a benefit to adjuvant hepatic intra-arterial chemotherapy. However, results of randomized controlled trials on the benefit of adjuvant systemic chemotherapy after resection of hepatic metastases have been mixed. In a multicenter randomized trial, Portier and associates[108] randomized 173 patients to hepatic resection alone (87 patients) or to hepatic resection plus adjuvant chemotherapy (5-FU–folinic acid) for 6 months (86 patients). Even though this chemotherapy regimen is no longer standard, the 5-year disease-free survival rate was 26.7% for patients who had surgery alone and 33.5% for patients who had surgery plus chemotherapy ($P = .028$). A nonsignificant trend toward improved overall survival was also observed in the chemotherapy arm. The results of this trial were pooled with another phase 3 trial that failed to accrue. This pooled analysis failed to show a statistically significant improvement in progression-free survival or overall survival.[109] In this analysis, there were 278 patients (138 in the surgery with chemotherapy arm and 140 in the surgery-alone arm). Median progression-free survival was 27.9 months in the chemotherapy arm compared with 18.8 months in the surgery arm (hazard ratio, 1.32; 95% confidence interval, 1.00-1.76; $P = .058$). Median overall survival was 62.2 months in the chemotherapy arm compared with 47.3 months in the surgery arm (hazard ratio, 1.32; 95% confidence interval, 0.95-1.82; $P = .095$).[109] Adjuvant chemotherapy was independently associated with both progression-free survival and overall survival in multivariable analysis.

In another multi-institutional randomized controlled trial (European Organization for Research and Treatment and Cancer, EORTC 40983 trial), Nordlinger and colleagues randomized 364 patients into two groups; 182 patients were treated with surgery alone, and 182 patients had surgery plus systemic chemotherapy.[110] Three cycles of systemic 5-FU–folinic acid plus oxaliplatin (FOLFOX4) were administered preoperatively and postoperatively in the chemotherapy group. Among eligible patients after randomization, the progression-free survival of patients at 3 years was 28.1% in the group with surgery alone and 36.2% in the group with surgery plus chemotherapy ($P = .041$). When analyzed by all patients, there was no significant difference in outcome. Long-term results of this trial have been released, and no difference in overall survival was observed with addition of chemotherapy.[111] Although this trial provides evidence that perioperative systemic chemotherapy can delay recurrence of disease, there is little difference in the recurrences at later time points. Also, the benefit of adjuvant chemotherapy may be related to better selection of patients. In summary, there is level 1 clinical evidence that adjuvant systemic chemotherapy, when combined with liver resection, modestly improves progression-free survival in patients with colorectal liver metastases.

Neoadjuvant chemotherapy for resectable metastases is also a common strategy to treat occult systemic disease and can be helpful in selecting the small group of patients (<10%) who progress while receiving chemotherapy and have a poor outcome after hepatectomy. A prospective randomized study by the National Surgical Adjuvant Breast and Bowel Project has begun accruing patients to study the role of adjuvant chemotherapy in these patients.

A convincing argument for adjuvant therapy with the use of hepatic arterial infusion (HAI) chemotherapy can be made.[112,113] The rationale for adjuvant hepatic artery chemotherapy is based on the fact that liver metastases derive most of their blood supply from the hepatic artery. Regional infusion of chemotherapeutic agents such as fluorodeoxyuridine has hepatic extraction rates of 90%, providing high local concentrations with minimal systemic toxicity. Furthermore, approximately 50% of all recurrences after hepatectomy involve the liver, so controlling the liver is likely to affect long-term outcome. There is clearly a higher response rate for liver tumors with HAI therapy compared with systemic therapy. A trial from MSKCC comparing HAI therapy with systemic chemotherapy to systemic chemotherapy alone has demonstrated significantly lower recurrence rates (9% and 36%) and a survival advantage at 2 years (86% versus 72%).[114] Other trials have shown HAI therapy with fluorodeoxyuridine to be more effective than hepatectomy alone, with significantly improved disease-free survival.

For patients with unresectable disease, preoperative systemic and HAI chemotherapy has been shown to convert some patients to resection candidates. A critical observation in these patients is that outcome after complete resection appears to be as good as in those who were resectable at initial presentation. Strategies to extend the limits of liver resection have used parenchyma-preserving segmental resections, two-stage operations, and thermal ablative techniques, such as cryoablation or RFA. Most recently, microwave ablation is being studied as a treatment for these patients, and long-term results suggest that recurrence rates increase with the size of the tumor and when ablation is performed for the tumor close to the vessels.[115] Recent results suggest that microwave ablation either alone or in combination with liver resection can provide good long-term results. Thus, multiple bilobar tumors can be extirpated by a combination of resection and ablation with preservation of sufficient hepatic parenchyma.

In summary, the treatment of hepatic colorectal metastases is evolving at a rapid pace, and improvements in hepatic surgery and chemotherapy have greatly improved prospects for patients. Chemotherapy has improved, but long-term survival with this modality alone is rare. Combinations of chemotherapy and complete resection of hepatic metastases are associated with long-term survival in up to 50% to 60% of patients. Long-term survival also appears to be possible in patients undergoing resection of extensive hepatic metastases and limited extrahepatic disease.[106] Complete resection of hepatic metastases appears to be a critically important treatment modality that is necessary for long-term survival.

Neuroendocrine Metastases

Liver metastases from neuroendocrine tumors are common but vary according to the primary tumor type. Examples of primary tumors that commonly metastasize to the liver are gastrinomas, glucagonomas, somatostatinomas, and nonfunctional neuroendocrine tumors. Insulinomas and carcinoid tumors metastasize to the liver less commonly.

There are two issues to consider in determining the appropriate therapy for metastatic neuroendocrine tumors. First, these are slow-growing, indolent tumors in which long-term survival is possible even in the absence of treatment. Thus, assessing the effects of any treatment is difficult. Second, these tumors often secrete functional neuropeptides that can create debilitating syndromes of hormonal excess, so the goal of treatment is focused more often on quality of life rather than on prolongation of life.

A number of effective nonsurgical therapies exist for neuroendocrine liver metastases. Long-acting somatostatin analogues are useful for alleviating hormonal symptoms and may have a cytostatic role as well. Liver tumors can also be treated by hepatic arterial embolization or thermoablative approaches. Combinations of these therapies can be effective in cytoreducing tumor loads and alleviating symptoms of hormonal excess.

Liver resection can play a role in patients whose tumor can be completely encompassed. Because these tumors are indolent, any therapy must be delivered with minimal morbidity. This has been the case in experienced hepatobiliary units.[116] Five-year survival rates in excess of 50% to 75% can be expected if a complete resection is accomplished. Retrospective comparisons have suggested that this survival is better than that in untreated patients, but selection bias accounts for at least some of this difference. Because of the rarity of this diagnosis, no prospective data exist. The other role of surgery is for those patients who have failed to respond to medical therapy and have recalcitrant symptoms of hormonal excess. If preoperative staging suggests that at least 90% of tumor can be removed without prohibitive operative risk, surgical cytoreduction is reasonable. Symptom improvement can be expected in most patients if adequate cytoreduction is achieved. Formal resections with wide margins are not necessary for neuroendocrine tumors, and techniques such as enucleation and wedge resection are reasonable options. Thermoablative approaches, such as cryoablation and RFA, are also attractive alternatives in this type of cytoreductive surgery. Laparoscopic RFA has recently been used, although long-term follow-up is not available.[117]

Noncolorectal, Non-Neuroendocrine Metastases

Other tumors can be manifested as isolated liver metastases, but these are uncommon situations and therefore data for these situations are sparse.[118,119] There are many tumors that can be manifested in this way, including breast, lung, melanoma, soft tissue sarcoma, Wilms tumor, ocular melanoma, upper gastrointestinal (gastric, pancreas, esophagus, gallbladder), adrenocortical, urologic (bladder, renal cell, prostate, testicular), and gynecologic (uterine, cervical, ovarian) tumors. General principles that should be considered in dealing with these tumors as isolated liver metastases are similar to those for metastatic colorectal cancer. Prognosis tends to be dismal if there is extrahepatic disease, multiple tumors, large tumors, or a short disease-free interval, and patients should be carefully selected for surgery on the basis of these factors.

Although there have been rare reports of long-term survival after resection of isolated liver metastases from upper gastrointestinal tumor, in general, these patients have a dismal prognosis and liver resection is not recommended. In most series, liver resection for genitourinary tumors has the best prognosis, and in well-selected patients, liver resection should be considered. Breast tumor, melanoma, and sarcoma patients rarely present with isolated liver metastases, and with a long disease-free interval or long-term stability on chemotherapy, liver resection should be considered. In general, liver resection for metastatic noncolorectal, non-neuroendocrine tumors has to be considered cytoreductive and should be used only in the most favorable situations (see earlier). Liver resection can also be an effective therapy for symptomatic tumors in patients who have a reasonable life expectancy and no other effective therapy.

Cystic Neoplasms

Simple Cyst

Simple cysts of the liver contain serous fluid, do not communicate with the biliary tree, and do not have septations. They are generally spherical or ovoid and can be as large as 20 cm. Large cysts can compress normal liver, inducing regional atrophy and sometimes compensatory contralateral hypertrophy. In 50% of cases, the cysts are singular. On histologic evaluation, a single layer of cuboidal or columnar cells without atypia lines these cysts. Simple cysts are generally regarded as congenital malformations.

Simple cysts are a relatively common finding in adults and are mostly asymptomatic incidental radiologic findings. On occasion, a large cyst will cause symptoms. Although CT demonstrates anatomic relationships, ultrasound is a helpful test of choice to confirm a single, thin-walled simple cyst. Hydatid disease, cystadenoma, and metastatic neuroendocrine tumor are the most important differential diagnoses to consider. A thick or nodular wall raises the suspicion of a cystadenoma but can also represent hemorrhage within the cyst. The most common complication is intracystic bleeding, but overall, complications are rare. The treatment of simple hepatic cysts is indicated only if they are symptomatic or there is diagnostic uncertainty. Because most cysts are asymptomatic, a thorough evaluation of the cause of the symptoms must be carried out before attributing them to the cyst. Nonsurgical treatment consists of aspiration and injection of a sclerosing agent. Few studies have documented long-term follow-up of sclerotherapy for hepatic cysts. Surgical therapy is achieved by fenestration or unroofing of the portion of the cyst that is extrahepatic. This can be performed at laparotomy with good long-term results or through laparoscopic approaches. The laparoscopic approach is favored, but long-term efficacy has not been well documented.[120] A meta-analysis including nine retrospective case-control studies involving 657 patients comparing laparoscopic fenestration with the open approach demonstrated that the laparoscopic approach was associated with shorter operative time, shorter hospital stay, and less operative blood loss with no difference in cyst recurrence rates.[121]

Cystadenoma and Cystadenocarcinoma

Cystadenoma of the liver is a rare neoplasm that generally is manifested as a large cystic mass, usually 10 to 20 cm. The cyst has a globular external surface with multiple protruding cysts and locules of various sizes. The fluid contained in these cysts is usually mucinous. On microscopic examination, atypical cuboidal or columnar cells resting on a basement membrane, with ovarian-like stroma, line the cysts. The epithelium often forms polypoid or papillary projections.

Cystadenoma of the liver mainly affects woman older than 40 years. Although many cystadenomas are asymptomatic, symptoms can include abdominal pain, anorexia, nausea, and abdominal distention. The diagnosis is usually suspected by a combination of cross-sectional imaging (CT or MRI) and ultrasound. Ultrasound usually demonstrates a cystic structure with varying wall thickness, nodularity, septations, and fluid-filled locules. Importantly, contrast-enhanced CT demonstrates enhancement of the cyst wall and septa. Hydatid disease must always be considered in the differential diagnosis. Cystadenomas tend to grow slowly but can eventually progress to their malignant counterpart, cystadenocarcinomas.

Cystadenocarcinoma is an extremely rare malignant neoplasm with little documentation of its natural history and outcome after resection. Malignant degeneration is typically suggested on imaging, with large projections and a markedly thickened wall. The treatment of cystadenoma or cystadenocarcinoma is complete excision, which can be done with an enucleation if there is no evidence of invasive malignant disease. Incomplete resection risks recurrence or the development of cystadenocarcinoma.

Polycystic Liver Disease

Liver cysts are commonly seen in patients with the autosomal dominant inherited adult polycystic kidney disease.[122] The cysts are histologically similar to simple cysts (see earlier). The main difference between the two entities is the number of cysts. When liver cysts are present in patients with adult polycystic kidney disease, they are always multiple in number. Also, there are usually numerous microscopic hepatic cysts as well as the grossly visible macrocysts. Despite the large number of liver cysts, hepatic parenchyma and function are usually preserved. Liver cysts are always preceded by kidney cysts, and their prevalence in adult polycystic kidney disease increases with age. In those younger than 20 years, the prevalence of liver cysts is 0%, whereas in those older than 60 years, it is 80%.

Liver cysts in patients with adult polycystic kidney disease are generally asymptomatic, but in a few patients, numerous large cysts may cause abdominal pain and distention. LFT results are almost always normal. Rare complications can occur; these include infection and intracystic bleeding. Ultrasound and CT reveal multiple simple cysts throughout the liver and kidneys. Treatment of polycystic liver disease is reserved for severe symptoms related to large cysts and complications. Treatment includes percutaneous aspiration with or without sclerotherapy, cyst fenestration (by laparotomy or laparoscopy), hepatic resection, and orthotopic liver transplantation. Liver transplantation is used only with progressive disease after fenestration or resection with liver or renal dysfunction. In the context of renal failure, a combined kidney and liver transplantation may be appropriate.

Bile Duct Cysts

Bile duct cysts or choledochal cysts are congenital dilations of the biliary tree that are usually diagnosed in childhood but can present in adulthood. Because of the risk of malignancy and recurrent cholangitis, treatment is excision with reestablishment of biliary-enteric continuity. Most bile duct cysts involve the extrahepatic biliary tree, but in type IV cysts, there is involvement of the extrahepatic bile duct and intrahepatic ducts. In contrast, Caroli disease (type V) is characterized by multiple intrahepatic cysts. Thus, bile duct cysts must be considered in the differential diagnosis of a patient with multiple hepatic cystic lesions. The intrahepatic lesions of type IV bile duct cysts and Caroli disease are multifocal dilations of the segmental bile ducts separated by portions of normal-caliber bile ducts. Approximately 50% of cases of Caroli disease are associated with congenital hepatic fibrosis; the cysts are diffusely located throughout the liver. In the other 50% of cases, the dilations may be confined to a portion of the liver, usually the left hemiliver. Recurrent bacterial cholangitis usually dominates the clinical course of these diseases, and death generally ensues within 5 to 10 years without adequate treatment. When intrahepatic bile duct cysts are localized, hepatic resection, with or without biliary reconstruction, is the treatment of choice. Treatment of diffuse hepatic involvement is poor; in complicated cases, the only probably effective treatment is transplantation.

Principles of Hepatic Resection

Although liver resections were performed in the late 1800s, it was not until 1952 that Lortat-Jacob was given credit for the first true anatomic right hepatectomy. This event ushered in the modern era of hepatic surgery. However, early series were plagued by high morbidity and mortality, which were largely related to massive intraoperative blood loss. Series from the 1970s and 1980s often reported mortality rates in excess of 10%, often as high as 20%, especially for major resections. This high mortality limited the use of liver resection, and there was reluctance to refer patients for such operations. During the last 3 decades, a number of advances have improved perioperative outcomes dramatically for patients undergoing major hepatic surgery. The understanding that most blood loss during a liver resection comes from the hepatic veins has prompted surgeons to perform these operations with a low central venous pressure. We perform partial hepatectomy with a central line in place, the patient in a mild Trendelenburg position, and fluid restriction and venodilators if necessary to maintain a central venous pressure lower than 5 mm Hg. The other major advance has been an improved understanding of the segmental anatomy of the liver, making intrahepatic dissection safer and more precise. There are numerous techniques to transect liver tissue and many methods to coagulate and to control vessels. The most important concept, however, is that dividing liver tissue is a dissection done by a surgeon with complete understanding of the liver's vascular anatomy.

In experienced centers, perioperative mortality is routinely 5% or less and depends on a number of factors. The three most critical factors related to perioperative morbidity are blood loss, the amount of normal liver resected, and the condition of the liver itself (e.g., cirrhosis). A partial hepatectomy must be performed with these factors in mind to minimize morbidity. In a review of more than 1800 liver resections during a 10-year period from MSKCC, the operative mortality was 3.1%.[123] The median blood loss was 600 mL, and two thirds of patients did not require a red blood cell transfusion. Overall, postoperative morbidity was 45%, but the median hospital stay was 8 days. Morbidity was mostly related to blood loss and the extent of resection. Minor resections were associated with a mortality of 1%. Most complications and deaths were seen in complex biliary tumors, cirrhotics with HCC, and extensive resections. Improving outcomes after partial hepatectomy continue, and experienced hepatobiliary centers have reported mortality rates that approach 1% to 2%, with fewer patients now requiring perioperative blood transfusions. As a result of the increasing safety of hepatic surgery, liver resection has become the treatment of choice for many malignant and benign hepatic conditions.

Bile leaks are a problem in cases requiring complex biliary reconstruction but can also occur in approximately 10% to 20% of hepatectomies without biliary reconstruction. Careful ligation of biliary radicals is of obvious importance in minimizing this complication. Because of the regenerative capacity of the liver, resections of up to 80% of normal noncirrhotic livers can be performed, with functional compensation within a few weeks. Because many resections encompass tumors and normal liver, the concepts of functional liver parenchyma and FLR volume are important because there is often compensatory hypertrophy of normal liver when tumors occupy a significant amount of the liver volume. The risk of hepatic dysfunction is minimal if the reduction of functional liver parenchyma is less than 50% but begins to rise when this figure approaches 20% to 25%. Patients with cirrhosis have much higher rates of postoperative liver dysfunction because of impaired regenerative capacity and impaired primary liver function. Liver failure, extrahepatic multiorgan failure, and death are serious hazards to performance of major liver resections in cirrhotics. In general, patients with Child class B or C cirrhosis or portal hypertension do not tolerate liver resections, and selection of patients is therefore critical. Ascites and infectious complications are also common problems after major liver resection. One strategy to minimize postoperative liver dysfunction and morbidity after major hepatectomy is to embolize the portal vein percutaneously on the side of the liver to be resected. In approximately 4 weeks, this induces atrophy of the liver parenchyma to be resected and hypertrophy of the FLR. In turn, this increases the relative volume of the FLR.

Techniques of liver resection differ according to the disease being treated. In benign hepatic diseases requiring resection, the indications for operation are usually symptoms or infection. Removal of normal liver should be kept to a minimum in these cases, and techniques such as enucleation are appropriate, although a major resection is occasionally necessary. For malignant disease, a margin of normal tissue is important, and formal anatomic resections yield the best results. Techniques such as wedge resection often result in higher rates of margin involvement and disease recurrence and should therefore be used carefully and sparingly.

Detailed knowledge of liver anatomy is essential to the practice of safe hepatic surgery (see earlier). Unfortunately, detailed and complicated descriptions of liver anatomy and common liver resections can be confusing to the student. A 2000 consensus conference conducted in Brisbane, Australia, with the assistance of the Americas Hepato-Pancreato-Biliary Association has published guidelines for this terminology (Table 53-11 and Fig. 53-40). In general, the term *lobectomy* is not preferred because there are no external markings on the liver denoting a lobe. When

TABLE 53-11	Nomenclature for Most Common Major Anatomic Hepatic Resections*		
SEGMENTS†	**COUINAUD, 1957**	**GOLDSMITH AND WOODBURNE, 1957**	**BRISBANE, 2000**
V-VIII	Right hepatectomy	Right hepatic lobectomy	Right hemihepatectomy
IV-VIII‡	Right lobectomy	Extended right hepatic lobectomy	Right trisectionectomy
II-IV	Left hepatectomy	Left hepatic lobectomy	Left hemihepatectomy
II, III	Left lobectomy	Left lateral segmentectomy	Left lateral sectionectomy
II, III, IV, V, VIII‡	Extended left hepatectomy	Extended left lobectomy	Left trisectionectomy

Adapted from the Terminology Committee of the International Hepato-Pancreatico-Biliary Association: The Brisbane 2000 terminology of liver anatomy and resections, 2000 <http://www.ahpba.org/assets/documents/Brisbane_Article.pdf>.
*The original terminology is based on the anatomic descriptions of Couinaud and of Goldsmith and Woodburne.
†See Figure 53-40A-E.
‡Another common name for these operations is right or left trisegmentectomy.

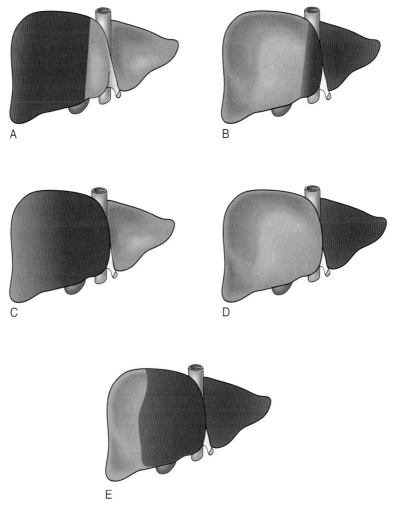

FIGURE 53-40 Commonly performed major hepatic resections are indicated by the *shaded areas.* **A,** Right hepatectomy, right hepatic lobectomy, or right hemihepatectomy (segments V to VIII). **B,** Left hepatectomy, left hepatic lobectomy, or left hemihepatectomy (segments II to IV). **C,** Right lobectomy, extended right hepatic lobectomy, or right trisectionectomy (trisegmentectomy; segments IV to VIII). **D,** Left lobectomy, left lateral segmentectomy, or left lateral sectionectomy (segments II to III). **E,** Extended left hepatectomy, extended left lobectomy, or left trisectionectomy (trisegmentectomy; segments II to V, VIII). See Table 53-11. (From Blumgart LH, Jarnagin W, Fong Y: Liver resection for benign disease and for liver and biliary tumors. In Blumgart LH, Fong Y, editors: *Surgery of the liver and biliary tract,* London, 2000, WB Saunders, pp 1639–1714.)

in doubt, one should always revert to the numeric segments of the liver if there is any confusion about the description of a liver resection. Recall that the right liver is composed of segments V through VIII, and *right hepatectomy* and *right hemihepatectomy* are appropriate terms for resection of these segments. Segments II through IV compose the left liver, and *left hepatectomy* and *left hemihepatectomy* are appropriate terms for resection of these segments. A right hepatectomy can be extended farther to the left to include segment IV, and a left hepatectomy can be extended farther to the right to include segments V and VIII. Terms such as *extended right-left hepatectomy, right-left trisectionectomy,* and *trisegmentectomy* are appropriate to describe these resections. Resection of segments II and III is a commonly performed sublobar resection and is often referred to as a left lateral segmentectomy or left lateral sectionectomy. Other common sublobar resections, such as that of the right posterior sector (segments VI

and VII) or the right anterior sector (segments V and VIII), are referred to as a right posterior sectorectomy-sectionectomy and right anterior sectorectomy-sectionectomy, respectively. Single or bisegmental resections can always be simply referred to by a numeric description of the segments to be resected.

A detailed discussion of the techniques of liver resection is beyond the scope of this chapter; in general, it requires specialty training, but general principles can be discussed. A liver resection must consider the disease to be treated and the goal of the operation, whether that is a margin-negative resection of a malignant neoplasm or the removal of benign tissue to alleviate symptoms. The most basic steps can be distilled down to inflow control (portal vein, hepatic artery, bile duct), outflow control (hepatic veins), and parenchymal transection, with preservation of a liver remnant of adequate size with intact inflow, biliary drainage, and venous outflow.

The most common approach to an anatomic resection, in the most common order, is mobilization of the liver to be resected, dissection of inflow and outflow structures, division of the inflow, division of the outflow, and parenchymal transection. Mobilization of the liver involves division of the right or left triangular ligaments, freeing up the liver from the diaphragm. Often, the liver must be mobilized completely off the vena cava, which it straddles, and this requires careful dissection and division of multiple retrohepatic caval venous branches. For major resections, the hepatic vein of the resected portion of liver is often encircled before the resection. There are various techniques to dissect, control, and divide inflow vessels. Classic inflow control is obtained by dissection of the liver hilum, with control of the portal vein and hepatic artery to the hemiliver to be resected. These can be suture ligated or divided with vascular staplers. Unless tumor proximity mandates, we advocate dividing the bile duct within the liver substance to minimize absolutely contralateral biliary injuries related to anatomic anomalies. Inflow control can also be obtained by dissection of the intrahepatic inflow pedicle to the anatomic section of liver to be resected. Recall that the inflow structures invaginate peritoneum at the hepatic hilum and run intrahepatically as an invested pedicle of the three inflow structures. The inflow pedicles can be encircled by making flanking hepatotomies or by splitting parenchyma down to the pedicle of interest. The pedicle can usually be divided with a vascular stapler, but suture ligation is sometimes necessary. Typically, the hepatic vein is divided in its extrahepatic position, which can also usually be done with a vascular stapler.

The hepatic vein can also be divided within the substance of the liver during parenchymal transection. There are a number of methods of parenchymal transection, ranging from complex ultrasonic irrigators to radiofrequency energy coagulators to a simple clamp-crushing technique. In experienced hands, these can all be used effectively to minimize blood loss, and it is important to develop a specific technique that one is comfortable performing. Ultimately, parenchymal transection is about dissecting intrahepatic anatomy, controlling vascular and biliary structures, minimizing blood loss, and avoiding injury to the FLR.

HEMOBILIA

A case of lethal hemobilia secondary to penetrating abdominal trauma was first described by Glisson in 1654. It was not until 1948 that Sandblom coined the term *hemobilia* in his seminal paper on the subject. Hemobilia is defined as bleeding into the biliary tree from an abnormal communication between a blood vessel and bile duct. It is a rare condition that is often difficult to distinguish from common causes of gastrointestinal bleeding. The most common causes of hemobilia are iatrogenic trauma, accidental trauma, gallstones, tumors, inflammatory disorders, and vascular disorders. Major hemobilia is relatively uncommon, whereas minor inconsequential hemobilia is a common consequence of gallstone disease or interventional radiologic hepatic procedures.

Causes

The most common cause of hemobilia is iatrogenic trauma to the liver and biliary tree. Before the 1980s, the ratio of hemobilia attributed to accidental trauma compared with iatrogenic trauma was 2 : 1, but iatrogenic trauma is now regarded as the cause of hemobilia in 40% to 60% of cases. Percutaneous liver biopsy results in hemobilia in less than 1% of cases, but percutaneous

transhepatic biliary drainage procedures have an incidence of 2% to 10%. Similarly, surgical exploration of the biliary tree can result in hemobilia from direct injury or arterial pseudoaneurysm. A number of cases of hemobilia after cholecystectomy have been reported. Hemobilia secondary to accidental trauma is more common with blunt than with penetrating abdominal trauma and occurs with a reported incidence of 0.2% to 3%. Risk factors for the development of hemobilia after accidental trauma are central hepatic rupture with a cavity, the use of packs, and inadequate drainage. The gallbladder can be a source of bleeding from trauma, gallstones, or acalculous cholecystitis. Primary vascular diseases, such as aneurysms, angiodysplasia, and hemangiomas, are rare causes of hemobilia. Malignant tumors of the liver, biliary tree, gallbladder, and pancreas as well as parasitic infections, hepatic abscesses, and cholangitis are uncommon causes of hemobilia.

Clinical Presentation

Portal venous bleeding into the biliary tree is rare and often self-limited unless the portal pressure is elevated. Minor hemobilia generally runs an uneventful asymptomatic clinical course. However, arterial hemobilia, the most common source, can be dramatic. Clinical sequelae of hemobilia are related to blood loss and the formation of potentially occlusive blood clots in the biliary tree. The classic triad of symptoms and signs of hemobilia is upper abdominal pain, upper gastrointestinal hemorrhage, and jaundice. In one report, all three were present in 22% of patients. The symptoms and signs of major hemobilia are melena (90% of cases), hematemesis (60% of cases), biliary colic (70% of cases), and jaundice (60% of cases). Upper gastrointestinal bleeding seen in conjunction with biliary symptoms must always raise the suspicion of hemobilia. One interesting aspect of hemobilia is the tendency for delayed presentations, up to weeks after the inciting causal event, as well as recurrent and brisk but limited bleeding during months and even years. Blood clots in the biliary tree can masquerade as stones if hemobilia goes unrecognized. These clots can cause cholangitis, pancreatitis, and cholecystitis.

Diagnostic Workup

Once hemobilia is suspected, the first evaluation should be upper gastrointestinal endoscopy, which rules out other sources of hemorrhage and may visualize bleeding from the ampulla of Vater. However, upper endoscopy is diagnostic of hemobilia in only approximately 10% of cases. If upper endoscopy is diagnostic and conservative management is planned, no further studies are necessary. Ultrasound or CT may be helpful in demonstrating intrahepatic tumor or hematoma. Evidence of active bleeding into the biliary tree may be seen on contrast-enhanced CT in the form of pooling contrast material, intraluminal clots, or biliary dilation. CT may also show risk factors associated with hemobilia, such as cavitating central lesions and aneurysms. Arterial angiography is now recognized as the test of choice when significant hemobilia is suspected and will reveal the source of bleeding in approximately 90% of cases. Cholangiography demonstrates blood clots in the biliary tree that may appear as stringy defects or smaller spherical defects that may be difficult to distinguish from stones.

Treatment and Outcomes

The treatment of hemobilia must be focused on stopping the bleeding and relieving biliary obstruction. Most cases of minor hemobilia can be managed conservatively with correction of coagulopathy, adequate biliary drainage (only if necessary), and close observation. In a review of 171 reported cases from 1996 to 1999,

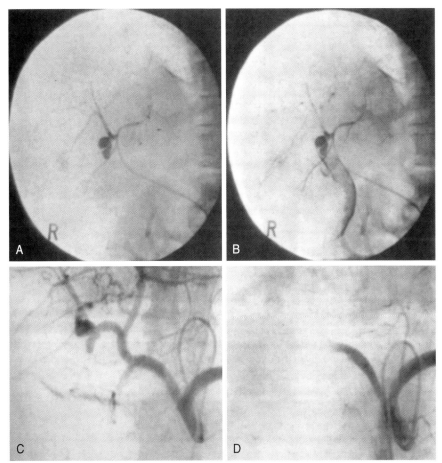

FIGURE 53-41 Classic Findings of Hemobilia. After a complicated cholecystectomy, an iatrogenic pseudoaneurysm developed and ruptured into the biliary tree. Exsanguinating hemobilia ensued; the diagnosis was made by endoscopy and then treated by arterial embolization. **A,** Arteriogram demonstrating a pseudoaneurysm of the hepatic artery at the hilum. **B,** A few seconds later, the contrast material is seen flowing down the hepatic duct, with evidence of clot in the biliary tree. **C** and **D,** The same aneurysm before **(C)** and after **(D)** successful embolization. (From Sandblom JP: Hemobilia and bilhemia. In Blumgart LH, Fong Y, editors: *Surgery of the liver and biliary tract*, London, 2000, WB Saunders, pp 1319–1342.)

43% of cases were successfully managed conservatively. The first line of therapy for major hemobilia was transarterial embolization, and success rates of 80% to 100% were reported. Angiography with transarterial embolization is indicated for major hemobilia requiring blood transfusion (Fig. 53-41).

Surgery is indicated when conservative therapy and transarterial embolization have failed. Surgical treatment of hemobilia is rarely necessary, and even in cases in which a laparotomy may be mandated for other reasons, transarterial embolization is still the therapy of choice for hemobilia because of its lower morbidity. Surgical approaches generally involve ligation of bleeding vessels, excision of aneurysms, or nonselective ligation of a main hepatic artery. Hepatic resection may be necessary for failed arterial ligation or for cases of severe trauma or tumor. Hemorrhage from the gallbladder or hemorrhagic cholecystitis mandates cholecystectomy. There have been isolated reports of successful management of hemobilia with endoscopic coagulation, somatostatin, and vasopressin. The management of hemobilia after percutaneous transhepatic biliary drainage usually consists of removal of the catheter or replacement with larger catheters but may require transarterial embolization.

At the time of Sandblom's report from the early 1970s, the mortality for hemobilia was at least 25%. A report from 1987 noted a mortality of 12%. In a review of cases from 1996 through 1999, only four deaths were reported. There has clearly been a reduction in mortality from hemobilia, which is probably related to two factors. First, the incidence of minor self-limited hemobilia has increased secondary to the rising number of percutaneous hepatic procedures. Second, improvements in selective angiography and transarterial embolization have greatly improved the treatment of major hemobilia.

Bilhemia

Bilhemia is an extremely rare condition in which bile flows into the bloodstream through the hepatic veins or portal vein branches. This flow occurs in the context of a high intrabiliary pressure exceeding that of the venous system. The cause can be gallstones eroding into the portal vein or accidental or iatrogenic trauma. The condition can be fatal secondary to embolization of large amounts of bile into the lungs. Usually, however, bile flow is low, and the fistulas close spontaneously. The clinical presentation is that of rapidly increasing jaundice, marked direct hyperbilirubinemia

TABLE 53-12	Serologic Evaluation of the Most Common Viral Hepatitides			
VIRUS	**ANTIGEN NAME**	**INTERPRETATION**	**ANTIBODY NAME**	**INTERPRETATION**
HAV	HAV antigen	Acute infection	Anti-HAV IgM	Acute infection
			Anti-HAV IgG	Immunity
HBV	HBsAg	Acute or chronic infection	Anti-HBs	Immunity
	HBeAg	HBV replication, infectivity	Anti-HBc	All phases of infection
			Anti-HBe	Late convalescence
HCV	None	—	Anti-HCV	Late convalescence or chronic infection

without elevation of hepatocellular enzyme levels (e.g., AST, ALT), and septicemia. This diagnosis is best determined by ERCP. Treatment is directed at lowering intrabiliary pressures through stents or sphincterotomy.

VIRAL HEPATITIS AND THE SURGEON

Epidemics of jaundice were noted in ancient civilizations and recorded by Hippocrates. During World War II, these epidemics were called catarrhal jaundice. More than 28,000 cases were documented at that time. Epidemiologic studies in the 1940s documented the difference between bloodborne hepatitis (hepatitis B) and enteric hepatitis (hepatitis A). The most important discovery was that of the Australia antigen by Blumberg and coworkers in 1965. This antigen proved to be the hepatitis B surface antigen (HBsAg) and provided a means for differentiating the two types of hepatitis and characterizing the epidemiology of this disease. This discovery also led to the development of HBV vaccines based on this antigen, with obvious and profound effects worldwide. Further research led to the discovery of the delta virus (hepatitis D) and hepatitis C, explaining cases of non-A, non-B hepatitis. Hepatitis E has been found to be a unique enteral form of infectious hepatitis; the hepatitis G virus, discovered in 1995, is still being defined.

Viral hepatitis is a major health problem and is the most common cause of liver disease worldwide. Although fulminant acute hepatitis is uncommon, there are more than 5 million people who suffer from chronic hepatitis. It is estimated that more than 15,000 patients die each year of viral hepatitis in the United States alone. Viral hepatitis is not a surgical disease, but it has important consequences for surgeons and surgical patients. For any surgeon performing hepatic surgery, the functional state of the liver is extremely important, and patients with chronic viral hepatitis require special attention before any surgical intervention. Also, chronic viral hepatitis is a common cause of HCC. Finally, the risk of transmission from patient to surgeon and vice versa is an issue with which all surgeons should be familiar.

Definition

Viral hepatitis is an infection of the liver by one of six known viruses that have diverse genetic compositions and structures. HAV, HCV, HDV, HEV, and HGV have RNA genomes, whereas HBV has a DNA genome that replicates through RNA intermediates. HAV and HEV are both responsible for forms of epidemic hepatitis and are transmitted through the fecal-oral route. HBV is the only one with the potential to integrate into host genomes, although this is not required for replication. HCV replicates in the cytoplasm of hepatocytes and has complex mechanisms of evading host immunity through hypervariable areas in its genome.

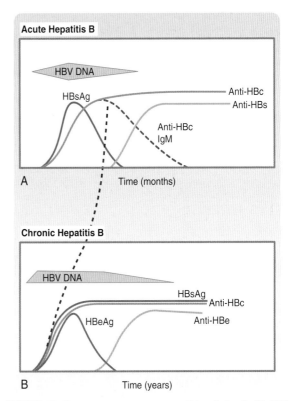

FIGURE 53-42 Serologic makers in acute **(A)** and chronic **(B)** HBV infection. (From Doo EC, Lian TJ: The hepatitis viruses. In Schiff ER, Sorrell MF, Maddrey WC, editors: *Schiff's diseases of the liver*, Philadelphia, 1999, Lippincott-Raven, pp 725–744.)

HDV requires the presence of HBV coinfection for replication and infectivity and can alter the clinical course of HBV infection. HGV was discovered more recently and has similarities to HCV but has no definitive association with clinical hepatitis.

Diagnosis

Table 53-12 summarizes the serologic tests and their implications for HAV, HBV, and HCV. The diagnosis of HAV infection relies on the determination of antibodies to HAV. Both IgM and IgG antibodies are present early in the infection, but only IgG persists long term. HAV antigens and tests for HAV RNA have been developed but are generally restricted to research laboratories.

HBV infection has been characterized by a number of antigens and antibodies (Fig. 53-42). HBsAg is the hallmark of the diagnosis of HBV infection and appears in the serum 1 to 10 weeks after infection; it usually disappears in 4 to 6 months, but persistence in the serum implies chronic infection. Anti-HBs antibodies usually appear during a window period after the disappearance of HBsAg and indicate recovery after HBV infection. Anti-HBs antibodies are also induced by the HBV vaccine. The hepatitis core antigen (HBcAg) is an intracellular antigen that is not detectable in serum. On the other hand, anti-HBc antibodies are detectable early after infection and persist after recovery and in chronic infections. Hepatitis B e antigen (HBeAg) is a secretory protein that is a marker of HBV replication and infectivity. It is usually present early and may persist for years in chronic infection but generally disappears within months in the absence of chronic infection. Seroconversion to anti-HBe antibodies is usually associated with resolution of infection. It has also been shown that many patients who have seroconverted often have measurable HBV DNA, albeit at low levels. Quantification of HBV DNA in the serum has become the most accurate way of assessing HBV activity. Evidence has shown that many patients thought to have resolved acute HBV infection may have persistent viral infection and may be at risk for ongoing hepatitis or reactivation.

The diagnosis of HCV infection relies on the detection of antibodies to a number of HCV antigens. Current immunoassays are highly specific and sensitive. No specific HCV antigen tests exist, but there are a variety of quantitative and qualitative tests for HCV RNA, which have become important in confirming the diagnosis in unclear cases and assessing responses to therapy.

HDV coinfection of HBV-infected patients is best diagnosed by detection of HDV RNA, which can be measured in serum. The HDV antigen can be detected in liver specimens. HEV infection can be diagnosed by measurement of antibodies in serum or by detection of the virus or its components in feces, serum, or the liver itself.

Epidemiology and Transmission

The incidence of hepatitis A has fallen dramatically since the introduction of effective vaccines, but vaccination is not routine in all countries. Hepatitis A is common in third-world countries, with seropositivity rates approaching 100% in some populations. Infection occurs in childhood and is facilitated by poor hygiene and sanitation. Infection rates are much lower in developed countries. In the United States, approximately 10% of children and 35% of adults have been infected with HAV. Despite vaccination availability, 6000 cases were reported in the United States in 2004, likely representing an estimated 60,000 cases nationwide. The primary route of HAV infection is the fecal-oral route. Most cases of HAV occur because of ingestion of contaminated water or food and person-to-person contact. Parenteral transmission is possible but uncommon. Sexual transmission has been documented in homosexual men.

Hepatitis B is a major worldwide health problem. There are more than 300 million carriers and 250,000 associated deaths annually. The prevalence of HBV infection has considerable geographic variation. Low prevalence areas such as the United States and western Europe have carrier rates of 0.1% to 2%. In these regions, transmission is generally through sexual intercourse or IV drug abuse. Carrier rates in intermediate-prevalence areas such as Japan and Singapore range from 3% to 5%. In high-prevalence areas such as Southeast Asia and sub-Saharan Africa, carrier rates range from 10% to 20%. Transmission in high-prevalence areas is largely perinatal and horizontal during childhood.

Transfusion-associated HBV infection was common in the 1960s, and the risk has been estimated to be as high as 50% at that time. Currently, screening programs and limitation of blood donation to voluntary donors have decreased the risk of acquiring HBV from a blood transfusion to 1 in 63,000. Percutaneous transmission through the use of any contaminated needle is a major route of HBV infection and is common in IV drug abusers. Sexual transmission is common in low-prevalence countries and is estimated to account for approximately 30% of cases in the United States. There is a particularly high incidence in male homosexuals and heterosexuals with multiple sexual partners. Perinatal HBV infection accounts for less than 10% of cases in the United States but is common in endemic regions, with rates of transmission of 90% in some areas. Horizontal transmission among children is common and is probably related to minor breaks in the skin and mucous membranes. HBV is the most commonly transmitted virus among health care personnel, and transmission is usually patient to patient or patient to worker. Needle-stick risk has been related to HBeAg positivity. Rare cases of physician to patient transmission have been reported.

Hepatitis C is the most common cause of chronic liver disease in the United States, with an estimated prevalence of 1.8% accounting for 3.9 million infected people. New infections typically occur at a younger age (20 to 39 years), and the most common risk factor is IV drug abuse. Health care workers have higher carrier rates than the general public. Transmission among health care workers is usually related to needle-stick incidents, and the risk of transmission is higher than that of HBV and HIV. In the past, blood transfusion was the major cause of HCV infection, accounting for at least 85% of cases. Currently, less than 2% of acute infections are caused by transfusions, and the risk of transfusion-associated transmission is estimated to be about 1 in 10,000. Although HCV has never been documented in semen, it is estimated that approximately 20% of HCV infections are caused by sexual transmission. Risk of sexual transmission appears to be related to the number of partners and presence of other sexually transmitted diseases. Monogamous sexual partners of HCV-infected people occasionally test positive for HCV in the absence of other risk factors, but this appears to be rare. Perinatal transmission has been documented but is also rare. No identifiable risk factors are found in 30% to 40% of HCV cases.

HDV infection occurs worldwide, with a variable distribution that parallels that of HBV infection. Approximately 5% of HBsAg-positive patients also harbor HDV infection. Transmission of HDV is parenteral and can occur only in patients previously infected with HBV.

HEV is endemic in Southeast Asia and central Asia and occurs with low frequency in other areas of the world. HEV infection outbreaks are usually large, affecting hundreds to thousands of people at once, and often follow large rains and flooding. There is a particularly high incidence and mortality in pregnant women. Transmission is fecal-oral and usually related to contaminated drinking water or food. Person-to-person transmission and vertical transmission are rare.

Pathogenesis and Clinical Presentation

The pathogenesis of hepatic injury from these viral infections is not completely understood. For all the viruses discussed in this section, hepatic inflammation appears to be caused by direct cytotoxicity or immune-related phenomena. A combination of these two mechanisms probably underlies the cause of hepatic damage.

Humans are the only host for HAV, and no reservoir of infection has been identified. After oral intake, HAV can survive the acidic gastric pH, but the mechanism of hepatic uptake is not known. HAV infection results in acute inflammation of the liver and has no associated chronic sequelae. The most recent data suggest that hepatocyte damage is most likely an immunopathologic response rather than direct hepatotoxicity. Most children with HAV infection younger than 2 years are asymptomatic, whereas in pediatric patients older than 5 years, 80% will develop symptoms. Fulminant hepatitis develops in 1% to 5% of cases, and mortality is generally below 1%.

Approximately 70% of patients with acute HBV infection have subclinical or anicteric hepatitis; the other 30% have icteric hepatitis. The incubation period for HBV infection ranges from 1 to 4 months. A prodromal serum sickness–like syndrome may develop, followed by a multitude of constitutional symptoms, such as malaise, anorexia, and nausea. The constitutional symptoms last about 10 days and are followed by jaundice in 30% of patients. Clinical symptoms usually disappear within 3 months. Fulminant hepatic failure develops in 0.1% to 0.5% of patients. Almost 80% of patients with fulminant HBV-related hepatitis will die unless liver transplantation is performed.

Risk of chronic HBV infection is related to immunocompetence and age. Immunocompetent adults have a risk of less than 5%, whereas 30% of children and 90% of infants will develop chronic disease. Most patients with chronic HBV infection are asymptomatic, but some may experience exacerbations of symptoms. Laboratory test results may be entirely normal in HBV carriers, or mild elevations of ALT and AST may be the only findings. Progression to cirrhosis is marked by hepatic synthetic dysfunction and often cytopenias, related to hypersplenism. Extrahepatic manifestations of HBV infection, caused by circulating immune complexes, occur in approximately 10% to 20% of patients; these include polyarteritis nodosa, glomerulonephritis, essential mixed cryoglobulinemia, and papular acrodermatitis. The sequelae of chronic HBV infection range from none to cirrhosis, HCC, hepatic failure, and death. It has been noted that patients thought to have previously cleared the infection can have a reactivation, especially during a period of immunosuppression. In nonendemic areas, the long-term risk appears to be low, but in endemic areas, chronic HBV infection is a significant cause of morbidity and mortality.

Acute HCV infection generally is manifested with mild elevation of hepatocellular enzyme levels. In general, 80% of cases occur 5 to 12 weeks after infection. Symptoms occur in less than 30% of patients and are usually so mild and nonspecific that they do not affect daily life. Jaundice occurs in less than 20% of patients, and fulminant hepatic failure caused by HCV is extremely uncommon. Chronic HCV infection develops in approximately two thirds of patients; the other third appear to clear the infection. Most patients with chronic HCV infection are asymptomatic without evidence of overt liver disease and present with only mildly elevated hepatocellular enzyme levels. Despite this quiet clinical course, patients with chronic HCV infection are at risk for development of cirrhosis and HCC. Estimates place the risk of cirrhosis at 2% to 20% at a 20- to 30-year interval. The risk for development of HCC from that point has been estimated at 1% to 4%/year. Progression of liver damage can be variable, and several factors appear to affect its rate. Factors associated with a more rapid progression include male gender, older age at infection, immunosuppression (e.g., HIV infection), coinfection with HBV, moderate alcohol intake, and obesity. Extrahepatic manifestations, such as autoimmune disorders and lymphoma, can occur with HCV infection and are likely related to circulating immune complexes.

The clinical presentation of HDV infection is related to a complex relationship between the degree of HBV and HDV infection. Simultaneous coinfection with high expression of HBV and HDV results in higher rates of acute fulminant hepatitis. Superinfection in a previous HBV carrier generally results in more rapidly progressive chronic liver damage. Some milder forms of acute HDV infection are associated with decreased expression of HDV and repression of HBV infection.

Hepatitis E has a histologic picture different from that of the other viral hepatitides in that a cholestatic type of hepatitis is seen in more than 50% of patients. HEV is introduced orally, and it is not known how the virus travels to the liver. The incubation period of HEV infection ranges from 2 to 9 weeks. The most common form of illness is acute icteric hepatitis; most series report jaundice in more than 90% of patients. Asymptomatic forms of the disease occur and are probably more common than the icteric form, but the actual frequency is unknown. The disease is usually self-limited, but fulminant hepatic failure can occur in a small percentage of patients. Overall, the mortality rate is probably significantly less than 1%. Pregnant women tend to have a more severe clinical course; mortality rates range from 5% to 25%.

Prevention

HAV infection prophylaxis relies on sanitary measures and administration of serum immunoglobulin. The development of safe and effective HAV vaccines, however, has made the use of preexposure immunoglobulin unnecessary. Serum immunoglobulin is still the therapy of choice for postexposure prophylaxis and may be safely given, along with active immunization. In the United States, the Centers for Disease Control and Prevention has recommended universal vaccination of children on the basis of the safety and efficacy of the vaccine in high-risk populations. Public health researchers are investigating vaccination schemes to eradicate HAV infection in high-risk populations throughout the world. However, cost-benefit analyses have not supported universal vaccination worldwide. Similarly, HEV infection prophylaxis has focused on sanitary measures, particularly strategies aimed at drinking water. Unfortunately, HEV immunoglobulin has not been successful in preexposure or postexposure prevention of HEV infection, whereas anti-HEV antibodies appear to be effective at attenuating the clinical syndrome. Vaccines for HEV infection have been developed and evaluated in clinical trials.

Remarkable advances have been made in the prevention of HBV infection. In the past, prevention of HBV infection was limited to passive immunization with immunoglobulin containing high titers of antibody to HBsAg. Currently, immunoglobulin immunization is used only in postexposure prophylaxis. HBsAg-containing vaccines have been developed, with good safety and efficacy profiles. These vaccines are used primarily for preexposure prophylaxis but can also be used in a postexposure setting along with immunoglobulin. HBV vaccination is recommended for high-risk groups such as health care workers. There are also programs for HBV vaccination to prevent perinatal transmission; currently, all children 11 or 12 years old should be vaccinated if this has not been done previously. HBV DNA–based vaccines have been developed, and a combined HBV and HAV vaccine was approved by the U.S. Food and Drug Administration in 2001. Although no vaccine is available for HDV infection, effective prevention of HBV infection prevents HDV infection.

The only effective preventive strategy for HCV infection relies on public health principles aimed at the major risk factors for transmission. Conventionally prepared anti-HCV immunoglobulin has been evaluated in a number of trials and has not been demonstrated to prevent transfusion-related non-A, non-B hepatitis. Screening of blood donors has rendered this issue irrelevant today. Unfortunately, because of various obstacles, a successful HCV vaccine has not been developed.

Treatment

Treatment of HAV or HEV infection is supportive in nature and is generally aimed at correcting dehydration and providing adequate calorie intake. Although fatigue may mandate significant periods of rest, hospitalization is usually not necessary, except in cases of fulminant liver failure.

The treatment of HBV infection is largely aimed at patients with chronic active disease. The two approved therapies are interferon alfa and the nucleoside analogue lamivudine. Interferon alfa is an immunomodulatory agent with some antiviral properties that can induce a virologic response in 35% to 40% of patients. However, long-term benefit with interferon therapy has not been proven. Many nucleoside analogues for the treatment of HBV infection have been developed and probably work through inhibition of DNA synthesis. They have similar viral response rates to interferon alfa, are inexpensive, are given orally, and have few side effects. On the other hand, nucleoside analogues often require long-term therapy (>1 year), and the development of resistant HBV mutants has been documented. Randomized trials have shown oral lamivudine to be effective at decreasing the risk of cirrhosis progression and HCC. Newer antiviral agents are in development and are likely to improve outcomes.

During the last 20 years, tremendous advances in the treatment of HCV infection have occurred. A benefit for interferon alfa in the treatment of non-A, non-B hepatitis was originally demonstrated in 1986, before the discovery of HCV. With current interferon alfa treatment regimens, complete viral response, defined as sustained loss of serum viral RNA, occurs in 12% to 20% of patients. The addition of ribavirin to interferon alfa has resulted in response rates of 35% to 45%. In the most recent trials, treatment with pegylated interferon alfa and ribavirin for 48 weeks resulted in viral clearance in 55% of patients. The specific genotype appears to be predictive of response, with some types resulting in response rates of 80% and others of 45%. Relapse can occur, but it usually occurs with monotherapy and shortened courses of therapy. Because therapy with interferon alfa has significant side effects, controversies such as indications for treatment, optimal doses, and duration of treatment are still being resolved.

SELECTED REFERENCES

Blumgart LH: *Video atlas: Liver, biliary and pancreatic surgery*, Philadelphia, 2011, Elsevier.

This video atlas includes an extensive library of narrated and captioned videos that present history, radiologic evidence, and operative procedures for hepatic and biliary surgery. It also includes laparoscopic approaches to liver resections.

Blumgart LH: *Surgery of the liver, biliary tract, and pancreas*, ed 5, Philadelphia, 2012, Elsevier.

A comprehensive and clinical review of hepatobiliary anatomy. The text is specifically oriented toward surgery of the liver and biliary tree. It covers anatomy, pathophysiology, immunology, molecular biology, genetics, diagnosis, and

treatment. In addition, it is accompanied by a DVD with detailed video clips of laparoscopic procedures, effectively allowing one to use it as an operative atlas.

Bruix J, Sherman M, American Association for the Study of Liver Disease: Management of hepatocellular carcinoma: An update. *Hepatology* 53:1020–1022, 2011.

This is an update on the original AASLD guidelines on the management of hepatocellular carcinoma.

Fong Y, Fortner J, Sun RL, et al: Clinical score for predicting recurrence after hepatic resection for metastatic colorectal cancer: Analysis of 1001 consecutive cases. *Ann Surg* 230:309–318, 1999.

At the time of publication, this was the largest single-institution series of liver resection for metastatic colorectal cancer. A very useful prognostic scoring system is presented and remains critically important in evaluating patients today.

Foster JH, Berman MM: *Solid liver tumors*, Philadelphia, 1977, WB Saunders.

A classic and comprehensive monograph that contains a complete history of liver surgery.

Herrera JL: Management of acute variceal bleeding. *Clin Liver Dis* 18:347–357, 2014.

This review article discusses the management of acute variceal bleeding with special emphasis on the appropriate role of various treatment modalities in the current era and when to escalate the therapy and move to the next stage.

House MG, Ito H, Gonen M, et al: Survival after hepatic resection for metastatic colorectal cancer: Trends in outcomes for 1,600 patients during two decades at a single institution. *J Am Coll Surg* 210:744–752, 2010.

This study analyzes factors associated with differences in long-term outcomes after hepatic resection for metastatic colorectal cancer. Despite worse clinical and pathologic features, survival rates after hepatic resection for colorectal metastases have improved, which might be attributable to improvements in patient selection, operative management, and chemotherapy.

Jang HJ, Yu H, Kim TK: Imaging of focal liver lesions. *Semin Roentgenol* 44:266–282, 2009.

Imaging modalities are key in diagnosing and differentiating various focal liver lesions. This monograph covers the critical elements of ultrasonography, computed tomography, and magnetic resonance imaging of focal liver lesions.

Jarnagin WR, Gonen M, Fong Y, et al: Improvement in perioperative outcome after hepatic resection: Analysis of 1,803 consecutive cases over the past decade. *Ann Surg* 236:397–406, 2002.

One of the largest series of hepatic resections that documents the remarkable improvement in perioperative outcomes.

Kelly K, Weber SM: Cystic diseases of the liver and bile ducts. *J Gastrointest Surg* 18:627–634, quiz 634, 2014.

This review article covers the diagnosis and management of cystic disease of the liver including hydatid disease.

Leung U, Fong Y: Robotic liver surgery. *Hepatobiliary Surg Nutr* 3:288–294, 2014.

This manuscript reviews the place and evolution of robotics in the current era of minimally invasive liver surgery.

Llovet JM, Ricci S, Mazzaferro V, et al: Sorafenib in advanced hepatocellular carcinoma. *N Engl J Med* 359:378–390, 2008.

The first randomized phase 3 clinical trial in patients with advanced hepatocellular carcinoma that showed a benefit of improved median survival and time to radiologic progression for patients treated with a chemotherapeutic agent compared with patients who were given a placebo.

Mittal S, El-Serag HB: Epidemiology of hepatocellular carcinoma: Consider the population. *J Clin Gastroenterol* 47(Suppl):S 2–S6, 2013.

A recent comprehensive and concise review of the subject.

Ochsner A, DeBakey M, Murray S: Pyogenic abscess of the liver. *Am J Surg* 40:292–319, 1938.

A classic landmark study on pyogenic abscesses of the liver. This was the first serious attempt to study hepatic abscesses and ushered in the modern era of treatment.

Sandhu BS, Sanyal AJ: Management of ascites in cirrhosis. *Clin Liver Dis* 9:715–732, 2005.

This is an excellent, comprehensive, and practical review of the treatment of ascites in patients with cirrhosis.

REFERENCES

1. Tsung A, Geller DA, Sukato DC, et al: Robotic versus laparoscopic hepatectomy: A matched comparison. *Ann Surg* 259:549–555, 2014.
2. Biernat J, Pawlik WW, Sendur R, et al: Role of afferent nerves and sensory peptides in the mediation of hepatic artery buffer response. *J Physiol Pharmacol* 56:133–145, 2005.
3. de Franchis R: Revising consensus in portal hypertension: Report of the Baveno V consensus workshop on methodology of diagnosis and therapy in portal hypertension. *J Hepatol* 53:762–768, 2010.
4. Garcia-Tsao G, Bosch J: Management of varices and variceal hemorrhage in cirrhosis. *N Engl J Med* 362:823–832, 2010.
5. Bureau C, Garcia-Pagan JC, Otal P, et al: Improved clinical outcome using polytetrafluoroethylene-coated stents for TIPS: Results of a randomized study. *Gastroenterology* 126:469–475, 2004.
6. Orloff MJ, Orloff MS, Orloff SL, et al: Three decades of experience with emergency portacaval shunt for acutely bleeding esophageal varices in 400 unselected patients with cirrhosis of the liver. *J Am Coll Surg* 180:257–272, 1995.
7. Bernard B, Lebrec D, Mathurin P, et al: Beta-adrenergic antagonists in the prevention of gastrointestinal rebleeding in patients with cirrhosis: A meta-analysis. *Hepatology* 25:63–70, 1997.
8. Villanueva C, Minana J, Ortiz J, et al: Endoscopic ligation compared with combined treatment with nadolol and isosorbide mononitrate to prevent recurrent variceal bleeding. *N Engl J Med* 345:647–655, 2001.
9. de la Pena J, Brullet E, Sanchez-Hernandez E, et al: Variceal ligation plus nadolol compared with ligation for prophylaxis of variceal rebleeding: A multicenter trial. *Hepatology* 41:572–578, 2005.
10. Funakoshi N, Segalas-Largey F, Duny Y, et al: Benefit of combination beta-blocker and endoscopic treatment to prevent variceal rebleeding: A meta-analysis. *World J Gastroenterol* 16:5982–5992, 2010.
11. Fong Y, Wong J: Evolution in surgery: Influence of minimally invasive approaches on the hepatobiliary surgeon. *Surg Infect (Larchmt)* 10:399–406, 2009.
12. Meddings L, Myers RP, Hubbard J, et al: A population-based study of pyogenic liver abscesses in the United States: Incidence, mortality, and temporal trends. *Am J Gastroenterol* 105:117–124, 2010.
13. Lai HC, Lin CC, Cheng KS, et al: Increased incidence of gastrointestinal cancers among patients with pyogenic liver abscess: A population-based cohort study. *Gastroenterology* 146:129–137, e1, 2014.
14. Salles JM, Salles MJ, Moraes LA, et al: Invasive amebiasis: An update on diagnosis and management. *Expert Rev Anti Infect Ther* 5:893–901, 2007.
15. Mezhir J, Fong Y, Jacks L, et al: Current management of pyogenic liver abscess: Surgery is now second-line treatment. *J Am Coll Surg* 975–983, 2010.
16. Wuerz T, Kane JB, Boggild AK, et al: A review of amoebic liver abscess for clinicians in a nonendemic setting. *Can J Gastroenterol* 26:729–733, 2012.
17. Haque R, Mollah NU, Ali IK, et al: Diagnosis of amebic liver abscess and intestinal infection with the TechLab *Entamoeba histolytica* II antigen detection and antibody tests. *J Clin Microbiol* 38:3235–3239, 2000.
18. Benedetti NJ, Desser TS, Jeffrey RB: Imaging of hepatic infections. *Ultrasound Q* 24:267–278, 2008.
19. Chavez-Tapia NC, Hernandez-Calleros J, Tellez-Avila FI, et al: Image-guided percutaneous procedure plus metronidazole versus metronidazole alone for uncomplicated amoebic liver abscess. *Cochrane Database Syst Rev* (1): CD004886, 2009.
20. Nunnari G, Pinzone MR, Gruttadauria S, et al: Hepatic echinococcosis: Clinical and therapeutic aspects. *World J Gastroenterol* 18:1448–1458, 2012.
21. Agayev RM, Agayev BA: Hepatic hydatid disease: Surgical experience over 15 years. *Hepatogastroenterology* 55:1373–1379, 2008.

22. Dziri C, Haouet K, Fingerhut A, et al: Management of cystic echinococcosis complications and dissemination: Where is the evidence? *World J Surg* 33:1266–1273, 2009.

23. Brunetti E, Kern P, Vuitton DA: Expert consensus for the diagnosis and treatment of cystic and alveolar echinococcosis in humans. *Acta Trop* 114:1–16, 2010.

24. Tamarozzi F, Vuitton L, Brunetti E, et al: Non-surgical and non-chemical attempts to treat echinococcosis: Do they work? *Parasite* 21:75, 2014.

25. Nasseri Moghaddam S, Abrishami A, Malekzadeh R: Percutaneous needle aspiration, injection, and reaspiration with or without benzimidazole coverage for uncomplicated hepatic hydatid cysts. *Cochrane Database Syst Rev* (2): CD003623, 2006.

26. Nguyen T, Powell A, Daugherty T: Recurrent pyogenic cholangitis. *Dig Dis Sci* 55:8–10, 2010.

27. Das AK: Hepatic and biliary ascariasis. *J Glob Infect Dis* 6:65–72, 2014.

28. Chen C, Huang M, Yang J, et al: Reappraisal of percutaneous transhepatic cholangioscopic lithotomy for primary hepatolithiasis. *Surg Endosc* 19:505–509, 2005.

29. Parray FQ, Wani MA, Wani NA: Oriental cholangiohepatitis—is our surgery appropriate? *Int J Surg* 12:789–793, 2014.

30. Mori T, Sugiyama M, Atomi Y: Gallstone disease: Management of intrahepatic stones. *Best Pract Res Clin Gastroenterol* 20:1117–1137, 2006.

31. Buell JF, Cherqui D, Geller DA, et al: The international position on laparoscopic liver surgery: The Louisville Statement, 2008. *Ann Surg* 250:825–830, 2009.

32. Sasaki A, Nitta H, Otsuka K, et al: Ten-year experience of totally laparoscopic liver resection in a single institution. *Br J Surg* 96:274–279, 2009.

33. Huurman VA, Schaapherder AF: Management of ruptured hepatocellular adenoma. *Dig Surg* 27:56–60, 2010.

34. Dhingra S, Fiel MI: Update on the new classification of hepatic adenomas: Clinical, molecular, and pathologic characteristics. *Arch Pathol Lab Med* 138:1090–1097, 2014.

35. Zucman-Rossi J, Jeannot E, Nhieu JT, et al: Genotype-phenotype correlation in hepatocellular adenoma: New classification and relationship with HCC. *Hepatology* 43:515–524, 2006.

36. Rebouissou S, Bioulac-Sage P, Zucman-Rossi J: Molecular pathogenesis of focal nodular hyperplasia and hepatocellular adenoma. *J Hepatol* 48:163–170, 2008.

37. Assy N, Nasser G, Djibre A, et al: Characteristics of common solid liver lesions and recommendations for diagnostic workup. *World J Gastroenterol* 15:3217–3227, 2009.

38. Curvo-Semedo L, Brito JB, Seco MF, et al: The hypointense liver lesion on T2-weighted MR images and what it means. *Radiographics* 30:e38, 2010.

39. Marrero JA, Ahn J, Rajender Reddy K: ACG clinical guideline: The diagnosis and management of focal liver lesions. *Am J Gastroenterol* 109:1328–1347, quiz 1348, 2014.

40. Katabathina VS, Menias CO, Shanbhogue AK, et al: Genetics and imaging of hepatocellular adenomas: 2011 update. *Radiographics* 31:1529–1543, 2011.

41. Bioulac-Sage P, Laumonier H, Couchy G, et al: Hepatocellular adenoma management and phenotypic classification: The Bordeaux experience. *Hepatology* 50:481–489, 2009.

42. Deneve JL, Pawlik TM, Cunningham S, et al: Liver cell adenoma: A multicenter analysis of risk factors for rupture and malignancy. *Ann Surg Oncol* 16:640–648, 2009.

43. Vetelainen R, Erdogan D, de Graaf W, et al: Liver adenomatosis: Re-evaluation of aetiology and management. *Liver Int* 28:499–508, 2008.

44. Wellen JR, Anderson CD, Doyle M, et al: The role of liver transplantation for hepatic adenomatosis in the pediatric population: Case report and review of the literature. *Pediatr Transplant* 14:E16–E19, 2010.

45. Cogley JR, Miller FH: MR imaging of benign focal liver lesions. *Radiol Clin North Am* 52:657–682, 2014.

46. Koffron A, Geller D, Gamblin TC, et al: Laparoscopic liver surgery: Shifting the management of liver tumors. *Hepatology* 44:1694–1700, 2006.

47. Harman M, Nart D, Acar T, et al: Primary mesenchymal liver tumors: Radiological spectrum, differential diagnosis, and pathologic correlation. *Abdom Imaging* 40:1316–1330, 2015.

48. Kamaya A, Maturen KE, Tye GA, et al: Hypervascular liver lesions. *Semin Ultrasound CT MR* 30:387–407, 2009.

49. Hsi Dickie B, Fishman SJ, Azizkhan RG: Hepatic vascular tumors. *Semin Pediatr Surg* 23:168–172, 2014.

50. Altekruse SF, Henley SJ, Cucinelli JE, et al: Changing hepatocellular carcinoma incidence and liver cancer mortality rates in the United States. *Am J Gastroenterol* 109:542–553, 2014.

51. Njei B, Rotman Y, Ditah I, et al: Emerging trends in hepatocellular carcinoma incidence and mortality. *Hepatology* 61:191–199, 2015.

52. El-Serag HB: Epidemiology of hepatocellular carcinoma in USA. *Hepatol Res* 37(Suppl 2):S88–S94, 2007.

53. El-Serag HB, Engels EA, Landgren O, et al: Risk of hepatobiliary and pancreatic cancers after hepatitis C virus infection: A population-based study of U.S. veterans. *Hepatology* 49:116–123, 2009.

54. Mittal S, El-Serag HB: Epidemiology of hepatocellular carcinoma: Consider the population. *J Clin Gastroenterol* 47(Suppl):S2–S6, 2013.

55. Corey KE, Kaplan LM: Obesity and liver disease: The epidemic of the twenty-first century. *Clin Liver Dis* 18:1–18, 2014.

56. Chiang CJ, Yang YW, Chen JD, et al: Significant reduction in end-stage liver diseases burden through national viral hepatitis therapy program in Taiwan. *Hepatology* 61:1154–1162, 2015.

57. Kim do Y, Han KH: Epidemiology and surveillance of hepatocellular carcinoma. *Liver Cancer* 1:2–14, 2012.

58. Riviere L, Ducroux A, Buendia MA: The oncogenic role of hepatitis B virus. *Recent Results Cancer Res* 193:59–74, 2014.

59. Hoshida Y, Fuchs BC, Bardeesy N, et al: Pathogenesis and prevention of hepatitis C virus–induced hepatocellular carcinoma. *J Hepatol* 61:S79–S90, 2014.

60. Tsai WL, Chung RT: Viral hepatocarcinogenesis. *Oncogene* 29:2309–2324, 2010.

61. Davila JA, Morgan RO, Shaib Y, et al: Diabetes increases the risk of hepatocellular carcinoma in the United States: A population based case control study. *Gut* 54:533–539, 2005.

62. Setiawan VW, Hernandez BY, Lu SC, et al: Diabetes and racial/ethnic differences in hepatocellular carcinoma risk: The Multiethnic Cohort. *J Natl Cancer Inst* 106:2014.

63. Turati F, Talamini R, Pelucchi C, et al: Metabolic syndrome and hepatocellular carcinoma risk. *Br J Cancer* 108:222–228, 2013.

64. Fowler KJ, Saad NE, Linehan D: Imaging approach to hepatocellular carcinoma, cholangiocarcinoma, and metastatic colorectal cancer. *Surg Oncol Clin N Am* 24:19–40, 2015.

65. Wald C, Russo MW, Heimbach JK, et al: New OPTN/UNOS policy for liver transplant allocation: Standardization of liver imaging, diagnosis, classification, and reporting of hepatocellular carcinoma. *Radiology* 266:376–382, 2013.

66. Bruix J, Sherman M, Llovet JM, et al: Clinical management of hepatocellular carcinoma. Conclusions of the Barcelona-2000 EASL conference. European Association for the Study of the Liver. *J Hepatol* 35:421–430, 2001.

67. Bruix J, Sherman M: Management of hepatocellular carcinoma. *Hepatology* 42:1208–1236, 2005.

68. EASL-EORTC clinical practice guidelines: Management of hepatocellular carcinoma. *J Hepatol* 56:908–943, 2012.

69. Bruix J, Sherman M: Management of hepatocellular carcinoma: An update. *Hepatology* 53:1020–1022, 2011.

70. Khalili K, Kim TK, Jang HJ, et al: Optimization of imaging diagnosis of 1-2 cm hepatocellular carcinoma: An analysis of diagnostic performance and resource utilization. *J Hepatol* 54:723–728, 2011.

71. Weitz J, D'Angelica M, Jarnagin W, et al: Selective use of diagnostic laparoscopy prior to planned hepatectomy for patients with hepatocellular carcinoma. *Surgery* 135:273–281, 2004.

72. Pawlik TM, Poon RT, Abdalla EK, et al: Critical appraisal of the clinical and pathologic predictors of survival after resection of large hepatocellular carcinoma. *Arch Surg* 140:450–457, discussion 457–458, 2005.

73. Schiffman SC, Woodall CE, Kooby DA, et al: Factors associated with recurrence and survival following hepatectomy for large hepatocellular carcinoma: A multicenter analysis. *J Surg Oncol* 101:105–110, 2010.

74. Yin L, Li H, Li AJ, et al: Partial hepatectomy vs. transcatheter arterial chemoembolization for resectable multiple hepatocellular carcinoma beyond Milan Criteria: A RCT. *J Hepatol* 61:82–88, 2014.

75. Mazzaferro V, Bhoori S, Sposito C, et al: Milan criteria in liver transplantation for hepatocellular carcinoma: An evidence-based analysis of 15 years of experience. *Liver Transpl* 17(Suppl 2):S44–S57, 2014.

76. Mazzaferro V, Regalia E, Doci R, et al: Liver transplantation for the treatment of small hepatocellular carcinomas in patients with cirrhosis. *N Engl J Med* 334:693–699, 1996.

77. Llovet JM, Fuster J, Bruix J: Intention-to-treat analysis of surgical treatment for early hepatocellular carcinoma: Resection versus transplantation. *Hepatology* 30:1434–1440, 1999.

78. Capussotti L, Ferrero A, Vigano L, et al: Liver resection for HCC with cirrhosis: Surgical perspectives out of EASL/AASLD guidelines. *Eur J Surg Oncol* 35:11–15, 2009.

79. Facciuto ME, Rochon C, Pandey M, et al: Surgical dilemma: Liver resection or liver transplantation for hepatocellular carcinoma and cirrhosis. Intention-to-treat analysis in patients within and outwith Milan criteria. *HPB (Oxford)* 11:398–404, 2009.

80. Llovet JM, Schwartz M, Mazzaferro V: Resection and liver transplantation for hepatocellular carcinoma. *Semin Liver Dis* 25:181–200, 2005.

81. Huang J, Yan L, Cheng Z, et al: A randomized trial comparing radiofrequency ablation and surgical resection for HCC conforming to the Milan criteria. *Ann Surg* 252:903–912, 2010.

82. Sangro B: Chemoembolization and radioembolization. *Best Pract Res Clin Gastroenterol* 28:909–919, 2014.

83. Malagari K, Pomoni M, Kelekis A, et al: Prospective randomized comparison of chemoembolization with doxorubicin-eluting beads and bland embolization with BeadBlock for hepatocellular carcinoma. *Cardiovasc Intervent Radiol* 33:541–551, 2010.

84. Llovet JM, Bruix J: Systematic review of randomized trials for unresectable hepatocellular carcinoma: Chemoembolization improves survival. *Hepatology* 37:429–442, 2003.

85. Llovet JM, Real MI, Montana X, et al: Arterial embolisation or chemoembolisation versus symptomatic treatment in patients with unresectable hepatocellular carcinoma: A randomised controlled trial. *Lancet* 359:1734–1739, 2002.

86. Lo CM, Ngan H, Tso WK, et al: Randomized controlled trial of transarterial lipiodol chemoembolization for unresectable hepatocellular carcinoma. *Hepatology* 35:1164–1171, 2002.

87. Llovet JM, Ricci S, Mazzaferro V, et al: Sorafenib in advanced hepatocellular carcinoma. *N Engl J Med* 359:378–390, 2008.

88. Lim II, Farber BA, LaQuaglia MP: Advances in fibrolamellar hepatocellular carcinoma: A review. *Eur J Pediatr Surg* 24:461–466, 2014.

89. Honeyman JN, Simon EP, Robine N, et al: Detection of a recurrent DNAJB1-PRKACA chimeric transcript in fibrolamellar hepatocellular carcinoma. *Science* 343:1010–1014, 2014.

90. Guglielmi A, Ruzzenente A, Valdegamberi A, et al: Hepatolithiasis-associated cholangiocarcinoma: Results from a multi-institutional national database on a case series of 23 patients. *Eur J Surg Oncol* 40:567–575, 2014.

91. Matsumoto K, Onoyama T, Kawata S, et al: Hepatitis B and C virus infection is a risk factor for the development of cholangiocarcinoma. *Intern Med* 53:651–654, 2014.

92. Reddy SK, Hyder O, Marsh JW, et al: Prevalence of nonalcoholic steatohepatitis among patients with resectable intrahepatic cholangiocarcinoma. *J Gastrointest Surg* 17:748–755, 2013.

93. Jamal MM, Yoon EJ, Vega KJ, et al: Diabetes mellitus as a risk factor for gastrointestinal cancer among American veterans. *World J Gastroenterol* 15:5274–5278, 2009.

94. Khan SA, Emadossadaty S, Ladep NG, et al: Rising trends in cholangiocarcinoma: Is the ICD classification system misleading us? *J Hepatol* 56:848–854, 2012.

95. Shaib YH, Davila JA, McGlynn K, et al: Rising incidence of intrahepatic cholangiocarcinoma in the United States: A true increase? *J Hepatol* 40:472–477, 2004.

96. Carpizo DR, D'Angelica M: Liver resection for metastatic colorectal cancer in the presence of extrahepatic disease. *Lancet Oncol* 10:801–809, 2009.

97. Maithel SK, D'Angelica MI: An update on randomized clinical trials in advanced and metastatic colorectal carcinoma. *Surg Oncol Clin N Am* 19:163–181, 2010.

98. Tomlinson JS, Jarnagin WR, DeMatteo RP, et al: Actual 10-year survival after resection of colorectal liver metastases defines cure. *J Clin Oncol* 25:4575–4580, 2007.

99. Beppu T, Miyamoto Y, Sakamoto Y, et al: Chemotherapy and targeted therapy for patients with initially unresectable colorectal liver metastases, focusing on conversion hepatectomy and long-term survival. *Ann Surg Oncol* 21(Suppl 3):S405–S413, 2014.

100. Smith DD, Schwarz RR, Schwarz RE: Impact of total lymph node count on staging and survival after gastrectomy for gastric cancer: Data from a large US-population database. *J Clin Oncol* 23:7114–7124, 2005.

101. Moulton CA, Gu CS, Law CH, et al: Effect of PET before liver resection on surgical management for colorectal adenocarcinoma metastases: A randomized clinical trial. *JAMA* 311:1863–1869, 2014.

102. Shubert CR, Habermann EB, Truty MJ, et al: Defining perioperative risk after hepatectomy based on diagnosis and extent of resection. *J Gastrointest Surg* 18:1917–1928, 2014.

103. Fong Y, Fortner J, Sun RL, et al: Clinical score for predicting recurrence after hepatic resection for metastatic colorectal cancer: Analysis of 1001 consecutive cases. *Ann Surg* 230:309–318, discussion 318–321, 1999.

104. Muratore A, Ribero D, Zimmitti G, et al: Resection margin and recurrence-free survival after liver resection of colorectal metastases. *Ann Surg Oncol* 17:1324–1329, 2010.

105. Are C, Gonen M, Zazzali K, et al: The impact of margins on outcome after hepatic resection for colorectal metastasis. *Ann Surg* 246:295–300, 2007.

106. Carpizo DR, Are C, Jarnagin W, et al: Liver resection for metastatic colorectal cancer in patients with concurrent extrahepatic disease: Results in 127 patients treated at a single center. *Ann Surg Oncol* 16:2138–2146, 2009.

107. Hwang M, Jayakrishnan TT, Green DE, et al: Systematic review of outcomes of patients undergoing resection for colorectal liver metastases in the setting of extra hepatic disease. *Eur J Cancer* 50:1747–1757, 2014.

108. Portier G, Elias D, Bouche O, et al: Multicenter randomized trial of adjuvant fluorouracil and folinic acid compared with surgery alone after resection of colorectal liver metastases: FFCD ACHBTH AURC 9002 trial. *J Clin Oncol* 24:4976–4982, 2006.

109. Mitry E, Fields AL, Bleiberg H, et al: Adjuvant chemotherapy after potentially curative resection of metastases from colorectal cancer: A pooled analysis of two randomized trials. *J Clin Oncol* 26:4906–4911, 2008.

110. Nordlinger B, Sorbye H, Glimelius B, et al: Perioperative chemotherapy with FOLFOX4 and surgery versus surgery alone for resectable liver metastases from colorectal cancer (EORTC Intergroup trial 40983): A randomised controlled trial. *Lancet* 371:1007–1016, 2008.

111. Nordlinger B, Sorbye H, Glimelius B, et al: Perioperative FOLFOX4 chemotherapy and surgery versus surgery alone for resectable liver metastases from colorectal cancer (EORTC 40983): Long-term results of a randomised, controlled, phase 3 trial. *Lancet Oncol* 14:1208–1215, 2013.

112. Kemeny N, Capanu M, D'Angelica M, et al: Phase I trial of adjuvant hepatic arterial infusion (HAI) with floxuridine (FUDR) and dexamethasone plus systemic oxaliplatin, 5-fluorouracil and leucovorin in patients with resected liver metastases from colorectal cancer. *Ann Oncol* 20:1236–1241, 2009.

113. Kemeny N, Jarnagin W, Gonen M, et al: Phase I/II study of hepatic arterial therapy with floxuridine and dexamethasone in combination with intravenous irinotecan as adjuvant treatment after resection of hepatic metastases from colorectal cancer. *J Clin Oncol* 21:3303–3309, 2003.

114. Kemeny N, Huang Y, Cohen AM, et al: Hepatic arterial infusion of chemotherapy after resection of hepatic metastases from colorectal cancer. *N Engl J Med* 341:2039–2048, 1999.

115. Leung U, Kuk D, D'Angelica MI, et al: Long-term outcomes following microwave ablation for liver malignancies. *Br J Surg* 102:85–91, 2015.

116. Que FG, Sarmiento JM, Nagorney DM: Hepatic surgery for metastatic gastrointestinal neuroendocrine tumors. *Adv Exp Med Biol* 574:43–56, 2006.

117. Mazzaglia PJ, Berber E, Milas M, et al: Laparoscopic radiofrequency ablation of neuroendocrine liver metastases: A 10-year experience evaluating predictors of survival. *Surgery* 142:10–19, 2007.

118. D'Angelica M, Jarnagin W, Dematteo R, et al: Staging laparoscopy for potentially resectable noncolorectal, nonneuroendocrine liver metastases. *Ann Surg Oncol* 9:204–209, 2002.

119. Groeschl RT, Nachmany I, Steel JL, et al: Hepatectomy for noncolorectal non-neuroendocrine metastatic cancer: A multi-institutional analysis. *J Am Coll Surg* 214:769–777, 2012.

120. Mimatsu K, Oida T, Kawasaki A, et al: Long-term outcome of laparoscopic deroofing for symptomatic nonparasitic liver cysts. *Hepatogastroenterology* 56:850–853, 2009.

121. Qiu JG, Wu H, Jiang H, et al: Laparoscopic fenestration vs open fenestration in patients with congenital hepatic cysts: A meta-analysis. *World J Gastroenterol* 17:3359–3365, 2003.

122. Gevers TJ, Drenth JP: Diagnosis and management of polycystic liver disease. *Nat Rev Gastroenterol Hepatol* 10:101–108, 2013.

123. Jarnagin WR, Gonen M, Fong Y, et al: Improvement in perioperative outcome after hepatic resection: Analysis of 1,803 consecutive cases over the past decade. *Ann Surg* 236:397–406, discussion 406–407, 2002.

54 CHAPTER

Biliary System

Patrick G. Jackson, Stephen R.T. Evans

第五十四章　胆道疾病

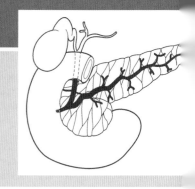

中文导读

　　本章共分5节：①胆道解剖和生理；②病理生理；③胆道良性疾病；④胆道恶性肿瘤和转移性肿瘤；⑤其他类型肿瘤。

　　第一节首先概括肝外胆管的解剖，重点阐述胆胰管汇合部和胆囊管汇合部的变异。其次介绍胆管的血流供应，阐述肝脏的Couinaud分段和肝内胆管的变异。最后讲述胆道生理，介绍胆汁的组成、合成、排泄、调节、功能、循环再利用等，重点讲述胆汁的肠肝循环。

　　第二节首先概述胆道疾病的常见症状，如疼痛、发热和黄疸。其次，简述诊断胆道疾病的实验室方法。然后，详细介绍诊断胆道疾病的影像学检查方法，包括腹部平片、超声、肝亚氨基二乙酸扫描、CT、MRI/MRCP、ERCP、PTC、术中胆道造影、超声内镜和PET-CT。最后，简述胆道疾病的常见致病菌。

　　第三节首先概述胆道结石的结石类型、结石发生的病理生理过程、外科和药物治疗方法。其次，分别介绍慢性胆囊炎和结石性胆囊炎的临床表现、诊断和治疗方法。再次，详细阐述胆总管结石的诊断和治疗，如ERCP、腹腔镜或开腹胆总管探查等。然后，简述胆源性胰腺炎、胆汁动力学障碍和Oddi氏括约肌功能障碍的病因和治疗方法。进而，阐述胆道结石的手术指征和手术方法，包括腹腔镜或开腹胆囊切除、腹腔镜或开腹胆总管探查等。再次，讲述胆道术后综合征，包括胆道损伤的临床表现、损伤类型、治疗方法和预后等；结石遗落腹腔可能导致的后果及预防手段；胆道术后疼痛的原因和处理；胆道残留结石、胆瘘、胆囊结石性肠梗阻、急性胆管炎，以及复发性化脓性胆管炎等的临床表现、诊断和治疗。最后，讲述非结石性胆道疾病，如急性无结石性胆囊炎、原发性硬化性胆管炎、胆管炎性狭窄、胆管囊肿、胆囊多发息肉样变、良性胆道新生物的临床表现、诊断和治疗。

第四节在胆囊癌部分，首先介绍胆囊癌的发病率、病因、病理和分期，临床表现和诊断方法；其次，重点阐述胆囊癌的手术指征和手术原则，包括胆囊切除术后意外胆囊癌、术前怀疑为胆囊癌和晚期胆囊癌的外科治疗；最后，简述不同分期胆囊癌病人的生存期。在胆管癌部分，首先介绍其风险因素、临床

表现、分期、Bismuth-Corlette分类、诊断方法和可切除性评估；其次介绍手术指征和手术方式，包括近端胆管癌和远端胆管癌的手术治疗、ERCP和PTC等姑息性治疗，以及化学治疗等药物治疗；最后，概述不同分期胆管癌病人的生存期。

第五节简述可以侵犯或压迫胆道系统从而导致相关胆道症状的肿瘤类型，如肝细胞肝癌、胰腺癌、结肠癌和淋巴瘤等。

〔秦仁义〕

ANATOMY AND PHYSIOLOGY

As anatomic variations in biliary anatomy are common, occurring in up to 30% of patients, understanding of both normal anatomy and the variations is important for the management of patients with biliary disease. The ampulla of Vater contains the distalmost portion of the common bile duct and inserts into the wall of the duodenum. The pancreatic duct also joins the ampulla and may fuse with the bile duct before passing through the wall of the duodenum or within the wall of the duodenum, or it may have a separate orifice within the ampulla (Fig. 54-1). The most inferior portion of the common bile duct is encompassed by the head of the pancreas. Superior to the intrapancreatic portion, the common bile duct is divided into retroduodenal and supraduodenal segments. The insertion of the cystic duct marks the differentiation of the common hepatic duct above and the common bile duct below.

The cystic duct drains the gallbladder, which is divided into the neck, infundibulum with Hartmann pouch, body, and fundus. Roughly the size and shape of a common light bulb, the gallbladder holds 30 to 60 mL of bile as an extrahepatic reservoir. The gallbladder is attached to the inferior surface of the liver and is enveloped by liver for a variable portion of its circumference. Although some gallbladders are almost enveloped by liver parenchyma, others hang on a mesentery, predisposing to volvulus. The attachment of the gallbladder to the liver, known as the gallbladder fossa, identifies the separation of the left and right lobes of the liver (Fig. 54-2). Where the gallbladder attaches to the liver, Glisson capsule does not form, and this common surface provides most of the venous drainage of the gallbladder. The cystic duct drains at an acute angle into the common bile duct and can range from 1 to 5 cm in length. There are a number of anatomic variations in insertion of the cystic duct, including into the right hepatic duct (Fig. 54-3). Within the neck of the gallbladder and cystic ducts lie folds of mucosa oriented in a spiral pattern, known as the spiral valves of Heister, which act to keep gallstones from entering the common bile duct in spite of distention and intraluminal pressure. The dependent portion of Hartmann pouch may overlie the common hepatic or right hepatic ducts, thus

placing these structures at risk during the performance of a cholecystectomy.

Above the cystic duct lies the common hepatic duct, draining the left and right hepatic duct systems. The confluence of these structures lies at the hilar plate, which is an extension of Glisson capsule. The absence of any vascular structures overlying the bile ducts at this location allows exposure of the bifurcation by incision of this layer at the base of segment IV, lifting the liver off these structures, known as lowering the hilar plate; this is generally used to expose the proximal extrahepatic biliary tree for resection or reconstruction.

Vascular Anatomy

The segmental anatomy of the liver parenchyma is based on the vascular supply and drainage, and the biliary drainage is described by the corresponding vascular segment. The hepatic parenchyma is divided into lobes, each of which is divided into lobar segments (Fig. 54-4) to define the basic hepatic anatomic resections. The left lobe is composed of medial and lateral segments. The right lobe is divided into posterior and anterior segments. Alternatively, the hepatic parenchyma can be divided into segments based on the specific hepatic venous drainage and portal inflow, allowing a more precise description of anatomic pathology as described by Couinaud.[1] The three hepatic veins divide the liver into four separate sectors. Each sector is then subdivided by the insertion of the portal vein, resulting in eight segments. In this classification system, the liver is composed of eight segments. Segment I refers to the caudate lobe. The left lobe of the liver, supplied by the left portal vein, constitutes segments II through IV. The left lobe is further subdivided by the falciform ligament, which separates segments II and III, also known as the left lateral segment, from segment IV. Within the left lateral segment, segment II lies superior to the insertion of the portal vein and segment III lies inferior to it. Segment IV is similarly divided into segment IVA above and segment IVB below the portal vein insertion. The right portal vein supplies the right lobe of the liver and divides it into the posterior and anterior sectors. Each sector is then subdivided on the basis of its relative location compared with the portal vein. Segment V is supplied by the inferior branch of the anterior sector, and

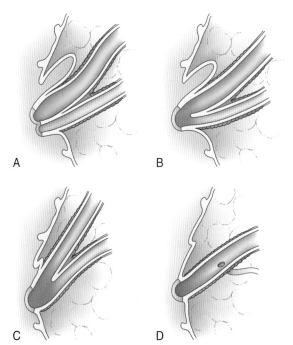

A

B

C

D

FIGURE 54-1 Patterns of biliary duct–pancreatic duct junction and insertion into the duodenal wall.

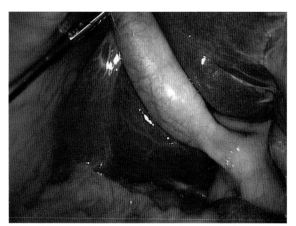

FIGURE 54-2 Laparoscopic photograph of the gallbladder in situ. The gallbladder is being suspended by the fundus to expose the infundibulum and porta hepatis.

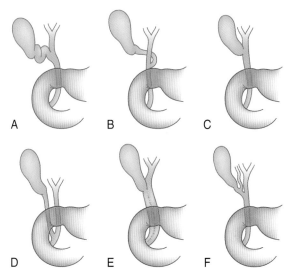

A

B

C

D

E

F

FIGURE 54-3 Variability in cystic duct anatomy. Knowledge of these variations is important to try to avoid inadvertent injury to the biliary tree during cholecystectomy.

segment VIII is supplied by the superior branch. In the posterior sector, segment VI is supplied by the inferior branch and segment VII is supplied by the superior branch. There are three major hepatic veins that drain into the inferior vena cava, in addition to a number of small veins that drain directly from the right lobe. The right hepatic vein constitutes most of the venous drainage from the right lobe and generally lies in the intersegmental fissure between the anterior and posterior sectors of the right lobe. The middle hepatic vein drains the medial segment of the left lobe and a small amount of the medial portions of segments V and VIII. In most cases, the middle hepatic vein fuses with the left hepatic vein that drains the left lateral segment.

As opposed to the hepatic parenchyma, where most perfusion comes from portal venous flow, the entire biliary tree is supplied solely by the arterial anatomy. This anatomic arrangement makes it particularly susceptible to ischemic injury at the intrahepatic and extrahepatic levels. The inferior bile duct, below the level of the duodenal bulb, receives its perfusion from tributaries of the posterosuperior pancreaticoduodenal and gastroduodenal arteries. The small branches coalesce to form the two vessels that run along the common bile duct at the 3- and 9-o'clock positions. With close dissection of the areolar tissue surrounding the bile duct, these vessels can be damaged, leaving the bile duct at risk for ischemic injury. The supraduodenal common bile duct, from the duodenal bulb to the cystic duct, and common hepatic ducts receive their blood supply from the right hepatic and cystic arteries. As the proper hepatic artery ascends on the anterior medial side of the porta, it divides into right and left hepatic arteries. In most cases, the right hepatic artery passes posterior to the common hepatic duct to supply the right lobe of the liver. After crossing the duct, the right hepatic artery passes through the triangle of Calot, bordered by the cystic duct, common hepatic duct, and edge of liver. In this triangle, the right hepatic artery gives off the cystic artery to the gallbladder and is at risk for injury during a cholecystectomy. An accessory or replaced right hepatic artery, when present, passes through the portacaval space and ascends to the right lobe along the lateral aspect of the common bile duct. A pulsatile structure on the most lateral aspect of the porta during a Pringle maneuver identifies this anomaly. In addition, it can be noted on computed tomography (CT) as a vessel passing transversely between the portal vein and inferior vena cava behind the head of the pancreas.

The cystic artery normally arises from the right hepatic artery, which can pass posterior or anterior to the common bile duct to supply the gallbladder. Similar to the variability of the cystic duct, the cystic artery may arise from the right hepatic, left hepatic, proper hepatic, common hepatic, gastroduodenal, or superior mesenteric artery. Although variable, the cystic artery generally lies superior to the cystic duct and is usually associated with a lymph node, known as Calot node (Fig. 54-5). Because this node provides some of the lymphatic drainage of the gallbladder, it can be enlarged in the setting of gallbladder disease, whether it is inflammatory or neoplastic.

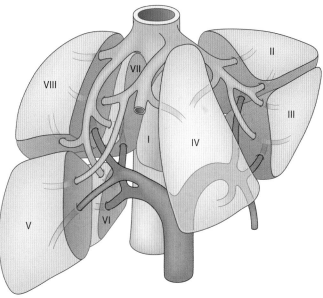

FIGURE 54-4 Couinaud Segmental Anatomy. Segment I is the caudate lobe. Segments II and III are supplied by the lateral branch of the left portal vein, with segment II lying above the passage of the portal vein and segment III below it. Segment IV is supplied by the medial branch of the left portal vein and is further subdivided into IVA above and IVB below the segmental portal vein. Segment V is supplied by the inferior distribution of the anterior branch of the right portal vein, and segment VIII receives flow from the superior distribution of this branch. Similarly, with respect to the posterior branch of the right portal vein, segment VI lies inferior to the portal vein, whereas segment VII lies superior.

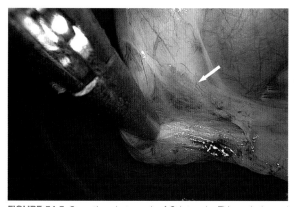

FIGURE 54-5 Operative photograph of Calot node. This node *(arrow)* is useful for identification of the common location of the cystic artery.

Both within the liver and immediately outside the parenchyma, the bile ducts generally lie superior to the corresponding portal veins, which in turn are superior to the arterial supply (Fig. 54-6). Retaining a longer extrahepatic segment before inserting into the liver, the left hepatic duct travels under the edge of segment IV before slipping superior and posterior to the left portal vein. During this transverse portion, it can receive a few subsegmental branches from segment IV. The left duct drains segments II, III, and IV, with the most distal branch draining segment IVA. Further superolateral, the ducts draining segment IVB arise, and further up the left duct are the ducts for segments II and III. These fused ducts can generally be found just posterior and lateral to the umbilical recess. The caudate lobe drains through smaller ducts that enter the right and left hepatic duct systems. The drainage of the right duct system includes segments V, VI,

VII, and VIII and is substantially shorter than the left duct, bifurcating almost immediately. The fusion of two sectoral ducts, posterior and anterior, creates this short right hepatic duct. The anterior sectoral duct runs in a vertical direction to drain segments V and VIII, whereas the posterior sectoral duct follows a horizontal course to drain segments VI and VII.

Physiology

Bile secretion from the liver serves two opposing functions, namely, excretion of toxins and metabolites from the liver and absorption of nutrients from the intestinal tract. Bile is secreted into bile canaliculi, which encircle each hepatocyte. Within the hepatic lobule, these canaliculi coalesce to form small bile ducts, eventually entering a portal triad. Four to six portal triads combine to create a hepatic lobule, the smallest functional unit of the liver, identified by its central terminal hepatic venule. On the opposite aspect from the canalicular surface of the hepatocyte lies the sinusoidal surface, which contacts the space of Disse. In this contact area, the hepatocyte is responsible for the absorption of circulating components of bile, an important step in the enterohepatic circulation of bile. Once the bile components are absorbed and secreted into the bile canaliculi, the tight junctions in the biliary tree keep these components within the bile secretory pathway. The secretion of bile components into the biliary tree is a major stimulus to bile flow, and the volume of bile flow is an osmotic process. Because bile salts combine to form spherical pockets, known as micelles, the salts themselves provide no osmotic activity. Instead, the cations that are secreted into the biliary tree along with the bile salt anion provide the osmotic load to draw water into the duct and to increase flow to keep bile electrochemically neutral. For this reason, bile maintains an osmolality approximately comparable to that of plasma.

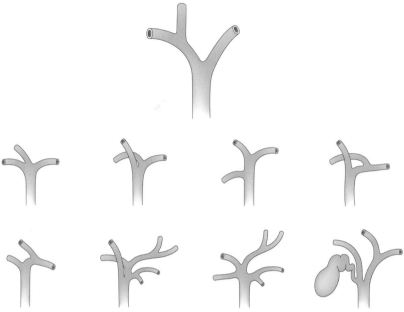

FIGURE 54-6 Hepatic lobar segmental biliary anatomy.

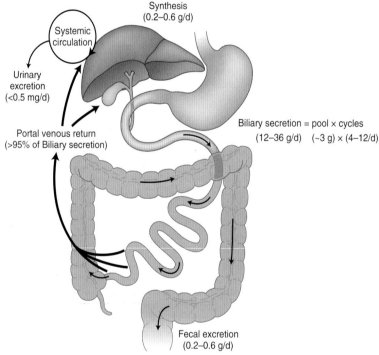

FIGURE 54-7 Enterohepatic circulation.

Although a small amount of bile flow is bile salt independent, serving to expel toxins and metabolites from the body, much of the flow is dependent on neural, humoral, and chemical stimuli. Vagal activity induces bile secretion, as does the gastrointestinal hormone secretin. Cholecystokinin (CCK), secreted by the intestinal mucosa, serves to induce biliary tree secretion and gallbladder wall contraction, thereby augmenting excretion of bile into the intestines.

Bile salts, such as cholic acid and deoxycholic acid, are originally created from cholesterol and secreted into bile canaliculi

as cholic acid and its metabolite, deoxycholic acid. The liver actually makes only a small amount of the total bile salt pool used on a daily basis because most bile salts are recycled after use in the intestinal lumen, known as the enterohepatic circulation (Fig. 54-7). After passage into the intestinal tract and reabsorption by the terminal ileum, bile acids are transported back to the liver for recycling bound to albumin. Less than 5% of bile salts are lost each day in the stool. When sufficient quantities of bile salts reach the colonic lumen, the powerful detergent activity of the bile salts can cause inflammation and diarrhea.

This can sometimes be seen after a cholecystectomy when the speed of the enterohepatic circulation of bile increases and may overwhelm the ability of the terminal ileum to absorb bile salts.

The passage of reabsorbed bile salts bound to albumin through the space of Disse allows uptake into the hepatocyte in an efficient process that involves sodium cotransport and sodium-independent pathways. In the less specific sodium-independent pathway, a number of organic anions are transported, including unconjugated and indirect bilirubin. The transport of bile salts across the canalicular membrane remains the rate-limiting step in bile salt excretion. Given the vast differences in concentration of bile salts, the transport of bile up an extreme concentration gradient is adenosine triphosphate dependent.

In addition to bile salts, bile contains proteins, lipids, and pigments. The major lipid components of bile are phospholipids and cholesterol. These lipids not only dispose of cholesterol from low- and high-density lipoproteins but also serve to protect hepatocytes and cholangiocytes from the toxic nature of bile. The sources of most biliary cholesterol are circulating lipoproteins and hepatic synthesis. Therefore, the biliary secretion of cholesterol actually serves to excrete cholesterol from the body.

Although cholesterol, bile salts, and phospholipids play an important role in nutritional homeostasis, bile also serves as a major route of exogenous and endogenous toxin disposal. One such example of the disposal system is that of bilirubin. Bile pigments, such as bilirubin, are breakdown products of hemoglobin and myoglobin. These are transported in the blood bound to albumin and transported into the hepatocyte. Here, they are transferred into the endoplasmic reticulum and conjugated to form bilirubin glucuronides, also known as conjugated or direct bilirubin. In healthy liver, bilirubin is conjugated and excreted to the intestine and converted by microbes to urobilinoids, which are reduced to the predominant pigment in feces, stercobilin, or reabsorbed.

In the fasting state, secreted bile will pass through the biliary tree into the intestine and be reabsorbed. In addition, bile will collect in the gallbladder, which serves as an extrahepatic storage site of secreted bile. To store bile secretions, the gallbladder is extremely efficient in water absorption and thus concentration of bile components. This absorption is an osmotic process performed through the active sodium transport. With the absorption of sodium and water across the gallbladder epithelium, the chemical composition of bile changes in the gallbladder lumen. Increases in cholesterol concentration, in addition to calcium, which is not as efficiently absorbed, then lead to decreased stability of phospholipid cholesterol vesicles. The reduced vesicle stability predisposes to nucleation of this stagnant pool of cholesterol and thus to cholesterol stone formation. The gallbladder neck and cystic duct also secrete glycoproteins to help protect the gallbladder from the detergent activity of bile. These glycoproteins also promote cholesterol crystallization.

The gallbladder fills through a retrograde mechanism. With an increase in the tonic activity of the sphincter of Oddi in the fasting state, pressure increases in the common bile duct. This increased pressure allows filling of the lower intraluminal pressure gallbladder, which is capable of storing up to 600 mL of the daily production of bile. The passage of fat, protein, and acid into the duodenum induces CCK secretion from duodenal epithelial cells. CCK, as its name suggests, then causes gallbladder contraction, with intraluminal pressures up to 300 mm Hg. Vagal activity also induces gallbladder emptying but is a less powerful stimulus to gallbladder contraction than CCK.

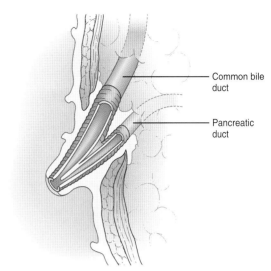

FIGURE 54-8 Sphincter of Oddi. Because the sphincter is responsible for control of most bile flow, this sphincter maintains a high tonic contraction but is inhibited by CCK.

Common bile duct

Pancreatic duct

The distal portion of the bile duct passes through the sphincter of Oddi (Fig. 54-8). The musculature of this sphincter is independent from that of the duodenal intestinal wall and responds differently to neurohumoral controls. This muscular sphincter, which normally maintains high tonic and phasic activity, is inhibited by CCK. With CCK-induced relaxation of the sphincter, bile flows more readily from the biliary tree. Coordinated with gallbladder contraction, the relaxation of this sphincter allows evacuation of up to 70% of the gallbladder contents within 2 hours of CCK secretion. During the fasting state, the oblique passage of the bile duct through the duodenal wall and the tonic activity of the sphincter prevent duodenal contents from refluxing into the biliary tree.

GENERAL CONSIDERATIONS IN BILIARY TREE PATHOPHYSIOLOGY

Symptoms

The Charcot triad of right upper quadrant pain, fever, and jaundice describes the three most common symptoms associated with biliary disease. With the blockage of any tubular structure, pain may come from acute increased intraluminal pressure or from inflammation. Obstruction will generally precede infection because stasis of bile is an inciting factor of biliary infection along with sufficient quantity of infectious inoculum in a susceptible host.

Pain

Postprandial abdominal pain is generally termed biliary colic, actually a misnomer because the pattern of pain is not colicky in nature. Because the nerve fibers to the gallbladder originate in the celiac axis, this pain can be epigastric in origin or may locate in the right upper quadrant as the inflammatory process affects the parietal peritoneum. As a meal containing fat or protein enters the duodenum, CCK is released, causing contraction of the gallbladder and increases in bile secretion. When the gallbladder lumen cannot fully empty because of a stone in the gallbladder neck, visceral pain fibers are activated, causing pain in the epigastrium or right upper quadrant. The same luminal obstruction of biliary colic but associated with sufficient stasis, pressure, and bacterial inoculum creates infection and thereby inflammation, therefore progressing to acute cholecystitis. With this infection and inflammation, the right upper quadrant pain of biliary colic will be accompanied by tenderness noted on palpation of the right upper quadrant. Specifically, the voluntary cessation of respiration when the examiner exerts constant pressure under the right costal margin, known as a Murphy sign, suggests inflammation of the visceral and parietal peritoneal surfaces and can be seen in diseases such as acute cholecystitis and hepatitis. Alternatively, biliary colic in the absence of infection and inflammation is not associated with any reproducible physical examination finding or systemic symptom.

Fever

Whereas biliary colic does not produce systemic manifestations, infection or inflammation in the gallbladder or biliary tree will usually cause fever. It can be seen in a number of inflammatory diseases, but fever associated with right upper quadrant pain is a hallmark of an infectious process in the biliary tree. With immediate and direct access to the metabolically active hepatic parenchyma, infection of the gallbladder and biliary tree induces cytokine secretion and thereby direct systemic manifestations.

Jaundice

Jaundice, caused by elevation of the serum bilirubin level, can be demonstrated in the sclera, the frenulum of the tongue, or the skin. Serum bilirubin levels above 2.5 mg/dL are necessary to detect scleral icterus routinely, and levels above 5 mg/dL will be manifested as cutaneous jaundice. Failure to excrete bile from the liver into the intestines is a prerequisite of jaundice. Therefore, although both are associated with fever and pain, acute cholecystitis does not cause the jaundice seen in infection of the biliary tree, known as ascending cholangitis. The constellation of fever, right upper quadrant pain, and jaundice, known as Charcot triad, suggests blockage of the biliary secretion from the liver, not just the gallbladder. With the addition of hypotension and altered mental status, known as Reynolds pentad, patients will demonstrate the systemic manifestations of shock from biliary origin. Jaundice is generally divided into surgical, from obstruction, and medical, from a hepatocellular process.

Laboratory Tests

Although termed liver function tests, the routine hepatic panel for most laboratories tests a number of aspects of metabolic and hepatic activity. The tests most useful for evaluation of biliary physiology include determination of levels of bilirubin and alkaline phosphatase, seen in any cholestatic process, and serum transaminases, suggesting evidence of hepatocellular injury. Bilirubin can be subdivided into the conjugated and unconjugated forms, thereby allowing delineation of cause based on cellular location of derangement. In other words, hyperbilirubinemia may be caused by increased synthesis of bilirubin, impaired hepatocyte uptake of unconjugated bilirubin, decreased intracellular conjugation, reduced intracellular transport and excretion of conjugated bilirubin, or obstruction of the biliary tree. Although this is an oversimplification of a complex process, derangements up to and including conjugation will be manifested as elevated unconjugated bilirubin levels.

Imaging Studies
Plain Films

Plain radiographs are of limited use in the overall evaluation of biliary tree disease. Gallstones are not regularly seen by plain films, and even when they are seen, it rarely changes therapy. Therefore, the role of plain radiographs in the evaluation of possible biliary disease is limited to exclusion of other diagnoses, such as a duodenal ulcer with free air, small bowel obstruction, or right lower lobe pneumonia causing right upper quadrant pain.

Ultrasound

Transabdominal ultrasound is a sensitive, inexpensive, reliable, and reproducible test to evaluate most of the biliary tree, being able to separate patients with medical jaundice, in which the source of hyperbilirubinemia is from hemoglobin breakdown through the process of conjugation, from those with surgical jaundice, in which the hyperbilirubinemia occurs from a blockage of excretion. Therefore, this modality is seen as the study of choice for the initial evaluation of jaundice or symptoms of biliary disease. The finding of a dilated common bile duct in the setting of jaundice suggests an obstruction of the duct from stones, usually associated with pain, or from a tumor, which is commonly painless (Fig. 54-9). Gallbladder diseases are regularly diagnosed by ultrasound because the superficial location of the gallbladder with no overlying bowel gas enables its evaluation by sound waves. Ultrasound has a high specificity and sensitivity for cholelithiasis, or gallstones. The density of gallstones allows crisp reverberation of the sound wave, showing an echogenic focus with a characteristic shadowing behind the stone (Fig. 54-10). Most gallstones, unless impacted, will move with positional changes in the patient. This feature allows their differentiation from gallbladder polyps, which are fixed, and from sludge, which will move more slowly and does not have the sharp echogenic pattern of gallstones. Pathologic changes seen in many gallbladder diseases can be identified by ultrasound. For example, the gallbladder wall thickening and pericholecystic fluid seen in cholecystitis are visible by ultrasound (Fig. 54-11). Porcelain gallbladder, with its calcified wall, will appear as a curvilinear echogenic focus along the entire gallbladder wall, with posterior shadowing (Fig. 54-12). In addition

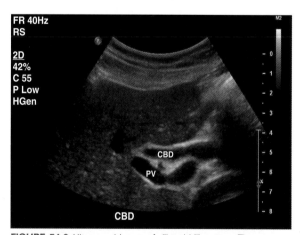

FIGURE 54-9 Ultrasound image of dilated biliary tree. The common bile duct (CBD) is dilated. As it travels parallel to the portal vein (PV), it is easy to identify. The depiction of the parallel stripes of duct and vein helps ensure that the common duct diameter is not overestimated by a tangential view, which would artificially increase the anteroposterior diameter.

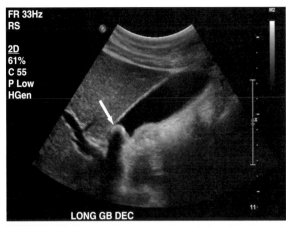

FIGURE 54-10 Ultrasound image of a gallstone in the gallbladder neck. The sharp echogenic wall of the gallstone *(arrow)*, with the characteristic posterior shadowing stripe under the stone, helps differentiate it from other intraluminal findings.

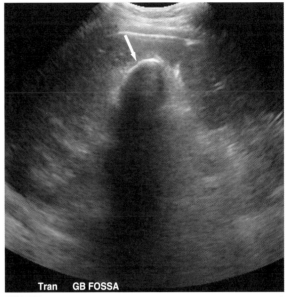

FIGURE 54-12 Ultrasound image of porcelain gallbladder. The curvilinear sharp echogenic focus *(arrow)* combined with substantial posterior shadowing helps confirm this diagnosis.

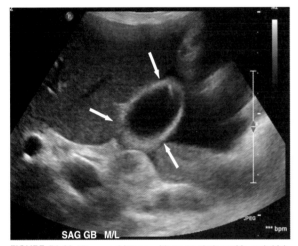

FIGURE 54-11 Ultrasound image with acute cholecystitis and thickened gallbladder wall *(arrows)*.

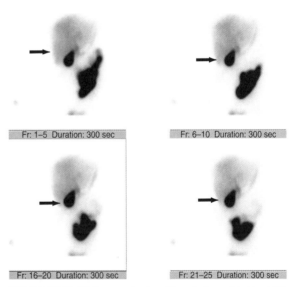

FIGURE 54-13 HIDA scan showing filling of the gallbladder. With gallbladder filling *(arrows)*, the diagnosis of acute cholecystitis is effectively eliminated.

to division of medical versus surgical jaundice, ultrasound can sometimes identify the cause of obstructive jaundice, showing common bile duct stones or even cholangiocarcinoma.

Hepatic Iminodiacetic Acid Scan

Although incapable of providing any precise anatomic delineation, biliary scintigraphy, also known as a hepatic iminodiacetic acid (HIDA) scan, can be used to evaluate the physiologic secretion of bile. The injection of an iminodiacetic acid, which is processed in the liver and secreted with bile, allows identification of bile flow. Therefore, the failure to fill the gallbladder 2 hours after injection demonstrates obstruction of the cystic duct, as seen in acute cholecystitis (Figs. 54-13 and 54-14). In addition, the scan will identify obstruction of the biliary tree and bile leaks, which may be useful in the postoperative setting. HIDA scans can also be used to determine gallbladder function because the injection of CCK during a scan will document physiologic ejection of the gallbladder. This may be useful in patients with biliary tract pain but without stones because some patients have pain from impaired emptying, known as biliary dyskinesia. As a nuclear

medicine test, the test demonstrates physiologic flow but does not provide fine anatomic detail, nor can it identify gallstones.

Computed Tomography

Although ultrasound is clearly the first test of choice for delineation of biliary disease, CT provides superior anatomic information and therefore is indicated when more anatomic delineation is required. Because most gallstones are radiographically isodense to bile, many will be indistinguishable from bile. However, because ultrasound is operator dependent and provides no anatomic reconstruction of the biliary tree, CT can be used to

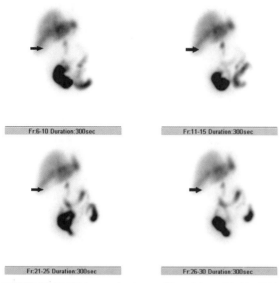

FIGURE 54-14 HIDA scan showing nonfilling of the gallbladder. With no filling of the gallbladder *(arrows)* even on delayed images, HIDA confirms occlusion of the cystic duct, the characteristic feature of acute cholecystitis.

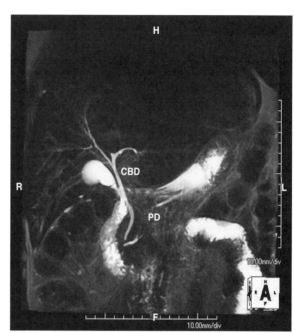

FIGURE 54-16 Normal MRCP image. Note the normal common bile duct (CBD) and pancreatic duct (PD).

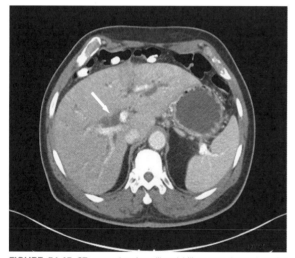

FIGURE 54-15 CT scan showing dilated biliary tree *(arrow)* at the portal confluence. This dilation continued down to the head of the pancreas.

identify the cause and site of biliary obstruction (Fig. 54-15). When it is performed for the evaluation of hepatic or pancreatic parenchyma or possible neoplastic processes, CT is invaluable in preoperative planning, and the use of arterial phase, portal venous phase, and delayed phase imaging, known as a triple-phase CT, has essentially replaced diagnostic angiography of the liver.

Magnetic Resonance Imaging and Magnetic Resonance Cholangiopancreatography

Magnetic resonance imaging uses the water in bile to delineate the biliary tree and thus provides superior anatomic definition of the intrahepatic and extrahepatic biliary tree and pancreas. Although management of most patients with biliary disease

does not require the fine detail of anatomic evaluation shown by cross-sectional imaging, magnetic resonance imaging is noninvasive, requires no radiation exposure, and can prove extremely useful in planning resection of biliary or pancreatic neoplasms or management of complex biliary disease. By use of the water content of bile, a cholangiopancreatogram can be created (Fig. 54-16), which makes it an excellent modality for cross-sectional imaging of the biliary tree.

Endoscopic Retrograde Cholangiopancreatography

Endoscopic retrograde cholangiopancreatography (ERCP) is an invasive test using endoscopy and fluoroscopy to inject contrast material through the ampulla to image the biliary tree (Fig. 54-17). Although it does carry a complication rate of up to 10%, its usefulness lies in its ability to diagnose and to treat many diseases of the biliary tree. For patients with malignant obstruction, ERCP can be used to provide tissue samples for diagnosis while also decompressing an obstruction, but it does not stage disease accurately. Many benign diseases, such as choledocholithiasis, can be easily treated by endoscopic means. ERCP has also proven extremely useful in the diagnosis and treatment of complications of biliary surgery.

Percutaneous Transhepatic Cholangiography

Interventional radiologic techniques can be used in the evaluation of biliary anatomy. Similar to ERCP, percutaneous transhepatic cholangiography (PTC) is an invasive procedure used to evaluate the biliary tree. A needle is passed directly into the liver to access one of the biliary radicals, and the tract is then used for insertion of transhepatic catheters. Useful for patients with intrahepatic biliary disease or in whom ERCP is not technically feasible, PTC can decompress biliary obstruction, stent obstructions nonoperatively, and provide anatomic information for biliary reconstruction (Fig. 54-18).

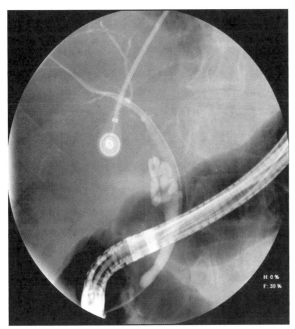

FIGURE 54-17 Normal ERCP image.

Intraoperative Cholangiography

Another imaging tool for the diagnosis of biliary tract abnormalities is intraoperative cholangiography. With the injection catheter inserted through the cystic duct during a cholecystectomy or through another point in the biliary tree, intraoperative cholangiography can help delineate anomalous biliary anatomy, identify choledocholithiasis, or guide biliary reconstruction. Some surgeons advocate routine cholangiography during cholecystectomy. Advocates for routine cholangiography note that common duct injuries can be identified and managed immediately when cholangiography is used routinely. However, because it adds operative time and fluoroscopic exposure to the operation, many surgeons use intraoperative cholangiography selectively during the performance of a cholecystectomy. Although debated, the routine use of intraoperative cholangiography does not reduce significantly the incidence of injury to the biliary tree during laparoscopic cholecystectomy. Indications for the selective use of cholangiography include pain on the day of operation, abnormal hepatic function panel, anomalous or confusing biliary anatomy, and alteration in anatomy that precludes the ability to perform ERCP after cholecystectomy, such as Roux-en-Y gastric bypass, dilated biliary tree, or any preoperative suspicion of choledocholithiasis (Box 54-1).

Endoscopic Ultrasound

Although of limited use in the evaluation of gallbladder disease or intrahepatic disease of the biliary tree, endoscopic ultrasound is valuable in the assessment of distal common bile duct and ampulla. With the close apposition of the distal common bile duct and pancreas to the duodenum, sound waves generated by endoscopic ultrasound provide detailed evaluation of the bile duct and ampulla; this has proved most useful in assessing tumors for invasion into vascular structures. Echoendoscopes are subdivided into those that scan perpendicular to the long axis of the endoscope, known as radial echoendoscopes, and those that scan parallel, known as linear echoendoscopes. Radial echoendoscopes are most

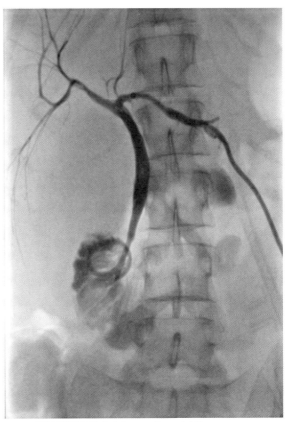

FIGURE 54-18 PTC image of hepatic biliary anatomy.

BOX 54-1 Indications for Selective Cholangiography

Pain at time of operation
Abnormal hepatic function panel
Anomalous or confusing biliary anatomy
Inability to perform postoperative ERCP
Dilated biliary tree
Any suspicion of choledocholithiasis

useful for providing a tomographic evaluation, whereas linear echoendoscopes can guide interventions such as needle biopsies under real-time ultrasound guidance (Fig. 54-19).

Fluorodeoxyglucose Positron Emission Tomography

Fluorodeoxyglucose positron emission tomography (FDG PET) exploits the metabolic difference between a highly metabolically active tissue, such as a neoplasm, and normal tissue. With the injection of a radiolabeled glucose molecule, FDG PET scans can differentiate benign and malignant lesions, detect recurrence, and identify metastatic disease. Unfortunately, FDG PET is incapable of demonstrating carcinomatosis and, given the high metabolism of the immune system, is of limited value in the setting of infection or inflammation.

Bacteriology

The biliary tree inserts into the duodenum and therefore cannot be considered truly sterile. Through a low bacterial load, and with

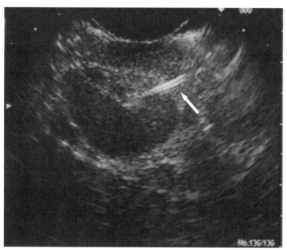

FIGURE 54-19 Linear endoscopic ultrasound with needle *(arrow)* biopsy of a lymph node.

the flow of bile, infection in the absence of obstruction is rare. However, with the presence of stones or obstruction, the likelihood of bacterial infection increases. The most common types of bacteria found in biliary infections are Enterobacteriaceae, such as *Escherichia coli, Klebsiella,* and *Enterobacter,* followed by *Enterococcus* spp.

Prophylactic antibiotics should be used in most patients undergoing interventions in the biliary tree, such as ERCP or PTC. To cover the most common bacterial species, a first- or second-generation cephalosporin or fluoroquinolone should suffice. For those undergoing elective laparoscopic cholecystectomy for biliary colic, no antibiotic prophylaxis is necessary. However, antibiotics should be used for any patient with suspected or documented infection of the biliary tree, such as acute cholecystitis or ascending cholangitis, and should be chosen to cover gram-negative bacteria and anaerobes.

BENIGN BILIARY DISEASE

Calculous Biliary Disease

By far, the most common disease state involving the gallbladder and biliary tree is that of cholelithiasis. Because the gallbladder concentrates bile, the concentration of solutes in the gallbladder differs from that in the rest of the biliary tree. This increase in solute concentration combined with stasis in the gallbladder between meals predisposes to stone formation in the gallbladder. Gallstones can be subclassified into two major subtypes, depending on the principal solute that precipitates into a stone. More than 70% of gallstones in America are formed by precipitation of cholesterol and calcium, with pure cholesterol stones accounting for only a small (<10%) portion. Pigment stones, further subclassified as black or brown stones, are caused by precipitation of concentrated bile pigments, the breakdown products of hemoglobin. Four major factors explain most gallstone formation: supersaturation of secreted bile, concentration of bile in the gallbladder, crystal nucleation, and gallbladder dysmotility. High concentrations of cholesterol and lipid in bile secretion from the liver constitute one predisposing condition to cholesterol stone formation, whereas increased hemoglobin processing is seen in most patients with pigment stones. Once in the gallbladder, bile is concentrated further through the absorption of water and sodium,

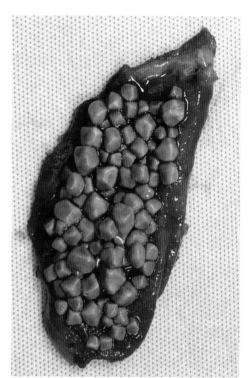

FIGURE 54-20 Gallbladder with characteristic yellow cholesterol stones.

increasing the concentrations of the bile solutes and calcium. Bile salts act to solubilize cholesterol. With respect to cholesterol stones (Fig. 54-20), cholesterol precipitates out into crystals when the concentration in the gallbladder vesicles exceeds the solubility of cholesterol (Fig. 54-21).[2] Crystal formation is further accelerated by pronucleating agents, including glycoproteins and immunoglobulins. Finally, abnormal gallbladder motility can increase stasis in the gallbladder, allowing more time for solutes to precipitate in the gallbladder. Therefore, increased stone formation can be seen in conditions associated with impaired gallbladder emptying, such as in prolonged fasting states, with use of total parenteral nutrition, after vagotomy, and with use of somatostatin analogues.

Pigment stones can be divided into black stones, as seen in hemolytic conditions and cirrhosis, and brown stones, which tend to be found in the bile ducts and are thought to be secondary to infection. The difference in color comes from incorporation of cholesterol into the brown stones. Because black pigment stones occur in hemolytic states from concentration of bilirubin, they are found almost exclusively in the gallbladder. Alternatively, brown stones occur within the biliary tree and suggest a disorder of biliary motility and associated bacterial infection.

Natural History

Most gallstones are asymptomatic, often being identified at the time of abdominal imaging for other reasons or during laparotomy. To become symptomatic, the gallstone must obstruct a visceral structure, such as the cystic duct. Biliary colic, caused by temporary blockage of the cystic duct, tends to occur after a meal, in which the secretion of CCK leads to gallbladder contraction. Stones that do not obstruct the cystic duct or pass through the entire biliary tree into the intestines without impaction do not

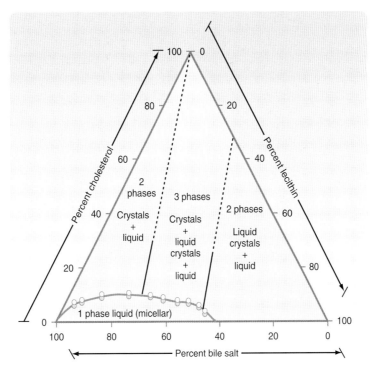

FIGURE 54-21 **Triangle of Solubility.** With the three major components of bile that determine cholesterol solubility and stability, each can be quantified by molar percentage to show a relative ratio to the other two. Cholesterol is completely soluble in only the small area in the left lower corner, where a clear micellar solution exists, below the *closed circles.* Just above this, in the area between the *open* and *closed circles,* cholesterol is supersaturated but stable and thus crystallized only with stasis. In the remainder of the triangle, cholesterol is significantly supersaturated and unstable. In this region, crystals form immediately. (From Admirand WH, Small DM: The physicochemical basis of cholesterol gallstone formation in man. *J Clin Invest* 47:1043–1052, 1968.)

cause symptoms. Only 20% to 30% of patients with asymptomatic stones will develop symptoms within 20 years, and because approximately 1% of patients with asymptomatic stones develop complications of their stones before onset of symptoms, prophylactic cholecystectomy is not warranted in asymptomatic patients.

Certain subsets of patients, however, constitute a higher risk pool, so prophylactic cholecystectomy should be considered. Among these are patients with hemolytic anemias, such as sickle cell anemia. These patients have an extremely high rate of pigment stone formation, and cholecystitis can precipitate a crisis. Patients with a calcified gallbladder wall (known as porcelain gallbladder), those with large (>2.5 cm) gallstones, and those with a long common channel of bile and pancreatic ducts all have a higher risk of gallbladder cancer and should consider cholecystectomy. In addition, patients with asymptomatic gallstones undergoing bariatric surgery may also benefit from cholecystectomy. Not only does rapid weight loss favor stone formation, but also, after gastric bypass, ERCP to remove common bile duct stones in ascending cholangitis is extremely challenging and usually unsuccessful. Finally, because severe infection can be life-threatening in the immunocompromised patient, some transplantation surgeons recommend prophylactic cholecystectomy before receipt of an organ transplant.

Nonoperative Treatment of Cholelithiasis

Medical treatment of gallstones is generally unsuccessful and is used rarely. Options include dissolution with oral bile salt therapy;

contact dissolution, which requires cannulation of the gallbladder and infusion of organic solvent; and extracorporeal shock wave lithotripsy. With the dissolution strategies, unacceptable recurrence rates of up to 50% limit their application to the most select group of patients. Extracorporeal shock wave lithotripsy has a lower recurrence rate, approximately 20%, and can be used in patients with single stones 0.5 to 2 cm in size. The widespread use, safety, and efficacy of laparoscopic cholecystectomy have relegated nonoperative therapy to patients for whom general anesthesia presents a prohibitively high risk.

Chronic Cholecystitis

Recurrent attacks of biliary colic, with only temporary occlusion of the cystic duct, can cause inflammation and scarring of the neck of the gallbladder and cystic duct. This process, called chronic cholecystitis, causes fibrosis as histologic evidence of repeated self-limited episodes of inflammation. The diagnosis of chronic cholecystitis lies along a continuum with biliary colic because it results from recurrent attacks. Therefore, the presentation is that of symptomatic cholelithiasis, or biliary colic. Pain occurring after ingestion of a fatty meal, with the attendant increase in CCK secretion in response to duodenal intraluminal fat, is classic for biliary colic, although only 50% of patients will report an association with food. Pain from stones tends to locate in the epigastrium or right upper quadrant and may radiate around to the scapula. These attacks of pain generally last a few hours. Pain lasting longer than 24 hours or associated with fever

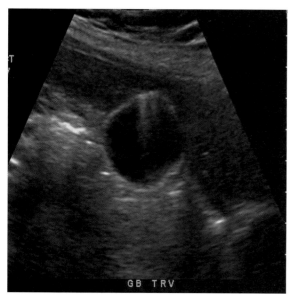

FIGURE 54-22 Ultrasound image of cholesterolosis.

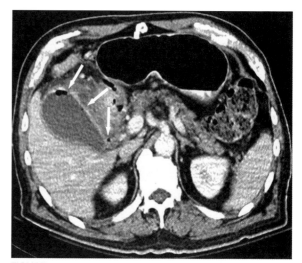

FIGURE 54-23 CT scan of emphysematous cholecystitis. Significant pericholecystic inflammatory changes and air in the gallbladder wall (*arrows*) are signs of emphysematous cholecystitis.

suggests acute cholecystitis. The pain of biliary colic, even in the absence of cholecystitis, may also cause other gastrointestinal symptoms, such as bloating, nausea, or even vomiting.

Symptomatic stones constitute a risk profile different from that of asymptomatic stones, with a higher likelihood of complications. Therefore, symptomatic cholelithiasis is an indication for cholecystectomy. To perform a cholecystectomy for symptomatic stones, one needs presence of symptoms and documentation of stones.

Diagnosis

The diagnosis of symptomatic cholelithiasis, the clinical manifestation of chronic cholecystitis, relies on a history consistent with biliary tract disease. Transabdominal ultrasonography reliably documents the presence of cholelithiasis. Ultrasound can provide other important information, such as common bile duct dilation, gallbladder polyps, porcelain gallbladder, or evidence of hepatic parenchymal processes. Cholesterolosis, or the accumulation of cholesterol found in gallbladder mucosal macrophages, can also be seen (Fig. 54-22). Even in the absence of frank stones, so-called sludge found in the gallbladder on ultrasonography, with appropriate symptoms, is consistent with biliary colic.

Treatment

Patients with sufficient symptoms from gallstones should undergo elective cholecystectomy. Cholecystectomy carries a low-risk profile but is not without complications, so an analysis of risks and benefits is important. Because patients with mild symptoms have a low rate of complications from gallstones (1% to 3%/year), observation and dietary and lifestyle changes are appropriate in this population. Patients with more severe or recurrent symptoms have a higher rate of complications of the disease (7%/year), so elective laparoscopic cholecystectomy is warranted. In more than 90% of patients, cholecystectomy is curative, leaving them symptom free.

Acute Calculous Cholecystitis

The pathophysiologic mechanism of acute cholecystitis is blockage of the cystic duct. When the blockage occurs from an obstructing

stone, the diagnosis is acute calculous cholecystitis. The differentiation of biliary colic from acute cholecystitis is unresolved blockage of the cystic duct. In biliary colic, the obstruction is temporary and self-limited. In acute cholecystitis, the obstruction does not resolve, and inflammation ensues, with edema and subserosal hemorrhage. Infection of the stagnant pool of bile is a secondary phenomenon; the primary pathophysiologic mechanism is unresolved cystic duct obstruction. Without resolution of the obstruction, the gallbladder will progress to ischemia and necrosis. Eventually, acute cholecystitis becomes acute gangrenous cholecystitis and, when complicated by infection with a gas-forming organism, acute emphysematous cholecystitis (Fig. 54-23).

Presentation

The inflammatory changes in the gallbladder wall are manifested as fever, right upper quadrant pain, tenderness to palpation, and guarding in the right upper quadrant. This process will cause an arrest of inspiration with gentle pressure under the right costal margin, a finding known as Murphy sign. Tenderness and the presence of Murphy sign help distinguish acute cholecystitis from biliary colic, in which there is no inflammatory process. Given that the common bile duct is not obstructed, profound jaundice in the setting of a picture of acute cholecystitis is rare and should raise the suspicion of cholangitis, with obstruction of the common bile duct, or Mirizzi syndrome, in which inflammation or a stone in the gallbladder neck leads to inflammation of the adjoining biliary system, with obstruction of the common hepatic duct. Mild elevations of alkaline phosphatase, bilirubin, and transaminase levels and a leukocytosis support the diagnosis of acute cholecystitis.

Diagnosis

Transabdominal ultrasonography is a sensitive, inexpensive, and reliable tool for the diagnosis of acute cholecystitis, with a sensitivity of 85% and specificity of 95%. In addition to identifying gallstones, ultrasound can demonstrate pericholecystic fluid (Fig. 54-24), gallbladder wall thickening, and even a sonographic Murphy sign, documenting tenderness specifically over the gallbladder. In most cases, an accurate history and physical

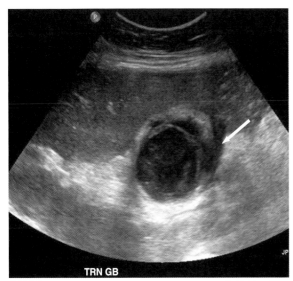

FIGURE 54-24 Ultrasound image of pericholecystic fluid. The thickened gallbladder wall with pericholecystic fluid *(arrow)* indicates acute cholecystitis.

examination, along with supporting laboratory studies and an ultrasound examination, make the diagnosis of acute cholecystitis. In atypical cases, an HIDA scan may be used to demonstrate obstruction of the cystic duct, which definitively diagnoses acute cholecystitis. Filling of the gallbladder during an HIDA scan essentially eliminates the diagnosis of cholecystitis. CT may show similar findings to ultrasound with pericholecystic fluid, gallbladder wall thickening, and emphysematous changes, but CT is less sensitive than ultrasound for the diagnosis of acute cholecystitis.

Treatment

Although the primary pathophysiologic event in acute cholecystitis is the obstruction of the cystic duct and infection is a secondary event that follows stasis and inflammation, most cases of acute cholecystitis are complicated by superinfection of the inflamed gallbladder. Therefore, patients are given nothing by mouth, and intravenous (IV) fluids and parenteral antibiotics are started. Given that gram-negative aerobes are the most common organisms found in acute cholecystitis, followed by anaerobes and gram-positive aerobes, broad-spectrum antibiotics are warranted. Parenteral narcotics are usually required to control the pain.

Cholecystectomy, whether open or laparoscopic, is the treatment of choice for acute cholecystitis. The timing of operative intervention in acute cholecystitis has long been a source of debate. In the past, many surgeons advocated for delayed cholecystectomy, with patients managed nonoperatively during their initial hospitalization and discharged home with resolution of symptoms. An interval cholecystectomy was then performed at approximately 6 weeks after the initial episode. More recent studies have shown that early in the disease process (within the first week), the operation can be performed laparoscopically with equivalent or improved morbidity, mortality, and length of stay as well as a similar conversion rate to open cholecystectomy.[3] In addition, approximately 20% of patients initially admitted for nonoperative management failed to respond to medical treatment before the planned interval cholecystectomy and required surgical intervention. Initial nonoperative therapy remains a viable option

for patients who present in a delayed fashion and should be decided on an individual basis.

Given the inflammatory process occurring in the porta hepatis, early conversion to open cholecystectomy should be considered when delineation of anatomy is not clear or when progress cannot be made laparoscopically. With substantial inflammation, a partial cholecystectomy, transecting the gallbladder at the infundibulum with cauterization of the remaining mucosa, is acceptable to avoid injury to the common bile duct. Some patients present with acute cholecystitis but have a prohibitively high operative risk. For these patients, a percutaneously placed cholecystostomy tube should be considered. Frequently performed with ultrasound guidance under local anesthesia with some sedation, cholecystostomy can act as a temporizing measure by draining the infected bile. Percutaneous drainage results in improvement in symptoms and physiology, allowing a delayed cholecystectomy 3 to 6 months after medical optimization. In patients with cholecystostomy tubes, when fluoroscopy shows a patent cystic duct, the cholecystostomy tube can be removed and the decision for cholecystectomy determined by the patient's ability to tolerate surgical intervention.

Choledocholithiasis

Choledocholithiasis, or common bile duct stones, is classified by the point of origin. Primary common duct stones arise de novo in the bile duct, and secondary common duct stones pass from the gallbladder into the bile duct. Primary choledocholithiasis is generally from brown pigment stones, which are a combination of precipitated bile pigments and cholesterol. Brown stones are more common in Asian populations and are associated with a bacterial infection of the bile duct. The bacteria secrete an enzyme that hydrolyzes bilirubin glucuronides to form free bilirubin, which then precipitates. Most common duct stones found in the United States are secondary, having originated in the gallbladder, and are termed retained common duct stones when they are found within 2 years after cholecystectomy.

Many common duct stones are clinically silent and may be identified only during cholangiography if it is performed routinely during cholecystectomy (Fig. 54-25). Without pain or an abnormal liver function panel, a setting in which selective cholangiography is not performed, 1% to 2% of patients after cholecystectomy will present with a retained stone. When it is performed routinely, intraoperative cholangiography identifies choledocholithiasis in approximately 10% of asymptomatic patients, suggesting that most choledocholithiasis remains clinically silent.[4,5]

When not clinically silent, common duct stones may be manifested with symptoms ranging from biliary colic to the clinical manifestations of obstructive jaundice, such as darkening of the urine, scleral icterus, and lightening of the stools. Jaundice with choledocholithiasis is more likely to be painful because the onset of obstruction is acute, causing rapid distention of the bile duct and activation of pain fibers. Fever, a common symptom, can be associated with right upper quadrant pain and jaundice, a constellation known as Charcot triad. This triad suggests ascending cholangitis that, if untreated, may progress to septic shock. The addition of hypotension and mental status changes, both evidence of shock from a biliary source, to Charcot triad is known as Reynolds pentad.

Diagnosis

In the setting of choledocholithiasis, abnormalities of the hepatic function panel are common but neither sensitive nor specific, and with superinfection, leukocytosis may also be present. Ultrasound

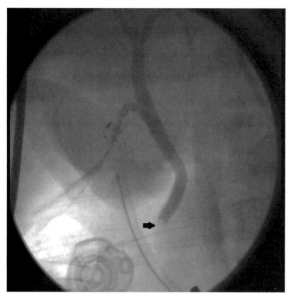

FIGURE 54-25 Intraoperative cholangiogram showing choledocholithiasis in an asymptomatic patient, with no filling of duodenum and outline of stone (arrow).

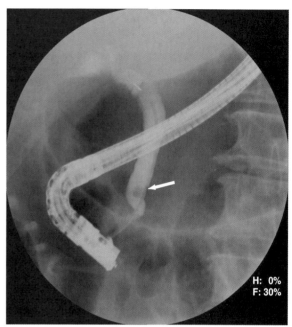

FIGURE 54-26 ERCP with choledocholithiasis. With retrograde injection of contrast material, a filling defect noted within the lumen of the common bile duct (arrow) identifies choledocholithiasis. ERCP can also be used to remove the stone through sphincterotomy and balloons or baskets.

may show choledocholithiasis or only biliary ductal dilation. In patients with biliary pain, gallstones, and jaundice, a dilated bile duct (>8 mm) is highly suggestive of choledocholithiasis, even if common duct stones are not documented ultrasonographically. Even without symptoms of biliary colic, a dilated bile duct in the presence of gallstones suggests choledocholithiasis.

ERCP is highly sensitive and specific for choledocholithiasis (Fig. 54-26) and can usually be therapeutic by clearing the duct of all stones in approximately 75% of patients during the first procedure and in approximately 90% with repeated ERCP. During the endoscopic procedure, a sphincterotomy is performed with a balloon sweep and extraction of the stone, all of which have a complication rate of 5% to 8%. Indications for preoperative ERCP before cholecystectomy include cholangitis, biliary pancreatitis, limited experience of the surgeon with common duct exploration, and patients with multiple comorbidities.

Alternatively, magnetic resonance cholangiopancreatography (MRCP) is highly sensitive (>90%) with an almost 100% specificity for the diagnosis of common duct stones (Fig. 54-27). As a noninvasive test, MRCP provides accurate imaging of the biliary tree, but in the setting of choledocholithiasis, it does not provide a therapeutic solution. A clear cholangiogram by MRCP eliminates the need for ERCP. However, choledocholithiasis identified by MRCP requires intervention by some other method. As many surgeons are not facile at laparoscopic common duct exploration, many have resorted to preoperative MRCP to determine the need for preoperative ERCP for duct clearance.[6] With inexperience in common duct exploration, choledocholithiasis found on cholangiography during laparoscopic cholecystectomy would necessitate postoperative ERCP and the small chance that endoscopic means could not clear the duct, necessitating reoperation.

PTC can also be used to diagnose and to treat choledocholithiasis. PTC is an invasive test with a complication rate similar to that of ERCP. Although requiring less skill, and at a lower cost, PTC is as effective in patients with a dilated biliary ductal system but less effective in the setting of a nondilated biliary tree.

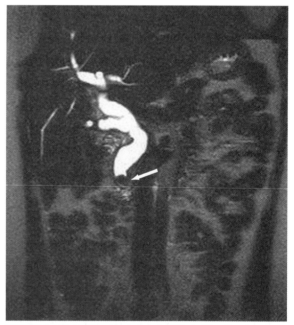

FIGURE 54-27 MRCP with choledocholithiasis. The dilated common bile duct ends abruptly, with a convex intraluminal filling defect (arrow) consistent with choledocholithiasis.

Ultrasound should be used routinely for evaluation of the gallbladder and biliary tree, but the remaining studies should be chosen selectively on the basis of the likelihood of finding common duct stones. Patients with highest risk, such as those with cholangitis or jaundice, should undergo ERCP. Those with lower risk can undergo laparoscopic cholecystectomy with cholangiography and possible laparoscopic common duct exploration or MRCP, depending on the surgeon's expertise. In general, choledocholithiasis identified but not removed during cholecystectomy mandates ERCP for stone extraction.

Treatment

Endoscopic retrograde cholangiopancreatography. Endoscopic sphincterotomy with stone extraction is effective for the treatment of choledocholithiasis. In the preoperative setting, it can clear the duct of stones, and when it is unsuccessful at removal of all stones, it will alter intraoperative decision making. Common reasons for endoscopic failure include large stones, intrahepatic stones, multiple stones, altered gastric or duodenal anatomy, impacted stones, and duodenal diverticula. Sphincterotomy with stone extraction does not eliminate the risk of recurrent biliary stone disease. When managed by ERCP and sphincterotomy, almost 50% of all patients have recurrent symptoms of biliary tract disease if they are not also treated by cholecystectomy.[7] More than one third of these patients eventually require cholecystectomy, suggesting that cholecystectomy should be offered to patients who present with choledocholithiasis. Interestingly, older patients (>70 years) have only a 15% rate of symptom recurrence, so cholecystectomy can be offered selectively to this population of patients.

Laparoscopic common bile duct exploration. At the time of cholecystectomy, intraoperative cholangiography will help identify choledocholithiasis. A laparoscopic common duct exploration can then be performed in an attempt to manage all calculous biliary tract disease in one setting, without the need for an additional anesthetic or procedure. Access to the common duct with a small-caliber cholangioscope is provided through the cystic duct or through a separate incision in the common duct itself. In the transcystic approach, the cystic duct is dilated, and a flexible cholangioscope is passed down into the common bile duct. For the transcystic approach in the setting of a narrow cystic duct, the duct can be dilated with a flexible dilator passed over a wire, using a Seldinger technique. Given the angle of insertion of the cystic duct into the common bile duct, stones in the common hepatic duct above the cystic duct insertion are not accessible through the transcystic route. Other contraindications for the transcystic approach include a small, friable cystic duct; numerous (more than eight) stones in the common bile duct; and large stones (>1 cm), which would be difficult or impossible to extract through the cystic duct orifice. In any of these settings, a separate incision can be made in the common bile duct, with the only contraindication being that of a small common duct that may become strictured on closure. Many studies show the high success rate of laparoscopic transcystic duct common bile duct exploration for choledocholithiasis.

Open common bile duct exploration. With greater use of endoscopic and laparoscopic methods, the frequency of open common duct exploration has decreased. Open exploration should be used when endoscopic and laparoscopic means are not feasible for documented common duct stones or when concomitant biliary drainage is required. Open exploration carries a low morbidity (8% to 15%) and mortality (1% to 2%), with a low rate of retained stones (<5%). Impacted stones at the ampulla present a difficult problem for ERCP and common duct exploration. With unsuccessful attempts to remove an impacted stone in the setting of a nondilated biliary tree, a transduodenal sphincteroplasty can provide drainage. In a similar setting but with a dilated biliary

tree, drainage of the biliary tree through a separate choledocho-enterostomy can be successful. The two options for drainage are a choledochoduodenostomy and Roux-en-Y choledochojejunostomy. Anastomosis to the duodenum can be performed rapidly with a single anastomosis (Fig. 54-28). This anatomic arrangement continues to allow endoscopic access to the entire biliary tree. The downside of this approach is that the bile duct distal to the anastomosis does not drain well and may collect debris that obstructs the anastomosis or the pancreatic duct, a process known as sump syndrome. Anastomosis to the jejunum in a Roux-en-Y arrangement provides excellent drainage of the biliary tree without a risk of sump syndrome but does not allow future endoscopic evaluation of the biliary tree (Fig. 54-29).

Intrahepatic stones, which are almost uniformly brown pigment stones, represent a different management challenge than secondary bile duct stones. Relatively uncommon in Western compared with Asian populations, these stones tend to occur specifically in patients with stasis of the biliary tree, such as those with strictures, parasites, choledochal cysts, or sclerosing cholangitis. Because these stones collect at sites above obstructions, the transhepatic approach to cholangiography is generally more successful. Percutaneous drainage catheters are left in place and upsized to perform percutaneous stone extraction. Long-term management of intrahepatic stones must be carefully tailored to the disease but frequently requires hepaticojejunostomy for better biliary drainage. Liberal use of choledochoscopy at the time of a drainage procedure ensures removal of all current stones. This approach allows a stone clearance rate of more than 90%.

Gallstone Pancreatitis

As a stone may pass through the common bile duct and into the duodenum, it traverses the ampulla. In the process, it may cause secondary injury to the pancreas. A generally accepted pathophysiologic mechanism involves temporary elevation of pancreatic ductal pressures, causing a secondary inflammation of the pancreatic parenchyma. Even a temporary elevation of intraluminal pressure can cause significant injury to the pancreas. As opposed to the gallbladder, in which relief of the obstruction is accompanied by pain resolution, the symptoms in pancreatitis continue in spite of passage of the stone. With the diagnosis of pancreatitis in which the cause is unclear, ultrasound will help identify gallstones and may show choledocholithiasis or a dilated bile duct. The offending stone usually passes spontaneously but may still cause severe pancreatitis. In most cases of gallstone pancreatitis, the pancreatitis is self-limited. If, by clinical assessment, the pancreatitis is severe, early ERCP to remove a stone that may not have passed is indicated and has been shown to reduce the morbidity of the episode of pancreatitis.[8] To prevent a future episode of gallstone pancreatitis, a laparoscopic cholecystectomy is warranted; this is generally recommended during the same hospitalization, just before discharge. Given the suspicion of choledocholithiasis, intraoperative cholangiography should be performed if no other imaging has been performed to confirm the passage of the gallstone.

Biliary Dyskinesia

Patients may present with classic symptoms of calculous biliary disease but have no ultrasonographic evidence of stones or sludge. In some of these cases, the dysfunction of the gallbladder creates pain, even in the absence of stones. These patients will have other diagnoses excluded by CT and upper endoscopy and should undergo a CCK-stimulated HIDA scan, in which the radiolabeled iminodiacetic acid will collect in the gallbladder. The

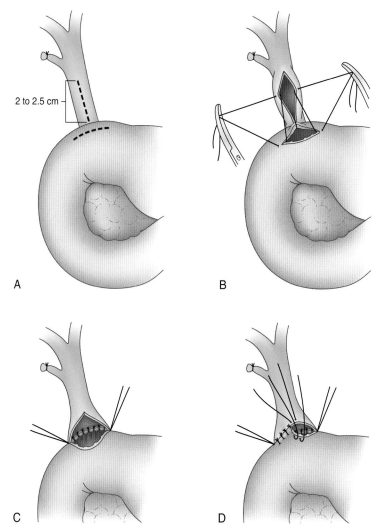

FIGURE 54-28 Choledochoduodenostomy. In the setting of a dilated common bile duct with inability to clear all the stones from the distal duct, an anastomosis can be performed between the common bile duct and adjacent duodenum. Although maintaining the possibility of future endoscopic therapy, this arrangement risks sump syndrome in the undrained distal duct.

patient is given an IV dose of CCK, and the percentage ejection of the gallbladder in response to CCK is calculated. An ejection fraction less than one third at 20 minutes after CCK administration in patients without stones is considered diagnostic of dyskinesia, which should be managed with cholecystectomy. The symptoms of dyskinesia are fairly responsive to cholecystectomy, with more than 85% of patients showing improvement or resolution. In nonresponders, ERCP with sphincterotomy may prove useful.

Sphincter of Oddi Dysfunction

Although there is considerable debate among surgeons and gastroenterologists as to the validity of this diagnosis, sphincter of Oddi dysfunction, which is manifested as biliary tract pain, with normal liver function test results and recurrent pancreatitis, may be caused by a structurally abnormal sphincter or a histologically normal but functionally abnormal one. The theoretical pathophysiologic event occurs with injury to the sphincter from trauma due to pancreatitis, gallstone passage, or congenital anomalies, which induces inflammation and subsequent fibrosis leading to elevated sphincter pressure. Alternatively, patients may have elevated sphincter pressure in the absence of fibrosis, suggesting a spasm of the muscular component. This subset of patients may have evidence of altered motility elsewhere in the gastrointestinal tract. The diagnosis of sphincter of Oddi dysfunction should be suspected in patients with biliary pain and a common duct diameter of more than 12 mm. The bile duct in these patients tends to increase in diameter in response to CCK, as does the pancreatic duct after secretin administration. Manometry has also been used to make the diagnosis, with sphincter pressure higher than 40 mm Hg predicting good response to therapy. Therapy consists of endoscopic sphincterotomy or transduodenal sphincteroplasty, with approximately equivalent results from the two approaches. In patients with objective evidence of sphincter of Oddi dysfunction, division of the sphincter will improve or resolve the pain in 60% to 80% of patients.

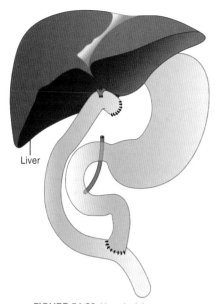

FIGURE 54-29 Hepaticojejunostomy.

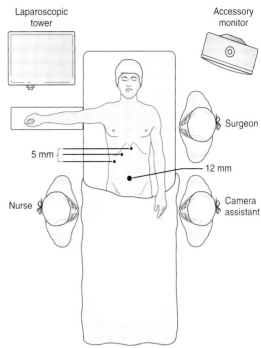

Surgery for Calculous Biliary Disease
Laparoscopic Cholecystectomy

Following the advent of laparoscopic surgery, with its accompanying smaller incisions, less pain, and shorter hospitalization, surgeons have performed an increasing number of laparoscopic cholecystectomies. Most cholecystectomies are performed for biliary colic, but the operation can be performed safely in the setting of acute inflammation. Laparoscopic cholecystectomy for acute cholecystitis carries longer operative times and a higher conversion rate to the open procedure than when it is performed in the elective setting, and it has a higher risk of common duct injury.[9] General anesthesia with muscle relaxation is required when a laparoscopic cholecystectomy is performed. Therefore, one contraindication to the procedure is the inability to tolerate general anesthesia. Others include end-stage liver disease with portal hypertension, precluding safe portal dissection, and coagulopathy. Because most pneumoperitoneum laparoscopy is performed using CO_2 and has a number of adverse physiologic effects, severe chronic obstructive pulmonary disease, with poor ability for gas exchange, and congestive heart failure are considered relative contraindications.

Preparation of the patient, induction of anesthesia, and sterile draping are performed as for an open cholecystectomy. Although use of a urinary catheter depends on the clinical setting, an orogastric tube is standard to decompress the stomach and help with exposure of the upper abdomen. After the establishment of a CO_2 pneumoperitoneum, a brief exploration is performed, and additional 5-mm ports are placed in the right anterior axillary line, right midclavicular line, and subxiphoid location (Fig. 54-30). The lateral port at the anterior axillary line is used to elevate the fundus of the gallbladder toward the right shoulder. This retraction provides exposure to the infundibulum and porta hepatis. The midclavicular trocar is used to grasp the gallbladder infundibulum, retracting it inferolaterally to open the triangle of Calot (Figs. 54-31 to 54-33). By distraction of Hartmann pouch laterally, the cystic duct no longer lies almost parallel to the common hepatic duct.

FIGURE 54-30 Laparoscopic Cholecystectomy Ports. The assistant uses the periumbilical port to provide access for the camera and the most lateral port to elevate the fundus and to expose the neck. The surgeon can then provide inferolateral traction on the infundibulum and open the critical view of safety.

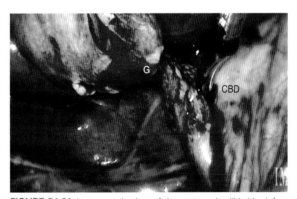

FIGURE 54-31 Laparoscopic view of the porta and gallbladder infundibulum, without inferolateral traction on the infundibulum. Note that the gallbladder infundibulum (G) lies immediately adjacent to the common bile duct (CBD).

The dissection is then carried along the infundibulum on the anterior and posterior surfaces to expose the base of the gallbladder. This dissection will eventually clear all fibrofatty tissue from the triangle of Calot. Inferolateral traction of the infundibulum then allows documentation of two structures entering the gallbladder, the cystic duct and cystic artery. A useful landmark for the cystic artery is the overlying lymph node, known as Calot node. To minimize bile duct injury, a strategy known as the critical view of safety can be employed. This process involves dissection of the infundibulum of the gallbladder and continuation of the dissection by taking down the cystic plate and separating the lower third of the gallbladder from its attachments to the liver. Once completed, the tubular structures attached to the gallbladder

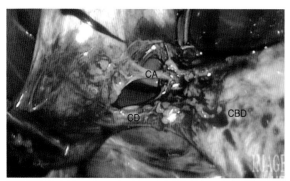

FIGURE 54-32 Laparoscopic view of the same patient as in Figure 54-31 but with inferolateral traction on the infundibulum. Note the angular change to the cystic duct (CD) compared with the common bile duct (CBD). The dissecting tool indicates the location of the right hepatic artery. The key element to this view in minimizing CBD injury is the identification of the cystic artery (CA) and duct entering the gallbladder, with the inferior aspect of segment V of the liver identified in the space on either side of the artery and duct.

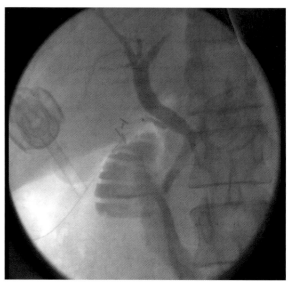

FIGURE 54-35 Normal cholangiogram.

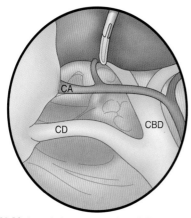

FIGURE 54-33 An artist's representation of Figure 54-32, showing hidden anatomy.

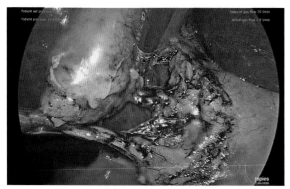

FIGURE 54-34 Wide critical view.

should be cleaned of all extraneous material. Rotating the gallbladder infundibulum laterally and then medially, there should be only two structures entering the gallbladder, and liver on the opposite side of the gallbladder should be visible through the open spaces around each structure (Fig. 54-34).[9] With sufficient dissection, clips are placed on the cystic artery and cystic duct. If

cholangiography is performed, the cystic duct is clipped only adjacent to the gallbladder, and the cystic duct is incised but not transected. A cholangiographic catheter is then fed through the incised duct, and fluoroscopic images are obtained with injection of contrast material into the cystic duct and biliary tree (Fig. 54-35). On obtaining a normal cholangiogram or when cholangiography is not performed, the cystic duct is doubly clipped on the common duct side and transected. The previously clipped artery is also transected, and the gallbladder is dissected off the liver bed using electrocautery. Because the venous drainage of the gallbladder is directly into the liver bed through venules, excellent hemostasis must be achieved during this dissection. The cystic duct and cystic artery clips are inspected just before completion of the dissection of the fundic attachments because the superior traction of the fundus has provided exposure to the porta and triangle of Calot. The gallbladder is then brought out of the abdominal cavity through the umbilical port. In the setting of acute cholecystitis or if the gallbladder was entered during dissection, a plastic bag should be used for retrieval. Any stones that are spilled during a cholecystectomy should also be retrieved.

Opinion is sharply divided about the performance of selective versus routine cholangiography, with supportive data for each approach. Routine cholangiography will identify unsuspected stones in less than 10% of patients, and the natural history of these asymptomatic stones suggests that they will remain asymptomatic. Although vigorously debated, the incidence of biliary injury is not significantly reduced with cholangiography. Even when it is performed routinely, cholangiograms are frequently misinterpreted.[10] In many cases of laparoscopic cholecystectomy performed for biliary colic, cholangiography will not alter management. Also, it increases the operative time and adds fluoroscopic exposure. Indications for cholangiography in the selective setting include unexplained pain at the time of cholecystectomy, any suspicion of current or previous choledocholithiasis without preoperative duct clearance, any question of anatomic delineation during cholecystectomy, elevated preoperative liver enzyme levels, dilated common bile duct in preoperative imaging, and suspicion of intraoperative biliary injury. Although the routine use of cholangiography has been decreasing, many authors advocate its use in the academic setting to ensure that trainees are facile in its performance.[6] Although it is just as accurate as cholangiography for the identification of choledocholithiasis, laparoscopic ultrasonography is highly operator dependent, requires additional instrumentation, and is not widely available.

Open Cholecystectomy

As laparoscopic cholecystectomy has become the procedure of choice for the treatment of most gallbladder disease, experience with open cholecystectomy has drastically declined. Open cholecystectomy is generally performed after conversion from the laparoscopic approach or as a step during another operation, such as a pancreaticoduodenectomy. The open cholecystectomy can be performed through a midline or right subcostal incision. Retraction of segment IV provides exposure of the cystic duct and artery. With similar inferolateral traction to the gallbladder infundibulum, the cystic duct is taken out of alignment from the common duct for its identification and division. Early identification and ligation of the cystic artery limit the blood loss during the procedure but may prove difficult because of inflammation. Another approach to the gallbladder infundibulum involves dissecting the fundus off the liver in a dome-down approach. Here, the attachments of the gallbladder are divided, allowing inferolateral traction of the entire gallbladder to open the triangle of Calot and to identify the appropriate duct and artery. This approach, although intermittently useful, must be used with caution as the extension of the dissection continues inferiorly, putting portal vein and other portal structures at risk.[11] When it is performed for severe cholecystitis, the dissection of the gallbladder of the liver bed may be associated with substantial blood loss, but with removal of the infected gallbladder and packing of the area, the bleeding is usually well controlled.

Laparoscopic Common Bile Duct Exploration

Given the risk of ascending cholangitis, gallstone pancreatitis, or cystic duct stump leak, all attempts must be made to remove known bile duct stones. Many factors are relevant to the decision as to which approach to duct clearance should be used. The experience of the surgeon or endoscopist is important in determining if operative clearance or postoperative ERCP will be most effective, with lowest morbidity. Anatomic aspects such as duct size and stone size and number should be considered. As experience with laparoscopic surgery has grown, laparoscopic approaches to bile duct clearance have become more prevalent. With a common bile duct stone identified fluoroscopically, the common duct can be irrigated, and glucagon is given to relax the sphincter of Oddi. If this technique fails to flush the stone, a balloon catheter or wire basket can be passed under fluoroscopic guidance to attempt stone extraction. If this is still unsuccessful, flexible choledochoscopy is indicated. The two common laparoscopic approaches to explore the common bile duct for stone removal are the transcystic approach and choledochotomy. In the transcystic approach, at the completion of cholangiography, a wire is fed down the cystic duct into the common bile duct. Through a Seldinger technique or use of a balloon catheter, the cystic duct is gently dilated to allow passage of a flexible choledochoscope. Alternatively, a flexible ureteroscope can be used. To pass the fiberoptic scope through the duct system, a water irrigation system is attached and allowed to constantly infuse out the end of the scope. If a laparoscopic screen is available, the choledochoscopic image is projected onto a corner it. With the surgeon feeding the choledochoscope into the cystic duct and the assistant adjusting the

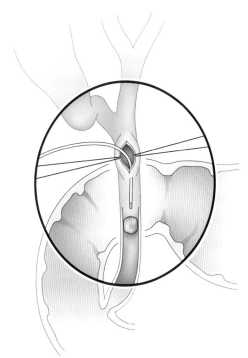

FIGURE 54-36 Laparoscopic choledochotomy for common bile duct exploration.

tip of the choledochoscope, keeping the lumen in the screen, the flexible choledochoscope is advanced to the distal bile duct. With identification of the offending stone, a wire basket is passed to ensnare the stone, withdrawing it and the choledochoscope together.

In the laparoscopic choledochotomy approach, a longitudinal incision is made in the common bile duct (i.e., below the cystic duct). To expose the common bile duct, two stay sutures are placed on either side of the planned choledochotomy (Fig. 54-36). The size of the incision should be at least as large as the diameter of the largest stone. The choledochoscope can then be fed down into the distal bile duct and stone extraction performed as described earlier. At the completion of the exploration, a T tube should be placed through the choledochotomy and the bile duct closed with 4-0 absorbable sutures. Completion cholangiography through the T tube documents stone removal.

In addition to being technically easier, because it does not require fine laparoscopic suturing, the transcystic approach avoids a T tube. Contraindications to the transcystic approach include numerous (more than eight) stones, a stone larger than 1 cm, intrahepatic stones, and a cystic duct that does not allow dilation and choledochoscope passage. Given the need for suture closure of the incision in the bile duct, the only contraindication to the choledochotomy approach is a small-caliber bile duct (<6 mm), which could be strictured by closure. Both approaches are successful at stone removal, with most studies showing a 75% to 95% rate of stone clearance. This is comparable to that of laparoscopic cholecystectomy, followed by postoperative ERCP, with the only difference being a shorter hospitalization and lower physician fees for patients undergoing common duct exploration as the cholecystectomy and clearance of stones are performed in one setting by a single physician.[12]

Open Common Bile Duct Exploration

With advanced laparoscopic, endoscopic, and percutaneous techniques, open exploration of the bile duct has become less common. When open surgery is otherwise required or previous surgery, such as gastric bypass, makes other techniques unsuccessful, clearance of choledocholithiasis must be performed by the open approach. The exposure to the bile duct is through a midline or right upper quadrant incision. A Kocher maneuver must be performed to expose the distal bile duct. Gentle palpation of the distal bile duct will frequently find the offending stone, which may be milked backward. As in the laparoscopic approach, stay sutures are placed and a choledochotomy is performed in the supraduodenal bile duct. Flushing of the duct with a soft rubber catheter will frequently remove the offending stones. Balloon catheters and, with fluoroscopic guidance, wire baskets may be useful to withdraw the stone. Flexible choledochoscopes are used to visualize the distal bile duct. With complete removal of stones, a T tube is placed and a cholangiogram obtained before closure to document clearance.

In the setting of common bile duct stones, some patients should be considered for a drainage procedure. With dilated bile ducts, multiple distal impacted stones, a distal duct stricture with stones, intrahepatic stones, or primary bile duct stones, drainage procedures provide more successful long-term outcomes. Options in this setting include choledochoduodenostomy and Roux-en-Y hepaticojejunostomy, with Roux-en-Y considered a superior drainage procedure. A side-to-side or end-to side choledochoduodenostomy is a fast and safe approach that allows future endoscopic intervention of the upper biliary tree, if necessary. In the side-to-side approach, however, by leaving of the distal bile duct in continuity, patients are at risk for sump syndrome, in which the distal bile duct that does not drain well may collect debris and even food stuffs. Occlusions of the ampulla, with subsequent pancreatitis, and anastomotic stricture with cholangitis have been reported. An alternative to duodenostomy is a Roux-en-Y choledochojejunostomy. By use of a 60-cm limb of jejunum for drainage, occlusion of the anastomosis by food debris is rare, but endoscopic treatment of the hepatic duct is impossible.

Impacted stones at the hepatic ampulla that cannot be removed through choledochotomy or several stones in a nondilated tree can be addressed by a transduodenal sphincteroplasty (Figs. 54-37 and 54-38). After completion of the Kocher maneuver, a longitudinal duodenotomy is made on the lateral wall. Compression of the lateral wall against the medial wall will allow palpation of the ampulla to plan placement of the duodenotomy appropriately. With identification of the ampulla, an incision is made at 11 o'clock, and each wall is elevated with stay sutures. The pancreatic duct usually enters at 5 o'clock on the ampulla and must be avoided. Sequential straight clamps are placed along the planned incision of the ampulla to guide visualization through hemostasis. With each step, the duodenal mucosa is sewn to the bile duct mucosa with absorbable 4-0 sutures. A 1.5-cm sphincterotomy is usually sufficient to allow stone removal and subsequent drainage. Closure of the longitudinal duodenotomy in transverse fashion avoids a future duodenal stricture.

Postcholecystectomy Syndromes
Bile Duct Injury

The most devastating complication of any right upper quadrant operation occurring with any significant frequency is iatrogenic bile duct injury. More than 80% of all iatrogenic bile duct injuries occur during cholecystectomy, and they can occur in the open or

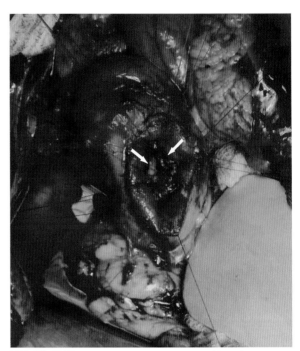

FIGURE 54-37 Transduodenal sphincteroplasty. Note the generous opening of the distal common duct with sequential duct to mucosa approximation *(arrows)*.

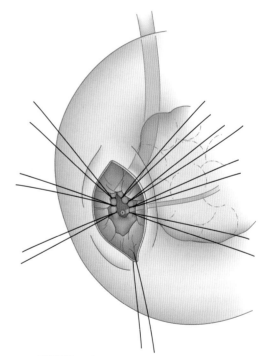

FIGURE 54-38 Transduodenal sphincteroplasty.

laparoscopic setting. Inflammation in the porta, variable biliary anatomy, inappropriate exposure, aggressive attempts at hemostasis, and inexperience of the surgeon are commonly cited risk factors. Although early reports suggested that surgical inexperience (performing fewer than 20 laparoscopic cholecystectomies) was highly correlated with bile duct injury, evidence has suggested that visual misperception accounts for 97% of iatrogenic biliary injuries and technical skill or knowledge accounts for only 3%.[6] With sufficient cephalad retraction of the gallbladder fundus, the cystic duct overlies the common hepatic duct, running in a parallel path. Without inferolateral traction of the gallbladder infundibulum to dissociate these structures, dissection of the apparent cystic duct may actually include the common hepatic duct, placing it in jeopardy. By retraction of Hartmann pouch inferolaterally and opening of the triangle of Calot, the cystic duct is displaced from the porta, no longer collinear with the hepatic duct. The use of a 30-degree laparoscope provides adequate visualization of the critical view of safety during laparoscopic cholecystectomy. Also, in many of these cases, a confirmation bias occurs, in which surgeons tend to rely on evidence that supports their perception while simultaneously discounting visual cues that suggest an alternative explanation. Confirmation bias helps explain why most bile duct injuries are identified in the postoperative setting, not intraoperatively.

The multifactorial nature of biliary injury highlights the concept that injury avoidance consists of many levels of protective mechanisms. The surgeon's knowledge of biliary anatomy and aberrant anatomy, use of an angled laparoscope, appropriate and directed traction and countertraction on the gallbladder, sufficient suspicion of findings that discount the current perspective, and low threshold for conversion to an open operation can help minimize the likelihood of biliary injury. Although the use of routine versus selective cholangiography is controversial, evidence has suggested that cholangiography does not completely avoid bile duct injury but may reduce the incidence and extent of injury and allow immediate recognition and management.[13] The original analysis of biliary reconstruction was based on the Bismuth classification and has been modified by Strasberg. Classification of bile duct injuries is determined by location of injury and helps guide later surgical reconstruction (Fig. 54-39).[14] Among postoperative bile duct strictures, types E1 and E2 involve the common hepatic duct but not the bifurcation, with type E1 maintaining more than 2 cm of common hepatic duct below the bifurcation and type E2 being within 2 cm of the confluence. Type E3 strictures occur at the confluence, preserving the extrahepatic ducts, and in type E4, the stricturing process includes the extrahepatic biliary tree. Type E5 strictures involve aberrant right hepatic duct anatomy, with injury to the aberrant duct and common hepatic duct.

Presentation. Bile duct injury may be identified intraoperatively but usually is manifested in the postoperative period. Leak of bile into the peritoneal cavity, with subsequent bile peritonitis, tends to be manifested earlier than bile duct stricture and its associated jaundice. In the setting of bile leakage, patients may present with fever, increasing abdominal pain, jaundice, or bile leakage from an incision. Alternatively, injury to the bile duct that does not leak bile will usually be manifested with jaundice, with or without pain. Overall, only 10% of postoperative bile duct strictures are recognized within the first week, and approximately 70% are diagnosed within 6 months of the original operation. Regardless of timing or presentation, adequate repair and subsequent outcome depend on diagnosis, sufficient delineation of anatomy, creation of a tension-free anastomosis, and liberal use of transanastomotic stents.[15]

Treatment

Recognized at the time of cholecystectomy. When bile duct injury is suspected intraoperatively, conversion to an open operation and use of cholangiography help delineate management.

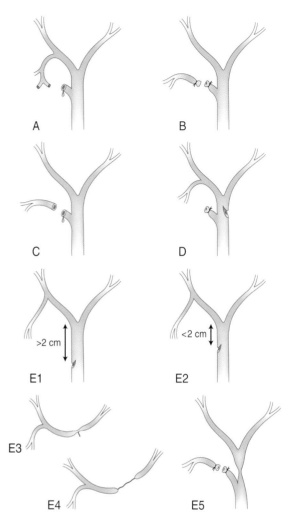

FIGURE 54-39 Strasberg classification of postoperative bile duct strictures.

Goals for the immediate treatment of bile duct injury include maintenance of ductal length, elimination of any bile leakage that would affect subsequent management, and creation of a tension-free repair.

In the adult, for ducts smaller than 3 mm that by cholangiography drain only a single segment or subsegment of liver, simple ligation should suffice for management. Ducts larger than 3 mm usually drain more than a single segment of liver and thus, if transected, should be reimplanted into the biliary tree. If the injury occurs to a larger duct but is not caused by electrocautery and involves less than 50% of the circumference of the wall, a T tube placed through the injury, which is effectively a choledochotomy, usually will allow healing without the need for subsequent biliary-enteric anastomosis. Any cautery-based injury, in which the extent of thermal damage may not be manifested immediately, or an injury involving more than 50% of the duct circumference requires resection of the injured segment with anastomosis to reestablish biliary-enteric continuity. Although it is unusual, when the defect is smaller than 1 cm and not near the hepatic duct bifurcation, mobilization with end-to-end anastomosis of the bile duct can provide acceptable reconstruction. This approach should be accompanied with transanastomotic T tube placement. The tube should be inserted through a separate choledochotomy and not exit the bile duct though the anastomosis. To ensure a tension-free anastomosis, a generous Kocher maneuver, mobilizing the duodenum and the head of the pancreas out of the retroperitoneum, is necessary.

More commonly, injuries occur adjacent to the bifurcation or involve more than a 1-cm defect between the ends of the bile duct. These injuries require reanastomosis to the gastrointestinal tract. In this setting, the distal end is oversewn and the proximal end débrided to normal tissue. The choice of reconstruction depends on location and extent of injury, history of previous attempts at repair, and preference of the surgeon. Low injuries to the bile duct can be reimplanted into the duodenum, although the new choledochoduodenostomy anastomosis risks a duodenal fistula, especially considering that these anastomoses may require significant mobilization to avoid anastomotic tension. Choledochoduodenostomy allows endoscopic intervention if necessary, but the Roux-en-Y approach to reconstruction is substantially more versatile and can be applied to injuries throughout the biliary tree. In addition, most injuries to the bile duct occur higher in the biliary tree, close to the hilum, thus not allowing tension-free anastomosis to the duodenum. Therefore, in almost all cases of bile duct injury, a resection of the injured segment with mucosa-to-mucosa anastomosis using a Roux-en-Y jejunal limb is preferred. Transanastomotic stenting has been shown to improve anastomotic patency, with longer duration of stenting providing a more favorable outcome. As concomitant vascular injuries are common, Doppler ultrasonography can confirm adequate hepatic arterial and portal venous flow to the hepatic parenchyma.

Recent data suggest that there is no significant difference in frequency of biliary injuries sustained at teaching hospitals compared with hospitals without residents.[16] Because most bile duct injuries and therefore most immediate repairs occur at centers where biliary reconstruction is performed infrequently, most immediate repairs go unreported in the literature. However, the importance of surgical judgment and experience in biliary reconstruction cannot be overemphasized. Although reports of previous failed attempts at reconstruction have not documented injuries successfully managed immediately, they do highlight the value of experience in the treatment of bile duct injuries.[17] Therefore, when one is confronted with a bile duct injury and no surgeon with experience in biliary reconstruction is available, the most appropriate management strategy is placement of a drain and immediate referral to an experienced center.

Identified after cholecystectomy

Diagnosis and management. Patients suffering a bile duct injury who present in the postoperative setting are generally found to have jaundice, with an elevated alkaline phosphatase level, or leakage from the injured duct. Leakage may be manifested as bilious drainage into a subhepatic drain placed at the time of operation or bilious drainage from a surgical incision. Without a site for external drainage, bile leakage can be manifested as a biloma, whether sterile or infected, or with biliary ascites.

The diagnosis of iatrogenic bile duct injury should be suspected in any patient who presents with new or increasing symptoms after a laparoscopic cholecystectomy. Changes in serum bilirubin and alkaline phosphatase levels can be seen, even in the first few days after injury. Symptoms of shoulder pain, postprandial pain, fever, and malaise tend to improve after the first few days because a laparoscopic cholecystectomy is generally well tolerated. Complaints that persist or increase over time should raise the suspicion of a bile duct injury.

> **BOX 54-2** **Goals of Therapy in Iatrogenic Bile Duct Injury**
>
> 1. Control of infection, limiting inflammation
>   - Parenteral antibiotics
>   - Percutaneous drainage of periportal fluid collections
> 2. Clear and thorough delineation of entire biliary anatomy
>   - MRCP or PTC
>   - ERCP (especially if cystic duct stump leak is suspected)
> 3. Reestablishment of biliary-enteric continuity
>   - Tension-free, mucosa-to-mucosa anastomosis
>   - Roux-en-Y hepaticojejunostomy
>   - Long-term transanastomotic stents if bifurcation or higher is involved

Patients suspected of having an iatrogenic bile duct injury should undergo imaging to assess for a fluid collection and to evaluate the biliary tree. Ultrasonography can achieve both these goals, but because percutaneous drainage may be required and anatomic delineation is valuable, cross-sectional imaging by CT will generally provide more useful data. Some surgeons advocate the use of radionuclide scanning to confirm bile leakage, but with any documentation of a leak, CT will be necessary to plan management. Also, ischemia is a common cause of bile duct stricture. In the setting of a bile duct injury, 20% or more of patients will have concomitant unrecognized vascular injuries.

In the delayed presentation of a bile duct injury, three major goals guide therapy (Box 54-2). First, control of infection with drainage of any fluid collections will minimize the inflammatory process. Inflammation in the porta hepatis leads to fibrosis, which acts only to increase stricture formation. Broad-spectrum antibiotics, decompression of the biliary tree, and drainage, whether percutaneous or operative, of any fluid collections will achieve this goal. With control of sepsis, there is no urgency for biliary reconstruction. In fact, with time, resolution of the periportal inflammation helps with the execution of a durable reconstruction. In addition, the retraction of an injured bile duct into the hilum of the liver as well as inflammation in this region makes successful repair in the immediate postoperative setting unlikely. Therefore, although immediate reexploration to manage the injury as expeditiously as possible is tempting, successful long-term management of bile duct injuries identified postoperatively depends on clear and deliberate preoperative planning of the reconstruction.

A second goal of management is clear and thorough delineation of the biliary anatomy with cholangiography. Without preoperative cholangiography, any attempts at repair are unlikely to be successful. The cholangiogram must indicate the intrahepatic anatomy and bile duct bifurcation. For patients with bile duct continuity, ERCP may be possible, but PTC is generally more useful. PTC will demonstrate the intrahepatic biliary tree, identify the location of the injury, provide drainage of bile, and possibly even allow the leak to close (Fig. 54-40). Percutaneous biliary catheters can also be left in place during reconstruction to assist in dissection and to provide drainage perioperatively. PTC can be combined with ERCP as necessary, depending on the site and extent of injury. Small bile leaks with bile duct continuity and cystic duct stump leaks can be successfully managed by endoscopic stenting and sphincterotomy.

The third goal of management is to reestablish durable biliary-enteric drainage. Although a combination of percutaneous and endoscopic biliary dilations and stenting may establish continuity, surgical reconstruction has the highest patency rates. To achieve

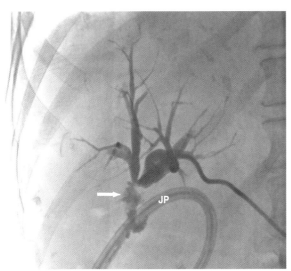

FIGURE 54-40 Percutaneous transhepatic cholangiogram of bile duct injury. Note the extravasation of contrast material *(arrow)* and the Jackson-Pratt drain (JP) placed at the time of initial operation.

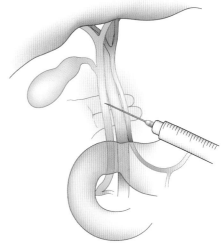

FIGURE 54-41 Needle aspiration of porta used to identify the common bile duct in the setting of substantial inflammation.

a successful and durable repair, the anastomosis must be performed between a minimally inflamed bile duct to intestines in a tension-free, mucosa-to-mucosa fashion. When the anastomosis is within 2 cm of the hepatic duct bifurcation or involves intrahepatic ducts, long-term stenting appears to improve patency. If the bifurcation is involved, stenting of both right and left ducts should be performed. When the reconstruction involves the common bile duct or common hepatic duct more than 2 cm from the bifurcation, stenting is not necessary; therefore, a preoperatively placed transhepatic drain or intraoperatively placed T tube will provide adequate decompression in the immediate postoperative period.

At the time of operation, the adhesions of the duodenum and colon to the liver should be separated. The porta hepatis can be encircled with a Penrose drain. Although the bile duct should lie on the lateral border of the porta hepatis, the marked fibrosis and inflammatory process may make its identification difficult. Preoperatively placed percutaneous biliary drainage catheters can assist in the dissection. Also, clips placed at the previous operation may be identified. If necessary, a small-caliber needle attached to a syringe can be used to aspirate and to identify the bile duct while avoiding inadvertent injury to a vascular structure (Fig. 54-41). Once identified, above the stricture only a limited segment of bile duct (<5 mm) is dissected free. Any further dissection of normal duct risks vascular compromise of the segment to be used in the anastomosis. Preservation of as much normal biliary tree as possible remains a goal of the reconstruction. Next, the bile duct can be opened and the percutaneously placed catheters advanced through the incision. At this point, a wire can be used to exchange the catheters for long-term Silastic stents, if appropriate, or the catheters can be left in place for transanastomotic decompression. The mucosa-to-mucosa anastomosis can be created in an end-to-side fashion to the Roux-en-Y jejunal limb. In the setting of substantial inflammation at the bifurcation, another reconstruction option involves anastomosis of the Roux limb to the left hepatic duct. As noted, the left hepatic duct retains a substantial extraparenchymal length, allowing an anastomosis in this portion of normal duct. Before this section is used for drainage of the

entire liver, cholangiography must confirm that the biliary bifurcation is widely patent, thus ensuring drainage of the right lobe across the bifurcation to the left duct system.

Interventional radiologic and endoscopic techniques. Although long-term patency rates are lower than those seen with surgical reconstruction, nonoperative techniques can be used when the injury has created a stricture in the biliary tree. When the duct remains in continuity, transhepatic management of bile duct strictures can be performed using fluoroscopy, with sedation and local anesthesia. With percutaneous access to the biliary tree, a wire is used to traverse the stricture. By use of balloon dilation techniques, the stricture is dilated, and a catheter is left in place to decompress the system, to allow healing, to document resolution, and, if necessary, to guide repeated dilations (Fig. 54-42). This approach is successful in up to 70% of patients.[18] Complications, although frequent, are generally limited and include cholangitis, hemobilia, and bile leaks requiring repeated intervention. Endoscopic balloon dilation of bile duct strictures is generally reserved for those with primary bile duct strictures or patients who have undergone choledochoduodenostomy for reconstruction because the Roux limb does not usually allow endoscopic strategies. Therefore, series are limited, but results are encouraging, with 88% of patients responding to therapy and a complication rate of 8% from pancreatitis and cholangitis.

Outcomes. Successful outcomes can be achieved in patients undergoing biliary-enteric reconstruction after bile duct injury, with many series showing more than 90% of patients free of jaundice and cholangitis. High success rates are generally achieved when injuries are identified early and patients are referred immediately to experienced centers. In several studies, referral to centers performing complex biliary surgery routinely was associated with better long-term success.[19] Surgical reconstruction provides a durable long-term management strategy.[20] Management of these injuries requires a multidisciplinary management and may need percutaneous techniques as well as surgical reconstruction. Sepsis at the time of reconstruction and biliary cirrhosis are predictors of stricture. In some studies, results were generally better if transanastomotic stents were used during reconstruction.[20] Chronic liver disease and hepatic fibrosis are associated with higher operative mortality and lower success rates. Although a devastating

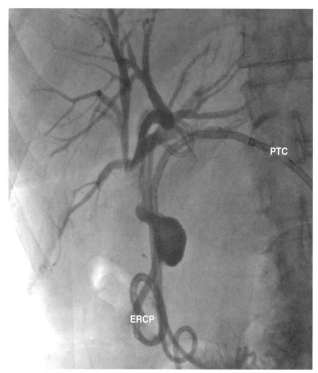

FIGURE 54-42 PTC catheter (PTC) traversing common bile duct iatrogenic injury. This catheter was used to guide ERCP stenting (ERCP) in a poor operative candidate with iatrogenic injury but common bile duct continuity.

complication, management is highly successful and restores health-related quality of life scores to preinjury levels.[21]

Lost Stones

In the era of laparoscopic cholecystectomy, inadvertent opening of the gallbladder with spillage of stones is not infrequent, occurring in 20% to 40% of cholecystectomies. Risk factors for intraoperative perforation of the gallbladder include cholecystitis, presence of pigmented stones, number of stones (>15), and performance of the operation by surgical resident. Unfortunately, stones lost during a cholecystectomy can have significant and even substantially delayed consequences, such as chronic abscess, fistula, wound infection, and bowel obstruction. Most dropped stones settle into Morison pouch or the retrohepatic space along the abdominal wall, which may develop into a chronic abscess in this location. The likelihood for development of complications from lost stones is difficult to quantify because surgeon documentation of gallbladder perforation is variable and a substantial delay frequently exists between cholecystectomy and complication from lost stones. On the basis of available studies, lost stones do not necessitate conversion to an open operation; treatment should include extensive irrigation, significant attempt to retrieve lost stones, course of antibiotics, documentation of the perforation in the operative notes, and clear communication with the patient of the small possibility of delayed presentation from erosion or abscess.[22]

Postcholecystectomy Pain

Although unusual, pain similar to biliary colic may persist or recur after cholecystectomy. A thorough evaluation of the biliary tree should be undertaken after cholecystectomy if the pain recurs.

Recurrence of pain, if it is associated with other system findings of jaundice, fever, or chills within days to weeks after cholecystectomy, suggests a secondary choledocholithiasis or a bile leak. Other biliary tree phenomena may cause a similar picture, such as sphincter of Oddi dysfunction. Postoperative bile duct strictures, which usually are manifested with jaundice, are generally identified within the first year after cholecystectomy and may be manifested with pain or fever if only one lobar duct is obstructed. In the setting of a normal liver panel, other causes of right upper quadrant pain should be investigated.

Retained Biliary Stones

Retained common bile duct stones, or secondary common duct stones, can be identified for up to 2 years after cholecystectomy. Secondary common duct stones, which, by definition, originate in the gallbladder and pass into the common duct, are usually cholesterol stones and frequently become symptomatic within weeks of a cholecystectomy. Patients will complain of sharp right upper quadrant pain, with jaundice. Fever, completing Charcot triad, is also common. Hyperbilirubinemia and an elevated alkaline phosphatase level should raise the suspicion of a retained stone. Ultrasound may not show intrahepatic biliary ductal dilation if the stone does not fully occlude the duct or the obstruction is early. Endoscopic removal of these stones through a generous sphincterotomy is almost universally successful (Fig. 54-43).

Biliary Leak

After a cholecystectomy, patients may suffer a leak from the cystic duct or an unrecognized duct of Luschka. Fever, chills, right upper quadrant pain, jaundice, leakage of bile from an incision or into a drain, or persistent anorexia or bloating should raise the

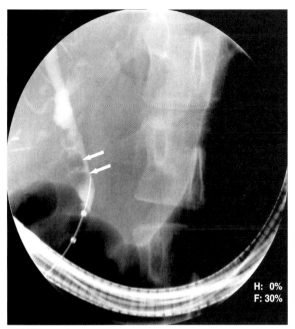

FIGURE 54-43 ERCP showing multiple retained common bile duct stones *(arrows)*.

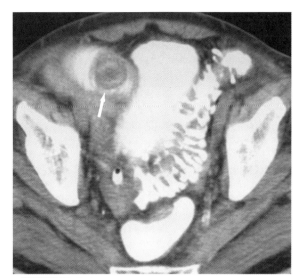

FIGURE 54-45 CT scan of stone *(arrow)* obstructing distal ileum.

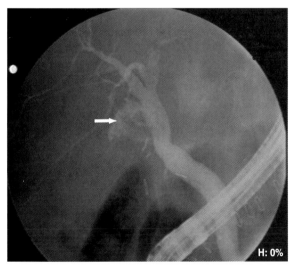

FIGURE 54-44 ERCP showing cystic duct stump leak *(arrow)*.

suspicion of a bile leak. Although it can be seen after any cholecystectomy, those performed for acute cholecystitis carry the greatest risk. With inflammation and fibrosis around an obstructed cystic duct, clips placed on the duct may not fully occlude it or may be dislodged as the inflammatory process resolves. Patients will generally present within 1 week of cholecystectomy as the bile collects and becomes clinically manifested. On presentation, CT should be performed and will show ascites or a right upper quadrant fluid collection consistent with a biloma. Not only is reexploration in this setting unsuccessful, but it further complicates later reconstruction attempts that may be necessary. Endoscopic cholangiography should be performed, with percutaneous drainage of any fluid collections (Fig. 54-44). If the leak is from a cystic duct stump, sphincterotomy with stenting of the common duct

will allow the leak to seal without need for surgical management.[20] Reexploration in this setting is reserved for patients with evidence of septic shock or those in whom the leakage is not percutaneously accessible. If percutaneous drainage is not feasible because of overlying bowel or the fluid is not localized and thus not amenable to percutaneous drainage, a laparoscopic washout of the abdomen and placement of subhepatic drains should be considered. No attempt should be made to fix the leak because any such intervention is almost always unsuccessful and carries a risk of further injury to the biliary tree. Persistence of a bile leak after longer than 6 weeks should raise the suspicion of an unrecognized bile duct injury, thus mandating complete cholangiography by MRCP and repeated ERCP. Similar to common bile duct injuries, surgical treatment of a duct leak is most successful once the inflammatory process has resolved.

Gallstone Ileus

Obstruction of the intestinal lumen from a gallstone carries the misnomer gallstone ileus, which is, in fact, a mechanical blockage. In order for a stone of sufficient size to obstruct the intestine, a large stone in the dependent portion of the gallbladder that has fistulized into the adjacent duodenum passes directly into the intestine. Most of these fistulas occur in older patients and may be caused by inflammation in the gallbladder or simply pressure necrosis. The blockage can be anywhere in the small intestine but occurs most commonly in the distal ileum as the ileum tapers before entering the cecum.

Presentation and diagnosis. Patients will present with clinical evidence of a mechanical small bowel obstruction in the absence of surgical history or hernias. A history of symptoms referable to the biliary tree is variable. Although most patients will have constant pain from the obstruction, others can present with only episodic discomfort because the gallstone only intermittently obstructs the intestinal tract. The most common site of stone impaction is in the distal ileum, a few centimeters proximal to the ileocecal valve, where the caliber of the ileum decreases (Fig. 54-45). Plain radiographs demonstrate air-fluid levels consistent with a small bowel obstruction, although the offending stone may or may not be identified. Pneumobilia, which may be identified only by CT scan, is a ubiquitous finding because the fistula that

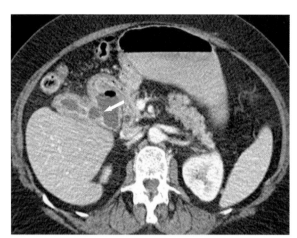

FIGURE 54-46 CT scan of cholecystoduodenal fistula *(arrow)*.

permitted a stone to pass into the duodenum allows air into the gallbladder and biliary tree (Fig. 54-46).

Treatment. Exploration and enterotomy are required to relieve the obstruction. A longitudinal incision is made on the antimesenteric border of the ileum, a few centimeters proximal to the impacted stone. The stone can then be milked back through the enterotomy. The site of impaction is at risk for ischemia and pressure necrosis, with eventual perforation. Therefore, any suggestion of nonviability of this region mandates resection. The remainder of the small intestine should be inspected because approximately 10% of patients will have multiple large stones that have passed through the fistula. Although some surgeons advocate surgical treatment of the biliary-enteric fistula at the same setting, the intense inflammatory process in the right upper quadrant may complicate the cholecystectomy and duodenal repair. In addition, because most of these patients are older, their overall physiologic status may not permit fistula repair in the emergent setting. One-stage repair should generally be performed in healthy patients without severe inflammatory changes in the right upper quadrant. Enterotomy with removal of the offending stone should suffice for patients with multiple comorbidities. Palpation of the remaining small intestine should be performed to exclude a second stone that could reobstruct the ileum. A second operation for the cholecystectomy can be considered to avoid the possibility of future biliary complications.

Acute Cholangitis

Acute cholangitis is due to an acute, ascending bacterial infection of the biliary tree caused by an obstruction. Although stones are a common cause, ascending cholangitis can be seen with any obstructing phenomenon, including a malignant neoplasm. The two absolute requirements for the development of acute cholangitis are bacteria in the biliary tree and obstruction of flow, with increased intraluminal pressure. The source of bactibilia in patients with acute cholangitis is unclear because culture of most bile is sterile. With obstruction from a stone, bactibilia can be identified in up to 90% of patients. The most common pathogens include *Klebsiella, E. coli, Enterobacter, Pseudomonas,* and *Citrobacter* spp.

The classic presentation of cholangitis is that of Charcot triad, with fever, jaundice, and right upper quadrant pain. All three findings are seen in less than 50% of patients, with jaundice being the most variable. When the infection begins to be manifested

with shock, the two additional findings of mental status changes and hypotension join Charcot triad to become Reynolds pentad. With the acute obstruction of a visceral tubular structure, the pain can be severe but is not usually associated with abdominal tenderness.

Diagnosis. As with any severe intra-abdominal infection, tachycardia and manifestations of shock are not uncommon. Leukocytosis with an abnormal liver panel is common. Hepatocellular injury from the infection and inflammation elevate serum transaminase and alkaline phosphatase levels. Ultrasound should be the first screening test and will commonly show dilation of the biliary tree. HIDA scans should be interpreted with caution because infection of the biliary tree reduces the secretion of these agents into the biliary tree. CT can be helpful in identifying the site of obstruction although not always the cause. Cholangiography through ERCP or PTC is critical not only to diagnosis but also to therapy. These two modalities can usually identify the location and cause of obstruction, drain the biliary tree, and obtain culture and biopsy specimens of a lesion if necessary.

Treatment. Acute cholangitis is a severe medical condition that can progress quickly to septic shock and death. Adequate hydration and IV antibiotics should be started immediately. Many patients will respond to medical therapy, so prompt diagnostic measures should be taken to identify the location and cause of obstruction. Others, however, will not respond to medical therapy and will progress to shock. These patients require emergent decompression of the biliary tree. Historically, this could be achieved only through a surgical route, with high morbidity and mortality. Endoscopic or percutaneous drainage achieves the same goal with less morbidity. Removal of the stone can be accomplished by endoscopic means, thus providing an advantage over percutaneous methods, which simply decompress the obstructed biliary tree. If endoscopic and percutaneous means are unavailable or unsuccessful, surgical drainage consists of common duct exploration with placement of a T tube. Given the unstable nature of the patient, definitive surgical treatment of the cause is deferred until the patient is stabilized, the cholangitis is treated, and the diagnosis is confirmed.

Recurrent Pyogenic Cholangitis

Recurrent pyogenic cholangitis is caused by cholangiohepatitis or intrahepatic stones and is usually found in East Asian populations. Biliary pathogens such as *Clonorchis sinensis* and *Ascaris lumbricoides* populate the biliary tree. These and other pathogens secrete an enzyme that hydrolyzes water-soluble bilirubin glucuronides to form free bilirubin, which then precipitates to form brown pigment stones. These stones may partially or fully obstruct the biliary tree, causing recurrent episodes of cholangitis and eventually abscesses or even cirrhosis. The chronicity of the infection and inflammation places these patients at risk for the development of cholangiocarcinoma. It is unclear whether the primary inciting event is infection causing inflammatory stricture or inflammatory stricture with subsequent infection of stagnant bile.

Presentation. Recurrent pyogenic cholangitis tends to occur in the third to fourth decade of life, affecting men and women equally. The clinical presentation is that of cholangitis with fever, right upper quadrant pain, and jaundice. Because the infection, inflammation, and stones commonly present in a segmental or lobar pattern, the jaundice tends to be mild. Serum studies are similar to other causes of cholangitis, with a leukocytosis and elevated bilirubin and high alkaline phosphatase levels. Diagnosis is usually made by a combination of CT or MRCP with ERCP

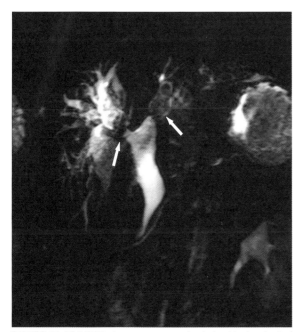

FIGURE 54-47 MRCP of recurrent pyogenic cholangitis. Intraluminal filling defects from stones are noted in both lobes *(arrows).*

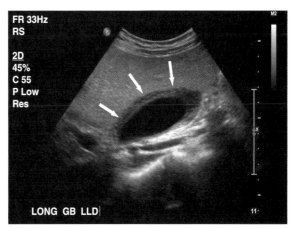

FIGURE 54-48 Ultrasound image of gallbladder with acute acalculous cholecystitis. The diffusely thickened gallbladder wall *(arrows)* is highly suggestive of cholecystitis.

(Fig. 54-47). Lobar or segmental atrophy or hypertrophy may be seen in chronic cases.

Treatment. In the setting of an acute attack, conservative treatment with parenteral antibiotics, IV fluids, and analgesics will usually suffice. Failure of this approach, with clinical deterioration, mandates biliary drainage by ERCP or percutaneous methods. Once the attack has subsided, a thorough investigation of biliary tree anatomy will help direct treatment. Definitive operative treatment is almost always required. The goals of surgical therapy are threefold: (1) remove all stones; (2) bypass, enlarge, or resect the strictures; and (3) provide adequate biliary drainage. The variability of presentation and location of disease has spurred the development of a number of operations to achieve these goals. The presence of intrahepatic strictures connotes a complicated case and may warrant resection, stricturoplasty, or hepaticocutaneous jejunostomy. When clearance of all stones is not possible or future need for endoscopic therapy is anticipated, the terminal end of the Roux limb for a hepaticojejunostomy can be brought out as a stoma to provide easy access for choledochoscopy. Given the risk of cholangiocarcinoma, disease affecting predominantly one lobe should be resected in patients with adequate hepatic reserve. In the absence of the development of cholangiocarcinoma, surgical management is highly successful.[23]

Noncalculous Biliary Disease
Acute Acalculous Cholecystitis
Any blockage of the cystic duct is known as acute cholecystitis. When this occurs in the absence of stones, the diagnosis is acute acalculous cholecystitis. Although the exact pathophysiologic mechanism is poorly understood, concentration of biliary solutes and stasis in the gallbladder clearly play important roles. Risk factors for the development of acalculous cholecystitis include older age, critical illness, burns, trauma, prolonged use of total parenteral nutrition, diabetes, and immunosuppression. The disease process is generally more fulminant than that of calculous

cholecystitis and may progress to gangrene and perforation of the gallbladder.

The presentation of acalculous cholecystitis can be similar to that of calculous disease, with fever, anorexia, and right upper quadrant pain. Because many of these patients are critically ill, history may be impossible to obtain and the physical examination may be unreliable. The workup of fever in the intensive care patient may reveal a thickened gallbladder wall, with pericholecystic fluid (Fig. 54-48). HIDA scans may make the diagnosis but can have a false-positive rate of up to 40%.

Treatment of acalculous cholecystitis is similar to that of calculous cholecystitis, with cholecystectomy being therapeutic. Given the substantial inflammation and high risk of gallbladder gangrene, an open procedure is generally preferred. However, many of these patients are critically ill and would not tolerate the physiologic insult of a laparotomy, explaining why the mortality rate of cholecystectomy for acalculous cholecystitis is up to 40%. Accordingly, percutaneous drainage of the distended and inflamed gallbladder is carried out in patients unable to tolerate a laparotomy. The cholecystostomy tube used to drain the gallbladder can be placed by ultrasound or CT guidance. Approximately 90% of patients will improve with percutaneous drainage, and the tube can eventually be removed. If follow-up imaging continues to demonstrate no stones, interval cholecystectomy is generally unnecessary.

Primary Sclerosing Cholangitis
Primary sclerosing cholangitis (PSC) is an idiopathic, likely autoimmune process affecting the intrahepatic and extrahepatic biliary trees. Although the cause is unknown, it is associated with other autoimmune diseases, such as ulcerative colitis and Riedel thyroiditis. As its name suggests, the disease causes inflammation and scarring in the biliary tree and must be distinguished from secondary sclerosing cholangitis, which involves a similar clinical picture but has an identifiable cause, such as malignant neoplasm, infection, or ischemia. The disease of PSC is characterized by progressive chronic cholestasis and advances at an unpredictable rate to biliary cirrhosis and eventually death from liver failure. Although historically the diagnosis was made only in the late stages of disease, understanding of the disease as well as increased frequency of liver function analyses and increased use of ERCP has contributed to earlier diagnosis, frequently in the asymptomatic phase.

The microscopic picture is one of inflammation, fibrosis, and cholestasis. In the absence of previous biliary manipulation, acute ascending cholangitis is uncommon in patients presenting with PSC.

Clinical presentation. The presentation of PSC is variable, but most patients present with fatigue, pruritus, and jaundice. This symptom complex spurs the physician to perform ERCP, although many patients have symptoms for 12 to 24 months before the diagnosis is made. The abnormalities seen on cholangiography confirm the diagnosis. Asymptomatic elevations of alkaline phosphatase levels can also occur and may be associated with evidence of hepatocellular injury and hyperbilirubinemia before clinical manifestations of symptoms. Abnormal liver function tests in a patient observed for inflammatory bowel disease should suggest PSC. Elevation of perinuclear antineutrophil cytoplasmic antibodies can be seen in 80% of patients. Disease severity does not correlate with perinuclear antineutrophil cytoplasmic antibody titer.

ERCP is the preferred route for cholangiography and can demonstrate the characteristic multifocal, diffusely distributed dilations and strictures of the intrahepatic and extrahepatic biliary trees. The sequential stricturing, proximal dilation, and more proximal stricturing create a pattern described as beading or chain of lakes. PTC is frequently unsuccessful because the proximal ducts are both fibrosed and generally not dilated. Other cholangiographic findings include multiple diverticulum-like outpouchings of the bile ducts and multiple short-segment strictures. MRCP can also be useful for diagnosis and monitoring of disease but does not allow interventions that may be necessary, such as brushing, balloon dilation, or stenting (Fig. 54-49). Liver biopsy tends to show an onionskin concentric periductal fibrosis. With disease progression, periportal fibrosis occurs, progressing to bridging necrosis and eventually biliary cirrhosis. Unfortunately, PSC is associated with cholangiocarcinoma, and distinguishing the strictures of PSC fibrosis from those of cholangiocarcinoma can be challenging.

Treatment. No specific effective medical therapy exists for PSC. Although some experimental trials of ursodeoxycholic acid have shown improvement in liver function test results and histologic appearance compared with controls, this did not result in any significant clinical improvement in the long term. Early in the disease, with mild symptoms, observation is a reasonable approach. Intervention must be specifically tailored to the pattern of disease and its clinical manifestations. Medical therapies are generally targeted to the underlying hepatobiliary disease process; these include choleretic agents such as ursodeoxycholic acid, immunosuppressive agents, and antifibrogenic agents such as colchicine. However, none of these agents has shown a consistent benefit. In the symptomatic patient, endoscopic therapy, consisting of balloon dilation of the dominant strictures, has been shown to alleviate pruritus, to reduce likelihood of cholangitis, and even to prolong survival.

With the lack of effective, durable medical therapy in this progressive and ultimately fatal disease, an aggressive surgical approach is advocated. Options include biliary reconstructive procedures and liver transplantation. Although it is associated with ulcerative colitis, proctocolectomy does not appear to affect biliary disease progression or survival in patients with both ulcerative colitis and PSC. Biliary reconstruction is an option for patients with a dominant stricture at the hepatic bifurcation, for which resection of this region with long-term Silastic stenting can be performed. With increased success of orthotopic liver transplantation, the use of biliary reconstructive procedures has decreased.

Orthotopic liver transplantation appears to be the only lifesaving option for patients with progressive hepatic dysfunction from PSC. The survival rate for patients undergoing liver transplantation for PSC is approximately equivalent to that of those undergoing transplantation for other noninfectious end-stage liver disease causes, with 5-year survival rates ranging from 75% to 85%.[24] Although the development of cholangiocarcinoma in a PSC liver is generally considered a contraindication to transplantation, some centers have shown excellent survival rates, up to 70% at 5 years, for patients with limited disease localized within the liver who undergo an extensive neoadjuvant protocol of chemotherapy and radiation followed by transplantation.[25] Because these results have not been reproduced universally, the use of liver transplantation for the treatment of cholangiocarcinoma occurring in the setting of PSC is limited to experimental protocols. After liver transplantation, many PSC patients develop strictures, raising the possibility of recurrence of disease in the donor liver. Biopsy may show identical findings to the original disease, but this is obviously complicated by the possibility of development of secondary sclerosing cholangitis from ischemia, infection, or rejection. Even with the development of strictures, disease progression does not usually follow the aggressive course for which PSC is known.

Biliary Strictures

Benign strictures of the bile duct have a number of causes and generally affect the extrahepatic biliary tree, although cholangiohepatitis can create intrahepatic biliary strictures as well. Any inflammatory process occurring along the length of the common bile duct can cause a stricture. For example, the fibrotic inflammatory process of chronic pancreatitis can create a stricture of the intrapancreatic portion of the bile duct. The cholangiographic pattern of this stricture is that of a long (2 to 4 cm), smooth, gradually tapered narrowing affecting the distal common bile duct.

Strictures may occur in the middle portion of the common duct and are frequently associated with a process in the gallbladder. Any inflammatory process involving the gallbladder and cystic duct can secondarily inflame the common bile duct, causing an obstruction. Alternatively, a large stone in Hartmann pouch

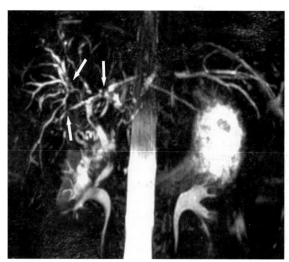

FIGURE 54-49 MRCP showing primary sclerosing cholangitis. Note the multilevel strictures *(arrows).*

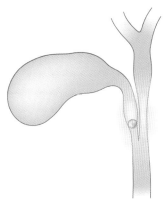

FIGURE 54-50 Mirizzi Syndrome. Obstruction of the bile duct from an inflammatory process is the hallmark of this syndrome; the cholecystocholedochal fistula may or may not be apparent.

can compress the adjacent bile duct and cause an apparent stricture. Both of these fall under the diagnosis of Mirizzi syndrome (Fig. 54-50). The prerequisites for this syndrome, characterized by gallbladder disease causing obstructive jaundice, include a cystic duct that courses parallel to the common hepatic duct, an impacted stone in the gallbladder neck or cystic duct, and an obstruction of the common hepatic duct caused by the stone or inflammatory response. The resultant inflammation can cause a cholecystocholedochal fistula. The treatment of Mirizzi syndrome is cholecystectomy, which may require repair of the common duct; when a large fistula exists, a choledochojejunostomy may be necessary.

Other strictures of the biliary tree include inflammatory strictures from long-standing choledocholithiasis, which tends to occur in the intrapancreatic portion of the bile duct, and stenosis of the sphincter of Oddi. ERCP with sphincterotomy, balloon dilation, and stent placement is generally regarded as primary treatment for benign bile duct strictures to make the diagnosis and potentially to treat the process. Endoscopic and percutaneous therapy can provide long-term success in more than 50% of patients. When this is unsuccessful, surgical management with anastomosis of the biliary tree to a Roux-en-Y jejunal limb has success rates of up to 90%.

Biliary Cysts

Cysts of the biliary tree are rare, occurring in fewer than 1/100,000 patients, but are more common in those of Asian descent and are three to eight times more common in women than in men. Biliary cysts, known as choledochal cysts, are considered a premalignant condition requiring surgical intervention. They are commonly diagnosed in infancy, but many present in adulthood. Although not proven, the commonly accepted theory of their pathogenesis relies on the presence of an anomalous pancreaticobiliary junction (APBJ; Figs. 54-51 and 54-52).

With APBJ, the pancreatic duct and biliary tree fuse to form a common channel before passage through the duodenal wall; APBJ is seen in up to 90% of patients with choledochal cysts. The fused duct forms a long common channel, which allows pancreatic secretions to reflux into the biliary tree. Because the pancreatic duct has higher secretory pressures than the biliary tree, exocrine pancreatic secretions reflux up into the bile duct and can inflame and damage the biliary tree, resulting in cystic degeneration.

The original classification for choledochal cysts by Alonso-Lej and colleagues has been modified by Todani and associates to

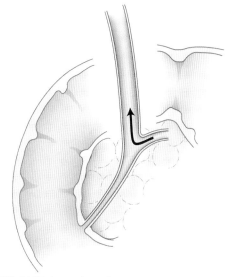

FIGURE 54-51 Anomalous Pancreaticobiliary Junction. With fusion of the common bile duct and pancreatic duct long before they pass through the duodenal wall, the pancreatic secretions can reflux into the common bile duct and may cause damage to the common duct through pressure or chemical injury.

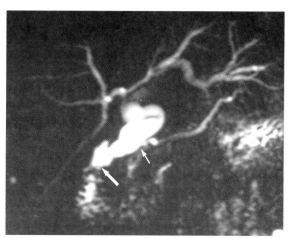

FIGURE 54-52 MRCP showing anomalous pancreaticobiliary junction with long common channel. The pancreatic duct fuses with the common bile duct (slender arrow), and the common channel enters the duodenum (bold arrow). Also noted in this illustration is the fusiform dilation of only the extrahepatic bile duct, as seen in a type I choledochal cyst.

include intrahepatic cystic disease (Fig. 54-53).[26] The most common choledochal cyst, type I, involves only the extrahepatic biliary tree and is generally a fusiform dilation. Type II cysts appear as a saccular diverticulum off the common bile duct and may be mistaken for an accessory gallbladder. Type III cysts appear as a cystic dilation of the intramural common bile duct, within the wall of the duodenum, and are also known as choledochoceles. Cysts involving the intrahepatic and extrahepatic biliary tree are known as type IVa, with type IVb being multiple cysts limited to the extrahepatic biliary tree. Type V cysts, also known as Caroli disease, involve the intrahepatic ducts only. Type V cysts may be solitary but usually occur diffusely in all segments. Although classified as a single disease, debate continues as to whether these constitute more than one pathologic entity.

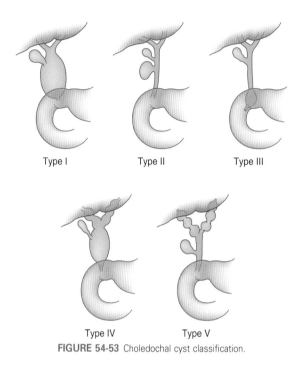

Type I   Type II   Type III

Type IV   Type V

FIGURE 54-53 Choledochal cyst classification.

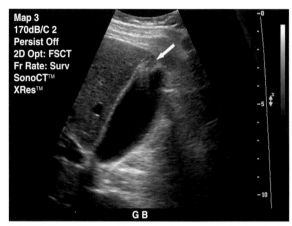

FIGURE 54-54 Ultrasound image of adenomyomatosis. Seen in the fundus of the gallbladder is a sessile thickening *(arrow)* with smaller microcysts within it, consistent with adenomyomatosis.

Presentation. The classic presentation of jaundice, right upper quadrant pain, and a palpable mass occurs rarely. Most patients have two of the three symptoms, with jaundice being the most consistent symptom, before undergoing any diagnostic imaging. Other symptoms include nausea, pruritus, and weight loss. Long-standing disease can induce a chronic injury to the liver with cirrhosis. Cholangitis, pancreatitis, hepatic fibrosis, and malignant disease have all been reported at the time of presentation. An unusual presentation is that of acute rupture of the cyst, with subsequent bile peritonitis.

Most cystic biliary lesions are originally identified and subsequently diagnosed by imaging because the common presenting symptoms are nonspecific. With the current liberal use of CT, the diagnosis of a choledochal cyst is suspected, but it is further classified by MRCP. With a choledochal cyst, the upper biliary tree is difficult to fill and therefore to evaluate by a retrograde route. Accordingly, MRCP helps create a complete cholangiogram. The distal bile duct is difficult to analyze by MRCP, so ERCP is more useful for defining the distal biliary tree and pancreatic duct–bile duct junction. Laboratory studies may identify cholestasis and jaundice. In late stages of disease, secondary hepatic injury and evidence of cirrhosis may be seen.

Because choledochal cysts are a premalignant condition, the original presentation of a choledochal cyst may be that of cholangiocarcinoma. The incidence of malignant disease in patients with biliary cysts ranges from 10% to 30%. The pathogenesis appears to be one of a field defect because the entire biliary tree is at risk, even in nondilated portions of the biliary tract, and complete excision of a benign choledochal cyst does not eliminate the risk of subsequent cholangiocarcinoma development. Malignant cyst degeneration is common and is thought to relate to chronic mucosal irritation from the refluxed pancreatic enzymes.

Treatment. Surgical management of choledochal cysts consists of resection of the entire cyst and appropriate surgical reconstruction. Historically, enteric drainage of the cyst was performed without resection, but this approach is complicated by recurrent

biliary stasis, infection, and development of malignancy. Type I cysts are treated by complete surgical excision, cholecystectomy, and Roux-en-Y hepaticojejunostomy. The proximal extent of resection should continue to the nondilated biliary tree and may require anastomosis to the left and right hepatic ducts. If there is substantial pericyst fibrosis, an intramural plane can be developed to excise the entire epithelium while leaving the fibrotic outer cyst wall in place. The distal duct is oversewn, with care taken not to injure the pancreatic duct. Type II cysts should be excised entirely, and in the presence of an APBJ, biliary-enteric diversion by Roux-en-Y hepaticojejunostomy is appropriate. Type III cysts are uncommon and may be approached transduodenally. Because the pathogenesis of type III cysts is not clear and may not involve APBJ, endoscopic drainage may suffice. In the setting of duodenal or biliary obstruction, transduodenal excision or sphincteroplasty can be performed. Surgical treatment of type IV cysts must be carefully individualized to the affected anatomy. Type IV cysts affecting only the extrahepatic bile ducts are managed similarly to type I cysts, with excision and hepaticojejunostomy. Those with intrahepatic extension involving only one lobe can be treated with partial hepatectomy and reconstruction. Surgical treatment of Caroli disease ranges from resection if the disease is unilobar to liver transplantation when diffuse disease is detected.

Polypoid Lesions of the Gallbladder

Benign masses of the gallbladder are common and consist of pseudotumors and adenomas. Pseudotumors are further divided into cholesterol polyps and adenomyomatosis. Cholesterol polyps appear as pedunculated echogenic lesions of the gallbladder, are usually smaller than 1 cm, and are frequently multiple. Alternatively, adenomyomatosis is seen as a sessile lesion, commonly in the fundus, with characteristic microcysts within the lesion, and is frequently larger than 1 cm (Fig. 54-54). Adenomas are benign growths in the wall of the gallbladder that may be difficult to differentiate from adenocarcinoma preoperatively because the only difference is that of transmural invasion, which can be challenging to detect by ultrasonography. Size larger than 10 mm is a risk factor for adenocarcinoma, along with growth, presence of gallstones, and age of the patient older than 60 years. The management of all symptomatic polypoid lesions of the gallbladder is laparoscopic cholecystectomy. Patients with a polypoid lesion and risk factors for adenocarcinoma or those suspected of having in situ or invasive cancer should undergo open cholecystectomy because perforation during laparoscopy may spread tumor cells throughout the peritoneal cavity. Asymptomatic lesions smaller than 10 mm with no other risk factors and no ultrasonographic features suggesting malignant disease can be observed with serial ultrasonography.

Benign Biliary Masses

Benign intraluminal growths of the biliary tree are unusual but mostly consist of adenomas. These lesions are soft fleshy growths occurring mostly in the periampullary bile duct arising from the glandular epithelium. The presentation is that of biliary obstruction, with jaundice and sometimes right upper quadrant pain. Treatment consists of complete resection with a small rim of normal epithelium because incomplete excision of affected epithelium carries a high risk of recurrence. These lesions occur in the periampullary duct, so a transduodenal approach can be used.

Inflammatory lesions of the biliary tree, known as pseudotumors or benign fibrosing disease, may be mistaken for cholangiocarcinoma. When this process follows surgical intervention on the biliary tree, the mass-like stricture may be the result of ischemia to the duct, with subsequent inflammation and fibrosis. Alternatively, pseudotumors may occur de novo; these commonly affect the extrahepatic biliary tree above the bifurcation.

MALIGNANT BILIARY DISEASE

Gallbladder Cancer

Gallbladder cancer is an aggressive malignant disease and carries an extremely poor prognosis. Patients have no specific presenting symptoms, and therefore presentation with late-stage disease is common. The poor prognosis corresponds to the high proportion of patients presenting with advanced disease. For patients with earlier stage disease, a more aggressive surgical approach is warranted.

Incidence

Gallbladder cancer generally is manifested in the sixth and seventh decades of life and is two to three times more common in women than in men. Ethnicity plays an important role in the development of gallbladder cancer, with the highest incidence in women from India and Pakistan. Among North American populations, Native Americans and immigrants from Latin America have the highest rates.

Cause

Although not proven scientifically, the prevailing theory of gallbladder cancer focuses on chronic inflammation with subsequent cellular proliferation. Therefore, the presence of gallstones is considered to be the primary risk factor, and larger stones (>3 cm) carry an increased risk of cancer development. More than 80% of patients with gallbladder cancer have cholelithiasis, and gallbladder cancer is approximately seven times more common in patients with gallstones than in those without stones. The type of stone does not correlate with incidence of gallbladder cancer. Other risk factors include entities that may also cause inflammation in the gallbladder wall, such as APBJ, choledochal cysts, and PSC.

Extensive calcification of the wall of the gallbladder can cause a brittle gallbladder wall, leading to what is termed porcelain gallbladder, and carries a risk of cancer development, as does the presence of a gallbladder polyp larger than 10 mm. Whereas the risk of gallbladder cancer is higher in patients with gallbladder wall

calcification, malignant disease in this setting is unusual, occurring in less than 10% of patients with porcelain gallbladder.[27]

Pathology and Staging

Gallbladder cancer is generally adenocarcinoma. Pathologic specimens show the progression from dysplasia to carcinoma in situ to invasive carcinoma, as has been described for other carcinomas; it is staged by the standard TNM staging system (Table 54-1).[28] A small subset of gallbladder cancers are of the papillary subtype and carry a significantly better prognosis as they tend to have an indolent course and are commonly limited to the gallbladder wall at the time of diagnosis (Fig. 54-55). Most gallbladder carcinomas, however, have systemic disease at the time of presentation, with nodal disease in 35% and distant metastases in 40%.

The draining nodal basin for gallbladder cancer includes the hepatoduodenal ligament. From there, affected lymph nodes may include periaortic nodes near the celiac axis or pancreaticoduodenal nodes around the superior mesenteric artery. Because the

TABLE 54-1 Staging for Gallbladder Cancer

Primary Tumor (T)

TX	Primary tumor cannot be assessed
T0	No evidence of primary tumor
Tis	Carcinoma in situ
T1	Tumor invades lamina propria or muscle layer
T1a	Tumor invades lamina propria
T1b	Tumor invades muscle layer
T2	Tumor invades perimuscular connective tissue; no extension beyond serosa or into liver
T3	Tumor perforates the serosa (visceral peritoneum) and/or directly invades the liver and/or one other adjacent organ or structure, such as the stomach, duodenum, colon, pancreas, omentum, or extrahepatic bile ducts
T4	Tumor invades main portal vein or hepatic artery or invades two or more extrahepatic organs or structures

Regional Lymph Nodes (N)

NX	Regional lymph nodes cannot be assessed
N0	No regional lymph node metastasis
N1	Metastases to nodes along the cystic duct, common bile duct, hepatic artery, and/or portal vein
N2	Metastases to periaortic, pericaval, superior mesenteric artery and/or celiac artery lymph nodes

Distant Metastasis (M)

M0	No distant metastasis
M1	Distant metastasis

Anatomic Stage and Prognostic Groups

Stage 0	Tis	N0	M0
Stage I	T1	N0	M0
Stage II	T2	N0	M0
Stage IIIA	T3	N0	M0
Stage IIIB	T1-3	N1	M0
Stage IVA	T4	N0-1	M0
Stage IVB	Any T	N2	M0
	Any T	Any N	M1

From Edge SB, Byrd DR, Compton CC, et al, editors: *AJCC cancer staging manual*, ed 7, New York, 2010, Springer, pp 213–214.

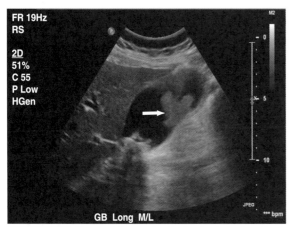

FIGURE 54-55 Ultrasound image showing intraluminal polypoid gallbladder wall mass *(arrow)* but without extraluminal extension.

venous drainage of the gallbladder includes direct venous tributaries into the liver parenchyma, these tumors may spread directly into segment IV of the liver. Transperitoneal spread is also common and can progress to carcinomatosis.

Clinical Presentation

Because 90% of gallbladder cancers originate in the fundus or body of the gallbladder, most do not produce symptoms until the disease is advanced (Fig. 54-56). Symptoms of acute cholecystitis, with obstruction of the neck of the gallbladder, may portend a better prognosis because patients with these symptoms may present with earlier stages of disease. Weight loss, jaundice, or an abdominal mass is associated with later stages of disease. Some patients describe symptoms of chronic cholecystitis in which the pain has recently changed in quality or frequency. Other common symptoms include chronic epigastric pain, early satiety, and a sense of fullness.

Diagnosis

Ultrasonography is generally the first examination used in the evaluation of right upper quadrant pain. Ultrasonographic findings of gallbladder cancer include an irregularly shaped lesion in the subhepatic space, heterogeneous mass in the gallbladder lumen, and asymmetrically thickened gallbladder wall (Fig. 54-57). The finding of a polyp larger than 10 mm should raise the suspicion of gallbladder cancer.

CT can be useful in the staging and therefore treatment of gallbladder cancer. Although the sensitivity of CT for detection of direct extension into the liver is poor, CT can demonstrate peritoneal metastases, hepatic parenchymal metastases, lymphadenopathy, and adjacent vascular involvement (Fig. 54-58). Cholangiography can help delineate the location of obstruction in patients with gallbladder cancer, but most of these patients are incurable. Triphasic CT can be used to identify hepatic arterial or portal venous involvement. In the setting of unresectability (portal vein encasement or extensive hepatic involvement) or incurability (hepatic or peritoneal metastases), percutaneous methods for confirmatory tissue diagnosis should be used.

Treatment

Resection of gallbladder cancer remains the only potential for cure. Patients with gallbladder cancer can be divided into four specific subgroups of presentation: patients with an incidental

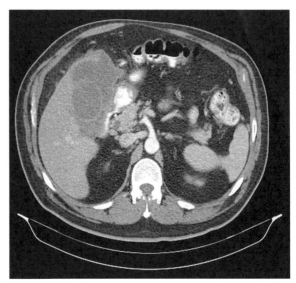

FIGURE 54-56 CT scan showing gallbladder cancer with invasion into the duodenum and liver parenchyma.

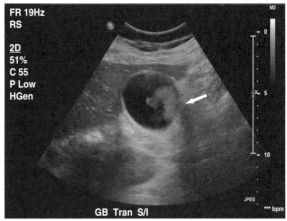

FIGURE 54-57 Ultrasound image of gallbladder mass with loss of continuity of gallbladder wall *(arrow)*, suggesting extraluminal growth.

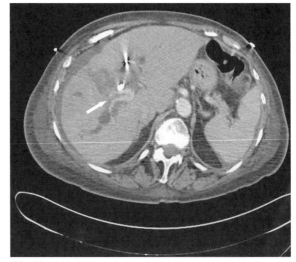

FIGURE 54-58 CT scan showing gallbladder mass with local invasion into portal vein *(arrow)*.

polyp on imaging, patients with an incidental finding of gallbladder cancer at the time of or after cholecystectomy, patients suspected of having gallbladder cancer preoperatively, and patients with advanced disease at presentation.

Patients with incidental findings

Gallbladder polyp. Because gallbladder polyps larger than 10 mm carry an increased risk of malignancy, cholecystectomy is the treatment of choice. It should be performed through an open approach because laparoscopic perforation in the setting of cancer may convert a potentially curable disease into an incurable one.

Gallbladder cancer after cholecystectomy. With the finding of carcinoma after cholecystectomy, subsequent treatment depends on depth of penetration of the gallbladder wall and surgical margins. With T1a lesions, in which the carcinoma penetrates the lamina propria but does not invade the muscle layer, cholecystectomy should suffice for therapy. The likelihood of nodal disease in this setting is less than 3%. For those penetrating the muscularis but not the deeper connective tissue or serosa, classified as T1b lesions, cholecystectomy is sufficient as long as the margins are negative. With T1b lesions and perineural, lymphatic, or vascular invasion, the likelihood of nodal disease increases significantly, and therefore an extended cholecystectomy is indicated. The extended cholecystectomy is directed at obtaining an R0 resection of the disease, including the draining lymph node basins. Therefore, removal of the pericholedochal, periportal, hepatoduodenal, right celiac, and posterior pancreaticoduodenal lymph nodes should be included. Resection of the cystic duct margin to uninvolved mucosa may require resection of the common bile duct with Roux-en-Y reconstruction. Because local extension into the hepatic parenchyma is common, 2 cm of apparently normal hepatic parenchyma from the gallbladder fossa is resected. As port site recurrences have been reported for patients with even in situ disease, all port sites should also be excised. In patients with T2 lesions, in which the cancer extends past the muscularis but not beyond the serosa, a similar approach with radical cholecystectomy is indicated because more than 40% of these patients have lymph node metastases and up to 25% have positive margins when treated with standard cholecystectomy alone. Because gallbladder cancer is generally unresponsive to other therapies, the presence of any residual disease after operative intervention predicts poor outcome.[29]

Patients suspected of having gallbladder cancer preoperatively. Patients in whom preoperative evaluation suggests possibly resectable gallbladder cancer without metastatic disease should be offered an attempt at resection, even though survival is poor compared with those found incidentally. These patients tend to present with advanced locoregional disease and may require an extended liver resection. Because surgical intervention provides the only potential for cure or prolongation of life, radical resection should be considered for adequate operative candidates. The operation begins with a diagnostic laparoscopy to identify small-volume peritoneal or hepatic metastases that would preclude a resection, thereby avoiding an unnecessary operation. In the setting of metastatic disease, nonoperative strategies should be used to palliate symptoms. Radical resection in the setting of T3 and T4 lesions includes at least segments IVB and V but more often requires a central hepatectomy, including all of segments IV, V, and VIII. If necessary to achieve R0 margin status, a right trisegmentectomy may be used. Direct extension of tumor into adjacent structures such as the hepatic flexure is not a contraindication to resection as long as negative margins can be obtained and all disease resected. Debulking without the possibility of complete resection has no role in the management of gallbladder cancer.

Patients with advanced disease at presentation. Many patients with gallbladder cancer will present with advanced disease, and therefore the goal of therapy is palliation of symptoms. Common symptoms requiring palliation include jaundice, pain, and intestinal obstruction. Jaundice can be managed by endoscopic biliary stenting, and self-expanding endobiliary metal stents can provide a durable solution, with less need for repeated interventions than with plastic stents. Pain is generally treated with oral narcotics but may progress to require parenteral opioids in the hospice setting. Percutaneous neurolysis of the celiac ganglion can help with the palliation of pain. Intestinal obstruction is usually gastric outlet obstruction from local extension of tumor and is generally managed by an endoscopic duodenal wall stent. Unfortunately, neither chemotherapy nor radiation therapy has shown a survival benefit in the management of gallbladder cancer.

Survival

Survival of patients diagnosed with gallbladder cancer is dependent on the stage of disease at presentation and whether surgical resection is performed. Independent factors affecting survival include T status, N status, histologic differentiation, and common bile duct involvement. Advances in surgical management and extent of resection have led to improvements in survival in surgical patients, although most patients present with late-stage disease and are not candidates for resection. Patients with T1a lesions, limited to the mucosa and lamina propria, have an excellent prognosis. Complete resection of T1b lesions to negative margins also affords an excellent prognosis. Survival of patients with T2 lesions depends on nodal status, and radical resection in this setting improves 5-year survival from approximately 20% to more than 60%. The 5-year survival of patients with T3 tumors is less than 20%, and patients with T4 lesions have a survival measured in months. Patients with metastatic disease at presentation have a median survival of 13 months. Because most patients with gallbladder cancer present with advanced disease, the overall survival of gallbladder cancer is less than 15%.

Bile Duct Cancer

Cholangiocarcinoma is a rare disease entity that carries a dismal prognosis. Historically, evaluation and management of cholangiocarcinoma required arbitrary division of the bile duct into thirds based on the location of obstruction. Lesions of the middle third, however, are decidedly rare, so investigations have recently focused on perihilar and intrahepatic lesions, known as proximal lesions, versus those involving the periampullary region, known as distal disease. More than two thirds of all cholangiocarcinomas involve the proximal biliary tree near the bifurcation, known as Klatskin tumor.

Risk Factors

Although most patients with cholangiocarcinoma have no identifiable cause, the risk of development of cholangiocarcinoma appears to correlate with chronic inflammation in the biliary tree and compensatory cellular proliferation. Therefore, many predisposing disease states carry an increased risk for development of cholangiocarcinoma. Congenital lesions, such as choledochal cysts, predispose to the development of cholangiocarcinoma from exposure of the biliary epithelium to toxic pancreatic secretions. Cholangiocarcinoma is more prevalent in Southeast Asia, where infection with the liver flukes *Clonorchis sinensis* and *Opisthorchis viverrini* creates chronic biliary inflammation, with obstructions and strictures. Recurrent pyogenic cholangitis is characterized by primary bile duct stone formation with infections and carries a risk of cholangiocarcinoma development. Finally, PSC, with its autoimmune multifocal strictures of the intrahepatic and extrahepatic biliary trees, carries an increased risk of cholangiocarcinoma. Although sporadic cases of cholangiocarcinoma tend to occur at the bifurcation, patients with PSC may have multifocal disease not amenable to resection. Medications and chemical carcinogens have been associated with the development of cholangiocarcinoma, including Thorotrast, oral contraceptives, asbestos, and cigarette smoke.

Staging and Classification

The three distinct pathologic subtypes include sclerosing, nodular, and papillary cholangiocarcinoma. Sclerosing cholangiocarcinoma tends to occur in the proximal bile ducts, causing periductal fibrosis in a concentric pattern and a circumferential duct occlusion. The papillary and nodular subtypes tend to occur in distal cholangiocarcinomas and are manifested with intraluminal growths. In the nodular subtype, a firm mass based in the duct wall can be seen growing into the duct lumen, whereas the more common papillary subtype appears as a polypoid lesion that is soft, with less periductal fibrosis and a better prognosis.

The staging of cholangiocarcinoma relies on the TNM staging system but is slightly different on the basis of anatomic location. The three staging subdivisions include intrahepatic (Table 54-2),

extrahepatic (Table 54-3), and distal bile duct (Table 54-4).[28] Similar to many adenocarcinomas, direct local invasion and local lymph node spread are common and portend a worse prognosis. Tumors confined to the bile duct (T1) and those extending outside the bile duct but not invading adjacent structures such as the hepatic artery or portal vein (T2) carry a significantly better prognosis than those invading any nearby structure. The two pathologic factors most influencing prognosis after resection are complete (R0) resection to negative margins and absence of lymph node metastases.

Clinical Presentation

The presentation of cholangiocarcinoma depends on the site of origin and manifestations of biliary obstruction at that site. Painless jaundice is a common symptom, but patients with unilobar obstruction of a bile duct may present with unilateral lobar

---

TABLE 54-2 Staging for Intrahepatic Bile Duct Cancer

Primary Tumor (T)

TX	Primary tumor cannot be assessed
T0	No evidence of primary tumor
Tis	Carcinoma in situ (intraductal tumor)
T1	Solitary tumor without vascular invasion
T2a	Solitary tumor with vascular invasion
T2b	Multiple tumors, with or without vascular invasion
T3	Tumor perforating the visceral peritoneum or involving local extrahepatic structures by direct extension
T4	Tumor with periductal invasion

Regional Lymph Nodes (N)

NX	Regional lymph nodes cannot be assessed
N0	No regional lymph node metastasis
N1	Regional lymph node metastasis present

Distant Metastasis (M)

M0	No distant metastasis
M1	Distant metastasis present

Anatomic Stage and Prognostic Groups

Stage 0	Tis	N0	M0
Stage I	T1	N0	M0
Stage II	T2	N0	M0
Stage III	T3	N0	M0
Stage IVA	T4	N0	M0
	Any T	N1	M0
Stage IVB	Any T	Any N	M1

From Edge SB, Byrd DR, Compton CC, et al, editors: *AJCC cancer staging manual*, ed 7, New York, 2010, Springer, pp 203–204.

TABLE 54-3 Staging for Perihilar Bile Duct Cancer

Primary Tumor (T)

TX	Primary tumor cannot be assessed
T0	No evidence of primary tumor
Tis	Carcinoma in situ
T1	Tumor confined to the bile duct, with extension up to the muscle layer or fibrous tissue
T2a	Tumor invading beyond the wall of the bile duct to surrounding adipose tissue
T2b	Tumor invades the adjacent hepatic parenchyma
T3	Tumor invades unilateral branches of the portal vein or hepatic artery
T4	Tumor invading main portal vein or its branches bilaterally; or the common hepatic artery; or the second-order biliary radicals bilaterally; or unilateral second-order biliary radicals with contralateral portal vein or hepatic artery involvement

Regional Lymph Nodes (N)

NX	Regional lymph nodes cannot be assessed
N0	No regional lymph node metastasis
N1	Regional lymph node metastasis (including nodes along the cystic duct, common bile duct, hepatic artery, and portal vein)
N2	Metastasis to periaortic, pericaval, superior mesenteric artery and/or celiac artery lymph nodes

Distant Metastasis (M)

M0	No distant metastasis
M1	Distant metastasis

Anatomic Stage and Prognostic Groups

Stage 0	Tis	N0	M0
Stage I	T1	N0	M0
Stage II	T2a-b	N0	M0
Stage IIIA	T3	N0	M0
Stage IIIB	T1-3	N1	M0
Stage IVA	T4	N0-1	M0
Stage IVB	Any T	N2	M0
	Any T	Any N	M1

From Edge SB, Byrd DR, Compton CC, et al, editors: *AJCC cancer staging manual*, ed 7, New York, 2010, Springer, p 221.

TABLE 54-4 Staging for Distal Bile Duct Cancer			
Primary Tumor (T)			
TX	Primary tumor cannot be assessed		
T0	No evidence of primary tumor		
Tis	Carcinoma in situ		
T1	Tumor confined to the bile duct histologically		
T2	Tumor invades beyond the wall of the bile duct		
T3	Tumor invades the gallbladder, pancreas, duodenum, or other adjacent organs without involvement of the celiac axis or superior mesenteric artery		
T4	Tumor involves the celiac axis or superior mesenteric artery		
Regional Lymph Nodes (N)			
N0	No regional lymph node metastasis		
N1	Regional lymph node metastasis		
Distant Metastasis (M)			
M0	No distant metastasis		
M1	Distant metastasis		
Anatomic Stage and Prognostic Groups			
Stage 0	Tis	N0	M0
Stage IA	T1	N0	M0
Stage IB	T2	N0	M0
Stage IIA	T3	N0	M0
Stage IIB	T1	N1	M0
	T2	N1	M0
	T3	N1	M0
Stage III	T4	Any N	M0
Stage IV	Any T	Any N	M1

From Edge SB, Byrd DR, Compton CC, et al, editors: *AJCC cancer staging manual*, ed 7, New York, 2010, Springer, p 229.

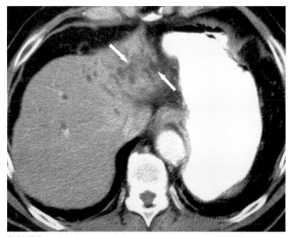

FIGURE 54-59 CT scan of cholangiocarcinoma with left lobar atrophy caused by obstruction of the left duct. Noted in the atrophied left lobe are dilated biliary radicals *(arrows)*.

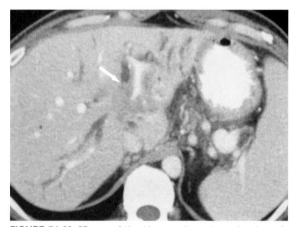

FIGURE 54-60 CT scan of Klatskin tumor *(arrow)* encasing the main portal vein, consistent with unresectable disease.

atrophy and subsequent contralateral lobar hypertrophy (Fig. 54-59). The resultant hepatic compensation can delay presentation until the later stages of disease. Therefore, cholangiocarcinoma causing obstruction at or below the hepatic bifurcation tends to be manifested at earlier stages than intrahepatic cholangiocarcinoma. With obstruction of the biliary tree, the common manifestations of direct hyperbilirubinemia, such as pruritus, dark urine, and steatorrhea, can be seen. Cholangiocarcinomas tend to extend in a submucosal route, with associated perineural invasion, but constant pain on presentation suggests more advanced disease.

Diagnosis and Assessment of Resectability

At the time of presentation, most patients will have manifestations of obstructive jaundice with hyperbilirubinemia and an elevated alkaline phosphatase level. Other markers of hepatic function, such as prothrombin time and albumin level, are generally unaffected until later in the disease or when the biliary obstruction is long-standing. Tumor markers, including carcinoembryonic antigen and carbohydrate antigen 19-9, are unreliable for diagnosis of cholangiocarcinoma but may be followed postoperatively in the surveillance of recurrence.

The radiologic evaluation of jaundice includes a right upper quadrant ultrasound examination, which may show intrahepatic biliary ductal dilation but does not usually identify the actual site of obstruction. With hilar cholangiocarcinomas, the gallbladder and visualized extrahepatic biliary tree are usually decompressed, whereas distal lesions will have extrahepatic biliary ductal dilation and gallbladder distention. Cross-sectional imaging by triphasic CT allows not only assessment of metastatic disease but also evaluation of resectability. The location of the tumor can be identified, and its relationship to vascular structures can also be assessed. Identification of aberrant anatomy and determination of segmental or lobar involvement by CT are helpful for preoperative planning.

Typically, CT alone is insufficient for the assessment of feasibility and appropriateness of resection. Cholangiography by MRCP, PTC, or ERCP helps determine the proximal extent of resection. Endoscopic cholangiography carries the additional risk of cholangitis by the introduction of enteric bacteria into an undrained portion of the biliary tree. Bilobar intrahepatic metastases and any extrahepatic disease are contraindications to resection, as is the involvement of bilateral secondary biliary radicals. Because complete (R0) resection is the only strategy that affords the possibility of cure, other contraindications to resection include encasement of the main portal vein (Fig. 54-60), bilateral hepatic lobar artery involvement, and lobar atrophy with involvement of the contralateral portal vein or biliary radicals. Involvement of unilobar vascular structures is managed with resection of the primary and affected lobe in continuity, and therefore it is not a contraindication.

Tissue diagnosis before resection in operative patients is unnecessary. With obstructive jaundice, bile cytology and brushings are unreliable, and thus a negative cytology report does not exclude malignant disease. Therefore, invasive attempts to establish a diagnosis before resection carry risk but do not alter subsequent management. Establishment of a tissue diagnosis is important only when the patient is not a surgical candidate. However, preoperative biliary drainage may be useful in select cases. In patients with distal cholangiocarcinoma, preoperative biliary drainage increases the rate of infectious complications of resection but is generally useful for those with preoperative hyperbilirubinemia (bilirubin level >10 mg/dL) and those with a prolonged time interval between presentation and resection. For patients with hilar cholangiocarcinoma, hepatic resection remains an important feature of the operative strategy. In the setting of complete biliary obstruction, hepatic resection carries an additional risk of bleeding, sepsis, and hepatic failure. Drainage of the obstructed but unaffected segments can enhance the postresection hypertrophy of the remaining liver but may increase perioperative infectious complications.

Treatment

Operative management. With the clinical suspicion of cholangiocarcinoma in adequate operative candidates without contraindications to resection, exploration should proceed, even in the absence of a confirmed tissue diagnosis. Between 7% and 15% of patients undergoing resection for suspected biliary malignant disease will prove to have benign disease. Alternatively, more than 50% of patients undergoing exploration will have findings precluding resection, such as peritoneal metastases, hepatic metastases, or locally advanced lesions.

Distal cholangiocarcinoma. Distal cholangiocarcinoma is managed by pancreaticoduodenectomy. Because these lesions tend to grow in a submucosal plane, a frozen section of the proximal bile duct margin helps ensure an R0 resection. An R0 resection remains one of the most important prognostic factors for this disease, with 5-year survival rates of up to 50% in node-negative patients with an R0 resection.

Proximal cholangiocarcinoma. Surgical management of proximal cholangiocarcinoma involves resection of regional nodal tissue and en bloc resection of the common bile duct with hepatic parenchyma as necessary to achieve negative margins. The Bismuth-Corlette classification of the tumor by assessment of the involvement of biliary radicals helps with operative planning (Fig. 54-61).[30] Types I and II lesions are treated with common duct resection, cholecystectomy, and a 5- to 10-mm margin of resection. Type II lesions may also require partial hepatic resection, which commonly includes resection of the caudate lobe.

Resection of the bile duct and nodal tissue requires skeletonization of the hepatic artery and portal vein. Reconstruction is performed using a Roux limb of jejunum. Types III and IV lesions may involve complex resection and reconstruction of the portal vein, hepatic artery, or both. With resection to secondary biliary radicals, transanastomotic stenting is used liberally to allow healing and even confirmation of anastomotic integrity.

A substantial improvement in long-term survival has correlated with the increasing use of hepatic resection to achieve negative margins. Negative margin status is the most important variable associated with outcome.[31] Five-year survival rates as high as 59% have been reported in selected series, and with vascular resection and reconstruction techniques, resectability rates have also increased. Increases in the magnitude of the operation have also correlated with an expected increase in surgical mortality, from 2% to 4% to 3% to 11%.

As noted previously, an extensive neoadjuvant therapy protocol followed by transplantation has shown promising results in tightly controlled trials. In spite of these findings, the role of transplantation in the management of cholangiocarcinoma remains experimental, and substantial debate remains about the routine use of an extremely limited resource in this disease process.

Palliation. In patients found to have unresectable or incurable disease preoperatively, all attempts to palliate their symptoms nonoperatively should be used. The goals of palliation should include relief of jaundice, alleviation of pain, and relief of duodenal obstruction, if necessary. Surgical palliation has not been shown to prolong survival or to reduce complication rates and thus should be reserved for candidates found to be unresectable or metastatic at time of operation. Depending on the location of the biliary obstruction, endoscopic or percutaneous routes of drainage can be used, and placement of a self-expandable metallic stent provides a durable solution. When plastic stents are used, additional manipulation or placement of subsequent stents may be required. For distal cholangiocarcinomas, ERCP is the preferred route of nonoperative biliary drainage, whereas PTC is more useful for proximal lesions. Drainage of atrophic lobes with stents does not improve palliation of disease. Pain can be treated with oral narcotics. IV narcotics and even percutaneous destruction of the celiac plexus have shown some benefit. For distal cholangiocarcinomas, in which duodenal obstruction may occur, endoscopic duodenal stenting can relieve the obstruction in this preterminal condition.

Medical treatment. Chemotherapy has not been shown to improve survival in patients with cholangiocarcinoma. In addition, radiation therapy has not been proven in a prospective fashion to affect survival. Therefore, neither chemotherapy nor radiation therapy is used routinely in the adjuvant or neoadjuvant setting. Although some retrospective studies have shown a small

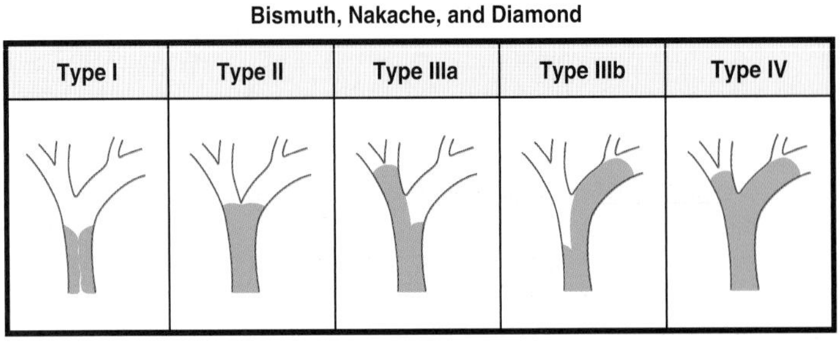

Bismuth, Nakache, and Diamond

Type I	Type II	Type IIIa	Type IIIb	Type IV

FIGURE 54-61 Bismuth-Corlette classification of tumor involvement.

survival advantage with adjuvant radiation, prospective studies of adjuvant radiotherapy have shown no benefit in completely resected patients. Radiation therapy may provide a small survival advantage as an adjunct to resection when microscopic residual disease remains. Most studies have reported a clinical response rate of less than 10%. Even in the absence of supportive data, adjuvant chemoradiation is used routinely at many centers but should be limited to patients with nodal disease, those with R1 resections, and those undergoing a clinical trial.

Outcomes

Long-term survival is highly dependent on stage at presentation and whether surgical resection to negative margins is achieved. With the use of common duct resection with partial hepatectomy, negative margin rates have increased to more than 75%. This has resulted in 5-year survival rates of 20% to 45% in most series. Although morbidity rates of 35% to 50% are common, mortality rates are generally low (<10%). In the setting of distal bile duct cancers, resection rates are generally higher, with approximately similar 5-year survival among patients undergoing R0 resections. Alternatively, because there is no reliable therapeutic alternative, the median survival of unresected patients ranges from 5 to 8 months.

Because negative margin status is easier to obtain by explanting the liver, some have advocated total hepatectomy with liver transplantation for treatment. Unfortunately, initial experience with therapeutic transplantation was plagued by early mortality and high recurrence rates. Even the most aggressive and radical resections with multivisceral transplantation have not shown a survival advantage. Therefore, without a specific clinical trial, cholangiocarcinoma is considered a contraindication to transplantation. However, some centers have attempted neoadjuvant chemoradiation followed by exploration for the evaluation of resectability and metastases, and finally transplantation, with improved survival over resection alone.[25] At present, the role of transplantation in the management of cholangiocarcinoma is at best controversial, and it should be limited to research protocols.

METASTATIC AND OTHER TUMORS

Any primary or secondary tumor affecting the liver can cause biliary obstruction. The most common examples include portal nodal disease from adenocarcinomas, such as hepatocellular carcinoma, pancreatic adenocarcinoma, and colorectal carcinoma. The metastatic nodes can compress the common bile duct at any point along its length. Lymphoma may affect the portal lymph node chain and, when isolated to periportal nodes, is notoriously difficult to differentiate from cholangiocarcinoma. Placement of temporary plastic stents to relieve the obstruction is usually the only therapeutic biliary intervention required because these lymphomas will generally respond to chemotherapy and the obstruction will usually resolve.

Primary lesions of the liver or metastatic disease may obstruct the biliary tree from direct compression or extension, as seen in hepatocellular carcinoma, but this phenomenon does not create an intraluminal biliary growth. Rarely, tumor cells may actually pass into the biliary tree and embolize distally. As the exfoliated cellular mass grows, it may be manifested with intraluminal biliary obstruction. Intrahepatic biliary cystadenomas and cystadenocarcinoma may obstruct the bile duct directly or by passage of the mucin that they produce.

SELECTED REFERENCES

Butte JM, Kingham TP, Gonen M, et al: Residual disease predicts outcomes after definitive resection for incidental gallbladder cancer. *J Am Coll Surg* 219:416–429, 2014.

This article evaluated the survival of gallbladder cancer after attempted surgical resection, noting the import of R0 resection status on survival.

Darwish Murad S, Kim WR, Harnois DM, et al: Efficacy of neoadjuvant chemoradiation, followed by liver transplantation, for perihilar cholangiocarcinoma at 12 US centers. *Gastroenterology* 143:88–98.e3, 2012.

This article evaluated the results of transplantation for cholangiocarcinoma after a rigorous neoadjuvant therapy protocol.

Fogel EL, Sherman S: ERCP for gallstone pancreatitis. *N Engl J Med* 370:150–157, 2014.

This article reviews the current status of the role of ERCP in the diagnosis and management of biliary pancreatitis, depending on severity.

Horwood J, Akbar F, Davis K, et al: Prospective evaluation of a selective approach to cholangiography for suspected common bile duct stones. *Ann R Coll Surg Engl* 92:206–210, 2010.

This article evaluates the criteria for selective cholangiography during routine cholecystectomy.

Pitt HA, Sherman S, Johnson MS, et al: Improved outcomes of bile duct injuries in the 21st century. *Ann Surg* 258:490–499, 2013.

This article reviewed a large series of iatrogenic bile duct injuries, highlighting the success of surgical intervention and the multidisciplinary approach to management.

Sirinek KR, Schwesinger WH: Has intraoperative cholangiography during laparoscopic cholecystectomy become obsolete in the era of preoperative endoscopic retrograde and magnetic resonance cholangiopancreatography? *J Am Coll Surg* 220:522–528, 2015.

This article highlights current practice patterns of imaging in the management of suspected choledocholithiasis, noting the application of MRCP as a screening tool for referral for ERCP before laparoscopic cholecystectomy.

Strasberg SM, Gouma DJ: 'Extreme' vasculobiliary injuries: Association with fundus-down cholecystectomy in severely inflamed gallbladders. *HPB* 14:1–8, 2012.

This article discusses the surgical pitfalls of a" dome down" approach to the inflamed gallbladder.

Strasberg SM, Hertl M, Soper NJ: An analysis of the problem of biliary injury during laparoscopic cholecystectomy. *J Am Coll Surg* 180:101–125, 1995.

This is the most cited article for classification of iatrogenic bile duct injuries and is considered the seminal comprehensive article on the topic.

REFERENCES

1. Couinaud C: Les envelopes vasculobiliares de foie ou capsule de Glisson: Leur interet dans la chirurgie vesiculaire, les resections hepatique et l'abord du hile du foie. *Lyon Chir* 49:589–615, 1954.
2. Admirand WH, Small DM: The physicochemical basis of cholesterol gallstone formation in man. *J Clin Invest* 47:1043–1052, 1968.
3. de Mestral C, Rotstein OD, Laupacis A, et al: Comparative operative outcomes of early and delayed cholecystectomy for acute cholecystitis: A population-based propensity score analysis. *Ann Surg* 259:10–15, 2014.
4. Verbesey JE, Birkett DH: Common bile duct exploration for choledocholithiasis. *Surg Clin North Am* 88:1315–1328, 2008.
5. Horwood J, Akbar F, Davis K, et al: Prospective evaluation of a selective approach to cholangiography for suspected common bile duct stones. *Ann R Coll Surg Engl* 92:206–210, 2010.
6. Sirinek KR, Schwesinger WH: Has intraoperative cholangiography during laparoscopic cholecystectomy become obsolete in the era of preoperative endoscopic retrograde and magnetic resonance cholangiopancreatography? *J Am Coll Surg* 220:522–528, 2015.
7. Lee JK, Ryu JK, Park JK, et al: Roles of endoscopic sphincterotomy and cholecystectomy in acute biliary pancreatitis. *Hepatogastroenterology* 55:1981–1985, 2008.
8. Fogel EL, Sherman S: ERCP for gallstone pancreatitis. *N Engl J Med* 370:150–157, 2014.
9. Strasberg SM, Hertl M, Soper NJ: An analysis of the problem of biliary injury during laparoscopic cholecystectomy. *J Am Coll Surg* 180:101–125, 1995.
10. Way LW, Stewart L, Gantert W, et al: Causes and prevention of laparoscopic bile duct injuries: Analysis of 252 cases from a human factors and cognitive psychology perspective. *Ann Surg* 237:460–469, 2003.
11. Strasberg SM, Gouma DJ: 'Extreme' vasculobiliary injuries: Association with fundus-down cholecystectomy in severely inflamed gallbladders. *HPB* 14:1–8, 2012.
12. Rogers SJ, Cello JP, Horn JK, et al: Prospective randomized trial of LC+LCBDE vs ERCP/S+LC for common bile duct stone disease. *Arch Surg* 145:28–33, 2010.
13. Nieuwenhuijs VB: Impact of routine intraoperative cholangiography during laparoscopic cholecystectomy on bile duct injury. *Br J Surg* 101:685, 2014.
14. Bismuth H, Majno PE: Biliary strictures: Classification based on the principles of surgical treatment. *World J Surg* 25:1241–1244, 2001.
15. Lillemoe KD: Current management of bile duct injury. *Br J Surg* 95:403–405, 2008.

16. Harrison VL, Dolan JP, Pham TH, et al: Bile duct injury after laparoscopic cholecystectomy in hospitals with and without surgical residency programs: Is there a difference? *Surg Endosc* 25:1969–1974, 2011.
17. Sicklick JK, Camp MS, Lillemoe KD, et al: Surgical management of bile duct injuries sustained during laparoscopic cholecystectomy: Perioperative results in 200 patients. *Ann Surg* 241:786–792, discussion 793–795, 2005.
18. Eum YO, Park JK, Chun J, et al: Non-surgical treatment of post-surgical bile duct injury: Clinical implications and outcomes. *World J Gastroenterol* 20:6924–6931, 2014.
19. Pottakkat B, Vijayahari R, Prakash A, et al: Factors predicting failure following high bilio-enteric anastomosis for post-cholecystectomy benign biliary strictures. *J Gastrointest Surg* 14:1389–1394, 2010.
20. Pitt HA, Sherman S, Johnson MS, et al: Improved outcomes of bile duct injuries in the 21st century. *Ann Surg* 258:490–499, 2013.
21. Ejaz A, Spolverato G, Kim Y, et al: Long-term health-related quality of life after iatrogenic bile duct injury repair. *J Am Coll Surg* 219:923–932.e10, 2014.
22. Pazouki A, Abdollahi A, Mehrabi Bahar M, et al: Evaluation of the incidence of complications of lost gallstones during laparoscopic cholecystectomy. *Surg Laparosc Endosc Percutan Tech* 24:213–215, 2014.
23. Co M, Pang SY, Wong KY, et al: Surgical management of recurrent pyogenic cholangitis: 10 years of experience in a tertiary referral centre in Hong Kong. *HPB* 16:776–780, 2014.
24. Carbone M, Neuberger JM: Autoimmune liver disease, autoimmunity and liver transplantation. *J Hepatol* 60:210–223, 2014.
25. Darwish Murad S, Kim WR, Harnois DM, et al: Efficacy of neoadjuvant chemoradiation, followed by liver transplantation, for perihilar cholangiocarcinoma at 12 US centers. *Gastroenterology* 143:88–98.e3, 2012.
26. Todani T, Watanabe Y, Narusue M, et al: Congenital bile duct cysts: Classification, operative procedures, and review of thirty-seven cases including cancer arising from choledochal cyst. *Am J Surg* 134:263–269, 1977.
27. Schnelldorfer T: Porcelain gallbladder: A benign process or concern for malignancy? *J Gastrointest Surg* 17:1161–1168, 2013.
28. Edge SB, Byrd DR, Compton CC, et al, editors: *AJCC cancer staging manual*, ed 7, New York, 2010, Springer.
29. Butte JM, Kingham TP, Gonen M, et al: Residual disease predicts outcomes after definitive resection for incidental gallbladder cancer. *J Am Coll Surg* 219:416–429, 2014.
30. Bismuth H, Nakache R, Diamond T: Management strategies in resection for hilar cholangiocarcinoma. *Ann Surg* 215:31–38, 1992.
31. Maithel SK, Gamblin TC, Kamel I, et al: Multidisciplinary approaches to intrahepatic cholangiocarcinoma. *Cancer* 119:3929–3942, 2013.

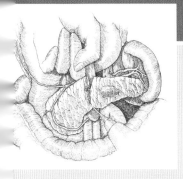

CHAPTER 55

Exocrine Pancreas

Vikas Dudeja, John D. Christein, Eric H. Jensen, Selwyn M. Vickers

第五十五章　胰腺外分泌疾病

OUTLINE

Anatomy
Embryology
Physiology
Acute Pancreatitis
Chronic Pancreatitis
Cystic Neoplasms of the Pancreas
Adenocarcinoma of the Exocrine Pancreas
Pancreatic Trauma

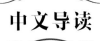

中文导读

　　本章共分为8节：①胰腺解剖；②胰腺胚胎学；③胰腺生理；④急性胰腺炎；⑤慢性胰腺炎；⑥胰腺囊性肿瘤；⑦胰腺腺癌；⑧胰腺创伤。

　　第一节从解剖学描述了胰腺的位置、形态及其毗邻关系；讲述了胰腺的动脉血供及静脉回流。强调熟练地掌握胰腺的解剖，将为胰腺疾病的外科治疗打下坚实的基础。

　　第二节从胚胎学阐述了胰腺发育过程，讲述了胰腺发育过程中PDX1和PTF1基因，以及Notch、Hedgehog、Wnt 3种信号通路的作用；介绍了胰腺分离、环状胰腺、异位胰腺3种胰腺先天发育异常及相关疾病。

　　第三节从生理学阐述了胰液的主要成分及其基本性状；胰酶的主要成分胰淀粉酶、胰脂肪酶、胰蛋白酶等；胰液分泌的神经及激素调控；胆囊收缩素CCK在胰液分泌调节过程中所发挥的重要作用。

　　第四节介绍了急性胰腺炎是外科常见的急腹症之一，大多数为轻症，易于治疗，呈自限性；但重型胰腺炎病情凶险、病死率高，是最棘手的外科急腹症。本节阐述了急性胰腺炎的病理生理学机制、病因、临床表现、诊断、治疗及并发症的防治等；特别深入剖析了急性重症胰腺炎这一临床常见而治疗过程复杂、并发症多、预后较差的疾病。

　　第五节介绍了慢性胰腺炎的临床表现和诊断；慢性胰腺炎的非手术治疗、介入-内镜治疗、手术治疗；重点介绍了慢性胰腺炎不同的手术治疗方案；同时指出慢性胰腺炎治疗上虽然有诸多方法，但疗效不佳，需要深入研究。

第六节讲述了胰腺囊性肿瘤这一类临床发病率相对低的疾病。胰腺囊性肿瘤主要包括黏液性囊腺瘤、浆液性囊腺瘤、导管内乳头状黏液肿瘤；对比介绍了三类囊性肿瘤的特性及其临床治疗方案。

第七节胰腺腺癌同样是本篇重点，在介绍流行病学、病因学的内容中，穿插讲解胰腺导管上皮瘤变进展成胰腺导管上皮腺癌的基因演进；重点突出地讲解了胰头肿瘤的手术治疗方案、手术技巧、消化道重建方式和胰腺体尾部肿瘤的手术治疗；同时对现代胰腺外科前沿争论进行了详尽阐述。

第八节主要介绍了胰腺外伤的分型，各型胰腺外伤的预后。

〔陈勇军〕

 Please access ExpertConsult.com to view the corresponding videos for this chapter.

ANATOMY

The average pancreas weighs between 75 and 125 g and measures 10 to 20 cm. It lies in the retroperitoneum just anterior to the first lumbar vertebra and is anatomically divided into four portions, the head, neck, body, and tail. The head lies to the right of midline within the C loop of the duodenum, immediately anterior to the vena cava at the confluence of the renal veins. The uncinate process extends from the head of the pancreas behind the superior mesenteric vein (SMV) and terminates adjacent to the superior mesenteric artery (SMA). The neck is the short segment of pancreas that immediately overlies the SMV. The body and tail of the pancreas then extend across the midline, anterior to Gerota fascia and slightly cephalad, terminating within the splenic hilum (Fig. 55-1).

Arterial Blood Supply

The pancreas is supplied by a complex arterial network arising from the celiac trunk and SMA. The head and uncinate process are supplied by the pancreaticoduodenal arteries (anterior and posterior), which arise from the hepatic artery through the gastroduodenal artery (GDA) superiorly and the SMA inferiorly. The neck, body, and tail receive arterial supply from the splenic arterial system. Several small branches originate from the length of the splenic artery, supplying arterial blood flow to the superior portion of the organ. The dorsal pancreatic artery arises from the splenic artery and courses posterior to the body of the gland to become the inferior pancreatic artery. The inferior pancreatic artery then runs along the inferior border of the pancreas, terminating at its tail.

Venous Drainage

The venous drainage mimics the arterial supply, with blood flow from the head of the pancreas draining into the anterior and posterior pancreaticoduodenal veins. The posterior superior pancreaticoduodenal vein enters the SMV laterally at the superior border of the neck of the pancreas. The anterior superior pancreaticoduodenal vein enters the right gastroepiploic vein just before its confluence with the SMV at the inferior border of the pancreas. The anterior and posterior inferior pancreaticoduodenal veins enter the SMV along the inferior border of the uncinate process. The remaining body and tail are drained through the splenic venous system.

EMBRYOLOGY

The exocrine pancreas begins development during the fourth week of gestation. Pluripotent pancreatic epithelial stem cells give rise to exocrine and endocrine cell lines as well as the intricate pancreatic ductal network. Initially, dorsal and ventral buds appear from the primitive duodenal endoderm (Fig. 55-2A). The dorsal bud typically appears first and ultimately develops into the superior head, neck, body, and tail of the mature pancreas. The ventral bud develops as part of the hepatic diverticulum and maintains communication with the biliary tree throughout development. The ventral bud will become the inferior part of the head and uncinate process of the gland. Between the fourth and eighth weeks, the ventral bud rotates posteriorly in a clockwise fashion to fuse with the dorsal bud (Fig. 55-2B). At approximately 8 weeks of gestation, the dorsal and ventral buds are fused (Fig. 55-2C).

The initiation of pancreas bud formation and differentiation of the ventral bud from the hepatic-biliary fates is dependent on the expression of pancreatic duodenal homeobox 1 (PDX1) protein and pancreas-specific transcription factor 1 (PTF1). In the absence of PDX1 expression in mice, pancreatic agenesis occurs, indicating its importance in the early phases of organogenesis. PTF1 expression is first detectable shortly after PDX1 in cells of the early endoderm, which will become the dorsal and ventral pancreas. By lineage analysis, 95% of acinar cells express PTF1. In PTF1 null mice, acini do not form. The notch signaling pathway is also critical to duct and acinar differentiation. In the absence of notch signaling, embryonic cells commit to endocrine lineage, suggesting that notch signaling is vital to exocrine differentiation. In addition to PDX1, PTF1, and notch signaling, complex interactions between mesenchymal growth factors such as transforming growth factor-β (TGF-β) and other signaling pathways, including hedgehog and Wnt, seem to play critical

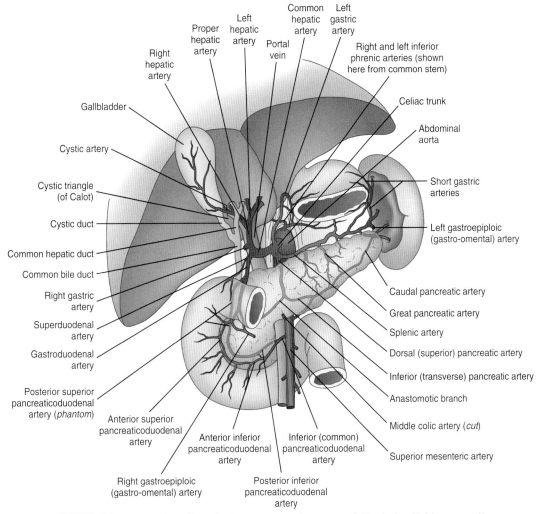

FIGURE 55-1 Anatomy. (Netter illustration from *www.netterimages.com.* © Elsevier Inc. All rights reserved.)

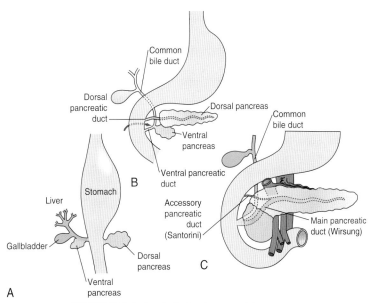

FIGURE 55-2 Embryologic development of the pancreas.

TABLE 55-1 Molecular Factors and Pathways Associated With Pancreatic Organogenesis

MUTATION	RELEVANCE
PDX1	Critical role in exocrine differentiation; knockout mice develop primitive pancreatic buds but agenesis of the organ
PTF1	Coexpression with PDX1 determines progenitor cells to pancreatic fate
Notch signaling pathway	Suppresses endocrine differentiation, promoting exocrine development
Hedgehog signaling pathway	Inhibition of hedgehog in PDX1-positive cells leads to initiation of endoderm differentiation into pancreas lineage
Wnt signaling pathway	Complex Wnt signaling is important in all aspects of pancreas development; lack of Wnt signaling results in absence of acinar tissue

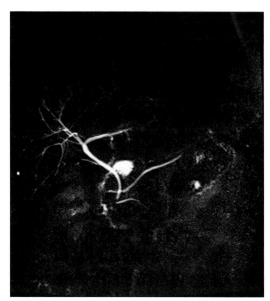

FIGURE 55-3 MRCP showing pancreas divisum, with the dorsal pancreatic duct draining through the minor papilla and the ventral pancreatic duct joining the biliary tree draining through the major papilla.

roles in pancreas development.[1] The precise interactions that lead to normal organogenesis continue to be defined. Table 55-1 summarizes the factors and pathways that affect pancreas development.

Pancreas Divisum

During normal organogenesis, the dorsal and ventral buds most commonly fuse to form a common duct, which enters the duodenum along with the common bile duct through the ampulla of Vater. Failure of the dorsal and ventral ducts to fuse during embryogenesis leads to pancreas divisum, a condition identified by a ventral pancreatic duct and common bile duct that enter the duodenum through a major papilla, whereas a dorsal pancreatic duct enters through a minor papilla that is slightly proximal (Fig. 55-3). Because most pancreatic exocrine secretions exit through the dorsal duct, pancreas divisum can lead to a condition of partial obstruction caused by a small minor papilla, leading to chronic backpressure in the duct. This relative outflow obstruction has been implicated in the development of relapsing acute or chronic pancreatitis. Although 10% of the population is affected by pancreas divisum, only rarely do affected individuals develop pancreatitis.

Annular Pancreas

Annular pancreas results from aberrant migration of the ventral pancreas bud, which leads to circumferential or near-circumferential pancreas tissue surrounding the second portion of the duodenum. This abnormality may be associated with other congenital defects, including Down syndrome, malrotation, intestinal atresia, and cardiac malformations. If symptoms of obstruction occur, surgical bypass through duodenojejunostomy is performed.

Ectopic Pancreas

Ectopic pancreas may arise anywhere along the primitive foregut but is most common in the stomach, duodenum, and Meckel's diverticulum. Clinically, ectopic nodules may result in bowel obstruction caused by intussusception, bleeding, or ulceration. They can sometimes be found incidentally as firm yellow nodules that arise from the submucosa. Although there have been rare case reports of adenocarcinoma arising in ectopic pancreas tissue, resection is not necessary unless symptoms occur.

PHYSIOLOGY

The human pancreas is a complex gland, with endocrine and exocrine functions. It is mainly composed of acinar cells (85% of the gland) and islet cells (2%) embedded in a complex extracellular matrix, which composes 10% of the gland. The remaining 3% to 4% of the gland is composed of the epithelial duct system and blood vessels.

Major Components of Pancreatic Juice

The main function of the exocrine pancreas is to provide most of the enzymes needed for alimentary digestion. Acinar cells synthesize many enzymes (proteases), such as trypsin, chymotrypsin, carboxypeptidase, and elastase, that digest food proteins. Under physiologic conditions, acinar cells synthesize these proteases as inactive proenzymes that are stored as intracellular zymogen granules. With stimulation of the pancreas, these proenzymes are secreted into the pancreatic duct and eventually the duodenal lumen. The duodenal mucosa synthesizes and secretes enterokinase, which is the critical enzyme in the enzymatic activation of trypsin from trypsinogen.[2] Trypsin also plays an important role in protein digestion by propagating pancreatic enzyme activation through autoactivation of trypsinogen and other proenzymes, such as chymotrypsinogen, procarboxypeptidase, and proelastase. Figure 55-4 summarizes the mechanisms of pancreatic exocrine secretion.

In addition to protease production, acinar cells also produce pancreatic amylase and lipase, also known as glycerol ester hydrolase, as active enzymes. With the exception of cellulose, pancreatic amylase hydrolyzes major polysaccharides into small oligosaccharides, which can be further digested by the oligosaccharidases present in the duodenal and jejunal epithelium. Pancreatic lipase hydrolyzes ingested fats into free fatty acids and 2-monoglycerides. In addition to pancreatic lipase, acinar cells produce other enzymes that digest fat, but they are secreted as proenzymes, like the

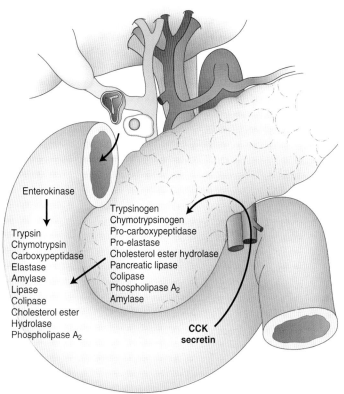

Enterokinase

Trypsin
Chymotrypsin
Carboxypeptidase
Elastase
Amylase
Lipase
Colipase
Cholesterol ester
Hydrolase
Phospholipase A$_2$

Trypsinogen
Chymotrypsinogen
Pro-carboxypeptidase
Pro-elastase
Cholesterol ester hydrolase
Pancreatic lipase
Colipase
Phospholipase A$_2$
Amylase

CCK
secretin

FIGURE 55-4 Physiology of the secretion of pancreatic enzymes. The presence of peptides and fatty acids from food triggers the release of cholecystokinin (CCK). CCK induces the release of pancreatic enzymes into the duodenal lumen. Conversely, S cells located in the duodenum release secretin in response to the acidification of the duodenum. Secretin induces the secretion of HCO_3^- from pancreatic cells into the duodenum.

proteases previously mentioned. These include colipase, cholesterol ester hydrolase, and phospholipase A2. The main function of colipase is to increase the activity of pancreatic lipase; cholesterol esters are cleaved by cholesterol ester hydrolase into free cholesterol and one fatty acid; and phospholipase A2 hydrolyzes phospholipids. Pancreatic acinar cells also secrete deoxyribonuclease and ribonuclease, enzymes required for the hydrolysis of DNA and RNA, respectively.

Pancreatic enzymes are inactive inside acinar cells because they are synthesized and stored as inactive enzymes. In addition to this autoprotective mechanism, acinar cells synthesize pancreatic secretory trypsin inhibitor, which also protects acinar cells from autodigestion because it counteracts premature activation of trypsinogen inside acinar cells. Pancreatic secretory trypsin inhibitor is encoded by serine protease inhibitor Kazal type 1 *(SPINK1)* gene. *SPINK1* gene mutations are associated with the development of chronic pancreatitis, especially in childhood.

The primary function of pancreatic duct cells is to provide the water and electrolytes required to dilute and to deliver the enzymes synthesized by acinar cells. Although the concentrations of sodium and potassium are similar to their respective concentrations in plasma, the concentrations of bicarbonate and chloride vary significantly according to the secretion phase.

The mechanism responsible for the secretion of bicarbonate was first described in 1988 on the basis of in vitro studies. According to this model, extracellular CO_2 diffuses across the basolateral

membrane of ductal cells. Once CO_2 is inside pancreatic duct cells, it is hydrated by intracellular carbonic anhydrase; as a result of this reaction, HCO_3^- and H^+ are generated. The apical membrane of pancreatic duct cells contains an anion exchanger that secretes intracellular HCO_3^- into the lumen of the cell and favors the exchange of luminal Cl^- inside the ductal epithelium. Studies have shown that this exchanger interacts with the cystic fibrosis transmembrane conductance regulator (CFTR). This may correlate with the inability of patients with cystic fibrosis to secrete water and bicarbonate. Although the nature of this exchanger has not been completely elucidated, it is possible that this anion exchanger is an SLC26 family member. This family contains different anion exchangers that transport monovalent and divalent anions, such as Cl^- and HCO_3^-. Some of these exchangers are known to interact with CFTR.

In addition to HCO_3^-, CO_2 hydration also generates H^+ ions, which are secreted by Na^+ and H^+ exchangers present in the basolateral membrane of ductal cells. These exchangers belong to the *SLC9* gene family. The main function of these exchangers is to maintain the intracellular pH within a physiologic range. In addition, the basolateral membrane of duct cells contains multiple Na^+,K^+-ATPases that provide the primary force that drives HCO_3^- secretion; the Na^+,K^+-ATPase maintains the Na^+ gradient used to extrude H^+ as well. Finally, K^+ channels present in the basolateral membrane of acinar cells maintain the membrane potential to allow recirculation of K^+ ions brought by the Na^+,K^+ pump inside

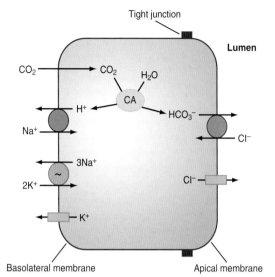

FIGURE 55-5 Cellular mechanism proposed for HCO_3^- secretion by pancreatic duct epithelium. (From Steward MC, Ishiguro H, Case RM: Mechanisms of bicarbonate secretion in the pancreatic duct. *Annu Rev Physiol* 67:377–409, 2005.)

the cell. Figure 55-5 illustrates HCO_3^- secretion inside pancreatic duct cells.

Once the HCO_3^- secreted by pancreatic duct cells reaches the duodenal lumen, it neutralizes the hydrochloric acid secreted by parietal cells. Pancreatic enzymes are inactivated at a low pH; therefore, pancreatic bicarbonate provides an optimal pH for acinar cell enzyme function. The optimal pH for the function of chymotrypsin and trypsin is 8.0 to 9.0; for amylase, the optimal pH is 7.0; and for lipase, it is 7.0 to 9.0.

Phases and Regulation of Pancreatic Secretion

Pancreatic exocrine secretion occurs during the interdigestive state and after the ingestion of food, which is also known as the digestive state. The same phases of secretion that have been identified in the stomach during the digestive state have also been described in pancreatic secretion. The first phase is the cephalic phase, in which the pancreas is stimulated by the vagus nerve in response to the sight, smell, or taste of food. This phase is generally mediated by the release of acetylcholine at the terminal endings of postganglionic fibers. The main effect of acetylcholine is to induce acinar cell secretion of enzymes. This phase accounts for 20% to 25% of the daily secretion of pancreatic juice.

The second phase of pancreatic secretion is known as the gastric phase. It is mediated by vagovagal reflexes triggered by gastric distention after the ingestion of food. These reflexes induce acinar cell secretion. It accounts for 10% of the pancreatic juice produced daily.

The most important phase of pancreatic secretion is the intestinal phase, which accounts for 65% to 70% of the total secretion of pancreatic juice. It is mediated by secretin and cholecystokinin (CCK). Acidification of the duodenal lumen induces the release of secretin by S cells. Secretin was the first polypeptide hormone identified more than 100 years ago. It is the most important mediator of the secretion of water, bicarbonate, and other electrolytes into the duodenum. Secretin receptors are located in the basolateral membrane of all pancreatic duct cells but cannot be

identified in other pancreatic components, such as islet cells, blood vessels, or extracellular matrix. Secretin receptors are members of the G protein–coupled receptor superfamily. The most important effect of secretin stimulation is an increase of intracellular cyclic adenosine monophosphate, which activates the HCO_3^--Cl^- anion exchanger in the apical membrane of pancreatic duct cells. It also increases the activity of the enzyme carbonic anhydrase, the excretion of H^+ outside the duct cell, and the activity of the CFTR.

The presence of lipid, protein, and carbohydrates inside the duodenum induces the secretion of CCK-releasing factor and monitor peptide. Both peptides induce release of CCK by I cells present in the duodenal mucosa. Whereas secretin is the main mediator of the secretion of water and bicarbonate in the intestinal phase, CCK is the main mediator of the secretion of pancreatic enzymes. CCK exerts a number of effects:

1. CCK travels through the bloodstream and induces the release of pancreatic enzymes by acinar cells.
2. CCK induces local duodenal vagovagal reflexes that cause the release of acetylcholine, vasoactive intestinal peptide, and gastrin-releasing peptide, which promotes the release of pancreatic enzymes.
3. CCK induces the relaxation of the sphincter of Oddi. Also, CCK potentiates the effects of secretin, and vice versa.

ACUTE PANCREATITIS

The incidence of acute pancreatitis (AP) has increased during the past 20 years. AP is responsible for more than 300,000 hospital admissions annually in the United States. Most patients develop a mild and self-limited course; however, 10% to 20% of patients have a rapidly progressive inflammatory response associated with prolonged length of hospital stay and significant morbidity and mortality. Patients with mild pancreatitis have a mortality rate of less than 1%, but in severe pancreatitis, this increases up to 10% to 30%. The most common cause of death in this group of patients is multiorgan dysfunction syndrome. Mortality in pancreatitis has a bimodal distribution; in the first 2 weeks, also known as the early phase, the multiorgan dysfunction syndrome is the final result of an intense inflammatory cascade triggered initially by pancreatic inflammation. Mortality after 2 weeks, also known as the late period, is often caused by septic complications.[3]

Pathophysiology

The exact mechanism whereby predisposing factors such as ethanol and gallstones produce pancreatitis is not completely known. Most researchers believe that AP is the final result of abnormal pancreatic enzyme activation inside acinar cells. Immunolocalization studies have shown that after 15 minutes of pancreatic injury, both zymogen granules and lysosomes colocalize inside the acinar cells. The fact that zymogen and lysosome colocalization occurs before amylase level elevation, pancreatic edema, and other markers of pancreatitis are evident suggests that colocalization is an early step in the pathophysiologic process and not a consequence of pancreatitis. Studies also suggest that lysosomal enzyme cathepsin B activates trypsin in these colocalization organelles. In vitro and in vivo studies have elucidated an intricate model of acinar cell death induced by premature activation of trypsin. In this model, once cathepsin B in lysosomes and trypsinogen in zymogen granules are brought in contact by colocalization induced by pancreatitis-inciting stimuli, activated trypsin then induces leak of colocalized organelles, releasing cathepsin B into the cytosol. It is the cytosolic cathepsin B that then induces apoptosis or necrosis, leading to acinar cell death. Thus, acinar cell death and to a degree the inflammatory response seen in AP can be prevented if acinar cells are pretreated with cathepsin B inhibitors. In vivo studies have also shown that cathepsin B knockout mice have a significant decrease in the severity of pancreatitis.[2]

Intra-acinar pancreatic enzyme activation induces autodigestion of normal pancreatic parenchyma. In response to this initial insult, acinar cells release proinflammatory cytokines, such as tumor necrosis factor-α (TNF-α) and interleukin (IL)-1, IL-2, and IL-6, and anti-inflammatory mediators, such as IL-10 and IL-1 receptor antagonist. These mediators do not initiate pancreatic injury but propagate the response locally and systemically. As a result, TNF-α, IL-1 and IL-7, neutrophils, and macrophages are recruited into the pancreatic parenchyma and cause the release of more TNF-α, IL-1 and IL-6, reactive oxygen metabolites, prostaglandins, platelet-activating factor, and leukotrienes. The local inflammatory response further aggravates the pancreatitis because it increases the permeability and damages the microcirculation of the pancreas. In severe cases, the inflammatory response causes local hemorrhage and pancreatic necrosis. In addition, some of the inflammatory mediators released by neutrophils aggravate the pancreatic injury because they cause pancreatic enzyme activation.[4]

The inflammatory cascade is self-limited in approximately 80% to 90% of patients. However, in the remaining patients, a vicious circle of recurring pancreatic injury and local and systemic inflammatory reaction persists. In a small number of patients, there is a massive release of inflammatory mediators to the systemic circulation. Active neutrophils mediate acute lung injury and induce the adult respiratory distress syndrome frequently seen in patients with severe pancreatitis. The mortality seen in the early phase of pancreatitis is the result of this persistent inflammatory response. A summary of the inflammatory cascade seen in AP is shown in Figure 55-6.

Risk Factors

Gallstones and ethanol abuse account for 70% to 80% of AP cases. In pediatric patients, abdominal blunt trauma and systemic diseases are the two most common conditions that lead to pancreatitis. Autoimmune and drug-induced pancreatitis should be a differential diagnosis in patients with rheumatologic conditions such as systemic lupus erythematosus and Sjögren syndrome.

Biliary or Gallstone Pancreatitis

Gallstone pancreatitis is the most common cause of AP in the West. It accounts for 40% of U.S. cases. The overall incidence of AP in patients with symptomatic gallstone disease is 3% to 8%. It is seen more frequently in women between 50 and 70 years of age. The exact mechanism that triggers pancreatic injury has not been completely understood, but two theories have been proposed.[5] In the obstructive theory, pancreatic injury is the result of excessive pressure inside the pancreatic duct. This increased intraductal pressure is the result of continuous secretion of pancreatic juice in the presence of pancreatic duct obstruction. The second, or reflux, theory proposes that stones become impacted in the ampulla of Vater and form a common channel that allows bile salt reflux into the pancreas. Animal models have shown that bile salts cause direct acinar cell necrosis because they increase the concentration of calcium in the cytoplasm; however, this has never been proven in humans.[2]

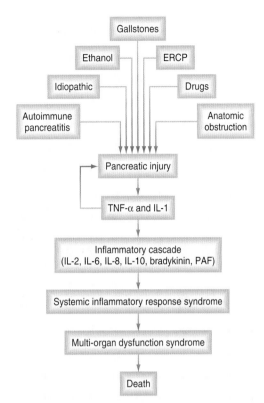

FIGURE 55-6 Pathophysiology of Severe Acute Pancreatitis. The local injury induces the release of TNF-α and IL-1. Both cytokines produce further pancreatic injury and amplify the inflammatory response by inducing the release of other inflammatory mediators, which cause distant organ injury. This abnormal inflammatory response is responsible for the mortality seen during the early phase of acute pancreatitis.

Alcohol-Induced Injury

Excessive ethanol consumption is the second most common cause of AP worldwide. It accounts for 35% of cases and is more prevalent in young men (30 to 45 years of age) than in women. However, only 5% to 10% of patients who drink alcohol develop AP. Factors that contribute to ethanol-induced pancreatitis include heavy ethanol abuse (>100 g/day for at least 5 years), smoking, and genetic predisposition. Compared with nonsmokers, the relative risk of alcohol-induced pancreatitis in smokers is 4.9.[6]

Alcohol has a number of deleterious effects in the pancreas. It triggers proinflammatory pathways such as nuclear factor κB (NF-κB), which increase the production of TNF-α and IL-1. It also increases the expression and activity of caspases. Caspases are proteases that mediate apoptosis. In addition, alcohol decreases pancreatic perfusion, induces sphincter of Oddi spasm, and obstructs pancreatic ducts through the precipitation of proteins inside the ducts.

Anatomic Obstruction

Abnormal flow of pancreatic juice into the duodenum can result in pancreatic injury. AP has been described in patients with pancreatic tumors, parasites, and congenital defects.

Pancreas divisum is an anatomic variation present in 10% of the population. Its association with AP is controversial. Patients with this variation have a 5% to 10% lifetime risk for development of AP caused by relative outflow obstruction through the minor papilla. Endoscopic retrograde cholangiopancreatography (ERCP) with minor papillotomy and stenting may be beneficial for such patients.

Infrequent anatomic obstructions that have been associated with AP include *Ascaris lumbricoides* infection and annular pancreas. Although pancreatic cancer is not uncommon, patients with pancreatic cancer usually do not develop AP.

Endoscopic Retrograde Cholangiopancreatography–Induced Pancreatitis

AP is the most common complication after ERCP, occurring in up to 5% of patients. AP occurs more frequently in patients who have undergone therapeutic procedures compared with diagnostic procedures. It is also more common in patients who have had multiple attempts of cannulation, sphincter of Oddi dysfunction, and abnormal visualization of the secondary pancreatic ducts after injection of contrast material. The clinical course is mild in 90% to 95% of patients.

Drug-Induced Pancreatitis

Up to 2% of AP cases are caused by medications. The most common agents include sulfonamides, metronidazole, erythromycin, tetracyclines, didanosine, thiazides, furosemide, 3-hydroxy-3-methylglutaryl-coenzyme A (HMG-CoA) reductase inhibitors (statins), azathioprine, 6-mercaptopurine, 5-aminosalicylic acid, sulfasalazine, valproic acid, and acetaminophen. More recently, antiretroviral agents used for the treatment of AIDS have been implicated in AP.

Metabolic Factors

Hypertriglyceridemia and hypercalcemia can also lead to pancreatic damage. Direct pancreatic injury can be induced by triglyceride metabolites. It is more common in patients with type I, II, or V hyperlipidemia. It should be suspected in patients with a triglyceride level higher than 1000 mg/dL. A triglyceride level higher than 2000 mg/dL confirms the diagnosis. Hypertriglyceridemia secondary to hypothyroidism, diabetes mellitus, and alcohol does not typically induce AP.

Hypercalcemia is postulated to induce pancreatic injury through the activation of trypsinogen to trypsin and intraductal precipitation of calcium, leading to ductal obstruction and subsequent attacks of pancreatitis. Approximately 1.5% to 13% of patients with primary hyperparathyroidism develop AP.

Miscellaneous Conditions

Blunt and penetrating abdominal trauma can be associated with AP in 0.2% and 1% of cases, respectively. Prolonged intraoperative hypotension and excessive pancreatic manipulation during abdominal surgery can also result in AP. Pancreatic ischemia in association with acute pancreatic inflammation can develop after splenic artery embolization. Other rare causes include scorpion venom stings and perforated duodenal ulcers.

Clinical Manifestations

The cardinal symptom of AP is epigastric or periumbilical pain that radiates to the back. Up to 90% of patients have nausea or vomiting that typically does not relieve the pain. The nature of the pain is constant; therefore, if the pain disappears or decreases, another diagnosis should be considered.

Dehydration, poor skin turgor, tachycardia, hypotension, and dry mucous membranes are commonly seen in patients with AP. Severely dehydrated and older patients may also develop mental status changes.

The physical examination findings of the abdomen vary according to the severity of the disease. With mild pancreatitis, the physical examination findings of the abdomen may be normal or reveal only mild epigastric tenderness. Significant abdominal distention, associated with generalized rebound and abdominal rigidity, is present in severe pancreatitis. The nature of the pain described by the patient may not correlate with the physical examination findings or the degree of pancreatic inflammation.

Rare findings include flank and periumbilical ecchymosis (Grey Turner and Cullen signs, respectively). Both are indicative of retroperitoneal bleeding associated with severe pancreatitis. Patients with concomitant choledocholithiasis or significant edema in the head of the pancreas that compresses the intrapancreatic portion of the common bile duct can present with jaundice. Dullness to percussion and decreased breathing sounds in the left or, less commonly, in the right hemithorax suggest pleural effusion secondary to AP.

Diagnosis

The cornerstone of the diagnosis of AP is the clinical findings plus an elevation of pancreatic enzyme levels in the plasma. A threefold or higher elevation of amylase and lipase levels confirms the diagnosis. The serum half-life of amylase is shorter than that of lipase. In patients who do not present to the emergency department within the first 24 to 48 hours after the onset of symptoms, determination of lipase levels is a more sensitive indicator to establish the diagnosis. Lipase is also a more specific marker of AP because serum amylase levels can be elevated in a number of conditions, such as peptic ulcer disease, mesenteric ischemia, salpingitis, and macroamylasemia.

Patients with AP are typically hyperglycemic; they can also have leukocytosis and abnormal elevation of liver enzyme levels. The elevation of alanine aminotransferase levels in the serum in the context of AP confirmed by high pancreatic enzyme levels has a positive predictive value of 95% in the diagnosis of acute biliary pancreatitis.[5]

Imaging Studies

Although simple abdominal radiographs are not useful for diagnosis of pancreatitis, they can help rule out other conditions, such as perforated ulcer disease. Nonspecific findings in patients with AP include air-fluid levels suggestive of ileus, cutoff colon sign as a result of colonic spasm at the splenic flexure, and widening of the duodenal C loop caused by severe pancreatic head edema.

The usefulness of ultrasound for diagnosis of pancreatitis is limited by intra-abdominal fat and increased intestinal gas as a result of the ileus. Nevertheless, this test should always be ordered in patients with AP because of its high sensitivity (95%) in diagnosing gallstones. Combined elevations of liver transaminase and pancreatic enzyme levels and the presence of gallstones on ultrasound have an even higher sensitivity (97%) and specificity (100%) for diagnosing acute biliary pancreatitis.

Contrast-enhanced computed tomography (CT) is currently the best modality for evaluation of the pancreas, especially if the study is performed with a multidetector CT scanner. The most valuable contrast phase in which to evaluate the pancreatic parenchyma is the portal venous phase (65 to 70 seconds after injection of contrast material), which allows evaluation of the viability of the pancreatic parenchyma, amount of peripancreatic inflammation, and presence of intra-abdominal free air or fluid collections. Noncontrast CT scanning may also be of value in the setting of renal failure by identifying fluid collections or extraluminal air.

Abdominal magnetic resonance imaging (MRI) is also useful to evaluate the extent of necrosis, inflammation, and presence of free fluid. However, its cost and availability and the fact that patients requiring imaging are critically ill and need to be in intensive care units limit its applicability in the acute phase. Although magnetic resonance cholangiopancreatography (MRCP) is not indicated in the acute setting of AP, it has an important role in the evaluation of patients with unexplained or recurrent pancreatitis because it allows complete visualization of the biliary and pancreatic duct anatomy. In addition, intravenous (IV) administration of secretin increases pancreatic duct secretion, which causes a transient distention of the pancreatic duct. For example, secretin MRCP is useful in patients with AP and no evidence of a predisposing condition to rule out pancreas divisum, intraductal papillary mucinous neoplasm (IPMN), or a small tumor in the pancreatic duct.

In the setting of gallstone pancreatitis, endoscopic ultrasound (EUS) may play an important role in the evaluation of persistent choledocholithiasis. Several studies have shown that routine ERCP for suspected gallstone pancreatitis reveals no evidence of persistent obstruction in most cases and may actually worsen symptoms because of manipulation of the gland. EUS has been proven to be sensitive for identifying choledocholithiasis; it allows examination of the biliary tree and pancreas with no risk of worsening of the pancreatitis. In patients in whom persistent choledocholithiasis is confirmed by EUS, ERCP can be used selectively as a therapeutic measure.

Assessment of Severity of Disease

The earliest scoring system designed to evaluate the severity of AP was introduced by Ranson and colleagues in 1974.[7] It predicts the severity of the disease on the basis of 11 parameters obtained at the time of admission or 48 hours later. The mortality rate of AP directly correlates with the number of parameters that are positive. Severe pancreatitis is diagnosed if three or more of the Ranson criteria are fulfilled. The main disadvantage is that it does not predict the severity of disease at the time of the admission because six parameters are assessed only after 48 hours of admission. The Ranson score has a low positive predictive value (50%) and high negative predictive value (90%). Therefore, it is mainly used to rule out severe pancreatitis or to predict the risk of mortality.[8] The original scoring symptom designed to predict the severity of the disease and its modification for acute biliary pancreatitis are shown in Boxes 55-1 and 55-2.

AP severity can also be addressed by the Acute Physiology and Chronic Health Evaluation (APACHE II) score. Based on the patient's age, previous health status, and 12 routine physiologic measurements, APACHE II provides a general measure of the severity of disease. An APACHE II score of 8 or higher defines severe pancreatitis. The main advantage is that it can be used on admission and repeated at any time. However, it is complex, not specific for AP, and based on the patient's age, which easily upgrades the AP severity score. APACHE II has a positive predictive value of 43% and a negative predictive value of 89%.[8]

Using imaging characteristics, Balthazar and associates[9] have established the CT severity index. This index correlates CT findings with the patient's outcome. The CT severity index is shown in Table 55-2.

BOX 55-1 Ranson Prognostic Criteria for Non-Gallstone Pancreatitis

At presentation
- Age >55 years
- Blood glucose level >200 mg/dL
- White blood cell count >16,000 cells/mm³
- Lactate dehydrogenase level >350 IU/liter
- Aspartate aminotransferase level >250 IU/liter

After 48 hours of admission
- Hematocrit*: decrease >10%
- Serum calcium level <8 mg/dL
- Base deficit >4 mEq/L
- Blood urea nitrogen level: increase >5 mg/dL
- Fluid requirement >6 liters
- PaO₂ <60 mm Hg

Ranson score ≥3 defines severe pancreatitis.

*Compared with admission value.

BOX 55-2 Ranson Prognostic Criteria for Gallstone Pancreatitis

At presentation
- Age >70 years
- Blood glucose level >220 mg/dL
- White blood cell count >18,000 cells/mm³
- Lactate dehydrogenase level >400 IU/liter
- Aspartate aminotransferase level >250 IU/liter

After 48 hours of admission
- Hematocrit*: decrease >10%
- Serum calcium level <8 mg/dL
- Base deficit >5 mEq/L
- Blood urea nitrogen level: increase >2 mg/dL
- Fluid requirement >4 liters
- PaO₂: Not available

Ranson score ≥3 defines severe pancreatitis.

*Compared with admission value.

In 1992, the International Symposium on Acute Pancreatitis defined severe pancreatitis as the presence of local pancreatic complications (necrosis, abscess, or pseudocyst) or any evidence of organ failure. Severe pancreatitis is diagnosed if there is any evidence of organ failure or a local pancreatic complication (Box 55-3).

C-reactive protein (CRP) is an inflammatory marker that peaks 48 to 72 hours after the onset of pancreatitis and correlates with the severity of the disease. A CRP level of 150 mg/mL or higher defines severe pancreatitis. The major limitation is that it cannot be used on admission; the sensitivity of the assay decreases if CRP levels are measured within 48 hours after the onset of symptoms. In addition to CRP, a number of studies have shown other biochemical markers (e.g., serum levels of procalcitonin, IL-6, IL-1, elastase) that correlate with the severity of the disease. However, their main limitation is their cost, and they are not widely available.

Treatment

Regardless of the cause or the severity of the disease, the cornerstone of the treatment of AP is aggressive fluid resuscitation with

TABLE 55-2 Computed Tomography Severity Index (CTSI) for Acute Pancreatitis

FEATURE	POINTS
Pancreatic Inflammation	
Normal pancreas	0
Focal or diffuse pancreatic enlargement	1
Intrinsic pancreatic alterations with peripancreatic fat inflammatory changes	2
Single fluid collection or phlegmon	3
Two or more fluid collections or gas, in or adjacent to the pancreas	4
Pancreatic Necrosis	
None	0
≤30%	2
30%-50%	4
>50%	6

CTSI 0-3, mortality 3%, morbidity 8%; CTSI 4-6, mortality 6%, morbidity 35%; CTSI 7-10, mortality 17%, morbidity 92%.

BOX 55-3 Atlanta Criteria for Acute Pancreatitis

Organ Failure, as Defined by
Shock (systolic blood pressure <90 mm Hg)
Pulmonary insufficiency (Pao$_2$ <60 mm Hg)
Renal failure (creatinine level >2 mg/dL after fluid resuscitation)
Gastrointestinal bleeding (>500 mL/24 hr)

Systemic Complications
Disseminated intravascular coagulation (platelet count ≤100,000)
Fibrinogen <1 g/liter
Fibrin split products >80 μg/dL
Metabolic disturbance (calcium level ≤7.5 mg/dL)

Local Complications
Necrosis
Abscess
Pseudocyst
  Severe pancreatitis is defined by the presence of any evidence of organ failure or a local complication.

isotonic crystalloid solution. The rate of administration should be individualized and adjusted on the basis of age, comorbidities, vital signs, mental status, skin turgor, and urine output. Patients who do not respond to initial fluid resuscitation or have significant renal, cardiac, or respiratory comorbidities often require invasive monitoring with central venous access and a Foley catheter.

In addition to fluid resuscitation, patients with AP require continuous pulse oximetry because one of the most common systemic complications of AP is hypoxemia caused by the acute lung injury associated with this disease. Patients should receive supplementary oxygen to maintain arterial saturation above 95%.

It is also essential to provide effective analgesia. Narcotics are usually preferred, especially morphine. One of the physiologic effects described after systemic administration of morphine is an increase in tone in the sphincter of Oddi; however, there is no

evidence that narcotics exert a negative impact on the outcome of patients with AP.

There is no proven benefit in treating AP with antiproteases (e.g., gabexate mesilate, aprotinin), platelet-activating factor inhibitors (e.g., lexipafant), or pancreatic secretion inhibitors.

Nutritional support is vital in the treatment of AP. Oral feeding may be impossible because of persistent ileus, pain, or intubation. In addition, 20% of patients with severe AP develop recurrent pain shortly after the oral route has been restarted. The main options to provide this nutritional support are enteral feeding and total parenteral nutrition (TPN). Although there is no difference in the mortality rate between both types of nutrition, enteral nutrition is associated with fewer infectious complications and reduces the need for pancreatic surgery. Although TPN provides most nutritional requirements, it is associated with mucosal atrophy, decreased intestinal blood flow, increased risk of bacterial overgrowth in the small bowel, antegrade colonization with colonic bacteria, and increased bacterial translocation. In addition, patients with TPN have more central line infections and metabolic complications (e.g., hyperglycemia, electrolyte imbalance). Whenever possible, enteral nutrition should be used rather than TPN.

Given the significant increase in mortality associated with septic complications in severe pancreatitis, a number of physicians advocated the use of prophylactic antibiotics in the 1970s. Recent meta-analyses and systematic reviews that have evaluated multiple randomized controlled trials have proved that prophylactic antibiotics do not decrease the frequency of surgical intervention, infected necrosis, or mortality in patients with severe pancreatitis. In addition, they are associated with gram-positive cocci infection, such as by *Staphylococcus aureus*, and *Candida* infection, which is seen in 5% to 15% of patients.[10]

Special Considerations

Endoscopic retrograde cholangiopancreatography. Early ERCP, with or without sphincterotomy, was initially advocated to reduce the severity of pancreatitis because the obstructive theory of AP states that pancreatic injury is the result of pancreatic duct obstruction. However, three randomized trials have demonstrated that ERCP is beneficial only for patients with severe acute biliary pancreatitis. Routine use of ERCP is not indicated for patients with mild pancreatitis because the bile duct obstruction is usually transient and resolves within 48 hours after the onset of symptoms. In addition to severe acute biliary pancreatitis, ERCP is indicated for patients who develop cholangitis and those with persistent bile duct obstruction demonstrated by other imaging modalities, such as EUS. Finally, in older patients with poor performance status or severe comorbidities that preclude surgery, ERCP with sphincterotomy is a safe alternative to prevent recurrent biliary pancreatitis.

Laparoscopic cholecystectomy. In the absence of definitive treatment, 30% of patients with acute biliary pancreatitis will have recurrent disease. With the exception of older patients and those with poor performance status, laparoscopic cholecystectomy is indicated for all patients with mild acute biliary pancreatitis. Studies have shown that early laparoscopic cholecystectomy, defined as laparoscopic cholecystectomy during the initial admission to the hospital, is a safe procedure that decreases recurrence of the disease.[5] Choledocholithiasis can be excluded by intraoperative cholangiography, ERCP, or laparoscopic common bile duct exploration.

For patients with severe pancreatitis, early surgery may increase the morbidity and length of stay.[11] Current recommendations suggest conservative treatment for at least 6 weeks before laparoscopic cholecystectomy is attempted in this setting. This approach has significantly decreased morbidity.[5]

Complications

Sterile and Infected Peripancreatic Fluid Collections

The presence of acute abdominal fluid during an episode of AP has been described in 30% to 57% of patients. In contrast to pseudocysts and cystic neoplasias of the pancreas, fluid collections are not surrounded or encased by epithelium or fibrotic capsule. Treatment is supportive because most fluid collections will be spontaneously reabsorbed by the peritoneum. Fever, elevated white blood cell count, and abdominal pain suggest infection of this fluid, and percutaneous aspiration is confirmatory. Percutaneous drainage and IV administration of antibiotics should be instituted if infection is present.

Pancreatic Necrosis and Infected Necrosis

Pancreatic necrosis is the presence of nonviable pancreatic parenchyma or peripancreatic fat; it can be manifested as a focal area or diffuse involvement of the gland. Contrast-enhanced CT is the most reliable technique to diagnose pancreatic necrosis. It is typically seen as areas of low attenuation (<40 to 50 HU) after the IV injection of contrast material. Normal parenchyma usually has a density of 100 to 150 HU. Up to 20% of patients with AP develop pancreatic necrosis. It is important to identify and to provide proper treatment of this complication because most patients who develop multiorgan failure have necrotizing pancreatitis; pancreatic necrosis has been documented in up to 80% of the autopsies of patients who died after an episode of AP.[3]

The main complication of pancreatic necrosis is infection. The risk is directly related to the amount of necrosis; in patients with pancreatic necrosis involving less than 30% of the gland, the risk of infection is 22%. The risk is 37% for patients with pancreatic necrosis that involves 30% to 50% of the gland and up to 46% if more than 70% of the gland is affected.[3] This complication is associated with bacterial translocation usually involving enteric flora, such as gram-negative rods (e.g., *Escherichia coli, Klebsiella,* and *Pseudomonas* spp.) and *Enterococcus* spp.

Infected pancreatic necrosis should be suspected in patients with prolonged fever, elevated white blood cell count, or progressive clinical deterioration. Evidence of air within the pancreatic necrosis seen on a CT scan confirms the diagnosis but is a rare finding. If infected necrosis is suspected, fine-needle aspiration (FNA) may be performed if the diagnosis is equivocal; from the aspirate, a positive Gram stain or culture establishes the diagnosis. Although positive cultures are confirmatory, a review has demonstrated that despite negative preoperative cultures, 42% of patients with so-called persistent unwellness will have infected necrosis.[12] Figure 55-7 illustrates the pathophysiologic process of pancreatic necrosis infection.

Once infection has been demonstrated, IV antibiotics should be given. Because of their penetration into the pancreas and spectrum coverage, carbapenems are the first option of treatment. Alternative therapy includes quinolones, metronidazole, third-generation cephalosporins, and piperacillin.

Historically, the definitive treatment of infected pancreatic necrosis is surgical débridement with necrosectomy, closed continuous irrigation, or open packaging (Fig. 55-8). The overall mortality rate after open necrosectomy has been as high as 25% to 30%[12] because of the severe nature of the disease as well as the high complication rate of an open débridement. Outcomes are

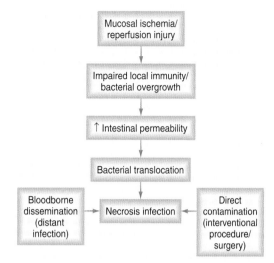

FIGURE 55-7 Pathophysiology of Pancreatic Necrosis Infection. The acute inflammatory injury that occurs during the first 48 to 72 hours causes mucosal ischemia and reperfusion injury. Both effects favor bacterial overgrowth because they alter local immunity. Mucosal ischemia also produces an increase in the permeability of intestinal cells, which is initiated 72 hours after the acute episode but typically peaks 1 week later. These transient episodes of bacteremia are associated with pancreatic necrosis infection. Less frequently, distant sources of infection, such as pneumonia and vascular or urinary tract infection associated with central lines and catheters, are associated with bacteremia and pancreatic necrosis. Finally, local contamination after surgery or interventional procedures such as ERCP is responsible for necrosis infection.

time dependent; patients who undergo surgery in the first 14 days have a mortality rate of 75%, and those who undergo surgery between 15 and 29 days and after 30 days have mortality rates of 45% and 8%, respectively.[13] As a result of the elevated morbidity and mortality rates with open débridement, endoscopic and laparoscopic techniques are being used more often. Both may ultimately provide similar outcomes, with hopes of reducing perioperative morbidity and mortality, although level I data are lacking. In general, the longer a patient can be medically optimized and managed with enteral nutrition and antibiotics (if indicated), the more mature a fluid collection (with or without necrosis), and therefore the extent of an endoscopic or operative débridement (if needed) will be better delineated and tolerated.

In 2010, the Dutch Pancreatitis Study Group performed a randomized trial evaluating open necrosectomy versus percutaneous drainage followed by minimally invasive retroperitoneal débridement for necrotizing and infected necrotizing pancreatitis. The results showed that long-term end-point complications and mortality rates were better compared with the open necrosectomy group.[14]

Currently, an endoscopic drainage with a large-bore stent and possible endoscopic débridement with or without percutaneous drainage may avoid open operations in some patients. If the endoscopic management fails, an open operation will usually be more straightforward and the results improved. When either route is taken, physiologic and nutritional support of the patient will have a large impact on outcome.

Pancreatic Pseudocysts

Pancreatic pseudocysts occur in 5% to 15% of patients who have peripancreatic fluid collections after AP. By definition, the capsule of a pseudocyst is composed of collagen and granulation tissue, and it is not lined by epithelium.[15] The fibrotic reaction typically requires at least 4 to 8 weeks to develop. Figure 55-9 shows CT scans of a large pseudocyst arising in the tail of the pancreas.

Up to 50% of patients with pancreatic pseudocysts will develop symptoms. Persistent pain, early satiety, nausea, weight loss, and elevated pancreatic enzyme levels in plasma suggest this diagnosis. The diagnosis is corroborated by CT or MRI. EUS with FNA is indicated for patients in whom the diagnosis of pancreatic pseudocyst is not clear. Characteristic features of pancreatic pseudocysts include high amylase levels associated with the absence of mucin and low carcinoembryonic antigen (CEA) levels.

Observation is indicated for asymptomatic patients because spontaneous regression has been documented in up to 70% of

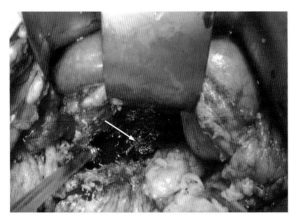

FIGURE 55-8 Infected Pancreatic Necrosis. This 45-year-old man had severe ethanol-induced pancreatitis. Four weeks after the initial episode, the patient developed fever (39.5° C [103° F]), hypotension, and leukocytosis (19,000 cells/mm³). The CT scan documented pancreatic necrosis involving 35% of the gland. After FNA, Gram staining documented the presence of gram-negative rods. The exploratory laparotomy indicated pancreatic necrosis involving mainly the body of the gland *(arrow)*. The patient was treated with necrosectomy, closed drainage, and IV meropenem. Final culture documented the presence of *Escherichia coli.* The patient was discharged home 56 days after the initial episode.

cases; this is particularly true for patients with pseudocysts smaller than 4 cm in diameter, located in the tail, and no evidence of pancreatic duct obstruction or communication with the main pancreatic duct.[15] Invasive therapies are indicated for symptomatic patients or when the differentiation between a cystic neoplasm and pseudocyst is not possible. Because most patients are treated with decompressive procedures and not with resection, it is imperative to have a pathologic diagnosis. Surgical drainage has been the traditional approach for pancreatic pseudocysts. However, there is increasing evidence that transgastric and transduodenal endoscopic drainage are safe and effective approaches for patients with pancreatic pseudocysts in close contact (defined as <1 cm) with the stomach and duodenum, respectively. In addition, transpapillary drainage can be attempted in pancreatic pseudocysts communicating with the main pancreatic duct. For patients in whom a pancreatic duct stricture is associated with a pancreatic pseudocyst, endoscopic dilation and stent placement are indicated.

Surgical drainage is indicated for patients with pancreatic pseudocysts that cannot be treated with endoscopic techniques and for patients who fail to respond to endoscopic treatment. Definitive treatment depends on the location of the cyst. Pancreatic pseudocysts closely attached to the stomach should be treated with a cystogastrostomy. In this procedure, an anterior gastrostomy is performed. Once the pseudocyst is located, it is drained through the posterior wall of the stomach using a linear stapler. The defect in the anterior wall of the stomach is closed in two layers. Pancreatic pseudocysts located in the head of the pancreas that are in close contact with the duodenum are treated with a cystoduodenostomy. Finally, some pseudocysts are not in contact with the stomach or duodenum. The surgical treatment for these patients is a Roux-en-Y cystojejunostomy. Surgical cyst enterostomy is successful in achieving immediate cyst drainage in more than 90% of cases. After initial resolution, pseudocyst formation may recur in up to 12% of cases during long-term follow-up, depending on the location of the cyst and underlying cause of the disease.[15]

Complications of pancreatic pseudocysts include bleeding and pancreaticopleural fistula secondary to vascular and pleural erosion, respectively; bile duct and duodenal obstruction; rupture into the abdominal cavity; and infection. Percutaneous drainage is indicated only for septic patients secondary to pseudocyst infection because it has a high incidence of external fistula.

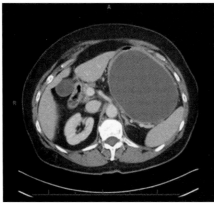
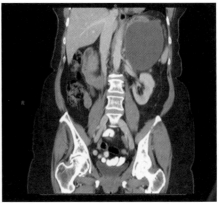

FIGURE 55-9 CT scans showing a large pseudocyst arising in the tail of the pancreas.

Pancreatic Ascites and Pancreaticopleural Fistulas

Although very rare, complete disruption of the pancreatic duct can lead to significant accumulation of fluid. This condition should be suspected in patients who have an episode of AP, develop significant abdominal distention, and have free intra-abdominal fluid. Diagnostic paracentesis typically demonstrates elevated amylase and lipase levels. Treatment consists of abdominal drainage combined with endoscopic placement of a pancreatic stent across the disruption. Failure of this therapy requires surgical treatment; it consists of distal resection and closure of the proximal stump.

Posterior pancreatic duct disruption into the pleural space has been described rarely. Symptoms that suggest this condition include dyspnea, abdominal pain, cough, and chest pain. The diagnosis is confirmed with chest radiography, thoracentesis, and CT scan. Figure 55-10 demonstrates a large, left-sided pleural effusion caused by a pancreatic-pleural fistula. Amylase levels above 50,000 IU in the pleural fluid confirm the diagnosis. It is more common after alcoholic pancreatitis and in 70% of patients is associated with pancreatic pseudocysts. Initial treatment requires chest drainage, parenteral nutritional support, and administration of octreotide. Up to 60% of patients respond to this therapy. Persistent drainage should also be treated with endoscopic sphincterotomy and stent placement. Patients who do not respond to these measures require surgical treatment, similar to that described for pancreatic ascites.

Vascular Complications

AP is rarely associated with arterial vascular complications. The most common vessel affected is the splenic artery, but the SMA, cystic artery, and GDA have also been found to be affected. It has been proposed that pancreatic elastase damages the vessels, leading to pseudoaneurysm formation. Spontaneous rupture results in massive bleeding. Clinical manifestations include sudden onset of abdominal pain, tachycardia, and hypotension. If possible, arterial embolization should be attempted to control the bleeding. Refractory cases require ligation of the vessel affected. The mortality ranges from 28% to 56%.

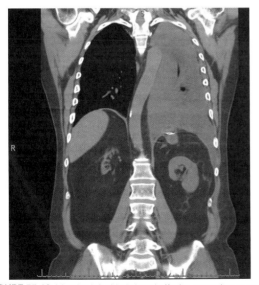

FIGURE 55-10 Massive left-sided pleural effusion secondary to a pancreaticopleural fistula.

Pancreatic inflammation can also produce vascular thrombosis; the vessel usually affected is the splenic vein, but in severe cases, it can extend into the portal venous system. Imaging demonstrates splenomegaly, gastric varices, and splenic vein occlusion. Thrombolytics have been described in the acute early phase; however, most patients can be managed with conservative treatment. Recurrent episodes of upper gastrointestinal bleeding caused by venous hypertension should be treated with splenectomy.

Pancreatocutaneous Fistula

The frequency of pancreatic fistulas is low. Only 0.4% of patients have this complication after an acute episode. However, the incidence of this complication increases in patients with other complications after AP: 4.5% in patients with pancreatic pseudocysts (4.5%) and 40% in patients with infected necrosis after surgical débridement.[12] Treatment is conservative for most patients.

CHRONIC PANCREATITIS

In contrast to AP, the histologic hallmark of chronic pancreatitis is the persistent inflammation and irreversible fibrosis associated with atrophy of the pancreatic parenchyma. These histologic features are associated with chronic pain and endocrine and exocrine insufficiency that significantly decrease the quality of life of these patients. Chronic pancreatitis affects between 3 and 10/100,000 persons.

Risk Factors

The specific cause and frequency of each condition vary among countries, hospital populations, and referral practices. In general, heavy alcohol consumption is the most common cause of chronic pancreatitis (70% to 80% of cases), especially in urban hospitals. Conditions such as chronic duct obstruction, trauma, pancreas divisum, cystic dystrophy of the duodenal wall, hyperparathyroidism, hypertriglyceridemia, autoimmune pancreatitis, tropical pancreatitis, and hereditary pancreatitis are rare and account for less than 10% of all cases. However, hereditary, chronic, and autoimmune pancreatitis are more common in referral centers. In up to 20% of patients, a clear cause cannot be documented and cases are considered to be idiopathic.

Alcohol Abuse

Prolonged alcohol abuse is the most important risk factor associated with chronic pancreatitis. The fact that only 3% to 7% of heavy drinkers develop chronic pancreatitis suggests that alcohol is only a cofactor and that other factors are required for development of this complication. Alcohol exerts multiple noxious effects in the pancreas: it increases the total protein concentration in the pancreatic juice, it promotes the synthesis and secretion of lithostathine by acinar cells, and it increases glycoprotein 2 secretion in pancreatic juice. These factors lead to protein precipitation and subsequent formation of protein plugs and eventually stones inside the pancreatic duct. As a result of the obstruction, acinar cells are no longer able to secrete pancreatic enzymes and are predisposed to autodigestion. In addition, several products of alcohol metabolism, such as fatty acid ethyl esters and reactive oxygen species, cause fragility of intra-acinar organelles, such as zymogen granules and lysosomes, which leads to abnormal pancreatic enzyme activation inside acinar cells. Acetaldehyde, another alcohol metabolite, causes direct acinar injury. Chronic alcohol consumption is associated with enhanced NF-κB activity, decreased perfusion in the microcirculation of the pancreas, and increased intracellular calcium levels.

The identification of pancreatic stellate cells (PSCs) in the late 1990s is one of the most important discoveries in the pathophysiology of chronic pancreatitis.[16] PSCs are specialized quiescent fibroblasts found at the base of acinar cells. Once stimulated, PSCs differentiate into activated myofibroblasts, which synthesize proteins that form the extracellular matrix. Examples of these proteins include collagen I and III, fibronectin, laminin, and matrix metalloproteinases. PSCs have responses similar to hepatic stellate cells; chronic necrosis and inflammation (necroinflammation) induce the release of inflammatory mediators, such as platelet-derived growth factor, TGF-β, TNF-α, IL-1, and IL-6, which are known to activate PSCs. Consequently, the synthesis of collagen and other components of pancreatic fibrosis is increased. It has been postulated that the chronic necroinflammation induced by ethanol activates PSCs and induces pancreatic fibrosis. Interestingly, it has also been shown that alcohol and some of its metabolites (e.g., acetaldehyde) cause activation of PSCs.

Although they have been evaluated only in preclinical studies, novel therapies that target the activation of PSCs are being investigated. It has been reported that antioxidants, angiotensin-converting enzyme inhibitors, peroxisome proliferator-activated receptor gamma ligands, and vitamin A inhibit the activity of PSCs.

Smoking

Epidemiologic studies have shown that smoking increases the risk of alcohol-induced chronic pancreatitis. Active smokers develop chronic pancreatitis at a younger age compared with nonsmokers. In addition, the risk of pancreatic calcifications and diabetes mellitus is increased in patients who smoke compared with nonsmokers.

Gene Mutations

Under physiologic conditions, pancreatic enzyme activation is strictly controlled. Mutations in proteins that regulate this activation increase the risk of chronic pancreatitis. Mutations in the cationic trypsinogen gene, also known as protease serine 1 (PRSS1) gene, are common in hereditary chronic pancreatitis. PRSS1 is located on chromosome 7 and regulates trypsinogen production; mutations in this gene are associated with intra-acinar trypsinogen activation. PRSS1 mutations have been documented in hereditary pancreatitis but are uncommon in other forms of chronic pancreatitis.

SPINK-1 is a peptide secreted by acinar cells that regulates the premature activation of trypsinogen. Because SPINK1 mutations are present in 1% to 2% of healthy patients but the prevalence of chronic pancreatitis is much lower, it has been hypothesized that SPINK1 mutations are not enough to trigger pancreatic inflammation. However, they lower the threshold for its development and influence the severity of the disease. SPINK1 mutations are more prevalent in alcoholic, hereditary, and idiopathic pancreatitis.

The secretion of bicarbonate and chloride in respiratory and pancreatic secretions is regulated by the CFTR gene. CFTR mutations affect the normal secretion of bicarbonate, decrease pancreatic juice volume, and augment the concentration of pancreatic enzymes inside the pancreatic duct. Homozygous CFTR mutations result in cystic fibrosis; heterozygous mild mutations predispose to pancreatic exocrine insufficiency and chronic pancreatitis.

The prevalence of CFTR gene mutations is higher in patients with alcoholic, idiopathic, and hereditary pancreatitis compared with the general population.

Animal studies in trypsin knockout mice suggest that even in the absence of trypsin, chronic noxious stimuli can induce chronic pancreatitis.[17] These results suggest that alternative pathways independent of trypsin may exist that can lead to chronic injury in pancreatitis, and elucidation of these pathways may lead to development of novel therapeutics.

Types of Chronic Pancreatitis
Autoimmune Pancreatitis

Autoimmune pancreatitis is a chronic inflammatory disorder that involves the pancreas. At least two different histologic variants have been defined. Type 1 is the most common; it is characterized by dense, periductal lymphoplasmacytic infiltrates, storiform fibrosis, and obliterative venulitis. Plasmatic cells typically stain positive for immunoglobulin G4. In type 2, the pancreas is infiltrated by neutrophils, lymphocytes, and plasma cells that destroy and obliterate the epithelium in the pancreatic duct. Autoimmune pancreatitis is more common in men than in women. Up to 80% of patients are older than 50 years. Patients with autoimmune pancreatitis can develop acute symptoms such as jaundice or AP, closely mimicking patients with pancreatic adenocarcinoma. However, most patients with chronic pancreatitis develop chronic abdominal discomfort associated with abnormal elevation of amylase and lipase levels.

Tropical Pancreatitis

Tropical pancreatitis is not common in the United States; it is more common in tropical areas within 30 degrees of the equator, particularly in India. Its pathophysiology has not been completely delineated, but it has been associated with cassava ingestion and SPINK1 mutations. Up to 45% to 50% of patients with tropical pancreatitis have SPINK1 mutations.

Idiopathic Pancreatitis

In up to 10% to 20% of patients with chronic pancreatitis, a clear cause that predisposed to the disease is not evident. Future identification of genetic defects associated with chronic pancreatitis may allow the identification of individuals at highest risk for development of this disease.

Clinical Manifestations

Pain is the primary manifestation of chronic pancreatitis. Initially precipitated by oral intake, the intensity, frequency, and duration of pain gradually increase with worsening disease. Quality of life of these patients is significantly affected because of decreased oral intake, interference with daily activities, and dependence on narcotic pain medications. Nausea and vomiting are not common early on; however, they may appear as the disease progresses.

Pancreatic inflammation and fibrosis not only affect the pancreatic ducts but also decrease the number and function of acinar cells. At least 90% of the gland needs to be dysfunctional before steatorrhea, diarrhea, and other symptoms of malabsorption develop. In severe cases, diseases associated with fat-soluble vitamin deficiency, such as bleeding, osteopenia, and osteoporosis, develop. Exocrine insufficiency occurs in 80% to 90% of patients with long-standing chronic pancreatitis.

Chronic pancreatitis also affects islet cell populations. As a result, 40% to 80% of patients will have clinical manifestations of diabetes mellitus. The prevalence depends on the predisposing condition and onset of symptoms. Diabetes mellitus typically occurs many years after the onset of abdominal pain and pancreatic exocrine insufficiency.

Jaundice or cholangitis occurs in 5% to 10% of patients because of fibrosis of the distal common bile duct. Extensive scarring in the head of the pancreas can also obstruct the duodenum, leading to severe nausea, vomiting, and abdominal pain. Upper gastrointestinal bleeding secondary to portal or splenic vein thrombosis is a rare manifestation of chronic pancreatitis.

Diagnosis
Imaging Studies

The diagnosis of chronic pancreatitis may be challenging early in the course of the disease because the correlation between symptoms and the structural changes seen on imaging studies is poor. The most common CT findings in chronic pancreatitis include dilated pancreatic duct (68%), parenchymal atrophy (54%), and pancreatic calcifications (50%; Fig. 55-11). Other findings include peripancreatic fluid, focal pancreatic enlargement, biliary duct dilation, and irregular pancreatic parenchyma contour. CT has a sensitivity of 56% to 95% and a specificity of 85% to 100% for the diagnosis of chronic pancreatitis. In addition to establishing the diagnosis, CT is particularly useful to assess complications, such as pancreatic duct disruption, pseudocysts, portal and splenic vein thrombosis, and splenic and pancreaticoduodenal artery pseudoaneurysms.

MRI is a reliable alternative to evaluate patients with chronic pancreatitis. The sensitivity for the diagnosis of pancreatic calcifications is lower, but MRI is useful to detect changes in the pancreatic parenchyma suggestive of chronic inflammation, such as changes in intensity, pancreatic atrophy, and irregularities in the contour. In addition, MRCP with secretin injection is particularly useful to evaluate intraductal strictures and pancreatic duct disruption.

Although ERCP was historically considered the "gold standard" for the diagnosis of chronic pancreatitis, the advent of secretin MRCP and EUS has significantly decreased its role as a diagnostic test. Current indications include patients for whom other diagnostic tests, including CT and MRCP, are contraindicated or have failed to corroborate the diagnosis. ERCP should

be considered a therapeutic modality in patients who develop pancreatic duct complications amenable to endoscopic therapy, such as stricture, stone, pseudocysts, and biliary stenosis.

EUS has emerged during the past 25 years as the most accurate technique to diagnose chronic pancreatitis in patients with minimal change disease or in the early stages. A panel of endosonographers has defined the criteria required for diagnosis of chronic pancreatitis, known as the Rosemont criteria (Box 55-4). Histologic evidence of inflammation, atrophy, and fibrosis is the gold standard for the diagnosis of chronic pancreatitis; however, current evidence does not support the use of EUS-guided FNA or Tru-Cut biopsies to diagnose this disease.[18]

Functional Tests

Measurement of the fecal elastase 1 level is the preferred noninvasive study to diagnose pancreatic exocrine insufficiency. It quantifies the amount of fecal elastase 1 using monoclonal or polyclonal anti–human elastase 1 antibodies. A fecal elastase 1 concentration above 200 μg/g feces is normal; a fecal elastase 1 concentration between 100 and 200 μg/g defines mild to moderate pancreatic insufficiency; and a fecal elastase 1 concentration below 100 μg/g establishes the diagnosis of severe pancreatic exocrine insufficiency.

The fecal fat and weight estimation test measures the stool content of fat after a nutritional intake of 100 g of fat per day during 3 days. If the stool fat content exceeds 7 g/day, the diagnosis of steatorrhea is established.

Treatment
Medical Treatment

The main goal in the treatment of these patients is palliation of symptoms. Optimal treatment requires that a multidisciplinary team follow a systematized and well-structured therapeutic plan. Patient counseling is an important component because current evidence suggests that this disease is irreversible, but disease progression can be delayed if the predisposing condition is eradicated. Patients should be strongly encouraged to stop drinking and smoking. Furthermore, other risk factors, such as hypertriglyceridemia, should be treated, and diet modification (i.e., low-fat diet)

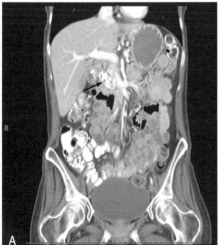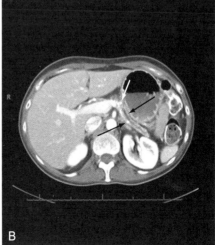

FIGURE 55-11 Typical CT findings associated with chronic pancreatitis. Shown are pancreatic duct dilation *(long arrow)* and intrapancreatic calcifications, which are also typical of chronic pancreatitis *(small arrow)*.

may benefit some patients.

Because most patients develop pain during the natural history of the disease, analgesic selection is a cornerstone of treatment. Nonsteroidal anti-inflammatory drugs are the first line of treatment. Moderate to severe pain that does not respond to nonsteroidal anti-inflammatory drugs should be treated with tramadol

or propoxyphene. Patients with severe pain that does not respond to these recommendations should be treated with potent long-acting narcotics. It cannot be overemphasized that adjuvant measures to prevent addiction, depression, and poor quality of life should be considered for patients with severe pain who require narcotics. Alternative drugs useful in the treatment of other conditions associated with chronic pain, such as tricyclic antidepressants, selective serotonin reuptake inhibitors, combined serotonin and norepinephrine reuptake inhibitors, and α2δ inhibitors, may also be considered.

There is no question about the digestive benefits of pancreatic enzyme replacement in patients with pancreatic exocrine insufficiency. However, it is controversial whether pancreatic enzyme replacement helps control the chronic pain seen in this condition. Therapeutic trials with pancreatic enzymes should last at least 6 weeks and should be given along with proton pump inhibitors because acid suppression improves the effects of uncoated pancreatic enzymes. For patients with unrelenting pain, celiac neurolysis has been attempted without sustained success in those with chronic pancreatitis. However, it is well established that during open operation, percutaneously, or through EUS, celiac block may diminish pain in those with unresectable or locally advanced pancreatic cancer.

Interventional Therapy: Endoscopic Treatment

ERCP is the primary modality for treating symptomatic pancreatic duct obstruction with dilation and polyethylene stent placement. A number of sessions are usually required because of symptom recurrence. Note that the differential diagnosis of pancreatic duct strictures includes pancreatic cancer. Only after a thorough evaluation, which includes CT, MRCP, or EUS, has completely ruled out the possibility of malignant disease should endoscopic treatment be considered. Surgical resection is indicated if any concern of malignant disease exists.

Endoscopic stone extraction should be considered for patients with pain and pancreatic duct dilation secondary to stones. Extracorporeal shock wave lithotripsy followed by therapeutic ERCP may be required for the treatment of large impacted stones. The success rate varies from 44% to 77% for this technique. In conjunction with stone extraction, pancreatic duct stenting may benefit patients by relieving obstruction. Although this relief may be temporary, during this interim a patient may be able to improve nutritional and functional status before further, perhaps more invasive therapy.

Biliary obstruction caused by chronic pancreatitis occurs in 10% of patients and is best treated with surgical bypass. Temporary relief of the obstruction with plastic stents is indicated for patients with cholangitis or for those who are severely malnourished.

Surgical Treatment

Several factors, including intractable pain, biliary or pancreatic duct obstruction, duodenal obstruction, pseudocyst or pseudoaneurysm formation, and the inability to rule out malignant disease, may prompt surgical intervention. The choice of surgical procedure depends on the symptoms requiring palliation and the presence or absence of pancreatic ductal dilation. In general, patients with a dilated pancreatic duct (defined as diameter >7 mm), or large duct disease, require a decompressing procedure; patients with a nondilated pancreatic duct, or small duct disease, require a resectional procedure. Several clinical scenarios that require surgical intervention are described here.

Pancreatic duct dilation secondary to duct stones or strictures. Pancreatic duct dilation is defined as a main pancreatic duct measuring at least 7 mm in diameter. Pancreatic duct dilation can be secondary to a single stone or stricture; however, it is often caused by multiple strictures and stones in the pancreatic duct. The pancreatic duct dilation observed on pancreatography for chronic pancreatitis is classically described as a chain of lakes, which reflects the presence of multiple dilations and stenoses. When it is accompanied by intractable pain, this condition is best treated with side-to-side Roux-en-Y pancreaticojejunostomy, also known as the modified Puestow procedure or lateral pancreaticojejunostomy.

The anterior surface of the pancreatic duct is opened, and the anterior surface of the duct is completely unroofed. This tissue may be sent for frozen section analysis to rule out underlying malignant disease. The proximal extent of tissue resection is within 1 cm of the duodenum, and the distal limit is within 1 to 2 cm of the end of the pancreas. Failure to cross the GDA into the neck and head of the pancreas may leave undrained pancreatic head or uncinate process ducts obstructed by stones or strictures, which may give incomplete relief or early recurrence of symptoms. After all stones are extracted, a standard Roux-en-Y is used to create a lateral pancreaticojejunostomy. The main advantage offered by this procedure is parenchymal conservation, which preserves endocrine and exocrine function. The modified Puestow procedure provides palliation of pain in 80% of cases; however, 30% of cases will recur, usually 3 to 5 years after surgery. Decompressive procedures temporarily relieve the ductal obstruction, but in most cases, they do not modify the natural history of the disease, and chronic pancreatitis progresses. Other factors associated with recurrence include smoking and alcohol ingestion after surgery, failure to decompress the head and uncinate process properly, and length of the pancreaticojejunostomy.[19]

In 1987, Andersen and Frey[20] described the local resection of the pancreatic head with longitudinal pancreaticojejunostomy as an alternative procedure. The surgical approach is similar to the Puestow procedure; however, once the anterior surface of the pancreatic duct has been completely exposed, the anterior portion of the head of the pancreas is also resected, leaving a 1-cm rim of pancreatic tissue along the duodenal margin. Figure 55-12 shows intraoperative images of a Frey procedure. This procedure is also an alternative for patients with a dilated pancreatic duct secondary to a benign stricture in the head of the pancreas associated with severe inflammation, scarring, or portal hypertension surrounding the head of the pancreas that precludes a safe pancreaticoduodenectomy. The main disadvantage is the removal of pancreatic parenchyma. A study has demonstrated that 62% of patients are completely free of pain and 95% of patients have satisfactory pain control after this procedure. In the same series, 34% of patients developed endocrine or exocrine pancreatic insufficiency.[21]

Pancreatic duct dilation secondary to a single stricture or stone. On occasion, a single stricture that is proximal to the papilla produces pancreatic duct dilation. As an alternative to a Puestow or Frey procedure, a pancreaticoduodenectomy can be performed to relieve the obstruction. This procedure is described later in the surgical treatment of pancreatic adenocarcinoma. It must be emphasized that this procedure is absolutely contraindicated if more than one obstruction is present in the duct. Single distal obstructions can occasionally be treated with a distal pancreatectomy. The main disadvantage of both procedures is that they can be associated with pancreatic insufficiency because normal parenchyma is removed.

Focal inflammatory mass without significant dilation of the pancreatic duct. In a small percentage of patients with chronic pancreatitis, a predominant mass in the head or, less commonly, in the tail of the pancreas without any evidence of pancreatic duct dilation is seen. Long-standing chronic pancreatitis is also a risk factor for development of pancreatic cancer; therefore, even in patients with a known history of chronic pancreatitis, finding a focal mass is concerning because it may represent an area of pancreatic adenocarcinoma that has developed in the setting of chronic pancreatitis. Resection is recommended for surgical candidates to avoid any error in diagnosis.

Once malignant disease is ruled out with percutaneous or EUS biopsy, resection of the pancreatic head may be done with either of two operations: pancreaticoduodenectomy or duodenum-preserving pancreatic head resection, otherwise known as the Beger procedure. The Beger procedure was designed to remove the pancreatic head while preserving the remainder of the foregut anatomy and therefore function. Once the pancreatic head is removed, a Roux-en-Y is created and anastomosed to the rim of pancreas or duodenum, pancreatic duct, and body and perhaps the bile duct if it was entered. Randomized controlled trials have demonstrated that the Beger procedure offers symptomatic relief that is equivalent to the pancreaticoduodenectomy and Frey procedure in appropriately selected patients.

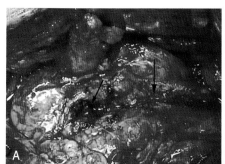 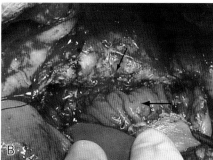

FIGURE 55-12 Frey procedure, intraoperative photographs. **A,** Significant dilation of the main pancreatic duct at the level of the head *(short arrow)* and body of the pancreas *(large arrow)* after the anterior surface of the pancreas has been opened. **B,** Side-to-side anastomosis between the pancreatic duct *(short arrow)* and jejunum *(large arrow)*.

Diffuse glandular involvement without dilation of the pancreatic duct. Decompressive procedures and local pancreatic resections are associated with an elevated failure rate in this group of patients. Patients who do not respond to medical and endoscopic therapies require surgical treatment. The most effective treatment to eliminate pain is total pancreatectomy. However, this procedure is invariably associated with diabetes mellitus. In contrast to type 1 diabetes mellitus, the severity and risk of hypoglycemia are increased in these patients.[22] In 1977, researchers at the University of Minnesota described islet autotransplantation after total pancreatectomy to prevent the effects of surgically induced diabetes. In the largest experience there, one third of patients who underwent this procedure were insulin independent, an additional one third required insulin intermittently, and the other third was fully dependent. According to this study, 90% had pain relief or reduction and 50% were able to discontinue narcotics. Similar results were demonstrated at the University of Cincinnati; up to two thirds of patients had complete or partial islet function, and 40% were insulin independent. Narcotics were discontinued in 66% of patients.[23] Although preliminary results have been encouraging, routine implementation of this operative intervention has been controversial. Major limitations associated with this procedure include the cost and lack of islet processing facilities.

As several other centers have established islet autotransplantation programs and laboratories, it has become clear that the treatment of patients with severe diffuse chronic pancreatitis should be coordinated by a multidisciplinary team. It is imperative to involve a pancreatic surgeon, pancreatologist, interventional endoscopist, radiologist, anesthesia pain specialist, and perhaps a neuropsychologist or psychiatrist. The multifaceted approach to the decision and the type of treatment is crucial to long-term success. The groups at the Medical University of South Carolina and at the University of Alabama at Birmingham[24] have shown that patients with depression or substance abuse, such as alcoholism, have a poor outcome compared with those patients without depression or alcoholism.

At the University of Minnesota,[25] a high rate of success for improvements in quality of life has been shown in pediatric patients after total pancreatectomy with islet autotransplantation. Similarly, the University of Cincinnati has described the benefit of genetic testing and the improvement in outcomes with early intervention once a genetic defect has been diagnosed.

Biliary strictures. Chronic scarring and fibrosis of the head of the pancreas result in external compression of the intrapancreatic portion of the common bile duct. Up to one third of patients with chronic pancreatitis develop radiologic evidence of bile duct dilation; however, significant biliary obstruction occurs in 6% of patients. Biliary strictures typically appear as a long symmetrical narrowing that involves the intrapancreatic portion of the common bile duct in MRCP or ERCP (Fig. 55-13). IV fluid and antibiotic therapy and temporary bile duct decompression with plastic stents is indicated for patients who present with cholangitis. Pancreaticoduodenectomy is indicated for patients in whom malignant disease cannot be excluded before surgery. A Roux-en-Y hepaticojejunostomy is an alternative treatment for patients without evidence of malignant disease or significant scarring that precludes resection of the head of the pancreas.

Duodenal stenosis. Up to 1.2% of patients with chronic pancreatitis develop duodenal strictures. Clinical manifestations include abdominal pain, nausea, vomiting, and significant weight loss. Differential diagnoses include other causes of gastric outlet obstruction secondary to upper gastrointestinal malignant neo-

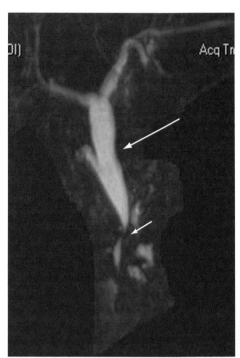

FIGURE 55-13 Bile duct stricture secondary to chronic pancreatitis. MRCP indicates common bile duct dilation *(large arrow)* secondary to a stricture at the level of the intrapancreatic portion of the common bile duct *(small arrow)*.

plasms and gastroparesis. Severely malnourished patients require IV hydration, nutritional support, and gastric decompression with a nasogastric tube. Permanent treatment requires a gastrojejunostomy.

Pancreatic pseudocyst. Pancreatic pseudocysts develop more frequently in patients with chronic pancreatitis compared with AP. Up to 30% to 40% of patients develop pseudocysts during the course of their disease. Only 10% of patients have spontaneous pancreatic pseudocyst regression. Spontaneous regression is less likely to occur in these patients because pancreatic pseudocysts arise more frequently in the setting of pancreatic duct obstruction. Indications for treatment include symptoms secondary to gastric, duodenal, or biliary compression or associated complications, such as bleeding, pancreaticopleural fistulas, rupture, or spontaneous bleeding. Alternative modalities in the treatment include endoscopic and surgical drainage (see earlier).

Traditionally, management of a symptomatic or persistent pseudocyst has been open operation and, depending on location, drainage through either cystogastrostomy or Roux-en-Y cystojejunostomy. With advancements in interventional endoscopy, drainage has proven successful with ERCP. More recently, drainage with EUS has been shown to be more successful because of improved visualization of vasculature as well as fluid collections and necrosis. Small-caliber plastic stents may be used for simple pancreatic fluid collections or larger metal stents for complex collections or those with infection or necrosis. At the University of Alabama at Birmingham, a prospective randomized trial of endoscopic versus operative cystogastrostomy showed equal efficacy but quicker improvement in quality of life and less hospital expenditure from the endoscopic approach for simple pancreatic pseudocysts.[26]

CYSTIC NEOPLASMS OF THE PANCREAS

Cystic tumors are the second most common exocrine pancreatic neoplasm, following only adenocarcinomas of the pancreas in incidence. Given the advances in modern cross-sectional imaging, the identification of cystic lesions of the pancreas is becoming common. Surgeons must be familiar with the characteristics and treatment of these lesions to determine individual management appropriately.

Types of Cystic Neoplasms
Mucinous Cystic Neoplasm

In the 1970s, the clinicopathologic spectrums of mucinous and serous cystic tumors were described. Mucinous cystic neoplasms (MCNs) are the most common cystic neoplasms of the pancreas. These tumors span the histologic spectrum from benign to invasive carcinomas. MCNs contain mucin-producing epithelium and are identified histologically by the presence of mucin-rich cells and ovarian-like stroma (Fig. 55-14). Staining for estrogen and progesterone is positive in most cases. Frequently seen in young women, the mean age at presentation is in the fifth decade. Men are rarely affected. MCNs are typically found in the body and tail of the pancreas but infrequently can occur elsewhere. Although incidental MCN is becoming increasingly common, up to 50% of patients present with vague abdominal pain. A history of pancreatitis may be found in up to 20% of patients, which explains the common misdiagnosis of pseudocyst.

The radiologic characteristic of an MCN on a CT scan is the presence of a solitary cyst, which may have fine septations and be surrounded by a rim of calcification (Fig. 55-15). Cross-sectional imaging may not be able to distinguish between benign and malignant MCNs; however, the presence of eggshell calcification, larger tumor size, or a mural nodule on cross-sectional imaging is suggestive of malignancy.

EUS and cyst fluid analyses play an important role in the diagnosis of MCN and other cystic neoplasms. FNA with cyst fluid analysis of MCNs demonstrates mucin-rich aspirate and high CEA levels (>192 ng/mL; log scale). Figure 55-16 illustrates the sensitivity and specificity of CEA in identifying mucinous neoplasms on the basis of fine-needle fluid aspiration. Unlike pseudocysts, MCNs typically have low levels of cyst fluid amylase. These fluid analyses provide accurate diagnosis in up to 80% of cases.[27] Table 55-3 summarizes the distinguishing features of cystic neoplasms of the pancreas.[28]

Pancreatic resection is the standard treatment for MCNs, given the potential for malignant transformation. In the absence of invasive malignant disease, resection is curative and no further surveillance is required. The prognosis of patients who undergo pancreatectomy for invasive MCNs is poor although more favorable than that of patients with ductal adenocarcinoma of the pancreas. Invasive MCNs exhibit slower growth, less frequent nodal involvement, and less aggressive clinical behavior compared with ductal adenocarcinoma; a 5-year survival of 50% to 60% can be expected after resection. Despite limited experience with invasive MCNs, most centers offer adjuvant systemic chemotherapy after surgical resection, especially when node-positive disease is present.

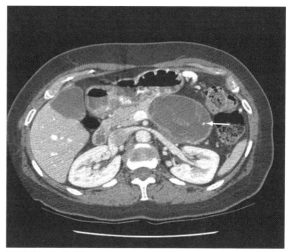

FIGURE 55-15 CT scan of the tail of the pancreas MCN showing a large multiloculated cyst in the absence of pancreatic ductal communication.

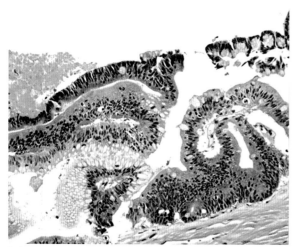

FIGURE 55-14 Ovarian-like stroma is a histologic feature often seen in MCN.

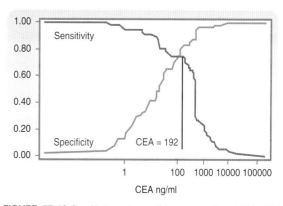

FIGURE 55-16 Sensitivity and specificity curves of cyst fluid CEA concentrations (ng/mL; log scale) for differentiating between mucinous and nonmucinous cystic lesions. An optimal cutoff value of 192 ng/mL correlated with the crossover of the sensitivity and specificity curves. (From Brugge WR, Lewandrowski K, Lee-Lewandrowski E, et al: Diagnosis of pancreatic cystic neoplasms: A report of the cooperative pancreatic cyst study. *Gastroenterology* 126:1330–1336, 2004.)

TABLE 55-3	Defining Characteristics of Pseudocysts and Pancreatic Cystic Neoplasms			
CHARACTERISTICS	**PSEUDOCYST**	**SCN**	**MCN**	**IPMN**
Epidemiology				
Gender	F = M	F ≫ M (4:1)	F ≫> M (10:1)	F = M
Age (years)	40-60	60-70	50-60	60-70
Imaging Findings				
Location	Evenly distributed	Evenly distributed	Head ≪ body/tail	Head > diffuse > body/tail
Appearance	Round, thick-walled large cyst; gland atrophy ± calcification	Multiple small cysts separated by internal septations with central starburst calcifications	Thick-walled, septated macrocyst with smooth contour; ± solid component, eggshell calcifications	Poorly demarcated, lobulated, polycystic mass with dilation of main or branch ducts
Communication with ducts	Yes	No	Very rare	Yes
Cyst Fluid Analysis				
Cytology	Inflammatory cells	Scant glycogen-rich cells, with positive periodic acid–Schiff stain	Sheets and clusters of columnar, mucin-containing cells	Tall, columnar, mucin-containing cells
Mucin stain	Negative	Negative	Positive	Positive
Amylase	Very high	Low	Low	High
CEA	Low	Low	High	High

From Tran Cao HS, Kellogg B, Lowy AM, et al: Cystic neoplasms of the pancreas. *Surg Oncol Clin N Am* 19:267–295, 2010.
IPMN, intraductal papillary mucinous neoplasm; *MCN*, mucinous cystic neoplasm; *SCN*, serous cystic neoplasm.

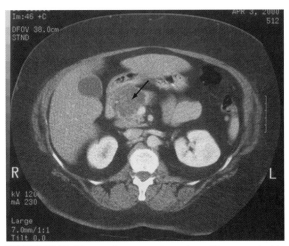

FIGURE 55-17 CT scan of serous cyst neoplasm. The *arrow* depicts the sunburst appearance and central calcification.

Serous Cystic Neoplasm

Compared with MCNs, serous cystic neoplasms (SCNs) have a predilection for the head of the pancreas and occur in patients with a higher median age. Patients commonly present with vague abdominal pain and less frequently with weight loss and obstructive jaundice. On gross inspection, SCNs are large, well-circumscribed masses. Microscopic examination reveals multi-loculated, glycogen-rich small cysts. Central calcification, with radiating septa giving the sunburst appearance, is a radiographic sign on CT in 10% to 20% of patients (Fig. 55-17). With the advent of EUS, these features can now be better delineated. Recently, differential cyst fluid protein expression was observed between SCNs and IPMNs, with accurate discrimination in 92%

of patients.[29] Although serous cystic tumors are generally considered benign, pancreatectomy is suggested when the diagnosis of malignant disease is uncertain or in symptomatic serous cystadenomas. Patients with a tumor larger than 4 cm are more likely to be symptomatic and to display a more rapid median growth rate than patients with tumors smaller than 4 cm. Thus, in select patients with large (>4 cm) or rapidly growing lesions, resection of an SCN is appropriate.

Intraductal Papillary Mucinous Neoplasm

IPMNs of the pancreas, first described by Ohashi, typically are manifested in the sixth to seventh decade of life. IPMNs encompass a wide spectrum of epithelial changes from benign adenoma to invasive adenocarcinoma.

IPMNs are further characterized by the extent to which they involve the pancreatic ducts. Neoplasia that affects only the small side branches is termed side branch or branch duct IPMN (BD-IPMN), whereas involvement of the main pancreatic duct is termed main duct IPMN (MD-IPMN). Side branch IPMNs that extend into the main duct are termed mixed-type IPMNs.

Branch duct intraductal papillary mucinous neoplasm. As the name implies, BD-IPMN involves dilation of the pancreatic duct side branches that communicate with but do not involve the main pancreatic duct. BD-IPMNs may be focal, involving a single side branch, or multifocal, with multiple cystic lesions throughout the length of the pancreas. Risk of malignant transformation has been described in BD-IPMNs and is related to multiple factors that have been stratified as worrisome and high risk. These factors have been identified through international consensus and are reported in the international consensus guidelines for the management of IPMN and MCN of the pancreas, most recently updated in 2012.[30]

Worrisome features of BD-IMPN based on imaging include cyst size larger than 3 cm, thickened enhancing cyst wall, main pancreatic duct size of 5 to 9 mm, nonenhancing mural nodule, abrupt change in caliber of main pancreatic duct with distal pancreatic atrophy, and lymphadenopathy. In addition, patients who present with clinical signs of pancreatitis due to a cystic lesion should be considered to have worrisome features. These features are summarized in Table 55-4.

High-risk imaging features of BD-IPMN include the presence of an enhancing solid component within the cyst and main pancreatic duct dilation of more than 1 cm. Patients who present with clinical signs of jaundice should also be considered at high risk.

All cysts with worrisome features on CT or MRI and any cyst larger than 3 cm with or without worrisome features should undergo EUS; all cysts with high-risk features should be resected. Recommendations for management of suspected BD-IPMN are summarized in Figure 55-18.[30]

TABLE 55-4	A Summary of Worrisome and High-Risk Features of Intraductal Papillary Mucinous Neoplasm	
WORRISOME FEATURES	**HIGH-RISK FEATURES**
Main duct 5-9 mm	Main duct >1 cm
Nonenhancing mural nodule	Enhancing solid component
Thickened, enhancing cyst wall	Jaundice
BD-IPMN size >3 cm	
Abrupt caliber change in main duct with upstream atrophy	
Lymphadenopathy	
Pancreatitis	

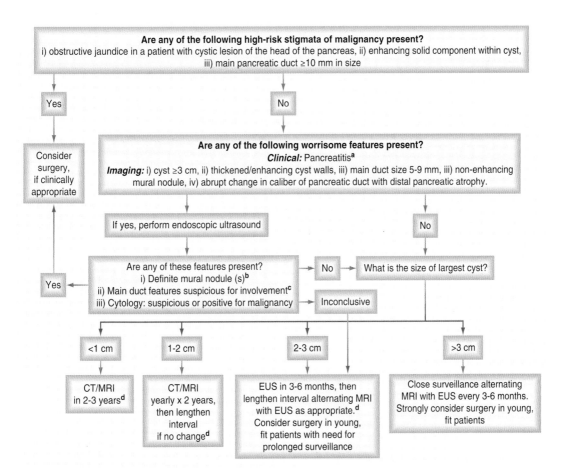

a. Pancreatitis may be an indication for surgery for relief of symptoms.
b. Differential diagnosis includes mucin. Mucin can move with change in patient position, may be dislodged on cyst lavage and does not have Doppler flow. Features of true tumor nodule include lack of mobility, presence of Doppler flow and FNA of nodule showing tumor tissue.
c. Presence of any one of thickened walls, intraductal mucin or mural nodules is suggestive of main duct involvement. In their absence main duct involvement is inconclusive.
d. Studies from Japan suggest that on follow-up of subjects with suspected BD-IPMN there is increased incidence of pancreatic ductal adenocarcinoma unrelated to malignant transformation of the BD-IPMN(s) being followed. However, it is unclear if imaging surveillance can detect early ductal adenocarcinoma, and, if so, at what interval surveillance imaging should be performed.

FIGURE 55-18 Recommendations for management of suspected BD-IPMN. (From Tanaka M, Fernandez-del Castillo C, Adsay V, et al: International consensus guidelines 2012 for the management of IPMN and MCN of the pancreas. *Pancreatology* 12:183–197, 2012.)

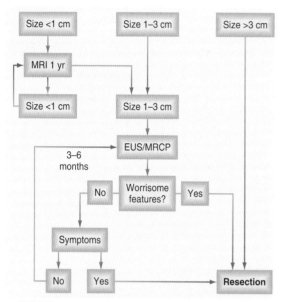

FIGURE 55-19 Algorithm for the management of BD-IPMN.

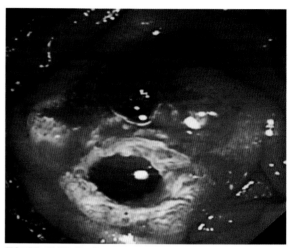

FIGURE 55-20 Classic endoscopic view of IPMN showing viscous fluid oozing from a patulous ampulla of Vater.

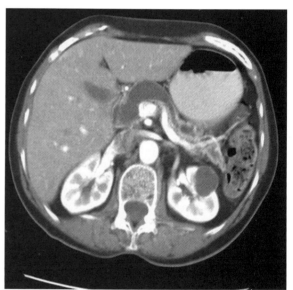

FIGURE 55-21 Cross-sectional imaging of MD-IPMN throughout the entire pancreatic gland and a prominent ampulla of Vater.

For asymptomatic lesions smaller than 3 cm, the risk of invasive malignant disease is small, and therefore serial surveillance has been proposed.[30] A clinical decision tree for the management of BD-IPMN is shown in Figure 55-19. For individuals incidentally found to have small (<1 cm) IPMNs with no worrisome features, surveillance with CT or MRI in 2 to 3 years is appropriate. For those with asymptomatic cysts between 1 and 2 cm, imaging at 1 year is appropriate, followed by less frequent evaluation if no change in size has occurred during the first 2 years of surveillance. Cysts that are 2 to 3 cm should be surveyed more frequently, at 3- to 6-month intervals, to ensure stability for the first year before lengthening of the interval is considered. Given the need for long-term surveillance, resection of cysts 2 to 3 cm may be considered in young, otherwise healthy individuals. Cysts larger than 3 cm warrant closer surveillance because of the increased risk of malignancy. EUS alternating with MRI every 3 to 6 months should be performed in cases in which surgical intervention may be of high risk. Surgery should be strongly considered in young patients with long life expectancy and individuals considered to be at low surgical risk. Any patient with symptoms or high-risk features related to BD-IPMNs (e.g., jaundice, mural nodule, dilated main pancreatic duct) should undergo surgical resection because the risk of malignant disease in symptomatic patients is heightened. Overall, the risk of invasive malignant disease in the setting of BD-IPMN is approximately 10% to 15%.

Main duct intraductal papillary mucinous neoplasm. In contrast to BD-IPMN, MD-IPMN indicates abnormal cystic dilation of the main pancreatic duct with columnar metaplasia and thick mucinous secretions, which can be seen oozing from a patulous papilla on endoscopic evaluation (Fig. 55-20). Involvement of the main pancreatic duct may be focal or diffuse; it is most relevant because of the significantly increased risk of malignant degeneration. Individuals with MD-IPMN have a 30% to 50% risk of harboring invasive pancreatic cancer at the time of presentation. Thus, surgical resection is the cornerstone of treatment. Figure 55-21 demonstrates MD-IPMN with dilation of the entire pancreatic duct.

Unlike patients with pancreatic ductal adenocarcinomas (PDACs), 50% of patients with IPMNs of the pancreas present with abdominal pain and up to 25% present with AP, which, not surprisingly, has led to the diagnosis of chronic pancreatitis in many series. Several investigators have studied clinical and pathologic markers as predictors of malignancy and found that jaundice, elevated serum alkaline phosphatase level, mural nodules, diabetes, and main pancreatic duct diameter of 7 mm or larger are strongly associated with invasive IPMNs.[31] Current guidelines suggest that main duct dilation of more than 5 mm is consistent with a diagnosis of MD-IPMN, whereas 5 to 9 mm is considered worrisome and more than 1 cm is considered high risk.[30] Given the overall high risk of malignant transformation, all patients with evidence of MD-IPMN should be considered for surgical resection if they are surgically fit.

On a molecular level, investigations using genomic array analysis of pancreatic cystic neoplasms have shown that IPMN has several distinct cytogenetic alterations that separate it as an entity from ductal adenocarcinoma of the pancreas.

The radiographic features of IPMNs on pancreatic CT scans may include a dilated main pancreatic duct, cysts of varying sizes, and possibly mural nodules (Fig. 55-21). MRCP and EUS are important secondary diagnostic studies for the evaluation of patients with suspected IPMN. MRCP may allow localization of mural nodules and pretreatment classification of suspected side branch or main duct types of IPMN. EUS can evaluate the pancreatic duct and assess the fluid and solid components of the neoplasm. Aspirated fluid is typically viscous and clear and contains mucin. Cytology studies demonstrate mucin-rich fluid with variable cellularity; columnar mucinous cells with variable atypia may also be seen. As in MCNs and BD-IPMNs, fluid aspirates characteristically reveal an elevated CEA level (>192 ng/mL; log scale). This elevation of the CEA level is not predictive of invasive malignant disease, only the presence of mucinous metaplasia.

Mixed-type intraductal papillary mucinous neoplasm. Mixed-type IPMN denotes a side branch IPMN that has extended to involve the main pancreatic duct to a varying degree. Concern for mixed-type IPMNs should be raised in individuals with side branch cysts who exhibit upstream dilation of the pancreatic duct because this is an indication of main duct involvement. The biologic behavior of mixed-type IPMNs most closely resembles that of MD-IPMNs, with a significant risk of invasive malignant disease at the time of presentation (30% to 50%). As for MD-IPMN, surgical resection is indicated for the treatment of mixed-type IPMN.

Treatment: Surgical Resection for Intraductal Papillary Mucinous Neoplasm

Partial pancreatectomy is the primary treatment for high-risk lesions; however, the optimal extent of pancreatic resection for some patients remains unknown. For BD-IPMN, resection should target the lesion of concern, and therefore surgical decision making is usually straightforward. For MD-IPMN, however, it is not always possible to determine the extent of microscopic abnormality within the duct. Many pancreatic surgeons recommend right-sided partial pancreatectomy with the knowledge that the disease is most often located in the head of the gland, even though ductal changes may extend to involve other parts of the pancreas.[32] Partial pancreatectomy also eliminates the risk of brittle diabetes, which accompanies total pancreatectomy. Although some investigators continue to advocate total pancreatectomy for the treatment of any IPMN, the evidence supporting this approach is decreasing with longer follow-up of patients treated by R0 and R1 partial pancreatectomy. It is appropriate to recommend partial pancreatectomy and to discuss management of the pancreatic margin preoperatively, advising the patient that approximately 15% of patients will require conversion to total pancreatectomy to achieve negative parenchymal resection margins. The surgical margins are assessed intraoperatively, and additional margins are obtained for high-grade dysplasia or invasive cancer.

Survival outcomes are significantly better in patients with IPMNs than in patients with PDACs. Sohn and associates[33] have analyzed a series of 136 patients with IPMNs; survival rates for patients with noninvasive IPMNs are 97% at 1 year, 94% at 2 years, and 77% at 5 years. When the group of patients with non-invasive IPMNs was analyzed further, no survival differences were found between patients with IPMNs and those with borderline IPMNs. On the contrary, there was a significant difference in

survival rate between patients with noninvasive IPMNs and those with invasive IPMNs. The 1-, 3-, and 5-year survival rates for patients with invasive IPMNs were 72%, 58%, and 43%, respectively. Therefore, survival is clearly dependent on the invasive component of the lesion.

It is increasingly clear that not all patients with IPMNs require surgery. Overall, for BD-IPMN, the risk of invasive malignant disease is approximately 2% to 3% per year.[34] A plan for watchful surveillance with delayed intervention in these patients is reasonable because the risk for malignant transformation with small, asymptomatic branch duct tumors is low, most patients are older, and the time required for development of invasive malignant disease may be longer than the patient's life expectancy.

ADENOCARCINOMA OF THE EXOCRINE PANCREAS

Epidemiology

In 2015, it is estimated that PDAC will affect approximately 48,960 individuals in the United States and 40,560 will die of the disease. In comparison, 2 decades ago in 1995, there were 24,000 new cases of pancreatic cancer. Whereas the increasing and aging population is the most likely cause of this increase, whether factors other than population size and age have contributed to this increase is not known. Although it is the ninth most common cancer diagnosis, pancreatic cancer ranks fourth in cancer deaths each year. Despite significant advances in the treatment of other cancers, the prognosis of pancreatic cancer remains dismal. Overall, less than 5% of individuals will survive 5 years beyond their diagnosis. One of the reasons for these dismal outcomes is that most patients with pancreatic cancer have locally advanced or distant metastatic disease at presentation. Efforts at early detection of pancreatic cancer may change these outcomes by detecting pancreatic cancer at an early and curable stage. In a recent study, the authors performed a quantitative analysis of the timing of evolution of metastatic clones in pancreatic cancer. This elegant study suggested that on average, 5 years are required for the acquisition of metastatic ability in pancreatic cancer, thus suggesting that a window of opportunity does exist when the cancer is a locoregional disease and potentially curable.[35] Men are affected slightly more commonly than women, with a 1.3 : 1 incidence ratio. African Americans have a slightly higher risk for development of pancreatic cancer and dying of their disease compared with whites. The risk of pancreatic cancer increases with age beyond the sixth decade; the mean age at diagnosis is 72 years.

Risk Factors
Environmental Risk Factors and Causes

Although the cause of pancreatic cancer remains unclear, several environmental risks have been associated with its increased incidence. The most notable risk factor is related to smoking. Several epidemiologic studies have shown an association of the amount and duration of smoking history with an elevated risk of pancreatic cancer. On average, smokers face a onefold to threefold increase in risk for development of pancreatic cancer compared with nonsmokers. This risk seems to be a linear association, with pancreatic cancer incidence directly related to the number of pack-years smoked (packs/day × number of years smoking). As with other cancers, the risk of pancreatic cancer persists many years beyond smoking cessation. Over the years, there have been several other factors, including chronic pancreatitis and occupational exposure, that were thought to contribute to an elevated risk of pancreatic cancer; however, population data have been somewhat controversial. It is likely that these factors are associated with an elevated risk, but the magnitude of the risk is uncertain. Obesity has recently become the focus of investigation; several authors have found that obese patients may be up to three times more likely to develop pancreatic cancer than nonobese individuals. It remains unclear whether obesity itself or one of the comorbidities related to obesity is associated with the higher incidence of pancreatic cancer seen in this population.

The relationship between diabetes and pancreatic cancer is a complicated one. Studies suggest that patients with new-onset diabetes have higher incidence of pancreatic cancer.[36] The association with pancreatic cancer is especially strong if the new diagnosis of diabetes is made in those who are elderly, have a lower body mass index, or have weight loss and in those who do not have family history of diabetes. In these patients with new-onset diabetes, diabetes may be caused by pancreatic cancer. However, the mechanism of pancreatic cancer–induced diabetes is unclear at this time. Other studies have suggested that long-term diabetes may increase the risk of pancreatic cancer. However, these observations may be confounded by the fact that factors like obesity are associated with both diabetes and pancreatic cancer. It is clear, though, that in elderly patients with new-onset diabetes in the presence of unusual symptoms like weight loss and abdominal symptoms, diagnosis of pancreatic cancer should be considered and may lead to early diagnosis of pancreatic cancer.

Hereditary Risk Factors

An inherited predisposition to pancreatic cancer is seen in a range of clinical settings. Several hereditary cancer syndromes (e.g., Peutz-Jeghers syndrome, familial atypical mole and multiple melanoma syndrome, hereditary breast and ovarian cancer syndrome) are known to be associated with increased risk of pancreatic cancer. Increased risk of pancreatic cancer is present in patients with inheritable inflammatory disease of the pancreas, namely, hereditary pancreatitis and cystic fibrosis. These patients with known genetic syndromes are responsible for about 20% of hereditary cases of pancreatic cancer. The term *familial pancreatic cancer* (FPC) applies to the remaining 80% of patients with an inherited predisposition but who do not have an identifiable genetic syndrome. Table 55-5 summarizes several known gene mutations and their clinical significance.

Hereditary pancreatitis (PRSS1 and SPINK1 gene mutation). It has long been noted that individuals with familial pancreatitis have an elevated risk of pancreatic cancer. Mutations in the cationic trypsinogen gene *(PRSS1)* are responsible for 80% of the cases of hereditary pancreatitis and lead to increased trypsin activity and chronic inflammation in the pancreas. The *SPINK1* gene codes for a serine protease inhibitor that inhibits active protein, and mutations in this gene have been associated with hereditary pancreatitis. Individuals with hereditary pancreatitis have a greater than 50-fold increase in their risk for development of pancreatic cancer compared with unaffected individuals.[37]

Peutz-Jeghers syndrome (STK11 gene mutation). Individuals with Peutz-Jeghers syndrome are distinguished by the development of gastrointestinal hamartomatous polyps and pigmented mucocutaneous lesions. The specific role of *STK11* is not defined, although it is thought to act as a tumor suppressor gene, with loss of heterozygosity leading to the development of gastrointestinal tumors. In addition to gastrointestinal cancers, individuals with Peutz-Jeghers syndrome are at a higher risk of lung, ovarian, breast, uterine, and testicular cancers. The risk of pancreatic

TABLE 55-5　Hereditary Risk Factors Associated With Development of Pancreatic Cancer

GENE	ASSOCIATED SYNDROME	CLINICAL SIGNIFICANCE
PRSS1	Familial pancreatitis	Mutation results in chronic pancreatitis and 40% lifetime risk of PDAC
STK11	Peutz-Jeghers syndrome	Mutation results in >100-fold increase in risk of PDAC
CDKN2A	Familial atypical mole and multiple melanoma syndrome	Mutation leads to increased risk of melanoma and >40-fold increase in risk of PDAC
CFTR	Cystic fibrosis	Thick secretions result in chronic pancreatitis and 30-fold increase in risk of PDAC
BRCA2	Hereditary breast and ovarian cancer	Mutation results in elevated risk of breast and ovarian cancer and 10-fold increase in risk of PDAC
MLH1	Lynch syndrome	Mismatch repair gene mutation leads to increased risk of colon cancer and eightfold increase in risk of PDAC
APC	Familial adenomatous polyposis	Mutation results in polyposis coli and colon cancer with fourfold increase in risk of PDAC

cancer in the setting of Peutz-Jeghers syndrome is more than 100 times greater than that in unaffected individuals.[37]

Cystic fibrosis (CFTR gene mutation). Although the cause remains unclear, those with cystic fibrosis (*CFTR* gene mutation) are up to 30 times more likely to develop pancreatic cancer than the general population. It is postulated that this elevated risk is caused by the chronic inflammatory condition of the pancreas resulting from a lifetime of thickened secretions and partial ductal obstruction.[37]

Familial atypical mole and multiple melanoma syndrome (CDKN2A gene mutation). *CDKN2A* encodes protein p16, which normally inhibits cell proliferation by binding to cyclin-dependent kinases (CDKs). Mutations of *CDKN2A* lead to uninhibited cell cycle activation and proliferation. Although *CDKN2A* is most noted for its associated increased risk of melanoma, individuals with *CDKN2A* mutations have up to a 20-fold increase in risk for the development of pancreas cancer.[37]

Hereditary breast and ovarian cancer (BRCA2 gene mutation). Although germline *BRCA* mutations are most recognized because of their association with breast cancer, 10% of individuals from high-risk pancreatic cancer families (at least two first-degree relatives with pancreas cancer) have been found to have *BRCA2* mutations. Germline mutations of the *BRCA2* gene lead to an elevated risk for pancreatic cancer, which is up to 10 times that of the general population.[37]

Lynch syndrome (mismatch repair gene mutations). Although most strongly associated with colon cancers caused by mutations in mismatch repair genes *(MLH1, MSH2, MSH6),* Lynch syndrome also leads to an increased risk of pancreatic cancer. The microsatellite instability noted in colon cancer cells has also been seen in pancreatic cancer cells from individuals with Lynch syndrome, indicative of a common genetic cause. It is estimated that the risk of pancreatic cancer is increased eightfold in individuals with Lynch syndrome.[37]

Familial adenomatous polyposis (APC gene mutation). Familial adenomatous polyposis results from mutation of the adenomatous polyposis coli gene *(APC)*, leading to the development of thousands of colonic polyps. It has been found that individuals affected by familial adenomatous polyposis are also significantly more likely to develop pancreas cancer, with a fourfold increase above that in the general population. These data remain observational because the cause of pancreatic cancer in this setting has not been defined.[37]

Familial pancreatic cancer (unknown gene). FPC is defined by families with two or more first-degree relatives with pancreatic adenocarcinoma that do not fulfill the criteria of other inherited tumor syndromes with an increased risk for the development of pancreatic adenocarcinoma. Compared with relatives of patients with sporadic pancreatic cancer, the risk for development of pancreatic cancer is markedly elevated in FPC kindreds. Family members of FPC kindreds are at an 18-fold increased risk for development of pancreatic cancer compared with the general population. Furthermore, this risk increases with increasing numbers of first-degree relatives with pancreatic cancer in FPC kindreds and if one of the affected individuals is diagnosed before 50 years of age. Segregation analysis suggests that the aggregation of pancreatic cancer in these families is due to unidentified, autosomal dominantly inherited genes with reduced penetrance. This entity is being increasingly appreciated, and guidelines for pancreatic cancer screening and management of identified suspicious lesions in this population are under evolution.

Pathogenesis of Sporadic Pancreatic Cancer

Although there are several inherited forms of PDAC, most cases are sporadic. As for many other cancers, a sequential pathway has been observed in the development of PDAC from pancreatic intraepithelial neoplasia (PanIN) to invasive cancer. A number of tumor suppressor genes and oncogenes have been identified that play a significant role in the pathogenesis of PDAC, including *PDX1, KRAS2, CDKN2A/p16, P53,* and *DPC4 (SMAD4).*

Genetic Progression of Pancreatic Intraepithelial Neoplasia to Invasive Pancreatic Ductal Adenocarcinoma

PanIN is defined histologically by progressive abnormality of the ductal epithelium from columnar metaplasia (PanIN-1A) through carcinoma in situ (PanIN-3). PanIN-1A is histologically characterized by the presence of columnar, mucin-producing ductal epithelium that maintains basally located homogeneous nuclei without atypia. The development of papillary architecture defines PanIN-1B, but it is otherwise identical to PanIN-1A. PanIN-2 denotes the progression from simple papillary growth to evidence of nuclear atypia not seen in PanIN-1B. Enlarged nuclei with nuclear crowding and loss of polarity are present. Prominent nuclear abnormalities with complete loss of polarity and marked cytologic atypia are characteristic of PanIN-3 (carcinoma in situ). Clusters of abnormal cells can usually be seen within the duct lumen.

The *KRAS2* oncogene is activated in more than 95% of pancreatic cancers and is thought to be the initiating event in tumorigenesis. *KRAS2* is activated by point mutation (codon 12, 13, or 61), which causes constitutive activation and loss of regulation of mitogen-activated protein kinase cell signal transduction. Mutation of the *KRAS2* oncogene is one of the earliest genetic abnormalities identified in the progression of PanIN to PDAC and has been noted in 36% of PanIN-1 cases, 44% of PanIN-2 cases, and 87% of PanIN-3 cases.

CDKN2A/p16, P53, and *DPC4* are tumor suppressor genes that also appear to play critical roles in the development of PDAC. *CDKN2A* encodes a protein, p16, that binds to cyclin-dependent kinases (CDK4, CDK6), resulting in cell cycle arrest. Mutation of *CDKN2A* and loss of p16 lead to a loss of cell cycle regulation. Like mutation of *KRAS,* mutation of *CDKN2A* (loss of p16 expression) has been identified in 30% of PanIN-1 cases, 55% of PanIN-2 cases, and 71% of PanIN-3 cases. Approximately 90% of PDACs demonstrate loss of p16 function. Also, *P53* encodes the protein p53, which regulates cell proliferation through cell cycle arrest and proapoptotic mechanisms. Although it is rare in PanIN, 79% of invasive PDACs demonstrate *P53* mutations, indicating its potential importance in the transition from noninvasive to invasive tumors. Similarly, *DPC4* mutations occur late in the pathway from PanIN to PDAC. Loss of *DPC4,* which normally functions as a downstream mediator related to TGF-β, leads to decreased inhibition of cell growth and proliferation. Loss of *DPC4* function has been observed in 20% to 30% of PanIN-3 and localized cancers, whereas 78% of widely metastatic tumors show loss of *DPC4.* Figure 55-22 demonstrates the molecular genetic alterations involved in the PanIN-PDAC pathway.

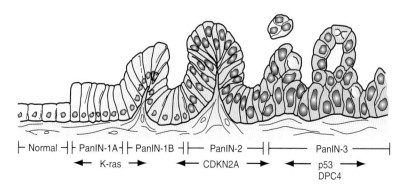

FIGURE 55-22 Molecular genetic progression from PanIN to invasive ductal adenocarcinoma. (Adapted from Wilentz RE, Iacobuzio-Donahoe CA, Argani P, et al: Loss of expression of DPC4 in pancreatic intraepithelial neoplasia: Evidence that DPC4 inactivation occurs late in neoplastic progression. *Cancer Res* 60:2002–2006, 2000.)

TABLE 55-6	Presenting Symptoms for Periampullary Tumors of the Pancreas
PRESENTING SYMPTOM	**FREQUENCY (%)**
Jaundice	75
Weight loss	51
Abdominal pain	39
Nausea/vomiting	13
Pruritus	11
Fever	3
Gastrointestinal bleeding	1

Clinical Presentation

The defining presenting symptom of patients with PDACs in the periampullary region is jaundice. Although painless jaundice has frequently been described, a significant number of patients present with pain in addition to jaundice, typically arising in the epigastrium and radiating to the back. Weight loss is also common at the time of presentation, affecting more than 50% of individuals. For tumors of the body and tail of the pancreas, pain and weight loss become more common at presentation. In the largest single-institution experience reported to date, Winter and coworkers[38] have described 1423 pancreaticoduodenectomies for PDAC. Table 55-6 lists the most common presenting symptoms and their frequency. As mentioned before, new-onset diabetes in an elderly patient with weight loss may be an early presenting symptom of pancreatic cancer. Except for jaundice, the physical examination findings are otherwise unremarkable for most patients with PDAC. A palpable distended gallbladder can be identified in approximately one third of patients with periampullary PDAC, an association first described by Courvoisier, a Swiss surgeon, in 1890. He noted that choledocholithiasis was commonly associated with a shrunken fibrotic gallbladder, whereas the slow progressive occlusion by other causes, including tumors, was more likely to result in ectasia of the organ. Although not diagnostic in itself, Courvoisier sign is familiar to medical students as a defining characteristic of PDACs. With widespread disease, a left supraclavicular node (Virchow node) may be palpable. Similarly, periumbilical lymphadenopathy may be palpable (Sister Mary Joseph node). In cases of peritoneal dissemination, perirectal tumor involvement may be palpable through digital rectal examination, referred to as Blumer shelf.

Diagnosis

Laboratory Evaluation

Laboratory evaluation of patients presenting with suspected PDAC should include hepatic function evaluation, including a coagulation profile and nutritional assessment. An elevated bilirubin level is expected, but careful attention should be paid to nutritional values, including prealbumin and albumin levels if surgical intervention is to be considered. Individuals with malnutrition should be given preoperative nutritional supplementation. Several tumor markers may be appropriate at the initial evaluation, including CEA, carbohydrate antigen 19-9 (CA 19-9), and α-fetoprotein. Of these, CA 19-9 is most sensitive for pancreatic adenocarcinoma, with a sensitivity of approximately 79% and a specificity of 82%. A notable limitation of CA 19-9 testing in the setting of periampullary tumors is the false elevation caused by biliary obstruction, which can be misleading. In addition, 10% to 15% of individuals do not have elevation of the CA 19-9 level,

a finding that has been associated with blood Lewis antigen–negative status. Accepting these limitations, CA 19-9 continues to be the most reliable tumor marker for pretreatment evaluation and post-treatment surveillance for pancreatic adenocarcinoma.

Imaging Studies

Multidetector CT is the imaging study of choice for the evaluation of lesions arising in the pancreas. CT allows an accurate determination of the level of biliary obstruction, the relationship of the tumor to critical vascular anatomy, and the presence of regional or metastatic disease. For suspected periampullary disease, a three-phase (noncontrast, arterial, and portal venous) CT scan with 3-mm slices and coronal and three-dimensional reconstruction should be routine. Because of its widespread availability and excellent sensitivity (85%), CT has become the imaging modality of choice for the evaluation of suspected pancreatic cancer. Pancreatic adenocarcinoma is typically seen as a hypoattenuating lesion during the portal venous phase of the imaging.

ERCP is frequently used in the assessment of the jaundiced patient because of its ability to perform a biopsy and to palliate jaundice, if necessary. Although palliative biliary stenting remains routine for PDAC tumors resulting in jaundice, its usefulness is questionable for patients who are candidates for surgical resection. Preoperative biliary decompression may increase the rate of wound infection caused by bactibilia, although overall morbidity and mortality are unchanged. In modern medical practice, ERCP should be reserved for cases requiring therapeutic or palliative intervention because other imaging modalities provide superior diagnostic abilities without the invasiveness of ERCP.

EUS is becoming widely used for the evaluation of suspected pancreatic disease. Perhaps its most important ability is to provide tissue diagnosis of suspected tumors through the use of FNA before initiation of systemic therapy. FNA has a sensitivity and specificity that are far superior to those of brush cytology, with a diagnostic accuracy of 92% to 95%. It may also play a crucial role in the molecular evaluation of tumor samples from patients undergoing neoadjuvant therapy. Although the use of EUS is increasing for the evaluation of peritumoral vasculature and regional lymph nodes, it has not been shown to provide any significant benefit over CT alone in the absence of a need for tissue diagnosis. EUS may be beneficial for the identification of small tumors that do not appear on CT scans and for the delineation of more clearly suspicious lesions smaller than 2 cm; it therefore plays an important complementary role.

For cases that require detailed assessment of luminal pancreatobiliary anatomy, MRCP should be considered. MRCP has become useful for the investigation of cystic lesions of the pancreas, with sensitivity and specificity slightly superior to CT alone. MRCP also provides several advantages over ERCP; it is noninvasive, has no risk of inciting pancreatitis, and provides three-dimensional reconstruction of the ductal system.

Biologic imaging. ^{18}F-fluorodeoxyglucose positron emission tomography (FDG PET) in combination with CT scanning has been increasingly used in the evaluation of pancreatic cancer. The ability of FDG PET to detect cancers is based on the principle that cells that are actively metabolizing will preferentially take up ^{18}F-labeled glucose compared with surrounding normal tissues. Several studies have noted the potential benefits of FDG PET with CT, including the ability to differentiate between benign and malignant pancreas tumors (autoimmune pancreatitis versus adenocarcinoma) and also to identify unsuspected disease, which alters clinical planning in more than 10% of cases. False-positive findings are also possible, most notably because of inflammatory conditions, and the risk-benefit ratio of FDG PET with CT has not yet been determined. Further studies will be necessary to clarify the role of FDG PET with CT in the evaluation of pancreatic cancer before its routine use should be advocated.

Staging

Pancreatic cancer staging is based on the American Joint Committee on Cancer tumor, node, metastasis (TNM) system (Table 55-7). After biopsy confirmation, typically by EUS-FNA, accurate staging is accomplished by multidetector CT scanning of the abdomen and pelvis with three-phase administration of contrast material and three-dimensional reconstruction. Chest radiography is sufficient for the evaluation of potential pulmonary metastasis and should be followed by CT of the chest if any suspicious lesions are noted. Individuals with stages IA to IIB tumors—tumor confined to the pancreas or peripancreatic tissue without evidence of celiac artery or SMA involvement and no evidence of metastasis—are considered potential candidates for surgical resection. Individuals with stage III (T4) disease involving the celiac

TABLE 55-7 Current American Joint Committee on Cancer Staging Guidelines for Pancreatic Cancer

Primary Tumor (T)

TX	Primary tumor cannot be assessed
T0	No evidence of primary tumor
Tis	Carcinoma in situ*
T1	Tumor limited to the pancreas, 2 cm or smaller in greatest dimension
T2	Tumor limited to the pancreas, more than 2 cm in greatest dimension
T3	Tumor extends beyond the pancreas but without involvement of the celiac axis or superior mesenteric artery
T4	Tumor involves the celiac axis or superior mesenteric artery (unresectable primary tumor)

Regional Lymph Nodes (N)

NX	Regional lymph nodes cannot be assessed
N0	No regional lymph node metastasis
N1	Regional lymph node metastasis

Distant Metastasis (M)

M0	No distant metastasis
M1	Distant metastasis

Anatomic Stage–Prognostic Groups

Stage 0	Tis	N0	M0
Stage IA	T1	N0	M0
Stage IB	T2	N0	M0
Stage IIA	T3	N0	M0
Stage IIB	T1	N1	M0
	T2	N1	M0
	T3	N1	M0
Stage III	T4	Any N	M0
Stage IV	Any T	Any N	M1

From Edge S, Byrd D, Compton C, et al, editors: *AJCC cancer staging manual*, ed 7, New York, 2010, Springer.
*This also includes the PanIN-3 classification.

artery or SMA or stage IV (metastatic disease) are not candidates for immediate surgery.

After CT imaging, tumors are classified into resectable, borderline resectable, or unresectable. Resectable tumors are defined as localized to the pancreas, with no evidence of SMV or portal vein involvement (i.e., no abutment, distortion, thrombus, or encasement) and a preserved fat plane surrounding the SMA and celiac artery branches, including the hepatic artery. Patients with imaging consistent with resectable disease should proceed with operative resection.

The appropriate definition of borderline resectable tumors continues to evolve. The National Comprehensive Cancer Network defines borderline resectable as tumors that exhibit one of the following characteristics: severe unilateral or bilateral SMV-portal impingement; less than 180-degree tumor abutment on the SMA; abutment or encasement of hepatic artery, if reconstructible; and SMV occlusion, if of a short segment and reconstructible. Historically, many of these patients would be considered to have locally advanced, unresectable (T4) disease, and the benefit of arterial resection in the setting of significant vascular involvement remains to be determined. Complex procedures required for the extirpation of borderline tumors should be performed only by experienced surgeons, ideally in the setting of a clinical trial.

Unresectable tumors are those that exhibit metastasis (including lymph node metastasis outside the field of resection), ascites, or vascular involvement beyond what has been detailed here.

Laparoscopy

Staging laparoscopy has been advocated by several authors as a means to reduce the frequency of nontherapeutic laparotomy for patients with unsuspected metastatic or locally advanced unresectable disease identified at the time of surgery. For patients who appear to have resectable disease on imaging studies alone, laparoscopy identifies additional unresectable disease in up to 30% of cases. Others have argued that with current imaging used properly, the benefit of additional laparoscopy only rarely alters surgical planning. Recently, there has been some consensus on a more selective use of laparoscopy for those at particularly high risk for occult disease, including those with large tumors (>3 cm), significantly elevated CA 19-9 level (>100 U/mL), uncertain findings on CT, or body or tail tumors. It may be clinically prudent also to consider laparoscopy for patients with clinical indicators of widespread disease, including significant weight loss, malnutrition, and pain.[39] There are no level I data available to define the role of staging laparoscopy, and therefore its use remains at the discretion of the surgeon. Furthermore, the role and place of peritoneal cytology are unclear at this time. However, patients with positive findings on peritoneal cytology have very poor prognosis and behave like patients with metastatic disease.[40]

Treatment

Surgical resection remains the only potentially curative treatment of pancreas cancer.

Surgery for Tumors of the Head of the Pancreas

For tumors involving the head of the pancreas, pancreaticoduodenectomy is the procedure of choice. Although first described in 1909 by Kausch, the technique became widely known after the first successful surgical resection was performed by Whipple and Parsons and presented to the American Surgical Association by Parsons in 1935. The first two attempts, in 1934, resulted in operative mortality; but in 1935, a two-stage procedure, which included biliary decompression followed by pancreaticoduodenectomy, was successful. The initial operative description included ligation of the pancreas remnant without reanastomosis.

The first one-stage Whipple procedure was reported by Trimble and colleagues at Johns Hopkins University in 1941.[41] The modern Whipple procedure maintained a perioperative mortality of 25% and morbidity of well above 50% up until the late 1970s. The advent of improved outcomes for this complex procedure can be attributed to many surgeons and institutions. Most notable on this list of early and seminal leaders in regard to improved mortality and outcome are Cameron (Johns Hopkins Hospital, Baltimore), Tredi (Mannheim Clinic, Mannheim, Germany), Warshaw (Massachusetts General Hospital, Boston), and Brennan (Memorial Sloan Kettering Cancer Center, New York). Each surgeon and center performed more than 100 procedures without any deaths in the 1980s and 1990s.

Surgical technique. The modern pancreaticoduodenectomy begins with exploration of the peritoneal surfaces for evidence of metastatic disease, which would deem the patient inoperable. The right colon is then fully mobilized and reflected medially (Cattell-Braasch maneuver), exposing the infrapancreatic SMV. A Kocher maneuver is performed to the level of the left lateral border of the aorta, with attention to clearance of the lymphatic tissue overlying the great vessels. The transverse mesocolon is separated off the head of the pancreas. Figure 55-23 shows complete mobilization of the head of the pancreas and gallbladder. The lesser sac is entered through the gastrocolic ligament, sparing the gastroepiploic vessels. The right gastroepiploic vein is ligated at its confluence with the SMV, allowing the SMV to be dissected from the inferior border and posterior neck of the pancreas. The middle colic vein may also be sacrificed, if necessary, to allow adequate dissection at this level.

Once the infrapancreatic SMV is dissected and the head of the pancreas is fully mobilized, the gallbladder is removed and the common hepatic duct is circumferentially dissected. Division of the common hepatic duct allows visualization of the suprapancreatic SMV. The duodenum is divided at least 2 cm distal to the pylorus using electrocautery or a blue load stapler. The hepatic

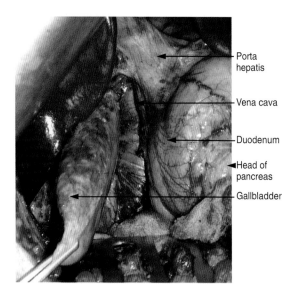

FIGURE 55-23 Complete mobilization of the head of the pancreas is shown. The vena cava is visible posteriorly. The gallbladder has been freed from the gallbladder fossa.

artery is exposed proximally and distally and assessed for replacement or aberrant anatomy. The GDA and right gastric artery are visualized. Before division of the GDA, the vessel is temporarily occluded, and blood flow through the distal common hepatic artery is ensured using a Doppler device. This maneuver is vital in patients with atherosclerosis of celiac origin to ensure that the hepatic blood supply is not dependent on collateral retrograde arterial flow from the SMA through the GDA. Once hepatic arterial flow is confirmed, the right gastric artery and GDA are ligated and divided. If flow in the hepatic artery is interrupted by occlusion of the GDA, resection may proceed only with preservation of the GDA or arterial resection and bypass, typically as an aortohepatic conduit.

The pancreas is then divided after four-point ligation of the inferior and superior pancreaticoduodenal arteries. Blunt dissection is used to separate the portal vein from the uncinate process. This dissection often includes ligation of a superior and inferior branch from the portal vein and SMV to the uncinate process. The jejunum is divided approximately 10 cm distal to the ligament of Treitz, and the short mesenteric vessels are divided to allow retromesenteric rotation of the jejunum and third and fourth portions of the duodenum. The head of the pancreas and attached small bowel are then retracted to the patient's right, and the remaining portal vein and uncinate dissection is completed.

With the portal vein completely free, the gland is retracted farther to the right to allow complete visualization of the uncinate process and SMA. The retroperitoneal tissue is dissected from the SMA, allowing complete removal of the caudate and periarterial lymphatic tissue. Figure 55-24A shows the anatomy after removal of the head of the pancreas, and Figure 55-24B highlights complete clearance of periarterial tissue from the SMA. If portal venous or SMV tumor involvement is encountered, as shown in Figure 55-25A and B, venous resection should be performed. Resections that compromise less than 50% of the venous diameter can be closed primarily (Fig. 55-25C); otherwise, segmental resection with primary anastomosis or interposition graft using internal jugular or femoral vein should be performed.

Reconstruction. Before reconstruction, frozen section evaluation of the surgical margins is performed. Once negative margins are ensured, the proximal jejunum is brought through the transverse mesocolon or the retromesenteric defect in preparation for pancreaticojejunostomy and hepaticojejunostomy. The pancreaticojejunostomy is created in two layers, anterior and posterior, with a duct-to-mucosa anastomosis (Fig. 55-26). An internal pancreatic stent can be left in place for ducts smaller than 5 mm. The hepaticojejunostomy anastomosis is then created 6 to 8 cm downstream from the pancreaticojejunostomy in an end-to-side fashion. If the duct is smaller than 5 mm, it is spatulated to improve patency. After this, an antecolic duodenojejunostomy is completed. External drains are selectively placed adjacent to the pancreaticojejunostomy and hepaticojejunostomy. Similarly, a feeding jejunostomy is placed in selected patients with significant preoperative malnutrition (albumin level <3.5 g/dL).

Surgery for Tumors of the Body and Tail of the Pancreas

Tumors arising in the body and tail of the pancreas are rarely resectable at the time of presentation, given the lack of symptoms with small tumors. Only 5% to 7% of individuals with body or tail PDACs will ultimately undergo surgery, and median survival is significantly shorter than with PDACs of the pancreatic head because of the more advanced nature of resected tumors. Although tumor involvement of the splenic artery or vein does not preclude

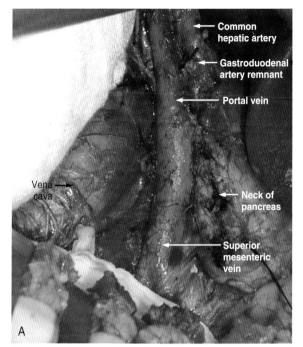

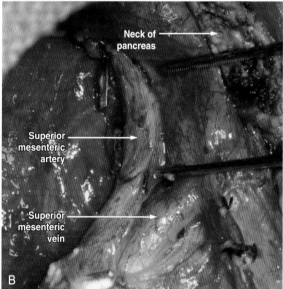

FIGURE 55-24 **A,** Surgical anatomy after pancreaticoduodenectomy. The SMV, portal vein, hepatic artery, and vena cava are visualized. Complete lymphatic clearance is noted. **B,** SMA dissection illustrating complete clearance of periarterial lymphatic tissue.

surgery, involvement of the celiac axis is a contraindication to resection. For resectable tumors, distal pancreatectomy and en bloc splenectomy should be performed. Distal pancreatectomy and splenectomy can be performed in a retrograde fashion whereby the spleen and pancreas are mobilized lateral to medial en bloc, thus providing access to splenic vasculature located superior and behind the pancreas. Alternatively, the dissection can proceed antegrade in a medial to lateral fashion. In this approach, the pancreatic neck is encircled and divided away from the tumor early in the procedure. This medial to lateral approach in

combination with extensive lymph node dissection has been termed radical antegrade modular pancreatosplenectomy.[42] The medial to lateral or antegrade approach is described here, but depending on the situation, a combination of these two approaches can be used.

After inspection of the peritoneal surfaces, the gastrocolic and splenocolic ligaments and short gastric vessels are divided to expose the pancreas and spleen. The inferior border of the pancreas is dissected, exposing the retroperitoneal plane behind the gland. This anatomic plane can be used to mobilize the body and tail of the pancreas anterior to Gerota fascia completely. At the superior border of the pancreas, the splenic artery is circumferentially dissected and divided at its origin from the celiac trunk. The splenic vein is carefully dissected from the posterior wall of the pancreas at its confluence with the SMV and divided. At this point, the distal pancreas and spleen are devascularized and the neck of the pancreas is divided. A medial to lateral dissection is completed, and the spleen is detached from its posterior peritoneal attachments to allow en bloc removal of the specimen and surrounding lymph node basin. Several techniques may be used to close the pancreatic duct remnant, with the most common being direct suture ligation or use of a linear stapling device. Either technique is appropriate, with similar risk for the development of pancreatic fistula.

Laparoscopic Distal Pancreatectomy

There has been growing interest in the use of minimally invasive surgery for the resection of tumors of the distal pancreas. Laparoscopic distal pancreatectomy (LDP) may offer advantages over open resection for select patients, with smaller incisions and shorter hospital stay. In a review of more than 800 LDPs, Borja-Cacho and colleagues[43] described an overall morbidity rate of 38% and hospital length of stay of 5 days, which compare favorably with large series after open pancreatectomy. Although LDP is increasingly used for benign conditions, its usefulness for the treatment of PDAC remains to be validated. There have been no randomized trials to evaluate LDP versus open resection, and few studies have reported outcomes of LDP for PDACs. Currently, LDP in the setting of PDACs should be considered experimental.

Outcomes

Perioperative Mortality: Long-Term Survival

Perioperative mortality has become a rare event after the Whipple procedure, occurring in less than 2% of cases at high-volume centers. Despite significant reduction in mortality, however, morbidity remains common, occurring after 30% to 50% of procedures.[38] Table 55-8 lists several of the most common postoperative morbidities and their frequencies.

After surgical resection and adjuvant therapy for pancreatic cancer, the median survival is approximately 22 months, with 5-year survival of 15% to 20%. Most patients experience relapse of disease in the form of metastatic disease (85%) and, less commonly, local recurrence (40%). In the absence of surgical resection, those with locally advanced disease who receive palliative chemotherapy may survive 10 to 12 months, whereas those with metastases rarely survive beyond 6 months. The role of adjuvant chemotherapy and radiation is described later in this chapter.

Morbidity

Delayed gastric emptying characterized by the need for prolonged nasogastric decompression or inability to tolerate oral intake is a

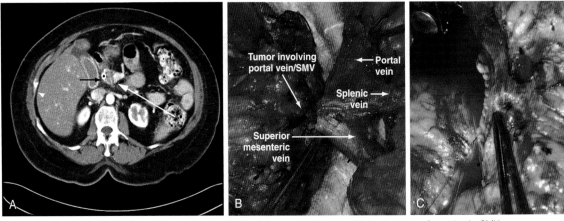

FIGURE 55-25 A, CT scan showing PDAC of the pancreatic head with involvement of portal vein–SMV confluence *(large arrow).* A metal biliary stent is in place *(small arrow).* **B,** Operative image demonstrating tumor involvement of the lateral aspect of the portal vein–SMV confluence. **C,** Primary closure of portal vein–SMV confluence after tumor removal with lateral vein resection.

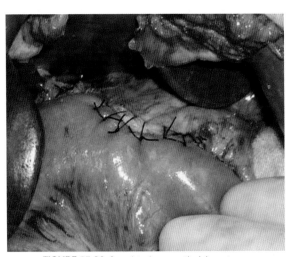

FIGURE 55-26 Completed pancreaticojejunostomy.

TABLE 55-9 International Study Group on Pancreatic Fistula Classification of Pancreatic Fistulas

PARAMETER	GRADE		
	A	B	C
Clinical conditions	Well	Often well	Ill-appearing, bad
Specific treatment	No	Yes/no	Yes
US/CT (if obtained)	Negative	Negative/positive	Positive
Persistent drainage (after 3 weeks)	No	Usually yes	Yes
Reoperation	No	No	Yes
Death related to POPF	No	No	Possibly yes
Signs of infections	No	Yes	Yes
Sepsis	No	No	Yes
Readmission	No	Yes/no	Yes/no

From Bassi C, Dervenis C, Butturini G, et al: Postoperative pancreatic fistula: An international study group (ISGPF) definition. *Surgery* 138:8–13, 2005.
POPF, postoperative pancreatic fistula.

TABLE 55-8 Morbidity After Pancreaticoduodenectomy

COMPLICATION	FREQUENCY (%)
Delayed gastric emptying	18
Pancreas fistula	12
Wound infection	7
Intra-abdominal abscess	6
Cardiac events	3
Bile leak	2
Overall reoperation	3

frequent complication after pancreaticoduodenectomy, occurring 5% to 15% of the time. Few studies have demonstrated an association of delayed gastric emptying with pylorus preservation, but this finding has not been confirmed by all. When patients have the inability to tolerate solid foods or a prolonged nasogastric tube requirement, it is critical to perform cross-sectional imaging to rule out a secondary cause, such as pancreatic leak or intra-abdominal abscess. An underlying structural abnormality, like stricture or other anastomotic complications, is ruled out with imaging and endoscopy. Enteral feeding with a feeding tube placed during surgery or percutaneously through endoscopy is used to maintain nutrition while waiting for stomach function to return.

Pancreatic leak or pancreatic fistula, which has been defined by the International Study Group on Pancreatic Fistula[44] as "output via an intraoperatively placed drain (or percutaneous drain) of any measurable volume on or after postoperative day 3, with amylase >3 times normal serum value," is a frequent complication after pancreaticoduodenectomy, occurring after 5% to 22% of surgeries. Perhaps the most predictive factor is the texture of the gland, with soft fatty glands at significantly higher risk of leak. Most fistulas are controlled by drainage catheters placed at the time of surgery and require no additional intervention. Rarely, uncontrolled fistulas require additional drain placement or operative exploration, sometimes mandating completion pancreatectomy to eliminate further abdominal contamination. The classification of pancreatic fistulas is given in Table 55-9.

Anastomotic leaks from the hepaticojejunostomy and duodenojejunostomy are rare and occur after less than 5% of procedures. Infectious complications (e.g., intra-abdominal abscess, wound infection) are slightly more common and may require intervention with percutaneous drainage or open wound dressing changes.

Pancreatic endocrine and exocrine insufficiency can occur after pancreaticoduodenectomy, but the risk of these events is unpredictable. For individuals with a normal gland, pancreatic insufficiency is rare. However, for those with preexisting chronic pancreatitis, fibrosis of the gland, or insulin resistance, exogenous enzyme and insulin replacement is usually needed.

Controversies

Pylorus-Preserving versus Non–Pylorus-Preserving Whipple Procedure

We have described the pylorus-preserving Whipple procedure, which is the operation of choice for a growing number of pancreatobiliary surgeons. It was initially proposed as a means to reduce postpancreatectomy dumping and bile reflux, which is common after a non–pylorus-preserving Whipple procedure. Although initial results were encouraging, none of the randomized controlled trials have suggested superiority of a pylorus-preserving over a non–pylorus-preserving Whipple procedure. We prefer pylorus preservation when possible but do not hesitate to proceed with a non–pylorus-preserving Whipple procedure in case of tumor involvement of the duodenum or concern for duodenal blood supply.

Pancreaticojejunostomy versus Pancreatogastrostomy

The pancreaticojejunostomy remains the Achilles heel of the Whipple procedure because of the frequency of pancreatic fistula. Several studies have reported successful outcomes with pancreatogastrostomy and reduced leak rates compared with pancreaticojejunostomy, but this finding has not been reproducible in several randomized trials, and most surgeons continue to prefer pancreaticojejunostomy.[45] In cases in which the pancreatic duct is not identified, invagination of the gland into the jejunal stump may also be performed.

Use of Somatostatin Analogues to Reduce Pancreatic Fistula

Although the mortality of pancreaticoduodenectomy has gone down, postoperative morbidity continues to be a significant problem. Pancreatic fistula is the major source of morbidity after the Whipple operation. Because pancreatic exocrine secretion is the proposed mechanism by which postoperative fistula occurs, inhibition of this secretion by means of somatostatin and its analogues has been evaluated in multiple trials with mixed results. Whereas European studies have shown that use of octreotide perioperatively leads to a decreased incidence of postoperative pancreatic fistula, North American trials have not confirmed these results. A trial evaluated the efficacy of pasireotide, a somatostatin analogue with a longer half-life (11 hours for pasireotide versus 2 hours for octreotide) and a broader binding profile (pasireotide binds to somatostatin-receptor subtypes 1, 2, 3, and 5, whereas octreotide binds only to receptor subtypes 2 and 5), in reducing pancreatic fistula, leak, or abscess of grade 3 or higher after pancreatic surgery (both pancreaticoduodenectomy and distal pancreatectomy). In this trial, pasireotide treatment significantly lowered the rate of grade 3 or higher postoperative pancreatic fistula, leak, or abscess (9% versus 21%; relative risk, 0.44; 95% confidence interval, 0.24-0.78; P = .006). This finding was seen consistently

in patients who underwent pancreaticoduodenectomy or distal pancreatectomy as well as in patients with dilated duct versus nondilated pancreatic duct.[46]

Extent of Lymphadenectomy

Given the fact that 75% to 80% of patients are found to have lymph node involvement at the time of the Whipple procedure and, overall, 80% to 85% of patients will experience tumor recurrence and cancer-related death, some have proposed that radical lymphadenectomy may improve outcomes. Regional pancreatectomy was first proposed by Fortner in 1973 and has been used widely in Japan, where significant improvements in survival of patients undergoing extended lymphadenectomy have been reported. In addition to peripancreatic, portal, and pyloric lymph nodes, extended lymphadenectomy includes retrieval of hilar and retroperitoneal lymph nodes, extending from the celiac origin to the level of the inferior mesenteric artery and including all tissue between the renal hilum laterally. Several randomized controlled trials have since been completed, with no evidence to suggest improved survival after extended lymphadenectomy. In fact, more than one trial has shown increased morbidity associated with extended lymphadenectomy, including delayed gastric emptying, pancreatic fistula, and dumping.[47] In view of the current evidence, standard pancreaticoduodenectomy is the operation of choice for localized pancreatic adenocarcinoma.

Laparoscopic and Robotic Pancreaticoduodenectomy

The first laparoscopic pancreaticoduodenectomy was performed in 1994 by Gagner and Pomp. Since then, several case reports and small series have demonstrated the feasibility of the minimally invasive approach. In the largest U.S. series to date, Kendrick and Cusati[48] have reported outcomes of 65 laparoscopic pancreaticoduodenectomies, with an overall morbidity rate of 42%: pancreatic fistula, 18%; delayed gastric emptying, 15%; bleeding, 8%; wound infection, 6%; reoperation, 5%; and mortality, 1.5%. These results indicate that laparoscopic pancreaticoduodenectomy has similar short-term outcomes to the open approach. Recently, the authors have presented the updated experience with 108 laparoscopic pancreaticoduodenectomies. Their data suggested that the median length of hospital stay was shorter with the laparoscopic approach. Furthermore, the authors observed that compared with the laparoscopic approach, a significantly higher proportion of patients had delay in delivery of adjuvant therapy with the open approach.[49] Pancreaticoduodenectomy is one of the most complex intra-abdominal operations, and to perform it laparoscopically, the operator needs advanced training in both hepatopancreatobiliary and laparoscopic approaches, not to mention years of high-volume experience. Given the complexity of the procedure and the fact that the major morbidities that follow pancreaticoduodenectomy are not related to the size of the incision, the laparoscopic Whipple procedure has not become widely adopted.

Robotics has emerged as both an alternative and an adjunct to laparoscopy. Given the limitations of current laparoscopic technology and the need for meticulous vascular control and complex reconstruction in pancreatic surgery, robotic pancreaticoduodenectomy has been proposed as an alternative to laparoscopic pancreaticoduodenectomy. There are only a few centers in the United States that are pursuing robotics as an approach to pancreaticoduodenectomy. The largest series on robotic pancreaticoduodenectomy is from the University of Pittsburgh. Zureikat and colleagues published their experience with 132 robotic pancreaticoduodenectomies.[50] However, as mentioned before, the major morbidity of pancreaticoduodenectomy does not emanate from the incision, and it is too early to predict whether robotic pancreaticoduodenectomy will ever be widely adopted. At this time, open pancreaticoduodenectomy remains the standard of care.

Antecolic versus Retrocolic Duodenojejunostomy

Delayed gastric emptying is a common occurrence after pancreaticoduodenectomy with an elusive cause. Emerging data suggest that creation of an antecolic duodenojejunostomy may improve gastric emptying compared with the retrocolic technique.

Drain versus No Drain

Given the high frequency of pancreatic fistula after pancreatic resection and morbidity associated with uncontrolled pancreatic leak, drains are routinely used after pancreatic resections. However, surgical drains are not without untoward effects, and their use has been associated with increased rates of intra-abdominal and wound infection, increased pain, and prolonged hospital stay. Use of surgical drains after pancreatic resection has been evaluated in randomized controlled trials. In a randomized controlled trial from Memorial Sloan Kettering Cancer Center comparing outcomes in patients undergoing pancreatic resection with and without placement of surgical drains, no difference in complication rate was observed between the two groups. Furthermore, presence of a drain failed to reduce the need for radiologic intervention or surgical exploration. However, a multi-institution randomized controlled trial comparing drain versus no drain in patients undergoing pancreaticoduodenectomy had to be terminated early as a result of increased morbidity as well as a fourfold increase in mortality in the no-drain group. In this trial, the use of a drain decreased the adverse clinical impact of pancreatic fistula. Good results without use of surgical drains have been achieved only at high-volume specialized centers that have vast experience in dealing with intra-abdominal complications after pancreaticoduodenectomy. These centers have access to advanced interventional radiology techniques as well as experienced endoscopists who can drain many of the intra-abdominal collections internally through the stomach. At this time, use of a surgical drain should be considered standard of care.

Adjuvant Therapy for Pancreatic Cancer
Chemotherapy and Radiation Therapy

During the last 30 years, there have been conflicting reports about the survival benefit of adjuvant therapy after surgical resection of localized pancreatic cancer, particularly with regard to radiation therapy. Although the use of chemotherapy is widely accepted, the usefulness of radiation therapy has been increasingly questioned. In the United States, chemotherapy and radiation therapy are still widely used, whereas European centers have stopped using radiation therapy as part of standard adjuvant therapy because of lack of evidence to support a survival benefit.

Several randomized trials have attempted to clarify the roles of chemotherapy and radiation therapy for adjuvant treatment of pancreatic cancer after surgical resection. Table 55-10 summarizes the findings of several important trials. In 1974, the Gastrointestinal Tumor Study Group (GITSG) began a prospective randomized trial comparing adjuvant 5-fluorouracil (5-FU) and 40-Gy radiation with observation after curative resection.[51] The trial was terminated prematurely because of low accrual and the observation that the chemoradiation arm had a significant survival

TABLE 55-10	Summary of Clinical Trials Defining Role of Adjuvant Therapy After Resection of Pancreatic Cancer
TRIAL	**CONCLUSIONS**
GITSG	Adjuvant chemoradiation with 5-FU and 40-Gy radiation therapy improves survival compared with observation alone.
ESPAC-1	Adjuvant chemotherapy improves survival; chemoradiation is deleterious.
CONKO-001	Adjuvant gemcitabine improves disease-free survival compared with observation.
RTOG 97-04	Gemcitabine before and after 5-FU–based chemoradiation provides similar overall survival compared with 5-FU but with significantly less toxicity.
ESPAC-3	Adjuvant chemotherapy alone with gemcitabine provides similar overall survival compared with 5-FU but with significantly less toxicity.

advantage. During an 8-year period, only 49 patients were accrued and randomized (43 patients were included in the final analysis because of withdrawal of 5 individuals and misdiagnosis of 1). Median survival was 20 months for the chemoradiation group compared with 11 months for the observation group. Despite its limitations, this was the first randomized controlled trial that demonstrated an overall survival benefit after chemoradiation.

The European Study Group for Pancreatic Cancer-1 (ESPAC-1) trial was a 2×2 factorial design that compared chemoradiotherapy alone (5-FU, 20 Gy during 2 weeks) versus chemotherapy alone (5-FU) versus chemoradiotherapy and chemotherapy versus observation.[52] At a median follow-up of 47 months, it was noted that the estimated 5-year survival for those who underwent chemoradiotherapy was significantly less than that for those who did not (10% versus 20%; $P = .05$). At the same time, those who received chemotherapy had a 5-year survival of 21% versus 8% for those who did not ($P < .009$). These findings led to the conclusion that although chemotherapy provided significant improvement in overall survival, the routine use of chemoradiation may be detrimental.

In 2007, the Charité Onkologie (CONKO-001) trial of 368 individuals enrolled during a 6-year period evaluated whether chemotherapy with gemcitabine (without radiation) could extend disease-free survival compared with observation.[53] Trial patients received six cycles of gemcitabine (days 1, 8, and 15 every 4 weeks for 6 months), and outcomes were compared with observation alone. Median disease-free survival was significantly improved in the gemcitabine group compared with the observation group (13.4 versus 6.9 months). There was a trend toward improved overall survival, but this did not meet statistical significance (median, 22.1 versus 20.2 months). This trial established the use of adjuvant gemcitabine for the treatment of pancreatic cancer.

The Radiation Therapy Oncology Group (RTOG 97-04) trial compared 5-FU versus gemcitabine chemotherapy before and after 5-FU–based chemoradiation.[54] The purpose of the study was to determine whether gemcitabine provided a survival benefit over 5-FU in combination with 5-FU–based chemoradiation. It was noted that although overall survival was similar (20.5 months for gemcitabine versus 16.9 months for 5-FU; $P = $ NS), the treatment-related toxicity was significantly higher in the 5-FU group. These data have led to the use of gemcitabine as the first-line agent for adjuvant chemotherapy, with or without radiation therapy.

The most recent international randomized controlled trial to be completed (ESPAC-3) was designed to evaluate overall survival comparing 5-FU (425 mg/m^2 IV bolus injection, given on days 1 to 5 every 28 days) versus gemcitabine (1000 mg/m^2 IV infusion, days 1, 8, and 15 every 4 weeks) after curative surgery. No observation arm was included because it was thought to be unethical, given the existing data suggesting a survival benefit of chemotherapy over observation alone. More than 1000 participants from 16 countries were randomized. Overall survival was similar between the groups (23.0 months for 5-FU, 23.6 months for gemcitabine), but gemcitabine was found to have less treatment-related toxicity, with fewer severe adverse events and better compliance. The current National Comprehensive Cancer Network guidelines recommend gemcitabine or 5-FU alone or in combination with 5-FU–based chemoradiation as adjuvant treatment after resection for PDAC. Given the overall poor prognosis, enrollment into clinical trials is encouraged.

Role of Neoadjuvant Therapy

It is clear that for the optimal outcome, patients with pancreatic cancer require multimodal treatment that includes a combination of surgery and chemotherapy with or without radiation treatment. The administration of chemotherapy, with or without radiation therapy, before planned surgical resection for pancreatic cancer is becoming increasingly common. The rationale for the neoadjuvant approach is multifaceted. After surgical resection, approximately 25% of patients do not receive adjuvant therapy because of refusal, surgical complications, or an inability to recover physiologically. Giving therapy before surgery ensures that all patients will receive multimodality therapy, and by delivery of therapy to an intact gland with an established blood supply, the efficacy of therapy may be maximized. In addition, by treatment of patients with measurable disease, response to therapy can be assessed more readily. Progression of disease during neoadjuvant treatment is indicative of aggressive tumor biology and may prevent these patients from undergoing extensive surgery, which is unlikely to provide any survival benefit. Finally, the administration of chemotherapy and radiation therapy before surgery has been viewed as a physiologic stress test and helps select patients who would be unlikely to tolerate the major stress of surgical resection. Neoadjuvant therapy may provide improved selection of patients, avoiding surgery for those who progress, but also improved negative margin rates and reduced lymph node metastasis.

Despite all these theoretical benefits, currently there is no level I evidence demonstrating advantage of the neoadjuvant strategy over the surgery first approach. Most of the data supporting the neoadjuvant approach are in the form of single- or multi-institutional retrospective studies. In a study from MD Anderson Cancer Center, the authors retrospectively reviewed and compared the outcomes of patients with resectable pancreatic adenocarcinoma who underwent neoadjuvant therapy followed by surgery with the outcomes of patients who were treated with the surgery first approach. In this study, 83% of patients with neoadjuvant therapy completed all components of therapy, including surgery with chemotherapy or radiotherapy, compared with 58% of patients treated with the surgery first approach. In this study, patients who completed all components of multimodal therapy had better outcomes compared with those who received only one component, whether surgery or chemotherapy. Although the rate

of complications in both groups was similar, patients who received neoadjuvant therapy and suffered postoperative major complication had longer survival compared with patients with the surgery first approach who had a major postoperative complication. This may suggest that neoadjuvant therapy protects patients with pancreatic cancer who undergo pancreatectomy for pancreatic cancer from early recurrence and death. Alternatively, these results may just be a reflection of the fact that the patients who underwent surgery first and developed a complication were unable to receive adjuvant therapy, which is an equally critical component of treatment. Although these results are intriguing, this study is retrospective, and overall survival was used instead of recurrence-free survival. The neoadjuvant approach has multiple advantages, but the issue of superiority over a surgery first approach can be settled only by a randomized controlled trial.

In select patients, the role of neoadjuvant therapy is clearer, particularly for those with significant venous or limited arterial involvement whose disease is classified as borderline resectable. In these patients, for whom upfront surgical exploration has a significant risk of exposing them to nontherapeutic laparotomy, the argument for neoadjuvant therapy is strengthened. For individuals with significant SMV–portal vein involvement (>180 degrees or short-segment encasement) or hepatic arterial or SMA abutment (<180 degrees) who have been traditionally considered to have unresectable disease, neoadjuvant therapy may play an important role in identifying the subset of patients most likely to derive benefit from aggressive multimodality therapy, including surgical resection with vascular reconstruction.[55] This type of aggressive treatment should be undertaken only by an experienced multidisciplinary team in the setting of a clinical trial.

Chemotherapy for Metastatic Pancreatic Adenocarcinoma

More than 80% of patients with pancreatic cancer present with locally advanced or metastatic disease and are primarily managed with chemotherapy. There has been some progress in the chemotherapy treatment of locally advanced or metastatic pancreatic adenocarcinoma. It is vital for the surgeons taking care of patients with pancreatic cancer to know these studies as regimens used to treat locally advanced and metastatic pancreatic adenocarcinoma slowly find their way into the treatment of patients with resectable pancreatic cancer in both adjuvant and neoadjuvant settings. Gemcitabine has been the standard of care for the treatment of metastatic pancreatic cancer since the late 1990s. Few chemotherapy regimens have shown greater efficacy than gemcitabine. Compared with gemcitabine alone, FOLFIRINOX (combination of 5-FU, oxaliplatin, irinotecan, and leucovorin) improves the median overall survival (gemcitabine, 6.8 months; FOLFIRINOX, 11.1 months) and progression-free survival (gemcitabine, 3.3 months; FOLFIRINOX, 6.4 months).[56] FOLFIRINOX is being used as the neoadjuvant regimen of choice in patients with borderline resectable pancreatic cancer and good performance status who can tolerate this aggressive regimen.

In a similar vein, the combination of gemcitabine with nab-paclitaxel improves overall and progression-free survival of patients with metastatic pancreatic cancer compared with gemcitabine alone.[57] The results with targeted therapies in pancreatic cancer have not been very promising as yet. The addition of erlotinib, which targets epidermal growth factor receptor–dependent growth pathways to gemcitabine, leads to statistically significant but marginal improvement in overall survival and progression-free survival in patients with metastatic pancreatic cancer.[58] Evaluation of gemcitabine-erlotinib combination as adjuvant therapy is currently ongoing. Randomized controlled trials evaluating addition of the vascular endothelial growth factor inhibitor bevacizumab or epidermal growth factor receptor inhibitor cetuximab to gemcitabine have not demonstrated improvement in outcomes of patients with metastatic pancreatic cancer compared with gemcitabine alone.

Palliative Therapy for Pancreatic Cancer

Given that 80% to 85% of those with pancreatic cancer have locally advanced or metastatic disease at the time of presentation and are therefore not candidates for surgical resection, it is imperative that all surgeons be familiar with nonoperative and operative palliative options. In general, nonoperative management should be pursued whenever possible to expedite systemic therapy and to optimize quality of life for these patients.

Biliary Obstruction

Palliation of biliary obstruction is commonly required for patients who are not candidates for surgical resection. ERCP with metal stent placement provides excellent palliation of jaundice, and at high-volume university centers, successful biliary drainage is possible in more than 90% of cases. In patients for whom endoscopic palliation is impossible, percutaneous biliary drainage with subsequent internalization may be required. For patients who are found at laparotomy to have unresectable disease or those for whom nonsurgical measures have failed, a surgical biliary-enteric bypass may be performed by Roux-en-Y hepaticojejunostomy, with excellent long-term patency.

Gastric Outlet Obstruction

Approximately 20% of patients with locally advanced pancreatic cancer will develop gastric outlet obstruction. For those with metastatic disease or disease found to be unresectable on the basis of imaging findings who have symptoms of gastric outlet obstruction, endoscopic luminal stenting should be carried out. Palliative endoscopic stenting has excellent short-term results, with almost immediate improvement in oral intake, but is limited in its ability to provide long-term patency. For this reason, patients who are found to have unresectable cancer at the time of laparotomy may benefit from preventive gastrojejunostomy, with no increase in perioperative morbidity. For patients who require surgical intervention, a double bypass consisting of a Roux-en-Y hepaticojejunostomy and gastrojejunostomy may be performed.

Pain Relief

Pain is a common component in the natural history of pancreatic cancer, affecting most patients with advanced disease. Palliation of pain is paramount for optimizing the quality of life for patients and should be a primary goal for physicians. The initial management of pain may include anti-inflammatories or long-acting opioids, taken orally or through a cutaneous patch. For patients with pain that is not well controlled or who suffer side effects of narcotic use, celiac nerve block should be considered. The procedure involves injecting a combination of 3 mL of 0.25% bupivacaine and 10 mL of absolute alcohol into each celiac plexus. For cases that are found at exploration to be unresectable, this can be performed intraoperatively, as described by Lillemoe and coworkers.[59] For those with unresectable disease based on staging evaluation who do not undergo surgical exploration, neurolysis can be achieved through EUS guidance, with pain relief expected in 80% of patients.[60] CT-guided percutaneous neurolysis may also be performed.

PANCREATIC TRAUMA

Pancreatic injuries are uncommon. The mechanism of injury varies according to the age of the patient. The most common mechanism in pediatric patients is abdominal blunt trauma. Direct compression of the epigastrium against the vertebral column and a blunt object (handlebar) is typically seen after bicycle injuries. The most common segment of the pancreas affected is the body. Penetrating injuries into the abdomen are the most common injuries seen in adults.[61]

Isolated pancreatic injuries are not common. Up to 90% of patients present with associated hepatic, gastric, splenic, renal, colonic, or vascular lesions.[61] The diagnosis and therapy in unstable patients with severe retroperitoneal injuries, gunshot wounds, or penetrating injury into the abdomen are usually straightforward, and they do not require further evaluation. Hemodynamically stable patients represent a challenge because isolated pancreatic injuries are normally associated with subtle or absent physical symptoms and signs. Undiagnosed pancreatic injuries are associated with significant complications, such as intra-abdominal abscess, fistula, and fluid collections, in 60% of patients.[62] Pancreatic injuries should always be considered after epigastric compression during a car or bicycle accident.

The modality of choice to evaluate patients with abdominal trauma is CT scanning of the abdomen. Findings such as peripancreatic hematomas, free fluid in the lesser sac, and abnormal thickening of Gerota fascia suggest pancreatic injury. Studies have shown that MRCP provides excellent visualization of the pancreatic duct, peripancreatic fluid contiguous to fractured segments of the pancreas, and hemorrhage after nonpenetrating trauma. Its main limitations include high cost, availability, and amount of time required to perform the study. Isolated pancreatic amylase measurement is not recommended because up to 40% of patients with transected pancreatic duct have normal serum amylase levels. Serial quantification levels increase the sensitivity of the assay. Abnormal amylase level elevations require further imaging.

The most reliable test to demonstrate pancreatic duct integrity is ERCP. However, its applicability is frequently limited by the risk of inducing pancreatitis, availability, and severity of the trauma.

Pancreatic injuries are classified according to the system described by the American Association for the Surgery of Trauma (Table 55-11). Definitive treatment is based on surgical findings.

TABLE 55-11 American Association for the Surgery of Trauma Pancreatic Injury Grading

GRADE		INJURY DESCRIPTION
I	Hematoma	Minor contusion without ductal injury
	Laceration	Superficial laceration without ductal injury
II	Hematoma	Major contusion without ductal injury or tissue loss
	Laceration	Major laceration without ductal injury or tissue loss
III	Laceration	Distal transection or pancreatic parenchymal injury with ductal injury
IV	Laceration	Proximal transection or pancreatic parenchymal injury involving the ampulla
V	Laceration	Massive disruption of the pancreatic head

From Subramanian A, Dente CJ, Feliciano DV: The management of pancreatic trauma in the modern era. *Surg Clin North Am* 87:1515–1532, 2007.

Major pancreatic resections have been described in stable patients with isolated pancreatic injury. However, pancreatic resections in unstable patients are associated with significant morbidity and mortality. Therefore, damage control surgery is indicated for complex injuries or unstable patients. Most pancreatic lesions can be temporarily controlled with drains. Once the physiologic insult has been controlled, definitive treatment should be considered, if indicated. Up to 75% of deaths occur within the 48 to 72 hours after trauma, and most are related to hypovolemic shock.[61]

SELECTED REFERENCES

Abrams RA, Lowy AM, O'Reilly EM, et al: Combined modality treatment of resectable and borderline resectable pancreas cancer: Expert consensus statement. *Ann Surg Oncol* 16:1751–1756, 2009.

A consensus statement about recommending multimodality therapy to optimize outcomes for patients with resectable and borderline resectable pancreatic cancer.

Andersen DK, Frey CF: The evolution of the surgical treatment of chronic pancreatitis. *Ann Surg* 251:18–32, 2010.

A historical review of surgical techniques for the management of chronic pancreatitis.

Beger HG, Rau BM: Severe acute pancreatitis: Clinical course and management. *World J Gastroenterol* 13:5043–5051, 2007.

A review of the pathophysiology of acute pancreatitis and clinical management strategies.

Gittes GK: Developmental biology of the pancreas: A comprehensive review. *Dev Biol* 326:4–35, 2009.

A comprehensive review of pancreatic embryology and development.

IAP/APA evidence-based guidelines for the management of acute pancreatitis. *Pancreatology* 4:e1–e16, 2013.

This manuscript provides evidence-based guidelines addressing multiple issues in the management of acute pancreatitis, including role and timing of ERCP and use of antibiotics.

Tanaka M, Chari S, Adsay V, et al: International consensus guidelines for management of intraductal papillary mucinous neoplasms and mucinous cystic neoplasms of the pancreas. *Pancreatology* 6:17–32, 2006.
Tanaka M, Fernandez-del Castillo C, Adsay V, et al: International consensus guidelines 2012 for the management of IPMN and MCN of the pancreas. *Pancreatology* 12:183–197, 2012.

The first version of the consensus guidelines (2006) for diagnosis and management of cystic neoplasms of the pancreas points out the issues, provides guidelines, and provides the evidence behind the guidelines. Even though these guidelines have been updated (2012), a review of the older version provides perspective on how the diagnosis and management of this common pancreatic problem have evolved.

Winter JM, Cameron JL, Campbell KA, et al: 1423 pancreaticoduodenectomies for pancreatic cancer: A single-institution experience. *J Gastrointest Surg* 10:1199–1210, 2006.

A historic review of the largest single-institution pancreaticoduodenectomy experience.

REFERENCES

1. Gittes GK: Developmental biology of the pancreas: A comprehensive review. *Dev Biol* 326:4–35, 2009.
2. Saluja AK, Lerch MM, Phillips PA, et al: Why does pancreatic overstimulation cause pancreatitis? *Annu Rev Physiol* 69:249–269, 2007.
3. Beger HG, Rau BM: Severe acute pancreatitis: Clinical course and management. *World J Gastroenterol* 13:5043–5051, 2007.
4. Elfar M, Gaber LW, Sabek O, et al: The inflammatory cascade in acute pancreatitis: Relevance to clinical disease. *Surg Clin North Am* 87:1325–1340, vii, 2007.
5. Larson SD, Nealon WH, Evers BM: Management of gallstone pancreatitis. *Adv Surg* 40:265–284, 2006.
6. Frossard JL, Steer ML, Pastor CM: Acute pancreatitis. *Lancet* 371:143–152, 2008.
7. Ranson JH, Rifkind KM, Roses DF, et al: Prognostic signs and the role of operative management in acute pancreatitis. *Surg Gynecol Obstet* 139:69–81, 1974.
8. Gravante G, Garcea G, Ong SL, et al: Prediction of mortality in acute pancreatitis: A systematic review of the published evidence. *Pancreatology* 9:601–614, 2009.
9. Balthazar EJ, Robinson DL, Megibow AJ, et al: Acute pancreatitis: Value of CT in establishing prognosis. *Radiology* 174:331–336, 1990.
10. Charbonney E, Nathens AB: Severe acute pancreatitis: A review. *Surg Infect (Larchmt)* 9:573–578, 2008.
11. Nealon WH, Bawduniak J, Walser EM: Appropriate timing of cholecystectomy in patients who present with moderate to severe gallstone-associated acute pancreatitis with peripancreatic fluid collections. *Ann Surg* 239:741–749, discussion 749–751, 2004.
12. Rodriguez JR, Razo AO, Targarona J, et al: Debridement and closed packing for sterile or infected necrotizing pancreatitis: Insights into indications and outcomes in 167 patients. *Ann Surg* 247:294–299, 2008.
13. Besselink MG, Verwer TJ, Schoenmaeckers EJ, et al: Timing of surgical intervention in necrotizing pancreatitis. *Arch Surg* 142:1194–1201, 2007.
14. van Santvoort HC, Besselink MG, Bakker OJ, et al: A step-up approach or open necrosectomy for necrotizing pancreatitis. *N Engl J Med* 362:1491–1502, 2010.
15. Lerch MM, Stier A, Wahnschaffe U, et al: Pancreatic pseudocysts: Observation, endoscopic drainage, or resection? *Dtsch Arztebl Int* 106:614–621, 2009.
16. Apte MV, Haber PS, Applegate TL, et al: Periacinar stellate shaped cells in rat pancreas: Identification, isolation, and culture. *Gut* 43:128–133, 1998.
17. Sah RP, Dudeja V, Dawra RK, et al: Cerulein-induced chronic pancreatitis does not require intra-acinar activation of trypsinogen in mice. *Gastroenterology* 144:1076–1085.e2, 2013.

18. Catalano MF, Sahai A, Levy M, et al: EUS-based criteria for the diagnosis of chronic pancreatitis: The Rosemont classification. *Gastrointest Endosc* 69:1251–1261, 2009.

19. O'Neil SJ, Aranha GV: Lateral pancreaticojejunostomy for chronic pancreatitis. *World J Surg* 27:1196–1202, 2003.

20. Andersen DK, Frey CF: The evolution of the surgical treatment of chronic pancreatitis. *Ann Surg* 251:18–32, 2010.

21. Keck T, Wellner UF, Riediger H, et al: Long-term outcome after 92 duodenum-preserving pancreatic head resections for chronic pancreatitis: Comparison of Beger and Frey procedures. *J Gastrointest Surg* 14:549–556, 2010.

22. Heidt DG, Burant C, Simeone DM: Total pancreatectomy: Indications, operative technique, and postoperative sequelae. *J Gastrointest Surg* 11:209–216, 2007.

23. Blondet JJ, Carlson AM, Kobayashi T, et al: The role of total pancreatectomy and islet autotransplantation for chronic pancreatitis. *Surg Clin North Am* 87:1477–1501, x, 2007.

24. Dunderdale J, McAuliffe JC, McNeal SF, et al: Should pancreatectomy with islet cell autotransplantation in patients with chronic alcoholic pancreatitis be abandoned? *J Am Coll Surg* 216:591–596, discussion 596–598, 2013.

25. Bellin MD, Freeman ML, Schwarzenberg SJ, et al: Quality of life improves for pediatric patients after total pancreatectomy and islet autotransplant for chronic pancreatitis. *Clin Gastroenterol Hepatol* 9:793–799, 2011.

26. Varadarajulu S, Bang JY, Sutton BS, et al: Equal efficacy of endoscopic and surgical cystogastrostomy for pancreatic pseudocyst drainage in a randomized trial. *Gastroenterology* 145:583–590.e1, 2013.

27. Brugge WR, Lewandrowski K, Lee-Lewandrowski E, et al: Diagnosis of pancreatic cystic neoplasms: A report of the cooperative pancreatic cyst study. *Gastroenterology* 126:1330–1336, 2004.

28. Tran Cao HS, Kellogg B, Lowy AM, et al: Cystic neoplasms of the pancreas. *Surg Oncol Clin N Am* 19:267–295, 2010.

29. Allen PJ, Qin LX, Tang L, et al: Pancreatic cyst fluid protein expression profiling for discriminating between serous cystadenoma and intraductal papillary mucinous neoplasm. *Ann Surg* 250:754–760, 2009.

30. Tanaka M, Fernandez-del Castillo C, Adsay V, et al: International consensus guidelines 2012 for the management of IPMN and MCN of the pancreas. *Pancreatology* 12:183–197, 2012.

31. Salvia R, Fernandez-del Castillo C, Bassi C, et al: Main-duct intraductal papillary mucinous neoplasms of the pancreas: Clinical predictors of malignancy and long-term survival following resection. *Ann Surg* 239:678–685, discussion 685–687, 2004.

32. Katz MH, Mortenson MM, Wang H, et al: Diagnosis and management of cystic neoplasms of the pancreas: An evidence-based approach. *J Am Coll Surg* 207:106–120, 2008.

33. Sohn TA, Yeo CJ, Cameron JL, et al: Intraductal papillary mucinous neoplasms of the pancreas: An updated experience. *Ann Surg* 239:788–797, discussion 797–799, 2004.

34. Levy P, Jouannaud V, O'Toole D, et al: Natural history of intraductal papillary mucinous tumors of the pancreas: Actuarial risk of malignancy. *Clin Gastroenterol Hepatol* 4:460–468, 2006.

35. Yachida S, Jones S, Bozic I, et al: Distant metastasis occurs late during the genetic evolution of pancreatic cancer. *Nature* 467:1114–1117, 2010.

36. Chari ST, Leibson CL, Rabe KG, et al: Probability of pancreatic cancer following diabetes: A population-based study. *Gastroenterology* 129:504–511, 2005.

37. Klein AP, Hruban RH, Brune KA, et al: Familial pancreatic cancer. *Cancer J* 7:266–273, 2001.

38. Winter JM, Cameron JL, Campbell KA, et al: 1423 pancreaticoduodenectomies for pancreatic cancer: A single-institution experience. *J Gastrointest Surg* 10:1199–1210, discussion 1210–1211, 2006.

39. Callery MP, Chang KJ, Fishman EK, et al: Pretreatment assessment of resectable and borderline resectable pancreatic cancer: Expert consensus statement. *Ann Surg Oncol* 16:1727–1733, 2009.

40. Ferrone CR, Haas B, Tang L, et al: The influence of positive peritoneal cytology on survival in patients with pancreatic adenocarcinoma. *J Gastrointest Surg* 10:1347–1353, 2006.

41. Trimble IR, Parsons JW, Sherman CP: One-stage operation for the cure of carcinoma of the ampulla of Vater and the head of the pancreas. *Surg Gynecol Obstet* 73:711–722, 1941.

42. Strasberg SM, Drebin JA, Linehan D: Radical antegrade modular pancreatosplenectomy. *Surgery* 133:521–527, 2003.

43. Borja-Cacho D, Al-Refaie WB, Vickers SM, et al: Laparoscopic distal pancreatectomy. *J Am Coll Surg* 209:758–765, quiz 800, 2009.

44. Bassi C, Dervenis C, Butturini G, et al: Postoperative pancreatic fistula: An international study group (ISGPF) definition. *Surgery* 138:8–13, 2005.

45. Wente MN, Shrikhande SV, Muller MW, et al: Pancreaticojejunostomy versus pancreaticogastrostomy: Systematic review and meta-analysis. *Am J Surg* 193:171–183, 2007.

46. Allen PJ, Gonen M, Brennan MF, et al: Pasireotide for postoperative pancreatic fistula. *N Engl J Med* 370:2014–2022, 2014.

47. Farnell MB, Aranha GV, Nimura Y, et al: The role of extended lymphadenectomy for adenocarcinoma of the head of the pancreas: Strength of the evidence. *J Gastrointest Surg* 12:651–656, 2008.

48. Kendrick ML, Cusati D: Total laparoscopic pancreaticoduodenectomy: Feasibility and outcome in an early experience. *Arch Surg* 145:19–23, 2010.

49. Croome KP, Farnell MB, Que FG, et al: Total laparoscopic pancreaticoduodenectomy for pancreatic ductal adenocarcinoma: Oncologic advantages over open approaches? *Ann Surg* 260:633–638, discussion 638–640, 2014.

50. Zureikat AH, Moser AJ, Boone BA, et al: 250 robotic pancreatic resections: Safety and feasibility. *Ann Surg* 258:554–559, discussion 559–562, 2013.

51. Kalser MH, Ellenberg SS: Pancreatic cancer. Adjuvant combined radiation and chemotherapy following curative resection. *Arch Surg* 120:899–903, 1985.

52. Neoptolemos JP, Stocken DD, Friess H, et al: A randomized trial of chemoradiotherapy and chemotherapy after resection of pancreatic cancer. *N Engl J Med* 350:1200–1210, 2004.

53. Oettle H, Post S, Neuhaus P, et al: Adjuvant chemotherapy with gemcitabine vs observation in patients undergoing curative-intent resection of pancreatic cancer: A randomized controlled trial. *JAMA* 297:267–277, 2007.

54. Regine WF, Winter KA, Abrams RA, et al: Fluorouracil vs gemcitabine chemotherapy before and after fluorouracil-based chemoradiation following resection of pancreatic adenocarcinoma: A randomized controlled trial. *JAMA* 299:1019–1026, 2008.

55. Abrams RA, Lowy AM, O'Reilly EM, et al: Combined modality treatment of resectable and borderline resectable pancreas cancer: Expert consensus statement. *Ann Surg Oncol* 16:1751–1756, 2009.

56. Conroy T, Desseigne F, Ychou M, et al: FOLFIRINOX versus gemcitabine for metastatic pancreatic cancer. *N Engl J Med* 364:1817–1825, 2011.

57. Von Hoff DD, Ervin T, Arena FP, et al: Increased survival in pancreatic cancer with nab-paclitaxel plus gemcitabine. *N Engl J Med* 369:1691–1703, 2013.

58. Moore MJ, Goldstein D, Hamm J, et al: Erlotinib plus gemcitabine compared with gemcitabine alone in patients with advanced pancreatic cancer: A phase III trial of the National Cancer Institute of Canada Clinical Trials Group. *J Clin Oncol* 25:1960–1966, 2007.

59. Lillemoe KD, Cameron JL, Kaufman HS, et al: Chemical splanchnicectomy in patients with unresectable pancreatic cancer. A prospective randomized trial. *Ann Surg* 217:447–455, discussion 456–457, 1993.

60. Puli SR, Reddy JB, Bechtold ML, et al: EUS-guided celiac plexus neurolysis for pain due to chronic pancreatitis or pancreatic cancer pain: A meta-analysis and systematic review. *Dig Dis Sci* 54:2330–2337, 2009.

61. Stawicki SP, Schwab CW: Pancreatic trauma: Demographics, diagnosis, and management. *Am Surg* 74:1133–1145, 2008.

62. Subramanian A, Dente CJ, Feliciano DV: The management of pancreatic trauma in the modern era. *Surg Clin North Am* 87:1515–1532, x, 2007.

56 CHAPTER

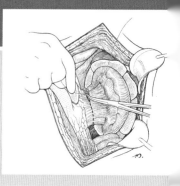

The Spleen

Benjamin K. Poulose, Michael D. Holzman

第五十六章　脾疾病

中文导读

本章共分5节：①脾脏的解剖；②脾脏的功能；③脾切除术；④脾切除术后晚期并发症；⑤脾切除病人的预防性治疗。

第一节主要介绍脾脏的解剖。包括脾脏的位置、邻近器官、周围韧带、与胰尾的关系；脾动脉的起源、走行及变异；脾小梁的组织结构；脾静脉的走行及回流。

第二节主要介绍脾脏的功能。包括脾脏在胚胎期的造血功能、过滤功能、免疫功能。重点介绍了脾切除后爆发性感染（overwhelming postsplenectomy infection, OPSI）的发病时间、病死率、致病原及其发病机制；脾脏产生的3种免疫因子及其功能；脾脏对红细胞、血小板的作用。

第三节主要介绍脾切除术。包括脾切除的适应证：①良性血液系统疾病；②恶性血液系统疾病；③脾脏非血液系统肿瘤；④其他各类良性疾病；⑤脾外伤。重点介绍择期腹腔镜脾切除术，包括选择腹腔镜手术的条件（疾病种类、脾脏大小等）、中转开腹的原因、术前评估、与开腹手术相比的优点及相对禁忌证等；然后介绍具体手术体位、麻醉方法、主刀与助手站位、打孔、探查、脾切除步骤、脾蒂离断方法、胰尾的保护、取出方法、引流等。简略介绍机器人脾切除术。

第四节主要介绍脾切除术后晚期并发症。简略介绍脾切除术后血小板增多与门静脉系统血栓形成。重点介绍脾切除后爆发性感染的发病时间、临床表现、病死率、后遗症、致病原及其危害。

第五节主要介绍脾切除病人的预防性治疗。重点介绍了多价肺炎球菌疫苗（PPV23）的特点，常见致病原，接种该疫苗的作用。详细描述了对于高危人群，PPV23再次接种的适应证。同时介绍了美国疾病控制和预防中心（Centers for Disease Control and Prevention, CDC）要求的针对脾切除术后各类不同的人群，其免疫接种的方案（包括PPV23和其他疫苗）。其次是抗生素的使用。主要介绍了预防性使用青霉素及其他抗生素存在的争议，以及抗生素的治疗性使用。

〔梅 试〕

SPLENIC ANATOMY

The spleen is an 80- to 300-g organ that initially develops from mesenchymal cells in the dorsal mesogastrium during week 5 of embryogenesis and settles into the left uppermost aspect of the abdomen. Its superior surface is roofed by the diaphragm, separating it from the pleura. However, the costodiaphragmatic recess extends to the inferiormost aspect of a normal-sized spleen. The spleen's visceral relationships include the greater curvature of the stomach, splenic flexure of the colon, apex of the left kidney, and tail of the pancreas (Fig. 56-1). It is protected by ribs 9, 10, and 11 and is suspended in its location by multiple peritoneal reflections, the splenophrenic, gastrosplenic, splenorenal, and splenocolic ligaments. In patients without portal hypertension, the splenophrenic and splenocolic ligaments are relatively avascular. The gastrosplenic ligament carries the short gastric vessels in its superior aspect and the left gastroepiploic in its inferior aspect. The splenorenal ligament houses the splenic artery and vein as well as the tail of the pancreas. The tail of the pancreas abuts the splenic hilum in 30% of individuals and is within 1 cm of the hilum in 70%.

The splenic artery, a branch of the celiac trunk, is a tortuous vessel that gives off multiple branches to the pancreas as it travels along its posterior aspect (Fig. 56-2). There are two common variations of the splenic artery as originally described by Michels: the magistral type, which branches into terminal and polar arteries near the hilum of the spleen; and the distributed type, which, as the name implies, gives off its branches early and distant from the hilum.[1] The magistral type of splenic arterial anatomy occurs in 30% of individuals compared with the distributed type (70%). There is typically a superior polar artery, which sometimes communicates with the short gastric arteries and the superior, middle, and inferior terminal arteries, and an inferior polar artery. Knowing these variable distributions is necessary in performing resections, especially a spleen-preserving procedure. Because of the variable nature of the splenic artery, one must be cautious when operating near this vessel and its tributaries.

The spleen is encased within a fibroelastic capsule. Trabeculae that compartmentalize the spleen pass from the splenic capsule. The spleen is also segmented by the divisions of the splenic vessels as they branch within the organ and merge with these trabeculae. The arterioles branch into even smaller vessels and leave these trabeculae to merge with the splenic pulp, where their adventitia is replaced by a covering of lymphatic tissue that continues until the vessels thin to capillaries. These lymphatic sheaths make up the white pulp of the spleen and are interspersed among the arteriolar branches as lymphatic follicles. The white pulp then interfaces with the red pulp at the marginal zone. It is in this marginal zone that the arterioles lose their lymphatic tissue and the vessels evolve into thin-walled splenic sinuses and sinusoids. The sinusoids then merge into venules, draining into veins that travel along the trabeculae to form splenic veins that mirror their arterial counterparts. The splenic vein leaves the splenic hilum and travels posteriorly to the pancreas, joining with pancreatic branches and often the inferior mesenteric vein to finally receive the superior mesenteric vein, forming the portal vein.

SPLENIC FUNCTION

During fetal development, the spleen has important hematopoietic functions, which include white and red blood cell production. This production is usurped by the bone marrow during the fifth month of gestation, and under normal conditions, the spleen has no significant hematopoietic function beyond this point. In certain pathologic conditions, such as myelodysplasia, the spleen may reacquire this function. Beyond hematopoiesis, the specialized vasculature in the spleen is directly related to its remaining functions, defense and cleansing. It is likely that the spleen's mechanical filtration contributes to control of infection by removing pathogens within cells (e.g., malaria) or circulating in the plasma. This filtration may be particularly important for removal of microorganisms for which the host does not have a specific antibody (Box 56-1).

The immune functions of the spleen become obvious after splenectomy, when patients are noted to be significantly at risk for infection. The most serious sequela is overwhelming postsplenectomy infection (OPSI), with meningitis, pneumonia, or bacteremia.[2] Older studies have demonstrated that the risk of OPSI is greatest within the first 2 years after splenectomy, but recent studies have confirmed that a lifelong risk remains. One third of cases occur more than 5 years after surgery, with the overall incidence reported to be 3.2% to 3.5%. For those who acquire OPSI, mortality is between 40% and 50%.[3] The risk is greatest in patients with thalassemia major and sickle cell disease. OPSI is typically caused by polysaccharide-encapsulated organisms, such as *Streptococcus pneumoniae, Neisseria meningitidis,* and *Haemophilus influenzae.* These and other organisms are identified and bound by antibodies and complement components in preparation for phagocytosis by macrophages in the spleen. After splenectomy, the antibodies continue to bind, but digestion by splenic macrophages is no longer possible.

In comparing the timing of pneumococcal vaccinations in postsplenectomy trauma patients and control subjects, asplenic patients have been noted to express similar postvaccination

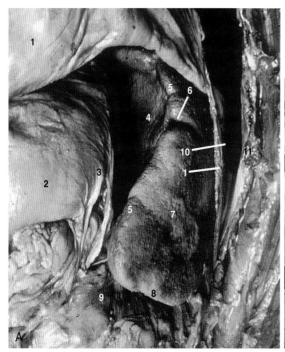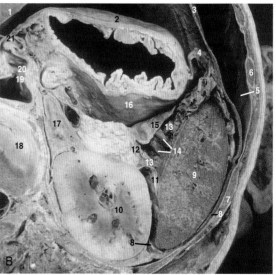

FIGURE 56-1 A, Spleen, from the front: (1) diaphragm, (2) stomach, (3) gastrosplenic ligament, (4) gastric impression, (5) superior border, (6) notch, (7) diaphragmatic surface, (8) inferior border, (9) left colic flexure, (10) costodiaphragmatic recess, and (11) thoracic wall. The left upper abdominal and lower anterior thoracic walls have been removed, and part of the diaphragm (1) has been turned upward to show the spleen in its normal position, lying adjacent to the stomach (2) and colon (9), with the lower part against the kidney (**B,** 9 and 10). **B,** Spleen, in a transverse section of the left upper abdomen: (1) left lobe of liver, (2) stomach, (3) diaphragm, (4) gastrosplenic ligament, (5) costodiaphragmatic recess of pleura, (6) ninth rib, (7) tenth rib, (8) peritoneum of greater sac, (9) spleen, (10) left kidney, (11) posterior layer of lienorenal ligament, (12) tail of pancreas, (13) splenic artery, (14) splenic vein, (15) anterior layer of lienorenal ligament, (16) lesser sac, (17) left suprarenal gland, (18) intervertebral disc, (19) abdominal aorta, (20) celiac trunk, and (21) left gastric artery. The section is at the level of the disc (18) between the twelfth thoracic and first lumbar vertebrae and is viewed from below looking toward the thorax. The spleen (9) lies against the diaphragm (3) and left kidney (10) but is separated from them by peritoneum of the greater sac (8). The peritoneum behind the stomach (2), forming part of the gastrosplenic (4) and ileorenal (15) ligaments, belongs to the lesser sac (16). (From McMinn RMH, Hutchings RT, Pegington J, Abrahams PH: *Color atlas of human anatomy*, ed 3, St Louis, 1993, Mosby–Year Book, pp 230–231.)

immunoglobulin G antibody levels; functional antibody levels, however, were lower.[4] Also, asplenic patients have been found to express subnormal immunoglobulin M levels, and their peripheral blood mononuclear cells exhibit a suppressed immunoglobulin response. The risk for development of OPSI or asplenic or hyposplenic overwhelming sepsis for reasons other than surgical removal of the spleen is linked to the patient's understanding of the risks of infection.[5] Registries that allow long-term follow-up and periodic teaching of current recommendations should be considered for this high-risk population.[6,7]

Other factors involved in the immune response, such as properdin and tuftsin, opsonins produced in the spleen, exhibit reduced serum levels after splenectomy. Properdin, a globulin protein also known as factor P, initiates the alternate pathway of complement activation; this increases the destruction of bacteria and foreign or otherwise abnormal cells. Tuftsin, a tetrapeptide, enhances the phagocytic activity of mononuclear phagocytes and polymorphonuclear leukocytes. Absence of a circulating mediator appears to result in suppressed neutrophil function. The spleen

also plays a key role in cleaving tuftsin from the heavy chain of immunoglobulin G; thus, circulating levels of tuftsin are subnormal in asplenic patients.

The filtration consists of two methods of blood flow within the spleen, the closed and open systems. In the closed system, blood flows directly from arteries to veins. In the open system, most of the spleen's blood flow occurs when blood flows through the arterioles and then trickles through a sieve-like parenchyma made up of reticuloendothelial cells into the splenic sinuses before draining into the venous system (Fig. 56-3). The cellular elements are directed toward these reticuloendothelial cells, in which cellular cleansing processes take place. These include removal of senescent cells, cellular inclusions (e.g., red blood cell nucleoli), and parasites and the sequestration of red blood cells (for maturation) and platelets (reservoir). The plasma is directed to the lymphoid tissue, where soluble antigens stimulate the production of antibodies.

Red blood cell morphology, and thus red blood cell function, is maintained by splenic filtration. Normal red blood cells are

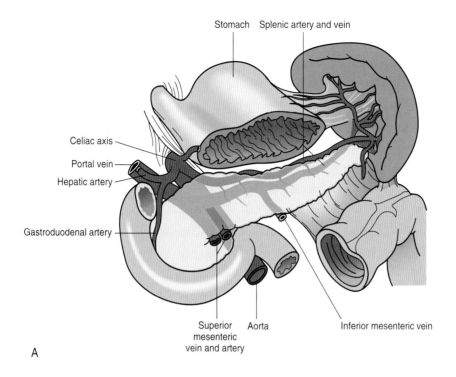

A

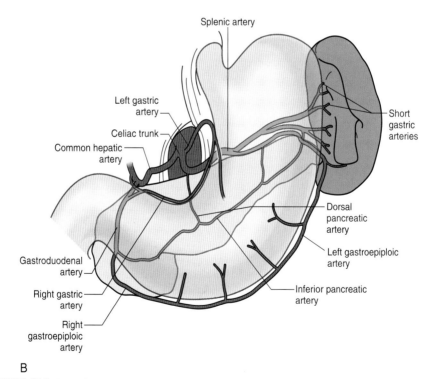

B

FIGURE 56-2 Anatomic relationships of the splenic vasculature. The magistral type of splenic artery anatomy **(A)** occurs in 30% of individuals. The more common distributed type of anatomy **(B)** occurs in 70% of individuals. (From Economou SG, Economou TS: *Atlas of surgical techniques*, Philadelphia, 1966, WB Saunders, p 562.)

biconcave and deform easily. This plasticity allows passage through the microvasculature and optimizes the exchange of oxygen and carbon dioxide. Imperfect red blood cells with inclusions such as nucleoli, Howell-Jolly bodies (nuclear remnant), Heinz bodies

(denatured hemoglobin), Pappenheimer bodies (iron granules), acanthocytes (spur cells), codocytes (target cells), and stippling cause these red blood cells to undergo cleansing in the spleen. Aged red blood cells with decreased plasticity (>120 days) become trapped and destroyed in the spleen.

Abnormal erythrocytes that result from sickle cell anemia, hereditary spherocytosis, thalassemia, or pyruvate kinase deficiency are also trapped and destroyed by the spleen. The overall effect is worsening anemia, splenomegaly, and sometimes autoinfarction of the spleen. Similarly, the spleen is involved in platelet destruction in immune thrombocytopenic purpura (ITP).

BOX 56-1   Biologic Substances Removed by the Spleen

Normal Subjects
Red blood cell membrane
Red blood cell surface pits and craters
Howell-Jolly bodies
Heinz bodies
Pappenheimer bodies
Acanthocytes
Senescent red blood cells
Particulate antigen

Patients With Disease
Spherocytes (hereditary spherocytosis)
Sickle cells, hemoglobin C cells
Antibody-coated red blood cells
Antibody-coated platelets
Antibody-coated white blood cells

Adapted from Eichner ER: Splenic function: Normal, too much and too little. *Am J Med* 66:311–320, 1979.

SPLENECTOMY

Splenectomy may be performed for a number of reasons and conditions.

Benign Hematologic Conditions
Immune Thrombocytopenic Purpura
ITP, classically known as idiopathic thrombocytopenic purpura, is characterized by a low platelet count despite normal bone marrow and the absence of other causes of thrombocytopenia that could be responsible for the finding. Autoantibodies are responsible for the disordered platelet destruction mediated by the overactivated platelet phagocytosis within the reticuloendothelial system. Within the bone marrow, normal (or sometimes increased)

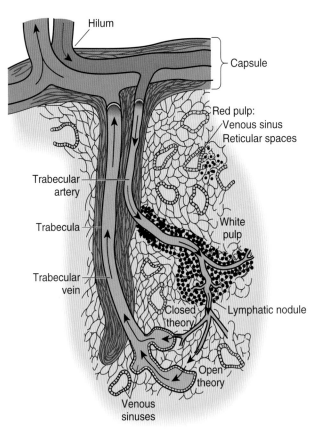

FIGURE 56-3 Structure of the sinusoidal spleen showing the open and closed blood flow routes. (From Bellanti JA: *Immunology. Basic processes.* Philadelphia, 1979, WB Saunders.)

amounts of megakaryocytes are present. There persists, however, a relative bone marrow failure in that production cannot match destruction to compensate sufficiently.

The typical presentation of ITP is characterized by purpura, epistaxis, and gingival bleeding. Less commonly, gastrointestinal bleeding and hematuria are noted. Intracerebral hemorrhage is a rare but sometimes fatal presentation. The diagnosis of ITP involves the exclusion of other relatively common causes of thrombocytopenia—pregnancy, drug-induced thrombocytopenia (e.g., heparin, quinidine, quinine, sulfonamides), viral infections, and hypersplenism (Box 56-2). Mild thrombocytopenia may be seen in approximately 6% to 8% of otherwise normal pregnancies and in up to 25% of women with preeclampsia. Drug-induced thrombocytopenia is thought to occur rarely, in approximately 20 to 40 cases/million users of common medications, such as trimethoprim-sulfonamide and quinine. Other medications, such as gold salts, have a higher incidence, almost 1% of users.[8] Viral infection (e.g., hepatitis C, HIV infection, rarely Epstein-Barr virus infection) can be responsible for thrombocytopenia independent of splenic sequestration. Once again, other processes must be ruled out, but health care providers can be confident of these causative factors if platelet counts improve with successful treatment of the responsible infection. Bacterial infection, specifically *Helicobacter pylori,* has also been linked to infection-related thrombocytopenia that improves with eradication. Other causes are listed in Box 56-2; spurious laboratory values caused by platelet clumping or the presence of giant platelets should not be ignored.

ITP is predominantly a disease of young women; 72% of patients older than 10 years are women, and 70% of affected women are younger than 40 years. ITP is manifested somewhat differently in children; both genders are affected equally, onset is sudden, thrombocytopenia is severe, and complete spontaneous remissions are seen in approximately 80% of affected children. Girls older than 10 years with more chronic purpura are those in whom the disease seems to persist.

Management of ITP depends primarily on the severity of the thrombocytopenia.[9] Asymptomatic patients with platelet counts higher than $50,000/mm^3$ may be observed without further intervention. Platelet counts of $50,000/mm^3$ and higher are rarely associated with clinical sequelae, even with invasive procedures. Patients with slightly lower platelet counts, between 30,000 and $50,000/mm^3$, may be observed but with more routine follow-up because they are at increased risk for progressing to severe thrombocytopenia. Initial medical treatment of patients with platelet counts below $50,000/mm^3$ and symptoms such as mucous membrane bleeding, high-risk conditions (e.g., active lifestyle, hypertension, peptic ulcer disease), or platelet counts below 20,000 to $30,000/mm^3$, even without symptoms, is glucocorticoid administration (typically, prednisone, 1 mg/kg body weight/day). Clinical response with increases in platelet levels to higher than $50,000/mm^3$ is seen in up to two thirds of patients within 1 to 3 weeks of initiating treatment. Of patients treated with steroids, 25% will experience a complete response. Patients with platelet counts higher than $20,000/mm^3$ who remain symptom free or who experience minor purpura as their only symptom do not require hospitalization. Hospitalization may be required for patients whose platelets counts remain below $20,000/mm^3$ with significant mucous membrane bleeding and is required for those who have life-threatening hemorrhage. Platelet transfusion is indicated only for those who experience severe hemorrhage. Intravenous immune globulin is important for the treatment of acute bleeding, in pregnancy, or for patients being prepared for operation, including splenectomy. The usual dose is 1 g/kg body weight/day for 2 days. This dose usually increases the platelet count within 3 days; it also increases the efficacy of platelet transfusions.

Should initial therapy for ITP fail, medical options for refractory ITP include oral prednisone, oral dexamethasone (40 mg/day for 4 days), rituximab ($375 mg/m^2$/wk intravenously for 4 weeks), and thrombopoietin receptor antagonists (eltrombopag, romiplostim). Successful response for months is observed in 28% to 44% of patients using rituximab; more transient responses are observed from thrombopoietin receptor antagonists.[10]

Before the establishment of glucocorticoids for treatment of ITP in 1950, splenectomy was the treatment of choice.[9] For those two thirds of patients in whom glucocorticoids result in the normalization of platelet counts, no further treatment is necessary. For patients with severe thrombocytopenia with counts below $10,000/mm^3$ for 6 weeks or longer, for those with thrombocytopenia refractory to glucocorticoid treatment, and for those who require toxic doses of steroid to achieve remission, the treatment of choice is to proceed to splenectomy. Splenectomy is also the treatment of choice for patients with incomplete response to glucocorticoid treatment and for pregnant women in the second trimester of pregnancy who have also failed to respond to steroid treatment or intravenous immune globulin therapy with platelet counts below $10,000/mm^3$ without symptoms or below $30,000/mm^3$ with bleeding problems. It is not necessary to proceed to splenectomy for patients who have platelet counts higher than $50,000/mm^3$, who have had ITP for longer than 6 months, who are not experiencing bleeding symptoms, and who are not engaged in high-risk activities. A review of short-term and long-term failure of laparoscopic splenectomy has reported an overall approximate failure rate of 28% at 5 years after splenectomy.[11]

BOX 56-2   Differential Diagnosis of Immune Thrombocytopenic Purpura

Falsely Low Platelet Count

In vitro platelet clumping caused by ethylenediaminetetraacetic acid (EDTA)–dependent or cold-dependent agglutinins
Giant platelets

Common Causes of Thrombocytopenia

Pregnancy (gestational thrombocytopenia, preeclampsia)
Drug-induced thrombocytopenia (common drugs include heparin, quinidine, quinine, sulfonamides)
Viral infections, such as HIV infection, rubella, infectious mononucleosis
Hypersplenism caused by chronic liver disease

Other Causes of Thrombocytopenia Mistaken for Immune Thrombocytopenic Purpura

Myelodysplasia
Congenital thrombocytopenias
Thrombotic thrombocytopenic purpura and hemolytic-uremic syndrome
Chronic disseminated intravascular coagulation

Thrombocytopenia Associated With Other Disorders

Autoimmune diseases, such as systemic lupus erythematosus
Lymphoproliferative disorders (chronic lymphocytic leukemia, non-Hodgkin lymphoma)

Adapted from George JN, El-Harake MA, Raskob GE: Chronic idiopathic thrombocytopenic purpura. *N Engl J Med* 331:1207–1211, 1994.

A systematic review of 436 published articles from 1966 to 2004 has reported that 72% of patients with ITP had a complete response to splenectomy. Relapse occurred in a median of 15% of patients (range, 1% to 51%), with a median follow-up of 33 months.[12]

In addition to relapse rates, predictors of successful splenectomy were examined. Of the variables in the multivariate model, age at the time of splenectomy was an independent variable that was most correlated with response.[12] Younger patients had improved responses. On preoperative indium In 111–labeled platelet scintigraphy, patients with platelets sequestered predominantly within the spleen had a significantly higher response rate than those noted to have hepatic sequestration.[13]

Most patients will exhibit improved platelet counts within 10 days postoperatively, and durable platelet responses are associated with patients who have platelet counts of 150,000/mm^3 by postoperative day 3 or more than 500,000/mm^3 by postoperative day 10. Even with splenectomy, however, some patients may relapse ($\approx$12%; range, 4% to 25%).[14] A review of 1223 ITP patients has estimated the long-term failure rate of laparoscopic splenectomy at approximately 8% and approximately 44/1000 patient-years of follow-up.[11] Another study has estimated the complete response of ITP patients after splenectomy to be 66%.[12]

Although a thorough search for accessory spleens is completed during the initial surgery, evaluation for a missed accessory spleen must be undertaken in patients who experience a relapse. In their evaluation of 394 patients treated with laparoscopic splenectomy, Katkhouda and colleagues[14] noted 15% of patients with accessory spleens. In those with accessory spleens, examination of a peripheral blood smear will lack the characteristic red blood cell morphology resulting from excision of the spleen. Radionuclide imaging may also be helpful in locating the presence and location of any accessory splenic tissue. Patients with chronic ITP in whom an accessory spleen is identified should have this removed, as long as the patient can withstand the surgical risk.

Other treatment options for these patients include observation of stable nonbleeding patients with platelet counts higher than 30,000/mm^3, long-term glucocorticoid therapy, and treatment with azathioprine or cyclophosphamide. Recent evidence regarding thrombopoietin receptor agonists may offer a novel medical therapy for patients with no response to steroids, intravenous immune globulin therapy, or splenectomy.[15]

Other conditions linked to thrombocytopenia include thrombotic thrombocytopenic purpura, chronic disseminated intravascular coagulation, congenital thrombocytopenia, myelodysplasia, autoimmune disorders (e.g., systemic lupus erythematosus), and lymphoproliferative disorders (e.g., chronic lymphocytic leukemia, non-Hodgkin lymphoma).

Approximately 10% to 20% of otherwise asymptomatic patients with HIV infection will develop ITP. Splenectomy is a safe treatment option for this cohort of patients and may actually delay HIV disease progression.[16,17]

Hereditary Spherocytosis

Hereditary spherocytosis is an autosomal dominant disease affecting the production of spectrin, a red blood cell cytoskeletal protein. Loss of this protein causes red blood cells to lack their characteristic biconcave shape. This affects the deformability of red blood cells because lack of this protein results in rigid erythrocytes that are small and sphere shaped. Also, these cells have increased osmotic fragility and are more susceptible to trapping and destruction by the spleen. The resulting clinical features are

anemia, occasionally with jaundice, and splenomegaly. Diagnosis is made by examination of a peripheral blood smear, increased reticulocyte count, increased osmotic fragility, and negative Coombs test result.

The resultant anemia can be successfully treated with splenectomy, but normalization of the erythrocyte morphology does not occur. Splenectomy should be delayed until the age of 5 years to preserve immunologic function of the spleen and to reduce the risk of OPSI. Just as with other hemolytic anemias, the presence of pigmented gallstones is common. The preoperative workup should include ultrasound evaluation; if gallstones are present, cholecystectomy may be performed at the same time as splenectomy.

Hereditary elliptocytosis, hereditary pyropoikilocytosis, hereditary xerocytosis, and hereditary hydrocytosis also result in anemia secondary to red blood cell membrane abnormalities. Splenectomy is indicated in cases of severe anemia with these conditions, except hereditary xerocytosis, which results in only mild anemia of limited clinical significance.

Hemolytic Anemia Caused by Erythrocyte Enzyme Deficiency

Pyruvate kinase deficiency and glucose-6-phosphate dehydrogenase (G6PD) deficiency are the predominant hereditary conditions associated with hemolytic anemia. Pyruvate kinase deficiency is an autosomal recessive disease that results in decreased red blood cell deformability and the formation of echinocytes, a type of spiculated red blood cell. This morphologic variant increases the likelihood that the cell will be trapped and destroyed by the spleen, which results in splenomegaly, hemolytic anemia, and associated transfusion requirements, which can be mitigated with splenectomy. Again, for reasons discussed earlier, splenectomy is delayed until 5 years of age.

In G6PD deficiency, however, splenectomy is rarely indicated. This X-linked condition is typically seen in people of African, Middle Eastern, or Mediterranean ancestry. Hemolytic anemia in these patients most often occurs after infection or exposure to certain foods, medications, or chemicals. Primary treatment, therefore, is avoidance of exacerbation of the condition.

Hemoglobinopathies

In addition to defects of cellular membranes or enzymes, hereditary anemias may also result from defects in hemoglobin molecules. Sickle cell disease and thalassemia are two disorders in which the hemoglobin molecules exhibit qualitative or quantitative defects. These lead to abnormally shaped erythrocytes, which may lead to splenic sequestration and subsequent destruction.

Sickle cell anemia results from a single amino acid substitution (valine for glutamic acid) in the sixth position of the β chain of hemoglobin A, which causes those hemoglobin chains, under reduced oxygen conditions, to become rigid and unable to deform within the microvasculature. This rigidity causes the red blood cells to assume the elongated crescent or sickle shape. Sickle cell disease results from homozygous inheritance of the defective hemoglobin (hemoglobin S), although sickling can also be seen when hemoglobin S is inherited along with other hemoglobin variants, such as hemoglobin C or sickle cell β-thalassemia. In African Americans, 8% are heterozygous for hemoglobin S (sickle cell trait), and approximately 0.5% are homozygous for hemoglobin S. During conditions of low oxygen tension, these hemoglobin S molecules crystallize, distorting the cell into a crescent shape. These misshapen cells are unable to pass through the microvasculature, which results in capillary occlusion, thrombosis, and ultimately microinfarction. This cascade of events frequently occurs in the spleen. These episodes of vaso-occlusion and progressive infarction result in autosplenectomy. The spleen, which is usually hypertrophied early in life, typically atrophies by adulthood, although splenomegaly may occasionally persist.

Other causes of hemolytic anemia are the thalassemias. These are inherited as autosomal dominant traits and result from a defect in hemoglobin synthesis that causes variable degrees of hemolytic anemia. Splenomegaly, hypersplenism, and splenic infarction, common in sickle cell disease, are also seen commonly in the thalassemias.

Hypersplenism and acute splenic sequestration are lifethreatening disorders in children with thalassemia and sickle cell disease. In these conditions, there may be rapid splenic enlargement, which results in severe pain and may require multiple blood transfusions. Patients with acute splenic sequestration crisis present with severe anemia, splenomegaly, and an acute bone marrow response, with erythrocytosis. There may be a concurrent decrease in hemoglobin levels, abdominal pain, and circulatory collapse. Resuscitation with hydration and transfusion may be followed by splenectomy in these patients. Hypersplenism related to sickle cell disease is characterized by anemia, leukopenia, and thrombocytopenia requiring transfusions; transfusions may be reduced by performing splenectomy. Symptomatic massive splenomegaly that interferes with daily activities may also be improved by splenectomy. Finally, in children with sickle cell disease who exhibit growth delay or even weight loss because of increased metabolic rate and whole body total protein turnover, splenectomy may relieve these symptoms.

Splenic abscesses may also be seen in patients with sickle cell anemia. These patients present with fever, abdominal pain, and a tender enlarged spleen. Most patients with splenic abscesses will have a leukocytosis as well as thrombocytosis and Howell-Jolly bodies, indicating a functional asplenia. *Salmonella* and *Enterobacter* spp. and other enteric organisms are commonly seen in those with a splenic abscess. These patients require resuscitation with hydration and transfusion and may require urgent splenectomy after stabilization.

Malignant Disease
Lymphomas

Hodgkin disease. Hodgkin disease is a malignant lymphoma that usually affects young adults in their 20s and 30s. Rarely, patients present with constitutional symptoms such as night sweats, weight loss, and pruritus; but more typically, asymptomatic lymphadenopathy usually involves the cervical nodes. Hodgkin disease is characterized histologically as lymphocyte predominant, nodular sclerosing, mixed cellularity, or lymphocyte depleted. The disease is pathologically staged according to the Ann Arbor classification. Stage I is disease in a single lymphatic site. Stage II is disease in two or more lymphatic sites on the same side of the diaphragm. Stage III indicates disease on both sides of the diaphragm and includes splenic involvement. Stage IV disease is disease in which there is dissemination into extralymphatic sites, such as liver, lung, or bone marrow. The addition of a subscript E to stage I, II, or III indicates single or contiguous extralymphatic spread; subscript S indicates splenic involvement. Patients who exhibit constitutional symptoms are denoted with a B (presence), and those without symptoms are denoted with an A (absence).

Historically, patients with Hodgkin disease underwent a staging laparotomy that included splenectomy to provide pathologic staging information required to determine appropriate therapy. This was particularly common in stage I and stage II disease to rule out splenic or subdiaphragmatic involvement. In addition to splenectomy, the procedure involves splenic hilar lymphadenectomy, liver biopsy, retroperitoneal node biopsy, and biopsy of a hepatoduodenal node and oophoropexy in premenopausal women. Staging methods have evolved to include imaging techniques—computed tomography (CT), ^{18}F-fluorodeoxyglucose positron emission tomography, and lymphangiography—thus making invasive staging methods almost obsolete. Staging laparotomy remains appropriate for select patients, such as those with early clinical disease stages (IA or IIA) in whom abdominal staging will significantly alter therapeutic management. Early-stage Hodgkin disease is often cured with radiation therapy alone. Laparotomy is no longer indicated for patients likely to relapse, those with evidence of intra-abdominal involvement on imaging, and those with B symptoms. These patients should receive systemic chemotherapy.

Non-Hodgkin lymphomas. Splenomegaly or hypersplenism is a common occurrence during the course of non-Hodgkin lymphoma (NHL). Splenectomy is indicated for NHL patients with massive splenomegaly leading to abdominal pain, early satiety, and fullness. It may also be indicated for patients who develop anemia, neutropenia, and thrombocytopenia associated with hypersplenism.

Splenectomy may also be instrumental in the diagnosis and staging of patients with isolated splenic disease. The most common primary splenic neoplasm is NHL. Less than 1% of patients present with splenomegaly without lymphadenopathy; however, 50% to 80% of patients with NHL have involvement of the spleen.[18] Patients with clinically isolated splenic disease are said to have malignant lymphoma with splenic involvement. Most patients have low-grade NHL, with frequent involvement of the splenic hilar lymph nodes, extrahilar nodes, bone marrow, or liver. Approximately 75% of these patients have clinically apparent hypersplenism. In patients with spleen-predominant features, survival is significantly improved after splenectomy compared with similar patients who did not undergo splenectomy.

Leukemia

Hairy cell leukemia. Hairy cell leukemia, a rare disease that accounts for approximately 2% of adult leukemias, is characterized by splenomegaly, pancytopenia, and neoplastic mononuclear cells in the peripheral blood and bone marrow. The cells that give the disease its name are B lymphocytes that have a ruffling of the cell membrane. This ruffling causes the cells to appear to have cytoplasmic projections under the light microscope. This disease affects older men, who present with palpable splenomegaly. Approximately 10% of patients require no treatment because of the indolent course of the disease. Treatment for cytopenias or splenomegaly typically begins with purine analogue chemotherapy.[19,20] For more refractory cancers, a second-line immunotherapy may be instituted. In others, however, the extent of splenomegaly or symptoms from hypersplenism, symptomatic anemia, infections from neutropenia, or hemorrhage from thrombocytopenia can lead to splenectomy. Most patients show improvement after the procedure, with a response lasting approximately 10 years after splenectomy, and some patients (≈40% to 60%) show normalization of blood counts after splenectomy.[21] Patients with diffusely involved bone marrow without massive splenomegaly are less responsive to splenectomy. Patients with hairy cell leukemia are also at a twofold to threefold risk for development of other malignant neoplasms after their diagnosis of hairy cell leukemia. Most of these second malignant neoplasms are solid tumors, such as skin cancers, lung cancer, prostate cancer, and gastrointestinal adenocarcinomas. Hairy cell leukemia behaves like a chronic leukemia; many patients can achieve a clinical remission, with a normal or near-normal life span.

Chronic lymphocytic leukemia. Chronic lymphocytic leukemia (CLL) is a clinically heterogeneous disease of B lymphocytes characterized by the progressive accumulation of relatively mature but functionally incompetent lymphocytes. CLL is seen with a slight predominance in men, mainly after the age of 50 years. CLL is staged according to the Rai system and correlates fairly well with survival. Low-risk CLL (formerly stage 0) involves bone marrow and blood lymphocytosis only; intermediate-risk CLL (formerly stages I and II) involves lymphocytosis and lymphadenopathy in any site or splenomegaly, hepatomegaly, or hepatosplenomegaly; and high-risk CLL (formerly stages III and IV) involves lymphocytosis and anemia or thrombocytopenia. The Rai system helps clinicians determine when therapy should be started. New molecular tests, such as that for ZAP-70, zeta chain–associated protein 70 (an intracellular protein rarely found in normal B cells), are increasingly helpful for determining prognosis.[22] Medical treatment, consisting of nucleoside analogues or combination therapy, is indicated for symptomatic patients or those exhibiting evidence of rapid disease progression. Monoclonal antibodies are also used in the treatment of CLL.

Bone marrow transplantation currently offers the only known cure for CLL. Splenectomy is indicated for patients with refractory splenomegaly and pancytopenia, which results in improvements in blood counts in 60% to 70% of patients.[23]

Chronic myelogenous leukemia. Chronic myelogenous leukemia (CML) is a myeloproliferative disorder that develops as a result of a neoplastic transformation of myeloid elements. CML is characterized by the progressive replacement of normal diploid elements of the bone marrow with mature-appearing neoplastic myeloid cells. Although CML can be asymptomatic at presentation, patients commonly present with fever, fatigue, malaise, effects of pancytopenia (infections, anemia, easy bruising), and occasionally splenomegaly. A chromosomal marker, the Philadelphia chromosome, is highly associated with CML and is caused by the fusion of fragments of chromosomes 9 and 22. This fusion results in expression of the BCR-ABL gene product, a tyrosine kinase, which then accelerates cell division and inhibits DNA repair.

CML may occur in patients from childhood to old age. It usually is manifested with an asymptomatic chronic phase but may progress to an accelerated phase associated with fever, night sweats, and progressive splenomegaly. The accelerated phase may be asymptomatic and may be detectable only by changes in peripheral blood or bone marrow. The accelerated phase may then progress to the blastic phase. This phase is also characterized by fever, night sweats, and splenomegaly but is also associated with anemia, infections, and bleeding.

The BCR-ABL gene product is the target for therapy with tyrosine kinase inhibitors and other chemotherapeutic modalities. Bone marrow transplantation is an option, but prognosis has improved dramatically with the advent of recent therapies, making transplantation less common. Studies evaluating the efficacy of newer therapies and combination therapies are ongoing. Symptomatic splenomegaly and hypersplenism in CML can be effectively treated with splenectomy, but there does not appear to be a survival benefit when it is performed during the early chronic phase.[24] Surgery is therefore reserved for patients with significant symptoms.

Nonhematologic Tumors of the Spleen

The spleen can also be the site of metastatic disease, seen in up to 7% of autopsies of cancer patients. The solid tumors that most frequently spread to the spleen are carcinomas of the breast and lung and melanoma. Any primary malignant neoplasm, however, can metastasize to the spleen.[25] Metastases are often asymptomatic but may be associated with splenomegaly and even splenic rupture; thus, splenectomy may provide palliation for carefully chosen patients with symptomatic splenic metastases.

Primary tumors of the spleen are commonly vascular neoplasms and include benign and malignant variants. Hemangiomas are frequent findings in spleens removed for other reasons. Angiosarcomas (or hemangiosarcomas) of the spleen usually occur spontaneously but have been linked to environmental exposures, such as to thorium dioxide and monomeric vinyl chloride. Patients with angiosarcomas may present with splenomegaly, hemolytic anemia, ascites, pleural effusions, or even spontaneous splenic rupture. These tumors are aggressive and have a poor prognosis. Lymphangiomas, by contrast, are endothelium-lined cysts that come to attention because of splenomegaly secondary to cyst enlargement. These are usually benign tumors; however, lymphangiosarcoma has been found within lymphangiomas. Splenectomy is appropriate for the diagnosis, treatment, and palliation of these conditions.

Miscellaneous Benign Conditions
Splenic Cysts

Splenic cysts have been seen with increasing frequency since the advent of CT and ultrasound scanning. They are classified as true cysts, which can be parasitic or nonparasitic, or as pseudocysts. Tumors of the spleen may also appear to be cystic; these include lymphangiomas and cavernous hemangiomas (see earlier).[26] Primary true cysts of the spleen account for approximately 10% of all nonparasitic splenic cysts, whereas most nonparasitic cysts are pseudocysts secondary to trauma. True cysts are lined with a squamous epithelium, and many are considered congenital. These epithelial cells are often positive for carbohydrate antigen 19-9 and carcinoembryonic antigen by immunohistochemistry. Patients with splenic epidermoid cysts may have elevated serum levels of one or both of these tumor markers. These cysts, however, are benign and apparently do not have malignant potential beyond that of the surrounding native tissue.

True splenic cysts are often asymptomatic and discovered incidentally. Patients may complain of abdominal fullness, early satiety, pleuritic chest pain, shortness of breath, and left shoulder or back pain. They may also experience renal symptoms from compression of the left kidney. On physical examination, an abdominal mass may be palpable. Rarely, splenic cysts are manifested with acute symptoms related to rupture, hemorrhage, or infection. Diagnosis is best made by CT, and operative intervention is indicated for those with symptomatic or large cysts. Total or partial splenectomy may provide appropriate treatment. Partial splenectomy has the advantage of preserving splenic function; 25% of the spleen appears to be sufficient to protect against pneumococcal pneumonia. Open and laparoscopic procedures allow total or partial splenectomy, cyst wall resection, or partial decapsulation.[26,27]

Most true splenic cysts are parasitic cysts and occur in areas of endemic hydatid disease (*Echinococcus* spp.). Radiographic imaging reveals cyst wall calcifications or daughter cysts, and although hydatid disease is uncommon in North America, this diagnosis must be excluded before invasive procedures are undertaken that might result in spillage of the cyst contents. Rupture of the cyst and expulsion of contents into the abdomen may precipitate anaphylactic shock and can also lead to intraperitoneal dissemination of the infection. Serologic testing is helpful for verifying the presence of these parasites. Splenectomy is the treatment of choice. As with hydatid cysts of the liver, the cysts may be sterilized by injection of a 3% sodium chloride solution, alcohol, or 0.5% silver nitrate. Even so, great care should be taken to avoid intraoperative rupture of the cyst.

Pseudocysts represent the remaining 70% to 80% of nonparasitic splenic cysts. A history of prior trauma can typically be elicited. Pseudocysts of the spleen are not lined with epithelium. Radiologic imaging usually reveals a smooth, unilocular, thick-walled lesion, sometimes with focal calcifications. Asymptomatic, small (<4 cm) pseudocysts do not require treatment and may involute with time. Symptomatic pseudocysts are manifested in a fashion similar to true splenic cysts; these are treated surgically with total or partial splenectomy, again remembering that partial splenectomy preserves splenic function. Percutaneous drainage has also been reported for splenic pseudocysts,[28] although, in a case series, recurrence was common and subsequent complications were deemed too high.[29]

Splenic Abscess

Splenic abscess is an unusual but potentially life-threatening illness, with a 0.7% incidence in autopsy series.[30] The mortality rate for splenic abscess ranges from 15% to 20% in previously healthy patients with single unilocular lesions to 80% for multiple abscesses in immunocompromised patients. Illnesses and other factors that predispose to splenic abscess include malignant neoplasms, polycythemia vera, endocarditis, prior trauma, hemoglobinopathies, urinary tract infections, intravenous drug use, and AIDS.

Approximately 70% of splenic abscesses result from hematogenous spread of the infective organism from another location, as in endocarditis, osteomyelitis, and intravenous drug use. Spread may also occur in a contiguous fashion from local infections of the colon, kidney, or pancreas. Gram-positive cocci (commonly *Staphylococcus, Streptococcus,* or *Enterococcus* spp.) and gram-negative enteric organisms are typically involved. *Mycobacterium tuberculosis, Mycobacterium avium,* and *Actinomyces* spp. have also been found. Fungal abscesses (e.g., *Candida* spp.) also occur, typically in immunosuppressed patients.

Splenic abscesses are manifested with nonspecific symptoms—vague abdominal pain, fever, peritonitis, and pleuritic chest pain. Splenomegaly is not typical. CT is the preferred method for diagnosis; however, the diagnosis can also be made with ultrasound.

Treatment of splenic abscesses depends on whether the abscess is unilocular or multilocular. In one third of adult patients, the abscess is multilocular. In one third of children, the abscess is unilocular. Unilocular abscesses are often amenable to percutaneous drainage, along with antibiotics,[31] with success rates reported at 75% to 90% for unilocular lesions. Multilocular lesions, however, are usually treated with splenectomy, drainage of the left upper quadrant, and antibiotics.[32] Laparoscopic splenectomy for abscess has been reported.[33]

Wandering Spleen

Wandering spleen is a rare finding seen in children and in women between the ages of 20 and 40 years. One of two causes is suspected. The first is theorized to result from a failure to form

normal splenic peritoneal attachments that suspend the organ securely within its usual anatomic position. Failure to form these attachments is thought to arise from lack of fusion of the dorsal mesogastrium to the posterior abdominal wall during embryogenesis. The second theory surmises that in multiparous women, hormonal changes and abdominal laxity lead to an acquired defect in splenic attachments. In either case, without these attachments, the splenic pedicle is unusually long and prone to torsion.

Intermittent abdominal pain, splenomegaly resulting from venous congestion, and severe persistent pain are suggestive of wandering spleen and tension or intermittent torsion of the splenic pedicle. A mobile mass may be palpable on physical examination. CT of the abdomen with intravenous administration of contrast material provides confirmation of the diagnosis, with the spleen located outside its usual position. A noncontrasted spleen or whorled appearance of the vascular pedicle provides additional evidence for the condition and may be helpful in choosing splenopexy or splenectomy.[34]

Other Considerations
Splenic Trauma
See Chapter 16.

Elective Laparoscopic Splenectomy

Laparoscopic splenectomy is now the preferred method for resecting the spleen. This technique was first described in 1991,[35] and many studies have supported its use in terms of outcomes and patient safety.[14] Disadvantages of the laparoscopic technique are longer operating times and difficulty in removing large organs; however, reduced hospital stay and more rapid postoperative recovery alleviate these limitations. Complications are typically linked to the patient's comorbidities.

Laparoscopic splenectomy has been reported for most splenic diseases and is the preferred method for most situations, barring trauma or cases of massive splenomegaly. In deciding whether to pursue laparoscopic methods for splenectomy, certain considerations should be taken into account, such as operative indication (e.g., benign or malignant disease), splenic size, and any potential contraindications to laparoscopy. Preoperative planning is aided by CT imaging especially regarding splenomegaly. Melman and Matthews[36] have noted that spleens measuring more than 22 cm in craniocaudal dimension or more than 19 cm in width and with an estimated weight of more than 1600 g will require hand-assisted laparoscopic procedures, if not open splenectomy. Laparoscopic splenectomy can be completed in approximately 90% of patients. The reported conversion to open splenectomy is between 0% and 20%. Most conversions are caused by intraoperative bleeding, lack of surgical experience, prohibitive adhesions,[37] massive splenomegaly,[28] and obesity.[2,17] As with other laparoscopic procedures, there is a learning curve, and with increasing experience, conversion to open splenectomy declines.[4,38] Recently published guidelines regarding laparoscopic splenectomy reiterate the importance of indications for the procedure, preoperative imaging for determining size and volume and presence of accessory splenic tissue, choices regarding hand-assisted techniques (early in cases of splenomegaly), contraindications (e.g., portal hypertension, major medical comorbidities), and splenic vaccinations.[39] Vaccinations for *N. meningitidis, S. pneumoniae,* and *H. influenzae* should be given 15 days before elective splenectomy or within 30 days of an emergent splenectomy to reduce the risk of OPSI (see earlier).

Postoperative recovery from laparoscopic splenectomy is rapid, as seen with laparoscopic cholecystectomy. The length of stay ranges from 1.8 to 6 days; shorter hospital stays are a major advantage of laparoscopic procedures.[18,20] A prospective randomized controlled trial comparing open and laparoscopic approaches was performed in patients with β-thalassemia major. This study reported a shorter median hospital stay in the laparoscopic patients but longer operative times and an increase in blood transfusions.[40] It is not known whether these results can be generalized to all patients with splenic disease. Several case series have also compared the laparoscopic with the open approach and consistently favored the laparoscopic approach, particularly in regard to earlier resumption of diet, decreased postoperative pain, and shorter hospital stay.[13]

Treatment outcomes are the primary concern in comparing these approaches. In published results to date, laparoscopic outcomes are equivalent to those of open splenectomy. In a review of laparoscopic splenectomy for malignant disease, Burch and associates[41] have reported that this population of patients benefits from laparoscopic splenectomy, similar to those with benign disease. Katkhouda and coworkers[14] have reported that in the treatment of ITP, laparoscopic and open splenectomy results appear to be similar.

As noted, laparoscopic surgery needs careful consideration for special populations. Portal hypertension and its risk of operative hemorrhage prohibit laparoscopic splenectomy. Laparoscopic splenectomy during pregnancy for refractory thrombocytopenia carries an associated fetal mortality rate of 31%. There is scant literature regarding this rare patient population, although laparoscopic splenectomy can be performed during pregnancy.[39,42]

The laparoscopic technique may be performed with the patient in the supine or lateral position or a combination. After induction of general anesthesia and endotracheal intubation, a nasogastric tube and urinary catheter are inserted. Standard antithrombotic precautions are taken. Positioning of the patient is crucial for the completion of a laparoscopic splenectomy. For all three positions, the patient is placed so that the kidney rest can be raised to maximize the space between the iliac crest and costal margin. The patient is positioned so that the table may be flexed to widen the working space. Finally, the patient is tilted in a reverse Trendelenburg position to facilitate retraction of the viscera caudally away from the left upper quadrant.

In the supine position, the surgeon stands to the patient's left, and the first assistant and camera assistant stand to the patient's right.[37] It may be easier for a right-handed surgeon to work from a position between the patient's legs, with the patient in a modified lithotomy position. The scrub nurse stands to the patient's left side, near the foot of the table. Alternatively, the patient may be placed in a 60-degree right lateral decubitus position using a beanbag and axillary roll. In this case, the patient's left arm is placed on an arm board or supported by a splint. With this approach, the surgeon and scrub nurse stand to the patient's right and the assistants stand to the patient's left. The spleen will thus be suspended from its diaphragmatic attachments; gravity retracts the stomach, omentum, and colon; and the splenic hilum will be under some degree of tension. For either approach, the video monitors are placed on either side of the table, at or above the level of the patient's shoulders.

Trocar access to the abdomen is gained, and pneumoperitoneum is established to a pressure of 12 to 15 mm Hg. Three to five 2- to 12-mm-diameter ports are used, with the camera port at the umbilicus or offset between the umbilicus and

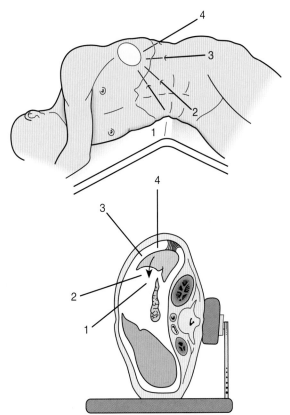

FIGURE 56-4 Right lateral decubitus position of the patient for laparoscopic splenectomy. The table is angulated, giving forced lateral flexion of the patient to open the costophrenic space. Trocars are inserted along the left costal margin more posteriorly. The spleen is suspended by its peritoneal attachments. The *numbered lines* show the position of laparoscopic ports. (From Gigot JF, Lengele B, Gianello P, et al: Present status of laparoscopic splenectomy for hematologic diseases: Certitudes and unresolved issues. *Semin Laparosc Surg* 5:147–167, 1998.)

costal margin. The other port sites are positioned as depicted in Figure 56-4.

The operation is begun with a thorough search of the abdominal cavity for the presence of accessory splenic tissue (Fig. 56-5); the stomach is retracted to the right side to facilitate examination of the gastrosplenic ligament. The splenocolic ligament, greater omentum, and phrenosplenic ligament are inspected next. The small and large bowel mesenteries, pelvis, and adnexal tissues are examined. Finally, the gastrosplenic ligament is opened, and the tail of the pancreas is confirmed to be free of splenic tissue.

Our preference has been to use the right lateral decubitus approach, with the operating room table bent 45 degrees from horizontal and the kidney rest elevated. The initial dissection is begun by mobilizing the splenic flexure of the colon. By use of sharp dissection, the splenocolic ligament is divided. The spleen can then be retracted cephalad; care should be taken not to rupture the splenic capsule during retraction. The lateral peritoneal attachments of the spleen are incised next, with use of scissors or ultrasonic shears. A 1-cm cuff of peritoneum is left along the lateral aspect of the spleen, which can then be grasped to facilitate medial retraction. The lesser sac is entered along the medial border

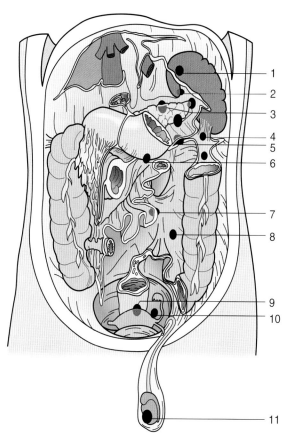

FIGURE 56-5 Usual location of accessory spleens: (1) gastrosplenic ligament, (2) splenic hilum, (3) tail of the pancreas, (4) splenocolic ligament, (5) left transverse mesocolon, (6) greater omentum along the greater curvature of the stomach, (7) mesentery, (8) left mesocolon, (9) left ovary, (10) Douglas pouch, and (11) left testis. (From Gigot JF, Lengele B, Gianello P, et al: Present status of laparoscopic splenectomy for hematologic diseases: Certitudes and unresolved issues. *Semin Laparosc Surg* 5:147–167, 1998.)

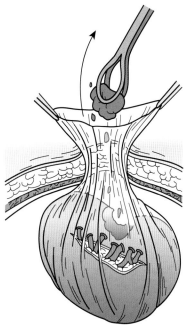

FIGURE 56-6 Extraction of the spleen within a heavy plastic bag, with instrumental morcellation of the organ with forceps. (From Gigot JF, Lengele B, Gianello P, et al: Present status of laparoscopic splenectomy for hematologic diseases: Certitudes and unresolved issues. *Semin Laparosc Surg* 5:147–167, 1998.)

of the spleen. Continuing the cephalad retraction, the short gastric vessels and main vascular pedicle can be identified. The tail of the pancreas is also visualized, and care is taken to avoid it as it nears the splenic hilum. The short gastric vessels are divided. A number of options are currently available for this, including ultrasonic dissectors, hemoclips, bipolar devices, LigaSure (Covidien, Boulder, Colo), and endovascular stapling devices. Hemoclips are used minimally around the area of the splenic hilum to prevent interference with future use of a stapling device, which could lead to significant bleeding from improperly ligated hilar vessels.

After the short gastric vessels are divided, the splenic pedicle is carefully dissected from the medial and lateral aspects. After the artery and vein are dissected, the vessels are divided by application of endovascular staplers or suture ligatures. In the more prevalent distributed mode, there are multiple vascular branches entering the spleen close to the hilum, so the dissection is carried out approximately 2 cm from the splenic capsule. Several branches may still be encountered, but these may be individually controlled more easily. A pedicle formed by the artery and vein that enters the hilum is known as the magistral type of arterial anatomy. If this is seen, the pedicle is transected en bloc using a linear vascular stapler. The tail of the pancreas, which is within 1 cm of the splenic hilum in 75% of patients and touches the hilum in 30%, should be well visualized as the stapler is applied to avoid injury.

The now-devascularized spleen is suspended only from a small cuff of avascular splenophrenic tissue at the superior pole. This tissue facilitates transfer of the spleen into a retrieval bag. To remove the detached spleen, the puncture-resistant nylon bag is grasped by its drawstring, which can be drawn through a port, usually the epigastric or supraumbilical site. The bag is opened slightly, providing access to the still intra-abdominal spleen. The spleen is then morcellated with ring forceps or finger fracture and removed piecemeal (Fig. 56-6). In the rare cases requiring pathologic examination of an intact spleen, an incision large enough to allow extraction of the spleen must be made. Care must be taken to avoid spillage of any splenic fragments into the abdominal cavity or wound. The laparoscope is then reinserted and the splenic bed assessed for hemostasis. Drains may be placed, if necessary. Pneumoperitoneum is then released, and the fasciae of all trocar ports larger than 5 mm are closed.

Robotic Splenectomy

There have been few reports of splenic disease treated robotically and only one report specifically comparing laparoscopic with robotic splenectomy. In their retrospective report, Bodner and colleagues[43] compared operative times, hospital stay, and cost. They concluded that although the robotic procedure is feasible and safe for the patient, cost and operative times are both higher in the robotic group. In another study, Corcione and associates[44] evaluated the use of a robotic system in common general surgical procedures. Although they noted some benefits (e.g., availability of three-dimensional vision, greater dexterity with instruments), they reported concerns about the ability to control bleeding with only two instruments available; in these cases, they were required to convert to a traditional laparoscopic procedure. Overall, the addition of the robot to a straightforward procedure such as laparoscopic splenectomy is currently deemed unnecessary.

LATE MORBIDITY AFTER SPLENECTOMY

Postsplenectomy thrombocytosis occurs particularly in patients with myeloproliferative disorders (e.g., CML, polycythemia vera, essential thrombocytosis), which can result in thrombosis of the mesenteric, portal, and renal veins and can be life-threatening because it can lead to hemorrhage and thromboembolism. The lifelong risk for deep venous thrombosis and pulmonary embolism has not been established but may be significant. Also, there have been case reports of acute myocardial infarction in postsplenectomy patients with thrombocytosis.

OPSI is the most common fatal late complication of splenectomy. Infection may occur at any time after splenectomy.[2] In one series, most infections occurred more than 2 years after splenectomy and 42% occurred more than 5 years after splenectomy, although the true incidence of OPSI has been difficult to determine because infection in postsplenectomy patients is likely to be underreported.

OPSI typically begins with a prodromal phase characterized by fever, rigors, and chills and other nonspecific symptoms, including sore throat, malaise, myalgias, diarrhea, and vomiting. Pneumonia and meningitis may be present. Many patients have no identifiable focal site of infection and present only with high-grade primary bacteremia. Progression of the illness is rapid, with the development of hypotension, disseminated intravascular coagulation, respiratory distress, coma, and death within hours of presentation. Despite antibiotics and intensive care, the mortality rate is between 50% and 70% for florid OPSI. Survivors also often have a long and complicated hospital course with multiple sequelae, such as peripheral gangrene requiring amputation, deafness from meningitis, mastoid osteomyelitis, bacterial endocarditis, and cardiac valvular destruction.

The most frequently involved organism in OPSI is *S. pneumoniae,* which is estimated to be responsible for between 50% and 90% of cases. Other organisms involved in OPSI include *H. influenzae, N. meningitidis, Streptococcus* and *Salmonella* spp., other pneumococcal organisms, and *Capnocytophaga canimorsus,* implicated in OPSI as a result of dog bites.

In an autopsy series by Pimpl and coworkers,[45] lethal pneumonia was identified twice as often in the postsplenectomy patients as in controls. Lethal sepsis with multiorgan failure was also identified in 6.9% of postsplenectomy patients compared with 1.5% of autopsies on the controls. One intriguing observation is that the risk for OPSI is greater for patients who have received splenectomy for malignant disease or hematologic conditions than for those who underwent splenectomy for trauma. The risk is also greater for young children (<4 years of age). The risk for fatal OPSI is estimated to be 1/300 to 350 patient-years of follow-up for children and 1/800 to 1000 patient-years of follow-up for adults. A review of selected reported splenectomy series of 7872 total cases, including children and adults, has revealed 270 episodes of sepsis (3.5%), with 169 septic fatalities (2.1%).[17] The incidence of nonfatal infection and sepsis is therefore likely to be significantly greater.

PROPHYLACTIC TREATMENT OF SPLENECTOMIZED PATIENTS

Immunization

Currently, the standard of care for postsplenectomy patients includes immunization with polyvalent pneumococcal vaccine (PPV23), *H. influenzae* type b conjugate, and meningococcal polysaccharide vaccine within 2 weeks of splenectomy if the patient did not receive these before surgery.[4] Despite this established standard, the literature reflects a diverse 11% to 75% postsplenectomy immunization rate. This may represent lack of understanding by patient and caregiver regarding the risk for postsplenectomy infection and sepsis.[46]

As noted, most cases of infection are caused by *S. pneumoniae, H. influenzae,* and *N. meningitidis* and thus are potentially preventable if appropriate prophylactic vaccinations are given. There are reports of other, less common organisms as the cause of postsplenectomy infection.[3] Continued education of patients, families, and caregivers must stress the need for prompt medical attention if these patients show signs of infection.

Many cases of delayed OPSI have been in nonimmunized immunocompetent patients, before the current PPV23 that was introduced in 1983, which replaced the 14-valent vaccine licensed in 1977. PPV23 is composed of purified preparations of pneumococcal capsular polysaccharide antigens of 23 types of *S. pneumoniae* (25 mg each) that cause 88% of the bacteremic pneumococcal disease in the United States.

The relationship between antibody titer and protection from invasive disease has not been established. Most healthy adults show a twofold or greater rise in type-specific antibody within 2 to 3 weeks of vaccination. However, it has been clearly documented that after vaccination with PPV23, antibody levels decline after 5 to 10 years and may fall to prevaccination levels. Even with vaccination, the development of a protective level of antibody against pneumococci is only about 50%. Currently available vaccines elicit a T cell–independent response and do not produce a sustained increase in antibody titers. Thus, the ability to define the need for revaccination based on serology continues to represent a clinical challenge.

Routine revaccination of immunocompetent persons is not recommended by the U.S. Centers for Disease Control and Prevention (CDC). Revaccination is, however, recommended for high-risk individuals. Candidates for revaccination with PPV23 include the following:

- Persons who received the 14-valent vaccine who are at highest risk for fatal pneumococcal infection (e.g., asplenic patients)
- Adults at highest risk who received the 23-valent vaccine 6 years prior
- Adults at highest risk who have shown a rapid decline in pneumococcal antibody levels (e.g., patients with nephrotic syndrome, those with renal failure, transplant recipients)
- Children at highest risk (e.g., those with asplenia, nephritic syndrome, sickle cell anemia) who would be 10 years old at revaccination

Only one PPV23 revaccination dose is recommended for these high-risk individuals, and it is administered 5 years after the initial dose. Rutherford and colleagues[47] have examined the efficacy and safety of pneumococcal revaccination after splenectomy for trauma. Of 45 patients offered revaccination 2 years or more after primary vaccination, 24 patients demonstrated a lack of understanding of the postsplenectomy state, confirming the poor understanding of patients of the postsplenectomy risk. After revaccination, 48% of patients demonstrated at least a twofold increase in at least one titer (serotypes 6 and 23 pneumococcus).

The CDC has concluded that despite physician and patient education, pamphlets, and MedicAlert bracelets, the patient's retention regarding the risks of the postsplenectomy state is poor. The CDC recommended that all splenectomy patients, including those with hereditary spherocytosis, be revaccinated and reeducated between 2 and 6 years after splenectomy. Recommendations include determination of pneumococcal antibody titers after immunization of every splenectomized patient because nonresponders to vaccination may be at high risk for OPSI. Subsequent follow-up of antibody titers is recommended at 3 to 5 years to evaluate for possible need for revaccination.

In an effort to improve host immunocompetence, partial splenic salvage or splenic autotransplantation has been considered because this may improve the humoral immune response to PPV23.[48] The difficulty with splenic salvage techniques is the lack of objective functional immune testing in humans. This is also true for patients who have undergone angiographic embolization for cessation of splenic hemorrhage in trauma. No studies are available regarding the risk of these patients for OPSI. Preclinical studies have examined the optimal site and amount of splenic tissue for autotransplantation. The most effective site of splenic autotransplantation was found to be the omental pouch, and approximately 50% of the spleen would be necessary for the prevention of pneumococcal sepsis. Although all efforts need to be made to preserve the spleen in trauma victims, the strategy of splenic autotransplantation seems to have limited applicability in humans.

Currently, it is suggested that educational intervention for patients who have undergone splenectomy is necessary; patients may require a number of instructional sessions. Communication with and educational efforts for primary care providers who assume medical care for asplenic patients are also extremely important because OPSI is preventable if appropriate precautions are taken. CDC immunization guidelines for 2010 have recommended the following vaccines for asplenic patients: tetanus (Td/Tdap); human papillomavirus; measles, mumps, rubella; varicella; zoster; influenza; pneumococcal polysaccharide; hepatitis A; hepatitis B; and meningococcal (Table 56-1).

The 2006 recommendations of the Surgical Infection Society for patients 2 to 64 years of age are *H. influenzae* type b conjugate vaccine, meningococcal vaccine, and 23-valent pneumococcal vaccine. Several sources have reported that the conjugate pneumococcal vaccine is more effective in asplenic patients than the polysaccharide vaccine and should be given immediately postoperatively as well as every 5 years to maintain efficacy. Shatz and associates[4] have evaluated antibody titers to pneumococcal vaccination in traumatic splenectomy patients randomized to receive the vaccine at 14 or 28 days postoperatively. Prior work by this group suggested that a delay in therapy might increase titer production; in the follow-up study, they determined that there was no statistically significant difference in antibody response between the two groups.

Despite lack of high-level evidence and because of the lifelong risk of OPSI, most recommend vaccines (*H. influenzae* type b conjugate vaccine, meningococcal vaccine, 23-valent pneumococcal vaccine) immediately for pneumococcal vaccination and at 14 days postoperatively or at least 2 weeks before elective splenectomy. Depending on the patient's reliability, these

TABLE 56-1	Centers for Disease Control and Prevention Vaccine Recommendations for Asplenic Patients
VACCINE	**RECOMMENDATION**
Tetanus (Td/Tdap)	One dose every 10 years
Human papillomavirus	Three doses for women through age 26 years (0, 2, 6 months)
Measles, mumps, rubella	One or two doses
Varicella	Two doses (0, 4-8 weeks)
Zoster	One dose
Influenza	One dose annually
Pneumococcal polysaccharide	One or two doses
Hepatitis A	Two doses (0, 6-12 months or 0, 6-18 months)
Hepatitis B	Three doses (0, 1-2 months, 4-6 months)
Meningococcal	One dose

vaccinations may be given before hospital discharge for emergent splenectomy. The current recommendations are summarized in Figure 56-7.

Antibiotics

Significant controversy still exists about antibiotic prophylaxis in postsplenectomy patients. The primary goal of this prophylaxis is to prevent OPSI, particularly that secondary to pneumococcal infection, which is reported to be the cause of OPSI in 50% to 90% of patients. However, OPSI secondary to penicillin-sensitive pneumococcal infection has been reported in children and adults receiving penicillin prophylaxis.

Regardless, prophylaxis with penicillin is routinely practiced in children, at least during the first 2 years after splenectomy, and some authors advocate this practice in adults, although evidence for this is scarce. Others recommend lifelong prophylaxis in adults and children. This length of treatment may be unacceptable to patients, and there is evidence that there is no difference in the incidence of sepsis in postsplenectomy sickle cell patients when the antibiotic prophylaxis is ceased after 5 years.[49] Other studies have reported significant differences in the incidence of sepsis, with and without antibiotic prophylaxis. Again, OPSI has been reported in patients taking prophylactic medications, and patients should be made aware that even with daily antibiotics, not all infections may be preventable.

A rational approach may be to provide a supply of oral antibiotics (standby antibiotics) to postsplenectomy adults, with instructions to begin taking the medication at the onset of a febrile illness or rigors if there is no access to immediate medical evaluation. There is evidence that the risk of OPSI is lowest in patients who exhibit the greatest understanding of the infectious risks of asplenia.[5] This highlights the importance of education of the patient, particularly at follow-up visits, to ensure compliance with antibiotic and vaccine prophylaxis.

Whether the patient elects to take antibiotic prophylaxis, and because of the risk of OPSI and the extreme level of associated mortality, any asplenic patient who presents with rigors or fever must be started immediately on aggressive empirical antibiotic coverage, even without culture data.

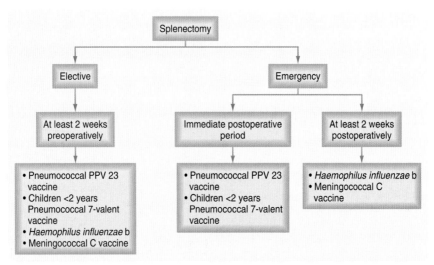

FIGURE 56-7 Splenectomy immunoprophylaxis flow chart. (From Harji DP, Jaunoo SS, Mistry P, Nesargikar PN: Immunoprophylaxis in asplenic patients. *Int J Surg* 7:421–423, 2009.)

SELECTED REFERENCES

Feldman LS: Laparoscopic splenectomy: Standardized approach. *World J Surg* 35:1487–1495, 2011.

This article provides a useful overview of indications and technique for laparoscopic splenectomy. It also provides useful tips on minimally invasive approaches to specific scenarios in splenic disease (e.g., splenomegaly, accessory spleens).

George JN, Woolf SH, Raskob GE, et al: Idiopathic thrombocytopenic purpura: A practice guideline developed by explicit methods for the American Society of Hematology. *Blood* 88:3–40, 1996.

Comprehensive summary and practice guidelines for the treatment of ITP established by the American Society of Hematology; provides a comprehensive review of the current treatment recommendations and outcomes for pediatric and adult patients with ITP.

Gigot JF, Jamar F, Ferrant A, et al: Inadequate detection of accessory spleens and splenosis with laparoscopic splenectomy. A shortcoming of the laparoscopic approach in hematologic diseases. *Surg Endosc* 12:101–106, 1998.

Despite being more than 10 years old, this article provides good technical tips for the surgeon. The article discusses numerous hematologic indications for splenectomy and their surgical outcome.

Habermalz B, Sauerland S, Decker G, et al: Laparoscopic splenectomy: The clinical practice guidelines of the European Association for Endoscopic Surgery (EAES). *Surg Endosc* 22:821–848, 2008.

Publication of an expert panel using a Delphi process to develop practice guidelines for laparoscopic splenectomy; covers indications, preoperative evaluation, management, and operative and postoperative issues.

Katkhouda N, Hurwitz MB, Rivera RT, et al: Laparoscopic splenectomy: Outcome and efficacy in 103 consecutive patients. *Ann Surg* 228:568–578, 1998.

Large series of patients with long-term follow-up demonstrating the safety and efficacy of laparoscopic splenectomy. The discussion section provides an extensive review of previously published series and compares open splenectomy with laparoscopic splenectomy.

Musallam KM, Khalife M, Sfeir PM, et al: Postoperative outcomes after laparoscopic splenectomy compared with open splenectomy. *Ann Surg* 257:1116–1123, 2013.

This study provides one of the few reliable comparative evaluations assessing the differences between open and laparoscopic splenectomy."

Spelman D, Buttery J, Daley A, et al: Guidelines for the prevention of sepsis in asplenic and hyposplenic patients. *Intern Med J* 38:349–356, 2008.

Reviews spectrum of causative organisms and recommended preventive strategies; consensus guidelines developed and discussed.

REFERENCES

1. Michels N: The variational anatomy of the spleen and splenic artery. *Am J Anat* 70:21–72, 1942.
2. Horowitz J, Smith JL, Weber TK, et al: Postoperative complications after splenectomy for hematologic malignancies. *Ann Surg* 223:290–296, 1996.
3. Spelman D, Buttery J, Daley A, et al: Guidelines for the prevention of sepsis in asplenic and hyposplenic patients. *Intern Med J* 38:349–356, 2008.
4. Shatz DV, Schinsky MF, Pais LB, et al: Immune responses of splenectomized trauma patients to the 23-valent

pneumococcal polysaccharide vaccine at 1 versus 7 versus 14 days after splenectomy. *J Trauma* 44:760–765, 1998.

5. El-Alfy MS, El-Sayed MH: Overwhelming postsplenectomy infection: Is quality of patient knowledge enough for prevention? *Hematol J* 5:77–80, 2004.

6. Spickett GP, Bullimore J, Wallis J, et al: Northern region asplenia register—analysis of first two years. *J Clin Pathol* 52:424–429, 1999.

7. Waghorn DJ: Overwhelming infection in asplenic patients: Current best practice preventive measures are not being followed. *J Clin Pathol* 54:214–218, 2001.

8. Aster RH, Bougie DW: Drug-induced immune thrombocytopenia. *N Engl J Med* 357:580–587, 2007.

9. George JN, Woolf SH, Raskob GE, et al: Idiopathic thrombocytopenic purpura: A practice guideline developed by explicit methods for the American Society of Hematology. *Blood* 88:3–40, 1996.

10. Thrombocytopenia, Chapter 175. In Goldman L, Schafer AI, editors: *Goldman's Cecil medicine*, ed 24, Philadelphia, 2012, Saunders/Elsevier.

11. Mikhael J, Northridge K, Lindquist K, et al: Short-term and long-term failure of laparoscopic splenectomy in adult immune thrombocytopenic purpura patients: A systematic review. *Am J Hematol* 84:743–748, 2009.

12. Kojouri K, Vesely SK, Terrell DR, et al: Splenectomy for adult patients with idiopathic thrombocytopenic purpura: A systematic review to assess long-term platelet count responses, prediction of response, and surgical complications. *Blood* 104:2623–2634, 2004.

13. Gigot JF, Jamar F, Ferrant A, et al: Inadequate detection of accessory spleens and splenosis with laparoscopic splenectomy. A shortcoming of the laparoscopic approach in hematologic diseases. *Surg Endosc* 12:101–106, 1998.

14. Katkhouda N, Hurwitz MB, Rivera RT, et al: Laparoscopic splenectomy: Outcome and efficacy in 103 consecutive patients. *Ann Surg* 228:568–578, 1998.

15. Kuter DJ, Bussel JB, Lyons RM, et al: Efficacy of romiplostim in patients with chronic immune thrombocytopenic purpura: A double-blind randomised controlled trial. *Lancet* 371:395–403, 2008.

16. Bernard NF, Chernoff DN, Tsoukas CM: Effect of splenectomy on T-cell subsets and plasma HIV viral titers in HIV-infected patients. *J Hum Virol* 1:338–345, 1998.

17. Hansen K, Singer DB: Asplenic-hyposplenic overwhelming sepsis: Postsplenectomy sepsis revisited. *Pediatr Dev Pathol* 4:105–121, 2001.

18. Morel P, Dupriez B, Gosselin B, et al: Role of early splenectomy in malignant lymphomas with prominent splenic involvement (primary lymphomas of the spleen). A study of 59 cases. *Cancer* 71:207–215, 1993.

19. Forconi F, Sozzi E, Cencini E, et al: Hairy cell leukemias with unmutated IGHV genes define the minor subset refractory to single-agent cladribine and with more aggressive behavior. *Blood* 114:4696–4702, 2009.

20. Saven A, Burian C, Koziol JA, et al: Long-term follow-up of patients with hairy cell leukemia after cladribine treatment. *Blood* 92:1918–1926, 1998.

21. Goodman GR, Bethel KJ, Saven A: Hairy cell leukemia: An update. *Curr Opin Hematol* 10:258–266, 2003.

22. Chiorazzi N, Rai KR, Ferrarini M: Chronic lymphocytic leukemia. *N Engl J Med* 352:804–815, 2005.

23. Cusack JC, Jr, Seymour JF, Lerner S, et al: Role of splenectomy in chronic lymphocytic leukemia. *J Am Coll Surg* 185:237–243, 1997.

24. Friedman RL, Fallas MJ, Carroll BJ, et al: Laparoscopic splenectomy for ITP. The gold standard. *Surg Endosc* 10:991–995, 1996.

25. Morgenstern L, Rosenberg J, Geller SA: Tumors of the spleen. *World J Surg* 9:468–476, 1985.

26. Sardi A, Ojeda HF, King D, Jr: Laparoscopic resection of a benign true cyst of the spleen with the harmonic scalpel producing high levels of CA 19-9 and carcinoembryonic antigen. *Am Surg* 64:1149–1154, 1998.

27. Breitenstein S, Scholz T, Schafer M, et al: Laparoscopic partial splenectomy. *J Am Coll Surg* 204:179–181, 2007.

28. Pachter HL, Hofstetter SR, Elkowitz A, et al: Traumatic cysts of the spleen—the role of cystectomy and splenic preservation: Experience with seven consecutive patients. *J Trauma* 35:430–436, 1993.

29. Wu HM, Kortbeek JB: Management of splenic pseudocysts following trauma: A retrospective case series. *Am J Surg* 191:631–634, 2006.

30. Gadacz TR: Splenic abscess. *World J Surg* 9:410–415, 1985.

31. Gleich S, Wolin DA, Herbsman H: A review of percutaneous drainage in splenic abscess. *Surg Gynecol Obstet* 167:211–216, 1988.

32. Green BT: Splenic abscess: Report of six cases and review of the literature. *Am Surg* 67:80–85, 2001.

33. Carbonell AM, Kercher KW, Matthews BD, et al: Laparoscopic splenectomy for splenic abscess. *Surg Laparosc Endosc Percutan Tech* 14:289–291, 2004.

34. Sayeed S, Koniaris LG, Kovach SJ, et al: Torsion of a wandering spleen. *Surgery* 132:535–536, 2002.

35. Delaitre B, Maignien B: Splenectomy by the laparoscopic approach. Report of a case. *Presse Med* 20:2263, 1991.

36. Melman L, Matthews BD: Current trends in laparoscopic solid organ surgery: Spleen, adrenal, pancreas, and liver. *Surg Clin North Am* 88:1033–1046, vii, 2008.

37. Flowers JL, Lefor AT, Steers J, et al: Laparoscopic splenectomy in patients with hematologic diseases. *Ann Surg* 224:19–28, 1996.

38. Romanelli JR, Kelly JJ, Litwin DE: Hand-assisted laparoscopic surgery in the United States: An overview. *Semin Laparosc Surg* 8:96–103, 2001.

39. Habermalz B, Sauerland S, Decker G, et al: Laparoscopic splenectomy: The clinical practice guidelines of the European Association for Endoscopic Surgery (EAES). *Surg Endosc* 22:821–848, 2008.

40. Konstadoulakis MM, Lagoudianakis E, Antonakis PT, et al: Laparoscopic versus open splenectomy in patients with beta thalassemia major. *J Laparoendosc Adv Surg Tech A* 16:5–8, 2006.

41. Burch M, Misra M, Phillips EH: Splenic malignancy: A minimally invasive approach. *Cancer J* 11:36–42, 2005.

42. Gernsheimer T, McCrae KR: Immune thrombocytopenic purpura in pregnancy. *Curr Opin Hematol* 14:574–580, 2007.

43. Bodner J, Kafka-Ritsch R, Lucciarini P, et al: A critical comparison of robotic versus conventional laparoscopic splenectomies. *World J Surg* 29:982–985, 2005.

44. Corcione F, Esposito C, Cuccurullo D, et al: Advantages and limits of robot-assisted laparoscopic surgery: Preliminary experience. *Surg Endosc* 19:117–119, 2005.

45. Pimpl W, Dapunt O, Kaindl H, et al: Incidence of septic and thromboembolic-related deaths after splenectomy in adults. *Br J Surg* 76:517–521, 1989.

46. Brigden ML: Detection, education and management of the asplenic or hyposplenic patient. *Am Fam Physician* 63:499–506, 508, 2001.

47. Rutherford EJ, Livengood J, Higginbotham M, et al: Efficacy and safety of pneumococcal revaccination after splenectomy for trauma. *J Trauma* 39:448–452, 1995.

48. Leemans R, Harms G, Rijkers GT, et al: Spleen autotransplantation provides restoration of functional splenic lymphoid compartments and improves the humoral immune response to pneumococcal polysaccharide vaccine. *Clin Exp Immunol* 117:596–604, 1999.

49. Falletta JM, Woods GM, Verter JI, et al: Discontinuing penicillin prophylaxis in children with sickle cell anemia. Prophylactic Penicillin Study II. *J Pediatr* 127:685–690, 1995.

CHEST

第十一篇　胸部

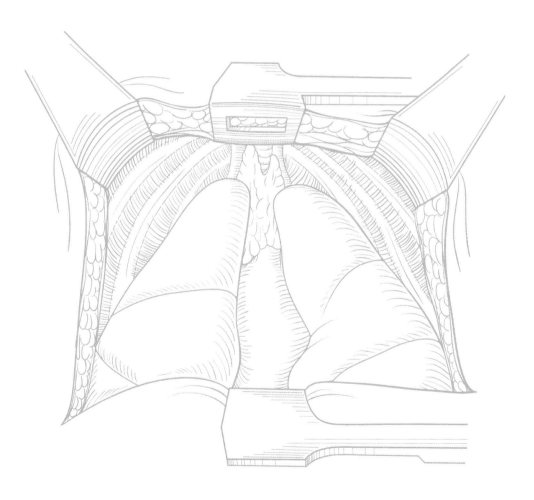

57 | CHAPTER

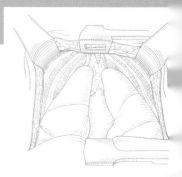

Lung, Chest Wall, Pleura, and Mediastinum

Joe B. Putnam, Jr.

第五十七章 肺、胸壁、胸膜和纵隔疾病

中文导读

　　本章共分16节：①解剖；②胸部手术病人选择；③肺；④肺癌；⑤气管；⑥肺部感染；⑦大咯血；⑧肺气肿和弥漫性肺疾病；⑨肺转移性肿瘤；⑩其他肺肿瘤；⑪胸壁；⑫胸廓出口综合征；⑬胸膜；⑭纵隔；⑮纵隔囊肿；⑯纵隔肿瘤。

　　第一节是解剖，胸腔的界限是颈部和腹部之间由肋骨、胸骨和椎骨放射状包围的区域，上方是胸廓入口，下方是膈肌。胸腔的主要结构包括肺、心脏大血管、气管、食管和膈肌。

　　第二节介绍了胸部手术病人选择应基于个体化的原则重点评估心肺功能，FEV1、FEV1/FVC、心肺运动试验、6分钟步行试验等均是重要的评估指标。

　　第三节介绍了先天性疾病包括先天性肺囊性病、先天性气管支气管畸形、先天性肺畸形、先天性血管异常等。

　　第四节介绍了肺癌的危险因素以及组织类型。根据国际抗癌联盟（Union for International Cancer

Control，UICC）与美国癌症联合会（American Joint Committee on Cancer，AJCC）的TNM分期标准，Ⅰ期和Ⅱ期肺癌可通过手术完全切除，可切除的ⅢA和ⅢB期肺癌需结合辅助治疗，Ⅳ期多属于转移性肺癌，通常采用铂类为基础的双药联合化学治疗，或基于EGFR、ALK等分子的靶向治疗，立体定向放射治疗对选定的不易切除的病人具有良好的效果。

　　第五节气管疾病包括气管狭窄、气管肿瘤、气管创伤等，可采用内镜下治疗或手术治疗。

　　第六节介绍了肺感染性疾病在特定条件下需要手术治疗的包括：支气管扩张症、肺脓肿、肺结核、肺

真菌病和肺寄生虫病。

第七节大咯血，指24小时失血量超过500～600mL，纤维支气管镜多可以诊断出血部位，治疗方法包括栓塞或必要时的手术。

第八节肺气肿和弥漫性肺疾病，肺气肿是终末气道的扩张和破坏。肺气肿合并肺大疱可能需行肺大疱切除手术，严重肺气肿病人可能需行肺移植术。

第九节介绍了孤立的肺转移瘤的综合治疗方式，在可切除的肺转移病人中，20%～30%的病人可以长期生存。

第十节介绍了其他肺肿瘤，包括了类癌、肺错构瘤、腺样囊性癌、肺母细胞瘤、肉瘤等。

第十一节胸壁疾病中，胸壁畸形包括漏斗胸、鸡胸、Poland综合征；胸壁肿瘤包括胸壁软组织和骨骼的原发性肿瘤、转移性胸壁肿瘤和胸内肿瘤直接侵犯，手术治疗包括肿瘤的切除和胸壁重建。

第十二节胸廓出口综合征，指由臂丛神经和锁骨下血管在胸廓出口受压迫所产生的症状，保守治疗无

效者可通过切除第1肋和前中斜角肌改善。

第十三节介绍了胸膜疾病，良性胸腔积液包括炎症性、结核性、乳糜性等，恶性胸腔积液多来源于肺癌、胸膜间皮瘤、淋巴瘤等。胸腔积液的外科治疗包括闭式引流、胸膜固定、纤维板剥脱、胸膜切除等。

第十四节介绍了纵隔疾病的症状和诊断方式，纵隔病变根据前上、中、后不同位置包括胸腺瘤、甲状腺肿瘤、纵隔囊肿、畸胎瘤、淋巴瘤、精原细胞肿瘤、神经源性肿瘤等。

第十五节纵隔囊肿包括多种来源于支气管、心包或胸腺的纵隔良性疾病，多数可通过微创手术治疗。

第十六节分别介绍了胸腺瘤、生殖细胞肿瘤、畸胎瘤、精原细胞瘤、非精原细胞肿瘤、神经源性肿瘤、神经母细胞瘤、神经节细胞瘤、副神经节瘤、淋巴瘤、内分泌肿瘤，多数纵隔肿瘤需行手术切除，部分胸腺肿瘤需行扩大切除，部分纵隔肿瘤术后需行辅助治疗。

〔付向宁〕

 Please access ExpertConsult.com to view the corresponding videos for this chapter.

The term *thorax* refers to the area between the neck and abdomen enclosed by the ribs, sternum, and vertebrae radially; the thoracic inlet superiorly; and the diaphragm inferiorly. The chest or thorax supports and protects the internal thoracic organs; provides for the negative inspiratory force that initiates ventilation and the positive expiratory force needed for vocalization; and creates a frame for the neck, upper extremities, thoracic structures, and abdomen. The major thoracic structures include the heart and lungs; chest wall including the overlying musculature, ribs, sternum, and vertebrae; diaphragm; trachea; esophagus; and great vessels.

ANATOMY

The thoracic organs are protected by the bony thorax and overlying chest musculature. The parietal pleura, the internal lining of the chest wall, is separated from the visceral pleura, the outer lining of the lung, by a small amount of pleural fluid. The parietal pleura covers the chest wall, mediastinum, diaphragm, and pericardium. The visceral pleura covers the lung and separates the lobes from one another. The pleural space is a potential space that may compress the lungs or heart with fluid, tumor, or infection. The right and left pleural spaces are separated from one another by the mediastinum.

The bony thorax is covered by three groups of muscles: the primary and secondary muscles for respiration and the muscles attaching the upper extremity to the body (Fig. 57-1). The primary muscles include the diaphragm and intercostal muscles. The intercostal muscles of the intercostal spaces include the external, internal, and transverse or innermost muscles. The 11 intercostal spaces, each associated numerically with the rib *superior* to it, contain the intercostal bundles (vein, artery, and nerve) that travel along the lower edge of each rib. All intercostal spaces are wider anteriorly, and each intercostal bundle falls away from the rib posteriorly to become more centrally located within each space. The intercostal muscle layers assist with respiration and protect the thoracic structures. The extrinsic muscles of the chest, latissimus dorsi muscle, serratus anterior muscle, pectoralis major and minor muscles, and cervical muscles (sternocleidomastoid, scalene muscles) attach to the bony thorax, protect the chest wall itself, and may assist with ventilatory efforts in patients with chronic obstructive pulmonary disease (COPD).

The secondary muscles consist of the sternocleidomastoid, serratus posterior, and levatores costarum. The third muscle group attaches the upper extremity to the body. The pectoralis major and minor muscles lie anteriorly and superficially. Posterior superficial musculature includes the trapezius and latissimus dorsi. Deep muscles include the serratus anterior and posterior, the levatores, and the major and minor rhomboids. These superficial and deep muscles help to hold the scapulae to the chest wall. In respiratory distress, the deltoid, pectoralis, and latissimus dorsi

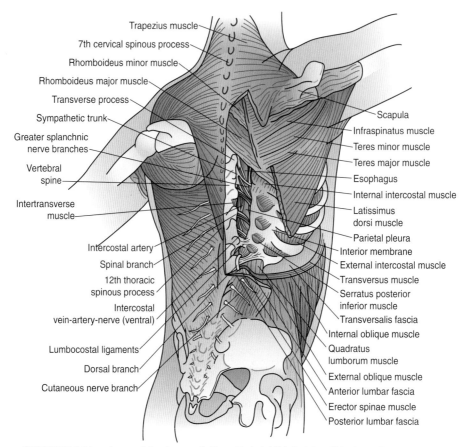

Trapezius muscle
7th cervical spinous process
Rhomboideus minor muscle
Rhomboideus major muscle
Transverse process
Sympathetic trunk
Greater splanchnic nerve branches
Vertebral spine
Intertransverse muscle
Intercostal artery
Spinal branch
12th thoracic spinous process
Intercostal vein-artery-nerve (ventral)
Lumbocostal ligaments
Dorsal branch
Cutaneous nerve branch

Scapula
Infraspinatus muscle
Teres minor muscle
Teres major muscle
Esophagus
Internal intercostal muscle
Latissimus dorsi muscle
Parietal pleura
Interior membrane
External intercostal muscle
Transversus muscle
Serratus posterior inferior muscle
Transversalis fascia
Internal oblique muscle
Quadratus lumborum muscle
External oblique muscle
Anterior lumbar fascia
Erector spinae muscle
Posterior lumbar fascia

FIGURE 57-1 Musculature of the chest wall. (From Ravitch MM, Steichen FM: *Atlas of general thoracic surgery*, Philadelphia, 1988, Saunders.)

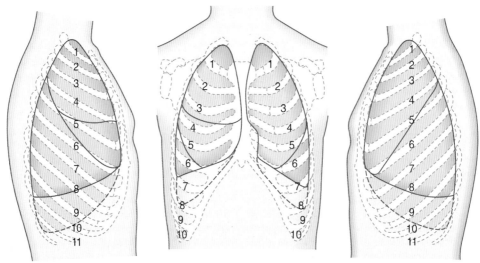

FIGURE 57-2 The relationships of the lobes of the lung to the ribs and the pleural reflections with respiration. The topographic anatomy and the relationship of the fissures of the lobes to specific ribs in inspiration and expiration are important in evaluation of routine posteroanterior and lateral chest films.

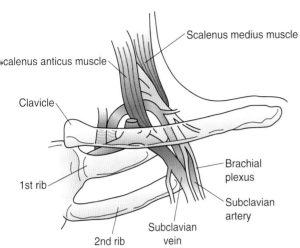

Scalenus medius muscle

Scalenus anticus muscle

Clavicle

1st rib

2nd rib

Subclavian vein

Brachial plexus

Subclavian artery

FIGURE 57-3 Relationship of the neurovascular bundle to the scalenus muscles, clavicle, and first rib. (From Urschel HC: Thoracic outlet syndromes. In Baue AE, Geha AS, Hammond GL, et al, editors: *Glenn's thoracic and cardiovascular surgery*, ed 6, Stamford, CT, 1996, Appleton & Lange, p 567.)

muscles form a tertiary system for ventilatory assistance through fixation of the upper extremities.

The bony thorax consists of 12 ribs peripherally extending from the vertebrae posteromedially to the sternum or costal arch anteriorly (Fig. 57-2). The 11th and 12th ribs are "floating ribs" and are not attached directly to the sternum. Ribs 1 to 5 are directly attached to the sternum by costal cartilages. The lower ribs (6 to 10) coalesce into the costal arch. The first rib is relatively flat and dense and travels from the first thoracic vertebra to the manubrium to create the thoracic inlet (Fig. 57-3). Through this relatively small area pass the great vessels, trachea, esophagus, and innervation to the upper extremity, diaphragm, and larynx. Trauma to this area, manifested by a first rib fracture, is the consequence of a significant mechanical force with likelihood of injury to one or more of these structures. Other structures within the thoracic inlet include the phrenic nerve, the recurrent laryngeal nerve in the tracheoesophageal groove (which recurs around the aorta at the ligamentum arteriosum on the left and around the innominate artery on the right), and the insertion of the thoracic duct posteriorly at the junction of the left subclavian with the left internal jugular veins. The remaining ribs gradually slope downward. Each rib is composed of a head, neck, and shaft. Each head has an upper facet, which articulates with the vertebral body above it, and a lower facet, which articulates with the corresponding thoracic vertebra to that rib, establishing the costovertebral joint. The neck of the rib has a tubercle with an articular facet; this articulates with the transverse process, creating the costotransverse joint and imparting strength to the posterior rib cage.

The sternum is flat, 15 to 20 cm long, and approximately 1.0 to 1.5 cm thick and comprises the manubrium, body, and xiphoid. The manubrium articulates with each clavicle and the first rib. The manubrium joins the body of the sternum at the angle of Louis, which corresponds to the anterior aspect of the junction of the second rib. The angle of Louis is a superficial anatomic landmark for the level of the carina. The anterior cartilaginous attachments of the true ribs to the sternum, along with intercostal muscles and the hemidiaphragms, allow for movement of the ribs with respiration.

The trachea in adults is approximately 12 cm long with 18 to 22 cartilaginous rings. The internal diameter is 2.3 cm laterally and 1.8 cm anteroposteriorly. The larynx ends with the inferior edge of cricoid cartilage. The cricoid is the only complete cartilaginous ring in the trachea. The trachea begins approximately 1.5 cm below the vocal cords and is not rigidly fixed to surrounding tissues. Vertical movement is easily possible. The most rigid point of fixation is where the aortic arch forms a sling over the left mainstem bronchus. The innominate artery crosses over the anterior trachea in a left inferolateral to high right anterolateral direction. The azygos vein arches over the proximal right mainstem bronchus as it travels from posterior to anterior to empty into the superior vena cava. The esophagus is closely applied to the membranous trachea and lies to the left of the midline of the trachea. The recurrent laryngeal nerves run in the tracheoesophageal groove on both the right and the left. The blood supply to the trachea is lateral and segmental from the inferior thyroid, the internal thoracic, the supreme intercostal, and the bronchial arteries. During trachea reconstruction, circumferential dissection greater than 1 to 2 cm may lead to vascular insufficiency with necrosis or anastomotic dehiscence.

Lung development begins at approximately 21 to 28 days' gestation. The true alveolar stage, with air sacs surrounded on all sides by capillaries, occurs from approximately 7 months to term. Alveolar proliferation continues after birth. There are approximately 20 million alveoli at birth, which increase to approximately 300 million by age 10 years, with no more increase after that time. There are 23 generations of bronchi between the trachea and terminal alveoli. Air accounts for 80% of the lung volume, blood accounts for 10%, and solid tissue accounts for approximately 10%. Alveoli make up approximately half of the entire lung volume.

The lungs are broadly divided into five lobes and multiple segments within each lobe (Fig. 57-4). The right lung is composed of three lobes: upper, middle, and lower. Two fissures separate these lobes. The major, or oblique, fissure separates the lower lobe from the upper and middle lobes. The minor or horizontal fissure separates the upper lobe from the middle lobe. The left lung has two lobes—the upper lobe and the lower lobe; the lingula corresponds embryologically to the right middle lobe. A single oblique fissure separates the lobes.

The bronchopulmonary segments are divisions of each lobe that contain anatomically separate arterial, venous, and bronchial supply. There are 10 bronchopulmonary segments on the right and 8 bronchopulmonary segments on the left.

The blood supply of the lung is twofold. Unoxygenated blood circulates from the right ventricle through the pulmonary artery to each lung. After oxygenation in the lung, the blood is returned to the left atrium through the pulmonary veins. Blood supply to the bronchi is from the systemic circulation by bronchial arteries arising from the superior thoracic aorta or the aortic arch, either as discrete branches or in combination with the intercostal arteries.

Lymphatic vessels are present throughout the lung parenchyma and pleura and gradually coalesce toward the hilar areas of the lungs. Generally, lymphatic drainage from the lung affects the ipsilateral lymph nodes; however, flow of lymph from the left lower lobe may drain to the right mediastinal (paratracheal) lymph nodes. Lymphatic drainage within the mediastinum moves cephalad. The pulmonary parenchyma does not contain a nerve supply.

The visceral pleura is separated from the parietal pleura by a small amount of pleural fluid, which allows nearly frictionless

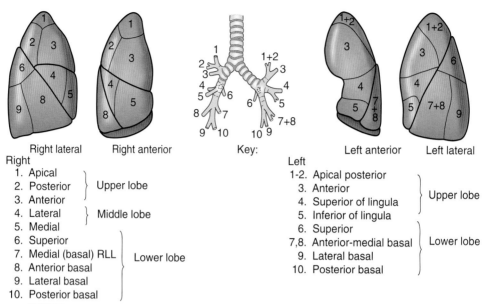

Right lateral   Right anterior   Key: Left anterior   Left lateral

Right
1. Apical   ⎫
2. Posterior   ⎬ Upper lobe
3. Anterior   ⎭
4. Lateral   ⎫ Middle lobe
5. Medial   ⎭
6. Superior   ⎫
7. Medial (basal) RLL ⎬ Lower lobe
8. Anterior basal ⎬
9. Lateral basal   ⎬
10. Posterior basal ⎭

Left
1-2. Apical posterior ⎫
3. Anterior   ⎬ Upper lobe
4. Superior of lingula ⎬
5. Inferior of lingula ⎭
6. Superior   ⎫
7,8. Anterior-medial basal ⎬ Lower lobe
9. Lateral basal   ⎬
10. Posterior basal   ⎭

FIGURE 57-4 Segments of the pulmonary lobes. *RLL,* Right lower lobe. (Adapted from Jackson CL, Huber JF: Correlated applied anatomy of the bronchial tree and lungs with a system of nomenclature. *Dis Chest* 9:319, 1943.)

movement during respiration. The blood supply of the parietal pleura comes from the systemic arteries and veins, including the posterior intercostal, internal mammary, anterior mediastinal, and superior phrenic arteries and corresponding systemic veins. The blood supply of the visceral pleura is both systemic and pulmonary. The lymphatic drainage of the parietal pleura is into regional lymph nodes, including intercostal, mediastinal, and phrenic nodes. Visceral pleural lymphatics follow the superficial lung lymphatics and drain into the mediastinal lymph nodes. The parietal pleura underlying the ribs has rich nerve endings from the intercostal nerves. Generous local anesthesia is necessary for chest tube insertion. The visceral pleura is innervated by vagal branches and the sympathetic system.

The anatomic boundaries of the mediastinum include the thoracic inlet superiorly, the diaphragm inferiorly, the sternum anteriorly, the vertebral column posteriorly, and medially to the parietal pleura. Thoracic tumors that penetrate through the pleura (by definition) invade the mediastinum. Traditionally, the mediastinum can be divided into anterosuperior, middle, and posterior compartments. No specific anatomic planes define these areas. Fat and lymph nodes are found throughout the mediastinum.

The anterosuperior compartment includes the thymus gland. The right and left lobes of the thymus extend into the cervical areas, and these portions of the thymus must be resected to provide for complete extirpation of the gland.

The middle mediastinum contains the heart; pericardium; great vessels including the descending, transverse, and descending aorta; superior and inferior vena cava; pulmonary artery and veins; trachea and bronchi; and phrenic, vagus, and recurrent laryngeal nerves. The phrenic nerve enters the thorax through the thoracic inlet on the anterior aspect of the anterior scalene muscle.

The vagus nerve enters the thoracic inlet through the carotid sheath. It lies anterior to the subclavian and posterior to the innominate artery on the right. The right recurrent laryngeal nerve loops or "recurs" around the innominate artery to innervate the right vocal cord. The vagus nerve then continues posteriorly

in the tracheoesophageal groove to innervate the trachea and continues down to innervate the esophagus. On the left side, the vagus nerve enters the thorax through the thoracic inlet, and as it exits the carotid sheath, it moves along the anterior aspect of the aortic arch. The recurrent laryngeal nerve arises from the vagus nerve and loops around under the ligamentum arteriosum and continues superiorly under the aorta and lies in the tracheoesophageal groove as it innervates the left recurrent laryngeal nerve. The left vagus continues posteriorly within the mediastinum along the esophagus to innervate both the trachea and the esophagus.

The posterior mediastinum contains structures between the heart/pericardium and trachea anteriorly and the vertebral column and paravertebral spaces posteriorly. The posterior mediastinum contains the esophagus, descending aorta, azygos and hemiazygos veins, thoracic duct, sympathetic chain, and lymph nodes. The thoracic duct originates from the cisterna chyli in the abdomen. It enters into the chest through the aortic hiatus in an anterolateral position and travels superiorly just to the right of midline in the chest along the anterolateral surface of the vertebral column. At approximately the level of T5, it crosses over to the left and continues superiorly to empty, posteriorly, into the junction of the left jugular and subclavian veins.

The inferior border of the mediastinum is the diaphragm, which separates the abdominal contents from the thorax. Hernias through the esophageal hiatus (paraesophageal hernias), through the foramen of Bochdalek (posteriorly), or through the foramen of Morgagni (anteriorly) may be initially identified as a mediastinal mass.

Each spinal root exits the neural foramina of the vertebral body and bifurcates to form a branch to the intercostal nerve to innervate the skin and intercostal musculature and a branch to the sympathetic ganglion. Intercostal nerves innervate the skin and musculature of the intercostal muscles. The spinal root divides as it exits the neural foramina. One branch goes to the intercostal nerve, and one lies in the posterior vertebral gutter to form the

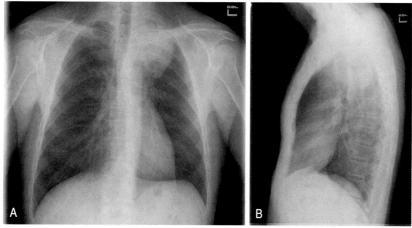

FIGURE 57-5 Initial chest x-ray. This patient is a 67-year-old man with weight loss of 10 pounds in 4 weeks and a 35 pack-year history of cigarette smoking. He quit smoking 10 year ago. He had left shoulder pain for 4 months with no dyspnea, cough, hemoptysis, or other symptoms. Massage and other musculoskeletal manipulation did not improve his symptoms. A chest x-ray with posteroanterior **(A)** and lateral views **(B)** demonstrates an 8.4-cm left upper lung mass. Some deviation of the distal trachea is noted.

sympathetic ganglion. The thoracic sympathetic trunk comprises several ganglia that lie along the ribs. The most superior ganglion is the stellate ganglion.

SELECTION OF PATIENTS FOR THORACIC OPERATIONS

The physiologic evaluation of the thoracic surgical patient must be individualized for each patient but generally emphasizes the pulmonary and cardiac function. The assessment of a patient's ability to tolerate lung resection from a cardiopulmonary standpoint is fundamental to patient selection for surgery. Patients with advanced pulmonary disease and severe pulmonary dysfunction may have prohibitive risk, which may exist in greater than one third of patients with otherwise resectable lung disease.[1]

Cigarette smoking is associated with increased postoperative pulmonary complications. If the patient is a smoker, he or she must stop smoking immediately. The physician must clearly communicate this message. Although there are few studies specific to pulmonary resection, there is evidence that smoking abstinence of 4 to 8 weeks' duration preoperatively is necessary to reduce the incidence of complications. Ideally, patients are smoke-free for a minimum of 2 weeks and preferably for 4 to 8 weeks before surgery,[2] although smoking cessation at any time is valuable.[3,4] Smoking cessation programs may be helpful for these patients, and patients may need pharmacologic assistance. This combination may have increased efficacy in smoking cessation efforts over counseling alone.[5]

Before the operation and in the perioperative period, deep venous thrombosis prophylaxis is provided by subcutaneous heparin, sequential compression stockings, or both.[6] Perioperative antibiotics are used to minimize complications from infections. Postoperative morbidity may also be minimized by adequate pain control to facilitate early ambulation. Routine use of a thoracic epidural catheter, or intercostal rib blocks with long-acting local anesthetics, or patient-controlled analgesia provide excellent pain control. Incentive spirometry assists in expanding the lung and reducing the incidence of pulmonary morbidity. Nasal bilevel

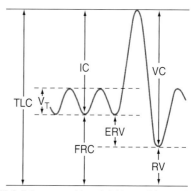

FIGURE 57-6 Spirometry with subdivisions of lung volumes. *ERV,* Expiratory reserve volume; *FRC,* functional residual capacity (i.e., lung volume at end expiration); *IC,* inspiratory capacity; *RV,* residual volume (i.e., lung volume after forced expiration from FRC); *TLC,* total lung capacity; *VC,* vital capacity (i.e., maximal volume of gas inspired from RV); V_T, tidal volume.

positive airway pressure for patients with obstructive sleep apnea may delay or eliminate the need for intubation or reintubation after pulmonary resection. Early mobilization is essential to avoid most perioperative complications.

Physiologic Evaluation

Before thoracic operations, patients may be evaluated by a combination of radiographic and physiologic studies.[1] A plain chest x-ray (CXR) is commonly obtained (Fig. 57-5). Spirometry measures the lung volumes (Fig. 57-6) and mechanical properties of lung elasticity, recoil, and compliance. Pulmonary function testing (Fig. 57-7) also evaluates gas exchange functions, such as carbon monoxide diffusing capacity (DLCO).

The predicted postoperative forced expiratory volume in 1 second (FEV_1) is the most commonly used as an indicator of postoperative pulmonary reserve. Depending on other evaluable factors, most patients with FEV_1 greater than 60% predicted can tolerate an anatomic lobectomy. If FEV_1 is less than 60% of predicted, further testing in an attempt to estimate postoperative

Section of Pulmonary Medicine
Pulmonary Function Report

Last Name: First Name:
Identification:
Age: 56 years   Room: Out-patient
Sex: Male   Race: Caucasian
Height: 65 inches   Physician:
Weight: 177 lbs   Operator:
Date
Time

Spirometry		Pred	Pre BD	%Pred	Post BD	%Pred	%Chg
FVC	[l]	3.48	3.07	88	3.07	88	0
FEV_1	[l]	2.83	2.23	79	2.26	80	1
FEV_1/VC	[%]	80.81	72.26	89	69.78	86	−3
FEF 25–75	[l/s]	3.01	1.37	45	1.46	49	7
PEF	[l/s]	7.57	6.43	85	7.10	94	10
FIVC	[l]	3.48	3.09	89	3.24	93	5
FIV_1	[l]		3.09		3.24		5
FIV_1/FVC	[%]		100.00		100.00		0

Lung Volumes		Pred	Measured	%Pred
SVC	[l]	3.48	3.04	87
TLC	[l]	5.51	5.54	101
RV	[l]	1.96	2.49	127
RV/TLC	[%]	35.9	45.0	125
FRC-Box	[l]	2.24	3.01	134

Diffusion SB		Pred	Measured	%Pred
DLCO SB	[ml/min/mm Hg]	22.59	23.81	105
DLCO Hb Corr	[ml/min/mm Hg]	22.6	24.2	107
VA	[l]		5.27	
DLCO/VA	[ml/min/mm Hg/l]	3.93	4.52	115
Hb	[g/100ml]		14.1	

Interpretation

Spirometry reveals an isolated reduction in mid-expiratory flows consistent with an obstructive small airways defect. Increased residual volume (RV) is consistent with air trapping. Following the inhalation of a bronchodilator, there is no improvement of the obstructive airway defect. The diffusing capacity is normal.

FIGURE 57-7 The pulmonary function report provides complete spirometry data based on predicted values for height and weight. In this patient, the forced expiratory volume in 1 second (FEV_1) is 2.26 liters after bronchodilators, which is 80% of predicted. The carbon monoxide diffusing capacity (DLCO) is measured as 23.81 ml/min/mm Hg, which is 105% of predicted. *FEF,* Forced expiratory flow; *FIV_1,* forced inspiratory volume in 1 second; *FIVC,* forced inspiratory vital capacity; *FRC,* functional reserve capacity; *FVC,* forced vital capacity; *Hb,* hemoglobin; *PEF,* peak expiratory flow; *SB,* single breath; *SVC,* slow vital capacity; *TLC,* total lung capacity; *VA,* alveolar volume; *VC,* vital capacity.

FEV_1 (predicted postoperative FEV_1 [ppo-FEV_1]) could be considered. The quantitative ventilation-perfusion lung scan is used to assist in the calculation of postoperative residual pulmonary function after resection. Patients with a ppo-FEV_1 of 35% to 40% should functionally tolerate the operation.

Quantitative radionucleotide lung perfusion (Fig. 57-8) provides a measurement of the relative function of each lobe and lung and allows an estimation of pulmonary function after lung resection:

ppo-FEV_1 = preop FEV_1 × (1 − fraction of perfusion
to region of planned resection)

A ppo-FEV_1 of 30% or less carries a greater risk for supplemental oxygen and ventilator dependence, but a decision to deny surgical resection to this group of patients must be considered on an individual basis because some will do better than expected with careful selection at experienced centers. Finally, in the immediate postoperative period, the ppo-FEV_1 is not likely to be realized secondary to limited ambulation, pain, or other emotional or physical factors.

DLCO can be measured by several methods, although the single-breath test is most commonly performed. DLCO measures the rate at which test molecules such as carbon monoxide move from the alveolar space to combine with hemoglobin in the red blood cells. DLCO is determined by calculating the difference between inspired and expired samples of gas. DLCO levels less than 40% to 50% are associated with increased perioperative risk.[7]

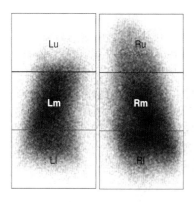

	Left lung		Right lung	
	%	Kct	%	Kct
Upper zone:	4.7	22.66	9.5	46.27
Middle zone:	24.0	116.91	28.3	138.05
Lower zone:	13.2	64.20	20.3	99.02
Total lung:	41.8	203.77	58.2	283.34

FIGURE 57-8 The quantitative perfusion lung scan report provides the lung volume and the perfusion to each lung. In a patient with a large left hilar tumor, perfusion may be reduced in the involved left lung compared with the uninvolved right lung. The predicted post–left pneumonectomy right lung function can be obtained by multiplying the right lung percent perfusion (58.2%) by the observed best FEV₁ (2.26 liters). The resulting value, 1.31 liter, 46.5% predicted, is the predicted postoperative FEV₁ (after left pneumonectomy). This value suggests that a left pneumonectomy would be functionally tolerated. *Ll,* Left lower zone; *Lm,* left middle zone; *Lu,* left upper zone; *Rl,* right lower zone; *Rm,* right middle zone; *Ru,* right upper.

The ratio of FEV_1 to forced vital capacity (FEV_1/FVC) describes the relationship between the FEV_1 and the functional lung volume. In obstructive disease, the ratio is low (FEV_1 is low, and FVC is high); in restrictive disease, the ratio is about normal because both FEV_1 and FVC are reduced.

Flow-volume loops derived from spirometry describe the relationship between lung volume and air flow as the lung volume changes during a forced expiration and inspiration. The typical test consists of tidal breathing at rest, followed by maximal inspiratory effort to total lung capacity, then maximal expiratory effort to residual volume, concluding with maximal inspiratory effort to total lung capacity.

Cardiopulmonary Exercise Testing

Cardiopulmonary exercise testing (CPET) can be extremely useful in the evaluation of marginal candidates (ppo-FEV_1 or predicted postoperative DLCO <50% predicted) or patients who appear more disabled than expected from simple spirometry measurements. CPET includes exercise electrocardiography, heart rate response to exercise, and measurements of minute ventilation and oxygen uptake per minute. CPET allows a calculation of maximal oxygen consumption ($\dot{V}O_2$max) and provides insight into overall cardiopulmonary function (the "cardiopulmonary axis") that cannot be ascertained from other objective studies. CPET may identify clinically occult cardiac disease and provide a more

accurate assessment of pulmonary function than spirometry and DLCO, which tend to overestimate functional loss after resection.

A patient's risk of perioperative morbidity and mortality may be stratified by $\dot{V}O_2$max. A level less than 11 to 15 mL/kg/min is associated with an increased risk, and $\dot{V}O_2$max less than 10 mL/kg/min indicates high risk.[8] In patients undergoing evaluation for lung volume reduction surgery or for lung transplantation, a 6-minute walk test is used for a measure of the cardiac and pulmonary reserve. Patients are told to walk as far and as fast as they can during this time period. Distances of more than 1000 feet suggest an uncomplicated course.

Measurement of diaphragm function by fluoroscopy, the "sniff test," is needed to determine symmetry of effort and to exclude paradoxical movement of the diaphragm. Paradoxical movement (elevation of one hemidiaphragm with active contraction/retraction of the other diaphragm) suggests paresis or paralysis. This finding may suggest a specific reason for breathlessness. Diaphragm plication may be therapeutic.

No single test result should be viewed as an absolute contraindication to surgical resection. Although the physiologic assessment for patients undergoing normal spirometry and minimal comorbidity is straightforward, patients with marginal preoperative indices must be considered on an individual basis.

Thoracic Incisions

The choice of incision depends on the operation, the patient's underlying physiologic condition, and the anticipated benefits and limitations of the planned approach. Video-assisted thoracic surgery (VATS), robotic surgery, and other minimally invasive surgical techniques have been developed to treat most thoracic problems, including lung cancer, mediastinal tumors, pleural diseases, and parenchymal diseases, and to diagnose and stage thoracic malignancies. Various small incisions are made for the camera and other instruments depending on the location of the tumor. The ribs are not spread. Improved lighting and optics create excellent exposure and visualization. Advantages of minimally invasive surgical techniques include minimizing pain and surgical trauma from the incisions, decreasing hospitalization, and improving convalescence.

A thoracotomy requires spreading the ribs with a retractor and is used for operations on a single thorax. The patient is placed in a lateral decubitus position. The location of the incision may be posterior, axillary, or anterior. Posteriorly, an oblique incision is used with or without sparing the latissimus dorsi muscle. The chest is typically entered through the fifth interspace for pulmonary resection. A vertical axillary incision is made anterior to the latissimus dorsi muscle, and the chest is entered through the fourth interspace. This approach provides excellent hilar visualization. The anterior or anterolateral thoracotomy is created by a curvilinear incision underneath the inferior border of the pectoralis major muscle at the inframammary fold. A median sternotomy is performed using a vertical incision from the sternal notch to the xiphoid. A sternal saw is then used to divide the sternum in the midline. With gentle retraction, the sternum can be spread approximately 8 to 10 cm to allow access to the mediastinum, heart, great vessels, and right and left thorax. The pleura can be opened on either side to explore the hemithorax. The sternum is usually closed with stainless steel wire.

The transverse sternotomy or "clamshell" incision is larger than a median sternotomy and more uncomfortable for the patient. This incision combines two anterior thoracotomy incisions in the inframammary fold with transverse division of the sternum at the fourth intercostal space. Both internal mammary arteries are ligated. This approach is ideal for accessing both the right and the left hilum and providing additional exposure for large mediastinal tumors, bilateral hilar dissections, bilateral lung transplantation, or posterior-based metastases in both lungs.

LUNG

Congenital Lesions of the Lung

Various congenital lung abnormalities can occur as a consequence of disturbed embryogenesis.[9] Bilateral agenesis of the lungs is fatal. Unilateral agenesis may occur more frequently on the left (~70%) than on the right (~30%), with more than a 2:1 male-to-female ratio.

Hypoplasia of the lungs may occur as a result of interference with the development of the alveolar system during the last 2 months of gestation. Bochdalek hernia is the most frequent cause of hypoplasia. Conditions associated with hypoplasia of the lungs include oligohydramnios, prune-belly syndrome (deficiency in the abdominal musculature, genitourinary abnormalities), scimitar syndrome (abnormal pulmonary vein draining into the inferior vena cava, demonstrated as a crescent along the right heart border on cardiac angiography), and dextrocardia. Isolated pulmonary hypoplasia is rare.

Hyaline membrane disease (or infant respiratory distress syndrome) is frequent in premature infants (24 to 28 weeks' gestation) and infants of diabetic mothers. At a gestational age of 24 to 28 weeks, infants have an immature surfactant system. Hyaline membrane disease develops in the alveoli, causing congestion and a lung with a deep purple gross appearance. Respiratory distress frequently ensues, requiring high concentrations of oxygen. CXRs demonstrate a ground-glass appearance from the interstitial edema. As needs for oxygen and ventilator pressure increase to counteract this interstitial edema, pneumothorax frequently occurs. Of these infants, 10% to 30% do not survive.

Congenital Cystic Lesions

Congenital cystic lesions generally occur as a result of separation of the pulmonary remnants from airway branchings. Clinically, approximately one third of patients do not have symptoms; one third have cough; and one third have infection or, rarely, hemoptysis. Treatment may be with antibiotics or, for more severe localized cases, with resection. Any cystic lesion that enlarges on serial radiographs needs to be considered for resection.[10]

A bronchogenic cyst arises from a tracheal or bronchial diverticulum (see also "Primary Mediastinal Cysts"). This diverticulum becomes completely separated from the trachea and is frequently found as an asymptomatic mass on routine CXRs. Computed tomography (CT) scan of the chest demonstrates this abnormality as a homogeneous, well-circumscribed mass adjacent to the trachea (Fig. 57-9). The bronchogenic cyst accounts for 10% of mediastinal masses in children and is located in the midmediastinum. Treatment consists of excision, even if the patient is asymptomatic, to confirm the diagnosis.

Cystic fibrosis is an autosomal recessive disorder that is found more commonly in whites. Approximately 20% of patients with cystic fibrosis survive to the age of 30 years. Lung failure is the most frequent cause of death. Excessively thick mucus leads to inspissation, recurrent infections, bronchitis, and bronchiectasis.

Pneumothorax secondary to air trapping is also found. Fibrosis and cystic changes on pathologic examinations are identified. A tension cyst may be a complication of cystic disease. A rapid increase in the size of the cyst may cause mechanical ventilation problems and mediastinal shift. Resection, usually lobectomy, corrects this problem. Pneumatoceles may develop as a result of childhood *Staphylococcus aureus* infection. They can be very large and may cause mechanical complications. These problems may resolve completely as the pneumonia resolves. Resection may be needed.

Congenital Bronchopulmonary Malformations

Lobar emphysema[9] is the most commonly resected congenital cystic lesion (50%). The onset of rapidly progressive respiratory distress usually occurs 4 to 5 days to several weeks after birth. It rarely occurs after 6 months of age. It affects the upper lobe predominately. Bronchiolitis is probably the most common cause overall. Treatment is lobectomy.

Congenital cystic adenomatoid malformations are the second most commonly resected congenital cystic lesion.[11] They are closely related to a hamartoma without cartilage. Terminal bronchioles proliferate, yielding the "adenomatoid" malformation. The lung has the appearance of Swiss cheese and feels like a large rubbery mass. With air trapping and overdistention, respiratory distress may occur, which is optimally relieved by lobectomy.

Pulmonary sequestration is an area of embryonic lung tissue, separate from the lung, which receives blood supply from an anomalous systemic artery from the aorta, not the pulmonary artery. This condition occurs secondary to an accessory lung bud caudal to the normal lung, but with a lack of absorption of primitive surrounding splanchnic vessels. During lung development, interlobar sequestration (75%) occurs early. Later, after the pleura forms, extralobar sequestration occurs (25%), primarily on the left side (66%), and is completely enclosed by its own pleura. The extralobar sequestration blood supply is usually from the thoracic or upper abdominal aorta to systemic (azygos or hemiazygos veins). Extralobar sequestration is more common in male patients. Resection is recommended. Intralobar sequestration occurs within the lower lobes predominantly (>95%) and is equally distributed between the right and left lower lobes. Intralobar sequestration blood supply is from the descending thoracic aorta that usually traverses the pulmonary ligament. Venous drainage is via the pulmonary veins. The thoracic aorta provides 95% of the systemic blood supply to the pulmonary sequestration.

Congenital Abnormalities of the Trachea and Bronchi

Esophageal atresia with tracheoesophageal fistula is the most frequent abnormality of the trachea in infants (see "Pediatric Surgery"). Bronchial atresia is the second most frequent congenital pulmonary lesion after tracheoesophageal fistula.[12] The lung tissue distal to the atresia expands and becomes emphysematous as a result of air entry through the pores of Kohn. With no exit for air or mucus because of this blind bronchial stump, emphysema from air trapping or development of a mucocele may occur. CXRs may demonstrate hyperinflation of a lobe or a segment. The oval density may be identified between the hyperinflated lung and the hilum. The left upper lobe is the most frequently involved of all lobes within the lung. Diagnosis may be confirmed with bronchography or CT. The surgeon must rule out a mucous plug, adenoma, vascular compression, or sequestration.

Tracheal agenesis is a rare phenomenon and is fatal. The trachea is absent from the larynx to the carina, and bronchi communicate with the esophagus.

Tracheal stenosis is also rare and consists of generalized hypoplasia, a funnel-like trachea, and bronchial and segmental malformations. The right upper lobe bronchus may come from the trachea directly and may be associated with an aberrant left pulmonary artery (so-called pulmonary artery sling). Completely circular vascular rings are common. Repair is by incision of the trachea vertically and widening of the tracheal lumen.

Tracheomalacia can be identified by diagnostic imaging (dynamic expiratory CT) or bronchoscopy. The surgeon should notice marked variation of the tracheal lumen with inspiration and expiration. Collapse of greater than half of the lumen during expiration is consistent with this condition. Respiratory difficulty ensues from the intermittently collapsing trachea. Relief of the extrinsic compression is needed. Stent placement in adults or posterior splinting or primary tracheobronchoplasty may be required.[13] This condition may have a congenital predisposition but is most often seen in adults with COPD.

Congenital Vascular Disorders

Congenital vascular disorders of the lungs may occur.[14] In Swyer-James and Macleod syndrome, there is idiopathic hyperlucent lung. This problem develops from chronic pulmonary infections such as bronchiectasis. As the consolidation persists, decreased pulmonary artery blood supply may cause an "autopneumonectomy" and a hyperlucent lung.

Scimitar syndrome is associated with hypoplastic right lung with drainage of the pulmonary vein to the inferior vena cava. The anomaly is usually corrected using extracorporeal cardiopulmonary support. A patch from the pulmonary vein to the left atrium via an atrial septal defect corrects this problem.

Pulmonary arteriovenous malformations may exist as one or more pulmonary artery–to–pulmonary vein connections,

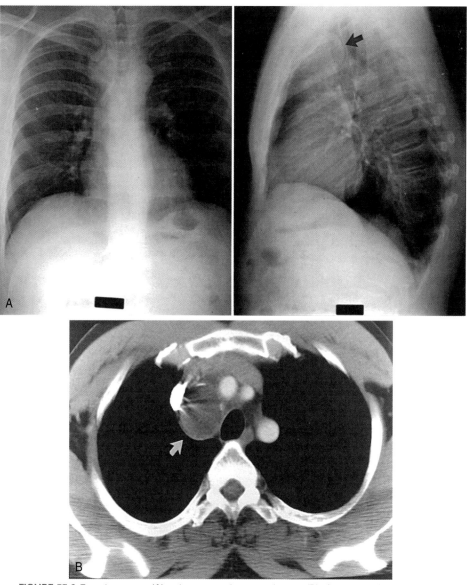

FIGURE 57-9 Two chest x-rays (A) and a computed tomography scan (B) of the chest of a patient with a bronchogenic cyst (arrow).

bypassing the pulmonary capillary bed. This connection results in a right-to-left shunt. Approximately one third of these patients have hereditary hemorrhagic telangiectasia (Osler-Weber-Rendu syndrome). Approximately half of the malformations are small (<1 cm) and tend to be multiple. Half are greater than 1 cm and usually less than 5 cm and tend to be subpleural. These lesions need to be considered in the differential diagnosis of any patient with hemoptysis that is unexplained on the basis of bronchoscopy or routine imaging. Either local resection or catheter embolization of these lesions can be curative.

A pulmonary vascular sling consists of an anomalous or aberrant left pulmonary artery, which causes airway obstruction, and is associated with other anomalies. The aberrant left pulmonary artery arises from the right (main) pulmonary artery and courses between the trachea and the esophagus to supply the left lung. More than 90% of patients have wheezing and stridor. Esophagoscopy shows the anomalous vessel anterior to the esophagus; bronchoscopy or bronchography demonstrates the vessel posterior to the trachea. Surgical correction requires exploration of the left chest, division of the artery, and oversewing of the vessel as far as possible distal within the mediastinum. Reanastomosis to the main pulmonary artery is then performed.

Vascular rings[15] constitute 7% of all congenital heart problems. The most common vascular ring is a double aortic arch, which occurs in 60% of these patients. The right, or posterior, arch is the larger arch and gives rise to the right carotid and right subclavian arteries. The ring wraps around both the trachea and the esophagus. A posterior indentation is noted in the esophagus on barium swallow. Simple division corrects the anomaly. A right aortic arch with a retroesophageal left subclavian artery and left ligamentum arteriosum occurs in approximately 25% to 30% of patients with vascular rings. Intracardiac defects occur with a double aortic arch. Most of these infants require operation within the first weeks or months of life. Most patients with vascular rings require only a careful history and barium swallow for diagnosis. Typically, bronchoscopy or esophagoscopy is not ordered because it may be harmful; aortography adds little additional information. Repair is performed through the left chest. Division of the smaller arch, usually the left one, is undertaken. The ligamentum is divided, and the trachea and the esophagus are freed from the surrounding tissues. When a retroesophageal right subclavian artery with left ligament occurs, the patient may complain of dysphagia, which is referred to as *dysphagia lusoria*. The differential diagnosis includes neuromotor diseases of the esophagus or stricture.

LUNG CANCER

Lung cancer is a significant global health problem. In the United States in 2015, there were estimated to be 221,200 new cases of lung cancer.[16] Lung cancer is the most frequent cause of death from cancer in men and women and accounts for 13.0% of all cancer diagnoses and 27.0% of all cancer deaths in the United States. Lung cancer deaths exceed the combined total deaths from breast, prostate, and colorectal cancer. Since 1987, more women have died of lung cancer than breast cancer. Lung cancer deaths in men have decreased by approximately 3% per year in men and by approximately 2% per year in women. Smoking cessation in women has lagged behind smoking cessation in men, and thus the incidence of lung cancer in women has not declined as much as the incidence in men (Fig. 57-10). The decline in lung cancer incidence and mortality rate likely reflects decreasing cigarette smoking and potentially earlier detection of smaller, asymptomatic lung cancers. African American men have both the highest incidence and the highest death rate from cancer of the lung and bronchus.

Lung cancer survival is stage specific. Overall, the 1-year 44%, and the 5-year relative survival rate is 17%. Localized (early-stage) lung cancer has a 5-year survival rate of 54%, although greater than 50% of all patients have advanced or distant disease at diagnosis, with 1-year and 5-year survivals of 26% and 4%, respectively.

Cigarette smoking is unequivocally the most important risk factor in the development of lung cancer. Other environmental factors may predispose to lung cancer. Environmental radon gas exposure is estimated to be the second most important risk factor. Other factors include asbestos, arsenic, chromium, nickel, organic chemicals, iatrogenic radiation exposure, air pollution, and secondary smoke from nonsmokers.

Radon is associated with approximately 18,000 lung cancer deaths a year.[17] Radon is a natural radioactive gas released from the normal decay of uranium in the soil. Inhalation is associated with health risk. Inexpensive test kits are available to determine the amount of radon present in homes.

Optimal treatment of lung cancer requires accurate diagnosis and clinical staging before treatment begins. The anatomic basis for staging (tumor, lymph nodes, and metastases) includes the physical properties of the tumor and the presence of regional or systemic metastases. The biologic basis for staging (molecular markers prognostic for survival as well as predictive for response to therapy) is expected to be incorporated into staging systems of the future. Clinical trials are available for patient enrollment to understand and evaluate various treatments better.[18] The National Cancer Institute National Clinical Trials Network conducts clinical trials for patients with lung cancer and other malignancies throughout the United States.[19]

Pathology

The pathology of lung cancer has been reviewed elsewhere.[20] Development of lung cancer follows a progression of histologic changes that results from smoking and includes (1) proliferation of basal cells, (2) development of atypical nuclei with prominent nucleoli, (3) stratification, (4) development of squamous metaplasia, (5) carcinoma in situ, and (6) invasive carcinoma.

Adenocarcinoma of the lung is the most frequent histologic type and accounts for approximately 45% of all lung cancers. Adenocarcinoma of the lung is derived from the mucus-producing cells of the bronchial epithelium. Microscopic features consist of cuboidal to columnar cells with adequate to abundant pink or vacuolated cytoplasm and some evidence of gland formation. Most of these tumors (75%) are peripherally located. Adenocarcinoma of the lung tends to metastasize earlier than squamous cell carcinoma (SCC) of the lung and more frequently to the central nervous system.

The pathology of adenocarcinoma has been revised.[21] Bronchoalveolar or bronchioloalveolar carcinoma and mixed type adenocarcinoma have been eliminated, and adenocarcinoma in situ (pure lepidic growth) and minimally invasive adenocarcinoma (predominantly lepidic growth with <5 mm invasion) have been created. A solitary focus is treated in a manner similar to adenocarcinoma. Multifocal disease generally is not amenable to surgical resection. For invasive adenocarcinomas, the predominant pattern includes lepidic, acinar, papillary, and solid growth.

SCC of the lung occurs in approximately 30% of patients with lung cancer. Approximately two thirds of these tumors are centrally located and tend to expand against the bronchus, causing extrinsic compression. These tumors are prone to undergo central necrosis and cavitation. SCC tends to metastasize later than adenocarcinoma. Microscopically, keratinization, stratification, and intercellular bridge formation are exhibited. SCC may be more readily detected on sputum cytology than adenocarcinoma.

A diagnosis of large cell undifferentiated carcinoma may be made in approximately 10% of all lung tumors. Specific cytologic features of SCC or adenocarcinoma are lacking. These tumors tend to occur peripherally and may metastasize relatively early. Microscopically, these tumors show anaplastic, pleomorphic cells with vesicular or hyperchromatic nuclei and abundant cytoplasm. Neuroendocrine histopathology in adenocarcinoma can also portend a poorer prognosis and is more common in the large cell variant.

Small cell lung cancer represents approximately 20% of all lung cancers; approximately 80% are centrally located. The disease is

characterized by an aggressive tendency to metastasize. It often spreads early to mediastinal lymph nodes and distant sites, especially bone marrow and brain. Small cell lung cancer appears to arise in cells derived from the embryologic neural crest. Microscopically, these cells appear as sheets or clusters of cells with dark nuclei and little cytoplasm. The term *oat cell carcinoma* for this disease is due to the oatlike appearance under the microscope. Neurosecretory granules are evident on electron microscopy. This tumor is staged as *limited stage* (disease restricted to an ipsilateral hemithorax within a single radiation port) and *extensive stage* (obvious metastatic disease). These tumors are often advanced at presentation with an aggressive tendency to metastasize. Chemoradiotherapy is generally used for treatment. Prophylactic cranial irradiation needs to be considered in a patient with limited or extensive stage disease that responds well to first-line therapy. Complete responses may occur in approximately 30% of patients; however, the 5-year survival rate is only 5%. Patients with clinical early-stage disease (e.g., <3 cm in size, no nodal metastases, and no extrathoracic metastases) may be considered for surgical resec-

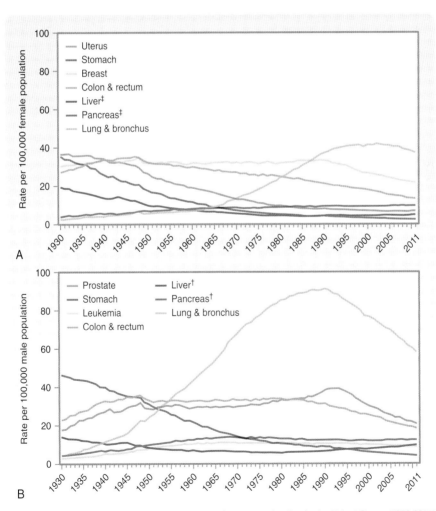

FIGURE 57-10 A, Age-adjusted cancer death rates for women, by site, in the United States (1930-2011) per 100,000, age-adjusted to the 2000 U.S. standard population. **B,** Age-adjusted cancer death rates for men, by site, in the United States (1930-2011) per 100,000, age-adjusted to the 2000 U.S. standard population. (From Siegel RL, Miller KD, Jemal A: Cancer statistics, 2015. *CA Cancer J Clin* 65:5–29, 2015.)

tion, followed by adjuvant systemic therapy. Staging before resection includes ^{18}F-fluorodeoxyglucose positron emission tomography (FDG-PET), brain CT or magnetic resonance imaging (MRI), and mediastinoscopy. Mediastinal metastases on clinical staging suggest advanced disease, which is best treated with chemoradiotherapy.

Lung cancers commonly metastasize to the pulmonary and mediastinal lymph nodes (lymphatic spread). Hematogenous spread of lung cancer commonly may result in metastases to the adrenal glands, brain, lung, and bone. Adenocarcinoma is more likely to metastasize to the central nervous system. Bone metastases are osteolytic. Extrathoracic metastases may occur without hilar nodes or mediastinal metastases.

Screening

Patients with lung cancer often present with advanced stage disease and symptoms. The pulmonary parenchyma does not contain nerve endings, and tumors may grow undetected until symptoms of pain, hemoptysis, or obstructive pneumonia arise. With the increased use of CT in the United States, smaller asymptomatic lung cancers are being identified.

Screening for lung cancer has been evaluated by the National Lung Screening Trial (NLST).[22,23] The NLST is a prospective randomized multicenter study evaluating annual low-dose helical CT with annual chest radiography. The 53,454 enrolled patients were randomly assigned between the two arms. The men and women screened were asymptomatic, and were older (age range, 55 to 74 years) with 30 pack-years or more of cigarette smoking at the beginning of the trial, and either were current smokers or had recently quit (within 15 years). The NLST found that patients randomly assigned to low-dose helical CT screening for 3 years (compared with CXR) had a reduced lung cancer–specific mortality and all-cause mortality. The death rate from lung cancer in this high-risk population was reduced by 20%, and all-cause mortality was reduced by 7%. The study showed the benefit is statistically significant, as 354 lung cancer deaths occurred in the CT group compared with 442 lung cancer deaths in the CXR group ($P = .0041$), leading to early study closure. Screening for early lung cancer detection using low-dose helical CT in average-risk asymptomatic individuals is recommended by the U.S. Preventive Services Task Force for selected current or former smokers 55 to 74 years old in good health with at least a 30-pack-year history of cigarette smoking.[24] Various professional organizations have incorporated the U.S. Preventive Services Task Force recommendations into their guidelines.[25]

These patients may discuss testing for early-stage lung cancer on an individual basis based on consultation and evaluation by their personal physicians—the informed shared decision-making model. This discussion with the patient should include the risks, benefits, and limitations associated with lung cancer screening with low-dose helical CT and should occur before a decision is made to start any lung cancer screening. Screening is not an alternative to smoking cessation. A clear and unambiguous statement is needed from the physician that smoking cessation is essential. Pharmacologic or other strategies need to be tailored to the individual patient. Screening of asymptomatic patients may identify nonspecific findings, such as overdiagnosis of benign nodules, which could result in patient anxiety as well as additional radiation exposure.

Diagnosis

The diagnosis of lung cancer can be challenging.[26] Many benign conditions mimic lung cancer. Physical examination should focus on the cardiorespiratory system. In addition, the presence of cancer in supraclavicular lymph nodes, identified by a careful examination of the cervical and supraclavicular lymph nodes, suggests advanced disease (N3 status for non–small cell lung cancer [NSCLC]), and therapy other than resection is recommended. Paraneoplastic syndromes are distant manifestations of lung cancer (not metastases) as revealed in extrathoracic nonmetastatic symptoms. The lung cancer causes an effect on these extrathoracic sites by producing one or more biologic or biochemical substances.

NSCLC typically occurs in patients who are 50 to 70 years old with a history of cigarette smoking. Patients develop symptoms based on the physical impact of tumor growth within the lung parenchyma. Symptoms such as cough, dyspnea, chest wall pain, and hemoptysis are related to the physical presence of the tumor and its interactions with the structures of the lung and chest wall.[27]

Pathologic confirmation of NSCLC can assist the patient and physician in discussions of risk and benefit for specific treatment options. Guidelines for management of the indeterminate pulmonary nodule, or "solitary" pulmonary nodule (SPN), are available.[28,29] Under certain circumstances, a SPN may be deemed benign with adequate confidence in the absence of a pathologic diagnosis. SPNs that are entirely calcified, or radiologically stable on CT of the chest over a minimum of 2 years, are very likely to be benign. Review of old radiographs or other prior imaging studies can assist in evaluation of changes in the mass.

In patients with a clinically suspicious SPN, histologic information may be needed to assess risk and benefit of various treatment options for the patient. Various options are available, and the least invasive strategy compatible with obtaining a diagnosis would be recommended. Diagnostic bronchoscopy, transthoracic needle aspiration, or navigational bronchoscopy[30] can be selected based on the size, location, and condition of the patient. In a physiologically fit patient with a suspicious yet undiagnosed SPN, nonanatomic wedge or sublobar resection provides a diagnosis. Confirmation of NSCLC by the pathologist should be followed by definitive resection in the same setting. For a SPN in the absence of a cancer diagnosis (that cannot be removed by wedge resection), a lobectomy can be considered for diagnosis (and treatment). A pneumonectomy is not performed without a cancer diagnosis.

One third of patients with NSCLC may have a pleural effusion at the time of presentation. Pleural fluid sampling with thoracentesis is required for cytologic examination. Malignant pleural effusion (MPE) is a contraindication to resection, but many pleural effusions in this setting may be sympathetic or reactive in origin.

Bronchoscopy is recommended before any planned pulmonary resection. The surgeon independently assesses (via bronchoscopy) the endobronchial anatomy to exclude secondary endobronchial primary tumors and to ensure that all known cancer will be encompassed by the planned pulmonary resection. Secretions can be cleared with suctioning and gentle irrigation. When pneumonectomy or bronchoplastic resection is contemplated for a central tumor, the surgeon's assessment at bronchoscopy is critical to the determination of whether complete (R0) resection can be achieved.

If the patient has hard palpable lymph nodes in the cervical or supraclavicular area, fine-needle aspiration or biopsy may provide an accurate diagnosis of N3 disease. Otherwise, a superficial lymph node biopsy or a scalene node biopsy could be performed to obtain tissue for further evaluation.

Staging

Staging is a description of the extent of the cancer based on similarities in survival for the group of patients with those characteristics. The staging system creates a shorthand description of the tumor, lymph nodes, and metastatic characteristics of the patient to facilitate the choice of optimal therapy and to evaluate outcomes based on the clinical and pathologic stage. The American Joint Committee on Cancer (AJCC) and the Union for International Cancer Control work to establish and promulgate staging system guidelines. The current international staging system for NSCLC[31] provides the basis for specific patient stage groupings and is used for initial treatment recommendations based on the clinical stage and on the pathologic stage after pulmonary resection.

The clinician's responsibility is to ensure the highest possible degree of certainty of the extent of the disease and to recommend the therapy or therapeutic combination of greatest efficacy based on this clinic stage. Optimal staging assists the clinician in providing the best recommendations for therapeutic interventions for the patient. The clinical stage is the physician's best and final estimate of the extent of disease based on all available information from invasive and noninvasive studies before the initiation of definitive therapy. The pathologic stage is the determination of the physical extent of the disease based on histologic examination of the resected tissues, including the hilar and mediastinal lymph nodes.

Evaluation of Tumor (T) Stage

As the tumor size increases, survival decreases. Diagnostic imaging commonly includes a CXR and CT scan of the chest and upper abdomen, including the liver and adrenals (Fig. 57-11). The CXR provides information on the size, shape, density, and location of the primary tumor and its relationship to the mediastinal structures. CT scan of the chest provides more detail on tumor characteristics and provides information on the relationship of the tumor to the mediastinum, chest wall, and diaphragm as well as invasion into the vertebrae or mediastinal structures (clinical T4). MRI may complement CT in these patients (T4). MRI of the brain may be reserved for patients with stage I or II cancer with new neurologic symptoms only (vertigo, headache), all patients with stage III and IV cancer, and patients with small cell carcinoma or superior sulcus tumors (Pancoast tumor) because these patients have a higher incidence of occult brain metastases.

Evaluation of Nodal (N) Stage

Determination of metastases to mediastinal lymph nodes constitutes a critical point in staging and treatment recommendations.[32,33] Mediastinal lymph node metastases are present in 26% to 32% of patients at the time of diagnosis and initially assessed with chest CT. Lymph nodes may be enlarged normally from infection (e.g., histoplasmosis, previous bronchitis, or pneumonia) or other inflammatory processes, such as granulomatous

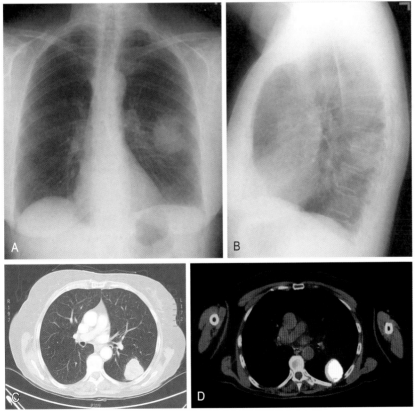

FIGURE 57-11 Radiographic evaluation for any patient with known or suspected lung cancer includes a plain chest x-ray, posteroanterior (**A**) and lateral (**B**) views. Evaluation of the plain films and computed tomography (CT) (**C**) guides subsequent evaluations. ¹⁸F-Fluorodeoxyglucose positron emission tomography (FDG-PET) with fused CT (**D**) provides the ability to correlate metabolic activity with physical findings. Although FDG-PET uses the increased metabolism in most neoplasms to create the FDG-PET image, other processes, such as infection, inflammation, or sequelae of trauma or fractures, can be identified as well. Sites of increased metabolism should be carefully evaluated for metastases.

disease. Mediastinal adenopathy is most often defined as lymph nodes with a maximal transverse diameter greater than 1 cm on axial tomographic images. In the absence of mediastinal nodes greater than 1 cm in diameter, the likelihood of N2 or N3 disease is low. If mediastinal nodes greater than 1 cm are identified, nodal tissue must be examined (e.g., with endoscopic bronchial ultrasound, cervical mediastinoscopy, endoscopic ultrasound, VATS) for histologic evidence of metastases before definitive resection.

CT has a reported sensitivity of 57% to 79% for mediastinal lymph node assessment in NSCLC, with a positive predictive value of 56%.[32] No CT size criteria are entirely reliable for the determination of mediastinal lymph node involvement. Larger mediastinal lymph nodes are more likely to be associated with metastasis (>70%); however, normal-sized lymph nodes (<1 cm) have a 7% to 15% chance of containing metastases.

PET may assist in evaluating the local extent and presence of known or occult metastases based on the differential increased metabolism of glucose by cancer cells compared with normal tissues (Fig. 57-12). A PET scan is not a cancer-specific study or a "cancer scan," as high cellular glucose metabolism is seen in inflammatory processes in addition to malignancy. FDG-PET scan is not a consistent diagnostic test for lung cancer.[34] Histologic confirmation of FDG avid mediastinal lymph node involvement is indicated to complete clinical staging before final treatment decisions. FDG-PET scan may identify areas of occult activity that must be evaluated for histologic evidence of NSCLC. FDG-PET coupled with CT may yield increased sensitivity and specificity in determining the stage of patients with lung cancer before treatment interventions.[35] Reed and colleagues[36] identified that PET and CT together were better than either one alone in determining a patient's suitability for resection. The negative predictive value of PET for mediastinal lymph node metastases from NSCLC was 87%.

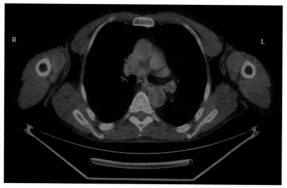

FIGURE 57-12 A subcarinal lymph node has mild ^{18}F-fluorodeoxyglucose (FDG) uptake. Based on these findings, additional invasive staging is warranted, including bronchoscopy and invasive staging of mediastinal lymph nodes. Endobronchial ultrasound with transtracheal needle aspiration can be performed with real-time ultrasound guidance to facilitate transtracheal needle placement. Biopsies of other stations can be performed as well. If needed, cervical mediastinoscopy is performed with biopsy of high paratracheal (2R and 2L), low paratracheal (4R and 4L), pretracheal (3A), and subcarinal (7) lymph nodes. If left-sided aortopulmonary lymph nodes were FDG avid, a Chamberlain procedure (anterior mediastinotomy) or video-assisted thoracic surgery with biopsy of aortopulmonary window lymph nodes or hilar lymph nodes could also be performed. Additional evaluation of the patient would be warranted if the patient would be considered a surgical candidate.

Invasive staging includes cervical mediastinoscopy or mediastinotomy (Chamberlain procedure), endoscopic bronchial ultrasound, or endoscopic ultrasound.[32] Cervical mediastinoscopy is traditionally indicated in patients with otherwise operable NSCLC with enlarged paratracheal or subcarinal lymph nodes, particularly if the cancer is proximal, if pneumonectomy is planned, or if the patient is at increased risk for the planned resection. Cervical mediastinoscopy is commonly performed for biopsy of bilateral paratracheal (level 2 and 4) and subcarinal (level 7) lymph nodes. A left anterior mediastinotomy is used to gain access to the mediastinum after resection of the second costosternal cartilage to evaluate the aortopulmonary window (level 5) or anterior mediastinum (level 6) lymph nodes. Cervical mediastinoscopy has a negative predictive value greater than 90%, may be performed as an outpatient procedure, and is associated with a low rate of significant complications. When pathologic "frozen section" evaluation fails to demonstrate malignant nodal involvement, mediastinoscopy may be followed by resection under the same anesthetic. The use of cervical mediastinoscopy regardless of radiographic evidence of nodal involvement ("routine mediastinoscopy") is not a cost-effective approach and adds little to the accuracy of staging in patients with an adequate noninvasive preoperative evaluation.[37]

Additional sampling techniques may be helpful. Endoscopic bronchial ultrasound may be more sensitive than mediastinoscopy.[38] Combining endoscopic bronchial ultrasound and surgical staging may provide greater sensitivity for mediastinal nodal metastases than surgical staging alone and avoid unnecessary thoracotomies.[39] VATS techniques can evaluate enlarged level 5 or 6 lymph nodes as well as enlarged level 8 or 9 or low level 7 lymph nodes. Endoscopic ultrasound–guided aspiration can be easily used for transesophageal needle aspiration of subcarinal and left aortopulmonary window lymph nodes.

Extrathoracic or distant metastases (M1b) are common in lung cancer. Beyond a thorough history and physical examination and standard staging techniques, additional evaluation for metastatic disease is indicated only for selected cases. In cases in which metastatic disease is suspected based on imaging techniques, a tissue diagnosis should be obtained to confirm the presence or absence of metastases. Nodules in the contralateral lung are characterized as metastatic disease (M1a) as are MPE and pleural carcinomatosis.

Up to 7% of patients have metastatic adrenal involvement at presentation. The standard CT evaluation of the chest should also include evaluation of the upper abdomen including the liver and the adrenal glands. Indeterminate adrenal lesions on CT may be further evaluated with MRI or with CT-guided percutaneous biopsy.

Current American Joint Committee on Cancer Seventh Edition Staging System

The International Association for the Study of Lung Cancer (IASLC) embarked on its lung cancer staging project to include all treatment and diagnostic groups, to collect data for analysis, and to reform future revisions.[40] The current AJCC seventh edition lung cancer staging reflects the impact of the IASLC lung cancer staging project.[41] The IASLC collected more than 100,000 NSCLC cases treated between 1990 and 2000. Each patient had a minimum of 5 years of follow-up, and all treatment modalities were included. Greater than 81,000 cases were submitted and eligible for analysis. These included 67,725 patients with NSCLC and 13,290 patients with small cell carcinoma. Survival was calculated by the Kaplan-Meier method. Prognostic groups were created using Cox regression analysis, and results were internally and externally validated.[42] Stage groupings were revised to reflect these analyses and internally and externally validated.[31] External validation was assessed against the Surveillance, Epidemiology, and End Results program database. The data collected were retrospective, and an audit of the data was not performed; however, information was provided by credible centers, which facilitated data collection, and analysis of a large patient population. Future directions will likely include prospective data collection[43] and proteomic and genomic characteristics.

The TNM definitions, nodal characteristics, and stage groupings of the TNM subsets with survival are shown in Table 57-1,

Box 57-1, and Table 57-2. Other schematics have been created for the lymph node map[44] and T characteristics.[45]

The mediastinal and regional lymph node classification schema is presented in Figure 57-13. This map presents a graphic representation of mediastinal and pulmonary lymph nodes in relation to other thoracic structures for optimal dissection and anatomic labeling by the surgeon.

Tumor (T)

In the IASLC lung cancer staging project, more than 18,000 patients had a T1 to T4 tumor with N0 lymph node dissection and R0 resection.[46] T1 was divided into T1a (≤2 cm) and T1b (>2 to 3 cm). T2 was divided into T2a (>3 to 5 cm) and T2b (>5

TABLE 57-1 T, N, and M Descriptors for Lung Cancer Staging

T (Primary Tumor)

TX — Primary tumor cannot be assessed, or tumor proven by the presence of malignant cells in sputum or bronchial washings but not visualized by imaging or bronchoscopy

T0 — No evidence of primary tumor

Tis — Carcinoma in situ

T1 — Tumor ≤3 cm in greatest dimension, surrounded by lung or visceral pleura, without bronchoscopic evidence of invasion more proximal than the lobar bronchus (i.e., not in the main bronchus)*
- T1a—Tumor ≤2 cm in greatest dimension
- T1b—Tumor >2 cm but ≤3 cm in greatest dimension

T2 — Tumor >3 cm but ≤7 cm or tumor with any of the following features (T2 tumors with these features are classified T2a if ≤5 cm)
- Involves main bronchus, ≥2 cm distal to the carina
- Invades visceral pleura
- Associated with atelectasis or obstructive pneumonitis that extends to the hilar region but does not involve the entire lung
- T2a—Tumor >3 cm but ≤5 cm in greatest dimension
- T2b—Tumor >5 cm but ≤7 cm in greatest dimension

T3 — Tumor >7 cm or one that directly invades any of the following: chest wall (including superior sulcus tumors), diaphragm, phrenic nerve, mediastinal pleura, parietal pericardium; or
- Tumor in the main bronchus <2 cm distal to the carina* but without involvement of the carina or
- Associated atelectasis or obstructive pneumonitis of the entire lung or
- Separate tumor nodule(s) in the same lobe

T4 — Tumor of any size that invades any of the following: mediastinum, heart, great vessels, trachea, recurrent laryngeal nerve, esophagus, vertebral body, carina; or
- Separate tumor nodule(s) in a different ipsilateral lobe

N (Regional Lymph Nodes)

NX — Regional lymph nodes cannot be assessed

N0 — No regional lymph node metastases

N1 — Metastasis in ipsilateral peribronchial and/or ipsilateral hilar lymph nodes and intrapulmonary nodes, including involvement by direct extension

N2 — Metastasis in ipsilateral mediastinal and/or subcarinal lymph node(s)

N3 — Metastasis in contralateral mediastinal, contralateral hilar, ipsilateral or contralateral scalene, or supraclavicular lymph node(s)

M (Distant Metastasis)

MX — Distant metastasis cannot be assessed

M0 — No distant metastasis

M1 — Distant metastasis
- M1a—Separate tumor nodule(s) in a contralateral lobe; tumor with pleural nodules or malignant pleural (or pericardial) effusion†
- M1b—Distant metastasis in extrathoracic organs

Adapted from Goldstraw P, Crowley J, Chansky K, et al: The IASLC Lung Cancer Staging Project: Proposals for the revision of the TNM stage groupings in the forthcoming (seventh) edition of the TNM Classification of malignant tumours. *J Thorac Oncol* 2:706–714, 2007; and Edge SB, Byrd DR, Compton CC, et al: *AJCC cancer staging manual*, ed 7, New York, 2010, Springer.

*The uncommon superficial spreading tumor of any size with its invasive component limited to the bronchial wall, which may extend proximally to the main bronchus, is also classified as T1.

†Most pleural (and pericardial) effusions with lung cancer are due to tumor. In a few patients, multiple cytopathologic examinations of pleural (pericardial) fluid are negative for tumor, and the fluid is nonbloody and is not an exudate. Where these elements and clinical judgment dictate that the effusion is not related to the tumor, the effusion should be excluded as a staging element, and the patient should be classified as T1, T2, T3, or T4.

BOX 57-1   Lymph Node Map Definitions

N2 Nodes*

1. Highest mediastinal nodes: Nodes lying above a horizontal line at the upper rim of the brachiocephalic (left innominate) vein where it ascends to the left, crossing in front of the trachea at its midline.
2. Upper paratracheal nodes: Nodes lying above a horizontal line drawn tangential to the upper margin of the aortic arch and below the inferior boundary of number 1 nodes.
3. Prevascular and retrotracheal nodes: Pretracheal and retrotracheal nodes may be designated 3A and 3P. Midline nodes are considered to be ipsilateral.
4. Lower paratracheal nodes: The lower paratracheal nodes on the right lie to the right of the midline of the trachea between a horizontal line drawn tangential to the upper margin of the aortic arch and a line extending across the right main bronchus at the upper margin of the upper lobe bronchus and contained within the mediastinal pleural envelope; the lower paratracheal nodes on the left lie to the left of the midline of the trachea between a horizontal line drawn tangential to the upper margin of the aortic arch and a line extending across the left main bronchus at the level of the upper margin of the left upper lobe bronchus, medial to the ligamentum arteriosum and contained within the mediastinal pleural envelope.

Regional (N2) Lymph Node Classification

5. Subaortic (aortopulmonary window): Subaortic nodes are lateral to the ligamentum arteriosum or the aorta or left pulmonary artery and proximal to the first branch of the left pulmonary artery and lie within the mediastinal pleural envelope.
6. Para-aortic nodes (ascending aorta or phrenic): Nodes lying anterior and lateral to the ascending aorta and the aortic arch or the innominate artery, beneath a line tangential to the upper margin of the aortic arch.
7. Subcarinal nodes: Nodes lying caudad to the carina of the trachea but not associated with the lower lobe bronchi or arteries within the lung.
8. Paraesophageal nodes (below carina): Nodes lying adjacent to the wall of the esophagus and to the right or left of the midline, excluding subcarinal nodes.
9. Pulmonary ligament nodes: Nodes lying within the pulmonary ligament, including nodes in the posterior wall and lower part of the inferior pulmonary vein.

N1 Nodes†

10. Hilar nodes: The proximal lobar nodes, distal to the mediastinal pleural reflection and the nodes adjacent to the bronchus intermedius on the right; radiographically, the hilar shadow may be created by enlargement of both hilar and interlobar nodes.
11. Interlobar nodes: Nodes lying between the lobar bronchi.
12. Lobar nodes: Nodes adjacent to the distal lobar bronchi.
13. Segmental nodes: Nodes adjacent to segmental bronchi.
14. Subsegmental nodes: Nodes around the subsegmental bronchi.

From Mountain CF, Dresler CM: Regional lymph node classification for lung cancer staging. *Chest* 111:1718–1723, 1997.
*All N2 nodes (single-digit designator) lie within the mediastinal pleural envelope.
†All N1 nodes lie distal to the mediastinal pleural reflection and within the visceral pleura.

TABLE 57-2   American Joint Committee on Cancer Seventh Edition TNM Stage Groupings

STAGE	T	N	M	PERCENT (%) 5-YEAR SURVIVAL CLINICAL STAGE	PATH STAGE
Occult cancer	TX	N0	M0	Not calculated	
Stage 0	Tis	N0	M0	Not calculated	
Stage IA	T1a/b	N0	M0	50	73
Stage IB	T2a	N0	M0	43	58
Stage IIA	T2b	N0	M0	36	46
	T1a/b; T2a	N1	M0		
Stage IIB	T2b	N1	M0	25	36
	T3	N0	M0		
Stage IIIA	Any T1; T2	N2	M0	19	24
	T3	N1/N2	M0		
	T4	N0/N1	M0		
Stage IIIB	T4	N2	M0	7	9
	Any T	N3	M0		
Stage IV	Any T	Any N	M1a/b	2	13

From Goldstraw P, Crowley J, Chansky K, et al: The IASLC Lung Cancer Staging Project: Proposals for the revision of the TNM stage groupings in the forthcoming (seventh) edition of the TNM Classification of malignant tumours. *J Thorac Oncol* 2:706–714, 2007; and Edge SB, Byrd DR, Compton CC, et al: *AJCC cancer staging manual*, ed 7, New York, 2010, Springer.

evaluated because of the small number of patients and inconsistent data. In the AJCC seventh edition, nodules in the same lobe were categorized as T3; nodules in a different lobe were categorized as T4; a nodule in a contralateral lobe would be designated as M1a, *unless* there was compelling evidence to suggest synchronous primary tumors.

T3 tumors may be characterized as a tumor with invasion into the pleura, pericardium, or diaphragm; an endobronchial tumor less than 2 cm from the carina; an obstructing tumor causing atelectasis of the entire lung; or, as mentioned before, two nodules in the same lobe. T4 tumors involve the mediastinal structures, such as the heart, great vessels, esophagus, and trachea, as well as the vertebral body or the carina. Two nodules, one each in two separate ipsilateral lobes, would also be characterized as T4.

Pleural metastases or MPE was changed from T4 (in the AJCC sixth edition) to M1 in the AJCC seventh edition. Patients previously categorized as a clinical T4 based on MPE, malignant pericardial effusions, or pleural nodules, are now categorized as clinical M1 based on poor survival more closely resembling patients with metastatic disease.

Lymph Nodes (N)

The nodal characteristics and designations did not change in the AJCC seventh edition.[47] T, N, and M characteristics as well as histologic type and survival were available for more than 67,000 patients. Clinical nodal staging information was available for 38,265 patients, and pathologic nodal staging information was available for 28,371 patients. Clinical staging studies included tests such as diagnostic imaging, CT, and mediastinoscopy.

to 7 cm). "T2c" would have been tumors greater than 7 cm; however, these patients had a survival that was statistically similar to survival of T3 patients, and so tumors greater than 7 cm were categorized as T3.

Other T2 descriptors, such as visceral pleural invasion and partial atelectasis (less than the entire lung), could not be

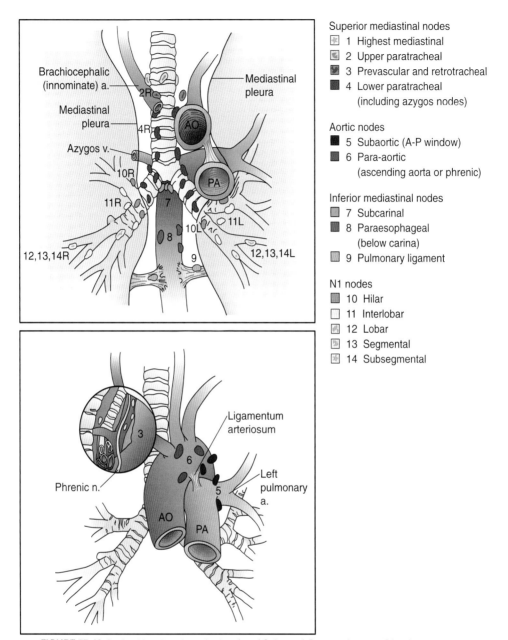

Superior mediastinal nodes
  1 Highest mediastinal
  2 Upper paratracheal
  3 Prevascular and retrotracheal
  4 Lower paratracheal
    (including azygos nodes)

Aortic nodes
  5 Subaortic (A-P window)
  6 Para-aortic
    (ascending aorta or phrenic)

Inferior mediastinal nodes
  7 Subcarinal
  8 Paraesophageal
    (below carina)
  9 Pulmonary ligament

N1 nodes
  10 Hilar
  11 Interlobar
  12 Lobar
  13 Segmental
  14 Subsegmental

FIGURE 57-13 Regional lymph node station location. *AO*, Aorta; *A-P*, aortopulmonary; *PA*, pulmonary artery. (From Mountain CF, Libshitz HI, Hermes KE: *Lung cancer: a handbook for staging, imaging, and lymph node classification*, Houston, TX, 1999, Mountain, pp 1–71.)

Thoracotomy for staging was excluded. PET was not widely used internationally in this cohort during this time. A new international lymph node map was proposed combining the integral aspects of the Japanese/Naruke and the North American/Mountain lymph node maps.[48] The authors proposed radiographic regions for the location of specific mediastinal lymph nodes, particularly for integration with CT, to guide the radiologic staging of patients with NSCLC.

Metastases (M)

Metastases were divided into M1a and M1b.[49] Patients with metastasis to the contralateral lung *only* were designated as M1a;

metastases to regions outside the lung/pleura were designated as M1b. A second nodule in the nonprimary ipsilateral lobe, previously designated as M1, was changed to T4M0. In this situation, the patient received the "benefit of the doubt" approach, as this might represent a second primary.

Results of Treatment of Lung Cancer

The choice of initial therapy (whether single-modality or multimodality therapy) depends on the patient's clinical stage at presentation and the availability of prospective protocols. However, treatment options may vary, even among different subsets of patients within the same clinical stage. Pretreatment staging is the critical step before initiating therapy. With current efforts, 5-year survival rates by pathologic stage are 73% for stage IA, 58% for stage IB, 46% for stage IIA, 36% for stage IIB, 24% for stage IIIA, 9% for stage IIIB, and 13% for stage IV.[31] Treatment for lung cancer can be roughly grouped into three major categories, as follows:

1. *Stage I and II* tumors are contained within the lung and may be completely resected with surgery. Stereotactic body radiation therapy has had good early results in selected patients not amenable to resection.[50]
2. *Stage IV* disease includes metastatic disease and is not typically treated by surgery except in patients requiring surgical palliation. Systemic therapies for metastatic disease are common. Targeted therapies have provided carefully screened patients with excellent results.
3. *Resectable stage IIIA and IIIB* tumors are locally advanced tumors with metastasis to the ipsilateral mediastinal (N2) lymph nodes (stage IIIA) or involving mediastinal structures (T4N0M0). These tumors, by their advanced nature, may be mechanically removed with surgery; however, surgery does not consistently control the micrometastases that exist within the general area of the operation or systemically. Combinations of chemotherapy and radiotherapy are used for locally advanced disease or before resection.

Lung carcinoma should be resected when the local disease can be controlled, the patient's physical condition can tolerate the planned resection and reconstruction, and the anticipated operative mortality is less than the stage-specific 5-year survival. Conditions such as superior vena cava syndrome, tumor invasion across the mediastinum into the main pulmonary artery, N3 nodal metastases, malignant pleural or pericardial disease, or extrathoracic metastases carry greater risk than benefit for resection in most patients. Some centers have had good results with resection and reconstruction of the trachea, atrium, great vessels, or other mediastinal or vertebral structures. These are complex operations requiring dedicated multidisciplinary teams during the preoperative phase and multispecialty teams in the operating room. Patients with tracheoesophageal fistula have a limited life expectancy, and palliative care with stent placement would be recommended.

Local Therapy for Early-Stage Non–Small Cell Lung Cancer

Stage I and II NSCLC can be treated safely with surgery and mediastinal lymph node dissection alone, and most patients have long-term survival.[51] Anatomic resection with lobectomy, with systematic mediastinal lymph node dissection/sampling, is the procedure of choice for lung cancer confined to one lobe (Fig. 57-14). The American College of Surgeons Oncology Group defined a systematic sampling strategy for specific mediastinal lymph nodes.[52] At a minimum, samples of nodal (not adipose) tissue from stations 2R, 4R, 7, 8, and 9 for right-sided cancers and stations 4L, 5, 6, 7, 8, and 9 for left-sided cancers should be obtained. Mediastinal lymphadenectomy should include exploration and removal of lymph nodes from stations 2R, 4R, 7, 8, and 9 for right-sided cancers and stations 4L, 5, 6, 7, 8, and 9 for left-sided cancers.

Lesser operations such as wedge resection or segmentectomy may be considered for patients at greater risk for lobectomy. A prospective trial found no local control advantage for patients with wedge resection with brachytherapy radioactive iodine-131 threads placed at the suture line compared with wedge resection

alone.[53] Patients with NSCLC that invades into the chest wall may undergo resection with lobectomy with en bloc chest wall resection.

Stereotactic body radiation therapy is another local control modality.[50] Treatment with 54 Gy in three fractions appears to be well tolerated with good early results. Prospective clinical trials, such as ACOSOG Z4099/RTOG 1021, were initiated to evaluate high-risk patients (unable to tolerate a lobectomy) with early-stage NSCLC randomly assigned to wedge resection or stereotactic body radiation therapy. This and other similar trials closed early without sufficient accrual to answer this important question.

Neoadjuvant and Adjuvant Therapy

Advanced stage lung cancer, particularly with nodal spread, cannot typically be considered a disease effectively treated with a single modality. Survival after resection may be improved in selected patients with adjuvant chemotherapy. The International Adjuvant Lung Trial[54] enrolled 1867 patients with completely resected stage I to III NSCLC. These patients were randomly assigned to observation or chemotherapy. Radiation therapy was at the discretion of the institution. The treatment group received one of four cisplatin-based doublet adjuvant regimens.[55] Survival was increased 5% in the adjuvant chemotherapy group. All patients staged IB and IIB should be considered for adjuvant chemotherapy after resection, and this should be discussed with a medical oncologist.

Surgery alone for stage IIIA (N2), IIIB, or IV lung cancer is infrequently performed; however, selected patients may benefit from a multidisciplinary approach to treatment.[56] Resection for isolated brain metastasis is warranted for improvement in symptoms, quality of life, and survival rate. The primary lung tumor can be treated according to T and N stage. Additional treatment beyond resection is needed.

Even with complete resection, patients with resectable NSCLC have poor survival. Preoperative therapy (induction or neoadjuvant) has been evaluated: Preoperative paclitaxel and carboplatin followed by surgery was compared with surgery alone in patients with early-stage NSCLC. Median overall survival was 41 months in the surgery-only arm and 62 months in the preoperative chemotherapy arm (hazard ratio, 0.79; 95% confidence interval, 0.60 to 1.06; $P = .11$). Median progression-free survival was 20 months for surgery alone and 33 months for preoperative chemotherapy (hazard ratio, 0.80; 95% confidence interval, 0.61 to 1.04; $P = .10$). Overall survival and progression-free survival were higher with preoperative chemotherapy, although the differences did not reach statistical significance.[57]

Induction chemoradiotherapy has been evaluated for treatment of clinical stage IIIA (N2) NSCLC.[58] In one phase III trial, concurrent chemotherapy and radiotherapy followed by resection was compared with standard concurrent chemotherapy and definitive radiotherapy without resection. The median overall survival was similar in both groups (~23 months). Progression-free survival was better in the surgery group (12.8 months median versus 10.5 months; $P = .017$). The authors reported pneumonectomy was associated with poor outcomes. In an exploratory analysis, overall survival was improved for patients who were found to have undergone induction chemoradiotherapy and lobectomy. In selected patients with resectable stage IIIA NSCLC, induction chemoradiotherapy followed by resection is an alternative treatment to chemoradiotherapy alone.[56]

Patients with local extension of lung cancer at the apex of the lung into the thoracic inlet may have characteristics of shoulder and arm pain, Horner syndrome, and occasionally paresthesia in the ulnar nerve distribution of the hand (fourth and fifth fingers) (Fig. 57-15). Patients with all these characteristics may be classified as having Pancoast syndrome. Pain comes from the C8 and T1 nerve roots. Sympathetic nerve involvement may result in Horner syndrome (miosis, ptosis, anhidrosis, and enophthalmos). Typically, the first, second, and third ribs are involved and require resection, but the bony spine and intraforaminal spaces can also be involved. MRI is necessary, in addition to CT, to plan the surgical procedure. Preoperative therapy includes chemoradiotherapy.[59,60]

Treatment of Metastatic Disease

Metastatic disease (stage IV NSCLC) is usually incurable.[61] Performance and quality of life decline. Patients and families should be informed of the diagnosis and potential outcomes of treatment. Treatment decisions should take into consideration the wishes of the patient and family, and realistic expectations should be set and monitored during therapy.

Combination chemotherapy with platinum doublets has been well tolerated and associated with a modest improvement in survival rates.[55] The addition of bevacizumab (a monoclonal antibody to the vascular endothelial growth factor receptor) to paclitaxel and carboplatin improved survival compared with treatment with paclitaxel and carboplatin alone.[62] Induction chemotherapy followed by radiation appears to improve survival rate in patients with locally advanced unresectable lung cancer. In these studies, cisplatin-based combination chemotherapy was shown to improve expected survival over and above survival achieved with radiation alone.

Additional strategies to identify the molecular characteristics of the tumor as part of the initial staging could also improve survival by creating better models for treatments of NSCLC. As a result of advances in tumor biology, predictive markers of response to epidermal growth factor receptor (EGFR) inhibitors[63]

SURGICAL PATHOLOGY REPORT

DIAGNOSIS:
1) LYMPH NODE, 4R, EXCISION: FRAGMENTS OF LYMPH NODE, NEGATIVE FOR MALIGNANCY.
2) LYMPH NODE, 2R, EXCISION: FRAGMENTS OF LYMPH NODE, NEGATIVE FOR MALIGNANCY.
3) LYMPH NODE, PRE-CARINAL, EXCISION: FRAGMENTS OF LYMPH NODE, NEGATIVE FOR MALIGNANCY.
4) LYMPH NODE, LEVEL 4, EXCISION: FRAGMENTS OF LYMPH NODE, NEGATIVE FOR MALIGNANCY.
5) LYMPHNODE, LEVEL 2L, EXCISION: FRAGMENTS OF LYMPH NODE, NEGATIVE FOR MALIGNANCY.
6) LYMPH NODE, LEVEL 7, EXCISION: FRAGMENTS OF LYMPH NODE, NEGATIVE FOR MALIGNANCY.
7) LYMPH NODE, LEVEL 8, EXCISION: INVOLVED BY METASTATIC ADENOCARCINOMA.
8) LYMPH NODE, LEVEL 11, EXCISION: 1 LYMPH NODE, NEGATIVE FOR MALIGNANCY (0/1).
9) LYMPH NODE, LEVEL 10, EXCISION: FRAGMENTS OF LYMPH NODE, NEGATIVE FOR MALIGNANCY.
10) LUNG, LEFT LOWER LOBE, LOBECTOMY: POORLY-DIFFERENTIATED ADENOCARCINOMA, SIMILAR TO PREVIOUS (SEE S10-37167), PREDOMINANTLY SOLID TYPE, 4.9 CM IN GREATEST EXTENT, INVADING INTO VISCERAL PLEURA; RESECTION MARGINS NEGATIVE FOR MALIGNANCY; LARGE VESSEL INVASION PRESENT; CENTRIACINAR EMPHYSEMA.
11) LYMPH NODE, LEVEL 5, EXCISION: FRAGMENTS OF LYMPH NODE, NEGATIVE FOR MALIGNANCY.

COMMENT: These findings correspond to AJCC 7th Edition pathologic Stage IIIA (pT2a, pN2, pM n/a).

    Lung Carcinoma Summary Findings

Specimen Type: lobectomy
Laterality: left
Tumor site: lower lobe
Tumor size: 4.9 x 4.1 x 3.8 cm
Tumor focality: unifocal
Histologic type: adenocarcinoma
Histologic Grade: poorly-differentiated
Visceral Pleura Invasion: present (confirmed with elastin stain)
Direct extension of tumor: limited to lung and visceral pleura
Venous (large vessel invasion): present
Arterial (large vessel invasion): negative
Lymphatic (small vessel invasion): negative
Treatment effect: n/a

Margins: 1.1 cm from parenchymal margin

Ancillary testing:
    EGFR mutational analysis: yes
    KRAS mutational analysis: yes
    Other (specify): ALK
Pathologic staging (pTNM): IIIA
    Primary tumor: pT2a
    Regional lymph nodes: pN2
    Distant metastasis: pM n/a

FIGURE 57-14 Structured pathology report after left lower lobectomy. Lung carcinoma summary findings are helpful in identifying factors critical for pathologic staging and factors that may influence subsequent survival. Ancillary testing for mutational analysis of epidermal growth factor receptor (EGFR), KRAS, and ALK is done routinely.

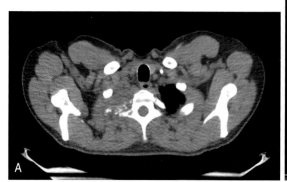
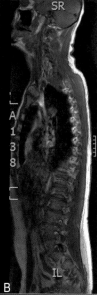

FIGURE 57-15 The patient is a 50-year-old man with a right superior sulcus tumor. Diagnostic imaging revealed a right apical mass and destruction of the posterior aspect of the second rib. Transthoracic biopsy was positive for poorly differentiated adenocarcinoma (non–small cell lung carcinoma). Endobronchial ultrasound for mediastinal staging was negative; cervical mediastinoscopy was also negative. Induction chemoradiotherapy was given with 48 Gy in 24 fractions over 1 month with chemotherapy (carboplatin AUC of 5 + pemetrexed 500 mg/m^2). **A,** Computed tomography (CT) scan of the chest demonstrates the mass is present in the apex of the chest with complete destruction of the posterior aspect of the right second rib and cortical erosion of the right T2 vertebral body secondary to the mass. The patient is left hand–dominant. **B,** Magnetic resonance imaging of the thoracic spine demonstrates a medial right apical lung mass, consistent with a Pancoast tumor involving the right lateral aspect of the T2 vertebral body, articular facet, and transverse process. There was also extension into the neural foramen and involvement of the nerve roots on the right at T1-2 and T2-3. There was no extension into the central canal or involvement of the spinal cord. CT scan of the head demonstrated no acute findings involving the brain. Complete resection was performed with a two-surgeon team, a thoracic surgeon and neurosurgeon. The patient required a right upper lobectomy with en bloc chest wall and vertebral body resection and mediastinal lymph node dissection. Spine stabilization was required.

and ALK (a chimeric protein originally identified in anaplastic large cell lymphoma) receptors have become available.[64] These studies focused efforts to target specific genetic mutations in a patient's specific lung cancer. Mutations in EGFR strongly predict the response to EGFR tyrosine kinase inhibitors. In addition, there is improved outcome for patients with adenocarcinoma treated with pemetrexed. Clinical trials have shown significant progression-free survival in patients with metastatic NSCLC treated with gefitinib and platinum-based doublet chemotherapy compared with chemotherapy alone.[65,66] Targeted therapies in addition to current chemotherapeutic regimens, or alone, may limit toxicity and improve outcomes compared with the current chemotherapeutic regimens. In 2015, the U.S. Food and Drug Administration approved gefitinib for first-line treatment of patients with metastatic NSCLC with the most common types of EGFR mutations (exon 19 deletions or exon 21 L858R substitution gene mutations).[67] In addition, several clinical trials are evaluating various antibodies that target the PD-1 pathway (programmed cell death protein 1) and the PDL1 (programmed death ligand-1) and provide a "checkpoint blockade" inhibiting further cancer progression.[68]

Quality-of-life issues arise in patients with metastatic NSCLC. Dyspnea from MPE, superior vena cava syndrome, tracheoesophageal fistula, bone metastases, and pain occur. Nutrition and hydration are significant issues. Palliation from symptoms may be accomplished with good results.[27,69]

TRACHEA

The position of the trachea can be up to 50% cervical with hyperextension in a young patient. The location of the carina is at the level of the angle of Louis anteriorly and the T4 vertebra posteriorly. Stenosis of the trachea implies significant functional impairment. A normal 2-cm trachea has a 100% peak expiratory flow rate. A 10-mm opening provides an 80% peak expiratory flow rate. At 5 to 6 mm, only a 30% expiratory flow rate is obtained. Tracheostomy is one of the most commonly performed operations. Percutaneous tracheostomy is frequently performed,[70] although open procedures may be selected. Infection and inflammation are uncommon causes of tracheal obstruction.

Primary neoplasms of the trachea[71] include SCC in approximately two thirds of patients and adenoid cystic carcinoma in other patients. SCC may be focal, diffuse, or multiple. The physical appearance may be exophytic or ulcerative. One third of these primary tracheal tumors have extensive local spread or metastases at initial presentation. Resection can be performed with excellent results.[72] Adenoid cystic carcinoma (previously called *cylindroma*) has a propensity for intramural and perineural spread. In adenoid cystic carcinoma, negative margins are important. Margin evaluation with frozen-section control is performed for stricture resection. Clinical features include dyspnea on exertion, wheezing, cough with or without hemoptysis, and recurrent pulmonary infections.

Involvement of the trachea because of local extension from bronchogenic carcinoma may contraindicate resection. Involvement of the trachea because of local extension of esophageal carcinoma may require palliative therapy or stent placement.

Tracheal Trauma

Penetrating injuries to the trachea are usually cervical and may involve the esophagus. Concurrent esophageal injury needs to be excluded by barium esophagography or esophagoscopy. Neck exploration may be required. Blunt trauma to the neck or trachea can produce lacerations, transections, or shattering injuries of both the cervical and the mediastinal trachea. Clinical features of a tracheal injury are suggested by subcutaneous air in the neck, respiratory distress, and hemoptysis. Diagnosis is made by bronchoscopy. Anesthetic management with laryngeal mask airway may be helpful for initial examination for full visualization of the airway before endotracheal intubation. Primary repair of tracheal injury may be accomplished with cervical exploration. Bronchial disruption may require thoracotomy for repair. Right thoracotomy provides excellent visualization of the carina and proximal left mainstem bronchus.

Postintubation tracheal stenosis may occur because of laryngeal or tracheal irritation from an indwelling endotracheal tube. Low-pressure cuffs on the endotracheal tube have reduced pressure necrosis. Tracheal stenosis may manifest with dyspnea on exertion, stridor or wheezing (which is easily noted), and sometimes episodes of obstruction by small amounts of mucus. Emergency management of obstruction may include sedation, humidified air, or racemic epinephrine by nebulizer. Dilation under general anesthesia may be helpful.

Acquired tracheoesophageal fistula can occur from cancer or from prolonged intubation with erosion posteriorly. Repair is with separation of the trachea and esophagus, repair of the fistulous tract, and interposition of normal tissue such as muscle between the two structures.

Tracheoinnominate fistula may result from prolonged cuff erosion inferiorly and anteriorly in the trachea. Inappropriate low stoma may further increase the likelihood of a direct erosion of the trachea by the innominate artery. The tip of the endotracheal tube may predispose to erosions or granulomas within the trachea. Tracheoinnominate fistula may manifest with a sentinel hemorrhage before sudden exsanguinating hemorrhage. Investigation of these sentinel hemorrhage episodes is critical. Evaluation in the operating room may provide for optimal situational control should additional interventions be required.

The surgical management of tracheal problems may be complex. General inhalational anesthesia is used, and induction may take a long time if the stenosis is tight. The patient should be maintained spontaneously breathing if possible. If the stenosis is less than 5 to 6 mm, dilation may be required before passing the endotracheal tube; the dilation may be performed with rigid bronchoscopy. If the stenosis is greater than 5 to 6 mm, the endotracheal tube may be positioned to a point above the stricture for induction. Stenoses that are subglottic must be dilated for intubation. The endotracheal tube often goes alongside tumors.

The cervical approach for tracheal resection is usually used for tumors of the upper half of the trachea plus all benign tracheal stenoses (because these usually occur as a result of endotracheal tube placement). Occasionally, an upper sternal split may be needed (Fig. 57-16). The posterolateral thoracotomy (fourth interspace) is used for tumors of the lower half of the trachea plus carinal reconstruction. Rigid bronchoscopy for diagnosis, biopsy, dilation, or morcellation of tumor or other treatment may be required if the tumor cannot be immediately resected (Fig. 57-17).

In general, the maximal amount of trachea that can be resected is approximately 5 cm, but this varies from person to person. Various techniques are used to mobilize the trachea to create a repair without undue tension on the anastomosis. The anterior cervical approach plus mobilization of the trachea and neck flexion can allow for 4 to 5 cm of trachea resection. A suprahyoid release may achieve 1 cm of additional length. Mobilization of the right hilum, together with division of the pericardium around the right hilum, may achieve an additional 1.4 cm.

Stenosis of the subglottic larynx or cricoid stenosis is a challenging technical procedure. The recurrent nerves innervate the larynx just superior to the posterolateral cricoid on each side. If the tracheal lesions involve only the anterior surface, the anterior cricoid can be removed and the distal trachea beveled to match the defect. This maneuver spares the recurrent laryngeal nerves. With circumferential involvement, it may be necessary to perform a laryngectomy.

Reconstruction of the lower trachea is performed in the right fourth intercostal space. Intubation of the distal trachea or the left mainstem is performed. Carinal reconstruction is usually performed for tumor and is the most feasible of alternative reconstructions chosen.

Contraindications to trachea repair include (1) inadequately treated laryngeal problem (which does not include single vocal cord paralysis); (2) need for ventilatory support or permanent tracheostomy for patients with amyotrophic lateral sclerosis, myasthenia gravis, or quadriplegia; (3) use of high-dose steroids; and (4) inflamed or recent tracheostomy. Poor pulmonary reserve is not a contraindication for repair in patients who have been weaned from the ventilator.

PULMONARY INFECTIONS

Pulmonary infections requiring surgical interventions are infrequent compared with pleural space infections. Clinical features are similar to pneumonia, including fever, cough, leukocytosis, pleuritic pain, and sputum production. The patient is specifically questioned about aspiration of a foreign body. Evaluation includes CXR and CT scan of the chest and upper abdomen. Bronchoscopy can be performed to clear secretions and, when the diagnosis is suspected, to rule out cancer, foreign body, bronchial stenosis, or stricture. Cultures may be obtained to facilitate antibiotic treatment. Medical treatment is optimized; this includes discontinuation of smoking and institution of postural drainage, bronchodilator medications, and oral antibiotics.

Bronchiectasis

Bronchiectasis is an infection of the bronchial wall and surrounding lung with sufficient severity to cause destruction and dilation of the air passages. As a result of the use of antibiotics, this condition is decreasing in frequency and severity. There are numerous predisposing factors, including cystic fibrosis; α_1-antitrypsin

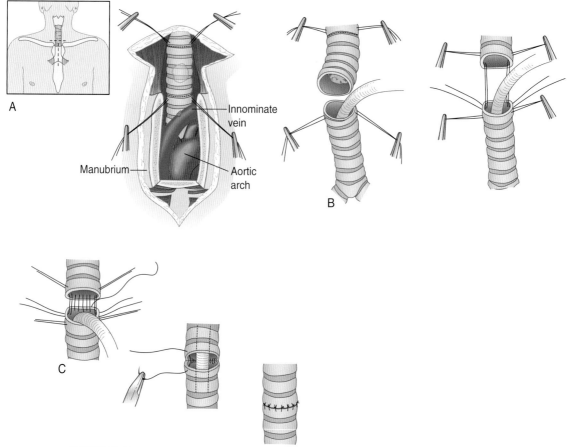

FIGURE 57-16 A, Exposure of the midtrachea through a cervical and partial sternal-splitting incision. The extent of the resection has been marked by sutures. **B,** After distal division, a sterile, armored endotracheal tube is placed. After proximal resection, two mattress sutures are placed in the edges of the cartilaginous rings. A simple running suture completes the membranous anastomosis. **C,** At this point, the original endotracheal tube is positioned in the distal trachea so that the anastomosis can be completed with interrupted simple sutures between cartilaginous rings.

deficiency; various immunodeficiency states; Kartagener syndrome (sinusitis, bronchiectasis, situs inversus, and hypomotile cilia); and bronchial obstruction from foreign body, extrinsic lymph nodes that compress the bronchus, neoplasm, or mucous plug. The distribution is primarily in the basal segments of the lower lobes. Destructive changes and dilation of the bronchi accompany the infection. Massive hemoptysis is rare. Symptoms frequently can be controlled with medical management, such as long-term antibiotic therapy and postural drainage. Disease limited to one lobe is best treated surgically. If bilateral bronchiectasis exists, medical management is continued.

Lung Abscess

The incidence of lung abscess is decreasing in frequency as a result of use of antibiotics. A lung abscess may occur from an infection behind a blocked bronchus. *Staphylococcus* bacteremia is frequently associated with lung abscess. Necrotizing pneumonia from *Klebsiella* spp. may rapidly destroy the involved lung with minimal surrounding reaction. Rupture of a lung abscess may yield empyema and pneumothorax. Lung abscess may also be superimposed on structural abnormalities, such as a bronchogenic cyst, sequestration, bleb, or tuberculous or fungal cavities. CXR

and CT scan of the chest may demonstrate an air-fluid level within the abscess cavity.

The differential diagnosis of a mediastinal or thoracic air-fluid level includes loculated empyema, epiphrenic diverticulum, tuberculous or fungal cavity, or a cavitary lung cancer (usually SCC). Tubercular and fungus cavities do not retain fluid, so no air-fluid level is present; however, they may contain debris or a fungus ball. *Aspergillus* spp. infection may manifest in this manner. Medical management is with antibiotics and pulmonary care (e.g., reexpansion). Bronchoscopy may be used for treatment to assist in drainage of the cavity either directly or via transbronchial catheterization of the cavity. Most patients (85% to 95%) respond to medical management with rapid decrease in fluid, collapse of the walls, and complete healing in 3 to 4 months. Patients with symptoms for longer than 3 months before treatment or cavities larger than 4 to 6 cm are less likely to respond.

Surgical therapy is indicated for persistent cavity ($\geq$2 cm and thick-walled), failure to clear sepsis after 8 weeks of medical therapy, hemoptysis, and exclusion of cancer. If a lung abscess ruptures into the pleural cavity, simple drainage may suffice, and the patient is managed for empyema or bronchopleural fistula. Lobectomy is typically required; the mortality rate is 1% to 5%.

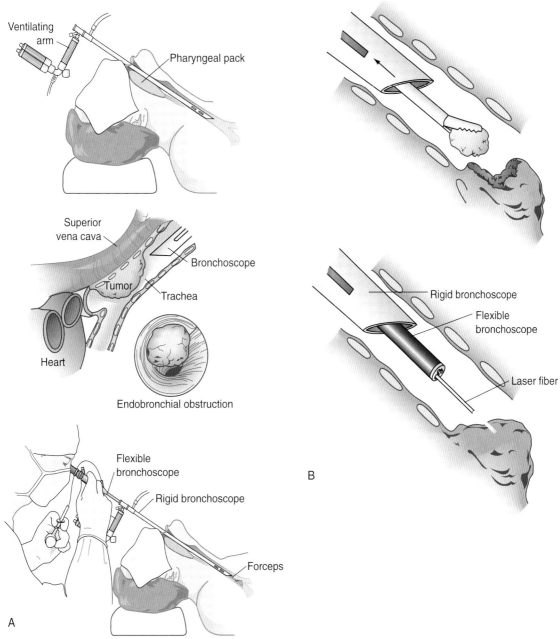

FIGURE 57-17 A, Proper technique for rigid bronchoscopy in a patient with a tracheal mass. *Top,* Pharyngeal packing used to protect the esophagus is shown. The surgeon should be cautious because this packing can move and may obstruct the larynx. Complete removal of the packing is done at the end of the operation. *Middle,* A nearly obstructing tumor is shown. *Bottom,* A flexible bronchoscope is placed into the rigid scope for the biopsy. This protects the airway. **B,** Technique for endoscopic resection of a tracheal mass with a rigid bronchoscope without *(top)* and with *(bottom)* use of the laser. (From Sugarbaker DJ, Mentzer SJ, Strauss G, et al: Laser resection of endobronchial lesions: Use of the rigid and flexible bronchoscopes. *Oper Tech Otolaryngol Head Neck Surg* 3:93, 1992.)

Occasionally, external drainage may be required in critically ill patients if pleural symphysis has occurred.

Other Bronchopulmonary Disorders

Bronchopulmonary disorders caused by inflammatory lymph node disease are usually caused by tuberculosis or histoplasmosis.

Lobar atelectasis, hemoptysis, or broncholithiasis can occur. Bronchial compressive disease typically occurs most commonly in the middle lobe. More than 20% of disorders are caused by cancer. This condition results in repeated infection in the same area of the lung, which usually responds to antibiotics. Bronchoscopy is essential to rule out cancer and foreign body and to evaluate for stricture. Medical management is required to treat infection. Surgery is indicated to treat bronchostenosis, irreversible bronchiectasis, or severe recurrent infection.

Broncholithiasis is a calcified node tightly adherent to a bronchus. An innocent hemoptysis may occur even with a negative CXR. Sudden bleeding caused by erosion of a small bronchial artery and mucosa by a spicule in the calcified node causes this hemoptysis. Bright red blood occurs and usually stops with sedation and antitussive therapy. This type of hemoptysis is almost never massive (≥600 mL in 24 hours). Bronchoscopy is possible during a bleeding episode to localize the site of the bleeding. Nasal or pharyngeal lesions or hematemesis from a gastrointestinal source should be excluded.

Organizing pneumonia may replace lung parenchyma with scar tissue or persistent atelectasis or consolidation. If the shadow or mass persists over 6 to 8 weeks, resection is performed to exclude carcinoma. The differential diagnosis includes pneumonia, congenital abnormality, and aneurysm of the aorta.

Mycobacterial Infections

Mycobacterium tuberculosis infects approximately 7% of patients exposed, and tuberculosis develops in 5% to 10% of patients who are infected. A primary infection develops. The exudative response progresses to caseous necrosis. Postprimary tuberculosis tends to occur in apical and posterior segments of the upper lobes and superior segments of the lower lobes. Healing occurs with fibrosis and contracture. Extensive caseation with cavitation may occur early. Coalescing areas of caseous necrosis may form cavities. There are frequently incomplete septations and lobulations. Erosions of septations supplied by bronchial arteries cause hemoptysis and may be secondarily infected.

Medical management is with isoniazid, rifampin, ethambutol, streptomycin, and pyrazinamide.[73] Bronchoscopy may be required for patients who do not respond to medical management. Cancer should be excluded for a newly identified mass on CXR even with a positive tuberculosis skin test and acid-fast bacillus–positive sputum.

Surgical therapy may be considered when medical therapy fails and persistent tuberculosis-positive sputum remains and when surgically correctable residua of tuberculosis may be of potential danger to the patient.[74,75] This is not the same management as for atypical mycobacteria; many of these patients remain clinically well even with positive sputum. Indications for surgery include the following:

1. Open positive cavity after 3 to 6 months of chemotherapy, especially if resistant mycobacteria.
2. Destroyed lung, atelectasis, bronchiectasis, or bronchostenosis that is amenable to resection.
3. Open negative cavities if thick-walled, slow response, or unreliable patient.
4. Exclusion of cancer.
5. Recurrent or persistent hemoptysis if greater than 600 mL of blood is lost in 24 hours or less.

Surgical options include resection with preservation of good lung tissue. Surgical complications are doubled if the sputum is positive for *M. tuberculosis* and decreased if remaining lung tissue is fully expanded within the chest. Infectious complications include empyema, bronchopleural fistula, and endobronchial spread of the disease and are associated with a higher mortality rate. Tuberculosis infection of the pleural space without lung destruction is primarily treated medically.

Thoracoplasty or muscle flap interposition may be used to control postresection empyema space. Collapse therapy, with thoracoplasty or plombage, is rarely used to manage parenchymal disease alone.

Fungal and Parasitic Infections

The surgical management of fungal infections includes diagnosis and management of complications of fungal disease. Frequently, cancer has to be excluded or other infectious or benign conditions have to be confirmed. Medical management may be considered as initial treatment of fungal diseases in the lung and as part of the patient's overall management.

Immunocompromised patients experience *Aspergillus* spp. infection as the most frequent opportunistic infection followed by *Candida* and *Nocardia* spp. and mucormycosis. Normal, or immunocompetent, patients may be affected by histoplasmosis, coccidioidomycosis, or blastomycosis. Immunocompromised and immunocompetent patients may be affected by actinomycosis and cryptococcosis. Although *Nocardia* and *Actinomyces* spp. are bacteria, they are usually discussed with fungal infections. Diagnosis is most often made by sputum examination using potassium hydroxide preparations (Fig. 57-18). Cultures may take some time for results to be obtained; Papanicolaou test cytology may be best. Silver methenamine stain is used for microscopic evaluation. Most infections are self-limited and do not require treatment. Intravenous or oral antifungal agents may be used for treatment of the diseases.

Aspergillosis is an opportunistic infection, characterized by coarse fragmented septa and hyphae (see Fig. 57-18*A*). There are three types of aspergillosis: aspergilloma, invasive pulmonary aspergillosis, and allergic bronchopulmonary aspergillosis. Aspergilloma is the most common form of aspergillosis. The fungus colonizes an existing lung cavity, commonly a tuberculosis cavity. CXR may demonstrate a crescent radiolucency next to a rounded mass. Cavities may form because of destruction of the underlying pulmonary parenchyma, and debris and hyphae may coalesce and form a fungus ball, which lies free in the cavity and can move with the patient's change in position. Invasion and destruction of parenchymal blood vessels occur within this cavity. Patients with aspergilloma fungus balls are at high risk for fatal hemorrhage; they are treated aggressively and undergo resection when possible.[76] Involvement and destruction of parenchymal blood vessels occur. Prophylactic resection is controversial, although some physicians recommend resection if isolated disease is present in low-risk patients. Surgery is indicated for treatment, for massive or recurrent hemoptysis, or to rule out neoplasm. The procedure of choice is lobectomy. The operation can be complex with a significant inflammatory response within the hilum. Invasive aspergillosis occurs in immunocompromised patients and manifests with chest pain, cough, and hemoptysis. The treatment is primarily medical, although lung biopsy may be necessary for diagnosis. Allergic aspergillosis is diagnosed by bronchoscopy and represents the allergic reaction to chronic colonization with the fungus. It is usually treated medically. Rarely, resection is performed for localized bronchiectasis.

Histoplasmosis is the most common of all fungal infections in the United States and is most frequently a serious systemic fungal disease. *Histoplasma capsulatum* is endemic to the Mississippi and Ohio River valleys as well as portions of the southwestern United States. A high percentage of patients are affected usually with a subclinical form of this disease. An inoculum (from the mycelial form found in soil, decaying materials, and bat or bird guano)

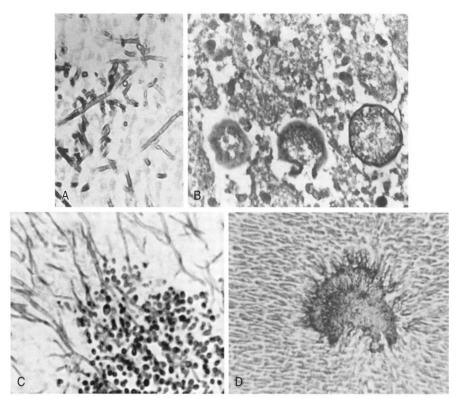

FIGURE 57-18 A, The coarse, fragmented, septate mycelia of *Aspergillus fumigatus.* **B,** Microscopic section of a coccidioidal granuloma (×400) shows spherules packed with endospores. **C,** *Candida albicans* with both the mycelial and the yeast forms. **D,** Actinomycotic granule shows branching filaments of a microscopic colony of *Actinomyces israelii.* (Gomori stain, ×250.) (**A** and **C,** From Takaro T: Thoracic mycotic infections. In *Lewis' practice of surgery,* New York, 1968, Hoeber Medical Division, Harper & Row; **B,** from Scott S, Takaro T: Thoracic mycotic and actinomycotic infections. In Shields TW, editor: *General thoracic surgery,* ed 4, Baltimore, 1994, Williams & Wilkins.)

can produce an acute pneumonic illness in immunocompetent hosts, which usually resolves without specific treatment. The yeast form exists in macrophages or within the cytoplasm of the alveoli. Pathologic examination demonstrates granulomas (e.g., tuberculosis) or caseating epithelioid granulomas. The lymphogenous reaction to *Histoplasma* causes mediastinal lymph node enlargement, middle lobe syndrome, bronchiectasis, esophageal traction diverticulum, broncholithiasis with hemoptysis, tracheoesophageal fistula, constrictive pericarditis, or fibrosing mediastinitis with superior vena cava syndrome or other problems relating to compression of mediastinal structures. In addition to the compressive symptoms, the lymphadenopathy caused by histoplasmosis may confound radiographic evaluation of the mediastinal lymph nodes in patients with lung cancer and may complicate lung resection.

Coccidioidomycosis is endemic to the Southwest and is localized in the soil. It is second only to histoplasmosis in frequency. Inhaling the organism results in a primary lung disease that is usually self-limited (see Fig. 57-18*B*). In endemic areas, coccidioidomycosis is a frequent cause of lung nodules, and resection may be required to rule out malignancy. Medical management is preferred. Surgery may be considered for treatment of cavitary disease or complications of cavitary disease.

Cryptococcosis is the second most common lethal fungus after histoplasmosis. Lungs are frequently involved. Central nervous system involvement with meningitis is the most frequent cause of death. Any patient diagnosed with pulmonary cryptococcosis undergoes lumbar puncture to rule out central nervous system involvement. Surgery may be required for open lung biopsy for diagnosis or to exclude lung cancer.

Mucormycosis is a rare, opportunistic, rapidly progressive infection; it occurs in immunocompromised patients, including patients with diabetes. The appearance is that of a black mold; it has wide nonseptate branching hyphae. The infection causes blood vessels to thrombose and lung tissue to infarct. Clinically, the rhinocerebral form occurs much more frequently than the pulmonary form of consolidation and cavities. Medical management involves cessation of steroids and antineoplastic drugs and initiation of amphotericin and control of diabetes. The disease is often too advanced for effective treatment. Aggressive surgical and medical treatment may improve what is usually a grave prognosis.

Candida is a small, thin-walled budding yeast that occurs in immunocompromised patients (see Fig. 57-18*C*). Lung involvement alone is rare. Surgery may be needed to confirm the diagnosis.

Pneumocystis carinii is an opportunistic infection that is positive on silver methenamine stain. Bronchoalveolar lavage is diagnostic in more than 90% of patients. However, lung biopsy may be required to confirm the diagnosis.

Surgery may also be used to manage the sequelae and complications of parasitic infections. Infections with *Entamoeba histolytica* are usually confined to the right lower thorax and are related to extension from a liver abscess below the diaphragm via direct extension or lymphatics to the right thorax. Metronidazole (Flagyl) is usually effective, although Flagyl and tube drainage may be required for treatment of empyema. Open resection is infrequently required. Similarly, infection with *Echinococcus* spp. may occur. The hydatid cyst may rupture, flooding the lung or producing a severe hypersensitivity reaction. A lung abscess could occur with compression of the airway, great vessels, or esophagus. Surgery, if feasible, may include simple enucleation via cleavage of planes between the cyst and the normal tissue. Aspiration and hypertonic saline 10% may be performed before enucleation. Positive pressure on the lung needs to be maintained until the cyst is out to prevent contamination, soilage, or hypersensitivity reaction. Nonoperative therapy for small asymptomatic calcified cysts may be considered. Paragonimiasis is another common infection and cause of hemoptysis in Asia. In endemic areas, prevalence may be 5%, and hemoptysis from paragonimiasis must be differentiated from tuberculosis or lung cancer.[77]

Actinomycosis is a bacterium that is not found free in nature. It produces a chronic anaerobic endogenous infection deep within a wound. "Sulfur granules" draining from infected sinuses are microcolonies (see Fig. 57-18*D*). The cervicofacial form is the most common. The thoracic form usually occurs as pulmonary parenchymal disease resembling cancer. The treatment is most commonly penicillin. Surgery may occasionally be required for radical excision of chest wall disease and empyema.

Nocardiosis is caused by an aerobic bacterium widely disseminated in soil and domestic animals; it was formerly rare, although it is increasing in immunocompromised patients. Nocardiosis resembles actinomycosis in invading the chest wall and produces subcutaneous abscesses and sinuses draining sulfur granules. Surgery is performed to exclude cancer, to obtain a diagnosis, or to treat complications of the disease. Medical therapy may include sulfonamides.

MASSIVE HEMOPTYSIS

Massive hemoptysis may be defined as greater than 500 to 600 mL of blood loss from the lungs in 24 hours.[78] However, the proximal airways may be occluded with only 150 mL of clotted blood, and even lower volume hemoptysis may be life-threatening.[79] The current mortality rate is approximately 13% and is related to drowning or suffocation rather than exsanguination. Diagnosis and treatment of massive hemoptysis typically include a CXR and emergency rigid bronchoscopy.[80] The major causes of massive hemoptysis are tuberculosis, bronchiectasis, and cancer. Flexible bronchoscopy is usually inadequate for treatment of hemoptysis, but it may be considered for diagnosis, localization of the source of the bleeding, or observation if active bleeding has stopped. Rigid bronchoscopy is recommended.[80,81] Mortality is high with urgent or emergency resection. Conservative management may consist of maintaining a functional and patent airway, bronchoscopy, clearing the airway of blood, cough suppression (with codeine), and monitoring until stabilized.

Angiographic catheterization for massive hemoptysis may be considered in patients with hemoptysis.[82,83] Risks include spinal cord ischemia and paralysis. Small particles of polyvinyl alcohol or other synthetic materials used for embolization occlude vessels

at a peripheral level. Embolization may be repeated.

EMPHYSEMA AND DIFFUSE LUNG DISEASE

Emphysema

Emphysema is defined as dilation and destruction of the terminal air spaces. These air cavities are blebs (subpleural air space separated from the lung by a thin pleural covering with only minor alveolar communications) or bullae (larger than a bleb with some destruction of the underlying lung parenchyma). Bullous emphysema (Fig. 57-19) is either congenital without general lung disease or a complication of COPD with more or less generalized lung disease. The challenge is to separate the disability related to the bullae from that caused by the chronic emphysema or chronic bronchitis. DLCO is a good index of the state of severity of the generalized lung disease. On pulmonary angiography, bullae are vacant and do not contain vessels. The bullae may compress normal lung with crowding of the relatively normal pulmonary vasculature. COPD may show abrupt narrowing and tapering of vessels. Surgical therapy includes resection of the bullae to leave functioning lung tissue. Simple removal of the bullae alone is required. Lobectomy is seldom indicated because good lung tissue is removed, which is frequently needed for independent function by these patients, who have significant lung impairment.

Treatment of emphysema is primarily medical, but there are surgical therapies. Although emphysema usually diffusely involves the lung, it may have a heterogeneous distribution within the lung. These areas may be identified by CT and perfusion scan. Often the disease predominates in the upper lobes and the superior segment of the lower lobes. Lung volume reduction surgery removes areas of greatest emphysematous involvement. The remaining lung tissue expands with improved elastic recoil, improved aeration and perfusion of the remaining lung, and improved chest wall mechanics. The National Emphysema Treatment Trial compared lung volume reduction surgery with the best medical therapy. Patients with predominantly upper lobe emphysema and low exercise capacity had lower mortality with lung volume reduction surgery than medical therapy.[84] In patients with non–upper lobe emphysema and high exercise capacity, mortality was higher in the operative group. Long-term results have been favorable.[85] Endoscopic therapies have been developed, including airway bypass and one-way valves. These devices are still in the investigational stage.

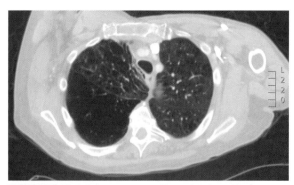

FIGURE 57-19 Bullous emphysema. The patient is a chronic smoker (>100 pack/years) and developed emphysema, which is progressing. The superior segment of the right lower lobe is completely destroyed, and the resultant bullae are compressing functioning lung parenchyma in the right and the left lung.

Lung transplantation is performed for COPD (including α_1-antitrypsin deficiency), pulmonary fibrosis, primary pulmonary hypertension, cystic fibrosis, and bronchiectasis. The survival rates after lung transplantation (all lungs) are approximately 78% at 1 year, 56% at 5 years, and 30% at 10 years.[86] Long-term immunosuppression is required. Unilateral lung transplantation is more readily tolerated than bilateral lung transplantation; however, bilateral lung transplantation is more frequently performed and has a survival advantage after 1 year.

Diffuse Lung Disease

The surgeon's role in diffuse lung disease is to obtain a diagnosis, typically by open lung biopsy after other methods (e.g., transthoracic needle aspiration; bronchoscopy with transbronchial biopsy) have failed. The CXR may demonstrate an alveolar pattern (fluffy with air bronchograms) or an interstitial pattern (ground-glass or granular appearance, indicating a diffuse increase in interstitial tissue) (Box 57-2). Patients may be mildly symptomatic, and biopsy may be needed to confirm or exclude a specific diagnosis before embarking on aggressive medical therapy, such as cyclophosphamide for Wegener granulomatosis, or patients may be critically ill and in the intensive care unit, requiring mechanical ventilation.

Sarcoidosis affects the lungs in 90% of patients with this diagnosis, causing symptoms of dyspnea and dry cough. Foci of non-caseating epithelioid granulomas may be found in any part of the body. In 40% to 50% of cases, patients have insidious respiratory complaints without constitutional symptoms. Severe progressive pulmonary fibrosis may develop in 10% to 20% of patients. Bilateral hilar mediastinal lymph nodes are involved in 60% to 80% of patients. Bronchoscopic lung biopsy is the initial diagnostic procedure. If required, biopsy of mediastinal lymph nodes may be performed. Steroids may be used for treatment.

Lung biopsy may be required for progressive interstitial parenchymal changes for which no diagnosis can be obtained. Lung biopsies can be performed using minimally invasive techniques. Biopsy specimens are sent for routine, fungal, and acid-fast bacillus culture. In immunocompromised patients, *Nocardia* cultures are considered. If possible, the surgeon should sample more than one area of the lung. One method is to resect the worst-appearing region on radiography and the most normal-appearing area. The normal-appearing lung may exhibit early-stage disease and may aid the pathologist in making the diagnosis. Frozen section is used only to confirm that adequate samples of the pathologic process were obtained. In the acute setting of a critically ill patient, an open lung biopsy is performed only when the results would significantly modify subsequent treatment, such as the initiation of protocol-based treatment for experimental antibiotics, or to withdraw futile care.

Adult Respiratory Distress Syndrome

Adult respiratory distress syndrome is a complex biologic and clinical process. Acute deterioration of pulmonary function occurs exclusive of pulmonary edema, pneumonia, or exacerbation of COPD. Approximately 50,000 cases occur each year in the United States, with a mortality rate of 30% to 40%.

The initial clinical presentation of dyspnea, tachypnea, hypoxemia, and mild hypocapnia is nonspecific. CXR may show diffuse bilateral infiltrates secondary to increased interstitial fluid. Pathologically, vascular congestion occurs with alveolar collapse, edema, and inflammatory cell infiltration. The underlying mechanism is increased pulmonary capillary permeability with extravasation of

intravascular fluid and protein into the interstitium and alveoli. The leukocyte is the most prominent mediator of this injury. Stimuli such as sepsis activate the complement pathway, causing recruitment of leukocytes to the site of the infection. The lung releases potent mediators, such as oxygen free radicals, arachidonic acid metabolites, and proteases. If the underlying disease is not controlled, these changes progress to vascular thrombosis and interstitial fibrosis and hyaline membrane deposition in the alveoli. This process causes hypoxemia; pulmonary hypertension; carbon dioxide retention; secondary infections; and eventually right heart failure, hypoxia, and death. Other criteria include

---

BOX 57-2   Classification of Diffuse Lung Diseases

Infections (more commonly cause focal disease, granuloma formation)
  Viruses—especially influenza, cytomegalovirus
  Bacteria—tuberculosis, all types of regular bacteria, Rocky Mountain spotted fever
  Fungi—all types can cause diffuse disease
  Parasites—*Pneumocystis* species infection, toxoplasmosis, paragonimiasis, among others
Occupational causes
  Mineral dusts
  Chemical fumes—NO_2 (silo filler's disease), Cl, NH_3, SO_2, CCl_4, Br, HF, HCl, HNO_3, kerosene, acetylene
Neoplastic disease
  Lymphangitic spread
  Hematogenous metastases
  Leukemia, lymphoma, bronchioloalveolar cell cancer
Congenital—familial
  Niemann-Pick disease, Gaucher disease, neurofibromatosis, and tuberous fibrosis
Metabolic and unknown
  Liver disease, uremia, inflammatory bowel disease
Physical agents
  Radiation, O_2 toxicity, thermal injury, blast injury
Heart failure and multiple pulmonary emboli
Immunologic causes
Hypersensitivity pneumonia
  Inhaled antigens
  Farmer's lung (actinomycosis)
  Bagassosis (sugar cane)
  Malt workers (*Aspergillus* spp.)
  Byssinosis (cotton)
Drug reactions
  Hydralazine, busulfan, nitrofurantoin (Macrodantin), hexamethonium, methysergide, bleomycin
Collagen diseases
  Scleroderma, rheumatoid disease, systemic lupus erythematosus, dermatomyositis, Wegener granulomatosis, Goodpasture syndrome
Other
  Sarcoidosis
  Histiocytosis
  Idiopathic hemosiderosis
  Pulmonary alveolar proteinosis
  Diffuse interstitial fibrosis, idiopathic pulmonary fibrosis
  Desquamative interstitial pneumonia
  Eosinophilic pneumonia (*Note:* some are caused by drugs, actinomycosis, and parasites)
  Lymphangioleiomyomatosis

impaired oxygenation with a PaO_2/FIO_2 ratio of less than 200 mm Hg. Pulmonary edema is present without cardiac failure, and pulmonary capillary wedge pressure is less than 18 mm Hg (noncardiac pulmonary edema).

Treatment is supportive and directed toward improving oxygenation. Maintaining an inspired oxygen concentration as low as possible and positive end-expiratory pressure (PEEP) as low as possible to maintain adequate oxygenation and carbon dioxide exchange is helpful.[87] Tidal volumes and PEEP are kept low; however, increased PEEP may be needed in selected patients to facilitate oxygenation.[88] Based on a more recent meta-analysis, prone or rotational therapy may improve outcomes of these patients.[89]

PULMONARY METASTASES

Isolated pulmonary metastases represent a unique manifestation of systemic spread of a primary neoplasm. Patients with metastases located only within the lungs may be more amenable to local or local and systemic treatment options than other patients with multiorgan metastases. Although primary tumors can be locally controlled with surgery or radiation, extraregional metastases are usually treated with systemic chemotherapy. Radiation therapy may be used to treat or palliate the local manifestations of metastatic disease, particularly when metastases occur within the bony skeleton and cause pain. Resection of solitary and multiple pulmonary metastases from sarcomas and various other primary neoplasms has been performed, with improved long-term survival rates in 40% of patients. Therefore, isolated pulmonary metastases are treatable.

Certain clinical characteristics (prognostic indicators) may be used to select patients with more favorable disease-free and overall survival expectations. Patients who have complete resection of all metastases have associated longer survival than patients whose metastases are unresectable. Long-term survival (>5 years) may be expected in approximately 20% to 30% of all patients with resectable pulmonary metastases. Optimal (and more consistent) survival statistics await improvements in local control, systemic therapy, or regional drug delivery to the lungs.

Surgical Treatment

Predictors for improved survival rate have been studied retrospectively for various tumor types. These predictors may allow the clinician to identify selected patients who would optimally benefit from pulmonary metastasectomy. Patients should have pulmonary parenchymal nodules consistent with metastasis, absence of uncontrolled or untreated extrathoracic metastases, control of the primary tumor, sufficient physiologic and pulmonary reserve to tolerate the operation, and the probability of complete resection. Regardless of histology, patients with pulmonary metastases isolated to the lungs that are completely resected have improved survival rates compared with patients with unresectable metastases. Resectability consistently correlates with improved post-thoracotomy survival rates for patients with pulmonary metastases. In one series of more than 5000 patients with metastases treated with resection, overall actuarial 5-year survival rate was 36%. Favorable clinical indicators included a disease-free interval of greater than 3 years, a SPN, and germ cell histology.[90] Soft tissue sarcomas of all types predominantly metastasize to the lungs. CT usually underestimates the number of metastases by 50% to 100%.

Resection can be accomplished safely. Open or minimally invasive procedures may be used. These procedures have minimal mortality and morbidity. Patients with pulmonary metastases may also undergo multiple procedures for reresection of metastases with prolonged survival expectations after complete resection. VATS procedures limit the ability of the surgeon to palpate the lung to identify occult metastases. Follow-up with radiographic screening at regular intervals is recommended to exclude recurrence.

MISCELLANEOUS LUNG TUMORS

Slow-growing lung tumors may arise from the epithelium, ducts, and glands of the bronchial tree and account for 1% to 2% of all lung neoplasms. Most are of low-grade malignant potential.

Carcinoid tumors (1% of lung neoplasms) arise from Kulchitsky (APUD [amine precursor uptake and decarboxylation]) cells in bronchial epithelium. They have positive histologic reactions to silver staining and to chromogranin. Special stains and examination can identify neurosecretory granules by electron microscopy. These typical carcinoid tumors (least malignant) are the most indolent of the spectrum of pulmonary neuroendocrine tumors that include atypical carcinoid, large cell undifferentiated carcinoma, and small cell carcinoma (most malignant).[91] Histologic findings include less than 2 to 10 mitoses per 10 high-power fields. Peripheral tumors are usually symptom-free, although central tumors may cause endobronchial obstruction with cough, hemoptysis, recurrent infection or pneumonia, bronchiectasis, lung abscess, pain, or wheezing. Symptoms may persist for many years without diagnosis, particularly if only an endobronchial component partially obstructs the airway. Carcinoid syndrome (flushing, tachycardia, wheezing, and diarrhea) is uncommon and occurs with large tumors or extensive metastatic disease. Bronchoscopy is usually positive, unless the nodule or mass is peripheral. Most carcinoids can be identified in this matter; although they tend to bleed, biopsy can usually be performed safely.

Atypical carcinoid may have lymph node or vascular invasion with metastasis. The location is in the mainstem bronchi (20%), lobar bronchi (70% to 75%), or peripheral bronchi (5% to 10%). They rarely occur in the trachea. Local invasion with involvement of peribronchial tissue occurs. At bronchoscopy, most carcinoids are sessile, although a few are polypoid. The histology is that of small uniform cells with oval nuclei and interlacing cords of vascular connective tissue stroma. Mitoses are infrequent, but occasionally bizarre cells are noted. Atypical carcinoids are more pleomorphic and have more mitoses (>2 to 10 mitoses per 10 high-power fields) than typical carcinoid. They have more prominent nucleoli but are more monotonous and have more cytoplasm than oat cell carcinoma. These tumors are more aggressive, with a 5-year survival rate of approximately 60%. Tumors tend to metastasize to the liver, bone, or adrenal. Electron microscopy can be used to identify neurosecretory granules.

Surgical resection is standard, with complete removal of the tumor and as much preservation of lung as possible.[92] Lobectomy is the most common procedure; endoscopic removal is performed only for rare polypoid tumors if thoracotomy is contraindicated. Survival rate is typically 85% at 5 to 10 years. Large cell neuroendocrine tumors and small cell cancer are not typically treated with surgery and may be best treated with combinations of chemotherapy and radiation; survival of these patients is poor.

Adenoid cystic carcinoma is a slow-growing malignancy involving the trachea and mainstem bronchi that is similar to salivary gland tumors.[93] Adenoid cystic carcinoma is more malignant than carcinoid tumors and has a slight female preponderance. The tumor typically involves the lower trachea, carina, and take-off of the mainstem bronchi. Stridor is often the presenting symptom of adenoid cystic tumors because these tumors are most often found in the trachea and mainstem bronchi. One third of patients have tumors that have metastasized at the time of treatment. These patients typically have involvement of the perineural lymphatics; regional nodes; or liver, bone, or kidneys. The tumor arises from ducts in the submucosa and extends proximally and distally in that plane. Microscopic examination demonstrates cells with large nuclei and a small cytoplasm and surrounding cystic spaces (pseudoacinar type); the medullary type has a Swiss cheese appearance. Treatment is wide en bloc resection with conservation of as much lung tissue as possible.[94] Radiation treatment alone may be effective in patients not amenable to surgical resection.

Benign tumors of the lung account for less than 1% of all lung neoplasms and arise from mesodermal origins (Box 57-3). Hamartomas are the most frequent benign lung tumor; they consist of normal tissue elements found in an abnormal location. Hamartomas are manifested by overgrowth of cartilage. Hamartomas are typically identified in patients 40 to 60 years old and have a 2:1 male-to-female predominance. They are usually peripheral and slow-growing. CXR demonstrates a 2- to 3-cm mass that is sharply demarcated and frequently lobulated. It is usually not calcified, but the "popcorn" appearance on CXR may provide the diagnosis

of hamartoma. Cystic adenomatoid malformation may represent adenomatous hamartomas, which occur in infants as cysts or immature elements in the lung.

Very low-grade malignancies include hemangiopericytoma and pulmonary blastoma that arises from embryonic lung tissue. Treatment is resection. Tumorlets are epithelial proliferative lesions that may resemble oat cell carcinoma or carcinoid. These are typically incidental findings noted on examination of resected lung specimens. They rarely metastasize.

Primary sarcomas of the lung occur rarely. Resection, similar to lung carcinoma, is feasible in 50% to 60% of patients.[95] Prognosis of patients with leiomyosarcoma is excellent, with approximately a 50% survival rate at 5 years; all other sarcomas have poor survival expectations.

Lymphoma of the lung most commonly occurs as disseminated lymphoma involving the lung. Disseminated lymphoma occurs in 40% of patients with Hodgkin disease and 7% of patients with non-Hodgkin disease. Primary lymphoma of the lung is rare. The diagnosis is usually made at surgery. A thorough evaluation for other primary sites of lymphoma is done if primary pulmonary lymphoma is suspected preoperatively.

CHEST WALL

Pectus Excavatum

Pectus excavatum is the most common chest wall deformity, occurring in 1 of 400 children with a male predominance (4:1).[96] More than 30% of cases have a family history of chest wall anomalies. Pectus excavatum refers to the sternal depression (depressed dorsally) caused by unequal growth rates or development of the lower ribs and costal cartilages (usually after the third rib). The sternum is not depressed equally or symmetrically and is also rotated. This syndrome may be associated with other musculoskeletal abnormalities. Most patients are asymptomatic, but some have decreased exercise capacity or pulmonary reserve. Patients are evaluated with plain CXRs, CT scans, pulmonary function studies, ventilation-perfusion lung scans, and other physiologic studies.

Surgical repair of pectus excavatum can be accomplished by various techniques, including sternal osteotomy, osteotomy with posterior strut or other stabilization (e.g., a metal plate), removing the sternum and turning it over with stabilization, placement of a prosthesis to fill the defect, and placement of an internal (posterior) sternal support (which is more effective in younger patients than older patients). Open techniques typically reflect the overlying pectoralis major and the rectus muscles. Involved costal cartilages are removed, leaving the perichondrium. The sternum is mobilized and stabilized. The muscles are reapproximated in the midline over the repair.

Pectus carinatum (also called *pigeon breast*) refers to the anterior protrusion of the sternum and costal cartilages and occurs with a male predominance (4:1). This condition is approximately five times less likely to occur than pectus excavatum.

Poland syndrome is a rare, nonfamilial disease of unknown cause that occurs in 1 in 30,000 births. Characteristics of this syndrome include absence of the pectoralis major muscle, absence or hypoplasia of the pectoralis minor muscle, absence of costal cartilages, hypoplasia of breast and subcutaneous tissue (including the nipple complex), and various hand anomalies.

Chest Wall Tumors

Chest wall tumors[97,98] are rare. The most frequent chest wall tumors are metastatic tumors related to metastasis to the chest

---

BOX 57-3   Miscellaneous Lung Tumors

Hamartoma
Epithelial origin tumors
　Papilloma—single or multiple, squamous epithelium, occurs in childhood, probably viral, may require bronchial resection but frequently recur
　Polyp—inflammatory-squamous metaplasia on a stalk; bronchial resection may be needed; these do not usually recur
Mesodermal origin tumors
　Fibroma—most frequent mesodermal tumor
　Chondroma
　Lipoma
　Leiomyoma—intrabronchial or peripheral; conservative resection
Granular cell tumors
　Rhabdomyoma
　Neuroma
　Hemangioma—subglottic larynx or upper trachea of infants; radiation therapy
　Lymphangioma—similar to cystic hygroma; upper airway obstruction in neonates
　Hemangioendothelioma—newborn lungs, often progressive and lethal
　Lymphangiomyomatosis—rare, slowly progressive; death from pulmonary insufficiency; fine, multinodular lesions, loss of parenchyma and honeycombing; usually women in their reproductive years
　Arteriovenous fistula—congenital, right-to-left shunt; cyanosis, dyspnea on exertion, clubbing, brain abscess; associated with hereditary hemorrhagic telangiectasia of lower lobes
Inflammatory tumors and pseudotumors
　Plasma cell granuloma
　Pseudolymphoma
　Xanthoma
Teratoma

wall from another primary tumor. Primary chest wall tumors are typically sarcomas of the chest wall (rib). Primary bone tumors can occur in the ribs, scapula, and sternum as well (Table 57-3).

Clinical presentation of chest wall tumors can range from an enlarging painless mass to a painful and fungating mass. Pain can occur with periosteal invasion. Local tumor extension onto the lung or mediastinum can create associated symptoms. Evaluation requires diagnostic imaging such as CXR, CT, and FDG-PET. MRI is effective for tumors involving the thoracic inlet or upper chest that may involve the brachial plexus or tumors that involve or abut the vertebral bodies. Histologic confirmation is required. A core needle biopsy is frequently effective. Excisional biopsy with minimal contamination of the surgical site may be required for a larger tumor. Consideration for future resection may dictate size and location of the incisional biopsy. Resection and

reconstruction with prosthesis or muscle flaps can be accomplished with excellent results. A multidisciplinary approach to treatment is complemented by a multispecialty team in the operating room.

Bone Tumors

Benign bone tumors include fibrous dysplasia of the bone, which accounts for approximately 30% of these tumors. Chondromas account for 15% to 20% of benign chest wall lesions and arise from the anterior costochondral junction. Osteochondroma occurs commonly in young men as an asymptomatic tumor originating from the cortex of the rib. Eosinophilic granuloma is a benign component of malignant fibrous histiocytosis and primarily affects men. Skull and rib involvement are common and appear as expansile lesions on radiographic evaluation. Excisional biopsy is indicated for solitary lesions, and radiotherapy is indicated for multiple lesions. Aneurysmal bone cysts occur in the ribs and may be associated with previous trauma. Radiographic characteristics include a blow-out lytic lesion (Fig. 57-20). Resection is recommended for diagnosis and for relief of pain.

Malignant bone tumors include chondrosarcoma, which is the most common malignant tumor of the chest wall, accounting for 20% of all bone tumors. Chondrosarcomas arise in the third and fourth decades of life. Radiographic characteristics include a poorly defined tumor mass that is destroying cortical bone. Resection with wide margins (3 to 5 cm) is the treatment of choice. The 5-year survival after complete resection is

TABLE 57-3	**Classification of Tumors of the Chest Wall**	
	BENIGN	**MALIGNANT**
Bony Tissue		
Bone	Osteoid osteoma	Osteosarcoma
	Aneurysmal bone cyst	Ewing sarcoma
Cartilage	Enchondroma	Chondrosarcoma
	Osteochondroma	
Fibrous	Fibrous dysplasia	Malignant fibrous histiocytoma
Marrow	Eosinophilic granuloma	Plasmacytoma
Vascular	Hemangioma	Hemangiosarcoma
Soft Tissue		
Adipose	Lipoma and variations	Liposarcoma
Muscle	Leiomyoma	Leiomyosarcoma
	Rhabdomyoma	Rhabdomyosarcoma
Neural	Neurofibroma	Neurofibrosarcoma
	Neurilemoma	Malignant schwannoma
		Askin tumor (primitive neuroectodermal tumor)
Fibrous	Desmoid	Fibrosarcoma

Adapted from Faber LP, Somers J, Templeton AC: Chest wall tumors. *Curr Probl Surg* 32:661–747, 1995.

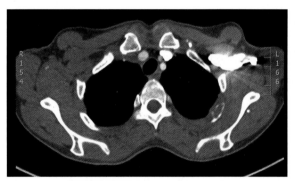

FIGURE 57-20 Aneurysmal bone cyst.

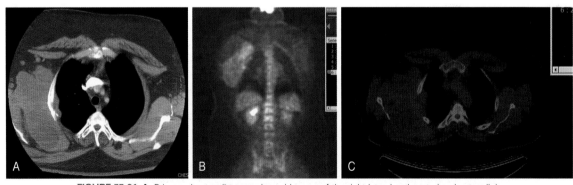

FIGURE 57-21 **A,** Primary chest wall tumor, desmoid tumor of the right lateral and posterior chest wall, is shown on computed tomography (CT) image. **B,** 18F-Fluorodeoxyglucose positron emission tomography (FDG-PET) demonstrates mild FDG avidity. No sites of metastases were identified. **C,** A fused image of CT and FDG-PET is shown. Resection of the tumor included chest wall musculature and chest wall. Reconstruction was performed with prosthetic material, and a muscle flap was required.

approximately 70%. Osteosarcoma (osteogenic sarcoma) most frequently arises in the long bones of adolescents and young adults. Primary osteosarcomas in the chest account for 10% to 15% of malignant tumors. The tumor grows rapidly, and radiographic characteristics include a sunburst pattern on CXR. Ewing sarcoma commonly arises in bones of the pelvis, humerus, or femur of young men. It is the third most common malignant chest wall tumor (5% to 10%). The radiographic characteristics include an onion-peel appearance with periosteal elevation and bony remodeling. With multimodality therapy, 5-year survival is 50%. Solitary plasmacytoma is a rare tumor that occurs in older men as a painful solitary tumor arising from plasma cells. Multiple myeloma is the same tumor arising in more than one location. Radiographic characteristics include a diffuse, moth-eaten or punched-out appearance of the bone. Systemic disease can be confirmed using serum protein electrophoresis, urinalysis (Bence-Jones protein), and bone marrow aspiration. Local radiotherapy for solitary plasmacytoma is recommended.

Soft Tissue Tumors

Soft tissue sarcomas are the most common malignant primary chest wall tumors.[98,99] Core needle or incisional biopsy is performed to establish the diagnosis (Fig. 57-21). Resection with wide local excision (3 to 5 cm) is required. These tumors should not be shelled out despite the presence of a pseudocapsule. Complete resection is associated with excellent local control and prolonged survival. Combinations of chemotherapy and radiation therapy may be used as components of the multidisciplinary treatment plan.

Metastatic Tumors

Metastatic neoplasms may involve the chest wall by direct extension, by lymphatic metastasis, or by hematogenous metastasis. Lung cancer and breast cancer can involve the chest wall by direct extension, and if identified, chest wall resection should be performed concurrently with resection of the primary neoplasm.

Reconstruction

Reconstruction of the chest wall depends on the size, location, and cosmetic and functional impairment that results from resection. Prevention of flail chest and maintenance of physiologic stability requires careful judgment regarding the choice of prosthetic reconstruction, autologous tissue coverage available including myocutaneous flaps, and free tissue flap transfer.

Chest Wall Infections

Chest wall infections may occur after thoracic surgery, thoracic trauma, or other interventions. Inflammatory breast carcinoma is not an infection but may mimic a chest wall infection. Biopsy may be needed to confirm the diagnosis. Mondor disease, thrombophlebitis of the superficial veins of the breast and anterior chest wall, is also not an infection. Ultrasound or biopsy may be necessary to confirm the diagnosis. Tietze syndrome or costochondritis is usually self-limited and can be treated with nonsteroidal anti-inflammatory drugs and rest. Because of the limited blood supply to the cartilage, infection in this area may be difficult to diagnose. Débridement and reconstruction may be necessary. Sternal wound infections are complications following median sternotomy or cardiac surgery. Spontaneous primary chest wall infections can arise from various sources as a consequence of immunosuppression, drug-resistant organisms including tuberculosis, or HIV infection.

Chest Wall Trauma

Trauma to the chest wall is common. CXR and chest CT scan are obtained often as part of the secondary survey in chest wall trauma. CT can identify rib, parenchymal, or other abnormalities. Blunt chest wall trauma commonly results in contusion of the chest wall tissues and the underlying lung parenchyma. Supportive care is warranted.

Rib fractures are perhaps the most common traumatic injury sustained after blunt chest wall trauma. Symptoms include pain on inspiration and localized point tenderness. Plain films can confirm the diagnosis. Fractures of the first or second ribs may occur after significant trauma or high-velocity injury. Because of the size and thickness of the first rib, tremendous force is needed to fracture this rib. This traumatic event is associated with aortic disruption. Contusion or injury to underlying structures should be suspected with any rib fracture. Contusion of the lung parenchyma and injury to the spleen, liver, diaphragm, or kidney can occur. Treatment with analgesia and nerve blocks can be helpful. Flail chest may occur with multiple rib fractures. Flail chest results in an unstable chest wall that develops paradoxical motion during respiration (e.g., depression during the negative inspiratory phase and extrusion during the positive expiratory phase). Flail chest is often associated with an underlying pulmonary contusion and should be supported with pain relief, stabilization of the chest wall, or even mechanical ventilation.

Sternal injuries are uncommon and may result from blunt trauma to the anterior chest, typically from a steering wheel injury during a motor vehicle accident. An underlying cardiac injury, such as aortic disruption, cardiac contusion, pericardial effusion, or arrhythmia, must be considered. Heart rhythm monitoring, serial cardiac observations with electrocardiography and cardiac enzymes, and echocardiography are used to exclude these injuries. Clavicular fractures may be associated with injury to the great vessels or the brachial plexus. Supportive care and stabilization are recommended.

THORACIC OUTLET SYNDROME

Thoracic outlet syndrome (TOS) refers to compression of the subclavian vessels and nerves of the brachial plexus in the region of the thoracic inlet. Symptoms most commonly develop secondary to neural compromise; however, vascular and neurovascular symptoms are reported.[100] Middle-aged women are most commonly affected by TOS. The subclavian vessels and the brachial plexus can be compressed at various locations as they pass between the thoracic inlet and the upper extremity (Fig. 57-22). From medial to lateral, these anatomic regions are as follows:
1. Interscalene triangle (artery and nerves)
2. Costoclavicular space (vein)
3. Subcoracoid area (artery, vein, nerves)

Diagnosis

The symptoms associated with TOS vary depending on the anatomic structure that is compressed. Neurogenic manifestations are reported in more than 90% of cases. Symptoms of subclavian artery compression include fatigue, weakness, coldness, upper extremity claudication, thrombosis, and paresthesia. Thrombosis with distal embolization rarely can occur, producing vasomotor symptoms (Raynaud phenomenon) in the hand or ischemic changes. Venous compression results in edema, venous distention, collateral formation, and cyanosis of the affected limb. Venous

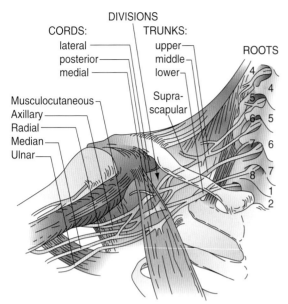

DIVISIONS

CORDS: TRUNKS:
lateral — upper—
posterior— middle— ROOTS
medial — lower—

Supra-
scapular

Musculocutaneous—
Axillary
Radial
Median
Ulnar—

4
4
5
6 5
6
7
8 7
1
2

FIGURE 57-22 Detailed view of brachial plexus. (From Urschel HC, Razzuk M: Upper plexus thoracic outlet syndrome: Optimal therapy. *Ann Thorac Surg* 63:935–939, 1997.)

TOS may be characterized by upper extremity edema, venous distention, or effort thrombosis, also known as *Paget-Schroetter syndrome.*

The diagnosis of neurogenic TOS is initially made clinically. Objective evaluation for TOS includes chest and cervical spine films. A cervical rib or bony degenerative cervical spine changes may be present.[101] CT, MRI, and cervical myelography are sometimes helpful to rule out narrowing of the intervertebral foramina or cervical disc pathology. Doppler studies or vascular imaging (angiography/venography) may be indicated if the extent of vascular impairment cannot be determined clinically or if an aneurysm or venous thrombosis is suspected. Neurogenic TOS needs to be confirmed with nerve conduction studies to localize the area of slowing of nerve conduction and to rule out other compression syndromes, such as carpal tunnel syndrome. Electromyelography and nerve conduction studies are helpful to rule out carpal tunnel syndrome. Patients with moderate to severe slowing of nerve conduction usually respond to nonoperative therapy. Vascular TOS must be confirmed with objective studies.[102]

Clinical maneuvers to evaluate a patient suspected to have TOS are performed to identify the loss or decrease of radial pulse or to reproduce neurologic symptoms. A clear objective validated definition for TOS is needed. Evocative tests to illicit symptoms include the following:

- Adson (scalene) test. The patient inspires maximally and holds his or her breath while the neck is fully extended and the head is turned toward the affected side. This maneuver narrows the space between the scalenus anticus and medius, resulting in compression of the subclavian artery and the brachial plexus. Decrease or loss of ipsilateral radial pulse suggests compression.
- Halsted (costoclavicular) test. The patient is instructed to place his or her shoulders in a military position (drawn backward and downward) to narrow the costoclavicular space between the first rib and the clavicle, causing neurovascular compression. Reproduction of neurologic symptoms or decrease or loss of ipsilateral radial pulse suggests compression.

- Wright (hyperabduction) test. The patient's arm is hyperabducted 180 degrees, which causes the neurovascular structures to be compressed in the subcoracoid region by the pectoralis tendon, the head of the humerus, or the coracoid process. Decrease or loss of ipsilateral radial pulse suggests compression.
- Roos test. The patient abducts the involved arm 90 degrees with external rotation of the shoulder. Maintaining this body position, the modified Roos test is performed by opening and closing the hand rapidly for 3 minutes in an attempt to reproduce symptoms. Additionally, neurogenic compromise may be detected using provocative tests, such as percussion of the nerve (Tinel sign) or flexion of the elbow or wrist (Phalen sign).

Management

Results of treatment of TOS are variable because there are inconsistent objective criteria for the diagnosis of TOS other than

---

BOX 57-4   Pleural Effusions

Cause of Transudative Effusions
Congestive heart failure
Cirrhosis
Nephrotic syndrome
Hypoalbuminemia
Fluid retention/overload
Pulmonary embolism
Lobar collapse
Meigs syndrome

Cause of Exudative Effusions
Malignant
  Primary lung or metastatic carcinoma
  Lymphoma
  Mesothelioma
Infectious
  Bacterial (parapneumonic)/empyema
  Tuberculosis
  Fungal
  Viral
  Parasitic
Collagen vascular disease related
  Rheumatoid arthritis
  Wegener granulomatosis
  Systemic lupus erythematosus
  Churg-Strauss syndrome
Abdominal/gastrointestinal disease related
  Esophageal perforation
  Subphrenic abscess
  Pancreatitis/pancreatic pseudocyst
  Meigs syndrome
Others
  Chylothorax
  Uremia
  Sarcoidosis
  After coronary artery bypass grafting
  Radiation/trauma
  Dressler syndrome
  Pulmonary embolism with infarction
  Asbestosis related

clinical diagnosis. Initial management of TOS is nonoperative. Physical therapy is needed. Repetitive upper extremity mechanical work and muscular trauma are eliminated. Indications for operation include failure of conservative management, progressive neurologic symptoms, prolonged ulnar or median nerve conduction velocities, narrowing or occlusion of the subclavian artery, and thrombosis of the axillary or subclavian vein. Operative management can provide excellent results.[103] Objective agreed-on outcome measures and clinical trials are needed to compare outcomes of surgery for TOS compared with no surgery.[104] Success rates with surgery only approach 70% at 5 years. Recurrent symptoms may prompt operation in up to one third of patients.

PLEURA

Pleural Effusions

The pleural space is a potential space defined normally by the small amount of pleural fluid separating the visceral and parietal pleura. Many benign and malignant pleural space problems can disrupt the balance of fluid production and absorption leading to various pleural space problems, including increased mass effect from air, fluid, or tumor on the ipsilateral lung parenchyma and heart, infection, or dyspnea and pulmonary dysfunction. The cause of pleural effusions is quite varied (Box 57-4).

The movement of fluid across the pleural membranes is governed by Starling's law of capillary exchange. The amount of pleural fluid is controlled by a balance of oncotic and hydrostatic pressure within the pleural space and the pleural capillaries. Under normal circumstances, the net pressure moves fluid from the parietal pleura into the pleural space. It is estimated that 5 to 10 liters of fluid are produced and transgress the pleural space over a 24-hour period. However, the normal volume of pleural fluid is quite small. The balance of forces favors fluid reabsorption from the pleural cavity across the visceral pleura. Under physiologic conditions, most pleural fluid is reabsorbed through lymphatics of the parietal pleura because protein that enters the pleural space cannot enter the relatively impermeable visceral pleura. The parietal pleura and its lymphatics have significant capacity for protein and fluid removal. A small imbalance of accumulation and absorption can lead to the development of a pleural effusion. The causative factors include increased hydrostatic pressure, increased negative intrapleural pressure, increased capillary permeability, decreased plasma oncotic pressure, and decreased or interrupted lymphatic drainage.

Pleural fluid is characterized as a transudate or an exudate. Transudative effusions are protein-poor and result in change in fluid balance in the pleural space. Exudative effusions are protein-rich and may be related to disruption of pleural or lymphatic reabsorption. After drainage, the fluid is evaluated by Light's criteria.[105] An exudate is defined as (1) pleural fluid protein–to–serum protein ratio greater than 0.5, (2) pleural fluid lactate dehydrogenase (LDH)–to–serum LDH ratio greater than 0.6, or (3) pleural fluid LDH 1.67 times the normal serum level or higher. In addition, pleural fluid should be assessed for its visual characteristics (serous, bloody, milky, turbid, or frankly purulent). Pleural fluid should be analyzed for cytology; cell counts; Gram stain; culture for aerobic, anaerobic, and fungal organisms; tuberculosis testing; and chemistry with simultaneous pleural and serum protein, glucose, LDH, and pH. The treatment goals for patients with pleural effusion include obtaining a diagnosis, relieving or eliminating symptoms such as dyspnea, optimizing patient function, minimizing or eliminating hospitalization, and minimizing costs of care.

Benign Pleural Effusions

Most benign pleural effusions are transudates, free-flowing, without loculation, and treatment should be directed toward the underlying cause, such as congestive heart failure, ascites, or malnutrition. Symptoms are typically dyspnea or cough. Pleural fluid can be identified on CXR; the presence of 300 mL of fluid causes blunting of the costophrenic angle on upright CXR. Clinical examination can detect 500 mL of fluid or greater. Initial thoracentesis should achieve complete drainage for diagnosis and treatment. In addition, radiographic evidence of complete re-expansion of the lung should be sought. Failure of the lung to expand completely suggests a "trapped" lung, which may require decortication, particularly if symptoms, such as dyspnea, persist. Relief of symptoms with thoracentesis usually indicates the pleural effusion as the cause. Occasionally, symptoms are not relieved by thoracentesis, and an alternative diagnosis is required.

Recurrent effusions can occur, and repeat thoracenteses may be required. Alternative therapies, such as chest tube insertion (tube thoracostomy) or thoracoscopic drainage with or without mechanical and chemical pleurodesis, can be considered. Visceral and parietal pleural apposition is required to achieve pleurodesis. Drainage of the effusion can be diagnostic and therapeutic. Sclerosing agents can be placed to facilitate pleural symphysis. This pleurodesis is most effectively accomplished with slurry of 5 g of talc in 100 mL of saline placed through the chest tube. Video-assisted thoracoscopic drainage of effusions can also be diagnostic and therapeutic. Pleural biopsy or wedge resection of the lung can be easily performed to facilitate diagnosis. Mechanical pleural abrasion or chemical pleurodesis with talc is typically used. The talc is insufflated within the hemithorax to cover all visceral pleural surfaces (e.g., talc poudrage). Pleurectomy is not commonly needed; however, persistent pleural effusions and trapped lung may not be amenable to more conservative measures. Decortication may be required.

Malignant Pleural Effusion

Patients with known or previous malignancy can develop MPE. In 25% of MPEs, a histologic diagnosis of cancer is not made within the fluid after two thoracenteses. Drainage is required for relief of dyspnea (Fig. 57-23).

MPE is an effusion with positive cytopathology. Not all pleural effusions associated with malignancy are caused by direct or metastatic pleural involvement. Other mechanisms for their development (bronchial or lymphatic obstruction, hypoproteinemia, and sympathetic accumulation from infradiaphragmatic involvement) exist. Although repeated cytologic evaluation of a pleural effusion achieves high positive and negative predictive values, this diagnostic procedure has important limitations. A cancer diagnosis is obtained after three thoracenteses in 70% to 80% of patients. Thoracoscopy is diagnostic in 92% of patients.

A patient with MPE has a median survival of 90 days.[106] Patients with breast cancer and MPE have a median survival of approximately 5 months; patients with lymphoma typically have a longer median survival.[107] Local treatment of MPE does not affect the systemic disease process but may provide significant symptomatic relief. Complications of treatments include hemothorax, loculation of fluid, empyema, failure of pleurodesis with recurrence of effusion, and lung entrapment caused by inexpansile lung. Open surgical pleurectomy and pleurodesis are reserved for patients who fail other therapies and who have a reasonably long life expectancy. A phase 3 study demonstrated that a long-term indwelling pleural catheter was as effective as chest tube drainage

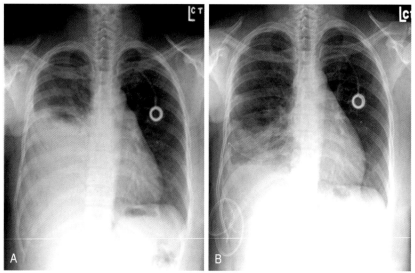

FIGURE 57-23 A, Malignant pleural effusion causing dyspnea. A long-term indwelling pleural catheter was placed as an outpatient procedure to facilitate drainage at home to prevent dyspnea. Hospitalization was not required. **B,** Following drainage. A long-term indwelling pleural catheter is effective in patients with trapped lung. Every-other-day drainage reduces impairment of the contralateral lung and prevents mediastinal shift.

with doxycycline pleurodesis.[108] Talc slurry following chest tube insertion and drainage of the effusion is as effective as VATS with talc pleurodesis.[109]

Empyema

Empyema is an infection of the pleural space and commonly an exudate.[110] Empyemas progress from an acute phase with fluid that is thin and can be drained completely with a chest tube or small bore catheter. This process typically worsens as the fluid becomes more turbid and thick and begins to loculate. Mucopurulent debris occurs within the pleural space and compresses the underlying lung parenchyma. The organizing or chronic phase is reflected in more lung entrapment with capillary ingrowth and creation of a pleural rind, which traps the lung.

An empyema typically occurs after a reactive pleural effusion as a consequence of a lung infection.[111] These infections historically were due to streptococcal or pneumococcal pneumonia; at the present time, gram-negative and anaerobic organisms are common causes of empyema. Tuberculous empyema can also be identified. Empyema can follow trauma or thoracic surgery (from residual pleural space or bronchopleural fistula), hematologic spread, rupture of a pulmonary or mediastinal abscess, or esophageal perforation.

Symptoms typically include constitutional symptoms of general malaise, fever, loss of appetite, and weight loss. Cough and dyspnea are common if lung infection is present. Evaluation includes CXR, posterior row anterior and lateral, and CT scan of the chest and upper abdomen.

Treatment of empyema depends on the extent of the disease and its location.[112] Complete and dependent drainage are required. Antibiotics and supportive care (e.g., fluids, nutrition, skin care) are commonly initiated. Use of fibrinolytic agents can be effective. Intrapleural tissue plasminogen activator and DNase when used together improve drainage of pleural fluid in patients with pleural infection or loculations and reduce the need for surgical drainage.[113]

Simple dependent and complete drainage is required for successful outcomes. This dependent drainage can be achieved easily with posterior rib resection and insertion of an empyema tube. This technique can be effective and can minimize operative time for patients who are critically ill or septic. Complete expansion of the lung may not be achieved at the time of the operation; however, with time and drainage, the lung typically reexpands, and the space closes. VATS decortication and thoracotomy with débridement or formal decortication in later stage empyema is reserved for treatment failures with persistent symptoms of dyspnea, loculations, or continued sepsis.

Bronchopleural fistula after lobectomy or pneumonectomy predisposes to empyema. Management of bronchopleural fistula requires evaluation of the underlying cause of the fistula, drainage of the infection, and obliteration of the residual pleural space along with general supportive care. Chronic empyema with a residual pleural space can be treated with drainage, gauze packing, or skin flap (Eloesser flap) with eventual muscle transposition and skin closure. Lung resection or pleuropneumonectomy is rarely required.

Chylothorax

Chylothorax occurs when chyle from the thoracic duct empties into the pleural space.[114] Chyle is a milky white fluid with a high concentration of triglycerides and chylomicrons and white blood cells. It is nutritionally rich and depends on the nutritional and dietary status of the patient. It may be clear. Chylothorax has multiple causes (Box 57-5).

Symptoms from chylothorax include dyspnea or cough. In addition, because of the nutritional consequences of chronic chyle leak (e.g., loss of fat, protein) and the volume of the leak (0.5 to 3.0 liters per day), fluid and nutritional replacement and correction of the underlying problem are necessary. The diagnosis may be made with thoracentesis or drainage of the fluid with a chest tube. Analysis of pleural fluid with chylomicrons confirms the diagnosis. Conservative measures, such as medium-chain triglyceride diet or total parenteral nutrition, are used initially. If conservative measures fail, operative intervention may be considered between days 7 and 14. Commonly ligation of thoracic duct where it enters the chest through the diaphragmatic hiatus is achieved via a right thoracotomy or thoracoscopy. Placement of olive oil or ice cream by nasogastric tube at the time of the operation may increase chyle drainage into the operative field and help to identify the area of thoracic duct disruption. Percutaneous techniques with needle cannulation and duct occlusion have been proposed.[115]

Pneumothorax

Pneumothorax is the accumulation of air within the pleural space and may occur as a result of trauma, surgery, needle aspiration, central line insertion, increased pressure from mechanical ventilation, or lung diseases (e.g., COPD, cystic or pulmonary fibrosis)

> **BOX 57-5 Chylothorax**
>
> Traumatic (chest and neck)
>   Blunt
>   Penetrating
> Iatrogenic
>   Catheterization, particularly subclavian vein
>   Postsurgical
>   Excision of cervical/supraclavicular lymph nodes
>   Radical lymph node dissections of the neck or chest
>   Lung, esophageal, or mediastinal resection
>   Thoracic aneurysm repair
>   Sympathectomy
>   Congenital cardiovascular surgery
> Neoplasms
>   Lymphoma, lung, esophageal, or mediastinal neoplasms
>   Metastatic carcinoma
> Infectious
>   Tuberculous lymphadenosis
>   Mediastinitis
>   Ascending lymphangitis
> Other
>   Lymphangioleiomyomatosis
>   Venous thrombosis
> Congenital

> **BOX 57-6 Pneumothorax**
>
> | | |
> |---|---|
> | Spontaneous | Traumatic |
> | Primary | Penetrating |
> | Secondary | Blunt |
> | • COPD | Iatrogenic |
> | • Bullous disease | Mechanical ventilation |
> | • Cystic fibrosis | Needle puncture: thoracentesis, |
> | • *Pneumocystis* related | FNA lung nodule, central line |
> | • Congenital cysts | insertion |
> | • IPF | Postsurgical |
> | • Pulmonary embolism | |
> | Catamenial | |
> | Neonatal | |
>
> *COPD*, Chronic obstructive pulmonary disease; *FNA*, fine-needle aspiration; *IPF*, Idiopathic pulmonary fibrosis.

---

or other conditions (e.g., catamenial pneumothorax) (Box 57-6). A primary spontaneous pneumothorax occurs as a consequence of subpleural blebs or other pulmonary disease. Tension pneumothorax occurs when air continues to enter the pleural space without decompression. This problem results in positive intrathoracic pressure causing compression of the lung and mediastinum, shift of the mediastinum into the contralateral chest, and decrease in ventilation and venous return. Cardiopulmonary collapse and death ensue. Immediate decompression with needle or chest tube insertion is lifesaving.

Symptoms of pneumothorax include pain and dyspnea. Patients with spontaneous pneumothorax are usually tall and thin young men. Diagnostic imaging includes CXR and occasionally CT. Apical blebs and bullae are common. CT scan can be performed to assess for the cause of spontaneous pneumothorax or the presence of other occult lung disease. Subcutaneous emphysema may or may not be present.

Treatment depends on size and symptoms. Smaller pneumothorax may be followed and may resolve spontaneously, particularly pneumothorax that occurs after needle aspiration for lung biopsy. Progression in the size of pneumothorax requires intervention with drainage. Initial spontaneous pneumothorax may be treated with small bore catheter drainage or chest tube and drainage with resolution of the air space and cessation of air leak. Persistent air leak (>72 hours) or failure of the lung to expand fully suggests additional intervention may be needed.

Operative intervention is recommended for patients who have a persistence or recurrence of spontaneous pneumothorax or who develop a contralateral pneumothorax. High-risk professions (e.g., scuba diver, airplane pilot) should be avoided. Operative repair typically includes thoracoscopy to identify apical blebs, which are resected with endoscopic staplers. Mechanical abrasion of the parietal pleura is performed. Pleurodesis with talc in patients with malignancy or in older patients may be considered.

Mesothelioma

Mesothelioma is a rare neoplasm that arises from mesothelial cells lining the parietal and visceral pleura and can manifest in a localized or diffuse manner. Pathology of pleural tumors has been reviewed elsewhere.[20] Mesothelioma develops from the mesothelial cells that line the pleural cavity. Histologic subtypes include epithelial, sarcomatoid, or mixed histology.[116] Epithelial histology alone has a more favorable prognosis.

The localized variant, the solitary fibrous tumor of the pleura, is a rare benign neoplasm that usually manifests as a well-defined, encapsulated tumor that is not associated with asbestos exposure. Historically, this variant was classified as a benign mesothelioma. Typically, the lesions are diagnosed as an asymptomatic mass on a chest radiograph. Complete surgical resection is the treatment of choice.

Diffuse malignant pleural mesothelioma manifests as a locally aggressive tumor commonly associated with asbestos exposure (75%). A long latency period between asbestos exposure and the development of the disease has been reported. Diagnostic imaging includes CXR, CT, and FDG-PET scan to determine the extent of tumor invasion and to evaluate occult metastases, including mediastinal metastases. Echocardiography is also performed to determine cardiac involvement. The diagnosis is made with pleural biopsy, which may include thoracentesis or pleural biopsy alone or incisional biopsies via thoracoscopy or open techniques.

Survival for this disease is poor, ranging from 4 to 12 months. Treatment has included chemotherapy,[117] standard and conformal radiation therapy, and extrapleural pneumonectomy. Combinations of therapies are commonly used. Extrapleural pneumonectomy and total pleurectomy are two commonly used surgical procedures.[118,119] In patients with epithelioid histology, negative margins, and negative mediastinal lymph nodes, 5-year survival is 46% after extrapleural pneumonectomy with adjuvant chemoradiotherapy.[120] Other techniques include preoperative chemotherapy followed by extrapleural pneumonectomy and conformal radiotherapy for the pleural surface. Survival is poor even with treatment. Improved therapies are needed.

MEDIASTINUM

Mediastinal abnormalities may manifest as an asymptomatic mass identified on screening CXR or with significant symptoms, including hypoxia, facial swelling, and acute respiratory distress. Symptoms are related to the involvement of the specific mediastinal structures. A definitive diagnosis is needed to optimize treatment planning.[121] Cytology from fine-needle aspiration or core biopsy or surgical biopsy may be needed to make the diagnosis and to determine optimal therapy. Generally, a mediastinal mass should be removed prophylactically to obtain a definitive diagnosis, achieve local control, and avoid future symptoms. If cancer is identified, adjuvant therapy given after complete resection may treat microscopic disease better than bulky disease.

Mediastinal masses differ between adults and children.[122] The most common mediastinal masses (Box 57-7) in adults are thymomas and thymic cysts (26.5%), neurogenic tumors (20.0%),

other cysts (16.1%), germ cell tumors (13.8%), and lymphomas (12.7%). In a combined series of 718 children with mediastinal masses, neurogenic tumors (41.6%), germ cell tumors (13.5%), primary cysts (13.4%), and lymphomas (13.4%) were diagnosed most frequently. Pericardial cysts and thymomas are uncommon in children.

Malignant mediastinal neoplasms account for 25% to 50% of mediastinal masses in adults. Lymphomas, thymomas, germ cell tumors, primary carcinomas, and neurogenic tumors are the most common. Primary carcinomas of the mediastinum constitute up to 10% of primary mediastinal masses and need to be differentiated from malignant thymomas, germ cell tumors, carcinoid tumors, lymphomas, mediastinal extension of bronchogenic carcinomas, and metastatic tumors, which may have a similar appearance by light microscopy.

Many mediastinal lesions occur in characteristic sites within the mediastinum (Fig. 57-24). Approximately half of all mediastinal masses are located in the anterosuperior mediastinum with the remainder divided between the posterior and middle mediastinum. In addition, the location of the mass explains some of the typical symptoms related to a mediastinal mass because of compression or invasion of adjacent mediastinal structures.

Anterosuperior Compartment

The anterosuperior compartment of the mediastinum borders the undersurface of the sternum ventrally, the pericardium dorsally, and the visceral pleura laterally (at the apposition of the pleura and pericardium). Tumors of the anterior mediastinum include thymomas, teratoma or germ cell tumors, a spectrum of lymphomas including Hodgkin disease, and thyroid goiter. In most cases, tissue (core biopsy) is required for diagnosis; fine-needle aspirate is usually inadequate.

Thymomas are usually the most frequently occurring neoplasm of the anterior mediastinum, and lymphomas are second. Germ cell neoplasms include benign and malignant teratomas, choriocarcinoma, seminoma, and embryonal cell neoplasm. Teratomas frequently occur in young adults. The gonads are the most common primary site, followed by the mediastinum. Most germ cell neoplasms are benign, but 20% are malignant. Malignant teratomas may produce high serum levels of α-fetoprotein (AFP) and carcinoembryonic antigen. Endocrine disease of the thyroid and parathyroid may occur in the anterior mediastinum as a result of their anatomic position in adults (substernal goiter) or embryologic development (Fig. 57-25). Carcinoid tumors may be found within the thymus. Primary carcinomas of the mediastinum are often unresectable and respond poorly to treatment.

Middle Compartment

The middle (or visceral) compartment extends from (and contains) the structures of the thoracic inlet (superiorly), the pericardium anteriorly, to the anterior surface of the vertebrae posteriorly. Lymphomas can occur in the middle mediastinum. Tumors of the heart and great vessels as well as tumors of the trachea, mainstem bronchi, and esophagus may be considered tumors of the middle compartment. Benign diseases, such as pericardial cysts and bronchogenic cysts, also occur here.

Posterior or Paravertebral Sulci Compartment

The posterior compartment is bounded by the middle compartment anteriorly and the costophrenic angle laterally. Neurogenic tumors are usually the most common primary tumors of the mediastinum, and approximately 25% of these tumors are

---

BOX 57-7   Mediastinum: Classification of Primary Mediastinal Tumors and Cysts

Thymoma
  Benign
  Malignant
Lymphoma
  Hodgkin disease
  Lymphoblastic lymphoma
  Large cell lymphoma
Germ cell tumors
  Teratodermoid (benign/malignant)
  Seminoma
  Nonseminoma
  • Embryonal
  • Choriocarcinoma
  • Endodermal
Primary carcinomas
  Mesenchymal tumors
  • Fibroma/fibrosarcoma
  • Lipoma/liposarcoma
  • Leiomyoma/leiomyosarcoma
  • Rhabdosarcoma
  • Xanthogranuloma
  • Myxoma
  • Mesothelioma
  • Hemangioma
  • Hemangioendothelioma
  • Hemangiopericytoma

  • Lymphangioma
  • Lymphangiomyoma
  • Lymphangiopericytoma
Endocrine tumors
  • Intrathoracic thyroid
  • Parathyroid adenoma/carcinoma
  • Carcinoid
Cysts
  Bronchogenic
  Pericardial
  Enteric
  Thymic
  Thoracic duct
  Nonspecific
Giant lymph node hyperplasia
  Castleman disease
Chondroma
Extramedullary hematopoiesis
Neurogenic tumors
  Neurofibroma
  Neurilemoma
  Paraganglioma
  Ganglioneuroma
  Neuroblastoma
  Chemodectoma
  Neurosarcoma

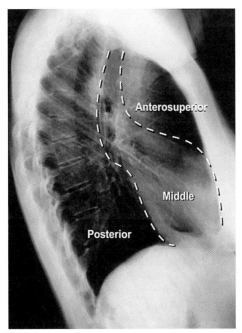

FIGURE 57-24 Lateral chest radiograph demonstrating the mediastinum divided into three anatomic subdivisions.

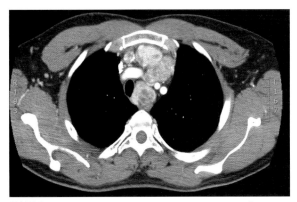

FIGURE 57-25 Thyroid carcinoma within the mediastinum. The tumor was resected via median sternotomy. No invasion was identified. A complete resection was accomplished.

malignant. These tumors are located within the paravertebral sulcus and may erode the adjacent vertebra or rib. Schwannomas and neurilemomas are the most common neurogenic tumors. Neurofibromas arise from the nerve sheath and fibers and occur in middle-aged patients. In children, ganglioneuroma is the most common neurogenic tumor. The tumor frequently attains a large size before presentation of symptoms. Increased levels of catecholamines may produce symptoms. Surgical resection of these neurogenic tumors is usually the procedure of choice.

Embryologic development of the neural crest cells forms the basis of neuroendocrine tumors in the mediastinum. Of pheochromocytomas, 1% occur within the mediastinum. Chemodectomas or paragangliomas may arise from chemoreceptor tissues around the aorta and great vessels, including the carotid. Symptoms may result from catecholamine production and are alleviated by surgical resection.

Clinical Manifestations and Diagnosis

Approximately one third of adult patients may develop symptoms from a mediastinal mass. Symptoms include chest pain, dyspnea, and cough. The symptoms may vary widely and relate to size (fatigue, weight loss); location; extent of compression or invasion of mediastinal structures (superior vena cava syndrome); and production of hormones, markers, or other biochemical materials (e.g., myasthenia gravis, fatigue, night sweats). Larger mediastinal tumors are more likely to produce symptoms. Benign lesions are more often asymptomatic. Superior vena cava syndrome (obstruction of the superior vena cava with head and neck and upper extremity swelling), cough, hoarseness (from involvement of the recurrent laryngeal nerve), dyspnea from tumor volume or phrenic nerve paralysis, and dysphagia occur with compression or invasion of mediastinal structures. Other manifestations include Horner syndrome and Pancoast syndrome.

Infections within the mediastinum are devastating. Because of the extensive thin areolar planes between major structures, infections within a limited portion of the mediastinum may spread vertically or horizontally to create an extensive infection. Synergistic aerobic and anaerobic infections from the perforated esophagus are particularly life-threatening. Treatment consists of surgical drainage and antibiotics.

Specific clinical syndromes may occur as a result of mediastinal tumors. Physical examination may reveal swelling of the head, neck, or upper extremities. Dyspnea may result from compression of the trachea, bronchus, or a portion of the lung parenchyma. Recurrent respiratory symptoms may occur for some time until a CXR is obtained and the abnormality is identified. Postobstructive pneumonitis or infection of benign pericardial or enteric duplication cysts may produce fever or sepsis. Myasthenia gravis may result from thymomas. In addition, thymomas may result in autoimmune problems, such as hypogammaglobulinemia, red cell aplasia, and smooth muscle degeneration. Mediastinal Hodgkin disease may produce an intermittent fever (Pel-Ebstein fever). Patients with hypertension from pheochromocytoma, thyrotoxicosis from goiter, hypercalcemia from ectopic mediastinal parathyroid adenoma or carcinoma, or hypogammaglobulinemia should be evaluated carefully; mediastinal findings may affect subsequent therapeutic recommendations.

Evaluation and Diagnostic Imaging

Diagnostic imaging typically includes a plain CXR taken in two planes (posteroanterior and left lateral), which provides basic information about the location of the mass within the mediastinum. Given the known propensity of specific lesions to occur in the anterior, visceral (middle), or paravertebral (posterior) sulcus based on the anatomy and embryologic development of cervicothoracic organs, a differential diagnosis may be obtained.

Diaphragm fluoroscopy, or "sniff test," is used to evaluate paradoxical motion of the diaphragm on rapid inspiration indicative of phrenic nerve paralysis. CT scan of the chest has replaced plain CXRs as the diagnostic procedure of choice for mediastinal masses. MRI may enhance the diagnostic abilities of chest CT. Anterior mediastinal masses, such as thymoma, can be evaluated for the extent of compression or possible invasion into the pulmonary artery, innominate vein, or superior vena cava. Evaluation of the extent of invasion into the brachial plexus, great vessels, vertebral body, neural foramina, and spinal column may be easily accomplished with MRI. Echocardiography and FDG-PET have been commonly used. High FDG uptake is more likely to correlate with invasion in both thymic carcinomas and invasive thymomas.

Mediastinal tumors may secrete specific hormones or biological markers. Parathyroid adenomas or functioning parathyroid carcinomas may secrete parathormone. Pheochromocytomas may secrete various catecholamines (in serum and urine), which may cause hypertension. Carcinomas may secrete carcinoembryonic antigen. Nonseminomatous germ cell neoplasms may secrete AFP or β-human chorionic gonadotropin (β-HCG). Skin tests for tuberculosis, histoplasmosis, and coccidioidomycosis may also yield positive results. Other diagnostic tests for mediastinal tuberculosis include sputum cytology, CXR, and urine cytology.

Histologic Diagnosis

A mediastinal mass cannot be treated until a diagnosis is made. Although radiographic diagnosis may suffice for mediastinal cysts, tissue for definitive diagnosis is needed for solid masses. Fine-needle aspiration or needle biopsy with CT guidance of a mediastinal mass may provide sufficient tissue for diagnosis for thymic carcinoma or other defined neoplasms. For lymphomas in particular as well as thymomas and neural tumors, larger amounts of tissue may be required for cellular analysis. In these patients, core needle biopsy, mediastinoscopy, or intrathoracic biopsy (via thoracoscopy or open thoracotomy) may be considered. Electron microscopy may be required for confirmation of specific histologies. For recurrent lymphomas, after chemotherapy, open techniques for incisional biopsy are often required.

Median sternotomy provides a direct visual approach to the mediastinum and may be used for management of a wide range of mediastinal disease. VATS techniques and robotic techniques of resection are increasingly used for treatment of these noninvasive tumors. More extensive approaches include the transverse sternotomy or "clam-shell" incision. Anesthetic considerations should include avoidance of airway obstruction, awake intubation, and avoidance of muscle paralytics or drugs such as fluoroquinolones with potential paralytic effects.

PRIMARY MEDIASTINAL CYSTS

Primary cysts of the mediastinum account for approximately 20% of mediastinal masses in most collected series.[122] Cysts are characterized from the organ of origin and may be bronchogenic, pericardial, enteric, or thymic or may be of an unspecified nature. More than 75% of cases are asymptomatic, and these tumors rarely cause morbidity; however, with proximity to vital structures within the mediastinum and increasing size, the cyst may cause significant problems. Benign cysts may be resected with minimally invasive techniques.

Bronchogenic cysts account for most primary cysts of the mediastinum (see Fig. 57-9). They originate as sequestrations from the ventral foregut, the antecedent of the tracheobronchial tree, and can be situated within the lung parenchyma or the mediastinum. Bronchogenic cysts are usually located proximal to the trachea or bronchi and may be just posterior to the carina. A connection to the bronchus rarely exists; however, when it occurs, these cysts may become infected. Diagnostic imaging may reveal an air-fluid level within the mediastinum. Two thirds of bronchogenic cysts are asymptomatic. In infants, cysts cause severe respiratory compromise by compressing the trachea or the bronchus. Resection is recommended.

Pericardial cysts are second in frequency to bronchogenic cysts and occur in the cardiophrenic angle mostly on the right side

(70%). These cysts may or may not communicate with the pericardium. Typically, clear fluid is encountered. The characteristics of pericardial cysts include location in the cardiophrenic angle, characteristic appearance, smooth borders, and attenuation approximating water for the cyst fluid. Needle aspiration and routine surveillance may be all that is needed. Resection may be used for diagnosis and to exclude malignant tumors.

Enteric cysts or duplication cysts arise from the primitive foregut, which develops into the upper division of the gastrointestinal tract. These cysts are usually attached to the esophagus. Symptoms occur as size increases with compression of the esophagus and dysphagia. Neuroenteric cysts are associated with anomalies of the vertebral column. Excision is recommended.

PRIMARY MEDIASTINAL NEOPLASMS

Thymoma

The pathology of thymoma has been reviewed elsewhere.[20] Thymoma is the most common neoplasm of the anterosuperior compartment. The peak incidence is in the third through fifth decades, but thymomas may occur throughout adulthood. Thymoma is rare in the first 2 decades of life. A thymoma may appear on a radiograph as a small, well-circumscribed mass or as a bulky lobulated mass confluent with adjacent mediastinal structures (Fig. 57-26). Symptoms at presentation are related to local mass effects causing chest pain, dyspnea, hemoptysis, cough, and superior vena cava syndrome or systemic syndromes caused by immunologic mechanisms. The most common syndrome is myasthenia gravis, although other syndromes include pure red blood cell aplasia, pure white blood cell aplasia, aplastic anemia, Cushing syndrome, hypogammaglobulinemia and hypergammaglobulinemia, dermatomyositis, systemic lupus erythematosus, progressive systemic sclerosis, hypercoagulopathy with thrombosis, rheumatoid arthritis, megaesophagus, and granulomatous myocarditis. Early surgical treatment of myasthenia gravis and small thymomas is common. When thymectomy is performed early in the course of myasthenia gravis, a greater percentage of thymomas are benign.

Benign and malignant disease is differentiated by the presence of gross invasion of adjacent structures, metastasis, or microscopic evidence of capsular invasion. Tumors less than 3 cm in size are frequently benign; however, determination of malignancy (invasion) can be challenging for patients with tumors between 3 and 5 cm. A malignant process may be present in tumors greater than 5 cm.

Whenever possible, the therapy for thymoma is excision without removing or injuring vital structures.[123] Even with well-encapsulated thymomas, extended thymectomy with eradication of all accessible mediastinal fatty areolar tissue is performed to ensure removal of all ectopic thymic tissue and to reduce the number of tumor recurrences. Protection and preservation of the phrenic nerves are integral components of thymectomy.

The perioperative management in patients with myasthenia gravis is crucial to prevent complications. Anticholinesterase inhibitors are discontinued to decrease the amount of pulmonary secretions and prevent inadvertent cholinergic weakness. Plasmapheresis is used routinely within 72 hours of thymectomy. In most patients, plasmapheresis is effective in controlling generalized weakness. Survival is based on stage. Stage I is characterized by a well-encapsulated tumor without evidence of gross or microscopic capsular invasion; in stage II, tumor exhibits pericapsular growth into adjacent fat or mediastinal pleura or microscopic invasion of the thymic capsule; in stage III, tumor invades adjacent organs;

stage IVa is characterized by intrathoracic metastases; and stage IVb is characterized by extrathoracic metastases (uncommon). Complete resection (R0) is required. For patients with stage I thymoma, resection alone is sufficient without the need for adjuvant therapy. For stage II and III disease, adjuvant radiation therapy is commonly used. Tumors greater than 5 cm, locally invasive tumors, unresectable tumors, and metastatic tumors are treated using protocols that include chemotherapy followed by surgical exploration with the goal of complete resection and postoperative (adjuvant) radiation therapy. Cisplatin-based regimens have excellent response rates.[124]

Invasive thymomas require radical resection of involved structures, which may include vascular reconstruction of the superior vena cava, innominate vein, or its branches.[125] Using this aggressive approach to obtain complete resection, a significant difference in 5-year survival rates is seen in patients with stage III thymomas (94%) compared with patients with incomplete resections (35%). Thymomas frequently show recurrence, and reoperation for recurrent disease has been recommended.

Germ Cell Tumors

Germ cell tumors arise from primordial germ cells that fail to complete the migration from the urogenital ridge and rest in the mediastinum. Treatment depends on histology.[126] The anterosuperior mediastinum is the most common extragonadal primary site of these tumors. Although these lesions are identical histologically to germ cell tumors originating in the gonads, they are not considered metastatic from primary gonadal tumors. The current recommendations for evaluating the testes of a patient with mediastinal germ cell tumor are careful physical examination and ultrasonography of the testes. Biopsy is reserved for positive findings. Blind biopsy or orchiectomy is contraindicated.

Teratomas

Teratomas are the most common mediastinal germ cell neoplasms and are located most commonly in the anterosuperior mediastinum. They are composed of multiple tissue elements that are derived from the three primitive embryonic layers foreign to the area in which they occur. The peak incidence is in the second and third decades of life. There is no gender predisposition. Radiographic evidence of normal tissue (e.g., well-formed teeth or globular calcifications, a fatty mass) in an abnormal location can be considered specific. The teratodermoid (dermoid) cyst is the simplest form of a teratoma and is composed of derivatives of the epidermal layer, including dermal and epidermal glands, hair, and sebaceous material. Teratomas are histologically more complex. The solid component of the tumor often contains well-differentiated elements of bone, cartilage, teeth, muscle, connective tissue, fibrous and lymphoid tissue, nerve, thymus, mucous and salivary glands, lung, liver, or pancreas. Malignant tumors are differentiated from benign tumors by the presence of primitive (embryonic) tissue or by the presence of malignant components. Immature teratomas contain combinations of mature epithelial and connective tissues with immature areas of mesenchymal and neuroectodermal tissues. Teratomas with malignant components are divided into categories based on the elements present.

Diagnosis and therapy rely on surgical excision. For benign tumors of large size or with involvement of adjacent mediastinal structures such that complete resection is impossible, partial resection has led to resolution of symptoms, frequently without relapse. For malignant teratomas, chemotherapy and radiation therapy, combined with surgical excision, are individualized for the type of malignant components contained in the tumors. The overall prognosis is poor for malignant teratomas.

Malignant Nonteratomatous Germ Cell Tumors

Malignant germ cell tumors occur predominantly in the anterosuperior mediastinum with a marked male predominance most commonly in the third and fourth decades of life.[127] Most patients have symptoms of chest pain, cough, dyspnea, and hemoptysis; the superior vena cava syndrome occurs commonly. A large anterior mediastinal mass is identified on diagnostic imaging. There is evidence of intrathoracic spread of disease. CT and MRI are helpful to define the extent of the disease and involvement of mediastinal structures. Serologic measurements of AFP and β-HCG are useful for differentiating seminomas from nonseminomatous tumors, assessing response to therapy, and diagnosing relapse or failure of therapy. Seminomas rarely produce β-HCG and never produce AFP; in contrast, more than 90% of nonseminomatous tumors secrete one or both of these hormones. This differentiation is important, as seminomas are radiosensitive, and nonseminomatous tumors are relatively radioinsensitive.

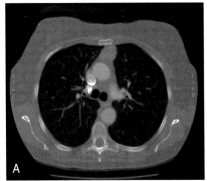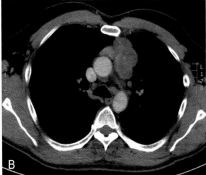

FIGURE 57-26 A, Computed tomography (CT) scan of the chest in a patient with myasthenia gravis and thymoma. The thymoma is small with a plane of separation between the tumor and the pericardium. **B,** Chest CT scan in a patient with a larger mediastinal mass. The location, character, and size are noted. Transthoracic core needle biopsy was performed. Germ cell tumor markers were normal. Pathology demonstrated thymoma. A 6.5-cm thymoma was subsequently resected. There was no invasion of the pericardium. A complete resection (R0) was accomplished.

Seminomas

Seminomas constitute 50% of malignant germ cell tumors. Seminomas usually remain intrathoracic. Symptoms are related to the mechanical effects of the tumor on adjacent mediastinal and pulmonary structures. The superior vena cava syndrome occurs in 10% to 20% of patients. These tumors are sensitive to irradiation and chemotherapy. Therapy is determined by the stage of the disease. Cytoreductive resection before chemotherapy or radiation therapy is unnecessary. Treatment consists of systemic and local therapy—chemotherapy with salvage surgery or combined chemoradiotherapy. Radiation therapy may be considered for early-stage disease but is not recommended for regional disease. Platinum-based chemotherapy is common. Occasionally, excision is possible without injury to vital structures and can be recommended. When complete resection is possible, the use of adjuvant therapy is unnecessary. When excision is impossible, a biopsy sample of sufficient size to establish the diagnosis is obtained.

Nonseminomatous Tumors

Malignant nonseminomatous germ cell tumors include choriocarcinomas, embryonal cell carcinomas, immature teratomas, teratomas with malignant components, and endodermal cell (yolk sac) tumors and occur mostly in men in their third or fourth decades. Diagnostic imaging reveals a large anterior mediastinal mass with frequent extension to the lung, chest wall, and mediastinal structures. Nonseminomatous germ cell neoplasms are more aggressive tumors and more frequently disseminated at the time of diagnosis, they are rarely radiosensitive, and more than 90% produce either β-HCG or AFP. All patients with choriocarcinoma and some patients with embryonal cell tumors have elevated levels of β-HCG. AFP is most commonly elevated in patients with embryonal cell carcinomas and yolk sac tumors. Mediastinal nonseminomatous germ cell tumors, but not testicular germ cell tumors, are associated with the development of rare hematologic malignancies, such as acute megakaryocytic leukemia, systemic mast cell disease, and malignant histiocytosis, as well as other hematologic abnormalities, including myelodysplastic syndrome and idiopathic thrombocytopenia refractory to treatment.

Treatment of these nonseminomatous tumors currently is with cisplatin and etoposide-based regimens. Advanced disease, invasion into thoracic structures, and metastasis preclude surgical resection. Serum markers, AFP or β-HCG, are followed to assess response to systemic treatment. If a complete serologic and radiologic response is achieved, patients are closely observed. If the disease progresses during therapy, salvage chemotherapy is initiated. Operative intervention may be required to establish a histologic diagnosis in patients without elevations in serum AFP or β-HCG or for salvage resection after tissue or serologic response to therapy.[126] The pathology of the resected postchemotherapy specimen appears to be the most significant predictor of survival. The presence of residual disease after chemotherapy portends a poor prognosis and the need for additional chemotherapy. When tumor necrosis or a benign teratoma is found during surgical exploration after chemotherapy, an excellent or intermediate prognosis is conferred, respectively.

Neurogenic Tumors

Neurogenic tumors are usually located in the posterior mediastinum and originate from the sympathetic ganglia (ganglioma, ganglioneuroblastoma, and neuroblastoma), the intercostal nerves (neurofibroma, neurilemoma, and neurosarcoma), and the paraganglia cells (paraganglioma). Although the peak incidence occurs in adults, neurogenic tumors make up a proportionally greater percentage of mediastinal masses in children. Although most neurogenic tumors in adults are benign, a greater percentage of neurogenic tumors are malignant in children.

The most common neurogenic tumor is neurilemoma or schwannoma, which originates from perineural Schwann cells. They are benign, slow-growing neoplasms that frequently arise from a spinal nerve root but can involve any thoracic nerve. These tumors are well circumscribed and have a defined capsule. They arise from the nerve sheath and extrinsically compress the nerve fibers. The peak incidence of these tumors is in the third through fifth decades of life; men and women are equally affected.

Many of these tumors are asymptomatic. Symptoms such as pain occur from compression or invasion of intercostal nerve, bone, and chest wall; cough and dyspnea resulting from compression of the tracheobronchial tree; Pancoast syndrome; and Horner syndrome resulting from involvement of the brachial and the cervical sympathetic chain. Approximately 10% of neurogenic tumors have extensions into the spinal column and are termed *dumbbell tumors* because of their characteristic shape with relatively large paraspinal and intraspinal portions connected by a narrow isthmus of tissue traversing the intervertebral foramen. Patients with paraspinal tumors should undergo MRI to evaluate the presence and extent of the tumor and its relationship to the neural foramen and the intraspinal space. During resection, the intraspinal component should be removed first via a posterior laminectomy. This approach minimizes the potential for spinal column hematoma, cord ischemia, and paralysis. A separate transthoracic approach is needed for resection of the intrathoracic component.

Neuroblastoma

Neuroblastomas originate from the sympathetic nervous system. The most common location for a neuroblastoma is in the retroperitoneum; however, 10% to 20% occur primarily in the mediastinum. These are highly invasive neoplasms that have frequently metastasized before diagnosis. Most of these tumors occur in children 4 years old or younger. A 24-hour urine collection to measure catecholamines is obtained in children with a posterior mediastinal mass. Therapy is determined by the stage of the disease: stage I, surgical excision; stage II, excision and radiation therapy; stages III and IV, multimodality therapy using surgical debulking, radiation therapy, and multiagent chemotherapy and a second-look exploration to resect residual disease when necessary. The usual chemotherapeutic agents are cisplatin, vincristine, doxorubicin, cyclophosphamide, and etoposide.

Ganglion Tumors

Ganglioneuroblastomas are composed of mature and immature ganglion cells. Treatment of ganglioneuroblastoma ranges from surgical excision alone to various chemotherapeutic strategies depending on histologic characteristics, age at diagnosis, and stage of disease. Ganglioneuromas are benign tumors that originate from the sympathetic chain and are composed of ganglion cells and nerve fibers. These tumors typically manifest at an early age and are the most common neurogenic tumors occurring during childhood. The usual location is the paravertebral region. These tumors are well encapsulated and, when cross-sectioned, frequently exhibit areas of cystic degeneration. Surgical excision provides cure.

Paraganglioma (Pheochromocytoma)

Mediastinal paragangliomas are rare tumors, representing less than 1% of all mediastinal tumors and less than 2% of all pheochromocytomas. Although most are found in the paravertebral sulcus, an increasing number occur in the branchial arch structures, coronary and aortopulmonary paraganglia, atria, and islands of tissue in the pericardium. Although adrenal pheochromocytomas often produce both epinephrine and norepinephrine, extra-adrenal paragangliomas rarely secrete epinephrine. Multiple paragangliomas occur in 10% of patients. These tumors are more common in patients with multiple endocrine neoplasia syndromes, a family history of disease, and Carney syndrome (pulmonary chondroma, gastric leiomyosarcoma, and functioning extra-adrenal paraganglioma). In patients who have had excision of an adrenal pheochromocytoma and continue to have symptoms, a search for an extra-adrenal lesion is undertaken, with careful attention to the mediastinum. Tumor localization has improved through the use of CT and iodine-131 metaiodobenzylguanidine scintigraphy, particularly when the tumors are hormonally active. When appropriate, surgical resection is the optimal therapy. In patients with tumors involving the middle mediastinum, cardiopulmonary bypass may be necessary to enable resection. Preoperative embolization to reduce perioperative bleeding may be considered. Although half of tumors appear malignant morphologically, metastatic disease rarely develops.

Lymphomas

Although the mediastinum is frequently involved in patients with lymphoma at some time during the course of their disease, it is infrequently the sole site of disease at the time of presentation. Hodgkin and non-Hodgkin lymphoma are distinct clinical entities with overlapping features. Patients usually have symptoms; chest pain, cough, dyspnea, hoarseness, and superior vena cava syndrome are the most common clinical manifestations. Nonspecific systemic symptoms of fever and chills, weight loss, and anorexia are frequently noted and are important in the staging of patients with Hodgkin lymphoma. Symptoms characteristic of Hodgkin lymphoma include chest pain after consumption of alcohol and Pel-Ebstein fever.

Surgical excision of all disease is rarely possible; the surgeon's primary role is to provide sufficient tissue for diagnosis and to assist in pathologic staging. A needle biopsy is often unsuccessful because larger tissue samples are needed to make a histologic diagnosis, particularly with nodular sclerosing lesions. Thoracoscopy, mediastinoscopy, or mediastinotomy and, rarely, thoracotomy or median sternotomy may be necessary to obtain sufficient tissue. The role of staging laparotomy has been minimized, and its only current indication is for patients with clinically limited disease who opt for limited treatment.

Patients with non-Hodgkin lymphoma usually have symptoms because of involvement of adjacent mediastinal structures. Superior vena cava syndrome is relatively common. Lymphoblastic lymphoma occurs predominantly in children, adolescents, and young adults and represents 60% of cases of mediastinal non-Hodgkin lymphoma.

After treatment of lymphomas, residual radiographic abnormalities within the mediastinum are commonly noted (64% to 88%). CT cannot differentiate fibrosis or necrosis from residual tumor. FDG-PET has shown promise as a noninvasive way to detect active mediastinal disease and predict relapse in patients with lymphoma, but tissue confirmation is required. Needle biopsy does not provide significant diagnostic material. Transthoracic incisional biopsy under general anesthesia is often needed given the significant fibrosis that remains after therapy.

Endocrine Tumors
Thyroid Tumors

Although substernal extension of a cervical goiter is common, totally intrathoracic thyroid tumors are rare and make up only 1% of all mediastinal masses in collected series. These tumors arise from heterotopic thyroid tissue, which occurs most commonly in the anterosuperior mediastinum but may also occur in the middle mediastinum between the trachea and the esophagus as well as in the posterior mediastinum. Although there may be a demonstrable connection with the cervical gland (usually a fibrous connective tissue band), a true intrathoracic thyroid gland derives its blood supply from thoracic vessels. Substernal extensions of a cervical goiter can usually be excised using a cervical approach.

Parathyroid Tumors

Although parathyroid glands may occur in the mediastinum in 10% of patients, they are usually accessible through the cervical incision. Most often, these adenomas are found in the anterosuperior mediastinum (80%) embedded in or near the superior pole of the thymus. This anatomic relationship is the result of the common embryogenesis of the inferior parathyroid glands from the third branchial cleft. The superior parathyroid glands and the lateral lobes of the thyroid gland are derived from the fourth branchial pouch. Because they migrate with the lateral lobes of the thyroid gland to a paraesophageal position, parathyroid adenomas can also be found in the posterior mediastinum.

Most frequently, the mediastinal parathyroid adenoma may be excised after a negative exploration of the cervical region through the existing cervical incision. Usually the vascular supply extends from cervical blood vessels. In patients with persistent hyperparathyroidism after cervical exploration, if localization studies show residual parathyroid in the mediastinum, mediastinal exploration using a median sternotomy or thoracoscopy is indicated.

Parathyroid carcinomas have been reported and are usually hormonally active. Patients differ in clinical presentation in that they often have higher serum calcium levels and manifest more severe symptoms of hyperparathyroidism. When possible, resection is the optimal therapy.

Neuroendocrine Tumors

Mediastinal neuroendocrine tumors, carcinoid tumors, arise from cells of Kulchitsky located in the thymus and commonly occur in men in their 40s and 50s; they are usually located in the anterosuperior mediastinum. These tumors are aggressive, and 20% have metastatic spread to mediastinal and cervical lymph nodes, liver, bone, skin, and lungs. More than 50% of thymic neuroendocrine tumors are hormonally active, often associated with Cushing syndrome because of production of adrenocorticotropic hormone, less frequently associated with multiple endocrine neoplasia syndromes, and only rarely associated with carcinoid syndrome (0.6%). If possible, resection is recommended; however, local invasion and metastasis often preclude complete excision. Adjuvant therapy is controversial, but irradiation should probably be added, particularly in patients with capsular invasion.

SELECTED REFERENCES

Arriagada R, Bergman B, Dunant A, et al: Cisplatin-based adjuvant chemotherapy in patients with completely resected non-small-cell lung cancer. *N Engl J Med* 350:351–360, 2004.

Adjuvant therapy after complete resection of non–small cell lung carcinoma has been shown to improve survival in selected patients. The International Lung Adjuvant Trial proved that adjuvant platinum-based chemotherapy improved survival compared with no treatment.

Diagnosis and Management of Lung Cancer: ACCP Guidelines (2nd Edition). *Chest* 132(Suppl 3):2007.

National Comprehensive Cancer Network: NCCN Clinical Practice Guidelines in Oncology. Non-small cell lung cancer, 2011 (<http://www.nccn.org/professionals/physician_gls/f_guidelines.asp>; Accessed August 20, 2015).

Guidelines for diagnosis, treatment, and surveillance are published by various organizations based on evidence and consensus of experts. Two sets of guidelines for the management of non–small cell lung cancer were published by the American College of Chest Physicians and the National Comprehensive Cancer Network.

Dresler CM, Olak J, Herndon JE, 2nd, et al: Phase III intergroup study of talc poudrage vs talc slurry sclerosis for malignant pleural effusion. *Chest* 127:909–915, 2005.

This prospective randomized study evaluated chest tube with talc slurry versus video-assisted thoracic surgery (VATS) with talc poudrage. Both groups benefited from the intervention, and neither intervention was superior. VATS has the advantage of complete drainage, pleural biopsy, and direct placement of talc.

Edge SB, Byrd DR, Compton CC, et al: *AJCC cancer staging manual,* ed 7, New York, 2010, Springer.

Goldstraw P, Crowley J, Chansky K, et al: The IASLC Lung Cancer Staging Project: Proposals for the revision of the TNM stage groupings in the forthcoming (seventh) edition of the TNM Classification of malignant tumours. *J Thorac Oncol* 2:706–714, 2007.

Pao W: Defining clinically relevant molecular subsets of lung cancer. *Cancer Chemother Pharmacol* 58(Suppl 1):s11–s15, 2006.

Staging for non–small cell lung carcinoma has changed significantly with the results of the International Association for the Study of Lung Cancer Staging Project. This data set was predominately surgery based but international in extent and both internally and externally validated. These results have formed the basis for the American Joint Committee on Cancer and Union for International Cancer Control staging systems. Future staging systems may evaluate the molecular characteristics of the tumor as both prognostic (of survival) and predictive (of response) characteristics.

Fernando HC, Schuchert M, Landreneau R, et al: Approaching the high-risk patient: Sublobar resection, stereotactic body radiation therapy, or radiofrequency ablation. *Ann Thorac Surg* 89:S2123–S2127, 2010.

Timmerman R, Paulus R, Galvin J, et al: Stereotactic body radiation therapy for inoperable early stage lung cancer. *JAMA* 303:1070–1076, 2010.

New methods of local control of non–small cell lung carcinoma are being studied. A review of local treatment options evaluated sublobar resection, stereotactic body radiation therapy, and radiofrequency. Clinical trials are underway to evaluate these treatment options prospectively.

National Lung Screening Trial Research Team, Aberle DR, Berg CD, et al: The National Lung Screening Trial: overview and study design. *Radiology* 258:243–253, 2011.

The National Lung Screening Trial tested screening for lung cancer and found that fewer lung cancer–related deaths occurred in the population screened with computed tomography compared with chest x-ray.

Walsh GL, Davis BM, Swisher SG, et al: A single-institutional, multidisciplinary approach to primary sarcomas involving the chest wall requiring full-thickness resections. *J Thorac Cardiovasc Surg* 121:48–60, 2001.

This article presents one of the largest series on primary chest wall tumors.

REFERENCES

1. Brunelli A, Kim AW, Berger KI, et al: Physiologic evaluation of the patient with lung cancer being considered for resectional surgery: Diagnosis and management of lung cancer, 3rd ed: American College of Chest Physicians evidence-based clinical practice guidelines. *Chest* 143:e166S–190S, 2013.
2. Thomsen T, Villebro N, Moller AM: Interventions for preoperative smoking cessation. *Cochrane Database Syst Rev* CD002294, 2010.
3. Mason DP, Subramanian S, Nowicki ER, et al: Impact of smoking cessation before resection of lung cancer: A Society of Thoracic Surgeons General Thoracic Surgery Database study. *Ann Thorac Surg* 88:362–370, discussion 370-371, 2009.
4. Zaman M, Bilal H, Mahmood S, et al: Does getting smokers to stop smoking before lung resections reduce their risk? *Interact Cardiovasc Thorac Surg* 14:320–323, 2012.
5. Cataldo JK, Dubey S, Prochaska JJ: Smoking cessation: An integral part of lung cancer treatment. *Oncology* 78:289–301, 2010.
6. Gould MK, Garcia DA, Wren SM, et al: Prevention of VTE in nonorthopedic surgical patients: Antithrombotic Therapy and Prevention of Thrombosis, 9th ed: American College of Chest Physicians Evidence-Based Clinical Practice Guidelines. *Chest* 141:e227S–277S, 2012.
7. Poonyagariyagorn H, Mazzone PJ: Lung cancer: Preoperative pulmonary evaluation of the lung resection candidate. *Semin Respir Crit Care Med* 29:271–284, 2008.
8. Beckles MA, Spiro SG, Colice GL, et al: The physiologic evaluation of patients with lung cancer being considered for resectional surgery. *Chest* 123:105S–114S, 2003.
9. Mendeloff EN: Sequestrations, congenital cystic adenomatoid malformations, and congenital lobar emphysema. *Semin Thorac Cardiovasc Surg* 16:209–214, 2004.

10. Fievet L, D'Journo XB, Guys JM, et al: Bronchogenic cyst: Best time for surgery? *Ann Thorac Surg* 94:1695–1699, 2012.

11. Sfakianaki AK, Copel JA: Congenital cystic lesions of the lung: Congenital cystic adenomatoid malformation and bronchopulmonary sequestration. *Rev Obstet Gynecol* 5:85–93, 2012.

12. Jaquiss RD: Management of pediatric tracheal stenosis and tracheomalacia. *Semin Thorac Cardiovasc Surg* 16:220–224, 2004.

13. Damle SS, Mitchell JD: Surgery for tracheobronchomalacia. *Semin Cardiothorac Vasc Anesth* 16:203–208, 2012.

14. Pegoli W, Mattei P, Colombani PM: Congenital intrathoracic vascular abnormalities in childhood. *Chest Surg Clin North Am* 3:529, 1993.

15. Maldonado JA, Henry T, Gutierrez FR: Congenital thoracic vascular anomalies. *Radiol Clin North Am* 48:85–115, 2010.

16. Siegel RL, Miller KD, Jemal A: Cancer statistics, 2015. *CA Cancer J Clin* 65:5–29, 2015.

17. Field RW: Environmental factors in cancer: Radon. *Rev Environ Health* 25:23–31, 2010.

18. U.S. National Institutes of Health: Information on clinical trials and human research studies, 2011 (<http://www.clinicaltrials.gov>; Accessed August 20, 2015).

19. An Overview of NCI's National Clinical Trials Network (<http://www.cancer.gov/research/areas/clinical-trials/nctn>; Accessed August 20, 2015).

20. Travis WD, Brambilla E, Muller-Hermelink HK, et al: *World Health Organization classification of tumours. Pathology and genetics of tumours of the lung, pleura, thymus, and heart*, Lyon, France, 2004, IARC Press.

21. Travis WD, Brambilla E, Noguchi M, et al: International Association for the Study of Lung Cancer/American Thoracic Society/European Respiratory Society: International multidisciplinary classification of lung adenocarcinoma: executive summary. *Proc Am Thorac Soc* 8:381–385, 2011.

22. National Lung Screening Trial Research T, Aberle DR, Berg CD, et al: The National Lung Screening Trial: Overview and study design. *Radiology* 258:243–253, 2011.

23. National Lung Screening Trial Research T, Aberle DR, Adams AM, et al: Baseline characteristics of participants in the randomized national lung screening trial. *J Natl Cancer Inst* 102:1771–1779, 2010.

24. Preventive Services Task Force: Lung cancer: Screening, 2013 (<http://www.uspreventiveservicestaskforce.org/Page/Document/UpdateSummaryFinal/lung-cancer-screening>; Accessed August 20, 2015).

25. Gould MK: Clinical practice. Lung-cancer screening with low-dose computed tomography. *N Engl J Med* 371:1813–1820, 2014.

26. Spiro SG, Gould MK, Colice GL, et al: Initial evaluation of the patient with lung cancer: Symptoms, signs, laboratory tests, and paraneoplastic syndromes: ACCP evidenced-based clinical practice guidelines (2nd edition). *Chest* 132:149S–160S, 2007.

27. Simoff MJ, Lally B, Slade MG, et al: Symptom management in patients with lung cancer: Diagnosis and management of lung cancer, 3rd ed: American College of Chest Physicians evidence-based clinical practice guidelines. *Chest* 143:e455S–497S, 2013.

28. Gould MK, Donington J, Lynch WR, et al: Evaluation of individuals with pulmonary nodules: When is it lung cancer? Diagnosis and management of lung cancer, 3rd ed: American College of Chest Physicians evidence-based clinical practice guidelines. *Chest* 143:e93S–120S, 2013.

29. Ost DE, Gould MK: Decision making in patients with pulmonary nodules. *Am J Respir Crit Care Med* 185:363–372, 2012.

30. Rivera MP, Mehta AC, Wahidi MM: Establishing the diagnosis of lung cancer: Diagnosis and management of lung cancer, 3rd ed: American College of Chest Physicians evidence-based clinical practice guidelines. *Chest* 143:e142S–165S, 2013.

31. Goldstraw P, Crowley J, Chansky K, et al: The IASLC Lung Cancer Staging Project: Proposals for the revision of the TNM stage groupings in the forthcoming (seventh) edition of the TNM Classification of malignant tumours. *J Thorac Oncol* 2:706–714, 2007.

32. Silvestri GA, Gonzalez AV, Jantz MA, et al: Methods for staging non-small cell lung cancer: Diagnosis and management of lung cancer, 3rd ed: American College of Chest Physicians evidence-based clinical practice guidelines. *Chest* 143:e211S–250S, 2013.

33. Detterbeck FC, Mazzone PJ, Naidich DP, et al: Screening for lung cancer: Diagnosis and management of lung cancer, 3rd ed: American College of Chest Physicians evidence-based clinical practice guidelines. *Chest* 143:e78S–92S, 2013.

34. Deppen SA, Blume JD, Kensinger CD, et al: Accuracy of FDG-PET to diagnose lung cancer in areas with infectious lung disease: A meta-analysis. *JAMA* 312:1227–1236, 2014.

35. Fischer B, Lassen U, Mortensen J, et al: Preoperative staging of lung cancer with combined PET-CT. *N Engl J Med* 361:32–39, 2009.

36. Reed CE, Harpole DH, Posther KE, et al: Results of the American College of Surgeons Oncology Group Z0050 trial: The utility of positron emission tomography in staging potentially operable non-small cell lung cancer. *J Thorac Cardiovasc Surg* 126:1943–1951, 2003.

37. Fernandez FG, Kozower BD, Crabtree TD, et al: Utility of mediastinoscopy in clinical stage I lung cancers at risk for occult mediastinal nodal metastases. *J Thorac Cardiovasc Surg* 149:35–41, 42.e1, 2015.

38. Harris CL, Toloza EM, Klapman JB, et al: Minimally invasive mediastinal staging of non-small-cell lung cancer: Emphasis on ultrasonography-guided fine-needle aspiration. *Cancer Control* 21:15–20, 2014.

39. Annema JT, van Meerbeeck JP, Rintoul RC, et al: Mediastinoscopy vs endosonography for mediastinal nodal staging of lung cancer: A randomized trial. *JAMA* 304:2245–2252, 2010.

40. Goldstraw P, Crowley JJ: The International Association for the Study of Lung Cancer International Staging Project on Lung Cancer. *J Thorac Oncol* 1:281–286, 2006.

41. Edge SB, Byrd DR, Compton CC, et al: *AJCC cancer staging manual*, ed 7, New York, 2010, Springer.

42. Groome PA, Bolejack V, Crowley JJ, et al: The IASLC Lung Cancer Staging Project: Validation of the proposals for revision of the T, N, and M descriptors and consequent stage groupings in the forthcoming (seventh) edition of the TNM classification of malignant tumours. *J Thorac Oncol* 2:694–705, 2007.

43. Giroux DJ, Rami-Porta R, Chansky K, et al: The IASLC Lung Cancer Staging Project: Data elements for the pro-

spective project. *J Thorac Oncol* 4:679–683, 2009.

44. American Joint Committee on Cancer: AJCC 7th Edition Staging Posters, 2012. http://cancerstaging.org/references-tools/quickreferences/Documents/Lung%20Cancer%20Staging%20Poster%20Updated.pdf

45. Rice TW, Murthy SC, Mason DP, et al: A cancer staging primer: Lung. *J Thorac Cardiovasc Surg* 139:826–829, 2010.

46. Rami-Porta R, Ball D, Crowley J, et al: The IASLC Lung Cancer Staging Project: Proposals for the revision of the T descriptors in the forthcoming (seventh) edition of the TNM classification for lung cancer. *J Thorac Oncol* 2:593–602, 2007.

47. Rusch VW, Crowley J, Giroux DJ, et al: The IASLC Lung Cancer Staging Project: Proposals for the revision of the N descriptors in the forthcoming seventh edition of the TNM classification for lung cancer. *J Thorac Oncol* 2:603–612, 2007.

48. Rusch VW, Asamura H, Watanabe H, et al: The IASLC lung cancer staging project: A proposal for a new international lymph node map in the forthcoming seventh edition of the TNM classification for lung cancer. *J Thorac Oncol* 4:568–577, 2009.

49. Postmus PE, Brambilla E, Chansky K, et al: The IASLC Lung Cancer Staging Project: Proposals for revision of the M descriptors in the forthcoming (seventh) edition of the TNM classification of lung cancer. *J Thorac Oncol* 2:686–693, 2007.

50. Timmerman R, Paulus R, Galvin J, et al: Stereotactic body radiation therapy for inoperable early stage lung cancer. *JAMA* 303:1070–1076, 2010.

51. Kozower BD, Sheng S, O'Brien SM, et al: STS database risk models: Predictors of mortality and major morbidity for lung cancer resection. *Ann Thorac Surg* 90:875–881, discussion 881-883, 2010.

52. Darling GE, Allen MS, Decker PA, et al: Randomized trial of mediastinal lymph node sampling versus complete lymphadenectomy during pulmonary resection in the patient with N0 or N1 (less than hilar) non-small cell carcinoma: Results of the American College of Surgery Oncology Group Z0030 Trial. *J Thorac Cardiovasc Surg* 141:662–670, 2011.

53. Fernando HC, Landreneau RJ, Mandrekar SJ, et al: Impact of brachytherapy on local recurrence rates after sublobar resection: Results from ACOSOG Z4032 (Alliance), a phase III randomized trial for high-risk operable non-small-cell lung cancer. *J Clin Oncol* 32:2456–2462, 2014.

54. Arriagada R, Bergman B, Dunant A, et al: Cisplatin-based adjuvant chemotherapy in patients with completely resected non-small-cell lung cancer. *N Engl J Med* 350:351–360, 2004.

55. Schiller JH, Harrington D, Belani CP, et al: Comparison of four chemotherapy regimens for advanced non-small-cell lung cancer. *N Engl J Med* 346:92–98, 2002.

56. Ramnath N, Dilling TJ, Harris LJ, et al: Treatment of stage III non-small cell lung cancer: Diagnosis and management of lung cancer, 3rd ed: American College of Chest Physicians evidence-based clinical practice guidelines. *Chest* 143:e314S–340S, 2013.

57. Pisters KM, Vallieres E, Crowley JJ, et al: Surgery with or without preoperative paclitaxel and carboplatin in early-stage non-small-cell lung cancer: Southwest Oncology Group Trial S9900, an intergroup, randomized, phase III trial. *J Clin Oncol* 28:1843–1849, 2010.

58. Albain KS, Swann RS, Rusch VW, et al: Radiotherapy plus chemotherapy with or without surgical resection for stage III non-small-cell lung cancer: A phase III randomised controlled trial. *Lancet* 374:379–386, 2009.

59. Deslauriers J, Tronc F, Fortin D: Management of tumors involving the chest wall including pancoast tumors and tumors invading the spine. *Thorac Surg Clin* 23:313–325, 2013.

60. Kappers I, van Sandick JW, Burgers JA, et al: Results of combined modality treatment in patients with non-small-cell lung cancer of the superior sulcus and the rationale for surgical resection. *Eur J Cardiothorac Surg* 36:741–746, 2009.

61. Socinski MA, Evans T, Gettinger S, et al: Treatment of stage IV non-small cell lung cancer: Diagnosis and management of lung cancer, 3rd ed: American College of Chest Physicians evidence-based clinical practice guidelines. *Chest* 143:e341S–368S, 2013.

62. Sandler A, Gray R, Perry MC, et al: Paclitaxel-carboplatin alone or with bevacizumab for non-small-cell lung cancer. *N Engl J Med* 355:2542–2550, 2006.

63. Pao W: Defining clinically relevant molecular subsets of lung cancer. *Cancer Chemother Pharmacol* 58(Suppl 1):s11–s15, 2006.

64. Pao W, Girard N: New driver mutations in non-small-cell lung cancer. *Lancet Oncol* 12:175–180, 2011.

65. Takeda K, Hida T, Sato T, et al: Randomized phase III trial of platinum-doublet chemotherapy followed by gefitinib compared with continued platinum-doublet chemotherapy in Japanese patients with advanced non-small-cell lung cancer: Results of a West Japan Thoracic Oncology Group trial (WJTOG0203). *J Clin Oncol* 28:753–760, 2010.

66. Mitsudomi T, Morita S, Yatabe Y, et al: Gefitinib versus cisplatin plus docetaxel in patients with non-small-cell lung cancer harbouring mutations of the epidermal growth factor receptor (WJTOG3405): An open label, randomised phase 3 trial. *Lancet Oncol* 11:121–128, 2010.

67. U.S. Food and Drug Administration: FDA approves targeted therapy for first-line treatment of patients with a type of metastatic lung cancer, July 13, 2015. (<http://www.fda.gov/NewsEvents/Newsroom/PressAnnouncements/ucm454678.htm>; Accessed August 20, 2015).

68. Harvey RD: Immunologic and clinical effects of targeting PD-1 in lung cancer. *Clin Pharmacol Ther* 96:214–223, 2014.

69. Ford DW, Koch KA, Ray DE, et al: Palliative and end-of-life care in lung cancer: Diagnosis and management of lung cancer, 3rd ed: American College of Chest Physicians evidence-based clinical practice guidelines. *Chest* 143:e498S–512S, 2013.

70. Dennis BM, Eckert MJ, Gunter OL, et al: Safety of bedside percutaneous tracheostomy in the critically ill: Evaluation of more than 3,000 procedures. *J Am Coll Surg* 216:858–865, discussion 865-857, 2013.

71. Honings J, Gaissert HA, Ruangchira-Urai R, et al: Pathologic characteristics of resected squamous cell carcinoma of the trachea: Prognostic factors based on an analysis of 59 cases. *Virchows Arch* 455:423–429, 2009.

72. Gaissert HA, Honings J, Gokhale M: Treatment of tracheal tumors. *Semin Thorac Cardiovasc Surg* 21:290–295,

2009.

73. Drugs for tuberculosis. *Treat Guidel Med Lett* 10:29–36, quiz 37-38, 2012.

74. Pezzella AT, Fang W: Surgical aspects of thoracic tuberculosis: A contemporary review—part 1. *Curr Probl Surg* 45:675–758, 2008.

75. Cummings I, O'Grady J, Pai V, et al: Surgery and tuberculosis. *Curr Opin Pulm Med* 18:241–245, 2012.

76. Passera E, Rizzi A, Robustellini M, et al: Pulmonary aspergilloma: Clinical aspects and surgical treatment outcome. *Thorac Surg Clin* 22:345–361, 2012.

77. Jeon K, Koh WJ, Kim H, et al: Clinical features of recently diagnosed pulmonary paragonimiasis in Korea. *Chest* 128:1423–1430, 2005.

78. Worrell SG, Demeester SR: Thoracic emergencies. *Surg Clin North Am* 94:183–191, 2014.

79. Dudha M, Lehrman S, Aronow WS, et al: Hemoptysis: Diagnosis and treatment. *Compr Ther* 35:139–149, 2009.

80. Sakr L, Dutau H: Massive hemoptysis: An update on the role of bronchoscopy in diagnosis and management. *Respiration* 80:38–58, 2010.

81. Shigemura N, Wan IY, Yu SC, et al: Multidisciplinary management of life-threatening massive hemoptysis: A 10-year experience. *Ann Thorac Surg* 87:849–853, 2009.

82. Chen J, Chen LA, Liang ZX, et al: Immediate and long-term results of bronchial artery embolization for hemoptysis due to benign versus malignant pulmonary diseases. *Am J Med Sci* 348:204–209, 2014.

83. Chun JY, Morgan R, Belli AM: Radiological management of hemoptysis: A comprehensive review of diagnostic imaging and bronchial arterial embolization. *Cardiovasc Intervent Radiol* 33:240–250, 2010.

84. Fishman A, Martinez F, Naunheim K, et al: A randomized trial comparing lung-volume-reduction surgery with medical therapy for severe emphysema. *N Engl J Med* 348:2059–2073, 2003.

85. Sanchez PG, Kucharczuk JC, Su S, et al: National Emphysema Treatment Trial redux: Accentuating the positive. *J Thorac Cardiovasc Surg* 140:564–572, 2010.

86. Hertz MI, Aurora P, Christie JD, et al: Scientific Registry of the International Society for Heart and Lung Transplantation: Introduction to the 2010 annual reports. *J Heart Lung Transplant* 29:1083–1088, 2010.

87. Malhotra A: Low-tidal-volume ventilation in the acute respiratory distress syndrome. *N Engl J Med* 357:1113–1120, 2007.

88. Briel M, Meade M, Mercat A, et al: Higher vs lower positive end-expiratory pressure in patients with acute lung injury and acute respiratory distress syndrome: Systematic review and meta-analysis. *JAMA* 303:865–873, 2010.

89. Tonelli AR, Zein J, Adams J, et al: Effects of interventions on survival in acute respiratory distress syndrome: An umbrella review of 159 published randomized trials and 29 meta-analyses. *Intensive Care Med* 40:769–787, 2014.

90. Pastorino U, Buyse M, Friedel G, et al: Long-term results of lung metastasectomy: Prognostic analyses based on 5206 cases. *J Thorac Cardiovasc Surg* 113:37–49, 1997.

91. Detterbeck FC: Clinical presentation and evaluation of neuroendocrine tumors of the lung. *Thorac Surg Clin* 24:267–276, 2014.

92. Horsch D, Schmid KW, Anlauf M, et al: Neuroendocrine tumors of the bronchopulmonary system (typical and atypi-cal carcinoid tumors): Current strategies in diagnosis and treatment. Conclusions of an expert meeting February 2011 in Weimar, Germany. *Oncol Res Treat* 37:266–276, 2014.

93. Maziak DE, Todd TR, Keshavjee SH, et al: Adenoid cystic carcinoma of the airway: Thirty-two-year experience. *J Thorac Cardiovasc Surg* 112:1522–1531, discussion 1531-1532, 1996.

94. Gaissert HA, Grillo HC, Shadmehr MB, et al: Long-term survival after resection of primary adenoid cystic and squamous cell carcinoma of the trachea and carina. *Ann Thorac Surg* 78:1889–1896, discussion 1896-1897, 2004.

95. Blackmon SH, Rice DC, Correa AM, et al: Management of primary pulmonary artery sarcomas. *Ann Thorac Surg* 87:977–984, 2009.

96. Huddleston CB: Pectus excavatum. *Semin Thorac Cardiovasc Surg* 16:225–232, 2004.

97. Shah AA, D'Amico TA: Primary chest wall tumors. *J Am Coll Surg* 210:360–366, 2010.

98. Walsh GL, Davis BM, Swisher SG, et al: A single-institutional, multidisciplinary approach to primary sarcomas involving the chest wall requiring full-thickness resections. *J Thorac Cardiovasc Surg* 121:48–60, 2001.

99. Gross JL, Younes RN, Haddad FJ, et al: Soft-tissue sarcomas of the chest wall: Prognostic factors. *Chest* 127:902–908, 2005.

100. Sanders RJ, Hammond SL, Rao NM: Diagnosis of thoracic outlet syndrome. *J Vasc Surg* 46:601–604, 2007.

101. Chang KZ, Likes K, Davis K, et al: The significance of cervical ribs in thoracic outlet syndrome. *J Vasc Surg* 57:771–775, 2013.

102. Klaassen Z, Sorenson E, Tubbs RS, et al: Thoracic outlet syndrome: A neurological and vascular disorder. *Clin Anat* 27:724–732, 2014.

103. Orlando MS, Likes KC, Mirza S, et al: A decade of excellent outcomes after surgical intervention in 538 patients with thoracic outlet syndrome. *J Am Coll Surg* 220:934–939, 2015.

104. Povlsen B, Belzberg A, Hansson T, et al: Treatment for thoracic outlet syndrome. *Cochrane Database Syst Rev* CD007218, 2010.

105. Light RW, Macgregor MI, Luchsinger PC, et al: Pleural effusions: The diagnostic separation of transudates and exudates. *Ann Intern Med* 77:507–513, 1972.

106. Putnam JB, Jr, Light RW, Rodriguez RM, et al: A randomized comparison of indwelling pleural catheter and doxycycline pleurodesis in the management of malignant pleural effusions. *Cancer* 86:1992–1999, 1999.

107. Heffner JE, Nietert PJ, Barbieri C: Pleural fluid pH as a predictor of survival for patients with malignant pleural effusions. *Chest* 117:79–86, 2000.

108. Warren WH, Kalimi R, Khodadadian LM, et al: Management of malignant pleural effusions using the pleurx catheter. *Ann Thor Surg* 85:1049–1055, 2007.

109. Dresler CM, Olak J, Herndon JE, 2nd, et al: Phase III intergroup study of talc poudrage vs talc slurry sclerosis for malignant pleural effusion. *Chest* 127:909–915, 2005.

110. Brims FJ, Lansley SM, Waterer GW, et al: Empyema thoracis: new insights into an old disease. *Eur Respir Rev* 19:220–228, 2010.

111. Light RW: Parapneumonic effusions and empyema. *Proc Am Thorac Soc* 3:75–80, 2006.

112. Molnar TF: Current surgical treatment of thoracic empyema in adults. *Eur J Cardiothorac Surg* 32:422–430, 2007.

113. Rahman NM, Maskell NA, West A, et al: Intrapleural use of tissue plasminogen activator and DNase in pleural infection. *N Engl J Med* 365:518–526, 2011.

114. Nair SK, Petko M, Hayward MP: Aetiology and management of chylothorax in adults. *Eur J Cardiothorac Surg* 32:362–369, 2007.

115. Lyon S, Mott N, Koukounaras J, et al: Role of interventional radiology in the management of chylothorax: A review of the current management of high output chylothorax. *Cardiovasc Intervent Radiol* 36:599–607, 2013.

116. Travis WD: Sarcomatoid neoplasms of the lung and pleura. *Arch Pathol Lab Med* 134:1645–1658, 2010.

117. Ellis P, Davies AM, Evans WK, et al: The use of chemotherapy in patients with advanced malignant pleural mesothelioma: A systematic review and practice guideline. *J Thorac Oncol* 1:591–601, 2006.

118. Yanagawa J, Rusch V: Surgical management of malignant pleural mesothelioma. *Thorac Surg Clin* 23:73–87, 2013.

119. Friedberg JS: The state of the art in the technical performance of lung-sparing operations for malignant pleural mesothelioma. *Semin Thorac Cardiovasc Surg* 25:125–143, 2013.

120. Sugarbaker DJ, Wolf AS: Surgery for malignant pleural mesothelioma. *Expert Rev Respir Med* 4:363–372, 2010.

121. Whitten CR, Khan S, Munneke GJ, et al: A diagnostic approach to mediastinal abnormalities. *Radiographics* 27:657–671, 2007.

122. Donahue JM, Nichols FC: Primary mediastinal tumors and cysts and diagnostic investigation of mediastinal masses. In Shields TW, LoCicero J, III, Reed CE, et al, editors: *General thoracic surgery*, ed 7, Philadelphia, 2009, Lippincott Williams & Wilkins, pp 2195–2199.

123. Falkson CB, Bezjak A, Darling G, et al: The management of thymoma: A systematic review and practice guideline. *J Thorac Oncol* 4:911–919, 2009.

124. Kim ES, Putnam JB, Komaki R, et al: Phase II study of a multidisciplinary approach with induction chemotherapy, followed by surgical resection, radiation therapy, and consolidation chemotherapy for unresectable malignant thymomas: Final report. *Lung Cancer* 44:369–379, 2004.

125. Wright CD: Extended resections for thymic malignancies. *J Thorac Oncol* 5:S344–S347, 2010.

126. Walsh GL, Taylor GD, Nesbitt JC, et al: Intensive chemotherapy and radical resections for primary nonseminomatous mediastinal germ cell tumors. *Ann Thorac Surg* 69:337–343, discussion 343-344, 2000.

127. Kesler KA, Einhorn LH: Multimodality treatment of germ cell tumors of the mediastinum. *Thorac Surg Clin* 19:63–69, 2009.

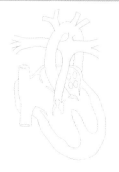

CHAPTER 58

Congenital Heart Disease

Charles D. Fraser, Jr., Lauren C. Kane

第五十八章　先天性心脏病

中文导读

　　本章共分为8节：①先天性心脏病外科发展历史及瓶颈；②先天性心脏病的诊疗流程；③先天性心脏病的解剖、术语及诊断；④先天性心脏病围手术期处理；⑤病变总论；⑥单心室；⑦其他心脏畸形；⑧小结。

　　第一节介绍了自19世纪40年代开始，随着氧合器技术的发展，外科医生逐步攻克了各种类型的心脏畸形，绝大多数罹患先天性心脏病的患儿有望获得手术治疗，延长生命，改善生活质量。

　　第二节概述了先天性心脏病的诊疗现状及相关思考。得益于遗传学和胎儿超声技术的快速发展，很多先天性心脏病在胎儿期即可诊断，有助于尽早进行医疗干预。先天性心脏病由于其病变复杂性的特点，需要多学科合作，为先天性心脏病患儿制定综合治疗方案。

　　第三节介绍了心脏解剖和心脏形态学描述系统，规范先天性心脏病术语。充分理解并掌握先天性心脏

病解剖和病理生理特点对于诊断和围手术期治疗具有重要指导意义。详细阐述了先天性心脏病的诊断方法，包括体格检查和各项辅助检查，重点介绍了各项检查的临床意义。

　　第四节主要讲述先天性心脏病围手术期治疗的要点及难点。结合不同种类先天性心脏病的病理生理特点，具体讲解了麻醉管理和术后药物治疗的特殊之处，针对性地指出麻醉过程中的关注要点及可能出现的各种疏忽及处理对策。

　　第五节全面介绍了各种常见先天性心脏病的胚胎学基础、解剖异常、病理生理学特点，结合具体病例

提纲挈领地介绍了不同术式的选择、手术要点和难点。

第六节介绍了单心室是较少见的先天性畸形，病人可能在新生儿期即表现出肺血不足、肺血过多或肺血均衡等多种不同状态，需要外科干预以提供足够的体循环供氧以及保护肺血管发育。主要介绍了单心室的外科治疗思路和策略。

第七节重点介绍了血管环和肺动脉吊带、冠脉血管发育异常、Ebstain畸形、二尖瓣狭窄等罕见心血管畸形的解剖特点、临床表现、诊断方法、手术时机的把握和手术方式。

第八节介绍了充分理解先天性心脏病病人的解剖学和病理学特征是制定合理治疗策略的必要条件，本章推荐的文献和书籍能更好地让广大专科医生理解各种先天性心脏病的特点和治疗方法。

〔魏　翔〕

This chapter is designed to provide medical students, general surgery residents, and practicing general surgeons with a working tool to aid in their understanding of the features of anatomy and physiology in patients presenting for general surgical procedures in the setting of repaired or unrepaired congenital cardiac lesions. The large scope and breadth of the evolving field of congenital heart surgery precludes an exhaustive treatise on all aspects of this specialty. Several excellent and thorough textbooks of congenital heart surgery are referenced in this chapter, and the reader is encouraged to use them for additional in-depth understanding of the lesions to be reviewed. A general surgeon practicing today needs to be well versed in the basics of cardiac anatomy, physiology, and specific derangements associated with the various known congenital cardiac lesions. Furthermore, few patients with complex congenital cardiac lesions may be considered cured of their cardiac problem, even after successful reconstructive surgery. Thus, it is imperative that a general surgeon who needs to perform a noncardiac operation on such a patient be familiar with the specific issues of ongoing concern in patients with congenital cardiac disease.

HISTORY AND OTHER CONSIDERATIONS

The era of surgical treatment for congenital cardiac anomalies was initiated in November 1944, when Alfred Blalock and associates Vivien Thomas and Helen Taussig combined their unique talents and vision to treat a young child dying of cyanotic congenital heart disease (CHD).[1] This palliative operation involved the surgical creation of a systemic–pulmonary artery connection in the patient, who had inadequate pulmonary blood flow. The procedure has since been recalled as miraculous and now more than 60 years later is known by the eponym Blalock-Taussig (BT) shunt. The striking success of this simple concept and the reproducible nature of the operation in children with otherwise fatal cardiac conditions have emboldened subsequent surgical innovators to venture inside the congenitally malformed heart. At first, the parent was asked to serve as a biologic oxygenator using the technique of controlled cross-circulation; soon thereafter, the mechanical, extracorporeal, heart-lung bypass pump was developed.[2,3] With the aid of this ability to support the patient's circulation during intracardiac exploration, surgeons have sequentially attacked almost every described congenital cardiac anomaly. The prospect of meaningful survival for patients born with otherwise devastating congenital cardiac lesions is now expected in most, if not all, cases.

As a result of this success story, there is now a large and growing population of adults with repaired or unrepaired CHD; estimates in the United States for 2010 placed the number of adult patients surviving with repaired or palliated congenital cardiac lesions at more than 1 million.[4] There has been an increase of greater than 50% in CHD prevalence since 2000, and by 2010, adults accounted for two thirds of patients with CHD in the general population.[5] This reality has been associated with new challenges in the ongoing medical maintenance of such patients, with particular focus on the care of patients with congenital cardiac lesions presenting for surgery for noncardiac illnesses. The evolving subspecialty of adult CHD points to the unique needs of this population of patients.

PATHWAYS FOR PRACTICING CONGENITAL HEART SURGERY

Before embarking on a review of the field, it is worthwhile to describe the setting in which patients with CHD seek and receive care in today's medical environment. With the development of sophisticated methods of fetal ultrasound, a large percentage of children requiring surgery for CHD are diagnosed during gestation (Fig. 58-1). A fetal diagnosis of complex CHD is extremely helpful to parents and the medical management team. Fetal diagnosis is particularly important in the setting of lesions dependent on persistent patency of the ductus arteriosus for postnatal survival. In these individuals, survival after delivery is predicated on the maintenance of ductal patency through the intravenous infusion of prostaglandin E1 (PGE1) initiated in the delivery suite, often through an umbilical vein catheter. Several studies have shown a decrease in morbidity, but there is inconclusive evidence that mortality rates are decreased.[6,7]

A growing number of congenital cardiac lesions are known to be associated with specific genetic mutations, many clearly inherited and some presumed to be sporadic. A chromosomal analysis

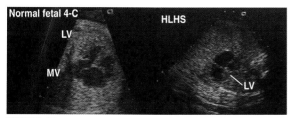

FIGURE 58-1 Normal fetal ultrasound (four chamber; *left*) and fetal ultrasound of a child with hypoplastic left heart syndrome *(right)*. *LV,* Left ventricle; *MV,* mitral valve.

is frequently performed in individuals found to have major structural cardiac abnormalities; this analysis may be performed during gestation through amniocentesis or after delivery. The chromosomal evaluation is beneficial to the family when planning the risk of such an occurrence in future offspring. For the clinician, knowledge of chromosomal abnormalities in their patients, such as DiGeorge sequence, velocardiofacial syndrome, and Marfan syndrome, aids in the delivery of acute medical management.

In general terms, the timing of surgery for various congenital cardiac conditions depends on the presenting symptoms and expectations for further associated complications. Neonates presenting with limited pulmonary blood flow or atretic pulmonary connections typically require surgery during the first few days of life and occasionally within hours of delivery. Lesions associated with excessive pulmonary blood flow result in early heart failure, which may manifest as poor feeding, tachypnea, or respiratory failure. These patients are operated on during early infancy to ameliorate their symptoms and prevent the development of pulmonary vascular disease.

Preterm and low-birth-weight infants with CHD have been presenting for surgical consideration with more frequency. This treatment strategy requires thoughtful planning and coordination among the surgery, anesthesia, cardiology, intensive care, and neonatology teams. At our institution, the Texas Children's Hospital, we successfully operated on an 800-g infant with transposition of the great arteries (TGA).

The specialty of congenital heart surgery is now recognized as a subspecialty of cardiothoracic surgery. Congenital heart surgeons were previously certified in cardiothoracic surgery by the American Board of Thoracic Surgery and received additional fellowship training in the United States or abroad in congenital heart surgery. As of 2009, the American Board of Thoracic Surgery offers a formal certification process for subspecialty training in congenital heart surgery. At the present time, there are 12 congenital cardiac surgery residency programs approved by the Accreditation Council for Graduate Medical Education.[8] Most pediatric cardiac surgery is performed in large, multispecialty children's hospitals in association with formal programs focused on the care of these complex patients. The management team includes pediatric cardiac anesthesiologists, perfusionists, and nursing staff. Focused pediatric cardiac intensive care units have been developed to optimize the patients' opportunity for recovery.

Historically, pediatric cardiologists have provided the medical management of patients born with CHD. Pediatric cardiology is also evolving. With advances in catheter-based technology, interventional pediatric cardiologists are now addressing lesions previously treated with surgery. Examples include device closure of

atrial septal defects (ASDs) and ventricular septal defects (VSDs), occlusion of patent ductus arteriosus (PDA), and dilation and stenting of stenotic vessels in the systemic and pulmonary circulation. For a more in-depth review of this specialty, see the excellent technical text by Mullins.[9]

The care for adults with CHD is in evolution. This issue is of particular relevance to the general surgeon faced with operating on an adult patient with significant CHD. One overriding message needs to be clear to the general surgeon in this setting: It must be assumed that in patients with previously repaired congenital cardiac lesions, even without overt cardiac symptoms, the potential for significant perioperative cardiorespiratory derangement exists. More simply stated, the presence of a surgical scar on the chest of a patient with known CHD does not suggest that the lesion has been cured. With this message firmly in mind, the general surgeon may find it challenging to determine the best source for a qualified consultation for such a patient. At the present time, many adult cardiologists are not adequately trained in CHD to provide competent consultation on adult patients with CHD.

Pediatric cardiologists are not educated in adult medicine and cardiology, and many feel uncomfortable providing consultation on adult patients with CHD. The subspecialty of adult CHD is currently becoming more formalized, but the number of physicians who have been educated specifically to care for these patients is still few. In 2015, the American Board of Internal Medicine offered the first certification examination in Adult Congenital Heart Disease. The Accreditation Council for Graduate Medical Education–accredited fellowship is expected to be available in 2019.[10] The practicing general surgeon needs to become familiar with the specific issues of concern for patients with CHD to ascertain that the patient's unique anatomic and physiologic issues have been evaluated properly. A pediatric cardiologist, in coordination with an adult cardiologist, must evaluate adult patients with CHD who present for care in a center without a designated qualified specialist. Of equal importance, the anesthesiologists and intensivists caring for an adult patient with CHD must have a working understanding of the complexities and nuances of the patient's cardiac condition. The anesthetic management of patients with CHD undergoing general surgical procedures is complicated and can become disastrous if managed improperly.

ANATOMY, TERMINOLOGY, AND DIAGNOSIS

Anatomy and Terminology

One of the most intimidating aspects for the student of CHD is developing a level of comfort with the terminology used for describing specific lesions. A thorough and sound understanding of normal cardiac anatomy is mandatory. There are several excellent texts on this subject; in particular, the text edited by Wilcox and coworkers[11] is especially concise and clear. One difficulty that challenges proper understanding of anatomy is the frequent use of abbreviations and eponyms for various congenital lesions—for example, congenitally corrected transposition of the great arteries (ccTGA), ventricular inversion, and L-transposition all describe the same heart, but none provides a complete anatomic description. Unless otherwise clear to all clinicians involved in the care of these complicated patients, the anatomic description needs to be segmental and complete to avoid mistakes and misinterpretations of structure.

In describing congenital cardiac lesions, a segmental approach is used to determine the relationship of the various structural elements. The situs describes the relationship of sidedness—situs solitus (normal), situs inversus (reversed), or situs ambiguus (indeterminate). The cardiac elements described include (in sequence) the atria, ventricles, and great vessels. The relationship of the connections must be understood; connections are concordant (e.g., the right atrium connecting to the right ventricle) or discordant (e.g., the right ventricle connecting to the aorta). The chamber sidedness must be clarified (e.g., a morphologic right atrium may be on the left side of the patient). The relationship and connections of the cardiac valves must then be assessed; connections may be normal, stenotic, atretic, or straddling. Of note to the general surgeon, abnormal sidedness of the cardiac structures is frequently associated with abnormal relationships of the thoracic and abdominal organs. A thorough assessment of the patient's anatomy is recommended before surgery. Commonly used tools in evaluation of anatomy include echocardiogram, computed tomography (CT), magnetic resonance imaging (MRI), and cardiac catheterization.

There are two widely accepted and applied schools of cardiac morphologic description. The Van Praagh nomenclature uses abbreviations to describe the relationship of the atria, ventricular looping, and position of the aorta sequentially. The first letter describes the situs of the atrial chambers (and usually the abdominal organs): "S" for situs solitus (normal), "I" for situs inversus (reversed), or "A" for situs ambiguus (indeterminate). The second letter describes the relationship of the embryologic looping of the ventricles: "D" for dextro looping or right-handed topology (normal) or "L" (levo) for left-handed topology. The third and last letter describes the relationship of the aortic valve to the pulmonary valve: "D" for right-sided and "L" for left-sided (Fig. 58-2).

The Anderson nomenclature is more wordy and longer but is perhaps simpler to understand. The descriptions are again of the sequential relationship of the structures. Starting with the atria, the connections and relationships are sequentially described. Thus, the atrial sidedness is described, followed by the sequence of connections to the ventricles and then great vessels. For example, "atrial situs solitus (normal) with atrioventricular discordance (reversed) and ventriculoarterial discordance (reversed)" describes the heart mentioned earlier as corrected transposition, or S,L,L by the Van Praagh classification (Fig. 58-3).

Diagnosis

As with all aspects of surgery, a wide variety of highly sophisticated diagnostic tools are available to examine cardiac structure and function. Despite the widespread availability and application of these tools, none has replaced or eliminated the necessity of a thorough history and physical examination. Most patients who have a history of CHD become very well informed about the specifics of their cardiac conditions, as do their parents. A detailed review of the patient's past medical history is mandatory. This review includes, when possible, securing records from all previous diagnostic and procedural reports. An incorrect assumption often is made about a patient's previous surgical history and anatomy, frequently in a setting in which a patient's old operative report or clinical summary could easily clarify the misunderstanding.

In adults with CHD, in particular, there are specific points of medical history that must be elucidated. A history of palpitations, syncope, and neurologic deficit must be investigated further. The incidence of significant dysrhythmias in certain categories of adults with CHD is high and, in many cases, warrants further investigation, including continuous monitoring (Holter), electrophysiologic study, or provocative testing.

Physical Examination

A complete physical examination in a patient with previously repaired CHD often yields critical information for the proper planning of a general surgical procedure. Patients need to be completely undressed and thoroughly examined. In many cyanotic patients, color changes may be prominent, particularly in the nail beds, lips, and mucous membranes. In other patients, cyanosis may be more subtle, giving the patient a gray or even pale appearance. Previous surgical incisions need to be noted and reconciled with the known medical history. Thoracotomy incisions on either side may indicate a previous BT shunt using the turned-down, divided subclavian artery or with a prosthetic interposition graft—the so-called modified BT shunt. In patients with a left aortic arch, a left thoracotomy incision is present if a previous coarctation repair has been carried out. Median sternotomy incisions or anterior thoracotomy incisions may indicate previous intracardiac or extracardiac surgery.

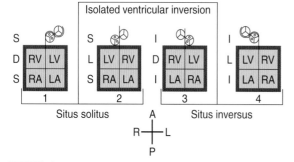

FIGURE 58-2 Model depicting cardiac morphology for normal hearts—that is, hearts with atrioventricular concordance and ventriculoarterial concordance—using Van Praagh nomenclature. The *vertical line* above the box denotes the position of the ventricular septum. (From Kirklin JW, Barratt-Boyes BG: General considerations: Anatomy, dimensions, and terminology. In *Cardiac surgery*, ed 2, New York, 1993, Churchill Livingstone.)

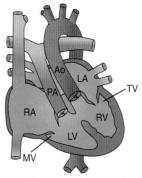

FIGURE 58-3 Congenitally corrected transposition of the great arteries. Atrial situs solitus (normal) with atrioventricular discordance and ventriculoarterial discordance using Anderson nomenclature, S,L,L by Van Praagh classification. *Ao*, Aorta; *LA*, left atrium; *LV*, left ventricle; *MV*, mitral valve; *RA*, right atrium; *RV*, right ventricle; *TV*, tricuspid valve.

A complete vascular examination is often overlooked in patients with CHD. It is important to assess pulses and obtain blood pressure measurements in all four extremities. Patients who have an existing or have previously had a BT shunt often have diminished or absent pulses in the upper extremity corresponding to the previous shunt. Also, patients with previous coarctation repairs may have diminished or absent pulses in the left upper extremity, especially if a subclavian flap angioplasty was performed (Waldhausen procedure). Furthermore, a history of previous coarctation repair does not guarantee that the lower extremity pulses and blood pressures will be normal. Moreover, patients who have undergone previous cardiac catheterization may have chronically stenosed or occluded femoral vessels. All these issues may be of significance for monitoring and vascular access in a patient undergoing a general surgical procedure.

Later in this chapter, the Fontan procedure for single-ventricle palliation is reviewed. Briefly, this operation results in significant systemic venous hypertension, often in 12 to 15 mm Hg. In patients with a Fontan circulation, physical examination may reveal hepatic congestion, ascites, pedal edema, venous varicosities, and jugular venous distention. In some patients, macronodular hepatic cirrhosis may be suspected on the basis of a firm fibrotic liver edge.

Entire textbooks have been dedicated to the physical examination of patients with cardiac disease, and a thorough discussion of this issue, particularly the specifics of cardiac auscultation, is beyond the scope of this chapter. In general, the cardiac examination includes an assessment of the patient's rhythm, point of maximal impulse, and character of any auscultated murmurs. Also, the absence of a significant cardiac murmur does not rule out significant cardiac pathology.

Diagnostic Tests

Pulse oximetry. Four-extremity pulse oximetry is an essential part of the clinical assessment of a patient with suspected CHD. Patients with ductal-dependent circulation to the lower body (severe aortic coarctation or aortic arch interruption) may present with differential cyanosis. This presentation indicates the ejection of desaturated systemic venous blood through the patent ductus to the descending aorta contrasted with fully saturated pulmonary venous blood ejected to the ascending aorta and the upper extremities. Baseline (room air) saturation must be documented in all patients for whom an operative intervention is anticipated to establish their normal range.

Plain radiography. Standard chest radiography with anteroposterior and lateral views is still an essential component of the assessment of a patient with CHD. Standard elements to be examined include a skeletal survey, assessment of the diaphragms and hepatic shadow, and location of the gastric bubble. The lung fields are assessed for pulmonary plethora (arterial or venous), air space disease, and the presence of effusions. The cardiac silhouette may reveal essential information, such as a cardiothoracic ratio indicative of cardiomegaly or pericardial effusion, the presence of atrial enlargement, the presence or absence of the pulmonary artery shadow, and arch sidedness (Fig. 58-4).

Electrocardiography. The electrocardiogram (ECG) is important in assessing patients with CHD. The rate and rhythm must be noted, including the presence or absence of P wave activity and axis. Many patients with CHD, especially patients with complex conditions such as heterotaxy syndrome, may exhibit deranged or absent sinus node activity, giving rise to a predominant junctional rhythm, which may significantly compromise cardiac output. The

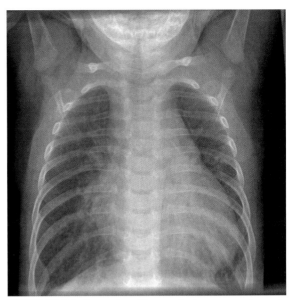

FIGURE 58-4 Cardiomegaly and increased pulmonary vascular markings in a patient with complete atrioventricular canal defect.

QRS duration and axis reveal information concerning conduction delay and abnormal ventricular forces. For example, patients with atrioventricular (A-V) canal defects are known to have left axis deviation. Furthermore, in patients undergoing repair of certain forms of CHD, there may be an early or late predisposition to malignant dysrhythmias. It is particularly important to elucidate a history of palpitations from a patient with repaired or unrepaired CHD; such a history may warrant further investigation with 24-hour continuous ECG monitoring (Holter).

Echocardiography. Noninvasive imaging is well established as the primary diagnostic modality for structural cardiac disease. For most patients, excellent anatomic detail may be obtained using two-dimensional transthoracic imaging. Standard images include subcostal, suprasternal, parasternal, and subxiphoid views and are oriented in long and short axis directions. Furthermore, significant hemodynamic information may be inferred using echo Doppler blood flow velocities and interpreted using the modified Bernoulli formula (pressure gradient = $4V^2$, where V is echocardiographic velocity in m/sec). To assess the patient's cardiac lesion properly, segmental analysis of the cardiac structures, connections, and valves must be performed. A quantitative estimate of ejection fraction, shortening fraction, and valvular inflow velocity aids in assessing cardiac function. For most patients with CHD, adequate diagnostic information is attainable through echocardiography in the hands of a qualified pediatric cardiologist.

Magnetic resonance imaging and computed tomography. Cardiac MRI and CT are adjuncts to echocardiography for noninvasive structural and functional assessment of the heart. MRI has been used with increasing frequency to provide anatomic detail in congenitally malformed hearts in which echocardiographic detail is lacking or unattainable. This modality has proved particularly useful for imaging the extracardiac great vessels and systemic and pulmonary venous connections and for providing accurate estimates of cardiac function, especially right ventricular ejection fraction. MRI has the added benefit of using nonionizing electromagnetic fields. CT may also be used for such imaging detail but has the potential detrimental association with significant radiation exposure. A CT scan of the chest averages 5 to 7 mSv, and CT coronary angiography averages 9 to 11 mSv.[12]

Cardiac catheterization. Cardiac catheterization was long considered the gold standard for diagnostic imaging of congenitally malformed hearts. With the current sophistication of echocardiography, this is no longer the case for most patients. Nonetheless, there are still circumstances in which diagnostic cardiac catheterization is necessary to obtain accurate anatomic detail. One such circumstance may be patients who have poor echocardiographic windows, although even this issue may be overcome using transesophageal echocardiography. More often, there are specifics of anatomic detail that neither echocardiography nor MRI can delineate, such as branch pulmonary artery (or segmental) stenosis, origin and course of aortopulmonary collateral vessels, and fistulous connections and intracardiac communications (septal defects) not clarified by other imaging modalities.

Usually, diagnostic cardiac catheterization is performed to obtain precise hemodynamic information needed to make an informed assessment of the consequences of the patient's cardiac lesions. Using oximetric measurements, pressure data, and thermodilution cardiac output determination, accurate assessment of the patient's hemodynamic profile is obtained. Measured or derived data include central venous pressure, atrial pressure, ventricular pressures (including end-diastolic pressure), shunt fraction (in the case of ASDs or VSDs), pulmonary artery pressures, pulmonary capillary wedge pressure, systemic arterial pressure, and segmental oximetry of cardiac structures, including systemic and pulmonary venous return (Fig. 58-5). Thus, critical information is obtained about the presence and degree of shunting, systemic and pulmonary vascular resistance (PVR), and cardiopulmonary function. In certain clinical settings, these data are mandatory to a successful clinical management strategy. This may

be particularly true for an adult patient with CHD requiring noncardiac surgery.

A thorough understanding of normal cardiorespiratory physiology is critical in interpreting data obtained by cardiac catheterization in a patient with CHD. Specifically, the normal pressure range, pulse waveforms, and oxygen saturations for the various cardiac chambers must be compared against data obtained in a deranged circulation. The various cardiac chambers have normal pulse waveforms. In the atria, there are characteristic waveforms—a wave corresponding to atrial contraction, c wave corresponding to A-V valve closure, and v wave corresponding to atrial filling from venous return against the closed A-V valve. Typical normal right atrial mean pressures range from 1 to 5 mm Hg, and left atrial pressures range from 2 to 10 mm Hg. Right ventricular pressure tracings in normal hearts demonstrate a more gradual upstroke when compared with the left ventricle. Filling or end-diastolic pressures are between 2 and 10 mm Hg in normal hearts. The normal right ventricular systolic pressure (and thus pulmonary artery systolic pressure) is 15 to 30 mm Hg, and the left ventricular systolic pressure is 90 to 110 mm Hg.

In normal hearts, there is a small, physiologically insignificant right-to-left shunt, which results from ventilation-perfusion mismatch in the lungs and coronary venous return directly to the left ventricle (thebesian venous return). This physiologic shunt represents less than 5% of the cardiac output and, in normal circumstances, does not produce detectable systemic arterial desaturation. Thus, significant systemic arterial desaturation represents a pathologic finding, consistent with pulmonary disease, intracardiac shunting, or both. As noted, the origin and degree of intracardiac shunting may be assessed by echocardiography. However, in certain circumstances, cardiac catheterization is necessary to measure cardiac oximetry, calculate shunt fraction, and derive systemic and PVR. Using a derivation of the Fick principle, the ratio of pulmonary blood flow (Qp) to systemic blood flow (Qs) can be determined as follows:

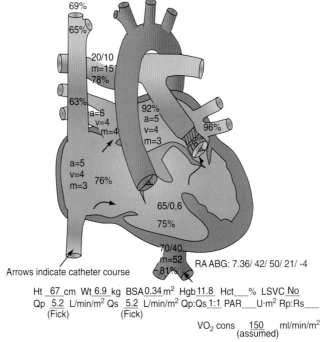

FIGURE 58-5 Hemodynamic information obtained after cardiac catheterization.

$$Qp/Qs = (SaO_2 \text{ sat} - (\overline{M}O_2 \text{ sat})/(\overline{P}O_2 \text{ sat}) - PaO_2 \text{ sat})$$

where SaO_2 sat is systemic arterial oxygen saturation, $\overline{M}O_2$ sat is mixed venous oxygen saturation, $\overline{P}O_2$ sat is pulmonary venous oxygen saturation, and PaO_2 sat is pulmonary arterial oxygen saturation.

Thus, in a patient with $\overline{M}O_2$ sat of 60%, $\overline{P}O_2$ sat of 100%, SaO_2 sat of 100%, and PaO_2 sat of 80%, the equation is as follows:

$$Qp/Qs = (100 - 60)/(100 - 80) = 40/20 = 2:1$$

Calculating vascular resistances may also be crucial in determining operability in a patient with CHD. In many settings, a precise measure of vascular resistance is unnecessary based on the clinical evidence. For example, in a small child with a large VSD seen on echocardiogram, the clinical findings of tachypnea, cardiomegaly, and failure to thrive confirm a large left-to-right shunt and infer acceptable PVR. However, in less clear circumstances, a precise calculation may be important in clinical decision making. The PVR may be calculated from cardiac catheterization data as follows:

Pulmonary vascular resistance (Rp)
= (mean pulmonary artery pressure [in mm Hg]
  − mean left atrial pressure [in 2 mm Hg])/
  (pulmonary blood flow [Qp, in liters/min/m])

In general, patients with an elevated PVR are further evaluated with pulmonary vasodilation—hyperventilation, hyperoxygenation, and inhaled nitric oxide—to determine whether the resistance is responsive. This information may be critical for patients who are otherwise marginal candidates.

Finally, cardiac catheterization has been evolving as the primary therapeutic method for many important structural cardiac defects. In many children's hospitals, including Texas Children's Hospital, most catheterizations now performed are for interventional procedures rather than diagnostic procedures. This fact may be particularly pertinent to a general surgeon faced with treating a patient with a previous catheter-based correction of a cardiac defect. For example, the patient may have had an ASD or VSD closed with an occluder device in the past. This information may have important ramifications for infectious exposure and vascular access.

PERIOPERATIVE CARE

Perioperative management of a patient with unrepaired or palliated CHD can be extremely challenging. Standard hemodynamic, respiratory, and pharmacologic manipulations appropriate for structurally normal hearts may be entirely inappropriate in settings of complex CHD; this is especially true in the operating room and intensive care settings. General rules include a thorough knowledge of the patient's intracardiac anatomy and expected physiology. It is possible to make significant management errors based on incorrect physiologic expectations in the setting of incomplete understanding of the patient's anatomy. For example, in a patient with unrepaired tetralogy of Fallot (TOF) and associated significant right ventricular outflow tract obstruction (RVOTO), it is expected that the patient will exhibit some degree of systemic arterial desaturation. However, a patient with repaired TOF, with no residual intracardiac shunts, needs to be fully saturated. This clinical scenario is a frequent one; a patient with a specific cardiac diagnosis, despite having undergone a successful correction, continues to be incorrectly presumed to have ongoing physiologic perturbation.

Anesthesia Pitfalls

Providing physiologic anesthetic management can be challenging in patients with CHD, especially in situations such as chronic single-ventricle palliation, unrepaired CHD, chronic cyanosis, and residual intracardiac pathology. Standard anesthetic management paradigms may be completely inappropriate and potentially disastrous in the setting of complex CHD. A thorough understanding of the patient's anatomy is mandatory, along with knowledge of the potential for unexpected response to anesthetic agents and ventilator settings. The field of pediatric and congenital cardiac anesthesia has evolved relative to this specific clinical need; the text by Andropoulos and colleagues[13] is an excellent resource.

Several points concerning anesthesia management warrant discussion. The first is vascular access for intraoperative and postoperative management. In patients with complex CHD, especially patients who have undergone previous complex surgical and catheterization procedures, obtaining appropriate vascular access may be challenging. Typically, a large-bore, multilumen central venous line is necessary for appropriate resuscitation and monitoring of right-sided filling pressures. In some patients, the placement of a thermodilution pulmonary artery catheter (oximetric) must be considered because one cannot presume that right-sided filling pressures correlate well with left heart volume or functional status (e.g., after a Fontan operation). Options for central access include percutaneous internal jugular or subclavian routes, with a secondary option of common femoral access to the inferior vena cava (IVC). Access may be difficult in the setting of previous catheterization or venous reconstruction; this situation may be addressed with the aid of ultrasound-guided catheter placement, which has become a standard in many cardiac operating room. Arterial access for continuous blood pressure monitoring and sampling is important for many patients. Percutaneous radial arterial cannulation can be readily achieved in most patients; however, upper extremity blood pressure values may be factitiously altered by previous systemic-to-pulmonary artery shunts, previous aortic arch surgery (especially coarctation), and abnormalities of vascular origin (e.g., aberrant subclavian origin from the descending aorta).

Ventilator management in the perioperative setting of CHD requires special understanding. In settings of large potential left-to-right shunts (e.g., unrepaired VSDs), hyperventilation and hyperoxygenation promote excessive pulmonary blood flow and potentially diminish systemic cardiac output. Positive pressure ventilation, particularly positive end-expiratory pressure, negatively influences hemodynamics in many patients, especially in palliated patients with a single ventricle after the Fontan procedure. Early extubation in these patients can be done to limit the deleterious effects of positive end-expiratory pressure on the Fontan circulation. Early data showed that early extubation improves outcomes for these patients and reduces overall hospital costs.[14] Finally, pharmacologic manipulation of systemic and PVR and cardiac performance is an important adjunct in the perioperative management of patients with CHD. In general, a low-dose infusion of epinephrine 0.05 mcg/kg/min (0.02-0.05 mcg/kg/min) with the addition of a phosphodiesterase inhibitor is an effective pharmacologic cocktail to promote a cardiac inotropic state, lower systemic and PVR, and limit tachycardia. Dopamine, vasopressin, sodium nitroprusside, and nitroglycerin are other frequently used agents. Appropriate perioperative analgesia and sedation are also important aspects of the patient's management.

Neurologic Outcomes

With expectations of almost 100% survival after surgery for CHD, emphasis has been placed on the long-term neurologic outcomes and quality of life of these patients. The potential for neurologic insult in children after CHD arises from the nature of their disease (e.g., cyanotic defects, low cardiac output state, genetic syndromes, effects of cardiopulmonary bypass, circulatory arrest). Evidence also suggests that patients with CHD may be genetically predisposed to neurologic insult. Gestational age has been found to be an important factor to consider in the optimization of neurologic outcomes.[15]

LESION OVERVIEW

Defects Associated With Increased Pulmonary Blood Flow

Persistent Arterial Duct (Patent Ductus Arteriosus)

A persistent arterial duct, or PDA, is a frequently encountered congenital cardiac condition. The arterial duct is necessary during gestation to shunt right ventricular blood away from the unventilated pulmonary vasculature; ductal flow is from the pulmonary artery to the aorta during gestation. At delivery, after the first breath of the neonate, ductal flow reverses and becomes left to right in most individuals. Over the first several hours or days of postnatal life, the PDA closes spontaneously and is completely closed in most infants by 2 to 3 weeks of age.

In the absence of other congenital cardiac lesions, a PDA becomes pathologic related to its presence and the degree of left-to-right shunting. A PDA may be present in association with other structural cardiac conditions and may sometimes be necessary for systemic or pulmonary blood flow. The amount of shunting produced relates to the size and geometry of the duct and the PVR. A PDA may be responsible for a large Qp/Qs and result in pulmonary overcirculation, left heart volume overload, and congestive heart failure (CHF). A large unrestricted PDA is associated with pulmonary hypertension; if left untreated, this proceeds to irreversible pulmonary vascular disease (Eisenmenger syndrome), ultimately proceeding to pulmonary and right heart failure, treatable only by pulmonary transplantation. Even with a small, pressure-restrictive PDA, there is an ongoing risk for pulmonary congestion and left heart volume overloading; endocarditis is always of concern even for small PDAs. Closure is recommended for all PDAs.

The gold standard of therapy for closure of PDA is surgery, usually accomplished through a left thoracotomy using ductal division, ligation, or clipping (Fig. 58-6). Surgery needs to be a low-risk procedure associated with minimal potential for persistence. Nonetheless, the invasive nature of this proven method has led to the development of alternative strategies for ductal occlusion. From a surgical perspective, many PDAs are amenable to thoracoscopic clipping through very small port incisions; robot-assisted PDA occlusion has been performed in many patients, with good results.[11] Medical treatment with indomethacin 0.1 mg/kg (0.1 mg/kg for <1 kg, 0.2 mg/kg ≥1 kg on day 1, then 0.1 mg/kg daily for days 2-7 oral or IV over 1 hr) can be attempted in a neonate but carries risk of necrotizing enterocolitis, intracranial hemorrhage, and renal toxicity. However, at the present time, most PDAs are occluded in the cardiac catheterization laboratory using occlusive devices. Even the repair of large defects in small infants has been successfully addressed. The long-term effects of the devices remaining in the vascular tree are not fully understood yet; however, successful device closure appears to be an extremely effective and durable therapy.

A PDA in an adult patient can be challenging. As noted, a long-standing large PDA may be associated with pulmonary vascular disease. A right-to-left shunt in a PDA is cause for significant

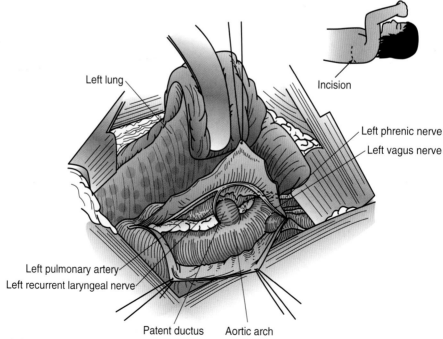

FIGURE 58-6 Anatomic relationships of a patent ductus arteriosus, exposed from a left thoracotomy. (From Castaneda AR, Jones RA, Mayer JE, Jr, et al: Patent ductus arteriosus. In *Cardiac surgery of the neonate and infant*, Philadelphia, 1994, Saunders.)

concern and warrants further investigation. In adults with PDAs, the arterial wall may calcify, making an attempt at ligation or division hazardous. In these patients, ductal occlusion may require resection of the adjacent descending aorta with patch grafting or short-segment graft replacement (Dacron).

Aortopulmonary Septal Defect (Aortopulmonary Window)

An aortopulmonary septal defect is a communication between the ascending aorta and, usually, the main pulmonary artery. This is a rare defect; it relates to the common embryologic origin of the arterial trunk and failure of complete separation into the aorta and pulmonary artery. Defects are classified by their location: Type I is proximal, just above the aortic sinuses; type II is more distal on the ascending aorta and often involves the origin of the right pulmonary artery; and type III is more distal and associated with a separate origin of the right pulmonary artery from the aorta (Fig. 58-7). An aortopulmonary septal defect may occur in isolation or in association with other conditions, including interrupted aortic arch (IAA) and anomalous origin of a coronary artery. Defects are typically large and responsible for a large left-to-right shunt with systemic pulmonary artery pressures. Children with this problem typically present with CHF, failure to thrive, and frequent respiratory infections. Echocardiography, MRI, or cardiac catheterization may be used to make the diagnosis.

All aortopulmonary septal defects are surgically closed; this lesion is not amenable to catheter-based closure, and such an attempt is hazardous. A small defect may be ligated through a thoracotomy or median sternotomy approach, but this method is not recommended because of significant risk for rupture or incomplete closure. Surgical closure is accomplished with cardiopulmonary bypass support. Options for closure include complete division and separate patch repairs of the great vessel defects or a sandwich type of closure, using a patch to construct a common intervening wall; both methods are effective (Fig. 58-8).

Atrial Septal Defect

An isolated ASD is one of the most common congenital cardiac lesions. The most frequently encountered ASD relates to a defect in the interatrial wall, as defined by the fossa ovalis. The defect develops as the result of incomplete closure of the embryologic patent foramen ovale; the defect is a result of incomplete closure of the septum primum. Although the terminology can be confusing, these defects are typically termed *secundum atrial septal defects.* They manifest in a wide variety of configurations, ranging from single small defects to multiple fenestrations to complete absence of the septum primum. The confines of the defect may extend from the IVC orifice up to the superior atrial wall adjacent to the aortic root (Fig. 58-9).

The primary pathophysiologic derangement in ASDs relates to a significant left-to-right shunt in the setting of normal PVR. However, even in the setting of a normal PVR, patients with ASDs are capable of transient right-to-left shunting, particularly during times of increased intrathoracic pressure. The effects of chronic, large left-to-right shunting (in some patients producing a Qp/Qs >3:1) include right heart volume overloading and enlargement. Most children are not overtly symptomatic but may exhibit some degree of exercise intolerance or frequent respiratory tract infection. Symptoms typically become more prevalent in adulthood and include dyspnea on exertion, palpitations, and, ultimately, evidence of right heart failure. Pulmonary vascular disease is not a typical finding in secundum ASDs, but one may demonstrate an ASD in a patient with primary pulmonary

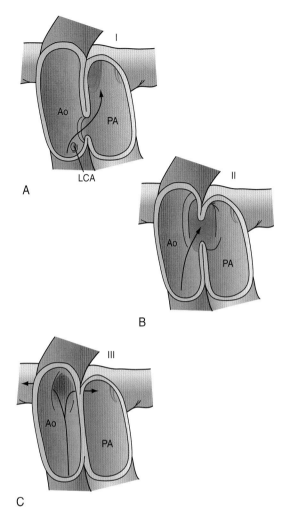

FIGURE 58-7 Native anatomy and classification of aortopulmonary septal defect. **A,** In type I, the communication is between the ascending aorta *(Ao)* and the main pulmonary artery *(PA)* on the posterior medial wall of the ascending aorta. The left main coronary artery *(LCA)* orifice may be close to the defect. **B,** In type II, the defect is more cephalic on the ascending aorta. **C,** In type III, the defect is more posterior and lateral in the aorta. The communication is with the right pulmonary artery, which may be completely separate from the main pulmonary artery. (Adapted from Fraser CD: Aortopulmonary septal defects and patent ductus arteriosus. In Nichols DG, Ungerleider RM, Spevak PJ, et al, editors: *Critical heart disease in infants and children,* Philadelphia, 2006, Mosby, pp 664–666.)

hypertension. A rare form of presentation relates to the potential of right-to-left shunting at the atrial level; the ever-present risk for paradoxical embolus and cerebrovascular accident must be considered when recommending ASD closure.

Most centers recommend ASD closure in patients before school age. Since the late 1950s, the standard therapy for ASDs has been surgical closure using cardiopulmonary bypass support. The defect is closed using direct suture closure, autologous pericardium, or prosthetic patch material (Fig. 58-10). This is an effective method, with a low associated perioperative risk, including the virtual absence of residual or recurrent defects.[16] Minimally invasive techniques for ASD closure have also gained popularity.

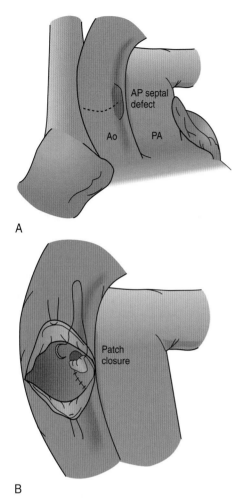

A

B

FIGURE 58-8 A, Surgical exposure of aortopulmonary *(AP)* septal defect includes a transverse incision in the ascending aorta *(Ao).* **B,** The aortopulmonary septal defect is closed by suturing a patch over the aortic side of the defect. *PA,* Pulmonary artery. (Adapted from Fraser CD: Aortopulmonary septal defects and patent ductus arteriosus. In Nichols DG, Ungerleider RM, Spevak PJ, et al, editors: *Critical heart disease in infants and children,* Philadelphia, 2006, Mosby, pp 664–666.)

The potential for closing defects using nonsurgical methods has led to the development of catheter-based therapies, which are now being widely applied to large numbers of patients worldwide for the treatment of ASD. The most commonly used device is the Amplatzer septal occluder device (St. Jude Medical, St. Paul, MN), made of nitinol metal mesh, which is placed percutaneously and delivered with echocardiographic and fluoroscopic guidance. Early reports indicated an acceptable procedure-related complication rate and successful closure rate.[17] However, the long-term effects of having such a device in mobile cardiac structures are not fully understood. More recent reports have documented an alarming incidence of device erosion through the atrial wall and into the adjacent ascending aorta as well as disruption of the conduction system.[18,19] A case report showing severe endocarditis involving a previously placed Amplatzer ASD device has highlighted the need for ongoing observation of the long-term consequences of placing large prosthetic devices into the circulation.[20]

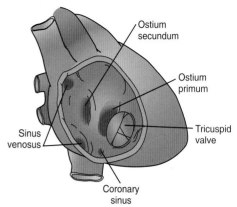

FIGURE 58-9 Types of atrial septal defects as viewed through the right atrium, ostium secundum, ostium primum, and sinus venosus. (Adapted from Redmond JM, Lodge AJ: Atrial septal defects and ventricular septal defects. In Nichols DG, Ungerleider RM, Spevak PJ, et al, editors: *Critical heart disease in infants and children,* Philadelphia, 2006, Mosby, p 580.)

Sinus venosus ASDs occur as the result of embryologic malalignment between the superior vena cava (SVC) or IVC. These defects are not associated with the ovale fossa and are frequently associated with partial anomalous pulmonary venous return. A superior sinus venosus ASD occurs high in the atrium, near the orifice of the SVC. This lesion is frequently associated with anomalous drainage of a portion of the right lung to the SVC. An inferior sinus venosus ASD is located low in the atrium, often extending into the IVC orifice. This lesion is typically associated with anomalous pulmonary venous drainage of the entire right lung to the IVC (potentially intrahepatic); pulmonary sequestration and an abnormal systemic artery perfusing the right lower lobe, with origin from the abdominal aorta, may also be present. In patients with total anomalous pulmonary venous return (TAPVR) to the IVC, the anomalous pulmonary vein may be obvious on a plain chest radiograph and has been described as appearing like a saber (scimitar syndrome), first described by Neill and colleagues.[21]

Surgery for sinus venosus ASDs is recommended for the same pathophysiologic reasons surgery is recommended for secundum ASDs. The repair is not amenable to catheter techniques, and surgery is more complicated than for an isolated secundum ASD. Superior sinus venosus defects with partial anomalous pulmonary venous return to the SVC may be treated with an intracardiac patch baffle; however, in the setting of high drainage of the anomalous pulmonary veins, an SVC translocation operation (Warden procedure) may be necessary. Surgery for an inferior sinus venosus ASD with a scimitar vein can be more complicated, potentially involving the need for a patch baffle within the intrahepatic IVC, which may require periods of hypothermic circulatory arrest.

Ventricular Septal Defect

A VSD is a pathologic communication involving a defect in the interventricular septum. Defects are classified in terms of their location and surrounding structures. Patients may be entirely asymptomatic, depending on the size and location of the VSD, along with associated lesions and PVR. In the setting of otherwise normal cardiac morphology and appropriate PVR, the net shunt in patients with VSD is left to right; the Qp/Qs depends on the size of the defect and pulmonary resistance. Large defects result

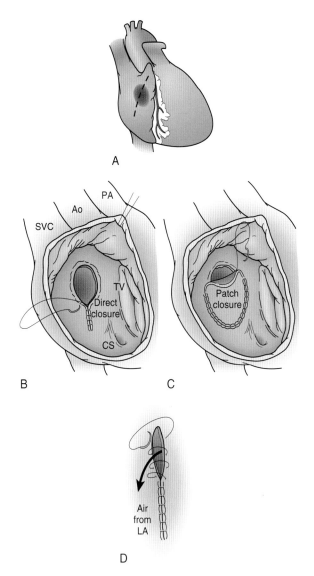

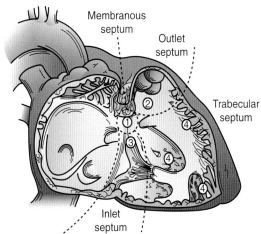

FIGURE 58-11 Location of ventricular septal defects (VSDs) in the ventricular septum (view of the ventricular septum from the right side). *1*, Perimembranous VSD; *2*, subarterial VSD; *3*, atrioventricular canal–type VSD; *4*, muscular VSD. (From Tchervenkov CI, Shum-Tim D: Ventricular septal defect. In Baue AE, Geha AS, Hammond GL, editors: *Glenn's thoracic and cardiovascular surgery*, ed 6, Stamford, CT, 1996, Appleton & Lange.)

FIGURE 58-10 Surgical closure for atrial septal defect. **A,** Right atriotomy. **B,** Direct suture closure. **C,** Patch closure. **D,** Deairing the left atrium *(LA)*. *Ao*, Aorta; *CS*, coronary sinus; *PA*, pulmonary artery; *TV*, tricuspid valve. (Adapted from Redmond JM, Lodge AJ: Atrial septal defects and ventricular septal defects. In Nichols DG, Ungerleider RM, Spevak PJ, et al, editors: *Critical heart disease in infants and children*, Philadelphia, 2006, Mosby, p 583.)

in large shunts; high right ventricular and pulmonary artery pressures; and significant pulmonary overcirculation, CHF, and left heart volume overload. In these settings, unrestrictive pulmonary blood flow exposes the patient to the risk for pulmonary vascular disease and Eisenmenger syndrome.

The ventricular septum can be best thought of in terms of the pathway of blood and associated cardiac anatomy. Thus, the right ventricular aspect of the septum has an inlet portion; midmuscular portion; apical, posterior, anterior, and outlet portions; and subaortic portion. This knowledge aids in the classification of VSDs. Furthermore, defects are understood relative to their embryologic origins and have varying propensities for spontaneous decreases in size or closure.

Perimembranous Ventricular Septal Defect

A perimembranous VSD occurs as a defect in the membranous portion of the interventricular septum; its associated margins include the annulus of the tricuspid valve, the muscular septum, and potentially the aortic annulus. The defects may be large and have associated prolapse of the noncoronary or right coronary aortic valve cusps. Perimembranous VSDs exhibit a potential for spontaneous closure, particularly small defects manifesting early in childhood.

Muscular Ventricular Septal Defect

Muscular VSDs occur in all aspects of the muscular interventricular septum. Margins of these defects are entirely muscle. The lesions may be isolated or involve multiple openings in the septum (so-called Swiss cheese septum). Small defects have great potential for regression or spontaneous closure.

Subarterial (Supracristal or Outlet) Ventricular Septal Defect

Subarterial VSDs occur in association with the annulus of the aortic valve, pulmonary valve, or both. The defects are almost always associated with significant prolapse of the adjacent aortic valve cusp, usually the right coronary cusp, which may lead to significant cusp distortion, aortic valve insufficiency, and cusp perforation. The only mechanism for spontaneous closure of these defects relates to the cusp prolapse and valve distortion and is generally not complete or a favorable arrangement. All these defects are surgically closed because of the ongoing risk for aortic valve injury (Fig. 58-11).

The indications for surgery to close VSDs relate to the size of the VSD, degree of shunting, and associated lesions. Small infants presenting with large VSDs, refractory heart failure, and large shunts undergo surgical closure of the defects in the newborn period, regardless of age or size. Other defects are addressed based on the ongoing concerns of left-to-right shunting, aortic valve cusp distortion, and risk for endocarditis. Asymptomatic patients with evidence of significant shunts and cardiomegaly are proposed for surgical therapy. Prophylactic closure of small defects in asymptomatic patients with normal cardiac size and function is advocated by some surgeons because of the lifelong risk for endocarditis and comparatively low risk for surgery.

Percutaneous VSD closure is an acceptable alternative to surgical closure of VSDs with very high procedural success.[22] The complex relationship of many defects, including close association with the aortic valve and cardiac conduction tissue, makes the existing technology less than ideal. At the present time, surgery remains the primary mode of therapy for VSD closure. Defects are approached with the aid of cardiopulmonary bypass support and may be closed with various materials, including autologous pericardium (our preference), Dacron, polytetrafluoroethylene, and homograft material. Surgical closure of VSDs is a low-risk procedure with a high expectation of complete closure. Challenging anatomic situations, such as Swiss cheese septum or multiple apical muscular VSDs, may be initially palliated by limiting pulmonary blood flow with a pulmonary artery band and deferring corrective surgery to later in life.

Atrioventricular Septal Defect (Atrioventricular Canal Defect)

Atrioventricular septal defects (AVSDs) are a complex constellation of cardiac lesions involving deficiency of the atrial septum, ventricular septum, and A-V valves. This lesion results from an embryologic maldevelopment involving the endocardial cushions; thus, the term *endocardial cushion defect* is often applied. AVSDs may be partial, involving no ventricular level component; intermediate or transitional, involving a small restrictive VSD; or complete, involving a large nonrestrictive VSD. The A-V valve tissue is always abnormal in AVSD, although there is great individual variability in terms of the severity of the valvular malformation and valve function. Complete AVSDs are frequently seen in patients with trisomy 21 but also occur in patients with normal chromosomes. The morphology of the septal defects in this condition is different from that previously discussed. The ASD in this defect is termed a *primum ASD* and is distinctly separate from the ovale fossa. There is displacement of the A-V node and bundle of His to the inferior aspect of the primum defect and A-V junction, a feature of critical importance during surgical repair. Patients with AVSD have an *inlet VSD*, which may extend into the subaortic region and have a component of septal malalignment. The chordal support of the A-V valves has a variable relationship to the interventricular septum. The relationship of the chordal support and superior bridging component of the left A-V valve has been used to classify complete AVSD, as described by Rastelli and associates[23]: type A, with superior leaflet and chordal support committed to the left side of the ventricular septum; type B, with straddling and shared chordal support; and type C, with a floating left superior leaflet component and chordal support on the right side of the ventricular septum (Fig. 58-12).

Patients with complete AVSD typically present in infancy with large left-to-right shunts, cardiomegaly, and CHF. Without surgical treatment, patients exhibit severe failure to thrive, a susceptibility to severe respiratory infections, and potential for early development of pulmonary vascular disease. Surgical repair is recommended in infancy (usually before 6 months of age) but may be necessary in the newborn period for neonates with refractory heart failure, especially in association with aortic arch anomalies. Patients with partial or intermediate defects may have the surgery deferred until later in childhood, depending on the degree

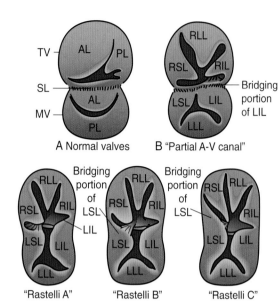

FIGURE 58-12 Rastelli classification type A, B, or C. The difference in valve morphology in a normal **(A)**, partial **(B)**, and complete **(C)** canal defect is illustrated. *AL,* Anterior leaflet; *A-V,* atrioventricular; *MV,* mitral valve; *PL,* posterior leaflet; *RIL,* right inferior leaflet; *RLL,* right lateral leaflet; *RSL,* right superior leaflet; *TV,* tricuspid valve. (From Kirklin JW, Pacifico AD, Kirklin JK: The surgical treatment of atrioventricular canal defects. In Arciniegas E, editor: *Pediatric cardiac surgery,* Chicago, 1985, Year Book Medical Publishers.)

of atrial level shunting and the presence of A-V valve regurgitation. AVSD may also manifest in unbalanced forms, with dominance of right-sided or left-sided components. In severely affected individuals, biventricular repair is not feasible, and patients are managed along a single-ventricle pathway. AVSD may also be found in association with TOF; this combination is associated with cyanosis, and repair is more challenging than for either condition considered in isolation.

Surgery is the primary mode of therapy for patients with AVSD. Operative goals include complete closure of ASDs and VSDs and effective use of available A-V valve tissue to achieve valve competence. As noted, the inferiorly displaced conduction tissue must be protected to avoid the complication of surgically induced A-V block (Fig. 58-13). Surgical intervention is performed with the use of the cardiopulmonary bypass machine. The atrial and ventricular septal components are closed with a common patch (single-patch method) or separate patches (two-patch technique). We believe the two-patch method to be superior in preserving A-V valve tissue (Fig. 58-14).[24] The critical component of the repair lies in the valve repair; typically, after suspending the valve tissue to the reconstructed septum, the line of coaptation between the superior and inferior leaflet components (cleft) is closed; however, care must be exercised to avoid valvular stenosis.

Perioperative care is predicated on an accurate and hemodynamically favorable repair. Patients with long-standing pulmonary overcirculation may have a potential for early perioperative pulmonary hypertensive crisis. This condition may require therapy, including oxygen, optimization of fluid balance, continuous sedation, hyperventilation, and, possibly, inhaled nitric oxide.

Adult Patients With Atrioventricular Septal Defect

Numerous patients with partial or transitional AVSD survive well into adulthood without surgery. These patients have variable presentations but may exhibit severe exercise intolerance; evidence of right heart dysfunction; some elevation of PVR; and, possibly, atrial dysrhythmias, including atrial fibrillation. In patients with late presentation of AVSD, cardiac catheterization is often

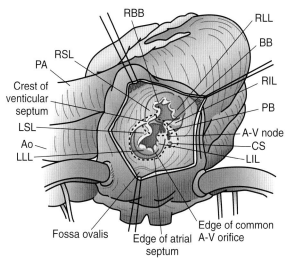

FIGURE 58-13 Position of the conducting system in complete atrioventricular canal defect. The anatomic relationships and morphology of the common atrioventricular *(A-V)* valve are shown. The view is through a right atriotomy. *Ao,* Aorta; *BB,* left bundle branch; *CS,* coronary sinus; *LIL,* left inferior leaflet; *LLL,* left lateral leaflet; *LSL,* left superior leaflet; *PA,* pulmonary artery; *PB,* penetrating bundle; *RBB,* right bundle branch; *RIL,* right inferior leaflet; *RLL,* right lateral leaflet; *RSL,* right superior leaflet. (From Bharati S, Lev M, Kirklin JW: *Cardiac surgery and the conducting system,* New York, 1983, Churchill Livingstone.)

recommended to rule out occult coronary artery lesions and to evaluate PVR. Nonetheless, in the absence of obvious surgical contraindication, surgery is recommended for adults with unrepaired AVSD to eliminate the chronic left-to-right shunt and repair the typically insufficient A-V valves.

Other patients present well into adulthood with previously repaired AVSDs. These patients may have a widely disparate constellation of findings, including atrial and ventricular dysrhythmias, valvular insufficiency or stenosis, and right heart dysfunction. In many of them, secondary reparative surgery may become necessary. Furthermore, in the setting of a patient with remotely repaired AVSD requiring noncardiac surgery, potential ongoing hemodynamic concerns that would affect the perioperative course must be expected.

Persistent Arterial Trunk (Truncus Arteriosus)

Truncus arteriosus or persistent arterial trunk results from failure of separation of the embryonic arterial trunk and semilunar valves. It is almost always associated with a large nonrestrictive VSD, is typically perimembranous, and is associated with varying degrees of truncal override of the interventricular septum, including 100% association of the trunk with the right ventricle. The condition is classified by the relationship of the origins of the pulmonary arteries. In type I truncus arteriosus, there is a demonstrable common main pulmonary artery with subsequent origins of the branch pulmonary arteries; in type II truncus arteriosus, the branch pulmonary arteries arise closely, but separately, from the trunk; in type III truncus arteriosus, the branch pulmonary arteries are widely separated in origin on the ascending aorta; and in type IV truncus arteriosus, no pulmonary arterial branch arises from the common trunk. Type IV truncus arteriosus is now recognized as a form of pulmonary atresia with VSD (Fig. 58-15).

In contrast to patients with aortopulmonary septal defects, patients with truncus arteriosus have a single outlet valve of highly variable morphology. The valve may have a normal appearance, with three well-formed and distinct cusps similar to those of a

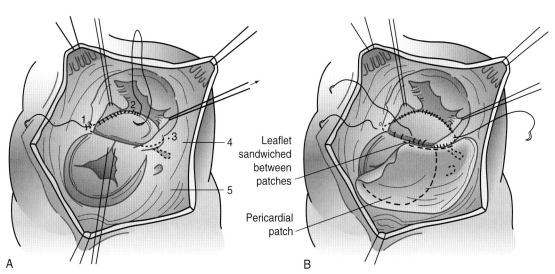

FIGURE 58-14 Two-patch closure of complete atrioventricular canal defect. **A,** A ventricular septal patch is placed first, and a separate patch is used to close the atrial septal defect (ASD) component. **B,** Note the position of the coronary sinus and conducting system relative to the ASD patch suture line to avoid injury to the atrioventricular node. (From Kirklin JW, Barratt-Boyes BG: *Cardiac surgery,* New York, 1986, Churchill Livingstone.)

Collett and Edwards

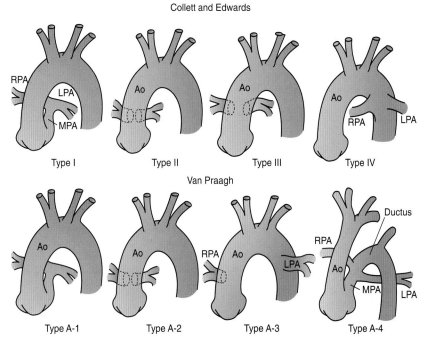

Van Praagh

FIGURE 58-15 Collett-Edwards and Van Praagh classification systems for persistent truncus arteriosus (see text for details). *Ao,* Aorta; *LPA,* left pulmonary artery; *MPA,* main pulmonary artery; *RPA,* right pulmonary artery. (Adapted from St Louis JD: Persistent truncus arteriosus. In Nichols DG, Ungerleider RM, Spevak PJ, et al, editors: *Critical heart disease in infants and children,* Philadelphia, 2006, Mosby, p 690.)

normal aortic valve. In other patients, the truncal valve may be severely malformed, with multiple cusps, dysmorphic leaflets, and abnormal commissural relationships. The truncal valve morphology and function have significant bearing on patient symptoms and the difficulty of surgery. Patients with truncus arteriosus frequently have coronary ostial abnormalities, including juxtacommissural origin and intramural course. There is an associated interruption of the aortic arch in 25% of newborns presenting with truncus arteriosus. Abnormalities of thymic genesis, T cell function, and calcium homeostasis may frequently be seen in this group of patients in association with a chromosome 22 deletion (DiGeorge syndrome).

Patients with truncus arteriosus present in the newborn period with unrestricted pulmonary blood flow and systemic pulmonary artery pressure. With the expected postnatal decrease in PVR, massive pulmonary overcirculation, and CHF, patients may exhibit a wide pulse pressure because of diastolic runoff of blood into the pulmonary vasculature. This situation is further exacerbated in the setting of significant truncal valve insufficiency, resulting in poor systemic perfusion and cardiovascular collapse. Some infants can be initially managed with medical decongestive therapy (e.g., diuretics, angiotensin-converting enzyme inhibitors, and digoxin) and fortified nutritional support (through gastric intubation); however, this is a precarious arrangement. In the few individuals who survive infancy, irreversible pulmonary vascular disease develops rapidly, and patients become inoperable. In other patients, refractory CHF results in poor weight gain, respiratory insufficiency, and susceptibility to infection. The profound hemodynamic compromise places many newborns with unrepaired truncus arteriosus at high risk for necrotizing enterocolitis. Patients with truncus arteriosus and IAA have ductal-dependent systemic blood flow and are dependent on intravenous PGE1 to

maintain ductal patency until they undergo repair. Given these considerations, it is recommended that most newborn patients undergo repair in the first several weeks of life.

The surgical repair is performed on cardiopulmonary bypass support. Components of the repair include division of the common trunk and reconstruction of confluent central branch pulmonary arteries. The large VSD is closed with a patch, typically through a right ventriculotomy. In patients with abnormal, insufficient truncal valves, a valve repair may be necessary. It is unusual to have to replace the truncal valve at the initial operation; most valves can be at least partially repaired to provide the patient with an adequate aortic valve. Right ventricle–pulmonary artery continuity must then be established. Most surgeons prefer to interpose a valved conduit between the right ventriculotomy and pulmonary artery bifurcation (Fig. 58-16).

Conduits are limited and include homografts (pulmonary artery or aorta, valved) or heterografts (bovine or porcine). Experience with a commercially available, glutaraldehyde-preserved, bovine jugular vein valved conduit (Contegra; Medtronic, Minneapolis, MN) had been encouraging.[25] However, there is a concerning increased incidence of endocarditis with Contegra valved conduits compared with other conduits, including homografts and heterografts. Successful repair of truncus arteriosus in infants using a direct hooded anastomosis between the pulmonary artery bifurcation and right ventriculotomy has also been reported.[26] No option available at the present time offers patients the lifetime solution of a connection capable of somatic growth along with a competent, durable pulmonary valve. Thus, it is expected that all infants undergoing successful truncus repair will require multiple subsequent cardiac surgeries as they outgrow their current right ventricle–pulmonary artery conduit. Experience with a percutaneously delivered, catheter-mounted

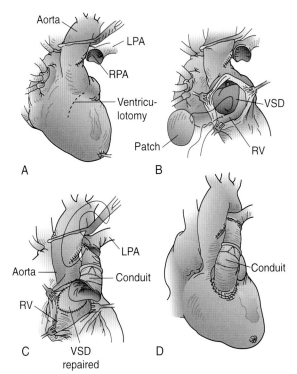

FIGURE 58-16 Surgical repair of truncus arteriosus. **A,** The origin of the truncus arteriosus is excised, and the truncal defect is closed with a direct suture. The incision is made high in the right ventricle *(RV).* **B,** The ventricular septal defect *(VSD)* is closed with a prosthetic patch. **C,** Placement of a valved conduit into the pulmonary arteries. **D,** Proximal end of conduit is anastomosed to the RV. *LPA,* Left pulmonary artery; *RPA,* right pulmonary artery. (From Wallace RB: Truncus arteriosus. In Sabiston DC, Jr, Spencer FC, editors: *Gibbons surgery of the chest,* ed 3, Philadelphia, 1976, Saunders.)

pulmonary valve has been encouraging as an interim solution for these patients in an effort to limit the number of required cardiac reoperations.[27]

A growing number of adults have survived childhood truncus arteriosus repair. All these patients require diligent longitudinal cardiology surveillance, and many will require reoperation. Issues of concern include late ventricular dysrhythmias, often related to surgical scarring from the previous right ventriculotomy; branch pulmonary artery stenosis; stenosis or insufficiency of the right ventricle–pulmonary artery conduit; truncal valve insufficiency; and right ventricular dysfunction.

Abnormalities of Venous Drainage
Total Anomalous Pulmonary Venous Return

TAPVR results from embryonic failure of connection of the fetal pulmonary venous sinus to the left atrium. This fatal condition has a spectrum of clinical presentations and may be associated with additional complex structural cardiac disease, including a single ventricle. In TAPVR, pulmonary venous return may take one of several pathways to return eventually to the right heart. Initial survival is predicated on an unobstructed pathway and unrestricted atrial-level communication so that sufficient intracardiac mixing affords the patient adequate systemic oxygenation. Patients with TAPVR are desaturated to varying degrees, depending on the adequacy of the anomalous pathway, atrial mixing, and

pulmonary function. The abnormal venous connection drains in several typical patterns.

In supracardiac TAPVR, the pulmonary veins drain to a vertical vein, which courses cephalad to join a systemic vein. In the most common variation, the vertical vein courses anterior to the left pulmonary artery to join the left innominate vein. This vein may course posterior to the left pulmonary artery, resulting in compression of the pulmonary venous pathway between the left pulmonary artery and left mainstem bronchus (so-called pulmonary artery vise). The vertical vein may also join the SVC or azygos vein. In intracardiac TAPVR, the pulmonary veins drain into the coronary sinus and, in most cases in which the coronary sinus is intact, into the right atrium. This variant is rarely obstructed and may not be diagnosed until later in life in some patients. In infracardiac TAPVR, the vertical veins descend in a caudal direction through the diaphragm to join the embryologic ductus venosus and then through the liver to join the IVC. This variation is almost always obstructed at some level (Fig. 58-17). In mixed TAPVR, the pulmonary venous pathway drains in several pathways to reach the heart. Frequently, in mixed TAPVR, one or several pulmonary veins connect to the SVC, with others draining to an infracardiac or supracardiac connection.

Obstructed total anomalous pulmonary venous return. Obstructed TAPVR is one of the few true surgical emergencies in congenital heart surgery. When the condition is suspected, it is diagnosed with transthoracic echocardiography. Obstructed TAPVR occurs when one of the drainage patterns noted earlier is obstructed, resulting in severe pulmonary venous hypertension. Secondary effects include pulmonary edema, pulmonary artery hypertension, and profound hypoxemia. Interstitial pulmonary emphysema and frank pneumothorax may develop while attempting vigorous ventilatory support in profoundly desaturated children. Patients with obstructed TAPVR may present within hours of birth in extremis and do not respond to resuscitative efforts. The only useful therapy is rapid surgical repair, regardless of the severity of the patient's preoperative status.

For other forms of TAPVR, elective surgical repair is recommended after the condition is diagnosed. Occasionally, the diagnosis is not made until later in childhood in patients with an unobstructed vertical vein and widely patent atrial communication. These patients undergo elective repair to relieve cyanosis, intracardiac mixing, and right heart volume overload.

Surgical repair of TAPVR requires cardiopulmonary bypass support; occasionally, periods of profound hypothermia and circulatory arrest are necessary. The principles of repair include identification of the pulmonary venous confluence and individual pulmonary veins. An anastomosis is constructed between the venous confluence and left atrium using a superolateral approach, with the heart reflected to the patient's right, or an incision directly through the interatrial septum and corresponding region of the posterior right atrial wall. The ASD and PDA that are typically present are closed as well (Fig. 58-18).

Cor triatriatum. Cor triatriatum is a rare condition in which the pulmonary veins enter a chamber posterior to the left atrium with a small connection to the right or left atrium. These patients exhibit evidence of pulmonary hypertension and variable desaturation. Surgical decompression is necessary to relieve the pulmonary venous obstruction; this is accomplished by resection of the membrane between the pulmonary venous chamber and left atrium.

A dreaded consequence of TAPVR occurs when there is a progressive, malignant sclerosing process involving the individual

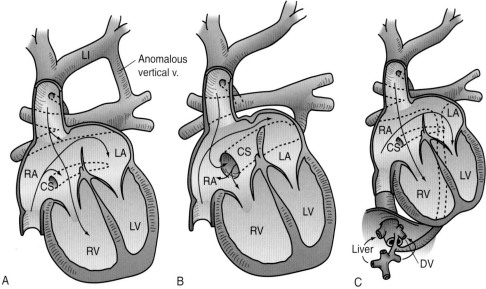

FIGURE 58-17 Types of total anomalous pulmonary venous connection. **A,** Supracardiac type with a vertical vein joining the left innominate *(LI)* vein. **B,** Intracardiac type with connection to the coronary sinus *(CS)*. **C,** Infracardiac type with drainage through the diaphragm via an inferior connecting vein. *DV,* Ductus venosus; *LA,* left atrium; *LV,* left ventricle; *RA,* right atrium; *RV,* right ventricle. (From Hammon JW, Jr, Bender HW, Jr: Anomalous venous connections: Pulmonary and systemic. In Baue AE, editor: *Glenn's thoracic and cardiac surgery,* ed 5, Norwalk, CT, 1991, Appleton & Lange.)

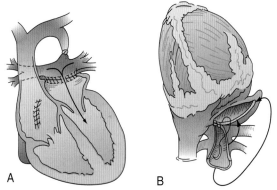

FIGURE 58-18 A, Repair of supracardiac total anomalous pulmonary venous connection (TAPVC) through a superior approach. **B,** Repair of infracardiac TAPVC. Elevating the apex of the heart to the right side exposes the left atrium and pulmonary confluence. Anastomosis is created as shown. (From Lupinetti FM, Kulik TJ, Beekman RH, et al: Correction of total anomalous pulmonary venous connection in infancy. *J Thorac Cardiovasc Surg* 106:880–885, 1993.)

pulmonary veins. This process may be initiated by inaccurate surgery resulting in obstruction of the venous confluence and individual veins, or it may progress independently of surgical manipulation. It may progress to intrapulmonary pulmonary venous stenoses. A technique to deal with individual pulmonary venous stenoses uses a pedicled flap of adjacent pericardium to augment the pulmonary venous orifices (sutureless technique), but this method is not applicable to all patients with pulmonary venous obstruction. Catheter-based dilation and stenting have been attempted in this setting with good acute relief of obstruction but have a high rate of reintervention and unknown

long-term success, with 50% survival at 5 years.[28] In the most severe cases, the only meaningful surgical option is lung transplantation.

Anomalous Systemic Venous Drainage

Congenital abnormalities of systemic venous drainage may occur in isolation or in association with other significant structural cardiac defects. In the setting of an otherwise normal heart, the anomaly is frequently not of physiologic significance. The most common example is a persistent left SVC draining to the coronary sinus. In the absence of an intracardiac communication or unroofing of the coronary sinus, this is of anatomic significance only. In many cases, a persistent left SVC occurs, with absence of a communicating innominate vein. This condition becomes important in situations of mechanical occlusion, which may be seen with trauma or chronic venous intubation with thrombosis. A persistent left SVC frequently is incidentally discovered after placement of a left internal jugular central line, which is apparently found to track into the heart on plain chest radiography. A persistent left SVC becomes more significant in patients requiring intracardiac or extracardiac surgery. If the left SVC drains to an unroofed coronary sinus in a patient undergoing atrial septation, the patient will be profoundly desaturated after surgery. This situation requires reconstruction of the coronary sinus or some other method to reroute the left SVC to the right atrium.

An interrupted IVC usually occurs in association with other structural cardiac disease. The IVC drainage in these settings is to the azygos (azygos continuation) or hemiazygos vein and ultimately the SVC. In these patients, the hepatic veins drain into the atrium as a common confluence or as individual veins. The physiologic significance of the interrupted IVC relates to the coexisting cardiac lesion and the necessity of appreciating the abnormality of systemic venous drainage in performing corrective

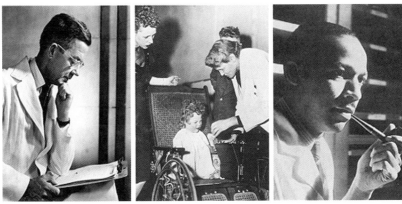

FIGURE 58-19 Drs. Alfred Blalock, Helen Taussig, and Vivien Thomas.

surgery. In patients requiring noncardiac surgery or catheter intervention, the presence of an interrupted IVC is noted when an attempt is being made to pass a venous catheter from the groin into the heart.

Cyanotic Congenital Heart Disease
Tetralogy of Fallot

TOF is a common form of cyanotic CHD and is probably the most studied lesion in the era of surgical correction for CHD. Many believe that The Johns Hopkins Hospital was the birthplace of cardiac surgery. Blalock performed the first successful palliative operation for TOF in November 1944, assisted by his laboratory technician.[1] Blalock was encouraged by Taussig, the matriarch of pediatric cardiology (Fig. 58-19). Until more recently, some degree of controversy has surrounded the relative degree of contribution by these three individuals in bringing this historical event to fruition. In actuality, all three were significant participants in this momentous medical advance. While working at Vanderbilt Medical School, Blalock had charged his young and capable laboratory technician, Vivien Thomas, with the development of a surgical model of pulmonary hypertension. Thomas and Blalock developed a method of anastomosing the left subclavian artery to the divided left pulmonary artery in a canine model. Specifically, Thomas worked out the technical details, including crafting the necessary surgical instruments, and mastered the operation. This work did not produce the desired effect; canine PVR is almost infinitely low, and the animals did not develop a hypertensive pulmonary vasculature. Nonetheless, the technique was developed and published approximately 10 years in advance of the clinical application in 1944.

Blalock subsequently became the Chair of Surgery at Johns Hopkins. Taussig had by that time established a reputation as a meticulous diagnostician of complex congenital heart lesions. She had a large clinic of critically ill children with disabling cyanosis—"blue babies." At her suggestion (and probably her insistence), Blalock was convinced to attempt a surgical palliation for TOF by constructing in a human the subclavian-to-pulmonary artery anastomosis that had been perfected in the research laboratory (Fig. 58-20). Blalock performed the operation in conditions and with instruments that would be considered extremely crude by today's standards. Thomas stood immediately behind Blalock during that operation and many subsequent cases, providing instruction and encouragement. The clinical success was an earth-shattering event; hundreds of patients subsequently traveled to Johns Hopkins for surgical treatment, and the era of cardiac

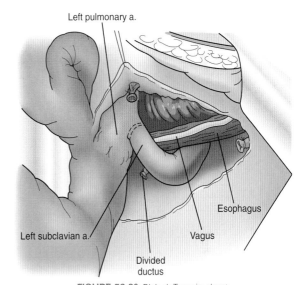

FIGURE 58-20 Blalock-Taussig shunt.

surgery was ushered in. (These historic accounts are factual, the result of personal interviews with many of those in attendance at that event, including Thomas, Taussig, J. Alex Haller, and Denton Cooley.)

The historic account of the development of the BT shunt has relevance to the practice of congenital heart surgery today. First, it is important that the facts surrounding this achievement are acknowledged. Second, this remarkably simple concept still remains a frequently applied technique for children with inadequate pulmonary blood flow. Finally, over almost 75 years of treatment of TOF, thousands of patients have been successfully treated, but most are not cured; many require subsequent reoperative cardiac surgery, even after complete repair.

The anatomic hallmark of TOF is anterior malalignment of the infundibular septum, which leaves a deficiency in the subaortic region—a malalignment VSD. This VSD is usually perimembranous, large, and pressure-nonrestrictive. The relative degree of malalignment influences the relationship of the aorta to the interventricular septum, producing varying degrees of aortic override. The deviated infundibular septum produces varying degrees of RVOTO. The path of pulmonary blood flow may be impeded at numerous levels, including the infundibulum, pulmonary valve and annulus, and main and branch pulmonary arteries. Secondary

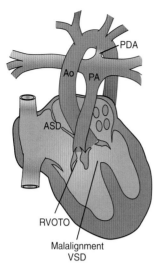

FIGURE 58-21 Anatomy of tetralogy of Fallot. A malalignment ventricular septal defect *(VSD)*, aortic override, right ventricular outflow tract obstruction *(RVOTO)*, and subsequent right ventricular hypertrophy. *Ao,* Aorta; *ASD,* atrial septal defect; *PA,* pulmonary artery; *PDA,* patent ductus arteriosus. (Adapted from Davis S: Tetralogy of Fallot with and without pulmonary atresia. In Nichols DG, Ungerleider RM, Spevak PJ, et al, editors: *Critical heart disease in infants and children,* Philadelphia, 2006, Mosby, p 756.)

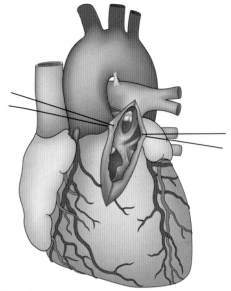

FIGURE 58-22 Long right ventriculotomy in a classic transventricular approach. (From Morales DL, Zafar F, Heinle JS: Right ventricular infundibulum sparing [RVIs] tetralogy of Fallot repair: A review of over 300 patients. *Ann Surg* 250:611–617, 2009.)

right ventricular hypertrophy occurs relative to the degree and duration of the obstruction and is progressive, contributing to the propensity for the lesion to worsen over time (Fig. 58-21).

The pathophysiology of TOF relates to shunting of desaturated, systemic venous blood through the VSD to mix with the systemic cardiac output. The greater the degree of obstruction to pulmonary blood flow, the larger the right-to-left shunt and the worse the desaturation. There are several modes of presentation. Newborns with TOF and severe RVOTO may present soon after birth with profound cyanosis; some require PGE1 to maintain ductal patency for adequate oxygenation. At the other end of the spectrum is children with little infundibular obstruction and normal pulmonary valve and branch pulmonary arteries. These patients may have net left-to-right flow through the VSD, occasionally to the extent that they experience pulmonary overcirculation and CHF (so-called pink TOF). Most children present between these extremes; an initially mild to moderate degree of infundibular stenosis progresses over time to become severe with worsening desaturation. A TOF spell occurs when there is an acute change in the cardiac inotropic state, often in the setting of agitation and dehydration. The infundibular stenosis acutely worsens, and patients become profoundly desaturated; this may be an extremely serious event, leading to brain damage or death. Acute treatment modalities include sedation, hydration, systemic afterload augmentation (α-adrenergic agonists), beta blockade to reduce the inotropic state, and endotracheal intubation with supplemental inspired oxygen.

The natural history of untreated TOF is dismal, with most children dying of progressive cyanosis before 10 years of age. Surgery is the mainstay of therapy. Medical and catheter-based therapy may be used to temporize, but TOF is a surgical disease. The principles of surgical correction include patch closure of the VSD and relief of all levels of the RVOTO and pulmonary artery stenosis. The classic method of TOF repair uses a longitudinal

incision through the right ventricular outflow tract (RVOT); this provides an excellent transventricular view of the VSD, which is closed with a patch. The pulmonary artery, pulmonary valve, and annulus are incised if stenotic, and then the RVOT is patched. This method was used for many years but has the complicating feature of the long ventriculotomy, with attendant right ventricular dysfunction and often severe pulmonic insufficiency (Fig. 58-22). An alternative method, the transatrial or transpulmonary approach, first proposed by Imai, has gained popularity. In this method, the VSD closure and RVOT resection are accomplished through a right atriotomy via the tricuspid valve. The main pulmonary artery and pulmonary annulus are incised only if stenotic, but there is no transmural infundibular incision. This method is technically more demanding than the classic method but may offer the patient improved long-term right ventricular function (Figs. 58-23 to 58-25). The approach has been further developed as a right ventricular infundibulum-sparing strategy that focuses on minimizing the right ventricular incision and preserving the pulmonary valve. The right ventricular infundibulum-sparing strategy includes an algorithm for optimal timing of the repair that considers the individual patient's weight, age, and overall clinical picture (Fig. 58-26). Midterm results with this approach have demonstrated preserved right ventricular function.[29]

The long-term sequelae of TOF repair have been unfolding. For most patients, successful childhood repair of TOF does not translate into a cure. As patients age after TOF repair, long-term complications may develop. Patients with long RVOT incisions (transannular) by necessity have severe pulmonary insufficiency and a noncontractile infundibulum. Over time, the effects of chronic right heart volume overload include right ventricular dilation and decreased function, often with progressive tricuspid insufficiency and elevated central venous pressure. These patients may present with hepatomegaly, peripheral edema, and severe exercise intolerance. Dysrhythmias may frequently occur; patients with large right ventriculotomies develop endocardial scarring, which may be the substrate for ventricular tachycardia. Chronic

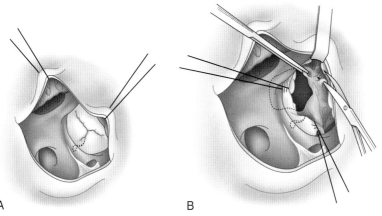

A   B

FIGURE 58-23 **A,** Surgeon's view through a transatrial incision in the transatrial/transpulmonary approach. **B,** Right ventricular outflow tract muscle resection through the right atriotomy. (From Morales DL, Zafar F, Heinle JS: Right ventricular infundibulum sparing [RVIs] tetralogy of Fallot repair: A review of over 300 patients. *Ann Surg* 250:611–617, 2009.)

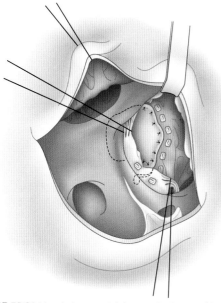

FIGURE 58-24 Ventricular septal defect patch closure with pledgets around the defect and onto the tricuspid valve annulus to avoid the conduction system. (From Morales DL, Zafar F, Heinle JS: Right ventricular infundibulum sparing [RVIs] tetralogy of Fallot repair: A review of over 300 patients. *Ann Surg* 250:611–617, 2009.)

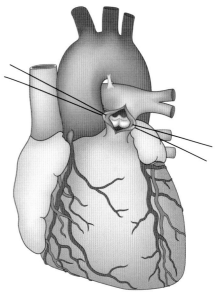

FIGURE 58-25 Mini–transannular incision in the transatrial-transpulmonary approach. (From Morales DL, Zafar F, Heinle JS: Right ventricular infundibulum sparing [RVIs] tetralogy of Fallot repair: A review of over 300 patients. *Ann Surg* 250:611–617, 2009.)

right atrial dilation may ultimately lead to atrial dysrhythmias, including atrial tachycardia and fibrillation. Relative to these and other potential issues after TOF repair, patients require careful and lifelong medical follow-up. Many need reintervention; this is frequently the case in patients with chronic, severe pulmonary insufficiency, which is indicated when right ventricular dilation and dysfunction become significant. In these patients, placing a competent pulmonary valve is necessary to relieve chronic right ventricular overload. These issues are of particular importance to a patient with repaired TOF presenting for noncardiac surgery. A careful assessment of the patient's cardiac anatomy and function is performed, including echocardiography, Holter monitoring, and occasionally cardiac catheterization.

Pulmonary Atresia and Intact Ventricular Septum

Pulmonary atresia with an intact ventricular septum manifests with profound desaturation and ductal-dependent pulmonary blood flow in newborns. The cardiac morphology in this condition varies widely. On the most severe end of the spectrum, patients have very small right ventricles, tiny tricuspid inlets, and often a right ventricle–dependent coronary circulation. In these cases, the right ventricle must remain hypertensive to provide flow to these segments of the coronary circulation. At the other end of the anatomic spectrum, patients have a relatively normal tricuspid valve and right ventricle. Most patients fall in between these extremes, with some degree of tricuspid valve and right ventricle underdevelopment.

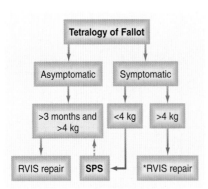

Tetralogy of Fallot

Asymptomatic | Symptomatic

>3 months and >4 kg | <4 kg | >4 kg

RVIS repair | SPS ← | *RVIS repair

FIGURE 58-26 Algorithm for the right ventricular infundibulum-sparing (RVIS) strategy. The goal of this strategy is to minimize the right ventricular incision and preserve the pulmonary valve. It is an individualized approach that considers the patient's weight, age, and overall clinical picture. *SPS,* systemic-to-pulmonary artery shunt. (From Morales DL, Zafar F, Heinle JS: Right ventricular infundibulum sparing [RVIs] tetralogy of Fallot repair: A review of over 300 patients. *Ann Surg* 250:611–617, 2009.)

Because patients are ductal-dependent at birth, an assessment must be made as to whether the right heart will be capable of ultimately supporting a biventricular circulation. If the coronary circulation is truly right ventricle–dependent, decompressing the right ventricle would result in coronary insufficiency. In these situations, a palliative BT shunt is created in anticipation of promoting the patient down a single-ventricle pathway. In other patients, the atretic pulmonary valve must be opened with percutaneous balloon dilation or open surgical valvotomy. Over time, the hypertensive, often apparently underdeveloped right ventricle will improve in size and function and become capable of supporting all or a significant proportion of the cardiac output. At initial presentation, many patients have a large patent foramen ovale or ASD; in patients with a restrictive ASD and marginal right heart, an atrial septostomy (balloon) allows for atrial-level right-to-left shunting until the right ventricle improves. Ultimately, if the right ventricle is adequate, the ASD can be closed.

Pulmonary Atresia With Ventricular Septal Defect

Pulmonary atresia with VSD is morphologically similar to TOF, with the exception of an atretic pulmonary valve. Patients may have confluent, normal-sized pulmonary arteries perfused by a PDA. In severe cases, the pulmonary arteries are discontinuous, and the lungs are variably perfused by diminutive native branch pulmonary arteries and muscularized collateral vessels originating from the descending aorta and brachiocephalic vessels. These major aortopulmonary collateral arteries (MAPCAs) have a propensity to develop severe stenoses as they are exposed to systemic arterial pressure. Many of these MAPCAs eventually occlude at an unpredictable rate during childhood. Because they may provide the only blood supply to some lung segments, patients become progressively desaturated.

The goal of surgical therapy for pulmonary atresia with VSD is biventricular repair to achieve normal cardiac workload and systemic arterial saturations. In patients with confluent native pulmonary arteries of adequate caliber, the VSD is surgically closed, and a valved conduit (homograft or heterograft) is interposed between the right ventricle and pulmonary bifurcation. In patients with pulmonary atresia with VSD and MAPCAs, the pulmonary arteries must be repaired by connecting the various

lung segments into a common trunk through a process termed *pulmonary artery unifocalization.* Depending on the source and size of the MAPCAs and native pulmonary arteries, this may be a challenging surgical procedure, but the goal is constructing a pulmonary tree as close to normal as possible so that biventricular repair is feasible (see earlier).

The long-term issues of repair of pulmonary atresia with VSD are similar to concerns described earlier for TOF. The addition of a right ventricle–pulmonary artery conduit guarantees the need for reoperation because no currently available conduit choice offers the potential for somatic growth or an indefinitely durable valve.

Valvular Pulmonic Stenosis

Patients with isolated valvular pulmonary stenosis are almost always treated in infancy with a percutaneous balloon pulmonary valvotomy. The intermediate-term results of this treatment are good; however, all patients are left with significant pulmonary valve insufficiency and eventually require pulmonary valve replacement.

Conotruncal Anomalies
Transposition of the Great Arteries

TGA is a common cyanotic congenital cardiac lesion. In this section, our discussion relates only to TGA in which there are two good ventricles identified as being capable of independent function as the right and left ventricle. TGA is commonly referred to as D-TGA, in relationship to the typically normal D (dextro) ventricular looping that occurs in association with the discordant ventriculoarterial connection and normal A-V connection. TGA occurs in the setting of an intact ventricular septum (TGA-IVS) or with associated VSD (TGA-VSD). In TGA-VSD, there may be associated aortic arch hypoplasia and coarctation. On the other extreme, there may be severe pulmonic and subpulmonic stenosis (left ventricular outflow tract obstruction [LVOTO]) or even pulmonary atresia (TGA-VSD with pulmonary atresia).

Patients with TGA-IVS typically present in the early newborn period with profound cyanosis associated with normal perinatal PDA closure. In the absence of a significant ASD, the cyanosis is severe and progresses to death if left untreated. Administration of intravenous PGE1 is almost uniformly successful in reestablishing ductal patency to improve the patient's arterial saturation by providing left-to-right shunting and improved pulmonary blood flow.

In most patients, a balloon atrial septostomy is performed (percutaneous through the umbilical vein or femoral vein) to allow atrial-level mixing (Fig. 58-27). This procedure is usually effective in allowing sufficient atrial-level mixing so that the patient is adequately saturated (70% to 80%).

After the procedure, the prostaglandin infusion can be discontinued. In TGA-VSD, there is often sufficient shunting at the level of the VSD to promote adequate systemic saturation; in patients with large VSDs, the predominant presenting symptom may be pulmonary overcirculation and CHF. Patients with TGA with pulmonary atresia have ductal-dependent pulmonary blood flow. In patients with TGA-VSD and aortic arch hypoplasia or coarctation, PGE1 may be necessary to maintain ductal patency and systemic perfusion. Echocardiography is the primary diagnostic modality for TGA.

The treatment of TGA has evolved significantly during the past 60 years of surgical therapy for CHD. Initial success was achieved by surgical reconstruction to create a physiologic repair. The atrial switch operation involves a series of intra-atrial baffles using a

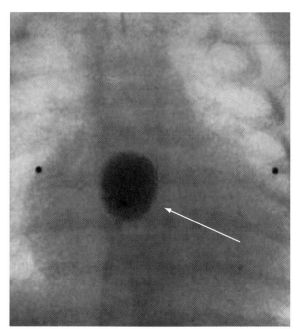

FIGURE 58-27 Angiogram during balloon atrial septostomy. The *arrow* points to the inflated balloon catheter at the atrial septum. The interventional cardiologist forcefully pulls the balloon across the patent foramen ovale to create an open, unobstructed secundum atrial septal defect.

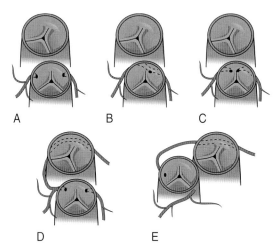

FIGURE 58-28 **(A-E)** Five basic coronary artery configurations, as described by Yacoub and Radley-Smith. (Adapted from Mee R: The arterial switch operation. In Stark J, de Leval M, editors: *Surgery for congenital heart defects*, ed 2, Philadelphia, 1994, Saunders, p 484.)

patch channel (Mustard procedure)[30] or infolding of the native atrial wall and interatrial septum (Senning procedure).[31] Both procedures achieve the same physiologic result: The systemic venous blood is redirected to the left ventricle (and the pulmonary circulation), and the pulmonary venous blood is redirected to the right ventricle. After a successful atrial switch, patients are fully saturated but are left with their morphologic right ventricle supporting the entire systemic cardiac output. In many (perhaps ultimately all) patients undergoing the atrial switch procedure, the right ventricle becomes dysfunctional over time, which is manifested by dilation, decreased ejection fraction, tricuspid insufficiency, and dysrhythmias. The observation of problems with the systemic right ventricle in patients after the atrial switch operation was the primary impetus behind the development and application of the arterial switch operation (ASO), which is now established as the surgical treatment of choice for patients with TGA. At the present time, operative survival rates for the ASO approach 100%.[32,33]

The ASO provides physiologic and anatomic correction of TGA by establishing ventriculoarterial concordance. The procedure involves transection and translocation of the malposed great vessels. The technically challenging requirement of the ASO relates to the translocation of the coronary arteries to the pulmonary root (the neoaorta). As noted, there are numerous possible branching patterns for the coronary arteries in TGA—some are easily transferred in the ASO, whereas others are more challenging (including single coronary ostium and intramural course) (Fig. 58-28).[34] Nonetheless, precise surgical techniques have been described and successfully applied to all coronary branching patterns. Given this as well as the known benefit of aligning the morphologic left ventricle with the systemic circulation, the ASO is offered to all patients with TGA regardless of the coronary branching pattern. There is no need for precise anatomic

definition before surgery; all patients undergo the ASO. In most patients undergoing this procedure, the pulmonary artery bifurcation is moved anterior to the reconstructed neoaorta to minimize the potential for pulmonary artery distortion and compression of the translocated coronary arteries—the Lecompte maneuver (Fig. 58-29). Although there are interinstitutional biases in terms of nuances of treatment for TGA, the following surgical strategies are generally agreed on for this group of patients.

Transposition of the great arteries–intact ventricular septum. After balloon atrial septostomy and weaning from PGE1, if possible, newborns with TGA-IVS undergo semielective ASO in the first few days to weeks of life. Rarely, patients present with profound desaturation refractory to balloon atrial septostomy and PGE1; in this setting, an emergent ASO is indicated. We have found this to be necessary in one patient during the past decade in an experience involving more than 200 ASOs performed in newborns. For other patients, the ASO needs to be performed in a timely but nonemergent setting. Even in the presence of adequate systemic saturation, the patient's morphologic left ventricle is functioning in a low-pressure work environment—supporting the pulmonary circulation. Thus, left ventricle mass and function involute rapidly in the first few weeks of life. By 6 weeks of life, the left ventricle may be incapable of supporting the normal systemic workload after the ASO. As such, the preferred timing for the operation is in the first 1 to 2 weeks of life.

Transposition of the great arteries–ventricular septal defect with or without arch hypoplasia. There are several modes of presentation for patients with TGA-VSD. In patients with small, pressure-restrictive VSD, the presenting symptoms are similar to those of TGA-IVS. These patients require the ASO early in life, along with VSD closure before left ventricle involution. In patients with TGA and nonrestrictive VSD, there may be adequate mixing to allow reasonable systemic arterial saturation. In this setting, the left ventricle remains pressure-loaded and does not involute; thus, the necessity of early promotion to the ASO is less time-compressed. Many newborns with TGA and a large VSD are relatively asymptomatic soon after birth; they go on to develop CHF in the first 1 to 2 months of life as the normal decrease in newborn pulmonary resistance occurs. Our preference for these patients is

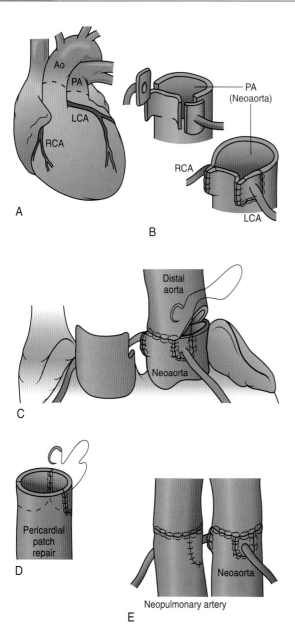

A

B

PA
(Neoaorta)

RCA

LCA

C

Distal
aorta

Neoaorta

D

Pericardial
patch
repair

E

Neoaorta

Neopulmonary artery

FIGURE 58-29 Arterial switch operation. **A,** The aorta (Ao) and pulmonary artery (PA) are transected above the sinuses of Valsalva. **B,** The coronaries are excised from the aorta and anastomosed to the pulmonary artery using a trapdoor technique. **C,** The distal aorta is brought behind the pulmonary artery (Lecompte maneuver) and anastomosed to the neoaorta. **D,** Separate pericardial patches are sutured to replace the excised coronary artery tissue from the aorta. **E,** Completed repair. *LCA,* Left coronary artery; *RCA,* right coronary artery. (Adapted from Karl TR, Kirshbom PM: Transposition of the great arteries and the arterial switch operation. In Nichols DG, Ungerleider RM, Spevak PJ, et al, editors: *Critical heart disease in infants and children,* Philadelphia, 2006, Mosby, p 721.)

to follow them closely for evidence of CHF and perform semielective ASO and VSD closure in the first 4 to 6 weeks of life. Some centers prefer to proceed with this surgery sooner; this appears to be a matter of surgeon preference and has not been shown to affect long-term outcome. In patients with TGA-VSD with arch

hypoplasia or coarctation, early surgery is required. In this setting, the preferred treatment involves one-stage, complete correction, including ASO, VSD closure, and aortic arch repair.

Transposition of the great arteries–ventricular septal defect with pulmonary stenosis–left ventricular outflow tract obstruction or pulmonary atresia. The issue of concern in this group of patients is the degree of LVOTO. In patients with TGA-VSD and organic LVOTO, with a relatively normal pulmonary valve, the treatment strategy is as described earlier, with ASO, VSD closure, and left ventricular outflow tract (LVOT) resection. The situation becomes more complex in the setting of severe pulmonary stenosis or pulmonary atresia. These patients may be ductal-dependent as newborns (pulmonary atresia) and require newborn complete correction or a palliative Blalock shunt in the newborn period, followed by biventricular repair later in infancy (our preference). The goal in these patients is to achieve biventricular repair to create an unobstructed connection between the morphologic left ventricle and systemic circulation. Several operations have been described and successfully used in this setting.

The Rastelli procedure involves an interventricular patch baffle, which commits the left ventricle to the aorta through the VSD. Typically, a right ventricle–pulmonary artery conduit is then placed to achieve pulmonary blood flow. Issues of concern include the potential for LVOTO (at or below the level of the VSD) and the certain need for future right ventricle–pulmonary artery conduit revision. The REV procedure is designed to minimize the potential of LVOT obstruction and to use all possible native tissue-tissue connections to limit the potential need for future surgery. This procedure involves resection of the muscular conus between the aorta and pulmonary roots, interventricular baffle of the left ventricle to the aorta, and translocation of the native main pulmonary artery to the right ventricle (by a Lecompte maneuver) without the use of an intervening conduit. The final option involves aortic root translocation, which includes resection of the entire native aortic root and coronary origins, resection of the intervening muscular conus, and posterior translocation of the aortic root to the surgically enlarged pulmonary root to achieve a direct connection between the left ventricle and aorta. The VSD is then closed, and a conduit is placed or a direct connection is created between the right ventricle and pulmonary arteries.

Transposition of the great arteries in adults. The long-term prognosis of adult patients who have undergone childhood repair of TGA is still incompletely understood; however, all these patients require lifelong surveillance and have the potential of developing significant anatomic and functional cardiac problems. Patients who were treated with the atrial switch operation have a morphologic right ventricle supporting their systemic circulation, which will predictably fail in many patients. Although fully saturated, these patients may present later in life with signs and symptoms of CHF and dysrhythmia. For severely affected individuals, the only realistic treatment option may ultimately be cardiac transplantation.

The long-term issues related to the ASO are less well understood. Despite technical advances in reconstructive methods, there is still a troubling incidence of postoperative supravalvular and branch pulmonic stenosis. The neoaortic root may dilate in some patients undergoing the ASO, leading to neoaortic insufficiency and coronary artery distortion. The fate of the surgically translocated coronary ostia is unclear; there is clearly a risk for late sudden cardiac death related to unsuspected coronary insufficiency noted elsewhere in this chapter. For an adult patient undergoing noncardiac surgery after previous surgery for complex congenital cardiac disease, including TGA, a high index of suspicion is warranted.

Double-Outlet Right Ventricle

Double-outlet right ventricle occurs when both great vessels are anatomically committed to the right ventricle. This condition may occur in association with a subaortic VSD, a noncommitted (remote) VSD, or a subpulmonary VSD (Taussig-Bing anomaly). As with other complex cardiac conditions, the goal of treatment relates to the presenting hemodynamic conditions and patient symptoms. The ultimate goal is to achieve a biventricular circulation when possible. Patients may present with severe cyanosis and require corrective or palliative therapy in the newborn period. Conversely, they may present with unrestricted pulmonary blood flow and develop CHF. The challenging issue of constructing a biventricular repair relates to achieving unobstructed outlets from the right and left ventricles. In patients with double-outlet right ventricle with subaortic VSD and RVOTO, reconstruction is similar to that for TOF. More remote VSDs may require enlargement with interventricular tunnel repair. For the Taussig-Bing anomaly, the relationship of the VSD to the pulmonary artery makes the ASO the procedure of choice. These patients often have RVOTO and aortic arch hypoplasia, which require attention at the time of complete correction. For rare individuals, the relationship of the great vessels and complexity of the VSD preclude a biventricular repair, and the patient must be treated as if he or she has a functional single ventricle.

Congenitally Corrected Transposition of the Great Arteries (L-Transposition)

ccTGA, or L-TGA, describes a constellation of conditions with the common feature of A-V and ventriculoarterial discordance. ccTGA may occur in association with VSD, pulmonic and subpulmonic stenosis, and displaced left A-V valve (Ebsteinoid left A-V valve). In ccTGA, the morphologic mitral valve is right-sided and associated with the morphologic left ventricle; the morphologic tricuspid valve is associated with the morphologic right ventricle. Patients with this condition are physiologically corrected in that in the absence of ventricular-level shunting, they are fully saturated—hence, the term *corrected transposition*. The age and mode of patient presentation in this condition depend on the contribution of associated defects and the function of the morphologic right ventricle, which acts as the systemic ventricle. Controversy exists regarding the timing and mode of surgical treatment for patients presenting with various manifestations of ccTGA.

Congenitally corrected transposition of the great arteries with intact ventricular septum. Patients with ccTGA-IVS may be entirely asymptomatic throughout childhood and early adulthood. Frequently, the diagnosis is made incidentally. In other patients, the disease manifests with symptoms of CHF in association with right ventricular dysfunction or left A-V valve insufficiency. There is also a high incidence of complete heart block in patients with ccTGA, and the first manifestation may be this dysrhythmia, with associated symptoms.

Treatment for patients presenting with CHF is a challenging management scenario. For patients with ccTGA and preserved right ventricular function, left A-V valve repair or replacement may be considered. In many of these patients, the valvular insufficiency may be more a manifestation of declining systemic RV function, with septal shift and annular dilation, rather than intrinsic valve pathology. In this setting, valve replacement would not correct the progression of right ventricular dysfunction. For patients with systemic right ventricular dysfunction, one option for treatment is a complex reconstruction known as a *double switch* (Fig. 58-30). This procedure includes an atrial switch in combination with an arterial switch to align the morphologic left ventricle with the systemic circulation. In almost all patients with ccTGA-IVS and right ventricular dysfunction (and in the absence of structural LVOTO), a period of left ventricle retraining is required before the double-switch procedure. This requirement relates to the fact that the left ventricle will have been functioning in the low-pressure pulmonary circulation and will be incapable of performing systemic work. Retraining or conditioning the left ventricle requires the surgical creation of pulmonary stenosis by the placement of a pulmonary artery band. Most surgeons agree that the left ventricle must work at or very near systemic blood pressure for many months (we favor a minimum of 6 months) before the double-switch operation. The double switch is a technically challenging operation, with significant perioperative risk. Because of the small numbers of patients treated worldwide with this complicated surgical strategy, there are only limited data of the acute and midterm results.[35] An issue of concern centers on the long-term ability of the retrained left ventricle to function as the systemic ventricle. Nonetheless, patients with ccTGA and depressed right ventricular function have a poor prognosis otherwise, and, as such, the complexity and risk of the double-switch operation appear justified. The only other surgical option for these patients is cardiac transplantation.

Congenitally corrected transposition of the great arteries with ventricular septal defect and pulmonic stenosis. Patients in this category are often well balanced and have mild cyanosis, with minimal symptoms in childhood, whereas others with more severe pulmonary stenosis or pulmonary atresia present early in life with symptomatic cyanosis. Treatment for an overtly cyanotic infant with ccTGA with pulmonary stenosis is initially palliative in the form of a Blalock shunt. The ultimate goal for all patients is a biventricular circulation, with normal arterial oxygen saturation. One option for these patients is to close the VSD surgically and place a conduit between the morphologic left ventricle and pulmonary arteries to relieve the pulmonary obstruction. This classic repair benefits the patient by separating the systemic and pulmonary circulations and allowing normal oxygen tension. The issue of concern in patients undergoing this repair is that the morphologic right ventricle must act independently as the systemic ventricle after repair. As noted, the ability of the right ventricle to support the systemic circulation may be questionable over the long-term in some patients. As such, an alternative strategy in these patients is to baffle the left ventricular outflow to the aorta through the VSD, then to perform an atrial switch to reroute the systemic and pulmonary venous return, and finally to place a conduit from the morphologic right ventricle to the pulmonary arteries. This option is a modification of the double-switch arrangement, affording the patient the benefit of a systemic left ventricle. Because the left ventricle has been working at systemic pressure before correction, a period of retraining is unnecessary.

Adult patients with ccTGA, with or without previous surgery, warrant careful attention before any noncardiac operation. These patients may have various complex ongoing cardiac issues, including rhythm disturbance, ventricular dysfunction, and valvular insufficiency.

Left Ventricular Outflow Tract Obstruction

LVOTO may manifest in isolation or in combination with other complex cardiac lesions. The physiologic consequences of severe

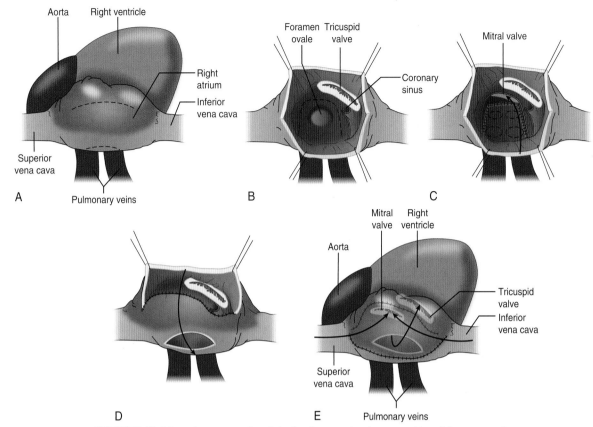

FIGURE 58-30 Schematic representation of the Senning procedure for transposition of the great arteries. **A,** Two separate incisions, one in the right atrium and the other in the left atrium near the insertion of the pulmonary veins. **B,** Location of the incision in the atrial septum. **C,** The atrial septum sewn down to the pulmonary veins preparing for oxygenated blood to be directed to the tricuspid valve. The inferior free wall of the right atrium is sewn along the cut edge of the atrial septum redirecting the deoxygenated blood to the mitral valve. **D,** The superior free wall of the right atrium is now sewn to the cut edge of the left atrium, redirecting the oxygenated blood from the pulmonary veins to the tricuspid valve. **E,** Schematic representation of the oxygenated blood and deoxygenated blood pathways. (Reprinted with permission from Texas Children's Hospital, 2016.)

LVOTO may be catastrophic, including diminished systemic cardiac output and tremendous left ventricular pressure overload. Newborns with severe LVOTO may present in shock with diminished peripheral perfusion, cardiomegaly, and pulmonary congestion. There is a significant risk for necrotizing enterocolitis in these infants. In older patients, gradual onset of LVOTO may be initially asymptomatic, only to manifest over time as decreasing exercise tolerance and declining left ventricular function. Patients with severe LVOTO and cardiomegaly are at high risk for myocardial ischemia and sudden cardiac death. The resting ECG often demonstrates left ventricular hypertrophy, with a strain pattern. If an exercise stress test is performed, it may demonstrate worrisome ST segment depression and ventricular dysrhythmias. Echocardiography is the primary diagnostic tool for patients with LVOTO. In rare cases, diagnostic cardiac catheterization may be considered to delineate the level of obstruction.

Valvular Aortic Stenosis

Congenital valvular aortic stenosis (AS) is a common cause of LVOTO. The degree of obstruction may range from mild in patients with a congenitally bicuspid aortic valve to severe in patients with critical AS with unidentifiable valve commissures and annular hypoplasia. Infants presenting with critical AS are often symptomatic early in the newborn period, presenting with shock and profoundly depressed ventricular function. At the present time, almost all patients are taken to the cardiac catheterization laboratory for balloon aortic valvotomy. This procedure may be lifesaving in relieving AS and allowing for recovery of ventricular function. However, for most patients, the procedure is palliative, with a significant incidence of recurrence of AS or development of significant aortic insufficiency after the procedure. In patients with AS refractory to balloon dilation, an open aortic valvotomy may be necessary (Fig. 58-31). A surgical valvotomy, especially in small infants with adequate annular dimension, can be accomplished by an accurate incision down a rudimentary commissure or raphe to improve cusp mobility.

Recurrent AS after previous ballooning may be amenable to repeat dilation; however, when associated with significant aortic insufficiency, the patient requires surgery. Severe aortic insufficiency after previous balloon dilation is usually related to an avulsed cusp. In these cases, valve repair may be possible, but replacement may become necessary. Published series have

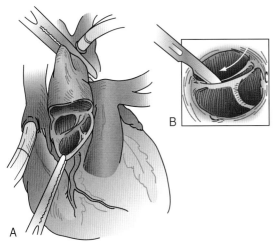

A

B

FIGURE 58-31 Close-up of the aortic valve demonstrating a surgical valvectomy. **A,** The valve is bicuspid, with a prominent raphe in the anterior valve leaflet. **B,** The orifice is enlarged by incising the fused commissure between the two leaflets. (From Chang AC, Burke RP: Left ventricular outflow tract obstruction. In Chang AC, Hanley FL, Wernovsky G, et al, editors: *Pediatric cardiac intensive care*. Baltimore, 1998, Williams & Wilkins.)

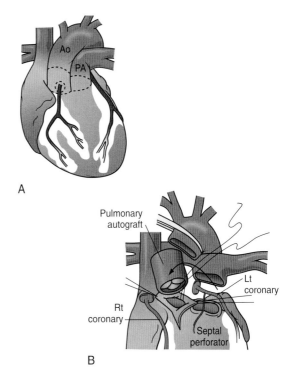

A

B

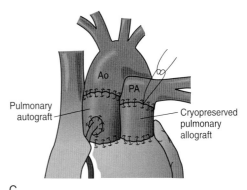

C

FIGURE 58-32 Ross procedure. **A,** The great arteries are transected above the sinotubular ridge. The coronary arteries are excised using coronary artery buttons. **B,** The pulmonary autograft is excised from the right ventricular outflow tract, and the proximal end of the autograft is anastomosed to the annulus. **C,** The coronary artery buttons are anastomosed to the pulmonary autograft. *Ao,* Aorta; *PA,* pulmonary artery. (Adapted from St Louis JD, Jaggers J: Left ventricular outflow tract obstruction. In Nichols DG, Ungerleider RM, Spevak PJ, et al, editors: *Critical heart disease in infants and children*, Philadelphia, 2006, Mosby, p 615.)

confirmed the usefulness of aortic valve repair procedures, which is a particularly attractive option for growing children.[36-38]

The decision to replace the aortic valve in growing children is clouded by the lack of an ideal aortic valve substitute—a valve capable of lifelong durability, appropriate somatic growth, easily implantable, and not requiring anticoagulation. Criteria for aortic valve replacement are beyond the scope of this chapter; however, severe valvular AS not amenable to catheter or open valvotomy is an appropriate indication. Options for aortic valve replacement in children include a mechanical prosthesis, heterograft, homograft, and pulmonary autograft. A mechanical prosthesis may be considered in childhood; however, the valve size must be sufficient to provide adequate function as the patient grows. Most surgeons and cardiologists recommend therapeutic anticoagulation in children with a mechanical valve prosthesis, but this can be challenging and potentially dangerous in growing children and adolescents. Many surgeons believe the risk for such medical treatment outweighs the potential benefit of a theoretically durable valve.

Heterograft aortic valve prostheses historically have been associated with limited durability in children and are not capable of somatic growth. Currently available heterograft prostheses have not undergone sufficient use in children to provide useful data concerning improved durability. Human cadaver aortic valves (aortic homograft) have been used extensively in children and young adults. These valves are usually implanted as a complete aortic root replacement, which requires coronary ostial implantation. Thus, surgery to place an aortic homograft is considerably more complex and with potentially higher risk. The positive features of an aortic homograft include improved durability compared with heterograft and avoidance of anticoagulation. Nonetheless, these valves eventually fail, necessitating a complicated reoperative aortic root replacement.

Pulmonary autograft aortic root replacement (Ross operation) involves translocation of the pulmonary valve to the aortic position with subsequent replacement of the pulmonary valve with a homograft or heterograft valved conduit (Fig. 58-32). The

theoretical advantages of the Ross procedure include the potential for somatic growth, avoidance of anticoagulation, and possibility of extended durability. Enthusiasm for this procedure has been tempered by the recognition that the need for extension cardiac dissection to harvest the autograft, along with a more complex implantation, is associated with increased operative risk. Furthermore, the unsupported pulmonary root may dilate in the presence of systemic arterial pressure, leading to progressive autograft aortic insufficiency. This observation has led to various modifications of the implantation technique to support the aortic annulus and the sinus segment. Given these considerations and the certain need for reoperation to replace the right ventricular–pulmonary artery conduit, great caution must be exercised in the application of the Ross operation.[39]

Fibromuscular Subaortic Stenosis

This condition is a progressive narrowing of the LVOT related to a dense fibrous membrane usually found in association with asymmetrical protrusion of the interventricular septum into the outflow tract. The membrane is often concentric and becomes densely adherent to the septum and mitral valve. The membrane progresses toward and eventually onto the undersurface of the aortic valve cusps, which leads to progressive LVOTO, aortic valve cusp retraction, and aortic insufficiency.

Echocardiography is the primary diagnostic tool when assessing the degree of obstruction and progression of subaortic stenosis. However, it is not accurate for assessing subtle degrees of cusp extension.[40] Cardiac catheterization is rarely needed to diagnose this condition; balloon dilation is of no use in treating LVOTO.

Surgery is the mainstay of treatment for subaortic stenosis, but there is disagreement about surgical indications. Most surgeons believe that new onset of any degree of aortic insufficiency in association with a subaortic membrane, regardless of the pressure gradient, is an indication for surgery. In other patients, an escalating LVOT gradient, associated left ventricular hypertrophy, and appropriate anatomic substrate are acceptable indications for operation.

The surgical procedure for subaortic stenosis involves a transaortic resection of the subaortic membrane, including all attachments to the mitral valve, septum, and aortic valve cusps. A septal myectomy is performed, along with membrane resection, in most patients (Fig. 58-33). Complications include membrane recurrence, injury to the bundle of His, and iatrogenic VSD creation.

Nonetheless, with careful technique, the risk for these complications is minimized.

Tunnel Subaortic Stenosis

Tunnel subaortic stenosis is a more severe form of LVOTO that is often associated with aortic annular hypoplasia and valvular AS. In severe cases, the LVOTO is not amenable to subaortic resection alone. In this situation, an aortic root–enlarging procedure may be necessary to relieve the obstruction (aortoventriculoplasty, or Konno procedure). This complex reconstruction generally is associated with the necessity of aortic valve replacement using one of the aforementioned options. Moreover, all degrees of LVOTO may be seen in association with numerous left heart obstructive lesions (Shone syndrome[41]) that may require extensive reconstruction.

Aortic Arch Anomalies
Aortic Coarctation

Coarctation of the aorta is one of the most frequently encountered congenital cardiac lesions. This condition has a wide range of presentations, from a severely symptomatic newborn with CHF and depressed ventricular function to an adult with proximal hypertension and minimal symptoms. Coarctation is classified relative to its association with the ligamentum arteriosus and aortic arch. An infantile or preductal aortic coarctation is seen in combination with a large PDA, which may have predominantly right-to-left flow to the lower descending aorta. In this setting, the patient is ductal-dependent for systemic blood flow until the coarctation is repaired, and a PGE1 infusion must be maintained to prevent ductal closure. A periductal or juxtaductal coarctation occurs in the region of the ductal insertion and is distal to the aortic isthmus, which may be normal or hypoplastic (Fig. 58-34).

Aortic coarctation with or without aortic arch hypoplasia is frequently associated with intracardiac anomalies, including

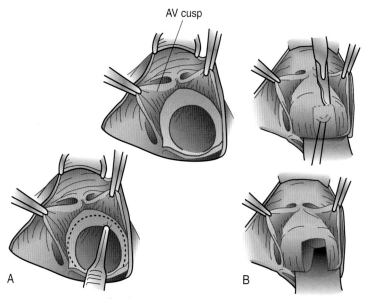

FIGURE 58-33 A, Excision of discrete subaortic stenosis. The aorta is opened obliquely, and the aortic valve leaflets are retracted to expose the subaortic membrane. The membrane is excised circumferentially *(dotted line)*. **B,** This is usually combined with a muscle resection. (From de Leval M: Surgery of the left ventricular outflow tract. In Stark J, de Leval M, editors: *Surgery for congenital heart defects*, ed 2, Philadelphia, 1994, Saunders.)

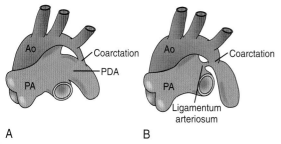

FIGURE 58-34 Coarctation of the aorta *(Ao)*. **A,** Infantile or preductal coarctation. **B,** Adult coarctation. *PA,* Pulmonary artery; *PDA,* patent ductus arteriosus. (From Backer CL, Mavroudis C: Coarctation of the aorta. In Mavroudis C, Backer CL, editors: *Pediatric heart surgery.* Philadelphia, 2003, Mosby, p 252.)

multiple left heart obstructive lesions (e.g., mitral stenosis, left ventricular hypoplasia or endocardial fibroelastosis, subaortic stenosis or AS) known as Shone syndrome.[41] Patients with large VSDs may present in infancy with severe aortic coarctation, with or without subaortic stenosis.

Aortic coarctation may be suspected on clinical examination by a significant upper extremity–lower extremity blood pressure gradient and diminished or absent femoral and pedal pulses. In older patients with well-developed intercostal collateral arteries, a continuous murmur may be auscultated over the posterior thorax. Echocardiography is now the primary diagnostic modality for aortic coarctation. MRI and CT angiography may also be useful in some patients. In rare cases, cardiac catheterization is required to define the anatomy, but this modality is now used more frequently for treatment, including balloon dilation with or without stenting.

Treatment strategies for aortic coarctation have evolved significantly since the first successful surgical treatment almost 70 years ago. Newborns presenting with severe aortic coarctation with or without associated ductal-dependent systemic blood flow are best treated by surgery. Initial enthusiasm regarding balloon dilation in these patients has diminished as it has become clear that there is a high incidence of recurrent coarctation after neonatal dilation.[42] Most congenital cardiac surgeons perform isolated coarctation repair through a left thoracotomy incision (third or fourth interspace) using resection of the coarctation and primary anastomosis. For patients with relative hypoplasia of the distal aortic arch, the anastomosis can be brought along the lesser curve of the aortic arch using an extended end-to-end method. For coarctation with a hypoplastic transverse arch, we favor the aortic arch advancement procedure at Texas Children's Hospital, which uses all native tissue repair to allow for growth.[43] Other methods include subclavian artery flap aortoplasty (Waldhausen method) and prosthetic patch aortoplasty. These latter methods are used less frequently than primary repair (Fig. 58-35). Catheter therapy as a primary treatment for aortic coarctation is a controversial therapy in the opinion of most surgeons. Although this methodology has been widely applied, its true comparability to surgery requires further prospective study. There are several issues of concern regarding angioplasty for coarctation. The balloon dilation results in transmural disruption of the aortic wall in many patients, and there is an acute and ongoing risk for aneurysm formation. To limit this risk and minimize the potential of recurrence, off-label use of stents has been done for treatment of coarctation. Obvious issues of concern include somatic growth and lifetime risk potential of a metal device in the descending aorta.

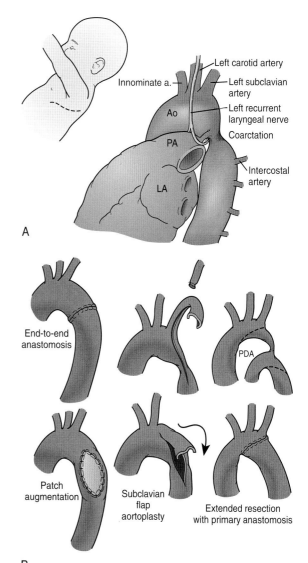

FIGURE 58-35 Surgical repair for aortic coarctation. **A,** Surgical incision and anatomic orientation. **B,** Four different methods are shown: end-to-end anastomosis, patch augmentation, subclavian flap aortoplasty, and extended resection with primary anastomosis. *Ao,* Aorta; *LA,* left atrium; *PA,* pulmonary artery. (Adapted from Hastings LA, Nichols DG: Coarctation of the aorta and interrupted aortic arch. In Nichols DG, Ungerleider RM, Spevak PJ, et al, editors: *Critical heart disease in infants and children,* Philadelphia, 2006, Mosby, p 635.)

Another controversial issue surrounds the concomitant treatment of coarctation and significant intracardiac pathology. Several series have demonstrated superior outcomes for simultaneous therapy in selected groups of patients, including neonates with large VSDs and coarctation with arch hypoplasia. Our approach to this condition has included one-stage complete repair of intracardiac defects along with aortic arch advancement through median sternotomy on cardiopulmonary bypass.

Interrupted Aortic Arch

IAA results from lack of proper fusion and involution of the fetal aortic arches. This is a fatal condition without treatment, and IAA

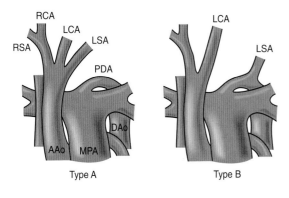

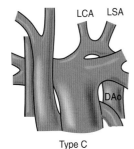

FIGURE 58-36 Classification of interrupted aortic arch. *AAo,* Ascending aorta; *DAo,* descending aorta; *LCA,* left common carotid artery; *LSA,* left subclavian artery; *MPA,* main pulmonary artery; *RCA,* right common carotid artery; *RSA,* right subclavian artery. (Adapted from Monro JL: Interruption of aortic arch. In Stark J, de Leval M, editors: *Surgery for congenital heart defects,* ed 2, Philadelphia, 1994, Saunders, p 299.)

is frequently associated with serious intracardiac pathology. IAA is classified based on the level of the interruption. Type A is distal to the left subclavian artery, type B occurs between left subclavian and common carotid arteries, and type C occurs proximal to the left subclavian artery (Fig. 58-36). There is a frequent finding of an aberrant right subclavian artery (retroesophageal) from the descending aorta. Survival for patients with IAA is initially predicated on ductal patency; thus, a PGE1 infusion is required to stabilize the patient. Diagnosis is confirmed by echocardiography; other methods, including cardiac catheterization, are needed infrequently.

IAA requires surgical treatment in the newborn period, which typically involves simultaneous repair of intracardiac lesions (Fig. 58-37). Repair may be accomplished with the aid of an aortic arch augmentation patch, although researchers at Texas Children's Hospital reported a series confirming that a primary tissue-tissue repair can be performed in most patients and minimizes the potential for recurrent aortic arch obstruction.[44]

SINGLE VENTRICLE

Single-ventricle physiology is a frequently encountered form of CHD. Patients may present as newborns with inadequate pulmonary blood flow, excessive pulmonary blood flow, or balanced circulations. The single ventricle may be of right, left, or indeterminate morphology. Surgical treatment is required to provide adequate systemic oxygen delivery, while protecting the pulmonary vasculature. The function of the single ventricle must be preserved to afford the patient the best possible long-term outcome.

The rapid evolution of successful palliation for patients with various forms of single-ventricle physiology since the late 1970s has led to a large and growing population of adults with a single ventricle. For most of these patients, lifelong cardiac attention is needed, and the potential for subsequent cardiac reoperation is high. Patients in this category who present for noncardiac surgery may be especially difficult to manage because of their challenging physiology.

An exhaustive discussion of the various forms of single ventricle is well beyond the scope of this chapter. This discussion is limited to common forms of single right and left ventricles to provide examples of the surgical management strategies for a single ventricle.

Tricuspid Atresia

Tricuspid atresia is the template of a single-ventricle lesion for which most current palliative strategies were developed. Patients with tricuspid atresia have a single morphologic left ventricle and may have normally related or transposed great vessels (Fig. 58-38). They may present with excessive pulmonary blood flow and require pulmonary artery banding early in infancy to relieve pulmonary overcirculation and CHF. Conversely, patients may have pulmonary stenosis or pulmonary atresia and require creation of a Blalock shunt to provide adequate pulmonary blood flow and systemic oxygenation.

As noted, the initial palliative goals in patients with tricuspid atresia include adequate systemic oxygenation, protection of ventricular function, and adequate pulmonary arterial growth. Patients with ductal-dependent pulmonary blood flow require a Blalock shunt in the newborn period. We prefer to construct the shunt to the morphologic right pulmonary artery through a right thoracotomy. This construction allows shunt flow to be governed by the size of the subclavian artery. Furthermore, the right pulmonary artery is typically longer and runs in a more horizontal plane compared with the left pulmonary artery; this facilitates avoiding distortion of a lobar branch. The goal of the shunt is to protect the pulmonary arteries, promote adequate pulmonary artery development, and support systemic arterial oxygenation for the first 4 to 6 months of life until the next planned stage of palliation (see later discussion of Glenn and Fontan operations). The shunt is not designed for long-term use; thus, in most patients, a small interposition graft (expanded polytetrafluoroethylene, 3.0 to 4.0 mm) is selected. In the early era of single-ventricle palliation, less well-controlled shunts were constructed, including classic Blalock (divided native subclavian artery-to-branch pulmonary artery), Pott's (side-to-side left pulmonary artery to descending aorta), and Waterston (side-to-side right pulmonary artery to ascending aorta) shunts (Fig. 58-39). These native tissue-tissue connections are capable of somatic growth but have the confounding risks for pulmonary overcirculation, pulmonary artery hypertension (potentially irreversible), and branch pulmonary artery distortion with hypoplasia. During the early stages of development of single-ventricle palliation, many patients were treated with these poorly controlled shunts. Thus, significant numbers of adult patients present with complications of these palliations including chronic cardiac volume overload and decreased ventricular function, severe pulmonary artery distortion or isolation pulmonary vascular disease, and profound cyanosis. These patients may present for surgery for noncardiac illness and are extremely difficult to manage.

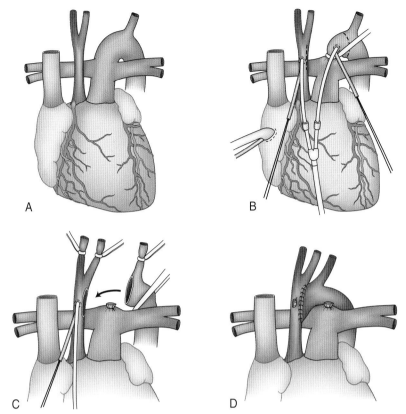

FIGURE 58-37 A, Type B interrupted aortic arch. **B,** Cannulation and site of incision for repair. The descending thoracic aorta is brought upward into the mediastinum **(C)** and then anastomosed to the ascending aorta in an end-to-side fashion **(D)**. (From Hirooka K, Fraser CD: One-stage neonatal repair of complex aortic arch obstruction or interruption. *Tex Heart Inst J* 24:317–321, 1997.)

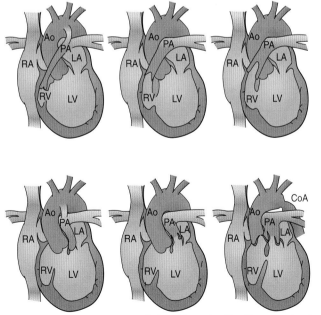

FIGURE 58-38 Anatomy of the various types of tricuspid atresia. *Top,* Normally related great vessels. *Bottom,* D-Transposition of the great vessels. *Ao,* Aorta; *CoA,* coarctation of the aorta; *LA,* left atrium; *LV,* left ventricle; *PA,* pulmonary artery; *RA,* right atrium; *RV,* right ventricle. (Adapted from Lok JM, Spevak PJ, Nichols DG: Tricuspid atresia. In Nichols DG, Ungerleider RM, Spevak PJ, et al, editors: *Critical heart disease in infants and children,* Philadelphia, 2006, Mosby, pp 800–801.)

CLASSIC RIGHT BLALOCK-TAUSSIG

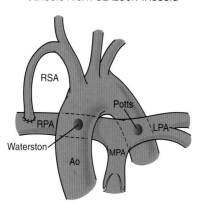

RIGHT MODIFIED BLALOCK-TAUSSIG

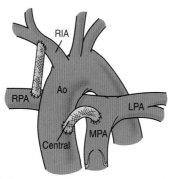

FIGURE 58-39 Systemic-to-pulmonary artery shunts. *Ao*, Aorta; *LPA*, left pulmonary artery; *MPA*, main pulmonary artery; *RIA*, right innominate artery; *RPA*, right pulmonary artery; *RSA*, right subclavian artery. (Adapted from Marino BS, Wernovsky G, Greeley WJ: Single-ventricle lesions. In Nichols DG, Ungerleider RM, Spevak PJ, et al, editors: *Critical heart disease in infants and children*, Philadelphia, 2006, Mosby, p 793.)

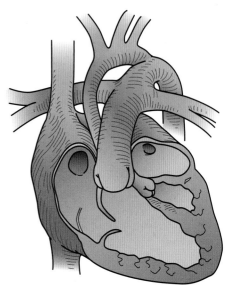

FIGURE 58-40 Anatomy of hypoplastic left heart syndrome. The tiny ascending aorta is seen arising from a markedly hypoplastic left ventricle. The ductus arteriosus is large, providing forward flow to the systemic circuit. The right ventricle is hypertrophied, and the pulmonary artery is enlarged. (From Wernovsky G, Bove EL: Single ventricle lesions. In Chang AC, Hanley FL, Wernovsky G, et al, editors: *Pediatric cardiac intensive care*, Baltimore, 1998, Williams & Wilkins.)

Hypoplastic Left Heart Syndrome

Hypoplastic left heart syndrome (HLHS) is the prototypical single right ventricle. Patients with this condition present with inadequate left heart structures ranging from mitral stenosis and AS with left ventricular hypoplasia to almost complete absence of the left heart structures with aortic and mitral atresia. In the case of aortic and mitral atresia, the ascending aorta is typically small (1 to 2 mm) and is perfused through retrograde aortic arch flow provided by the PDA. In HLHS, ductal closure results in rapid cardiovascular collapse, with profound systemic hypoperfusion and hypoxia, followed quickly by death. Therefore, in cases of prenatal diagnosis, patients must be born in a facility qualified to institute appropriate medical management immediately, including the establishment of suitable vascular access (umbilical artery catheter) and institution of intravenous PGE1 to maintain ductal patency. Patients with HLHS undiagnosed at birth typically have an early grace period of a few hours, but with the initiation of ductal closure, these children become critically ill and require aggressive resuscitation for survival. Although most children with HLHS are otherwise normal, without treatment, HLHS is a uniformly fatal condition (Fig. 58-40).

After delivery, medical treatment is directed at maintaining ductal patency and balancing systemic and pulmonary blood flow. Balancing the circulations becomes increasingly challenging with the normal decline in neonatal PVR, resulting in massive pulmonary overcirculation. As the overcirculation progresses, infants become tachypneic and may exhibit decreased systemic perfusion. Necrotizing enterocolitis is a significant risk in these children, and if there is any question of visceral malperfusion, many centers avoid enteral nutrition in an effort to minimize this potential. Other medical maneuvers include deliberate hypoventilation, low inspired oxygen concentration, and additional carbon dioxide in an attempt to increase PVR and limit pulmonary flow. These options are of limited use in newborns with HLHS; over days to weeks, the infants become progressively ill, with pulmonary congestion and marginal systemic cardiac output. Patients who are maintained have the potential of developing increased PVR as they age, and there is a known association with advanced age (>30 days) and increased operative mortality.

Surgery in the newborn period is the only realistic option for long-term survival in infants born with HLHS. Outcomes for surgical palliation of HLHS have come to be synonymous with the reputation of the treating center and surgeons. As with tricuspid atresia, patients with HLHS require a staged palliative approach. In the experiences of all centers, the first stage is the most challenging and risk-laden. The various first-stage options are described in the following sections.

Neonatal Cardiac Transplantation

Transplantation is a theoretically attractive option in infants with HLHS that replaces the malformed heart with a structurally normal one. Leonard Bailey has been an influential champion of this approach and was the first to report exciting results with transplantation in newborns with HLHS.[45] Furthermore, although there is an ever-present risk for rejection and infection in children with heart transplants, long-term meaningful survival is possible, and the quality of life of the recipients is good. The option of cardiac transplantation is limited by the small numbers of suitable donor hearts, and most children with HLHS are unable to survive the wait time for a donor graft. This situation has led most centers, including Texas Children's Hospital, to abandon cardiac transplantation as the primary mode of therapy for most neonates with HLHS.

Norwood Reconstruction

After initial work and success at Boston Children's Hospital, Norwood and colleagues[46] gained international attention at the Children's Hospital of Philadelphia for developing and implementing a reconstructive technique to palliate newborns with HLHS; this methodology now carries the widely used eponym of the Norwood procedure. This procedure was gradually refined as experience accrued. The most common method involves surgical connection of the divided main pulmonary artery to the reconstructed aortic arch. In almost all children with HLHS, there is associated aortic arch hypoplasia with coarctation. A critical feature of the operation is to reconstruct the aortic arch to provide unrestricted systemic blood flow. Most surgeons use some form of prosthetic material, usually pulmonary artery homograft patching. Some surgeons have reported accomplishing the arch reconstruction without the necessity of additional material. After reconstructing the aortic arch, the divided main pulmonary artery is anastomosed to the arch and small ascending aorta to create a neoaortic confluence providing systemic output from the right ventricle. The challenging feature of the reconstruction involves

the accurate connection of this often-miniscule ascending aorta to the confluence of the arch and main pulmonary artery stump. The risk for torsion and coronary insufficiency is high. The final element of the classic Norwood reconstruction is the creation of a controlled source of pulmonary blood flow in the form of a modified BT shunt (Fig. 58-41).

Sano Modification of the Norwood Operation

Achieving survival after the Norwood operation is challenging, involving innumerable technical and medical details. At best, after a Norwood procedure, the patient is fragile, with a delicate balance between systemic and pulmonary blood flow. This fact and the observation of widely disparate outcomes for the procedure have led to many important advances in the treatment of these children. One issue relates to the difficulty of balancing the systemic to pulmonary artery shunt, which lowers diastolic blood pressure (and coronary perfusion pressure) and volume loads the heart. Sano and associates[47] from Okayama University in Japan were the first to report a series of infants undergoing a successful Norwood procedure with the modification of a right ventricle–pulmonary artery conduit rather than a Blalock shunt. The theoretical advantage of this approach is the increase in diastolic pressure, creating a physiology more similar to a banded circulation rather than shunted circulation. Early reports with this method were encouraging, although patients appeared to become more rapidly desaturated as they aged compared with the shunted patients. The long-term effects of the right ventriculotomy on cardiac function are unknown. In one report, patients undergoing the Norwood operation were randomly assigned to receive a right ventricle-to-pulmonary artery shunt or modified Blalock-Taussig shunt.

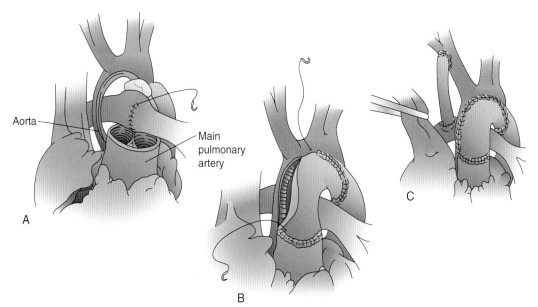

FIGURE 58-41 Norwood procedure for first-stage palliation of hypoplastic left heart syndrome. **A,** The main pulmonary artery is divided proximal to the bifurcation, the ductus arteriosus is ligated and divided, and the aortic arch is opened from the level of the transected main pulmonary artery to a point distal to the ductal insertion in the descending aorta. **B,** A segment of homograft is cut to an appropriate size and shape. This is sutured into place, creating an unobstructed outflow from the right ventricle to the pulmonary artery and aorta. **C,** Polytetrafluoroethylene tube graft is placed from the innominate artery to the right pulmonary artery. The atrial septectomy is done while the patient is under circulatory arrest. (From Castaneda AR, Jonas RA, Mayer JE, et al: Hypoplastic left heart syndrome. In *Cardiac surgery of the neonate and infant*, Philadelphia, 1994, Saunders.)

Transplantation-free survival was higher 12 months after random-ization in the right ventricle-to-pulmonary artery shunt group, as was the rate of unplanned reinterventions and complications.[48] Midterm results are being analyzed and preliminarily show pos-sible midterm survival benefit.

Hybrid Procedure

The notion of a combined therapy between interventional cardiol-ogy and surgery for the first-stage palliation of HLHS has achieved significant attention. The idea is to minimize the risk of the first operation by banding the branch pulmonary arteries and deliver-ing a stent into the ductus to maintain patency. This hybrid arrangement is designed to allow newborn survival so that a more complete reconstruction may be performed later in infancy in a larger child. There appears to be a significant learning curve with this approach, as with any new procedure, and the incidence of complications warrants further study. Data have shown that the prevalence of necrotizing enterocolitis after the hybrid procedure is significant and comparable to reports after the Norwood pro-cedure.[49] In addition, concerning features include the effect of the banding on long-term pulmonary artery growth, the fact that cardiac perfusion is still retrograde through the aortic arch, and the risk profile of the more extensive reconstruction later in life. The true place for this mode of therapy is unclear at the present time, but it represents an important direction of advancement to optimize the opportunity of survival for these children.

Fontan Operation

The long-term goal of single-ventricle palliation is to optimize ventricular function and promote systemic oxygen delivery. As noted earlier, patients with a single ventricle who are shunted or banded have ongoing concerns, including systemic desaturation, continued intracardiac mixing, and chronic cardiac volume over-load. The current strategy for addressing these concerns uses a direct connection between the branch pulmonary arteries and systemic venous return, as initially proposed by Fontan in the early 1970s.[50] The Fontan operation is now the treatment of choice for children born with all varieties of single ventricle and provides acceptable long-term palliation in suitable patients. However, the Fontan circulation is not normal and even in the best of circumstances results in significant alteration in normal cardiorespiratory physiology.

The Fontan circulation is established by connecting the sys-temic venous return directly into isolated branch pulmonary arteries without an intervening power source. Thus, blood flow in the Fontan circuit is passive, being promoted only by the pressure differential between the systemic venous system and pulmonary venous atrium. An impediment to flow in the systemic-to-pulmonary pathway results in a poor Fontan outcome. Estab-lished criteria for creating an effective Fontan circulation include the ability to connect the systemic venous return surgically to the pulmonary arteries in an unobstructed manner, normal pulmo-nary artery architecture and resistance, normal pulmonary venous drainage and low left atrial pressure, absence of significant A-V valve regurgitation, good ventricular function (and low ventricular end-diastolic pressure), an unobstructed systemic arterial outlet, and good aortic valve function. Compromise of any of these ele-ments may compromise the quality of the Fontan circulation.

The Fontan operation has undergone several technical modifi-cations in the almost 40 years of successful application to patients with single-ventricle physiology. Many patients underwent an atriopulmonary connection in which the open right atrial

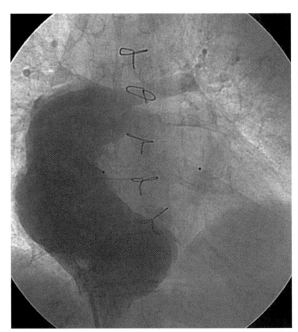

FIGURE 58-42 Angiogram of a dilated right atrium in a patient with an atriopulmonary Fontan connection.

appendage was directly anastomosed to the pulmonary artery bifurcation with surgical closure of the ASD. Many of these patients present as adults with extreme dilation of the right atrium, with resulting sluggish flow, hepatic congestion, and atrial dysrhythmias (Fig. 58-42). Today, the most widely practiced modification of the Fontan operation is the total cavopulmonary connection. First described by DeLeval, this operation involves connection of the divided SVC to the superior and inferior aspects of the right pulmonary artery (typically offset), along with the creation of a channel to direct the IVC flow into the pulmonary arteries. The channel may be created using a surgically created lateral tunnel in the right atrium (Fig. 58-43) or interposing a conduit between the IVC and pulmonary arteries (extracardiac Fontan) (Fig. 58-44).

The change from a volume-loaded circulation in patients with a single ventricle who are shunted or banded to a Fontan circula-tion results in acute volume unloading of the systemic ventricle. In the chronic overloaded heart, this acute change may be poorly tolerated, with resultant diastolic dysfunction and decreased ven-tricular compliance. To deal with this problem, patients with a single ventricle typically undergo an intervening stage of palliation in the form of a bidirectional, superior cavopulmonary anastomo-sis (Glenn shunt). The bidirectional Glenn shunt is constructed by anastomosing the cephalad end of the divided SVC to the superior aspect of the right pulmonary artery (Fig. 58-45). Other sources of pulmonary blood flow are typically eliminated, and the heart is volume-unloaded; however, systemic cardiac output is maintained because the IVC return is preserved. After the Glenn shunt, the patients are not fully saturated; typically, patients have saturations of approximately 80%. Over time, the unloaded ven-tricle remodels, and the patient is promoted to reoperation and completion of the Fontan circulation.

Perioperative care of a patient after a Fontan procedure can be challenging. The acute changes in cardiac volume loading may negatively affect cardiac output. Even in patients with supposedly

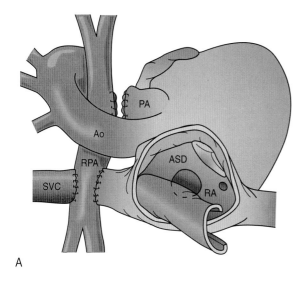

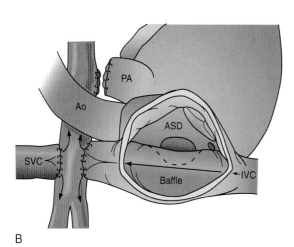

FIGURE 58-43 A and **B,** Lateral tunnel Fontan procedure. *Ao,* Aorta; *ASD,* atrial septal defect; *IVC,* inferior vena cava; *PA,* pulmonary artery; *RA,* right atrium; *RPA,* right pulmonary artery; *SVC,* superior vena cava. (Adapted from Lok JM, Spevak PJ, Nichols DG: Tricuspid atresia. In Nichols DG, Ungerleider RM, Spevak PJ, et al, editors: *Critical heart disease in infants and children,* Philadelphia, 2006, Mosby, p 813.)

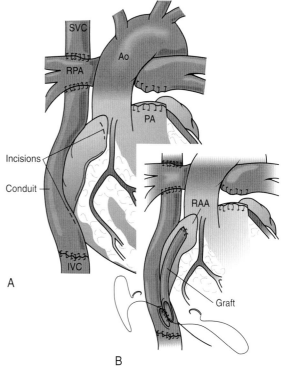

FIGURE 58-44 A, Extracardiac Fontan procedure. **B,** Creation of a fenestration in an extracardiac Fontan procedure using a graft between the extracardiac conduit and right atrial appendage *(RAA)*. *Ao,* Aorta; *IVC,* inferior vena cava; *PA,* pulmonary artery; *RPA,* right pulmonary artery; *SVC,* superior vena cava. (Adapted from Lok JM, Spevak PJ, Nichols DG: Tricuspid atresia. In Nichols DG, Ungerleider RM, Spevak PJ, et al, editors: *Critical heart disease in infants and children,* Philadelphia, 2006, Mosby, p 814.)

ideal Fontan connections, the central venous pressure acutely increases to 12 to 15 mm Hg. Consequences of this increased venous pressure include pleural effusions, hepatic congestion, and ascites. In marginal Fontan candidates, some surgeons routinely place an intentional leak, or fenestration; the goal here is to preserve systemic ventricular volume loading and decrease systemic venous congestion at the expense of some degree of desaturation caused by the right-to-left shunting. The practice of routine fenestration after the Fontan operation has been examined, and some early data have shown that excellent outcomes can be achieved with highly selective application of a fenestration, which mitigates the risks associated with such a procedure, including hypoxia and systemic embolism.[51] Any impediment to passive pulmonary blood flow will inhibit Fontan flow and result in right heart failure. Positive pressure ventilation, especially elevated levels of

positive end-expiratory pressure, impedes pulmonary blood flow in the Fontan patient. Conversely, early extubation and effective spontaneous ventilation will improve pulmonary blood flow in the Fontan patient. Data have suggested that early extubation in the operating room for patients after the Fontan procedure improves hemodynamics, decreases the length of stay for patients, and decreases hospital costs.[14]

The chronic complications of living with a Fontan circulation are still unfolding and include chronic hepatic congestion and cirrhosis, protein-losing enteropathy, atrial dysrhythmias, and venous stasis disease. Management of patients with failing Fontan circulations is especially challenging. These patients are at high risk for severe cardiac compromise while undergoing general anesthesia with positive pressure ventilation or any procedure involving large fluid shifts, including abdominal surgery. Patients with chronic hepatic congestion may develop a coagulopathy related to a decrease in factor production.

MISCELLANEOUS ANOMALIES

Vascular Rings and Pulmonary Artery Slings
Vascular Rings
Vascular rings are abnormalities of the aortic arch and its branches, compressing the trachea, esophagus, or both. The ring may be

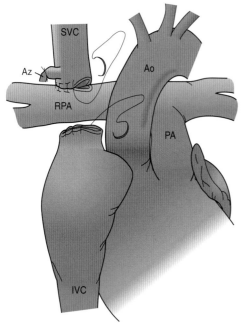

FIGURE 58-45 Bidirectional Glenn shunt. *Ao,* Aorta; *Az,* azygos vein; *IVC,* inferior vena cava; *PA,* pulmonary artery; *RPA,* right pulmonary artery; *SVC,* superior vena cava. (Adapted from Lok JM, Spevak PJ, Nichols DG: Tricuspid atresia. In Nichols DG, Ungerleider RM, Spevak PJ, et al, editors: *Critical heart disease in infants and children,* Philadelphia, 2006, Mosby, p 809.)

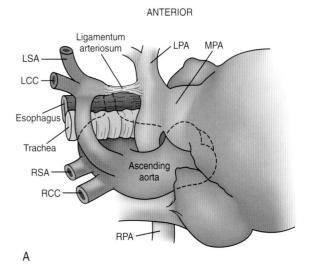

A

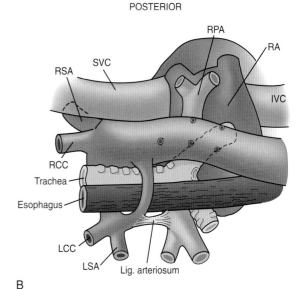

B

FIGURE 58-46 Double aortic arch, posterior **(A)** and superior **(B)** views. *IVC,* inferior vena cava; *LCC,* Left common carotid artery; *LPA,* left pulmonary artery; *LSA,* left subclavian artery; *MPA,* main pulmonary artery; *RA,* right atrium; *RCC,* right common carotid artery; *RSA,* right subclavian artery; *SVC,* superior vena cava. (Adapted from Jonas RA: *Comprehensive surgical management of congenital heart disease.* New York, 2004, Oxford University Press, p 499.)

complete or partial. Categorization of the defects is useful for description:

- Complete vascular rings
  - Double arch: Equal arches or left or right arch dominant (Fig. 58-46)
  - Right arch: Left ligamentum arteriosus from anomalous left subclavian artery
  - Right arch: Mirror image branching, with left ligamentum from descending aorta
- Partial vascular rings
  - Left arch: Aberrant right subclavian artery
  - Left arch: Innominate artery compression

The double aortic arch is the most common form of complete ring. Two arches arise from the ascending aorta, forming a true ring. The left arch is usually smaller. The right arch–left ligamentum complex is formed from persistence of the right fourth arch and regression of the left fourth arch. The anomalously arising left subclavian artery is often associated with a diverticulum at its base (Kommerell diverticulum). In partial rings, the most common form is an aberrant right subclavian artery arising distal to the left subclavian artery with a left arch. The right subclavian artery passes behind the esophagus from left to right. Innominate artery compression arises from a more posterior and leftward origin of the innominate artery from a left arch, leading to anterior compression of the trachea.

Pulmonary Artery Slings

A pulmonary artery sling occurs when the left pulmonary artery arises from the right pulmonary artery, passing leftward between the trachea and the esophagus. The ligamentum arteriosum attachment from the main pulmonary artery to the undersurface

of the aorta forms a vascular ring around the trachea but not the esophagus. The trachea may be compressed, the cartilage may be soft, or there may be intrinsic stenosis of the trachea in the form of complete cartilage rings.

Diagnosis and Indications for Intervention

Symptoms reflect the degree of tracheal and esophageal compression from complete rings as well as the presence of coexistent tracheomalacia or stenosis. Upper respiratory symptoms predominate, with a characteristic brassy cough, recurrent respiratory infections, failure to thrive, and sometimes esophageal motility problems. In children, documentation of a ring is an indication for surgery. Older patients are often asymptomatic. Initially, the diagnosis is based on a high index of suspicion, and barium swallow is the first investigation. Echocardiography can document an abnormal head and neck vessel branching pattern, excluding intracardiac abnormalities. MRI provides complete anatomic detail.

Surgery

Most vascular rings are accessible through a left posterolateral thoracotomy; the exception is a left arch with right-sided ligamentum. Division of the ring and, in the case of double arch, preservation of the dominant arch is performed. Preservation of the recurrent laryngeal nerve is important. Initial experience with endoscopic robotically assisted repair of vascular rings has also been reported. Pulmonary artery slings are approached through the midline; the use of cardiopulmonary bypass facilitates tracheal reconstruction and relocation of the right pulmonary artery (Fig. 58-47). Repair can be achieved with low risk. Symptoms may take months to resolve, with slow resolution of the underlying tracheomalacia.

Coronary Artery Anomalies

Anomalies occur as a result of anomalous origin, termination, courses, and aneurysm formation. Of these variables, only an anomalous left coronary artery rising from the pulmonary artery (ALCAPA) and coronary artery fistulas are discussed here.

Anomalous Left Coronary Artery Rising From the Pulmonary Artery

An ALCAPA is a rare, often lethal lesion in early infancy. Untreated, the mortality rate approaches 90%.

Anatomy and pathophysiology. Developmentally, failure of the normal connection of the left coronary artery bud to the aorta results in an abnormal connection to the pulmonary artery. The abnormal origin can be situated in the main pulmonary artery or proximal branches. Associated abnormalities are rare but important to recognize because lowering of the pulmonary artery pressure by PDA ligation or closure of a VSD can be fatal if the ALCAPA is not noted. In utero, with equal pulmonary arterial and aortic pressures, satisfactory perfusion of the ALCAPA can occur. After birth, the pulmonary artery pressure falls, and left coronary artery perfusion decreases. Ischemia causes impaired ventricular function and myocardial infarcts and leads to left ventricular dilation. Papillary muscle dysfunction causes mitral regurgitation. Early coronary collateral development may prevent ongoing infarction.

Diagnosis and indications for intervention. ALCAPA is suspected in any infant with mitral regurgitation, ventricular dysfunction, or dilated cardiomyopathy. Infants present with low cardiac output and systemic heart failure. Feeding may also precipitate sudden death and angina in infants. Sudden death has been described in older children. The ECG may reflect ischemic changes. The echocardiogram is usually diagnostic. However, because this diagnosis is often confused with dilated cardiomyopathy, there is an argument in favor of catheterizing all patients with dilated cardiomyopathy in whom the coronary artery anatomy cannot be clearly defined on echocardiography. Secondary findings of dilated cardiac chambers and segmental wall motion abnormalities together with mitral regurgitation prompt a search for an ALCAPA. Diagnosis of an ALCAPA is an indication for intervention.

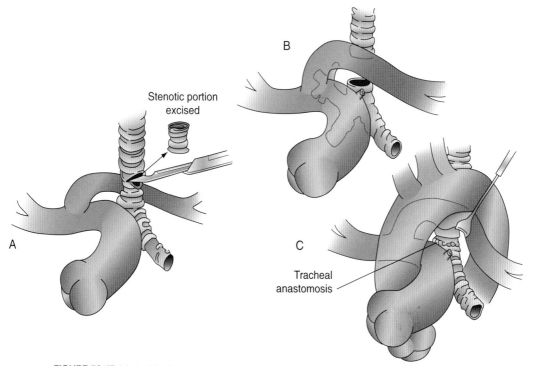

Stenotic portion excised

A

B

C

Tracheal anastomosis

FIGURE 58-47 Method for the management of a pulmonary artery sling with associated tracheal stenosis, using cardiopulmonary bypass. **A,** Tracheal resection of the involved segment. **B,** Anterior translocation of the left pulmonary artery after transection of the trachea. **C,** Direct anastomosis of the trachea. (From Castaneda AR, Jonas RA, Mayer JE, et al: Vascular rings, slings, and tracheal anomalies. In *Cardiac surgery of the neonate and infant*, Philadelphia, 1994, Saunders.)

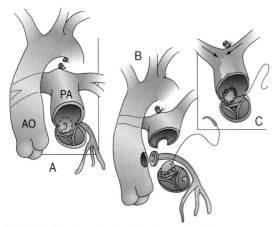

FIGURE 58-48 Direct reimplantation of anomalous left coronary artery rising from the pulmonary artery (ALCAPA). **A,** Excision of ALCAPA from the pulmonary artery *(PA)*. **B,** Aortic reimplantation of the coronary ostium into the aorta. **C,** Reconstruction of the PA with autologous pericardium. *AO,* Aorta. (From Vouhe PR, Tamisier D, Sidi D, et al: Anomalous left coronary artery from the pulmonary artery: Results of isolated aortic reimplantation. *Ann Thorac Surg* 54:621–626, 1992.)

Surgery. A degree of ventricular dysfunction is usually present. Preoperative inotropic support and optimization of hemodynamics may be required before surgical intervention. Severe cardiomyopathy rarely may necessitate cardiac transplantation. Current experience indicates that creation of a dual coronary system is safe and reproducible and offers the best opportunity for recovery of function.[52] Operative considerations include optimal myocardial protection and prevention of left heart distention. Direct reimplantation of the ALCAPA into the ascending aorta is the procedure of choice (Fig. 58-48). Sometimes, limited mobility of the coronary artery precludes reimplantation, and a surgically created aorta–pulmonary artery–coronary artery tunnel is created; this is known as the *Takeuchi procedure.* Ligation of the ALCAPA is not recommended.

Postoperative management is directed toward maintaining adequate coronary perfusion and cardiac output. Mechanical support of the heart may be temporarily required. Mitral regurgitation usually improves, and valve replacement is rarely necessary. Current intervention has a low operative mortality. Risks for nonsurvival relate to preoperative ventricular dysfunction and cardiogenic shock. The Takeuchi repair is associated with tunnel complications such as obstruction, leak, aortic valve damage, and RVOTO in the long-term.

Coronary Arteriovenous Fistula and Aneurysms

Isolated coronary artery fistula is more rare than ALCAPA. Drainage of coronary artery fistula is reported to terminate more commonly in the right side of the heart or pulmonary artery than in the left side of the heart. A shunt from the high-pressure coronary artery system into a low-pressure cardiac chamber may result in coronary steal and some degree of cardiac volume overload. Coronary artery aneurysms are associated with Kawasaki disease.

Diagnosis and indications for intervention. Presentation depends on the amount of functional compromise produced by the ischemia and volume overload. Echocardiography may be able to delineate the anomaly, but coronary angiography is diagnostic. Details of coronary anatomy are essential for determining intervention. Interventional catheterization is useful for the obliteration of fistulas and terminal aneurysms.

Surgery. If the lesion is not amenable to transcatheter intervention, surgery is indicated. Options include suture ligation without bypass, cardiopulmonary bypass, and aneurysmectomy with closure of the fistula. Early and late mortality rates are low. Risk factors for death and ventricular dysfunction relate to coronary artery insufficiency and infarction after fistula ligation or aneurysmectomy.[53]

Ebstein Anomaly of the Tricuspid Valve

Ebstein anomaly of the tricuspid valve is a rare defect in which the tricuspid valve attachments are displaced into the right ventricle to varying degrees. Ebstein anomaly includes a spectrum of abnormalities involving a degree of displacement of the tricuspid valve, variable right ventricular size, and variable pulmonary outflow obstruction. Associated abnormalities are ASD, pulmonary atresia, and ccTGA. The posterior and septal leaflets of the tricuspid valve are variably displaced to the apex of the right ventricle, which results in an atrialized portion of the right ventricle. The anterior leaflet remains large and sail-like. The major hemodynamic issue is tricuspid incompetence with decreased pulmonary blood flow and, if an ASD is present, right-to-left shunting causing cyanosis. Long-standing tricuspid incompetence leads to volume overload of an abnormal right ventricle. Variable pulmonary outflow tract obstruction limits effective pulmonary blood flow. If adequate pulmonary blood flow requires continued ductal patency, the need for neonatal intervention is almost certain.

Diagnosis and Intervention

The more severe forms of Ebstein anomaly manifest with cyanosis in infancy. Critically ill neonates tend to have a severe form of the disease, with a grossly inefficient right ventricle compounded by the high pulmonary resistance of the neonate or by pulmonary valve atresia. The mortality rate in this group is high. Older patients present in heart failure and may have cyanosis. Supraventricular dysrhythmias and the pre-excitation syndrome (Wolff-Parkinson-White syndrome) are associated with Ebstein anomaly. Echocardiography is diagnostic. Critically ill neonates have poor survival rates, and surgery is indicated only after stabilization with PGE1 and controlled ventilation. In older patients, cyanosis and heart failure are indications to intervene, although earlier intervention in asymptomatic patients, before excessive right ventricular dilation, is being more actively pursued.

Surgery

In critically ill neonates, after stabilization, palliation with a systemic-to-pulmonary artery shunt may be required. The Starnes operation has allowed salvage in previously hopeless cases. This operation consists of patch closure of the tricuspid orifice, atrial septectomy, and a systemic-to-pulmonary artery shunt.[54] In patients with less severe forms of this disease, tricuspid valve repair or replacement is also an option. Surgical techniques for the treatment of Ebstein anomaly have been evolving, and outcomes are improving for this challenging group of patients (Fig. 58-49).[55]

Mitral Valve Anomalies

Most abnormalities of the mitral valve are associated with other complex lesions (e.g., Shone complex). More commonly, mitral disease in children is inflammatory in nature—that is, rheumatic disease or infective endocarditis. It may also be associated with collagen vascular disease and Marfan syndrome.

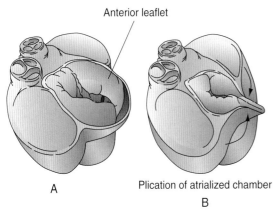

Anterior leaflet

A

Plication of atrialized chamber

B

FIGURE 58-49 Repair of Ebstein malformation using the Carpentier method. **A,** The anterior and posterior leaflets of the tricuspid valve are detached from the annulus. **B,** The atrium is plicated, reducing the annular diameter. The detached leaflets are reattached to the annulus. (From Castaneda AR, Jonas RA, Mayer JE, et al: Ebstein's anomaly. In *Cardiac surgery of the neonate and infant*, Philadelphia, 1994, Saunders.)

Mitral Stenosis

Mitral stenosis is caused by obstruction at a supravalvular, valvular, or subvalvular level, singly or in combination. Supravalvular stenosis is caused by a ring of fibrous tissue above the annulus of the mitral valve or attached to the proximal leaflets. Valvular stenosis involves the leaflets, with commissural fusion occurring with or without hypoplasia of the valve ring. Hypoplasia of the mitral valve is often associated with left ventricular hypoplasia. Frequently, the leaflets and subvalvular apparatus are also dysplastic. Fusion of the leaflets can lead to an accessory orifice and produce mitral stenosis at a purely valvular level (so-called double-orifice mitral valve). Three types of subvalvular stenosis have been recognized—parachute mitral valve, hammock valve, and absence of one or both papillary muscles. Mitral regurgitation is a result of secondary annular dilation, congenital isolated clefts of the valve, and prolapse of the leaflets from abnormal chordae or papillary muscle insertion.

Echocardiography is diagnostic. Intervention includes balloon valvuloplasty, particularly for selected forms of rheumatic mitral stenosis, and surgical intervention. Intervention is timed to avoid irreversible sequelae related to chronic volume overload or pulmonary hypertension. Surgical intervention is aimed at preserving the mitral valve, and valvuloplasty techniques have a valuable place in children. Prosthetic valves are the least desirable option. Bioprosthetic or tissue valves need to be avoided in children. Supra-annular placement of the prosthesis may be necessary. Repeat placement is ensured.

SUMMARY

This chapter provides a basic overview of the major congenital cardiac lesions and a framework for the diagnosis and treatment of these conditions. For most patients, the diagnosis of CHD, whether surgically treated or not, carries lifelong implications. For patients with CHD presenting for noncardiac surgery, a thorough understanding of the patient's unique anatomy and physiology is mandatory when planning a rational management strategy. The reader is directed to several excellent texts on CHD for a more thorough review of each of the lesions reviewed in this chapter.

SELECTED REFERENCES

Bailey LL, Nehlsen-Cannarella SL, Doroshow RW, et al: Cardiac allotransplantation in newborns as therapy for hypoplastic left heart syndrome. *N Engl J Med* 315:949–951, 1986.

This classic reference describes the first report of cardiac transplantation in newborns with hypoplastic left heart syndrome (HLHS). Although limited in its applicability because of limited donor organs, neonatal cardiac transplantation has provided children born with HLHS a new option for survival.

Blalock A, Taussig HB: The surgical treatment of malformations of the heart in which there is pulmonary stenosis or pulmonary atresia. *JAMA* 128:189–202, 1945.

This landmark article describes the surgical procedure that initiated the era of elective cardiac surgery. The study reported the initial experience with palliative surgical treatment of patients with pulmonary stenosis or pulmonary atresia using the Blalock-Taussig shunt.

Fontan F, Baudet E: Surgical repair of tricuspid atresia. *Thorax* 26:240–248, 1971.

This article represents a milestone in the evolution of surgical management of patients with single-ventricle physiology. It described the first corrective operation for patients with tricuspid atresia. Although previous palliative procedures, provided by various systemic-to-pulmonary artery shunts, improved the clinical condition of patients, systemic blood was still a mixture of oxygenated and deoxygenated blood. The Fontan operation redirected superior and inferior vena cava blood flow to the lungs so that only oxygenated blood returned to the heart and subsequently to the systemic circulation.

Kirklin JW, Dushane JW, Patrick RT, et al: Intracardiac surgery with the aid of a mechanical pump-oxygenator system (gibbon type): Report of eight cases. *Mayo Clin Proc* 30:201–206, 1955.

This landmark article demonstrated that open repairs of congenital cardiac defects using mechanical pump oxygenator systems could be performed with minimal risk to patients.

Mustard W: Successful two-stage correction of transposition of the great vessels. *Surgery* 55:469–472, 1964.

This classic reference describes one of the initial surgical approaches to the treatment of transposition of the great arteries (D-TGA). Although the arterial switch operation is now the surgical treatment of choice for D-TGA, there are many adult patients with congenital heart disease who have been palliated with the Mustard operation. Understanding the operation and resulting physiology is critical to general surgery management strategies for noncardiac operations.

Nichols DG, Ungerleider RM, Spevak PJ, et al, editors: *Critical heart disease in infants and children*, ed 2, Philadelphia, 2006, Mosby.

This text provides a comprehensive and current review of heart disease in infants and children. It contains numerous surgical drawings and diagnostic images to supplement the didactic material.

Norwood WI, Lang P, Casteneda AR, et al: Experience with operations for hypoplastic left heart syndrome. *J Thorac Cardiovasc Surg* 82:511–519, 1981.

In this landmark article, Norwood and colleagues reported the outcomes of what was then a new reconstructive surgical technique to palliate newborns with hypoplastic left heart syndrome (HLHS). Until the Norwood operation, the only option for survival of patients with HLHS was cardiac transplantation. At most centers today, the Norwood operation is the primary mode of therapy for most neonates with HLHS.

Sano S, Ishino K, Kawada M, et al: Right ventricle-pulmonary artery shunt in first-stage palliation of hypoplastic left heart syndrome. *J Thorac Cardiovasc Surg* 126:504–509, 2003.

This classic reference describes the right ventricle–to–pulmonary artery conduit used in the Norwood procedure. This novel procedure, named after the author, Sano, allowed for more hemodynamic stability postoperatively from the Norwood procedure and improved intrastage survival.

Senning A: Surgical correction of transposition of the great vessels. *Surgery* 45:966–980, 1959.

This classic reference describes the initial surgical approach to management of transposition of the great arteries (D-TGA). Although the arterial switch operation is currently the surgical treatment of choice for D-TGA, there are many adult patients with congenital heart disease in the community who have had the Senning operation. Understanding the operation and resulting physiology is critical to general surgery management strategies for noncardiac operations.

Starnes VA, Pitlick PT, Bernstein D, et al: Ebstein's anomaly appearing in the neonate. A new surgical approach. *J Thorac Cardiovasc Surg* 101:1082–1087, 1991.

This classic reference describes the first report of a new surgical approach to Ebstein anomaly in neonates. The procedure was named after the surgeon, Starnes. This approach has provided children born with severe Ebstein anomaly a new option for survival.

Warden HE, Cohen M, Read RC, et al: Controlled cross circulation for open intracardiac surgery: Physiologic studies and results of creation and closure of ventricular septal defects. *J Thorac Surg* 28:331–341, 1954.

This landmark article described the technique of cross-circulation to facilitate cardiopulmonary bypass and intracardiac repair of congenital heart lesions. Warden and colleagues documented the successful use of cross-circulation to correct defects such as ventricular septal defect.

Wilcox B, Cook A, Anderson R: *Surgical anatomy of the heart*, ed 3, Cambridge, England, 2004, Cambridge University Press.

This text provides an excellent reference manual for understanding the complex anatomy of the heart. It contains color photographs and diagrams and is an invaluable resource for any student of cardiac surgery.

REFERENCES

1. Blalock A, Taussig HB: The surgical treatment of malformations of the heart in which there is pulmonary stenosis or pulmonary atresia. *JAMA* 128:189–202, 1945.
2. Warden HE, Cohen M, Read RC, et al: Controlled cross circulation for open intracardiac surgery: Physiologic studies and results of creation and closure of ventricular septal defects. *J Thorac Surg* 28:331–341, discussion 341–343, 1954.
3. Kirklin JW, Dushane JW, Patrick RT, et al: Intracardiac surgery with the aid of a mechanical pump-oxygenator system (gibbon type): Report of eight cases. *Proc Staff Meet Mayo Clin* 30:201–206, 1955.
4. Marelli A, Gilboa S, Devine O, et al: Estimating the congenital heart disease population in the United States in 2010—what are the numbers? *J Am Coll Cardiol* 59:E787–E787, 2012.
5. Marelli AJ, Ionescu-Ittu R, Mackie AS, et al: Lifetime prevalence of congenital heart disease in the general population from 2000 to 2010. *Circulation* 130:749–756, 2014.
6. Levey A, Glickstein JS, Kleinman CS, et al: The impact of prenatal diagnosis of complex congenital heart disease on neonatal outcomes. *Pediatr Cardiol* 31:587–597, 2010.
7. Morris SA, Ethen MK, Penny DJ, et al: Prenatal diagnosis, birth location, surgical center, and neonatal mortality in infants with hypoplastic left heart syndrome. *Circulation* 129:285–292, 2014.
8. American Board of Thoracic Surgery. <https://www.abts.org/root/home.aspx>; (Accessed August 6, 2015).
9. Mullins CE: *Cardiac catheterization in congenital heart disease: Pediatric and adult*, Malden, MA, 2006, Blackwell Futura.
10. American Board of Internal Medicine. <www.abim.org>; (Accessed August 6, 2015).
11. Wilcox BR, Cook AC, Anderson RH: *Surgical anatomy of the heart*, ed 3, Cambridge, 2004, Cambridge University Press.
12. Morin RL, Gerber TC, McCollough CH: Radiation dose in computed tomography of the heart. *Circulation* 107:917–922, 2003.
13. Andropoulos DB, Stayer SA, Russell IA: *Anesthesia for congenital heart disease*, ed 2, Hoboken, NJ, 2010, Wiley-Blackwell.
14. Morales DL, Carberry KE, Heinle JS, et al: Extubation in the operating room after Fontan's procedure: Effect on practice and outcomes. *Ann Thorac Surg* 86:576–581, discussion 581–582, 2008.
15. Licht DJ, Shera DM, Clancy RR, et al: Brain maturation is delayed in infants with complex congenital heart defects.

J Thorac Cardiovasc Surg 137:529–536, discussion 536–527, 2009.

16. Hopkins RA, Bert AA, Buchholz B, et al: Surgical patch closure of atrial septal defects. *Ann Thorac Surg* 77:2144–2149, author reply 2149–2150, 2004.

17. Knepp MD, Rocchini AP, Lloyd TR, et al: Long-term follow up of secundum atrial septal defect closure with the Amplatzer septal occluder. *Congenit Heart Dis* 5:32–37, 2010.

18. Clark JB, Chowdhury D, Pauliks LB, et al: Resolution of heart block after surgical removal of an Amplatzer device. *Ann Thorac Surg* 89:1631–1633, 2010.

19. Piatkowski R, Kochanowski J, Scislo P, et al: Dislocation of Amplatzer septal occluder device after closure of secundum atrial septal defect. *J Am Soc Echocardiogr* 23:1007.e1–1007.e2, 2010.

20. Slesnick TC, Nugent AW, Fraser CD, Jr, et al: Images in cardiovascular medicine. Incomplete endothelialization and late development of acute bacterial endocarditis after implantation of an Amplatzer septal occluder device. *Circulation* 117:e326–e327, 2008.

21. Neill CA, Ferencz C, Sabiston DC, et al: The familial occurrence of hypoplastic right lung with systemic arterial supply and venous drainage "scimitar syndrome". *Bull Johns Hopkins Hosp* 107:1–21, 1960.

22. Balzer D: Current status of percutaneous closure of ventricular septal defects. *Pediatr Therapeut* 2:112–114, 2012.

23. Rastelli GC, Weidman WH, Kirklin JW: Surgical repair of the partial form of persistent common atrioventricular canal, with special reference to the problem of mitral valve incompetence. *Circulation* 31(Suppl 1):31–35, 1965.

24. Bakhtiary F, Takacs J, Cho MY, et al: Long-term results after repair of complete atrioventricular septal defect with two-patch technique. *Ann Thorac Surg* 89:1239–1243, 2010.

25. Morales DL, Braud BE, Gunter KS, et al: Encouraging results for the Contegra conduit in the problematic right ventricle-to-pulmonary artery connection. *J Thorac Cardiovasc Surg* 132:665–671, 2006.

26. Chen JM, Glickstein JS, Davies RR, et al: The effect of repair technique on postoperative right-sided obstruction in patients with truncus arteriosus. *J Thorac Cardiovasc Surg* 129:559–568, 2005.

27. Vezmar M, Chaturvedi R, Lee KJ, et al: Percutaneous pulmonary valve implantation in the young 2-year follow-up. *JACC Cardiovasc Interv* 3:439–448, 2010.

28. Balasubramanian S, Marshall AC, Gauvreau K, et al: Outcomes after stent implantation for the treatment of congenital and postoperative pulmonary vein stenosis in children. *Circ Cardiovasc Interv* 5:109–117, 2012.

29. Morales DL, Zafar F, Heinle JS, et al: Right ventricular infundibulum sparing (RVIS) tetralogy of Fallot repair: A review of over 300 patients. *Ann Surg* 250:611–617, 2009.

30. Mustard WT: Successful two-stage correction of transposition of the great vessels. *Surgery* 55:469–472, 1964.

31. Senning A: Surgical correction of transposition of the great vessels. *Surgery* 45:966–980, 1959.

32. Dibardino DJ, Allison AE, Vaughn WK, et al: Current expectations for newborns undergoing the arterial switch operation. *Ann Surg* 239:588–596, discussion 596–598, 2004.

33. Angeli E, Formigari R, Pace Napoleone C, et al: Long-term coronary artery outcome after arterial switch operation for transposition of the great arteries. *Eur J Cardiothorac Surg* 38:714–720, 2010.

34. Yacoub MH, Radley-Smith R: Anatomy of the coronary arteries in transposition of the great arteries and methods for their transfer in anatomical correction. *Thorax* 33:418–424, 1978.

35. Ly M, Belli E, Leobon B, et al: Results of the double switch operation for congenitally corrected transposition of the great arteries. *Eur J Cardiothorac Surg* 35:879–883, discussion 883–884, 2009.

36. Bacha EA, McElhinney DB, Guleserian KJ, et al: Surgical aortic valvuloplasty in children and adolescents with aortic regurgitation: Acute and intermediate effects on aortic valve function and left ventricular dimensions. *J Thorac Cardiovasc Surg* 135:552–559, 559.e551–553, 2008.

37. d'Udekem Y: Aortic valve repair in children. *Ann Cardiothorac Surg* 2:100–104, 2013.

38. Brown JW, Rodefeld MD, Ruzmetov M, et al: Surgical valvuloplasty versus balloon aortic dilation for congenital aortic stenosis: Are evidence-based outcomes relevant? *Ann Thorac Surg* 94:146–153, discussion 153–155, 2012.

39. Shinkawa T, Bove EL, Hirsch JC, et al: Intermediate-term results of the Ross procedure in neonates and infants. *Ann Thorac Surg* 89:1827–1832, discussion 1832, 2010.

40. Booth JH, Bryant R, Powers SC, et al: Transthoracic echocardiography does not reliably predict involvement of the aortic valve in patients with a discrete subaortic shelf. *Cardiol Young* 20:284–289, 2010.

41. Shone JD, Sellers RD, Anderson RC, et al: The developmental complex of "parachute mitral valve," supravalvular ring of left atrium, subaortic stenosis, and coarctation of aorta. *Am J Cardiol* 11:714–725, 1963.

42. Cowley CG, Orsmond GS, Feola P, et al: Long-term, randomized comparison of balloon angioplasty and surgery for native coarctation of the aorta in childhood. *Circulation* 111:3453–3456, 2005.

43. Mery CM, Guzman-Pruneda FA, Carberry KE, et al: Aortic arch advancement for aortic coarctation and hypoplastic aortic arch in neonates and infants. *Ann Thorac Surg* 98:625–633, discussion 633, 2014.

44. Morales DL, Scully PT, Braud BE, et al: Interrupted aortic arch repair: Aortic arch advancement without a patch minimizes arch reinterventions. *Ann Thorac Surg* 82:1577–1583, discussion 1583–1584, 2006.

45. Bailey LL, Nehlsen-Cannarella SL, Doroshow RW, et al: Cardiac allotransplantation in newborns as therapy for hypoplastic left heart syndrome. *N Engl J Med* 315:949–951, 1986.

46. Norwood WI, Lang P, Casteneda AR, et al: Experience with operations for hypoplastic left heart syndrome. *J Thorac Cardiovasc Surg* 82:511–519, 1981.

47. Sano S, Ishino K, Kado H, et al: Outcome of right ventricle-to-pulmonary artery shunt in first-stage palliation of hypoplastic left heart syndrome: A multi-institutional study. *Ann Thorac Surg* 78:1951–1957, discussion 1957–1958, 2004.

48. Ohye RG, Sleeper LA, Mahony L, et al: Comparison of shunt types in the Norwood procedure for single-ventricle lesions. *N Engl J Med* 362:1980–1992, 2010.

49. Luce WA, Schwartz RM, Beauseau W, et al: Necrotizing enterocolitis in neonates undergoing the hybrid approach to complex congenital heart disease. *Pediatr Crit Care Med* 12:46–51, 2011.

50. Fontan F, Baudet E: Surgical repair of tricuspid atresia. *Thorax* 26:240–248, 1971.

51. Salazar JD, Zafar F, Siddiqui K, et al: Fenestration during Fontan palliation: Now the exception instead of the rule. *J Thorac Cardiovasc Surg* 140:129–136, 2010.

52. Alsoufi B, Sallehuddin A, Bulbul Z, et al: Surgical strategy to establish a dual-coronary system for the management of anomalous left coronary artery origin from the pulmonary artery. *Ann Thorac Surg* 86:170–176, 2008.

53. Valente AM, Lock JE, Gauvreau K, et al: Predictors of long-term adverse outcomes in patients with congenital coronary artery fistulae. *Circ Cardiovasc Interv* 3:134–139, 2010.

54. Starnes VA, Pitlick PT, Bernstein D, et al: Ebstein's anomaly appearing in the neonate. A new surgical approach. *J Thorac Cardiovasc Surg* 101:1082–1087, 1991.

55. Brown ML, Dearani JA, Danielson GK, et al: The outcomes of operations for 539 patients with Ebstein anomaly. *J Thorac Cardiovasc Surg* 135:1120–1136, 1136.e1121–1127, 2008.

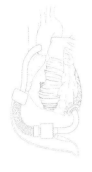

CHAPTER 59

Acquired Heart Disease: Coronary Insufficiency

Shuab Omer, Lorraine D. Cornwell, Faisal G. Bakaeen

第五十九章　后天性心脏病：冠状动脉供血不足

中文导读

　　本章共分9节：①冠状动脉解剖学和生理学；②冠状动脉搭桥手术史；③冠状动脉粥样硬化病的临床表现及诊断；④冠状动脉血管重建术的适应证；⑤冠状动脉旁路移植术的辅助治疗；⑥术后护理；⑦可供选择的心肌血运重建方法；⑧冠状动脉搭桥术的机械并发症；⑨特殊人群病人的冠状动脉搭桥术。

　　第一节主要介绍了冠状动脉的基本解剖以及其生理过程，冠状动脉是供给心脏血液的主要动脉，主要分为左前降支、回旋支、右冠状动脉。了解冠状动脉的基本解剖以及生理过程为冠心病的诊断及治疗提供了很好的理论基础。

　　第二节主要介绍了心脏冠状动脉搭桥术的手术发展史以及冠心病的高危因素，并详细介绍了冠心病主要发病机制和发展过程。

　　第三节介绍了冠心病的临床表现及诊断方法。冠

脉造影除了可以决定是否进行手术或经皮冠状动脉介入治疗（percutaneous coronary intervention, PCI）外，还可以准确看到冠状动脉病变的特征，为后续可能的冠状动脉搭桥术提供依据。同时也有一些血管内超声、混合成像等新技术，各有利弊，需要权衡选择。

　　第四节主要介绍了冠状动脉血管重建术的适应证，利用循证医学证据，综合性分析了药物治疗、PCI、冠状动脉搭桥术3种冠心病治疗方案，分析了不同的治疗方案在不同类型的冠心病病人中的具

体区别及应用。同时介绍了体外循环、胸骨正中切开术、移植血管的选择问题以及冠状动脉搭桥手术当中需要注意的一系列问题。

第五节主要介绍了经食管超声心动图在冠状动脉搭桥中的具体应用以及正性肌力药物、主动脉内球囊反搏（intra-aortic ballon pump, IABP）在冠心病中的应用。需要注意上述药物或器械的适应证和禁忌证。

第六节主要描述了冠状动脉搭桥术后护理的重要性以及术后护理需要注意的细节。详细介绍了这些并发症的高危因素以及出现后的处理办法，同时强调了药物治疗在冠状动脉搭桥术后管理的重要性以及药物

的使用方法。

第七节主要介绍了冠心病治疗的新方法，如体外循环下心肌纤维阻滞、体外循环不停跳搭桥、非体外循环冠状动脉搭桥术、微创动脉搭桥、完全内镜冠状动脉搭桥术、经心肌激光血运重建等。同时介绍了冠状动脉搭桥术再次手术的技术问题。

第八节主要介绍冠心病的机械并发症：室壁瘤、室间隔缺损、二尖瓣反流的发病率、诊断以及治疗方法。

第九节主要介绍了特殊人群的冠状动脉搭桥术。

〔王海灏〕

Ischemic heart disease (IHD) is the predominant public health problem worldwide. In the United States, 1 in 3 adults (about 83.6 million) has cardiovascular disease; 15.4 million of these persons have coronary artery disease (CAD).[1] Despite improved survival among CAD patients,[2] CAD is responsible for approximately 380,000 deaths in the United States every year, with an age-adjusted mortality rate of 113 per 100,000 population.[3] CAD is the leading cause of death in both men and women, and IHD accounts for most of the mortality and morbidity associated with CAD.[1] The costs of caring for patients with IHD are enormous, with hundreds of billions of dollars spent every year in the United States in taking care of these patients. Although recent advances in percutaneous intervention have reduced the number of referrals for surgical intervention, coronary artery bypass grafting (CABG) still remains the most effective treatment for CAD and is the most commonly performed open cardiac procedure in the United States.

CORONARY ARTERY ANATOMY AND PHYSIOLOGY

Anatomic Considerations

The coronary arteries, the predominant blood supply to the heart, arise from the sinuses of Valsalva. They are the first arterial branches of the aorta, and two are usually present. The coronary arteries are designated right and left according to the embryologic chamber that they predominantly supply. The left coronary artery (LCA) arises from the left coronary sinus, which is located posteromedially; the right coronary artery (RCA) arises from the right coronary sinus, which is located anteromedially. The LCA, also called the left main coronary artery, averages approximately 2 to 3 cm in length and courses in a left posterolateral direction, winding behind the main pulmonary artery trunk and then splitting into the left anterior descending (LAD) and left circumflex arteries. The LAD courses in an anterolateral direction to the left of the pulmonary trunk and runs anteriorly over the interventricular septum. The diagonal branches of the LAD supply the anterolateral wall of the left ventricle (LV). The LAD is considered the most important surgical vessel because it supplies more than

50% of the LV mass and most of the interventricular septum. The LAD has several septal perforating branches that supply the interventricular septum from its anterior aspect. The LAD extends over the interventricular septum up to the apex of the heart, where it may form an anastomosis with the posterior descending artery (PDA), which is typically a branch of the right coronary system (Fig. 59-1).

The circumflex artery passes through the atrioventricular (AV) groove and follows a clockwise course. Where the circumflex artery courses through the AV groove, it gives off branches that extend toward but do not quite reach the apex of the heart. These branches, the obtuse marginal branches, are designated numerically from proximal to distal. The circumflex coronary artery usually terminates as the left posterolateral branch after taking a perpendicular turn toward the apex.

The term *ramus intermedius* is used to designate a dominant coronary vessel that arises from the occasional trifurcation of the LCA. This branch can be intramyocardial and difficult to locate at times.

The RCA supplies most of the right ventricle as well as the posterior part of the LV. The RCA emerges from its ostium in the right coronary sinus and passes deep in the right AV groove. At the superior end of the acute margin of the heart, the RCA turns posteriorly toward the crux and usually bifurcates into the PDA over the posterior interventricular sulcus and right posterolateral artery. The RCA also supplies multiple right ventricular branches (i.e., the acute marginal branches). On occasion, the PDA arises from both the RCA and LCA, and the circulation is considered to be codominant. The AV node artery arises from the RCA in approximately 90% of patients. The sinoatrial node artery arises from the proximal RCA in 50% of patients. Although the source of the PDA is often used clinically to define dominance of circulation in the heart, anatomists define it according to where the sinoatrial node artery arises. Table 59-1 summarizes the hierarchy of the coronary artery anatomy.

All the epicardial conductance vessels and septal perforators from the LAD give rise to a multitude of branches, termed

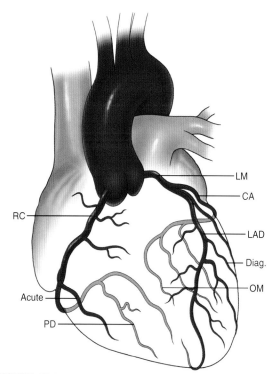

FIGURE 59-1 Anatomy of normal coronary artery vasculature. *CA,* circumflex artery; *LAD,* left anterior descending; *LM,* left main; *OM,* obtuse marginal; *PD,* posterior descending; *RC,* right coronary.

Labels on figure: LM, CA, RC, LAD, Diag., OM, Acute, PD

TABLE 59-1   Anatomic Architecture of Coronary Arteries

NAMED VESSELS	BRANCHES
Left main coronary artery	Left anterior descending
	Circumflex coronary
	Ramus intermedius
Left anterior descending	Diagonal arteries
	Septal perforators
Circumflex coronary artery	Obtuse marginal branches
	Left posterolateral artery
Right coronary artery	Acute marginal artery
	Posterior descending artery
	Right posterolateral artery

resistance vessels, that penetrate into the ventricular wall. These vessels play a crucial role in oxygen and nutrient exchange with the myocardium by forming a rich capillary plexus. This plexus offers a low-resistance sink that allows arterial blood flow to increase unimpeded when oxygen demand rises. This is important because the myocardial vascular bed extracts oxygen at its full capacity, even in low-demand circumstances, thereby allowing no margin for further oxygen extraction when demand is high.

An intricate network of veins drains the coronary circulation, and the venous circulation can be divided into three systems: the coronary sinus and its tributaries, the anterior right ventricular veins, and the thebesian veins. The coronary sinus predominantly drains the LV and receives 85% of coronary venous blood. It lies within the posterior AV groove and empties into the right atrium.

> **BOX 59-1   Unique Features of Coronary Blood Flow**
>
> - Autoregulated over wide pressure ranges
> - Blood flow: 0.7-0.9 mL per gram of myocardium per minute
> - 75% oxygen extraction
> - Coronary sinus blood is the most deoxygenated blood in the body
> - 4- to 7-fold increase in flow with increased demand
> - 60% blood flow occurs during diastole
> - Flow-limited oxygen supply

The anterior right ventricular veins travel across the right ventricular surface to the right AV groove, where they enter directly into the right atrium or form the small cardiac vein, which enters into the right atrium directly or joins the coronary sinus just proximal to its orifice. The thebesian veins are small venous tributaries that drain directly into the cardiac chambers and exit primarily into the right atrium and right ventricle. Understanding of the anatomy of the coronary sinus is essential for placement of the retrograde cardioplegia cannula during cardiopulmonary bypass (CPB).

Physiology and Regulation of Coronary Blood Flow

Aortic pressure is a driving force in the maintenance of myocardial perfusion. During resting conditions, coronary blood flow is maintained at a fairly constant level over a wide range of aortic perfusion pressures (70 to 180 mm Hg) through the process of autoregulation.

Because the myocardium has a high rate of energy use, normal coronary blood flow averages 225 mL/min (0.7 to 0.9 mL per gram of myocardium per minute) and delivers 0.1 mL/g/min of oxygen to the myocardium. Under normal conditions, more than 75% of the delivered oxygen is extracted in the coronary capillary bed, so any additional oxygen demand can be met only by increasing the flow rate. This highlights the importance of unobstructed coronary blood flow for proper myocardial function. Box 59-1 summarizes the unique features of coronary blood flow.

In response to increased load, such as that caused by strenuous exercise, the healthy heart can increase myocardial blood flow fourfold to sevenfold. Blood flow is increased through several mechanisms. Local metabolic neurohumoral factors cause coronary vasodilation when stress and metabolic demand increase, thereby lowering the coronary vascular resistance. This results in increased delivery of oxygen-rich blood, mimicking the phenomenon of reactive hyperemia. When a transient occlusion to the coronary artery is released (e.g., during the performance of a beating-heart operation), blood flow immediately rises to exceed the normal baseline flow and then gradually returns to its baseline level. The autoregulatory mechanism responsible is guided by several metabolic factors, including carbon dioxide, oxygen tension, hydrogen ions, lactate, potassium ions, and adenosine. Adenosine, a potent vasodilator and a degradation product of adenosine triphosphate, accumulates in the interstitial space and relaxes vascular smooth muscle. This results in vasomotor relaxation, coronary vasodilation, and increased blood flow. Another substance that plays an important role is nitric oxide, which is produced by the endothelium. Without the endothelium, coronary arteries do not autoregulate, suggesting that the mechanism for vasodilation and reactive hyperemia is endothelium dependent.

Extravascular compression of the coronaries during systole also plays an important role in the regulation of blood flow. During systole, the intracavitary pressures generated in the LV wall exceed intracoronary pressure, and blood flow is impeded. Hence, approximately 60% of coronary blood flow occurs during diastole. During exercise, increased heart rate and reduced diastolic time can compromise flow time, but this can be offset by vasodilatory mechanisms of the coronary vessels. Buildup of atherosclerotic plaques and fixed coronary occlusion significantly impair coronary arterial compensatory mechanisms while heart rate is elevated. This forms the basis for exercise-induced stress tests, in which abnormal physiologic responses to increased physical activity unmask underlying CAD.

HISTORY OF CORONARY ARTERY BYPASS SURGERY

One of the first attempts at myocardial revascularization was made by Arthur Vineberg from Canada. He operated on a series of patients who presented with symptoms of myocardial ischemia and implanted the left internal mammary artery (LIMA) into the myocardium by creating a pocket. The operation did not entail a direct anastomosis to any coronary vessel and was performed on a beating heart through a left anterolateral thoracotomy. Michael DeBakey performed a successful aortocoronary saphenous vein graft in 1964. Mason Sones, who is credited with inventing cardiac catheterization, helped establish CABG surgery as a planned and consistent therapy in patients with angiographically documented CAD.

The development of the heart-lung machine and its successful clinical use by John Heysham Gibbon in the 1950s, along with the advancement of cardioplegia techniques in later years by Gerald Buckberg, allowed surgeons to perform coronary anastomosis on an arrested (nonbeating) heart with a relatively bloodless field, thus increasing the safety and accuracy of the coronary bypass. In the 1990s, the advent of devices that could atraumatically stabilize the heart provided another pathway for the development of off-pump techniques of myocardial revascularization. Today, an armamentarium of techniques ranging from conventional on-pump CABG to minimally invasive robotic and percutaneous approaches is available to manage CAD. Table 59-2 summarizes the timeline of major historical events in the development of surgery for myocardial revascularization.

TABLE 59-2 Evolution of Surgical Coronary Artery Interventions: Timeline

1950	A. Vineberg	Direct implantation of mammary artery into myocardium
1953	J. H. Gibbon	First successful use of cardiopulmonary bypass machine
1962	F. M. Sones	Successful cineangiography
1964	M. E. DeBakey	First successful coronary artery bypass grafting
1964	T. Sondergaard	Introduced routine use of cardioplegia for myocardial protection
1964	D. A. Cooley	Routine use of normothermic arrest for all cardiac cases
1968	R. Favoloro	First large series showing success of coronary artery bypass grafting
1973	V. Subramanian	Beating-heart coronary artery bypass grafting
1979	G. Buckberg	First use of blood cardioplegia as preferred method for arrested myocardial protection

ATHEROSCLEROTIC CORONARY ARTERY DISEASE

Coronary atherosclerosis is a process that begins early in the patient's life. Epicardial conductance vessels are the most susceptible and intramyocardial arteries, the least. Risk factors for atherosclerosis include elevated plasma levels of total cholesterol and low-density lipoprotein cholesterol, cigarette smoking, hypertension, diabetes mellitus, advanced age, low plasma levels of high-density lipoprotein cholesterol, and family history of premature CAD.

Epidemiologic evidence suggests that coronary artery atherosclerosis is closely linked to the metabolism of lipids, specifically low-density lipoprotein cholesterol. The development of lipid-lowering drugs has resulted in a significant reduction in mortality. In one observational study of patients who received statin therapy and were known to have CAD, statin treatment was associated with improved survival in all age groups.[4] The greatest survival benefit was found in those patients in the highest quartile of plasma levels of high-sensitivity C-reactive protein, a biomarker of inflammation and CAD.[5] Animal and human studies have demonstrated that statin therapy also modifies the lipid composition within plaques by lowering the amount of low-density lipoprotein cholesterol and stabilizing the plaque through various mechanisms, including reduced macrophage accumulation, collagen degradation, reduced smooth muscle cell protease expression, and decreased tissue factor expression.

Pathogenesis

The primary cause of CAD is endothelial injury induced by an inflammatory wall response and lipid deposition. There is evidence that an inflammatory response is involved in all stages of the disease, from early lipid deposition to plaque formation, plaque rupture, and coronary artery thrombosis. Vulnerable or high-risk plaques that are prone to rupture have the following characteristics: a large, eccentric, soft lipid core; a thin fibrous cap; inflammation within the cap and adventitia; increased plaque neovascularity; and evidence of outward or positive vessel remodeling.

Thinner fibrous caps are at a higher risk for rupture, probably because of an imbalance between the synthesis and the degradation of the extracellular matrix in the fibrous cap that results in an overall decrease in the collagen and matrix components (Fig. 59-2). Increased matrix breakdown caused by matrix degradation by an inflammatory cell-mediated metalloproteinase or reduced production of extracellular matrix results in thinner fibrous caps. Not all plaque ruptures are symptomatic; whether they are depends on the thrombogenicity of the plaque's components. Tissue factor within the lipid core of the plaque, secreted by activated macrophages, is one of the most potent thrombogenic stimuli. Rupture of a vulnerable plaque may be spontaneous or caused by extreme physical activity, severe emotional distress, exposure to drugs, cold exposure, or acute infection.

Fixed Coronary Obstructions

More than 90% of patients with stable IHD (SIHD) have advanced coronary atherosclerosis caused by a fixed obstruction. Atherosclerotic plaques of the coronary arteries are concentric (25%) or eccentric (75%). Eccentric lesions compromise only a portion of the lumen; through vascular remodeling, the arterial lumen may remain patent until late in the disease process. The impact of an arterial stenosis on coronary blood flow can be appreciated in the context of Poiseuille's law. Reductions in

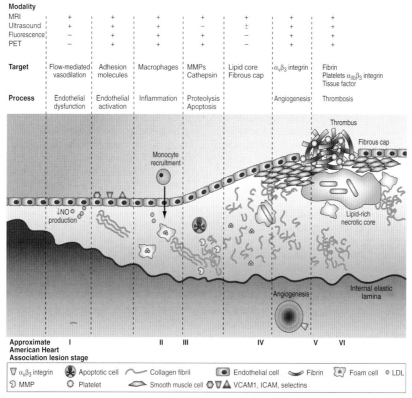

Modality							
MRI	+	+	+	+	+	+	+
Ultrasound	+	+	+	–	±	+	+
Fluorescence	–	+	+	+	–	+	+
PET	–	+	+	+	–	+	+
Target	Flow-mediated vasodilation	Adhesion molecules	Macrophages	MMPs Cathepsin	Lipid core Fibrous cap	$\alpha_v\beta_3$ integrin	Fibrin Platelets $\alpha_{IIb}\beta_3$ integrin Tissue factor
Process	Endothelial dysfunction	Endothelial activation	Inflammation	Proteolysis Apoptosis		Angiogenesis	Thrombosis

Thrombus
Fibrous cap
Monocyte recruitment
↓NO production
Lipid-rich necrotic core
Angiogenesis
Internal elastic lamina

Approximate American Heart Association lesion stage   I   II   III   IV   V   VI

▽ $\alpha_v\beta_3$ integrin   Apoptotic cell   Collagen fibril   Endothelial cell   Fibrin   Foam cell   ○ LDL
MMP   Platelet   Smooth muscle cell   ○▽▲ VCAM1, ICAM, selectins

FIGURE 59-2 Components of Atherosclerotic Plaque. Thinning of the fibrous cap eventually results in plaque rupture and extrusion of highly thrombogenic lipid-laden material into the coronary artery. This causes an acute occlusion of the coronary artery, resulting in myocardial infarction. (Adapted from Choudhury RP, Fuster V, Fayad ZA: Molecular, cellular and functional imaging of atherothrombosis. *Nat Rev Drug Discov* 3:913–925, 2004.)

luminal diameter up to 60% have minimal impact on flow, but when the cross-sectional area of the vessel has decreased by 75% or more, coronary blood flow is significantly compromised. Clinically, this loss of flow often coincides with the onset of exertional angina. A 90% reduction in luminal diameter results in resting angina.

CLINICAL MANIFESTATIONS AND DIAGNOSIS OF CORONARY ARTERY DISEASE

Clinical Presentation

Clinically, IHD has two predominant modes of presentation:
• Stable angina
• Acute coronary syndrome: ST-segment elevation myocardial infarction (STEMI) and its complications, non–ST-segment myocardial infarction (NSTEMI), and unstable angina (UA)

Anginal pain is the main presenting symptom of IHD. It typically lasts minutes. The location is usually substernal, and pain can radiate to the neck, jaw, epigastrium, or arms. Anginal pain is precipitated by exertion or emotional stress and relieved by rest. Sublingual nitroglycerin also usually relieves angina within 30 seconds to several minutes.

On presentation, angina must be classified as stable or unstable.[6] Patients are said to be having UA if the pain is increasing (in frequency, intensity, or duration) or occurring at rest. Such patients should be transferred promptly to an emergency department.

Patients, especially female and elderly patients, sometimes present with atypical symptoms, such as nausea, vomiting, midepigastric discomfort, or sharp (atypical) chest pain. In the WISE (Women's Ischemic Syndrome Evaluation) study, 65% of women with ischemia presented with atypical symptoms.[7]

The term *acute coronary syndrome* has evolved to refer to a constellation of clinical symptoms that represent myocardial ischemia. It encompasses both STEMI and NSTEMI. Myocardial infarction (MI) often is manifested as crushing chest pain that may be associated with nausea, diaphoresis, anxiety, and dyspnea. Symptoms of the hypoperfusion that follows MI may include dizziness, fatigue, and vomiting. Heart rate and blood pressure may be initially normal, but both increase in response to the duration and severity of pain. Loss of blood pressure is indicative of cardiogenic shock and indicates a poorer prognosis. At least 40% of the ventricular mass must be involved for cardiogenic shock to occur.

Mechanical complications of MI include acute ventricular septal defect (VSD), papillary muscle rupture, and free ventricular rupture. They usually occur approximately 7 to 10 days after the initial MI.

Physical Examination

Some clinical findings are generic and are related to the systemic manifestations of atherosclerosis. Eye examination may reveal a copper wire sign, retinal hematoma or thrombosis secondary to vascular occlusive disease, and hypertension. Corneal arcus and

BOX 59-2 Sequelae of Coronary Artery Disease: Clinical Manifestations

- Abnormal neck vein pulsations, which may be seen in patients with second- or third-degree heart block or CHF
- Bradycardia—a subtle presentation of ischemia involving the right coronary territories and a possible sign of heart block
- Weak or thready pulse suggestive of ectopic or premature ventricular beats
- Third heart sound that is noted with elevated left ventricular filling pressures/CHF
- Fourth heart sound, which is commonly heard in patients with acute and chronic CAD
- Mitral regurgitant heart murmurs caused by ischemic papillary muscles
- Ejection systolic murmur indicative of aortic stenosis, which can contribute to coronary ischemia
- Holosystolic murmurs caused by ventricular septal rupture
- Manifestations of CHF, such as rales, hepatomegaly, right upper abdominal quadrant tenderness, ascites, and marked peripheral and presacral edema

BOX 59-3 Stress Tests to Identify Coronary Artery Disease

Exercise Stress ECG
- Bruce protocol
- Five 3-minute bouts of treadmill exercise
- Determines the ischemia threshold
- 12 metabolic equivalents of energy expenditure needed for complete test
- Low cost and short duration
- Highly sensitive in multivessel disease

Limitations
- Suboptimal sensitivity
- Low detection rate of one-vessel disease
- Nondiagnostic with abnormal baseline ECG
- Poor specificity in premenopausal women
- Many cannot accomplish the 12 metabolic equivalents for a complete test or an appropriate heart rate response

Exercise and Pharmacologic Stress SPECT Perfusion Imaging
- Simultaneous evaluation of perfusion and function
- Higher sensitivity and specificity than exercise ECG
- Quantitative image analysis

Limitations
- Long procedure time with ^{99m}Tc
- Higher cost
- Radiation exposure
- Poor-quality images in obese patients

Exercise and Pharmacologic Stress Echocardiography
- Higher sensitivity and specificity than exercise ECG
- Comparable value with dobutamine stress
- Short examination time
- Identification of structural cardiac abnormalities
- Simultaneous evaluation of perfusion with contrast agents
- No radiation

Limitations
- Decreased sensitivity for detection of one-vessel disease or mild stenosis
- Highly operator dependent
- No quantitative image analysis
- Poor imaging in some patients
- Infarct zone poorly defined

xanthelasma are features noticed in cases of hypercholesterolemia. Other clinical manifestations are caused by sequelae of CAD (Box 59-2).

A thorough vascular evaluation is essential for any patient who presents with CAD because atherosclerosis is a systemic process. In addition, if surgery is being planned, the extremities should be evaluated for any previous surgical scars or fractures that could potentially preclude conduit harvest.

Diagnostic Testing
Biochemical Studies
Patients suspected of having an acute coronary syndrome should undergo appropriate blood testing. Levels of creatine kinase muscle and brain subunits (CK-MB) and troponin T or I should be assessed at least 6 to 12 hours apart. Additional laboratory tests include a complete blood count, comprehensive metabolic panel, and lipid profile (total cholesterol, triglycerides, low-density lipoprotein cholesterol, high-density lipoprotein cholesterol). Elevated brain natriuretic peptide and C-reactive protein levels suggest a worse outcome.

Chest Radiography
The chest radiograph is helpful in identifying causes of chest discomfort or pain other than CAD. Chest radiography does not detect CAD directly; it only identifies sequelae, such as cardiomegaly, pulmonary edema, and pleural effusions, that are indicative of heart failure. From a surgical standpoint, preoperative chest radiography is important because it can identify obvious abnormalities, such as porcelain aorta, lung masses, effusion, and pneumonias, that may affect further workup or prompt a change in operative strategy.

Resting Electrocardiography
A 12-lead resting electrocardiogram (ECG) should be obtained in all patients with suspected IHD or sequelae thereof. The ECG is evaluated for evidence of LV hypertrophy, ST-segment depression or elevation, ectopic beats, or Q waves. In addition, arrhythmias (atrial fibrillation or ventricular tachycardia) and conduction defects (left anterior fascicular block, right bundle branch block, left bundle branch block) are suggestive of CAD and MI. Persistent ST-segment elevation or an evolving Q wave is consistent with myocardial injury and ongoing ischemia. Fifty percent of

patients with significant CAD nonetheless have normal electrocardiographic results, and 50% of ECG recordings obtained during chest pain at rest will be normal, indicating the inaccuracy of the test. Patients with SIHD tend to have a worse prognosis if they have the following abnormalities on a resting ECG: evidence of prior MI, especially Q waves in multiple leads or an R wave in V_1 indicating a posterior infarction; persistent ST-T wave inversions, particularly in leads V_1 to V_3; left bundle branch block, bifascicular block, second- or third-degree AV block, or ventricular tachyarrhythmia; or LV hypertrophy.[8-10]

Functional (Stress) Tests
In patients with suspected stable ischemic CAD, functional or stress testing is used to detect inducible ischemia. These are the most common noninvasive tests used to diagnose SIHD (Box 59-3). All functional tests rely on the principle of inducing cardiac

ischemia by using exercise or pharmacologic stress agents, which increase myocardial work and oxygen demand, or by causing vasodilation-elicited heterogeneity in induced coronary flow. Whether ischemia is induced, however, depends on the severity of both the stress imposed (e.g., submaximal exercise can fail to produce ischemia) and the flow disturbance. Approximately 70% of coronary stenoses are not detected by functional testing. Because abnormalities of regional or global ventricular function occur later in the ischemic cascade, they are more likely to indicate severe stenosis; thus, such abnormalities have a higher diagnostic specificity for SIHD than do perfusion defects, such as those seen on nuclear myocardial perfusion imaging (MPI).

Exercise versus pharmacologic testing. In patients capable of performing routine activities of daily living without difficulty, exercise testing is preferred to pharmacologic testing because it induces greater physiologic stress than drugs can. This may make exercise testing the better means of detecting ischemia as well as providing a correlation to a patient's daily symptom burden and physical work capacity not offered by pharmacologic stress testing.

The treadmill protocols initiate exercise at 3.2 to 4.7 metabolic equivalents (METs) of work and increase by several METs every 2 to 3 minutes of exercise (e.g., modified or standard Bruce protocol). Performance of most activities of daily living requires approximately 4 to 5 METs of physical work. Patients unable to perform moderate physical activity and those with disabling comorbidities should undergo pharmacologic stress imaging instead.

Diagnostic accuracy of stress testing for SIHD

Exercise electrocardiography (Bruce protocol). The criterion for diagnosis of ischemia is an ECG showing 1-mm horizontal or downsloping (at 80 ms after the J point) ST-segment depression at peak exercise. The diagnostic sensitivity and specificity of this sign is 61% (range, 70% to 77%). It is lower in women than in men[11,12] and lower than that of stress imaging modalities.

Exercise and pharmacologic stress echocardiography. These tests rely on detecting new or worsening wall motion abnormalities and changes in global LV function during or immediately after stress. In addition to the detection of inducible wall motion abnormalities, most stress echocardiography includes screening images to evaluate resting ventricular function and valvular abnormalities.

Pharmacologic stress echocardiography is usually performed using dobutamine with an end point of producing wall motion abnormalities. Vasodilator agents such as adenosine can be used to the same effect.

The diagnostic sensitivity is 70% to 85% for exercise and 85% to 90% for pharmacologic stress echocardiography.[13,14] The use of intravenous ultrasound contrast agents, by improving endocardial border delineation, can result in improved diagnostic accuracy.

Exercise and pharmacologic stress nuclear myocardial perfusion imaging. Myocardial perfusion single-photon emission computed tomography (SPECT) generally is performed with rest and with stress. Technetium Tc 99m agents are generally used; one of these, thallium Tl 201, has limited applications (e.g., viability) because of its higher radiation exposure. Pharmacologic stress is generally induced with vasodilator agents administered by continuous infusion (adenosine, dipyridamole) or bolus injection (regadenoson).

The diagnostic end point of nuclear MPI is a reduction in myocardial perfusion after stress. The diagnostic accuracy for detection of obstructive CAD of exercise and pharmacologic stress

nuclear MPI has been studied in detail.[15-17] Studies suggest that nuclear MPI's sensitivity ranges from 82% to 88% for exercise and 88% to 91% for pharmacologic stress, and its diagnostic specificity ranges from 70% to 88% and 75% to 90% for exercise and pharmacologic stress nuclear MPI, respectively.

For myocardial perfusion SPECT, global reductions in myocardial perfusion, such as in the patients with left main or three-vessel CAD, can result in balanced reduction and an underestimation of ischemic burden.

Echocardiography

From a surgical standpoint, most patients with SIHD should undergo preoperative echocardiography. Echocardiography provides information not only for surgical planning but also regarding prognosis. A resting LV ejection fraction (LVEF) of 35% is associated with an annual mortality rate of 3% per year. Resting two-dimensional Doppler echocardiography provides information on cardiac structure and function, including identifying the mechanism of heart failure and differentiating systolic from diastolic LV dysfunction. Echocardiography can identify LV or left atrial dilation, identify aortic stenosis (a potential non-CAD cause of angina-like chest pain), measure pulmonary artery pressure, quantify mitral regurgitation, identify LV aneurysm, identify LV thrombus (which increases the risk of death), and measure LV mass and the ratio of wall thickness to chamber radius—all of which predict cardiac events and mortality.[18-20]

Multidetector Computed Tomography

From a surgical standpoint, multidetector computed tomography (CT) has two pertinent applications in the management of CAD: to detect CAD and to inform the planning of grafting sites for CABG by providing additional information about coronary lesions, especially calcification and the course of coronary arteries. It also gives additional pertinent information about aortic disease and calcification, which might profoundly influence surgical decision making. However, the timing of cardiac CT should be carefully weighed against the risk of renal failure as a result of contrast nephropathy. Although revascularization decisions are currently made on the basis of coronary angiography, there have been tremendous improvements in temporal and spatial resolution of cardiac CT that make it useful for this purpose as well. Coronary computed tomography angiography (CCTA) can now provide high-quality images of the coronary arteries.[21] When it is performed with 64-slice CT, CCTA has a sensitivity of 93% to 97% and a specificity of 80% to 90% for detecting obstructive CAD.[22-28] Factors such as image quality, extent of coronary calcification, and body mass index adversely affect accuracy; in addition, coronary stenosis measurements are not well correlated between CT angiography and traditional angiography. This is an important fact to consider because current recommendations state that only vessels with stenosis greater than 50% to 70% should be bypassed.

The potential advantages of CCTA over standard functional testing for CAD screening include the high negative predictive value of CCTA for obstructive CAD. This can reassure caregivers that it is a sensible strategy to provide guideline-directed medical therapy (GDMT) and to defer consideration of revascularization. Among the greatest potential advantages of CCTA over conventional angiography, in addition to documentation of stenotic lesions, is that CCTA can assess remodeling and identify nonobstructive plaque, including calcified, noncalcified, and mixed plaque.[29,30]

Magnetic Resonance Imaging

Myocardial first-pass perfusion magnetic resonance imaging has been considered a good alternative to nuclear cardiac ischemia and viability testing. However, the procedure has not gained widespread popularity because special training and expertise are required to perform this type of imaging and to interpret the results.

Cardiac Catheterization and Intervention

Coronary catheterization is the "gold standard" for diagnosis of CAD. Coronary angiography defines coronary anatomy, including the location, length, diameter, and contour of the epicardial coronary arteries; the presence and severity of coronary luminal obstructions; the nature of the obstruction; the presence and extent of angiographically visible collateral flow; and coronary blood flow.

The classification for defining coronary anatomy that is still used today was developed for the Coronary Artery Surgery Study (CASS)[31] and further modified by the Balloon Angioplasty Revascularization Investigation (BARI) study group.[32] This scheme assumes that there are three major coronary arteries: the LAD, the circumflex, and the RCA, with a right-dominant, left-dominant, or codominant circulation. The extent of disease is defined as one-vessel, two-vessel, three-vessel, or left main disease; a luminal diameter reduction of at least 70% is considered to be significant stenosis (Figs. 59-3 and 59-4). Left main disease, however, is defined as stenosis of at least 50% (Fig. 59-5). Despite being recognized as the traditional gold standard for clinical assessment of coronary atherosclerosis, this test is not without limitations. There is marked variation in interobserver reliability, and investigators have found only 70% overall agreement among readers with regard to the severity of stenosis; this was reduced to 51% when restricted to coronary vessels rated as having some stenosis by any reader. Also, angiography provides only anatomic data and is not a reliable indicator of the functional significance of a given coronary stenosis unless a technique such as fractional flow reserve (FFR) is used to provide information about the physiologic effects of the stenosis. FFR is measured by passing a sensor guidewire into the LAD or circumflex vessels for LCA lesions. Thereafter, the flow reserve in the artery is checked by using adenosine to induce hyperemia in the coronary system, which is discussed in the next section on FFR. In addition, angiography cannot distinguish between vulnerable and stable plaques. In angiographic studies performed before and after acute events and early after MI, plaques causing UA and MI commonly were found to be 50% obstructive before the acute event and were therefore

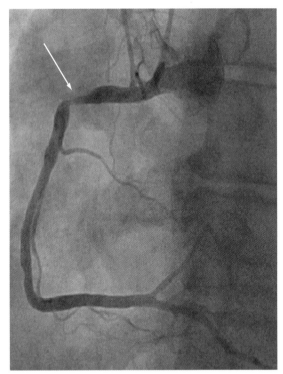

FIGURE 59-4 Right coronary angiogram showing hemodynamically significant lesion *(arrow)*. The right coronary artery terminates as a posterior descending artery in the right dominant system.

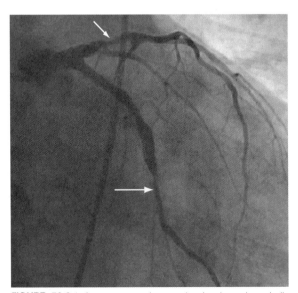

FIGURE 59-3 Left coronary angiogram showing hemodynamically severe lesions in the left anterior descending artery *(small arrow)* and the circumflex artery *(large arrow)*.

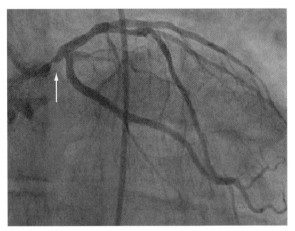

FIGURE 59-5 Coronary angiogram showing critical left main coronary artery stenosis *(arrow)*.

angiographically "silent."[31,32] Diagnostic testing methods to identify vulnerable plaque and therefore the patient's risk of MI are being intensely studied, but no gold standard has yet emerged. Despite these limitations of coronary angiography, the extent and severity of CAD as revealed angiographically remain important predictors of long-term patient outcomes.[33,34]

In the CASS registry[35] of medically treated patients, the 12-year survival rate of patients with normal coronary arteries was 91% compared with 74% for those with one-vessel disease, 59% for those with two-vessel disease, and 40% for those with three-vessel disease.

Importantly, besides informing the decision whether to intervene surgically or with percutaneous coronary intervention (PCI), the salient characteristics of coronary lesions (e.g., stenosis severity, length, and complexity and presence of thrombus), the number of lesions threatening regions of contracting myocardium, the effect of collaterals, and the volume of jeopardized viable myocardium also can afford some insight into the potential consequences of subsequent vessel occlusion and therefore the haste with which surgery should be scheduled. For example, a patient with a noncontracting inferior or lateral wall and severe proximal stenosis of a large LAD artery is presumably at substantial risk for development of cardiogenic shock if the LAD artery were to become occluded. Thus, such a patient should be scheduled relatively quickly for surgery.

Right-sided heart catheterization is used to measure central venous, right atrial, right ventricular, pulmonary artery, and pulmonary wedge pressures as well as cardiac output. It can also be used to identify intracardiac shunts, to assess arrhythmias, and to initiate temporary cardiac pacing. Preoperative right-sided heart catheterization is used selectively and is generally not necessary unless right ventricular dysfunction or pulmonary vascular disease is suspected.

PCI techniques in current use include balloon dilation, stent-supported dilation, atherectomy and plaque ablation with a variety of devices, thrombectomy with aspiration devices, specialized imaging, and physiologic assessment with intracoronary devices.

Coronary artery stents were the first substantial breakthrough in the prevention of restenosis after angioplasty. Although stent recoil and compression are not completely insignificant problems, the greatest cause of lumen loss in stented coronary arteries is neointimal hyperplasia. This is the principal mechanism of in-stent stenosis and results from inappropriate cell proliferation—hence, the advent of cytotoxic drug-eluting stents (DES).

Fractional Flow Reserve

Angiography can underestimate the severity of CAD, especially LCA disease. This underestimation may be due to the lack of a reference segment or to very ostial or distal disease. Therefore, in cases with intermediate lesions, FFR has emerged as a helpful modality.[36,37]

FFR is measured by passing a sensor guidewire into the LAD or circumflex vessels for LCA lesions. Thereafter, the flow reserve in the artery is checked by using adenosine to induce hyperemia in the coronary system. An FFR below 0.75 is considered to signify ischemia-producing lesions. Some studies have used a threshold of 0.8.

Intravascular Ultrasonography

Intravascular ultrasonography (IVUS) provides high-quality cross-sectional images of the coronary system.[38] It is done by inserting an IVUS wire into the LAD or circumflex artery and gradually pulling it out while obtaining real-time images of the coronary system. In indeterminate lesions of the LCA, an IVUS minimum luminal diameter of 2.8 or a minimum luminal area of 6 mm^2 suggests a physiologically significant lesion.

Hybrid Imaging

Hybrid imaging has the potential of taking coronary artery assessment one step further by combining the advantages of two different modalities to give both anatomic and physiologic information in one snapshot. Hybrid imaging can combine positron emission tomography (PET) and CT or SPECT and CT, thus allowing combined anatomic and functional testing. In addition, novel scanning techniques make it possible to use CCTA alone to assess perfusion and FFR, in addition to coronary anatomy.[39-41] Interestingly, these combined assessments can produce a fused image in which physiologic information about flow is combined with information about the anatomic extent and severity of CAD, plaque composition, and arterial remodeling. Robust evidence to support the use of hybrid imaging is lacking at this point, despite its reported accuracy in predicting cardiac events with both ischemic and anatomic markers.[42] The strength of combined imaging is that it provides anatomic information to guide the interpretation of ischemic and scarred myocardium as well as information to guide therapeutic decision making. Hybrid imaging also can overcome technical limitations of myocardial perfusion SPECT or myocardial perfusion PET by providing anatomic correlates to guide interpretative accuracy,[43] and it can provide the functional information that an anatomic technique like CCTA or magnetic resonance angiography lacks; however, use of hybrid techniques requires increasing the radiation dose.

INDICATIONS FOR CORONARY ARTERY REVASCULARIZATION

Per the most current American College of Cardiology/American Heart Association guidelines, the only class Ia indication for PCI is acute STEMI. In all other indications, CABG has superior class based on current evidence (Table 59-3). These guidelines are based on the existing literature, which spans 4 decades. Many of the studies on which current recommendations are based were conducted in the 1970s and 1980s.

Coronary Artery Bypass Grafting versus Contemporaneous Medical Therapy

In the 1970s and 1980s, three landmark randomized controlled trials (RCTs) established the survival benefit of CABG compared with medical therapy without revascularization in certain patients with SIHD: the Veterans Affairs Cooperative Study,[44] European Coronary Surgery Study,[45] and CASS.[35] Subsequently, a 1994 meta-analysis of seven studies in which 2649 patients were randomly assigned to medical therapy or CABG[36] showed that CABG offered a survival advantage over medical therapy for patients with LCA or three-vessel CAD. The studies also established that CABG is more effective than medical therapy for relieving anginal symptoms. These studies have been replicated only once during the past decade. In MASS II (Medicine, Angioplasty, or Surgery Study II), patients with multivessel CAD who were treated with CABG were less likely than those treated with

TABLE 59-3   Guidelines for Coronary Revascularization

CORONARY ARTERY LESIONS	RECOMMENDATIONS
Unprotected left main	
CABG	I
PCI	IIa—For SIHD when both of the following are present:
	• Cardiac catheterization reveals a low risk of PCI procedural complications with a high likelihood of good long-term outcome (low SYNTAX score 22, ostial or trunk left main).
	• Significantly increased risk of adverse surgical outcomes (STS-predicted risk of operative mortality 5%)
	IIa—For UA/NSTEMI if not a CABG candidate
	IIa—For STEMI when distal coronary flow is TIMI flow grade 3 and PCI can be performed more rapidly and safely than CABG
	IIb—For SIHD when both of the following are present:
	• Cardiac catheterization reveals a low to intermediate risk of PCI procedural complications and an intermediate to high likelihood of good long-term outcome (low-intermediate SYNTAX score of 33, bifurcation left main)
	• Increased risk of adverse surgical outcomes (moderate—severe COPD, disability from prior stroke, or prior cardiac surgery; STS-predicted operative mortality 2%)
	III: Harm—For SIHD in patients (versus performing CABG) with unfavorable anatomy for PCI and who are good candidates for CABG
3-vessel disease with or without proximal LAD artery disease	
CABG	I
	IIa—It is reasonable to choose CABG over PCI in patients with complex 3-vessel CAD (SYNTAX score 22) who are good candidates for surgery
PCI	IIb—Of uncertain benefit
2-vessel disease with proximal LAD artery disease	
CABG	I
PCI	IIb—Of uncertain benefit
2-vessel disease without proximal LAD artery disease	
CABG	IIa—With extensive ischemia
	IIb—Of uncertain benefit without extensive ischemia
PCI	IIb—Of uncertain benefit
1-vessel proximal LAD artery disease	
CABG	IIa—With LIMA for long-term benefit
PCI	IIb—Of uncertain benefit
1-vessel disease without proximal LAD artery involvement	
CABG	III: Harm
PCI	III: Harm
LV dysfunction	
CABG	IIa—LVEF 35% to 50%
	IIb—LVEF 35% without significant left main CAD
PCI	Insufficient data
Survivors of sudden cardiac death with presumed ischemia-mediated VT	
CABG	I
PCI	I
No anatomic or physiologic criteria for revascularization	
CABG	III: Harm
PCI	III: Harm

Class I   Benefit >>> Risk. Procedure should be performed.
Class IIa   Benefit >> Risk. Additional studies with focused objectives needed. It is reasonable to perform procedure.
Class IIb   Benefit ≥ Risk. Additional studies with broader objectives and additional registry data may be needed. Procedure treatment may be considered.
Class III   No Benefit
   or
Class III   Harm
From reference 45a.
CABG, coronary artery bypass graft (major adverse events occurred less frequently with CABG); *CAD,* coronary artery disease; *COPD,* chronic obstructive pulmonary disease; *LAD,* left anterior descending; *LIMA,* left internal mammary artery; *LV,* left ventricle; *LVEF,* left ventricular ejection fraction; *PCI,* percutaneous coronary intervention; *SIHD,* stable ischemic heart disease; *STEMI,* ST-elevation myocardial infarction; *STS,* Society of Thoracic Surgeons; *SYNTAX,* Synergy between Percutaneous Coronary Intervention with Taxus and Cardiac Surgery; *TIMI,* Thrombolysis In Myocardial Infarction; *UA/NSTEMI,* unstable angina/non–ST-elevation myocardial infarction; *VT,* ventricular tachycardia.

medical therapy to have a subsequent MI, to need additional revascularization, or to experience cardiac death in the 10 years after randomization.[37] Surgical techniques and medical therapy have improved substantially during the intervening years. Some critics state that if CABG were compared with GDMT in RCTs today, the relative benefits in terms of survival and angina relief observed several decades ago might no longer be observed. However, it should also be understood that the concurrent administration of GDMT, which most post–cardiac surgery patients now receive, may also substantially improve long-term outcomes in patients treated with CABG in comparison with those receiving medical therapy alone. Thus, the survival difference might still favor CABG over GDMT.

Percutaneous Coronary Intervention versus Medical Therapy

Although contemporary interventional treatments have lowered the risk of restenosis compared with earlier techniques, meta-analyses have not shown that the use of bare-metal stents (BMS) confers a survival advantage over balloon angioplasty[38,39] or that the use of DES confers a survival advantage over BMS.[40] Evaluation of trials of PCI conducted during the last 30 years shows that despite improvements in PCI technology and pharmacotherapy, PCI has not reduced the risk of death or MI in patients without recent acute coronary syndrome. The findings from individual studies and systematic reviews of PCI versus medical therapy can be summarized as follows:

- PCI reduces the incidence of angina.
- PCI has not been demonstrated to improve survival in stable patients.
- PCI may increase the short-term risk of MI.
- PCI does not lower the long-term risk of MI.

Coronary Artery Bypass Grafting versus Balloon Angioplasty or Bare-Metal Stents

From a review of multiple RCTs comparing CABG with balloon angioplasty or BMS, the following conclusions can be drawn[41]:

- Survival was similar for CABG and PCI (with balloon angioplasty or BMS) at 1 year and 5 years. Survival was similar for CABG and PCI in patients with one-vessel CAD (including those with disease of the proximal portion of the LAD artery) or multivessel CAD.
- Incidence of MI was similar at 5 years.
- Procedural stroke occurred more commonly with CABG than with PCI (1.2% versus 0.6%).
- Relief of angina was more effective with CABG than with PCI at 1 year and 5 years.
- At 1 year after the index procedure, repeated coronary revascularization was performed less often after CABG than after PCI (3.8% versus 26.5%). This was also found after 5 years of follow-up (9.8% versus 46.1%). This difference was more pronounced with balloon angioplasty than with BMS.

Coronary Artery Bypass Grafting versus Drug-Eluting Stents

Multiple observational studies comparing CABG and DES implantation have been published, but most of them had short (12 to 24 months) follow-up periods. Only one large RCT

comparing CABG and DES implantation has been published, called the Synergy between Percutaneous Coronary Intervention with Taxus and Cardiac Surgery (SYNTAX) trial,[42] in which 1800 patients (of a total of 4337 who were screened) were randomly assigned to undergo DES implantation or CABG. Major adverse cardiac events (a composite of death, stroke, MI, or repeated revascularization during the 3 years after randomization) occurred less frequently in CABG patients (20.2%) than in DES patients (28.0%; $P = .001$). The rates of death and stroke were similar; however, MI (3.6% for CABG, 7.1% for DES) and repeated revascularization (10.7% for CABG, 19.7% for DES) were more likely to occur with DES implantation. In SYNTAX, the extent of CAD was assessed by using the SYNTAX score, which is based on the location, severity, and extent of coronary stenoses, with a low score indicating less complicated anatomic CAD. In post hoc analyses, a low score was defined as 22 or lower; intermediate, 23 to 32; and high, 33 or higher. The occurrence of major adverse cardiac events correlated with the SYNTAX score for DES patients but not for those undergoing CABG. At 12-month follow-up, the primary end point was similar for CABG and DES in those with a low SYNTAX score. In contrast, major adverse cardiac events occurred more often after DES implantation than after CABG in those with an intermediate or high SYNTAX score. At 3 years of follow-up, the mortality rate was greater in patients with three-vessel CAD treated with PCI than in those treated with CABG (6.2% versus 2.9%). The differences in major adverse cardiac events of those treated with PCI or CABG increased with an increasing SYNTAX score. Although the utility of using a SYNTAX score in everyday clinical practice remains uncertain, it seems reasonable to conclude from SYNTAX and other data that outcomes of patients undergoing PCI or CABG in those with relatively uncomplicated and lesser degrees of CAD are comparable, whereas in those with complex and diffuse CAD, CABG appears to be preferable.

Left Main Coronary Artery Disease
CABG or PCI versus Medical Therapy for Left Main CAD

CABG confers a survival benefit over medical therapy in patients with LCA CAD. Subgroup analyses from RCTs performed 3 decades ago demonstrated a 66% reduction in relative risk of death with CABG, with the benefit extending to 10 years.[36,46]

Studies Comparing PCI versus CABG for Left Main CAD

Of all patients undergoing coronary angiography, approximately 4% are found to have LCA CAD, 80% of whom have significant (70% diameter) stenoses in other epicardial coronary arteries. Published cohort studies have found that major clinical outcomes for ostial LCA are similar with PCI or CABG 1 year after revascularization and that mortality rates are similar at 1 year, 2 years, and 5 years of follow-up; however, the risk of needing target vessel revascularization is significantly higher with stenting than with CABG.

Three RCTs have looked at this topic: the SYNTAX trial, the Study of Unprotected Left Main Stenting versus Bypass Surgery (LE MANS) trial,[43] and the Premier of Randomized Comparison of Bypass Surgery versus Angioplasty Using Sirolimus-Eluting Stent in Patients with Left Main Coronary Artery Disease (PRE-COMBAT) trial. The results from these three RCTs suggest (but do not definitively prove) that major clinical outcomes in *selected* patients with LCA CAD are similar with CABG and PCI at 1- to 2-year follow-up, but repeated revascularization rates are higher after PCI than after CABG. RCTs with extended follow-up of 5 years are required to provide definitive conclusions about the optimal treatment of LCA CAD.

Revascularization Options for LCA CAD

Although CABG has been considered the gold standard for unprotected LCA CAD revascularization, PCI has more recently emerged as a possible alternative mode of revascularization in carefully selected patients. Lesion location is an important determinant when PCI is considered for unprotected LCA CAD. Stenting of the LCA ostium or trunk is more straightforward than treatment of distal bifurcation or trifurcation stenoses, which generally requires a greater degree of operator experience and expertise.[47] In addition, PCI of bifurcation disease is associated with higher restenosis rates than PCI of disease confined to the ostium or trunk. Although lesion location influences technical success and long-term outcomes after PCI, location exerts a negligible influence on the success of CABG. In subgroup analyses, patients with LCA CAD and a SYNTAX score of 33 with more complex or extensive CAD had a higher mortality rate with PCI than with CABG. Physicians can estimate operative risk for all CABG candidates by using a standard instrument, such as the risk calculator from the Society of Thoracic Surgeons (STS) database. These considerations are important factors when one is choosing among revascularization strategies for unprotected LCA CAD and have been factored into revascularization recommendations. Use of a Heart Team approach has been recommended in cases in which the choice of revascularization is not straightforward. The patient's ability to tolerate and to comply with dual antiplatelet therapy is also an important consideration in revascularization decisions.

Experts have recommended immediate PCI for unprotected LCA CAD in the setting of STEMI.[48] The impetus for such a strategy is greatest when LCA CAD is the site of the culprit lesion, antegrade coronary flow is diminished (e.g., Thrombolysis In Myocardial Infarction [TIMI] flow grade 0, 1, or 2), the patient is hemodynamically unstable, and it is believed that PCI can be performed more quickly than CABG. When possible, the interventional cardiologist and cardiac surgeon should decide together on the optimal form of revascularization for these patients, although it is recognized that they are usually critically ill and therefore not amenable to a prolonged deliberation or discussion of treatment options.

Proximal Left Anterior Descending Artery Disease

Multiple studies have suggested that CABG confers a survival advantage over contemporaneous medical therapy for patients with disease in the proximal segment of the LAD artery. Cohort studies and RCTs as well as collaborative analyses and meta-analyses have shown that PCI and CABG result in similar survival rates in these patients.

Completeness of Revascularization

Most patients undergoing CABG receive complete or nearly complete revascularization, which seems to influence long-term prognosis positively.[49,50] In contrast, complete revascularization is accomplished less often in patients receiving PCI (e.g., in 70% of patients), and the extent to which the incomplete initial revascularization influences outcome is less clear. Rates of late survival and survival free of MI appear to be similar in patients with and without complete revascularization after PCI. Nevertheless, the need for subsequent CABG is usually higher in those whose initial revascularization procedure was incomplete (compared with those with complete revascularization) after PCI.

Left Ventricular Systolic Dysfunction

Several older studies and a meta-analysis of the data from these studies reported that patients with LV systolic dysfunction (predominantly mild to moderate in severity) had better survival with CABG than with medical therapy alone. For patients with more severe LV systolic dysfunction, however, the evidence that CABG results in better survival compared with medical therapy is lacking. In the Surgical Treatment for Ischemic Heart Failure (STICH) trial of CABG and GDMT in patients with an LVEF of 35% with or without viability testing, both treatments resulted in similar rates of survival (i.e., freedom from death from any cause, the study's primary outcome) after 5 years of follow-up. The data suggest the possibility that outcomes would differ if the follow-up were longer; as a result, the study is being continued to provide follow-up for up to 10 years.[51,52]

Only limited data are available comparing PCI with medical therapy in patients with LV systolic dysfunction. The data that exist at present on revascularization in patients with CAD and LV systolic dysfunction are more robust for CABG than for PCI, although data from contemporary RCTs in this population of patients are lacking. Therefore, the choice of revascularization method in patients with CAD and LV systolic dysfunction is best based on clinical variables (e.g., coronary anatomy, presence of diabetes mellitus, presence of chronic kidney disease), magnitude of LV systolic dysfunction, preferences of the patient, clinical judgment, and consultation between the interventional cardiologist and the cardiac surgeon.

Revascularization Options for Previous CABG

In patients with recurrent angina after CABG, repeated revascularization is most likely to improve survival in patients at highest risk, such as those with obstruction of the proximal LAD artery and extensive anterior ischemia. Patients with ischemia in other locations and those with a patent LIMA to the LAD artery are unlikely to experience a survival benefit from repeated revascularization.[53] Cohort studies comparing PCI and CABG among post-CABG patients report similar rates of midterm and long-term survival after the two procedures. In patients with previous CABG who are referred for revascularization for medically refractory ischemia, factors that may support the choice of repeated CABG include vessels unsuitable for PCI, multiple diseased bypass grafts, availability of the internal mammary artery (IMA) for grafting of chronically occluded coronary arteries, and good distal targets for bypass graft placement. Factors favoring PCI over CABG include limited areas of ischemia causing symptoms, suitable PCI targets, patent graft to the LAD artery, poor CABG targets, and comorbid conditions.

Unstable Angina/Non–ST-Segment Elevation Myocardial Infarction

The main difference between treating a patient with SIHD and a patient with UA/NSTEMI is that the impetus for revascularization is stronger in the treatment of UA/NSTEMI because myocardial ischemia occurring as part of an acute coronary syndrome is potentially life-threatening, and associated angina symptoms are more likely to be reduced with a revascularization procedure than with GDMT.[54] Thus, the indications for revascularization are strengthened by the acuity of presentation, the extent of ischemia, and the likelihood of achieving full revascularization. The choice of revascularization method is generally dictated by the same considerations used to decide between PCI or CABG for patients with SIHD.

ST-Segment Elevation Myocardial Infarction–Acute Myocardial Infarction

Percutaneous Coronary Intervention versus Medical Management for Acute Myocardial Infarction

In general, PCI confers a greater survival advantage than thrombolytics as an initial treatment for STEMI–acute myocardial infarction (AMI), and the use of delayed PCI as an adjunct to therapy, including therapy with thrombolytics, does not affect survival. In the Global Use of Strategies to Open Occluded Coronary Arteries in Acute Coronary Syndromes (GUSTO) IIb trial,[55] the 30-day rate of the composite end point of death, nonfatal MI, and nonfatal disabling stroke was 9.6% for PCI patients and 13.7% for recipients of thrombolytics.

Prospective observational data collected from the Second National Registry of Myocardial Infarction between June 1994 and March 1998 included data from a cohort of 27,080 consecutive patients with AMI associated with ST-segment elevation or left bundle branch block. These patients were all treated with primary angioplasty. The study revealed that the adjusted odds of mortality were significantly higher (62% versus 41%) for patients with door-to-balloon times longer than 2 hours. The longer the door-to-balloon time, the higher the mortality risk, emphasizing that door-to-balloon time has a significant impact on outcomes for patients with AMI.[56]

On the basis of this evidence, PCI facilities have been required to establish a target door-to-balloon time of no longer than 90 minutes. Depending on the available facilities in a particular region, it is the responsibility of emergency medical services personnel to determine whether that goal can be achieved by transferring the patient to a PCI-capable facility. If this cannot be accomplished, a medical management strategy should be considered, with the goal being a door-to-needle time of 30 minutes or less.[46]

Role of Coronary Artery Bypass Grafting

Although an increasing number of patients undergo catheterization early after AMI, the initial treatment is directed by the interventionalist, which has significantly diminished the role of emergency CABG. In general, patients who undergo CABG early after AMI are sicker, and efforts to improve myocardial function are typically refractory to medical therapy. These patients typically have a higher incidence of comorbidities and are more likely to require intra-aortic balloon pump (IABP) insertion. The optimal timing of CABG after AMI is not well established. A review of California discharge data identified 9476 patients who were hospitalized for AMI and subsequently underwent CABG. Of these, 4676 (49%) were in the early CABG group and 4800 (51%) were in the late CABG group. The mortality rate was highest (8.2%) among patients who underwent CABG on day 0 and declined to a nadir of 3.0% among patients who underwent CABG on day 3. The mean time to CABG was 3.2 days. Early CABG was an independent predictor of mortality, suggesting that CABG may best be deferred for 3 days or more after admission for AMI in nonurgent cases.[57]

The SHOCK (Should We Emergently Revascularize Occluded Coronaries for Cardiogenic Shock) trial has shown the survival advantage of emergency revascularization versus initial medical stabilization in patients in whom cardiogenic shock developed after AMI. A subanalysis that compared the effects of PCI and CABG on 30-day and 1-year survival showed that survival rates were similar at both time points. Among SHOCK trial patients

randomly assigned to undergo emergency revascularization, those treated with CABG had a greater prevalence of diabetes and worse CAD than those treated with PCI. However, survival rates were similar.[58]

In patients with AMI, CABG is usually performed in conjunction with an operation to treat a specific complication, such as refractory postinfarction angina, papillary muscle rupture with mitral regurgitation, and infarction VSD. The rationale for urgent or emergent surgery is often based on high early mortality risk from mechanical complications.

Preoperative Evaluation

The success of coronary artery revascularization depends on proper workup and patient selection. Currently, a multidisciplinary approach with cardiologists and cardiac surgeons is needed to give the patient the most appropriate form of revascularization based on guidelines (Fig. 59-6). Comorbidities that affect CABG outcomes and that are typically incorporated into risk models include age, gender, urgency of the procedure, ejection fraction, need for mechanical circulatory support, MI, smoking status, use of immunosuppressive drugs, prior coronary interventions, hypertension, diabetes, peripheral vascular disease (PVD), and cerebrovascular disease. In addition, the severity of angina, as designated by the Canadian Cardiovascular Society classification of angina, and the New York Heart Association classification of congestive heart failure (CHF) are important risk variables.

The following are essential components of a preoperative workup for CABG patients:

- Detailed history and physical examination, including conduit evaluation
- Review of medications, including angiotensin-converting enzyme inhibitors, beta blockers, antiplatelet agents, and anticoagulants
- Carotid duplex ultrasonography in patients who have clinical bruit or are at high risk for cerebrovascular disease
- Cardiac echocardiography to evaluate ventricular function and the structural integrity of valves and chambers
- Cardiac viability study in patients with depressed LVEF, chronic total occlusions, frailty, and high-risk operations to decide between PCI and CABG
- Cardiac catheterization to delineate the coronary anatomy
- Chest radiography
- Coagulation and platelet profile, comprehensive metabolic panel, and complete blood count

Depending on the findings of these tests, patients may need additional workup. In emergency circumstances, several of these tests may be skipped so that immediate revascularization can be performed.

Technique of Myocardial Revascularization: Conventional On-Pump Cardiopulmonary Bypass

Box 59-4 outlines all the major steps of an on-pump CABG operation.

Positioning and Draping

General anesthesia with a single-lumen endotracheal tube is the anesthetic technique of choice. After anesthetic induction and placement of necessary access and monitoring lines, the patient is positioned supine, with or without a roll underneath the shoulder blades according to the surgeon's preference. The arms are tucked beside the patient with appropriate padding to minimize the

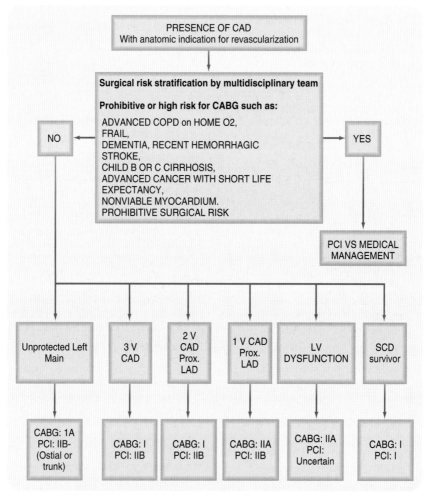

FIGURE 59-6 Surgical decision-making tree for coronary revascularization.

BOX 59-4   Major Steps in On-Pump Coronary Artery Bypass Grafting

- Induction of anesthesia and establishment of intraoperative monitoring adjuncts
- Positioning and draping
- Median sternotomy or appropriate approach
- Harvest and evaluation of blood conduits
- Heparinization and cannulation for cardiopulmonary bypass
- Establishment of cardiopulmonary bypass
- Myocardial arrest and protection
- Identification of target vessels and construction of distal anastomoses
- Restoration of myocardial electromechanical activity
- Creation of proximal anastomoses
- Weaning from cardiopulmonary bypass
- Evaluation for and establishment of necessary adjuncts—inotropes, IABP, pacing wires
- Reversal of anticoagulation and establishment of hemostasis
- Evaluation of surgical sites and establishment of surgical drainage
- Closure of sternotomy

chance of any nerve injury. A warming blanket is typically placed underneath the patient to assist in rewarming after controlled hypothermia during CPB. The entire chest, abdomen, and lower extremities are prepared. Circumferential preparation of the lower extremities is important because the leg may have to be maneuvered during harvesting of the saphenous vein conduit. If radial artery harvesting is being contemplated, the arm also has to be circumferentially prepared and positioned 90 degrees from the bedside on an arm board. Because most patients have a multilumen central line in the internal jugular vein or a Swan-Ganz catheter, the anesthesiologist must have continuous access to these lines, but without compromising the domain of the surgeon. Anchor points on the drapes are designated appropriately to allow CPB circuit lines to be secured without compromising sterility.

Cardiopulmonary Bypass

CPB is the establishment of extracorporeal oxygenation and perfusion of the human body by diverting all returning venous blood from the body to the heart-lung machine and returning the oxygenated blood in a controlled, pressurized manner. In essence, most blood flow to the heart and lungs is bypassed. Establishment

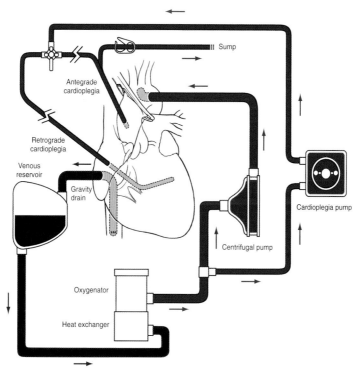

FIGURE 59-7 Schematic of Total Cardiopulmonary Bypass Circuit. All returning venous blood is siphoned into a venous reservoir and is oxygenated and temperature regulated before being pumped back through a centrifugal pump into the arterial circulation. The most common site for inflow cannulation is the ascending aorta; alternative sites include the femoral arteries and the right axillary artery in special circumstances. A parallel circuit derives oxygenated blood that is mixed with cold (4°C) cardioplegia solution in a 4:1 ratio and administered in antegrade or retrograde fashion to induce cardiac arrest. Cardioplegia solution is administered antegrade into the aortic root and retrograde through the coronary sinus. During the retrograde administration of cardioplegia solution, the efflux of blood from the coronary ostium is siphoned off through the sump drain, a return parallel circuit connected to the venous reservoir (not shown) that also helps to keep the heart decompressed during the arrest phase.

of CPB is a critical step for any major cardiac procedure and allows complete control of the operation.

The basic components of an extracorporeal heart pump circuit are venous cannulas to drain the returning venous blood, venous reservoir that collects blood by gravity, oxygenator and heat exchanger, perfusion pump, blood filter in the arterial line, and arterial cannula (Fig. 59-7). The blood conduits are designed to minimize turbulence, cavitation, and changes in blood flow velocity, which are detrimental to the integrity of component blood cells. Because the circuit contains a dead space created by the tubing and pump, a certain volume of nonblood solution is necessary to prime the pump and tubing. The priming solution consists of a balanced salt solution and, often, a starch solution. Homologous blood or fresh-frozen plasma may be added if the patient is anemic or if a bleeding problem is anticipated. The circuit has multiple access ports or sites from which to obtain blood samples for laboratory studies and into which to infuse blood, blood products, crystalloids, or drugs.

Supplemental components include a cardiotomy suction system to collect undiluted or clean blood from open cardiac chambers and the surgical field. This blood is filtered, de-aired, and returned to the bypass pump. Diluted field blood and blood that has mixed with inflammatory cytokines or fat is collected through a separate device that concentrates washed red cells before returning them directly to the patient.

A cardioplegia infusion device consists of a separate pump, reservoir, and heat exchanger. It is used to deliver cold, potassium-enriched blood or crystalloid solutions into the coronary circulation to arrest and to protect the heart.

Use of CPB requires suppression of the clotting cascade with heparin because the surgical wound and components of the bypass pump are powerful stimuli for thrombus formation. A strict anticoagulation protocol should be enforced before CPB is initiated. The pump prime is premixed with 4 U/mL heparin, and the patient is systemically heparinized with 300 U/kg before cannulation. An activated clotting time obtained approximately 3 minutes after heparin administration should be more than 400 seconds before cannulation is begun and should be maintained for more than 450 seconds throughout CPB, with intermittent doses given as needed during the operation.

The usual pumps are roller head pumps, which consist of circumferential tubing that is compressed by a roller on the outside, thereby forcing blood in one direction. This pump mechanism is associated with higher rates of hemolysis compared with centrifugal pumps, so roller head pumps are used only in cardiotomy suction and cardioplegia pumps. The main systemic pump is a centrifugal pump that consists of a vortex polyurethane-embedded magnetic cone housed in a conical chamber. The vortex spins at approximately 2000 to 5000 rpm, thereby generating enough centrifugal force to pump blood. Because the flow is

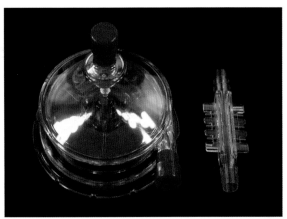

FIGURE 59-8 Main centrifugal pump used in most cardiopulmonary bypass circuits. The entire unit is sterile molded and contains a finless cone that spins at 2000 to 5000 rpm, generating a powerful yet non-turbulent vortex. A flow meter (shown) must be used with these pumps because the ultimate volume of flow depends on outflow resistance rather than on pump speed. The conventional roller head pumps are still used for the auxiliary circuits, such as cardiotomy suction and cardioplegia circuits.

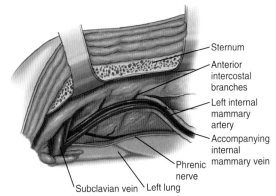

FIGURE 59-9 Surgeon's View of the Left Internal Mammary Artery (LIMA) as It Is Being Harvested. A mammary retractor is used to elevate the left hemithorax to provide adequate visualization. The LIMA is dissected away from the chest wall as a pedicle with its accompanying venae comitantes. Low-voltage electrocautery with no-touch technique is crucial for the atraumatic harvest of this important conduit. Understanding of its relation to the phrenic nerve and subclavian veins is important to avoid injury to these structures during LIMA harvest.

entirely caused by a nonturbulent vortex generated by a finless cone, this mechanism is almost atraumatic to the blood cells and is therefore associated with less hemolysis than the roller head pump mechanism (Fig. 59-8).

Neurologic Protection During Cardiopulmonary Bypass

The incidence of stroke after CPB is approximately 2.5%, but neurocognitive deficits are more frequent. Thus, several steps should be taken during CPB to minimize the risk of neurologic insult, including maintaining adequate cerebral perfusion, minimizing fat microemboli by eliminating the unnecessary use of cardiotomy suction, minimizing aortic manipulation by using single-clamp techniques when feasible, and instituting moderate hypothermia.

The oxygen consumption of a patient on CPB at normal temperatures averages 80 to 125 mL/min/m^2, similar to that of an anesthetized adult not on bypass. However, with the use of hypothermia, the oxygen consumption is markedly lower, and the flow rate can be reduced to less than 2.2 L/min/m^2. This is because the mean oxygen consumption of the body decreases by 50% for every 10°C decrease in body temperature. Below 28°C, a flow rate of 1.6 L/min/m^2 may be safe for as long as 2 hours. Significant disadvantages of using systemic hypothermia to accommodate lower flow rates include the extra time required to rewarm the patient and associated changes in the reactivity of blood elements, particularly platelets. These changes may increase the rewarmed patient's propensity for bleeding.

Median Sternotomy

The most common approach for performing CABG is a median sternotomy, although anterolateral thoracotomy is used in certain circumstances. A traditional sternotomy incision commences at the midpoint of the manubrium and is carried down to the xiphoid. The sternum is split through the middle with a sternal saw. It is essential that gentle upward force and a backward tilt be applied to the saw to prevent it from engaging the lung or soft tissues in the anterior mediastinum. Once the sternotomy is completed, the periosteum of the posterior table is cauterized, and a

passive hemostatic agent such as bone wax or a reconstituted mixture of vancomycin may be used to prevent bleeding from the marrow. The most important consideration during the sternotomy is staying in the midline because the most common cause of sternal dehiscence is an off-midline sternotomy and the consequent technically suboptimal closure. Other potential problems associated with the sternotomy include indirect injury to the liver and direct injury to the heart, innominate vein, and lungs.

Conduit Choice and Harvesting

Left internal mammary artery. In a seminal study from the Cleveland Clinic, Loop and colleagues[59] have shown improved 10-year survival in patients who received a LIMA graft; patients who received a saphenous vein graft (SVG) had 1.6 times the risk of death that LIMA graft recipients had. The long-term patency rate of the LIMA graft has been shown to be approximately 95% and 90% at 10 and 20 years, respectively. The best patency rates are achieved when the LIMA is used as an in situ pedicled graft and is anastomosed to the LAD.

Bilateral internal mammary artery. Observational studies from major CABG centers suggested that the use of bilateral IMA (BIMA) grafts improves survival and significantly reduces the need for reoperation without increasing mortality. However, early results from a randomized trial demonstrated that compared with SVGs, BIMA grafts are associated with a higher (twofold) incidence of deep sternal wound infection. BIMA grafts are best used by experienced surgeons in younger, nondiabetic, nonobese patients. Four major studies that tilted the balance in favor of BIMA grafts were the two Cleveland Clinic studies (1999 and 2004), in which propensity scores were used to match single and bilateral IMA graft recipients; the Oxford meta-analysis (2001); and a retrospective study from Japan (2001). Skeletonization of the IMA grafts may reduce the wound complication rate.

The IMA is harvested after the sternotomy is completed. A specially designed mammary retractor is used to elevate the appropriate hemithorax, typically the left for harvesting the LIMA. Adequately exposing the undersurface of the sternum is essential for successful harvest of the IMA (Fig. 59-9). The artery may be harvested as a pedicle that includes the two venae comitantes and surrounding soft tissue from the level of the subclavian vein to the level of the bifurcation of the artery into the superior epigastric and musculophrenic branches. The alternative method of harvesting is the skeletonized harvest, in which only the IMA is dissected away from the chest wall.

The basic principle of harvesting the IMA relies exclusively on the no-touch technique, use of low-voltage electrocautery, and clipping of the anterior intercostal branches. Care must be taken during the harvest to identify the course of the phrenic nerves and to avoid injury to them. This is particularly important while harvesting the right IMA because the phrenic nerve is more closely related to it at the level of the second or third intercostal space. The IMA is a fragile vessel, and direct handling or undue traction should be avoided because it may cause traumatic dissection of the vessel. The distal end of the IMA should be divided only after the patient is fully heparinized to avoid thrombosis of the conduit. Once the IMA is divided, the distal end is spatulated appropriately to fashion the anastomosis.

Greater saphenous vein. Grafts made from this vein have a patency rate of 90% at 1 year.[60] Beyond 5 years after surgery, graft atherosclerosis develops in a substantial number of SVGs. By 10 years, only 60% to 70% of SVGs are patent, and 50% of those have angiographic evidence of atherosclerosis.

While the sternotomy is being done, a separate team begins harvesting saphenous or radial artery conduits. Saphenous vein harvesting can be performed by open or endoscopic techniques. The conventional method of open vein harvesting involves making a long incision along the entire length of the harvested vein. Alternatively, a bridging technique can be used in which multiple 1- to 2-inch incisions are made, with intact bridges of skin between them. The most common complications associated with long open incisions are pain, slow wound healing, and dehiscence, which is compounded by the fact that a significant number of CABG patients have diabetes or PVD. The use of endoscopic or bridging techniques significantly alleviates but does not entirely eliminate these problems. There are some centers that avoid endoscopic vein harvesting entirely on the assumption that the technique is too traumatic to the vein itself, may be associated with intimal trauma, and may impair the long-term patency of the conduit. However, studies have shown reduced graft patency in endoscopically harvested veins. These reports were based on post hoc analyses of data from trials designed to address other aspects of coronary revascularization. Once the vein is extracted and the branches are ligated, the graft is soaked in a heparin solution while awaiting implantation. The veins are typically used in a reversed fashion and hence may not require valvotomy. A typical configuration of a three-vessel coronary artery bypass graft is shown in Figure 59-10.

Alternative conduits may be needed in patients who have had previous coronary bypass, peripheral vascular surgery with the use of vein conduits, or lower extremity amputations and in those who have unusable saphenous vein conduits because of severe varicosities of the saphenous vein. Other manifestations of venous insufficiency or disease may also pose problems. In addition, patients who have severely calcified ascending aortas may not be amenable to a vein-based aortocoronary bypass because anastomosis to the ascending aorta is complicated. In these cases, alternative bypass strategies include total arterial revascularization with BIMA pedicles (Fig. 59-11). In addition, the IMA may be used as the main conduit from which further arterial conduits may be Christmas-treed in an off-pump setup so that any aortic manipulation is avoided.

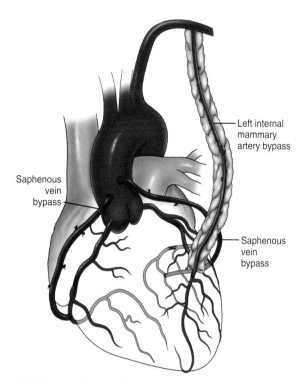

FIGURE 59-10 Typical Configuration for a Three-Vessel Coronary Artery Bypass. The left internal mammary artery is anastomosed to the left anterior descending artery. Aortocoronary bypasses are created with reversed saphenous vein to the distal right coronary artery and an obtuse marginal branch of the circumflex coronary artery. The circumflex coronary artery is usually avoided as a target for bypass because its location well inside the atrioventricular groove makes it difficult to visualize.

Labels in figure: Left internal mammary artery bypass; Saphenous vein bypass; Saphenous vein bypass

Other conduits

Radial artery. The radial artery graft is easily harvested and can reach all coronary territories, making it an attractive option for an arterial conduit. Both the Radial Artery Patency Study and the Radial Artery versus Saphenous Vein Patency study showed radial artery grafts to have better patency than SVGs on 5-year angiographic follow-up. However, the radial artery is associated with a significantly higher incidence of string sign. In addition, to date, no study has shown a survival advantage of radial artery over SVG grafting. Also, patency is much worse if the radial grafts are not placed on critically stenotic vessels.

Gastroepiploic artery. The gastroepiploic artery is rarely used today, although some centers in Asia still use gastroepiploic grafts and continue to report acceptable outcomes associated with them. Evidence from RCTs and a recent meta-analysis suggests that the saphenous vein has better early (6-month) and midterm (3-year) graft patency than the right gastroepiploic artery when it is used for RCA revascularization.

Total Arterial Revascularization

More than 95% of all CABG operations performed in the United States and more than 90% of those performed in the United Kingdom and Australia involve only one arterial graft.[61,62] The LIMA and SVG remain the standard CABG grafts; SVGs account for most of the conduits used. Of these SVGs, 40% to 50% become occluded at 10 years, and more than 75% are occluded

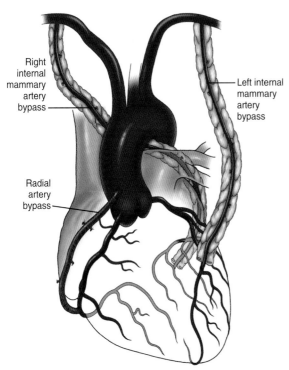

Right internal mammary artery bypass

Left internal mammary artery bypass

Radial artery bypass

FIGURE 59-11 Total arterial revascularization by use of bilateral mammary artery and radial artery conduits. The right internal mammary artery, bypassed to an obtuse marginal branch, is routed behind the aorta, and the pulmonary artery is routed through the transverse sinus.

at 15 years. In an effort to ameliorate these shortcomings of SVGs, some centers have been heavily emphasizing total arterial revascularization in which the LIMA, right IMA, and radial arteries are used.

Results from retrospective series have shown some survival benefit with total arterial revascularization, as would be expected. However, there are certain pragmatic reasons that total arterial revascularization has not totally replaced the use of SVGs:

• Concern about arterial spasm: Most arterial grafts are prone to spasm, and their use necessitates vasodilator administration, both locally and systemically, for a prolonged period. This can interfere with achieving stable hemodynamics in the immediate postoperative period.
• Use of arterial grafts appropriate only for severely stenotic arteries: Most experts would not use an arterial graft other than the LAD unless the stenosis was at least 80% and probably 90% or more because of the risk of competitive flow. It is well known that venous grafts work with less critical lesions.
• Inadequate length: As an in situ graft, the right IMA is not long enough to reach the PDA, distal RCA, mid or distal circumflex, or distal LAD and cannot be used easily as a sequential graft. It can, however, be used as a free graft.
• Concern about sternal nonunion and mediastinitis: There is a higher risk of sternal nonunion and mediastinitis with the use of BIMA grafts versus SVGs. Most experts will not use BIMA grafts in patients with diabetes, severe PVD, use of steroids, severe chronic obstructive pulmonary disease, or morbid obesity. Also, in the event that BIMA is used, most would recommend the skeletonized technique of BIMA harvest with preservation of the intercostal blood supply.

• Longer operative times: Using BIMA grafts obviously prolongs operative times.

Because of all these practical considerations, total arterial revascularization has not become as popular as would be expected, and most surgeons would offer total arterial revascularization only to younger patients because of their longer life expectancy.

Cannulation for Cardiopulmonary Bypass

Cannulation for establishment of CPB commences after conduit harvest and preparation are completed, the pericardium is opened, and the thymus is divided along the embryologic fusion plane. The patient is fully heparinized at a dose of 3 mg/kg. A purse-string is created on the anterior surface of the distal ascending aorta at the cannulation site. The aortic purse-string should involve only a partial thickness of the aorta, incorporating the adventitia and media but entirely avoiding the intimal layer. It is essential that the cannulation site be free of calcified plaques or atheroma to minimize the chance of embolization and cannulation site bleeding. Manual palpation, the commonly practiced method of assessment, is unreliable. Doppler transesophageal or epiaortic ultrasonographic guidance should be used whenever aortic disease is suspected. Also, the presence of calcium elsewhere in the ascending aorta may preclude safe clamp application. Although cannulation of the aorta may be a simple task, loss of control of the aortic cannulation site or inadvertent dissection could lead to a disastrous situation.

With a sharp scalpel, the adventitia is teased, and a full-thickness stab incision is made. The aortic cannula is inserted with the outflow bevel aimed toward the aortic arch. Tourniquet snares are used to secure the cannula in position and are tied. After the cannula is de-aired, it is connected to the arterial line of the CPB circuit. Alternative sites of arterial cannulation include the femoral artery and right axillary artery, which are used in reoperations or cases in which concomitant complex aortic and arch reconstruction may be required. Axillary artery cannulation is usually achieved with an 8-mm graft anastomosed end to side to the axillary artery.

For venous cannulation, a purse-string is then placed around the right atrial appendage. The tip of this appendage is amputated, and a dual-stage venous cannula is inserted and positioned with the tip at the level of the diaphragm. The basket of the dual-stage cannula should rest in the main chamber of the right atrium to capture drainage from the superior vena cava into the right atrium (Figs. 59-12 and 59-13).

Cardiac Arrest and Myocardial Protection

The initiation of CPB allows the heart to be stopped. To achieve cardiac arrest, a large dose of potassium solution (cardioplegia) is injected into the coronary vessels. This requires the coronary blood flow to be completely isolated from the systemic circulation, which is done by applying a cross-clamp to the ascending aorta proximal to the aortic cannula.

There are several different delivery options for cardioplegia solutions. One involves taking a balanced approach; the cardioplegia solution is administered antegrade through the ascending aorta proximal to the cross-clamp and then retrograde through a coronary sinus catheter inserted through a purse-string suture placed in the right atrium by use of special cannulas (Fig. 59-14). The extensive collateralization among the coronary veins and arteries and the paucity of valves in the coronary vein system ensure a relatively homogeneous distribution of cardioplegia solution when the retrograde approach is used. Patients with high-grade

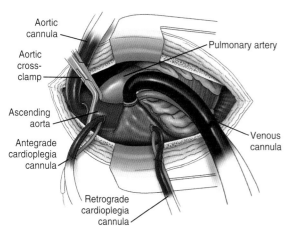

FIGURE **59-12** **Surgeon's View of the Heart After Cannulation.** The cross-clamp isolates the aortic root and coronary vessels from the rest of the systemic circulation. This allows administration of cardioplegia solution in a closed circuit and prevents the systemic blood from washing the cardioplegia solution out of the coronary system during the arrest phase. Applying the cross-clamp prevents active blood flow through the coronary arteries and thus allows the surgeon to perform the distal anastomoses in a bloodless field.

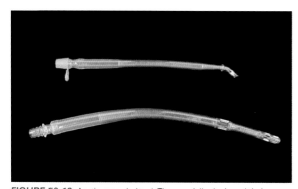

FIGURE **59-13** Aortic cannula *(top)*: The specially designed tip is angulated to allow laminar flow of blood into the aortic arch. Dual-stage venous cannula *(bottom)*: The first stage is the fenestrated basket that usually rests at the level of the hepatic veins and captures all venous return from the inferior vena cava. The second-stage basket is located such that it remains within the right atrium and captures venous return from the superior vena cava, azygos vein, coronary sinus, and direct collateral drainage into the right atrium. The venous drainage is a passive siphon aided by gravity.

proximal lesions, especially those with suboptimal collateral vessels, may benefit from the application of both techniques. After the initial administration of cardioplegia solution, additional doses are usually administered every 15 to 20 minutes.

An antegrade cardioplegia line with a Y-connector to the circuit is inserted into the ascending aorta. This allows antegrade administration of cardioplegia solution and also sumping and decompression of the ascending aorta while cardioplegia solution is administered retrogradely into the coronary sinus. The sump drain also functions to keep the coronary arteries free of any blood, thus providing the surgeon with a bloodless field in which to fashion the distal anastomoses. In addition, the sump drain performs the important function of decompressing the LV while the heart is arrested (see Figs. 59-7 and 59-12).

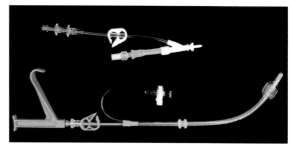

FIGURE **59-14** Retrograde cardioplegia cannula *(bottom)* used to administer cardioplegia solution into the coronary sinus. The self-inflating balloon distends, forming a seal only when cardioplegia solution is administered. Antegrade cardioplegia cannula *(top)* used to administer cardioplegia solution into the aortic root. The side port functions as a sump.

The most important task for ensuring myocardial protection is establishing complete diastolic arrest with an unloaded heart. In this state, the myocardial consumption of adenosine triphosphate is extremely low and allows maximal preservation of myocytes. In conventional CABG with total CPB, the decompression of the ventricle by off-loading, systemic cooling, topical cooling, and diastolic arrest of the heart with potassium cardioplegia solution serves to decrease myocardial oxygen consumption. Approximately 40% of the myocardial metabolic demand is eliminated when total CPB is established before diastolic arrest and cooling are instituted.

Target Identification and Distal Anastomosis

Once successful diastolic arrest of the heart is accomplished, the target coronary arteries to be bypassed are identified. Some of the epicardial conductance vessels are intramyocardial and therefore may not be directly visible. Once a target vessel is identified, it is opened with a sharp blade. Typically, the arteriotomy is approximately 5 mm long. The conduit, which is prepared and spatulated, is then grafted in an end-to-side fashion with running 7-0 Prolene suture. This component of the operation is technically the most challenging and requires precision. The flow and integrity of each vein conduit are tested by flushing it with cold blood or cardioplegia solution mix. The LIMA to left descending artery anastomosis is usually the last one to be performed (Fig. 59-15) because it is best to avoid manipulating the heart once this anastomosis is completed in case avulsion of the LIMA conduit occurs. Bypassing the PDA and obtuse marginal targets requires lifting the apex of the heart out of the pericardium.

Typically, a single segment of conduit is anastomosed to each planned distal target. On occasion, a single conduit can be used to supply blood to two targets, which is known as a sequential anastomosis. This is a good technique to use when there is a shortage of available vein conduits or when the target vessels are small; in these cases, use of this technique ensures a higher rate of blood flow through the vein conduit, reducing the risk of graft thrombosis (Fig. 59-16).

As the last distal anastomosis is being completed, the patient is warmed back to physiologic temperature. The cross-clamp is released after the final dose of warm cardioplegia solution is administered, which helps in scavenging the accumulated free radicals in the myocardium. A partial clamp is then applied to the ascending aorta, and the proximal anastomoses are constructed in an end-to-side fashion with running 5-0 Prolene suture. If there

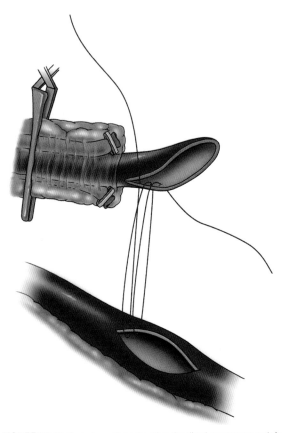

FIGURE 59-15 Technique of constructing the distal anastomoses: left internal mammary artery to left anterior descending artery, magnified surgeon's view. A 5-mm longitudinal arteriotomy is made on the coronary artery to be bypassed. The distal end of the left internal mammary artery is spatulated to an appropriate size match. A 7-0 Prolene suture is used to create the anastomosis with a parachuting technique.

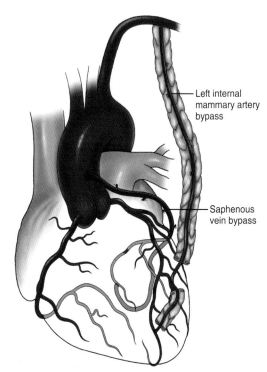

FIGURE 59-16 Alternative Configuration for a Three-Vessel Coronary Artery Bypass. The left internal mammary artery is anastomosed sequentially to a diagonal branch and to the distal left anterior descending artery. Aortocoronary bypasses are constructed with reversed saphenous vein in sequential configuration to the left posterolateral artery and an obtuse marginal branch of the circumflex coronary artery. The ideal configuration depends on the extent and distribution of the coronary blockages.

are concerns about the quality of the aorta, use of a partial clamp is typically avoided in favor of a single-clamp technique, which involves constructing the proximal anastomoses on an arrested heart, as for the distal anastomoses.

In patients in whom the ascending aorta is calcified or a free IMA pedicle needs to be used, a branching pattern of proximal anastomoses is made. This conserves vein length to a certain extent but also minimizes the number of aortotomies, especially if the ascending aorta is short or a concomitant aortic procedure has been performed. The ascending aorta is allowed to de-air as the aortic clamp is released, after which the vein grafts are de-aired.

Separation from Cardiopulmonary Bypass

Separation from CPB commences once the following physiologic criteria have been met:

- Resumption of rhythmic electromechanical activity
- Attainment of physiologic temperature above 36.5°C
- Availability of adequate reserve blood volume
- Restoration of normal systemic potassium levels
- Resumption of ventilation with an acceptable arterial blood gas level

A few other actions that may be considered at this point are placement of temporary pacing wires and insertion of an IABP, if

needed. Typically, the CPB flows are progressively decreased as the following parameters are closely observed:

- Data from the Swan-Ganz catheter
- Direct visual observations of cardiac function and chamber volume
- The transesophageal echocardiogram

Most patients have a transient systemic inflammatory response, causing vasodilation that becomes more pronounced as they are warmed. Thus, restoration of volume with intravascular fluids or administration of vasopressors may be necessary to maintain systemic blood pressure. Inotropic agents may be used if ventricular function is not adequate. Separating patients from CPB is primarily the surgeon's responsibility but requires dynamic communication with the perfusionist and anesthesiologist.

After CPB is discontinued, the venous cannula is removed and the purse-string is tied down. Once it is confirmed that the heart is providing satisfactory perfusion, protamine is administered. Close monitoring is needed because adverse reactions to protamine range from transient hypotension to fatal anaphylaxis. Such reactions necessitate the resumption of CPB.

Hemostasis

As protamine is being administered, hemostasis is expeditiously accomplished. As the patient rewarms, blood vessels that had been hemostatic may dilate and rebleed. Persistent bleeding should alert the surgeon to the following possible causes: aspects of the surgical technique; platelet dysfunction; inadequate protamine reversal; and hypothermia. The administration of blood and blood products may be necessary.

Sternal Closure and Completion of Surgery

The chest tube and temporary pacing wires should be checked for appropriate positioning. The sternum is approximated with stainless steel wires. The soft tissues and skin are closed in layers with absorbable sutures.

ADJUNCTS TO CORONARY ARTERY BYPASS GRAFTING

Transesophageal Echocardiography

Use of transesophageal echocardiography (TEE) enables the assessment of ventricular wall motion abnormalities and the detection of any chamber or valve anomalies that may change the strategy of the operation. Examples of TEE findings that may affect the conduct of the operation include an incidentally discovered large patent foramen ovale or fibroelastoma of the valves. New-onset or worsening mitral regurgitation after CABG suggests inferior wall ischemia and may indicate reevaluation of the bypass grafts or valve repair or replacement. Also, TEE helps in assessing ejection fraction and the volume status of the heart after surgery.

Inotropes and Pharmacotherapy

Cardioplegic arrest causes transient myocardial ischemia and lactic acid accumulation. After perfusion is reestablished, the ventricles are stiffer and require higher filling pressures to maintain adequate stroke volume. Also, CPB may cause significant third spacing and vasodilation. Thus, epinephrine as an inotropic agent is ideal to maintain adequate contractility in the initial recovery phase and during separation from CPB. Alpha agonists such as norepinephrine, phenylephrine, and vasopressin may be used to counteract the effects of inflammatory vasodilation. In patients with depressed myocardial function, such as left- or right-sided heart failure, dobutamine or a phosphodiesterase inhibitor such as milrinone may be required to enhance myocardial contractility and to decrease afterload or pulmonary vascular resistance. Because hypotension is a common side effect of these drugs, the systemic volume must be adequate, and an alpha agonist may be required. Calcium channel blockers or nitroglycerin may be needed in patients with preexisting hypertension.

It is essential to maintain a mean arterial pressure higher than 60 mm Hg in the initial postoperative period, but hypertension should be avoided because it puts stress on a myocardium that is trying to recover and increases the risk of bleeding from anastomotic suture lines. Blood pressure management requires a thorough understanding of physiologic and pharmacologic principles. It is a balancing act geared toward maintaining adequate systemic pressure, cardiac output, and peripheral perfusion while minimizing myocardial stress. Urine output is the most reliable indicator of peripheral organ perfusion.

Intra-Aortic Balloon Pump

For patients whose profound myocardial dysfunction is unresponsive to volume resuscitation and significant pharmacologic therapy, IABP support may be indicated. The IABP is a special Silastic balloon with a capacity of 40 to 60 mL that is positioned in the descending aorta just beyond the origin of the left subclavian artery. The balloon is designed to be actively inflated and deflated during each cardiac cycle; its timing is controlled by a specially designed computer with input from an arterial line tracing or ECG. Intra-aortic balloon counterpulsation has the benefit of decreasing myocardial work and oxygen consumption while increasing coronary perfusion.

The balloon is actively deflated just before systolic contraction begins, thereby decreasing LV impedance and assisting in the ejection of blood. The balloon then actively inflates at the time of aortic valve closure, that is, it is timed to occur at the dicrotic notch of the arterial line tracing. This increases the diastolic perfusion pressure and improves coronary blood flow, both of which decrease the time-tension index and increase the diastolic pressure-time index, thereby increasing the myocardial oxygen supply-to-demand ratio. The use of IABP is absolutely contraindicated in patients with aortic regurgitation and aortic dissection. It is relatively contraindicated in patients with PVD or aortic aneurysm.

POSTOPERATIVE CARE

Postoperative care in the intensive care unit (ICU) begins with a thorough physical and hemodynamic assessment. Mediastinal chest tube drainage should be recorded and assessed hourly. Initial ventilator settings should be set to match those in the operating room. Further adjustments in ventilator settings are made according to the postoperative blood gases. High positive end-expiratory pressure should be avoided in patients with hemodynamic instability. The ideal mode of ventilation is that with which the surgical or intensive care team is comfortable. A portable chest radiograph is obtained to confirm the position of the endotracheal tube, central lines, Swan-Ganz catheter, and IABP and to identify any pneumothorax, atelectasis, pulmonary edema, or pleural effusions. Initial laboratory studies should include hemoglobin, hematocrit, electrolyte, blood urea nitrogen, creatinine, and arterial blood gas levels and platelet count, prothrombin time, and partial thromboplastin time.

The patient should have an ECG monitor that can assess ST-T wave abnormalities; an arterial line to measure arterial blood pressure; and a line to measure central venous pressure, pulse oximetry, and core temperature. In select patients, pulmonary artery pressures and cardiac output are monitored continuously with a Swan-Ganz catheter. Neurologic assessment should be completed as soon as the patient wakes up to ensure that no cerebrovascular accident has occurred.

The primary considerations during the first 12 hours after the operation should be maintaining adequate blood pressure and cardiac output, correcting coagulation defects and electrolyte levels, stabilizing intravascular volume, and normalizing the peripheral vascular resistance. This often involves administration of crystalloid solutions, blood or blood products, inotropic agents, calcium, and vasodilators or vasoconstrictors.

Some of the goals in the postoperative period are as follows:
- Avoiding marked elevations in blood pressure
- Maintaining adequate perfusion pressure (60-80 mm Hg)
- Maintaining core body temperature higher than 36.5°C by warming the patient with forced hot air blankets
- Maintaining adequate cardiac output and a cardiac index of 2.2 L/min/m^2
- Keeping mixed venous oxygenation at 60%
- Reducing afterload, as appropriate, to minimize myocardial work

- Volume resuscitation with crystalloid or blood products, as necessary
- Maintaining hemoglobin level higher than 8 g/dL, or higher than 10 g/dL in older patients or those with severe cerebrovascular disease
- Maintaining homeostatic pH. Metabolic acidosis may be caused by hypoperfusion from low cardiac output, poor resuscitation, hypovolemia, or end-organ ischemia from embolism.
- Monitoring neurologic and peripheral vascular status
- Maintaining a sinus or perfusing rhythm at a rate of 70 to 100 beats/min
- Monitoring for and treating postoperative cardiac arrhythmias
- Ensuring adequate pain control to minimize fluctuations in blood pressure and myocardial stress
- Keeping blood glucose levels below 180 mg/dL. Standardized insulin-infusion regimens should be initiated, if needed.

Pulmonary Care

It is desirable to separate patients from the ventilator as soon as they awaken, are hemodynamically stable with minimal chest tube drainage, and can maintain a satisfactory spontaneous tidal volume and respiratory rate. Coughing and deep breathing exercises with appropriate sternal precautions are essential for postoperative recovery. Suboptimal postoperative pulmonary function may indicate additional therapy, including the use of bronchodilators, mucolytics, and chest physical therapy. Although β-adrenergic bronchodilators and *N*-acetylcysteine are useful adjuncts, they also can induce atrial fibrillation.

After extubation, it is important to provide the patient with sufficient pain relief to minimize emotional distress, poor coughing, and reluctance to begin ambulation. Unrelieved pain can also be a source of tachycardia, hypertension, myocardial ischemia, atelectasis, hypoxia, and pneumonia.

Discharge from the Intensive Care Unit

Before the patient leaves the ICU, unnecessary lines and catheters should be removed. Chest tubes are removed approximately 48 hours postoperatively, when the combined drainage is less than 200 mL per shift and chest radiography reveals no effusion. Removal of temporary atrial and ventricular pacing wires is often deferred to the third postoperative day.

Outcomes
Hospital Mortality

Seven core variables—emergency of operation, age, prior heart surgery, gender, LVEF, percentage stenosis of LCA, and number of major coronary arteries with more than 70% stenosis—have the greatest impact on CABG mortality. Other variables are important but have minimal impact when added to these core variables; these include recent MI (<1 week), angina severity, ventricular arrhythmia, CHF, mitral regurgitation, diabetes, PVD, renal insufficiency, and creatinine level.

In cardiac surgery, operative mortality has traditionally included 30-day and in-hospital mortality. The mortality figure for CABG is 1% to 3% in most modern series. Risk-adjusted outcomes have become the gold standard for reporting and comparing cardiac surgery outcomes. The STS database is the largest and most authoritative voluntary national database to date. The STS has developed a risk calculator that estimates morbidity and mortality for a given patient's risk profile. The observed-to-expected mortality ratio for a given surgeon or institution can then be determined.

Long-Term Survival

Survival after CABG is related to cardiac and noncardiac comorbidities. Risk factors for atherosclerosis, particularly cigarette smoking, hypercholesterolemia, hypertension, and diabetes, are associated with decreased survival.

In no longitudinal study has CABG obliterated the negative impact of abnormal LV function on late survival. Incomplete revascularization is associated with decreased survival, whereas complete revascularization, the use of the LIMA, and, in some studies, the use of BIMA are associated with improved survival.

The CASS documented overall survival of 96%, 90%, 74%, 56%, and 45% at 1, 5, 10, 15, and 18 postoperative years, respectively. These figures are inferior to those for the age-matched U.S. population and for modern series of patients who receive single or bilateral mammary grafts.

Morbidity

Tamponade. Pericardial tamponade is caused by the formation of pericardial clot and compression of the heart. The condition should be suspected if there is evidence of low cardiac output, hypotension coincident with tachycardia, and elevated central venous pressure. The quantity of mediastinal drainage is an unreliable predictor of tamponade, although an abrupt decline in mediastinal chest tube drainage should raise suspicion of tamponade caused by absence of an exit path for the blood. Widening of the mediastinum on chest radiography and echocardiographic evidence of a pericardial effusion should confirm the diagnosis.

If a Swan-Ganz catheter is in place and right- and left-sided heart pressures are monitored, the central venous pressure and pulmonary capillary wedge pressure are usually elevated and equal. The earliest manifestation of tamponade is an acute drop in mixed venous oxygen saturation. After the diagnosis is made, the patient should be returned to the operating room for evacuation of the clot and relief of the compression. If the patient's condition is rapidly deteriorating, the sternotomy incision may have to be reopened at the bedside.

Postoperative bleeding. The combination of heparinization, hypothermia, CPB, and protamine reversal is associated with increased risk for bleeding after CABG. Post-CABG bleeding that requires transfusion or reoperation is associated with a significant increase in morbidity and mortality risk. A minority of patients having cardiac procedures (15% to 20%) consume more than 80% of all blood products transfused at operation. Blood must be viewed as a scarce resource that carries significant risks and unproven benefits. There is a high-risk subset of patients who require multiple preventive measures to reduce the chance of postoperative bleeding. Nine variables stand out as important indicators of risk (Box 59-5).

Available evidence-based blood conservation techniques include the following:

- Administration of drugs that increase preoperative blood volume (e.g., erythropoietin) or decrease postoperative bleeding (e.g., ε-aminocaproic acid). Aprotinin is currently banned in the United States because some studies have associated it with increased mortality, stroke, and renal failure when it is administered to cardiac surgery patients.
- Intraoperative blood salvage and blood-sparing interventions
- Interventions that protect the patient's own blood from the stress of operation (e.g., autologous predonation, normovolemic hemodilution)
- Institution-specific blood transfusion algorithms supplemented with point-of-care testing

---

BOX 59-5   **Risk Factors for Postoperative Bleeding**

- Advanced age
- Low preoperative red blood cell volume (preoperative anemia or small body size)
- Preoperative antiplatelet or antithrombotic drugs
- Reoperative or complex procedures
- Emergency operations
- Noncardiac patient comorbidities
- Renal failure
- Chronic obstructive pulmonary disease
- Congestive heart failure

BOX 59-6   **Causes of Immediate Postoperative Bleeding**

Surgical
  - Conduit
  - Anastomoses
  - Cannulation sites
  - Mammary bed
  - Thymic veins
  - Pericardial edge
  - Sternal wire sites
Platelet dysfunction
Inadequate protamine reversal
Hypothermia

Despite efforts at blood conservation to limit perioperative bleeding and blood transfusions, 2% to 3% of patients will require reexploration for bleeding, and as many as 20% will have excessive bleeding and blood transfusion postoperatively. Bleeding of more than 500 mL in the first hour or persistent bleeding of more than 200 mL/hr for 4 hours is an indication for mediastinal exploration. Exploration is also indicated if a large hemothorax is identified on chest radiography or pericardial tamponade occurs. Usually, a specific bleeding site is not identified. Box 59-6 summarizes the common causes of immediate postoperative bleeding.

Neurologic complications. There are two types of neurologic deficits after CABG: type I deficit, which is a focal neurologic deficit; and type II deficit, which is manifested as nonspecific encephalopathy. In a 1996 multi-institutional prospective study, 6% of patients had these adverse outcomes, which were evenly distributed between the two types of deficit. Associated mortality was 20% for type I, which was twice the mortality for type II deficit. Age (especially >70 years) and hypertension are consistent risk factors for both types. History of previous neurologic abnormality, diabetes, and atherosclerosis of the aorta are risk factors for type I. Significant atherosclerosis of the ascending aorta mandates a surgical approach that will minimize the possibility of atherosclerotic emboli. Patients with concomitant carotid stenosis are at an elevated risk for neurologic complications. One approach used in such patients involves a staged procedure in which the more symptomatic and more critical vascular bed is addressed first. Otherwise, a combined approach may be used, but this poses a greater overall risk.

Mediastinitis. The incidence of deep sternal wound infection is 1% to 4% in CABG patients. Risk factors include obesity, reoperation, diabetes, and duration and complexity of operation. Using a BIMA graft can increase the risk of sternal wound complications in high-risk patients. The use of perioperative antibiotics and a strict protocol aimed at controlling the blood glucose level to less than 180 mg/dL by continuous intravenous infusion of insulin has been shown to reduce the incidence of mediastinitis significantly. Early débridement and muscle flap closure improve outcome. More recently, good outcomes have also been reported with the use of wound vacuum-assisted closures after adequate débridement.

Renal dysfunction. Mangano and coworkers have reported a 7.7% incidence of postoperative renal dysfunction (PRD) in CABG patients and mortality rates of 0.9%, 19%, and 63% in patients without PRD, patients with PRD but without need for dialysis, and patients who required dialysis, respectively. The 63% figure was confirmed in a large Veterans Administration study.

Medical Adjuncts for Postoperative Management

The following drugs are considered essential components of the postoperative management of CABG patients:

- Aspirin administration, 81 to 325 mg orally or rectally, is begun on the same day after CABG, unless the patient is bleeding because of platelet dysfunction. This is a quality-of-care index and has been shown to improve long-term graft patency.
- Beta blocker administration should begin after all inotropes have been discontinued. The goal is to maintain a heart rate of 60 to 80 beats/min and adequate mean perfusion pressures.
- Afterload reduction is important in all patients with a low LVEF. Afterload reduction is commenced after all inotropes are discontinued and adequate beta blockade is achieved. The angiotensin-converting enzyme inhibitors are first-line drugs for afterload reduction. Creatinine levels should be monitored.
- For antiarrhythmic treatment, amiodarone is used in many cardiac centers as prophylaxis against or treatment of atrial fibrillation. This drug should be used with caution in patients with preexisting interstitial lung disease and those taking warfarin. A prolonged Q-T interval is a contraindication.
- Administration of furosemide, a diuretic, is begun on the first postoperative day; the goal is to maintain a negative fluid balance. Chest radiography, creatinine levels, physical examination, and input-output charts help guide the dose of furosemide.

ALTERNATIVE METHODS FOR MYOCARDIAL REVASCULARIZATION

Cardiopulmonary Bypass With Hypothermic Fibrillatory Arrest

Hypothermic fibrillatory arrest is a good on-pump alternative to conventional cardioplegic arrest and avoids the use of the aortic cross-clamp. Although cardioplegic arrest offers maximal myocardial protection while providing a stable, immobile target for the distal anastomoses, not all patients are amenable to cardioplegia-based arrest. In patients with an extensively calcified aorta, cross-clamp application may be precarious and associated with an elevated incidence of stroke.

In these cases, a hypothermic fibrillatory arrest strategy may be used in which aortic manipulation is minimized. Once CPB is initiated, the patient is cooled to 28°C. The heart typically begins fibrillating at approximately 32°C. An LV sump is usually introduced through the right superior pulmonary vein to ensure LV decompression. Handling of the distal and proximal targets is similar to off-pump CABG (OPCAB) techniques because the coronary arteries are still fully perfused while the anastomoses are being performed. Vessel loops or occluders may be needed. In patients with extensive aortic calcification, there may not be any room to place an aortic cannula in or a proximal vein graft on the ascending aorta. In these cases, the right axillary artery may be used for arterial perfusion, and the saphenous vein can be anastomosed to the innominate artery if it is free of disease, or a total arterial vascularization approach should be considered with the use of one or both mammary arteries.

Once the anastomoses are completed, the patient is rewarmed to physiologic temperature and the heart is defibrillated into sinus rhythm. The use of hypothermic fibrillatory arrest is contraindicated in patients with significant aortic valve incompetence because the ventricle would distend with the regurgitant blood once fibrillation sets in, and no stroke volume is generated. Increased ventricular wall tension and energy consumption could lead to myocardial ischemia.

On-Pump Beating-Heart Bypass

On-pump beating-heart bypass is a selective strategy used for patients who have a very low LVEF and have suffered a recent MI. The logic behind this approach is that the myocardium is severely compromised and would poorly tolerate further ischemic compromise. Despite currently available techniques for myocardial protection, cardioplegic arrest is always associated with a certain degree of ischemia. This is especially true in patients with severe CAD and a stunned myocardium, in whom uniform protection of the ventricle with cardioplegia may be difficult to achieve, and an on-pump beating-heart strategy can be considered. The coronary arteries continue to be perfused, and exposure and handling of the anastomoses are similar to those for OPCAB. The use of CPB offloads the ventricle and offers a safety margin to manipulate the heart and to visualize all the targets that need to be bypassed. Use of IABP should be considered for most of these patients because their hemodynamic state is precarious to begin with.

Off-Pump Coronary Artery Bypass Grafting

The main rationale for using OPCAB was to avoid the adverse effects of CPB related to the systemic inflammatory response caused by contact of blood components with the surface of the bypass circuit. This hypothesis, although not supported by much sound scientific clinical data, spawned the belief that CPB contributed to various adverse outcomes, including postoperative bleeding, neurocognitive dysfunction, thromboembolism, fluid retention, and reversible organ dysfunction. Because OPCAB eliminated the use of a CPB circuit and could potentially reduce some of these pump-associated complications, there was a great enthusiasm for OPCAB. In fact, throughout Asia and particularly in India, 95% of CABG operations are still performed off-pump.

In a recent nationwide review of the STS database by Bakaeen et al, the use of off-pump procedures peaked in 2002 (23%) and again in 2008 (21%), followed by a progressive decline in off-pump frequency to 17% by 2012. Interestingly, after 2008, off-pump rates declined among both high-volume and intermediate-volume centers and surgeons, and currently in the United States, this technique is used in fewer than one in five patients who undergo surgical coronary revascularization. A minority of surgeons and

centers, however, continue to perform OPCAB in most of their patients.

This decline in OPCAB is presumably due not only to the procedure's technical complexity and steep learning curve but also, and more important, to the decreased long-term patency, higher rate of incomplete revascularization, and inferior long-term survival associated with OPCAB.

Data from multiple studies have not supported the belief that OPCAB decreases inflammatory mediator release. Some investigators have shown that even though complement activation may be reduced, there is no difference in production of cytokines and chemokines that modulate neutrophils and platelets.[63,64] In addition, myocardial ischemia by itself activates complement such as C5b-9. Thus, great caution should be used in interpreting studies regarding activation of the inflammatory cascade.

Three recent RCTs—the ROOBY trial, the SMART trial, and the CORONARY trial—have also shown worse outcomes with OPCAB than with CABG. In addition, the GOPCADE trial showed no benefit of OPCAB in elderly patients.

The Randomized On/Off Bypass (ROOBY) trial was a prospective RCT of CABG and OPCAB that involved 2203 patients at 18 Veterans Affairs medical centers. There was no difference in 30-day mortality or short-term major adverse cardiovascular events. The OPCAB patients received significantly fewer grafts per patient. One-year rates of cardiac-related death (8.8% versus 5.9%; $P = .01$) and major adverse events (9.9% versus 7.4%; $P = .04$) were significantly higher in the OPCAB group. Furthermore, graft patency was significantly lower in the OPCAB group (82.6% versus 87.8%; $P < .001$). The results did not differ when the operation was performed by a resident or attending physician or by a high- or low-volume surgeon. Critics noted that women were excluded from the study, and there were no data regarding low-density lipoprotein levels, the use of statins and aspirin, or whether glycemic control was practiced in these patients.

The Surgical Management of Arterial Revascularization Therapy (SMART) trial examined long-term survival and graft patency in a prospective RCT involving 297 patients who underwent isolated elective CABG or OPCAB. After 7.5 years of follow-up, there was no difference in mortality or late graft patency between OPCAB and on-pump CABG. Although recurrent angina was more common in the OPCAB group, this difference did not reach statistical significance. Hence, this study, performed by one of the world's experts in OPCAB surgery, could not demonstrate any superiority of OPCAB over on-pump CABG.

Another prospective study, the Coronary Artery Bypass Surgery Off or On Pump Revascularization Study (CORONARY) trial, involved 4752 patients randomly assigned to either CABG or OPCAB at 79 centers in 19 countries. There were no significant differences in the incidence of recurrent angina between the OPCAB (0.9%) and CABG (1.0%) groups, but the need for repeated revascularization was higher in the OPCAB group, and the difference approached statistical significance (1.4% OPCAB versus 0.8% CABG; $P = .07$).

The CORONARY trial included twice as many participants as the ROOBY trial. Each off-pump procedure was performed by an experienced surgeon who had more than 2 years of experience and had performed more than 100 OPCAB cases. Trainees were not allowed to be the primary surgeon. The rate of crossover from the off-pump to the on-pump group was lower in the CORONARY trial (7.9% versus 12.4%), suggesting a higher level of surgical expertise. Despite the improved technical experience of highly qualified off-pump surgeons, the need for revascularization remained higher in the off-pump group.

In the German Off-Pump Coronary Artery Bypass Grafts in Elderly Patients (GOPCADE) trial, patients aged 75 years and older scheduled for isolated bypass surgery were randomly assigned to on-pump or off-pump surgery. The trial was undertaken to attempt to define the potential benefits of OPCAB in an elderly group of high-risk patients with multiple comorbidities. The study involved 2539 patients from 12 centers. The primary end point was the composite of death or major adverse events (MI, cerebrovascular accident, acute renal failure requiring renal replacement therapy, or need for repeated revascularization) within 30 days and within 12 months after surgery. The secondary end points included operating room time, duration of mechanical ventilation, transfusion requirements, and ICU and hospital length of stay.

There was no difference in the primary composite end point (7.0% off-pump versus 8.0% on-pump; $P = .40$). However, additional revascularization procedures within 30 days were more frequent in the off-pump group (1.3% versus 0.3%; $P = .03$). Patients in the off-pump group were less likely to receive blood products; however, the study had no protocols to determine when transfusions should be given. There was no difference in any of the other secondary end points. The mean number of grafts was significantly lower in the off-pump group (2.7 versus 2.8; $P < .001$). The investigators concluded that OPCAB did not improve outcomes in these elderly high-risk patients. Furthermore, concerns were raised that the increased need for early repeated revascularization and the decreased number of grafts in the off-pump group would lead to an increased incidence of future cardiovascular events, thus exposing these elderly patients to increased morbidity and mortality.

These findings have dampened the enthusiasm for OPCAB at most centers. However, it is our practice to offer OPCAB to patients with single-vessel CAD in the LAD system.

The technique and operative strategy of OPCAB differ significantly from those of on-pump CABG. Certain adjuncts are needed to provide adequate exposure of the coronary vessels. Because the heart is fully contractile and maintaining systemic perfusion, the manipulation should proceed in a planned and systematic manner. Both the pleural spaces are opened to allow the heart to rotate into either side to allow the surgeon to visualize the targets, especially the lateral and inferior wall. The more critical areas of the myocardium are revascularized first, which minimizes ischemia time, improves myocardial reserve, and permits more complex manipulation of the heart for the other targets. Mammary artery–based pedicles are typically approached first because these do not require a proximal anastomosis, thus providing immediate coronary blood flow to the bypassed vessel.

Once the target vessel is selected, a small area of the coronary artery is exposed proximal and distal to the planned area of anastomosis to allow placement of vessel loops or bulldog clamps for proximal and distal control. A coronary occluder may also be used. Two stabilizers are used to stabilize the myocardium (Fig. 59-17). The fork-octopus has a suction padded tip and is attached to a multifunctional arm. The fork is positioned so that the limbs straddle the coronary target, and suction is applied, which attaches the device to the myocardium while the arm is secured in position. The other device consists of a suction cup that is applied to the apex of the heart and is used to lift it out of the chest to expose its posterior aspect. A sling attached to the posterior pericardium

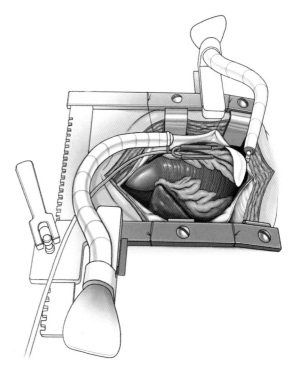

FIGURE 59-17 Off-pump coronary artery bypass with vacuum-assisted multiarticulating arms to position and to stabilize the myocardium. This minimizes the movement of the heart, allowing the surgeon to feasibly perform the distal anastomoses. Here, the stabilizer is positioned in preparation for creating a bypass to the left anterior descending artery.

allows the heart to be elevated out and enhances visualization of the posterior targets.

Full heparinization is not needed; in general, 50% of the usual dose is used. Success of the operation requires coordinated efforts between the surgeon and anesthesiologist so that adequate systemic perfusion is maintained throughout the operation while allowing a comfortable milieu in which the surgeon can operate. Short-acting beta blockers to slow the heart rate and alpha constrictors to maintain systemic perfusion pressures are important adjuncts for this procedure.

The postoperative management of OPCAB patients is significantly different from that of patients who undergo conventional CABG, primarily because of the reduced inflammatory effects, which are more prominent in patients who have undergone CPB. The OPCAB patients do not manifest the vasodilatory response or massive fluid shifts seen with CPB. Rather, these patients are more like those who have undergone major general surgery and require early deep venous thrombosis and balanced postoperative fluid management. In our practice, all patients who undergo OPCAB are given aspirin and clopidogrel (Plavix) on the day of surgery.

Minimally Invasive Direct Coronary Artery Bypass

Minimally invasive direct coronary artery bypass (MIDCAB) describes any technique of coronary artery bypass that uses a minimally invasive approach, such as an anterolateral thoracotomy (Fig. 59-18), ministernotomy, or subxiphoid approach, without the use of a robot. Most MIDCABs are performed on the beating heart and involve vascularization of the anterior wall.

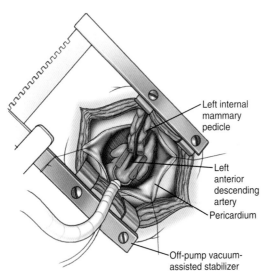

Left internal mammary pedicle

Left anterior descending artery

Pericardium

Off-pump vacuum-assisted stabilizer

FIGURE 59-18 Left thoracotomy approach for performing off-pump left internal mammary to left anterior descending bypass. This is commonly used in the minimally invasive direct coronary artery bypass (MIDCAB) approach. Multiarticulating stabilizers are essential for this technique.

A meta-analysis of all published outcome studies of MIDCAB grafting performed from January 1995 through October 2007 has revealed early and late (>30 days) death rates of 1.3% and 3.2%, respectively. Of the grafts that were studied angiographically immediately after surgery, 4.2% were occluded and 6.6% had a significant stenosis (50% to 99%). At 6-month follow-up, 3.6% were occluded and 7.2% had significant stenosis. Long-term follow-up results and further prospective RCTs comparing MIDCABs with standard revascularization procedures in large patient cohorts are needed. Although MIDCAB offers several advantages, such as the avoidance of sternotomy and CPB, it is subject to the same limitations as OPCAB in addition to its own technical challenges and limited revascularization territory.

Robotics: Totally Endoscopic Coronary Artery Bypass

With the popularity of robotic technology in other surgical specialties, robotic totally endoscopic coronary artery bypass (TECAB) has been in vogue for several years. Robotically assisted microsurgical systems have the theoretical advantage of enhancing surgical dexterity and minimizing the invasiveness of otherwise conventional coronary artery surgery. The da Vinci system (Intuitive Surgical, Mountain View, Calif) is the most commonly used system. It consists of three major components: surgeon-device interface module, computer controller, and specific patient interface instrumentation. It allows real-time surgical manipulation of tissue, advanced dexterity in multiple degrees of freedom, and optical magnification of the operative field, all through minimal access ports. The technology has seen significant use in valve repair operations and other surgical specialties as well.

With regard to coronary artery bypass, TECAB can be performed on-pump or totally off-pump, and multivessel TECAB is currently a reality. However, operating times and conversion rates are much higher with this technology. More important, it is technically more difficult and expensive, and it has a steep learning curve. Long-term data regarding its durability and safety are unavailable at this point.

In the largest TECAB series to date (about 500 cases), success and safety rates were 80% (n = 400) and 95% (n = 474), respectively. Intraoperative conversion to larger thoracic incisions was required in 49 (10%) patients. The median operative time was 305 minutes (range, 112-1050 minutes), and the mean lengths of stay in the ICU and in the hospital were 23 hours (range, 11-1048 hours) and 6 days (range, 2-4 days), respectively. Independent predictors of success were single-vessel TECAB (P = .004), arrested-heart TECAB (P = .027), non–learning curve case (P = .049), and transthoracic assistance (P = .035). The only independent predictor of safety was EuroSCORE (P = .002). Interestingly, the mean time per anastomosis was 27 minutes (range, 10-100 minutes), which is significantly longer than an average surgeon would take to accomplish an open anastomosis (i.e., well below 10 minutes per anastomosis). Also, the LIMA injury rate was high (n = 24; 5%).[65] All these data point to less than perfect procedures and technology that require further development before they can replace open CABG, which has an excellent track record and is an elegant, fast, and reproducible procedure.

The current limitations of robotic TECAB include its lack of applicability to all patients, prolonged operating room time, limited access to all vessels, cost, and limited training opportunities. However, over time, robotic surgery is likely to become a niche specialty for a subset of surgeons who treat a specific population of patients.

Transmyocardial Laser Revascularization

Patients with chronic, severe angina refractory to medical therapy who cannot be completely revascularized with percutaneous catheter intervention or CABG present clinical challenges. Transmyocardial laser revascularization (TMLR), either as sole therapy or as an adjunct to CABG surgery, may be appropriate for some of these patients. The STS Evidence-Based Workforce has reviewed available evidence and recommends the use of TMLR for patients with an LVEF greater than 0.30 and Canadian Cardiovascular Society class III or class IV angina that is refractory to maximal medical therapy. These patients should have reversible ischemia of the LV free wall and CAD corresponding to the regions of myocardial ischemia. In all regions of the myocardium, the CAD must not be amenable to CABG or PCI.

The TMLR procedure uses a high-energy laser beam to create myocardial transmural channels that were originally thought to provide direct access to oxygenated blood in the LV cavity. This is no longer considered to be the mechanism whereby TMLR reduces the symptoms of IHD. Although some local neovascularization has been documented, the magnitude of changes does not account for any substantive increases in myocardial perfusion. One mechanism that has been proposed relates to a local effect on cardiac neuronal signaling. It has been hypothesized that local tissue injury by TMLR damages ventricular sensory neurons and autonomic efferent axons, which leads to local cardiac denervation and anginal relief. Regardless of the mechanism, TMLR therapy is associated with a reproducible improvement in symptoms. Patients who undergo TMLR show a persistent improvement in Canadian Cardiovascular Society angina class. This improvement is observed in 60% to 80% of patients within 6 months after the operation.

Hybrid Procedures

It is generally accepted that the LIMA to LAD anastomosis is the single most important component of CABG and confers long-term benefits unmatched by those of any other intervention. State-of-the-art PCIs with DES have produced outcomes competitive with those of vein grafts to non-LAD targets. This has led to an integrated approach to coronary revascularization, termed the hybrid procedure. The hybrid procedure consists of a minimally invasive LIMA to LAD anastomosis in conjunction with PCI of non–LAD-obstructed coronary arteries.

This approach has met with initial success, but many potential pitfalls exist. The procedural costs may be greater than those of either CABG or DES implantation alone. The timing and staging of the procedures are uncertain, and limited data are available on long-term outcomes.

Technical Aspects of Reoperative Coronary Artery Bypass Grafting

Within 5 years, 15% of CABG patients experience a recurrence of symptoms, typically angina. This increases to approximately 40% within 10 years. Recurrent symptoms almost always indicate either progression of disease in the native coronary circulation or graft disease. In most cases, the indications for coronary angiography, PCI with or without stenting, or repeated CABG are the same as for the first operation. Patients who are considered candidates for reoperative CABG are usually older, have more diffuse CAD, and have diminished ventricular function. Factors that increase the risk for reoperation include the absence of an IMA graft, younger age at the time of the index operation, prior incomplete revascularization, CHF, and New York Heart Association class III or class IV angina.

The technical aspects of reoperative CABG differ significantly from those of the index procedure. Reentry into the chest and dissection of the old grafts are sometimes challenging. Preparation for femoral cannulation for femorofemoral bypass or axillary cannulation should be considered with preemptive availability of blood products. Redo sternotomy is typically completed with an oscillating saw or after the heart is dissected away from the sternum through a subxiphoid approach. Injury to the right ventricle or to the aorta or vein grafts is of potential concern. A poorly placed LIMA graft from the prior operation is also at risk during the sternotomy. If a cardiac or vascular injury is identified, an assistant holds the sternum together to prevent further bleeding, and expeditious cannulation of alternative sites is begun with the institution of CPB. Preoperative CT scans are helpful in planning the operation.

Once the sternotomy is completed, the rest of the adherent cardiac structures are dissected away from the underside of the sternum to allow placement of a sternal retractor. No retractor should be placed unless the heart is adequately dissected away; this will result in disruption of the aorta or right ventricle, which may be difficult to control.

The next steps are geared toward establishing sites for cannulation. The right atrium and aorta are dissected first; then, the rest of the heart is dissected away from the pericardium, which may be performed on CPB. The areas of previous cannulation and vein grafts are the most adherent regions, whereas the diaphragmatic aspect is least adherent and provides a good starting point to gain entry into the correct plane.

Manipulation of the old grafts should be kept to a minimum to avoid distal coronary bed microembolization. Isolation of the LIMA pedicle is often necessary and should be carefully performed, with the ability to start bypass rapidly if an inadvertent injury occurs (Fig. 59-19). The rest of the operation proceeds in

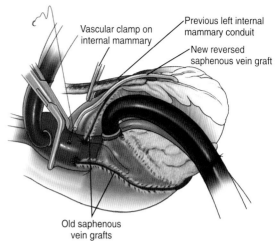

FIGURE 59-19 Redo Coronary Artery Bypass Grafting. The cannulation is similar to that used in a first-time coronary artery bypass operation in most cases. However, identification of coronary targets is much more difficult because of scarring. The course of the prior grafts is useful in identifying the targets. In addition to clamping of the aorta above the previous vein grafts, the left internal mammary pedicle should be dissected and clamped separately, if feasible. A single-clamp technique is preferred because it avoids the tedious and potentially dangerous dissection around the proximal aorta that may be needed to place a partial side-biting clamp.

a similar fashion to primary CABG and can be performed on-pump or off-pump. In some cases, the procedure can be performed through a left anterolateral thoracotomy approach. Typically, this approach is used in patients with previous mediastinitis or multiple sternotomies or when an extensive area of the heart is adherent to the sternum, precluding a safe entry. The vein conduit is anastomosed to the descending aorta in these cases (Fig. 59-20).

To summarize, some of the unique difficulties that can be encountered in redo CABG are as follows:
- Injury to heart during sternotomy
- Injury to mammary pedicle
- Limited space on ascending aorta for placement of new grafts
- Inability to identify distal targets because of scars and adhesions
- Limited availability of conduits
- Increased risk of perioperative MI because atheroembolic embolization from diseased vein grafts and diffuse CAD preclude optimal cardioplegia
- Increased bleeding because of higher inflammatory response and more raw surface
- Injury to pulmonary artery during cross-clamping of the aorta

In most published series, the mortality rate of reoperative CABG patients exceeds that of primary CABG patients.

MECHANICAL COMPLICATIONS OF CORONARY ARTERY DISEASE

Left Ventricular Aneurysm

The incidence of ventricular aneurysm after AMI has been declining because of early interventional therapies. Of LV aneurysms, 90% are the result of a transmural MI secondary to an acute

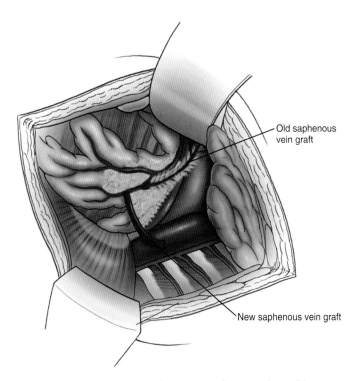

Old saphenous
vein graft

New saphenous vein graft

FIGURE 59-20 **Left Thoracotomy Approach for Recurrent Coronary Artery Disease.** This approach avoids the hazards of a difficult redo sternotomy and is used as an alternative in some cases. New saphenous vein graft: descending thoracic aorta to obtuse marginal bypass.

occlusion of the LAD. Patients may develop an aneurysm (pseudoaneurysm) as early as 48 hours after infarction, but most patients develop one within weeks. Approximately two thirds of patients who develop ventricular aneurysms remain asymptomatic.

The 10-year survival rate is 90% for asymptomatic patients and 50% for symptomatic patients. The most common causes of death are arrhythmias (>40%), CHF (>30%), and recurrent MI (>10%). The risk of thromboembolism is low, so long-term anticoagulation is not recommended unless there is a mural thrombus. The diagnosis is usually made by echocardiography. Thallium imaging or PET is useful for determining the extent of the aneurysm and viability of adjacent regions.

Surgery for LV aneurysm is indicated if the patient is scheduled to undergo CABG for symptomatic CAD, there is contained rupture or evidence of a false aneurysm, or the patient has a thromboembolic event despite anticoagulation. The 5-year postoperative survival rate has been reported to range between 60% and 80%. In general, surgical repair or resection in conjunction with CABG results in angina relief and resolution of heart failure symptoms for most patients.

Surgical ventricular restoration is a technical term that describes the surgical resection of the aneurysm and reconstruction of the native ventricular geometric shape. This is ideally performed with CPB and without cardioplegic arrest, as long as the aortic valve is competent. The aneurysm is usually recognized by the paradoxical movement of the walls compared with the rest of the viable LV myocardium. The aneurysm is opened, and a purse-string Fontan stitch is placed at the junction of the viable and nonviable myocardium, which can be manually palpated on the beating heart. A Dacron or bovine pericardial patch is used to exclude the aneurysm, and the aneurysm is closed over the patch. Two

potentially acute complications that require surgical intervention are postinfarction VSD and postinfarction mitral regurgitation caused by papillary muscle rupture.

Ventricular Septal Defect

This occurs in less than 1% of patients and is associated with acute LAD occlusion. The defect is more common in men than in women (3:2) and typically is manifested within 2 to 4 days of the infarction. However, a VSD that occurs in the first 6 weeks after an infarct is still considered acute. The VSD is usually located in the anterior or apical aspect of the ventricular septum. Approximately 25% of affected patients have a posterior VSD caused by an inferior wall MI due to occlusion of the RCA system or a distal branch LCA. A full-thickness infarct is a prerequisite for VSD formation. A new, loud, systolic cardiac murmur after an MI suggests the diagnosis; echocardiography is effective for determining the size and character of the VSD as well as the degree of left-to-right shunting. Right-sided heart catheterization typically shows an increase in oxygen saturation levels in the right ventricle and pulmonary artery. The defect is usually approximately 1 to 2 cm in size.

After the diagnosis is established, patients should undergo immediate left-sided heart catheterization to characterize the degree of CAD and the magnitude of LV dysfunction and to detect any mitral valve insufficiency. Approximately 60% of patients with an infarction VSD have significant CAD in an unrelated vessel. The mortality rate in untreated patients is high; 25% of patients die within 24 hours of refractory heart failure. Survival rates of patients at 1 week, 1 month, and longer than 1 year are 50%, 20%, and less than 3%, respectively.

Patients who are considered candidates for surgery should be treated early with closure of the defect and concomitant CABG.

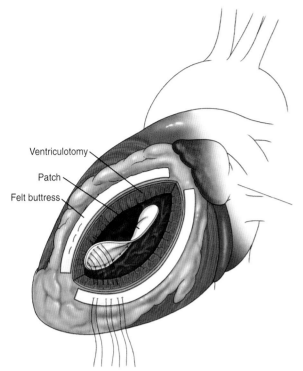

FIGURE 59-21 Infarct exclusion technique for repair of acute ventricular septal defect secondary to acute myocardial infarction. A ventriculotomy is made through the zone of infarct, and all necrotic muscle is débrided. The repair is accomplished with a patch placed on the left ventricular aspect of the septum. Felt buttresses are used to reinforce the closure of the ventriculotomy, and it is essential that all sutures be incorporated into healthy myocardium to ensure durability of the repair.

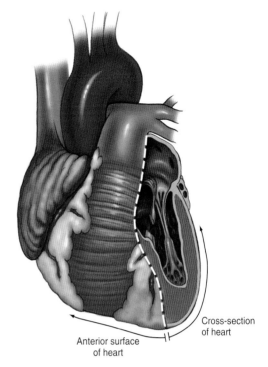

FIGURE 59-22 Mechanical Complication of Acute Myocardial Infarction. Acute papillary muscle rupture (shown here) and acute ventricular septal defect are two sequelae in a patient with extensive zones of infarct. Acute papillary muscle rupture results in acute mitral regurgitation that is manifested as cardiogenic shock and immediate pulmonary decompensation. If the patient is a surgical candidate, mitral valve replacement is the only option.

In the absence of refractory heart failure and hemodynamic instability, the survival rate may be as high as 75%. The infarct exclusion technique is used to repair the VSD and is one of the most technically challenging procedures. The LV is opened longitudinally on the infarct, and the defect is evaluated. Multiple VSDs may be present, and necrotic myocardium is débrided to viable tissue. A prosthetic Dacron patch or bovine pericardium is then sutured to the LV side of the septal defect and brought out through the ventriculotomy, where it is incorporated into the closure (Fig. 59-21). In this method, the posterior aspect of the patch is thus anchored to the remnant viable septum, and the anterior aspect is incorporated with the free ventricular wall, forming the neo–interventricular septum. Felt strips are used to buttress the closure.

In addition to the traditional repair of postinfarction VSD, there has been recent enthusiasm about transcatheter closure of postinfarction VSD. This obviates a pump run in an otherwise tenuous patient. In both the patients treated surgically and with transcatheter closure, temporary circulatory support in the form of extracorporeal membrane oxygenation or ventricular assist device can be lifesaving.

Mitral Regurgitation

Approximately 40% of patients who sustain an AMI develop chronic ischemic mitral regurgitation (IMR) detectable by color flow Doppler echocardiography. In 3% to 4% of cases, the degree of mitral regurgitation is moderate or severe.

The cause of chronic IMR is ischemic papillary muscle dysfunction and LV dilation associated with mitral annular dilation and restriction of the posterior leaflet. The operation for chronic IMR is usually performed on an elective basis. It consists of complete myocardial revascularization and mitral valve repair with the use of an annuloplasty ring.

Acute IMR may result from papillary muscle necrosis and rupture caused by occlusion of the overlying epicardial arteries that give rise to the penetrating vessels that supply the papillary muscles. The posterior papillary muscle is involved three to six times more often than the anterior muscle (Fig. 59-22), and either the entire trunk of the muscle or one of the heads to which chordae attach may rupture partially or totally.

In most cases, prompt surgical intervention provides the best chance for survival. Predictors of in-hospital death include CHF, renal insufficiency, and multivessel CAD. Emergent surgical treatment usually involves mitral valve replacement and concomitant CABG. The hospital mortality rate may be as high as 50% in acute cases. Mitral repair should not be attempted in such cases because it may not be feasible in papillary muscle rupture; it requires prolonging the cross-clamp time (compared with replacement), which is not ideal in acute cases. Operations on patients with acute mechanical complications from MI are challenging; the surgeon has to anticipate and be prepared for placement of an LV assist device if the patient cannot be separated from CPB (Fig. 59-23).

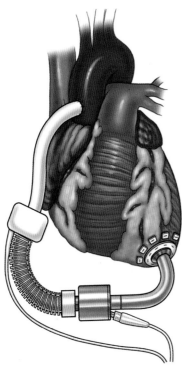

FIGURE 59-23 An axial flow left ventricular assist device, which can be used as temporary mechanical support or a bridge to transplantation for a patient in end-stage cardiomyopathy due to coronary artery disease not amenable to bypass surgery. The inflow of blood into the pump is from the apex of the left ventricle. The blood is then pumped into the ascending aorta through specially designed grafts that are incorporated into the pump. The axial flow pumps are less bulky and relatively easy to implant. They have only a single moving part, which is the axial impeller.

CORONARY ARTERY BYPASS GRAFTING AND SPECIAL POPULATIONS OF PATIENTS

Patients With Diabetes

Mortality and morbidity rates after CABG are higher in diabetic patients than in the general population. The BARI trial showed that diabetic patients with multivessel disease benefit more from CABG than from any other treatment. Similarly, the FREEDOM trial also demonstrated superiority of CABG over PCI.

Older Patients

Approximately 10% of patients who undergo CABG are older than 80 years. Older age is an independent predictor of surgical morbidity and mortality and a nonroutine discharge status. Although CABG should not be denied to patients on the basis of age alone, it should be considered during risk assessment. Appropriate arrangements should be made beforehand with the expectation that only one in five postoperative patients will be able to go home without additional support.

Women

Although women in every age group have a lower incidence of CAD than men, CAD is still the leading cause of death in women in the United States. Historically, serious manifestations and associated complications of CAD in women were considered

uncommon. Examination of the STS database in two separate studies has revealed that the operative mortality rate is higher in women, 3.15% versus 2.61% in men.

With evolving strategies, studies have been designed to evaluate specific aspects of coronary artery bypass that would benefit women. For example, OPCAB has produced favorable outcomes in women. A review of 42,477 patients in the STS National Cardiac Database revealed that women have a significantly greater adjusted risk of death and prolonged ventilation and longer length of stay than do men who undergo on-pump CABG. In contrast, among OPCAB cases, women had a lower risk of reexploration than men did and a similar risk of death, MI, and prolonged ventilation and hospital stay.

Patients With Renal Disease

Renal insufficiency is also an independent risk factor for mortality after CABG. A preoperative serum creatinine level higher than 1.4 to 2.5 mg/dL is independently associated with a twofold increase in mortality. In a retrospective study of 59,576 patients who underwent CABG or PCI, CABG had a survival benefit in patients with a serum creatinine level higher than 2.5 mg/dL. The 1-, 2-, and 3-year survival rates were 84.1%, 77.4%, and 65.9%, respectively, for CABG compared with 70.8%, 51.9%, and 46.1% for PCI. This effect was more dramatic in diabetic patients. Long-term survival is also affected by preoperative renal dysfunction, especially if the patient's creatinine clearance is less than 30 mL/min. Although CABG in patients with renal insufficiency or failure is associated with increased morbidity and mortality, CABG is nonetheless associated with better survival than PCI in such patients.

Obese Patients

The incidence of postoperative renal failure, prolonged ventilation, and sternal wound infection is significantly higher in obese patients than in normal-weight patients. Both extremes of weight are risk factors for CABG-related mortality.

ACKNOWLEDGMENTS

We would like to acknowledge Scott Weldon and Michael DeLaflor for graphic services, Johnny Airheart for photographic support, Dr. Chinnapapu Muthusamy for assistance with review questions, and Dr. Stephen N. Palmer for editorial assistance.

SELECTED REFERENCES

Chu D, Bakaeen FG, Dao TK, et al: On-pump versus off-pump coronary artery bypass grafting in a cohort of 63,000 patients. *Ann Thorac Surg* 87:1820–1826, 2009.

> This study was a nationwide comparison of on-pump versus off-pump coronary artery bypass surgery in the United States. The study highlighted the fact that off-pump coronary artery bypass does not produce lower postoperative mortality or stroke rates than conventional on-pump coronary artery bypass. Furthermore, off-pump coronary artery bypass was associated with longer hospital stays and higher hospital costs.

Edwards FH, Carey JS, Grover FL, et al: Impact of gender on coronary bypass operative mortality. *Ann Thorac Surg* 66:125–131, 1998.

This study analyzed the outcomes of more than 300,000 patients from the Society of Thoracic Surgeons database and used multivariate analysis and risk model stratification to examine the outcomes of female patients. Female gender was shown to be an independent predictor of higher mortality in low- to moderate-risk patients but not in high-risk patients.

Influence of diabetes on 5-year mortality and morbidity in a randomized trial comparing CABG and PTCA in patients with multivessel disease: The Bypass Angioplasty Revascularization Investigation (BARI). *Circulation* 96:1761–1769, 1997.

Follow-up results from the initial randomized controlled trial established that patients with treated diabetes mellitus who were assigned to undergo CABG had a striking reduction in mortality compared with patients who underwent percutaneous transluminal coronary angioplasty. This benefit was attributed predominantly to the use of the left internal mammary artery conduit in CABG.

Loop FD, Lytle BW, Cosgrove DM, et al: Influence of the internal-mammary-artery graft on 10-year survival and other cardiac events. *N Engl J Med* 314:1–6, 1986.

This retrospective study of 5931 CABG patients operated on at a single institution compared the outcomes of patients who had an internal mammary artery graft with those of patients who had only vein grafts. The findings of this landmark study established the superiority of the internal mammary artery over any other conduit. During a 10-year period, patients who had only vein grafts had a 1.6 times higher risk of mortality than those who had mammary grafts.

Lopes RD, Hafley GE, Allen KB, et al: Endoscopic versus open vein-graft harvesting in coronary-artery bypass surgery. *N Engl J Med* 361:235–244, 2009.

This retrospective study evaluated the effects of endoscopic vein harvesting on the rate of vein graft failure and on clinical outcomes. Endoscopic vein harvesting was shown to be independently associated with vein graft failure and adverse clinical outcomes compared with open vein harvesting.

Parisi AF, Khuri S, Deupree RH, et al: Medical compared with surgical management of unstable angina: 5-year mortality and morbidity in the Veterans Administration Study. *Circulation* 80:1176–1189, 1989.

This prospective, multicenter Veterans Administration randomized controlled trial compared surgical and medical management and established that for patients with triple-vessel coronary disease, surgical intervention better promotes survival than medical management.

Peduzzi P, Kamina A, Detre K: Twenty-two-year follow-up in the VA Cooperative Study of Coronary Artery Bypass Surgery for Stable Angina. *Am J Cardiol* 81:1393–1399, 1998.

This study compared the 22-year results of initial CABG surgery with saphenous vein grafts with those of initial

medical therapy with regard to survival, the incidences of myocardial infarction and reoperation, and symptomatic status in 686 patients with stable angina who participated in the Veterans Affairs Cooperative Study of Coronary Artery Bypass Surgery. This trial provided strong evidence that initial bypass surgery did not improve survival for low-risk patients and did not reduce the overall risk of myocardial infarction. The early survival benefit with surgery in high-risk patients did not translate to comparable long-term survival rates for both treatment groups.

Serruys PW, Morice MC, Kappetein AP, et al: Percutaneous coronary intervention versus coronary-artery bypass grafting for severe coronary artery disease. *N Engl J Med* 360:961–972, 2009.

This was a landmark contemporary study of PCI with drug-eluting stents versus CABG. The primary end point was a major adverse cardiac or cerebrovascular event (i.e., death from any cause, stroke, myocardial infarction, or repeated revascularization) during the 12-month period after randomization. Rates of major adverse cardiac or cerebrovascular events at 12 months were significantly higher in the PCI group (17.8% versus 12.4% for CABG; P = .002), in large part because of an increased rate of repeated revascularization (13.5% versus 5.9%; P < .001); as a result, the criterion for noninferiority was not met. At 12 months, the rates of death and myocardial infarction were similar between the two groups; stroke was significantly more likely to occur with CABG (2.2% versus 0.6% with PCI; P = .003). The investigators concluded that CABG remains the standard of care for patients with three-vessel or left coronary artery disease because the use of CABG, compared with PCI, resulted in lower rates of the combined end point of major adverse cardiac or cerebrovascular events at 1 year.

Serruys PW, Ong AT, van Herwerden LA, et al: Five-year outcomes after coronary stenting versus bypass surgery for the treatment of multivessel disease: The final analysis of the Arterial Revascularization Therapies Study (ARTS) randomized trial. *J Am Coll Cardiol* 46:575–581, 2005.

The final results of the ARTS were summarized and showed that the overall rate of major adverse cardiac and cerebrovascular events was higher in patients who underwent coronary artery stenting than in CABG patients. This difference was driven by the increased need for repeated revascularization in the stent group.

Shroyer AL, Grover FL, Hattler B, et al: On-pump versus off-pump coronary-artery bypass surgery. *N Engl J Med* 361:1827–1837, 2009.

This study was a randomized, multicenter Veterans Affairs trial that compared conventional CABG with off-pump coronary artery bypass (OPCAB) in 2203 patients. The primary end point was a composite of death from any cause, repeated revascularization, or nonfatal myocardial infarction within 1 year after surgery. At 1-year follow-up, the OPCAB patients had worse composite outcomes and poorer graft patency. The presumed benefit of fewer neuropsychological adverse outcomes was not found in OPCAB patients.

White HD, Assmann SF, Sanborn TA, et al: Comparison of percutaneous coronary intervention and coronary artery bypass grafting after acute myocardial infarction complicated by cardiogenic shock: Results from the Should We Emergently Revascularize Occluded Coronaries for Cardiogenic Shock (SHOCK) trial. *Circulation* 112:1992–2001, 2005.

> *This randomized controlled trial was designed to compare CABG surgery with PCI in patients who presented with cardiogenic shock. The trial evaluated 30-day and 1-year mortality and found comparable results between the two groups, even though the CABG patients had a higher prevalence of diabetes and worse coronary artery disease preoperatively.*

REFERENCES

1. Lloyd-Jones D, Adams RJ, Brown TM, et al: Executive summary: Heart disease and stroke statistics—2010 update: A report from the American Heart Association. *Circulation* 121:948–954, 2010.
2. Ford ES, Capewell S: Coronary heart disease mortality among young adults in the U.S. from 1980 through 2002: Concealed leveling of mortality rates. *J Am Coll Cardiol* 50:2128–2132, 2007.
3. Murphy SL, Xu J, Kochanek K: Deaths: Preliminary data for 2010. *Natl Vital Stat Rep* 60:1–52, 2012.
4. Maycock A, Muhlestein JB, Horne BD, et al: Statin therapy is associated with reduced mortality across all age groups of individuals with significant coronary disease, including very elderly patients. *J Am Coll Cardiol* 40:1777–1785, 2002.
5. de Winter RJ, Windhausen F, Cornel JH, et al: Early invasive versus selectively invasive management for acute coronary syndromes. *N Engl J Medicine* 353:1095–1104, 2005.
6. Jneid H, Anderson JL, Wright RS, et al: 2012 ACCF/AHA focused update of the guideline for the management of patients with unstable angina/non-ST-elevation myocardial infarction (updating the 2007 guideline and replacing the 2011 focused update): A report of the American College of Cardiology Foundation/American Heart Association Task Force on Practice Guidelines. *J Am Coll Cardiol* 60:645–681, 2012.
7. Pepine CJ, Balaban RS, Bonow RO, et al: Women's Ischemic Syndrome Evaluation: Current status and future research directions: Report of the National Heart, Lung and Blood Institute workshop: October 2-4, 2002: Section 1: Diagnosis of stable ischemia and ischemic heart disease. *Circulation* 109:e44–e46, 2004.
8. Daly C, Norrie J, Murdoch DL, et al: The value of routine non-invasive tests to predict clinical outcome in stable angina. *Eur Heart J* 24:532–540, 2003.
9. Daly CA, De Stavola B, Sendon JL, et al: Predicting prognosis in stable angina—results from the Euro heart survey of stable angina: Prospective observational study. *BMJ* 332:262–267, 2006.
10. Hammermeister KE, DeRouen TA, Dodge HT: Variables predictive of survival in patients with coronary disease. Selection by univariate and multivariate analyses from the clinical, electrocardiographic, exercise, arteriographic, and quantitative angiographic evaluations. *Circulation* 59:421–430, 1979.
11. Kwok Y, Kim C, Grady D, et al: Meta-analysis of exercise testing to detect coronary artery disease in women. *Am J Cardiol* 83:660–666, 1999.
12. Shaw LJ, Mieres JH, Hendel RH, et al: Comparative effectiveness of exercise electrocardiography with or without myocardial perfusion single photon emission computed tomography in women with suspected coronary artery disease: Results from the What Is the Optimal Method for Ischemia Evaluation in Women (WOMEN) trial. *Circulation* 124:1239–1249, 2011.
13. Imran MB, Palinkas A, Picano E: Head-to-head comparison of dipyridamole echocardiography and stress perfusion scintigraphy for the detection of coronary artery disease: A meta-analysis. Comparison between stress echo and scintigraphy. *Int J Cardiovasc Imaging* 19:23–28, 2003.
14. Marcassa C, Bax JJ, Bengel F, et al: Clinical value, cost-effectiveness, and safety of myocardial perfusion scintigraphy: A position statement. *Eur Heart J* 29:557–563, 2008.
15. Fleischmann KE, Hunink MG, Kuntz KM, et al: Exercise echocardiography or exercise SPECT imaging? A meta-analysis of diagnostic test performance. *JAMA* 280:913–920, 1998.
16. Sabharwal NK, Stoykova B, Taneja AK, et al: A randomized trial of exercise treadmill ECG versus stress SPECT myocardial perfusion imaging as an initial diagnostic strategy in stable patients with chest pain and suspected CAD: Cost analysis. *J Nucl Cardiol* 14:174–186, 2007.
17. Underwood SR, Anagnostopoulos C, Cerqueira M, et al: Myocardial perfusion scintigraphy: The evidence. *Eur J Nucl Med Mol Imaging* 31:261–291, 2004.
18. Badran HM, Elnoamany MF, Seteha M: Tissue velocity imaging with dobutamine stress echocardiography—a quantitative technique for identification of coronary artery disease in patients with left bundle branch block. *J Am Soc Echocardiogr* 20:820–831, 2007.
19. Leischik R, Dworrak B, Littwitz H, et al: Prognostic significance of exercise stress echocardiography in 3329 outpatients (5-year longitudinal study). *Int J Cardiol* 119:297–305, 2007.
20. Levy D, Garrison RJ, Savage DD, et al: Prognostic implications of echocardiographically determined left ventricular mass in the Framingham Heart Study. *N Engl J Med* 322:1561–1566, 1990.
21. Mark DB, Berman DS, Budoff MJ, et al: ACCF/ACR/AHA/NASCI/SAIP/SCAI/SCCT 2010 expert consensus document on coronary computed tomographic angiography: A report of the American College of Cardiology Foundation Task Force on Expert Consensus Documents. *Catheter Cardiovasc Interv* 76:E1–E42, 2010.
22. Budoff MJ, Dowe D, Jollis JG, et al: Diagnostic performance of 64-multidetector row coronary computed tomographic angiography for evaluation of coronary artery stenosis in individuals without known coronary artery disease: Results from the prospective multicenter ACCURACY (Assessment by Coronary Computed Tomographic Angiography of Individuals Undergoing Invasive Coronary Angiography) trial. *J Am Coll Cardiol* 52:1724–1732, 2008.
23. Hamon M, Biondi-Zoccai GG, Malagutti P, et al: Diagnostic performance of multislice spiral computed tomography of coronary arteries as compared with conventional invasive coronary angiography: A meta-analysis. *J Am Coll Cardiol* 48:1896–1910, 2006.

24. Janne d'Othee B, Siebert U, Cury R, et al: A systematic review on diagnostic accuracy of CT-based detection of significant coronary artery disease. *Eur J Radiol* 65:449–461, 2008.

25. Meijboom WB, Meijs MF, Schuijf JD, et al: Diagnostic accuracy of 64-slice computed tomography coronary angiography: A prospective, multicenter, multivendor study. *J Am Coll Cardiol* 52:2135–2144, 2008.

26. Miller JM, Rochitte CE, Dewey M, et al: Diagnostic performance of coronary angiography by 64-row CT. *N Engl J Med* 359:2324–2336, 2008.

27. Schuijf JD, Bax JJ, Shaw LJ, et al: Meta-analysis of comparative diagnostic performance of magnetic resonance imaging and multislice computed tomography for noninvasive coronary angiography. *Am Heart J* 151:404–411, 2006.

28. Stein PD, Beemath A, Kayali F, et al: Multidetector computed tomography for the diagnosis of coronary artery disease: A systematic review. *Am J Med* 119:203–216, 2006.

29. Motoyama S, Sarai M, Harigaya H, et al: Computed tomographic angiography characteristics of atherosclerotic plaques subsequently resulting in acute coronary syndrome. *J Am Coll Cardiol* 54:49–57, 2009.

30. Shmilovich H, Cheng VY, Tamarappoo BK, et al: Vulnerable plaque features on coronary CT angiography as markers of inducible regional myocardial hypoperfusion from severe coronary artery stenoses. *Atherosclerosis* 219:588–595, 2011.

31. Ambrose JA, Tannenbaum MA, Alexopoulos D, et al: Angiographic progression of coronary artery disease and the development of myocardial infarction. *J Am Coll Cardiol* 12:56–62, 1988.

32. Little WC, Constantinescu M, Applegate RJ, et al: Can coronary angiography predict the site of a subsequent myocardial infarction in patients with mild-to-moderate coronary artery disease? *Circulation* 78:1157–1166, 1988.

33. Eleven-year survival in the Veterans Administration randomized trial of coronary bypass surgery for stable angina. The Veterans Administration Coronary Artery Bypass Surgery Cooperative Study Group. *N Engl J Med* 311:1333–1339, 1984.

34. Ringqvist I, Fisher LD, Mock M, et al: Prognostic value of angiographic indices of coronary artery disease from the Coronary Artery Surgery Study (CASS). *J Clin Invest* 71:1854–1866, 1983.

35. Passamani E, Davis KB, Gillespie MJ, et al: A randomized trial of coronary artery bypass surgery. Survival of patients with a low ejection fraction. *N Engl J Med* 312:1665–1671, 1985.

36. Yusuf S, Zucker D, Peduzzi P, et al: Effect of coronary artery bypass graft surgery on survival: Overview of 10-year results from randomised trials by the Coronary Artery Bypass Graft Surgery Trialists Collaboration. *Lancet* 344:563–570, 1994.

37. Hueb W, Lopes N, Gersh BJ, et al: Ten-year follow-up survival of the Medicine, Angioplasty, or Surgery Study (MASS II): A randomized controlled clinical trial of 3 therapeutic strategies for multivessel coronary artery disease. *Circulation* 122:949–957, 2010.

38. Brophy JM, Belisle P, Joseph L: Evidence for use of coronary stents. A hierarchical bayesian meta-analysis. *Ann Intern Med* 138:777–786, 2003.

39. Trikalinos TA, Alsheikh-Ali AA, Tatsioni A, et al: Percutaneous coronary interventions for non-acute coronary artery disease: A quantitative 20-year synopsis and a network meta-analysis. *Lancet* 373:911–918, 2009.

40. Kastrati A, Mehilli J, Pache J, et al: Analysis of 14 trials comparing sirolimus-eluting stents with bare-metal stents. *N Engl J Med* 356:1030–1039, 2007.

41. Bravata DM, Gienger AL, McDonald KM, et al: Systematic review: The comparative effectiveness of percutaneous coronary interventions and coronary artery bypass graft surgery. *Ann Intern Med* 147:703–716, 2007.

42. Serruys PW, Morice MC, Kappetein AP, et al: Percutaneous coronary intervention versus coronary-artery bypass grafting for severe coronary artery disease. *N Engl J Med* 360:961–972, 2009.

43. Buszman PE, Kiesz SR, Bochenek A, et al: Acute and late outcomes of unprotected left main stenting in comparison with surgical revascularization. *J Am Coll Cardiol* 51:538–545, 2008.

44. VA Coronary Artery Bypass Surgery Cooperative Study Group: Eighteen-year follow-up in the Veterans Affairs Cooperative Study of Coronary Artery Bypass Surgery for stable angina. *Circulation* 86:121–130, 1992.

45. Varnauskas E: Twelve-year follow-up of survival in the randomized European Coronary Surgery Study. *N Engl J Med* 319:332–337, 1988.

45a. Fihn SD, Gardin JM, Abrams J, et al: 2012 ACCF/AHA/ACP/AATS/PCNA/SCAI/STS guideline for the diagnosis and management of patients with stable ischemic heart disease: a report of the American College of Cardiology Foundation/American Heart Association Task Force on practice guidelines, and the American College of Physicians, American Association for Thoracic Surgery, Preventive Cardiovascular Nurses Association, Society for Cardiovascular Angiography and Interventions, and Society of Thoracic Surgeons. *Circulation* 126:e354–e471, 2012.

46. Antman EM, Hand M, Armstrong PW, et al: 2007 Focused update of the ACC/AHA 2004 guidelines for the management of patients with ST-elevation myocardial infarction: A report of the American College of Cardiology/American Heart Association Task Force on Practice Guidelines: Developed in collaboration with the Canadian Cardiovascular Society endorsed by the American Academy of Family Physicians: 2007 Writing Group to review new evidence and update the ACC/AHA 2004 guidelines for the management of patients with ST-elevation myocardial infarction, writing on behalf of the 2004 Writing Committee. *Circulation* 117:296–329, 2008.

47. Chieffo A, Park SJ, Valgimigli M, et al: Favorable long-term outcome after drug-eluting stent implantation in nonbifurcation lesions that involve unprotected left main coronary artery: A multicenter registry. *Circulation* 116:158–162, 2007.

48. Lee MS, Bokhoor P, Park SJ, et al: Unprotected left main coronary disease and ST-segment elevation myocardial infarction: A contemporary review and argument for percutaneous coronary intervention. *JACC Cardiovasc Interv* 3:791–795, 2010.

49. Jones EL, Craver JM, Guyton RA, et al: Importance of complete revascularization in performance of the coronary bypass operation. *Am J Cardiol* 51:7–12, 1983.

50. Omer S, Cornwell LD, Rosengart TK, et al: Completeness of coronary revascularization and survival: Impact of age and off-pump surgery. *J Thorac Cardiovasc Surg* 148:1307–1315.e1, 2014.

51. Bonow RO, Maurer G, Lee KL, et al: Myocardial viability and survival in ischemic left ventricular dysfunction. *N Engl J Med* 364:1617–1625, 2011.

52. Velazquez EJ, Lee KL, Deja MA, et al: Coronary-artery bypass surgery in patients with left ventricular dysfunction. *N Engl J Med* 364:1607–1616, 2011.

53. Subramanian S, Sabik JF, 3rd, Houghtaling PL, et al: Decision-making for patients with patent left internal thoracic artery grafts to left anterior descending. *Ann Thorac Surg* 87:1392–1398, discussion 1400, 2009.

54. Choudhry NK, Singh JM, Barolet A, et al: How should patients with unstable angina and non-ST-segment elevation myocardial infarction be managed? A meta-analysis of randomized trials. *Am J Med* 118:465–474, 2005.

55. Berger PB, Ellis SG, Holmes DR, Jr, et al: Relationship between delay in performing direct coronary angioplasty and early clinical outcome in patients with acute myocardial infarction: Results from the global use of strategies to open occluded arteries in Acute Coronary Syndromes (GUSTO-IIb) trial. *Circulation* 100:14–20, 1999.

56. Cannon CP, Gibson CM, Lambrew CT, et al: Relationship of symptom-onset-to-balloon time and door-to-balloon time with mortality in patients undergoing angioplasty for acute myocardial infarction. *JAMA* 283:2941–2947, 2000.

57. Weiss ES, Chang DD, Joyce DL, et al: Optimal timing of coronary artery bypass after acute myocardial infarction: A review of California discharge data. *J Thorac Cardiovasc Surg* 135:503–511, 511.e1–511.e3, 2008.

58. White HD, Assmann SF, Sanborn TA, et al: Comparison of percutaneous coronary intervention and coronary artery bypass grafting after acute myocardial infarction complicated by cardiogenic shock: Results from the Should We Emergently Revascularize Occluded Coronaries for Cardiogenic Shock (SHOCK) trial. *Circulation* 112:1992–2001, 2005.

59. Loop FD, Lytle BW, Cosgrove DM, et al: Influence of the internal-mammary-artery graft on 10-year survival and other cardiac events. *N Engl J Med* 314:1–6, 1986.

60. Comparison of coronary bypass surgery with angioplasty in patients with multivessel disease. The Bypass Angioplasty Revascularization Investigation (BARI) Investigators. *N Engl J Med* 335:217–225, 1996.

61. Tabata M, Grab JD, Khalpey Z, et al: Prevalence and variability of internal mammary artery graft use in contemporary multivessel coronary artery bypass graft surgery: Analysis of the Society of Thoracic Surgeons National Cardiac Database. *Circulation* 120:935–940, 2009.

62. Tatoulis J, Buxton BF, Fuller JA: The right internal thoracic artery: Is it underutilized? *Curr Opin Cardiol* 26:528–535, 2011.

63. Castellheim A, Hoel TN, Videm V, et al: Biomarker profile in off-pump and on-pump coronary artery bypass grafting surgery in low-risk patients. *Ann Thorac Surg* 85:1994–2002, 2008.

64. Hoel TN, Videm V, Mollnes TE, et al: Off-pump cardiac surgery abolishes complement activation. *Perfusion* 22:251–256, 2007.

65. Bonaros N, Schachner T, Lehr E, et al: Five hundred cases of robotic totally endoscopic coronary artery bypass grafting: Predictors of success and safety. *Ann Thorac Surg* 95:803–812, 2013.

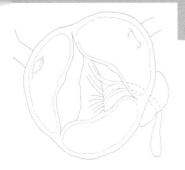

CHAPTER 60

Acquired Heart Disease: Valvular

Todd K. Rosengart, Jatin Anand

第六十章　后天性心脏病：心脏瓣膜疾病

中文导读

本章共分为6节：①心脏瓣膜外科发展历史；②心脏瓣膜的解剖；③心脏瓣膜疾病的病理和病因学；④心脏瓣膜疾病的病理生理学变化；⑤心脏瓣膜疾病的临床表现；⑥心脏瓣膜疾病的手术治疗方法。

第一节回顾了心脏瓣膜外科发展历史。人类对心脏瓣膜疾病外科治疗的探索可追溯到100多年前的经胸二尖瓣闭式分离术。如今，随着抗凝技术和机械瓣膜耐久性能提升，以及经皮介入瓣膜置换等新技术的开展，众多以前无法医治的瓣膜病人获得了满意的疗效。

第二节详细介绍了心脏瓣膜的解剖位置、胚胎发育过程、瓣膜装置的解剖结构、瓣膜的组织成分及各组心脏瓣膜的生理功能及其运转机制；同时对与瓣膜手术相关的外科解剖也进行了重点描述，以免在进行瓣膜修复及置换等操作时损伤冠状动脉、房室结及希氏束等重要解剖结构。

第三节首先对最常见的病因——风湿热造成心脏瓣膜病的发病过程、机制及其后果进行了阐释。随后对二尖瓣狭窄、主动脉瓣狭窄、二尖瓣关闭不全及主动脉瓣关闭不全等四种常见病理改变的病因、发病机制进行了详尽的描述。最后对二尖瓣环钙化、心内膜炎、继发性三尖瓣病变等也进行了介绍。

第四节介绍的内容包括:心脏瓣膜的两种基本病变——狭窄及关闭不全对心脏及大血管的血流动力学影响；瓣膜病变带来的容量及压力负荷过重导致心脏功能受损的病理生理学机制；本节还介绍了心力衰竭的定义、基本病因及分类，其中着重介绍了前向心力衰竭和后向心力衰竭的病理生理学改变及其机制。

第五节对二尖瓣狭窄、二尖瓣关闭不全、主动脉瓣狭窄、主动脉瓣关闭不全及三尖瓣关闭不全等几种较常见瓣膜病变的定义、分型、病理生理学改变、诊断方法、自然病程及治疗原则等进行了详尽的描述，同时对联合瓣膜病也作了简要介绍。

第六节对传统及小切口二尖瓣和主动脉瓣修复及

置换手术的暴露方式、病变瓣膜切除、瓣膜修复及人工瓣膜缝合技术等进行了详细的描述；对不同种类人工心脏瓣膜的特点也进行了介绍和比较；同时还对经皮主动脉瓣置换和经皮二尖瓣钳夹术等新技术进行了介绍。

〔陈　涛〕

The heart contains four one-way valves that regulate the flow of blood into and out of its chambers. Normal cardiac pumping activity is dependent on the proper functioning of these valves. The atrioventricular (AV) valves (mitral and tricuspid valves), when closed, allow stepwise pressure gradients to be maintained between the atria and ventricles; the semilunar valves (aortic and pulmonic valves) likewise allow pressure gradients between the ventricles and great arteries.

The heart beats 100,000 times per day on average and more than 2.5 billion times throughout an average life span. Given the great number of open-close cycles to which the heart valves are subjected and the relative infrequency of cardiac valvular heart disease (reported at a prevalence of <2% of the population[1]), it must be concluded that the cardiac valvular structures are exceedingly well designed to meet the hemodynamic demands to which they are exposed.

The cardiac valves may nevertheless succumb to injury or degeneration from a number of pathophysiologic processes. The advent in the past century of open surgical valve repair and replacement procedures and more recently of percutaneous interventions to repair or to replace damaged valves has meant life and health to countless millions of individuals with cardiac valve disease. Today, for example, approximately 90,000 patients in the United States and 280,000 worldwide undergo valve replacement each year.

HISTORY OF HEART VALVE SURGERY

The possibility of human intervention to abort the fulminant sequelae of cardiac valve disease was well recognized at least a century ago. The ravages of heart failure secondary to mitral stenosis caused by rheumatic disease became an obvious initial target for such interventions, which were first considered in detail as early as the late 19th century. Conceptualization of such interventions was at first limited to blind procedures incorporating remote manipulation of the valve through surgically created apertures in the heart wall. Later, beginning in the middle of the 20th century, the development of the heart-lung machine provided open access to the interior of the heart and the possibility of precise manipulations of the heart valves under direct vision in a still, bloodless field.

Sir Thomas Lauder Brunton, a Scottish physician, was in 1902 one of the first to describe a technique for closed mitral repair, proposing access to the mitral valve by passing a dilator through the left ventricular (LV) wall. This idea was shunned by his colleagues and never attempted.

After significant experimentation in the research laboratories of the Peter Bent Brigham Hospital in Boston, Elliot Cutler and Peter Levine followed up on Brunton's early surgical theory and performed the first surgical correction of the mitral valve in 1923. Their technique involved the blind insertion of a neurosurgical tenotomy knife through a transventricular approach to divide the stenotic valve commissures. Although their first clinical attempt at valve repair was successful, subsequent procedures had less promising results, and this specific technique was also abandoned.

A new era of cardiac intervention was ushered in soon after Cutler and Levine's false start by the innovation of closed digital commissurotomy. In this procedure, the operator's index finger was inserted into the left atrial (LA) appendage through a purse-string suture and across the mitral valve as a means for mechanical dilation. The first successful clinical report was by Henry Souttar of England in 1925. Although the procedure was technically successful, it was still not until 1948, when Charles Bailey of Philadelphia and Dwight Harken of Boston both reported successful closed digital mitral commissurotomies, that the procedure became a widespread technique for treatment of mitral stenosis (Fig. 60-1).

Techniques for blinded aortic valvular surgery were also attempted as early valve interventions, with varying degrees of success. In 1912, Theodore Tuffier of Paris reported the first clinical attempt to dilate a stenotic aortic valve, reportedly by pushing his finger against the aorta and invaginating the aortic wall through the valve. This report met with considerable skepticism, but then mechanical dilation using an instrument passed retrograde through the innominate artery was reported by Russell Brock of London in 1940. Although this technique led to poor results and was abandoned, it opened the door to new, more compelling possibilities.

In 1948, Horace Smithy of Charleston, South Carolina, performed the first successful aortic valvotomy using a valvulotome inserted through a purse-string suture in the LV apex. Three years later, Charles Bailey of Philadelphia reported the first successful aortic valvotomy using a transventricular expanding dilator, and "closed" approaches to treatment of cardiac valve disease continued to proliferate until further advances overtook these early endeavors.

Two major milestones occurring in the middle of the 20th century marked the beginning of the modern era of successful heart valve surgery: the development of a prosthetic valve and the

possible for an ever-expanding spectrum of patients previously considered inoperable, with ever-improving results.

VALVE ANATOMY

The four human heart valves follow similar early embryologic development, beginning as early as 4 weeks of gestation with the formation of the valve primordia in the primitive heart tube. This development is closely linked to the division of the heart tube into its chambers, including septation of the outflow tract (truncus arteriosus) and fusion of the AV canal cushions (Fig. 60-2).

The majority of the cells that migrate into the valve primordia originate from the endocardial cushion, although epicardial and neural crest cells also appear to contribute. Between 20 and 39 weeks of gestation, the valve primordia grow and elongate, thinning to form leaflets and cusps. In late gestation and early after birth, the valve leaflets become stratified into highly organized collagen-, proteoglycan-, and elastin-rich compartments (Fig. 60-3). Valve maturation and remodeling continue into the juvenile stages of life.

In the fully formed heart, the bileaflet mitral and the trileaflet (tricuspid) AV valves are positioned at the inflow to the left and right ventricles, and the three-leaflet aortic and pulmonic semilunar valves are seated atop the outflow tracts of these ventricles, respectively. The AV valves are tethered at their origin to fibrous annular rings (the annuli fibrosi). In comparison, the aortic and pulmonic semilunar valves do not have discrete, ring-like annuli, instead attaching in a curvilinear fashion to the wall of the aorta or pulmonary artery at their junction with the left or right ventricular (RV) outflow tracts, respectively.

The three *cusps* of the semilunar valves (aortic and pulmonic) have a semilunar shape from which they derive their name (Fig. 60-4). Each cusp is in turn made up of four components: the hinge region, where the cusp connects to the annulus; the belly, which makes up the majority of the cusp; the coapting surface at the cusp periphery; and the lunulae, which are thin, crescent-shaped segments of the cusp surrounding a central fibrous nodule at the midpoint of its free edge (termed the nodes of Arantius in the aortic valve).

The mitral valve proper has two *leaflets* possessing approximately equal surface area (Fig. 60-5). The square-shaped anterior leaflet originates from approximately the anterior third of the valve annulus. The posterior mitral leaflet is less wide ("tall") but is longer than the anterior leaflet, attaching to approximately two thirds of the annulus. The anterior and posterior leaflets have three scallops each (e.g., A1, P1), based on indentations found in the posterior leaflet (Fig. 60-5). In comparison, the tricuspid valve is composed of anterior, posterior, and septal leaflets, of which the anterior leaflet is the largest and the septal leaflet the smallest.

All four cardiac valves are supported by internal plates of dense collagen and elastin-rich connective tissue that are continuous with the fibrous cardiac skeleton at the base of the heart. This highly organized extracellular matrix is compartmentalized into three layers: the fibrosa, made of fibrillar collagen; the spongiosa, made of proteoglycans; and either the ventricularis of the semilunar valves or the atrialis of the AV valves, made of elastin fibers (see Fig. 60-3).

In contrast to the free-standing semilunar valves, the mitral and tricuspid valve leaflets and their adjoining fibrous annuli are also part of a complex anatomic unit including fibrous chordae tendineae that arise from the leaflet free edges (marginal or

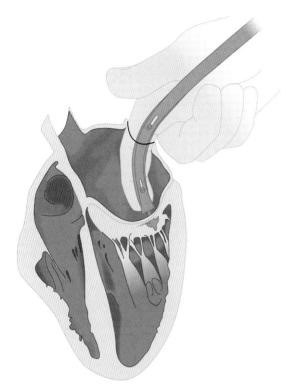

FIGURE 60-1 Closed Mitral Commissurotomy. Dwight Harken developed a closed mitral commissurotomy procedure to correct rheumatic mitral stenosis that became the first widespread approach to treatment of valvular heart disease. (From Muller WH, Jr: The surgical treatment of mitral stenosis. *Calif Med* 75:285–289, 1951.)

advent of cardiopulmonary bypass. The first successful implantation of a prosthetic valve was reported by Charles Hufnagel of Georgetown University in 1952. Given the then absence of a means to access the aortic valve in situ, Hufnagel innovated the implantation of a caged-ball valve into the *descending aorta* in a series of patients with aortic insufficiency. In this ingenious design, the forward flow of blood pushed the ball out of the orifice to open the valve during systole, while regurgitant flow was prevented when the ball fell back into the orifice to seal the valve during diastole. Although this extra-anatomic device served to prevent aortic regurgitation, the replacement of cardiac valves in situ would still need to await the advent of cardiopulmonary bypass.

Following the first successful clinical use of the heart-lung machine by Gibbon in 1953 to repair an atrial septal defect, Harken in 1960 finally reported the first successful in situ aortic valve replacement, using a caged-ball device inserted in place of an excised aortic valve. That same year, Albert Starr, working with Lowell Edwards in Oregon, replaced the mitral valve using a similar caged-ball prosthesis of their own design. What followed was an explosion of improvements in prosthetic valve design and implantation techniques that led to applications in millions of patients worldwide during the next 50 years.

Advances in heart valve surgery have spanned ever-improved tissue valve preservation techniques, mechanical valve antithrombotic and durability properties, mitral and now aortic valve repair techniques, and the modern era of percutaneous interventions. These improvements have made survival from cardiac valve disease

Partitioning of the heart into four chambers

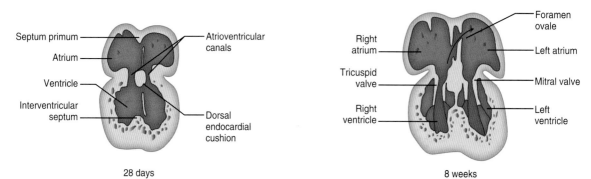

28 days

8 weeks

FIGURE 60-2 Embryology of the Cardiac Valves. The development of the valve primordia is closely linked to the division of the heart tube into its chambers, including septation of the outflow tract (truncus arteriosus) and fusion of the atrioventricular canal cushion.

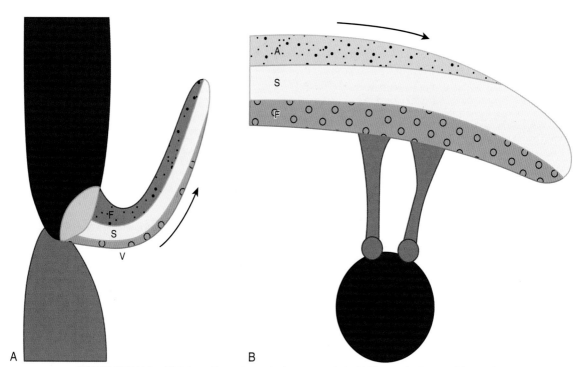

A   B

FIGURE 60-3 Valve Histology. The mature valve is composed of a highly organized extracellular matrix, which is compartmentalized into three layers: the fibrosa (F), made of fibrillar collagen; the spongiosa (S), made of proteoglycans; and either the ventricularis (V) of the semilunar valves or the atrialis (A) of the atrioventricular valves, made of elastin fiber. (From Combs MD, Yutzey KE: Heart valve development: Regulatory networks in development and disease. *Circ Res* 105:408–421, 2009.)

primary chordae) or undersurface (intermediate or secondary chordae), with basal (tertiary) chordae also arising from the posterior leaflet base and annulus. These chordae attach to intraventricular papillary muscles, which in turn arise from the ventricular myocardium.

The mitral valve is supported by an anterior and posterior papillary muscle that sends chordae to the anterior and posterior leaflets. In comparison, the tricuspid valve is supported by a large anterior papillary muscle that sends chordae to the anterior and posterior leaflets and a variable medial or posterior papillary

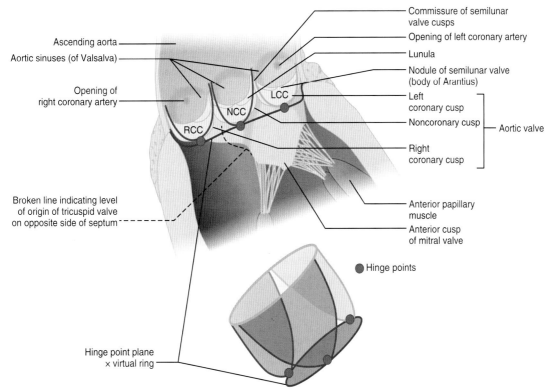

FIGURE 60-4 Anatomy of the Semilunar Valves. Each valve is composed of three cusps arising directly from the juncture of the great vessel and ventricular outflow tract walls. (From Kasel AM, Cassese S, Bleiziffer S, et al: Standardized imaging for aortic annular sizing: Implications for transcatheter valve selection. *JACC Cardiovasc Imaging* 6:249–262, 2013.)

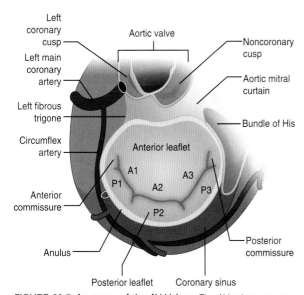

FIGURE 60-5 Anatomy of the AV Valves. The AV valves are composed of leaflets arising from a distinct fibrous annulus. The depicted mitral valve is composed of an anterior and posterior leaflet, each subdivided into three scallops. (From http://www.sciamsurgery.com/sciamsurgery/institutional/figTabPopup.action?bookId=ACS&linkId=part11_ch01_fig20&type=fig.)

muscle that provides chordae to the posterior and septal leaflets. The RV septal wall also provides chordae to the anterior and septal tricuspid leaflets, but there is no formal septal papillary muscle.

As suggested by their contrasted anatomy, the semilunar and AV valves differ in their mechanisms of maintaining coaptation. The semilunar valve cusps are dependent largely on coaptation mechanisms intrinsic to the cusps themselves, falling passively to the central arterial lumen in diastole and there sealing the orifice by coapting with the corresponding midpoint nodules on adjoining cusps. The AV valves are tethered in their closed position by their chordal attachments to the papillary muscles, which contract during systole to maintain leaflet coaptation and to prevent leaflet prolapse into the atria (Fig. 60-6).

Surgical Anatomic Relationships

The central location of the aortic valve at the base of the heart imparts to it important anatomic as well as clinical surgical relationships to the other cardiac chambers and valves. The coronary arterial circulation originates at the sinuses of Valsalva, gentle dilations of the aorta just distal to the valve proper that impart important facilitation to valve closure and coronary and blood flow. The right and left coronary arteries arise from the right and left sinuses, respectively. The aortic valve cusps are named with respect to these sinusoidal and coronary relationships, that is, the right coronary, left coronary, and noncoronary (posterior) cusps.

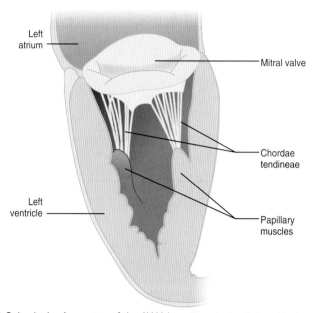

FIGURE 60-6 Subvalvular Apparatus of the AV Valves. The mitral and tricuspid valves are supported by a robust subvalvular apparatus featuring the chordae tendineae that tether the leaflets and annuli to the papillary muscles, which contract during systole to maintain leaflet coaptation and to prevent leaflet prolapse into the atria. (From Filsoufi F, Carpentier A. TheMitralValve.org.)

(The pulmonic valve cusps are analogously termed the right, left, and anterior cusps.)

In direct continuity with the left and noncoronary cusps of the aortic valve, from about 5 to 8 o'clock in the traditional surgical perspective, is the anterior leaflet of the mitral valve. The noncoronary cusp of the aortic valve and the anterior leaflet of the mitral valve are therefore at risk of injury during mitral and aortic valve surgery, respectively. Likewise, the AV node lies embedded in the top of the ventricular membranous septum, just beneath the commissure between the noncoronary and right coronary aortic leaflets, from 3 to 5 o'clock in the surgical perspective. Only the remaining circumference of the aortic annulus is relatively free anatomically from surgical injury during aortic valve surgery.

The mitral valve bears two additional anatomic relationships of important surgical consideration. The posterior (mural or lateral) leaflet is in continuity with the posterior LV wall. Deep (posterior) to the posterior leaflet lies the AV groove, within which lies the circumflex coronary artery, which is thereby at risk of surgical injury. The AV node likewise lies deep to the posteromedial commissure of the mitral valve.

Tricuspid valve surgery entails risks to two additional structures, found superior to the valve in the right atrium. The coronary sinus ostium lies adjacent to the commissure of the septal and posterior leaflets of the valve and can be inadvertently oversewn if it is not carefully identified. The AV node lies in the apex of a triangular area first described by Koch, which is bounded by the septal annulus of the tricuspid valve anteriorly, the tendon of Todaro posteriorly, and the central fibrous body containing the bundle of His superiorly, leading to the coronary sinus inferiorly (Fig. 60-7). A suture placed within the triangle may lead to complete heart block.

Because the pulmonic valve lies superior and distal to the heart proper in the embryonic conus, in contrast to the other valves, it

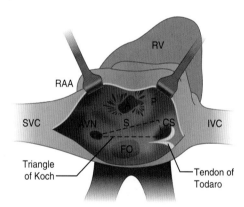

FIGURE 60-7 Surgical Anatomy of the Tricuspid Valve. The AV node lies in the apex of a triangular area first described by Koch, which is bounded by the septal annulus of the tricuspid valve anteriorly, the tendon of Todaro posteriorly, and the central fibrous body containing the bundle of His superiorly, leading to the coronary sinus inferiorly. *A,* anterior tricuspid valve leaflet; *AVN,* atrioventricular node; *CS,* coronary sinus ostium; *FO,* foramen ovale; *IVC,* inferior vena cava; *P,* posterior tricuspid valve leaflet; *RAA,* right atrial appendage; *RV,* right ventricle; *S,* septal tricuspid valve leaflet; *SVC,* superior vena cava. (From Rogers JH, Bolling SF: The tricuspid valve: Current perspective and evolving management of tricuspid regurgitation. *Circulation* 119:2718–2725, 2009.)

shares limited surgical anatomic considerations of significance.

PATHOLOGY AND ETIOLOGY OF VALVULAR HEART DISEASE

The cardiac valves may become impaired through two fundamental forms of dysfunction: valvular stenosis, an obstruction to forward flow due to incomplete opening of the valve; and valvular insufficiency, in which backward flow (regurgitation) occurs through a valve when its cusps or leaflets do not fully coapt. Valvular stenosis is almost always caused by a primary abnormality of the cusp or leaflet from a chronic disease process, but regurgitation may be caused by an acute or chronic disease process affecting the valve itself or may be secondary to a structural abnormality of associated supporting structures, such as the great arteries, annuli fibrosi, chordae tendineae, papillary muscles, or ventricular myocardium (Table 60-1). Both stenosis and insufficiency may exist simultaneously in any one valve.

In the developed world, aortic valvular stenosis (AS) is the most common form of valvular heart disease requiring surgical intervention, followed by mitral regurgitation (MR). AS is most often the result of degenerative changes to the aortic valve, resulting in fibrosis and calcification in older patients. Because of the aging population, the prevalence of AS continues to rise, and it

is now found in 4% of the population older than 85 years. The most common cause of MR is degenerative changes to the mitral valve apparatus, which are typically found in younger patients (Table 60-1).

Although degenerative disease is a more prevalent cause of valve disease in the developed world, rheumatic fever probably remains the most common (albeit decreasing) cause of valvular dysfunction worldwide. Despite the increasing application of antibiotics to treat rheumatic fever, rheumatic heart disease (RHD) will still occur in 30% of those with the acute illness. RHD is still prevalent in part because of the decades-long lag time between the occurrence of rheumatic fever in the first decade of life (mean age, 8 to 12 years) and the subsequent manifestation of rheumatic valvular disease as a sequel in the third or fourth decade of life.[2] The basis of RHD is a chronic inflammatory insult against laminin, a valvular basement membrane protein typically exposed by an initial group A beta-hemolytic streptococcal infec-

TABLE 60-1   Etiology of Valve Disease

	LEAFLETS	ANNULUS	CHORDAE TENDINEAE	VENTRICULAR WALL/ PAPILLARY MUSCLE	AORTIC ROOT
Mitral Stenosis					
Rheumatic valve disease	++	++	++	± (PM fusion/shortening)	NA
Endocarditis (vegetation)	±	–	–	–	NA
Congenital*	++	–	–	±	NA
Supravalvular (thrombus, myxoma)	++	–	–	–	NA
Mitral Regurgitation					
Mitral valve prolapse (myxomatous/ connective tissue disorder)	++	++	++	–	NA
Rheumatic fever	++	–	±	–	NA
Endocarditis	++	±	++	+	NA
Congenital anomaly[†]	++	–	±	–	NA
Systemic lupus erythematosus[‡]	++	±	±	± (PM)	NA
Mitral annular calcification	±	++	–	–	NA
Myocardial ischemia/infarction	–	±	–	++	NA
Hypertrophic cardiomyopathy				++	NA
Aortic Stenosis					
Degenerative disease (trileaflet)	++	+	NA	–	–
Bicuspid valve disease	++	+	NA	–	–
Rheumatic valve disease	++	+	NA	–	–
Endocarditis (vegetation)	++	+	NA	–	–
Other congenital anomaly[§]	++	+	NA	++	+
Hypertrophic cardiomyopathy	–	–	–	++	NA
Aortic Insufficiency					
Degenerative/connective tissue disease[‖]	++	++	NA	–	++
Rheumatic disease	++	–	NA	–	–
Inflammatory disease[¶]	+	–	NA	–	++
Endocarditis	++	+	NA	–	+
Congenital (bicuspid, unicuspid)	++	–	NA	–	+
Aortic dissection/aortic aneurysm	–	++	NA	–	++

++ common; + fairly common; ± possibly involved; – rarely involved. *NA*, not applicable; *PM*, papillary muscle.
*Parachute mitral valve, supramitral ring.
[†]Cleft leaflet, endocardial cushion defect, parachute mitral valve.
[‡]Libman-Sacks lesion.
[§]Unicuspid/unicommissural valve, hypoplastic annulus/root, subaortic membrane/stenosis.
[‖]Marfan syndrome, myxomatous degeneration, osteogenesis imperfecta, Ehlers-Danlos syndrome.
[¶]Ankylosing spondylitis, Reiter syndrome, Takayasu disease, giant cell aortitis.

tion and subsequently targeted through a cross-reactive antibody formation process known as molecular mimicry.

RHD is the most common cause of regurgitant valve lesions, primary multivalvular disease, and mixed (stenotic and regurgitant) lesions. Although RHD may be manifested as MR acutely, chronic disease most commonly is manifested as mitral valve stenosis (MS) or mixed valve lesions and affects women in two thirds of cases. RHD next most frequently directly leads to AS, although indirect upstream hemodynamic stresses caused by MS (see later) make tricuspid regurgitation (TR) a common secondary valvular abnormality.

RHD is the most common cause of MS, and it is uncommon to have rheumatic valvular disease without mitral valve involvement. In 50% of cases, rheumatic mitral valve disease presents as a pathognomonic, mixed stenotic and regurgitant "fish mouth" funnel valve lesion, often associated with fusion and shortening of the leaflets and chordae tendineae (Fig. 60-8). Congenital anomalies, such as parachute deformities and supramitral rings, are far more unusual causes of MS in the adult.

Stenotic disease of the aortic valve is relatively equally divided between that affecting initially normal trileaflet valves and that arising in congenitally bicuspid valves. It occurs as a degenerative process at increasing frequency with age, with more than 90% of AS seen in patients older than 60 years and more than 80% of patients with trileaflet AS presenting for surgery after the age of 60 years.[3] The progression of degenerative (calcific) AS (previously termed senile or wear-and-tear disease) is now thought to be an actively regulated phenomenon related to atherosclerotic disease, wherein turbulent blood flow at leaflet attachment points induces endothelial injury, which leads to accumulation of lipids, infiltration of macrophages and T cells, and transformation of cells to an osteoblastic phenotype.[4] It is believed that this process leads to aortic leaflet calcification, which may involve the aortic and mitral annuli as well as the mitral leaflets.

AS occurs in 20% to 30% of patients born with bicuspid aortic valves, which are more commonly found in males than in females and are present in 1% to 2% of the population, making this anomaly the most prevalent of the congenital valve lesions. Less commonly, unicuspid aortic valves or other congenital anomalies of the LV outflow tract may also be manifested as AS early in life.

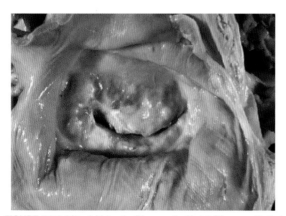

FIGURE 60-8 Mitral Valve in Rheumatic Heart Disease. Typical rheumatic mitral valve disease presenting as a pathognomonic, mixed stenotic and regurgitant "fish mouth" funnel valve lesion, often associated with fusion and shortening of the leaflets and chordae tendineae. (From http://library.med.utah.edu/WebPath/CVHTML/CV061.html.)

Degenerative disease of bicuspid aortic valves is manifested as AS about 2 decades earlier than it is with tricuspid valves, peaking in the fifth and sixth decades of life. Increased hemodynamic stresses associated with the abnormally configured bicuspid valve leaflets are thought to accelerate degenerative valve changes in this anomaly.

Although AS is the most common pathologic presentation of a congenitally bicuspid valve, regurgitant lesions may also occur, typically at a much younger age and with a lower rate of progression requiring surgical intervention. Importantly, mendelian inheritance of a bicuspid aortic valve anomaly is also associated with dilation of the proximal ascending aorta because of pathologic alterations of the aortic media in up to 50% of patients with bicuspid aortic valves.

MR leads to surgical intervention far less often than does AS, but MR is actually the most frequently occurring form of valve dysfunction, with at least trivial MR present in most healthy adults. MR necessitating surgical intervention is related to degenerative disease in 60% to 70% of cases, to ischemic disease in 20% of cases, and to endocarditis or rheumatic disease in 2% to 5%.[5] Congenital anomalies, such as cleft leaflets and AV canal or endocardial cushion defects, may lead to MR as well. Carpentier described a functional classification of MR based on abnormal patterns of leaflet motion (Table 60-2), which together with MR etiology and the specific valve lesion can be used to plan treatment and to predict prognosis.

A wide variety of connective tissue diseases may lead to degenerative disease of the mitral valve, most prominently including Marfan syndrome. Myxomatous disease describes a common pathologic end point of connective tissue disruption that typically is manifested as MR in the third and fourth decades of life. This process is characterized by glycosaminoglycan infiltration of the valve leaflets, thickening of the spongiosa, and separation of collagen bundles in the fibrosa.

Myxomatous disease of the mitral valve typically leads to excessive, "billowing" valve leaflets, annular dilation, and chordae enlargement or elongation and consequent abnormal systolic leaflet "prolapse" into the atrium. This syndrome typically occurs in young women and is termed Barlow disease after the clear identification in 1963 of the cause of this "click-murmur syndrome."[6] Mitral disease is the most common manifestation of myxomatous disease, but it may also present as aortic and tricuspid valve disease. It is often differentiated from fibroelastic deficiency syndrome, which is typically characterized by thinned leaflets and chordal rupture presenting in older patients. Prolapse or flail of the middle posterior leaflet cusp (P2) due to chordae rupture is a common manifestation of this syndrome.[7]

MR may also be caused by secondary, "functional" disorders, in which the morphology of the valve itself is normal. Typically, functional MR is a result of myocardial ischemic events or infarction or ventricular enlargement, which leads to outward (lateral) and apical displacement of the posteromedial papillary muscle and malapposition of the leaflets because of "tethering" of the leaflets by the chordae (Carpentier type IIIb lesion).

Ischemia or rupture of a papillary muscle secondary to coronary ischemia or acute myocardial infarction, particularly in the inferior distribution, can also lead to functional MR (Carpentier type II). This typically involves the posterior muscle, leading to prolapse or flail of the posterior leaflet because the blood supply to the posterior papillary muscle is from only a single (terminal) branch of the posterior descending coronary artery, compared with dual blood supply to the anterolateral papillary muscle from

TABLE 60-2   Carpentier Classification of Mitral Valve Regurgitation

CARPENTIER CLASSIFICATION	DYSFUNCTION	LESIONS	ETIOLOGY
Type I	Normal leaflet motion	Annular dilation Leaflet perforation/tear	Dilated cardiomyopathy Endocarditis
Type II	Excessive leaflet motion (prolapse)	Elongation/rupture of chordae Elongation/rupture of papillary muscle	Degenerative valve disease Fibroelastic deficiency Barlow disease Marfan disease Rheumatic (acute) Endocarditis Trauma Ischemic cardiomyopathy
Type IIIa	Restricted leaflet motion (diastole and systole)	Leaflet thickening/retraction Leaflet calcification Chordal thickening/retraction/fusion Commissural fusion	Rheumatic (chronic) Carcinoid heart disease
Type IIIb	Restricted leaflet motion (systole)	Left ventricular dilation/aneurysm Papillary muscle displacement Chordae tethering	Ischemic/dilated cardiomyopathy

Carpentier AF: Cardiac valve surgery—the "French correction." *J Thorac Cardiovasc Surg* 86:323–337, 1983.
Carpentier AF, Lessana A, Relland JY, et al: The "physio-ring": An advanced concept in mitral valve annuloplasty. *Ann Thorac Surg* 60:1177–1186, 1995.

the left anterior descending and circumflex arteries.

Aortic valve insufficiency (AI) may be caused by myxomatous disease leading to thinning, enlargement, perforation, or prolapse of the aortic valve cusps themselves. AI may also be caused by dilation of the aortic root, which prevents proper aortic valve coaptation by increasing intravalvular closing distances. Root enlargement is typically caused by hypertension or connective tissue disorders, such as cystic medial necrosis, Marfan syndrome, Ehlers-Danlos syndrome, or Loeys-Dietz syndrome, either directly or as a result of aortic dissection.

Bicuspid valve disease is also frequently associated with aortic root enlargement, potentially either through a currently unidentified common genetic defect causing abnormalities in aortic wall elasticity or through hemodynamic "blast" effects of abnormal flow through the bicuspid valve orifice. Less common causes of aortic root enlargement and aortic dissection include trauma, syphilitic aortitis, rheumatoid arthritis, lupus erythematosus, and other systemic vasculopathies, such as Takayasu and giant cell aortitis and osteogenesis imperfecta.

Mitral annular calcification (MAC) is an extremely common degenerative change found in older patients that is typically without functional sequelae. It may be associated with similar changes involving the aortic or mitral valves. However, on occasion, MAC can produce MR by reducing annulus pliability and systolic contraction, which prevents appropriate leaflet coaptation. Less frequently, MAC may be associated with mitral or aortic valve disorders through a more widespread degenerative process.

Endocarditis can also lead to valve destruction and insufficiency or, less frequently, to valve orifice obstruction by endocarditic vegetations—masses of platelets, fibrin, microcolonies of microorganisms, and inflammatory cells. Platelets and fibrin initially become deposited on normal or deformed valves as part of a normal healing process after normal disruptions of the valvular endothelium, typically caused by hemodynamic or metabolic injury. Endocarditis results from subsequent seeding onto the valve of a microbiologic organism, most commonly staphylococci, streptococci, and enterococci, after bacteremia or fungemia.

The incidence of endocarditis varies from 3 to 10 episodes per 100,000 person-years and carries a relatively high mortality compared with other valve lesions.[8] It may affect previously normal valves, but it typically affects valves deformed by congenital or rheumatic disease, degenerative processes such as calcification, or previously replaced prosthetic valves. Infectious endocarditis is usually left sided, reflecting the normal distribution of such pre-existing valvular disease.

Acute endocarditis, increasingly affecting normal valves, may follow an aggressive course with valvular perforation or more extensive destruction of the leaflet or surrounding support structures, resulting in acute valvular regurgitation. Although endocarditis is typically relatively indolent, endocarditis is the most common cause of death secondary to acute AI in the adult population. With subacute presentations, valve insufficiency may result from residual leaflet deformities caused by fibrotic healing of endocarditic lesions. The growth of large vegetations may also uncommonly lead to improper leaflet coaptation and insufficiency.

Nearly all of the pathophysiologic mechanisms causing left-sided valve disease may analogously lead to primary right-sided valve disease, but the most common presentation of right-sided valve disease is functional TR caused by RV failure arising from left-sided dysfunction and pulmonary hypertension. Less commonly, functional TR may also be caused by RV infarction or ischemia. Less frequently, transvalvular pacemaker or cardioverter-defibrillator leads can also cause mild or even higher grade TR.

Tricuspid stenosis (TS) occurs infrequently in developed countries because rheumatic disease accounts for more than 90% of such lesions. Carcinoid syndrome is the most common of a group of unusual disorders that lead to the deposition of pathologic materials in the tricuspid and pulmonic leaflets as a far less frequent cause of primary TR, TS, or pulmonic valve disease. Congenital anomalies causing pulmonic valve stenosis are often associated with tetralogy of Fallot, TS, and TR, typically occurring as part of Ebstein anomaly, three of the most common of the congenital disorders leading to right-sided valve disease.

PATHOPHYSIOLOGY OF VALVULAR HEART DISEASE

Two fundamental pathophysiologic derangements may affect the heart valves: stenosis and insufficiency. The hemodynamic hallmark of cardiac valve stenosis is the occurrence of a pressure gradient between an upstream pumping chamber and a downstream receiving chamber or artery caused by the resistance to normal laminar blood flow introduced by the stenotic valve during the time that the valve is normally open. The hemodynamic hallmark of regurgitant valvular disease is the retrograde flow of blood from downstream structures (ventricle or great vessel) into an upstream chamber during the diastolic interval during which the malfunctioning valve should normally be closed. Uncompensated, both stenotic and regurgitant lesions cause an increase in upstream chamber afterload and consequent wall stress—predominating either during ventricular systolic ejection against the resistance of stenotic valves or with increased chamber filling by regurgitant volumes peaking at the end of diastole, respectively.

Two compensatory mechanisms provide robust reserves in cardiac function before the volume and pressure overload stresses of valve disease translate into significant cardiac physiologic derangements. The first, described by the Frank-Starling law (Fig. 60-9), produces increases in ventricular contractile force as a function of end-diastolic volume (EDV), or preload, which enhances stroke volume and ventricular emptying. The second involves stress-induced ventricular hypertrophy, which leads to increased wall thickness. By decreasing chamber radius (volume) or increasing wall thickness, respectively, each of these processes can improve wall stress, as described by Laplace's law: wall stress α = (pressure × radius)/(2 × wall thickness). Decreased wall stress, in turn, translates into decreased myocardial work and oxygen demand and improved cardiac function.

The microanatomic basis of the Frank-Starling relationship relates to the orientation between cardiomyocyte sarcomeric actin and myosin fibers, which become ideally aligned to generate contractile force as cardiac muscle is stretched from a "zero-load" status. At a sarcomere length of 2.2 μm, contractile proteins become optimally sensitized to calcium fluxes, resulting in maximized sarcomere contractility as well as rates of contraction and relaxation. As valve-induced cardiomyopathies progress, however, contractile function diminishes at a given level of stretch on the macroanatomic and microanatomic level, and eventually heart failure ensues.

Heart Failure

Heart failure is defined as the inability of the heart to adequately fill or to pump blood in quantities sufficient to support the metabolic demands of the body under tolerable preload (volume filling) conditions. In the setting of cardiac valvular disease, congestive heart failure ultimately occurs when increases in ventricular volume loading (EDV) or decreases in myocardial contractile function (i.e., change in pressure over time [dp/dt]) exceed the adaptive range of Frank-Starling pressure responses or when

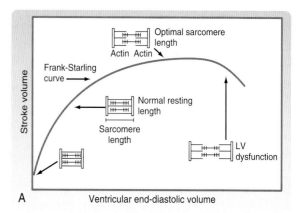

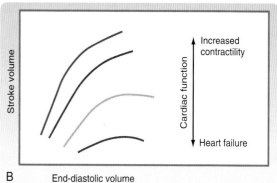

FIGURE 60-9 Frank-Starling Curve. The Frank-Starling law describes a generally linear relationship between increasing end-diastolic volume, or preload, and generated ventricular pressure. **A,** Shifts in volume change generated pressure or stroke volume along a given pressure-volume curve. **B,** Cardiomyopathy shifts the curve downward. (From http://cardiovascres.oxfordjournals.org/content/cardiovascres/77/4/627/F1.large.jpg.)

excessive ventricular hypertrophy exceeds available nutritive blood supply, causing myocardial ischemia.

Precipitous, fulminant or even fatal heart failure may occur despite relatively normal intrinsic ventricular function in the setting of acute valvular dysfunction when there is insufficient time for compensatory mechanisms to adapt to excessive hemodynamic stresses. More typically, with the chronic progression of valvular dysfunction, heart failure develops after a prolonged, asymptomatic period during which hemodynamic stresses are initially well compensated. In this scenario, profound changes in cardiac functional anatomy (i.e., hypertrophy, enlargement) occur before the onset of symptoms. In modern treatment models, interventions are therefore increasingly indicated before the onset of symptoms.

Heart failure secondary to valvular disease reflects both impaired ventricular relaxation (diastolic failure) and impaired ventricular contractility (systolic failure). Diastolic failure occurs secondary to excessive myocardial hypertrophy that may outstrip blood supply or causes decreased ventricular compliance and consequently increased end-diastolic pressure (EDP). Systolic failure may occur as a result of cumulative myocardial injury and fibrosis as excessive myocardial hypertrophy outstrips blood supply, but it also occurs when excessive volume overload drives ventricular pressure-volume relationships "off the [right] end" of the Frank-

Starling curve (Fig. 60-9), and a self-reinforcing cycle of increased EDVs and wall stress further decrease contractility and diminish ejection pressures by overstretched sarcomeres.

Heart failure may also be subdivided into "backward" and "forward" failure. In backward failure, increased LVEDP resulting from the mechanisms described before is transmitted through the left atrium back to the pulmonary vasculature. Pulmonary congestion results at approximately 25 mm Hg when increased pulmonary intravascular pressure exceeds oncotic pressure. Pulmonary congestion and vascular engorgement lead to a reduction in vital capacity as air in the lungs is displaced by interstitial and intra-alveolar edema fluid. Ventilation-perfusion mismatches further result in increased dead space and alveolar-arterial gradients, and hypoxemia results. The lungs simultaneously become less compliant and the work of breathing increases, tidal volume decreases, and respiratory frequency increases to compensate. Dyspnea occurs through a complex interaction of skeletal muscle fatigue, vascular chemoreceptors measuring blood gas levels, and intrapulmonary, chest wall, and skeletal muscle stretch receptors.

Long-standing increases in LVEDP can eventually lead to pulmonary hypertension. Pulmonary hypertension, representing an increase in RV afterload, can eventually precipitate right-sided failure. Right-sided heart failure leads to increased central venous pressure, peripheral venous congestion, and ultimately peripheral organ (e.g., hepatic and renal) failure as a result of decreased capillary–central venous pressure gradients and impaired peripheral emptying.

Typical backward/right-sided heart failure symptoms of orthopnea (dyspnea on recumbency) and paroxysmal nocturnal dyspnea (intermittent nighttime dyspnea associated with recumbency) occur when increases in venous return associated with gravity-neutral recumbency exacerbate pulmonary congestion as otherwise peripherally pooled blood returns to the central circulation.

Forward heart failure—inadequate cardiac output resulting as ventricular systolic dysfunction progresses—leads to further increases in end-systolic volume as ejection fraction (EF) decreases, which in turn leads to further exacerbation of the decompensatory processes described before. Right-sided forward failure impairs left-sided heart filling, furthering inadequate LV ejection and forward output. Left-sided forward failure can be manifested by end-organ hypoperfusion symptoms, such as fatigue, and can trigger a number of systemic components of heart failure that are initially adaptive but typically lead to a number of the maladaptive sequelae of heart failure.

With left-sided forward failure, decreased inhibitory inputs from the carotid and aortic arch baroreceptors and cardiopulmonary mechanoreceptors as well as increased excitatory inputs from peripheral chemoreceptors and mechanoreceptors lead to an increase in sympathetic tone. Together with increased circulating plasma norepinephrine, adrenergic activation causes an increase in heart rate (chronotropy), conduction velocity (dromotropy), contractility (inotropy), and rate of relaxation (lusitropy) as compensatory responses to decreased cardiac output.

Decreased effective arterial blood volume resulting from left-sided forward failure causes renal hypoperfusion, decreased filtered sodium at the macula densa, and increased renal sympathetic tone, all contributing to increased release of renin from the juxtaglomerular apparatus. Renin-angiotensin system activation leads to sodium retention, activation of thirst centers in the brain, and secretion of aldosterone, increasing cardiac preload from salt and water retention.

Both adrenergic and renin-angiotensin system activation leads to vasoconstriction, hypertension, and increased afterload. With elevated preload and afterload, ventricular wall stress increases, leading to further myocyte hypertrophy. Eventually, myocyte hypertrophy, necrosis, apoptosis, and fibrosis combine with desensitization of β-adrenergic receptors and other maladaptive changes in gene expression and biomolecular mechanisms, such as those affecting intracellular calcium handling, to further propagate decreasing cardiac function.

VALVE DISEASE SYNDROMES

Mitral Stenosis

The nondiseased mitral valve orifice has a cross-sectional area of 4 to 6 cm². Under normal conditions, there is no gradient across the mitral valve, and LA pressure is typically less than 10 to 15 mm Hg. MS, typically occurring as a result of rheumatic disease, causes a pressure gradient to develop across the diseased mitral valve. More specifically, as the mitral valve orifice narrows to a cross-sectional area of 2 to 2.5 cm² (mild MS), resistance to flow leads to increased LA blood volume "pooling." Increased LA pressure generated by Frank-Starling mechanics maintains adequate diastolic flow across the resistive valve orifice.

When progressive MS leads to a transvalvular gradient of more than 5 to 10 mm Hg, typically corresponding to a valve orifice of less than 1.5 cm², MS is classified as severe. The resultant increase in LA pressure is transmitted upstream to the pulmonary veins, capillaries, and arteries. At an LA pressure of 25 mm Hg, pulmonary edema typically develops.

With chronically increased pulmonary pressure, arterial vasoconstriction and vascular remodeling lead to fixed pulmonary hypertension. Elevated pulmonary arterial systolic pressure higher than 60 mm Hg imparts significant RV afterload and may ultimately lead to RV dilation, TR, and RV failure as well. MS, on the other hand, is the most sparing of left-sided valvular lesions in regard to sparing intrinsic left ventricle function. LVEDP is normal or below normal in 85% of cases, and LV chamber size is normal or smaller than normal in most cases. Cardiac output is impaired in one third of cases, but primarily because of restricted LV inflow.

Several changes in cardiac hemodynamics can acutely exacerbate this pathophysiologic process. Any increase in cardiac output, as with exercise, will lead to an increase in transvalvular pressure gradients according to the law of Poiseuille: flow α = Δp/resistance, where Δp signifies pressure gradient. At a given cardiac output, decreased diastolic filling time caused by increased heart rates, such as with exercise or the onset of atrial fibrillation, will cause a similar increase in transvalvular gradient as more flow must occur per unit time.

Chronically increased transmitral pressure gradients caused by MS typically lead to atrial hypertrophy and dilation. Associated LA fibrosis and disorganization of the atrial muscle fibers cause abnormal atrial conduction velocities and refractory times. Increased automaticity, ectopic foci, and reentry circuits eventually lead to supraventricular tachycardias and atrial fibrillation in nearly 40% of patients with MS. Loss of the "kick" generated by normal atrial contraction, responsible for 30% of ventricular diastolic filling, results in a 20% decrease in cardiac output and necessitates increased atrial pressure to allow adequate ventricular loading. Atrial fibrillation consequently causes increased diastolic pressures and volume overload, potentially leading to worsening congestion.

Diagnosis of Mitral Stenosis

Symptoms and signs. MS patients may remain asymptomatic for many years. As valvular stenosis gradually worsens, however, symptoms characteristic of low cardiac output and pulmonary venous congestion eventually develop, including fatigue, dyspnea, orthopnea, and paroxysmal nocturnal dyspnea. Ultimately, peripheral edema and other congestive symptoms caused by volume overload and right-sided heart failure ensue. Increased heart rate caused by atrial fibrillation or supraventricular tachycardia, exercise, or other factors may exacerbate or precipitate earlier symptoms.

Patients with MS who develop atrial fibrillation may complain of palpitations and symptomatic tachycardia. More ominously, thromboembolization will occur in 20% of patients with MS and may be its first symptom in 10% of cases, presenting as stroke, myocardial ischemia or infarction, renal infarction, and gut or limb ischemia. Half of all thromboembolic events will involve the cerebral circulation. Rarely, a large, pedunculated atrial thrombus may form and obstruct the valve inlet, resulting in hemodynamic collapse and sudden death.

With advanced disease, LA enlargement may cause hoarseness from left recurrent laryngeal nerve compression onto the pulmonary artery, dysphagia from esophageal compression, or persistent cough from bronchial compression. Pulmonary venous congestion may induce hemoptysis from sudden rupture of a dilated bronchial vein. RV failure and TR can cause abdominal pain and swelling from hepatomegaly and ascites or even florid peripheral edema.

Physical examination. The characteristic physical finding of MS is a low-pitched, rumbling diastolic murmur that is best heard at the apex with the patient in the left lateral decubitus position. In patients who are in sinus rhythm, the murmur increases in intensity during late diastole (known as presystolic accentuation) because of the increased flow across the stenotic valve with atrial contraction. As severity of MS progresses, the diastolic rumble may be of longer duration or even holodiastolic. The Graham Steell diastolic murmur of MS can result from pulmonary regurgitation caused by pulmonary hypertension and right-sided overload.

A high-pitched "opening snap" or an accentuated first heart sound caused by forceful opening or closing, respectively, of an inflexible but still mobile mitral leaflet may be heard with early MS. As MS progresses, LA pressure rises and the mitral valve opens earlier in diastole. As pulmonary arterial pressure increases, a loud pulmonic component of second heart sound (P2) may be appreciated.

Advanced MS is typically associated with rales developing with the onset of pulmonary edema. As RV failure develops, an RV heave, jugular venous distention, hepatomegaly, ascites, and lower extremity edema may be found.

Diagnostic testing. The earliest appreciable changes of MS discernible by routine chest radiography include evidence of an enlarged left atrium seen as a straightening of the left cardiac border, a double shadow in the cardiac silhouette, and an elevated left mainstem bronchus. Prominent pulmonary vessels may also be appreciated. If stenosis is severe, congested pulmonary lymphatics in the lower lung fields may be present as horizontal linear opacities, known as Kerley B lines. Mitral valve calcification may also be visible. Stigmata of heart failure, such as opacification of the lung fields and pleural effusions, may follow.

The electrocardiographic recording of MS patients is often grossly normal, although 90% of patients will demonstrate evidence of LA enlargement as a widened, notched P wave (P mitrale). Atrial arrhythmias may also be appreciated if present. With advanced MS, RV hypertrophy may be associated with right axis deviation.

Echocardiography, as with other valve lesions, is the primary diagnostic method to determine the presence and severity of MS and associated abnormalities. Commissural fusion, leaflet immobility, and leaflet as well as annular and subvalvular thickening and calcification can be well assessed by transthoracic and especially by transesophageal echocardiography. Newer, three-dimensional echocardiography provides further definition of valve morphology and function, although the role for this technology has not as yet been fully defined.

Doppler echocardiography has largely replaced cardiac catheterization in accurately assessing the hemodynamic parameters of MS as well as other valve lesions. Doppler blood velocity measurement allows mean and peak transvalvular mitral pressure gradient determination as a function of the simplified Bernoulli equation: $p = 4v^2$. Orifice area can be measured by planimetry (tracing the valve opening orifice on a still echocardiographic image) or as a derivative of velocity measurements, based on continuity equations. Mitral valve area can also be calculated on the basis of the pressure half-time, the time in which the transvalvular velocity decreases by half. Pressure half-time will become prolonged with increasing severity of stenosis.

Natural History

Ten-year patient survival is greater than 80% in the asymptomatic patient with MS, and interventional treatment is consequently not recommended in this setting. In comparison, 10-year survival for symptomatic patients with severe MS who forgo intervention is less than 15%, and mean survival is less than 3 years in patients with MS and severe pulmonary hypertension. All MS patients are therefore recommended to receive careful clinical surveillance, including serial echocardiography.

Treatment

Medical management. Medical management of patients with symptomatic MS includes the use of diuretics to reduce LA pressure and vascular congestion. Beta blockers and calcium-blocking agents are recommended to provide heart rate control and to help maintain sinus rhythm. Anticoagulation therapy is guided by $CHADS_2$ scoring in patients developing atrial fibrillation (Table 60-3) and in patients without atrial fibrillation but who have suffered a prior embolic event or have a documented LA thrombus.[9]

Interventional management. Early operation is associated with improved long-term survival compared with patients in whom intervention is delayed until the development of class III symptoms, in whom 5-year survival is 62%, and compared with class IV patients, in whom 5-year survival is 15%.[10] Mechanical relief of MS is accordingly indicated for symptomatic patients with severe MS (mitral valve area 1.5 cm²) or even in asymptomatic patients with critical MS (orifice area < 1 cm²) or those who have significant elevation of mean transvalvular gradient (>15 mm Hg) or pulmonary capillary wedge pressure (>25 mm Hg) during provocative testing.[9,11] The onset of atrial fibrillation and systemic embolization, especially if recurrent, are other considerations for intervention.

Options for mechanical intervention include percutaneous balloon mitral commissurotomy (PBMC), open mitral commissurotomy (OMC) and surgical repair, and replacement of the mitral valve.

Percutaneous balloon mitral commissurotomy. The first clinical application of mitral commissurotomy by a balloon catheter was reported by Inoue and colleagues in 1984.[12] This endovascular procedure introduces a balloon catheter into the left atrium through transseptal puncture or retrograde transaortic delivery with subsequent dilation of the mitral valve. Randomized clinical trials have clearly established the safety and efficacy of PBMC compared with surgical commissurotomy, and PBMC has largely replaced surgical interventions in patients with appropriate (Wilkins) echocardiographic criteria (Table 60-4), which include the presence of mobile, noncalcified, thin valves with minimal fusion, scarring, or calcification of the subvalvular apparatus and the absence of moderate to severe MR or LA thrombus.[9]

Successful PBMC, defined as a valve area of more than 1.5 cm^2 with no MR higher than grade 2/4, is achieved in more than 80% of appropriately selected patients undergoing this procedure. Mortality risk is 0.5%, and there is a less than 10% risk of cardiac or peripheral vascular complications, embolization, or creation of severe MR.[11] Although reintervention is often ultimately required, more than half of patients can expect to remain free from surgery at 20 years.[13]

Open mitral commissurotomy. Although it is seldom performed in lieu of PBMC or valve replacement, OMC is the primary form of surgical repair for patients with MS in whom intervention is needed but PBMC is contraindicated or for patients in whom previous percutaneous intervention has failed. OMC under cardiopulmonary bypass provides for careful inspection of the mitral valve apparatus, débridement of calcium deposits, sharp division of fused commissures and leaflets, mobilization of scarred chordae, removal of LA thrombus, and ligation of the LA appendage as indicated. It can be performed through a median sternotomy or minimally invasive access. The mortality rate for open commissurotomy is less than 2%, and the 10-year freedom from reoperation rate after OMC is approximately 90%.[14,15]

Mitral valve replacement. For patients in whom PBMC or OMC is contraindicated, mitral valve replacement with a bioprosthetic or mechanical valve is today a safe procedure providing excellent long-term results (Table 60-5). Regardless of whether a mechanical or tissue valve is employed, there is well-documented evidence that preservation of the subvalvular apparatus is critical for the maintenance of optimal LV geometry and function and improving 30-day and long-term survival.[9,16]

Mitral Regurgitation

Pathologic changes to any portion of the mitral valve apparatus or its function may cause improper systolic coaptation between the anterior and posterior mitral leaflets with subsequent valvular regurgitation. Importantly, disease of the mitral annulus or leaflets proper, termed primary MR and classified as type I or type II disease in the Carpentier system (see Table 60-2), is distinct in terms of pathophysiology, natural history, and treatment approach from functional MR, which is typically caused by abnormal LV function and classified as a Carpentier type IIIb lesion.

The severity of MR depends on the size of the mitral orifice, the pressure gradient between the left ventricle and left atrium, and the systemic afterload. Because LV pressure exceeds LA pressure well before it exceeds systemic pressure, mitral valve incompetency may allow a significant amount of regurgitant volume (up to half of the ventricular preload) into the left atrium well before the opening of the aortic valve and forward flow into the aorta.

In the acute phase of MR, retrograde flow into the small, low-compliance left atrium receiving chamber may be poorly tolerated, and high atrial pressures may be transmitted into the pulmonary vasculature. Pulmonary hypertension with fulminant heart failure can ensue and even prove to be fatal. When the onset of MR is more insidious, the left atrium has time to dilate and hypertrophy, and a chronic compensated state without pulmonary hypertension may be sustained for many years. On the other

---

TABLE 60-3 CHADS$_2$ Score for Atrial Fibrillation Stroke Risk and Recommended Anticoagulation

CHADS$_2$ SCORE	POINTS
Congestive heart failure	1
Hypertension	1
Age ≥ 75 years	1
Diabetes mellitus	1
Stroke or TIA history	2

Points are additive for each risk factor. Score of 0, low risk; 1, moderate risk; 2-6, high risk. Recommended therapy for low risk is aspirin, 75 to 325 mg daily; for moderate risk, warfarin or aspirin; for high risk, warfarin (international normalized ratio, 2-3).
TIA, transient ischemic attack.

TABLE 60-4 Wilkins Score for Assessing Appropriateness of Percutaneous Balloon Mitral Commissurotomy

WILKINS SCORE GRADE	MOBILITY	THICKENING	CALCIFICATION	SUBVALVULAR THICKENING
1	Highly mobile valve with only leaflet tips restricted	Leaflets nearly normal in thickness (4-5 mm)	A single area of increased echocardiographic brightness	Minimal thickening just below the mitral leaflets
2	Leaflet mid and base portions have normal mobility	Midleaflets normal, considerable thickening of margins (5-8 mm)	Scattered areas of brightness confined to leaflet margins	Thickening of chordal structures extending to one-third the chordal length
3	Valve continues to move forward in diastole, mainly from the base	Thickening extending through the entire leaflet (5-8 mm)	Brightness extending into the midportions of the leaflets	Thickening extended to distal third of the chords
4	No or minimal forward movement of the leaflets in diastole	Considerable thickening of all leaflet tissue (>8-10 mm)	Extensive brightness throughout much of the leaflet tissue	Extensive thickening and shortening of all chordal structures extending down to the papillary muscles

Sum of the four items ranges between 4 and 16. With a score of 8 or less, percutaneous balloon mitral valvuloplasty is likely to be successful. If the score is higher than 8, surgery is recommended.

TABLE 60-5 Outcomes of Surgery for Valvular Heart Disease

VALVE SURGERY	VALVE LESION	OPERATIVE MORTALITY	SURVIVAL AFTER SURGERY	FREEDOM FROM REOPERATION
Aortic valve replacement	Aortic stenosis	1%-3%[a]	85% at 10 years[b]	75% (lifetime; biologic) 97% (lifetime; mechanical)[c]
	Aortic insufficiency	1%-4%[a]	63% at 10 years[d]	75% (lifetime; biologic) 97% (lifetime; mechanical)[c]
Aortic valve repair	Aortic insufficiency	1%-4%[a]	95% at 13 years[d]	83% to 93% at 8 years[e]
Mitral valve replacement	Mitral stenosis	3%-10%[a]	15%-62% at 5 years[f]	92% at 10 years[g]
	Primary mitral regurgitation	4%[h]	60% at 10 years[g]	92% at 10 years[g]
	Functional mitral regurgitation	3%-5%[i,j]	66% at 5 years[k]	70%-85% at 4 years[l]
Mitral valve repair	Primary mitral regurgitation	0%-1%[l]	87% at 10 years[g]	94% at 10 years[g]
	Functional mitral regurgitation	~5%[m]	50%-75% at 5 years[k,n]	63% at 10 years[l]
Percutaneous balloon mitral commissurotomy	Mitral stenosis	0.5%-2%[a]	80% at 9 years[o]	50% at 20 years[p]
Open mitral commissurotomy	Mitral stenosis	<2%[o]	96% at 10 years[q]	98% at 9 years[j]

[a]Vahanian A, Alfieri O, Andreotti, et al: Guidelines on the management of valvular heart disease (version 2012): The Joint Task Force on the Management of Valvular Heart Disease of the European Society of Cardiology (ESC) and the European Association for Cardio-Thoracic Surgery (EACTS). *Eur J Cardiothorac Surg* 42:S1–S44, 2012. Patients younger than 70 years.
[b]Kvidal P, Bergström R, Hörte LG, et al: Observed and relative survival after aortic valve replacement. *J Am Coll Cardiol* 35:747–756, 2000.
[c]van Geldorp MW, Eric Jamieson WR, Ye J, et al: Patient outcome after aortic valve replacement with a mechanical or biological prosthesis: Weighing lifetime anticoagulant-related event risk against reoperation risk. *J Thorac Cardiovasc Surg* 137:881–886, 2009.
[d]Chaliki HP, Mohty D, Avierinos JF, et al: Outcomes after aortic valve replacement in patients with severe aortic regurgitation and markedly reduced left ventricular function. *Circulation* 106:2687–2693, 2002.
[e]Talwar S, Saikrishna C, Saxena A, et al: Aortic valve repair for rheumatic aortic valve disease. *Ann Thorac Surg* 79:1921–1925, 2005.
[f]Olesen KH: The natural history of 271 patients with mitral stenosis under medical treatment. *Br Heart J* 24:349–357, 1962.
[g]Gillinov AM, Blackstone EH, Nowicki ER, et al: Valve repair versus valve replacement for degenerative mitral valve disease. *J Thorac Cardiovasc Surg* 135:885–893, 2008.
[h]Gammie JS, Sheng S, Griffith BP, et al: Trends in mitral valve surgery in the United States: Results from the Society of Thoracic Surgeons Adult Cardiac Surgery Database. *Ann Thorac Surg* 87:1431–1439, 2009.
[i]Lorusso R, Gelsomino S, Vizzardi E, et al: Mitral valve repair or replacement for ischemic mitral regurgitation? The Italian Study on the Treatment of Ischemic Mitral Regurgitation (ISTIMIR). *J Thorac Cardiovasc Surg* 145:128–139, 2013.
[j]DiBardino DJ, ElBardissi AW, McClure RS, et al: Four decades of experience with mitral valve repair: Analysis of differential indications, technical evolution, and long-term outcome. *J Thorac Cardiovasc Surg* 139:76–84, 2010.
[k]Calafiore AM, Di Mauro M, Gallina S, et al: Mitral valve surgery for chronic ischemic mitral regurgitation. *Ann Thorac Surg* 77:1989–1997, 2004.
[l]Tourmousoglou C, Lalos S, Dougenis D: Is aortic valve repair or replacement with a bioprosthetic valve the best option for a patient with severe aortic regurgitation? *Interact Cardiovasc Thorac Surg* 18:211–218, 2014.
[m]Braunberger E, Deloche A, Berrebi A, et al: Very long-term results (more than 20 years) of valve repair with Carpentier's techniques in nonrheumatic mitral valve insufficiency. *Circulation* 104:I8–I11, 2001.
[n]Oliveira JM, Antunes MJ: Mitral valve repair: Better than replacement. *Heart* 92:275–281, 2006.
[o]Song JK, Kim MJ, Yun SC, et al: Long-term outcomes of percutaneous mitral balloon valvuloplasty versus open cardiac surgery. *J Thorac Cardiovasc Surg* 139:103–110, 2010.
[p]Bouleti C, Iung B, Himbert D, et al: Reinterventions after percutaneous mitral commissurotomy during long-term follow-up, up to 20 years: The role of repeat percutaneous mitral commissurotomy. *Eur Heart J* 34:1923–1930, 2013.
[q]Antunes MJ, Vieira H, Ferrão de Oliveira J: Open mitral commissurotomy: The 'golden standard.' *J Heart Valve Dis* 9:472–477, 2000.

hand, LA dilation may be accompanied by atrial fibrillation with the potential for thrombosis and episodic embolization.

Critical compensatory changes in LV hemodynamics are characteristic of chronic MR. Regurgitant volumes returning to the left ventricle during diastole result in increased LVEDV and supranormal EFs, based on standard Frank-Starling mechanics as well as the presence of LV ejection into the relatively low-resistance/low-afterload left atrium. Although net forward blood flow is reduced, this supranormal ejection serves to marginally unload the left ventricle and normalize LVEDV. Wall stress resulting from increased LVEDV also leads to compensatory myocardial hypertrophy and restoration of normal wall tension per Laplace's law.

Whereas a hypertrophied or hyperdynamic left ventricle is typical of acute or compensated chronic MR, the finding of diminished EF despite the afterload reduction associated with MR is suggestive of a decompensated state with rightward or downward shifts in Frank-Starling curve pressure-volume relationships (Fig. 60-9). In this setting, net forward flows continue to decrease and LVEDV increases. Consequent LA and LV dilation leads to an increase in mitral orifice size. A self-perpetuating cycle of worsening heart failure with worsened MR eventually takes hold. LV failure may then lead to pulmonary hypertension and right-sided heart failure.

Diagnosis of Mitral Regurgitation

Symptoms and signs. Acute decompensated MR may cause the sudden onset of dyspnea secondary to pulmonary venous hypertension and congestion. An associated decrease in forward cardiac output may cause hypotension or even hemodynamic collapse. More typically, patients with chronic, mild MR may be asymptomatic for most of their lives. When MR more gradually becomes moderate to severe, typical symptoms of left-sided heart failure, atrial fibrillation, or even right-sided heart failure may become manifested.

Physical examination. Palpation of patients with MR may reveal a hyperdynamic, laterally displaced cardiac impulse. Auscultation typically reveals a holosystolic, high-pitched, blowing apical murmur that radiates to the axilla. Isolated posterior leaflet dysfunction may cause the murmur to radiate to the sternum or aortic area, whereas isolated anterior leaflet dysfunction may cause the murmur to radiate to the back or head. Other findings may include a diminished first heart sound, wide splitting of the second heart sound due to early aortic valve closure, and a third heart sound due to increased blood flow across the mitral valve.

Diagnostic testing. Echocardiography is the primary method for diagnosis and monitoring of MR, although cardiac magnetic resonance imaging can also provide useful regurgitant volume and cardiac function data. Routine chest radiography may demonstrate an enlarged cardiac silhouette and LA enlargement or signs of pulmonary congestion associated with heart failure. Electrocardiography may reveal atrial fibrillation or signs of LA enlargement (P mitrale) and QRS or ST-T interval changes reflective of ventricular hypertrophy or bundle branch conduction abnormalities.

Transthoracic and in particular transesophageal echocardiography studies allow precise visualization of the mechanisms responsible for inducing MR and classification according to the Carpentier system (see Table 60-2), including single-leaflet or bileaflet prolapse or flail, enlarged or billowing leaflets, annular dilation, chordal rupture, papillary muscle rupture, and restricted leaflet motion and tethering caused by an enlarged or infarcted ventricle. Leaflet disruption or perforation, valvular vegetations, or annular abscesses secondary to infective endocarditis may also be visualized.

Doppler analysis provides important prognostic data on regurgitant jet localization and quantification, typically measured by the proximal isovolumetric surface area (PISA) metric. The PISA measurement is based on the principle that flow through an orifice (mitral valve) will produce a hemispheric area of flow convergence proximal to the orifice (on the ventricular side of the leaking mitral valve). Measuring the radius of this zone allows estimated calculation of the regurgitant flow, effective regurgitant orifice area, and regurgitant volume on the basis of the equation flow = velocity × area.

Natural History

Acute MR is poorly tolerated and typically requires urgent intervention. In the absence of intervention, severe pulmonary edema, cardiac decompensation, and development of pulmonary hypertension often lead to rapid deterioration and poor outcomes.

It was long thought that the asymptomatic MR patient was not at decreased survival risk, but a rich body of new data now clearly demonstrates that even in the asymptomatic patient, the presence of severe MR with ventricular dysfunction, pulmonary hypertension, or atrial fibrillation carries a diminished prognosis. For example, it has been shown prospectively that asymptomatic patients with severe MR have significantly reduced 5-year survival with medical management compared with the general population.[17] Even moderate primary MR has now been shown to be associated with an annual mortality risk of 3%, representing excessive risk in the context of outstanding results now achievable with mitral repair.[5]

Patients with functional MR, typically occurring on the basis

of ischemic disease, carry a far worse prognosis than patients with primary MR.[5] Retrospective data from the STICH trial examining patients undergoing coronary artery bypass grafting (CABG) with diminished EF demonstrated that mortality during approximately 4.5 years was about twofold greater in patients with moderate to severe MR compared with those with mild or no MR.[18]

Treatment

Medical treatment. The medical management of acute MR involves intravenous vasodilator therapy, typically with nitroprusside. The resultant decrease in aortic pressure and afterload enhances forward cardiac output and decreases regurgitant flow into the LA. When vasodilator use is limited by systemic hypotension, intra-aortic balloon counterpulsation effectively lowers systolic afterload and increases forward flow. Prompt mitral valve surgery is typically needed in acute MR, particularly in the symptomatic or hemodynamically compromised patient.

In symptomatic patients with chronic MR, standard vasodilator and diuretic medical therapy can be useful in improving ventricular hemodynamics and reducing pulmonary congestion. Diuretics may be particularly effective in reducing volume overload and ventricular distention and thus annular orifice size and regurgitant MR fractions. Contrary to popular practice, however, there is no evidence to support the use of vasodilator or other afterload-reducing medications in an attempt to delay the need for surgery in asymptomatic patients with chronic MR and normal LV systolic function.[9] In fact, vasodilators may decrease LV size and therefore reduce the mitral valve closing force, potentially increasing mitral valve prolapse and worsening rather than decreasing the severity of regurgitation.

For patients with functional MR, medical therapy should specifically address underlying ventricular dysfunction. Treatment should include carefully titrated use of nitrates, diuretics, angiotensin-converting enzyme inhibitors or angiotensin receptor antagonists, beta blockers (carvedilol is preferred), and aldosterone antagonists in the presence of heart failure.[11]

Surgical treatment. The onset of symptoms is a class I indication for surgical intervention in the setting of severe MR, but even patients with asymptomatic severe MR have a class II indication if mitral repair can be performed, given the risk for the insidious development of LV dysfunction in these individuals and a deteriorated prognosis (Table 60-6). Some evidence suggests that these considerations hold for moderate MR as well.[9]

Because a supranormal EF is typically associated with severe MR before the onset of ventricular dysfunction, an EF less than 60% or an LV end-systolic volume greater than 40 to 45 mm should also prompt consideration of surgery, even in the asymptomatic patient with severe MR (class I indication). The presence of pulmonary hypertension and the new onset of atrial fibrillation represent other indications for repair of MR lesions (Table 60-6).

Importantly, it has been traditional to defer surgical treatment of functional MR, especially in the setting of CABG, under the presumption that improvements in the ischemic milieu after CABG would lead to the resolution of functional MR. Although the literature remains contradictory, data from studies such as the STICH trial suggest, however, that deferring intervention for moderate to severe MR leads to worse outcomes in the setting of concomitant CABG.[18] Isolated intervention for correction of functional MR likewise remains controversial, with no clear evidence of survival benefit as yet identified.

Mitral valve repair is the procedure of choice in the 90% of individuals with primary MR amenable to this approach when

TABLE 60-6   Indications for Intervention for the Treatment of Valvular Heart Disease (excerpted)

VALVE LESION	PROCEDURE	INDICATION	INDICATION CLASS	LEVEL OF EVIDENCE
Mitral stenosis	Percutaneous balloon mitral commissurotomy (PBMC)[a]	Symptomatic patients with severe MS (MVA 1.5 cm²)	I	A[c]
		Asymptomatic patients with very severe MS (MVA 1.0 cm²) or	IIa	C
		Severe MS (MVA 1.5 cm²) and new onset of AF	IIb[c]	C
		Severely symptomatic patients (NYHA class III/IV) with severe MS (MVA 1.5 cm²) who have suboptimal valve anatomy and are at high risk for surgery	IIb[c]	C
		Symptomatic patients with MVA >1.5 cm² if there is evidence of hemodynamically significant MS during exercise	IIb	C
	Mitral valve surgery[b]	Severely symptomatic patients (NYHA class III/IV) with severe MS (MVA 1.5 cm²)	I	B
		Severe MS (MVA 1.5 cm²) in patients who have had recurrent embolic events while receiving adequate anticoagulation[d]	IIb	C
Mitral regurgitation, chronic primary	Mitral valve surgery	Symptomatic patients with severe primary MR:	I	B
		With severe primary MR and LVEF >30%	I	B
		Undergoing cardiac surgery for other indications; may be considered with LVEF ≤30%	IIb	C
		Asymptomatic patients with severe primary MR and LV dysfunction (LVEF 30%-60% and/or LVESD ≥40 mm[e])	I	Be
	Mitral valve repair	Severe primary MR	I	B
		Limited to the posterior leaflet		
		Involving the anterior leaflet or both leaflets when a successful and durable repair can be accomplished		
		Reasonable in asymptomatic patients with severe primary MR with preserved LV function (LVEF >60% and LVESD <40 mm) in whom the likelihood of a successful and durable repair without residual MR is >95%	IIa	B
		With an expected mortality rate of <1% when performed at a Heart Valve Center of Excellence		
		With nonrheumatic disease and (1) new onset of AF or (2) resting pulmonary hypertension (systolic pulmonary arterial pressure >50 mm Hg)		
		Moderate primary MR in patients undergoing cardiac surgery for other indications	IIa	C
Mitral regurgitation, chronic severe secondary	Mitral valve surgery	Reasonable as concomitant procedure when undergoing CABG or AVR[f]	IIa[f]	C
	Mitral valve repair	Severely symptomatic patients (NYHA class III/IV)	IIb[f]	B[f]
		May be considered for patients with chronic moderate secondary MR who are undergoing other cardiac surgery	IIb[f]	C
Aortic stenosis	AVR	Severe high-gradient AS in patients who have symptoms by history or on exercise testing	I	B
		Severe AS and LVEF <50% in asymptomatic patients	I	B[g]
		Severe AS (stage C or D) when undergoing other cardiac surgery	I	B[g]
		Reasonable for asymptomatic patients with very severe AS (aortic velocity ≥5.0 m/s) and low surgical risk	IIa	B
		Reasonable in asymptomatic patients with severe AS and decreased exercise tolerance or an exercise fall in blood pressure	IIa	B[g]
		Reasonable in symptomatic patients with low-gradient severe AS with reduced LVEF with aortic velocity ≥4.0 m/s (or mean pressure gradient ≥40 mm Hg) with a valve area ≤1.0 cm² on dobutamine study	IIa[g]	B[g]
		Reasonable with moderate AS (aortic velocity 3.0-3.9 m/s) who are undergoing other cardiac surgery	IIa	C
		May be considered for asymptomatic patients with severe AS and rapid disease progression and low surgical risk	IIb[g]	C

Continued

TABLE 60-6 Indications for Intervention for the Treatment of Valvular Heart Disease (excerpted)—cont'd

VALVE LESION	PROCEDURE	INDICATION	INDICATION CLASS	LEVEL OF EVIDENCE
	TAVR	Recommended in patients who meet an indication for AVR who have a prohibitive surgical risk and a predicted post-TAVR survival >12 months	I	B
		Reasonable alternative to surgical AVR in patients who meet an indication for AVR and who have high surgical risk	IIa	B
Aortic insufficiency	AVR	Symptomatic patients with severe AI regardless of LV systolic function	I	B
		Asymptomatic patients with chronic severe AI and LV systolic dysfunction (LVEF <50%)	I	B
		Severe AR while undergoing cardiac surgery for other indications	I	C
		Reasonable for asymptomatic patients with severe AI with LVEF ≥50% but with severe LV dilation (LVESD >50 mm)	IIa	B[h]
		Reasonable for moderate AI for patients undergoing other cardiac surgery	IIa	C
		Consider for asymptomatic patients with severe AI and LVEF ≥50% with progressive severe LV dilation (LVEDD >65 mm) if surgical risk is low	IIb	C

Adapted from References 9 and 11.

AF, atrial fibrillation; *AI*, aortic insufficiency; *AR*, aortic regurgitation; *AS*, aortic stenosis; *AVR*, aortic valve replacement; *CABG*, coronary artery bypass grafting; *LV*, left ventricular; *LVEDD*, left ventricular end-diastolic diameter; *LVEF*, left ventricular ejection fraction; *LVESD*, left ventricular end-systolic diameter; *MR*, mitral regurgitation; *MS*, mitral stenosis; *MVA*, mitral valve area; *NYHA*, New York Heart Association; *TAVR*, transcatheter aortic valve replacement.

[a]PBMC is indicated if valve morphology is favorable based on Wilkins score (Table 60-4) in the absence of contraindications.

[b]If appropriate risk and not candidates for PBMC.

[c]In the ESC/EACTS guidelines, PBMC for symptomatic patients with favorable characteristics is Class I, Level of Evidence B. In the ESC/EACTS guidelines, PBMC is indicated in symptomatic patients with contraindication or high risk for surgery—Class I, Level C. In the ESC/EACTS guidelines, PBMC should be considered in asymptomatic patients without unfavorable characteristics and high thromboembolic risk (previous history of embolism, dense spontaneous contrast in the left atrium, recent or paroxysmal atrial fibrillation)—Class IIa, Level C.

[d]With excision of the left atrial appendage.

[e]In the ESC/EACTS guidelines, indicated in asymptomatic patients with LV dysfunction (LVESD ≥45 mm and/or LVEF ≤60%)—Class I, Level C.

[f]In the ESC/EACTS guidelines, indicated in patients with severe MR undergoing CABG and LVEF >30%—Class I, Level C. In the ESC/EACTS guidelines, surgery should be considered in symptomatic patients with severe MR, LVEF <30%, option for revascularization, and evidence of viability— Class IIa, Level C. In the ESC/EACTS guidelines, surgery should be considered in patients with moderate MR undergoing CABG— Class IIa, Level C.

[g]In the ESC/EACTS guidelines, indicated for asymptomatic patients with severe AS and systolic LV dysfunction (LVEF <50%) not due to another cause—Class I, Level C; indicated for severe AS if undergoing CABG, surgery of the ascending aorta or another valve—Class I, Level C; considered in asymptomatic patients with severe AS and abnormal exercise test showing fall in blood pressure below baseline—Class IIa, Level C; considered in symptomatic patients with severe AS and LV dysfunction without flow reserve—Class IIb, Level C.

[h]In the ESC/EACTS guidelines, considered for asymptomatic patients with resting EF >50% with severe LV dilation—Class IIa, Level C.

they are treated at high-volume, experienced centers. A wide variety of well-validated, relatively easy to perform procedures are available to repair regurgitant mitral valves. Valve repair minimizes the risks of prosthetic valve complications, such as endocarditis, as well as a potential need for long-term anticoagulation.[9] Importantly, operative mortality should be close to 0%, and 10-year freedom from reoperation or recurrent moderate to severe MR should exceed 90% with successful repair documented by (mandatory) intraoperative transesophageal echocardiography and when the repair also includes the mandatory use of a reinforcing annuloplasty ring (see Table 60-5).

When valve replacement is required for MR, it is generally associated with an operative mortality rate about double that of patients undergoing repair, although these data are solely from retrospective studies (see Table 60-5).[19] However, valve replacement may be preferable to repair for functional MR in light of discouraging recent survival and freedom from reoperation with repair.[20] Recurrent moderate to severe MR has been reported in at least 20% to 30% of mitral repairs for functional MR, even with the use of annuloplasty rings designed specifically to correct

the apicolateral posterior leaflet displacement associated with this syndrome.[21] Alternative procedures to restore ventricular-annular dimensions using papillary muscle anchoring and other similar techniques remain largely investigational.[22]

Aortic Stenosis

The normal aortic valve orifice measures 3 to 5 cm^2. Aortic valve stenosis to less than half this size causes hemodynamic obstruction and a transvalvular pressure gradient. Increased ventricular pressure, generated through Frank-Starling mechanisms (see earlier), leads to an increase in myocardial wall tension, and the left ventricle undergoes compensatory concentric hypertrophy through parallel replication of sarcomeres. Wall tension thereby normalizes according to the law of Laplace, and a compensated state preserving the systolic function of a hypertrophied but nondilated left ventricle may persist for many years.

Progressive AS is associated with several pathophysiologic sequelae. Two thirds of patients with severe AS develop myocardial ischemia as a result of the elevated myocardial oxygen demand and the increased work of a hypertrophied ventricle generating increased ejection pressures over prolonged systolic intervals against the increased afterload of the narrowed aortic valve. Myocardial ischemia, particularly in the subendocardial region, is accentuated by the reduction of perfusion gradients during diastolic coronary flow intervals. AS patients likewise demonstrate severely impaired coronary arterial flow reserve—decreased from normal values of up to 800% to often less than double the resting coronary flow. Consequent cell death and myocardial fibrosis can lead to a cardiomyopathy and exacerbate AS-induced heart failure.

Myocardial hypertrophy can also precipitate ventricular diastolic dysfunction, which typically occurs before the onset of systolic dysfunction. Decreased ventricular compliance leads to increased LVEDP, prolonged LV relaxation time, and shortened diastolic filling time. These increased pressures are transmitted back through the left atrium and pulmonary circulation, leading to pulmonary congestion. Pulmonary hypertension and right-sided heart failure may develop in severe cases. Eventually, maximal ventricular hypertrophy is reached and an adequate pressure gradient can no longer be achieved, resulting in inadequate cardiac outputs and overt, self-reinforcing systolic LV failure.

Increased LA pressure and consequent LA dilation also increase the risk for atrial arrhythmias. The loss of normal atrial contraction severely compromises filling of the noncompliant ventricle, leading to a sometimes precipitous decrease in cardiac output. Reduced forward flow can further increase LVEDP and aggravate the symptoms of heart failure.

Presyncope and syncope are unusual sequelae of AS related to inadequate (cerebral) organ perfusion, typically caused by inadequate forward flow through the restrictive aortic valve. Symptoms are typically associated with periods of peripheral vasodilation, such as during exercise or in changing from a recumbent to standing positioning when increased cardiac output is required to maintain peripheral vascular filling.

Diagnosis of Aortic Stenosis

Symptoms and signs. Patients with AS will typically remain asymptomatic for an extended time. The onset of symptoms occurs when the valve orifice area decreases to approximately 1 cm^2, which marks a critical point in the natural history of the disease. The classic symptoms of AS typically progress from the appearance of *angina* and (pre-)*syncope* to the occurrence of *dyspnea* associated with heart failure (mnemonic: ASD). Whereas angina is the presenting symptom of AS in 35% of patients, syncope is a relatively sporadic event that is the presenting symptom in 15% of patients. Although heart failure typically appears late in the course of AS, dyspnea or other heart failure symptoms are presenting signs in 50% of patients.

Physical examination. The diagnosis of AS is frequently made before the onset of symptoms. The typical finding is a crescendo-decrescendo ejection murmur best heard along the left sternal border and that radiates to the upper right sternal border and carotid arteries. The apical impulse in AS is forceful and slightly enlarged. If heart failure develops, the apical impulse may become laterally displaced. The characteristic carotid upstroke of AS has a slow rate of rise and a reduced peak (pulsus parvus et tardus) and may have an associated thrill.

As AS progresses, its murmur peaks progressively later in systole and may actually decrease in intensity because of diminished stroke volume. The second heart sound may become singular because the aortic and pulmonic components are superimposed, or the aortic valve component may be absent because of the immobility of the calcified valve. A third or fourth heart sound may become audible in patients in sinus rhythm.

Diagnostic testing. Nonspecific findings of AS on chest radiography include a boot-shaped heart typical of concentric hypertrophy of the left ventricle, calcification of the valvular cusps, and poststenotic dilation of the aorta. As heart failure ensues, cardiomegaly and pulmonary vascular congestion may be seen. The right-sided heart border may become more prominent in severe failure. Electrocardiographic changes are similar to those seen for MR.

Echocardiography allows the precise assessment of aortic valve anatomy, calcification, and effective orifice size, measured by planimetry. Ventricular hypertrophy and function can also be assessed. As with MS, Doppler echocardiography allows measurement of transvalvular pressure gradients and valve area as a derived function (e.g., Doppler velocity >4 m/sec = valve area <1 cm^2). Pressure gradients may be decreased in AS patients with low cardiac output, leading to miscalculated (falsely increased) aortic valve areas. Low-dose dobutamine may be used during echocardiography to increase cardiac output and to assess the true severity of the AS lesion in these patients.

Cardiac catheterization may occasionally be needed to measure pressure gradients in ambiguous cases. Simultaneous pressure readings can be obtained in such instances with one pressure measuring port in the body of the left ventricle and a second device in the proximal aorta. Valvular area may then be determined by the Gorlin formula. Catheterization may be needed to assess the presence of coronary artery disease, coexistent in up to 50% of AS patients.

Natural History

Calcific AS is a progressive disease marked by a long, asymptomatic latent period. The duration of the asymptomatic period varies greatly between individuals. Ross and Braunwald's classic 1968 report first described the onset of symptoms of heart failure, syncope, or angina in patients with AS as a marker of impending death (Fig. 60-10).[23] Although mean survival after the appearance of angina is about 5 years, it is less than 3 years after the onset of syncope and only 1 to 2 years once heart failure symptoms develop. Since Ross and Braunwald's report, other studies have confirmed that nearly 50% of patients will die within 3 to 5 years after the onset of symptoms from AS.[24,25] Sudden death may occur in symptomatic patients at a rate of 2%/month but appears to be rare (<1% per year) in asymptomatic patients.[24] Significantly, echocardiography-based population studies have demonstrated that aortic jet velocity can effectively predict progression to symptoms and surgery.[24]

Treatment

Medical management. Medical therapy is important in the treatment of early signs and symptoms of heart failure and other common comorbidities, such as hypertension. Treatment of hypertension may also serve to unload the AS ventricle, helping to relieve adverse ventricular remodeling. Although there are no medical therapies currently proven to alter the natural history of calcific AS, multiple ongoing investigations are seeking to slow disease progression through an apparent endothelial injury/atherosclerosis AS pathway.

Surgical treatment. Because the natural history of untreated symptomatic AS is grave, mechanical relief of AS is recommended as a class I indication in all symptomatic patients, and a careful history noting the onset of symptoms in AS patients is essential (see Table 60-6). Aortic valve surgery improves symptoms,

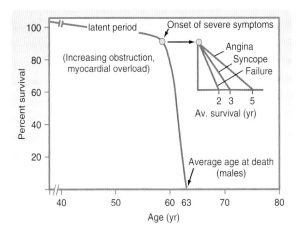

FIGURE 60-10 Symptoms and Survival in AS. Ross and Braunwald's classic 1968 report first described the onset of symptoms of heart failure, syncope, and angina in patients with AS as a marker of impending death. (From Ross J, Jr, Braunwald E: Aortic stenosis. *Circulation* 38:61–67, 1968.)

increases life expectancy, and often improves or normalizes systolic function and has transformed the outlook for this disease.

Surgical intervention now also carries a class I indication in the asymptomatic patient with severe AS and evidence of LV dysfunction (LVEF <50%). Other class IIb indications have also been proposed for patients with severe asymptomatic disease who demonstrate rapid disease progression and are at low surgical risk, given evidence that these patients will likely go on to develop symptoms and that the risk of death without surgery remains significant even before the onset of symptoms.[9,11] Ongoing investigations are attempting to identify other subgroups of patients who are at high risk for disease progression and who may benefit from valve replacement rather than watchful waiting. For example, exercise or dobutamine stress echocardiography has been shown to elicit abnormal physiology or symptoms in as many as 30% of patients tested.[26]

Surgery for AS almost always requires valve replacement, with either a mechanical or tissue valve (see later), and is associated with excellent immediate and long-term outcomes (see Table 60-5), especially when it is conducted before the onset of ventricular dysfunction. Earlier efforts at valve débridement met with disastrous intermediate-term outcomes with delayed onset of regurgitation and led to the general abandonment of this technique. Patients in whom surgical valve replacement is considered too risky may alternatively be candidates for percutaneous, catheter-based valve replacement (see later section on transcatheter aortic valve replacement).

Aortic Insufficiency

Competency of the aortic valve, like that of the mitral valve, is dependent on the coordinated function of a complex and dynamic anatomy. It includes the valve cusps, annulus, sinuses of Valsalva, and sinotubular junction above the sinuses. Aortic regurgitation, or aortic insufficiency (AI), may be induced by pathologic processes that may alter any one or more of these components or their anatomic relationships with each other.

Acute AI, usually the consequence of endocarditis or aortic dissection, produces sudden increases in LVEDV caused by acute regurgitant flow into a relatively small, nonadapted, noncompli-

ant ventricle. Even greater increases in LVEDP result, and equalization of systemic and ventricular pressure may occur. Transmission of increased LVEDP into the pulmonary circuit may produce fulminant pulmonary edema, particularly in the setting of coexisting MR. Increased wall tension typically leads to myocardial ischemia, especially if aortic dissection extends to the coronary ostia, and hemodynamic collapse or early death may ensue.

Chronic AI, like chronic MR, is an insidious process that triggers a number of compensatory mechanisms to maintain net forward stroke volume, and patients with chronic AI often remain well compensated for many years. Ventricles can ultimately weigh as much as three times normal and have a capacitance of more than 200 mL to accommodate massive regurgitant volumes. Marked decreases in systemic diastolic pressure, with reciprocal increases in pulse pressure, are typically found with massive regurgitant flow back into the ventricle. The sum effect of myocardial hypertrophy and LV enlargement in AI patients is a dramatically enlarged heart known as cor bovinum, characterized by the largest EDV and mass of any form of heart disease.

These changes associated with chronic AI begin with increases in afterload and wall stress caused by mild or moderate regurgitant flow and increases in LVEDV less severe than those associated with acute AI. Compensation occurs through Frank-Starling shifts in contractility (see earlier) and stress-induced eccentric ventricular hypertrophy characterized by sarcomere replication in series and elongation of myofibers. This hypertrophy tends to preserve ventricular compliance and to minimize increases in LVEDP while still decreasing wall tension. Increases in heart rate and decreases in peripheral vascular resistance that reduce diastolic filling time and decrease afterload also act to decrease regurgitant flow.

Over time, however, progressive increases in LVEDV eventually exhaust preload reserve and overwhelm compensation mechanisms. Progressive increases in LVEDV and LVEDP lead to ventricular dilation, increased wall tension, and increased myocardial oxygen demand. Decreased systemic diastolic pressure and increased intramyocardial wall tension decrease coronary perfusion gradients and further exacerbate myocardial ischemia. Ultimately, ischemia may lead to myocardial fibrosis and cardiomyopathy. When the ventricle can no longer maintain adequate forward flow, overt heart failure ensues.

Diagnosis and Treatment of Aortic Insufficiency

Symptoms and signs. Severe acute AI may be difficult to recognize clinically, although acute AI patients may present with dyspnea, hemodynamic instability, or shock. Frequently, symptoms reflecting the underlying cause of the AI, such as fever from endocarditis or chest pain from aortic dissection, may mask AI symptoms and obscure a correct diagnosis.

Although chronically compensated AI patients remain asymptomatic for long periods, symptoms of heart failure often eventually develop. Those with severe AI may also experience angina pectoris, nocturnal angina, and palpitations during stress or exertion.

Physical examination. Acute AI may yield few if any diagnostic signs other than those of fulminant heart failure or hemodynamic collapse. In comparison, chronic AI typically offers many physical findings, primarily related to the increases in stroke volume, systolic blood pressure, and pulse pressure associated with this condition. These include peripheral pulses that rise abruptly and rapidly collapse (water-hammer pulse), a bounding carotid pulse (Corrigan pulse), head bobbing with each heartbeat (de Musset sign), pulsation of the uvula (Müller sign), a "pistol shot" auscultated with compression of the femoral artery (Traube sign), and capillary pulsations seen with fingernail compression using a glass slide (Quincke sign).

Cardiac examination typically reveals an apical impulse that is diffuse, hyperdynamic, and displaced inferiorly and laterally. It may be associated with a systolic thrill at the base of the heart, suprasternal notch, and carotid arteries due to high stroke volume. Auscultation reveals a high-frequency blowing, decrescendo diastolic murmur best heard with the diaphragm at the left sternal border with the patient sitting up, leaning forward, and at end-exhalation. The murmur is increased by maneuvers such as squatting or hand-grip, which increase diastolic pressure. The examiner may appreciate a mid and late diastolic apical rumble (Austin Flint murmur), which is thought to be secondary to vibration of the anterior mitral leaflet caused by a posteriorly directed AI jet. The second heart sound may be soft or absent, and a third heart sound may be present.

Diagnostic testing. Chest radiography in patients with acute AI may reveal only pulmonary edema, and electrocardiography may reveal evidence of LV strain, but echocardiography may be the only test useful in diagnosis of this condition. With chronic AI, chest radiography typically shows a significantly enlarged cardiac silhouette. The ascending aorta may be enlarged if AI is due to an aortic aneurysm. Electrocardiography will typically show signs of increased LV mass, with left axis deviation and increased QRS amplitude with strain patterns and conduction abnormalities.

Echocardiography allows the comprehensive evaluation of aortic apparatus abnormalities as well as the character and magnitude of the regurgitant jet. Severe AI, for example, may be diagnosed by a jet width of 65% or more of the LV outflow tract, vena contracta (the narrowest central flow region of a jet that occurs at or just downstream to the orifice of a regurgitant valve) of more than 0.6 cm, regurgitant fraction of 50% or more, or an effective regurgitant orifice area (derived from the PISA radius) of 0.3 cm^2 or more. Echocardiography also allows assessments of LV size and compliance important to prognostic calculations.

Natural History

Whereas acute AI may lead to the sudden onset of heart failure or hemodynamic collapse, patients with chronic AI typically enjoy years of asymptomatic, compensated LV function. The combined likelihood of onset of adverse events for such patients (LV dysfunction, onset of symptoms, or death) is less than 5% per year. Overall, the freedom from ventricular dysfunction or death incidence rate in asymptomatic patients is about 75% at 5 years, but this incidence decreases to 60% at 10 years.[27] Furthermore, once the end-systolic diameter of the left ventricle is greater than 50 mm, adverse event rates increase to about 20% per year.[9,11,27] Once symptoms develop in AI patients, mortality rates rise to more than 10% per year.[27]

Treatment

Medical management. Medical therapy should be considered only a temporizing measure for patients with acute severe AI and acute volume overload, hypotension, or pulmonary edema who will require emergent surgery. In this scenario, vasodilators and inotropes may be valuable in augmenting forward flow and reducing LVEDP. Beta blockers used for aortic dissection should be employed with great caution in other causes of acute AI because they block compensatory tachycardia and could cause a significant drop in blood pressure. Importantly, intra-aortic balloon counterpulsation is contraindicated in patients with AI because it will worsen regurgitation and compromise forward output.

Patients with chronic severe AI may benefit from medical management with the primary goal of reducing systolic hypertension, therefore reducing wall stress and improving ventricular function. Vasodilator therapy is also indicated in patients with severe AI who have symptoms or LV dysfunction, although surgical intervention should not be delayed if it is indicated.[9,11] Furthermore, although vasodilating drugs may improve hemodynamic abnormalities and forward flow, their effect in favorably prolonging the asymptomatic period in patients with chronic severe AI and normal ventricular function is uncertain.[9,11] Medical treatment of symptomatic patients with AI is appropriate only until surgical intervention can be undertaken.

Surgical treatment. Urgent or emergent surgical intervention to repair or to replace the aortic valve and to address underlying pathologic mechanisms (e.g., endocarditis, aortic dissection) is nearly always indicated in patients with acute severe AI. Surgery is also indicated (class I) for symptomatic patients with severe chronic AI (see Table 60-6). Importantly, on the basis of improved current understandings of the natural history of chronic AI, aortic valve surgery now also carries a class I indication for asymptomatic chronic severe AI patients with LV systolic dysfunction (LVEF <50%) and a class IIa and class IIb indication, respectively, for asymptomatic severe AI with normal LV systolic function (LVEF ≥50%) but with severe LV dilation (LV end-systolic diameter >50 mm) or progressive severe LV dilation (LV end-diastolic diameter >65 mm).

Valve replacement with mechanical or biologic prostheses has yielded excellent results in correcting isolated AI (see Table 60-5); however, during the past 2 decades, increasing numbers of centers are employing repair strategies in selected patients, as described later.[28] For patients with aortic root disease, these procedures are typically combined with root repair or replacement and coronary reimplantation, as discussed elsewhere in this text.

In selected patients, the aortic valve may alternatively be replaced with a pulmonary autograft, with heterograft substitution of the native pulmonic valve (Ross procedure). Excellent results with this procedure have been demonstrated in highly experienced centers, especially for younger (<30 years) patients in whom traditional valve replacement procedures carry high risks of valve-related complications over time. However, given the lack of reproducibility of these results more generally because of technical challenges, this procedure is likely best performed for selected patients undergoing surgery at experienced centers.[9]

Tricuspid Regurgitation and Other Right-Sided Valve Disease

Functional TR is by far the most prevalent right-sided valve disease. It typically occurs as the result of left-sided valve disease or heart failure, and like primary right-sided valve disease, it is due to pathophysiologic mechanisms very similar to left-sided equivalents. Unlike in left-sided disease, altered RV mechanics and geometry associated with RV failure may cause irreversible dilation of the saddle-shaped ellipsoid of a healthy tricuspid annulus into a more planar circular shape, leading to persistence of TR despite the correction of inciting hemodynamics. Increased central venous pressure resulting from tricuspid valve disease can lead to venous congestion, hepatic enlargement, ascites, and peripheral edema as well as right atrial enlargement and arrhythmias. Decreased RV output can lead to LV underfilling and inadequate left-sided output.

Diagnosis of Tricuspid Valve Disease

Symptoms and signs. Because patients with tricuspid disease almost invariably have coexisting left-sided valve disease, it is difficult to separate symptoms of tricuspid disease from those of multivalvular disease, and tricuspid valve disease itself may frequently be asymptomatic. Dyspnea, fatigue, and exercise intolerance may, however, result as heart failure develops.

Physical examination. A classic holosystolic murmur that increases with inspiration (Carvallo sign) and that may be heard along the sternal border is typical of TR. With TS, an opening snap followed by a diastolic rumble may be heard at the right sternal border. The physical examination of patients with tricuspid valve disease may otherwise reveal only jugular venous distention with a prominent systolic *v* wave. With progressive central venous congestion, physical findings that may be out of proportion to symptoms may include pleural effusions, hepatic enlargement (with a pulsatile liver typical of TR), abdominal tenderness, ascites, and peripheral edema.

Diagnostic testing. Because of the overlay of concomitant left-sided disease, echocardiography is the sole reliable testing modality useful in assessing tricuspid disease, similar in application to that for assessing mitral disease. Estimation of pulmonary arterial systolic pressure based on the velocity of the TR jet measured by continuous-wave Doppler is a useful prognostic criterion. An annular diameter of more than 40 mm defines significant tricuspid annular dilation, an important consideration in selecting appropriate treatment of TR.[29]

Natural History

Decreased survival is associated with increasing TR severity, regardless of other indices of cardiac function.[30] Although patients who undergo surgical treatment of left-sided valve disease may experience improved or resolved functional TR, such improvement is highly unpredictable, and survival for patients with uncorrected moderate to severe TR is less than 50% at 4 years.[30] The natural history of other right-sided valve lesions is poorly documented because such lesions typically require surgical correction as congenital anomalies or with rheumatic disease of the mitral and aortic valves.

Treatment

Medical management. The medical treatment of tricuspid valve disease involves optimization of RV preload and afterload, using diuretics and angiotensin-converting enzyme inhibitors, respectively. If atrial fibrillation is present, rate control may optimize diastolic filling. With functional TR, medical treatment to reduce pulmonary hypertension may also improve cardiac output.

Surgical treatment. The timing and method for surgical treatment of functional TR are controversial. Until recent years, the notion that functional TR would improve or disappear after the primary left-sided heart disease was treated led to recommendations of avoiding tricuspid surgery. However, the improvement of functional or primary forms of severe TR has not been predictable after left-sided heart surgery. Left uncorrected, secondary TR may worsen in about 25% of patients, which has functional and survival implications because of irreversible progression of RV damage and organ failure.[30]

Adding tricuspid repair during left-sided heart surgery does not significantly increase operative risk. However, reoperation due to persistent TR after left-sided heart surgery carries a perioperative mortality of 10% to 25%. Therefore, severe TR has emerged as a class I indication for concomitant tricuspid valve surgery in patients who are undergoing left-sided heart surgery.[9,11] Concomitant repair is also probably indicated in those with mild or greater TR and either tricuspid annular dilation or evidence of right-sided heart failure.[30]

Tricuspid valve repair is generally preferred to replacement whenever possible. For severe TR due to isolated annular dilation, annuloplasty using a prosthetic ring has been shown in a number of studies to have better long-term results than traditional suture annuloplasty.[31] Valve replacement should be considered for functional TR due to leaflet tethering and RV remodeling.

Symptomatic patients with isolated TS do not benefit from medical management and are best treated with valve replacement. Those with TS and left-sided valve disease should likewise undergo concomitant correction during the same operation.[9,11] Percutaneous tricuspid valvulotomy may be considered, but outcomes are less optimistic than those seen with MS and may induce significant TR.[32]

Mixed Valve Disease

Patients with mixed valve disease typically present with a predominant lesion that dictates symptoms and pathophysiologic changes. There are limited data on the natural history of mixed valve disease, and therefore the optimal timing of serial evaluation is not clear. Therapy should be targeted to the predominant lesion while considering the severity of concomitant valve disease.

Patients with multivalvular disease present even more complex diagnostic and therapeutic challenges. The coexistence of aortic valve disease and MR, for example, will mitigate LV changes induced by aortic valve disease but worsen pulmonary and right-sided complications. Limited data are available to guide treatment in these cases, and indications for interventions should be based on symptoms and objective analysis of surgical outcome rather than on severity indices for the individual lesions.[11]

OPERATIVE APPROACHES

Surgery for valvular heart disease is today associated with excellent short- and long-term outcomes, with some evidence suggesting even better outcomes for surgery performed at high-volume centers.[33] The risk of operative mortality, which in the modern era is generally less than 5% for all types of valve disease, can now be accurately predicted by several widely available multivariable risk calculation scoring systems, such as those provided by the Society of Thoracic Surgeons and the European Association for Cardiothoracic Surgery.

In general, operative mortality is predicted by risk factors such as age, female gender, emergency surgery, symptoms, concomitant procedures, decreased EF, and comorbidities, such as diabetes mellitus, renal dysfunction or pulmonary disease, peripheral vascular disease, or prior operation (Table 60-7). Typically, MR is associated with the poorest operative mortality risk, followed by AI, with surgery for AS and MS offering the best operative mortality outcomes. Complications most frequently associated with surgery for valvular heart disease include infection, bleeding, stroke, conduction block (potentially requiring permanent pacemaker placement), and heart failure (Table 60-8).

Long-term outcomes and resolution of ventricular hemodynamic pathophysiology can likewise generally be predicted by the duration or severity of symptoms as well as by the extent of ventricular dysfunction or the presence and severity of pulmonary

TABLE 60-7 European System for Valvular Surgery Operative Risk Evaluation (EuroSCORE)

	DEFINITION	SCORE
Patient-Related Factors		
Age	Per 5 years or part thereof over 60 years	1
Sex	Female	1
Chronic pulmonary disease	Long-term bronchodilators or steroids	1
Extracardiac arteriopathy	Claudication; carotid occlusion or >50% stenosis; intervention on abdominal aorta, limb arteries, carotids	2
Neurologic dysfunction	Severely affecting ambulation or day-to-day functioning	2
Previous cardiac surgery	Requiring opening of the pericardium	3
Serum creatinine concentration	>200 mmol/liter preoperatively	2
Active endocarditis	Antibiotic treatment for endocarditis at the time of surgery	3
Critical preoperative state	Ventricular tachycardia, fibrillation, aborted sudden death; preoperative cardiac massage, ventilation, inotropic support, IABP, or acute renal failure (anuria or oliguria <10 mL/hr)	3
Cardiac-Related Factors		
Unstable angina	Rest angina requiring intravenous nitrates preoperatively	2
LV dysfunction	Moderate or LVEF 30-50%	1
	Poor or LVEF <30%	3
Recent myocardial infarct	Within 90 days	2
Pulmonary hypertension	Systolic pulmonary artery pressure >60 mm Hg	2
Operation-Related Factors		
Emergency	Carried out on referral before next working day	2
Other than isolated CABG	Major cardiac procedure other than or in addition to CABG	2
Surgery on thoracic aorta	For disorder of ascending, arch, or descending aorta	3
Postinfarct septal rupture		4

Adapted from Roques F, Nashef SA, Michel P, et al: Risk factors and outcome in European cardiac surgery: Analysis of the EuroSCORE multinational database of 19030 patients. *Eur J Cardiothorac Surg* 15:816–822, 1999.
Interpretation: low risk, 0-2; medium risk, 3-5; high risk, 6 or more.
CABG, coronary artery bypass graft surgery; *IABP*, intra-aortic balloon counterpulsation; *LV*, left ventricular; *LVEF*, left ventricular ejection fraction.

TABLE 60-8 Complications Associated With Valvular Heart Surgery

OUTCOME	AVR	MVR
Prolonged ventilation	7%	10.8%
Renal failure	3.7%	5.2%
Reoperation for bleeding	4.1%	4.7%
Permanent stroke	1.6%	2.2%
Deep sternal infection	0.5%	0.3%
Postoperative hospital stay*	8.5 ± 8.4	9.9 ± 10.3
Overall hospital stay*	10.6 ± 9.6	12.8 ± 12.6

Adapted from data from the Society of Thoracic Surgeons national database (N = 49,073 patients). Edwards FH, Peterson ED, Coombs LP, et al: Prediction of operative mortality after valve replacement surgery. *J Am Coll Cardiol* 37:885–892, 2001.
AVR, aortic valve replacement; *MVR*, mitral valve replacement.
*Mean days ± standard deviation.

hypertension.[9,11] Complete hemodynamic recovery from valvular disease, including resolution of ventricular hypertrophy and enlargement, may be seen as early as the first several weeks postoperatively but may progress for up to a year after surgery. The long-term complications frequently associated with valve surgery are thromboembolic events including stroke, reoperation for valve deterioration or perivalvular leaks, bleeding associated with anticoagulant medications, and endocarditis (Table 60-8).

Conduct of Surgery

A full midline median sternotomy has traditionally been the predominant means to obtain wide exposure for heart valve surgery. More recently, partial upper or lower sternotomies or small third or fourth interspace thoracotomies have been popularized as minimally invasive access approaches, using either direct visualization with specialized instruments or indirect, robotic surgical techniques (Fig. 60-11). In all cases, intraoperative transesophageal echocardiography is essential in the assessment of valve anatomy and function.

Cardiopulmonary bypass and hypothermic cardioplegic arrest of the heart are standard to performance of open heart procedures on the cardiac valves. Bicaval cannulation is typically used for mitral or tricuspid valve surgery. Minimally invasive approaches generally use peripheral cannulation of the femoral or axillary arteries for cardiopulmonary bypass, although direct aortic cannulation may also be possible.

Mitral Valve Replacement and Repair

The mitral valve is typically exposed through a left lateral atriotomy made just anterior to the pulmonary veins (Fig. 60-12). Alternatively, a right atriotomy and a second incision through the atrial septum also provide excellent exposure to the mitral valve. Even greater exposure can be provided by a "superior septal" approach joining the right atrial and septostomy incisions onto the dome of the left atrium, but this approach requires more extensive closure. Once the mitral valve has been exposed and appropriate retraction applied, typically including rotation of the heart toward the left side of the chest, the surgeon carefully

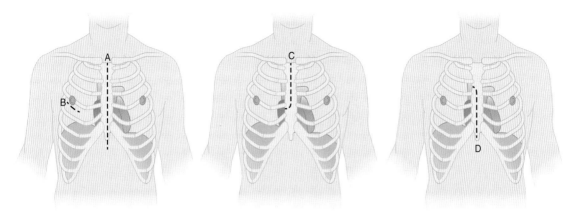

FIGURE 60-11 Surgical Access for Valvular Heart Surgery. Median sternotomy (A) versus minimally invasive access through minithoracotomy (B) or partial upper (C) or lower (D) sternotomy. (From Byrne JG, Leacche M, Vaughan DE, et al: Hybrid cardiovascular procedures. *JACC Cardiovasc Interv* 1:459–468, 2008.)

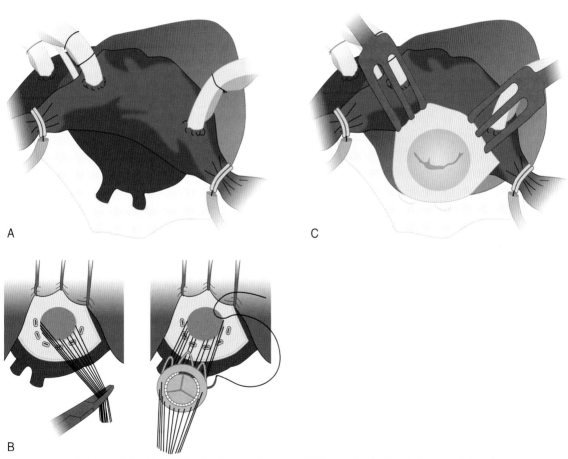

FIGURE 60-12 Mitral Valve Replacement Surgery. **A,** The mitral valve is typically exposed through a left lateral atriotomy made just anterior to the pulmonary veins. **B,** After partial excision of the native valve, pledgeted horizontal mattress sutures are placed circumferentially into the valve annulus and then into the cloth sewing ring of the prosthesis. **C,** Valve lowered into position and sutures securely tied. (From Glower DD: Surgical approaches to mitral regurgitation. *J Am Coll Cardiol* 60:1315–1322, 2012.)

inspects all components of the mitral valve apparatus to select valve repair versus replacement.

Mitral Valve Replacement

If valve replacement is necessary, minimal resection (typically of a portion of the anterior leaflet) should be performed, making best efforts to preserve the subvalvular apparatus in continuity with the valve leaflets and annulus. Calcified or fused fibrotic leaflet or annular tissue is excised as needed to allow implantation of an adequately sized valve prosthesis without perivalvular leak.

Typically, after sizing of the annulus with a plastic avatar and selection of an appropriate prosthesis, nonabsorbable braided pledgeted horizontal mattress sutures are placed circumferentially into the valve annulus and then into the cloth sewing ring of the prosthesis (Fig. 60-12B). The sutures are tied securely to make sure there is no perivalvular defect that would allow a regurgitant leak, and the atriotomy is closed after de-airing of the heart (Fig. 60-12C).

Mitral Valve Repair

A wide variety of surgical techniques may be employed to repair primary MR lesions. Most commonly, flail or prolapsing (typically posterior [P2]) segments of the valve can be excised through a limited (triangular) or more extensive (quadrangular) resection, and leaflet continuity is restored simply by suturing the resected leaflet edges back together (Fig. 60-13A). Often, relaxing incisions along the posterior leaflet base (sliding annuloplasty) may be used to take tension off this repair or to decrease the "height" of the posterior leaflet. This helps prevent postresection MR resulting from systolic anterior motion of the anterior mitral leaflet, which may become displaced toward the aortic outflow tract after inadequate resections.

More recently, a number of authors have validated the use of artificial chordae, instead of or in addition to valve resection, to help support normal leaflet function. Typically made of polytetrafluoroethylene and now available as presized lengths selected on the basis of pre-repair measurements, these are sutured between the papillary muscles and leaflet edges to correct flail or prolapsing leaflet segments.

An annuloplasty ring is almost always implanted, in a manner analogous to valve implantation, to supplement resectional repairs, or it may be used alone to address MR arising from a dilated annulus (Fig. 60-13B). Insertion of an annuloplasty ring dramatically helps re-form normal annular geometry to "compress" the anterior and posterior leaflets together, providing a minimum

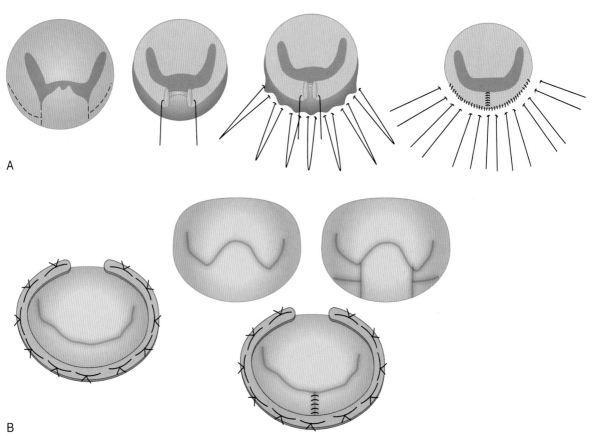

FIGURE 60-13 Mitral Valve Replacement Surgery. A, Exposure of the left atrium is obtained from the right side of the heart by developing Sondergaard's plane at the interatrial groove. **B,** The mitral valve is exposed through a left lateral atriotomy made just anterior to the pulmonary veins. **C,** After partial excision of the native valve, pledgeted horizontal mattress sutures are placed circumferentially into the valve annulus and then into the cloth sewing ring of the prosthesis. The valve is then lowered into position and the sutures securely tied.

coaptation length of 6 to 8 mm between anterior and posterior leaflets.

Annuloplasty rings are generally sized to approximate the surface area of the anterior mitral leaflet but may be "undersized" to maximize leaflet coaptation while care is taken to avoid an inadequately sized ring, which can create systolic anterior motion from redundancy in the anterior leaflet. The author typically uses complete, semirigid rings to maximally stabilize the annulus, but more flexible or partial rings are preferred by many surgeons and may provide comparable results.

A number of specially configured rings have also been developed to correct the apical and lateral displacement of the posterior valve leaflet associated with functional MR. In general, intermediate- and long-term results with these repair strategies have been discouraging. More complex techniques to correct papillary muscle–annular relationships have been proposed.[22]

Surgical Aortic Valve Replacement and Aortic Valve Repair

Exposure of the aortic valve is typically obtained through a transverse or "hockey stick" incision of the proximal ascending aorta (Fig. 60-14A). For valve replacement, the native aortic valve cusps are carefully excised to avoid perforation of the aortic wall, and a thorough decalcification of residual annular tissue is performed to improve prosthetic valve fit. Implantation of a mechanical or bioprosthetic valve is similar to that described for the mitral valve (Fig. 60-14B,C). Homografts or "free-style" stentless aortic valve homografts may sometimes be used, often to provide improved implant hemodynamics. The details of these more complex implant techniques may be referenced elsewhere.[34]

The repair technique for AI has more recently been developed and attained an increasingly well-validated long-term track record. Commonly known as the David procedure (in credit to the surgeon who initially conceived the operation, Tirone David), the valve-sparing root replacement is a complex operation meant to restore the normal relationships of the aortic root by reimplanting the native valve inside of a Dacron graft that replaces the dilated ascending aorta causing AI.[35] The operation involves excision of the aortic sinuses and detachment of the coronary arteries, aortic replacement with a Dacron graft, securing of the aortic valve inside of the graft above and below the annulus, and reimplantation of the coronary vessels. Overall 20-year freedom from reoperation rates in excess of 90% have been reported with this procedure.[36]

Prosthetic Valves

The prosthetic heart valves most often implanted are made from a synthetic material (mechanical valves; Fig. 60-15A), allogeneic biologic tissue (bioprosthetic valves; Fig. 60-15B), or (cadaveric) homografts. Each has distinct advantages and disadvantages. Anticoagulation with a vitamin K antagonist (warfarin) and monitoring of the international normalized ratio are recommended in nearly all patients with mechanical prosthetic valves and typically for the first 3 months after bioprosthetic mitral implants (Table 60-9). Aspirin may be added to warfarin therapy to reduce rates of major embolism, stroke, and overall mortality. In comparison, bioprosthetic or homograft valves carry a greater risk of structural deterioration and need for reoperation. Health care professionals must carefully advise their patients on these considerations in their valve selection process.

The current generation of mechanical valves, nearly all bileaflet pyrolytic carbon in design, can be expected to provide an extremely

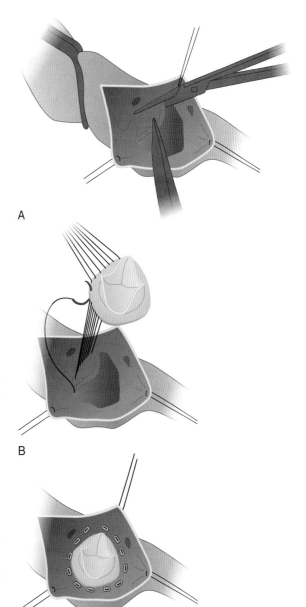

A

B

C

FIGURE 60-14 Aortic Valve Replacement Surgery. Exposure of the aortic valve is typically obtained through a transverse or "hockey stick" incision of the proximal ascending aorta. **A,** The aortic valve is excised. **B,** Pledgeted horizontal mattress sutures are placed circumferentially into the valve annulus and then into the cloth sewing ring of the prosthesis. **C,** The prosthetic valve is lowered into position and the sutures are securely tied.

low incidence of structural deterioration but a 0.6% to 2.3% per patient-year incidence of thromboembolic complications, even with warfarin anticoagulation.[37] The need for anticoagulation with warfarin in turn is associated with approximately a 1% annual risk of bleeding complications. Both bleeding and thromboembolic complications may be reduced through more frequent (e.g., weekly) surveillance of international normalized ratio or home testing.[38]

Bioprosthetic valves are almost universally fabricated from pre-

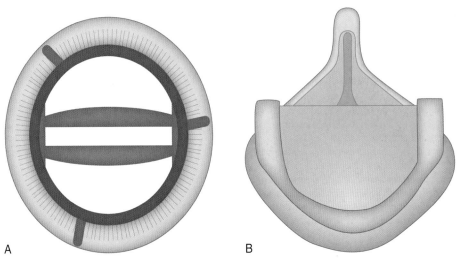

A   B

FIGURE 60-15 Prosthetic Valves. Prosthetic heart valves most often implanted are made from synthetic material (**A**), such as pyrolytic carbon (mechanical valve), or allogeneic biologic tissue (**B**), such as bovine pericardium (bioprosthetic valve). (From http://circ.ahajournals.org/content/119/7/1034/F1.expansion.html.)

TABLE 60-9   Anticoagulation Recommendation With Prosthetic Valves

| VALVE TYPE | ANTICOAGULATION RECOMMENDATION | | | |
	ASPIRIN*	WARFARIN (INR GOAL)	DURATION	INDICATION CLASS
Mechanical				
MVR	+	(3.0)	Long-term	I
AVR (+ risk factors)[†]	+	(3.0)	Long-term	I
AVR (− risk factors)[†]	+	(2.5)	Long-term	I
Bioprosthetic				
MVR		(2.5)	3 months	IIa
AVR		(2.5)	3 months	IIb
MVR	+	−	Long-term	IIa
AVR	+	−	Long-term	IIa
TAVR	+[‡]		6 months	IIb

Adapted from Nishimura RA, Otto CM, Bonow RO, et al: 2014 AHA/ACC guideline for the management of patients with valvular heart disease: A report of the American College of Cardiology/American Heart Association Task Force on Practice Guidelines. *J Thorac Cardiovasc Surg* 148:e1–e132, 2014.
AVR, aortic valve replacement; *INR*, international normalized ratio; *MVR*, mitral valve replacement; *TAVR*, transcatheter aortic valve replacement.
*Recommended aspirin dose, 75-100 mg daily.
[†]Risk factors: atrial fibrillation, previous thromboembolism, left ventricular dysfunction, hypercoagulable condition, older-generation valve.
[‡]For TAVR, lifelong aspirin plus clopidogrel 75 mg daily for 6 months.

served (bovine) pericardium or from porcine valves specially harvested for this use. Anticoagulation is typically not needed with the implantation of bioprosthetic valves beyond an initial 3-month period to allow sewing ring endothelialization to occur, unless other indications such as atrial fibrillation exist.[37]

Modern antimineralization and tissue preservation techniques involving treatment of valves with alpha-oleic acid reduce cusp calcification and typically provide approximately 90% freedom from structural valve deterioration and reoperation at 10 years in patients older than 65 years.[39] Failure rates may be higher in younger patients as a result of greater hemodynamic stresses or metabolic (calcium turnover) rates, but many surgeons now recommend implantation of bioprosthetic valves in patients younger than the recommended cutoff of 60 to 70 years of age (class IIa), accepting the risk of reintervention by open or percutaneous technique

as being less than the lifelong risk of anticoagulation/mechanical valve thromboembolism. Relative contraindications to anticoagulation, including pregnancy, may influence choice of prosthesis.

Regardless of implant type, similar excellent early and long-term survival outcomes have been achieved after valve implantation (see Tables 60-5 and 60-8), and the technical considerations in implantation are generally considered similar between valve types, except for xenograft stentless aortic bioprosthetic roots and homografts. In particular, improved valve designs have largely eliminated differences in the hemodynamic profile of bioprostheses versus historically better-performing mechanical valves.

Patient-prosthesis mismatch describes a syndrome arising from an undersized (aortic) prosthetic effective orifice area compared with the patient's body surface area (0.65 cm^2/m^2). Inadequate prosthetic valve effective orifice area can lead to residual transvalvular gradients, resulting in persistent ventricular hypertrophy, impaired ventricular remodeling, and excessive late cardiac events. Charts are available to select the appropriately sized prosthesis as a function of body surface area. Patient-prosthesis mismatch is unusual with the excellent hemodynamic performance of current valves, but native annulus/root enlargement can be performed to accommodate a sufficiently large prosthesis.

Finally, prosthetic valve endocarditis (PVE) occurs with an incidence that is 50 times greater than the risk of endocarditis in the general population. Excision and re-replacement are typically indicated for PVE, especially when PVE is caused by virulent organisms such as *Staphylococcus aureus* or fungi, although antibiotic therapy alone may occasionally be used to sterilize lesions in high-risk individuals. Even with appropriate antibiotic therapy and surgical intervention, PVE carries a mortality rate approaching 40% at 1 year. Accordingly, practitioners and patients with prosthetic valves as well as individuals at increased risk for native valve endocarditis should be well versed in and strictly adhere to recommendations for antibiotic prophylaxis against endocarditis.

Transcatheter Aortic Valve Replacement and Other Emerging Technologies

Transcatheter aortic valve replacement (TAVR) describes a new procedure coupling balloon aortic valvuloplasty, which of itself does not provide long-term relief of AS, with implantation of an expandable bioprosthesis delivered and expanded into the aortic annulus using catheter technology. This technology has rapidly evolved since early reports of the clinical applicability of catheter-based pulmonic and aortic valve replacements in 2000 and 2002.[40,41] Compelling evidence of the efficacy of TAVR was provided by the PARTNER (Placement of Aortic Transcatheter Valves) trial, the world's first randomized, controlled study of this new procedure.[42,43] On the basis of data from PARTNER, the Food and Drug Administration (FDA) granted approval for TAVR in 2011 for inoperable (>50% predicted mortality or irreversible morbidity) patients and in 2012 for high-risk (>10% predicted mortality) patients with a predicted postprocedural survival longer than 12 months. Involvement of a Heart Team, consisting of both cardiologists and cardiac surgeons, in evaluation and treatment of TAVR patients is a critical, FDA-mandated component of TAVR protocols.

More specifically, PARTNER A demonstrated that TAVR mortality rates were noninferior to surgery (24% versus 27% at 1 year and 34% versus 35% at 2 years). PARTNER B demonstrated a 40% mortality reduction at 1 year after TAVR compared with standard therapy (31% versus 51%; $P < .001$). This mortality benefit persisted at 2 years (43% versus 68%), although the risk of stroke was significantly higher (14% versus 6% at 2 years) in the TAVR group.[44]

TAVR is being applied today with improving results to increasing numbers of high-risk and even moderate-risk AS patients. These outcomes have been aided by the introduction of new, smaller caliber valves and catheters and ventricular transapical deployment techniques that have decreased vascular complications and improved patient selection and deployment strategies (including rapid ventricular pacing during deployment to minimize prosthesis displacement).

Despite these encouraging data, surgical aortic valve replacement still remains the "gold standard" for low- and intermediate-

risk patients, especially because long-term durability data are not yet available for TAVR. In addition, the risk of stroke continues to increase with TAVR compared with surgical aortic valve replacement over time, presumably because of vascular injury or thromboembolic material from the native calcified valve that remains exposed to the circulation.[43,44] Complications such as complete heart block, left bundle branch block, and paravalvular regurgitation are also higher after TAVR than after surgical aortic valve replacement, and these complications have been linked to higher long-term mortality.[42-46]

Percutaneous Mitral Interventions

Percutaneous therapies for mitral valve disease are also being developed, although they lag TAVR, in part because of the greater difficulty in successfully accessing the mitral as opposed to the aortic annulus. Most therapies are adaptations of current surgical techniques, including the Alfieri stitch (edge-to-edge leaflet repair) and annuloplasty.

The MitraClip System, clinically introduced in 2003, has seen the greatest advancement of all percutaneous mitral valve therapies, receiving FDA approval for high-risk patients in 2013. With use of a catheter-based clip delivery system, an intra-atrial septal puncture is performed to gain access to the left atrium and to cross the mitral valve. The catheter then grasps the mitral valve leaflet edges and places a clip that emulates the edge-to-edge leaflet repair (Fig. 60-16). Although the reduction of severe MR is less effective than with surgical therapy, this technology has brought therapeutic options with demonstrable hemodynamic improvement to many who are not surgical candidates.[47]

Other experimental mitral valve therapies include "indirect annuloplasty" strategies using compression devices placed inside the coronary sinus (because of its anatomic proximity to the mitral annulus) designed to apply radial forces onto the annulus to decrease the size of an enlarged mitral orifice in functional regurgitation. Results with this approach have been inconsistent.

Sutureless valves are another emerging technology that has already seen significant advancement in clinical trials. These valves are placed surgically, under direct vision, but with an implantation technique similar to current catheter-based technology. Because sutureless valves do not require meticulous sewing to the native annulus, their major benefits include decreased cardiopulmonary bypass and aortic cross-clamp times, reduced risk of iatrogenic injury to structures surrounding the diseased valve, and preserved options to perform concomitant open procedures such as CABG.[48,49] Reports of shorter intubation times, fewer days in the intensive care unit, and decreased incidence of postoperative atrial fibrillation, pleural effusion, and respiratory insufficiency have recently emerged.[50] Much like for transcatheter valve replacements, long-term outcomes data will be important in guiding the appropriate use of this new technology.

ACKNOWLEDGMENT

The authors would like to acknowledge Ana María Rodríguez, PhD, for her outstanding assistance in providing editorial support.

SELECTED REFERENCES

Carpentier A: Cardiac valve surgery—the "French correction".

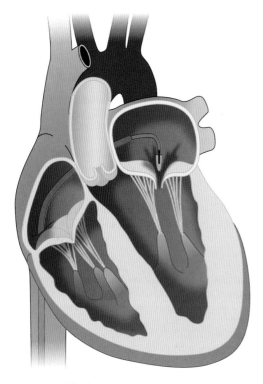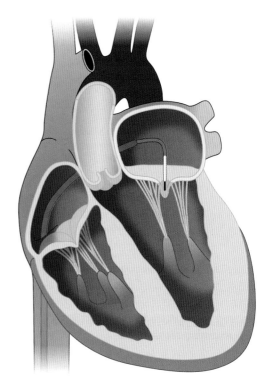

FIGURE 60-16 Percutaneous Mitral Valve Repair. Using a catheter-based clip delivery system, the operator grasps the mitral valve leaflet edges and places a clip that emulates the edge-to-edge leaflet repair. (From http://www.cathlabdigest.com/files/mitra1.png.)

J Thorac Cardiovasc Surg 86:323–337, 1983.

> This seminal work by Alain Carpentier for the first time described a comprehensive strategy for repairing regurgitant lesions of the mitral valve. It remains a relevant classic today.

David TE, Feindel CM: An aortic valve-sparing operation for patients with aortic incompetence and aneurysm of the ascending aorta. *J Thorac Cardiovasc Surg* 103:617–622, 1992.

> In this seminal article, David and Feindel reported their initial cohort of patients treated with a novel technique for aortic valve-sparing root replacement. David has shown excellent results 20 years later in several hundred patients. This technique is used around the world as retaining the native valve avoids prosthetic structural valve degeneration or the need for anticoagulation.

Leon MB, Smith CR, Mack M, et al: Transcatheter aortic-valve implantation for aortic stenosis in patients who cannot undergo surgery. *N Engl J Med* 363:1597–1607, 2010.

> This is the original prospective randomized study report from the PARTNER investigators demonstrating the feasibility of percutaneous aortic valve replacement.

Nishimura RA, Otto CM, Bonow RO, et al: 2014 AHA/ACC guideline for the management of patients with valvular heart

disease: A report of the American College of Cardiology/American Heart Association Task Force on Practice Guidelines. *J Thorac Cardiovasc Surg* 148:e1–e132, 2014.

> These are the most recent American College of Cardiology/American Heart Association Task Force guidelines on current knowledge and treatment of valvular heart disease.

Ross J, Braunwald E: Aortic stenosis. *Circulation* 38:61–67, 1968.

> This classic article first described the onset of symptoms of heart failure, syncope, or angina in patients with aortic stenosis as a marker of impending death and indicated a mean survival of 5 years after onset of angina, 3 years after onset of syncope, and 1 to 2 years after onset of heart failure symptoms.

REFERENCES

1. Nkomo VT, Gardin JM, Skelton TN, et al: Burden of valvular heart diseases: A population-based study. *Lancet* 368:1005–1011, 2006.
2. Seckeler MD, Hoke TR: The worldwide epidemiology of acute rheumatic fever and rheumatic heart disease. *Clin Epidemiol* 3:67–84, 2011.
3. Roberts WC, Ko JM: Frequency by decades of unicuspid, bicuspid, and tricuspid aortic valves in adults having isolated

aortic valve replacement for aortic stenosis, with or without associated aortic regurgitation. *Circulation* 111:920–925, 2005.

4. Rajamannan NM, Evans FJ, Aikawa E, et al: Calcific aortic valve disease: Not simply a degenerative process: A review and agenda for research from the National Heart and Lung and Blood Institute Aortic Stenosis Working Group. Executive summary: Calcific aortic valve disease—2011 update. *Circulation* 124:1783–1791, 2011.

5. Enriquez-Sarano M, Akins CW, Vahanian A: Mitral regurgitation. *Lancet* 373:1382–1394, 2009.

6. Barlow J, Pocock W, Marchand P, et al: The significant late systolic murmurs. *Am Heart J* 66:443–452, 1963.

7. Anyanwu AC, Adams DH: Etiologic classification of degenerative mitral valve disease: Barlow's disease and fibroelastic deficiency. *Semin Thorac Cardiovasc Surg* 19:90–96, 2007.

8. Habib G, Hoen B, Tornos P, et al: Guidelines on the prevention, diagnosis, and treatment of infective endocarditis (new version 2009): The Task Force on the Prevention, Diagnosis, and Treatment of Infective Endocarditis of the European Society of Cardiology (ESC). Endorsed by the European Society of Clinical Microbiology and Infectious Diseases (ESCMID) and the International Society of Chemotherapy (ISC) for Infection and Cancer. *Eur Heart J* 30:2369–2413, 2009.

9. Nishimura RA, Otto CM, Bonow RO, et al: 2014 AHA/ACC guideline for the management of patients with valvular heart disease: A report of the American College of Cardiology/American Heart Association Task Force on Practice Guidelines. *J Thorac Cardiovasc Surg* 148:e1–e132, 2014.

10. Olesen KH: The natural history of 271 patients with mitral stenosis under medical treatment. *Br Heart J* 24:349–357, 1962.

11. Vahanian A, Alfieri O, Andreotti F, et al: Guidelines on the management of valvular heart disease (version 2012): The Joint Task Force on the Management of Valvular Heart Disease of the European Society of Cardiology (ESC) and the European Association for Cardio-Thoracic Surgery (EACTS). *Eur J Cardiothorac Surg* 42:S S1–S44, 2012.

12. Inoue K, Owaki T, Nakamura T, et al: Clinical application of transvenous mitral commissurotomy by a new balloon catheter. *J Thorac Cardiovasc Surg* 87:394–402, 1984.

13. Bouleti C, Iung B, Himbert D, et al: Reinterventions after percutaneous mitral commissurotomy during long-term follow-up, up to 20 years: The role of repeat percutaneous mitral commissurotomy. *Eur Heart J* 34:1923–1930, 2013.

14. Song JK, Kim MJ, Yun CS, et al: Long-term outcomes of percutaneous mitral balloon valvuloplasty versus open cardiac surgery. *J Thorac Cardiovasc Surg* 139:103–110, 2010.

15. Antunes MJ, Vieira H, Ferrão de Oliveira J: Open mitral commissurotomy: The 'golden standard.' *J Heart Valve Dis* 9:472–477, 2000.

16. Sá MP, Ferraz PE, Escobar RR, et al: Preservation versus non-preservation of mitral valve apparatus during mitral valve replacement: A meta-analysis of 3835 patients. *Interact Cardiovasc Thorac Surg* 15:1033–1039, 2012.

17. Enriquez-Sarano M, Avierinos JF, Messika-Zeitoun D, et al: Quantitative determinants of the outcome of asymptomatic mitral regurgitation. *N Engl J Med* 352:875–883, 2005.

18. Deja MA, Grayburn PA, Sun B, et al: Influence of mitral regurgitation repair on survival in the surgical treatment for ischemic heart failure trial. *Circulation* 125:2639–2648, 2012.

19. Dayan V, Soca G, Cura L, et al: Similar survival after mitral valve replacement or repair for ischemic mitral regurgitation: A meta-analysis. *Ann Thorac Surg* 97:758–765, 2014.

20. Acker MA, Parides MK, Perrault LP, et al: Mitral-valve repair versus replacement for severe ischemic mitral regurgitation. *N Engl J Med* 370:23–32, 2014.

21. McGee EC, Gillinov AM, Blackstone EH, et al: Recurrent mitral regurgitation after annuloplasty for functional ischemic mitral regurgitation. *J Thorac Cardiovasc Surg* 128:916–924, 2004.

22. Pantoja JL, Ge L, Zhang Z, et al: Posterior papillary muscle anchoring affects remote myofiber stress and pump function: Finite element analysis. *Ann Thorac Surg* 98:1355–1362, 2014.

23. Ross J, Jr, Braunwald E: Aortic stenosis. *Circulation* 38:61–67, 1968.

24. Pellikka PA, Sarano ME, Nishimura RA, et al: Outcome of 622 adults with asymptomatic, hemodynamically significant aortic stenosis during prolonged follow-up. *Circulation* 111:3290–3295, 2005.

25. Bach DS, Cimino N, Deeb GM: Unoperated patients with severe aortic stenosis. *J Am Coll Cardiol* 50:2018–2019, 2007.

26. Gillam LD, Marcoff L, Shames S: Timing of surgery in valvular heart disease: Prophylactic surgery vs watchful waiting in the asymptomatic patient. *Can J Cardiol* 30:1035–1045, 2014.

27. Bekeredjian R, Grayburn PA: Valvular heart disease: Aortic regurgitation. *Circulation* 112:125–134, 2005.

28. David TE: Surgical treatment of aortic valve disease. *Nat Rev Cardiol* 10:375–386, 2013.

29. Van de Veire NR, Braun J, Delgado V, et al: Tricuspid annuloplasty prevents right ventricular dilatation and progression of tricuspid regurgitation in patients with tricuspid annular dilatation undergoing mitral valve repair. *J Thorac Cardiovasc Surg* 141:1431–1439, 2011.

30. Nath J, Foster E, Heidenreich PA: Impact of tricuspid regurgitation on long-term survival. *J Am Coll Cardiol* 43:405–409, 2004.

31. De Bonis M, Taramasso M, Lapenna E, et al: Management of tricuspid regurgitation. *F1000Prime Rep* 6:58, 2014.

32. Yeter E, Ozlem K, Kiliç H, et al: Tricuspid balloon valvuloplasty to treat tricuspid stenosis. *J Heart Valve Dis* 19:159–160, 2010.

33. Goodney PP, O'Connor GT, Wennberg DE, et al: Do hospitals with low mortality rates in coronary artery bypass also perform well in valve replacement? *Ann Thorac Surg* 76:1131–1137, 2003.

34. El-Hamamsy I, Clark J, Stevens LM, et al: Late outcomes following freestyle versus homograft aortic root replacement: Results from a prospective randomized trial. *J Am Coll Cardiol* 55:368–376, 2010.

35. David TE, Feindel CM: An aortic valve-sparing operation for patients with aortic incompetence and aneurysm of the ascending aorta. *J Thorac Cardiovasc Surg* 103:617–622, 1992.

36. David TE: Aortic valve sparing operations: Outcomes at 20 years. *Ann Cardiothorac Surg* 2:24–29, 2013.

37. Pibarot P, Dumesnil JG: Prosthetic heart valves: Selection of the optimal prosthesis and long-term management. *Circula-*

tion 119:1034–1048, 2009.

38. Garcia-Alamino JM, Ward AM, Alonso-Coello P, et al: Self-monitoring and self-management of oral anticoagulation. *Cochrane Database Syst Rev* (4):CD003839, 2010.

39. Flameng W, Rega F, Vercalsteren M, et al: Antimineralization treatment and patient-prosthesis mismatch are major determinants of the onset and incidence of structural valve degeneration in bioprosthetic heart valves. *J Thorac Cardiovasc Surg* 147:1219–1224, 2014.

40. Cribier A, Eltchaninoff H, Bash A, et al: Percutaneous transcatheter implantation of an aortic valve prosthesis for calcific aortic stenosis: First human case description. *Circulation* 106:3006–3008, 2002.

41. Bonhoeffer P, Boudjemline Y, Saliba Z, et al: Percutaneous replacement of pulmonary valve in a right-ventricle to pulmonary-artery prosthetic conduit with valve dysfunction. *Lancet* 356:1403–1405, 2000.

42. Leon MB, Smith CR, Mack M, et al: Transcatheter aortic-valve implantation for aortic stenosis in patients who cannot undergo surgery. *N Engl J Med* 363:1597–1607, 2010.

43. Smith CR, Leon MB, Mack MJ, et al: Transcatheter versus surgical aortic-valve replacement in high-risk patients. *N Engl J Med* 364:2187–2198, 2011.

44. Kodali SK, Williams MR, Smith CR, et al: Two-year outcomes after transcatheter or surgical aortic-valve replacement. *N Engl J Med* 366:1686–1695, 2012.

45. Généreux P, Webb JG, Svensson LG, et al: Vascular complications after transcatheter aortic valve replacement: Insights from the PARTNER (Placement of AoRTic TraNscathetER Valve) trial. *J Am Coll Cardiol* 60:1043–1052, 2012.

46. Houthuizen P, Van Garsse LA, Poels TT, et al: Left bundle-branch block induced by transcatheter aortic valve implantation increases risk of death. *Circulation* 126:720–728, 2012.

47. Munkholm-Larsen S, Wan B, Tian DH, et al: A systematic review on the safety and efficacy of percutaneous edge-to-edge mitral valve repair with the MitraClip system for high surgical risk candidates. *Heart* 100:473–478, 2014.

48. Shrestha M, Folliquet TA, Pfeiffer S, et al: Aortic valve replacement and concomitant procedures with the Perceval valve: Results of European trials. *Ann Thorac Surg* 98:1294–1300, 2014.

49. Englberger L, Carrel TP, Doss M, et al: Clinical performance of a sutureless aortic bioprosthesis: Five-year results of the 3f Enable long-term follow-up study. *J Thorac Cardiovasc Surg* 148:1681–1687, 2014.

50. Pollari F, Santarpino G, Dell'Aquila AM, et al: Better short-term outcome by using sutureless valves: A propensity-matched score analysis. *Ann Thorac Surg* 98:611–617, 2014.

VASCULAR

第十二篇　血管与淋巴

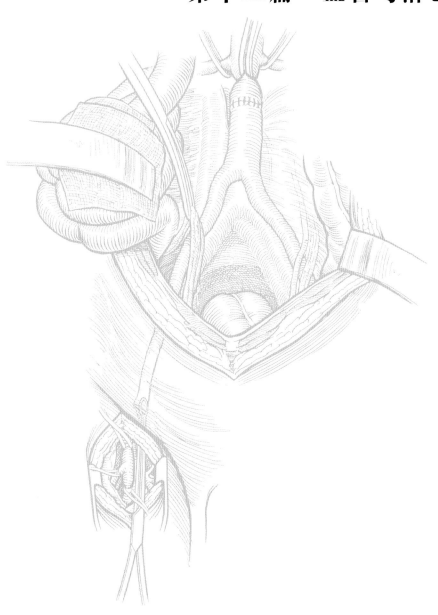

61 CHAPTER

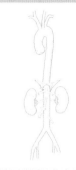

The Aorta

Margaret C. Tracci, Kenneth J. Cherry

第六十一章　主动脉疾病

OUTLINE

Aneurysmal Disease
Aortoiliac Occlusive Disease
Aortic Dissection

中文导读

　　本章分为3节：①动脉瘤疾病；②主髂动脉闭塞性疾病；③主动脉夹层。

　　第一节从解剖学及病因学阐释了动脉瘤的概念，以及动脉瘤破裂的危险因素、诊断、筛选以及监测标准、药物治疗、手术治疗、血管腔内修复技术。其中外科治疗主要介绍了术前评估、腹主动脉瘤开放术式、动脉瘤破裂的管理以及术后管理。腹主动脉瘤腔内隔绝术以其缩短住院天数、降低30天发病率和死亡率的显著优势而得到更多应用。最后还介绍了胸主动脉瘤、胸主动脉挫伤、累及内脏的动脉瘤的诊断与治疗。

　　第二节由第一例主髂动脉闭塞症的动脉重建，引出主髂动脉闭塞症手术方式的进展，接着介绍了主髂动脉闭塞症的评估方法，并着重强调了这类疾病的特例：心血管疾病的评估。血管腔内治疗应用日益广泛并将成为主髂动脉闭塞症治疗的主要方法，但是开放术式主（全股动脉旁路移植术、腋股动脉旁路移植术、股股动脉旁路移植术、髂股动脉旁路移植术、主髂动脉内膜切除术）仍然是目前主要治疗方式。同时对动脉移植物感染的外科处理方法进行了详细的介绍。

　　第三节从主动脉夹层的发生机制来阐释其概念及分型。Stanford A型主动脉夹层主要介绍了其临床诊断要点、检查及治疗手段。Stanford B型主动脉夹层则从其发生、发展、危险因素来阐述，CT、MRI及血管造影在协助诊断过程中各有利弊。急性复杂的B型主动脉夹层病人实施传统开放性手术往往伴随较高的发病率和致死率，急性非复杂B型主动脉夹层预后也不容乐观。新型动脉模型为新的治疗方法提供了可能。

〔王　伟〕

Please access ExpertConsult.com to view the corresponding video for this chapter.

The aorta is a broad topic encompassing the diagnosis and management of aneurysms, occlusive disease, and dissections of the abdominal and thoracic aorta. In the past 2 decades, endovascular therapy has offered a frequently less morbid approach to each of these disease entities. The rapid adoption of endovascular techniques and technologies has clearly revolutionized the management of aortic disease. Endovascular aneurysm repair (EVAR) is now performed much more frequently than open repair and appears to have had an impact on the mortality rate attributable to aortic aneurysm.[1] Thoracic EVAR (TEVAR) is now the recommended first treatment option. The new TransAtlantic Inter-Society Consensus guidelines (TASC III) will recommend endovascular therapy as the first option for almost all degrees of aortoiliac occlusive disease (AIOD). Nevertheless, 2013 data suggest that aortic disease is identified as the cause of nearly 10,000 deaths per year,[2] and others have noted that this number is likely to be significantly higher because of the failure to identify aortic disease in deaths that occur out of the hospital and without autopsy.

We have tried to make this chapter relevant to general surgery residents training in the second decade of the 21st century, with particular attention to the fact that with a shift toward endovascular therapy, the exposure of surgical residents to open reconstructive techniques for management of both the thoracic and the abdominal aorta has declined noticeably. Relatively few centers still offer rich experience in open aortic surgery and, in particular, the most complex cases, and yet mastery of aortic surgery remains a necessity. Dense calcium, involvement of visceral vessels, infections, trauma, small arteries, and failed endografts may and do necessitate formal open reconstruction. We hope that concurrent changes in the training regimen not only will allow the maintenance of standards with regard to the surgeon's skill set and outcomes but also will enable future generations to continue to drive advances in the state of the art of vascular surgery.

ANEURYSMAL DISEASE

Aneurysms, typically defined as an increase in size of more than 50% above the normal arterial diameter, may occur anywhere along the aorta, from the aortic root to the bifurcation. Aneurysms may be further characterized on the basis of anatomy or etiology. Anatomically, fusiform aneurysms exhibit smooth, circumferential dilation as opposed to saccular aneurysms, which, as their name suggests, appear as a focal outpouching of the arterial wall. Whereas true aneurysms involve all three layers of the vessel wall, false aneurysm or pseudoaneurysm describes a focal defect in the artery with an associated collection of blood contained by adventitia and periarterial tissue; it may be degenerative, infectious, or traumatic in etiology. The majority of aneurysms addressed in this chapter are degenerative in nature. Less frequently, aneurysms may be associated with infection (mycotic aneurysms), inflammation, or autoimmune or connective tissue disease. These cases merit special consideration in their evaluation and management. Aneurysmal enlargement of the aorta is associated with factors that result in weakening of the arterial wall and increased local hemodynamic forces. These may include heritable conditions, such as Marfan syndrome, familial thoracic aortic aneurysm and dissection, and vascular-type Ehlers-Danlos, as well as less well defined entities that contribute to the significantly elevated incidence of aneurysm in patients with a family history of aneurysm. Factors that contribute to the degradation of collagen and elastin are also associated with aneurysmal disease, and research in this area has focused on the role of matrix metalloproteinases and other mediators of tissue enzyme function. Ongoing avenues of investigation in this area also include the role of the immune response and hormone milieu.[3] Aneurysms do also occur as a degenerative complication after aortic dissection.

The incidence of abdominal aortic aneurysm (AAA), based on large screening studies, is estimated to range from 3% to 10%. A number of risk factors, in addition to genetic or familial disorders, for the development, expansion, and rupture of AAAs have been identified (Table 61-1). Risk factors for development of an AAA include age, male gender, concurrent aneurysms, family history, tobacco use, hypertension, hyperlipidemia, and height. Female gender, black race, and diabetes appear to be protective.[4-14]

Gender differences extend to the presentation, associations, and natural history of aneurysms. Men with AAA, for instance, are more likely to present with concurrent iliac or femoropopliteal aneurysms.[15] Women are more likely to experience rupture and consistently demonstrate poorer outcomes after repair, perhaps because of a significantly higher incidence of challenging anatomy.[16,17]

Risk of Rupture

Predicting the behavior of an aneurysm over time is difficult. Published risk factors for rupture include chronic obstructive pulmonary disease (COPD), current tobacco use, larger initial AAA diameter, female gender, cardiac or renal transplantation, and certain patterns of wall stress.[4,18-26]

The most widely adopted surrogate for rupture risk is maximal cross-sectional aneurysm diameter (Table 61-2), although the implications for rupture risk of a particular aortic diameter remain debated. Some data suggest that surgeons tend to overestimate rupture risk.[27] In addition, an observational study suggested that even broadly accepted estimates of risk may overstate the rupture rates of untreated AAA and noted, in patients deemed medically unfit for elective repair, that the risk of death from non–aneurysm-related causes exceeded the risk of death from rupture.[28]

In addition, despite a relative paucity of natural history data regarding growth rate and rupture, most clinicians do consider the rate of enlargement a risk factor for rupture. A rate of growth of more than 5 mm in 6 months or more than 1 cm per year has been widely adopted as an indication for repair, independent of aneurysm size. Size is an imperfect predictor of rupture risk; autopsy studies have discovered evidence of rupture in up to 12% of aneurysms less than 5 cm in diameter.[29] A number of investigational models attempt to quantify rupture risk by calculations of wall stress, observation of particular wall or thrombus characteristics, or the combination of multiple factors thought to contribute to increased wall stress or decreased strength.

Diagnosis

Abdominal aneurysm may be detected on physical examination as a palpable pulsatile mass, most commonly supraumbilical and in the midline. The location may be variable, however, as aortic tortuosity can result in a lateral or infraumbilical location. The sensitivity of physical examination is, as one might expect, dependent on the aneurysm's size and the patient's habitus.

TABLE 61-1   Risk Factors for Aneurysm Development, Expansion, and Rupture

SYMPTOM	RISK FACTORS
AAA development	Tobacco use
	Hypercholesterolemia
	Hypertension
	Male gender
	Family history (male predominance)
AAA expansion	Advanced age
	Severe cardiac disease
	Previous stroke
	Tobacco use
	Cardiac or renal transplantation
AAA rupture	Female gender
	↓ FEV_1
	Larger initial AA diameter
	Higher mean blood pressure
	Current tobacco use (length of time smoking ≫ amount)
	Cardiac or renal transplantation
	Critical wall stress–wall strength relationship

Adapted from Chaikof EL, Brewster DC, Dalman RL, et al: The care of patients with an abdominal aortic aneurysm: The Society for Vascular Surgery practice guidelines. *J Vasc Surg* 50:S2–S49, 2009.

TABLE 61-2   Estimated Annual Rupture Risk

AAA DIAMETER (cm)	RUPTURE RISK (%/yr)
<4	0
4-5	0.5-5
5-6	3-15
6-7	10-20
7-8	20-40
>8	30-50

Adapted from Brewster DC, Cronenwett JL, Hallett JW Jr, et al: Guidelines for the treatment of abdominal aortic aneurysms. Report of a subcommittee of the Joint Council of the American Association for Vascular Surgery and Society for Vascular Surgery. *J Vasc Surg* 37:1106–1117, 2003.

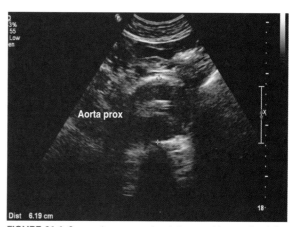

FIGURE 61-1 Gray-scale cross-sectional ultrasound image of an infrarenal aortic aneurysm measuring 6.19 cm in maximal anteroposterior diameter.

The detection and characterization of aneurysms are greatly aided by modern imaging techniques. Ultrasound examination has been demonstrated to afford excellent sensitivity and specificity (Fig. 61-1). Ultrasound may be limited by the patient's habitus or bowel gas, but as it avoids the complications associated with invasive testing, radiation, and contrast media, it is an excellent choice for screening. Ultrasound is not an ideal method for detecting rupture; it is unable to image all portions of the aortic wall, and the nonfasting status of emergently examined patients may further preclude ideal image acquisition. It has been estimated that ultrasound may fail to detect up to 50% of aneurysm ruptures.

Computed tomography (CT) provides excellent imaging of AAA, with greater reproducibility of diameter measurements than by ultrasound. CT, particularly with the adjunctive use of iodinated contrast agents to perform CT angiography (CTA), provides a wealth of anatomic information; it detects vessel calcification, thrombus, and concurrent arterial occlusive disease and permits multiplanar and three-dimensional reconstruction and analysis for operative planning (Fig. 61-2). Drawbacks include substantial radiation exposure, particularly in the setting of serial examinations, and the use of iodinated contrast media in a population with a high incidence of comorbid kidney disease.[4]

Magnetic resonance imaging (MRI) and magnetic resonance angiography (MRA) are, like CT, sensitive in the detection of AAA (Fig. 61-3). Unlike CT, MRI does not demonstrate aortic wall calcification, which may be important in operative planning. Although the study does not require the use of iodinated contrast material, MRA uses gadolinium, which has been associated with the development of nephrogenic systemic fibrosis in patients with low glomerular filtration rate. The availability of MRI may also be limited by the presence of incompatible metallic implants or foreign bodies. The ability to acquire dynamic images throughout the cardiac cycle may ultimately prove clinically useful.[30]

Screening and Surveillance Recommendations

Screening recommendations for AAA are informed by the sensitivity and specificity of ultrasound screening, the detection yield of screening based on various risk factor selection criteria, and cost. A major recent compilation of evidence-based recommendations for screening and surveillance of AAA is provided by the 2009 Practice Guidelines developed by the Clinical Practice Council of the Society for Vascular Surgery. The Society for Vascular Surgery committee charged with reviewing available data regarding screening made a strong recommendation for one-time screening of all men aged 65 years and older or men 55 years and older with a family history of AAA. Screening of women is also strongly recommended for those aged 65 years and older with a family history of AAA or a personal smoking history. The evidence basis of these recommendations was deemed to be strong in the former case and moderate in the latter.[4]

The U.S. Preventive Services Task Force issued a more limited recommendation for one-time screening of men between 65 and 75 years of age who have a personal smoking history.[31]

Screening of women remains controversial. Although there is evidence that women may exhibit a stronger association between smoking and aneurysm, it is known that the incidence of aneurysm in women who have smoked exceeds that of men who have never smoked, and mortality data reflect that gender differences in aneurysm-related mortality narrow with advanced age.[4] Payer policies regarding reimbursement may not track either of these recommendations. Medicare, for instance, as a result of the Screening Abdominal Aortic Aneurysms Very Efficiently (SAAAVE) Act, reflects an intermediate approach in offering a screening benefit for men with a personal smoking history and men or women with a family history of AAA, although only as a part of the initial Welcome to Medicare physical examination.

Once an aneurysm has been detected, the Society for Vascular Surgery Clinical Practice Council recommends further screening intervals as follows, based on aneurysm size (maximum external aortic diameter) and associated risk of rupture[4]:

    <2.6 cm: no further screening recommended
    2.6-2.9 cm: reexamination at 5 years
    3-3.4 cm: reexamination at 3 years
    3.5-4.4 cm: reexamination at 12 months
    4.5-5.4 cm: reexamination at 6 months

The recommendation for follow-up of aortic diameters less than 3 cm is controversial and has been criticized on the basis of cost-effectiveness analyses. It is based on findings that a significant proportion of 65-year-old men (13.8%) with an initial aortic diameter of 2.6 to 2.9 cm developed aneurysms exceeding 5.5 cm at 10 years. Given current life expectancy projections, it is evident that a subset of patients deemed "normal" at screening will go on to develop large aneurysms.[32]

Medical Therapy

Once an aneurysm has been diagnosed, the optimization of medical therapy serves a dual purpose: to potentially minimize the rate of aneurysm expansion or rupture and to medically prepare for potential repair. Many avenues have been investigated in the search for effective medical treatment to prevent the progression of aortic aneurysm, leading to a recent editorial statement that "the bottom line is that no drug can currently be recommended for the indication of reducing AAA enlargement."[33] A highly anticipated, randomized trial of doxycycline, an antibiotic and inhibitor of matrix metalloproteinase activity, not only failed to demonstrate benefit but found increased AAA enlargement primarily in the first 6 months of follow-up.[34] Investigation is ongoing, particularly with regard to the role of anti-inflammatory agents.

Currently, many continue to incorporate beta blockade in an effort to control blood pressure and dP/dT that may contribute to harmful wall stress. Studies using propranolol demonstrated mixed results and low patient compliance. Angiotensin-converting enzyme inhibitors and angiotensin receptor blockers have yielded mixed results in clinical studies, but their use is based on the goal of blood pressure management as well as on evidence for their utility in the management of patients with aortic disease associated with Marfan syndrome.[35] HMG–coenzyme A reductase inhibitor (statin) therapy has been associated with reduced rates of AAA enlargement and is otherwise appropriate in a population with a high prevalence of concurrent atherosclerotic disease. Antiplatelet therapy using aspirin does, like beta blockers and statins, offer secondary preventive benefit in this population and should be considered. Perhaps the most important intervention, in both regards, is smoking cessation. Current tobacco use has been associated with an increased rate of aneurysm expansion. Smoking cessation may also yield benefits with regard to perioperative morbidity and mortality in the event that the aneurysm ultimately requires repair.

Surgical Treatment

Surgical treatment is generally recommended for aneurysms more than 5.5 cm in maximal diameter, those demonstrating more than 5 mm of growth in 6 months or more than 1 cm in a year, and aneurysms with a saccular rather than the typical fusiform anatomy. Gender differences in a variety of factors have led some to advocate for consideration of aneurysm repair at a smaller size in women. It has been observed that the average size of "normal" aorta tends to be slightly smaller in women. Evaluation of several indices relating aortic diameter to body build, such as body surface area or wrist circumference, also suggests that measures

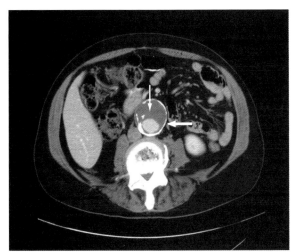

FIGURE 61-2 CTA axial plane image of an infrarenal abdominal aortic aneurysm demonstrating aortic wall calcification (*thick arrow*) and intraluminal thrombus (*thin arrow*).

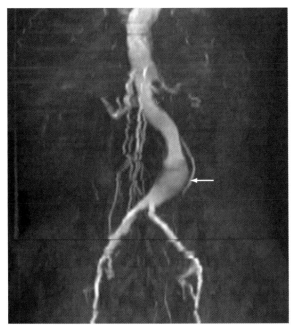

FIGURE 61-3 MRA coronal view of an infrarenal aneurysm (*arrow*).

other than aortic diameter alone may be more accurate in predicting AAA.[36] These observations are consistent with evidence suggesting more rapid aneurysm growth and rupture at smaller sizes in women (average diameter of 5 cm rather than one of 6 cm in male patients).[37,38] The presence of significant aneurysm-related anxiety associated with awareness of the presence of an unrepaired aneurysm has also been cited as affecting quality of life and presenting a potential consideration in managing aneurysms below 5.5 cm in diameter.[38]

Preoperative Evaluation

The preoperative evaluation of patients with AAA comprises operative planning as well as identification and management of important medical comorbidities, such as coronary artery disease, renal insufficiency, peripheral arterial occlusive disease, diabetes, and obstructive lung disease. As coronary artery disease is the primary cause of mortality after either open or endovascular repair of AAA, a great deal of attention has been focused on the preoperative evaluation and management of comorbid coronary artery disease. The guiding principles in this evaluation have traditionally been the identification of information that will alter management and the institution of therapy that will improve cardiac-related mortality. In 2007, the American College of Cardiology/American Heart Association (ACC/AHA) published guidelines regarding the preoperative cardiac evaluation of patients undergoing noncardiac vascular surgery.[39] These guidelines stratify patients according to the presence or absence of symptomatic cardiac disease, the presence of significant clinical risk factors (mild angina, prior myocardial infarction, compensated congestive heart failure, diabetes mellitus, or renal insufficiency), and the level (quantified in metabolic equivalents) of the patient's functional capacity. Resting electrocardiography is typically performed before high-risk surgery, such as open aneurysm repair, but it is no longer recommended by the ACC/AHA or European Society of Cardiology for patients without clinical risk factors who are undergoing low-risk surgery. Echocardiography may be used to evaluate the cardiac function of those with a history of heart failure or current dyspnea. Heart failure is a significant consideration; left ventricular ejection fraction less than 35% has been found to have 50% sensitivity and 91% specificity for predicting perioperative cardiac events.[40]

The decision to proceed with noninvasive testing in patients without symptoms of active cardiac disease should be based on the patient's functional capacity and the presence of three or more significant additional risk factors. Coronary angiography should be considered in patients with evidence of active cardiac disease based on screening questions or evidence of ischemia on noninvasive stress testing. Adjunctive medical therapy may also serve to reduce the risk of perioperative cardiac events. Perioperative beta blockade, statin use, and aspirin use are widely accepted, and there is also evidence to support the use of other antihypertensives during this period (Fig. 61-4). An important caveat has been added to the perioperative use of beta blockade, with the 2009 American College of Cardiology Foundation/American Heart Association Focused Update on Perioperative Beta Blockade advising continuation of previously prescribed beta blockers in the perioperative period and titration of beta blockers to desired heart rate and blood pressure, noting that routine perioperative high-dose beta blockers without titration may be harmful.[41] The withdrawal of statins in the perioperative period may be associated with an increased risk of coronary events.[42]

Renal insufficiency related to renovascular or medical renal disease is a well-established risk factor for morbidity and mortality after AAA repair. Coexisting renal artery occlusive disease may be present in 20% to 38% of patients with AAA.[43] In addition, both open and endovascular repair of AAA may result in further deterioration in the renal function of patients with preexisting renal disease. Concurrent repair of clinically significant renal occlusive disease is appropriate at the time of either open repair or EVAR. A number of strategies for intraoperative renal protection have been proposed. Current recommendations include adequate hydration, perioperative discontinuation of angiotensin-converting enzyme inhibitors and angiotensin receptor blockers, and avoidance of hypotension. There is also evidence of increased perioperative mortality associated with postoperative nonresumption of angiotensin-converting enzyme inhibitors.[44] There is mixed evidence regarding the benefits of antioxidants (mannitol, ascorbic acid, vitamin E, N-acetylcysteine, and allopurinol) and some data supporting the beneficial effects of infused fenoldopam.[45,46] When suprarenal clamp placement is necessary, the authors endorse the use of cold saline perfusion of the kidneys, preclamp administration of furosemide and mannitol, and selective use of fenoldopam. An additional consideration, particularly in patients with preexisting renal dysfunction, is contrast-induced nephropathy associated with administration of iodinated contrast agents for CT imaging or angiography. Current data support intravenous hydration with sodium bicarbonate or normal saline and possibly the use of antioxidants, such as ascorbic acid or N-acetylcysteine. When EVAR is contemplated, carbon dioxide may be used as an imaging agent to alleviate or to minimize the need for iodinated agents as the rate of contrast-induced nephropathy is related to the amount of agent administered as well as age and prior renal function.

Data are mixed with regard to the impact of pulmonary disease, particularly COPD, on mortality after AAA repair. However, there is evidence that optimal management of comorbid COPD may improve morbidity and mortality.[47] The authors support obtaining a preoperative pulmonary function assessment, including arterial blood gases, to assess risk and to guide management in the perioperative period. Patients with poor pulmonary function must be made aware of the increased risk that they will require prolonged ventilatory support postoperatively and the attendant possibility that tracheostomy will be required during this period. Smoking cessation before surgery may be beneficial and can be aided by counseling and a variety of pharmacologic therapies. Although several studies have suggested that initiating smoking cessation less than 2 weeks before surgery may actually be associated with worse outcomes, a meta-analysis suggests that smoking cessation at any time within 8 weeks of surgery is not associated with a higher rate of either overall complications or pulmonary complications postoperatively.[48]

The preoperative evaluation should also include a chest radiograph, complete blood count, blood chemistries, and coagulation studies as well as urinalysis. The chest radiograph may demonstrate evidence of infection, thoracic aortic disease, or malignant disease, all of which should be thoroughly investigated before AAA repair. The use of various anticoagulant agents is common in patients with AAA, and management is tailored to the indication for use. Vitamin K antagonists should be stopped 5 to 7 days before surgery and bridging anticoagulation provided, if indicated, with low-molecular-weight or unfractionated heparin. Thienopyridines are typically stopped 7 to 10 days before surgery, although patients receiving thienopyridine therapy for drug-eluting coronary stents necessitate careful consideration of the

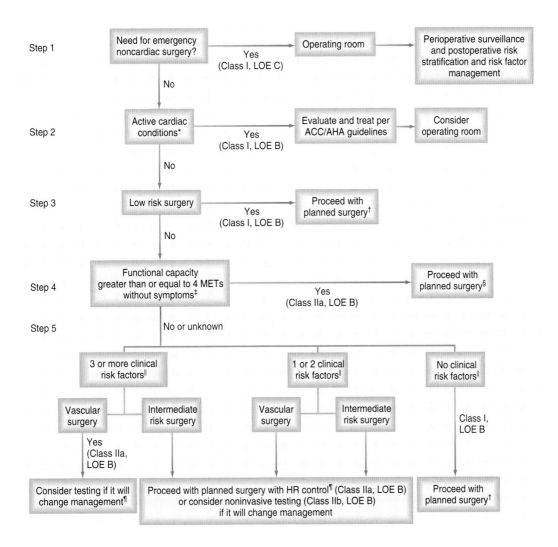

*See Table 2 for active clinical conditions.
†See Class III recommendations in Section 5.2.3, Noninvasive Stress Testing.
‡See Table 3 for estimated MET level equivalent.
§Noninvasive testing may be considered before surgery in specific patients with risk factors if it will change management.
‖Clinical risk factors include ischemic heart disease, compensated or prior heart failure, diabetes mellitus, renal insufficiency, and cerebrovascular disease.
¶Consider perioperative beta blockade (see Table 12) for populations in which this has been shown to reduce cardiac morbidity/mortality.
ACC/AHA indicates American College of Cardiology/American Heart Association; HR, heart rate, LOE, level of evidence; and MET, metabolic equivalent.

FIGURE 61-4 Cardiac evaluation and care algorithm for noncardiac surgery based on active clinical conditions, known cardiovascular disease, or cardiac risk factors for patients 50 years of age or older. (From Fleisher LA, Beckman JA, Brown KA, et al: ACC/AHA 2007 guidelines on perioperative cardiovascular evaluation and care for noncardiac surgery: A report of the American College of Cardiology/American Heart Association Task Force on Practice Guidelines [Writing Committee to Revise the 2002 Guidelines on Perioperative Cardiovascular Evaluation for Noncardiac Surgery]: Developed in collaboration with the American Society of Echocardiography, American Society of Nuclear Cardiology, Heart Rhythm Society, Society of Cardiovascular Anesthesiologists, Society for Cardiovascular Angiography and Interventions, Society for Vascular Medicine and Biology, and Society for Vascular Surgery. Circulation 116:e418–e499, 2007.)

merits of delaying surgery until therapy is discontinued in light of the additional bleeding risk associated with these drugs. Aspirin is typically continued perioperatively as it may confer some degree of benefit with regard to cardiac complications in the perioperative period.

Careful evaluation of preoperative imaging is crucial in planning repair. Anatomic variations, such as a retroaortic renal vein, variant inferior vena cava, or horseshoe kidney, may significantly affect the selection of surgical approach and, if not appreciated preoperatively, can lead to disastrous complications. CT imaging affords the additional advantage of demonstrating vascular calcification, thus permitting the surgeon to assess the feasibility of clamping the aorta and iliac arteries at various levels (Fig. 61-5). Occlusion balloons may be substituted for arterial clamp placement, most frequently at the iliac arteries, should severe calcification render clamp placement untenable. Finally, the size and patency of branch vessels, such as the inferior mesenteric, accessory renal, iliac, and lumbar arteries, can be assessed and may further contribute to preoperative planning.

Technique of Open Surgical Repair of Abdominal Aortic Aneurysms

Open surgical repair of AAA may be accomplished by either a transperitoneal or a retroperitoneal approach. The choice of technique is guided by technical advantages and disadvantages afforded by each as well as by the surgeon's experience and preference. Transperitoneal repair through a midline laparotomy incision is the most widely used approach to the usual infrarenal aneurysm and offers a rapid exposure, excellent access to renal and iliac vessels, and the ability to fully examine the abdominal contents. Adjunctive measures to improve exposure at or above the level of the renal arteries may include ligation and division of the tributaries (gonadal, lumbar, and adrenal) of the left renal vein, if the vein is to be preserved, or division of the proximal left renal vein itself. Although data are mixed regarding the effect of left renal vein ligation on postoperative renal function, it is essential that these tributaries be preserved to provide collateral outflow should renal vein ligation be planned. Alternatively, repair of the left renal vein after ligation has been reported.

The infrarenal transperitoneal repair begins with the perioperative administration of an antibiotic, typically a first-generation cephalosporin, and scrupulous skin preparation from the nipples to the thighs. If a ruptured aneurysm is being treated, skin preparation and draping are accomplished before the induction of general anesthesia to permit rapid exposure and control should induction incite hemodynamic collapse. The patient is draped, and a generous midline laparotomy incision is made from the xiphoid to just above the pubis. Extension of this incision along the xiphoid may facilitate supraceliac exposure, if necessary. If repair is elective and preoperative imaging has demonstrated iliac disease necessitating extension of a bifurcated graft to the femoral artery on one or both sides, the femoral artery dissection should be accomplished before laparotomy (Fig. 61-6).

If supraceliac clamp placement is anticipated, the left lobe of the liver is mobilized by division of the triangular ligament, and the esophagus is identified and reflected to the patient's left. Placement of a nasogastric tube facilitates identification and protection of the esophagus. The crural fibers of the diaphragm are divided proximal to the celiac artery to provide adequate exposure and mobilization of the aorta for supraceliac clamp placement. Once these steps have been accomplished, the neck of the aneurysm may be approached. In some cases, the proximal clamp may be moved down to a suprarenal or infrarenal position at this stage, permitting perfusion of visceral and, ideally, renal vessels. The surgeon may then proceed with iliac dissection and clamp placement.

The surgeon's preference guides the decision with regard to intravenous administration of heparin in rupture. Typical systemic administration of heparin in the elective setting consists of 100 units/kg, administered intravenously and permitted to circulate before clamp placement.

Elective repair permits controlled exposure of the iliac arteries

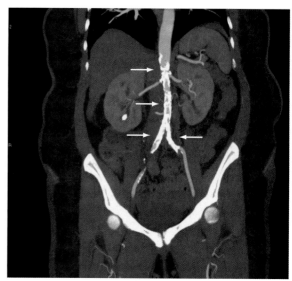

FIGURE 61-5 Reconstruction of coronal CTA image demonstrating heavy calcification *(arrows)* extending from above the renal arteries distally through both common iliac arteries.

and aneurysm neck before heparinization and clamp placement. Exposure of the infrarenal neck of the aneurysm requires careful mobilization of the duodenum, distal to the ligament of Treitz, to the patient's right side. The retroperitoneum may then be opened to the level of the iliac bifurcation. Mobilization of the left renal vein facilitates exposure and control of the neck of the aneurysm. At this time, a decision should be made about the necessity of division of either the left renal vein or its tributaries. The iliac arteries may be exposed by careful dissection in the avascular anterior plane, with attention to preservation of the ureter, which will typically cross at the level of the iliac bifurcation, and the pelvic sympathetics, which cross the bifurcation and proximal left common iliac artery. Extensive dissection of the bifurcation and proximal common iliac arteries is not typically necessary as clamp placement in the mid or distal common iliacs is more typical when the aneurysm terminates at or proximal to the aortic bifurcation, permitting repair with a simple tube graft. When aneurysmal or occlusive disease of the iliacs requires replacement of the common iliac, clamps may be placed at the proximal internal (hypogastric) and external iliac arteries. Soft iliac arteries may be controlled with vessel loops placed in a Potts fashion or using a Rumel tourniquet. However, the authors prefer to use vascular clamps to avoid circumferential dissection of the iliac arteries, where possible, and the attendant risk of venous injury, which can lead to catastrophic bleeding. Severely calcified iliac arteries may be controlled with occlusive balloons, although the proximal ends may require endarterectomy to permit either anastomosis or oversewing.

Once adequate dissection has been accomplished to permit proximal and distal control and systemic heparin administered, clamps may be placed and the aneurysm sac opened. There are a variety of opinions for the order of clamp placement. Some think that initial proximal clamp placement minimizes the risk of distal embolization; others maintain that initial distal clamp placement permits staging of the hemodynamic effect of clamp placement. The sac should be opened just below the aneurysm neck and the opening extended along the right side of the anterior surface of the aneurysm, leaving the orifice of the inferior mesenteric artery in situ. Lumbar arteries and the middle sacral artery may be ligated from within the sac to prevent backbleeding. An inferior mesenteric artery with brisk, pulsatile backbleeding or one that is chronically occluded, as often occurs in aneurysms, may be safely oversewn at its origin. Poor backbleeding suggests inadequate collateralization and is an indication for reimplantation of the inferior mesenteric artery into either the main graft or the left iliac limb.

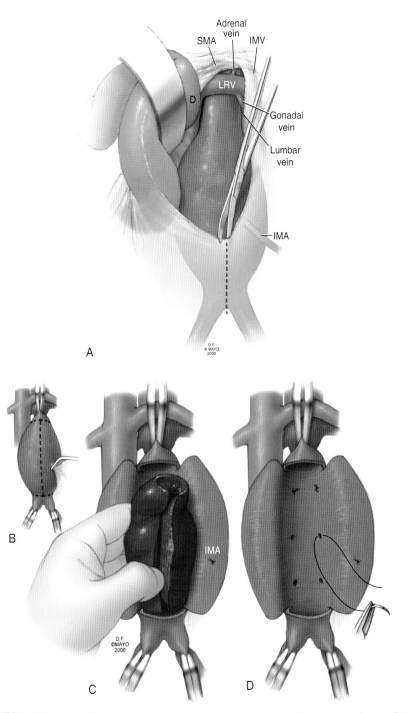

FIGURE 61-6 Technique of open operative repair of an infrarenal abdominal aortic aneurysm using a straight tube graft **(H)** or a bifurcated aortoiliac or aortofemoral **(I)** configuration. Note the attention to closure of the aneurysm sac over the completed repair, with additional closure of retroperitoneal tissues to exclude the duodenum fully **(J)**. *D*, duodenum; *IMA*, inferior mesenteric artery; *IMV*, inferior mesenteric vein; *LRV*, left renal vein; *SMA*, superior mesenteric artery. (Courtesy Mayo Foundation for Medical Education and Research.)

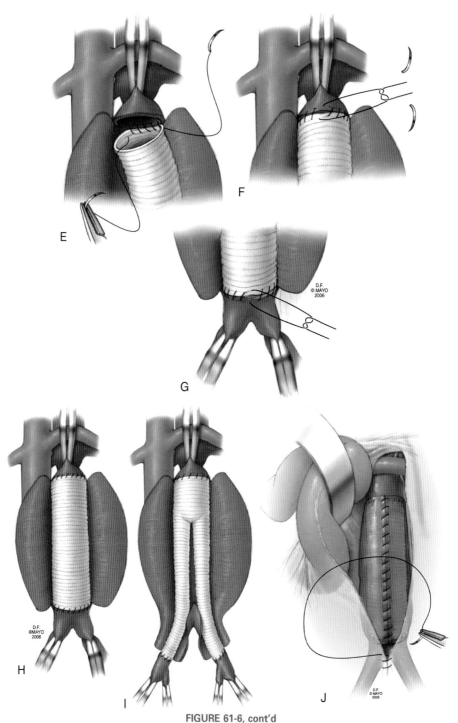

FIGURE 61-6, cont'd

Once backbleeding has been controlled, the proximal anastomosis may be addressed, typically in an end-to-end running fashion using nonabsorbable monofilament suture such as Prolene and an appropriately sized woven or knitted polyester graft. An aneurysm terminating at or before the aortic bifurcation may be repaired with a simple tube graft, whereas involvement of the iliac vessels may necessitate a bifurcated graft and distal anastomoses to either the iliac or femoral arteries. Once the proximal anasto-

mosis is complete, it should be examined by placing a second clamp below the anastomosis and carefully removing the proximal clamp. Any areas of bleeding may be readily addressed with repair sutures at this time, before immobilization of the graft by the distal anastomosis. If a tube graft is sufficient, the distal anastomosis may similarly be completed in a running fashion. Iliac anastomoses may frequently be performed at the level of the iliac bifurcation, incorporating both internal and external iliac arteries as a common orifice. If femoral anastomosis is performed, a ret-roperitoneal tunnel should be created bluntly in the avascular, anatomic plane anterior to the native external iliac artery, passing beneath the ureter. The limb may then be passed to the groin incision using either a blunt clamp passed gently through the tunnel from groin to retroperitoneum or a sterile tape or drain passed along the same course.

Before completion of the distal anastomosis, the distal iliac or femoral vessels should sequentially be permitted to backbleed to flush out any thrombus or atherosclerotic debris, the proximal clamp briefly removed to flush the graft, and the graft flushed with heparinized saline. The proximal and distal clamps may then be removed. It is imperative that the surgical and anesthesia teams communicate well during this process as clamping and unclamp-ing of the aorta produce profound hemodynamic effects. The patient should be well resuscitated before unclamping as this act is frequently attended by a significant hypotension. Slightly staging release of the iliac arteries or limbs, in the case of a bifur-cated graft, may alleviate this somewhat. Sodium bicarbonate to counteract acidosis and the use of vasopressor agents may also be required at this time. The inferior mesenteric artery may be reim-planted at this time, if necessary, most commonly as a Carrel patch. If hemostasis appears to be adequate at all anastomoses and the patient is normotensive, protamine may be administered at 0.5 to 1 mg per 100 units of heparin given.

Once aortic replacement has been accomplished, attention should be turned to graft coverage. The aneurysm sac and retro-peritoneum may be approximated over the graft to effectively exclude the abdominal contents and, in particular, the third portion of the duodenum, which typically rests just anterior to the proximal, infrarenal suture line. The abdominal and, if present, groin incisions should be closed meticulously. Hernias, as previ-ously noted, occur relatively frequently after open aneurysmor-rhaphy. Wound breakdown, particularly at the groin, can be costly and difficult for the patient and significantly increases the risk of catastrophic graft infection. The authors do not routinely drain groin incisions.

The retroperitoneal approach is thought, by some, to reduce physiologic stress on the patient and to result in fewer postopera-tive pulmonary complications as well as a reduction of postopera-tive ileus.[49] Both approaches are associated with a significant rate of wound healing complications. Midline incisions for AAA repair are complicated by radiographically apparent abdominal wall defects in approximately 20% of cases in a recent series, although clinically significant hernias are less frequent. Persistent postopera-tive pain, flank wall laxity, and hernia have been described com-plicating retroperitoneal repair, and some investigators have reported more frequent occurrence of these complications with use of the retroperitoneal technique. With regard to operative exposure, the retroperitoneal approach does afford greater access to the visceral segment of the abdominal aorta and may be aided, where required, by thoracic extension of the incision and exposure with or without division of the diaphragm.

A retroperitoneal aortic exposure may be accomplished with the patient in a modified right lateral decubitus position with the thorax rotated but hips relatively flat to permit access to both groins (Fig. 61-7). A curvilinear incision is made from the costal margin to below the umbilicus, depending on the extent of expo-sure required and the patient's habitus. The retroperitoneal plane may be entered at the lateral border of the rectus sheath. The rectus abdominis may be reflected either medially or laterally. Some surgeons prefer lateral reflection as this may result in less

difficulty with postoperative body wall laxity. Care is taken to avoid entering the peritoneum. Much of the initial portion of this dissection may be carried out bluntly, with the aid of a tonsil sponge on a ring or Kelly forceps. The abdominal contents, envel-oped in peritoneum, may be swept medially. The ureter will be visualized and swept medially. The left kidney may be either ele-vated or left in situ, although the authors generally prefer to medialize the kidney, which also serves to mobilize the left renal vein. The gonadal tributary, however, must generally be identified, ligated, and divided. Proximally, the spleen is carefully mobilized within its peritoneal covering to expose the underside of the dia-phragm. The fibers of the left crus of the diaphragm, when divided, expose the supraceliac and visceral portions of the aorta. The left renal artery should be readily accessible, and the celiac and superior mesenteric arteries may be mobilized by careful dis-section. The right renal artery is frequently difficult to isolate before aortotomy. Distally, the iliacs are carefully exposed in the avascular plane by gently mobilizing overlying structures, includ-ing the ureters. Again, the full exposure of the right iliac is typi-cally more difficult by this approach, depending on the patient's habitus. The extensive exposure of the supraceliac and visceral portions of the aorta permits full access and nuanced decision making about clamp placement, which may be suprarenal, supra-mesenteric, or supraceliac. Visceral and renal vessels may be con-trolled by clamp placement, vessel loops, or, after aortotomy, use of occlusion balloons, with great care taken in handling to avoid dissection or embolization. Occlusive disease or aneurysmal involvement of renal or visceral vessels may be readily addressed by this approach. According to the patient's indications and the surgeon's preference, cardiopulmonary bypass may be used as an adjunct and provides the ability to actively perfuse the renal and visceral vessels should a complex or prolonged reconstruction be anticipated.

Once adequate exposure has been achieved, proximal and distal clamps may be placed. As in the transperitoneal approach, repair is typically accomplished by endoaneurysmorrhaphy, using end-to-end proximal and distal anastomoses to replace the dis-eased portion of aorta as an interposition. Once again, the aneu-

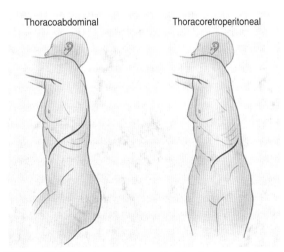

FIGURE 61-7 Patient positioning and incision for thoracoabdominal and thoracoretroperitoneal exposures. Note the open configuration of the hips in the latter, facilitating bilateral access to the iliac and femoral arteries.

rysm thrombus is removed at the time of aortotomy, and lumbar arteries are ligated within the sac. The same principles of back-bleeding and flushing of the graft before completion of the distal anastomosis apply. This approach does also permit a variety of approaches to reconstruction of the juxtarenal, pararenal, and paravisceral aorta. Branch vessels may be incorporated together by careful beveling of the graft, reimplanted individually as Carrel patches, or reconstructed using short bypass grafts. In treating thoracoabdominal aneurysms, the incision may be extended into the chest at the appropriate rib space and the diaphragm circumferentially divided to afford enough exposure to extend the repair to virtually any level of the descending aorta. The rib may be circumferentially dissected and divided posteriorly to further improve thoracic exposure as needed. When hemostasis is achieved, the sac may again be closed over the graft, although the retroperitoneally placed graft is not as vulnerable to erosion and aortoduodenal fistula as that placed transperitoneally (Fig. 61-8).

Medial visceral rotation, introduced by Mattox for trauma and adapted to aortic reconstruction by Stoney, is a third technique that may, through an abdominal incision, afford exposure of the entire abdominal aorta. This technique may be used for type IV or high paravisceral aneurysms and is best suited for patients who are not obese or asthenic, with narrow costal margins extending to the iliac crest.

Management of the Ruptured Aneurysm

Patients who survive to present to the hospital with a ruptured AAA may range from relatively stable to circulatory collapse. Optimal outcomes rely on the establishment of an institutional system for management of this critical aortic emergency that facilitates the early notification of the operative team, the availability of appropriate equipment (including an inventory of implants) and staff to support endovascular or open repair, and a system for rapid anatomic assessment. Several key principles of management must be considered. First, the appropriate hemodynamic parameters are those of permissive hypotension, with systolic blood pressures as low as 50 to 70 mm Hg considered adequate in a conscious patient, and avoidance of aggressive volume resuscitation. Management of a hemodynamically unstable patient or one in whom aortic control is expected to be delayed, prolonged, or complex, whether open or endovascular, may use percutaneous balloon control of the proximal aorta.[50] When possible, contrast-enhanced CTA should be performed preoperatively, although techniques that rely exclusively on angiography have been described. This may establish whether endovascular repair is possible or preferred, in addition to delineating anatomy and identifying associated aneurysmal or occlusive disease.

In the operating room, consideration should be given to the method and timing of anesthesia. Endovascular repair may be performed initially or in its entirety under local anesthesia. When open repair and general anesthesia are required, it is prudent to complete positioning, sterile preparation, and draping of the field before induction of anesthesia. In treating a ruptured aneurysm, a supraceliac control clamp should greatly facilitate resuscitation and provide a measure of hemodynamic stability. A formal protocol for resuscitative endovascular balloon occlusion of the aorta has been developed and can be of great utility in the unstable patient with ruptured aneurysm as well as other forms of hemorrhagic shock. This balloon may be placed percutaneously to establish proximal control in anticipation of open or endovascular repair.[51] Initial wire access to the suprare-

nal aorta should be followed by passage of a stiff guidewire and placement of a sheath of sufficient size (14 Fr) to accommodate a large, compliant occlusion balloon and length (40 cm) to support the inflated balloon in a suprarenal position against aortic pulsation.

Postoperative Management

In the immediate postoperative period, patients are typically admitted to an intensive care unit, with continuous cardiopulmonary monitoring. Adequate pain control, appropriate resuscitation, adequate oxygenation, and heart rate control all serve to minimize the risk of postoperative myocardial infarction. Epidural anesthesia and patient-controlled analgesia are both excellent options for postoperative pain management, and epidural anesthesia may actually decrease postoperative complications.[52] The use of appropriate prophylaxis for deep venous thrombosis is important and is not precluded by the use of an epidural catheter. Attention to early mobilization and nutrition of the patient are also essential to recovery.

Although late events after open surgical repair are relatively rare, a program of surveillance is typical to detect complications such as the formation of anastomotic or para-anastomotic aneurysms, which may occur up to 20% of the time at 15 years after repair.[53,54] The authors typically image patients with CT initially, then at 5-year intervals after repair. Ultrasound may also be used for surveillance but is operator dependent and lacks the sensitivity of CT for detecting anastomotic or para-anastomotic changes.

Ruptured aneurysm may pose a significant challenge in the postoperative period, whether it is approached in an open or endovascular fashion. The incidence of serious complications, such as colon ischemia, renal failure, and spinal cord infarction, is significantly higher than after elective repair and is associated with increased mortality. Surgeons must remain vigilant as colon ischemia may be manifested subtly and must have a low threshold for sigmoidoscopy if it is suspected. Ischemia and reperfusion may also contribute to injury to the lungs, development of lower extremity compartment syndrome with rhabdomyolysis, and abdominal compartment syndrome. The abdominal compartment syndrome may necessitate decompressive laparotomy after successful endovascular repair.

Endovascular Repair

EVAR was first reported by Parodi and colleagues in 1991[55] and has been widely adopted since the first Food and Drug Administration (FDA)–approved devices for EVAR, the AneuRx (Medtronic, Minneapolis, Minn) and the Ancure (Guidant Corporation, Menlo Park, Calif), became available in 1999. In 2006, the Agency for Healthcare Research and Quality published a comparison of EVAR and open surgical repair for AAA that concluded that "EVAR has shorter length of stay, lower 30-day morbidity and mortality but does not improve quality of life beyond 3 months or survival beyond 2 years."[56] These advantages, although limited, have been sufficient to make EVAR more frequently performed in recent years than open surgical repair for aneurysms with suitable anatomy.[57] The advantages of EVAR extend to treatment of ruptured aneurysms, for which multiple studies have confirmed that endovascular repair is associated with lower in-hospital morbidity and mortality.[58] Several anatomic considerations guide patient suitability for EVAR, including the anatomy of the aneurysm neck (size, length, shape, and angulation) and the iliac arteries (caliber, tortuosity, and aneurysmal involvement). The capabilities of currently available devices, as summarized in

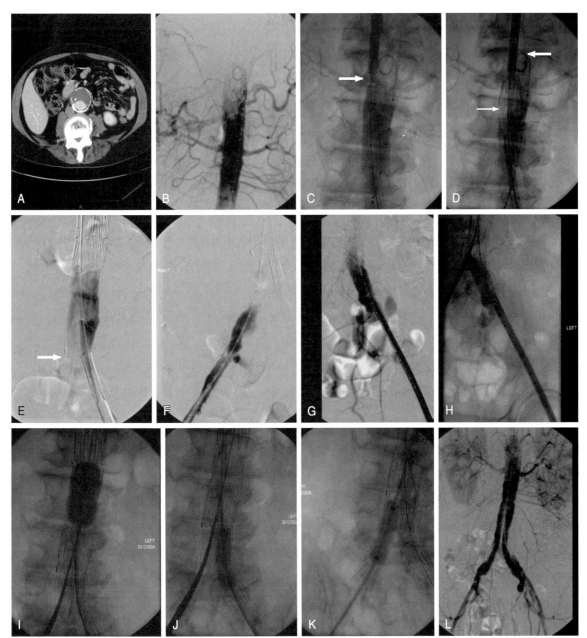

FIGURE 61-8 Technique of EVAR. **A,** Initial aortogram profiling the renal arteries. **B,** Device has been advanced over a stiff wire to the level of the renal arteries. **C,** Note radiopaque markers indicating the beginning of fabric coverage *(arrow)*. **D,** Device sheath withdrawn, permitting partial opening of the proximal graft *(thin arrow)*. Note that the top cap continues to constrain the suprarenal fixation wires *(thick arrow)*. **E,** The contralateral iliac limb gate *(arrow)* has been cannulated; contrast material is introduced with use of a rim catheter to confirm successful cannulation before placement of iliac extension. **F-H,** Angiography of both iliac arteries with marker catheters in place to permit deployment of iliac extensions, with preservation of both internal iliac arteries. **I-K,** Balloon molding of the proximal graft, overlap segments of the main graft and iliac limbs, and distal seal zones of the iliac limbs to facilitate proximal, distal, and intercomponent seals. **L,** Completion aortogram demonstrating successful exclusion of the aneurysm and no evidence of endoleak, which would be manifested as continued filling of the aneurysm sac by contrast material.

their approved indications for use, are listed in Table 61-3. The majority of available devices are modular bifurcated grafts consisting of an aortic main body to be used with a variable number of iliac or proximal aortic extension components. Aortouni-iliac devices are also available and may be used, generally in conjunction with femoral-femoral bypass grafting, either primarily or to salvage a failed bifurcated device. Branched devices designed to preserve the hypogastric artery in the setting of an aneurysmal common iliac artery are available in Europe and in clinical trials in the United States.*

TABLE 61-3 Endovascular Repair Devices: Indications for Use

DEVICE (MANUFACTURER)	STENT OR GRAFT MATERIAL	SHEATH OR DEVICE DIAMETER (MAIN BODY)	AORTIC DIAMETER* (mm)	ILIAC DIAMETER (mm)	MAXIMUM ANGULATION	MINIMUM NECK LENGTH	OTHER
AneuRx (Medtronic)	Nitinol, polyester	21 Fr	20-28 (graft)	12-24 (graft)	45-degree neck	15 mm	Initial FDA approval 1999; No suprarenal fixation or barbs; Sheath not required
Talent (Medtronic)	Nitinol, polyester	22 Fr	18-32 (aorta), 22-36 (graft)	8-22 (iliac), 8-24 (graft)	60-degree neck	10 mm	Suprarenal fixation stent; Tapered and flared limbs available; Uni-iliac Talent Converter device available
Endurant (Medtronic)	Nitinol, polyester	18 Fr, 20 Fr	19-32 (aorta), 23-36 (graft)	8-25 (iliac), 10-28 (graft)	60-degree neck	10 mm	Barbed suprarenal fixation stent; Like Talent, approved for 10-mm neck; Thin fabric, low delivery profile
Zenith (Cook Medical)	Stainless steel, polyester	18 Fr, 20 Fr, 22 Fr	18-32 (aorta), 22-36 (graft)	7.5-20 (iliac), 9-24 (graft)	60-degree neck	15 mm	Barbed suprarenal fixation stent; Tapered limb configurations available; Zenith Renu aortouni-iliac graft available; Graft sizing based on outer diameter
Excluder (W.L. Gore)	Nitinol, ePTFE	18 Fr, 20 Fr	19-29 (aorta), 23-31 (graft)	8-13.5 (ipsilateral graft), 12-14.5 (ipsilateral graft), 8-18.5 (contralateral graft), 12-20 (contralateral graft), 10-20 (extender)	60-degree neck	15 mm	Available ipsilateral limb sizes vary with size of primary graft; Contralateral limb components may be used as iliac extenders; Proximal nitinol anchors
Powerlink (Endologix)	Cobalt-chromium, ePTFE	19 Fr, 21 Fr	18-32 (aorta), 22, 25, 28 (graft), 25, 28, 34 (aortic cuff)	10-23 (iliac), 13-16 (graft), 16-25 (extensions)	60-degree neck, 90-degree iliac	15 mm	Anatomic fixation on aortic bifurcation; Seal achieved with suprarenal or infrarenal proximal aortic cuff; IntuiTrak system avoids need to cannulate contralateral gate
AFX (Endologix)	Cobalt-chromium, ePTFE	17 Fr	18-32 (aorta), 22, 25, 28 (graft), 25, 28, 34 (aortic cuff)	10-23 (iliac), 13-16 (graft), 16-25 (extensions)	60-degree neck, 90-degree iliac	15 mm	Similar to Powerlink in design; Multiple limb configurations; Low-profile delivery system for bifurcated graft and proximal cuff
OvationPrime (Trivascular/Endologix)	Cobalt-Chromium/ ePTFE	14 Fr	16-30 (aorta)	8-25 (iliac)	60-degree neck (45-degree if neck <10 mm)	<10 mm†	Uses polymer-filled sealing ring technology for proximal seal; Offers integrated crossover lumen as alternative to retrograde cannulation of contralateral gate
Aorfix (Lombard)	Nitinol/woven polyester	22 Fr	19-29 (aorta), 24-31 (graft)	9-19 (iliac), 10-20 (graft)	90-degree neck	20 mm	Combination circular and helical stents to accommodate extreme angulation; Proximal fishmouth configuration

*Recommended methods of vessel sizing and guidelines for graft oversizing vary by device.
†Proximal seal based on diameter at 13 mm from lowest renal, as sealing O-ring centered 13 mm from leading edge.

Whereas early morbidity and mortality (0.5% to 1.54% versus 3% to 4.8%) are lower with EVAR, there is overall a higher rate of re-intervention (albeit primarily endovascular) after endovascular than after open aneurysm repair and, after 2 to 3 years, no significant difference in the overall mortality rate.[1,59] This relatively new technology has borne an entirely new set of complications. Early, periprocedural complications include endoleak; access-related complications, which occur in up to 3% of cases and include hematoma, pseudoaneurysm, arterial occlusion or dissection, and iliac artery rupture or transection; peripheral embolization; renal insufficiency; local wound complications; inadvertent renal or hypogastric artery occlusion; and rare occurrences, such as colon or spine ischemia. Late complications include rupture, which occurs rarely but at a higher rate than after open repair; graft limb occlusion; endoleak or sac enlargement; and graft infection.[60] Some of these, such as access site complications, have diminished in frequency over time as operator experience has improved and newer generations of devices have incorporated smaller diameters and hydrophilic coatings.

Endoleak is the most common indication for re-intervention after EVAR. Type I endoleak is defined as failure to achieve a satisfactory seal at either the proximal (type Ia) or distal (type Ib) seal zone, representing a failure to exclude the aneurysm sac. In general, a type I endoleak should be addressed at the time of detection. More aggressive balloon inflation within the seal zone, placement of additional graft components to extend the seal zone, and placement of balloon-expandable stents within the seal zone to improve wall apposition through increased radial force are among the most common endovascular therapies for type I endoleak. One FDA-approved device uses helical EndoAnchors (Aptus Endosystems, Sunnyvale, Calif) delivered with a deflectable sheath to address both type I endoleak and migration.[61] Embolization using endovascular coils or liquid embolic agents such as Onyx has also been described.

Type II endoleaks are the most common form and represent continued filling of the aneurysm sac by lumbar branches or the inferior mesenteric artery. Further treatment is indicated if a persistent type II endoleak is accompanied by an increase in sac size. Treatment may include embolization of feeding branches by selective catheterization (transarterial technique) or direct sac puncture (translumbar technique) or laparoscopic or open surgical ligation of these vessels. Efforts have recently focused on identifying preoperative imaging characteristics predictive of persistent type II endoleaks or those that will result in sac enlargement. Aneurysm sac diameter at the level of the inferior mesenteric artery and the number of patent lumbar arteries have been associated with persistent type II endoleak and delayed or recurrent presentation, the presence of inferior mesenteric artery–lumbar artery type of endoleak, and the diameter of the largest feeding or draining artery with sac enlargement.[62-64] Whereas embolization of patent aortic branches at the time of the index procedure seems to decrease the rate of type II endoleak, rupture due to type II endoleak remains rare and difficult to predict; therefore, the role of preemptive branch vessel embolization is controversial.[65,66] Additional techniques, such as perigraft sac embolization, are being investigated.[67]

Type III endoleaks represent failure of an individual component or of the seal between components of a modular graft system. As with type I leaks, all type III endoleaks should be treated, typically by relining the offending area with new graft components. Type IV endoleaks represent seepage through porous graft material and are typically self-limited, resolving when procedural anticoagulation is reversed. Finally, an entity known as endotension is sometimes considered a fifth type of endoleak. This represents persistent growth of the aneurysm sac in the absence of a detectable leak. It is proposed that this phenomenon is due to either the passage of serous ultrafiltrate across an excessively porous fabric or, as some believe, the existence of an undetected endoleak of one of the prior types.

It has also been noted that as operators have gained experience with EVAR, a growing proportion of procedures are performed outside the approved instructions for use. There has, during the same period, been a trend toward treating a greater proportion of patients 80 years of age or older. When demographic and anatomic factors were reviewed, it was noted that only 42% of patients met the conservative definition of instructions for use, whereas 69% met the most liberal definition. Independent predictors of post-EVAR sac enlargement at 5 years were the presence of endoleak, age of 80 years or older, aortic neck diameter of 28 mm or more, aortic neck angulation of 60 degrees or more, and common iliac artery diameter of more than 20 mm, suggesting that factors associated with the gradual liberalization of anatomic criteria over time are associated with sac enlargement and, by implication, worse outcomes.[68] As techniques and devices extend the proximal seal zone into the visceral segment and beyond, one may expect that the trend toward treatment outside instructions for use with infrarenal devices may be reversed.

Device migration, either intraprocedurally or over time, may occur. In the EVAR setting, migration may be facilitated by unfavorable aneurysm neck anatomy. Manufacturers have attempted to address this issue by mechanisms including increased radial force, use of barbs or suprarenal fixation, or use of "anatomic fixation" at the aortic bifurcation. Device failure resulting from fracture of metallic components or fabric failure may also occur. The iliac limbs of these devices are also subject to thrombosis and occlusion, possibly at a higher rate than bifurcated grafts placed during open surgical repair.[69]

It is recommended that contrast CT surveillance be conducted at 1 month, 6 months, and 12 months after graft implantation and annually thereafter. Concern about accumulated lifetime radiation exposure and the use of nephrotoxic contrast agents has driven the expansion of the role of color Doppler and contrast-enhanced duplex ultrasonography in graft surveillance.[70,71] Implantable sensor technology has been approved by the FDA to monitor pressure within the aneurysm sac and may evolve to augment or even to supplant current imaging techniques for postoperative aneurysm surveillance.

Thoracic Aortic Aneurysm

Aneurysms of the descending thoracic aorta may be classified as type A, B, or C, depending on whether the aneurysm involves the proximal, mid, or distal third of the descending aorta, respectively (Fig. 61-9). Thoracoabdominal aneurysms are typically distinguished according to the Crawford classification system (Fig. 61-10). As with aneurysms of the abdominal aorta, rupture risk is closely associated with aneurysm size and, to a lesser extent, female gender. Current guidelines recommend repair of the descending thoracic aorta at 5.5 cm.

---

*Gore Excluder Iliac Branch Endoprosthesis, Cook Zenith Branch Iliac Endovascular Graft. *http://www.goremedical.com/eu/excluder/*, *http://zenithglobal.cookmedical.com/zenith-abdominal.html*. Accessed September 29, 2015.

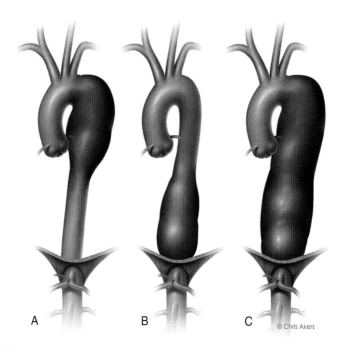

A   B   C   © Chris Akers

FIGURE 61-9 Classification, descending thoracic aortic aneurysm. **A,** Type A, distal to the left subclavian artery to the sixth intercostal space. **B,** Type B, sixth intercostal space to above the diaphragm (twelfth intercostal space). **C,** Type C, entire descending thoracic aorta, distal to the left subclavian artery to above the diaphragm (twelfth intercostal space). (Courtesy Chris Akers, 2006.)

Open Repair of Thoracic and Thoracoabdominal Aneurysms

The level of entry into the thoracic cavity for repair of thoracic or thoracoabdominal aneurysm is guided by the proximal extent of the aneurysm. Incision at the fifth or sixth interspace provides excellent exposure of the proximal descending aorta; at the eighth or ninth interspace, the mid-descending aorta; and at the tenth or eleventh interspace, the infradiaphragmatic portion of the aorta. Cardiopulmonary bypass combined with the selective use of distal aortic and visceral perfusion and hypothermic circulatory arrest have yielded exemplary results in experienced hands.[72]

Endovascular Management of Thoracic Aneurysms

In 2005, the FDA approved the GORE TAG Thoracic Endoprosthesis (W.L. Gore & Associates, Flagstaff, Ariz) for treatment of the descending thoracic aorta. Since that time, open surgical therapy for aneurysms of the descending thoracic aorta has largely been supplanted by TEVAR for anatomically suitable lesions.[73]

As with abdominal aortic endografts, initial and subsequent studies have demonstrated a significantly lower rate of short-term morbidity and mortality than with open repair. Unlike EVAR, TEVAR appears to offer a significant, long-term aneurysm-related mortality advantage. The most frequent complications of TEVAR are related to injuries to femoral or iliac access vessels. As the diameters of delivery devices for thoracic endografts may be considerably larger than those required for EVAR, many surgeons have developed a distinctly conservative approach to device access, performing open femoral artery exposure or addressing diminutive iliac vessels through the use of iliac or aortic conduits, open aortic or iliac exposure and direct puncture, or the use of endovascular iliac conduits to prevent injury. Recently, several investigators have pioneered the technique of caval-aortic access for delivery of larger diameter devices to the thoracic aorta or aortic

valve.[74] The combination of operator experience and the development of lower profile and hydrophilic delivery systems has, over time, reduced the rate of access-related complications of TEVAR.[75]

Because of the passage of endovascular wires, catheters, and other devices through the aortic arch, TEVAR carries the additional risk of embolic stroke.[76] Nevertheless, TEVAR has consistently yielded lower rates of early mortality and common postoperative complications than in open repair, with Bavaria and colleagues reporting perioperative mortality rates of 2.1% versus 11.7%, spinal cord ischemia rates of 3% versus 14%, respiratory failure rates of 4% versus 20%, and renal insufficiency rates of 1% versus 13% in low-risk patients after endovascular and open repair, respectively.[77]

Several anatomic considerations guide the selection of patients for TEVAR. As with EVAR, the size and configuration of the proximal aneurysm neck must suit the configuration and capabilities of available grafts. Commercially available thoracic endograft diameters currently range from 21 to 46 mm, creating limitations in patients with large proximal necks or small-caliber aortas. Tapered configurations are also available. The radius of the aortic arch and proximal descending aorta can also challenge device conformability and may result in a "bird's beak" deformity on deployment and, potentially, device collapse with consequent compromise of the aortic lumen (Fig. 61-11). In addition, coverage of one or more supra-aortic vessels may be required to achieve an adequate proximal landing and seal zone for the graft, necessitating decisions about extra-anatomic reconstruction. Most commonly, the left subclavian artery origin is covered. Justifications for surgical reconstruction of the subclavian artery, generally by carotid–subclavian artery bypass or subclavian artery transposition, include prevention of arm claudication, preservation of flow to a dominant left vertebral artery, and perhaps most important,

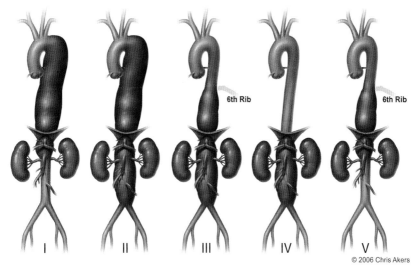

© 2006 Chris Akers

FIGURE 61-10 Normal thoracoabdominal aorta aneurysm classification: extent I, distal to the left subclavian artery to above the renal arteries; extent II, distal to the left subclavian artery to below the renal arteries; extent III, from the sixth intercostal space to below the renal arteries; extent IV, from the twelfth intercostal space to the iliac bifurcation (total abdominal aortic aneurysm); extent V, below the sixth intercostal space to just above the renal arteries (modified Crawford classification). (Courtesy Chris Akers, 2006.)

maximization of collateral spinal cord perfusion. More recently, endovascular fenestration of the left subclavian artery by a laser technique has been reported. Ultimately, branched devices such as the GORE TAG Thoracic Branch Endoprosthesis are being trialed to extend the proximal seal zone into the aortic arch. Endoleaks, primarily type I, complicate a significant proportion of TEVAR procedures. Some close spontaneously, perhaps because of reversal of intraprocedural heparin anticoagulation. Others require repair by the same techniques used for endoleaks encountered after EVAR.[78]

As with open repair of thoracic and thoracoabdominal aneurysms, prevention of spinal cord ischemia, which may be manifested as temporary or permanent, unilateral or bilateral paraparesis or paraplegia, is of great importance. Delayed rather than immediate postoperative spinal cord ischemia seems to be more common after TEVAR than after open surgical repair, and these patients may be more likely to experience functional improvement after injury.[79] Risk factors for spinal cord ischemia include the length of aortic coverage, coverage of the distal thoracic aorta, compromise of multiple collateral territories, preoperative renal insufficiency, and hypotension.[80] Whereas institutional protocols vary, particularly with regard to selection of patients for cerebrospinal fluid drain placement, the mainstays of prevention of spinal cord ischemia and the treatment of delayed-onset symptoms remain avoidance of hypotension, blood pressure augmentation (target mean arterial pressure > 90 mm Hg), and cerebrospinal fluid drainage to minimize ischemia related to cord compression in the setting of elevated cerebrospinal fluid pressure after ischemia-reperfusion.

Endovascular Repair of Aneurysms Involving the Visceral Segment: Snorkels, Fenestrations, and Branched Grafts

Endovascular therapy for juxtarenal, suprarenal, and thoracoabdominal aneurysms was, until recently, limited to a few centers

with access to investigational fenestrated devices or with substantial experience in either creating customized fenestrated devices (Fig. 61-12) or using debranching (antegrade grafts from the thoracic aorta or retrograde iliac grafts to the renovisceral vessels, permitting stent graft coverage of the perivisceral segment) or "snorkel" or "chimney" techniques (use of covered stents extending from the branch vessels beyond the proximal or distal extent of an aortic stent graft) to maintain perfusion to branch vessels.[81,82]

At present, a broader range of centers have gained critical experience in the use of surgeon-modified grafts or snorkel techniques for the treatment of aneurysms involving the visceral segment of the aorta.[83] In 2012, the FDA issued the first U.S. approval for a fenestrated device for the treatment of juxtarenal and pararenal aneurysms, the custom-made Zenith Fenestrated AAA Endovascular Graft (Cook Medical, Bloomington, Ind). This approval mandated a rigorous physician training program including an intensive 2-day training session for the initial group of implanting physicians, selected for their extensive EVAR experience, followed by physician proctoring. Additional branched or fenestrated devices have gained European CE Mark approval or are in investigational stages either in the United States or abroad. There is particular interest in the development of "off-the-shelf" devices that would permit accommodation of the majority of anatomic configurations without the 3- to 4-week manufacturing period required to obtain the custom-manufactured grafts. Devices currently in U.S. clinical trials include the Cook Zenith p-Branch and Endologix (Irvine, Calif) Ventana and the Cook Zenith t-Branch Thoracoabdominal Endovascular Graft, which incorporates four caudally oriented branches into an off-the-shelf design for the treatment of thoracoabdominal aneurysms. The Gore Excluder Thoracoabdominal Branch Endoprosthesis, which began enrolling in clinical trials outside the United States in November 2014 and anticipates initiating enrollment at six U.S. sites in September 2015, includes four visceral branches that are precannulated to facilitate branch vessel selection. The features of the next generation of thoracoabdominal grafts address many of

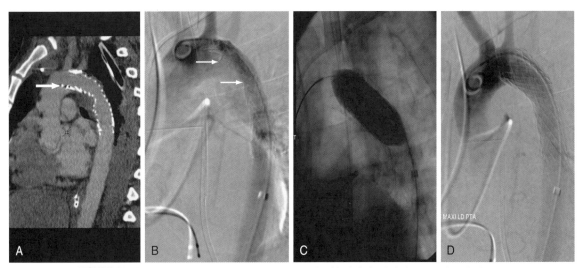

FIGURE 61-11 A, CT scan demonstrating thoracic endograft with bird's beak deployment along the lesser curve of the aorta, leaving the leading edge of the endograft projecting into the lumen *(arrow)*. **B,** Thoracic aortogram demonstrating subsequent collapse of the endograft caused by pressure on the protruding proximal portion of the endograft, resulting in distal hypoperfusion *(arrows)*. **C** and **D,** Deployment of a balloon-expandable Palmaz stent to reopen the proximal graft.

the drawbacks of current custom-made fenestrated grafts and, certainly, of the surgeon-modified branched or fenestrated and various snorkel configurations.

Blunt Thoracic Aortic Injury

In the modern era, the majority of blunt aortic injury is related to motor vehicles and involves the thoracic aorta. True transections are rapidly fatal, generally before arrival at the hospital; some estimates of prehospital mortality are as high as 80% to 90%. Patients may, however, arrive relatively stable with injuries ranging from contained pseudoaneurysms to intramural hematoma to relatively subtle intimal disruptions. The current "gold standard" for imaging of aortic trauma is contrast-enhanced CTA. The most frequent site of injury is the aortic isthmus, and it is typically a transverse tear that can encompass partial or full aortic circumference and may be either partial or transmural. It is thought that injury at this location is a result of rapid deceleration, which creates severe torsion and shearing forces where relatively mobile segments of the aorta become fixed, such as the ligamentum arteriosum, aortic root, and diaphragm.

Particularly in the setting of other distracting or disabling injuries, the history and physical examination may be unrevealing. Chest radiography may demonstrate mediastinal widening, apical pleural cap, loss of the aortopulmonary window, rightward deviation of the mediastinal structures or instrumentation, or depression of the left mainstem bronchus. CT is sensitive and may distinguish between mediastinal hematoma with a preserved periaortic plane and true periaortic hematoma. One must also distinguish between ductus remnants or diverticula and acute injury.

Since the first report of endovascular repair of a traumatic injury to the thoracic aorta in 1997, data have rapidly accumulated to support preferential use of endovascular stent graft over traditional open repair because of consistently reduced rates of mortality (8% to 9% versus 19%), paraplegia (0.5% to 3% versus 3% to 9%), and end-stage renal disease (5% versus 8%) as well

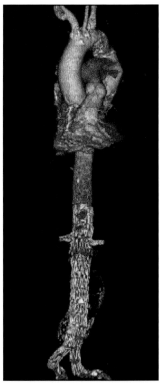

FIGURE 61-12 CT reconstruction demonstrating successful placement of an endovascular graft with fenestrations at the level of the renal arteries, permitting renal stent placement and use of a proximal seal zone above the renal arteries, with preservation of renal perfusion. (Courtesy Dr. Gilbert R. Upchurch, Jr.)

as a comparable stroke rate (2.5% versus 1%).[84,85] In practice, endovascular repair was adopted rapidly despite initial concerns about its durability, accounting for 65% of blunt thoracic aortic injury repairs within a decade of the initial publication. During this time, despite technical challenges related to the smaller aortic sizes, endovascular repair offers the additional benefits of reduced hemodynamic impact, lower complication rate, and less overall morbidity. The lower risk nature of the procedure itself may permit earlier aortic repair in patients with significant concurrent injuries.

AORTOILIAC OCCLUSIVE DISEASE

In 1950, the first aortic reconstruction for AIOD (Leriche syndrome) was performed by Jacques Oudot in France. This was performed through a retroperitoneal approach using homograft. Following the investigational and clinical work of Arthur Voorhees at Columbia University, prosthetic grafts of Vinyon-B and nylon were used for reconstruction of aortic occlusive as well as aneurysmal disease. Both of these materials had significant problems associated with them. Wylie introduced aortoiliac endarterectomy to the United States in 1952, and that technique was the most commonly used during the 1950s. In 1958, DeBakey introduced Dacron grafts, and aortofemoral grafting with Dacron became the most widely used technique for open reconstruction, although aortoiliac endarterectomy was still performed at certain centers, notably San Francisco, Boston, and Portland, Oregon. It is still useful for patients with aortoiliac disease confined to the aorta and common iliac arteries, especially those patients with small aortas and iliac arteries, for whom endovascular repair may not be optimal. Axillofemoral artery grafting and femoral-femoral artery grafting were introduced to provide inflow procedures for poor-risk patients and patients with unilateral iliac disease, respectively.

Endovascular repair for occlusive disease of the aorta and iliac arteries was introduced in the 1990s. The use of kissing stents and the size of the common iliac arteries especially have allowed this modality to work extremely well for the majority of patients with AIOD. The TASC document on management of peripheral arterial disease (TASC I) was published in January 2000.[86,87] These guidelines were developed to help in the rational choice of an open or endovascular approach to aortoiliac disease in particular patients. At present, endovascular treatment is the treatment of choice for type A lesions. It is also the most commonly used modality for type B. For type C lesions with more extensive disease of the external iliacs or bilateral occlusions of the common iliacs, surgical treatment has been more often recommended. For type D lesions, that is, extensive disease of the common and external iliac arteries, surgery has been the treatment of choice. Nonetheless, multiple authors have documented good success with endovascular treatment even for TASC C and D lesions.[88-90]

The next iteration of the TASC recommendation is shortly expected, and it is likely that endovascular treatment will be the recommended first-line treatment for all patients. It is difficult, however, to imagine endovascular therapy to be as good or as long lasting for AIOD for these extensive lesions, especially in young patients. It is worth noting the proportion of aortofemoral bypass patients whose concomitant femoral disease requires endarterectomy at the time of the index operation.[91] These patients as well as patients with a significant aortic component of their AIOD

may not be well served by endovascular therapy alone. It is also difficult to imagine its utility for juxtarenal aortic occlusion, with its "dunce's cap" of chronic thrombus extending upward between the renal arteries, without a disproportionate increase in renal failure. Hybrid techniques, such as the combination of femoral endarterectomy with the placement of iliac stents, may address some of the limitations of the percutaneous-only approach.

Concomitant with the change in TASC definitions has been a marked increase in the use of endovascular techniques in comparison to open techniques. This increase corresponds to improvements in the delivery systems and stents that are employed as well as to improved skill sets of vascular radiologists, cardiologists, and vascular surgeons. Upchurch and colleagues documented an increase of 850% in endovascular use by 2000 with a concomitant 16% decrease in open cases. There was a 34% increase in treated disease without an increase in the prevalence of the disease.[92] These trends have continued and amplified; endovascular repair for AIOD is performed much more commonly than open repair.

The classic indications for AIOD were claudication, rest pain, and threatened limb viability, manifested by tissue loss, nonhealing ulcers, or frank gangrene. Rest pain and threatened limb viability implied extensive disease of either the deep femoral artery or the femoropopliteal segments in addition to the aortoiliac disease. The advent of endovascular techniques has, as stated before, broadened the indications, with mild claudication being treated much more frequently than in the past. There is certainly more justification for stenting of short-segment iliac stenoses than there is for performing aortofemoral bypass grafting for them.

Nonetheless, open surgery remains the gold standard for long-term patency. Chiu and associates in Birmingham, England, performed a meta-analysis of aortofemoral bypass grafting, iliofemoral bypass grafting, and aortoiliac endarterectomy. Their analysis yielded 29 studies including 5738 patients for aortofemoral bypass grafting, 11 studies incorporating 778 patients for iliofemoral bypass grafting, and 11 studies including 1490 patients for endarterectomy. Operative mortality was 4.1% for aortofemoral bypass grafting, 2.7% for iliofemoral bypass grafting, and 2.7% for aortoiliac endarterectomy. Morbidity was 16%, 18.9%, and 12.5%, respectively. Five-year primary patency rates were 86.3%, 85.3%, and 88.3%, respectively.[93] A meta-analysis published in 2009 suggests that formal aortic reconstruction is still the procedure of choice in terms of long-term patency. That durability may be more appealing to younger, healthier patients than return trips for further endovascular intervention. Similarly, an earlier meta-analysis covering the years 1970 to 1996 showed constant patency rates for aortic bifurcation grafts and declining mortality and morbidity over time. Mortality after 1975 was 3.3%.[94]

Axillofemoral artery bypass grafting is reserved for extremely poor risk patients with rest pain or tissue loss. Its suspect patency makes it a poor choice for claudicants. It is of course used as one of the mainstays of reconstruction for infected aortic grafts or aorta-enteric fistulas. This modality is offered to a different, higher risk group than is aortofemoral bypass grafting. Hertzer reported a 12% mortality compared with 5.6% for femoral-femoral grafting and 2.3% for aortic reconstruction. Within that group, mortality was only 1.2% for aortofemoral bypass grafting but 5.6% for aortoiliac endarterectomy or aortoiliac grafting.[95]

Iliofemoral grafting yields patency rates superior to femoral-femoral bypass in the treatment of unilateral external iliac occlusive disease not amenable to endovascular therapy or when endovascular therapy has failed. Ricco and Probst compared the two operative methods in 143 patients. Primary 5-year patency for iliofemoral grafting was 92.7% versus 73.2% for femoral-femoral grafting.[96]

As in all vascular beds, endovascular repair of the aortoiliac segments requires much more re-intervention than its open counterpart, but the mortality is lower. At some "aortic centers," there is no difference in mortality, but on average, open mortality is about 4%. Hertzer reported mortality of 2.3% for direct aortic reconstructions in an elegant paper.[95] Both Hertzer and Reed and colleagues found increased limb occlusion in patients with small arteries, especially women.[97] Primary assisted and secondary patency rates for endovascular repair nearly equal the primary patency rates of open reconstruction, and this has indeed been the rationale for the widespread application of endovascular techniques for most patients with AIOD, accepting repeated intervention as a necessary component of treatment.

Multiple authors have written about the endovascular treatment of TASC C and D lesions as well as aortic occlusion. Klonaris and colleagues recommended primary stenting for all aortic occlusive disease, including occlusion. Their study, however, did not include juxtarenal aortic occlusions as opposed to more distal aortic obstruction.[98]

Jongkind and colleagues reviewed all published articles of patients undergoing endovascular treatment of TASC C and D lesions from 2000 to 2009. There were 1711 patients identified. Technical success was achieved in 86% to 100% of those studies. Clinical symptoms were improved in 83% to 100%. Mortality ranged from 1.2% to 6.7% and complication rates varied, being reported between 3% and 45%. Primary patency ranged from 60% to 86% and secondary patency from 80% to 98%.[88]

Ichihashi and colleagues reported technical success in 99% of their 125 patients with TASC C and D lesions. Complications were significantly higher than for their TASC A and B patients (9% versus 3%). Their 5-year patency was 83%, among the very highest reported.[89]

Ye and associates performed a meta-analysis of TASC C and D patients undergoing endovascular reconstruction. TASC C patients had a 93.7% technical success rate and a 1-year primary patency of 89.6%. TASC D patients had 90.1% technical success and 87.3% 1-year patency.[90] Indes and colleagues, reviewing the Nationwide Inpatient Sample for 4119 patients, found that endovascular procedures were associated with lower cost, lower complication rates, and shorter length of stay. Mortality was not different statistically, being 1.8% for endovascular procedures and 2.5% for open procedures.[99] There is a third option for aortic reconstruction, and that is laparoscopic aortic surgery. Its greatest proponents have been in Europe, particularly France, and Québec. This has not gained widespread popularity in the United States.[100]

Presentation and Evaluation

Patients with AIOD may present with claudication. It is a much more likely presentation for AIOD than is rest pain or tissue loss. Rest pain or tissue loss, as stated previously, indicates disease of the deep femoral artery or the femoral popliteal segments in addition to the aorta and iliac segments. Physical examination historically has been accurate in these patients. A decreased femoral pulse is indicative of at least common femoral disease or more proximal aortoiliac disease. With the advent of the obesity epidemic in this country, physical examination of femoral pulses is not as accurate as it once was. Consequently, vascular laboratory examination is of even more importance than in the past. Wave patterns as well as ankle-brachial indices are necessary to localize the disease to

aortoiliac segments, femoral-popliteal segments, or both. It is also vital in identifying the contribution of AIOD to patients with multiple diseases contributing to their lower extremity problems, including neurogenic claudication, spinal stenosis, and hip arthritis, either alone or in combination with arterial disease.

With a tentative diagnosis of AIOD, the most commonly used modality to visualize the arteries is CTA. There are some patients in whom the calcium load is so great that either MRA or conventional arteriography is necessary to determine whether areas of calcific involvement are highly stenotic. Those surgeons for whom endovascular treatment is uniformly their first choice may proceed directly to conventional arteriography with planned endovascular intervention at the same time.

As with all vascular patients, cardiac risk is the greatest one at operation. Consequently, most authors recommend that all of these patients undergo cardiac function evaluation by stress testing. Those patients with myocardium at risk are usually treated by cardiologists or cardiac surgeons before embarking on an aortic reconstruction in an elective situation. Hertzer showed a marked decrease in cardiac mortality when patients underwent preoperative cardiac evaluation and treatment.[95]

As endovascular techniques gain wider acceptance, the most common indication for formal aortic reconstruction may be claudication or severe ischemia in the setting of failed multiple attempts at endovascular repair. These occluded stents make the operation more complex, with the need for suprarenal aortic clamping and more extended profundaplasties in many cases.

Technique of Open Reconstruction
Aortofemoral Bypass Grafting

For aortofemoral bypass grafting (Fig. 61-13), the patient is prepared from the nipples to the knees. If concomitant distal bypass grafting will be necessary, the patient is prepared to the toes. This would be done for tissue loss with multilevel disease only. Epidural catheters may be used to alleviate postoperative pain. Bilateral groin incisions are made. These are usually done in a vertical or slight curvilinear fashion. The common, superficial, and deep femoral arteries are dissected free. These need to be dissected distally to where they are soft and suitable for anastomosis. Most surgeons use a midline incision for the aortic exposure, although a transverse incision or a retroperitoneal approach can be used. The authors favor standard midline with infracolic exposure. The abdominal contents are mobilized so that the retroperitoneum can be entered. If the mobilized viscera can be kept inside the abdominal cavity rather than being placed on the abdominal wall, the patient's gastrointestinal functional recovery is usually a bit quicker. The retroperitoneum is entered. Care is taken to stay to the patient's right of the inferior mesenteric vein to avoid violating the left mesocolon. The aorta is dissected free below the renal arteries. The surgeon needs to remember that this disease extends from the renal arteries and not from the lower-lying renal vein level. The vein may be mobilized by division and ligation of its tributaries. In general, the exposure required for occlusive disease is less than is necessary in aneurysmal disease. The aorta is exposed down to the level of the inferior mesenteric artery. Retroperitoneal tunnels connecting this wound with the groin wounds are made. On the left side, a counterincision in the gutter lateral to the white line of Toldt may be necessary. The tunnels should be made posterior to the ureters. It is our habit to create the left tunnel posterior to the inferior mesenteric artery as well to allow the left limb of the graft to be isolated from the gastrointestinal tract by

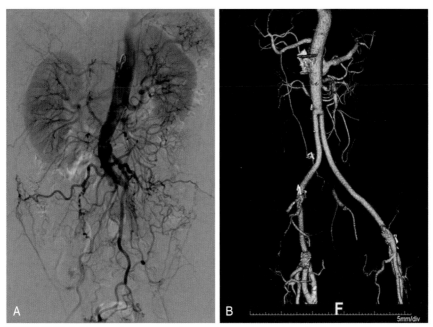

FIGURE 61-13 A, Preoperative aortogram demonstrating occlusion of the distal aorta and iliacs with extensive collateralization. **B,** Postoperative three-dimensional CT reconstruction demonstrating revascularization with an aortofemoral bypass graft.

the left mesocolon after completion of reconstruction. The patient is heparinized.

Control is obtained of the aorta below the renal arteries and of the distal aorta. The aorta is divided. Distally, a portion of it is resected on an angular bias and the distal aorta oversewn. That area of excision should be done proximal to the inferior mesenteric artery. This allows comfortable placement of an end-to-end graft. An appropriately chosen graft is fashioned to fit and sewn to the end of the proximal aorta using running 3-0 or 4-0 permanent suture. If one extremity has been less symptomatic that the other, that side is reconstructed first as it is less used to ischemia. The graft is brought through the tunnel into the groin, and control is obtained of the femoral arteries. An arteriotomy is made running from the common femoral artery down to the appropriate level. In many cases, this would be down to a point on the deep femoral artery. If endarterectomy of the common and deep femoral arteries is necessary, it is undertaken at this point. The graft is fashioned to fit and sewn end to side using either running 4-0 or 5-0 permanent suture. Appropriate backbleeding and forward bleeding is allowed before that. The opposite is done in a similar manner. When flow is restored into the limbs, it is restored first to the common, then to the deep, and last to the superficial femoral artery.

In general, end-to-end anastomoses are performed. These may lessen the chance of aortoenteric fistula. They have better flow characteristics than end-to-side proximal anastomoses. If the patient has bilateral external iliac artery occlusions, either a proximal end-to-side aortic anastomosis or a formal reconstruction of one of the internal iliac arteries is necessary to ensure continued blood flood into the pelvis.

The retroperitoneum should be carefully closed in layers to exclude the graft from the gastrointestinal tract. If there is insufficient tissue, an omental flap should be created and placed over

the graft to isolate it from the duodenum.

Axillofemoral Bypass Grafting

Axillobifemoral bypass grafting (Fig. 61-14) was introduced in the 1960s to provide inflow to patients who were poor physiologic candidates for aortic reconstruction. Its use has been extended to those patients having aortic graft infections or otherwise hostile abdomens for whom an in-line aortic reconstruction is considered too hazardous.

The patient is prepared from the shoulders down to the knees. It is our practice to extend the upper extremity on the side on which the graft is to be based 90 degrees. This will prevent the graft from being too taut when the patient moves the extremity. Reports of pseudoaneurysms and indeed ruptures secondary to short grafts have been published. A transverse incision is made in the deltopectoral groove. The axillary artery is exposed as medial as is possible. The more medial the anastomosis, the less excursion of the graft with use of the upper extremity. The pectoralis minor tendon may be incised to facilitate this exposure. If the tendon is not incised, the tunnel should be posterior to the tendon and then brought to the midaxillary line. In general, the right side is chosen if at all possible as the right subclavian artery is less prone to atherosclerotic disease than the left. Furthermore, if a later formal aortic reconstruction is planned, a right axillofemoral graft is much less a hindrance than one on the left, especially if a retroperitoneal approach is planned. Bilateral groin incisions are made. If the tunnel connecting the ipsilateral groin incision to the axillary incision can be created without a counterincision, this maneuver should be performed in that manner. If not, a counterincision can be made in the patient's flank. The counterincision seems to be prone to infection, and we try to avoid its use. Grafting is then done in the usual manner. The long portion of the graft should be at least 8 mm and preferably 10 or 12 mm in

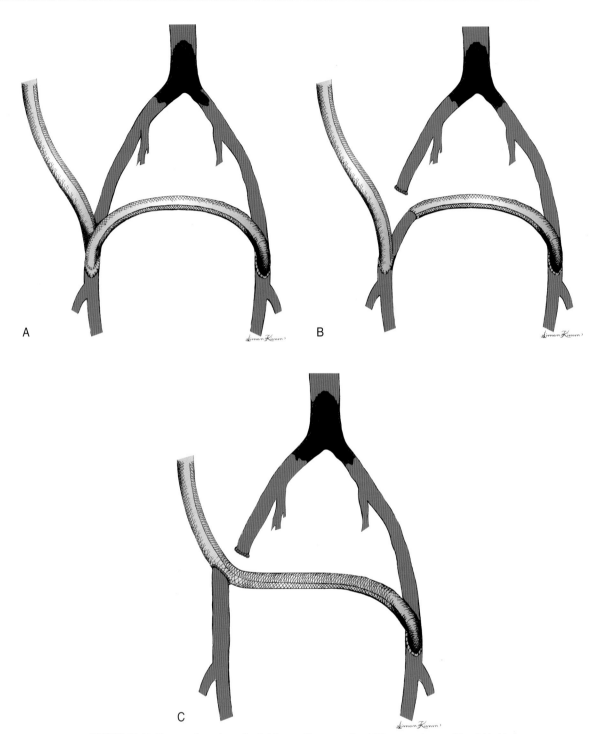

FIGURE 61-14 Three configurations of axillobifemoral bypass grafts. All three are shown with a right-sided axillofemoral graft component. **A,** The most common configuration. **B** and **C,** Modifications described by Blaisdell and associates **(B)** and Rutherford and Rainer **(C),** designed to prevent competitive inflow from a patent ipsilateral iliac system. (From Cronenwett J, Johnston KW, editors: *Rutherford's vascular surgery*, ed 7, Philadelphia, 2011, Elsevier.)

diameter to prevent a functional aortic stenosis. Mortality figures are higher for these patients than for patients having aortic reconstruction, ranging from 10% to 15%. This is because this is a population of much sicker patients. Five-year primary patencies vary greatly, but approximately 50% failure can be expected during the course of 5 years.

Femoral-Femoral Artery Bypass Grafting

Femoral arteries are exposed in the standard manner. Most surgeons now use a bucket-handle approach rather than trying to create a completely antegrade sigmoid-shaped reconstruction. This is done superior to the pubis at the subcutaneous level. Either polyester or expanded polytetrafluoroethylene can be used. Grafts of at least 7 or 8 mm are usually preferred. Patency of this has not been nearly as good as was first expected, ranging from 60% to 80% at 5 years. See Figure 61-15.

Iliofemoral Artery Bypass Grafting

In-line reconstruction of isolated external iliac artery lesions is preferable to femoral-femoral artery grafting if the patient's physiology and anatomy will allow. A flank incision is made and the retroperitoneal plane developed. The proximal anastomosis is performed to the common iliac artery or to the distal aorta as is necessary and then brought through that tunnel into the groin. Patency rates for this at 5 years are in the 90% range. See Figure 61-16.

Aortoiliac Endarterectomy

This operation is usually done through a midline incision. In contradistinction to exposure for aortic grafting, for endarterectomy, the aorta, the common iliac arteries, and the origins of the internal and external iliac arteries all need to be circumferentially exposed. In addition to the clamping of the aorta and the iliac arteries, it is also best to clamp the lumbar arteries with small clamps to prevent annoying backbleeding, which impedes accurate endarterectomy. The patient is heparinized. Control is obtained of the aorta and the iliac arteries. A vertical aortotomy is made. With use of an elevator, an endarterectomy of the aorta down to the origins of the common iliacs is performed. At this point, either transverse incisions, which is our preference, or vertical incisions may be made at the distal common iliac arteries. The endarterectomy plane is begun here. There may be a tongue of atherosclerosis extending into the origin of the external iliac and the internal iliac. These are elevated. A stripper, such as a Wylie stripper, is used. Classically, this is passed in a retrograde manner. It may be that in some patients with deep pelvises, passing in an antegrade manner is more advantageous. An appropriate-sized stripper is picked, and the endarterectomy of the iliac artery is completed. The atherosclerotic plaque from both the aorta and the iliac arteries may be brought out as a single specimen if retrograde iliac endarterectomy has been performed. The arterial incisions are closed primarily with fine permanent suture after appropriate flushing and ascertainment of good end points. When flow is restored, interestingly enough, the aorta remains essentially the same size and the common iliac arteries balloon up much like pantaloons. The retroperitoneum and abdomen are then closed in standard manner. See Figure 61-17.

Complications of Open Aortic Surgery

A number of complications may arise after operations to repair the aorta, whether for aneurysmal or occlusive disease.[101] These may be site-specific complications, such as wound infection or hematoma, also commonly seen with endograft approaches. Of more concern and major morbidity are the intra-abdominal and systemic complications. Cardiac ischemia is the most frequent complication of open aortic surgery, and in the very best of hands one can expect that 50% of deaths related to aortic reconstruction will be attributable to the heart. Only a minority of patients with occlusive disease have normal coronary arteries. Stress testing, cardiac angiography, and coronary intervention (catheter based or, more rarely, open) have reduced mortality for direct aortic operations. Some specialty centers with aggressive heart evaluation

management schemes have reported mortality in the range of 1% to 2.5%.[95]

Renal insufficiency is a common complication and may result from embolization from clamping, prolonged ischemia with suprarenal clamping, intrinsic renal artery disease, hypovolemia, or hypoperfusion. It is exacerbated by paravisceral aortic repair and intraoperative complications. It most probably relates directly to the patient's preoperative renal and cardiac status. Accurate assessment of the patient's anatomy and a precise preoperative plan for clamping site and sequence are necessary to minimize the incidence of perioperative renal insufficiency.

Pulmonary dysfunction is a frequent and serious complication. This, too, is more prevalent with proximal and paravisceral aortic procedures. Transverse abdominal incisions, epidural analgesia, and retroperitoneal approaches may mitigate pulmonary complications.

Abdominal wall hernia is a common late complication of open aneurysm repair, occurring at a much higher rate (10% to 33%) than after other open operations requiring midline laparotomy, suggesting that there are patient factors associated with the pathology of AAA that predispose this population to hernia. However, attention to fascial closure remains important to minimize this complication; a prospective study has demonstrated a relatively low 11.6% rate of midline hernia, with a suture length to wound length ratio of less than 4:1 predictive of hernia development. This study, contrary to earlier findings, did not note a statistically significant difference between the aneurysm and occlusive disease groups.[102] Retroperitoneal exposures crossing the flank are prone to subsequent abdominal wall laxity, which is not a true hernia but remains bothersome to patients.

Graft limb thrombosis occurs in 5% to 10% of patients and is associated with female gender, younger patients, and extra-anatomic bypass graft.[96,97]

An anastomotic pseudoaneurysm may be a sterile process or the result of infection. These pseudoaneurysms occur more frequently at the femoral anastomosis than at iliac and aortic anastomoses, which may reflect the higher rate of wound complications and graft infection in this region and the more clinically apparent nature of degeneration at the femoral site. Anastomotic pseudoaneurysms may result from degeneration of the suture line. True aneurysms tend to be para-anastomotic in nature, forming in the aorta proximal to or the iliac or femoral arteries distal to an aortic graft. True aneurysms occur more frequently in patients treated for aneurysmal than occlusive disease. Hypertension, COPD, smoking, hyperlipidemia, suture type, technical failures, and postoperative wound complications may be associated with this phenomenon.

Detection of anastomotic pseudoaneurysms in the iliac or aortic positions is highly reliant on imaging. Prospective studies using routine imaging of arterial grafts in a variety of anatomic positions have demonstrated higher rates of anastomotic pseudoaneurysm than those relying on clinical detection. Routine surveillance with ultrasound, for instance, demonstrated intra-abdominal anastomotic pseudoaneurysms in 10% of patients and 6.3% of aortic anastomoses after abdominal aortic graft placement at a mean interval of 12 years from operation.[54] CT and MRI provide excellent visualization of pseudoaneurysm and aneurysmal degeneration of the para-anastomotic area (Fig. 61-18).

Although some anastomotic pseudoaneurysms are sterile, it is prudent to begin evaluation and treatment with a presumption of infection. Diagnosis should include history (fever, chills, malaise, or weight loss), physical examination (erythema, fluctuant mass,

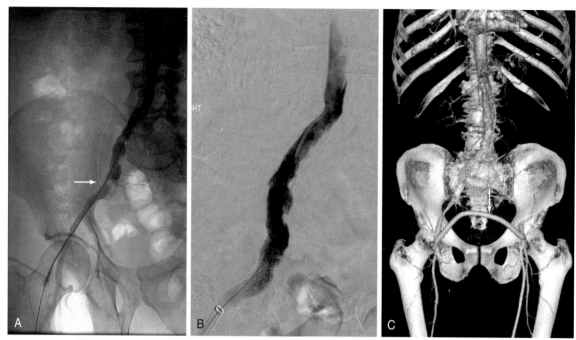

FIGURE 61-15 A, Preoperative angiogram demonstrating occlusion of the left iliac system in severe focal atherosclerotic disease of the right iliac artery *(arrow).* **B,** Magnified view of the right iliac system after angioplasty and stent placement to establish adequate inflow for femoral-femoral bypass graft. **C,** Three-dimensional CT reconstruction demonstrating completed right to left femoral-femoral bypass graft *(arrow).*

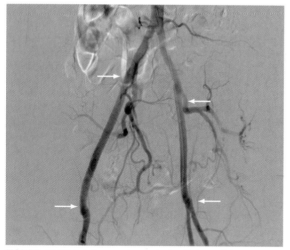

FIGURE 61-16 Arteriogram demonstrating iliofemoral bypasses extending from the bilateral common iliac to common femoral arteries *(arrows).*

induration, drainage, or tenderness to palpation), and laboratory evaluation (complete blood count, blood and fluid cultures, C-reactive protein level, or erythrocyte sedimentation rate). With regard to imaging, ultrasound may demonstrate the pseudoaneurysm itself as well as perigraft fluid suggestive of infection. CT and MRI may more completely characterize these findings (Fig. 61-19). The use of nuclear medicine modalities, such as indium In 111 or technetium Tc 99m tagged white blood cell scans, has greatly improved the surgeon's ability to evaluate for infection in

a noninvasive manner (Fig. 61-20). Whereas positive cultures are definitive, many of the organisms common in graft infections are fastidious and may yield multiple negative cultures despite clear clinical evidence of infection. When diagnostic investigation yields evidence of infection, thorough débridement of infected material accompanied by in situ or extra-anatomic arterial reconstruction is the mainstay of management. Surgical management of anastomotic pseudoaneurysm is dictated by the presence or absence of infection, the nature of presentation, and the surgeon's experience and preference. In an uninfected field, débridement and interposition grafting may suffice. Whereas aneurysmal degeneration at or near the graft anastomoses historically necessitated open repair, a growing proportion are now successfully managed by endovascular techniques.[103] In any event, expeditious treatment is appropriate for a large, enlarging, or symptomatic lesion.

Surgical Treatment of Aortic Graft Infection

Infection should be managed by removal of the entire affected graft with débridement of all infected or devitalized tissue, traditionally accompanied by extra-anatomic reconstruction. Staging of this process by performing the extra-anatomic bypass and then either proceeding to débridement or permitting a recovery interval of up to several days greatly improved the historically substantial morbidity and mortality associated with primary graft resection followed by reconstruction.[104] Further investigation has suggested that in instances of infection limited to a single limb of the graft, satisfactory results may be achieved by limiting resection to the involved limb or limb segment, followed by in situ or extra-anatomic reconstruction and, according to the surgeon's preference, combined with sterile antibiotic irrigation of the field through operatively placed drains.[105] However, recurrent graft

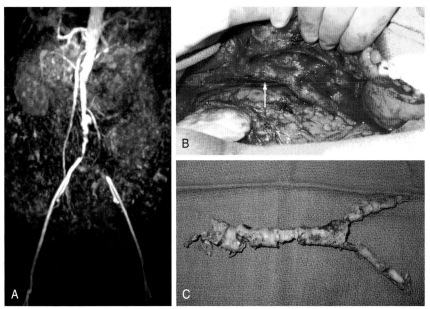

FIGURE 61-17 **A,** Preoperative MRA demonstrating severe atherosclerotic disease involving the infrarenal aorta and both common iliac arteries. **B,** Intraoperative photograph of completed aortoiliac endarterectomy showing suture line of primary closure *(arrow)*. **C,** Photograph of intact specimen demonstrating contiguous near-occlusive plaque.

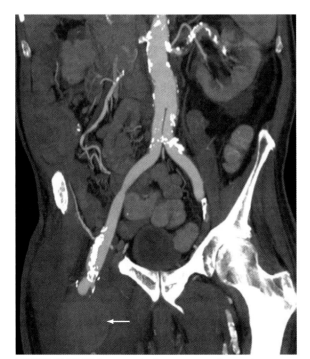

FIGURE 61-18 CT demonstrating large anastomotic pseudoaneurysm arising at the right femoral anastomosis of an aortofemoral graft.

infection, graft thrombosis, and the nearly invariably fatal complication of aortic stump infection or disruption continue to contribute to significant morbidity, mortality, and limb loss after this operation. Thorough débridement, layered closure, and vascularized pedicle flap coverage of the aortic stump are considered of paramount importance in avoiding the last complication.

In situ reconstruction may be accomplished by using rifampin-soaked or silver-coated polyester graft, cryopreserved arterial allograft, or saphenofemoral vein allograft.[106-109] The first of these is the most expeditious but yields a higher rate of reinfection as well as poor results in grossly purulent operative fields. Those espousing its use tend to embrace adjuncts such as wrapping the new graft and anastomoses in vascularized pedicle flaps, antibiotic irrigation therapy, or creation of clean retroperitoneal tunnels. The neoaortoiliac system venous autograft reconstruction described by Clagett is a lengthy procedure that places significant demands on both the patient and the operative team but yields the lowest reported rate of reinfection. Reported results using cryopreserved arterial allograft for in situ reconstruction have been mixed but generally reflect an intermediate rate of reinfection.[106] Endovascular treatment of anastomotic disruptions is generally limited to cases without evidence of infection and may use covered stent exclusion of the pseudoaneurysm or embolization of the pseudoaneurysm, generally with coils or occlusion devices. Aortoenteric fistula represents the most severe manifestation of aortic graft infection. It rarely occurs as a primary process, generally due to erosion of an untreated aneurysm into the duodenum. Most commonly, the lesion is at the point of contact of the third portion of the duodenum with the proximal graft anastomosis. Aortoenteric fistula has been reported in association with aortic stent graft placement. This complication generally is manifested with herald upper or lower gastrointestinal bleeding, which, if left untreated, may be followed by exsanguinating hemorrhage. Aortoenteric fistula should be suspected when gastrointestinal bleeding develops in a patient with a history of abdominal aortic surgery or endograft. Although endoscopy may confirm the diagnosis, demonstrating either an erosion or frank exposure of graft most frequently in the duodenum, CT is a more sensitive diagnostic study. The placement of synthetic or endovascular grafts in the setting

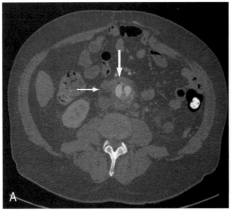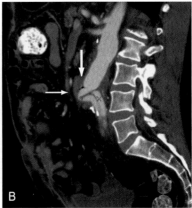

FIGURE 61-19 Axial **(A)** and sagittal **(B)** CT views of an infected aortofemoral graft after repair of an infra-renal aneurysm. Foci of gas *(thick arrows)* and extensive inflammation *(thin arrows)* are visible surrounding the graft. Of note, the tortuosity of the limbs of this graft represents a technical error.

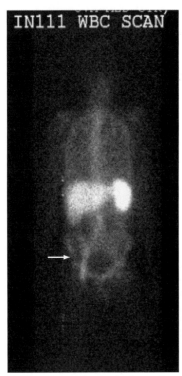

FIGURE 61-20 ¹¹¹In-tagged white blood cell scan image at 20 hours of delay demonstrates abnormal uptake in the region of the right limb of an aortofemoral graft *(arrow)*.

of infected pseudoaneurysm, graft infection, primary aortic infection, or aortoenteric fistula is perhaps best viewed as a temporizing measure and is attended by high rates of re-intervention, morbidity, and mortality.[110] Repair of aortoenteric fistula or primary aortic infection follows many of the same principles as for infected graft removal: consideration of staged extra-anatomic bypass, appropriate selection of conduit if in situ reconstruction is elected, establishment of safe proximal control, wide débridement of infected material, coverage of in situ graft with a pedicle flap such as omentum, and appropriate use of antibiotic and antifungal therapy.

AORTIC DISSECTION

Aortic dissection occurs when a defect in the intimal layer of the vessel permits blood to create a false channel within the aortic wall, typically between media and adventitia. The aorta is divided into true and false lumens, separated by a septum referred to as the dissection flap. A number of conditions, including connective tissue disorders such as Marfan syndrome, hypertension, and pregnancy, are associated with the development of aortic dissection, as are activities such as cocaine abuse and power weightlifting.[111]

A number of important distinctions must be made once the diagnosis of aortic dissection is made. The DeBakey and Stanford classification systems define dissections on the basis of anatomic extent. DeBakey type I (involving both ascending and thoracoabdominal aorta) and type II (limited to the ascending aorta) dissections correspond to the Stanford type A (any involvement of the ascending aorta); DeBakey type IIIa (confined to the descending thoracic aorta) and type IIIb (involving the descending thoracic and abdominal aorta) correspond to the Stanford type B (not involving the ascending aorta; Figs. 61-21 and 61-22).

Type A dissection typically is manifested acutely with chest or back pain, commonly described as ripping or tearing in nature. This may be accompanied by profound hypotension, particularly in the setting of pericardial tamponade or disruption of the aortic valve, and distal hypoperfusion as seen in type B dissections. Distal pulse deficits or other evidence of malperfusion in a patient presenting with sudden-onset, severe chest or back pain should immediately prompt evaluation for aortic dissection. CT and echocardiography both provide the ability not only to diagnose dissection but to rapidly assess the status of the proximal aorta, permitting the critical distinction between type A and type B lesions. Acute type A dissection is generally considered a surgical emergency. Repair necessitates the use of adjuncts such as cardiopulmonary bypass and hypothermic circulatory arrest and, on occasion, replacement of the aortic valve in addition to replacement of the ascending aorta.[73]

Type B dissection is further characterized as acute (≤14 days from onset of symptoms) or chronic (>14 days from initial symptoms) and, within these categories, as uncomplicated or complicated. Acute type B dissections will also frequently be manifested with tearing chest or back pain, often in the setting of severe hypertension. Malperfusion of the spine and renal, visceral, or lower extremity vessels may complicate the presentation. Rarely, patients may present with frank rupture. Anatomically, type B dissections generally originate from a primary tear in the proximal descending thoracic aorta just distal to the origin of the left subclavian artery. Extension is typically antegrade, extending as far as the iliac or femoral arteries, although retrograde extension may occur. Fenestrations or openings in the dissection flap may permit communication between true and false lumens at intervals along the length of the dissection.

Penetrating atherosclerotic ulcer and intramural hematoma are also considered to be variants of aortic dissection. Penetrating atherosclerotic ulcer represents focal intimal ulceration of the aorta within a region of preexisting atherosclerotic disease. These lesions may eventually extend into the media and evolve into a true dissection. Intramural hematoma occurs when intramural thrombus is found without evidence of associated intimal disruption, possibly as a result of disrupted vasa vasorum within the aortic wall. Like penetrating atherosclerotic ulcer, intramural hematoma may evolve into dissection should a frank intimal tear develop.[112]

CT remains the mainstay of diagnostic imaging as it provides excellent anatomic data, ability to localize the entry tear and fenestrations, assessment of branch vessel patency, and detection of extravasation of contrast material consistent with rupture (Fig. 61-23). Electrocardiography-gated techniques have recently enabled the acquisition of motion-free images of the proximal aorta. CT imaging is widely available, and excellent studies may be obtained rapidly with modern multidetector helical scanners, often in a matter of a few minutes. As in abdominal aortic imaging, the effect of iodinated contrast material on renal function remains the principal drawback of CT.

MRI is substantially more time-consuming to obtain and may be limited by patient factors, such as the presence of metallic debris or medical implants, that preclude its use. Electrocardiography gating of contrast-enhanced MRI can provide exceptional motion-free images of the proximal aorta. In addition, unlike contrasted CT, MRI permits appreciation of direction of blood flow as well as the calculation of values such as peak flow and velocity.

Catheter angiography provides excellent information about

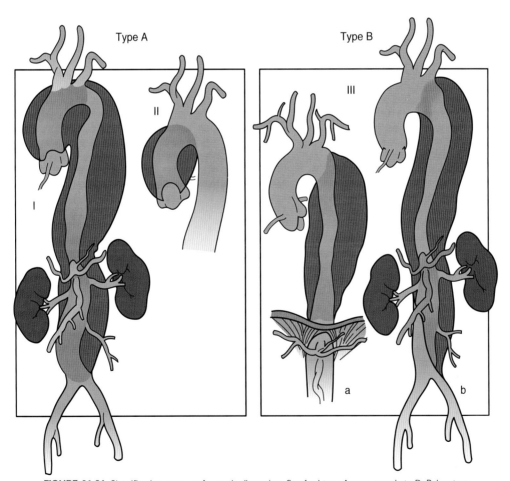

FIGURE 61-21 Classification systems for aortic dissection. Stanford type A corresponds to DeBakey type I (involving the ascending and descending aorta) and type II (involving the ascending aorta). Stanford type B corresponds to DeBakey type III (origin of the dissection distal to the left subclavian artery and involving the descending aorta only or the descending and abdominal aorta).

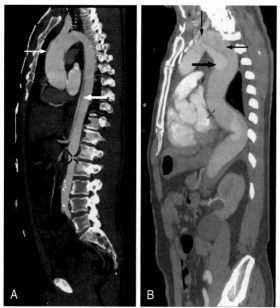

FIGURE 61-22 A, Stanford type A dissection with dissection flap visible in both the ascending *(thin arrow)* and descending *(thick arrow)* aorta. **B,** Stanford type B dissection demonstrating proximal entry tear fenestration distal to the left subclavian artery *(thin vertical arrow)* and differential filling of true *(thick arrow)* and false *(thin horizontal arrow)* lumens.

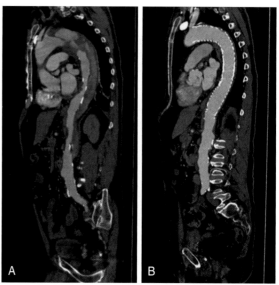

FIGURE 61-23 Reformatted CT images demonstrating a type B dissection before **(A)** and after **(B)** placement of a thoracic endograft. Note coverage of the proximal fenestration, with resulting false lumen thrombosis and aortic remodeling.

aortic and branch anatomy and involvement; it has the ability to visualize dissection flap anatomy and fenestrations (particularly with the adjunct of intravascular ultrasound) and to evaluate dissection physiology through measuring true and false lumen pressures and pressure differentials across fenestrations. In addition, angiography permits intervention on the coronary vessels, aorta, and branch vessels at the same setting.

The treatment of type B dissection is in evolution, particularly since the advent of endovascular therapy. Traditionally, intensive medical management has been the mainstay of therapy for uncomplicated dissection; dissections complicated by rupture, aneurysmal expansion, and evidence of malperfusion or, according to some sources, intractable pain have been managed surgically.[113] Aortic branch vessels to the lower extremities, viscera, and spine may originate from either true or false lumen. Malperfusion may result from dynamic compression of the true lumen by the false lumen, thrombosis of one or both lumens, or static obstruction due to extension of the dissection into the branch vessel. It may be manifested as new-onset renal dysfunction, abdominal pain and mesenteric ischemia, lower extremity ischemia, or neurologic function ranging from paresthesia to paraplegia.

Open surgical therapy for type B dissection may consist of replacement of the descending aorta or fenestration of the abdominal aorta to address visceral or limb malperfusion. Whereas replacement addresses the risk of further aortic enlargement or rupture within the replaced segment of aorta, fenestration addresses malperfusion exclusively. This procedure, which is rarely performed, involves creating a transverse (if interposition graft is anticipated) or longitudinal aortotomy in the dissected but nonaneurysmal paravisceral aorta to excise a portion of the dissection flap to permit perfusion of the mesenteric and renal arteries or in the infrarenal aorta to reperfuse the lower limbs. Similar effect

may be achieved in an endovascular fashion by traversing the dissection flap at the level of the desired fenestration and using an angioplasty balloon to enlarge the opening. Angioplasty may be used alone or with subsequent stent placement within the fenestration.[114]

Historically, open surgical therapy for acute, complicated type B dissection has been associated with high rates of morbidity and mortality. A review of data from the International Registry of Acute Aortic Dissection (IRAD) yielded a 29.3% overall rate of in-hospital mortality among patients treated surgically for acute, complicated type B dissection, whereas Panneton and colleagues reported a 43% rate of operative mortality for emergency open surgical fenestration. In the IRAD report, 69% of the patients were treated with replacement of the descending aorta, 28% with partial or complete replacement of the aortic arch, and 9% with surgical fenestration. Surgical or endovascular approaches to revascularization of malperfused branch territories were used in 20% and 9% of patients, respectively.[114,115] Open repair for chronic dissection may yield more favorable results; a recent series of 69 patients reflected an exemplary 5.8% 30-day mortality rate, 3% stroke rate, and 6% rate of spinal cord ischemia, and a recent systematic review found that other contemporary series also suggested acceptable results.[116,117]

In 1999, Dake and colleagues reported the placement of endovascular stent grafts for acute aortic dissection as an alternative to traditional surgical therapy. The principle of endovascular stent graft therapy is coverage of the entry tear, depressurizing the false lumen; this results in expansion of the true lumen and thrombosis of the false lumen with subsequent remodeling of the aorta, with an increase in the diameter of the true lumen and a decrease in the diameter of the false lumen and, ideally, the overall aortic diameter (Fig. 61-24).[118] In the setting of chronic dissection, progressive thickening of the intimal flap has generally occurred and distal "reentry" fenestrations are well established, rendering false lumen thrombosis more difficult to induce than in acute dissection and probably decreasing the overall occurrence of favorable remodeling.[112]

Adjunctive techniques, such as fenestration or direct stent placement to restore flow to obstructed branch vessels, are also important components of modern therapy for dissection. As in the endovascular management of thoracic aortic aneurysm, cervical reconstruction of the supra-aortic branches may facilitate coverage of portions of the aortic arch to achieve an adequate proximal seal zone for the device.

At present, the standard of care for acute, uncomplicated type B dissection is in flux. Whereas medical therapy remains the standard of care, the dismal natural history of medically managed type B dissection is clear, as the majority of patients fail to respond to therapy over time. A review of a cohort of 298 patients presenting with acute type B dissection and managed medically demonstrated early failure (within the first 15 days) in 37 patients (12%), resulting in 25 interventions and 15 deaths. During the study period, there were 174 failures (58.4%), primarily related to aneurysmal degeneration, resulting in a total of 87 interventions and 119 deaths. Ultimately, intervention-free survival was only 55% at 3 years and dropped to 41% by 6 years.[119] In the setting of these prospects, the potential for aortic remodeling and the pre-

vention of aneurysmal dilation over time has prompted growing interest in early stent grafting in this population. A randomized trial of TEVAR and optimal medical treatment versus optimal medical treatment alone (INSTEAD-XL trial) has recently reported landmark analysis suggesting a benefit for TEVAR for all end points, including all-cause mortality, aorta-specific mortality, and disease progression, between 2 and 5 years, with favorable results in each category significantly associated with stent graft–induced false lumen thrombosis.[120]

The quest for aortic remodeling has spurred additional investigation, including new approaches such as the combination of a covered proximal stent graft with a distal bare-metal aortic stent as part of the STABLE trial.[121] A version of this device, the Cook Zenith Dissection Endovascular System, is commercially available in European markets. Another potentially important development in this area is the application of fenestrated and branched graft techniques to address aneurysmal degeneration of the abdominal aorta and even the aortic arch.[122]

Procedural complications of endovascular stent graft therapy for dissection generally parallel those of TEVAR. There are, however, several complications largely specific to the treatment

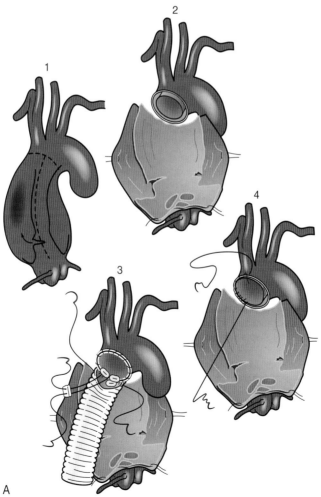

A

FIGURE 61-24 **A,** Ascending aorta dissection repair. Under circulatory arrest, the ascending aorta and transverse arch are opened, exposing the dissection (1, 2). The false lumen is obliterated (3). The graft is sutured to the transverse arch in an open distal anastomosis (4).

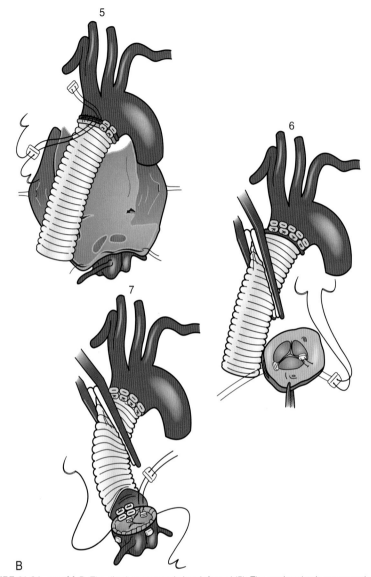

FIGURE 61-24, cont'd B, The distal anastomosis is reinforced (5). The aortic valve is resuspended (6). The proximal anastomosis is constructed (7).

of dissection, including retrograde dissection (converting a type B into a type A dissection), creation or worsening of malperfusion, and continued false lumen filling with inability to induce thrombosis.

REFERENCES

1. Schermerhorn ML, Giles KA, Sachs T, et al: Defining perioperative mortality after open and endovascular aortic aneurysm repair in the US Medicare population. *J Am Coll Surg* 212:349–355, 2011.
2. Deaths: Final data for 2013. NCVR Volume 64, Number 2. CDC. <http://www.cdc.gov/nchs/data/nvsr/nvsr64/nvsr64_02.pdf>. Accessed September 23, 2015.
3. Wassef M, Upchurch GR, Jr, Kuivaniemi H, et al: Challenges and opportunities in abdominal aortic aneurysm research. *J Vasc Surg* 45:192–198, 2007.
4. Chaikof EL, Brewster DC, Dalman RL, et al: The care of patients with an abdominal aortic aneurysm: The Society for Vascular Surgery practice guidelines. *J Vasc Surg* 50:S2–S49, 2009.
5. Allardice JT, Allwright GJ, Wafula JM, et al: High prevalence of abdominal aortic aneurysm in men with peripheral vascular disease: Screening by ultrasonography. *Br J Surg* 75:240–242, 1988.
6. O'Kelly TJ, Heather BP: General practice-based population screening for abdominal aortic aneurysms: A pilot study. *Br J Surg* 76:479–480, 1989.
7. Bengtsson H, Norrgard O, Angquist KA, et al: Ultrasonographic screening of the abdominal aorta among siblings of patients with abdominal aortic aneurysms. *Br J Surg* 76:589–591, 1989.
8. Shapira OM, Pasik S, Wassermann JP, et al: Ultrasound screening for abdominal aortic aneurysms in patients with

atherosclerotic peripheral vascular disease. *J Cardiovasc Surg (Torino)* 31:170–172, 1990.

9. Webster MW, Ferrell RE, St Jean PL, et al: Ultrasound screening of first-degree relatives of patients with an abdominal aortic aneurysm. *J Vasc Surg* 13:9–13, discussion 13-14, 1991.

10. Bengtsson H, Sonesson B, Lanne T, et al: Prevalence of abdominal aortic aneurysm in the offspring of patients dying from aneurysm rupture. *Br J Surg* 79:1142–1143, 1992.

11. MacSweeney ST, O'Meara M, Alexander C, et al: High prevalence of unsuspected abdominal aortic aneurysm in patients with confirmed symptomatic peripheral or cerebral arterial disease. *Br J Surg* 80:582–584, 1993.

12. Lindholt JS, Juul S, Henneberg EW, et al: Is screening for abdominal aortic aneurysm acceptable to the population? Selection and recruitment to hospital-based mass screening for abdominal aortic aneurysm. *J Public Health Med* 20: 211–217, 1998.

13. Lederle FA, Johnson GR, Wilson SE, et al: Prevalence and associations of abdominal aortic aneurysm detected through screening. Aneurysm Detection and Management (ADAM) Veterans Affairs Cooperative Study Group. *Ann Intern Med* 126:441–449, 1997.

14. van der Graaf Y, Akkersdijk GJ, Hak E, et al: Results of aortic screening in the brothers of patients who had elective aortic aneurysm repair. *Br J Surg* 85:778–780, 1998.

15. Lawrence PF, Lorenzo-Rivero S, Lyon JL: The incidence of iliac, femoral, and popliteal artery aneurysms in hospitalized patients. *J Vasc Surg* 22:409–415, discussion 415-416, 1995.

16. Biebl M, Hakaim AG, Hugl B, et al: Endovascular aortic aneurysm repair with the Zenith AAA Endovascular Graft: Does gender affect procedural success, postoperative morbidity, or early survival? *Am Surg* 71:1001–1008, 2005.

17. Velazquez OC, Larson RA, Baum RA, et al: Gender-related differences in infrarenal aortic aneurysm morphologic features: Issues relevant to Ancure and Talent endografts. *J Vasc Surg* 33:S77–S84, 2001.

18. Brown LC, Powell JT, UK Small Aneurysm Trial Participants: Risk factors for aneurysm rupture in patients kept under ultrasound surveillance. *Ann Surg* 230:289–296, discussion 296-297, 1999.

19. Brown PM, Zelt DT, Sobolev B: The risk of rupture in untreated aneurysms: The impact of size, gender, and expansion rate. *J Vasc Surg* 37:280–284, 2003.

20. Cronenwett JL, Murphy TF, Zelenock GB, et al: Actuarial analysis of variables associated with rupture of small abdominal aortic aneurysms. *Surgery* 98:472–483, 1985.

21. Norman PE, Powell JT: Abdominal aortic aneurysm: The prognosis in women is worse than in men. *Circulation* 115:2865–2869, 2007.

22. Englesbe MJ, Wu AH, Clowes AW, et al: The prevalence and natural history of aortic aneurysms in heart and abdominal organ transplant patients. *J Vasc Surg* 37:27–31, 2003.

23. Sonesson B, Sandgren T, Lanne T: Abdominal aortic aneurysm wall mechanics and their relation to risk of rupture. *Eur J Vasc Endovasc Surg* 18:487–493, 1999.

24. Hall AJ, Busse EF, McCarville DJ, et al: Aortic wall tension as a predictive factor for abdominal aortic aneurysm rupture: Improving the selection of patients for abdominal aortic

aneurysm repair. *Ann Vasc Surg* 14:152–157, 2000.

25. Fillinger MF, Marra SP, Raghavan ML, et al: Prediction of rupture risk in abdominal aortic aneurysm during observation: Wall stress versus diameter. *J Vasc Surg* 37:724–732, 2003.

26. Fillinger MF, Raghavan ML, Marra SP, et al: In vivo analysis of mechanical wall stress and abdominal aortic aneurysm rupture risk. *J Vasc Surg* 36:589–597, 2002.

27. Lederle FA: Risk of rupture of large abdominal aortic aneurysms. Disagreement among vascular surgeons. *Arch Intern Med* 156:1007–1009, 1996.

28. Parkinson F, Ferguson S, Lewis P, et al: Rupture rates of untreated large abdominal aortic aneurysms in patients unfit for elective repair. *J Vasc Surg* 61:1606–1612, 2015.

29. Darling RC, Messina CR, Brewster DC, et al: Autopsy study of unoperated abdominal aortic aneurysms. The case for early resection. *Circulation* 56:II161–II164, 1977.

30. Engellau L, Albrechtsson U, Dahlstrom N, et al: Measurements before endovascular repair of abdominal aortic aneurysms. MR imaging with MRA vs. angiography and CT. *Acta Radiol* 44:177–184, 2003.

31. U.S. Preventive Services Task Force: Abdominal aortic aneurysm: Screening. <http://www.uspreventiveservicestaskforce.org/uspstf/uspsaneu.htm>. Accessed August 2, 2011.

32. McCarthy RJ, Shaw E, Whyman MR, et al: Recommendations for screening intervals for small aortic aneurysms. *Br J Surg* 90:821–826, 2003.

33. Lederle FA: Abdominal aortic aneurysm: Still no pill. *Ann Intern Med* 159:852–853, 2013.

34. Meijer CA, Stijnen T, Wasser MN, et al: Doxycycline for stabilization of abdominal aortic aneurysms: A randomized trial. *Ann Intern Med* 159:815–823, 2013.

35. Baxter BT, Terrin MC, Dalman RL: Medical management of small abdominal aortic aneurysms. *Circulation* 117:1883–1889, 2008.

36. Sconfienza LM, Santagostino I, Di Leo G, et al: When the diameter of the abdominal aorta should be considered as abnormal? A new ultrasonographic index using the wrist circumference as a body build reference. *Eur J Radiol* 82:e532–e536, 2013.

37. Hannawa KK, Eliason JL, Upchurch GR, Jr: Gender differences in abdominal aortic aneurysms. *Vascular* 17(Suppl 1):S30–S39, 2009.

38. Suckow BD, Schanzer A, Hoel AW, et al: A novel quality of life instrument for patients with an abdominal aortic aneurysm. *J Vasc Surg* 61:43S–44S, 2015.

39. Fleisher LA, Beckman JA, Brown KA, et al: ACC/AHA 2007 guidelines on perioperative cardiovascular evaluation and care for noncardiac surgery: A report of the American College of Cardiology/American Heart Association Task Force on Practice Guidelines (Writing Committee to Revise the 2002 Guidelines on Perioperative Cardiovascular Evaluation for Noncardiac Surgery): Developed in collaboration with the American Society of Echocardiography, American Society of Nuclear Cardiology, Heart Rhythm Society, Society of Cardiovascular Anesthesiologists, Society for Cardiovascular Angiography and Interventions, Society for Vascular Medicine and Biology, and Society for Vascular Surgery. *Circulation* 116:e418–e499, 2007.

40. Shah TR, Veith FJ, Bauer SM: Cardiac evaluation and management before vascular surgery. *Curr Opin Cardiol* 29:499–505, 2014.

41. Fleischmann KE, Beckman JA, Buller CE, et al: 2009 ACCF/AHA focused update on perioperative beta blockade: A report of the American College of Cardiology Foundation/American Heart Association Task Force on Practice Guidelines. *Circulation* 120:2123–2151, 2009.

42. Schouten O, Hoeks SE, Welten GM, et al: Effect of statin withdrawal on frequency of cardiac events after vascular surgery. *Am J Cardiol* 100:316–320, 2007.

43. Corriere M, Edwards M, Hansen KJ: Abdominal aortic aneurysm and renal artery stenosis. *Vasc Dis Manage* 5:16–21, 2008.

44. Lee SM, Takemoto S, Wallace AW: Association between withholding angiotensin receptor blockers in the early postoperative period and 30-day mortality: A cohort study of the Veterans Affairs Healthcare System. *Anesthesiology* 123: 288–306, 2015.

45. Hersey P, Poullis M: Does the administration of mannitol prevent renal failure in open abdominal aortic aneurysm surgery? *Interact Cardiovasc Thorac Surg* 7:906–909, 2008.

46. Wijnen MH, Vader HL, Van Den Wall Bake AW, et al: Can renal dysfunction after infra-renal aortic aneurysm repair be modified by multi-antioxidant supplementation? *J Cardiovasc Surg (Torino)* 43:483–488, 2002.

47. Upchurch GR, Jr, Proctor MC, Henke PK, et al: Predictors of severe morbidity and death after elective abdominal aortic aneurysmectomy in patients with chronic obstructive pulmonary disease. *J Vasc Surg* 37:594–599, 2003.

48. Myers K, Hajek P, Hinds C, et al: Stopping smoking shortly before surgery and postoperative complications: A systematic review and meta-analysis. *Arch Intern Med* 171:983–989, 2011.

49. Sicard GA, Toursarkissian B: Midline versus retroperitoneal approach for abdominal aortic aneurysm surgery. In Calligaro KD, Dougherty MJ, Hollier LH, editors: *Diagnosis and treatment of aortic and peripheral arterial aneurysms*, Philadelphia, 1999, WB Saunders, pp 135–148.

50. Berland TL, Veith FJ, Cayne NS, et al: Technique of supraceliac balloon control of the aorta during endovascular repair of ruptured abdominal aortic aneurysms. *J Vasc Surg* 57:272–275, 2013.

51. Stannard A, Eliason JL, Rasmussen TE: Resuscitative endovascular balloon occlusion of the aorta (REBOA) as an adjunct for hemorrhagic shock. *J Trauma* 71:1869–1872, 2011.

52. Nishimori M, Ballantyne JC, Low JH: Epidural pain relief versus systemic opioid-based pain relief for abdominal aortic surgery. *Cochrane Database Syst Rev* (3):CD005059, 2006.

53. Ylonen K, Biancari F, Leo E, et al: Predictors of development of anastomotic femoral pseudoaneurysms after aortobifemoral reconstruction for abdominal aortic aneurysm. *Am J Surg* 187:83–87, 2004.

54. Edwards JM, Teefey SA, Zierler RE, et al: Intraabdominal paraanastomotic aneurysms after aortic bypass grafting. *J Vasc Surg* 15:344–350, discussion 351-353, 1992.

55. Parodi JC, Palmaz JC, Barone HD: Transfemoral intraluminal graft implantation for abdominal aortic aneurysms. *Ann Vasc Surg* 5:491–499, 1991.

56. Wilt TJ, Lederle FA, Macdonald R, et al: Comparison of endovascular and open surgical repairs for abdominal aortic aneurysm. *Evid Rep Technol Assess (Full Rep)* 144:1–113, 2006.

57. Dimick JB, Upchurch GR, Jr: Endovascular technology, hospital volume, and mortality with abdominal aortic aneurysm surgery. *J Vasc Surg* 47:1150–1154, 2008.

58. Ali MM, Flahive J, Schanzer A, et al: In patients stratified by preoperative risk, endovascular repair of ruptured abdominal aortic aneurysms has a lower in-hospital mortality and morbidity than open repair. *J Vasc Surg* 61:1399–1407, 2015.

59. Chang DC, Parina RP, Wilson SE: Survival after endovascular vs open aortic aneurysm repairs. *JAMA Surg* 2015. [Epub ahead of print].

60. Heyer KS, Modi P, Morasch MD, et al: Secondary infections of thoracic and abdominal aortic endografts. *J Vasc Interv Radiol* 20:173–179, 2009.

61. Mehta M, Henretta J, Glickman M, et al: Outcome of the pivotal study of the Aptus endovascular abdominal aortic aneurysms repair system. *J Vasc Surg* 60:275–285, 2014.

62. Muller-Wille R, Schotz S, Zeman F, et al: CT features of early type II endoleaks after endovascular repair of abdominal aortic aneurysms help predict aneurysm sac enlargement. *Radiology* 274:906–916, 2015.

63. Zhou W, Blay E, Jr, Varu V, et al: Outcome and clinical significance of delayed endoleaks after endovascular aneurysm repair. *J Vasc Surg* 59:915–920, 2014.

64. Guntner O, Zeman F, Wohlgemuth WA, et al: Inferior mesenteric arterial type II endoleaks after endovascular repair of abdominal aortic aneurysm: Are they predictable? *Radiology* 270:910–919, 2014.

65. Alerci M, Giamboni A, Wyttenbach R, et al: Endovascular abdominal aneurysm repair and impact of systematic preoperative embolization of collateral arteries: Endoleak analysis and long-term follow-up. *J Endovasc Ther* 20:663–671, 2013.

66. Sidloff DA, Gokani V, Stather PW, et al: Type II endoleak: Conservative management is a safe strategy. *Eur J Vasc Endovasc Surg* 48:391–399, 2014.

67. Quinones-Baldrich W, Levin ES, Lew W, et al: Intraprocedural and postprocedural perigraft arterial sac embolization (PASE) for endoleak treatment. *J Vasc Surg* 59:538–541, 2014.

68. Schanzer A, Greenberg RK, Hevelone N, et al: Predictors of abdominal aortic aneurysm sac enlargement after endovascular repair. *Circulation* 123:2848–2855, 2011.

69. Greenhalgh RM, Brown LC, Powell JT, et al: Endovascular versus open repair of abdominal aortic aneurysm. *N Engl J Med* 362:1863–1871, 2010.

70. Gurtler VM, Sommer WH, Meimarakis G, et al: A comparison between contrast-enhanced ultrasound imaging and multislice computed tomography in detecting and classifying endoleaks in the follow-up after endovascular aneurysm repair. *J Vasc Surg* 58:340–345, 2013.

71. Nagre SB, Taylor SM, Passman MA, et al: Evaluating outcomes of endoleak discrepancies between computed tomography scan and ultrasound imaging after endovascular abdominal aneurysm repair. *Ann Vasc Surg* 25:94–100, 2011.

72. Kouchoukos NT, Masetti P, Murphy SF: Hypothermic cardiopulmonary bypass and circulatory arrest in the management of extensive thoracic and thoracoabdominal aortic aneurysms. *Semin Thorac Cardiovasc Surg* 15:333–339, 2003.

73. Hiratzka LF, Bakris GL, Beckman JA, et al: 2010 ACCF/

AHA/AATS/ACR/ASA/SCA/SCAI/SIR/STS/SVM guidelines for the diagnosis and management of patients with Thoracic Aortic Disease: A report of the American College of Cardiology Foundation/American Heart Association Task Force on Practice Guidelines, American Association for Thoracic Surgery, American College of Radiology, American Stroke Association, Society of Cardiovascular Anesthesiologists, Society for Cardiovascular Angiography and Interventions, Society of Interventional Radiology, Society of Thoracic Surgeons, and Society for Vascular Medicine. *Circulation* 121:e266–e369, 2010.

74. Greenbaum AB, O'Neill WW, Paone G, et al: Caval-aortic access to allow transcatheter aortic valve replacement in otherwise ineligible patients: Initial human experience. *J Am Coll Cardiol* 63:2795–2804, 2014.

75. Vandy FC, Girotti M, Williams DM, et al: Iliofemoral complications associated with thoracic endovascular aortic repair: Frequency, risk factors, and early and late outcomes. *J Thorac Cardiovasc Surg* 147:960–965, 2014.

76. Gutsche JT, Cheung AT, McGarvey ML, et al: Risk factors for perioperative stroke after thoracic endovascular aortic repair. *Ann Thorac Surg* 84:1195–1200, discussion 1200, 2007.

77. Bavaria JE, Appoo JJ, Makaroun MS, et al: Endovascular stent grafting versus open surgical repair of descending thoracic aortic aneurysms in low-risk patients: A multicenter comparative trial. *J Thorac Cardiovasc Surg* 133:369–377, 2007.

78. Adams JD, Tracci MC, Sabri S, et al: Real-world experience with type I endoleaks after endovascular repair of the thoracic aorta. *Am Surg* 76:599–605, 2010.

79. DeSart K, Scali ST, Feezor RJ, et al: Fate of patients with spinal cord ischemia complicating thoracic endovascular aortic repair. *J Vasc Surg* 58:635–642.e2, 2013.

80. Czerny M, Eggebrecht H, Sodeck G, et al: Mechanisms of symptomatic spinal cord ischemia after TEVAR: Insights from the European Registry of Endovascular Aortic Repair Complications (EuREC). *J Endovasc Ther* 19:37–43, 2012.

81. Duwayri Y, Jim J, Sanchez L: Alternative techniques to abdominal debranching. *Vasc Dis Manage* 7:E210–E213, 2010.

82. Greenberg R, Eagleton M, Mastracci T: Branched endografts for thoracoabdominal aneurysms. *J Thorac Cardiovasc Surg* 140:S171–S178, 2010.

83. Donas KP, Lee JT, Lachat M, et al: Collected world experience about the performance of the snorkel/chimney endovascular technique in the treatment of complex aortic pathologies: The PERICLES registry. *Ann Surg* 262:546–553, 2015.

84. Fox N, Schwartz D, Salazar JH, et al: Evaluation and management of blunt traumatic aortic injury: A practice management guideline from the Eastern Association for the Surgery of Trauma. *J Trauma Acute Care Surg* 78:136–146, 2015.

85. Murad MH, Rizvi AZ, Malgor R, et al: Comparative effectiveness of the treatments for thoracic aortic transection [corrected]. *J Vasc Surg* 53:193–199.e1–21, 2011.

86. Dormandy JA, Rutherford RB: Management of peripheral arterial disease (PAD). TASC Working Group. TransAtlantic Inter-Society Consensus (TASC). *J Vasc Surg* 31:S1–S296, 2000.

87. Norgren L, Hiatt WR, Dormandy JA, et al: Inter-Society Consensus for the Management of Peripheral Arterial Disease (TASC II). *J Vasc Surg* 45(Suppl S):S5–S67, 2007.

88. Jongkind V, Akkersdijk GJ, Yeung KK, et al: A systematic review of endovascular treatment of extensive aortoiliac occlusive disease. *J Vasc Surg* 52:1376–1383, 2010.

89. Ichihashi S, Higashiura W, Itoh H, et al: Long-term outcomes for systematic primary stent placement in complex iliac artery occlusive disease classified according to TransAtlantic Inter-Society Consensus (TASC)-II. *J Vasc Surg* 53:992–999, 2011.

90. Ye W, Liu CW, Ricco JB, et al: Early and late outcomes of percutaneous treatment of TransAtlantic Inter-Society Consensus class C and D aorto-iliac lesions. *J Vasc Surg* 53:1728–1737, 2011.

91. Kashyap VS, Pavkov ML, Bena JF, et al: The management of severe aortoiliac occlusive disease: Endovascular therapy rivals open reconstruction. *J Vasc Surg* 48:1451–1457, 1457.e1-3, 2008.

92. Upchurch GR, Dimick JB, Wainess RM, et al: Diffusion of new technology in health care: The case of aorto-iliac occlusive disease. *Surgery* 136:812–818, 2004.

93. Chiu KW, Davies RS, Nightingale PG, et al: Review of direct anatomical open surgical management of atherosclerotic aorto-iliac occlusive disease. *Eur J Vasc Endovasc Surg* 39:460–471, 2010.

94. de Vries SO, Hunink MG: Results of aortic bifurcation grafts for aortoiliac occlusive disease: A meta-analysis. *J Vasc Surg* 26:558–569, 1997.

95. Hertzer NR, Bena JF, Karafa MT: A personal experience with direct reconstruction and extra-anatomic bypass for aortoiliofemoral occlusive disease. *J Vasc Surg* 45:527–535, discussion 535, 2007.

96. Ricco JB, Probst H: Long-term results of a multicenter randomized study on direct versus crossover bypass for unilateral iliac artery occlusive disease. *J Vasc Surg* 47:45–53, discussion 53-54, 2008.

97. Reed AB, Conte MS, Donaldson MC, et al: The impact of patient age and aortic size on the results of aortobifemoral bypass grafting. *J Vasc Surg* 37:1219–1225, 2003.

98. Klonaris C, Katsargyris A, Tsekouras N, et al: Primary stenting for aortic lesions: From single stenoses to total aortoiliac occlusions. *J Vasc Surg* 47:310–317, 2008.

99. Indes JE, Mandawat A, Tuggle CT, et al: Endovascular procedures for aorto-iliac occlusive disease are associated with superior short-term clinical and economic outcomes compared with open surgery in the inpatient population. *J Vasc Surg* 52:1173–1179, 1179.e1, 2010.

100. Cau J, Ricco JB, Corpataux JM: Laparoscopic aortic surgery: Techniques and results. *J Vasc Surg* 48:37S–44S, discussion 45S, 2008.

101. Cherry KJ: Complications following reconstructions of the pararenal aorta and its branches. In Towne JB, Hollier LH, editors: *Complications in vascular surgery*, ed 2, New York, 2004, Marcel Dekker, pp 275–287.

102. Gruppo M, Mazzalai F, Lorenzetti R, et al: Midline abdominal wall incisional hernia after aortic reconstructive surgery: A prospective study. *Surgery* 151:882–888, 2012.

103. Sachdev U, Baril DT, Morrissey NJ, et al: Endovascular repair of para-anastomotic aortic aneurysms. *J Vasc Surg* 46:636–641, 2007.

104. Reilly LM, Stoney RJ, Goldstone J, et al: Improved management of aortic graft infection: The influence of operation

sequence and staging. *J Vasc Surg* 5:421–431, 1987.

105. Oderich GS, Bower TC, Cherry KJ, Jr, et al: Evolution from axillofemoral to in situ prosthetic reconstruction for the treatment of aortic graft infections at a single center. *J Vasc Surg* 43:1166–1174, 2006.

106. Brown KE, Heyer K, Rodriguez H, et al: Arterial reconstruction with cryopreserved human allografts in the setting of infection: A single-center experience with midterm follow-up. *J Vasc Surg* 49:660–666, 2009.

107. Noel AA, Gloviczki P, Cherry KJ, Jr, et al: Abdominal aortic reconstruction in infected fields: Early results of the United States cryopreserved aortic allograft registry. *J Vasc Surg* 35:847–852, 2002.

108. Batt M, Magne JL, Alric P, et al: In situ revascularization with silver-coated polyester grafts to treat aortic infection: Early and midterm results. *J Vasc Surg* 38:983–989, 2003.

109. Clagett GP, Bowers BL, Lopez-Viego MA, et al: Creation of a neo-aortoiliac system from lower extremity deep and superficial veins. *Ann Surg* 218:239–248, discussion 248–249, 1993.

110. Lonn L, Dias N, Veith Schroeder T, et al: Is EVAR the treatment of choice for aortoenteric fistula? *J Cardiovasc Surg (Torino)* 51:319–327, 2010.

111. Cherry KJ, Dake MD: Aortic dissection. In Hallett JW, Mills JL, Earnshaw JJ, et al, editors: *Comprehensive vascular and endovascular surgery*, ed 2, Philadelphia, 2009, Mosby, pp 517–531.

112. Swee W, Dake MD: Endovascular management of thoracic dissections. *Circulation* 117:1460–1473, 2008.

113. Estrera AL, Miller CC, 3rd, Safi HJ, et al: Outcomes of medical management of acute type B aortic dissection. *Circulation* 114:I384–I389, 2006.

114. Panneton JM, Teh SH, Cherry KJ, Jr, et al: Aortic fenestration for acute or chronic aortic dissection: An uncommon but effective procedure. *J Vasc Surg* 32:711–721, 2000.

115. Trimarchi S, Nienaber CA, Rampoldi V, et al: Role and results of surgery in acute type B aortic dissection: Insights from the International Registry of Acute Aortic Dissection (IRAD). *Circulation* 114:I357–I364, 2006.

116. Tian DH, De Silva RP, Wang T, et al: Open surgical repair for chronic type B aortic dissection: A systematic review. *Ann Cardiothorac Surg* 3:340–350, 2014.

117. Kouchoukos NT, Kulik A, Castner CF: Open thoracoabdominal aortic repair for chronic type B dissection. *J Thorac Cardiovasc Surg* 149:S125–S129, 2015.

118. Dake MD, Kato N, Mitchell RS, et al: Endovascular stent-graft placement for the treatment of acute aortic dissection. *N Engl J Med* 340:1546–1552, 1999.

119. Durham CA, Cambria RP, Wang LJ, et al: The natural history of medically managed acute type B aortic dissection. *J Vasc Surg* 61:1192–1198, 2015.

120. Nienaber CA, Kische S, Rousseau H, et al: Endovascular repair of type B aortic dissection: Long-term results of the randomized investigation of stent grafts in aortic dissection trial. *Circ Cardiovasc Interv* 6:407–416, 2013.

121. Hofferberth SC, Newcomb AE, Yii MY, et al: Combined proximal stent grafting plus distal bare metal stenting for management of aortic dissection: Superior to standard endovascular repair? *J Thorac Cardiovasc Surg* 144:956–962, discussion 962, 2012.

122. Kitagawa A, Greenberg RK, Eagleton MJ, et al: Fenestrated and branched endovascular aortic repair for chronic type B aortic dissection with thoracoabdominal aneurysms. *J Vasc Surg* 58:625–634, 2013.

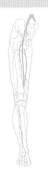

CHAPTER 62

Peripheral Arterial Disease

Charlie C. Cheng, Faisal Cheema, Grant Fankhauser,
Michael B. Silva, Jr.

第六十二章　周围动脉疾病

中文导读

本章共分为8节：①流行病学；②血管疾病基础科学；③周围动脉疾病的诊断和治疗；④其他病因引起的肢体急慢性缺血；⑤肾动脉疾病；⑥内脏动脉瘤：脾动脉、肠系膜上动脉及肾动脉；⑦颈动脉疾病；⑧透析通路。

第一节讲述了周围动脉疾病的定义及流行病学。周围动脉疾病指各种病因引起的周围动脉病变，主要包括狭窄、堵塞及瘤样扩张。动脉粥样硬化导致的动脉狭窄或闭塞是最为常见的周围动脉疾病。

第二节讲述了动脉管壁的基本结构，动脉疾病最常见的病理生理改变及好发部位。动脉粥样硬化是最常见的病变，其主要危险因素包括高脂血症、糖尿病及吸烟等。动脉硬化主要发生于血管分叉等血流剪切

应力较大的地方。

第三节为作者重点阐述的内容。诊治周围动脉疾病先要评估病人全身状况。制定治疗方案时要在疗效与风险之间进行平衡。症状及体征可以确定周围动脉疾病引发肢体缺血的严重程度，确定是否需要手术治疗。影像学检查可以对病变进行定性及定位，并可评估血管形态，为手术治疗提供较为精确的指引。开放手术、腔内手术各有优缺点，后者目前还无法全面取

代前者。本章还阐述了腔内医疗器械的进展，手术并发症及处理方法。

　　第四节主要介绍了雷诺综合征、血栓闭塞性脉管炎、巨细胞动脉炎等少见病的诊断及治疗。

　　第五节重点介绍了肾动脉狭窄引起的肾性高血压的诊断及治疗。引发肾性高血压、肾功能减退或肾显著血流动力学改变的肾动脉狭窄均需手术治疗，以腔内手术为主。

　　第六节阐述了内脏动脉瘤的常见发病人群及手术治疗指征。手术方式依据瘤体的位置及血管形态决定，可选择手术切除或腔内治疗。

　　第七节主要讲了动脉硬化引起的颈动脉狭窄与缺血性脑卒中之间的关系，解除颈动脉狭窄对防治缺血性脑卒中的意义。颈动脉狭窄的主要手术方式为颈动脉内膜剥脱术。近年来，颈动脉腔内手术取得了较大的发展，但目前主要适应于开放手术风险较大的病人。

　　第八节介绍主要的透析通路有3种：中心静脉通路、自体动静脉瘘、人工血管通路。前者为临时性通路，后两者为永久性通路。文中讲解了各种透析通路的建立方法、适应证及并发症的处理。

〔王　其〕

The specialty of vascular surgery has matured dramatically during the past decade. With the advent of new devices and techniques and the expansion of catheter and guidewire skills, the management of almost all vascular pathologic processes has been undergoing a process of reevaluation. Surgeons have traditionally been called on to make diagnoses and to manage patients with emergent, urgent, and elective vascular surgical conditions. Although other medical disciplines are participating in this process to a greater degree, the surgeon with advanced open skills and complete facility with endovascular techniques is ideally suited to manage these patients. As our population ages and the prevalence of vascular disease increases, along with the growing awareness of potential therapeutic benefits by an educated populace, it is incumbent on the vascular specialist to be facile with a widening set of tools and techniques—medical, surgical, and endovascular—to meet the needs of our patients.

This chapter covers epidemiology, basic science, diagnostic workup, and medical treatment of peripheral vascular disease. Treatments of acute and chronic limb ischemia, open and endovascular, are discussed. Management of the diabetic foot, with an emphasis on amputations, is included. Less common causes of limb ischemia are presented for completion. The rapidly changing treatment paradigm of carotid stenosis is discussed, as is that of renovascular hypertension. Management of peripheral and splanchnic aneurysms is reviewed. Finally, arteriovenous access for the patient with end-stage renal disease is presented in detail because this remains an important component of contemporary general and vascular surgical practice.

EPIDEMIOLOGY

Peripheral artery occlusive disease, commonly referred to as peripheral arterial disease (PAD) or peripheral vascular disease

(PVD), refers to the obstruction or deterioration of arteries other than those supplying the heart and within the brain. There are a number of pathologic processes that manifest their effects on the arterial circulation.

The common denominator among these processes is the impairment of circulation and resultant ischemia to the end organ involved. Highly prevalent in our society, arterial occlusive disease, in its myriad iterations, constitutes the leading overall cause of death. In addition to death from myocardial infarction or stroke, significant disability and loss of function from PAD result in an enormous cost in impaired quality of life for our aging population and a direct financial cost to our health care system.

The incidence of symptomatic PAD increases with age, from approximately 0.3%/yr for men aged 40 to 55 years to approximately 1%/yr for men older than 75 years. In the United States, PAD affects 12% to 20% of Americans aged 65 years and older.

PAD is more prevalent in nonwhite populations, and this is not completely explained by an increased incidence of comorbid diseases.[1] An ankle-brachial index (ABI) less than 0.90 is almost twice as common in non-Hispanic blacks as in whites. Risk is increased in smokers and in patients with hypertension, dyslipidemia, hypercoagulable states, renal insufficiency, and diabetes mellitus (Fig. 62-1). The prevalence of PAD is strikingly higher in a younger diabetic population, affecting one in three diabetics older than 50 years. Diagnosis is critical because people with PAD have a risk of heart attack or stroke four to five times higher than that of the age-matched population (Fig. 62-2). The risk of PAD also increases in individuals who are older than 50 years, male, or obese and in those with a family history of vascular disease, heart attack, or stroke. Other risk factors that are being studied include levels of various inflammatory mediators, such as C-reactive protein and homocysteine.

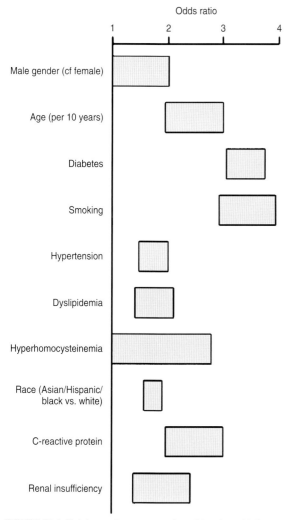

Odds ratio

- Male gender (cf female)
- Age (per 10 years)
- Diabetes
- Smoking
- Hypertension
- Dyslipidemia
- Hyperhomocysteinemia
- Race (Asian/Hispanic/black vs. white)
- C-reactive protein
- Renal insufficiency

FIGURE 62-1 Risk factors for symptomatic peripheral arterial disease.

BASIC SCIENCE OF VASCULAR DISEASE

Vascular Wall Microanatomy

The arterial wall consists of three concentric layers:

1. The innermost layer is the intima. This is structurally a tube of endothelial cells in which the long axis of each cell is oriented longitudinally. The cells are aligned in a single layer and interface with the blood, providing metabolic reactivity and signaling by transport of mediators through their internal cellular architecture. The intima is separated from the media by the internal elastic membrane.

2. The media is the major structural support for the artery. It is composed predominantly of circumferentially arranged smooth muscle cells, collagen, elastin, and proteoglycans. Proteoglycans are formed of disaccharides bound to protein; they serve as binding or cement material in the interstitial spaces. The blood supply for the inner part of the media is by direct diffusion through the intima, whereas the outer part is supplied by smaller penetrating arteries, known as vasa vasorum. The media is separated from the outermost layer, the adventitia, by the external elastic membrane.

3. The adventitia contains fibroblasts, collagen, and elastic tissue and is the strength layer of the artery.

Atherosclerosis

Atherosclerosis is the most common pathologic change associated with PAD. A number of terms are used to describe this process that are similar and yet distinct in spelling and meaning and are often confused. The principal root, *athera*, is from the Greek word meaning gruel; an atheroma can be translated literally as a lump of gruel. Atherosclerosis is a hardening of an artery specifically caused by an atheromatous plaque. The term *atherogenic* is used for substances or processes that cause atherosclerosis. *Arteriosclerosis* is a general term describing any hardening (and loss of elasticity) of medium or large arteries (from the Greek *arteria*, meaning artery, and *sclerosis*, meaning hardening); arteriolosclerosis is any hardening (and loss of elasticity) of arterioles (small arteries).

A number of causative factors have been identified for atherosclerosis. Hyperlipidemia, hypercholesterolemia, hypertension, diabetes mellitus, and exposure to infectious agents or toxins, such as from cigarette smoking, are all important and independent risk factors. The common mechanism is thought to be endothelial cell injury, smooth muscle cell proliferation, inflammatory reactivity, and plaque deposition.

Several components are found in atherosclerotic plaque—lipids, smooth muscle cells, connective tissue, and inflammatory cells, often macrophages. Lipid accumulation is central to the process and distinguishes atheromas from other arteriopathies. In advanced plaques, calcification is seen and erosive areas or ulcerations can occur, exposing the contents of the plaque to circulating prothrombotic cells. There is an important correlation between plaque morphology and clinical sequelae. The plaque's lipid core may become a necrotic mix of amorphous extracellular lipid, proteins, and prothrombotic factors covered by a layer of smooth muscle cells and connective tissue of variable thickness, the fibrous cap. If the thin fibrous cap ruptures and the contents of the lipid core are exposed to circulating humoral factors, the body, perceiving the ulceration as an injury, may lay down platelets and initiate clot formation. In this manner, a relatively low grade, hemodynamically insignificant narrowing can precipitate an acute thrombosis and result in a dramatically significant ischemic event, such as a myocardial infarction.

Plaque morphology can be evaluated by ultrasound and magnetic resonance imaging (MRI). The heterogeneous plaque with a thin fibrous cap or ulceration, often described as unstable or vulnerable, is more likely to be virulent in nature, with an increased risk for embolization of particulate and thrombotic material. Ischemia, therefore, can result from a number of possible plaque behaviors, such as encroachment on the lumen (stenosis or narrowing) with hypoperfusion, stagnation, and thrombosis; rupture of the fibrous cap inducing thrombus formation in the lumen, with outright occlusion; and embolization of thrombotic debris into the downstream circulation.

Although atherosclerosis is a systemic disorder, there is an interestingly predictable pattern of distribution of atheromatous plaques throughout the arterial tree that is likely a result of consistent hemodynamic stresses associated with human anatomic design. Plaques tend to occur at bifurcations or bends associated with repetitive external stresses. Areas at which shear stress increases from disturbances in flow or turbulence, with lateralizing vectors and eddy formation, are prone to atheromatous degeneration. The infrarenal abdominal aorta, iliac bifurcations, carotid bifurcations, superficial femoral arteries as they exit at Hunter

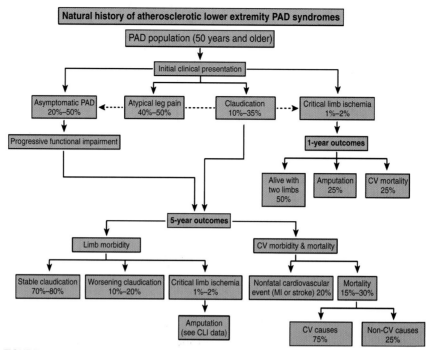

FIGURE 62-2 Outcomes of atherosclerotic peripheral arterial disease at 5 years. (From Hirsch AT, Haskal ZJ, Hertzer NR, et al; American Association for Vascular Surgery/Society for Vascular Surgery; Society for Cardiovascular Angiography and Interventions; Society for Vascular Medicine and Biology; Society of Interventional Radiology; ACC/AHA Task Force on Practice Guidelines: ACC/AHA Guidelines for the Management of Patients with Peripheral Arterial Disease [lower extremity, renal, mesenteric, and abdominal aortic]: A collaborative report from the American Associations for Vascular Surgery/Society for Vascular Surgery, Society for Cardiovascular Angiography and Interventions, Society for Vascular Medicine and Biology, Society of Interventional Radiology, and the ACC/AHA Task Force on Practice Guidelines [writing committee to develop guidelines for the management of patients with peripheral arterial disease]—summary of recommendations. *J Vasc Interv Radiol* 17:1383–1397, 2006.)

canal, and ostia of the coronary, renal, and mesenteric arteries are all common sites of plaque formation. Conversely, the upper extremity arteries and common carotid, renal, and mesenteric arteries, beyond their origins, are often much less involved.

EVALUATING AND TREATING THE PATIENT WITH PERIPHERAL ARTERIAL DISEASE

Patients are typically referred to the vascular specialist for clarification of a diagnosis and determination of a strategy for treatment. The process involves clinical assessment, establishing the particulars of the patient's medical history and performing a physical examination; diagnostic studies to clarify and to localize the problem and potentially to elucidate the functional severity of the condition; and ultimately balancing the severity of the patient's condition with the potential risks and benefits of therapeutic intervention.

History and Physical Examination

Rapidly advancing technology in imaging and endovascular therapies epitomize the cutting edge, the "high-tech" side of vascular surgery, but the foundation of this field is profoundly "low-tech." The history and physical examination process can often identify the location and relative severity of the patient's vascular disease accurately.

The most common presenting symptom in lower extremity vascular disease is pain. Characterizing the pain—location; precipitating, aggravating, and relieving factors; and frequency, duration, and evolution—can allow one to diagnose or to exclude most arterial and venous diseases with a high degree of sensitivity, even before examining the patient. Clarifying the nature of the pain as a starting point allows one to segregate patients into two broad categories of presentation for PAD, chronic arterial insufficiency and acute arterial occlusion.

Chronic Arterial Insufficiency

The clinical presentation ranges from asymptomatic to gangrenous tissue loss. Intermittent claudication is a common presentation in the outpatient setting and usually signifies mild to moderate vascular occlusive disease. Classically, pain occurs with activity or ambulation and is relieved with rest. Because of the frequency of superficial femoral arterial disease, the usual location of the pain is in the calf, but claudication may also involve the thighs or the buttocks because the arterial disease may be located in the aortoiliac segment. The arterial disease is usually one level above the symptomatic muscle group. The differential diagnosis of leg pain is broad, and the treatment modalities are equally disparate. Table 62-1 outlines an approach to the differential diagnosis of claudication.

Patients who are limited in ambulation because of arthritis, severe lung disease, or heart failure or who are diabetic with

TABLE 62-1 Differential Diagnosis of Intermittent Claudication

CONDITION	LOCATION OF PAIN OR DISCOMFORT	CHARACTERISTIC DISCOMFORT	ONSET RELATIVE TO EXERCISE	EFFECT OF REST	EFFECT OF BODY POSITION	OTHER CHARACTERISTICS
Intermittent claudication	Buttock, thigh, or calf muscles and rarely the foot	Cramping, aching, fatigue, weakness, or frank pain	After some degree of exercise	Quickly relieved	None	Reproducible
Nerve root compression (e.g., herniated disc)	Radiates down leg, usually posteriorly	Sharp lancinating pain	Soon, if not immediately after onset	Not quickly relieved (also often present at rest)	Relief may be aided by adjusting back position	History of back problems
Spinal stenosis	Hip, thigh, buttocks (follows dermatome)	Motor weakness more prominent than pain	After walking or standing for variable lengths of time	Relieved by stopping only if position changed	Relief by lumbar spine flexion (sitting or stooping forward)	Frequent history of back problems, provoked by intra-abdominal pressure
Arthritic, inflammatory process	Foot, arch	Aching pain	After variable degree of exercise	Not quickly relieved (and may be present at rest)	May be relieved by not bearing weight	Variable, may relate to activity level
Hip arthritis	Hip, thigh, buttocks	Aching discomfort, usually localized to hip and gluteal region	After variable degree of exercise	Not quickly relieved (and may be present at rest)	More comfortable sitting, weight taken off legs	Variable, may relate to activity level, weather changes
Symptomatic Baker cyst	Behind knee, down calf	Swelling, soreness, tenderness	With exercise	Present at rest	None	Not intermittent
Venous claudication	Entire leg, but usually worse in thigh and groin	Tight, bursting pain	After walking	Subsides slowly	Relief speeded by elevation	History of iliofemoral deep venous thrombosis, signs of venous congestion, edema
Chronic compartment syndrome	Calf muscles	Tight, bursting pain	After much exercise (e.g., jogging)	Subsides very slowly	Relief speeded by elevation	Typically occurs in heavily muscled athletes

Adapted from Dormandy JA, Rutherford RB: Management of peripheral arterial disease (PAD). TASC Working Group. TransAtlantic Inter-Society Consensus (TASC). *J Vasc Surg* 31:S1–S296, 2000.

neuropathy may not experience leg pain and may present initially with advanced disease. Worsening perfusion leads to critical limb ischemia, which may be manifested by rest pain. This is described as pain that occurs at rest; it may wake the patient from sleep. This is usually in the dorsum of the foot and is relieved with dangling the leg over the edge of the bed. The patient may also have tissue loss with ulcerations or nonhealing wounds of the foot (Table 62-2).

Initial evaluation must include a detailed medical history of comorbid conditions. In addition to coronary artery disease, carotid artery stenosis, and prior stroke, risk factors for atherosclerosis (e.g., diabetes, hypertension, dyslipidemia, tobacco abuse, hyperhomocysteinemia) should be queried and their level of optimization understood. Because medical management is a cornerstone of vascular therapy, a review of the patient's medications is imperative, with attention to the potential need for antiplatelet agents, beta blockers, angiotensin-converting enzyme inhibitors, and statins as a matter of course. Previous exposure to heparin, protamine, and NPH insulin should be noted. Allergies to contrast agents or iodine should be documented.

The surgical history and physical examination include details of surgical incisions as indicative of prior surgical intervention. Many patients will have undergone coronary artery bypass

TABLE 62-2 Clinical Classification of Peripheral Arterial Disease: Fontaine and Rutherford Systems

FONTAINE CLASSIFICATION		RUTHERFORD CLASSIFICATION	
STAGE	CLINICAL	GRADE	CLINICAL
I	Asymptomatic	0	Asymptomatic
IIa	Mild claudication	1	Mild claudication
IIb	Moderate to severe claudication	2	Moderate claudication
		3	Severe claudication
III	Ischemic rest pain	4	Ischemic rest pain
IV	Ulceration or gangrene	5	Minor tissue loss
		6	Major tissue loss

grafting; the presence of a left internal mammary–left anterior descending coronary graft and previous great saphenous vein harvest can change the surgical plan for peripheral revascularization. Frequent or recent coronary catheterization (or peripheral angiography) can suggest challenging groin access with significant scar tissue. Procedure reports should be reviewed for details of access closure or incidental findings of peripheral artery stenoses. Previous surgery, whether neck, abdominal, spine, joint, or vascular operations, can affect decision making, and efforts to gain the details of these are important. A family history of a first-degree relative with abdominal aortic aneurysm, stroke, or early myocardial infarction should be sought.

A vascular review of symptoms documents the presence or absence of transient ischemic attack (TIA) or stroke, such as unilateral weakness or sensory deficit, difficulty with speech or swallowing, word-finding difficulties or memory changes, dizziness, drop attacks, blurry vision, arm fatigue, weight loss or pain after eating, renal insufficiency or poorly controlled hypertension, impotence, claudication, rest pain, or tissue loss. As for all patients, a detailed understanding of the patient's functional status helps delineate goals of therapy and perioperative risk. Patients who are limited in their activities of daily living by their vascular disease or other comorbidities cannot provide an accurate picture of their cardiac function and will likely require further cardiac workup. History of tobacco abuse as well as all clinical efforts for encouraging smoking cessation must be documented.

The physical examination begins with vital signs, which often reveal hypertension and tachycardia. Blood pressure in both arms should be documented. The presence or absence of carotid bruits, cardiac murmurs, abdominal bruits, flank bruits, or groin bruits should be noted. The abdomen should be palpated for the aortic pulsation. Incision scars should be noted. Bilateral carotid, radial, ulnar, femoral, popliteal, dorsalis pedis, and posterior tibial pulses should be palpated and characterized. If pulses are not palpable, a continuous-wave Doppler examination can be used to check for signals. Common physical findings of PAD include hair loss and dry, shiny skin with nail hypertrophy. In critical limb ischemia, the classic findings of dependent rubor and pallor with elevation of the limb can be observed. In cases of severe rest pain, patients may have peripheral edema because they are unable to take their legs from the dependent position without pain. The feet should be meticulously inspected for wounds and signs of skin breakdown. A neurologic examination documenting equivalent strength and sensation in the limbs and cranial nerves should be performed.

Routine laboratory work should include a complete blood count, chemistry (to evaluate renal function and glucose concentration), and a lipid panel. An albumin level can be helpful in delineating the adequacy of a patient's nutritional status, if this is in question. The hemoglobin A1c level indicates the patient's level of glycemic control during the previous 120 days.

A baseline electrocardiogram should be obtained. Any previous cardiac testing, including echocardiography, stress echocardiography, dobutamine-adenosine sestamibi scan, and coronary catheterization, should be reviewed and documented.

Physiologic Testing and Imaging

The vascular laboratory is a powerful tool in the armamentarium of the surgeon. Noninvasive testing confirms and localizes disease, provides end points to demonstrate improvement after intervention, enables long-term follow-up of bypass grafts and percutaneous interventions, and can detect silent disease recurrence. Tests commonly performed in the laboratory include the ABI with multisegmental pressures and waveforms, toe-brachial index, pulse volume recording, photoplethysmography, and arterial duplex examination. The vascular laboratory represents one of the last arenas in which a nonimaging indirect measure of physiology is still widely used as a diagnostic tool.

Regardless of plans for intervention, it is recommended that asymptomatic patients at risk for PAD and those with symptoms undergo ABI testing. This examination can be performed simply with a manual blood pressure cuff at the ankle and a continuous-wave Doppler probe. With the patient in a supine position, after several minutes of rest to allow limb pressure to return to baseline, the cuff is inflated at the ankle, with the Doppler probe held at the location of the distal dorsalis pedis or posterior tibial signal. The systolic pressure is recorded as the pressure in the cuff when the Doppler signal returns. This process can be performed with multiple cuffs, allowing segmental pressure determination (Fig. 62-3), which is helpful in localizing the level of the obstructing lesion. The ABI for a limb is calculated using the higher of the two ankle pressures divided by the higher of the two brachial pressures (Tables 62-3 and 62-4). Patients with an ABI of 0.90 or less have a threefold to sixfold increased risk of cardiovascular mortality.

Continuous-wave Doppler analog waveforms can be obtained along with the segmental pressures. Photoplethysmography uses an infrared light–emitting source and a photosensor; it is based on the principle that red light is decreased with increased blood flow in tissues to generate a pressure and waveform within the

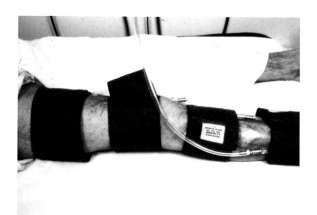

FIGURE 62-3 Segmental pressure is measured with the same technique as ankle pressure, but with cuffs placed at the upper part of the thigh, at the lower part of the thigh, below the knee, and at the ankle. (From Kohler TR, Sumner DS: Vascular laboratory: Arterial physiologic assessment. In Cronenwett JL, Johnston W, editors: *Rutherford's vascular surgery*, ed 7, Philadelphia, 2010, Saunders.)

TABLE 62-3 **Clinical Correlation of Different Levels of Ankle-Brachial Index**	
ABI*	**PRESENTATION**
1.11 ± 0.10	Normal
0.59 ± 0.15	Intermittent claudication
0.26 ± 0.13	Ischemic rest pain
0.05 ± 0.08	Tissue loss

From Moneta GL, Zaccardi MJ, Olmsted KA: Lower extremity arterial occlusive disease. In Zierler RE, editor: *Strandness's duplex scanning in vascular disorders*, ed 4, Philadelphia, 2010, Lippincott Williams & Wilkins, Wolters Kluwer Health, pp 133–147.
*The diagnosis of peripheral arterial disease is given to ABI < 0.9. ABI > 1.3 is interpreted as abnormal because of incompressible tibial arteries, frequently seen in diabetes and end-stage renal failure.

digit. The data generated from these studies should include bilateral brachial artery, high thigh, low thigh, calf, dorsalis pedis, posterior tibial, and toe pressures with waveforms (Fig. 62-4). A decrease in pressure of 20 to 30 mm Hg between adjacent segments is indicative of a significant lesion. The normal Doppler arterial waveform demonstrates triphasic flow with a sharp systolic upstroke, reversal of flow in early diastole from vessel compliance, and low-amplitude forward flow throughout diastole. With obstructive disease, the initial feature lost is the reversal of the flow component, leading to multiphasic (previously called biphasic) flow. Severe disease leads to blunting of the arterial waveform, with decreased amplitude and decreased slope of the upstroke. With worsening symptoms, there is increased diastolic flow, resulting in monophasic flow. A change in waveform can be interpreted, along with a decrease in pressure, as indicative of disease at that level. Limitations of ABI and segmental pressure determinations include mural calcification, such as in diabetes mellitus and end-stage renal disease, leading to elevated pressures that do not accurately reflect intra-arterial perfusion pressure. With a noncompressible vessel, a toe-brachial index higher than 0.70 with an absolute digit pressure higher than 50 mm Hg, with a normal waveform, is indicative of preserved flow because digit arteries are relatively resistant to the intramural calcification. The high thigh pressure cannot always distinguish among common

TABLE 62-4 Calculation of Ankle-Brachial Index

PARAMETER	RIGHT	LEFT
Brachial blood pressure	150 mm Hg	100 mm Hg
Dorsalis pedis	50 mm Hg	25 mm Hg
Posterior tibia	25 mm Hg	50 mm Hg
ABI	0.30	0.30

Example: The ABI is calculated using the higher of the two ankle pressures (as indicative of limb perfusion) and the higher brachial pressure (as indicative of systemic pressure). In this example, the left and right ABI values are both 0.30.

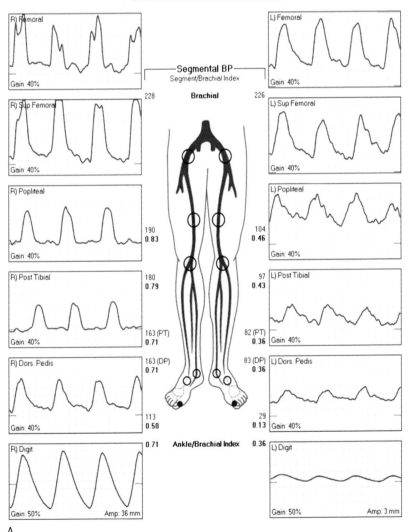

FIGURE 62-4 **A,** Patient with severe left leg claudication and diabetes. Segmental pressures demonstrate left iliofemoral obstruction.

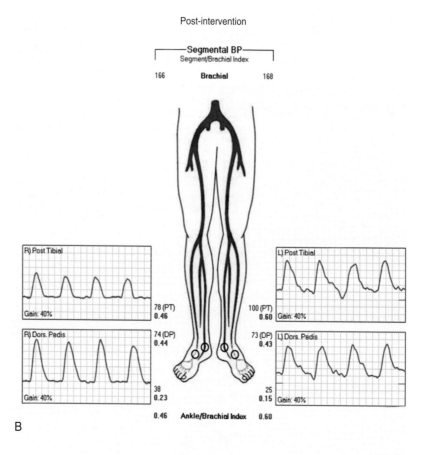

Post-intervention

Segmental BP
Segment/Brachial Index

166   Brachial   168

R) Post Tibial

Gain: 40%

78 (PT)
0.46

100 (PT)
0.60

L) Post Tibial

Gain: 40%

R) Dors. Pedis

Gain: 40%

74 (DP)
0.44

73 (DP)
0.43

L) Dors. Pedis

Gain: 40%

38
0.23

25
0.15

0.46   Ankle/Brachial Index   0.60

B

FIGURE 62-4, cont'd B, After left iliofemoral bypass and common iliac artery stent placement, the ankle-brachial index is significantly improved and the patient is asymptomatic.

iliac, external iliac, or common femoral disease. A proximal stenosis can decrease flow to the extent that accuracy is lost in interpreting gradients downstream.

Symptomatic patients with palpable distal pulses or a normal resting ABI should undergo exercise testing with measurement of the postexercise ABI. The decrease in peripheral vascular resistance that occurs with exercise-induced vasodilation will increase the drop in pressure seen across a stenotic lesion. Patients undergo resting ABI testing, followed by treadmill exercise until symptoms occur; repeated ABI testing may then reveal a decrease in ankle pressure of 20 mm Hg or a decrease in the ABI of 0.20. These changes and a failure of the ABI to return to preexercise baseline within 3 minutes are interpreted as a positive result.

Arterial duplex ultrasonography provides B-mode (gray-scale) imaging, pulsed Doppler spectral waveforms, and color flow data for analysis; in experienced hands, it can provide sensitive and specific information about the abdominal aorta and visceral, renal, iliac, and distal limb vessels. Peak systolic velocities and end-diastolic velocities are recorded. Waveforms are generated and analyzed. Color flow is useful for demonstrating patent vessels in low-flow states and for distinguishing antegrade from retrograde flow. As in continuous-flow Doppler analysis, a change in

waveform from triphasic to monophasic, or an increase in peak systolic velocity followed by a drop in velocity, indicates a hemodynamically significant lesion. A ratio of the peak systolic velocity within the stenosis to the peak systolic velocity of the proximal normal segment of 2.0 or more correlates with a stenosis of 50% or more. Visualization of intra-abdominal segments requires the patient to be fasting before the examination to eliminate bowel gas; studies can be limited by body habitus. Severe calcification of the distal vessels can impede imaging of flow (Figs. 62-5 and 62-6).

Imaging Studies

When intervention is planned, further imaging to delineate the location and nature of disease is needed. The "gold standard" for these purposes has been angiography. Because of the invasive nature of this test, with attendant risks of complications, imaging was previously reserved as a preoperative study for patients determined to be operative candidates because of the severity of their disease and their suitability for surgery. This algorithm has changed somewhat in contemporary practice. Most angiography is therapeutic rather than diagnostic, with lesions that are deemed amenable for endovascular intervention addressed in the same setting

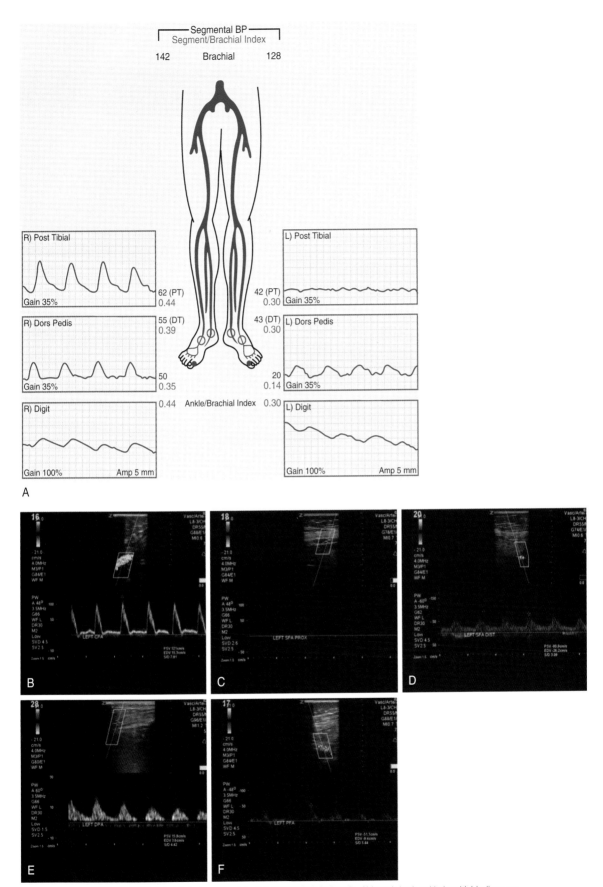

FIGURE 62-5 Arterial duplex scanning, left critical limb ischemia. Although both ankle-brachial indices are abnormal **(A),** the right limb waveforms are multiphasic and the left-sided waveforms are monophasic. Arterial duplex images show normal left common femoral artery **(B)** and no flow in the proximal superficial femoral artery **(C);** however, flow in the distal superficial femoral artery **(D)** and dorsalis pedis artery **(E)** is present because of collateral flow from the profunda femoris **(F).**

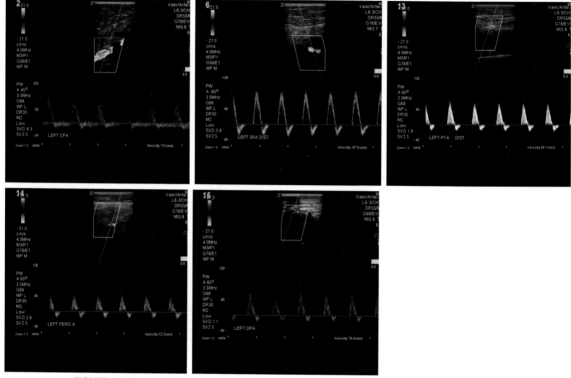

FIGURE 62-6 Postintervention images of the same patient as in Figure 62-5 show intact flow throughout the superficial femoral artery and improved distal flow.

as the initial angiogram. Alternatively, computed tomography angiography (CTA) or magnetic resonance angiography (MRA) may enable the acquisition of the same vascular road map before a planned intervention.

Angiography. Access is usually through the contralateral common femoral or left brachial artery. A complete diagnostic study is performed in four steps:

1. Abdominal aortography, with a multi–side hole catheter placed at the level of the diaphragm, images the abdominal aorta, celiac artery, superior mesenteric artery, inferior mesenteric artery, renal artery, and aortic bifurcation.
2. Pelvic angiography, with a multi–side hole catheter at the aortic bifurcation, images the bilateral common iliac, hypogastric, and external iliac arteries; common femoral arteries; and proximal superficial femoral artery (SFA) and profunda femoris artery (Fig. 62-7).
3. The contralateral common femoral artery is then selected by use of an end-hole catheter, and images of the contralateral SFA, profunda, popliteal, tibial, and pedal vessels are obtained in one to three low-bolus runs.
4. The access sheath is then pulled back to the level of the distal ipsilateral external iliac artery to image the ipsilateral limb.

Trans-stenotic pressure gradients and multiplanar images can clarify the significance of an ambiguous lesion. Complete assessment of the aortic and iliac inflow and bilateral lower extremities requires 75 to 100 mL of contrast material.

Risks of diagnostic angiography and all endovascular procedures include groin hematoma, retroperitoneal bleeding, pseudoaneurysm, arteriovenous fistula, and arterial dissection. Even a small amount of bleeding after brachial artery access can cause symptomatic brachial sheath hematoma and neural compromise

requiring exploration and evacuation. These risks are reduced by the routine use of ultrasound-guided access and micropuncture techniques.

The risk of contrast nephropathy is limited by prudent use of contrast material; selective catheterization, which decreases the volume of the contrast bolus required to opacify the vessels; and use of lower ionic load or iso-osmolar contrast agents. Patients are counseled to increase oral hydration in preparation for and after arteriography. Metformin and angiotensin-converting enzyme inhibitors as well as diuretics are held before the procedure and for 48 hours after the procedure. There is some evidence for preoperative medication with acetylcysteine, 1200 mg orally twice daily, before and after arteriography, as well as intravenous (IV) fluid hydration using half-normal saline with 1.5 ampules of sodium bicarbonate or dextrose in water solution with three ampules of sodium bicarbonate. Patients with a history of allergy to contrast media should be premedicated according to institutional guidelines with steroids and histamine blockers (e.g., diphenhydramine).

Risk of radiation exposure for diagnostic procedures is limited, but with the growing complexity of endovascular interventions, cumulative exposure is a potential concern for the patient and for the physician exposed during the therapeutic procedure. Monitoring is essential and routine.

Computed tomography angiography. The widespread use of multidetector CT scanners has improved the speed, volume coverage, and slice thickness of images so that a single bolus of contrast material can be imaged as it passes through the arterial system. One advantage of CTA (Fig. 62-8A) is the depiction of the entire vessel, with the ability to appreciate thrombus and calcification; arteriography typically characterizes only the lumen of the artery.

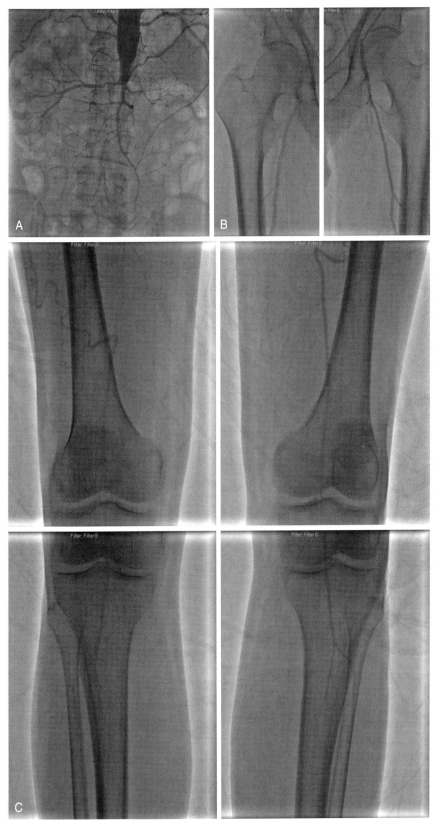

FIGURE 62-7 Aortogram with bilateral lower extremity runoff, nonsubtracted. **A,** Occluded aorta with left renal artery occlusion. **B,** Reconstitution of bilateral common femoral arteries, flush superficial femoral artery occlusions. **C,** Reconstitution of right above-knee popliteal artery, left superficial femoral artery. Below the knee, proximal bilateral tibial flow appears intact.

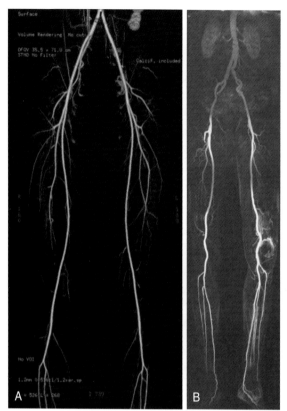

FIGURE 62-8 A, CTA scan with volume rendering demonstrates normal common iliac, external iliac, common femoral, deep and superficial femoral, popliteal, and proximal tibial arteries. **B,** MRA scan demonstrating distal tibial disease. (Courtesy Dr. Douglas Hughes, University of Texas Medical Branch at Galveston, Department of Radiology.)

Thin slices of 0.625 mm allow three-dimensional reconstructions and multiplanar reformatting that is not routinely achieved with conventional arteriography. CTA disadvantages are similar to those of arteriography, with the potential for complications from the use of iodinated contrast agents and significant accumulation of radiation exposure.

Magnetic resonance angiography. Advocates of contrast-enhanced MRA with gadolinium (Fig. 62-8*B*) report a high sensitivity and specificity of this modality for demonstrating the degree of stenosis and lesion length and even superiority in identifying distal target vessels compared with conventional arteriography. Disadvantages of MRA technology include the need for cooperation of the patient, discomfort of the patient, longer studies, expense, contraindications with certain metallic implants, and renal toxicity reported with use of the contrast agent gadolinium. Its use is contraindicated in renal disease because of the risk of nephrogenic systemic fibrosis. This is a rare complication associated with the administration of gadolinium-based agents to patients with renal failure or renal insufficiency having a glomerular filtration rate of 30 mL/min or lower. Patients develop fibrosed nodules of the skin, eyes, and joints. Severe contracture limiting movement or involvement of the heart, liver, and lungs has been described.

Carbon dioxide angiography. Angiography using carbon dioxide as a contrast medium can be helpful in patients with severe chronic renal insufficiency. Carbon dioxide temporarily displaces the blood in the artery being imaged. Carbon dioxide rapidly dissolves, but 3 to 5 minutes must be allowed to pass between injections. The limitations of this contrast agent include poor detail, especially for small distal vessels. The bolus may cause significant discomfort for the patient. Sequelae of carbon dioxide embolus, with gas trapping leading to mesenteric ischemia, have been described. Carbon dioxide is not used for arch or cerebral arteriography.

Intravascular ultrasound. With improvements in high-frequency smaller transducers, the use of catheter-based intravascular ultrasound (Fig. 62-9) has increased. Intravascular ultrasound provides a transverse, 360-degree image of the lumen of the vessel to be imaged throughout its length and provides qualitative data about the wall anatomy. It has been used in peripheral interventions for opening chronic total occlusions and has been instrumental in the endovascular treatment of aortic dissection. As a diagnostic tool, adjuncts such as color flow Doppler enable the delineation between flow and thrombus, whereas virtual histology, in which color is assigned to plaque components of fibrous, fibrofatty, calcified, and necrotic lipid core densities, has been shown to correlate well with actual histology in assessment of coronary and carotid artery disease. The use of intravascular ultrasound, however, increases the length of procedures, and its expense limits its applicability.

Treatment
Medical Treatment
Despite the aging of our population and increasing numbers of people afflicted by atherosclerotic arterial disease, morbidity from myocardial infarction and stroke is decreasing. This is likely secondary to advances in medical management and increasing awareness by affected individuals about the availability of medications that can limit the progression of the disease process. The American Heart Association has published guidelines for risk modification that have grown increasingly aggressive in efforts to treat this important public health concern. In contemporary surgical practice, lipid modification, antiplatelet and antihypertensive control, and smoking cessation strategies are all becoming standard management issues for the patient with vascular disease. Table 62-5 summarizes the American Heart Association guidelines for risk factor modification.

Risk factors contributing to PAD are the same as those for atherosclerosis:

- Smoking. Tobacco use in any form is the single most important modifiable cause of PVD internationally. Smokers have up to a 10-fold increase in relative risk for PVD in a dose-related effect. Exposure to second-hand smoke from environmental exposure has also been shown to promote changes in endothelium, the precursor to atherosclerosis.
- Dyslipidemia. Decreased high-density lipoprotein cholesterol and elevations of total cholesterol, low-density lipoprotein cholesterol, and triglyceride levels have been correlated with accelerated PAD. Correction of dyslipidemia by diet, exercise, or medication is associated with a major improvement in short-term rates of heart attack and stroke. This benefit is gained even though current evidence does not demonstrate a major reversal of peripheral or coronary atherosclerosis.
- Hypertension. Elevated blood pressure is correlated with an increased risk for development of PAD and associated coronary and cerebrovascular events (e.g., heart attack, stroke).
- Diabetes mellitus. The presence of diabetes mellitus involves a twofold to fourfold increased risk of PVD by causing

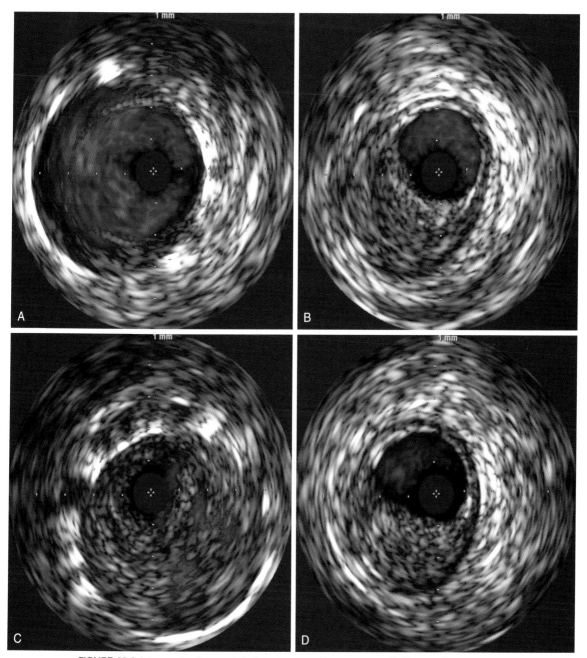

FIGURE 62-9 Intravascular ultrasound. **A,** Patent common iliac artery stent. **B,** Common iliac artery stent thrombosis. **C,** External iliac artery plaque. **D,** External iliac artery plaque. (Courtesy Dr. Syed Gilani, University of Texas Medical Branch at Galveston, Department of Cardiology.)

endothelial and smooth muscle cell dysfunction in peripheral arteries. Diabetics account for up to 70% of nontraumatic amputations performed, and a known diabetic who smokes has an approximately 30% risk of amputation within 5 years.

Revascularization: Surgical Treatment

Intermittent claudication. Patients with intermittent claudication are treated by risk factor modification to decrease their risk of myocardial infarction and cerebrovascular accident. A trial of cilostazol and supervised exercise is recommended; these therapies, combined with risk factor modification (particularly smoking cessation), have been shown to improve walking distance. Patients are reassured that they are at limited risk of limb loss, approximately 2% to 3% at 5 years. Although significant disability may occur as a result of intermittent claudication, symptoms remain stable because of the development of collateral flow or perhaps alterations in gait that favor nonischemic muscle groups. However, 25% of intermittent claudication patients will see deterioration in their clinical course, usually during the first year after diagnosis; the best predictor of this decline is the initial ABI. Patients with an initial ABI of less than 0.50 have a hazard ratio of more than 2 compared with patients with an ABI higher than 0.50.

TABLE 62-5 Medical Therapy for Peripheral Arterial Disease

DISORDER	RECOMMENDED PHARMACOLOGIC AGENT	PURPOSE OF CARDIOVASCULAR RISK REDUCTION	CLASS OF RECOMMENDATIONS	LEVEL OF EVIDENCE	COMMENTS
Dyslipidemia	Statin	Statin therapy, with target LDL <100 mg/dL	I	B	
		Statin therapy, with target LDL <70 mg/dL	II	B	High-risk patients with multiple and/or poorly controlled risk factors: DM, continued tobacco abuse, metabolic syndrome (TG ≥200 mg/dL + HDL ≤40 mg/dL + non-HDL ≥130 mg/dL), acute coronary syndrome
	Gemfibrozil	May be useful in PAD patients with low HDL, normal LDL, high TG	II	C	Gemfibrozil reduces risk of nonfatal MI or cardiovascular death by 22% in CAD patients with low HDL; effects on PAD unknown
Hypertension		140/90 mm Hg in nondiabetics, 130/80 mm Hg in DM and CRI	I	A	Reduces risk of MI, CHF, cardiovascular death and stroke
	Beta blocker	Effective, not contraindicated	I	A	Reduces risk of MI and death in CAD patients; does not impair walking distance
	ACE inhibitors	Reasonable in symptomatic PAD to decrease risk of cardiovascular events	IIa	B	In patients with symptomatic PAD, ramipril reduces risk of MI, stroke, or vascular death by ≈25%
		May be used in asymptomatic PAD to decrease risk of cardiovascular events	IIb	C	No evidence for efficacy of ACE inhibitors in patients with asymptomatic PAD
Diabetes		Proper foot care; skin lesions, ulcerations should be addressed urgently in all diabetic patients with lower extremity PAD	I	B	
		Hemoglobin A1c <7%	IIa	C	Can be effective to reduce microvascular complications, potentially improve cardiovascular outcome
Atherosclerosis	Aspirin	75-325 mg PO qd; reduces risk of MI, stroke, and vascular death	I	A	Reduces risk of events by 26% to 32%
	Clopidogrel	75 mg PO qd; effective alternative to aspirin to reduce risk of MI, stroke, vascular death	I	B	Reduces risk of events by 23.8%
Smoking		Clinicians to advise smoking cessation, offer medical therapy	I	B	Physician's advice with frequent follow-up: 1-year success rate, 5% Without physician's interventions: 1-year success rate, 0.1% With nicotine replacement: 1-year success rate, 16% With bupropion: 1-year success rate, 30%

Adapted from Hirsch AT, Haskal ZJ, Hertzer NR, et al: ACC/AHA 2005 Practice Guidelines for the management of patients with peripheral arterial disease (lower extremity, renal, mesenteric, and abdominal aortic): A collaborative report from the American Association for Vascular Surgery/Society for Vascular Surgery, Society for Cardiovascular Angiography and Interventions, Society for Vascular Medicine and Biology, Society of Interventional Radiology, and the ACC/AHA Task Force on Practice Guidelines (Writing Committee to Develop Guidelines for the Management of Patients With Peripheral Arterial Disease): Endorsed by the American Association of Cardiovascular and Pulmonary Rehabilitation; National Heart, Lung, and Blood Institute; Society for Vascular Nursing; TransAtlantic Inter-Society Consensus; and Vascular Disease Foundation. *Circulation* 113:e463–e654, 2006.

ACE, angiotensin-converting enzyme; *CAD,* coronary artery disease; *CHF,* congestive heart failure; *CRI,* chronic renal insufficiency; *DM,* diabetes mellitus; *HDL,* high-density lipoprotein; *LDL,* low-density lipoprotein; *MI,* myocardial infarction; *PAD,* peripheral arterial disease; *TG,* triglyceride.

Intermittent claudication patients with an initial ankle pressure of 40 to 60 mm Hg have an annual limb loss rate of 8.5%.

Patients who present initially with low ankle pressures or absent femoral pulses or patients who return with unabated, severe, lifestyle-limiting symptoms that have not adequately responded to nonoperative measures are considered for intervention (Fig. 62-10).

Critical limb ischemia. Patients who present initially with rest pain or who progress from claudication to rest pain undergo the same detailed history and physical examination with risk factor modification as patients presenting with milder disease. However, because rest pain is associated with a significant risk of limb loss without intervention, patients are immediately offered imaging and revascularization if prohibitive perioperative risk does not preclude this.

Similarly, patients who present with nonhealing wounds of the feet, dry gangrene, or necrotizing infection are offered an expeditious workup to plan a revascularization that will reestablish in-line blood flow to the foot. In case of tissue loss with infection, an immediate decision about the need for operative débridement or amputation before revascularization must be made. In case of severe sepsis with hemodynamic instability or evidence of multisystem organ failure, patients may require amputation before revascularization. However, if a patient with systemic toxicity from the infection responds rapidly to IV administration of antibiotics, revascularization before débridement may minimize tissue loss (Fig. 62-11).

Diabetic foot. PVD is common among patients with diabetes (Fig. 62-12). Intermittent claudication is twice as common among diabetic patients as among nondiabetic patients. An increase in

hemoglobin A1c by 1% can result in more than a 25% risk of PAD. Major amputation rates are 5 to 10 times higher in diabetics than in nondiabetics. Because of these causal relations, the American Diabetes Association recommends ABI screening every 5 years in patients with diabetes.[2]

The care of diabetic patients should start with preventive measures, and it is important to avoid infections in patients with insensate feet because of neuropathy. These patients need to wear properly fitted shoes at all times for protection. Orthotic inserts should be used to distribute weight evenly to avoid pressure on the metatarsal heads of the foot.

Diabetic patients may be unaware of the presence of infections or ulcerative lesions because of peripheral neuropathy and a decreased ability to sense pain. In this population, infections can progress rapidly, with significant tissue damage from a combination of delayed presentation and compromised immune function.

On presentation, a careful physical examination is important to plan for appropriate treatment. The overlying cellulitis is assessed, and any possible underlying abscess is examined by palpation for crepitus or detection of drainage of purulent fluid. Cellulitis should not be confused with dependent rubor caused by severe ischemia in patients with PAD. The presence of an abscess requires immediate drainage before revascularization.

The status of arterial circulation is documented. The presence or absence of lower extremity pulses in the common femoral, popliteal, and pedal arteries is examined. The pulses may be difficult to palpate because of swelling from foot infection; noninvasive arterial ultrasound can be useful in assessing the extent of arterial disease.

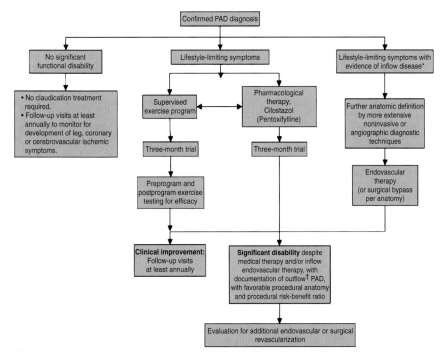

FIGURE 62-10 Treatment Algorithm for Peripheral Arterial Disease. (From Hirsch AT, Haskal ZJ, Hertzer NR, et al: ACC/AHA 2005 Practice Guidelines for the Management of Patients With Peripheral Arterial Disease (Lower Extremity, Renal, Mesenteric, and Abdominal Aortic). *Circ* 113:e463–e654, 2006.) *Inflow disease should be suspected in individuals with gluteal or thigh claudication and femoral pulse diminution or bruit and should be confirmed by noninvasive vascular laboratory diagnostic evidence of aortoiliac stenoses. †Outflow disease represents femoropopliteal and infrapopliteal stenoses, (the presence of occlusive lesions in the lower extremity arterial tree below the inguinal ligament from the common femoral artery to the pedal vessels). PAD indicates peripheral arterial disease.

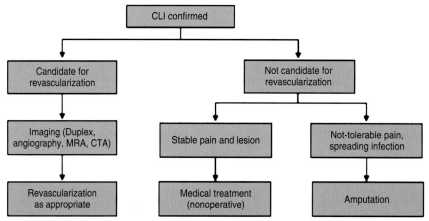

FIGURE 62-11 Algorithm for treatment of the critical limb ischemia (CLI) patient. (From Norgren L, Hiatt WR, Dormandy JA, et al: Inter-Society Consensus for the Management of Peripheral Arterial Disease [TASC II]. *J Vasc Surg* 45[Suppl]:S5–S67, 2007.)

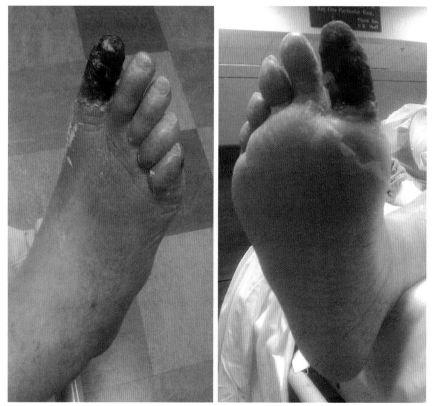

FIGURE 62-12 Diabetic patient who presented with chronic dry gangrene of the right great toe, with dependent rubor of the forefoot.

Insulin-dependent diabetic patients may have calcified walls of the medium and small arteries that can falsely elevate the segmental pressures of the leg. In this situation, digital pressures of the toes can be accurately measured, and a pressure higher than 30 mm Hg is predictive of healing after local amputation and débridement.

Plain radiographs with multiple views of the foot can assist in assessing the extent of foot infection. Gas in soft tissue signifies deep tissue infection and the need for urgent surgical débridement. Advanced osteomyelitis can be detected; however, plain films may not show early bone infection. MRI of the foot is a sensitive imaging modality for detecting soft tissue infection and early osteomyelitis.

Routine laboratory work is sent and evaluated for subtle signs of sepsis. Sudden worsening of glycemic control or a rise in creatinine level is seen frequently, often without leukocytosis.

In infections with only cellulitis and no underlying soft tissue involvement, patients are treated with IV antibiotic therapy. If the cellulitis does not resolve in several days, there may not be adequate antibiotic coverage, and the presence of deep tissue infection is considered. The choice of the antibiotics used and the foot need to be reevaluated; reimaging of the foot may be necessary.

The cause of persistent cellulitis and nonhealing infection is usually underlying deep infection or osteomyelitis. Other patients may present with gangrene, open joint or exposed bone, or abscess. In these patients, surgical débridement is required in addition to antibiotic therapy. Small open wounds can be treated with simple débridement, but often there is deep tissue involvement that is not visible on the surface. For removal of all nonviable tissue and wide drainage, amputation may be required. If there is extensive infection of the foot with gas, calf pain, or systemic sepsis, the patient may require amputation as an initial therapy. After surgical débridement, patients are treated with aggressive wound care by dressing changes and continued, broad-spectrum antibiotic therapy until intraoperative culture sensitivities are finalized and allow the use of targeted antimicrobials. Wounds are evaluated closely for persistent infection that may require additional surgical intervention. In patients with adequate arterial circulation, the wound can be closed secondarily after resolution of the infection.

All patients with evidence of concomitant arterial occlusive disease are considered for lower extremity revascularization with open bypass surgery or endovascular stenting or angioplasty to optimize wound healing and limb salvage.

Lower Extremity Amputations

Amputation, unfortunately, in the minds of most surgeons and their patients, represents a failure of therapy or care. Consent for this operation, regardless of the level, is usually imbued with an emotional gravity that few other, even more complex, dangerous,

life-altering procedures carry. Not infrequently, amputations in the vascular patient are prone to breakdown and the need for revision is common, thereby prolonging the patient's time in the hospital, lengthening the recovery process, decreasing the chances of functional recovery, and contributing to a high rate of depression. It is therefore incumbent on the surgeon to ensure that all steps are taken to optimize healing and to minimize the risks of local and systemic complications.

The perioperative mortality rate for below-knee amputation is 5% to 10%, and that of above-knee amputation is even higher, 10% to 15%, testifying to the limited reserves of patients facing these procedures.[3] Wound healing in below-knee amputation is poor; almost one third of patients require débridement or healing by secondary intention or conversion to above-knee amputation (Fig. 62-13). Despite optimistic preoperative counseling, functional recovery with ambulation is poor for above-knee amputation patients.

The determination of the appropriate level for amputation has been studied extensively (Table 62-6). In an effort to preserve limb length and to decrease the metabolic demands of ambulation, toe and transmetatarsal amputations are usually attempted. Aside from clinical judgment, segmental arterial pressures, Doppler waveforms, and toe pressures have been studied. Diabetes, combined with a toe pressure of lower than 30 mm Hg, has been correlated with failure of healing of minor amputations. Transcutaneous oxygen pressure ($TcPO_2$) measurement, easily obtained through a small sensor placed on the skin in the area of proposed amputation, has an accuracy of higher than 87% for predicting

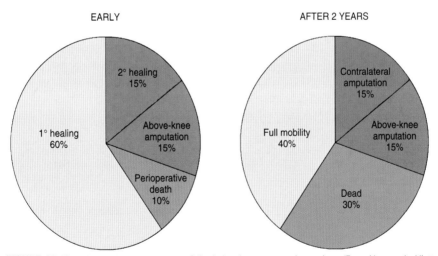

FIGURE 62-13 Early and 2-year outcomes of the below-knee amputation patient. (From Norgren L, Hiatt WR, Dormandy JA, et al: Inter-Society Consensus for the Management of Peripheral Arterial Disease [TASC II]. *J Vasc Surg* 45[Suppl]:S5–S67, 2007.)

TABLE 62-6 Prediction of Wound Healing by Vascular Studies

STUDY	THRESHOLD (mm Hg)	WOUND HEALING (%) BELOW THRESHOLD	WOUND HEALING (%) ABOVE THRESHOLD	SENSITIVITY (%)	SPECIFICITY (%)
SPP	40	10	69	72	88
$TcPO_2$	30	14	63	60	87
TBP	30	12	67	63	90
ABP	80	11	45	74	70

ABP, ankle blood pressure; *SPP*, skin perfusion pressure; *TBP*, toe blood pressure; *TcPO₂*, transcutaneous oxygen pressure.

wound healing. A reading higher than 40 mm Hg is associated with successful healing, whereas TcPO$_2$ less than 20 mm Hg is associated with failure. Absolute ankle pressure higher than 60 mm Hg has been shown to predict the healing of below-knee amputations with an accuracy of 50% to 90%.[4]

Ray amputation. For ray amputation, a tennis racquet incision around the base of the affected toe is made. For first toe amputations, the handle of the racquet is oriented along the medial aspect of the metatarsal head; for the fifth toe, it is oriented laterally. For toes 2 to 4, the incision is along the dorsal midline (Fig. 62-14). Neighboring digital vessels are carefully preserved as the soft tissues are divided. The extensor tendons are divided under tension and permitted to retract. The bone is divided proximal to the metatarsal head. If sesamoid bones are encountered, these are removed. Plantar soft tissue is divided; flexor tendons are similarly allowed to retract after being divided under tension. Soft tissue is closed over the metatarsal head with absorbable sutures. Minimal handling of the skin prevents ischemic trauma. The skin is approximated without tension or left open for closure by secondary intention.

The great toe and first metatarsal bone are important for normal gait because weight is transferred from the posterolateral foot during heel strike toward the medial toes, and the transfer of weight forward occurs principally through force transmitted during push off through the first metatarsal and great toe. Because of the significant rate of repeated ulceration and need for revision in up to 60% of patients requiring a great toe ray amputation, some have advocated proceeding directly to transmetatarsal amputation in these patients.

Partial transmetatarsal amputation can be performed when two digits are involved and the foot is deemed salvageable. However, multiple ray amputations will narrow the foot, resulting in instability and change in gait that may lead to repeated ulceration, wound breakdown, and the need for revision.

Transmetatarsal amputation. A curvilinear incision is made above the metatarsal heads, with an intentionally longer flap fashioned on the plantar surface (Fig. 62-15). Soft tissues anterior to the bone are divided, including the tendons of the extensor muscles. Digital arteries are suture ligated as needed. A periosteal elevator is applied to elevate the soft tissues just to the point of division. An oscillating saw is used to divide the metatarsals behind their heads. The plantar tendons and soft tissues are divided distal to the level of bone amputation. This posterior soft tissue is used as a flap for wound coverage. The wound is irrigated

with a mechanical lavage system and inspected for hemostasis. The soft tissue is reapproximated over the bone with absorbable sutures. The skin is reapproximated, with minimal manipulation and without tension, with interrupted nylon vertical mattress sutures. Non–weight-bearing status is encouraged for at least 4 weeks. In case of infection, a guillotine procedure may be performed and a vacuum dressing applied, with placement of a split-thickness skin graft after the wound bed has adequately granulated.

Alternatively, more proximal transmetatarsal amputation incisions include the Lisfranc and Chopart amputations (Fig. 62-16). The Syme amputation is rarely used because it is thought to provide the patient with less functional ambulation than a transtibial amputation. There is evidence to support multiple revisions and preservation of length in diabetic patients. In one study, 56% of patients failed to heal their initial transmetatarsal amputations. Of these, 9 of 41 underwent major amputation; 32 underwent midfoot amputations and achieved functional ambulation. Toe pressure higher than 50 mm Hg had a positive predictive value

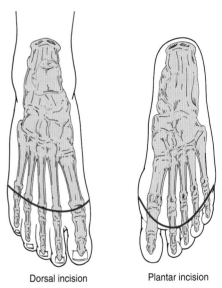

FIGURE 62-15 Surgical approach to transmetatarsal amputation. (From Eidt JF, Kalapatapu VR: Techniques and results. In Cronenwett JL, Johnston W, editors: *Rutherford's vascular surgery*, ed 7, Philadelphia, 2010, Saunders, pp 1772–1790.)

Dorsal incision   Plantar incision

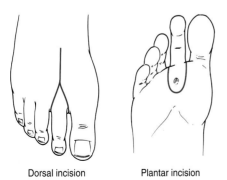

Dorsal incision   Plantar incision

FIGURE 62-14 Surgical approach to ray amputation. (From Eidt JF, Kalapatapu VR: Techniques and results. In Cronenwett JL, Johnston W, editors: *Rutherford's vascular surgery*, ed 7, Philadelphia, 2010, Saunders, pp 1772–1790.)

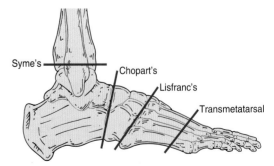

FIGURE 62-16 Alternative distal amputation approaches. (From Eidt JF, Kalapatapu VR: Techniques and results. In Cronenwett JL, Johnston W, editors: *Rutherford's vascular surgery*, ed 7, Philadelphia, 2010, Saunders, pp 1772–1790.)

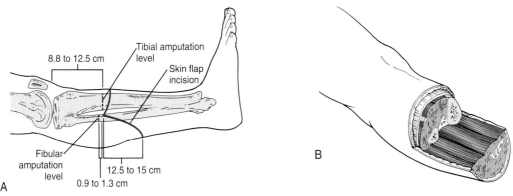

FIGURE 62-17 Surgical approach to posterior flap for below-knee amputation. (From Eidt JF, Kalapatapu VR: Techniques and results. In Cronenwett JL, Johnston W, editors: *Rutherford's vascular surgery*, ed 7, Philadelphia, 2010, Saunders, pp 1772–1790.)

of 91% for determining healing of transmetatarsal-midfoot amputations.[5]

Below-knee amputation. There are multiple skin incisions described for below-knee amputation (Fig. 62-17). The most common is the long posterior flap. A tourniquet may be used to decrease blood loss, which can be substantial, even in the vascular patient. Approximately 10 cm below the tibial tuberosity, an anterior incision of two thirds of the circumference is created. The great saphenous vein is ligated and divided. All muscle and soft tissue structures anterior to the tibia are divided. Vascular bundles are suture ligated with care because they are likely to be extremely calcified. Nerves are tied under tension, divided, and allowed to retract. The tibia is divided with an oscillating saw and beveled anteriorly. The fibula is divided approximately 2 cm proximal to the tibia after detachment of the anterior, lateral, and posterior compartment muscles. The posterior flap incision is created with the length approximately one third of the circumference of the leg. The muscle flap is created just deep to the tibia, including the soleus and gastrocnemius muscles. After irrigation and inspection for hemostasis, the fascia is reapproximated with interrupted absorbable sutures. The skin is reapproximated with monofilament vertical mattress sutures or staples. A dressing of gauze wrap and elastic bandage is applied. A splint is created or a well-padded knee immobilizer is applied to prevent knee contracture.

In case of severe necrotizing foot infection, emergent guillotine transtibial amputation can be performed just proximal to the ankle, followed by formal revision to a below-knee amputation once the infectious process has resolved.[6]

Cryoamputation or physiologic amputation has been described to isolate the infected or acutely ischemic limb and to prevent it from causing systemic effects in an already critically ill individual.

Above-knee amputation. In general, the longer the stump, the better. A fish-mouth incision is created (Fig. 62-18). The great saphenous vein is ligated and divided. The sartorius, rectus femoris, and vastus lateralis are divided. The femoral artery and vein are separately suture ligated and divided. Laterally, the vastus lateralis and intermedius are divided. The periosteal elevator is used to clear the femur at the level of the skin; the bone is divided by use of a pneumatic saw and beveled anteriorly. The profunda femoris artery and vein or their branches are ligated and divided. The sciatic nerve is cut under tension and allowed to retract. After irrigation and inspection of hemostasis, the fascia of the muscles

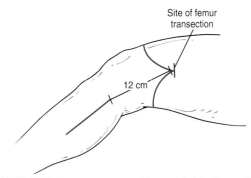

FIGURE 62-18 Surgical approach to fish-mouth incision for transfemoral above-knee amputation. (From Eidt JF, Kalapatapu VR: Techniques and results. In Cronenwett JL, Johnston W, editors: *Rutherford's vascular surgery*, ed 7, Philadelphia, 2010, Saunders, pp 1772–1790.)

is approximated over the bone with absorbable interrupted sutures, and the skin is closed.

Complications of above-knee amputation include hip contracture; this and the poor rates of ambulation are related to unopposed action of the hip flexors. Preservation of adductor function is improved with myodesis; the length of the adductor magnus may be preserved and anchored to the lateral aspect of the femur through drill holes.

Trans-knee amputations may be used as an alternative to above-knee amputation in younger patients for improved functional capability.

Surgical Revascularization Procedures

There are fewer areas in medicine today in which treatment algorithms are changing more rapidly than in arterial occlusive disease. Currently, the decision for revascularization is based on the risks for the surgical intervention balanced against the expected benefits, including the durability of the treatment and options for further intervention if there is recurrence of symptoms. Rapid advances in endovascular techniques and devices have made the therapeutic decision-making process increasingly complex; opinions about which therapies should be used first are varied. In an effort to characterize patients and their lesions and to provide guidance about open versus endovascular alternatives, the TransAtlantic Inter-Society Consensus (TASC) document on management of peripheral arterial disease was written and published in January 2000. As practice patterns matured, a second TASC II document was released later in the decade, in 2007. These documents provided classifications of aortoiliac and femoropopliteal disease and strategies for their treatment (Tables 62-7 and 62-8). TASC II recommendations state the following:

TASC A and D lesions: Endovascular therapy is the treatment of choice for type A lesions and surgery is the treatment of choice for type D lesions.

    TASC B and C lesions: Endovascular treatment is the preferred treatment for type B lesions and surgery is the preferred treatment for good-risk patients with type C lesions. The patient's comorbidities, fully informed patient

preference and the local operator's long-term success rates must be considered when making treatment recommendations for type B and type C lesions.

Arguably, as long as endovascular intervention does not negatively affect a patient's option to have an open surgery in the event of restenosis or reocclusion, endovascular intervention can be attempted for even complex lesions.

Open Surgical Management

Aortoiliac disease. Most patients with aortoiliac occlusive disease are treated with endovascular management. When the extent of disease or involvement of the common femoral arteries necessitates an open approach, patients typically undergo

TABLE 62-7   TransAtlantic Inter-Society Consensus (TASC) Classification of Aortoiliac Lesions

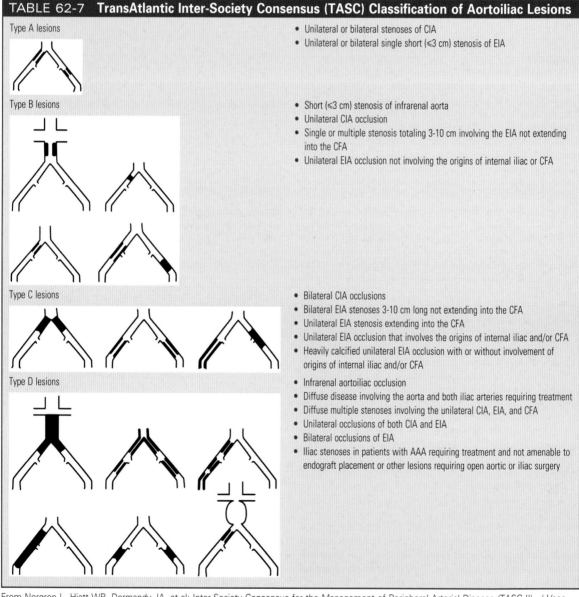

Type A lesions	• Unilateral or bilateral stenoses of CIA • Unilateral or bilateral single short (≤3 cm) stenosis of EIA
Type B lesions	• Short (≤3 cm) stenosis of infrarenal aorta • Unilateral CIA occlusion • Single or multiple stenosis totaling 3-10 cm involving the EIA not extending into the CFA • Unilateral EIA occlusion not involving the origins of internal iliac or CFA
Type C lesions	• Bilateral CIA occlusions • Bilateral EIA stenoses 3-10 cm long not extending into the CFA • Unilateral EIA stenosis extending into the CFA • Unilateral EIA occlusion that involves the origins of internal iliac and/or CFA • Heavily calcified unilateral EIA occlusion with or without involvement of origins of internal iliac and/or CFA
Type D lesions	• Infrarenal aortoiliac occlusion • Diffuse disease involving the aorta and both iliac arteries requiring treatment • Diffuse multiple stenoses involving the unilateral CIA, EIA, and CFA • Unilateral occlusions of both CIA and EIA • Bilateral occlusions of EIA • Iliac stenoses in patients with AAA requiring treatment and not amenable to endograft placement or other lesions requiring open aortic or iliac surgery

From Norgren L, Hiatt WR, Dormandy JA, et al: Inter-Society Consensus for the Management of Peripheral Arterial Disease (TASC II). *J Vasc Surg* 45(Suppl S):S5–S67, 2007.
AAA, abdominal aortic aneurysm; *CFA*, common femoral artery; *CIA*, common iliac artery; *EIA*, external iliac artery.

TABLE 62-8 TransAtlantic Inter-Society Consensus (TASC) Classification of Femoropopliteal Lesions

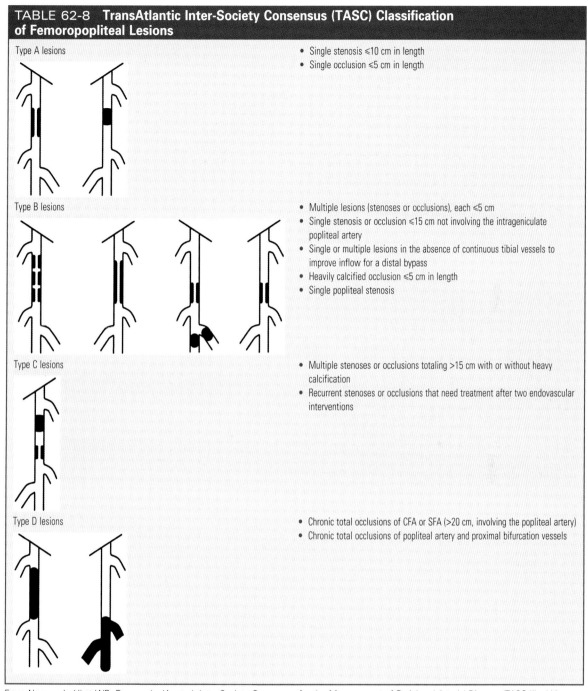

Type A lesions
- Single stenosis ≤10 cm in length
- Single occlusion ≤5 cm in length

Type B lesions
- Multiple lesions (stenoses or occlusions), each ≤5 cm
- Single stenosis or occlusion ≤15 cm not involving the intrageniculate popliteal artery
- Single or multiple lesions in the absence of continuous tibial vessels to improve inflow for a distal bypass
- Heavily calcified occlusion ≤5 cm in length
- Single popliteal stenosis

Type C lesions
- Multiple stenoses or occlusions totaling >15 cm with or without heavy calcification
- Recurrent stenoses or occlusions that need treatment after two endovascular interventions

Type D lesions
- Chronic total occlusions of CFA or SFA (>20 cm, involving the popliteal artery)
- Chronic total occlusions of popliteal artery and proximal bifurcation vessels

From Norgren L, Hiatt WR, Dormandy JA, et al: Inter-Society Consensus for the Management of Peripheral Arterial Disease (TASC II). *J Vasc Surg* 45(Suppl S):S5–S67, 2007.
CFA, common femoral artery; *SFA,* superficial femoral artery.

aortobifemoral bypass with a prosthetic graft through the transabdominal or retroperitoneal approach (Fig. 62-19). Preoperative imaging should delineate the target vessels, usually the common femoral or profunda femoris arteries. Proximal anastomoses can be performed in end-to-end or end-to-side configuration. For patients with external iliac occlusive disease, the end-to-side configuration is more commonly used because it may preserve perfusion to the pelvis through the diseased but patent common iliac, sacral, and lumbar collaterals. Arguments for end-to-end anastomosis include improved flow dynamics and the potential for decreased friction between the overlying bowel and graft. In the past, it was common practice to cut the body of the graft to leave minimal redundancy; however, it has become more popular to leave a longer segment of graft body and shorter limbs to ease the endovascular up-and-over approaches in the future. Minimal dissection in the area of the left common iliac artery is performed

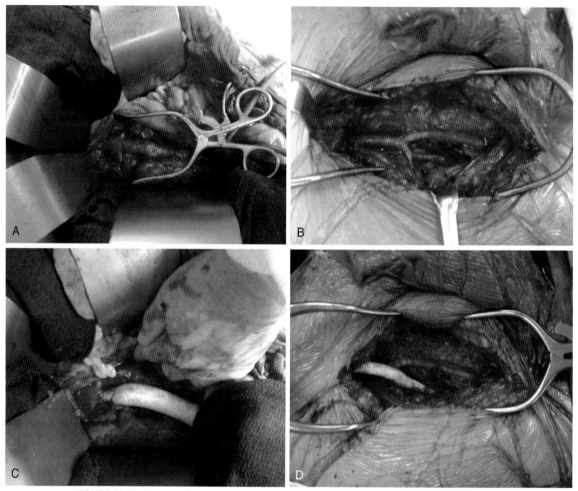

FIGURE 62-19 The patient from Figure 62-7 underwent aortobifemoral bypass. **A,** Note bilateral renal arteries. The left renal vein has been divided. **B,** Exposure of the right common femoral, profunda, and superficial femoral arteries. **C,** End-to-side aortic anastomosis using PTFE bifurcated graft. **D,** End-to-side profunda anastomosis. The patient had palpable distal pulses at the close of the procedure, despite long-term bilateral superficial femoral artery occlusion, and excellent collateral flow.

to protect the nervi erigentes and to avoid the complication of retrograde ejaculation. It is usual practice to close the retroperitoneum over the graft to protect it from the overlying bowel, which can potentially cause aortoenteric fistula through friction.

Alternative inflow sources include the thoracic aorta, axillary artery, and contralateral femoral artery if disease is unilateral.

Lower extremity occlusive disease. Patients with significant lesions involving the common femoral artery and origin of the profunda artery are usually best served with open groin exploration, common femoral artery endarterectomy, and profundaplasty or iliofemoral bypass. If concomitant iliac artery or SFA disease is present, patients may undergo combination procedures with iliac stent placement through open femoral access or SFA revascularization by femoropopliteal bypass or SFA stenting.

Vascular control is achieved with minimal force or traction. Heparin, 80 to 100 units/kg, is given for anticoagulation during periods of vascular occlusion. Anastomoses are constructed with care using small, evenly placed bites to include all layers of the vessel wall. Intraoperative completion arteriography is performed

in all small, distal tibial vessel bypasses as well as in larger arterial bypasses, such as femoropopliteal bypass, to assess technical adequacy and outflow. The anastomoses, graft, and runoff vessels are carefully examined in multiple planes and any defects corrected before closure.

The two main types of conduits used for lower extremity bypasses are the great saphenous veins and polytetrafluoroethylene (PTFE) grafts. The great saphenous veins should be used preferentially in all bypasses, especially in those reconstructions using below-knee popliteal and small tibial arteries as the distal target vessels. PTFE grafts can be used for bypasses to above-knee popliteal arterial segments with satisfactory patency rates.

To date, the disappointing patency rates for prosthetic grafts in below-knee and tibial bypasses have discouraged their use. Recently, a new PTFE graft with heparin coating on the luminal surface has been shown to be more resistant to thrombosis. Although these grafts may have an advantage over non–heparin-coated grafts, an adequately sized (4 mm or larger) saphenous vein remains preferable to synthetic conduits because of its innate antithrombotic properties.

The great saphenous vein can be placed in situ or reversed because of the presence of valves. The advantage of the reversed saphenous vein graft is that the valves do not need to be rendered incompetent with the use of a valvulotome. For the in situ vein graft, there is better size match—larger thigh vein for the common femoral artery and smaller leg vein for the tibial artery. Care must be used in passing the valvulotome to avoid tearing of the delicate vein. Neither of these configurations has been shown to be superior and surgeons use both, depending on their personal preference.

In the absence of a usable great saphenous vein, the cephalic and basilic veins from the upper extremities as well as the small saphenous vein of the leg should be evaluated. However, these veins have thinner walls and may have diseased segments that appear normal on external inspection. Furthermore, when several veins are joined to form a composite graft to achieve adequate length, there is the potential for technical complications and reduced overall patency. There is some evidence that the use of a vein patch with a prosthetic femorodistal bypass improves patency. Other conduits include cryopreserved arteries and veins, which have been shown to be more resistant to infection in the setting of gross infection.

For endarterectomy patch angioplasty, there are prosthetic patches of PTFE or Dacron. Bovine pericardial patches are also available. Alternatively, an endarterectomized segment of the native occluded SFA can be used for common femoral or profunda artery patch angioplasty or as a short-segment bypass conduit.

Femoropopliteal bypass. The femoropopliteal bypass is used in patients with superficial femoral and popliteal arterial occlusion with a popliteal artery segment distal to the occlusion that is patent, with luminal continuity with any tibial arterial branches. Bypasses can be performed even if one or more of the tibial arteries are occluded in the leg.

A longitudinal groin incision is used to access the common femoral artery. The popliteal artery is exposed medially from the thigh or the leg. In above-knee popliteal bypasses, an incision is made proximal to the knee for exposure of the artery near the adductor hiatus or Hunter canal, distal to the occlusive disease. In below-knee popliteal bypass, the popliteal space is accessed. The more superficial popliteal vein is retracted with a Silastic loop to assist with dissection of the underlying popliteal artery. If the saphenous vein is to be used, skin incisions are placed directly over the vein. A single long incision or multiple smaller skip incisions can be used. Alternatively, endoscopic vein harvesting can be performed. The graft is tunneled and placed in the anatomic space, under the sartorius muscle, unless an in situ saphenous vein graft is used.

Infrapopliteal bypass. The infrapopliteal bypass is used for arteries beyond the popliteal artery when there is arterial disease that involves the popliteal or proximal tibial artery. The target tibial artery will have luminal continuity to the foot without obstruction. With femoropopliteal and infrapopliteal bypasses, a tibial artery with stenosis of less than 50% distal to the distal anastomosis is acceptable, and neither the absence of a complete plantar arch nor the presence of vascular calcification is considered a contraindication to revascularization. The common femoral artery is generally used as the inflow for these bypasses. Shorter bypasses are preferred because of improved patency, so the SFA or popliteal artery may provide inflow if there is no proximal arterial disease. Bypasses to the arteries near the ankle or the foot can be performed if there is no patent artery more proximally.

Exposure of the posterior tibial artery is through a medial calf incision. The soleus muscle attachments to the tibia are taken down to expose the posterior tibial artery. Division of the overlying tibial veins exposes the tibial peroneal trunk. Further separation of the soleus muscle from the tibia provides access to terminal branches, the peroneal and posterior tibial arteries. For bypass to the anterior tibial artery, an additional anterolateral incision in the leg is made, midway between the tibia and fibula. Separation of the anterior tibial muscle and the extensor longus muscle exposes the neurovascular bundle. Further posterior dissection allows access to the interosseous membrane, and an incision is made to allow tunneling of the bypass graft. Exposure of the peroneal artery can be made through a medial incision, laterally by fibulectomy, or posteriorly by mobilization of the Achilles tendon.

Complications. Complications of surgery include superficial and deep wound infections, including those that involve the graft itself. One of the dreaded complications of aortic bypass is aorto-duodenal fistula, which has high mortality rates. The treatment is extra-anatomic bypass and graft removal, with débridement of the retroperitoneal tissues. An alternative to extra-anatomic bypass grafting is in situ bypass using bilateral superficial femoral veins, cryopreserved aortoiliac arteries, or antibiotic-soaked Dacron graft as conduit. In case of severe sepsis, an endograft system can be placed as a temporizing measure, with endograft and graft explantation when the patient is more stable. Other complications include groin hematoma, lymphatic leak or lymphocele, femoral nerve entrapment, limb swelling, and knee contracture.

Endovascular Management

Endovascular techniques require familiarity with a variety of devices, such as wires of varying lengths, thicknesses, and flexibility with hydrophobic or hydrophilic coatings; catheters with differing curves to negotiate angles with varying degrees of flexibility; sheaths to provide scaffolding support; balloons to dilate lesions; and bare-metal and covered stents to provide continuous outward radial force, to prevent arterial recoil, and to manage occlusive disease or dissections (Fig. 62-20).

A multitude of endovascular devices and techniques are available to the surgeon to treat PAD and aneurysmal disease, but there is little consensus about the best choice. The following are all viable alternatives to reestablish continuity of blood flow; each method has its enthusiastic proponents.

Subintimal angioplasty. First described in 1987,[7] the subintimal angioplasty technique involves use of a wire to create an arterial dissection purposely, beginning at the proximal segment of the arterial occlusion. With use of this plane, a chronic total occlusion can be circumvented. Once the wire has passed beyond the lesion, it reenters the true arterial lumen. The false lumen is treated with balloon angioplasty to increase its diameter. Although technical success rates have been favorable, long-term patency and limb salvage rates have not been impressive. In a review of 472 patients treated for principally TASC C and D lesions, 63% of patients presented with critical limb ischemia and the remaining with disabling claudication.[8] Stenotic lesions were not included. The mean increase in ABI was 0.27, from 0.50 ± 0.16 to 0.77 ± 0.23. The primary patency rates were disappointing at 45%, 30%, and 25% at 12, 24, and 36 months, respectively. Patency was higher in limbs treated for claudication, whereas reduced patency was significantly associated with femorotibial occlusions and critical limb ischemia. At 3 years, primary patency was 30% for claudication and 21% for critical limb ischemia.

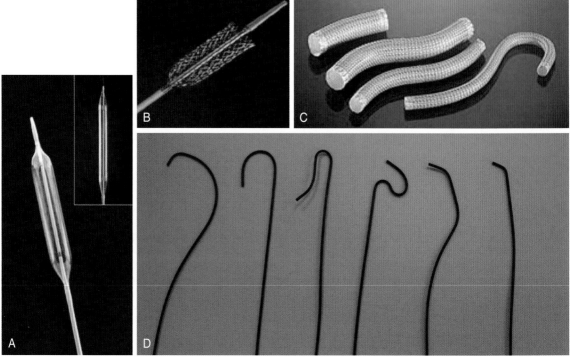

FIGURE 62-20 **A,** Balloon. **B,** Bare-metal stent. **C,** Stent grafts. **D,** Catheters.

Bare-metal stents were used in 20.3% of successful cases, but stent use was not associated with improved patency. Limb salvage for critical limb ischemia was a respectable 88% at 12 months, 81% at 24 months, and 75% at 36 months. Claudication was improved in 96.8% of limbs and sustained in 67% at 36 months. Overall, the results of subintimal angioplasty as a stand-alone procedure for critical limb ischemia have been underwhelming; adjuncts such as stents and stent grafts are often used to increase patency.

Balloon angioplasty. Balloon angioplasty, originally described in 1974, first requires crossing the arterial lesion transluminally with a guidewire and then inflating a balloon advanced over the wire at the location of the lesion. The treatment is considered successful if the residual stenosis is less than 30% or there is no pressure gradient across the area treated.

In the femoropopliteal segments, Clark and colleagues[9] reported a multicenter experience with 219 limbs in 205 patients. Patients were observed prospectively with clinical outcomes as well as objective testing by angiography or duplex ultrasound. The primary patencies at 12, 24, 36, 48, and 60 months for all limbs were 87%, 80%, 69%, 55%, and 55%, respectively. A negative predictor of long-term patency was found to be poor tibial runoff, specifically single tibial vessel runoff with 50% to 99% stenosis or occlusion. Diabetes or renal failure was also associated with lower patency.

In the tibioperoneal segment, Dorros and associates[10] reported a nonrandomized series of 312 patients with 417 vessels and 657 lesions. Overall technical success was 92% (98% in stenotic and 77% in occlusive lesions); 13 patients required stenting for intimal flap or dissection refractory to prolonged inflation. Claudication was relieved in 98% of patients with stenoses and in 86% of patients presenting with occlusions. Resolution of critical limb ischemia was noted in 98% of patients when stenotic lesions were

treated and in 77% of patients with occlusions. In a subsequent report of the 5-year experience for the same patients, there were 284 limbs in 235 patients with 529 lesions.[11] Follow-up was obtained in 215 (97%) successfully treated patients; 8% of the limbs required bypass surgery and 9% required amputation, yielding an overall limb salvage rate of 91% at 5 years.

Kudo and associates[12] published a 10-year experience of angioplasty for critical limb ischemia with 138 limbs in 111 patients. The most distal lesions treated were 33% in the iliac, 30% in the femoropopliteal, and 37% in the below-knee group. By Kaplan-Meier analysis, the primary patency and limb salvage rates for the femoropopliteal and below-knee groups at 3 years were 59.4% and 92.7% and 23.5% and 77.3%, respectively. Significant independent risk factors for outcomes included multiple-segment, more distal, and TASC D lesions.

Stenting. Sabeti and colleagues[13] have reported their experience with stainless steel and nitinol self-expanding stents for the treatment of femoropopliteal diseases in a retrospectively reviewed nonrandomized study. In their studies, 175 consecutive patients presented with claudication (150 patients) and critical limb ischemia (25 patients). Stents were placed electively after balloon angioplasty failure caused by residual stenosis or flow-limiting dissection. The cumulative patency rates at 6, 12, and 24 months were 85%, 75%, and 69%, respectively, for nitinol stenting versus 78%, 54%, and 34%, respectively, for stainless steel stenting. The authors noted significantly improved primary patency rates for nitinol stents.

The same authors also reported their early experience with long lesions (median length was 16 cm) in the femoropopliteal segment using only nitinol stents after primary failure of balloon angioplasty. The overall cumulative freedom from restenosis at 6 and 12 months was 79% and 54%, respectively. This was not affected by stent length or the number of stents used.

They later randomly assigned 104 patients with stenotic or occlusive SFA lesions to undergo primary stenting (51 patients) or angioplasty (53 patients), with optional stenting (32% receiving stents).[14] The mean length of the lesions was 13.2 cm for the stent group and 12.7 cm for the angioplasty group. At 6 months, the rate of restenosis was 24% in the stent group and 43% in the angioplasty group. These results were sustained at 2 years; the restenosis rate was 45.7% for the stent group versus 69.2% for the angioplasty group. During this period, re-intervention was also lower in the primary stenting group (37% versus 53.8%).

With advances in technology, angioplasty and stenting of infrapopliteal lesions are gaining acceptance. Kickuth and coworkers[15] reported their initial experience with a low-profile, self-expanding nitinol stent. They treated 35 patients, 19 with lifestyle-limiting claudication and 16 with critical limb ischemia. Selective stenting was performed after failed balloon angioplasty caused by residual stenosis, elastic recoil, or flow-limiting dissections. Stent placement was performed in 22 patients with distal popliteal artery lesions and in 13 patients with tibioperoneal artery lesions. Technical success was achieved in all patients. Follow-up studies were performed with duplex ultrasound and angiography. The 6-month primary patency rate was 82%. The authors noted the feasibility of treating infrapoplitcal lesions with the new nitinol stent.

A meta-analysis was reported by Mwipatayi and colleagues[16] comparing balloon angioplasty with stenting for the treatment of femoropopliteal lesions. Seven randomized controlled trials between September 2000 and January 2007 comparing angioplasty with stenting were used for this meta-analysis. Of a total of 934 patients, 482 patients were treated with stenting and the rest (452) with balloon angioplasty. The mean length treated was 4.3 cm in the angioplasty group and 4.6 cm in the stent group. The use of stents did not improve the patency rate at 1 year, which varied from 63% to 90%. However, limitations include length of follow-up, various stents used, and inconsistent use of optimal medical therapy.

Stent graft. One of the most widely used stent grafts (Fig. 62-21) in the treatment of chronic lower extremity ischemia is the Viabahn endoprosthesis (Gore Medical, Flagstaff, Ariz). It is constructed with an expanded PTFE liner attached to an external nitinol stent. The inner surface is bonded with heparin. This stent graft is extremity flexible, allowing it to conform closely to the anatomy of the SFA.

Railo and coworkers[17] first reported preliminary results in 15 patients with femoropopliteal lesions. The clinical presentation varied from claudication to acute leg ischemia as well as one ruptured popliteal artery aneurysm. Primary patency rates at 1 month, 12 months, and 24 months were 100%, 93%, and 84%, respectively. There was no limb loss during the follow-up period.

In a 6-year experience, Fischer and associates[18] evaluated outcomes for 57 patients treated for stenoses (13%) or occlusions (87%) of the SFA. The average length of treated lesions was 10.7 cm; 10% suffered early thrombosis of the graft within 30 days. The mean follow-up was 55 months (range, 8 to 78 months). The primary patency rates for 30 days, 1 year, 3 years, and 5 years were 90%, 67%, 57%, and 45%, respectively. In an earlier long-term study, Bleyn and coworkers[19] treated 67 patients with a mean lesion length of 14.3 cm. The 5-year primary patency rate was 47%.

Comparison of Viabahn treatment with different modalities has been reported by several authors. Saxon and associates[20] compared stent graft with percutaneous transluminal angioplasty alone in a multicenter, prospective randomized study. The stent graft group had a significantly higher technical success rate (95% versus 66%; $P < .0001$) and higher 1-year primary patency rate (65% versus 40% for percutaneous transluminal angioplasty alone).

In a prospective randomized study, Kedora and coworkers[21] compared Viabahn with above-knee surgical bypass with synthetic graft material; 86 patients with 100 limbs were randomized to 50 limbs each for the stent graft and bypass. The mean length of artery stented was 25.6 cm. ABIs and duplex ultrasonography were used for follow-up. At 3, 6, 9, and 12 months, the primary patency rates were 84%, 82%, 75.6%, and 73.5% for stent grafts, respectively; for bypass, they were 90%, 81.8%, 79.7%, and 74.2%, respectively. The authors also noted similar re-intervention and secondary patency rates.

Cutting balloon. The cutting balloon was originally designed for use in the coronary artery for lesions resistant to compliant balloon angioplasty or in-stent restenotic lesions. The balloon features three or four atherotomes, or microsurgical blades, mounted longitudinally on the surface of a noncompliant balloon. The blades score the lesion and dilate the vessels with less force than in conventional balloon angioplasty.

Atherectomy. Endovascular atherectomy allows the physical removal of atherosclerotic plaque material from the blood vessel, with a theoretical benefit of removing the obstructing plaque rather than merely displacing it, as with angioplasty and stenting. Excisional atherectomy catheters remove and collect the atheroma, whereas ablative devices fragment the atheroma into small particles. Rotational cutters turn at speeds up to 8000 rpm, shaving the atherosclerotic plaque material from the luminal surface of the arterial wall and collecting it in a storage chamber. The 1-year patency rates range from 22% to 84%, with limb salvage rates of 62% to 86%.[22]

An example of ablative atherectomy includes the laser atherectomy, a cold-tipped laser that delivers bursts of ultraviolet xenon energy in short pulse durations. Its reported key feature is the ability to debulk tissue without damaging surrounding tissue, minimizing restenosis. Compared with balloon angioplasty alone, no difference was reported in 1-year patency or technical success.[23] The largest trial was the LACI (Laser Angioplasty for Critical Limb Ischemia) phase 2 study that involved 14 sites in the United States and Germany.[24] There were 145 patients with 155 limbs and 423 lesions: 41% SFA, 15% popliteal, 41% infrapopliteal, and 70% a combination of stenoses. Technical success was achieved in 86% of limbs, with most lesions TASC C and D. Limb salvage at 6 months was 93%.

Acute Limb Ischemia

A popular mnemonic for describing the presentation of an acutely ischemic leg is referred to as the five or six *p*'s, depending on one's willingness to include *p*oikilothermia; *p*ain, *p*allor, *p*ulselessness, *p*aresthesias, and *p*aralysis are often cited as indicative of acute arterial ischemia. These symptoms and findings, however, are often variable in degree and not necessarily predictive of the extent of disease or degree of ischemia. A similar presentation may be seen in the setting of blunt or penetrating trauma, in which the native, nondiseased blood supply is suddenly interrupted. It is the acuity of the insult that leads to this constellation of symptoms; the chronically ischemic limb may have become so over a duration of time that allowed collateral flow to develop. The patient with acute ischemia may have less developed collateral circulation and less tolerance to prolonged ischemia.

The cause of acute limb ischemia is usually thromboembolism in the intervention-naïve patient. The source of the embolism can

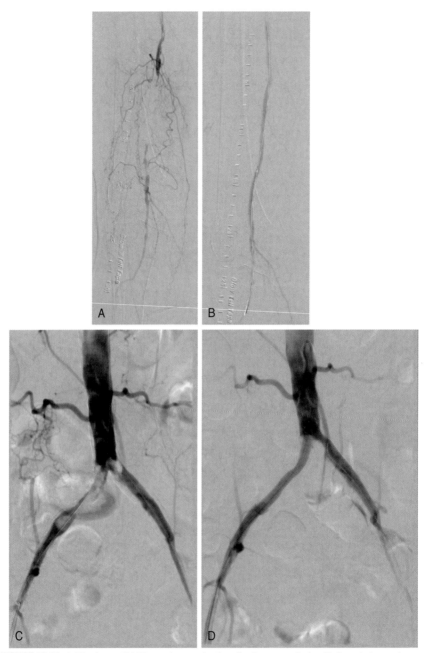

FIGURE 62-21 **A,** Distal superficial femoral to proximal popliteal artery occlusion. **B,** Completion angiogram after recanalization and stent placement. **C,** Bilateral common iliac artery thrombus, acute. **D,** Successful treatment with stent graft. Flow was restored without distal embolization.

be the heart, in which case atrial fibrillation is a commonly observed comorbidity. Alternative embolic sources include the valvular leaflets, and the aorta and iliac arteries may house thrombus, with or without concurrent aneurysmal disease. Patients presenting with a surgical history of previous bypass or stent placement may have an acute occlusion from graft or stent failure or may have disease progression. This history and the location of the occlusive lesion will affect surgical decision making. Acute limb ischemia constitutes a surgical emergency. As in most cases of vascular disease, there are endovascular and open surgical methods for addressing the problem.

As in all cases, a detailed history and physical examination are needed for a clinical diagnosis of the severity of disease:
- Category I limbs are viable and not immediately threatened.
- Category IIa limbs are threatened but salvageable if treated.
- Category IIb limbs are salvageable if treated as an emergency.
- Category III limbs have irreversible ischemia and are not salvageable.

Therefore, patients whose limbs are viable and do not appear immediately threatened (category I) as well as patients whose limbs are threatened but salvageable without paralysis but with mild sensory changes (category IIa) are potential candidates for

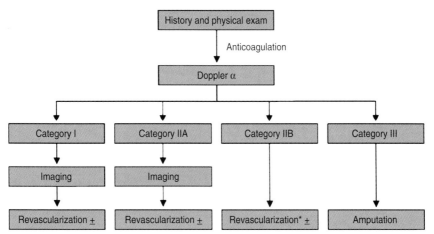

FIGURE 62-22 Treatment Algorithm for Acute Limb Ischemia. (From Norgren L, Hiatt WR, Dormandy JA, et al: Inter-Society Consensus for the Management of Peripheral Arterial Disease [TASC II]. *J Vasc Surg* 45 [Suppl]:S5–S67, 2007.) Category I—Viable; Category IIA—Marginally Threatened; Category IIB—Immediately Threatened; α Confirming either absent or severely diminished ankle pressure/signals; *In some centers imaging would be performed.

thrombolytic therapy. Patients with threatened limbs with more significant neurologic changes (category IIb) require a more urgent intervention and may best be served with an operative intervention. Patients with irreversible ischemia and a nonsalvageable limb usually require primary amputation (Fig. 62-22).

Patients with viable or minimally threatened limbs are candidates for thrombolytic therapy. They must have no contraindication to thrombolysis, which would include an active bleeding diathesis, recent gastrointestinal bleeding (<10 days), intracranial or spinal surgery, and intracranial trauma within the previous 3 months. Also, patients with a recent cerebrovascular accident, within 2 months, represent an absolute contraindication to thrombolysis. Relative major contraindications include major nonvascular surgery or trauma within the previous 10 days, uncontrolled hypertension, puncture of noncompressible vessels, intracranial tumors, and recent eye surgery. Minor contraindications to thrombolysis include hepatic failure, bacterial endocarditis, pregnancy, and diabetic hemorrhagic retinopathy.

An alternative to thrombolysis is open thrombectomy. Patients are begun on heparin on presentation. Proximal and distal control on the femoral versus below-knee popliteal artery is obtained. A longitudinal arteriotomy is created, and the thrombectomy balloon is passed proximally and distally with care until excellent forward bleeding and reasonable backbleeding are seen. Fluoroscopy can be used to assist in the thrombectomy procedure, with contrast material used in the embolectomy balloon and within the artery. Once the clot is successfully removed, the artery is flushed proximally and distally with heparinized saline before the clamps are replaced. Patch angioplasty should be considered to avoid narrowing of the artery. Completion angiography is helpful for confirming removal of most of the thrombus and identifying a culprit lesion. Four-compartment fasciotomy may be necessary, depending on the duration of ischemic insult.

Complications of open thrombectomy include intimal damage and dissection. Complications of thrombolysis include bleeding, which in minor cases is from the arterial access, venipuncture sites, or Foley catheter, but it can be severe and lead to hemothorax, gastrointestinal bleeding, and symptomatic intracranial hemorrhage.

If no culprit lesion is found, the patient should undergo a hypercoagulable workup. Oral anticoagulation should be considered.

OTHER CAUSES OF ACUTE AND CHRONIC LIMB ISCHEMIA

Nonatherosclerotic Arteriopathies

Other causes of arterial occlusive disease, although far less common than atherosclerosis in the West, should be considered for patients who do not fit the risk factor profile outlined earlier.

Raynaud Syndrome

Episodic digital ischemia was first described by Maurice Raynaud in 1862. Raynaud phenomenon is characterized by recurrent episodic vasospasm of the digits precipitated by a stimulus such as environmental cold or emotional stress, manifesting as tricolor changes—white, blue, and red. It initially produces pallor from cold exposure and vasoconstriction, subsequent cyanosis from hypoxia, and then rubor from the hyperemic response associated with rewarming. The digits return to normal 10 to 15 minutes after removal of the stimulus, and the fingers remain normal between ischemic episodes. Fingers of both hands are usually involved, extending to the metacarpophalangeal joint, with sparing of the thumb. The lower extremities are rarely involved. The clinical spectrum is broad, ranging from milder forms managed by avoidance to cold to more severe symptoms of ulceration and tissue loss from vascular occlusions beyond vasospasm. Secondary Raynaud phenomenon can be associated with various connective tissue diseases, such as scleroderma, or exposure to drugs, toxins, or repetitive trauma.

The prevalence of Raynaud syndrome varies with climate, approaching 20% to 25% in cool, damp regions such as Scandinavia and the Pacific Northwest. It usually occurs in young women, with a median age at onset of 14 years, and rarely after the age of 40 years. In these patients, 25% have a family history of Raynaud syndrome in a first-degree relative.

The evaluation of patients for Raynaud syndrome should include complete blood cell count determination of erythrocyte sedimentation rate, antinuclear antibody titer, and rheumatoid factor. Routine vascular laboratory testing with digital photoplethysmography and digital blood pressures can help distinguish patients with obstructive disease from those with an abnormal vasoconstrictive response. A digital hypothermic cold challenge test has been described, with an overall sensitivity and accuracy of approximately 90%.

The hallmark of conservative treatment is the avoidance of cold and emotional stimuli. All patients with Raynaud syndrome should refrain from tobacco use. The most widely used pharmacologic agents are calcium channel blockers. Patients with digital ulcers can usually be healed with aggressive local wound care and débridement. Surgical intervention is reserved for patients with proximal atherosclerotic or aneurysmal disease in an effort to eliminate any embolic source or potential physical impediment to perfusion.

Buerger Disease

Thromboangiitis obliterans, or Buerger disease, predominantly affects young male smokers in their 30s, presenting with distal limb ischemia and localized digital gangrene. There is an increasing incidence in women that likely parallels changes in smoking patterns. There is an increased incidence in patients of eastern European or Japanese heritage. Diagnostic hallmarks include age at onset before 45 years, exposure to tobacco, absence of arterial lesions proximal to the knee or elbow, and absence of other atherosclerotic risk factors.

Thromboangiitis obliterans is a polyarteritis nodosa vasculitis, with surgical specimens showing involvement of arteries and veins. Occlusive lesions are seen typically in small and medium-sized arteries. It usually occurs in the distal portions of the upper and lower extremities distal to the elbow and knee. Patients frequently have rest pain, ulceration, and, often, digital gangrene. Objective confirmation can be obtained with four-limb digital plethysmography, showing obstructive arterial waveforms in all digits. Arteriography typically reveals extensively diseased infrageniculate vessels and diffuse plantar arterial occlusions. The reconstitution of distal arterial segments is provided by tortuous, pathognomonic, corkscrew collaterals.

Treatment requires absolute tobacco cessation, which often results in clinical remission. Finger ulcers can frequently be healed with aggressive local wound care. Up to one third of patients with lower extremity disease will eventually require major amputation. Distal arterial bypass or endovascular intervention should be considered when it is anatomically feasible for critical limb ischemia, but the distal to proximal pattern of disease progression often precludes successful surgical revascularization. Currently, there is no effective pharmacologic treatment.

Vasculitis

The term *vasculitis* refers to a primary inflammatory process involving blood vessels with resultant transmural injury, necrosis, and obstruction or obliteration of the lumen. Vessels of any size and location can be affected. A useful classification system for vasculitis may be based on the size of the vessels involved by the inflammatory process: large-, medium-, or small-vessel vasculitis.

Large-Vessel Vasculitis

The large-vessel vasculitides includes giant cell arteritis (GCA), also referred to as temporal arteritis, and Takayasu arteritis. Although both vasculitides can affect the aorta and its major branches, GCA primarily involves the extracranial branches of the carotid artery. GCA usually occurs in older patients, whereas Takayasu arteritis afflicts younger female patients, with a higher prevalence in those of Asian or eastern European heritage. Both conditions are associated with the development of aneurysms of the thoracic and abdominal aorta and the progression of occlusive disease in the carotid, upper extremity, visceral, and renal arteries.

Giant cell arteritis (temporal arteritis). GCA usually occurs in patients older than 55 years. It is two to three times more common in women than in men. The average annual incidence is 18 cases/100,000 in older women. It primarily affects branches of the external carotid artery (ECA), although it may involve any large artery of the body. Patients may describe a history of a febrile myalgic process, with aching and stiffness of the hip, back, and shoulders lasting 4 weeks or more. Constitutional symptoms include headaches, malaise, anorexia, and weight loss. A characteristic presentation is severe pain over the temporal artery that is frequently bilateral, with tenderness and nodularity of the artery. Up to 20% of patients may develop permanent unilateral blindness; one third of them progress to contralateral blindness within an additional week's time.

Treatment should be prompt, consisting of high-dose corticosteroids. Patients suspected of having GCA should undergo temporal artery biopsy before the initiation of steroid therapy. Bilateral sequential temporal artery biopsies may be needed. The erythrocyte sedimentation rate is elevated in 75% of patients, although the C-reactive protein level may be a more sensitive indicator.

Early initiation of steroid therapy can result in prevention of blindness and restoration of pulses. Revascularization is rarely needed because of the collateral vessels that develop; it is relatively contraindicated during the acute phase of GCA.

Takayasu disease. Takayasu disease most commonly occurs in young, Asian female patients ranging in age from 3 to 35 years (85%). Patients present initially with fever, anorexia, and myalgia, followed by a second stage of multiple arterial occlusive symptoms, depending on the location of disease involvement.

The disease frequently affects the aorta, its major branches, and the pulmonary artery. Lesions are usually stenotic but may also be manifested as aneurysmal degeneration. Four patterns of cardiovascular manifestations have been described. Type I is localized to the arch and the arch vessels. Type II involves the descending thoracic and abdominal aorta. Type III involves the arch vessels and abdominal aorta and its branches. Type IV involves the pulmonary arteries.

Patients are best treated with conservative medical management. Surgical or endovascular intervention is used for symptomatic stenotic disease but is undertaken only when the active inflammatory process has been brought under control.

Medium-Vessel Vasculitis

Polyarteritis nodosa. Polyarteritis nodosa is a disseminated disease with transmural arterial necrosis of the medium-sized arteries. It occurs typically in the fourth to sixth decade and is more common in men than in women by a 2:1 margin. The arteries of the kidney, liver, heart, and gastrointestinal tract are commonly affected. It is characterized by the formation of multiple visceral aneurysms, with attendant risk of rupture. Alternatively, the inflammatory process of polyarteritis nodosa may lead to arterial occlusions, manifesting as enteric perforation, gastrointestinal bleeding, or appendicitis.

Immunosuppressive therapy has greatly improved the 5-year survival from 15% to 80%. Patients with mild symptoms can be treated with steroid therapy alone. However, patients with poor prognostic indicators, such as renal insufficiency, require immunosuppressive therapy in addition to steroids.

Kawasaki disease. Kawasaki disease is an acute vasculitis with a predilection for involving the coronary arteries in children younger than 5 years, with a peak incidence at 1 year of age. Boys are affected more commonly than girls. The distinguishing feature of advanced Kawasaki disease is the formation of diffuse fusiform and saccular coronary artery aneurysms. Systemic arteritis can also occur, commonly affecting the iliac arteries in addition to the coronaries.

Death may result from acute myocardial infarction or arrhythmia following thrombosis of a coronary artery aneurysm. Alternatively, aneurysm rupture may occur. Treatment with aspirin and immune globulin therapy has decreased the mortality during the past 2 decades and reduced the incidence of coronary artery aneurysmal degeneration. If refractory, more complete immunosuppressive therapy should be considered.

Behçet disease. Behçet disease commonly is manifested as iritis associated with oral and genital mucocutaneous ulcerations. It primarily affects patients from the Mediterranean area and Japan. The vasculitis component of Behçet disease involves the venous and arterial systems. Venous thrombosis is the most common vascular disorder with Behçet disease. Arterial lesions, although less frequent, are associated with a higher incidence of mortality. The usual cause of mortality in these patients is aortic aneurysmal degeneration and rupture.

Patients with Behçet disease and venous thrombosis are managed with lifelong oral anticoagulation. Immunosuppressive therapy is used for nonarterial symptoms, such as mucocutaneous lesions and eye disease. Traditional aneurysm repair with interposition grafting has been associated with a high incidence of thrombosis and anastomotic pseudoaneurysms. Endovascular aneurysm repair is emerging as the treatment of choice.

Cogan syndrome. Cogan syndrome is a rare disease consisting of interstitial keratitis and vestibuloauditory symptoms. It may occasionally consist of aortitis, with subsequent aortic valvular insufficiency. Cogan syndrome commonly affects young patients in their third decade. High-dose steroid therapy can be used to reverse visual and auditory complications. Surgical intervention may be needed for aortic valve replacement, mesenteric revascularization, or thoracoabdominal aortic aneurysm repair.

Small-Vessel Vasculitis

Antineutrophil cytoplasmic antibody–associated vasculitides. The major forms of small-vessel vasculitis are associated with the presence of antineutrophil cytoplasmic antibodies, autoantibodies formed against enzymes found in primary granules of neutrophils. Antineutrophil cytoplasmic antibody–associated vasculitides include Wegener granulomatosis, microscopic polyangiitis, and Churg-Strauss syndrome and often have circulating antineutrophil cytoplasmic antibodies. Wegener granulomatosis is the most common form. The overall incidence of antineutrophil cytoplasmic antibody–associated vasculitides in the population is 10 to 20 per million/year, affecting men and women equally, with a peak onset in the 60s. Patients present with constitutional symptoms that include fever and weight loss. Wegener granulomatosis is characterized by renal and respiratory tract involvement. Microscopic polyangiitis is characterized by rapid progressive glomerulonephritis in almost all patients. Churg-Strauss syndrome is characterized by allergic rhinitis and asthma, eosinophilic infiltrative disease, and small-vessel vasculitis. Diagnostic testing should include assessment for inflammatory markers and for liver and renal function as well as assays for antineutrophil cytoplasmic antibodies, antinuclear antibodies, and rheumatoid factor. Small-vessel vasculitis can be documented by microscopic examinations of biopsy specimens from affected tissues, such as skin and kidney. Treatment involves three stages using corticosteroids and immunosuppressive therapy—induction of remission, maintenance of remission, and treatment of relapses.

Vasculitis Associated With Connective Tissue Diseases

Vasculitis is frequently associated with scleroderma, rheumatoid arthritis, and systemic lupus erythematosus. Scleroderma is characterized by small-vessel occlusion within the arterioles of the skin, gastrointestinal tract, kidneys, lung, and heart. Rheumatoid arthritis typically involves digital arteries and small vessels of the vasa nervorum. Lupus patients commonly have Raynaud syndrome but may also have atherosclerosis of large vessels. Treatment consists of steroid and immunosuppressive therapies.

Heritable Arteriopathies
Cystic Medial Necrosis

Cystic medial necrosis, formerly known as medial degeneration, is associated with collagen vascular disorders, Ehlers-Danlos syndrome, and Marfan syndrome, with elastolysis degrading aortic medial collagen and elastin. Aortic dissection is the result. Although it is also seen in normal aging, cystic medial necrosis is accelerated by hypertension and atherosclerosis.

Pseudoxanthoma Elasticum

Pseudoxanthoma elasticum is an inherited disease, with most patients demonstrating an autosomal recessive inheritance. The prevalence is 1 in 70,000 to 160,000. Patients present with baggy skin and yellow-orange cutaneous papules in intertriginous areas. Symptoms may include intermittent claudication, angina, and abdominal pain caused by involvement of cerebral, coronary, visceral, and peripheral vessels. Arterial disease can be seen in young patients (20s to 30s) without risk factors for atherosclerosis. Digital plethysmography shows abnormal pulse waveforms from loss of the elastic recoil of vessels. Arterial stenosis and occlusion with extensive calcification can be seen radiographically. Surgical and endovascular management options are the same as for atherosclerotic occlusive disease.

Arteria Magna Syndrome

Arteria magna syndrome is a disease characterized by arterial elongation, dilation, and tortuosity. It occurs in younger patients with no evidence of atherosclerosis, with a familial incidence in first-degree relatives. There is a propensity for arterial aneurysm formation in multiple sites. Arteriograms show characteristic arterial widening and tortuosity, slow arterial flow velocity, and multiple aneurysms. The low-velocity arterial flow makes arteriography difficult to perform, requiring a large volume of contrast material and multiple injections with delayed timing. These patients should be screened annually for the development of aneurysms in the aorta and iliac, femoral, and popliteal arteries. Symptomatic aneurysms or those whose diameter is 2 to 2.5 times that of the parent arteries should be repaired. Complications of arterial occlusions are almost always caused by thrombosis or embolization. A number of surgical interventions are often needed for aneurysms at multiple sites.

Congenital Conditions Affecting the Arteries
Persistent Sciatic Artery

The sciatic artery in the embryo is a vessel that arises from the umbilical artery and supplies the lower extremity. During development, this artery is replaced by the femoral artery from the external iliac artery, and the remnants of the sciatic artery remain as the inferior gluteal artery, distal popliteal artery, and peroneal artery. Rarely, this sciatic artery persists as a large artery that is located in the posterior thigh, exiting the pelvis to continue as the popliteal artery. The SFA may coexist or be hypoplastic or absent. On occasion, this may be detected in an individual with an absent femoral pulse but palpable distal pulses. However, the persistent sciatic artery usually is not detected until patients are in their 50s and symptoms typical of PVD develop. Up to 25% of patients may present with pulsatile buttock masses caused by aneurysmal degeneration. Surgical intervention is indicated for ischemic and aneurysmal complications. Options include arterial ligation, endovascular coiling for occlusion of an isolated aneurysm, and iliopopliteal or femoropopliteal bypasses.

Popliteal Entrapment Syndromes

This syndrome is based on an anomalous anatomic relationship between the popliteal artery and surrounding gastrocnemius muscle that may occur during embryonic development. The most common variant (50%) is the medial location of the popliteal artery to the normally placed medial head of the gastrocnemius muscle. The second most common variant (25%) is the medial location of the popliteal artery to the abnormally attached medial head of the gastrocnemius muscle. In other variants, the normally located popliteal artery may be compressed by muscle slips of the medial head of the gastrocnemius muscle or fibrous bands. Symptoms are caused by obstruction of the popliteal artery with gastrocnemius contraction. The typical patient is a younger man (younger than 30 years; 90%) without risk factors for PVD; 20% of patients have the disorder bilaterally. Popliteal entrapment syndrome should be suspected in younger patients with calf claudication.

Diagnosis with noninvasive arterial duplex ultrasound and photoplethysmography is difficult and findings are nonspecific. Arteriography may be nonspecific. MRI is the diagnostic modality of choice because it will show the anomalous relationships between the popliteal artery and gastrocnemius muscle. Treatment is indicated for symptomatic patients and requires surgical intervention. Removal of the medial gastrocnemius head may be sufficient for patients with minimal arterial disease. Patients with arterial stenosis or aneurysmal degeneration should be treated with arterial bypass using autogenous veins.

Adventitial Cystic Disease

Adventitial cystic disease is another rare condition that should be considered in younger patients with claudication. The arterial stenosis is caused by compression of the lumen from synovial-like cysts in the subadventitial layer of the arterial wall. It is commonly located in the popliteal artery but may also be found in the iliac and femoral arteries. Patients present in their 40s, and 80% are men. Diagnosis may be made with ultrasonography, CT, or MRI. Arteriography may show a scimitar sign, with luminal compression by the cyst. The artery is normally placed, with no signs of atherosclerotic disease. Treatment with CT- or ultrasound-guided needle aspiration may be used for small cysts, although there may be a 10% rate of recurrence. Arterial bypass with an autogenous vein is used for patients with large cysts causing arterial compression or occlusion.

Peripheral Artery Aneurysms
Femoral and Popliteal Artery Aneurysms

Femoral and popliteal artery aneurysms account for more than 90% of peripheral aneurysms, with popliteal artery aneurysms being the most common (70%). However, they are still relatively uncommon. The estimated incidence of femoral and popliteal aneurysms is approximately 7/100,000 men and 1/100,000 women. Femoral aneurysms usually involve the common femoral artery but may occasionally extend or be limited to the SFA in the midthigh. Femoral and popliteal aneurysms are commonly associated with other aneurysms, with approximately 80% of patients having multiple aneurysms. In patients with common femoral aneurysms, 90% have an aortoiliac aneurysm and 60% have bilateral femoral aneurysms. In patients with popliteal aneurysms, 70% have an aortoiliac aneurysm and 50% have bilateral popliteal aneurysms. Femoral and popliteal aneurysms show a high incidence of thromboembolic complications, which can result in limb loss.

The diagnosis of femoral and popliteal aneurysms is suspected in patients with widened pulses that are easily palpated. These aneurysms should be considered in patients presenting with foot embolization or acute limb ischemia. CT and ultrasonography can accurately diagnose the femoral and popliteal aneurysms. Ultrasonography should be used for patients with aortoiliac aneurysms to search for these peripheral aneurysms. Arteriography is important for visualization of the aneurysms and runoff to plan for surgical intervention.

Femoral and popliteal aneurysms should be considered for treatment when the diagnosis is made. Because of the high incidence of thromboembolic events, these aneurysms are repaired, regardless of size. Even small aneurysms can cause ischemic limb complications. Surgical intervention of the femoral aneurysms consists of resection of the aneurysms with interposition grafts. Treatment of the popliteal aneurysms usually involves bypass using autogenous veins, with exclusion of the aneurysm to prevent embolization. Patients with ischemic limbs from embolic complications may require thrombolytic therapy to establish arterial outflow before bypass surgery. Endovascular repair with covered stents is emerging as the treatment of choice for popliteal aneurysms (Fig. 62-23).

Evaluating the Success of Revascularization Procedures

Although there is a lack of consensus about the best endovascular modality to use for most patients, there is certainly a need for routine follow-up and close involvement of all patients treated for claudication and critical limb ischemia. The ultimate success of any intervention performed, endovascular or open surgical bypass, can be improved by a continued relationship with the patient and regular examination. Smoking cessation counseling and adjuvant techniques, such as medications and nicotine replacement, are used routinely to help patients with this important aspect of their treatment. Lifelong administration of oral antiplatelet agents (81 mg aspirin daily and 75 mg clopidogrel daily) and aggressive lipid modification in all patients who have had a vascular intervention are routine.

Duplex arterial ultrasound has gained wide acceptance as the modality of choice for surgical bypass graft surveillance, and it has become the standard for observing patients treated with endovascular therapy. Contemporary practice guidelines include a baseline duplex ultrasonography scan before intervention, another after the intervention to document improvement (the timing of this scan varies from 1 day to 2 weeks after the intervention), and then additional scans at 3 and 6 months after the procedure to assess for continued efficacy. Duplex ultrasonography is then performed at 6-month intervals thereafter. Evaluation of continued

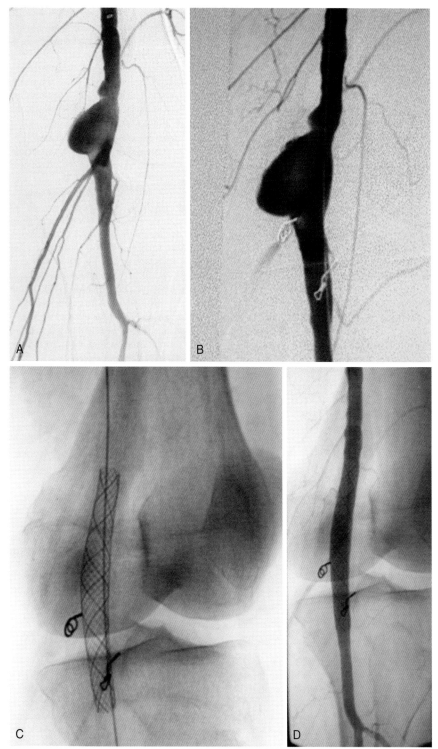

FIGURE 62-23 A, Popliteal aneurysm. **B,** Collateral feeding branches treated with coil embolization. **C,** Stent placement to exclude flow into aneurysm sac. **D,** Completion angiogram showing successful repair.

subjective clinical improvement and determination of ABIs are essential and simple adjunctive measures that should be performed at each visit. Most studies discussed earlier used duplex ultrasonography as their method of imaging follow-up. Although very early studies and coronary trials used routine postprocedure

contrast angiography (at 6 months and 1 year), the ready availability, lower risk, and proven sensitivity and specificity of duplex ultrasonography have made it the preferred method of follow-up over contrast angiography. Once a problem has been identified, routine surveillance with duplex ultrasonography and selective angiography is the standard for open and endovascular intervention.

The benefit of graft surveillance by duplex ultrasonography in lower extremity bypass has been established. Reports have shown that all vein grafts progress to occlusion when stenosis of more than 70% diameter reduction is detected by ultrasound surveillance. Buth and coworkers further established the duplex criteria needed to identify high-risk lesions: peak systolic velocity at the site of the lesion exceeding 300 to 350 cm/sec or a velocity ratio exceeding 3.5 or 4.[25] The ratio is calculated using the peak systolic velocity at the site of the lesion divided by the peak systolic velocity of a normal graft segment proximal to the lesion.

Using these duplex criteria, Mills and colleagues[26] studied the natural history of autogenous infrainguinal vein grafts with intermediate and critical stenosis. A peak systolic velocity higher than 300 cm/sec or velocity ratio of more than 4 was used to detect critical stenosis. In grafts with the unrevised critical stenosis, almost 80% progressed to occlusion, all within 4 months of ultrasound detection. For grafts with intermediate stenosis, the occlusion rate was no different from that of grafts without stenosis, and serial surveillance was safe and effective.

Calligaro and associates[27] have established the usefulness of surveillance in prosthetic grafts; 85 prosthetic bypasses in 59 patients were studied in a graft surveillance protocol. There were 35 femoropopliteal, 16 femorotibial, 15 iliofemoral, 13 axillofemoral, and 6 femorofemoral bypasses. The benefit of duplex ultrasound was compared with other noninvasive studies, such as changes in symptoms or pulses and ABI. Follow-up was performed 1 week and every 3 months after the initial bypass or after graft revision, for a mean of 11 months. Duplex ultrasound was able to predict 81% of graft failures versus 24% with use of nonultrasound findings. In the presence of a normal study, the likelihood of a graft failure was 7% with use of duplex criteria versus 21% with nonultrasound studies. In contrast, Carter and coworkers[28] concluded that surveillance is a valid method for detecting high-risk lesions in vein grafts but failed in prosthetic and femorocrural grafts. It was noted that prosthetic grafts and femorocrural bypasses tended to occlude without any prior documented stenosis, whereas vein grafts were more likely to develop progressive stenosis before occlusion.

Lesion characteristics detected during ultrasound surveillance may also be used to determine the type of re-intervention needed. Gonsalves and colleagues[29] noted factors based on temporal and duplex data. Percutaneous transluminal angioplasty is recommended for short (<2 cm) stenoses in good-caliber veins (≥3.5 mm) found more than 3 months after the bypass procedure. Direct surgical repair or replacement is recommended for early (<3 months) and long-segment stenoses in small-caliber veins.

Although the use of duplex ultrasonography in endovascular follow-up is intuitive and consistent with the usefulness observed in the management of surgical bypass, few large studies have looked at its ability to predict failure and impact on long-term results. Tielbeek and coworkers[30] used duplex ultrasonography surveillance, clinical examination, and ABI on femoropopliteal lesions successfully treated with endovascular interventions. Impending failure was diagnosed with a peak systolic velocity ratio of more than 2.5. Failure was diagnosed as occlusion or recurrent stenosis requiring intervention for severe symptoms. Treatment failure was predicted by duplex ultrasonography, with a sensitivity of 86% and a specificity of 75%. Interestingly, ABI decrease was even more predictive, with a sensitivity of 93% and specificity of 90%.

Critical limb ischemia is often a hallmark of the beginning of the end game in the battle for survival in patients with diffuse atherosclerotic disease. With a known 5-year survival of less than 50%, this population is extremely disadvantaged. The surgeon's best chance for helping this group of patients lies in providing the least invasive intervention that will provide pain relief, tissue healing, and limb salvage. Close follow-up with appropriate counseling is essential, as is intensive medical management with repeated interventions performed as clinical conditions warrant. These measures offer the best strategy for limb salvage and improved mortality for patients with vascular disease. However, the final determinant of success is the patient's perception of enhancement in the quality of his or her remaining years of life.

RENAL ARTERY DISEASE

Renovascular hypertension occurs as a consequence of decreased blood flow through a stenotic renal artery. The renin-angiotensin system is a potent regulator of blood pressure. Renin is an enzyme produced in the juxtaglomerular cells of the afferent arterioles of the kidney. It is released into the bloodstream in response to reduced renal blood flow. Once it is systemic, renin acts on a plasma substrate to produce angiotensin I. Angiotensin I is converted to angiotensin II in the pulmonary circulation by angiotensin-converting enzyme. Angiotensin II, in addition to being a potent vasoconstrictor of smooth muscle in the arterial walls, stimulates the secretion of aldosterone from the adrenal cortex. Aldosterone enhances sodium absorption in the renal tubules, with an attendant increase in water retention and overall volume expansion. Angiotensin-converting enzyme inhibitors, which prevent the conversion of angiotensin I to the vasoactive angiotensin II, are a commonly used class of antihypertensive drugs.

In patients with unilateral renal artery stenosis, renin is elaborated and the blood pressure rises in response to arterial constriction and volume retention. The opposite unaffected kidney may successfully respond by excreting the excess intravascular volume. This condition, of elevated renin levels in the presence of unilateral renal artery stenosis and the contralateral kidney producing compensatory euvolemia, is known as renin-dependent hypertension. In patients with bilateral renal artery stenosis, renin levels rise and volume expands and is maintained. Elevated renin levels may initiate a negative feedback response from the afferent arteriole endothelium, with a resultant normal or decreased serum renin level but a persistent expansion of intracellular and intravascular volume. Thus, bilateral renal artery stenosis results in what is referred to as volume-dependent hypertension. The natural history of renal artery stenosis is a progressive decline in renal function and worsening hypertension refractory to medical management, presumably from a combination of ischemia and repetitive embolization. Atherosclerosis is the most common cause of renal artery stenosis, and renal atrophy has been observed in patients with atherosclerotic renal disease and progression of stenoses.[31,32] Hypertension directly attributable to renal artery stenosis is identified in less than 5% of all patients treated for hypertension. However, the prevalence of renal artery stenosis increases in certain populations, such as patients with atherosclerotic peripheral or coronary artery disease, young patients presenting with hypertension, and patients with a combination of hypertension refractory to medical management and concomitant renal insufficiency. Renal insufficiency and ischemic nephropathy can be a direct result of renal artery stenoses. As many as 40% of patients with end-stage renal disease requiring dialysis have been found to have a significant renal artery stenosis on evaluation with duplex ultrasound.[33]

Diagnosis

The diagnosis of renal artery stenosis can be made by duplex ultrasonography examination of the renal arteries. Duplex ultrasonography combines direct visualization of the renal arteries (B mode) with hemodynamic measurements in the renal arteries (Doppler-derived velocity). Furthermore, ultrasonography allows direct measurement of renal size. The procedure identifies the abdominal aorta at the level of the renal arteries and records blood velocity at this site, followed by identification and measurement of blood velocity in the renal arteries. Other measurements include those of renal parenchymal velocities from the upper, middle, and lower poles of the kidneys as well as renal size. The important parameter is the ratio of velocity in the renal artery to that of the aorta. If the ratio is more than 3.5, this is likely to be associated with a stenosis of more than 60%. If the renal artery velocity is more than 180 cm/sec, this is also considered abnormal. The test is limited by the experience of the operator and by the patient's habitus (being more difficult in obese patients) and bowel gas. Thus, Doppler ultrasonography of the kidneys is best performed in the early morning, after fasting. Reported sensitivity and specificity range from 90% to 95% and 60% to 90%, respectively. In one study, if renal arteriograms were obtained on all patients with a positive finding on Doppler ultrasound, a 2.7% false-positive rate was found. A further use of Doppler ultrasonography may be in predicting which patients would benefit from revascularization. The renal resistive index (RRI) is obtained from Doppler ultrasonography. It can be expressed by the following:

$$RRI = 1 - \frac{\text{End-diastolic velocity}}{\text{Maximal systolic velocity}} \times 100$$

The RRI has been predictive in determining the response of blood pressure to revascularization. An RRI higher than 0.80 has identified patients with renal artery stenosis in whom angioplasty or surgery did not improve blood pressure or renal function. Finally, the presence of asymmetrical kidney size may be a clue to underlying renal artery stenosis and renal ischemia.

Magnetic Resonance Angiography

This technique can be used for the diagnosis of proximal (and thus largely atherosclerotic) renal artery stenosis. Gadolinium is used as a contrast agent for patients with a glomerular filtration rate of more than 30 mL/min. Reconstructions of images are used to obtain detailed views of the renal arteries. Limitations include the high cost, limited availability, and substantial expertise needed to analyze images. Results for CTA are similar, again with the disadvantage of requiring contrast material, with the attendant risk of nephropathy.

Other imaging studies in addition to MRA, such as contrast angiography, may also be diagnostic but are associated with increased cost and morbidity. In practice, however, many renal artery stenotic lesions are discovered incidentally during studies performed for other reasons.

Serologic renin measurements of blood obtained by venous sampling were once commonly used to validate the significance of an identified renal artery stenosis. These required that a catheter be inserted into the venous system and blood samples obtained from each renal vein and the vena cava. In patients with unilateral renal artery stenosis, a renin ratio of the affected kidney to the opposite kidney of 1.5 or higher is highly suggestive of the stenosis

functionally activating the renin system. In a large series, an abnormal ratio was 92% predictive of curability with revascularization; however, 65% of patients with nonlateralizing renin ratios also had curable disease. In an effort to improve the sensitivity and specificity of the test, the renal-systemic renin index has been used. This allows determination of the functional significance of bilateral lesions. The index is obtained by subtracting the systemic (infrarenal vena cava) plasma renin activity from the plasma renin activity in the renal veins and dividing by the systemic plasma renin activity. An index above 0.24 indicates excessive renin production from that kidney, whereas lower levels are indicative of renin suppression. However, given the invasive nature of these tests and the low specificity, renal vein renin sampling is usually reserved for diagnostic dilemmas.

Treatment

Difficult to control hypertension (e.g., the patient is taking three or more antihypertensive medications) or decreased renal function and a hemodynamically significant stenosis are the most commonly used indications for intervention.

Open Renal Artery Bypass

Open renal artery bypass is rarely performed as an isolated procedure with the advent of renal artery stenting. Surgical procedures used to correct renal artery stenosis included aortorenal bypass with vein grafts, arterial autografts (for children) or prosthetic grafts, aortorenal endarterectomy, hepatic artery–renal artery bypass, gastroduodenal–renal artery bypass, and splenic artery–renal artery bypass. These procedures, although durable and revered by surgeons, are obviously maximally invasive and can be associated with significant morbidity. They have been almost universally supplanted by angioplasty and stenting procedures.

Renal Artery Stenting

Value, limitations, and techniques. Percutaneous therapy for renovascular occlusive disease has become the preferred alternative to open renal revascularization. In the appropriately selected patient, angioplasty and stenting of renal artery stenoses have been shown to be safe and effective options for severe hypertension and ischemic nephropathy. Catheter-based treatment, especially when it is performed with lower profile systems, can be performed with minimal morbidity and a reliably high degree of initial technical success. The long-term beneficial effects on blood pressure control and renal function have been debated but appear to be valid.

Renal angioplasty was first performed in 1978 by Grüntzig and colleagues,[34] and there have been many series demonstrating the success of this interventional procedure. With the advent of the stent, durability, efficacy, and ultimately acceptance of catheter-based management of renal artery lesions have increased. Stents were initially used for cases of immediate technical failure, such as residual anatomic stenoses of more than 30%, residual pressure gradients or postangioplasty dissections, or recurrent stenoses after prior angioplasty. Routine stenting of renal artery stenoses (as an adjunct to balloon angioplasty), especially in treatment of ostial lesions, has become an accepted practice. The incidence of recurrent stenosis has been shown to be significantly decreased with angioplasty and stent placement versus angioplasty alone.[35]

Although the number of patients completely cured of renovascular hypertension after renal artery stenting has been reported to be as low as 5% or less,[36] up to 80% of patients treated demonstrate measurable improvement in blood pressure control.[35-39] Henry and associates[37] have reported a series of 210 patients with chronic hypertension and a diastolic blood pressure higher than 90 mm Hg who underwent renal artery angioplasty and stenting. A favorable response was seen in 80% of patients, with 35% reported as cured of hypertension. In this study, a hypertensive cure was defined as diastolic blood pressure less than 90 mm Hg achieved without the administration of antihypertensive medications. In another series of patients treated with stenting for renal artery stenosis associated with hypertension, impaired renal function, or both, only 4.2% achieved a complete cure, but an additional 79% benefited from an improvement in hypertensive control.[36] A meta-analysis of 14 studies involving renal angioplasty and stenting has found an overall 20% cure rate for hypertension, with 49% of patients experiencing an improvement in hypertensive control.[35] This meta-analysis recognized the variability in reporting criteria for a cure among the different renal angioplasty and stent series.

Improvement in serum creatinine level may be seen in approximately 30% of patients after renal angioplasty and stenting.[37] However, a higher percentage of patients demonstrate a clinical benefit of creatinine stabilization when renal artery stents are placed for ischemic nephropathy.[36,40] Rundback and coworkers[41] have reported a series of 45 patients with azotemia who received a renal stent for treatment of a renal stenosis. A clinical benefit was defined as improvement or stabilization of creatinine levels. Life-table analysis demonstrated a benefit at 12, 24, and 36 months in 72%, 62%, and 54% of patients, respectively. In patients with significant renal artery stenosis and a solitary functioning kidney, renal artery stenting has been shown to be a safe alternative to surgery. Bush and colleagues[42] have reported a series of 27 patients, each with a solitary functioning kidney and azotemia, who underwent endovascular treatment of significant renal artery stenosis. An improvement or stabilization of renal function was seen in 74% of patients.

There is variability among series in terms of renal stent patency rates. The reported incidence of recurrent stenoses of renal stents has ranged from as low as 1.5%[43] to as high as 25%[44] at 6 months. Several series of renal artery stenting have shown a patency of up to 5 years by life-table analysis. Rodriquez-Lopez and associates[45] have performed a life-table analysis of 108 patients undergoing renal angioplasty and primary stent placement and found 74% primary and 85% secondary patency rates. A larger series of patients with renal artery stents placed for failed angioplasty, recurrent stenosis, dissection, or ostial lesions was reported by Henry and colleagues.[37] This series demonstrated a 79% primary and 98% secondary patency at 5 years by life-table analysis.

Duplex surveillance is accurate for identifying recurrent renal artery stenosis.[46] The stenosis within a stent is most often caused by myointimal hyperplasia. Treatment usually consists of repeated angioplasty, and occasionally a new stent is required. Bax and colleagues[47] have reported a series of 15 patients with 20 stents with recurrent stenoses; 18 stents were successfully treated with angioplasty alone, and only two required the placement of a second stent. The 1-year success rate of the repeated interventions was 75%. Balloon-expandable covered stents may be helpful for recurrent in-stent restenosis in the future.

The morbidity and mortality of a major operative procedure can be avoided with endovascular treatment of renal artery stenoses. Mackrell and associates[48] have reported their experience with 165 patients who underwent endovascular or surgical intervention for renal artery stenosis. They noted a shift from open surgical revascularization of renal artery stenosis to endovascular treatment. In comparing endovascular treatment with surgical renal revascularization and combined aortic and renal revascularization, all had excellent technical success rates, but the surgical group had a significantly higher morbidity (5.6% versus 15% and 23%, respectively) and mortality rate (0% versus 9.1% and 8.1%).

With combined aortic and renal open reconstructions, the complexity of surgery is increased. Endovascular repair has become popular for the treatment of abdominal aortic aneurysms with suitable aortic anatomy. A renal artery stenosis in the presence of an abdominal aortic aneurysm can be treated before or after the aortic endograft is placed. A benefit to placing the renal stent before the endograft is to allow the stent to serve as a radiopaque marker for the origin of the renal artery. This may help in positioning and placement of the endograft below the renal arteries. One must be cautious not to entrap the endograft or the delivery system on the stent if it protrudes out into the aortic lumen.

The technical success of renal artery stent placement is high in most of the series, with technical failures usually caused by poor positioning or deployment of the stent. Access to the renal artery is an important consideration for renal artery stenting. The angulation of the renal arteries relative to the aorta and the short distance of the renal artery beyond the stenosis for secure guidewire placement can make renal stenting from a femoral artery access point challenging. A brachial or axillary approach is sometimes required to overcome the angulation of the renal artery or to avoid significant aortic and iliac disease. Radial artery access with angioplasty and stenting of the renal artery has been described.[49]

One early technical limitation of renal artery stenting was the large size of the 0.035-inch guidewire-based balloons and stents. These platforms required a 7 Fr or 8 Fr sheath, and tracking the stent into an angulated renal artery was difficult or sometimes not possible from a femoral approach. Miniaturization of balloons and stents was first shown to be safe and effective in coronary use[50] and, in some cases, resulted in shorter procedural times and use of less contrast material.[51] The required guiding sheath size is reduced with the lower profile balloons and stents that use 0.014- and 0.018-inch guidewire platforms. The lower profile angioplasty balloons and stents have a better ability to negotiate difficult angles. These factors have led to the routine use of 0.014-inch systems for renal artery stenosis. The following is a stepwise guide to our preferred technique for renal artery angioplasty and stenting with use of the lower profile angioplasty balloons and stents.

Renal Angioplasty and Stent Procedure

See Figure 62-24.

Renal artery access and guide sheath positioning. Arterial access, femoral or brachial, is an important initial decision that has been made easier with the lower profile balloon, stent, and sheath systems. Retrograde common femoral access is the first choice, usually secondary to table and patient positioning constraints. Brachial access is used only in certain circumstances, such as severe aortoiliac occlusive disease, aortic aneurysms, and extreme caudal renal artery angulation. In most cases, an antero-posterior aortogram is first obtained, with a pigtail catheter in the suprarenal position. Oblique angulation is sometimes required to better visualize the renal origins. To limit contrast material, a selective catheterization can be made without the aortogram if one has been previously obtained. Alternative contrast agents, such as carbon dioxide and gadolinium, have been successfully used in renal angiography and renal artery interventions.[52,53] Most renal arteries can be accessed simply with an angled catheter; however, some will require a more complex-shaped catheter, such as a cobra, shepherd's hook, or Simmons catheter. A selective renal

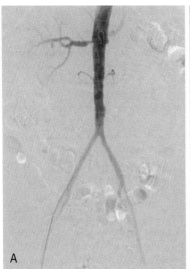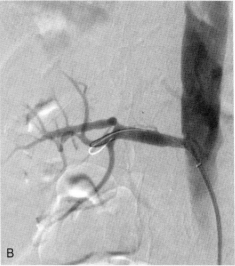

FIGURE 62-24 Renal artery stent. **A,** Right renal artery stenosis. **B,** Lesion improved after stent placement.

angiogram is then obtained with hand injections of contrast material or careful power injections. All phases of the renal circulation are visualized, including the arterial, parenchymal, and venous phases.

A 0.035-inch guidewire is then positioned in the tertiary renal branches. Maintaining guidewire position and stability becomes difficult because of the relatively short length of the renal artery. A 6 Fr guide sheath is advanced into the proximal renal artery. With use of a 4 Fr or 5 Fr glide catheter to help maintain guidewire crossing of the renal stenosis, a 0.035-inch guidewire is then exchanged for a 0.014-inch guidewire.

Renal angioplasty. Over the 0.014-inch guidewire, an angioplasty balloon is advanced across the stenosis. The balloon should be approximately the size of the native normal renal artery beyond the stenosis, not a segment with poststenotic dilation. Typically, the initial angioplasty is performed with a 4-mm semicompliant balloon. The compliant nature of the balloon gives a range of diameters above and below 4 mm, depending on the inflation pressure. While the balloon is inflated, a saved image is obtained to compare the size of the angioplasty balloon with the native artery. This comparison will be taken into account in deciding whether a larger angioplasty balloon is needed and what size stent to choose.

Stent placement. A postangioplasty angiogram is then obtained and the renal artery is assessed for residual stenosis or significant dissection; if this is present, a stent is placed. All renal artery lesions involving the origin will require a stent. A balloon-expandable stent from a low-profile 0.014- and 0.018-inch system is used (0.018-inch balloons and stents can also be delivered over a 0.014-inch guidewire). Contrast material may be puffed through the sheath positioned in the aorta near the ostium of the renal artery to confirm proper positioning of the renal stent. The stent is deployed by expanding the angioplasty balloon to its predetermined deployment pressure. Higher pressures may be required to expand the stent further. However, the rated burst pressure should not be exceeded.

Completion angiography. Before removal of the guidewire and sheath, a completion angiogram with a flush catheter in the aorta

is obtained. This presents an interesting question: How can a good-quality completion study be obtained to include the renal artery origin without losing guidewire access? This can easily be done using a tandem wire technique. The sheath is withdrawn into the infrarenal aorta while maintaining guidewire position across the stented segment of renal artery. A second guidewire is advanced into the aorta; a 4 Fr pigtail catheter is placed over this wire and through the same sheath in the suprarenal position to obtain good detail of the renal artery origin.

Technical Tips

- The renal arteries often originate anteriorly or posteriorly, and the initial diagnostic evaluation of the renal artery origins may be improved with oblique image intensifier views.
- Catheter selection for initial access to the renal artery will depend on the patient's anatomy. Although most branch vessels can be accessed with just an angled Glidecath, a formed catheter such as a cobra or Simmons catheter may be required.
- Arterial perforation is possible with inadvertent guidewire advancement into the renal parenchyma; thus, one should be conscious of the tip of the wire throughout the entire procedure.
- The saved image of the fully expanded initial angioplasty balloon will help estimate the native artery diameter and optimal stent size.
- Care must be taken not to overdilate and risk rupture of the renal artery.
- Stents placed for ostial lesions should extend into the aorta by approximately 2 mm.
- Always read the package insert for the balloon and stent system for sheath and guidewire compatibility, balloon compliance, and the nominal deployment and rated burst pressures.

Renal artery stenting may be an effective treatment of renovascular hypertension and ischemic nephropathy that avoids the morbidity and mortality of open surgical treatment. The role of renal stents after angioplasty can be debated; however, there is good evidence for stenting of all ostial lesions. A more traditional approach to stenting may be used for nonostial stenosis, with the stent reserved for angioplasty failures. Lesions caused by fibromuscular dysplasia usually do not require adjuvant stenting because they respond well to primary angioplasty. The technical success of renal stenting is high, with most technical failures caused by imprecise stent placement. A lower profile 0.014- or 0.018-inch platform for percutaneous renal artery interventions will reduce the sheath size necessary for access and has replaced the more cumbersome 0.035-inch platforms.

SPLANCHNIC ANEURYSMS: SPLENIC, MESENTERIC, AND RENAL ARTERY ANEURYMS

The most common splanchnic artery aneurysm (Fig. 62-25) is the splenic artery aneurysm, accounting for 60% of all splanchnic artery aneurysms. However, it is still rare, with an incidence of 0.78% in patients undergoing abdominal arteriography; it is found incidentally in 0.1% to 10% of autopsies. Splenic aneurysms are more common in women than in men, with a ratio of

4 : 1. Pregnancy is associated with up to 50% of all ruptures. The overall mortality from rupture is approximately 25%. However, rupture during pregnancy is associated with high maternal (80%) and fetal (90%) mortality. The most common risk factors associated with splenic aneurysms are female gender, history of multiple pregnancies, and portal hypertension.

Splenic aneurysms are commonly diagnosed incidentally during arteriographic and CT studies performed for other indications. A signet ring calcification in the left upper quadrant may be seen on plain abdominal radiographs. Ultrasonography, CT, and MRI are useful for aneurysm surveillance in asymptomatic patients.

Patients with splenic aneurysms may report a history of left upper quadrant or epigastric pain. The term *double rupture* has been used to describe these aneurysms, but it is relatively rare. There is initial contained bleeding in the lesser sac, followed by free hemorrhage into the peritoneal cavity, causing hypovolemic shock. Treatment should be considered in aneurysms larger than 2 cm in diameter. Because of the high mortality rate, treatment

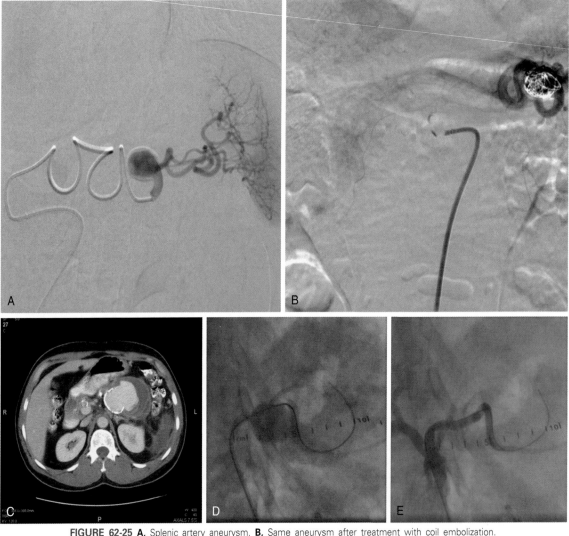

FIGURE 62-25 A, Splenic artery aneurysm. **B,** Same aneurysm after treatment with coil embolization. **C,** CT scan demonstrating ruptured splenic aneurysm. **D,** Arteriogram demonstrates sac with wire passing through aneurysm into intact distal artery. **E,** Flow into sac excluded with stent graft.

is warranted for pregnant women and those of childbearing age. Simple ligation or excision of the aneurysm is preferred to splenectomy. Endovascular repair is emerging as the treatment of choice, with embolization or exclusion with a covered stent.

Hepatic aneurysms are the second most common splanchnic aneurysms, accounting for 20%. These are usually discovered incidentally. Management recommendations are for immediate repair in symptomatic patients or when pseudoaneurysm is suspected, such as those lesions related to iatrogenic injury; otherwise, asymptomatic aneurysms are repaired when the diameter is more than 2 cm. The surgical approach depends on the location of the lesion; options include ligation of common hepatic artery lesions, open aneurysmorrhaphy, and aneurysmectomy with reconstruction. In favorable anatomy, endovascular exclusion can be successful with either covered stents or coil embolization.

Superior mesenteric artery aneurysms account for 5.5% of splanchnic aneurysms; the majority are mycotic and symptomatic, presenting with abdominal pain, nausea, vomiting, or gastrointestinal bleeding. Because of the high mortality risk associated with rupture or intestinal ischemia, superior mesenteric artery aneurysms are repaired regardless of size. Surgical options, which depend on patient factors as well as the anatomy, include ligation, open aneurysmorrhaphy or resection, and endovascular repair with either covered stent grafts or coil embolization.

Celiac axis aneurysms are rarer still and constitute 5% of all splanchnic aneurysms. These are associated with infection, trauma, and dissection as well as with degenerative disease. Similar to splenic lesions, these may initially be manifested with rupture into the lesser sac with epigastric pain and hypotension, followed by shock due to free rupture into the abdominal cavity. Because of the high mortality, all symptomatic lesions as well as asymptomatic lesions larger than 1.5 cm in diameter are repaired immediately. Ligation may be well tolerated. Open or endovascular intervention should be selected on the basis of the patient's anatomy.

The true incidence of renal artery aneurysms is difficult to estimate, ranging from 0.09% to 0.9% on the basis of autopsy studies or radiographic series. Pathogenic contributors include fibromuscular dysplasia, atherosclerotic disease, and trauma. The majority of true aneurysms are saccular and often occur at the main renal artery bifurcation, complicating surgical repair; 10% bilaterality is seen. Fibromuscular dysplasia, particularly medial dysplasia, is known to cause multiple stenoses with poststenotic dilation, effecting the "string of beads" appearance on imaging. The majority are asymptomatic; symptomatic patients present with rupture. Indications for repair include symptomatic lesions, lesions larger than 2 cm, and lesions in women of childbearing age. Options for repair depend on the location of the lesion. Fibromuscular dysplasia is treated with balloon angioplasty alone. The rare aneurysm that occurs along the straight portion of the artery can be treated with either coil embolization or covered stent placement or both. Aneurysms that occur at major branch points, in which one of the branches cannot be sacrificed, require open repair. The complexity of this approach varies from simple aneurysmorrhaphy to resection with reconstruction with inflow from the aorta (or the hepatic, splenic, or iliac arteries), explantation of the kidney for back table repair, and nephrectomy.

CAROTID ARTERY DISEASE

Stroke is the third leading cause of death and is the leading cause of serious disability in the United States. There are about 700,000 strokes per year, with almost 175,000 deaths (25%) occurring within 1 year after the stroke. Approximately 85% of strokes have an ischemic cause; 15% are caused by primary hemorrhage, such as intraparenchymal bleeding from hypertension. Of the ischemic strokes, 20% to 30% are secondary to emboli from atherosclerotic cerebrovascular disease. In patients with greater than 50% stenosis, 20% of patients were shown to have embolic events in transcranial Doppler studies. The incidence and frequency increase with increased stenosis and recent symptomatic neurologic events. The most common location for atherosclerosis in the cerebrovascular circulation is the carotid bifurcation; thus, many strokes are preventable with carotid intervention.

Pathophysiology

The development of atherosclerotic plaque in the extracranial arteries is the leading cause of ischemic stroke in North America and Europe. It accounts for approximately 90% of extracranial cerebrovascular disease; the remaining 10% is caused by disease processes such as fibromuscular dysplasia and arteritis. Atherosclerotic lesions usually occur at the proximal internal carotid artery (ICA) and carotid bifurcation along the wall opposite the origin of the ECA. The enlargement of the carotid bifurcation at the carotid bulb creates a well-defined region of low wall shear stress, flow separation, and loss of unidirectional flow. In this region of low shear stress with sluggish flow, there is prolonged exposure and interaction of plasma lipids and vessel walls, which may account for the localized plaque at the carotid bulb. In contrast, regions with high shear stress, such as the inner border of the carotid sinus, are usually free of atherosclerosis. After the development of a hemodynamically significant stenosis, the atherosclerotic plaque may cause stroke by one of three principal mechanisms: embolization of atherosclerotic particle, thrombotic occlusion, or hypoperfusion.

Clinical Presentation

Symptoms of carotid artery disease include TIAs, amaurosis fugax, and stroke. A TIA is defined as a brief acute loss of focal cerebral function, generally less than 24 hours in duration. There is no persistent deficit after each TIA, but there are often multiple attacks. The loss of function can be localized to a region of brain that is supplied by one vascular system, such as the right or left carotid artery. Most TIAs are brief, lasting 2 to 15 minutes, and are rapid in onset. Symptoms include unilateral motor and sensory loss, aphasia (difficulty finding words), and dysarthria (difficulty speaking because of motor dysfunction). Motor function loss may be manifested as weakness, paralysis, dysarthria, or clumsiness of the upper or lower extremities or face that is contralateral to the affected carotid artery. Sensory function loss may be manifested as numbness or paresthesia of the contralateral upper or lower extremities or face. Aphasia occurs when the speech center, usually located in the dominant hemisphere, is affected. If the neurologic deficit lasts longer than 24 hours but there is return of full neurologic function with 48 to 72 hours, it is termed a reversible ischemic neurologic deficit. A patient with persistent neurologic deficit is considered to have a stroke. In contrast, fleeting episodes lasting only a few seconds are usually not considered to be TIAs.

Amaurosis fugax is the transient unilateral loss of vision. It is caused by an embolus to the ophthalmic artery, the first branch of the ICA. Patients describe the event as a shade descending or ascending over the entire eye, half of the eye, or a quadrant of one eye. The location of the affected visual field depends on whether the embolization is to the superior or inferior retinal artery. If the entire retinal artery is transiently affected, the patient may complain of complete loss of vision in one eye. Similar to TIAs, most incidents of amaurosis fugax are sudden in onset and last for minutes. However, there may be occasional patients with permanent blindness.

A patient may also be asymptomatic when diagnosed with hemodynamically significant carotid artery disease. An audible carotid bruit may be heard in the neck during routine physical examination. It should be noted that severe carotid disease may not have an audible bruit because of markedly reduced blood flow. A screening carotid duplex ultrasound examination should be performed in asymptomatic patients with bruits or high-risk patients without bruits.

Diagnosis

Once a patient is diagnosed with TIA, amaurosis fugax, or stroke, expedient workup with confirmation of carotid artery disease and treatment are needed because the risk of a stroke is greatest within the first 3 months after the initial event. This risk returns to baseline at approximately 6 months. The most useful test for the diagnosis of extracranial carotid artery disease is duplex ultrasound. Carotid duplex ultrasonography (Fig. 62-26) allows accurate indirect determination of the severity of the carotid stenosis by measuring velocity. As the stenosis increases and the lumen narrows, there is an increase in the blood velocity to maintain distal flow. Many studies have confirmed the correlation of increased velocity with severity of disease. CTA and MRA (Fig. 62 27) can also be used to determine the degree of carotid stenosis

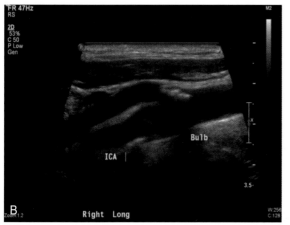

RIGHT	(S)	(D)	Percent	Plaque
ECA	266	0		
DICA	56	24		
MICA	80	28		
PICA	867	443		
DCCA	56	11		
MCCA	62	8		
PCCA	77	12		
SUBCL	155	0		

Max ICA Stenosis 80-99%
ICA/CCA Ratio 11.3

LEFT	(S)	(D)	Percent	Plaque
ECA	249	0		
DICA	97	28		
MICA	83	31		
PICA	149	37	50-79%	
DCCA	147	36		
MCCA	101	27		
PCCA	103	20		
SUBCL	176	0		

Max ICA Stenosis 50-79%
ICA/CCA Ratio 1.0

FIGURE 62-26 A, Carotid duplex velocities demonstrating severe right internal carotid artery stenosis. **B,** Soft plaque is seen within the right internal carotid artery on gray-scale imaging.

at the bifurcation. In addition, they are useful to study potential tandem lesions that may be present in the proximal supra-aortic trunk or intracranial vessels and to assess the configuration of the aortic arch. These studies are also useful for confirmation of duplex findings and planning of intervention with a carotid endarterectomy (CEA) or stenting. Contrast arteriography (Fig. 62-28) is occasionally performed. It is most useful for patients with normal findings on duplex studies or for whom a noninvasive study is in disagreement with the clinical presentation. In addition to findings similar to those of CTA and MRA, contrast arteriography can be used to identify intracranial vascular disease or unusual nonatherosclerotic arteriopathies, such as fibromuscular dysplasia.

Treatment
Carotid Endarterectomy

Indications. CEA is the removal of the atherosclerotic plaque from the carotid bifurcation. In the North American Symptomatic Carotid Endarterectomy Trial (NASCET), the effectiveness of CEA was evaluated for symptomatic patients with carotid artery stenosis ranging from 30% to 99% in the United States and Canada. Patients with TIA, amaurosis fugax, or nondisabling stroke were randomized to best medical therapy or CEA. In the first study of patients with 70% stenosis or greater, CEA reduced the incidence of ipsilateral stroke from 26% to 9% at 2 years. The incidence of a major or fatal ipsilateral stroke was 13.1% for the medical group and 2.5% for the surgical group. In a subsequent report, the results of patients with symptomatic mild (30% to 49%) and moderate (50% to 69%) ipsilateral stroke were reported. The 5-year risk of ipsilateral stroke in patients with moderate stenosis was 22.2% for the medical group and 15.7% for the surgical group. For patients with mild stenosis, the risk of ipsilateral stroke was equivalent for the medical and surgical groups. The NASCET outcome showed that symptomatic patients with severe stenosis (70% to 99%) gained substantial benefit from surgical intervention during a brief period of less than 2 years. The results also favored surgery in symptomatic patients with 50% to 69% stenosis. The best medical therapy at the time of the NASCET trial did not include clopidogrel (Plavix) or statin anticholesterol agents, both of which have been shown to decrease the risk of stroke.

CEA has also been shown to be effective in asymptomatic patients. The Asymptomatic Carotid Atherosclerosis Study (ACAS) randomized asymptomatic patients with 60% to 99% stenosis to best medical treatment or CEA. The 5-year risk of ipsilateral stroke and any perioperative stroke or death was 11% for the medical group and 5.1% for the surgical group. The perioperative complication rate was low, 2.3%, with approximately 50% of the risk associated with mandatory preoperative contrast arteriography for patients randomized to CEA. Therefore, the actual surgical complication rate was only 1.5%. The largest trial was the Asymptomatic Carotid Surgery Trial (ACST), with equal randomization of 3120 patients to CEA or medical treatment. The results were similar, with a 5-year stroke risk of 11.8% in the medical group and 5.4% in the surgical group. The perioperative complication rate was also low, 3.1%.

The results of landmark studies of CEA have confirmed that surgery provides better protection from ipsilateral stroke in patients with symptomatic or asymptomatic disease. The Stroke Council of the American Heart Association convened a consensus conference on the indications for CEA. The recommendation recognized four categories: (1) proven—the strongest indication,

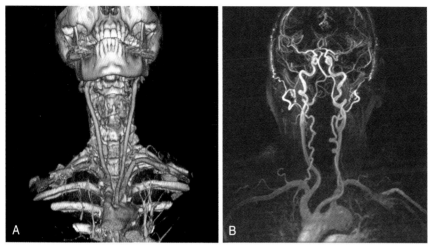

FIGURE 62-27 **A,** Arch and cervical carotid CTA reconstruction. **B,** Arch, cervical, and intracranial MRA scans with gadolinium. (Courtesy Dr. Douglas Hughes, University of Texas Medical Branch at Galveston, Department of Radiology.)

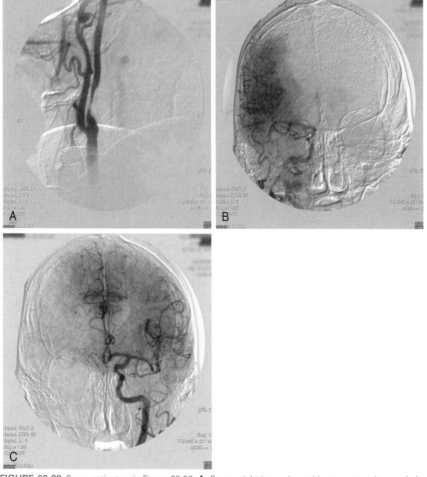

FIGURE 62-28 Same patient as in Figure 62-26. **A,** Severe right internal carotid artery stenosis, correlating with carotid duplex findings. **B,** Intracerebral anteroposterior angiogram of right common carotid artery injections demonstrates no filling of the anterior circulation. **C,** Injection of the left internal carotid artery demonstrates filling of the right anterior circulation.

usually supported by results of prospective, randomized trials; (2) acceptable but not proven—a good indication for operation supported by promising but not scientifically certain data; (3) uncertain—data insufficient to define the risk-benefit ratio; and (4) proven inappropriate—current data adequate to show that the risk of surgery outweighs any benefits. The recommendations are further classified for patients with symptomatic or asymptomatic carotid disease.

For symptomatic good-risk patients treated by a surgeon whose surgical morbidity and mortality rate is less than 6%, the indications for CEA are as follows:

Proven indications
- One or more TIAs in the last 6 months and carotid stenosis ≥70%
- Mild stroke with carotid stenosis ≥70%

Acceptable but not proven indications
- TIAs in the past 6 months and stenosis of 50% to 69%
- Progressive stroke and stenosis ≥70%
- Mild or moderate stroke in the past 6 months and stenosis of 50% to 69%
- CEA ipsilateral to TIAs and stenosis ≥70%, combined with required coronary bypass grafting

Uncertain indications
- TIAs with stenosis ≤50%
- Mild stroke with stenosis ≤50%
- Symptomatic acute carotid thrombosis

Proven inappropriate indications
- Moderate stroke with stenosis ≤50%, not receiving aspirin
- Single TIA, stenosis ≤50%, not receiving aspirin
- High-risk patient with multiple TIAs, stenosis ≤50%, not receiving aspirin
- High-risk patient, mild or moderate stroke, stenosis ≤50%, not receiving aspirin
- Global ischemic symptoms with stenosis ≤50%
- Acute internal carotid dissection, asymptomatic, receiving heparin

For asymptomatic good-risk patients treated by a surgeon whose surgical morbidity and mortality rates are each less than 3%, the indications for CEA are as follows:
- Proven indications: Stenosis ≥60%
- Acceptable but not proven indications: None defined
- Uncertain indications: High-risk patient or surgeon with a morbidity-mortality rate >3%, combined carotid-coronary operation, or nonstenotic ulcerative lesions
- Proven inappropriate indications: Operations with a combined stroke morbidity-mortality rate ≥5%

Technique. The patient is positioned supine on a shoulder roll, with the neck extended and the head turned to the contralateral side. A longitudinal incision is placed parallel and along the anterior border of the sternocleidomastoid muscle. Alternatively, an oblique incision can be made along the skin lines of the neck. The longitudinal incision may provide better exposure, whereas the oblique incision may result in a more cosmetic scar when healed. With the longitudinal exposure, the incision can be extended proximally to the sternal notch or distally to the mastoid process for exposure of the proximal common or distal ICA, respectively. The platysma is divided. The sternocleidomastoid muscle is mobilized away from the carotid sheath and retracted posteriorly. The internal jugular vein may be exposed along the anterior border until the large common facial vein is identified. The common facial vein is divided; the carotid bifurcation is usually located underneath. The internal jugular vein may be mobilized laterally

to provide exposure to the carotid bifurcation. The vagus nerve (cranial nerve X) is found posterolateral to the common carotid artery (CCA) in the carotid sheath. Therefore, dissection of the CCA is performed anteriorly to avoid nerve injury. However, care must still be exercised to identify the occasional anomalous anterior course of the vagus nerve and the presence of a rare nonrecurrent laryngeal nerve that branches directly from the vagus to innervate the vocal cord. The nonrecurrent laryngeal nerve usually occurs on the right side of the neck.

Meticulous dissection of the carotid artery is necessary to avoid embolization. Movement of the carotid bulb should be minimized; the initial dissection should be limited to the normal ICA and ECA distal to the diseased segment and the CCA proximal to the diseased segment. During mobilization of the ICA superiorly, the hypoglossal nerve (cranial nerve XII) needs to be identified and protected (Fig. 62-29). Dissection near the carotid bifurcation and carotid body may cause reflex bradycardia and hypotension. This can be prevented with the injection of 1% lidocaine into the carotid body.

On occasion, there may be patients with a high carotid bifurcation or an extensive lesion, and maximum exposure of the ICA may be needed. Several techniques can be used to provide this exposure. The skin incision is first extended all the way superiorly to the mastoid process and the sternocleidomastoid muscle is mobilized to its tendinous insertion on the mastoid process. At this level of dissection, the spinal accessory nerve (cranial nerve XI) is identified and protected. Additional exposure of the ICA can be achieved with the division of the posterior belly of the digastric muscle. If further exposure of the ICA superiorly is necessary, the styloid process can be transected and the mandible displaced anteriorly. At this level of dissection, the glossopharyngeal nerve (cranial nerve IX) crosses the ICA near the base of the skull. Injury to this nerve can be avoided by dissecting close to the anterior surface of this artery. In retracting the wound superiorly, care should also be exercised to avoid other nerve injuries. There can be temporary compression injury to the greater auricular nerve laterally and the marginal mandibular branch of the facial nerve medially.

Once the carotid arteries are fully exposed, vessel loops are placed around the arteries and heparin is given for full anticoagulation. To avoid embolization, the ICA is clamped first, followed by control of the CCA and ECA. The CCA is opened, and a longitudinal arteriotomy is extended through the plaque into the normal ICA distally. If a shunt is to be used, it is inserted at this time. The decision whether to shunt can be made using electroencephalographic or back-pressure criteria. Using back-pressure criteria, an arterial pressure transducer is set up. A 22-gauge needle bent at a 45-degree angle is carefully inserted into the CCA, with the distal needle in the lumen of the ICA. The pressure of the ICA is measured with the ECA and CCA clamped. If the back-pressure is a mean arterial pressure of 65 mm Hg or higher, there is adequate collateral cerebral circulation and a shunt can be avoided. Alternative methods of cerebral blood flow evaluation include intermittent neurologic checks on the awake patient undergoing CEA with local anesthesia only and transcranial duplex or electroencephalographic monitoring of the patient undergoing CEA under general anesthesia.

The endarterectomy is started in the CCA. The optimal plane for endarterectomy is the plane between the inner and outer medial layers. This results in the removal of the intima, the plaque, and a portion of the media. The remaining arterial wall thus consists of the adventitia and residual media. The plaque is divided

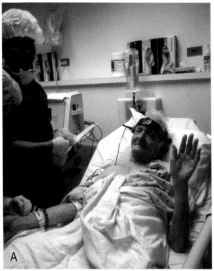
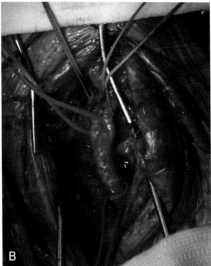
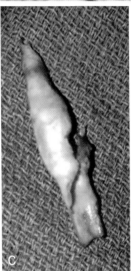

FIGURE 62-29 A, Patient preparing for carotid endarterectomy with intraoperative transcranial duplex monitoring. **B,** Carotid exposure with hypoglossal nerve at top of incision. **C,** Carotid plaque with calcified and friable components.

proximally in the CCA, and the endarterectomy is extended distally into the carotid bulb. The vessel loop around the ECA is loosened, and endarterectomy of the ECA is performed by simple eversion. Removal of the plaque is continued distally into the ICA. Endarterectomy of the distal ICA is feathered to its transition to the normal distal intima. If the distal plaque cannot be feathered, the residual intima is sharply transected and secured in place with tacking sutures. After completion of the endarterectomy, the residual wall is copiously irrigated with heparinized saline solution, and any remaining debris or medial fibers are removed to prevent embolization. The ICA, ECA, and CCA are allowed to backbleed.

The arteriotomy is closed with a patch. There is evidence showing that patch angioplasty has better results with a reduced risk of restenosis, especially in female patients, patients with small ICAs, and patients who continue to smoke. Once the arteriotomy is completed, flow is first established to the ECA with release of clamps to the ECA and CCA. After several heartbeats

to flush debris out of the ECA, flow is then reestablished into the ICA.

If desired, heparin reversal is given with protamine.

Postoperative care. At the completion of the endarterectomy, a gross neurologic examination of the patient is performed in the operating room. If no deficit is found, the patient is transferred to the recovery room. Patients are monitored closely during the postoperative period. Although they were formerly cared for in the intensive care unit routinely, most patients now can be transferred to a regular room if they are neurologically intact and hemodynamically normal in the postanesthesia care unit. Usually, patients are discharged safely the next day. Important factors to be monitored are the patient's neurologic status, blood pressure, and incision to evaluate for hematoma.

If, at the completion of the procedure, there is neurologic deficit, the patency of the ICA is evaluated with noninvasive carotid duplex ultrasound. Initial flap or occlusion of the ICA on duplex imaging requires immediate reoperation. If the ICA is patent, arteriography is performed to detect possible clots or defects. Any lesion is treated with reoperation. If there is no lesion on the arteriogram in a patent ICA, the patient is treated conservatively with anticoagulation, antiplatelet agents, or both. However, if the patient continues to have repeated or worsening neurologic events, immediate reoperation may be needed.

Blood pressure monitoring and control during the postoperative period are of paramount importance to prevent stroke. Immediately after CEA, 20% of patients may have significant hypertension and 30% may have hypotension. Up to 9% of these patients were found to have neurologic deficits, whereas there was no neurologic morbidity in normotensive patients. In addition, blood pressure fluctuation has adverse effects on myocardial function. Systolic blood pressure should be kept below 140 mm Hg for normotensive patients and below 160 mm Hg for chronically hypertensive patients. Diastolic pressure is maintained below 100 mm Hg. Hypertension should be treated immediately; sodium nitroprusside can be used. Hypotension is initially treated with fluid to correct the volume deficit; if it is refractory, vasoconstrictors can be initiated.

The use of antiplatelet therapy and intraoperative heparin anticoagulation can cause wound hematoma after endarterectomy; the incidence of reoperation for hematoma drainage is less than 1%. Usually, there is diffuse ooze from the wound rather than bleeding from the suture line. A large hematoma may cause compression on the ICA and adjacent cranial nerves and wound infection. If there is airway compromise, the incision needs to be opened at the bedside for drainage of the hematoma. The incidence may be decreased with the routine use of a Silastic drain.

It is not unusual for patients to complain of headache after CEA; they may complain of these symptoms at approximately 3 to 5 days postoperatively. This is likely caused by reperfusion syndrome from dysfunction in the cerebral circulation autoregulation once the blood flow is restored after endarterectomy. It is usually self-limited and resolves spontaneously. However, if there is associated neurologic deficit, CT should be performed.

Complications. Stroke is the most feared complication of CEA; it occurs in 1% to 3% of patients, depending on the indication for the surgery. Causes include embolization from a friable or ulcerated plaque during carotid dissection, inadequate cerebral perfusion during endarterectomy, thrombosis from a flap or technical error, and reperfusion syndrome. Most of the reported low rates of stroke are from specialized centers, and a more realistic complication rate from the community data for combined stroke morbidity and mortality ranges from 6% to 20%. The Stroke Council of the American Heart Association has set standards for upper acceptable limits of stroke and death as a function of indications for endarterectomy. For patients with asymptomatic carotid disease, the combined operative stroke morbidity and mortality should not be more than 3%; for TIA, 5%; for history of previous stroke, 7%; and for recurrent carotid stenosis, 10%.

Injury to the cranial nerves can cause postoperative morbidity. The incidence has been found to be approximately 16%; incidence increased to 39% if further evaluation was performed by a speech pathologist. Only 60% of these patients were symptomatic, and most of these symptoms were temporary. After 6 weeks, the incidence was between 1% and 4%. Dysfunction of the superior laryngeal and recurrent laryngeal nerves is the most common cranial nerve injury encountered. This is likely caused by retraction injury or direct trauma by forceps during surgery, which can lead to paralysis of the vocal cord in the paramedian position, resulting in hoarseness and loss of an effective cough mechanism.

Unilateral injury can be asymptomatic, but airway obstruction can be caused if there is bilateral injury. If staged bilateral CEA is planned, routine direct visualization of the vocal cord by laryngoscopy is recommended after the first endarterectomy. Staged surgery is delayed if there is cord paralysis. Wound retraction can also cause injury to the hypoglossal nerve during superior exposure for high carotid bifurcation. This is manifested by tongue deviation to the ipsilateral side, but it can occasionally cause speech impairment and mastication problems.

Carotid Angioplasty and Stent Procedure

Many randomized trials have shown that CEA is effective in preventing stroke in symptomatic and asymptomatic patients with significant internal carotid stenosis. It has been accepted that CEA is the gold standard of treatment for these patients. However, there remain a group of patients who have been identified as high risk for CEA. Carotid angioplasty with stenting (CAS) has emerged as a safe and effective alternative to CEA for patients with indications for carotid intervention. During the past decade, CAS has seen a rapid evolution in technique and technology with the introduction of self-expanding nitinol stents, smaller delivery systems, and embolic protection devices (EPDs).

Early single-center studies performed from 1990 to 1999 showed significantly higher rates of stroke and death for CAS than for CEA in 30-day outcomes for symptomatic patients. The risk of major stroke or death was 3.9% after CAS and 2.2% after CEA, and the risk of any stroke or death was 7.8% for CAS and 4% for CEA. During these studies, most CAS procedures were performed without an EPD. When early studies were designed to randomize patients between CAS and CEA, many had to be terminated prematurely because of inferior results with CAS. These studies showed that patients with unprotected CAS without EPD had a higher stroke rate than with CEA and protected CAS and that unprotected CAS was not equivalent to CEA. The Stenting and Angioplasty with Protection in Patients at High Risk for Endarterectomy (SAPPHIRE) trial was the first randomized study to show the benefits of using EPD in CAS and that protected CAS was not inferior to CEA in high-risk patients. Most recently, in 2010, preliminary results from the Carotid Revascularization Endarterectomy versus Stent Trial (CREST) became available.[54] This was the first multicenter prospective, randomized clinical trial funded by the National Institutes of Health to compare the safety and efficacy of CAS and CEA in symptomatic and asymptomatic patients. Preliminary end points were any clinical stroke, myocardial infarction, or death and any ipsilateral stroke during the entire follow-up period. There were 2502 patients (asymptomatic, 47%; symptomatic, 53%), with a median follow-up period of 2.5 years. In regard to the primary composite end point, there was no difference between CAS and CEA (7.2% for CAS versus 6.8% for CEA; $P = .51$). There was a statistically significant difference in 30-day stroke rate, 4.1% for CAS and 2.3% for CEA. The risk of myocardial infarction was significantly lower for CAS, 1.1%, compared with CEA, 2.3%. At median follow-up of 2.5 years, there was no difference in stroke rate between CAS and CEA.

The data from CREST have shown similar composite outcomes between the two procedures, which led the investigators to conclude that both CAS and CEA had similar composite outcomes, with differences in periprocedural stroke and myocardial infarction. It is likely that there will be more demand from the public for this less invasive modality for the treatment of high-grade carotid disease. Of note, CAS procedures performed during the second half of this 10-year trial had a significantly lower incidence of complications compared with those CAS procedures performed during the first half of the study. These findings indicate improvements in device design and operator experience over time and suggest that future results may continue to improve with this technique.

Indications and contraindications. CAS is currently indicated for symptomatic high-risk patients. Indications for symptomatic patients with high-grade carotid stenosis were outlined in the consensus conference of the Stroke Council of the American Heart Association (see earlier). At the time of this printing, the Centers for Medicare and Medicaid Services continue to deny coverage for carotid stent procedures for asymptomatic patients as well as for symptomatic patients who are deemed good-risk candidates for CEA.

There is a group of patients who are considered at high risk for open surgical CEA. They can be divided into two main categories: those with anatomic conditions and those with physiologic conditions. High-risk anatomic conditions include the following: restenosis after previous CEA caused by association with higher risk of cranial nerve injury; "hostile" neck from previous neck radiation, radical neck dissection, permanent tracheostomy, or frozen neck; high or low lesions above C2 or below the clavicle, respectively; and other carotid lesions, including tandem lesions within the same carotid artery and contralateral high-grade ICA disease. High-risk physiologic conditions include the following: class III or class IV angina or congestive heart failure; severe chronic obstructive pulmonary disease (forced expiratory volume ≤1 or the need for home oxygen); and cardiac disease necessitating open heart surgery within 4 weeks.

Contraindications to CAS include coils or kinking of the CCA or ICA and excessive calcification of the carotid disease. Difficult access because of iliac disease and a tortuous and calcified arch or tandem CCA stenoses may also contribute to difficulties in stent delivery.

Technique

Carotid artery access and guide sheath positioning. Just as in CEA, patients are medically optimized with antihypertensives, statins, and smoking cessation. Patients who have not been taking clopidogrel are given an oral loading dose of 600 mg and then maintained on 75 mg by mouth daily. Retrograde common femoral artery access is usually the first choice, primarily secondary to table and patient positioning constraints. Brachial access is used only in certain circumstances, such as severe aortoiliac occlusive disease. In most cases, diagnostic arteriography and the intervention are performed at separate times. Diagnostic arch aortography with four-vessel extracranial and bilateral cerebral arteriography is first performed for the evaluation of the carotid disease and cerebral circulation and for procedural planning. The aortogram is obtained with a pigtail catheter in the ascending aorta in left anterior oblique angulation. The bilateral CCAs are then catheterized for arteriograms of the ICA and cerebral circulation. The subclavian arteries are catheterized for the evaluation of vertebral arteries. After diagnostic arteriography, the patient is discharged on the same day.

For patients requiring treatment, the intervention is performed at a later time. Based on the diagnostic arteriogram, appropriately shaped catheters and sheaths are chosen. To limit contrast material, a selective catheterization can be made on the basis of a previous arch aortogram. Most CCAs can be accessed simply with an angled catheter; however, some will require a more complex-shaped catheter, such as a Simmons catheter. Selective carotid angiography is then performed with careful hand injections of contrast material. A 0.035-inch guidewire is positioned in the ECA and catheterized by the angled catheter. An angiogram is used to confirm the location of the ECA. A stiff wire is then placed in this artery, and the catheter and short groin sheath are removed and exchanged for a long 6 Fr sheath. The tip of the sheath is advanced to the distal CCA. The stiff wire is removed from the patient.

Placement of embolic protection device. With the long sheath near the carotid bulb, a careful angiogram with hand injection is obtained to determine the anatomy of the disease and location of the ICA. The wire with the EPD is advanced across the disease and into the distal ICA, just before the horizontal petrous segment. The EPD is deployed. Flow through the EPD and its apposition to the wall are evaluated.

Carotid stent placement. An angiogram is then obtained, noting the location of the carotid disease. The stent is advanced carefully across the disease, and it is deployed from the ICA into the CCA, covering the ECA origin (Fig. 62-30). Prestenting angioplasty is not routinely performed unless it is necessary to create a space needed for placement of the stent in near-occlusive lesions. The self-expanding nitinol stent is typically 8 to 10 mm in diameter by 30 mm in length. It is sized to the largest portion of the vessel, usually the distal CCA. A small stent that does not oppose the carotid wall may become a nidus for thrombus formation. Current stents are designed to be used in small delivery systems with a rapid exchange or monorail platform.

Carotid angioplasty. After stenting, poststenting angioplasty is performed. The patient receives 0.5 mg of atropine or 0.1 mg of glycopyrrolate intravenously immediately before angioplasty to blunt the effect of pressure from the balloon on the carotid bulb. An angioplasty balloon is advanced over the 0.014-inch guidewire across the location of the narrowest area of the stent. The balloon should approximate the size of the native normal ICA beyond the stenosis, not a segment with poststenotic dilation. Typically, the initial angioplasty is performed with a 5-mm semicompliant balloon. The balloon is inflated slowly until apposition is achieved and then deflated slowly. Transcranial Doppler imaging may be used to monitor for embolic debris. Experience with this procedure has shown that the greatest number of emboli are released with balloon deflation.

Completion angiogram. Before removal of the guidewire and sheath, a completion angiogram is obtained to confirm adequate resolution of the carotid disease and to ensure flow through the ICA. Spasm of the ICA distal to the stent can be treated with a vasodilator, such as nitroglycerin or papaverine. However, most spasms resolve with removal of the EPD. Once the EPD is removed, another angiogram is obtained to confirm vasodilation of the vessel and flow. A closure device is then used to close the arteriotomy. If a patient has neurologic functional changes, a cerebral angiogram is obtained and compared with previous diagnostic angiograms. Nonvisualization of cerebral arteries after stenting that were previously seen on a diagnostic angiogram is of concern for an embolic event, and an intervention must be carried out (Fig. 62-31).

Neurologic deficits that occur as a result of stent placement are not the same as those that occur with carotid surgery.[55] Rather than an immediate intraprocedural event, a substantial number of the periprocedural events that occur with CAS occur hours to days after the procedure. In one study, 26% of the periprocedural neurologic events occurred more than 1 day (and up to 14 days) after the procedure and after discharge of the patient.[56] In another

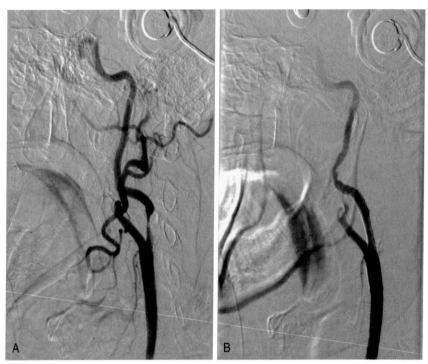

FIGURE 62-30 Carotid stent. **A,** Severe internal carotid artery stenosis. **B,** Improved flow after internal carotid artery stent placement.

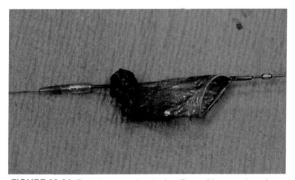

FIGURE 62-31 Embolic protection device; filter with acute thrombus.

study, 71% of the periprocedural deficits (10 of 14) after carotid stent placement in 111 patients occurred after the procedure was completed rather than during the procedure.[57] This presents logistic challenges if intracranial thrombolysis ever becomes the standard method for managing this problem because it often occurs after catheters and intra-arterial access devices have been removed; in some cases, the patient may already have been discharged. The patient would have to return and be treated in a timely manner. The site at which the carotid stent was placed would require repeated instrumentation (crossing with guidewires and catheters), with the attendant added risk of additional embolization.

Conclusions. The CREST trial demonstrated a significant learning curve with CAS. In CAS, selection of patients is the key to early success. Patients who are good stent candidates because of high medical comorbidities may not always have favorable anatomy for stent placement and will likely have an elevated risk of periprocedural complications, even from a percutaneous procedure. Some patients with complex anatomy who are otherwise good candidates for CAS may have to be treated by alternative means if they are seen early in the program's development, while the physician is accumulating experience. The best early candidates for CAS are patients with focal recurrent stenosis. Performance of CAS requires excellent imaging; the procedure is facilitated by the use of a floating radiolucent table. Specific equipment and tools for carotid arteriography, balloon angioplasty, and stent placement differ somewhat from those used for other vascular beds. The components for carotid intervention must be determined, understood, requested, and assembled before proceeding. There is growing consensus that CAS may be an effective alternative treatment for high-grade carotid artery disease that avoids the morbidity and mortality of open surgical treatment. Outside of clinical trials, it is currently indicated for symptomatic high-risk patients. With the results from CREST recently published, it is likely that approved indications will be expanded to include normal-risk, high-grade symptomatic and asymptomatic patients. Vascular surgeons have traditionally assumed a leadership role in the management of carotid disease. If we are to continue to provide our patients with the full breadth of therapeutic alternatives, it is imperative that we develop the necessary skills to perform safe and effective CAS procedures while maintaining our open surgical expertise with CEA. Further rigorous scientific investigation will allow us to elucidate the subtle characteristics of patients and their lesions that may better inform our recommendations for one of these two competing treatment options.

DIALYSIS ACCESS

Dialysis Outcomes Quality Initiative Guidelines

Three types of access are commonly placed for hemodialysis: (1) autogenous fistula (AF); (2) prosthetic bridging graft (BG); and

(3) indwelling central venous catheter. The ideal access delivers a flow rate sufficient for effective dialysis, is easily cannulated, has a long life, and has a low complication rate.

Currently, AFs are preferred to prosthetic grafts and central venous catheters because of their higher primary patency rates and lower frequency of stenosis, thrombosis, and infection.[58] Previously, prosthetic conduit was often used for the initial hemodialysis access. Justification for a preference for prosthetic grafts included technical ease of procedure, avoidance of prolonged maturation times, ease of cannulation, differences in reimbursement, and disbelief in the superiority of AFs.[59] The reluctance to perform native fistulas was also fueled by the wide range of reported rates of patency and maturation to a functional access with traditional single-incision direct arteriovenous fistulas, such as the wrist radiocephalic fistula. Maturation rates of arteriovenous fistulas range from 25% to 90%.[60-62]

The U.S. Renal Data System, which accumulates and reviews data from the nation's dialysis centers, reported in 1995 that the frequency of native AF construction in the United States was less than 30% of total access procedures performed, with some regions having AF placement rates of less than 10%.[63] In 1996, the Dialysis Outcomes Quality Initiative (DOQI) Vascular Access Work Group met at the request of the National Kidney Foundation to address all aspects of current medical and surgical issues associated with hemodialysis and to publish a set of practice guidelines.[64] This was updated in 2000.[58]

To attain the goals recommended by the DOQI, surgeons are expected to increase their rates of autogenous arteriovenous fistulas to at least 50% of all new permanent hemodialysis accesses constructed. An important objective of the DOQI is to have a prevalence of AFs in 40% of all hemodialysis patients.

Nomenclature

In 2002, the Committee on Reporting Standards for Arterio-Venous Accesses of the Society for Vascular Surgery and the American Association for Vascular Surgery published standardized definitions related to arteriovenous access procedures and recommended reporting standards for patency and complications.[65] *Autogenous* refers to the native vein. An autogenous arteriovenous access is an access created by a connection between an artery and vein, and the vein serves as the access site for needle cannulation. A *transposition* is an access performed with a transposed vein. The peripheral portion of the vein is moved from its original position, usually through a superficial subcutaneous tunnel, and connected to the artery. The more central venous segment in a transposed access is left in its anatomic position. In contrast, the term *translocated* is used to describe an access constructed from a segment of vein that has been completely mobilized, disconnected proximally and distally, and placed in a location remote from its origin. The recommended nomenclature for the autogenous transposition procedures can be found in Table 62-9.

Configuration descriptors provide information about the anastomotic connection and course of the conduit. An access has a direct or indirect configuration. A direct access describes the connection between native artery and vein and involves such configurations as end-to-side, side-to-side, and end-to-end anastomoses.[65] In an indirect access, an autogenous or prosthetic graft is interposed between the native artery and vein. Additional descriptors may be used, such as transposed, translocated, straight, and looped.

Primary patency refers to the interval from the time of access placement to the intervention designed to maintain or to

TABLE 62-9 Recommended Nomenclature for Transposition Access Procedures	
RECOMMENDED NOMENCLATURE	**TRADITIONAL NOMENCLATURE**
Forearm	
Autogenous radial-basilic forearm transposition	Superficial venous transposition in the forearm, basilic vein to radial artery
Autogenous ulnar-basilic forearm transposition	Superficial venous transposition in the forearm, basilic vein to ulnar artery
Autogenous radial-cephalic forearm transposition	Superficial venous transposition in the forearm, cephalic vein to radial artery
Autogenous brachial-cephalic forearm transposition	Superficial venous transposition in the forearm, cephalic vein to brachial artery
Upper Arm	
Autogenous brachial-basilic upper arm transposition	Basilic vein transposition
Lower Extremity	
Autogenous femoral–greater saphenous looped access transposition	Greater saphenous vein end-to-side to femoral artery fistula

Adapted from Sidawy AN, Gray R, Besarab A: Recommended standards for reports dealing with arteriovenous hemodialysis accesses. *J Vasc Surg* 35:603–610, 2002.

reestablish patency or access thrombosis or the time of measurement of patency. *Assisted primary patency* refers to the interval from the time of access placement until access thrombosis or the time of measurement of patency, including interventions designed to maintain the function of a patent access. *Secondary patency* refers to the interval from the time of access placement until access abandonment or thrombosis or the time of patency measurement, including interventions to reestablish function in a thrombosed access.[65]

Superficial Venous System of the Upper Extremity

An understanding of the venous anatomy of the upper extremity is essential for the planning of permanent hemodialysis access. Although there is an anatomic commonality among patients that represents a starting point for inspection, anatomic variations and segmental venous stenoses and occlusions from previous medical or surgical interventions are important to identify by thorough preoperative assessment.

Cephalic Vein

The cephalic vein arises from the radial aspect of the veins draining the dorsum of the hand and travels around the radial border of the forearm. On the proximal aspect of the volar forearm, the median cubital vein arises. This vein communicates with the deep veins in the forearm and then crosses the antecubital fossa to join the basilic vein. As it crosses the elbow, the cephalic vein is found in an anatomic groove between the brachioradialis and biceps muscles. The cephalic vein travels superficially to the musculocutaneous nerve and then ascends in the groove along the lateral border of the biceps muscle. In the upper third of the arm, the cephalic vein passes between the pectoralis major and deltoid muscles, crosses the axillary artery, and joins the axillary vein just below the clavicle. The accessory cephalic vein arises from the ulnar side of the dorsum of the hand or the posterior aspect of the forearm and usually joins the cephalic vein below the elbow.

Basilic Vein

The basilic vein originates on the ulnar aspect of the dorsum of the hand and travels in the subcutaneous space up the ulnar side of the forearm, shifting from the posterior surface distally toward a more anterior orientation below the elbow. The median antecubital vein joins the basilic vein in the antecubital fossa and then travels in the groove between the biceps and pronator teres muscles to cross the brachial artery. In this region, the vein is crossed anteriorly and posteriorly by branches of the median cutaneous nerve. As it courses proximately along the medial border of the biceps muscle, the basilic vein descends below the deep fascia to travel parallel to the brachial artery and vein. The union of the basilic and brachial veins in the axilla forms the axillary vein.

Median Antebrachial Vein

The median antebrachial vein drains the palmar surface of the hand and is located on the ulnar side of the anterior forearm. In the proximal forearm, it joins the basilic vein or median antecubital vein.

Initial Evaluation for New Access

The first step in establishing hemodialysis access is to select the best available site, based on optimal arterial inflow and venous outflow, observing the preference of an AF over a BG, the forearm over the upper arm, and the nondominant over the dominant upper extremity. Visual inspection and physical examination of the upper extremity are performed but may be inadequate to assess certain factors, especially vein size, quality, and adequacy of central venous outflow. For this reason, duplex ultrasound scanning is used for all patients.

The examination is initiated at the wrist of the nondominant upper extremity, and a tourniquet is placed at the midforearm. After dilation of the superficial veins by gentle tapping and stroking, the veins are insonated with a 5- or 7-MHz scanning probe. They are evaluated for diameter, compressibility, and continuity with upper arm veins. Patency of the deep system and continuity with patent axillary and subclavian veins are also verified. However, central venous stenosis or thrombosis does not preclude the use of that arm; multiple large collateral veins are able to provide outflow and support an AF.

The largest diameter superficial vein of good quality is mapped with skin markings. Suitability criteria for access include the following:
- Target vein diameter of more than 2.5 mm for an AF and more than 4.0 mm for a BG
- Continuity with the deep and central system
- Absence of stenosis in the vein itself

When favorable venous anatomy is found, the arterial system is then evaluated for target artery diameter and patency of the palmar arch. Reduced pressure measurements compared with the other arm or abnormal Doppler waveforms indicate proximal arterial stenosis and preclude use of that arm for access unless the problem is successfully addressed. The basic requirements are as follows:
- An arterial luminal diameter of more than 2.0 mm
- Absence of obliterating calcification
- Palmar arch patency

Evaluation of central venous outflow stenosis or occlusion is an integral part of the duplex ultrasound examination. Central venous stenosis usually results from previous use of central catheters, especially in the subclavian vein.

If a unilateral central vein problem is found, the contralateral extremity becomes the preferred choice regardless of the issue of extremity dominance. If bilateral central vein problems exist but are amenable to endovascular treatment, this should be attempted on the least diseased side.

If a subsequent duplex scan confirms effective treatment of the central vein problem, this arm can be selected for access. If not, the patient may require a nonstandard complex access solution (see later). Patients with multiple large collateral veins from chronic central venous disease can still have AF attempted if a suitable vein is available.

The anticipated duration of dialysis determines the type of catheter access selected.
- Patients expected to require dialysis for less than 3 weeks are candidates for noncuffed central venous catheter access for dialysis; these dual-lumen catheters may be placed at the bedside without fluoroscopic guidance.
- For patients expected to require dialysis for longer than 3 weeks, cuffed tunneled catheters are placed.
- For patients undergoing placement of an AF who require immediate dialysis, a cuffed tunneled catheter is placed concurrently, typically in the contralateral internal jugular vein, to provide access while the AF matures.

The internal jugular vein is preferred to the subclavian vein; the contralateral deep venous system is accessed when possible to avoid catheter obstruction of venous outflow or catheter-induced venous stenosis during the period of AF maturation. Duplex scans aid in the selection of a patent normal vein for catheter placement. Femoral catheters can also be used on a temporary basis if the deep central venous system of the upper extremity is intractably compromised.

Central Venous Catheters

A cuffed central venous catheter is placed in all patients requiring immediate dialysis after AF formation so that adequate maturation time (6 to 12 weeks) can be provided before cannulation of the AF. Because a BG can generally be used within 3 weeks, temporary noncuffed catheters can be used in this group.

The contralateral internal jugular vein is the preferred site, if it is available, because it limits ipsilateral venous outflow obstruction and would not be associated with the development of subclavian vein stenosis. Alternative sites may be used:
- Ipsilateral internal jugular vein. This choice poses some risk of venous outflow obstruction because the catheter physically rests across the confluence of the internal jugular vein and the now high-flow subclavian vein, but it has the benefit of limiting subclavian vein stenosis.
- Contralateral subclavian vein. Perhaps there would be less outflow obstruction but greater potential for negative long-term sequelae if stenosis results.
- Ipsilateral subclavian vein. This is the least attractive alternative, with potential for outflow obstruction and stenosis.

The routine use of upper extremity duplex ultrasound imaging for access planning identifies many patients who have veins suitable for AF formation but that are too deep for successful cannulation or that are too remote from the optimal arterial inflow to allow direct anastomosis without tension. Superficial venous transposition in the forearm increases AF rates in these patients.[66] This technique involves extensive dissection of a vein identified by duplex scan as being suitable in diameter, with ligation of side branches and transposition to a subcutaneous tunnel along the volar aspect of the forearm, bringing the vein to the inflow artery. This position is optimal for comfortable arm positioning during dialysis.

Types of Venous Transpositions
Upper Arm Venous Transposition

The basilic vein in the upper arm is often a good conduit for dialysis access because of its relatively large size and location in the deeper tissue planes. The traumatic consequences of repeated venipunctures observed in more superficial veins are not seen in the basilic vein because of its deeper position. Classically, the brachiobasilic transposition was regarded as a secondary option after a failed forearm fistula or graft.[67] The creation of an access using the proximal basilic vein was devised on the basis of the theoretical benefits of using a superficial vein spared repeated venipunctures, with a relatively large diameter and length. As with all venous transpositions, only one anastomosis is required, and anatomic continuity with the axillary vein is maintained. The transposition of the basilic vein to the brachial artery was described by Dagher in 1976. Four years after the original description of 24 brachiobasilic fistulas, the 5-year follow-up of a series of 90 fistulas was reported, with a 73.5% patency rate. The long-term patency remained good; a 70% functional patency rate at 8 years in 176 fistulas was reported.[68]

In certain subgroups of patients, such as those with small cephalic veins, PVD, and diabetes, the maturation rate of the radiocephalic fistula has been poor. The brachiobasilic transposition has been a good second option for these patients. Hakaim and associates[61] have reported on the superior fistula maturation in brachiobasilic transpositions (73%) compared with primary radiocephalic arteriovenous fistulas (30%). Ascher and coworkers[69] have reviewed their experience using arm veins to create brachiocephalic and brachiobasilic arteriovenous fistulas. They found no significant difference between primary patency rates at 1 year (72% for brachiocephalic versus 70% for brachiobasilic). Because of excellent patency with these fistulas, this group proposed an algorithm for the placement of arteriovenous fistulas. If a radiocephalic fistula is not feasible, a brachiocephalic fistula should first be attempted. If the brachiocephalic fistula fails or is not possible, a brachiobasilic fistula should be placed before an arteriovenous graft. In an attempt to maximize the AF rate, we favor a similar algorithm, with the addition of the superficial venous transposition of the forearm before performance of the brachial artery–based fistulas, that is, radiocephalic fistula, followed by forearm basilic venous transposition, followed by brachiocephalic fistula, followed by brachiobasilic fistula.

Long-term patency with transposed brachiobasilic fistulas that have matured has been good, with reported primary patency rates as high as 90% at 1 year and 86% at 2 years.[70] In 2003, Taghizadeh and associates[71] reported a series of 75 brachiobasilic transpositions performed during 5 years, with a mean follow-up of 14 months. In their series, 92% of fistulas matured to allow hemodialysis access. The cumulative patency was 66% at 1 year, 52% at 2 years, and 43% at 3 years. Overall, complications developed in 55% of fistulas; these included thrombosis (33%), stenosis (11%), local infection (6%), arm edema (5%), hemorrhage (3%), aneurysm (1%), and steal syndrome (1%).

The overall patency rate for autogenous brachial-basilic transpositions is superior to that of PTFE upper arm dialysis grafts. A review of all basilic vein transpositions and brachial PTFE arteriovenous fistulas created during a 5-year period has demonstrated

a statistically significant difference in primary patency rate at 1 year (90% versus 70%; $P < .01$) and 2 years (86% versus 49%; $P < .001$).[70] In this study, complications occurred approximately twice as frequently with the PTFE grafts than with the venous transpositions.

Forearm Venous Transpositions

The radiocephalic fistula, performed through a single incision, was initially described in 1966 by Brescia and coworkers.[72] This primary arteriovenous fistula was a dramatic improvement over the other, less durable modes of hemodialysis access available at the time and soon became the preferred approach to long-term dialysis access. The hemodialysis population has changed, and the dialysis patient who has a suitable vein close to the radial artery is becoming uncommon. Therefore, venous transposition procedures in the forearm have become important for enabling these patients to have a primary arteriovenous fistula.

Physical examination and visual inspection alone poorly identify suitable arteries and veins in the upper extremity. Duplex ultrasound examination allows a more thorough evaluation of the superficial venous system, increasing the number of patients who can have a forearm fistula.[66] The duplex scan can identify veins in the forearm that may have been spared repeated venipunctures because of their deeper subcutaneous location. The size of these veins may be suitable for arteriovenous creation, but if left in situ, their position in the deeper subcutaneous tissues and their anatomic position on the forearm make needle cannulation for hemodialysis technically more difficult. These usable veins on the posterior aspect of the forearm, such as the basilic vein, if not transposed, require uncomfortable and awkward positioning of the arm for dialysis. Therefore, once identified by duplex scanning, these veins are mobilized and transposed to a more favorable location on the forearm through a superficial subcutaneous plane.

To increase the number of primary AFs, Silva and colleagues,[66] in 1997, described the routine use of duplex scanning for preoperative access planning for superficial venous transposition of forearm veins for autogenous hemodialysis access. They reported a series of 89 patients in whom arteries and veins were identified with duplex scanning as suitable for primary arteriovenous fistulas. After the superficial venous transposition procedure, 91% of the fistulas matured, to be used for hemodialysis access. The primary patency rate was 84% at 1 year and 69% at 2 years. (The beneficial impact of preoperative duplex ultrasound assessments was reported in 1998.[60]) This group demonstrated a dramatic improvement in their AF rate with the institution of the protocol of routine use of duplex scanning for preoperative access planning. Their AF rate was 14% before the institution of the protocol and 63% after the protocol was established. Table 62-10 demonstrates the three general areas in which the superficial veins are found and the rates at which they were used in the study. Note that the minority (15%) of the transpositions were accomplished through a single incision, with the artery and vein in proximity. Approximately 50% of transposed veins arose from the volar surface of the forearm, and a third were harvested from the dorsal aspect of the forearm.

Lower Extremity Venous Transpositions

The upper extremity is the preferred site for hemodialysis access, with the lower extremity generally being reserved for use once upper extremity options have been exhausted. If the extremity is not suitable for fistula creation, a prosthetic graft can be placed. However, there is a concern about increased thrombosis and

TABLE 62-10 Superficial Venous Transpositions of the Forearm

TRANSPOSITION PERFORMED	% OF TOTAL
Type A	15
Artery and vein in immediate proximity	
Single incision	
Superficial subcutaneous transposition only	
Type B	33
Dorsally located vein transposed to volar surface artery	
Separate incisions	
Superficial subcutaneous transposition	
Type C	52
Volar vein transposed to midforearm volar surface	
Separate incisions	
Superficial subcutaneous transposition	

From Silva MB Jr, Hobson RW 2nd, Pappas PJ, et al: Vein transposition in the forearm for autogenous hemodialysis access. *J Vasc Surg* 26:981–986, 1997.

infection rates in thigh hemodialysis grafts, which have been reported as high as 55% and 35%, respectively. Tashjian and associates,[73] reviewing their experience with 73 femoral artery–based hemodialysis grafts, found a primary patency rate of 71% and a secondary patency rate of 83% at 1 year. The infection rate in this series was 22%.

Venous transpositions in the lower extremity using the great saphenous vein and superficial femoral vein have been described.[74] The transposed great saphenous veins and superficial femoral veins in the leg have theoretical benefits similar to those of venous transpositions in the upper extremity. The venous conduits are long and generally of good caliber and are less prone to infection than prosthetic grafts. Importantly, only one anastomosis is required because the more central venous segment maintains its native connection with the common femoral vein.

The superficial femoral vein, part of the deep venous system, has a diameter in the range of 6 to 10 mm, has relatively thick walls, and has been used for a wide variety of vascular reconstructions.[75] Gradman and coworkers have reported a retrospective analysis of 25 patients who underwent arteriovenous construction with use of superficial femoral veins. Of these patients, 18 underwent superficial femoral vein transposition and 7 were given a composite loop fistula of superficial femoral vein and PTFE. The cumulative primary fistula patency rate was 78% at 6 months and 73% at 1 year. The cumulative secondary patency rate was 91% at 5 months and 86% at 1 year. There were no fistula infections, but the rate of major wound complications was 28%. Eight patients required secondary procedures for symptomatic steal syndrome, and one patient ultimately needed an above-knee amputation after the development of ipsilateral compartment syndrome.[74]

The saphenous vein has been used for arterial reconstructions in almost all vascular beds and in the construction of arteriovenous access in the upper and lower extremities. The great saphenous vein has been used to create an AF in the upper thigh in a looped configuration and an arterial anastomosis with the common femoral artery or SFA.[76]

Techniques of Venous Transposition

Assessment of the Patient and Selection of Optimal Site

The evaluation and preoperative assessment of the patient are the most important steps in the establishment of durable hemodialysis

access. First, the best available site is selected on the basis of optimal arterial inflow and venous outflow. According to the DOQI guidelines, the preference is for an AF over a prosthetic graft, for the forearm over the upper arm, and for the nondominant arm over the dominant arm.

Preference for the nondominant arm relates to convenience for the patient, allowing the dominant arm to be used for activity during dialysis. When duplex ultrasound surveillance identifies a suitable vein and artery in the nondominant forearm, an AF constructed between them becomes the procedure of choice. Duplex ultrasonography is also used to select the optimal anastomotic site. If the radial or ulnar arteries are disadvantaged, a suitable vein in the forearm may be dissected and looped back to the brachial artery in the antecubital space. All autogenous forearm possibilities are exhausted before proceeding to autogenous upper arm alternatives because this maximizes future possible sites.

Absence of suitable veins in both forearms necessitates construction of the access in the upper arm. Again, duplex ultrasonography is valuable in identifying a superficial (preferred) or deep (second-choice) arm vein that can be transposed to a volar subcutaneous location for creation of an AF with the brachial artery. The dominant upper arm is used if the arteries and veins in the nondominant upper arm are unsuitable.

If there are no suitable veins for an AF, outflow through the deeper venous system in the arm is examined to identify a possible site of placement of a prosthetic BG. A looped BG configuration is used in the nondominant forearm when an appropriate antecubital vein and brachial artery are present.

The dominant forearm is the next site of choice. If both forearms are unsuitable, the nondominant upper arm, followed by the dominant upper arm, is the next option. To maximize the number of BG possibilities, a prosthetic graft is initially placed between the brachial artery and the brachial vein in the distal upper arm, followed by the vein in the mid arm and the proximal arm, and finally the axillary vein.

Duplex ultrasonography is used to identify and to mark the best possible location for the anastomosis and to confirm adequate central venous runoff. When possible, avoid placement of prosthetic BGs in patients who are significantly immunocompromised because of the significant risk of infection and the complexities involved with removal of the BG and restoration of prograde arterial flow.

Superficial Venous Transposition of the Forearm

The superficial venous transposition of the forearm is performed using local 1% lidocaine infusion supplemented with IV sedation. Lidocaine with epinephrine is avoided because of its vasoconstrictive properties.

A longitudinal incision is made directly over the cephalic or basilic vein, beginning at the distal extent of the previously mapped and marked vein. The incision proceeds toward the antecubital fossa for a distance of at least 15 cm. Multiple short skip incisions can also be used. A 3-0 silk suture ligature is used to ligate the portion of vein remaining in its distal bed, and the vein is transected at the wrist. The vein is dissected free from its surrounding tissue so that it may be completely transposed to a superficial tunnel in the midportion of the volar aspect of the forearm. Most venous branches along the length of the vein are ligated and divided; however, those that will not interfere with transposition are left intact to maximize outflow. Heparinized saline is flushed through the open end of the vein with digital compression for occlusion of outflow at the antecubital fossa; this results in substantial dilation of the freed segment of vein. The vein is wrapped in a heparin- and saline-soaked sponge, and attention is then turned to the arterial dissection.

The segment of artery that has been preoperatively identified as suitable for inflow is exposed. Usually, the radial artery is identified between the brachial radialis and flexor carpi radialis tendons. The superficial branch of the radial nerve is located lateral to the radial artery, and this nerve is separated from the radial artery by the brachial radialis muscle. The nerve is sensory at this level, and care must be taken not to injure it. Concomitant veins run parallel to the artery on either side. These should be carefully dissected free from the artery, facilitating identification of the numerous small arterial branches. Although there are usually no arterial branches on the anterior aspect of the artery, several paired arterial branches usually leave the radial artery on each side, and they must be addressed. These may be ligated, with the ligature placed approximately 2 mm away from the radial artery to avoid impingement once dilation has occurred. Vessel loops are placed proximally and distally along the artery for vascular control.

A tunneling instrument is passed through the subcutaneous tissues to develop a superficial tunnel. The vein is marked on the anterior surface along its length with a sterile marking pen to facilitate passage through the tunnel without twisting or kinking. Once the vein has been passed through the subcutaneous tunnel and hemostasis has been ensured, the patient is typically given 3000 units of heparin intravenously, and a 1- to 2-mm arteriotomy is made with a No. 11 scalpel blade on the volar surface of the artery. The arteriotomy is extended to approximately 15 to 20 mm with fine Potts scissors. With an 18-gauge angiocatheter, the artery is heparinized locally by injection of heparinized saline distally and then proximally while the vessel loops are simultaneously opened.

An end-to-side anastomosis is performed with 7-0 polypropylene or Gore-Tex PTFE suture (Gore Medical). Before completion of the anastomosis, vascular dilators are used to size the vein and radial artery. This step has the benefit of allowing enlargement of blood vessels in spasm from vessel loops and manipulation.

After the anastomosis is constructed, it is essential that a thrill be felt within the vein. Absence of a thrill indicates a probable technical or anatomic defect and requires further investigation, with exploration of the anastomosis. Wounds are closed with a running subcuticular absorbable stitch. Care is taken to maintain strict atraumatic technique during handling of the skin edges to limit wound complications. Adhesive strips and tape applied directly to the skin are not used.

Superficial Venous Transposition of the Arm

The transposition of the cephalic or basilic vein is performed with local anesthesia using 1% lidocaine and IV sedation or regional anesthesia using an interscalene nerve block. The entire arm and ipsilateral axilla and shoulder are prepared in a sterile fashion. For the cephalic vein transposition, the vein is found in an anatomic groove between the brachioradialis and biceps muscles. It travels superficially to the musculocutaneous nerve and then ascends in the groove along the lateral border of the biceps muscle. A longitudinal incision over the cephalic vein is used for exposure. For the basilic vein transposition, the vein is identified anterior to the medial epicondyle of the humerus, and through a longitudinal incision along the medial aspect of the upper arm to the axilla, the basilic vein is exposed. The median cutaneous nerve is close to the basilic vein and should be preserved.

All venous branches are ligated and divided. The cephalic vein is mobilized for at least 15 cm. The basilic vein is mobilized to its junction with the brachial vein. The brachial artery can be exposed through the same incision or through a separate incision. Vessel loops are loosely encircled around the brachial artery proximally and distally.

Next, the cephalic or basilic vein is divided near the antecubital fossa and flushed and distended with heparinized saline. A sterile marking pen is used to mark the vein along its entire length to help avoid twisting during passage through the subcutaneous tunnel created anteriorly between the axilla and antecubital fossa. Approximately 3000 units of heparin is administered intravenously, and proximal and distal control of the brachial artery is obtained with the vessel loops. An end-to-side anastomosis with the brachial artery is constructed with 6-0 polypropylene sutures. After completion of the anastomosis, the fistula is inspected for a thrill. If a thrill is not present, a technical or structural problem is suspected that will require correction. The subcutaneous tissues and skin are closed with absorbable suture.

Follow-Up

Adequate arterialization of the vein usually occurs within 8 to 12 weeks. Hand exercises are advocated to encourage fistula maturation.

The AF access is studied by duplex ultrasound approximately 6 weeks after placement to assess maturation and to mark sites most suitable for initial cannulation by the dialysis center staff. For a new AF, dialysis should be initiated through a 16- or 17-gauge needle and for longer sessions at minimal rates of flow.

At least three successful hemodialysis sessions should be accomplished before removal of the central venous catheter. If flow rates are insufficient for successful dialysis or if follow-up duplex ultrasonography identifies a problem in the access, the access is considered a failure, and the patient is referred for evaluation and treatment (see next section).

Patients With Failing or Failed Access

For patients with a failing or failed access, the first step is a thorough duplex ultrasound evaluation of the access and underlying arterial and venous anatomy to ascertain the cause of failure, correctability, or salvage and alternative sites. In particular, patients with a prosthetic BG should be evaluated for graft salvage and for the identification of a possible site for placement of a new AF in case the BG salvage is not successful.

Patients with a failing dialysis catheter typically present with suboptimal flow on dialysis or, less commonly, upper extremity swelling secondary to pericatheter deep venous thrombosis. A duplex ultrasound scan can easily identify the latter, in which case endovascular treatment to reestablish deep venous outflow after catheter removal is considered. Subsequent imaging is directed at assessing the efficacy of treatment and identifying an alternative insertion site.

In patients with poor catheter flow rates but no evidence of central venous compromise, transcatheter thrombolytic therapy has been effective. Tissue plasminogen activator instilled directly through the catheter access port and allowed to dwell for some time has been effective.

Catheters compromised by malpositioning of the tip or encapsulation in a fibrin sheath can be treated endovascularly. If catheter salvage is unsuccessful, the catheter is exchanged. Over-the-wire techniques may be used for noncuffed catheters but can be challenging with cuffed catheters having exit sites remote from the insertion site. This technique may result in similarly poor flow rates if the problem is a suboptimal subcutaneous tunnel, either acutely angled or compromised by proximity to the clavicle. Usually, a new percutaneous placement is performed at the site identified as optimal by duplex ultrasound scans.

Information available from duplex ultrasound examination of a threatened or failed AF or BG is essential for directing treatment. Results of salvage are significantly worse with fistulas or grafts that have thrombosed than with those that are patent but have an identifiable stenosis. Thrombolytic therapy and surgical thrombectomy have poor 6-month primary efficacy rates. Nonetheless, the value of sustaining each access site in today's dialysis population usually warrants an attempt at salvage.

Thrombolysis and surgical thrombectomy are aimed at removal of the clot as a prerequisite to identifying the underlying anatomic anomaly. Post-thrombectomy access imaging in the surgical suite is imperative. Appropriate adjunctive management of the offending lesion follows—first with endovascular options, if warranted, and surgical revision if this proves unsuccessful.

Prospective monitoring of the access for hemodynamically significant stenoses, combined with correction, improves patency and decreases the incidence of thrombosis. A number of techniques have been proposed to monitor for stenoses. These include intra-access flow, static or dynamic venous pressure measurements, measurements of recirculation using urea concentration or dilution techniques, and observation for changes in characteristics of pulse or thrill in the access and prolongation of bleeding after needle withdrawal. Most of these techniques suggest increasing resistance at the venous anastomosis, which is the most common site of myointimal hyperplastic problems.

The DOQI guidelines suggest that persistent abnormalities in any of these parameters mandate venography. A comprehensive duplex scan can also serve as the initial examination. The decision to proceed with endovascular or surgical treatment is determined by the type of lesion identified and the physician's experience.

In modern vascular practice, endovascular balloon dilation of venous outflow stenoses in a BG or segmental stenoses in an AF is the initial choice of treatment. This must eliminate the hemodynamically significant stenosis and restore normal flow for it to be considered a success (Fig. 62-32).

Postprocedure evaluation by duplex ultrasound scan at 1 month to assess efficacy is recommended. Repeated angioplasty may be performed if indicated. In our practice, two failures of endovascular treatment for the same lesion within a 3-month period prompt open surgical intervention.

Surgical revision can be guided by the duplex scan and by subsequent contrast studies obtained during attempted endovascular revision. Surgical revision is focused on eliminating the causative lesion and preserving the maximal usable segment of vein for future use.

Recalcitrant stenoses in an AF can be treated by patch angioplasty or segmental resection and interposition of a translocated reversed segment of vein or, frequently, by mobilization of the matured vein and primary repair. Arterial or venous stenoses near or involving the anastomosis can be treated with patch angioplasty or, alternatively, with mobilization and formation of a new arteriovenous connection.

For focal defects in a BG, such as midgraft stenosis or pseudoaneurysm, direct excision and interposition of a new segment may be indicated. The BG venous outflow lesion resistant to endovascular treatment may be treated with surgical patch angioplasty or a jump graft to a segment of uninvolved vein with good outflow.

Any failed or failing graft that undergoes successful revision and salvage is reassessed at 1 month by duplex ultrasound examination. To achieve the reported 60% 1-year success rates after endovascular or surgical intervention, further intervention is typically required.

Secondary Interventions in Autogenous Fistulas

Few published series have focused on re-intervention of failing or nonmaturing autogenous arteriovenous fistulas, and most of those that have been reported focused on the traditional radiocephalic arteriovenous fistula. Recognizing this, Hingorani and colleagues[77] have reviewed their experience with salvage procedures in the management of nonfunctioning or nonmaturing arteriovenous fistulas, which included fistulas based in the upper arm. The distribution of fistulas that required salvage procedures was 37% radiocephalic, 47% brachiocephalic, and 16% brachiobasilic. In 46 patients (49 fistulas), 75 procedures, both open and endovascular, were performed; 17 patients underwent 26 balloon angioplasties and 20 patients had vein patch angioplasty. The group performed 12 fistula revisions to a more proximal level and 4 vein interposition grafts. Although the total number of subsequent procedures required for percutaneously treated fistulas was higher than that for open repair, there was no statistical difference

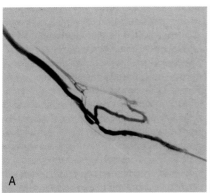
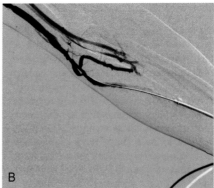

FIGURE 62-32 Endovascular-assisted arteriovenous fistula maturation. **A,** Severe stenosis of radiobasilic arteriovenous fistula. **B,** After balloon angioplasty, flow improved, and the patient was able to undergo dialysis within 2 weeks using the arteriovenous fistula.

between primary patency rates. It was concluded that salvage procedures may allow maturation and extend the life span of arteriovenous fistulas for hemodialysis.

The beneficial effects of secondary interventions on the maturation and maintenance of autogenous arteriovenous fistulas have been demonstrated by Berman and Gentile.[78] They placed 170 AFs in 163 patients (115 brachiocephalic, 47 radiocephalic, and 8 brachiobasilic). Secondary procedures were required for failure to mature in nine patients and for failure of previously functioning fistulas in six patients. A functional access was achieved in 90% of patients; these researchers demonstrated a 10% improvement in accomplishing or maintaining functional autogenous access through secondary procedures.

In the series of 89 patients with superficial venous transposition of forearm veins after duplex mapping for establishment of hemodialysis access, Silva and coworkers[66] reported a total of 18 failed fistulas. With surgical revision, four were successfully salvaged and six were converted to ipsilateral prosthetic grafts (three forearm, three upper arm). In addition, access was established on the other arm in five patients (three AFs, two prosthetic grafts).

Complex Access

Complex access solutions are required when all upper extremity access sites have been exhausted or when extensive central venous obliteration is not responsive to endovascular treatment. If the central venous system is patent, placement of a cuffed catheter is the simplest alternative.

In patients with refractory central subclavian vein occlusion and a patent ipsilateral internal jugular vein, the jugular vein turndown procedure may be performed.[79] The cephalad portion of the jugular vein at the angle of the mandible is divided; after mobilization, the jugular vein is anastomosed to the patent axillary vein segment, just proximal to the subclavian occlusion, to provide runoff for the upper arm. Resection of the central portion of the clavicle may be performed to facilitate a favorable anatomic lie of the vein graft. Other nonstandard access configurations, such as axillary artery to axillary vein body wall prosthetic grafts (loop configuration if ipsilateral, crossover or collar graft if contralateral), may be considered. Axillary arterial to right atrial BGs and axillary arterial to arterial prosthetic configurations have been used when extensive central venous obliteration is encountered, but these options are compromised by their potential for increased morbidity.

If upper extremity options are unsatisfactory and the superior central venous system is occluded, lower extremity access options can be used. Transposition of the saphenous vein in a loop configuration to the SFA or common femoral artery has been performed. Alternatively, a prosthetic BG can be placed in a loop configuration from the common femoral vein to the SFA or common femoral artery. A prosthetic BG can also be created from one femoral artery to a contralateral femoral vein and tunneled subcutaneously across the lower anterior abdominal wall. With a percutaneous approach to the femoral vein, a cuffed catheter can be tunneled into the anterior thigh. In patients with lower extremity venous thrombosis, a translumbar approach to the inferior vena cava has been used with a lateral tunnel for the cuffed catheter.

Vascular Access Complications

Infection is the second leading cause of death in dialysis patients, causing 10% of deaths, exceeded only by cardiovascular disease. Most of the systemic infections are directly related to infections

from vascular access. The increased rate of infection in dialysis patients is caused by immunodeficiency and poor wound healing associated with chronic renal failure. *Staphylococcus aureus* is the most common cause of infection, and the use of aseptic technique is the best way to prevent bacterial colonization and vascular access site infection. Infection of an autogenous arteriovenous fistula is rare; it can be treated with appropriate antibiotics and local wound care, with drainage of abscess. Infection of a prosthetic arteriovenous graft is more common and is caused by contamination from skin flora during implantation or direct inoculation of the graft by an access needle from inadequately prepared skin. Treatment is with excision of the prosthetic material. The use of perioperative antibiotics has been shown to be effective in reducing infections. Cephalosporins can significantly decrease postoperative wound infections, and vancomycin can reduce graft infections.

The most common complication of vascular access is thrombosis of the venous fistula or prosthetic graft. The cause of most graft failures is the development of intimal hyperplasia at the venous anastomosis or venous outflow tract. This can account for 85% of graft failures, with 55% of thromboses caused by venous anastomosis and 30% caused by venous outflow occlusion or long-segment stenosis. For venous fistula, the specific offending location is not as clear. The lesion can be located at the arterial anastomosis or within the fistula. Flow in the vascular access can be restored with open surgical thrombectomy or endovascular thrombolysis and angioplasty. Venous outflow or anastomotic lesions need to be treated to prevent a high graft failure rate of 70% at 6 months. An improved patency rate of more than 70% at 6 months can be achieved with surgical anastomotic revision or endovascular stenting.

Aneurysmal degeneration of fistula can develop over time. These massively dilated venous segments can involve the skin, placing the patient at risk of significant bleeding. The low resistance of the enlarged fistula can lead to steal syndrome. Treatment is with interposition grafts and removal of the enlarged portion (Fig. 62-33).

Arterial insufficiency, or steal syndrome, can develop in patients with vascular access. The creation of this access results in a low-resistance circulation that shunts arterial inflow into this

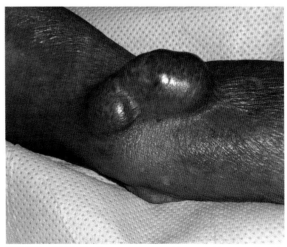

FIGURE 62-33 Fistula aneurysm without evidence of skin involvement.

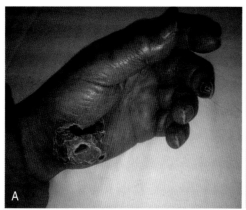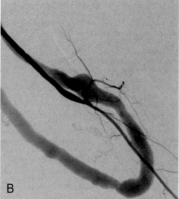

FIGURE 62-34 A, Patient with tissue loss of the hand because of steal. He underwent arterial duplex ultrasound examination and angiography before distal revascularization and interval ligation **(B),** with immediate symptomatic improvement.

low-pressure venous outflow. In addition, the flow in the artery distal to the access origin may become retrograde and is no longer antegrade. The effect is that the vascular access steals arterial flow, which may compromise distal limb perfusion. This physiologic steal phenomenon can be demonstrated in 75% to 90% of patients; however, only 1% to 6% are symptomatic. Symptoms may include a cold and painful hand or foot; with significant flow compromise, patients may develop tissue loss in their fingers or toes (Fig. 62-34). In patients with forearm vascular access using radial artery as inflow, such as radiocephalic or radiobasilic fistulas, ligation of the artery just distal to the fistula restores flow in the palmar arch through the ulnar artery. In patients with vascular access in the upper arm, the distal revascularization with interval ligation procedure is used to revascularize the distal limb while preserving the vascular access. The procedure is a bypass from the inflow artery proximal to the access to the artery distal to the access. The arterial segment between the vascular access and distal anastomosis of the bypass is ligated to prevent steal. The low-pressure zone around the access origin may shunt blood flow from the bypass into the access rather than restoring distal flow. An autogenous conduit should be used for this bypass if possible.

CONCLUSION

Ultimately, the goals of the DOQI are to minimize the deep effects on the end-stage renal disease patient's quality of life that hemodialysis dependence entails. Increasing rates of autogenous arteriovenous access increase patency rates, decrease complications, and therefore decrease the number of unplanned interventions and hospitalizations that this population is required to endure. This vision cannot be realized with traditional arteriovenous access alone. Early referral to vascular surgery, institutional strategies of preoperative noninvasive vascular assessments, and use of venous transposition procedures can be effective in increasing autogenous access in the dialysis population. A system of prospective monitoring for the development of hemodynamically significant stenosis can improve long-term assisted patency. A multidisciplinary approach involving the nephrologist, vascular surgeon, and hemodialysis center nurses as well as the patient and the patient's social support system is required to optimize the care of this population of complex patients.

SELECTED REFERENCES

Adam DJ, Beard JD, Cleveland T, et al: Bypass versus angioplasty in severe ischaemia of the leg (BASIL): Multicentre, randomised controlled trial. *Lancet* 366:1925–1934, 2005.

> This randomized trial showed that in patients with severe limb ischemia due to infrainguinal disease and who are suitable for surgery and angioplasty, strategies of bypass surgery first and balloon angioplasty first are associated with broadly similar outcomes in terms of amputation-free survival, and in the short-term, surgery was more expensive than angioplasty.

Barnett HJ, Taylor DW, Eliasziw M, et al: Benefit of carotid endarterectomy in patients with symptomatic moderate or severe stenosis. North American Symptomatic Carotid Endarterectomy Trial Collaborators. *N Engl J Med* 339:1415–1425, 1998.

> NASCET was a randomized prospective trial confirming the superiority of CEA over medical management for patients with high-grade symptomatic carotid disease.

Brott TG, Hobson RW, 2nd, Howard G, et al: Stenting versus endarterectomy for treatment of carotid-artery stenosis. *N Engl J Med* 363:11–23, 2010.

> CREST, the definitive randomized prospective trial comparing carotid stenting and CEA, lasted more than 10 years and produced the best results from both therapies ever reported in such a trial. Results from carotid stenting were dramatically improved during the second half of the trial compared with the first half, suggesting the evolutionary nature of endovascular procedures and an identifiable learning curve for new technologies.

CAPRIE Steering Committee: A randomised, blinded, trial of clopidogrel versus aspirin in patients at risk of ischaemic events (CAPRIE). *Lancet* 348:1329–1339, 1996.

This blinded randomized trial showed clopidogrel to be more effective and safer than aspirin in reducing the combined risk of ischemic stroke, myocardial infarction, or vascular deaths in patients with atherosclerosis.

Endarterectomy for asymptomatic carotid artery stenosis: Executive Committee for the Asymptomatic Carotid Atherosclerosis Study. *JAMA* 273:1421–1428, 1995.

ACAS was a randomized prospective trial confirming the superiority of CEA over medical management for the treatment of asymptomatic carotid disease.

Hirsch AT, Haskal ZJ, Hertzer NR, et al: ACC/AHA 2005 Practice Guidelines for the management of patients with PAD (lower extremity, renal, mesenteric, and abdominal aortic): A collaborative report from the American Association for Vascular Surgery/Society for Vascular Surgery, Society for Cardiovascular Angiography and Interventions, Society for Vascular Medicine and Biology, Society of Interventional Radiology, and the ACC/AHA Task Force on Practice Guidelines (Writing Committee to Develop Guidelines for the Management of Patients With Peripheral Arterial Disease): Endorsed by the American Association of Cardiovascular and Pulmonary Rehabilitation; National Heart, Lung, and Blood Institute; Society for Vascular Nursing; TransAtlantic Inter-Society Consensus; and Vascular Disease Foundation. *Circulation* 113:e463–e654, 2006.

The ACC/AHA guidelines are a consensus document describing targets for medical management of vascular disease, including current thoughts on prevention.

Norgren L, Hiatt WR, Dormandy JA, et al: Inter-Society Consensus for the Management of Peripheral Arterial Disease (TASC II). *J Vasc Surg* 45(Suppl):S5–S67, 2007.

This consensus document describes an approach for choosing open revascularization versus endovascular therapy for patients on the basis of lesion characteristics.

REFERENCES

1. Criqui MH, Vargas V, Denenberg JO, et al: Ethnicity and peripheral arterial disease: The San Diego Population Study. *Circulation* 112:2703–2707, 2005.
2. Norgren L, Hiatt WR, Dormandy JA, et al: Inter-Society Consensus for the Management of Peripheral Arterial Disease (TASC II). *J Vasc Surg* 45(Suppl S):S5–S67, 2007.
3. Feinglass J, Pearce WH, Martin GJ, et al: Postoperative and late survival outcomes after major amputation: Findings from the Department of Veterans Affairs National Surgical Quality Improvement Program. *Surgery* 130:21–29, 2001.
4. Taylor SM, Kalbaugh CA, Blackhurst DW, et al: Preoperative clinical factors predict postoperative functional outcomes after major lower limb amputation: An analysis of 553 consecutive patients. *J Vasc Surg* 42:227–235, 2005.
5. Stone PA, Back MR, Armstrong PA, et al: Midfoot amputations expand limb salvage rates for diabetic foot infections. *Ann Vasc Surg* 19:805–811, 2005.
6. Fisher DF, Jr, Clagett GP, Fry RE, et al: One-stage versus two-stage amputation for wet gangrene of the lower

extremity: A randomized study. *J Vasc Surg* 8:428–433, 1988.
7. Bolia A, Sayers RD, Thompson MM, et al: Subintimal and intraluminal recanalisation of occluded crural arteries by percutaneous balloon angioplasty. *Eur J Vasc Surg* 8:214–219, 1994.
8. Scott EC, Biuckians A, Light RE, et al: Subintimal angioplasty: Our experience in the treatment of 506 infrainguinal arterial occlusions. *J Vasc Surg* 48:878–884, 2008.
9. Clark TW, Groffsky JL, Soulen MC: Predictors of long-term patency after femoropopliteal angioplasty: Results from the STAR registry. *J Vasc Interv Radiol* 12:923–933, 2001.
10. Dorros G, Jaff MR, Murphy KJ, et al: The acute outcome of tibioperoneal vessel angioplasty in 417 cases with claudication and critical limb ischemia. *Cathet Cardiovasc Diagn* 45:251–256, 1998.
11. Dorros G, Jaff MR, Dorros AM, et al: Tibioperoneal (outflow lesion) angioplasty can be used as primary treatment in 235 patients with critical limb ischemia: Five-year follow-up. *Circulation* 104:2057–2062, 2001.
12. Kudo T, Chandra FA, Ahn SS: The effectiveness of percutaneous transluminal angioplasty for the treatment of critical limb ischemia: A 10-year experience. *J Vasc Surg* 41:423–435, discussion 435, 2005.
13. Sabeti S, Schillinger M, Amighi J, et al: Primary patency of femoropopliteal arteries treated with nitinol versus stainless steel self-expanding stents: Propensity score–adjusted analysis. *Radiology* 232:516–521, 2004.
14. Schillinger M, Sabeti S, Dick P, et al: Sustained benefit at 2 years of primary femoropopliteal stenting compared with balloon angioplasty with optional stenting. *Circulation* 115:2745–2749, 2007.
15. Kickuth R, Keo HH, Triller J, et al: Initial clinical experience with the 4-F self-expanding XPERT stent system for infra-popliteal treatment of patients with severe claudication and critical limb ischemia. *J Vasc Interv Radiol* 18:703–708, 2007.
16. Mwipatayi BP, Hockings A, Hofmann M, et al: Balloon angioplasty compared with stenting for treatment of femoro-popliteal occlusive disease: A meta-analysis. *J Vasc Surg* 47:461–469, 2008.
17. Railo M, Roth WD, Edgren J, et al: Preliminary results with endoluminal femoropopliteal thrupass. *Ann Chir Gynaecol* 90:15–18, 2001.
18. Fischer M, Schwabe C, Schulte KL: Value of the Hemobahn/Viabahn endoprosthesis in the treatment of long chronic lesions of the superficial femoral artery: 6 years of experience. *J Endovasc Ther* 13:281–290, 2006.
19. Bleyn J, Schol F, Vanhandenhove I, et al: Endovascular reconstruction of the superficial femoral artery. In Becquemin JP, Alimi YS, Watelet J, et al, editors: *Controversies and updates in vascular cardiac surgery, 14*, Torino, Italy, 2004, Edizioni Minerva Medica, pp 87–91.
20. Saxon RR, Dake MD, Volgelzang RL, et al: Randomized, multicenter study comparing expanded polytetrafluoroethylene–covered endoprosthesis placement with percutaneous transluminal angioplasty in the treatment of superficial femoral artery occlusive disease. *J Vasc Interv Radiol* 19:823–832, 2008.
21. Kedora J, Hohmann S, Garrett W, et al: Randomized comparison of percutaneous Viabahn stent grafts vs prosthetic femoral-popliteal bypass in the treatment of superficial

femoral arterial occlusive disease. *J Vasc Surg* 45:10–16, discussion 16, 2007.

22. Keeling WB, Shames ML, Stone PA, et al: Plaque excision with the Silverhawk catheter: Early results in patients with claudication or critical limb ischemia. *J Vasc Surg* 45:25–31, 2007.

23. Scheinert D, Laird JR, Jr, Schroder M, et al: Excimer laser–assisted recanalization of long, chronic superficial femoral artery occlusions. *J Endovasc Ther* 8:156–166, 2001.

24. Laird JR, Zeller T, Gray BH, et al: Limb salvage following laser-assisted angioplasty for critical limb ischemia: Results of the LACI multicenter trial. *J Endovasc Ther* 13:1–11, 2006.

25. Buth J, Disselhoff B, Sommeling C, et al: Color-flow duplex criteria for grading stenosis in infrainguinal vein grafts. *J Vasc Surg* 14:716–726, discussion 726–728, 1991.

26. Mills JL, Sr, Wixon CL, James DC, et al: The natural history of intermediate and critical vein graft stenosis: Recommendations for continued surveillance or repair. *J Vasc Surg* 33:273–278, discussion 278–280, 2001.

27. Calligaro KD, Doerr K, McAffee-Bennett S, et al: Should duplex ultrasonography be performed for surveillance of femoropopliteal and femorotibial arterial prosthetic bypasses? *Ann Vasc Surg* 15:520–524, 2001.

28. Carter A, Murphy MO, Halka AT, et al: The natural history of stenoses within lower limb arterial bypass grafts using a graft surveillance program. *Ann Vasc Surg* 21:695–703, 2007.

29. Gonsalves C, Bandyk DF, Avino AJ, et al: Duplex features of vein graft stenosis and the success of percutaneous transluminal angioplasty. *J Endovasc Surg* 6:66–72, 1999.

30. Tielbeek AV, Rietjens E, Buth J, et al: The value of duplex surveillance after endovascular intervention for femoropopliteal obstructive disease. *Eur J Vasc Endovasc Surg* 12:145–150, 1996.

31. Guzman RP, Zierler RE, Isaacson JA, et al: Renal atrophy and arterial stenosis. A prospective study with duplex ultrasound. *Hypertension* 23:346–350, 1994.

32. Caps MT, Zierler RE, Polissar NL, et al: Risk of atrophy in kidneys with atherosclerotic renal artery stenosis. *Kidney Int* 53:735–742, 1998.

33. Mailloux LU, Napolitano B, Bellucci AG, et al: Renal vascular disease causing end-stage renal disease, incidence, clinical correlates, and outcomes: A 20-year clinical experience. *Am J Kidney Dis* 24:622–629, 1994.

34. Grüntzig A, Kuhlmann U, Vetter W, et al: Treatment of renovascular hypertension with percutaneous transluminal dilatation of a renal-artery stenosis. *Lancet* 1:801–802, 1978.

35. Leertouwer TC, Gussenhoven EJ, Bosch JL, et al: Stent placement for renal arterial stenosis: Where do we stand? A meta-analysis. *Radiology* 216:78–85, 2000.

36. Gill KS, Fowler RC: Atherosclerotic renal arterial stenosis: Clinical outcomes of stent placement for hypertension and renal failure. *Radiology* 226:821–826, 2003.

37. Henry M, Amor M, Henry I, et al: Stents in the treatment of renal artery stenosis: Long-term follow-up. *J Endovasc Surg* 6:42–51, 1999.

38. Webster J, Marshall F, Abdalla M, et al: Randomised comparison of percutaneous angioplasty vs continued medical therapy for hypertensive patients with atheromatous renal artery stenosis. Scottish and Newcastle Renal Artery Stenosis Collaborative Group. *J Hum Hypertens* 12:329–335, 1998.

39. van Jaarsveld BC, Krijnen P, Pieterman H, et al: The effect of balloon angioplasty on hypertension in atherosclerotic renal-artery stenosis. Dutch Renal Artery Stenosis Intervention Cooperative Study Group. *N Engl J Med* 342:1007–1014, 2000.

40. Rocha-Singh KJ, Ahuja RK, Sung CH, et al: Long-term renal function preservation after renal artery stenting in patients with progressive ischemic nephropathy. *Catheter Cardiovasc Interv* 57:135–141, 2002.

41. Rundback JH, Gray RJ, Rozenblit G, et al: Renal artery stent placement for the management of ischemic nephropathy. *J Vasc Interv Radiol* 9:413–420, 1998.

42. Bush RL, Martin LG, Lin PH, et al: Endovascular revascularization of renal artery stenosis in the solitary functioning kidney. *Ann Vasc Surg* 15:60–66, 2001.

43. Henry M, Amor M, Henry I, et al: Stent placement in the renal artery: Three-year experience with the Palmaz stent. *J Vasc Interv Radiol* 7:343–350, 1996.

44. Dorros G, Jaff M, Jain A, et al: Follow-up of primary Palmaz-Schatz stent placement for atherosclerotic renal artery stenosis. *Am J Cardiol* 75:1051–1055, 1995.

45. Rodriguez-Lopez JA, Werner A, Ray LI, et al: Renal artery stenosis treated with stent deployment: Indications, technique, and outcome for 108 patients. *J Vasc Surg* 29:617–624, 1999.

46. Zeller T, Frank U, Muller C, et al: Duplex ultrasound for follow-up examination after stent-angioplasty of ostial renal artery stenoses. *Ultraschall Med* 23:315–319, 2002.

47. Bax L, Mali WP, Van De Ven PJ, et al: Repeated intervention for in-stent restenosis of the renal arteries. *J Vasc Interv Radiol* 13:1219–1224, 2002.

48. Mackrell PJ, Langan EM, 3rd, Sullivan TM, et al: Management of renal artery stenosis: Effects of a shift from surgical to percutaneous therapy on indications and outcomes. *Ann Vasc Surg* 17:54–59, 2003.

49. Kessel DO, Robertson I, Taylor EJ, et al: Renal stenting from the radial artery: A novel approach. *Cardiovasc Intervent Radiol* 26:146–149, 2003.

50. Schobel WA, Mauser M: Miniaturization of the equipment for percutaneous coronary interventions: A prospective study in 1,200 patients. *J Invasive Cardiol* 15:6–11, 2003.

51. Rakhit RD, Matter C, Windecker S, et al: Five French versus 6 French PCI: A case control study of efficacy, safety and outcome. *J Invasive Cardiol* 14:670–674, 2002.

52. Spinosa DJ, Matsumoto AH, Angle JF, et al: Renal insufficiency: Usefulness of gadodiamide-enhanced renal angiography to supplement CO_2-enhanced renal angiography for diagnosis and percutaneous treatment. *Radiology* 210:663–672, 1999.

53. Ailawadi G, Stanley JC, Williams DM, et al: Gadolinium as a nonnephrotoxic contrast agent for catheter-based arteriographic evaluation of renal arteries in patients with azotemia. *J Vasc Surg* 37:346–352, 2003.

54. Brott TG, Hobson RW, 2nd, Howard G, et al: Stenting versus endarterectomy for treatment of carotid-artery stenosis. *N Engl J Med* 363:11–23, 2010.

55. Sheehan MK, Baker WH, Littooy FN, et al: Timing of postcarotid complications: A guide to safe discharge planning. *J Vasc Surg* 34:13–16, 2001.

56. Wholey MH, Wholey MH, Tan WA, et al: Management of neurological complications of carotid artery stenting. *J Endovasc Ther* 8:341–353, 2001.

57. Qureshi AI, Luft AR, Janardhan V, et al: Identification of patients at risk for periprocedural neurological deficits

associated with carotid angioplasty and stenting. *Stroke* 31: 376–382, 2000.

58. III. NKF-K/DOQI Clinical Practice Guidelines for Vascular Access: Update 2000. *Am J Kidney Dis* 37:S137–S181, 2001.

59. Huber TS, Ozaki CK, Flynn TC, et al: Prospective validation of an algorithm to maximize native arteriovenous fistulae for chronic hemodialysis access. *J Vasc Surg* 36:452–459, 2002.

60. Silva MB, Jr, Hobson RW, 2nd, Pappas PJ, et al: A strategy for increasing use of autogenous hemodialysis access procedures: Impact of preoperative noninvasive evaluation. *J Vasc Surg* 27:302–307, discussion 307–308, 1998.

61. Hakaim AG, Nalbandian M, Scott T: Superior maturation and patency of primary brachiocephalic and transposed basilic vein arteriovenous fistulae in patients with diabetes. *J Vasc Surg* 27:154–157, 1998.

62. Mendes RR, Farber MA, Marston WA, et al: Prediction of wrist arteriovenous fistula maturation with preoperative vein mapping with ultrasonography. *J Vasc Surg* 36:460–463, 2002.

63. U.S. Renal Data System: USRDS 1995 Annual Data Report. *Am J Kidney Dis* 26:S12–S166, 1995.

64. NKF-DOQI Clinical Practice Guidelines for Vascular Access: National Kidney Foundation–Dialysis Outcomes Quality Initiative. *Am J Kidney Dis* 30:S150–S191, 1997.

65. Sidawy AN, Gray R, Besarab A, et al: Recommended standards for reports dealing with arteriovenous hemodialysis accesses. *J Vasc Surg* 35:603–610, 2002.

66. Silva MB, Jr, Hobson RW, 2nd, Pappas PJ, et al: Vein transposition in the forearm for autogenous hemodialysis access. *J Vasc Surg* 26:981–986, discussion 987–988, 1997.

67. LoGerfo FW, Menzoian JO, Kumaki DJ, et al: Transposed basilic vein–brachial arteriovenous fistula. A reliable secondary-access procedure. *Arch Surg* 113:1008–1010, 1978.

68. Dagher FJ: The upper arm AV hemoaccess: Long term follow-up. *J Cardiovasc Surg (Torino)* 27:447–449, 1986.

69. Ascher E, Hingoran A, Gunduz Y, et al: The value and limitations of the arm cephalic and basilic vein for arteriovenous access. *Ann Vasc Surg* 15:89–97, 2001.

70. Coburn MC, Carney WI, Jr: Comparison of basilic vein and polytetrafluoroethylene for brachial arteriovenous fistula. *J Vasc Surg* 20:896–902, discussion 903–904, 1994.

71. Taghizadeh A, Dasgupta P, Khan MS, et al: Long-term outcomes of brachiobasilic transposition fistula for haemodialysis. *Eur J Vasc Endovasc Surg* 26:670–672, 2003.

72. Brescia MJ, Cimino JE, Appel K, et al: Chronic hemodialysis using venipuncture and a surgically created arteriovenous fistula. *N Engl J Med* 275:1089–1092, 1966.

73. Tashjian DB, Lipkowitz GS, Madden RL, et al: Safety and efficacy of femoral-based hemodialysis access grafts. *J Vasc Surg* 35:691–693, 2002.

74. Gradman WS, Cohen W, Haji-Aghaii M: Arteriovenous fistula construction in the thigh with transposed superficial femoral vein: Our initial experience. *J Vasc Surg* 33:968–975, 2001.

75. Huber TS, Ozaki CK, Flynn TC, et al: Use of superficial femoral vein for hemodialysis arteriovenous access. *J Vasc Surg* 31:1038–1041, 2000.

76. May J, Tiller D, Johnson J, et al: Saphenous-vein arteriovenous fistula in regular dialysis treatment. *N Engl J Med* 280:770, 1969.

77. Hingorani A, Ascher E, Kallakuri S, et al: Impact of reintervention for failing upper-extremity arteriovenous autogenous access for hemodialysis. *J Vasc Surg* 34:1004–1009, 2001.

78. Berman SS, Gentile AT: Impact of secondary procedures in autogenous arteriovenous fistula maturation and maintenance. *J Vasc Surg* 34:866–871, 2001.

79. Puskas JD, Gertler JP: Internal jugular to axillary vein bypass for subclavian vein thrombosis in the setting of brachial arteriovenous fistula. *J Vasc Surg* 19:939–942, 1994.

63 CHAPTER

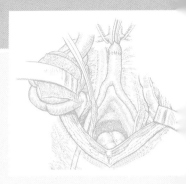

Vascular Trauma

Michael J. Sise, Carlos V.R. Brown, Howard C. Champion

第六十三章　血管损伤

OUTLINE

Mechanism of Injury and
　Pathophysiology
Clinical Presentation
Diagnosis
Minimal Vascular Injury and
　Nonoperative Management
Endovascular Management

Open Surgical Management
Specific Injuries
Postoperative Management
Outcomes and Follow-Up
Training and Preparation for
　Successful Management

中文导读

　　本章共分为10节：①血管损伤的机制和病理生理；②临床表现；③诊断；④轻微血管损伤和非手术治疗；⑤血管腔内治疗；⑥开放手术治疗；⑦特定部位血管损伤；⑧术后管理；⑨结局及随访；⑩成功治疗的培训及准备。

　　第一节阐述血管损伤的机制及病理生理变化。血管损伤可由钝性或者穿透性损伤引起。穿透伤通常是分散的或者局部的，而钝性伤更加弥散，不仅累及血管结构，还累及骨骼、肌肉和神经。穿透性损伤分为低速伤和高速伤，高速武器比低速武器造成更加严重的组织损害。血管创伤可导致出血、血栓形成或者血管痉挛。此外，还可导致亚急性、慢性或者隐匿性损伤，最常见的是动静脉瘘和假性动脉瘤。

　　第二节讲述血管损伤广泛多样的临床表现，包括从严重的出血性休克到细微的发现。

　　第三节讲述血管损伤的诊断。血管损伤后出血可导致低血容量性休克而危及生命，因此首先应遵循创伤高级

生命支持的原则（advanced trauma life support, ATLS），初步评估病情，保证呼吸道通气及建立静脉通路。这些完成并开始复苏后，应开始第二阶段评估，获得完整的病史并进行详细的体格检查。如判断血管损伤严重，应直接送入手术室。血管造影和CT血管成像常用来评估血管损伤，彩色多普勒超声并不常用于急性血管损伤的评估。

　　第四节讲述轻微血管损伤及非手术治疗。轻微血管损伤包括内膜损伤、局部痉挛导致的血管狭窄以及小的假性动脉瘤。大量证据表明非手术治疗大多数无症状的病变是安全有效的，但需要持续监测。

　　第五节首先介绍了杂交手术室的设置及应用。然

后分别讲述了血管腔内技术在躯干血管损伤、脑血管损伤、四肢血管损伤中的应用，以及哪些医生可以做血管介入治疗。

第六节分别介绍了血管开放手术的术前准备、血管显露及控制、血管损伤控制、血管修复及移植物的选择、术中成像及无创评估、组织覆盖的作用、筋膜切开术的作用、直接截肢的作用以及常见的错误和误区。

第七节讲述了特定部位血管损伤的特点及处理，包括头部、颈部及胸廓出口血管损伤，胸廓内大血管损伤，腹部血管损伤，上肢血管损伤和下肢血管损伤，同时讲述了肢体骨筋膜室切开的手术技巧。

第八节讲述术后管理，关键在于加强对病人的血管检查，及时发现病情的变化。

第九节讲述血管损伤导致截肢的主要原因是神经损伤，肢体功能恢复的情况往往取决于其合并损伤的严重性。对于血管修复后的病人需要定期随访。

第十节讲述成功治疗的培训及准备，包括普通外科医师培训，血管专业医师培训和血管创伤治疗的现状，强调开放血管手术能力培训的重要性，同时介绍了教育和培训的方法和机会。

〔董水林〕

Despite the widespread implementation of trauma systems with designated trauma centers, the prompt recognition and effective management of vascular trauma still have significant challenges in the care of injured patients. Although the incorporation of lessons learned from combat casualty care in the wars in Afghanistan and Iraq has improved overall outcomes after vascular injury, the risk to life and limb remains significant and the margin for error is very thin. Either delay in recognition of or failure to adequately manage vascular injuries remains alarmingly common in trauma centers. An organized approach with well-planned and implemented practice guidelines is essential to convert an error-prone process into one of prompt diagnosis and safe and effective treatment.

Effective management of vascular injuries requires trauma team members with both skill and experience in open vascular techniques and the capability to perform timely endovascular techniques. These skills cannot be taken for granted and must be carefully managed to provide injured patients timely access to the right physicians with the right skills. The widespread preference for endovascular techniques for elective vascular surgery coupled with fewer and fewer open vascular surgery cases has produced a shortage of surgeons who feel capable of and comfortable in performing open vascular repairs for vascular trauma. The steadily decreasing volume of open vascular procedures in both general surgery residencies and vascular fellowships has significantly eroded the skill level of both trauma surgeons and the vascular surgeons who support them in managing vascular injuries. The need for innovative solutions to restore the skill level among trauma and vascular surgeons is compelling.

This chapter reviews the pathophysiology, clinical presentation, diagnostic workup, management, and outcome of vascular injuries. Education and training solutions to restore the skills required to manage vascular injuries are also presented. The educational objectives of this review are the following: to elucidate the mechanisms of vessel injury and the resulting clinical manifestations; to provide an organized approach to rapid assessment of injured patients for the presence of vascular injuries in the neck, torso, and extremities; to present management guidelines to assist in the decision of which treatment options best apply and how to effectively implement them; to identify the clinically important sequelae of vascular injuries and the appropriate measures required to maximize functional recovery; and to review the available education and training opportunities to maintain the open surgical skills that are essential to effective management of vascular trauma.

MECHANISM OF INJURY AND PATHOPHYSIOLOGY

Vascular injury can be produced by either a blunt or a penetrating mechanism. Penetrating injury tends to be more discrete and to produce focal injuries; blunt trauma is more diffuse, producing injuries not only to the vascular structures but also to the bone, muscle, and nerves. Blunt injury not only affects major arteries, it also disrupts smaller vessels that would normally provide collateral flow. As a result, ischemia may be worsened. Knife wounds produce focal injury along their track. Gunshot wounds produce injury of varying degrees dependent on the characteristics of both the weapon and the projectile.

Penetrating gunshot wound injury is generally classified as low velocity (<2500 ft/sec, typically a handgun wound) or high velocity (>2500 ft/sec, such as a military rifle wound).[1] High-velocity military-style weapons produce significantly more tissue damage than low-velocity weapons because of the high amount of kinetic energy (energy = mass × velocity^2). The bullet creates a cavity by the rapidly expanding and rapidly contracting tissue surrounding the bullet's course that can reach a size equal to 30 times the diameter of the projectile at right angles to the missile track. Tearing of the adjacent tissue can be devastating. Impact with bone can lead to further damage from secondary bullet and bone fragment impact on the adjacent tissue. Civilian gunshot injuries involve predominantly low-velocity projectiles and create more focal injuries with little cavitation.[2]

Shotgun wounds, depending on the proximity to the gun barrel, the gunpowder load, and the size of the shot, cause highly variable injury patterns. The spread and force of the shot determine the extent of injury. Close-range gunshot wounds are defined as within 6 feet; intermediate, 6 to 18 feet; and long range, beyond 18 feet.[3] Close-range injures are devastating and often lethal. Intermediate-range injuries are often severe, and longer range injuries may be mild.

Vascular trauma produces a spectrum of findings from life-threatening hemorrhage from major vessel laceration to no overtly detectable findings in minimal injuries. Hemorrhage is produced when all of the vessel layers (intima, media, and adventitia) are disrupted or lacerated. If the bleeding is controlled locally, a hematoma is produced, which may or may not be pulsatile. If bleeding is not contained, exsanguination can occur. Completely transected extremity vessels often retract and constrict secondary to spasm of the muscular middle layer of the vessel wall. The surrounding adventitia is highly thrombogenic. Subsequently, hemorrhage may cease secondary to thrombosis. Paradoxically, partially transected arteries and veins cannot retract and thrombose and may cause much more extensive hemorrhage.

Arterial thrombosis occurs if there is damage to the intima, exposing the underlying media and causing local thrombus formation, which may propagate and either occlude the lumen or embolize distally. In addition, the injured intima can prolapse into the lumen as a result of blood flow dissecting this layer into the lumen, producing partial or complete obstruction. Trauma to surrounding bone structures may cause external compression of the vessel, interrupting flow and producing thrombosis. Spasm occurs if there is external trauma to the vessel, such as stretching or contusion, which can stimulate the release of mediators (such as hemoglobin) that cause constriction of the vascular smooth muscle. Spasm, by reducing the cross-sectional area of the vessel, reduces flow.

Vascular trauma can produce subacute, chronic, or occult injuries. The most common of these are arteriovenous fistula and pseudoaneurysm. An arteriovenous fistula typically occurs after penetrating trauma that causes injury to both an artery and a vein in proximity. The high-pressure flow from the artery will follow the path of least vascular resistance into the vein, producing local, regional, and systemic signs and symptoms. These include local tenderness and edema, regional ischemia from "steal," and congestive heart failure if the fistula enlarges.[4] A pseudoaneurysm is a result of a puncture or laceration of an artery that bleeds into and is controlled by the surrounding tissue. Pseudoaneurysms can enlarge and produce local compressive symptoms, erode adjacent structures, or, rarely, be a source of distal emboli.[4] They can initially be clinically occult but with time become symptomatic.[4]

CLINICAL PRESENTATION

Vascular injuries have a broad spectrum of clinical manifestations varying from profound hemorrhagic shock to subtle findings, such as an asymptomatic bruit. Patients who present in hemorrhagic shock must be assumed to have a major vascular injury until proven otherwise.[5] There are five anatomic areas to consider, each with specific considerations. In the head and neck, external hemorrhage is required for vascular injuries to result in shock. Relatively small and tightly organized tissue planes preclude significant internal hemorrhage. In the chest, each hemithorax can accommodate lethal amounts of hemorrhage from cardiac, pulmonary, or great vessel arterial and venous injuries. Abdominal and pelvic vascular injuries can also result in lethal hemorrhage,

particularly from the aorta and iliac arteries. As in the head and neck, extremity vascular injuries generally cause hemorrhagic shock only if there is significant external hemorrhage. The patient with hypotension and a lack of chest, abdomen, and pelvic findings may have what appears to be a trivial neck or extremity laceration that initially communicated with a major vessel injury. A hemorrhage sufficient to produce hypotension can be followed by thrombosis. It is therefore necessary to obtain a history from the prehospital personnel about the amount of blood at the scene or the initial presence of severe wound hemorrhage. It is also necessary to thoroughly examine the patient for additional wounds and to carefully assess each of them.[5]

Extremity vascular trauma may be immediately apparent on presentation because of external hemorrhage, hematoma, or obvious limb ischemia. A history of penetrating trauma associated with hypotension, pulsatile bleeding, or a large quantity of blood at the scene suggests vascular injury. Blunt trauma is also capable of causing significant vascular injury that can be overlooked when serious head, chest, or abdominal injuries are present. Extremity fractures may result in vascular injury. Supracondylar humerus fracture can be associated with brachial artery injury, and knee dislocation carries a significant risk of popliteal artery injury.[6] Crush injuries of the extremity without fracture may also result in vascular injury.

A relatively small number of vascular injuries are manifested in a delayed fashion without initial findings. These are limited to thrombosis of a previously partially disrupted but initially patent vessel, distal emboli from an intimal tear of the arterial wall with formation of platelet debris, and, least commonly, rupture or expansion of a pseudoaneurysm that was initially small and contained by the outer arterial wall and local tissue.[4] Local signs of hematoma, diminished pulses, and patterns of associated injuries should point to the presence of these vascular injuries. A thorough history and physical examination and appropriate adjunctive imaging studies will result in effective initial diagnosis and a decrease in the frequency of these delayed presentations.

Because such a broad spectrum of clinical findings are associated with vascular trauma, it is best to assume that vascular injury is present until proven otherwise in all patients with hemorrhagic shock and all patients with extremity fractures.[5]

DIAGNOSIS

Physical Examination

Vascular injury can produce systemic symptoms of hypotension, tachycardia, and altered mental status by hypovolemic shock caused by hemorrhage. As a result, vascular injury can be life-threatening, and attention must initially be directed to the primary survey using the principles of advanced trauma life support.[5] The airway must be assessed, adequate oxygenation and ventilation ensured, and intravenous access achieved. Once this is completed and resuscitation is under way, the secondary survey is undertaken. A thorough history and careful physical examination are then performed. This examination must include a careful inspection of the injured sites and wounds, a complete sensory and motor assessment, and a pulse examination of each extremity. The presence of a hematoma, bruit, or thrill must be noted. If distal pulses are diminished or absent, ankle or wrist systolic blood pressure should be determined with a continuous-wave Doppler device and compared with the uninjured side. A significant difference in systolic blood pressure (>10 mm Hg) between extremities may be an indication of vascular injury. Patients with "hard" findings of vascular injury (Table 63-1) should be taken directly to the operating room.

In patients with "soft" findings (Table 63-1), vascular imaging can be used to rule out the need for operation. In addition, patients with hard findings but with multilevel injuries in the same extremity may also need imaging. Catheter arteriography is both sensitive and specific in the diagnosis of extremity vascular injuries (Fig. 63-1). However, computed tomography (CT) angiography with the latest generation scanners is readily available and highly accurate and obviates the delay caused by mobilizing the angiography suite for catheter angiography (Fig. 63-2).[7-9] Although this imaging technique requires an infusion of contrast material, it does not require arterial catheterization, is easily performed, and is less costly and less time-consuming than conventional angiography.[7] The important distinction, however, is the ability to perform endovascular techniques with catheter access in the angiography suite or properly equipped operating room. Therefore, an orchestration of CT imaging and catheter imaging to meet the patient's needs and to manage vascular injuries in a timely and effective manner is essential.

Severely injured patients who must be taken to the operating room for treatment of life-threatening associated injuries, such as penetrating thoracic injury or ruptured spleen, may not be able to undergo CT angiography. In such cases, it is not prudent to delay operative therapy to obtain formal vascular imaging. An arteriogram can be obtained in the operating room by cannulating the artery proximal to the suspected vascular injury, injecting 20 to 25 mL of a full-strength radiographic contrast agent, and taking a radiograph or using fluoroscopy (Fig. 63-3).[10] If doubt remains about the presence of a vascular injury and the imaging studies and other diagnostic tests are inconclusive, there is a role for operative exploration and direct assessment of the artery. Routine operative exploration in the stable patient with soft signs, however, has a 5% to 30% incidence of morbidity, occasional mortality, and low diagnostic yield.[11] These patients are better served with formal vascular imaging.

Duplex color flow imaging is not used for the acute assessment of vascular injury. Wounds, swelling, air in the tissue, and dressings or splints impair the ability to obtain satisfactory images. Duplex imaging does have a role in the follow-up of treated lesions (i.e., to assess patency of bypass grafts or to detect luminal stenosis at an anastomosis) or in the follow-up of nonoperative

TABLE 63-1 History and Physical Examination Findings of Vascular Injury
Hard Findings
Indicate need for immediate intervention for vascular injury
• Pulsatile bleeding
• Expanding hematoma
• Palpable thrill or audible bruit
• Evidence of extremity ischemia
• Pallor
• Paresthesia
• Paralysis
• Pain
• Pulselessness
• Poikilothermia
Soft Findings
Consider further imaging and evaluation for vascular injury
• History of moderate hemorrhage
• Proximity fracture, dislocation, or penetrating wound
• Diminished but palpable pulse
• Level of peripheral nerve deficit in proximity to major vessel
• Wounds in proximity to extremity or neck vessels in patients with unexplained hemorrhagic shock

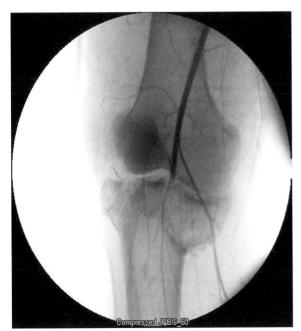

FIGURE 63-1 Catheter arteriogram demonstrating an acute occlusion of right popliteal artery secondary to blunt injury with associated tibial plateau fracture.

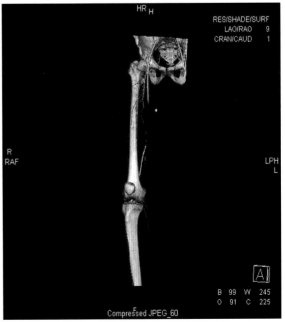

FIGURE 63-2 CT angiogram with VTR view of a gunshot wound to the right superficial femoral artery resulting in segmental thrombosis.

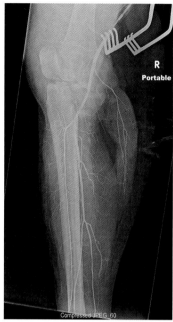

FIGURE 63-3 Intraoperative plain film (direct injection arteriogram) in the patient described in Figure 63-2 with blunt injury of the knee. Exploration of the popliteal artery with fasciotomy of the posterior compartments released compression of the artery with return of flow. This intraoperative arteriogram confirms a normal popliteal artery.

management of minimal vascular injury, such as small pseudoaneurysms or arteriovenous fistulas.

MINIMAL VASCULAR INJURY AND NONOPERATIVE MANAGEMENT

The widespread application of CT angiography in the evaluation of injured extremities results in the detection of clinically insignificant lesions.[12] There is now an extensive body of experience with lesions that are not limb-threatening. These minimal vascular injuries include intimal irregularity, small nonocclusive intimal flaps, focal spasm with minimal narrowing, and small pseudoaneurysms. They are often asymptomatic and usually do not progress.[6,12]

A small, nonocclusive intimal flap is the most commonly encountered clinically insignificant minimal vascular injury. The likelihood that it will progress to cause either occlusion or distal embolization is approximately 10% or less.[6,12] This progression, if it occurs, will be early in the postinjury course. Spasm is another common minimal vascular injury. This finding should resolve promptly after initial discovery. Failure of the return of normal extremity perfusion pressure indicates that a more serious vascular injury is present and intervention is needed. Small pseudoaneurysms are more likely to progress to the point of needing repair and must be actively observed with Duplex color flow imaging. Arteriovenous fistulas always enlarge over time and should be promptly repaired.

There is extensive evidence supporting nonoperative therapy for many asymptomatic lesions. However, successful nonoperative therapy requires continuous surveillance for subsequent progression, occlusion, or hemorrhage. Operative therapy is required for

thrombosis, symptoms of chronic ischemia, and failure of small pseudoaneurysms to resolve.[12]

ENDOVASCULAR MANAGEMENT

Endovascular techniques are an important component of effective management of vascular injuries.[13,14] They are, however, one tool among many that are required to manage the full spectrum of these injuries. Endovascular therapy for atherosclerotic arterial disease has become the first choice in management. Endoluminal stent deployment for occlusive lesions and stent graft for aortic aneurysms have become widely accepted. However, there is a strong tendency to generalize from this elective experience in elderly patients with atherosclerosis to the treatment of younger patients with acute vascular injuries. The evidence to support these approaches in preference to traditional open techniques is not well developed, and there have been problems.[6,15] The striking decrease in open vascular surgical experience among general surgeons and vascular surgeons trained in the 21st century creates a lack of comfort and competence in performing open vascular repairs.[16,17] A balanced approach using each of these techniques where they best apply supported by clinical evidence is essential to good outcomes in patients with vascular trauma.

Endovascular Operating Rooms

There is a widespread proliferation of "hybrid" operating rooms. These high-technology suites have both advanced imaging capability and traditional operating room properties. They require a major commitment of resources and personnel to be effective. They are ideal for complex elective endovascular cases. Not all trauma centers have hybrid operating rooms, or if they do, they cannot staff them on an emergency basis for the often after-hours management of vascular trauma.

Many centers create "hybrid operating rooms of opportunity" with high-resolution digital subtraction C-arm fluoroscopy equipment, mobile cabinets with the appropriate catheters and stent grafts, and on-call technical staff. They can create hybrid suite capabilities in an operating room large enough for the C-arm and the rolling cabinets with a standard orthopedic surgery operating table that accommodates fluoroscopy. An unstable trauma patient taken directly to the operating room with a major vascular injury or solid organ hemorrhage can be placed on an orthopedic surgery table and then be managed with all the functionality of a dedicated hybrid operating room. Many trauma centers already provide these mobile capabilities to their vascular surgeons performing elective endovascular abdominal aortic aneurysm repair. All trauma centers need to develop this capacity for their trauma patients.

Endovascular Management of Torso Vascular Injuries

Endovascular techniques offer a variety of options for hemorrhage control in the torso. Intra-arterial catheter-directed embolization has become a mainstay of the management of solid organ hemorrhage in the abdomen.[18,19] Whether it is used as the sole treatment or in combination with open procedures, this approach has been effective in liver, spleen, and kidney injuries. Less commonly used intra-arterial balloon occlusion for proximal control is a promising adjunct to open repair.[20,21] The availability of retrograde endovascular balloon occlusion of the aorta is growing and will soon be common practice in the same clinical setting of exsanguinating abdominal hemorrhage in which an aortic cross-clamp in the chest is needed. In trauma centers with the appropriately trained surgeons and proper equipment, these techniques are quick, accurate, and easily performed. The major obstacle to widespread popularity has been the reluctance of surgeons either to adopt catheter skills or to partner with interventional radiologists to bring these techniques to the trauma operating room. This reluctance to adopt new and promising technology must be avoided, and trauma surgeons need either to add surgeons or radiologists with endovascular capabilities to their specialty physician call panels or to obtain the training themselves.

The early use of catheter-directed control of hemorrhage associated with pelvic fracture is an effective method of limiting blood loss and improving outcome.[22] This approach is well tolerated and has proved superior to open attempts at hemorrhage control by packing in most patients. Unstable patients benefit from an immediate trip to the operating room. If intraoperative endovascular capability is present, a combined approach may offer the best results.

Enthusiasm for stent graft management of great vessel injuries in the chest has steadily grown.[23,24] The success of stent grafts for the treatment of aneurysm disease in the infrarenal aorta has led to the use of similar devices to treat contained thoracic aortic lacerations after blunt trauma. The initial results have been encouraging, but they are not without complications (Table 63-2).[24,25] Lifelong CT imaging is necessary because of the possibility of delayed endoleak and the possible loss of device fixation as the aorta enlarges over time. There is a promising role for covered stents in proximal branches of the aorta in both the thorax and abdomen. In stable injuries at risk for delayed hemorrhage or thrombosis, carefully placed stents have the potential to lower morbidity compared with open procedures that require extensive operative dissection for exposure and control. Endoluminal management with stent grafts appears most effective in those torso injuries that are surgically inaccessible with the potential for significant hemorrhage in stable patients (Fig. 63-4). These techniques should be used only in centers with an active elective endovascular practice that has experience in treating trauma patients.

Endovascular Management of Cerebrovascular Vascular Injuries

Endovascular techniques offer advantages in anatomic regions where direct operative control is difficult or impossible. For example, hemorrhage from a penetrating injury at the base of the skull is extremely difficult to control (Fig. 63-5). Catheter-directed placement of coils, balloons, or hemostatic agents in the injured carotid or vertebral artery could be lifesaving. Stent placement initially appeared less effective than anticoagulation in partially occluded injuries without associated hemorrhage.[26] However, the role of stents in cerebrovascular trauma has yet to be defined and may prove safe.[27,28] This use of endoluminal cerebrovascular interventions requires significant expertise and experience. If such experience does not exist at the receiving hospital, consideration should be given to transfer of the patient to a medical center with experience in this mode of therapy.

Endovascular Management of Extremity Vascular Injuries

The use of stent grafts in extremity vascular injuries is becoming more common.[13] The long-term results, however, have not been documented, and caution should be used in considering this type of treatment. In hemodynamically stable patients with contained hemorrhage, difficult to access proximal subclavian or iliac arterial injuries may be effectively treated with covered stents. In the extremities distal to these areas, autologous vein interposition grafts have excellent long-term patency rates and remain the "gold standard" for vascular repairs.

Catheter-directed therapies for controlling hemorrhage from large branch vessels in the extremities are often effective and sufficient to manage these injuries. Endoluminal treatment is used sparingly for pseudoaneurysms of extremity arteries. Small pseudoaneurysms are likely to resolve without any intervention, and large pseudoaneurysms are best treated with open techniques because the risk of arterial thrombosis or distal embolization is high with this endovascular intervention (Fig. 63-6).

Who Should Perform Endovascular Repairs?

Successful management of vascular injuries requires that the most qualified person do the indicated intervention in the appropriate patient in the appropriate place at the appropriate time. Endovascular surgery is an operative procedure and, like all operations, should be performed by readily available trained clinicians who not only are cognizant of the technical aspects of a procedure but are also knowledgeable about the disease for which the procedure is being performed. In many centers, this person is the interventional radiologist. Other centers have catheter-trained vascular surgeons, and a few others have trauma surgeons who are capable of performing endovascular procedures. Catheter skills training is being integrated in many surgical critical care fellowships and may subsequently become more available in the near future at many trauma centers. (See later section on training and preparation.)

Endoluminal management of vascular trauma does not require a full endovascular hybrid operating room, as explained before. Planning and preparation, however, are essential for the endovascular capability, which more often than not is needed in the middle of the night. Preparing a team who can perform these techniques and who can organize the appropriate equipment with brief notice requires commitment, dedication, collaboration, and training.

TABLE 63-2 Comparison of Endovascular and Open Blunt Thoracic Aortic Injury Repairs			
	RELATIVE DEGREE OF RISK		
TECHNIQUE	CLAMP AND SEW	PARTIAL BYPASS	ENDOVASCULAR
Complications			
Physiology impact	High	Medium	Low
Blood loss	Medium	Medium	Low
Operative time	Medium	High	Low
Paraplegia	High	Medium	Low
Clinical Variables			
High surgical risk	High	Medium	Low
Severe lung injury	High	Medium	Low
Severe head injury	High	High	Low
Challenging aortic anatomy	Medium	Low	High

From Neschis DG, Scalea TM, Flinn WR, et al: Blunt aortic injury. *N Engl J Med* 359:1708–1716, 2008.

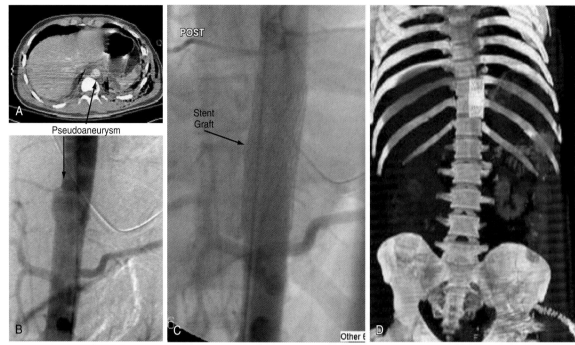

FIGURE 63-4 Endovascular repair of a difficult to expose aortic injury with pseudoaneurysm at the diaphragm from blunt-force trauma. **A,** CT angiogram showing cross-sectional view of pseudoaneurysm and associated thoracic spine fracture. **B,** Catheter arteriogram demonstrating the pseudoaneurysm. **C,** Deployed stent graft. **D,** CT scan of level of aortic stent graft in mid torso (VTR view).

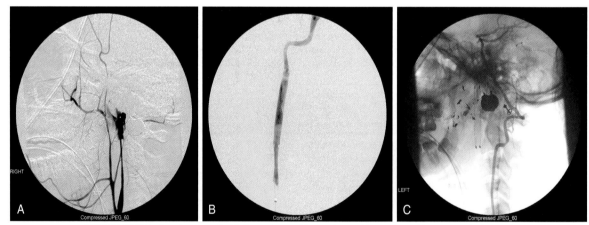

FIGURE 63-5 A, Gunshot wound with laceration and hemorrhage of internal carotid artery at the base of the skull. **B,** Covered stent placed at site of internal carotid artery injury. **C,** After placement of a covered stent in the internal carotid artery at base of the skull.

OPEN SURGICAL MANAGEMENT

Preparation for Operative Management

Operative procedures to manage vascular injuries should be limited to those surgeons who are capable, experienced, and qualified. Board certification in vascular surgery is not enough to qualify a surgeon as capable to handle these injuries, just as the lack of certification does not necessarily disqualify a surgeon. Many surgeons who perform elective vascular surgery are not sufficiently experienced in the management of vascular trauma. Conversely, there are many trauma surgeons who are very skilled in vascular technique by virtue of their interest and experience. The results of major open vascular repairs are dependent on the skill level of the vascular trauma–capable surgeon independent of board preparation. In a multicenter review of close to 700 major extremity vascular injuries, board-certified general surgeons and board-certified vascular surgeons had nearly identically high limb salvage rates for major vascular surgical repairs.[29] Every trauma center needs to develop a call panel of surgeons with the skill and knowledge to perform the full spectrum of vascular trauma repairs.

Successful operative management of vascular injuries requires a systematic approach with careful preparation. This begins with

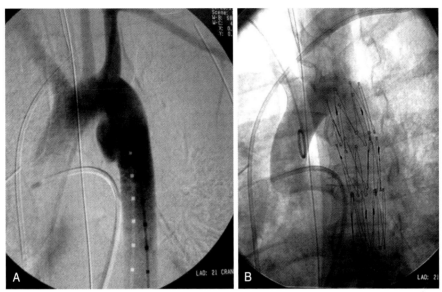

FIGURE 63-6 A, Acute traumatic pseudoaneurysm of the thoracic aorta. **B,** Fluoroscopy image after stent graft deployment.

airway control, adequate intravenous access, and availability of blood products. The administration of these blood products, however, should not begin before obtaining control of hemorrhage unless the patient is profoundly hypotensive.[5] If the blood pressure is below 80 to 90 mm Hg, the goal should be to provide adequate volume restoration with type O-negative packed cells and type AB fresh-frozen plasma infusion to support transport to the operating room for definitive hemorrhage control without delay. Volume infusion that raises the blood pressure above a systolic pressure of 90 to 100 mm Hg may increase bleeding and have a negative impact on outcome, particularly if the infusion delays transport to the operating room.[5]

Broad-spectrum preoperative antibiotics (and tetanus toxoid, if it is a penetrating wound) should be administered, and if there is an isolated extremity injury without significant hemorrhage, a bolus of 5000 units of heparin should also be given intravenously. Systemic heparinization should be avoided in patients with torso injuries, head injuries, or multiple extremity injuries. The most commonly omitted step in preparation is a failure to document preoperative extremity neurologic status. The presence of a neurologic deficit after operative vascular repair without knowing the preoperative status presents a difficult management challenge. A new neurologic deficit after vascular repair merits investigation and, possibly, reoperation. Therefore, a thorough preoperative neurologic examination and careful documentation are essential to effective management.

The operative management of extremity vascular injuries must be carefully orchestrated with the overall care of the patient. The choice between definitive repair and damage control should be made as soon as possible in patients with life-threatening torso injuries or severe head injuries. This includes coordinating two surgical teams to work simultaneously to care for the torso injury and the extremity vascular injury at the same time. Associated injuries to the soft tissue and bone require a coordinated assessment and treatment with orthopedic and plastic surgery consultants. These specialists should be involved as early as possible to facilitate any additional imaging or diagnostic procedures before proceeding to the operating room. The conduct of the operation

should also be discussed with these colleagues. For example, the use of damage control procedures with shunt placement followed by orthopedic stabilization can remove the sense of urgency to restore blood flow. Extensive soft tissue injuries may compromise the proper coverage of vascular repairs and fracture fixation. The advice and assistance of a plastic and reconstructive surgeon can be helpful in obtaining coverage of exposed grafts and fractures.

Vascular Exposure and Control

Always place the patient with major hemorrhage or suspected vascular injury on a fluoroscopy-capable operating room table to allow the endovascular therapy option for hemorrhage control or vascular repair. A generous sterile field should be prepared to allow adequate exposure of vessels to obtain proximal and distal control. In torso injuries, this includes preparing the chest and abdomen to the table laterally on both sides and both legs in case distal access or an autologous conduit is needed. For proximal vascular injuries of the extremities (at the groin crease or axilla), the chest or abdomen should be prepared to obtain proximal control out of the zone of injury. An uninjured leg should also be prepared for harvesting of autologous venous conduit.

Proximal control is the first priority in the exposure of vascular injuries. In the torso, chest injuries with life-threatening hemorrhage are best approached through a fourth intercostal space anterolateral thoracotomy that can be extended across the sternum into the third intercostal space of the right side of the chest to create a "clamshell" incision.[30] Thoracic outlet and proximal neck vascular injuries may require median sternotomy with extension above the clavicle up along the ipsilateral sternocleidomastoid muscle. For abdominal vascular injury, a generous xiphoid to pubis incision is needed for adequate exposure.[31] Proximal control for aortic injuries can be obtained just below the aortic hiatus of the diaphragm or may require a left anterolateral thoracotomy to clamp the distal thoracic aorta. If retrograde endovascular balloon occlusion of the aorta is available, it should be considered for temporary proximal thoracic aorta occlusion in the presence of high intra-abdominal aortic injury.[21]

In the proximal extremity injuries with active hemorrhage, the first incision site is chosen to give the fastest exposure of inflow vessels for clamping. For proximal upper extremity injuries, this may include incisions over the infraclavicular region of the chest to expose the axillary artery. For injuries in the groin, prepare to enter the lower quadrant of the abdomen for access to the external iliac vessels. In mid and distal extremity vascular injuries associated with active hemorrhage, tourniquets can rapidly obtain control in the trauma resuscitation room. In the operating room, have one team member precisely compress the bleeding site with a gloved hand and a sponge, remove the tourniquet, and prepare the extremity. A 5000-unit heparin bolus is then given, if appropriate, and the extremity is prepared and draped and a sterile tourniquet is placed proximal to the wound and inflated. The injury site can then be explored in a controlled fashion and clamps or vessel loops placed above and below the vascular injury. In certain injuries, distal arterial occlusion and retrograde intraluminal insertion of a Fogarty catheter with a stopcock to maintain balloon inflation will provide rapid hemorrhage control.[6]

Incisions used to manage vascular injuries are often the same as those used to manage elective cases but are generally more generous. The use of smaller incisions may lead to error in identifying the extent of vascular injury, adequately controlling branch vessel hemorrhage, and identifying associated venous lacerations. This is particularly true for popliteal artery and vein injuries. A limited approach with separate medial above- and below-knee incisions will not adequately expose the site of injury. A medial incision from the proximal popliteal space to the distal popliteal space with division of the medial head of the gastrocnemius muscle and the semimembranosus and semitendinosus muscles with full exposure of the popliteal artery and vein and the tibial nerve provides adequate exposure. This ensures adequate vascular control and the opportunity for successful repair. Closure of the wound to include approximation of the divided muscles yields an excellent functional result. Dividing the inguinal ligament in the groin, dividing the pectoralis major in the axilla, and removing the midclavicle may rarely be necessary. In each of these areas, rapid endovascular balloon occlusion offers an excellent adjunct to proximal control. In the presence of life-threatening hemorrhage that cannot be controlled by any other approach, these structures should not stand in the way of adequate exposure and control.

Vascular Damage Control

Damage control has gained wide acceptance in trauma surgery and is directed at rapid control of hemorrhage and closure of enteric wounds so that the patient can be warmed and resuscitated. The choice between definitive time-consuming vascular repair and temporary measures that achieve control must be made early in care of patients with vascular injury and hypovolemic shock. This is particularly important when an extremity vascular injury is associated with major torso injuries. Ligation and placement of intraluminal shunts are the mainstays of vascular damage control.[32,33]

Ligation should be reserved for vessels with adequate distal collateral flow. In the torso, this includes the subclavian and innominate arteries, the celiac artery, and the inferior mesenteric artery. In the upper extremity, proximal injuries of the axillary artery and distal injuries to either the radial or ulnar artery may be ligated, provided there is evidence of adequate distal collateral flow assessed by either physical examination or continuous-wave Doppler interrogation. Similarly, in the lower extremity, ligation

of a single tibial artery or the peroneal artery can be performed after a similar assessment. If distal perfusion is compromised, an intraluminal shunt should be inserted, rather than ligating the vessel. Superior mesenteric artery (SMA) ligation is associated with a high risk of bowel necrosis, and damage control is best accomplished with placement of an intraluminal shunt. In the extremities, ligation of the brachial, external iliac, superficial femoral, or popliteal artery has a high likelihood of producing limb-threatening ischemia and should be avoided, if possible.

A variety of commercially available shunts can be used for damage control. If these are not available, sterile intravenous tubing is of adequate size to "shunt" both the artery and the vein, if necessary. Venous shunt placement (instead of ligation) may improve extremity perfusion and lower the risk of compartment syndrome. Damage control shunt placement begins with obtaining adequate proximal and distal control. Thrombus should be cleared with a Fogarty embolectomy catheter, followed by the instillation of regional heparinized saline (5000 units heparin/500 mL saline). The shunt should be placed in a straight line and be long enough to remain safely held in place in the proximal and distal vessel with a tied umbilical tape or 2-0 silk tie at each end. Long, looped shunts run the risk of becoming dislodged during subsequent dressing changes and should be avoided. The ties securing the shunt cause intimal damage, and those portions of the artery must be resected at the time of definitive vascular repair.

The condition of the patient determines the timing of definitive vascular repair after damage control. Hemorrhage must be controlled, coagulopathy and acidosis corrected, and temperature normalized.

Choice of Repair and Graft Material

Vessel injuries that cannot be repaired by primary end-to-end technique will require an interposition graft. The most desirable graft is autologous great saphenous vein harvested from an uninjured leg.[6] Native vein graft is preferable because it has elastic properties that make it compliant with the normal pulsatile flow of an artery; it has a diameter that approximates that of an extremity artery, producing an adequate size match for grafting in the arm and leg; it is not thrombogenic; and it has superior long-term patency in elective vascular surgery compared with prosthetic material when it is used with smaller vessels (popliteal and tibial). Cephalic vein and lesser saphenous vein have been suggested as suitable second choices, but cephalic vein is less muscular than the great saphenous and, like the lesser saphenous, may present problems with harvesting in a trauma patient.[6] Also, upper extremity venous access becomes compromised when the cephalic vein is used.

Saphenous vein may not be suitable in all instances because of inadequate size or because it has been traumatized or harvested previously. In such cases, a prosthetic conduit may be needed. Initial experiences with the use of prosthetic material (Dacron) in traumatic vascular injuries were not good. Rich and Hughes reported a complication rate of 77% (infection and thrombosis were the most common) in 26 patients.[34] However, more recent experience with newer graft material (polytetrafluoroethylene [PTFE]) has shown improved patency (70% to 90% short term) and rare infection (even in contaminated wounds).[35] Early rates of patency with PTFE grafts are equivalent to those with vein for injuries proximal to the popliteal artery and in the brachial artery. Distal to these levels, PTFE is inferior to vein for popliteal and more distal vessels and in the arm and leg. PTFE grafts of less than 6 mm should not be used.[35] PTFE and vein grafts must be covered or there is a significant risk of hemorrhage from desiccation of the vein with subsequent autolysis or breakdown of the anastomosis.[21,35]

Intraoperative Imaging and Noninvasive Evaluation

The successful management of vascular injury requires knowing precisely the status of blood flow in the area of the vessel injury. Preoperative imaging with catheter angiography or CT angiography is not always possible. In addition, when a vascular repair has been completed, the presence of thrombus, kinking, or unexpected technical problems may cause early failure. Intraoperative imaging is therefore an important part of assessing the injured vessels and the repair site.[6] Either single-injection radiography or fluoroscopy is effective in providing images in the operating room (see Fig. 63-6). Intraoperative duplex scanning is also effective but requires significant training and experience for it to be performed adequately. Hand-held continuous-wave Doppler interrogation can be helpful but requires considerable experience to be used effectively. Ankle or wrist pressure measurements may be misleading because of regional vasospasm in the proximal injured extremity, resulting in a reduced distal pressure compared with the uninjured leg. Intraoperative radiographic imaging remains the most accurate and useful method to detect technical problems with a vascular repair or to determine the presence of thrombus in the runoff vessels distal to a repair. Routine completion arteriography after vascular repairs will yield findings of clinical importance in approximately 10% of patients.[6]

Role of Tissue Coverage

All vascular repairs must be covered to prevent desiccation and disruption. In crushed or badly mangled extremities, this can be a difficult challenge. Rotation of regional muscle or skin flaps may be required. The early involvement of a plastic and reconstructive surgeon is essential to obtain tissue coverage when there is extensive soft tissue injury or loss. Local muscle can be advanced into the wound at the initial operation. If there is a large contaminated wound and local muscle viability is questionable, early reexploration and preparation for a free flap should be considered. On occasion, tissue loss may be so extensive that an extra-anatomic course for an interposition graft may be required. Attention to coverage is also essential in damage control procedures to avoid shunt dislodgment during dressing changes.

Role of Fasciotomy

Failure to perform an adequate fasciotomy after revascularization of an acutely ischemic limb is the most common cause of preventable limb loss.[6] Calf compartment syndrome is the most common indication for fasciotomy. Forearm and thigh compartment syndromes are less common. Any muscle group can develop compartment syndrome, including those in the hands and feet.

Compartment syndrome may be manifested immediately or delayed to 12 to 24 hours after reperfusion. If it is not promptly diagnosed and treated, the risk of limb loss or limb dysfunction is high. Calf compartment syndrome most commonly results from prolonged ischemia or a crush injury. Frequent physical examinations augmented with compartment pressure measurements are necessary to detect this complication in its early stage. The first clinical finding is loss of light touch sensation in the distribution of the nerve in the compartment. The diagnosis of compartment syndrome should be suspected in any patient complaining of increasing pain after injury. The physical findings include a tense compartment, pain on passive range of motion,

progressive loss of sensation, and weakness. The loss of arterial pulses is a late finding, which usually indicates a poor prognosis. Neurologic signs and symptoms, although helpful, are neither sensitive nor specific in the upper extremity after arterial injury because associated peripheral nerve injury often exists. Early diagnosis must be predicated on measurement of compartment pressures. The normal tissue compartment pressure ranges from 0 to 9 mm Hg. Much controversy exists about what constitutes a pathologic elevation. However, the safest approach is to perform fasciotomy when compartment pressure exceeds 25 mm Hg.[6,36,37]

A compartment syndrome can also develop in either the upper arm (triceps, deltoid, or along the axillary sheath) or the forearm. The forearm compartment syndrome is more common. Increased tissue pressure can follow either blunt or penetrating trauma because of hematoma, post-traumatic transudation of serum into the interstitial space, venous thrombosis, or reperfusion after ischemia.[36] The possibility of a compartment syndrome must always be a consideration in a patient who has been injured, particularly one with prolonged ischemia before reperfusion.

Role of Immediate Amputation

A very limited role for primary amputation exists in the management of complex extremity vascular injuries. Patients with extensive soft tissue loss, neurologic deficit, extensive fractures, and vascular injuries should be evaluated collaboratively with orthopedic, neurosurgical, and plastic and reconstructive surgery colleagues to determine if primary amputation is the best initial management. Scoring systems to predict the need for amputation have not been useful.[38,39] Because of the emotional impact of amputation and because marginally viable tissue often takes hours to demarcate or declare, it may be best to proceed with initial intraoperative evaluation and documentation (pictures, radiographs, and consultation), damage control using intravascular shunts for the vascular injuries, and a second look in 24 hours. The interval of time allows communication with the patient and the family and a more planned approach. Immediate amputation should also be considered in patients with extensive soft tissue, bone, and neurovascular disruption who have life-threatening torso injuries as mentioned earlier in the discussion of damage control techniques. If immediate amputation is required, extensive documentation of the extremity injury with photographs placed in the chart will be helpful in later explaining the decision to the patient and family and will help with their acceptance of this drastic surgical procedure.

Common Errors and Pitfalls

The management of vascular injuries is challenging. An organized approach is necessary to avoid the common errors and pitfalls. One of the most common errors is the lack of recognition of an extremity vascular injury in a patient with multiple torso injuries. Failure to recognize and adequately treat compartment syndrome is another error that is all too common and has devastating consequences. In torso injuries to the great vessels, failure to adequately expose and control the injured site can lead to a rapid death from exsanguination. Finally, failure to recognize the need for damage control techniques and a rapid completion of the operation in an unstable patient can also be deadly. The three most common factors in generating errors in caring for the injured are fatigue, distraction, and familiarity.[40] Each of these factors is inherent to process of care at busy trauma centers. An organized approach mitigates these factors and intercepts errors in progress before they are completed and the patients suffer.

SPECIFIC INJURIES

Head, Neck, and Thoracic Outlet

Vascular injuries of the head, neck, and thoracic outlet are often challenging to manage. Penetrating trauma can injure large vessels, such as the innominate and subclavian arteries, which can lead to exsanguination. Blunt trauma to the carotid and vertebral arteries, collectively known as blunt cerebrovascular injuries, is often occult and, if not diagnosed and treated rapidly, can lead to cerebral ischemia, infarction, and possibly death.

The principles of management of penetrating trauma to this region are based on the location of the injury relative to the three zones of the neck: zone 1, inferior to the cricoid cartilage; zone 2, cricoid cartilage to the angle of the mandible; and zone III, cephalad from the angle of the mandible. In a stable patient with a suspected vascular injury in either zone 1 or zone 3, vascular imaging is mandatory to confirm the suspicion of vascular injury and to plan proximal and distal control.[41] Vascular imaging is also recommended for stable patients with penetrating trauma in zone 2, but exploration should be undertaken expeditiously for patients with an expanding hematoma or impending airway compromise (manifested by hoarseness and tracheal deviation).[41] In the unstable patient, a Foley urinary catheter with the balloon inflated can be inserted into the wound to achieve temporary tamponade of injuries in these regions. Conventional angiography can have a dual role for injuries in zone 1 or zone 3. It not only can provide the diagnosis but also may provide a venue for endoluminal management—coiling of bleeding vessels or pseudoaneurysms in zone 3 or placement of covered stents in zone 1.

Blunt cerebrovascular injuries are often occult and asymptomatic. Therefore, rapid diagnostic screening is essential and provides the underpinning of successful management. Initially, blunt cerebrovascular injuries were thought to be rare, occurring in about 0.1% of patients; but with use of the screening criteria developed by the group at Denver General Hospital, the incidence is actually 10 to 20 times that.[27] Factors associated with these injuries include displaced midface fractures, basilar skull fracture with carotid canal involvement, cervical spine fracture, closed head injury consistent with diffuse axonal injury and Glasgow Coma Scale score below 6, and blunt neck trauma from hanging or seat belt injuries. Both carotid and vertebral artery injuries occur from stretching or tearing of the intima of the vessels produced by rapid extreme extension or flexion of the neck or by direct blunt-force injury. The carotid artery is particularly vulnerable where it lies close to the second and sixth cervical transverse processes. The vertebral artery is also vulnerable to stretch injuries and fractures of the transverse process of the cervical vertebrae that involve the foramen transversarium. Cerebrovascular injuries vary from minor intimal irregularities to arterial rupture and severe hemorrhage (Table 63-3).[27]

Patients who fulfill the Denver criteria should undergo CT angiography of the neck.[26,27] The treatment of blunt carotid and

vertebral artery injuries is anticoagulation in patients who do not have a contraindication.[26] Aspirin is the only alternative in patients who cannot be safely anticoagulated. The use of endovascular techniques has a very limited role as discussed before. However, in patients with carotid injuries at the base of the skull or injuries of the vertebral artery, covered stents or embolization offers the best results (see Fig. 63-5).

Vascular injuries of the thoracic outlet are challenging because they involve large-caliber vessels that can be difficult to expose and to control. Unstable patients with vascular injury in the region of the thoracic outlet must be expeditiously taken to the operating room. Stable patients should have preoperative imaging with catheter or CT angiography to locate the injury and to determine its extent. This will allow planning for endoluminal treatment or open exposure.[42,43] Operative control may require a simple supraclavicular incision, a sternotomy, or a combination of the two incisions, depending on the location and extent of the injury. Clamp application on the proximal subclavian and carotid arteries must be precise to avoid injury to the vagus, phrenic, or recurrent laryngeal nerves, all of which reside in this anatomic region. Sternotomy is frequently used for proximal innominate, proximal right subclavian, and proximal right carotid arterial injuries. Left subclavian artery proximal control is best obtained through a posterolateral thoracotomy for definitive repair. However, for supraclavicular injuries, a third intercostal space anterolateral thoracotomy provides exposure for proximal control. Distal control of the carotid arteries is obtained by extending the median sternotomy superiorly along the border of the ipsilateral sternocleidomastoid muscle. Distal subclavian arterial control is obtained through a supraclavicular incision. Resection of the clavicle results in little or no morbidity and can be performed quickly to control hemorrhage if needed. Suturing of the subclavian and axillary arteries must be done with extreme caution. Undue tension or traction will result in a tear of these vessels.[44] Endovascular balloon occlusion, when it is rapidly available, is an excellent adjunctive measure for proximal control.

Intrathoracic Great Vessels

Penetrating injuries of the intrathoracic great vessels (aorta, superior and inferior venae cavae, pulmonary arteries and veins) usually cause death at the time of injury from exsanguination. The small number of patients with penetrating injuries of the intrathoracic great vessels who arrive to the trauma center alive often present hemodynamically unstable and require emergent operative intervention. Repair of intrathoracic great vessel injuries may be achieved through sternotomy, left or right anterolateral thoracotomy, or, in many cases, bilateral (or clamshell) anterolateral thoracotomy.[30] Although many of these structures are exposed through a posterolateral thoracotomy in the elective setting, patients who present in hemorrhagic shock and without a distinct diagnosis should be managed with more versatile incisions, such as median sternotomy and anterolateral thoracotomy.

Injuries to the ascending aorta and the superior or inferior vena cava are best exposed and treated through a median sternotomy.[30] These injuries should be controlled with digital pressure and then placement of a side-biting clamp to allow suture repair of the injury and may require cardiopulmonary bypass to achieve repair. Injuries of the descending aorta are ideally approached through a left posterolateral thoracotomy. However, most of these injuries will be discovered during emergent left anterolateral thoracotomy and will need to be quickly repaired. Injuries of the pulmonary arteries and veins can be approached

TABLE 63-3	Spectrum of Severity of Blunt Cerebrovascular Arterial Injury
Grade I	Luminal irregularity with <25% luminal narrowing
Grade II	Dissection of hematoma with ≥25% luminal narrowing
Grade III	Pseudoaneurysm
Grade IV	Occlusion
Grade V	Transection with extravasation

through a sternotomy or anterolateral thoracotomy, depending on their proximity to the heart.[30] If possible, these injuries should be repaired primarily. However, destructive injuries to the pulmonary arteries and veins may necessitate pneumonectomy for definitive control.

Blunt injuries to the intrathoracic great vessels consist primarily of blunt thoracic aortic injury (BTAI). BTAI occurs as a result of high-energy blunt trauma. The most common mechanisms of injury resulting in BTAI are high-speed motor vehicle crashes and falls from a height. The aorta is typically injured in a location where it is relatively fixed (root of the aorta, ligamentum arteriosum, diaphragmatic hiatus), and the majority (85% to 90%) of patients die at the scene. Patients with BTAI who arrive at the hospital alive have typically sustained multisystem associated injuries. BTAI must be ruled out when there is a high-energy mechanism injury or a chest radiograph shows a widened mediastinum. However, definitive diagnosis of BTAI is established with a high-resolution CT scan of the chest. Injuries vary from an intimal injury to pseudoaneurysm or a contained periaortic hematoma just distal to the left subclavian artery.[7,9]

Once the diagnosis of BTAI is confirmed, the initial management is focused on blood pressure control and addressing associated immediately life-threatening injuries. Blood pressure is best controlled with a short-acting intravenous beta blocker (e.g., esmolol) that can be titrated to a systolic blood pressure of less than 110 mm Hg while also keeping heart rate below 100 beats/min.[30] If beta blockade does not achieve blood pressure goals, other intravenous agents, such as calcium channel blockers, nitroglycerin, and nitroprusside, may be used. Whereas some stable minimal BTAIs may be managed nonoperatively, most will require definitive repair through the open or endovascular approach. Regardless of the approach, most BTAIs should be repaired in a delayed fashion after the patient is stable. Early repair of these injuries has been associated with increased mortality.[30]

Open repair of BTAI has been the mainstay of treatment for decades. Open repair is achieved through a left posterolateral thoracotomy, cardiopulmonary bypass, and placement of a synthetic aortic interposition graft. Endovascular repair of BTAI has become increasingly more common during the past decade (Fig. 63-7). Although there are no prospective, randomized trials comparing open versus endovascular management of BTAI, there have been two multicenter American Association for the Surgery of Trauma trials showing lower morbidity (spinal cord ischemia, stroke) and mortality with the endovascular approach.[24,25] However, patients who undergo endovascular repair require lifelong surveillance because there is no information about long-term sequelae of endovascular grafts in the aortic position in young patients. In addition, many young patients do not have favorable anatomy for endovascular repair and still require the open approach. More recent series of open repair with spinal cord protection from partial cardiopulmonary bypass have a competitively low rate of paraplegia.[25] The widespread preference for thoracic endovascular aortic repair may suffer from the famous British thoracic surgeon Ronald Belsey's observation that "the follow-up clinics are the shoals upon which founder many attractive theories in surgery."[45] Late graft failure due to endoleak and possible collapse within aortas susceptible to the elongation and widening that occur with age may be a future source of major morbidity and mortality. As of 2016, there is not conclusive evidence that thoracic endovascular aortic repair in young patients is superior to well-performed open repairs with partial bypass for spinal cord protection.[25]

Abdominal Vascular Injury

Abdominal vascular injury most often results from penetrating trauma, and all are treated through a generous midline laparotomy.[31] Many of these injuries will require supraceliac control of the aorta to achieve adequate visualization to complete exposure and repair. Penetrating injuries to the abdominal aorta are best exposed and repaired with a left medial visceral rotation that exposes the aorta from the diaphragmatic hiatus to the iliac bifurcation (see Fig. 63-7). The injury can typically be controlled with direct digital pressure, which allows time for placement of vascular clamps proximal and distal to the site of injury.[31] Abdominal aortic injuries may be repaired primarily after stab wounds, but gunshot wounds will often require a patch repair or interposition graft. Uncommonly, patients will sustain a blunt abdominal aortic injury without life-threatening hemorrhage, and these injuries are best repaired by endovascular techniques.

The inferior vena cava is exposed with a right medial visceral rotation that exposes the vena cava from iliac vein confluence to inferior edge of the liver (see Fig. 63-7).[31] Injury to the vena cava is best controlled with direct digital pressure, with subsequent proximal and distal control using sponge sticks or vessel loops. Lumbar tributaries and renal veins may also need to be controlled to clearly visualize and repair the injury. Injuries to the anterior or lateral surfaces of the vena cava can most often be repaired primarily as long as the repair does not narrow the lumen more than 50%. Penetrating injuries to the vena cava may be through-and-through and require repair of a posterior injury as well. Injuries to the posterior vena cava may be repaired through the anterior injury, or the vena cava may be mobilized after ligating and dividing lumbar veins. Complex injuries may require patch repair, interposition graft, shunting with delayed reconstruction, or ligation.[31] Complexity of repair will depend on physiologic status of the patient and location of the injury. Hemodynamically unstable patients with ongoing hemorrhage are not candidates for complex repairs and should have the vena cava ligated or shunted. Hemodynamically stable patients with injuries at or above the level of the renal veins may be candidates for complex reconstruction, but ligation is still an option for the exsanguinating patient.[31]

The right common, external, and internal iliac arteries are best exposed by widely mobilizing the cecum, whereas injuries to the left iliac arteries are exposed by completely mobilizing the sigmoid colon.[31] Keep in mind the course of the ureter on both sides as it crosses the iliac vessels. Injuries to the common and external iliac arteries are initially controlled with digital pressure to allow proximal and distal control with vascular clamps or vessel loops. Injuries to the common and external iliac arteries may be repaired primarily but will often require a synthetic interposition graft. The common and external iliac arteries should never be ligated; if a patient is hemodynamically unstable, these injuries should be shunted and repaired in a delayed fashion. However, injuries to the internal iliac artery can be routinely ligated.[31]

Iliac veins are exposed in the same manner as for iliac arteries. Exposure is made more challenging by the location of the confluence of the iliac veins with the inferior vena cava directly posterior to the right common iliac artery. It will need to be widely mobilized to allow access to the confluence of the iliac veins. However, we do not advocate division of the right iliac artery to achieve exposure of the iliac vein confluence. Once the common, external, and internal iliac veins are exposed, the injury is best controlled with direct digital pressure, then proximal and distal control may be achieved with vessel loops. If possible, simple injuries to the iliac veins should be repaired with primary venorrhaphy. However,

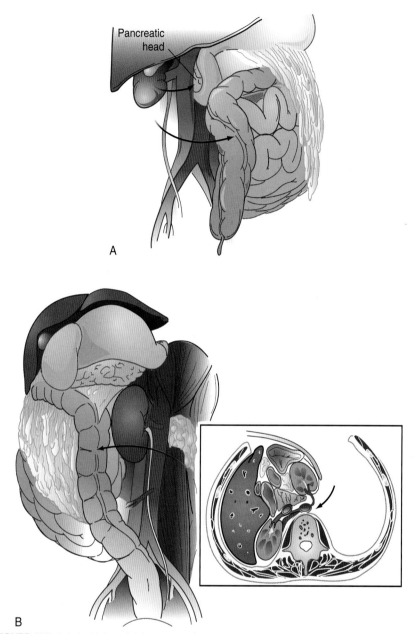

FIGURE 63-7 A, Left-sided medial visceral rotation for exposure of great vessels in the retroperitoneum. **B,** Right-sided medial visceral rotation for exposure of vena cava and renal veins in the retroperitoneum.

complex repairs of destructive injuries to the iliac veins should not be attempted, and these injuries should be ligated.[31]

Injuries to the mesenteric vessels are some of the most challenging injuries to expose and to repair. In the elective setting, the celiac trunk is often approached through the lesser sac; but in the setting of trauma, this may prove difficult because of a large lesser sac hematoma that obscures the usual landmarks. In the setting of trauma, the celiac trunk is best exposed through a wide left medial visceral rotation that mobilizes the spleen and tail of pancreas but leaves the left kidney in situ.[31] Once exposed, most injuries to the celiac trunk should be ligated because repair is difficult and ligation is well tolerated in the majority of patients. Although the SMA and celiac trunk take off from the aorta within

1 to 2 cm of each other, the exposure and treatment algorithm for SMA injuries is different. Management of SMA injuries will depend on location based on the Fullen classification: zone I, beneath the pancreas; zone II, between pancreaticoduodenal and middle colic branches; zone III, beyond middle colic branch; zone IV, enteric branches. Injuries that present with a large contained central hematoma at the root of the mesentery are best approached with a left medial visceral rotation. Active hemorrhage is controlled by manual compression followed by left medial visceral rotation.[31] This will allow exposure and control of the aorta proximal and distal to the SMA or direct clamping of the SMA as it comes off the aorta. Once this control has been achieved, attention is turned anteriorly for definitive exposure and repair of the SMA injury.

Zone I and zone II SMA injuries can be exposed and repaired through the lesser sac by dividing the gastrocolic ligament. The pancreas will need to be retracted inferiorly to expose the origin of the SMA or superiorly to expose the proximal SMA. Uncommonly, in active bleed SMA injuries behind the pancreas, it may need to be divided to completely visualize and control that segment of the SMA. Zone III and zone IV injuries should be approached by reflecting the transverse colon and its mesentery superiorly with or without taking down the ligament of Treitz. All zones of SMA injuries (except distal zone IV injuries) should always be repaired, with a primary repair, end-to-end anastomosis, or interposition graft of reversed saphenous vein.[31] If the patient is in extremis, the SMA may be shunted with plan for delayed repair. The superior mesenteric vein (SMV) can be exposed in the same fashion as the SMA. SMV injuries should be repaired or reconstructed when possible, although shunting with delayed repair is also an option. The SMV may be ligated for patients in extremis who would otherwise exsanguinate. Injuries to the inferior mesenteric artery may be ligated if there is adequate collateral flow from the middle colic branch of the SMA and the inferior and middle hemorrhoidal branches of the internal iliac arteries. The inferior mesenteric vein may be safely ligated if required.

The portal vein runs close to the inferior vena cava and is the most posterior structure within the portal triad, closely associated with the common bile duct and hepatic artery. Portal vein injuries are initially controlled with direct manual pressure. A right medial visceral rotation, including a generous Kocher maneuver, is performed to expose and to visualize the lateral and inferior portal vein. The common bile duct and hepatic artery will need to be mobilized to expose the anterior surface of the portal vein. Similar to SMA and SMV exposure, the neck of the pancreas may need to be divided to visualize the entirety of the portal vein.[31] These injuries should be managed in the same fashion as SMV injuries with repair or reconstruction in the majority of cases, shunting and delayed repair if necessary, and ligation only for patients in extremis who would otherwise exsanguinate.

Penetrating renal vascular injuries are easily exposed on either side after medial visceral rotation. Gerota fascia is opened, and the kidney is bluntly mobilized into the wound. Once the kidney is mobilized, the vascular injury can be controlled with direct manual pressure while proximal and distal control is obtained with vessel loops. Renal artery injuries can be managed with primary repair, end-to-end anastomosis, vein patch, interposition graft, or nephrectomy (after confirming a normal contralateral kidney by palpation). Treatment of renal artery injuries is based on complexity of the injury and physiologic status of the patient. Renal vein injuries can be repaired with primary venorrhaphy or ligation. On the right, ligation of the renal vein will require a nephrectomy, and patch angioplasty or interposition graft should be considered in stable patients. The left renal vein may be safely ligated near the inferior vena cava because of collateral flow through the adrenal, gonadal, and lumbar veins.[31] Combined injuries to the renal artery and vein should be treated with nephrectomy in unstable patients. Renal artery injuries rarely occur after blunt trauma. These injuries may be managed nonoperatively with expected involution of the affected kidney or nephrectomy. It is uncommon to successfully salvage renal function with vascular reconstruction of complete blunt renal artery occlusion. Management must consider several factors, including overall status of the patient, warm ischemia time, and need for laparotomy for associated intra-abdominal injuries.

Upper Extremity

Penetrating injury often presents with a history of either arterial hemorrhage or ongoing bleeding. Blunt injury usually causes thrombosis and the signs of acute arterial occlusion with resultant ischemia. Significant neurologic injury, usually involving the median nerve, is present in 60% of patients with upper extremity arterial injury.[6,46] Concomitant venous injury is common. In the setting of multisystem injury, arterial occlusion in the upper extremity is easily missed. Delay in diagnosis resulting in prolonged ischemia is an important contributing factor to preventable limb loss or long-term disability from irreversible ischemic nerve injury. All significant vascular injuries of the upper extremity result in clinical findings that are apparent on thorough physical examination. Unfortunately, associated severe torso or lower extremity injuries distract the trauma team from the injured and ischemic upper extremity. Delays in diagnosis and treatment are common in collected series of patients with upper extremity arterial injury and are more common after blunt-force trauma.[6,46]

The diagnosis of upper extremity arterial injury is often made on physical examination alone, particularly in penetrating injuries. Noninvasive evaluation of the injured upper extremity adds little to a thorough history and physical examination. Patients with obvious arterial or venous laceration from penetrating trauma or those with blunt trauma and hard findings (see Table 63-1) should be taken directly to the operating room. The arterial bed of the upper extremity is extremely reactive to vasoconstriction produced by hypovolemic shock, pain, and drugs including cocaine and methamphetamine. Absent pulses in the presence of complex fractures or crush injuries of the upper extremity need to be assessed with imaging (either multidetector CT or conventional angiography) if normal perfusion does not return after resuscitation and the administration of adequate pain medications.

There is currently not a role for endovascular therapy in the brachial artery and forearm vessels. Traditional operative exposure, catheter thrombectomy, and repair remain the best approach to optimize results.[6,46] In patients unstable from associated torso injuries, damage control with arterial shunt placement followed by repair when the patient is hemodynamically stable is the best management option. Vascular injuries in the upper extremity are often associated with significant musculoskeletal, neurologic, and soft tissue injuries. When this occurs, a multidisciplinary approach is often required with orthopedics, neurosurgery, and plastic surgery. Venous injuries of the upper extremity can be ligated unless there is extensive soft tissue injury and loss of venous collaterals. In that setting, some form of venous reconstruction should be considered.

On occasion, bleeding from a partially transected arm or forearm vessel can be significant. The senior surgeon should make certain that adequate control is obtained and maintained during resuscitation, transportation to the operating room, and surgical preparation and draping. Although they have proved lifesaving in the field for management of hemorrhage from extremities, tourniquets should be used sparingly in the trauma bay and only placed and carefully monitored for adequacy of compression and duration of application by the senior surgeon present.

The patient should be widely prepared and draped with generous inclusion of the entire upper extremity, the shoulder, and the anterior-superior aspect of the chest to allow incisions for proximal control.[6] An uninjured leg should also be prepared and draped from inguinal region to toes to allow saphenous vein harvest. Adjunctive measures, such as bolus intravenous systemic heparinization, administration of a continuous infusion of low-molecular-weight dextran, and administration of intravenous antibiotics, should be considered and used where appropriate. In patients with multisystem injuries, especially head injury, local or regional infusion of heparin should be used in place of systemic administration. Loupe magnification and coaxial lighting ("headlight") are technical adjuncts that may be useful in suturing small blood vessel with fine suture.

Surgical exposure requires generous incisions placed to maximize exposure and to provide appropriate options for further exploration and repair. The brachial artery is best exposed through a longitudinal incision along the medial aspect of the upper arm over the groove between the triceps and biceps muscles. The incision can be extended distally with an S-shaped extension across the antecubital fossa from ulnar to radial aspect and onto the forearm to expose the origins of the forearm vessels.[6,46] Proximal brachial artery injuries may require control of the infraclavicular axillary artery. Vascular repair requires attention to detail in all phases. Balloon catheter thrombectomy and flushing with heparinized saline followed by débridement of damaged arterial wall are essential to successful repair. Lacerated veins should be ligated unless there is extensive soft tissue injury and collateral venous flow is compromised. In such cases, the vein should be repaired. In repairing both venous and arterial injuries, the vein should be repaired first. If the duration of arterial occlusion and ischemia is a concern, temporary intraluminal shunts may be placed in the artery. Primary arterial repair of undamaged ends of vessel (end-to-end anastomosis) should be performed only if the repair is tension free. Saphenous vein interposition should be chosen whenever vessel injury is extensive or if primary tension-free repair is not possible. PTFE needs to remain a second choice to autologous vein in the management of injuries distal to the axillary artery.[2,6,46]

Forearm fasciotomy, particularly in the setting of prolonged ischemia, must always be considered before completion of the operation, and compartment pressures should be measured at the completion of the operation. If normal pressures are obtained, fasciotomy is not necessary, but pressure measurements should be repeated frequently because compartment syndrome can occur in the postoperative period as a consequence of reperfusion.[37,46]

There is a limited but important role for "primary" or early amputation in the management of upper extremity vascular injuries. Patients with extensive soft tissue loss or with scapulothoracic dissociation who have severe neurologic deficits, extensive fractures, and vascular injuries should be evaluated collaboratively with orthopedic, neurosurgery, and plastic surgery colleagues to determine if early amputation is appropriate. The best approach is intraoperative, multidisciplinary assessment, damage control, and plan for reoperative assessment in 24 to 48 hours. This will allow discussions with the patient and family and a second look.

Combined ulnar and radial artery injury in the forearm requires repair of at least one vessel. The ulnar artery is usually larger in the proximal forearm and is a better target for direct repair or saphenous vein bypass. Distally, the vessel repair should be performed in whichever vessel is largest or amenable to simple repair.[6,46]

Isolated ulnar or radial artery injuries can be managed with simple ligation only if there is absolute certainty that flow through the remaining vessel is adequate. Close inspection of the forearm and hand with palpation of pulses augmented by continuous-wave (hand-held) Doppler interrogation is essential.[6]

Lower Extremity

Vascular injuries in the legs are more common in military series (30% to 40%) than in civilian practice (20%).[2,47] Although penetrating injuries are more common, blunt vascular trauma in the lower extremity remains a significant challenge. In the thigh and the leg, fractures and dislocations can be associated with vascular injuries. The popliteal artery is at particularly high risk of injury after dislocation of the knee.[2,47]

Findings at presentation vary from significant hemorrhage from a wound (i.e., open fracture, stab, or gunshot) to occult arterial occlusion from blunt injury. A systematic approach with a thorough extremity vascular examination is essential to avoid errors in recognition and delays in treatment.

Exposure is obtained with incisions used for elective surgical procedures. The common femoral artery is best exposed through a longitudinal incision overlying its course from the inguinal ligament inferiorly for 8 to 12 cm. Proximal control may require exposure of the external iliac artery, best accomplished through an oblique muscle-splitting lower quadrant abdominal incision carried into retroperitoneum, where the artery and vein can be controlled. Superficial femoral artery (SFA) injuries are best exposed through a longitudinal groin incision similar to that used for femoral bifurcation exposure for the proximal portion. The mid-SFA is approached through an oblique incision over the sartorius muscle. The junction of the SFA and popliteal can be exposed by extending this incision, dividing the adductor tendon.

Popliteal injuries are exposed through a generous medial incision. Exposure of the artery in the area at the knee joint requires division of the medial head of the gastrocnemius muscle and the semimembranosus and semitendinosus muscles. The distal popliteal artery is exposed with an incision along the posterior margin of the tibia.

Repair of lower extremity vascular injuries usually requires an interposition graft. This is particularly true in the popliteal artery. Reverse saphenous vein from the contralateral extremity is the first choice for interposition grafts. In the common femoral artery, PTFE is an acceptable choice for interposition if the saphenous vein is not of sufficient size, but it should not be used in the below-knee popliteal arteries.[35]

Injuries below the popliteal artery at the level of the tibial vessels are best managed by ligation if two of the three calf vessels are patent and there is adequate collateral flow. In the presence of both anterior and posterior tibial vessel occlusion, the peroneal artery is usually not sufficiently connected to the distal arterial bed by collaterals, and repair of one of the injured vessels should be performed. The choice of which vessel to repair is based on both the extent of associated soft tissue injury and the patency of the distal segments of those vessels.

Damage control techniques with arterial and venous shunt placement with delayed definitive repair are an important part of managing lower extremity vascular injury associated with major torso injuries and hemodynamic instability (Fig. 63-8). All efforts should be made early postoperatively to achieve adequate stability as rapidly as possible to allow a timely return to the operating room for definitive vascular repair before shunt thrombosis and prolonged ischemia.

Operative Techniques for Extremity Fasciotomy

Fasciotomy of the forearm compartments requires release of individual muscle bundles. Generous incisions are required to release the dorsal and volar compartments and the mobile wad. Fasciotomy in the leg requires release of the anterior and lateral compartments on the anterior lateral aspect of the calf and the deep and superficial posterior compartments through incisions on the lateral and medial aspects of the calf (Fig. 63-9). These incisions should be generous in their length to accommodate subsequent muscle swelling and to avoid further compression.[6]

Thigh compartment syndrome is uncommon. The most common cause is thigh crush injury associated with femur fracture. Fasciotomy should release the three compartments: lateral, medial, and posterior. Two incisions, one lateral for the lateral compartment and one medial for the other two compartments, are sufficient. These need to be generous in their length. Compartment syndromes occur in the hands and feet, and these are best managed by orthopedic surgeons or hand surgeons.[6]

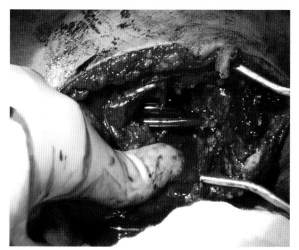

FIGURE 63-8 Damage control for multiple gunshot wounds with shunt placement in the popliteal artery and vein in a patient with associated major torso hemorrhage.

POSTOPERATIVE MANAGEMENT

The cornerstone of postoperative management is close follow-up to detect a change in the vascular examination findings. This includes frequent assessment of the vital signs, the distal extremity pulse, the continuous-wave Doppler signal, the capillary refill, and the neurologic examination findings of the injured extremity. If there is concern about any portion of the examination, an immediate return to the operating room may avert a potentially limb-threatening problem. Because failure of a vascular repair due to thrombosis can occur during the first 48 hours after the repair, careful follow-up with frequent examinations should continue for at least that length of time.

Reperfusion edema or intracompartmental hemorrhage can lead to a delayed onset of a compartment syndrome.[37] Physical examination alone may not detect the presence of compartment syndrome. Frequent postoperative compartment pressure measurements are the only way to accurately assess the injured extremity in patients who are not conscious and cooperative. The presence of a new postoperative extremity neurologic deficit is an important indicator of ongoing ischemia and should prompt assessment of both the patency of the vascular repair and the pressure within muscle compartments.

OUTCOMES AND FOLLOW-UP

The most common cause of amputation after vascular injury is the neurologic insult from either direct trauma to the nerve or ischemia. This should be remembered as one contemplates repair of a vascular injury in a "flail extremity" (permanently denervated secondary to irreversible neurologic injury).[38,39] Functional outcome after vascular repair is related to the severity of the associated injuries of muscle, bone, and nerve. Regular follow-up of patients with vascular repairs should continue to assess patency of the repair and to determine the presence of late complications.

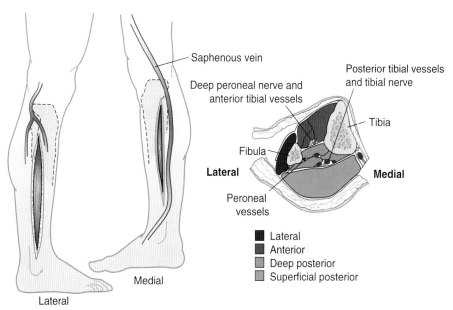

FIGURE 63-9 Calf muscle compartments and incisions for fasciotomy.

These include aneurysmal dilation or segmental stenosis of vein grafts, venous insufficiency from venous ligation, thrombosis of a pseudoaneurysm, and arteriovenous fistula. Ideally, these patients should be seen in yearly follow-up. Pulse examination and, if indicated, noninvasive imaging should be performed on a regular basis. Imaging with CT angiography or catheter angiography should be used if there is a suspicion of a complication.

Torso vascular injuries have relatively few late complications. Venous interposition grafts, when used, should be observed with periodic noninvasive imaging and, if indicated, CT angiography. Aortic and iliac arterial repairs should be observed similarly, and surveillance should ascertain signs and symptoms of arterial occlusive disease, such as upper or lower extremity claudication. Patients with synthetic interposition grafts should be counseled on the need for antibiotic prophylaxis during subsequent dental work or invasive procedures. Although late infections are uncommon, patients should be made aware of this possibility and counseled to notify all of their health care providers of the presence of a vascular prosthesis.

TRAINING AND PREPARATION FOR SUCCESSFUL MANAGEMENT

Vascular surgery carries a high risk of technical surgical error compared with many other areas of surgery. The optimal treatment of vascular trauma remains challenging and is rapidly evolving. Establishing goals for training in vascular trauma cannot be discussed without understanding the trends of increasing endovascular approaches and declining numbers of open repairs. Although one can acquire the didactic knowledge base from reading chapters such as this, the acquisition of decision-making abilities and surgical skills is based on experience that is becoming more and more difficult to obtain during surgical training. The average general surgical resident completes surgical residency having managed less than one vascular trauma case.[48,49] The average high-volume major trauma center in the United States manages approximately 10 to 15 vascular training cases a year. Fellowship-trained vascular surgeons receive vastly more exposure to chronic vascular disease and endovascular techniques than training in the rapid exposure of major vessels for proximal and distal control, let alone their open surgical management. The number of trauma surgeons contemporarily trained in endovascular techniques is extremely low. Many military general surgeons deployed to Afghanistan and Iraq for combat surgical care of wounded warriors site deficiencies in open vascular surgeries as their number one concern (personal communication to the authors).

General Surgery Training

The shrinking volume of open elective and emergency vascular surgery operations combined with resident work hour limitations has created significant obstacles to obtaining adequate experience in vascular surgical technique.[48] As opposed to residents graduating 2 decades ago, today's general surgeons rarely have enough experience to make them competent and capable of independently performing vascular surgery. Currently, there are a significant number of general surgeons who include vascular surgical cases in their practices. However, almost all completed their training before 2000 and the advent of the extensive use of endovascular techniques. These surgeons honed skills on open aortic aneurysm repairs, aortobifemoral bypass, and femoral popliteal bypass procedures.

The numbers of vascular surgery cases done by residents appears to be rising according to the Residency Review Committee. However, a closer look reveals the harsh reality that the case logs include a growing number of endovascular and venous procedures and an alarming decrease in open arterial procedures.[48-50] There has been as much as a 65% decrease in open arterial reconstruction case volume for graduate general surgery residents.[48,49] Open aortic surgery experience is much more uncommon, with many residents participating in five or fewer open aortic cases. Most surgery residents, however, claim endovascular aortic aneurysm repair (EVAR) among their vascular surgery numbers. Dialysis access cases have ironically become one of the last bastions of giving residents training in vascular techniques. The above-knee elective femoral popliteal bypass on mildly or moderately diseased vessels has all but disappeared. Most lower extremity bypasses are performed to very small distal vessels, and residents are often not able to perform these anastomoses.

Vascular Fellowship Training

The shrinking volume of open cases has also had an impact on vascular fellowship training. EVAR has become the treatment of choice for elective aneurysm repair, and emergency EVAR capabilities for ruptured abdominal aortic aneurysm have become a widespread practice. Consequently, there is real concern about the lack of open aortic cases available for training vascular surgery fellows. A conservative estimate of the number of cases required to give a surgeon adequate experience to competently handle the difficult ruptured aorta is well above 20 to 30 cases. The old saying that it takes up to 50 to 100 aortic repairs before the surgeon's fear transforms to profound respect for the aorta is probably accurate. Very few training programs come close to that volume. In reality, with widespread use of EVAR as the first-line therapy for elective abdominal aortic aneurysm repair, most graduating fellows will not see 100 open cases in the first 10 to 15 years of practice. The "fear factor" remains a considerable issue for these surgeons to contend with.

The decrease in open case volume during training and the significant rise in endovascular experience have produced a generation of vascular fellowship graduates who are more comfortable with closed techniques versus open techniques in many areas. This translates to a reluctance to convert to open technique and a discomfort with situations such as vascular trauma in which endovascular techniques may not be an option.

Vascular Trauma Realities

In a multi-institutional study presented in September 2012 at the annual meeting of the American Association for the Surgery of Trauma, Shackford and colleagues reported that more than 60% of complex extremity vascular reconstructions performed at 12 trauma centers across the country between 1995 and 2010 were performed by general surgeons.[29] The outcome of these repairs by general surgeons was not significantly different from the outcome of repairs performed by fellowship-trained cardiac and vascular surgeons. The overall amputation rate was low. All 12 hospitals were mature trauma centers with well-organized surgical specialty support. The average age of the surgeons who performed these repairs suggested that they all had adequate exposure during their surgical residency. What all the surgeons from the centers in this study had in common was a commitment to maintaining the skills needed to manage vascular injuries. The results of this approach were successful management of these complex injuries.

The conventional wisdom at successful trauma centers has always been to have the right surgeon available to do the right operation in a timely fashion. This has been especially important in repair of vascular injuries. Whether this capability will continue to be widely available remains to be seen. Few recent graduates of general surgery residencies feel confident in managing vascular injuries or other vascular emergencies. The alarming lack of open abdominal vascular procedures in most fellowship training programs has similarly eroded the confidence and competence of recently trained vascular surgeons. The paucity of capable vascular surgical emergency backup represents a threat to most of our trauma and emergency centers.

Need for Remedial Training and Review

We cannot expect the current general surgery and vascular surgery training programs to mitigate this lack of technical and cognitive competence without adding additional educational content focusing on areas of limited experience. The alternatives to hands-on operative experience remain limited. Simulation, although promising, has yet to accomplish the vision that it can replace actual experience as an adequate teaching opportunity. Maximizing open experience by resident participation in abdominal organ harvest by the transplantation team has been somewhat helpful.

There are two approaches in residency and fellowship training programs that hold promise. One is to actively audit general surgery and vascular fellowship trainee case logs to detect which resident should be the next participant in a major abdominal vascular procedure. These cases are precious training opportunities and should be shared evenly with all trainees. At this operation, the resident must be taught by actually performing the procedure, not simply watching. Attending surgeons must have the patience and forbearance to actually allow the trainee to perform the operation. Preparation with thoughtful didactic material focusing on these key operations should occur early in the trainee's rotation so that the operative experience has maximum educational impact. Postprocedure debriefing with a thorough discussion of decision points, troubleshooting, and management of different versions of the anatomy and pathologic findings needs to be rigorously performed.

The second important educational opportunity is participation in courses such as the American College of Surgeons–sponsored Advanced Surgical Skills for Exposure in Trauma (ASSET) and Advanced Trauma Operative Management (ATOM). These courses combine appropriate focused didactic material with either cadaver or live animal dissection. They are highly successful in improving both the knowledge and skill set of the participants. Equally important is the increase in confidence all participants report.

Additional courses developed through international cooperation are extremely promising. The Definitive Surgical Trauma Care course was developed by the International Association for Trauma and Surgical Intensive Care. The Definitive Surgical Trauma Skills course was developed by the Royal College of Surgeons of England with the Royal Defence Medical College and the Uniformed Services University of the Health Sciences in the United States. Completing either of these two courses provides excellent surgical training in trauma surgery decision making, vascular exposures, and vascular repairs.

The Need for Action

The rapidly disappearing knowledge and experience base of major open vascular surgical technique threatens all trauma centers'

ability to provide effective care for patients with major vascular injury and other vascular emergencies. Not taking action ensures a crisis in the near future that will result in poor outcomes. New education strategies are called for. Combining the maximal education value of a decreasing number of key open cases with appropriate courses that use cadaver and live animal operative experience will partially mitigate this looming deficit of open operative cases. Simulation is a cornerstone of training and maintenance of competence in commercial aviation. Simulation in surgery has yet to achieve its promise to augment real operative experience. However, in the future, it may become an important method for both acquiring and maintaining skills.

SELECTED REFERENCES

Biffl WL, Cothren CC, Moore EE, et al: Western Trauma Association critical decisions in trauma: Screening for and treatment of blunt cerebrovascular injuries. *J Trauma* 67:1150–1153, 2009.

> This practice recommendation from the Western Trauma Association offers an evidence-based approach to the diagnosis of blunt cerebrovascular injuries.

Feliciano DV, Mattox KL, Graham JM, et al: Five-year experience with PTFE grafts in vascular wounds. *J Trauma* 25:71–82, 1985.

> This is a landmark report establishing the acceptability of PTFE in vascular trauma repairs. It remains the best work in this area.

Gilani R, Tsai PI, Wall MJ, Jr, et al: Overcoming challenges of endovascular treatment of complex subclavian and axillary artery injuries in hypotensive patients. *J Trauma Acute Care Surg* 73:771–773, 2012.

> This report of eight patients, the majority of whom were hypotensive from major upper torso injuries, has major ramifications for the ability to use emergency endovascular techniques to control hemorrhage and to repair significant vascular injuries. This approach represents a promising future of a blended open and endovascular approach to vascular injuries.

Mattox KL, Feliciano DV, Burch J, et al: Five thousand seven hundred sixty cardiovascular injuries in 4459 patients. Epidemiologic evolution 1958 to 1987. *Ann Surg* 209:698–705, 1989.

> This is the largest epidemiologic study in the literature on civilian vascular injuries, and it remains the best work on the subject.

Neschis DG, Scalea TM, Flinn WR, et al: Blunt aortic injury. *N Engl J Med* 359:1708–1716, 2008.

> This review of series of both open and endovascular repairs of blunt thoracic injury provides a valuable overview of the risks versus benefits of each technique.

Patel MB, Guillamondegui OD, May AK, et al: Twenty-year analysis of surgical resident operative trauma experiences. *J Surg Res* 180:191–195, 2013.

This report gives a sobering perspective on the dwindling open surgical experience for surgical residents and highlights the need for alternative training modalities.

Patterson BO, Holt PJ, Cleanthis M, et al: Imaging vascular trauma. *Br J Surg* 99:494–505, 2012.

This systematic review was performed of literature relating to radiologic diagnosis of vascular trauma from 2000 to 2010. This excellent review conclusively established the superiority of CT angiography for the diagnosis of vascular injuries.

Reuben BC, Whitten MG, Sarfati M, et al: Increasing use of endovascular therapy in acute arterial injuries: Analysis of the National Trauma Data Bank. *J Vasc Surg* 46:1222–1226, 2007.

This report was a harbinger of the shift away from open vascular repairs and, from the perspective of 2016, was a predictor of the loss of open surgical experience and skills in the management of vascular injuries.

Sirinek KR, Levine BA, Gaskill HV, 3rd, et al: Reassessment of the role of routine operative exploration in vascular trauma. *J Trauma* 21:339–344, 1981.

This report was the basis for the cessation of operative exploration in stable patients in favor of angiography. In its time, it was a landmark paper and vastly improved the workup of patients with suspected vascular injury.

Stannard A, Eliason JL, Rasmussen TE: Resuscitative endovascular balloon occlusion of the aorta (REBOA) as an adjunct for hemorrhagic shock. *J Trauma* 71:1869–1872, 2011.

This report on the use of REBOA serves as a thorough update on the current practice and points out future directions in the development of this important aid for hemorrhage control.

REFERENCES

1. Amato JJ, Rich NM, Billy LJ, et al: High-velocity arterial injury: A study of the mechanism of injury. *J Trauma* 11:412–416, 1971.
2. Mattox KL, Feliciano DV, Burch J, et al: Five thousand seven hundred sixty vascular injuries in 4459 patients. Epidemiologic evolution 1958 to 1987. *Ann Surg* 209:698–707, 1989.
3. *Prehospital trauma life support*, ed 7, Chicago, 2012, American College of Surgeons.
4. Rich NM: Historic review of arteriovenous fistulas and traumatic false aneurysms. In Rich NM, Mattox KL, Hirshberg A, editors: *Vascular trauma*, Philadelphia, 2004, Elsevier Saunders, pp 457–524.
5. *Advanced trauma life support for doctors*, ed 9, Chicago, 2012, American College of Surgeons.
6. Sise MJ, Shackford SR: Peripheral vascular injury. In Mattox KL, Moore EE, Feliciano DV, editors: *Trauma*, ed 7, New York, 2013, McGraw-Hill, pp 817–847.
7. Patterson BO, Holt PJ, Cleanthis M, et al: Imaging vascular trauma. *Br J Surg* 99:494–505, 2012.
8. Seamon MJ, Smoger D, Torres DM, et al: A prospective validation of a current practice: The detection of extremity vascular injury with CT angiography. *J Trauma* 67:238–244, 2009.
9. White PW, Gillespie DL, Feurstein I, et al: Sixty-four slice multidetector computed tomographic angiography in the evaluation of vascular trauma. *J Trauma* 68:96–102, 2009.
10. O'Gorman RB, Feliciano DV, Bitondo CG, et al: Emergency center arteriography in the evaluation of suspected peripheral vascular injuries. *Arch Surg* 152:323–325, 1984.
11. Sirinek KR, Levine BA, Goskill HV, et al: Reassessment of the role of routine operative exploration in vascular trauma. *J Trauma* 21:339–344, 1981.
12. Dennis JW: Minimal vascular injury. In Rich NM, Mattox KL, Hirshberg A, editors: *Vascular trauma*, ed 2, Philadelphia, 2004, Elsevier Saunders, pp 85–96.
13. Reuben BC, Whitten MG, Sarfati M, et al: Increasing use of endovascular therapy in acute arterial injuries: Analysis of the National Trauma Data Bank. *J Vasc Surg* 46:1222–1226, 2007.
14. Worni M, Scarborough JE, Gandhi M, et al: Use of endovascular therapy for peripheral arterial lesions: An analysis of the National Trauma Data Bank from 2007 to 2009. *Ann Vasc Surg* 27:299–305, 2013.
15. Cothren CC, Moore EE, Ray CE, Jr, et al: Carotid artery stents for blunt cerebrovascular injury: Risks exceed benefits. *Arch Surg* 140:480–486, 2005.
16. Patel MB, Guillamondegui OD, May AK, et al: Twenty-year analysis of surgical resident operative trauma experiences. *J Surg Res* 180:191–195, 2013.
17. Schanzer A, Steppacher R, Eslami MH, et al: Vascular surgery training trends from 2001-2007: A substantial increase in total procedure volume is driven by escalating endovascular procedure volume and stable open procedure volume. *Vasc Surg* 49:1330–1344, 2009.
18. Richardson JD, Franklin GA, Lukan JK, et al: Evolution in the management of hepatic trauma: A 25 year perspective. *Ann Surg* 232:324–330, 2000.
19. Dent D, Alsabrook G, Erikson BA, et al: Blunt splenic injuries: High non-operative management rate can be achieved with selective embolization. *J Trauma* 56:1063–1067, 2004.
20. Martinelli T, Thony F, Decléty P, et al: Intra-aortic balloon occlusion to salvage patients with life-threatening hemorrhagic shocks from pelvic fractures. *J Trauma* 68:942–948, 2010.
21. Stannard A, Eliason JL, Rasmussen TE: Resuscitative endovascular balloon occlusion of the aorta (REBOA) as an adjunct for hemorrhagic shock. *J Trauma Acute Care Surg* 71:1869–1872, 2011.
22. Velmahos GC: Pelvis. In Mattox KL, Moore EE, Feliciano DV, editors: *Trauma*, ed 7, New York, 2013, McGraw-Hill, pp 655–668.
23. Mattox KL, Whigham C, Fisher RG, et al: Blunt trauma to the thoracic aorta: Current challenges. In Lumsden AB, Lin PH, Chen C, et al, editors: *Advanced endovascular therapy of aortic disease*, London, 2007, Blackwell Publishing, pp 127–133.
24. Demetriades D, Velmahos GC, Scalea TM, et al; American Association for the Surgery of Trauma Thoracic Aortic Injury Study Group: Operative repair or endovascular stent graft in blunt traumatic thoracic aortic injuries: Results of an

American Association for the Surgery of Trauma Multicenter Study. *J Trauma* 64:561–570, 2008.
25. Neschis DG, Scalea TM, Flinn WR, et al: Blunt aortic injury. *N Engl J Med* 359:1708–1716, 2008.
26. Cothren CC, Biffl WL, Moore EE, et al: Treatment for blunt cerebrovascular injuries: Equivalence of anticoagulation and antiplatelet agents. *Arch Surg* 144:685–690, 2009.
27. Biffl WL, Cothren CC, Moore EE, et al: Western Trauma Association critical decisions in trauma: Screening for and treatment of blunt cerebrovascular injuries. *J Trauma* 67:1150–1153, 2009.
28. DuBose J, Recinos G, Teixeira PG, et al: Endovascular stenting for the treatment of traumatic internal carotid injuries: Expanding experience. *J Trauma* 65:1561–1566, 2008.
29. Shackford SR, Kahl JE, Calvo RY, et al: Limb salvage after complex repairs of extremity arterial injuries is independent of surgical specialty training. *J Trauma Acute Care Surg* 74:716–724, 2013.
30. Wall MJ, Tsai P, Mattox KL: Heart and thoracic vascular injuries. In Mattox KL, Moore EE, Feliciano DV, editors: *Trauma*, ed 7, New York, 2013, McGraw-Hill, pp 485–511.
31. Dente CJ, Feliciano DV: Abdominal vascular injury. In Mattox KL, Moore EE, Feliciano DV, editors: *Trauma*, ed 7, New York, 2013, McGraw-Hill, pp 633–654.
32. Ding W, Wu X, Li J: Temporary intravascular shunts used as a damage control surgery adjunct in complex vascular injury: Collective review. *Injury* 39:970–977, 2008.
33. Subramanian A, Vercruysse G, Dente C, et al: A decade's experience with temporary intravascular shunts at a civilian level I trauma center. *J Trauma* 65:316–324, 2008.
34. Rich NM, Hughes CW: The fate of prosthetic material used to repair vascular injuries in contaminated wounds. *J Trauma* 12:459–467, 1972.
35. Feliciano DV, Mattox KL, Graham JM, et al: Five-year experience with PTFE grafts in vascular wounds. *J Trauma* 25:71–82, 1985.
36. Kim JY, Buck DW, Forte AJ, et al: Risk factors for compartment syndrome in traumatic brachial artery injuries: An institutional experience in 139 patients. *J Trauma* 67:1339–1344, 2009.
37. Branco BC, Inaba K, Barmparas G, et al: Incidence and predictors for the need for fasciotomy after extremity trauma: A 10-year review in a mature level I trauma center. *Injury* 42:1157–1163, 2011.
38. Ly TV, Travison TG, Castillo RC, et al: Ability of lower-extremity injury severity scores to predict functional outcome after limb salvage. *J Bone Joint Surg Am* 90:1738–1743, 2008.
39. Busse JW, Jacobs CL, Swiontkowski MF, et al: Complex limb salvage or early amputation for severe lower-limb injury: A meta-analysis of observational studies. *J Orthop Trauma* 21:70–76, 2007.
40. Dekker S: *The field guide to understanding human error*, Hampshire, UK, 2006, Ashgate Publishing Ltd.
41. Feliciano DV, Vercruysse GA: Neck. In Mattox KL, Moore EE, Feliciano DV, editors: *Trauma*, ed 7, New York, 2013, McGraw-Hill, pp 414–442.
42. Du Toit DF, Lambrechts AV, Stark H, et al: Long-term results of stent graft treatment of subclavian artery injuries: Management of choice for stable patients? *J Vasc Surg* 47:739–743, 2008.
43. Gilani R, Tsai P, Wall MJ: Overcoming challenges of endovascular treatment of complex subclavian and axillary artery injuries in hypotensive patients. *J Trauma Acute Care Surg* 73:771–773, 2012.
44. Carrick MM, Morrison CA, Pham HQ: Modern management of traumatic subclavian artery injuries: A single institution's experience in the evolution of endovascular repair. *Am J Surg* 199:28–34, 2010.
45. Cooper JD: The history of surgical procedures for emphysema. *Ann Thorac Surg* 63:312–319, 1997.
46. Franz RW, Goodwin RB, Hartman JF, et al: Management of upper extremity arterial injuries at an urban level I trauma center. *Ann Vasc Surg* 23:8–16, 2009.
47. Franz RW, Shah KJ, Halaharvi D, et al: A 5-year review of management of lower extremity arterial injuries at an urban level I trauma center. *J Vasc Surg* 53:1604–1610, 2011.
48. Keir J: Changes in caseload and the potential impact on surgical training: A retrospective review of one hospital's experience. *BMC Med Ed* 6:6–10, 2006.
49. Kairys JC, McGuire K, Crawford AG, et al: Cumulative operative experience is decreasing during general surgery residency: A worrisome trend for surgical trainees? *J Am Coll Surg* 206:804–811, 2008.
50. Grabo DJ, DiMuzio PJ, Kairys JC, et al: Have endovascular procedures negatively impacted general surgery training? *Semin Vasc Surg* 19:168–171, 2006.

64 CHAPTER

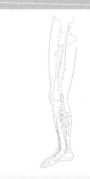

Venous Disease

Julie A. Freischlag, Jennifer A. Heller

第六十四章　静脉疾病

OUTLINE

Anatomy
Venous Insufficiency
Deep Venous Thrombosis
Superficial Thrombophlebitis
Conclusion

中文导读

　　本章共分为5节：①静脉解剖学；②静脉功能不全；③深静脉血栓；④血栓性浅静脉炎；⑤小结。

　　第一节详细介绍了下肢静脉的体表定位、引流区域，对于深静脉、浅静脉和交通静脉进行了分类阐述，着重突出了大隐静脉、小隐静脉、胫前静脉、胫后静脉、腘静脉等内容。同时介绍了静脉组织学和功能，重点讲述静脉壁的组织学结构及静脉管径的影响，也介绍了静脉系统作为重要容量血管的调节机制和静脉瓣膜在其中发挥的作用。

　　第二节讲述了静脉功能不全可分为先天性、原发性和继发性，其中原发性静脉功能不全临床最常见，也是本节的重点。作者详细介绍了原发性静脉功能不全的解剖分类，发病机制（主要是力学异常），危险因素及其作用机制、症状以及相应的体征，各种影像检查的选择，静脉功能不全的诊断评价和分型，

不同治疗方案的适应证及注意事项。其中，重点论述了浅静脉功能不全的治疗及相应并发症，包括非手术治疗、毛细血管扩张症的治疗、轴静脉功能不全的外科手术治疗、静脉内热消融治疗、超声引导下硬化治疗、分支静脉曲张的治疗等。对继发性静脉功能不全的治疗，作者重点论述了深静脉功能不全手术和直接静脉重建手术。

　　第三节讲述了深静脉血栓包括下肢深静脉血栓和上肢深静脉血栓。重点阐述了下肢深静脉血栓的病因、发病率和临床诊断、实验室检验和影像学检查、预防及治疗。本节也讨论了下腔静脉滤器和可回收下腔静脉滤器的植入适应证和潜在风险。

　　第四节讲述了血栓性浅静脉炎可分为原发性和特发性，前者常伴有危险因素如近期分娩、静脉瘀滞、

静脉曲张、静脉给药等，而后者则需要考虑是否存在高凝状态或潜在的恶性肿瘤。对累及深静脉的血栓性浅静脉炎需抗凝治疗，对局限性血栓性浅静脉炎需选择适当的治疗方案。

第五节讲述了静脉疾病具有广泛而多元的特点，充分理解静脉的生理学特征能够帮助制定合理的治疗方案和未来的研究策略。

〔涂振霄〕

 Please access ExpertConsult.com to view the corresponding videos for this chapter.

An understanding of venous physiology provides the surgeon with valuable information with which to formulate a diagnostic and treatment plan. Technologic advances have broadened the therapeutic armamentarium. This chapter provides the reader with a thorough overview of the physiology and pathophysiology of the venous system. Pathognomonic features of superficial and deep venous disorders are described with discussion of appropriate diagnostic modalities and therapeutic interventions.

ANATOMY

To determine whether a pathophysiologic process is present, knowledge of venous anatomy is essential. Venous drainage of the legs is the function of two parallel and associated units, the deep and superficial veins. A third system, the perforating veins, interconnects the superficial and deep veins. The nomenclature of the venous system of the lower limb was revised in 2002, and the most relevant changes are addressed here.[1] The revised nomenclature is delineated in Tables 64-1 and 64-2.

Superficial Venous System

The superficial veins of the lower extremity form a network that connects the superficial dorsal veins of the foot and deep plantar veins. The dorsal venous arch, into which empty the dorsal metatarsal veins, is continuous with the great saphenous vein medially and the small saphenous vein laterally (Fig. 64-1).

The great saphenous vein arises from dorsal veins of the foot. The great saphenous vein extends cephalad and travels over the medial aspect of the tibia and in parallel to the saphenous nerve. As the great saphenous vein ascends through the thigh, multiple accessory branches are demonstrated, and variability of the number and location of these branches is the norm. The great saphenous vein travels within its own fascia, called the saphenous sheath. This structure is superior to the deep fascia of the leg. Although a classic feature, the great saphenous vein can be contained completely within the saphenous sheath or exit the fascia and reenter at another point in its course along the extremity. In some cases, patients exhibit an incomplete saphenous sheath, which makes identification of the great saphenous vein difficult. The great saphenous vein terminates into the saphenofemoral junction, where it is joined by the confluence of the superficial circumflex iliac veins, the external pudendal veins, and the superficial epigastric veins. It then ascends in the superficial compartment and empties into the common femoral vein after entering the fossa ovalis (Fig. 64-2).

The small saphenous vein arises from the dorsal venous arch at the lateral aspect of the foot and ascends posterior to the lateral malleolus, rising cephalad in the midposterior calf. The small saphenous vein continues to ascend, penetrates the superficial fascia of the calf, and then terminates into the popliteal vein. However, this anatomy is extremely variable. Most commonly, the small saphenous vein terminates within a lateral branch of the thigh, bypassing the classic saphenopopliteal junction. The sural nerve lies parallel to the small saphenous vein. This relationship becomes more intimate at the distal calf. A common vein branch, the vein of Giacomini, connects the small saphenous vein with the great saphenous vein.

Deep Venous System

The plantar digital veins in the foot empty into a network of metatarsal veins that compose the deep plantar venous arch. This continues into the medial and lateral plantar veins, which then drain into the posterior tibial veins. The dorsalis pedis veins on the dorsum of the foot form the paired anterior tibial veins at the ankle.

The paired posterior tibial veins, adjacent to and flanking the posterior tibial artery, run under the fascia of the deep posterior compartment. These veins enter the soleus and join the popliteal vein, after joining with the paired peroneal and anterior tibial veins. There are large venous sinuses within the soleus muscle—soleal sinuses—that empty into the posterior tibial and peroneal veins. Bilateral gastrocnemius veins empty into the popliteal vein distal to the point of entry of the small saphenous vein into the popliteal vein.

The popliteal vein enters a window in the adductor magnus, at which point it is termed the femoral vein, previously known as the superficial femoral vein. The femoral vein ascends and receives venous drainage from the profunda femoris vein, or deep femoral vein, and after this confluence, it is the common femoral vein. As the common femoral vein crosses the inguinal ligament, it becomes the external iliac vein.

Venous System Perforators

Perforating veins connect the superficial venous system to the deep venous system by penetrating the fascial layers of the lower extremity. These perforators run in a perpendicular fashion to the axial veins previously described. Although the total number of perforator veins is variable, up to 100 have been documented. The perforators enter at various points in the leg—the foot, medial and lateral calf, and mid and distal thigh (Fig. 64-3). Some have been named by the surgeons who first identified them: Crockett

TABLE 64-1 Superficial Veins

ANATOMIC TERMINOLOGY	PROPOSED TERMINOLOGY
Greater or long saphenous vein	Great saphenous vein
	Superficial inguinal veins
External pudendal vein	External pudendal vein
Superficial circumflex vein	Superficial circumflex iliac vein
Superficial epigastric vein	Superficial epigastric vein
Superficial dorsal vein of clitoris or penis	Superficial dorsal vein of clitoris or penis
Anterior labial veins	Anterior labial veins
Anterior scrotal veins	Anterior scrotal veins
Accessory saphenous vein	Anterior accessory great saphenous vein
	Posterior accessory great saphenous vein
	Superficial accessory great saphenous vein
Smaller or short saphenous vein	Small saphenous vein
	Cranial extension of small saphenous vein
	Superficial accessory small saphenous vein
	Anterior thigh circumflex vein
	Posterior thigh circumflex vein
	Intersaphenous veins
	Lateral venous system
Dorsal venous network of the foot	Dorsal venous network of the foot
Dorsal venous arch of the foot	Dorsal venous arch of the foot
Dorsal metatarsal veins	Superficial metatarsal veins (dorsal and plantar)
Plantar venous network	Plantar venous subcutaneous network
Plantar venous arch	
Plantar metatarsal veins	Superficial digital veins (dorsal and plantar)
Lateral marginal vein	Lateral marginal vein
Medial marginal vein	Medial marginal vein

TABLE 64-2 Deep Veins

ANATOMIC TERMINOLOGY	PROPOSED TERMINOLOGY
Femoral vein	Common femoral vein
	Femoral vein
Profunda femoris vein or deep vein of thigh	Profunda femoris vein or deep femoral vein
Medial circumflex femoral vein	Medial circumflex femoral vein
Lateral circumflex femoral vein	Lateral circumflex femoral vein
Perforating veins	Deep femoral communicating veins (accompanying veins of perforating arteries)
	Sciatic vein
Popliteal vein	Popliteal vein
	Sural veins
	Soleal veins
	Gastrocnemius veins
	Medial gastrocnemius veins
	Lateral gastrocnemius veins
	Intergemellar vein
Genicular veins	Genicular venous plexus
Anterior tibial veins	Anterior tibial veins
Posterior tibial veins	Posterior tibial veins
Fibular or peroneal veins	Fibular or peroneal veins
	Medial plantar veins
	Lateral plantar veins
	Deep plantar venous arch
	Deep metatarsal veins (plantar and dorsal)
	Deep digital veins (plantar and dorsal)
	Pedal vein

perforators, which connect the posterior arch and posterior tibial veins; Boyd perforators, which connect the great saphenous and gastrocnemius veins; and hunterian and Dodd perforators, which connect the great saphenous and superficial femoral veins. The perforator veins have an important function. Their valve system aids in preventing reflux from the deep to the superficial system, particularly during periods of standing and ambulation.

Normal Venous Histology and Function

The venous wall is composed of three layers, the intima, media, and adventitia. Vein walls have less smooth muscle and elastin than their arterial counterparts. The venous intima has an endothelial cell layer resting on a basement membrane. The media is composed of smooth muscle cells and elastin connective tissue. The adventitia of the venous wall contains adrenergic fibers, particularly in the cutaneous veins. Central sympathetic discharge and brainstem thermoregulatory centers can alter venous tone, as can other stimuli, such as temperature changes, pain, emotional stimuli, and volume changes.

The histologic features of veins vary, depending on the caliber of the veins. The venules, the smallest veins, range from 0.1 to

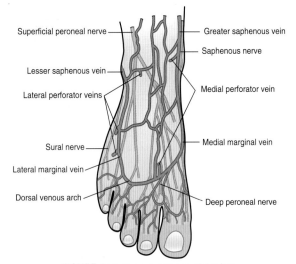

FIGURE 64-1 Venous drainage of the foot.

1 mm and contain mostly smooth muscle cells, whereas the larger extremity veins contain relatively few smooth muscle cells. These larger caliber veins have limited contractile capacity in comparison to the thicker walled great saphenous vein. The venous valves prevent retrograde flow; it is their failure or valvular incompetence that leads to reflux and its associated symptoms. Venous valves are

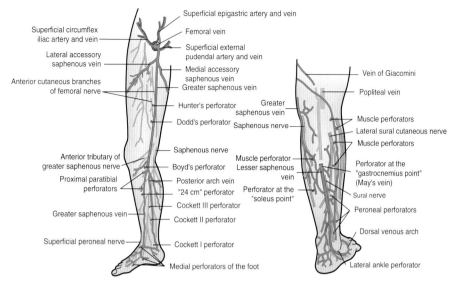

FIGURE 64-2 Venous drainage of the lower limb.

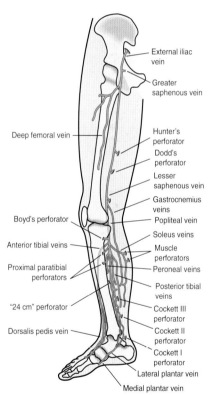

FIGURE 64-3 Perforating veins of the lower limb.

most prevalent in the distal lower extremity, whereas as one proceeds proximally, the number of valves decreases to the point that no valves are present in the superior vena cava and inferior vena cava (IVC).

Most of the capacitance of the vascular tree is in the venous system. Because veins do not have significant amounts of elastin, veins can withstand large volume shifts with comparatively small changes in pressure. A vein has a normal elliptical configuration until the limit of its capacitance is reached, at which point the vein assumes a round configuration.

The calf muscles augment venous return by functioning as a pump. In the supine state, the resting venous pressure in the foot is the sum of the residual kinetic energy minus the resistance in the arterioles and precapillary sphincters. Thus, a pressure gradient is generated to the right atrium of approximately 10 to 12 mm Hg. In the upright position, the resting venous pressure of the foot is a reflection of the hydrostatic pressure from the upright column of blood extending from the right atrium to the foot.

The return of the blood to the heart from the lower extremity is facilitated by the muscle pump function of the calf, a mechanism whereby the calf muscle, functioning as a bellows during exercise, compresses the gastrocnemius and soleal sinuses and propels the blood toward the heart. The normally functioning valves in the venous system prevent retrograde flow; when one or more of these valves become incompetent, symptoms of venous insufficiency can develop. During calf muscle contraction, the venous pressure of the foot and ankle drops dramatically. The pressures developing in the muscle compartments during exercise range from 150 to 200 mm Hg, and when there is failure of perforating veins, these high pressures are transmitted to the superficial system.

VENOUS INSUFFICIENCY

There are three categories of venous insufficiency—congenital, primary, and secondary. Congenital venous insufficiency comprises predominantly anatomic variants that are present at birth. Examples of congenital venous anomalies include venous ectasias, absence of venous valves, and syndromes such as Klippel-Trénaunay syndrome. Primary venous insufficiency is an acquired idiopathic entity. This is the largest clinical category and represents most of the superficial venous insufficiency encountered in the office. Secondary venous insufficiency arises from a post-thrombotic or obstructive state and is caused by a deep venous thrombus or primary chronic obstructive process.

Primary Venous Insufficiency

There are three main anatomic categories of primary venous insufficiency—telangiectasias, reticular veins, and varicose veins. Telangiectasias, reticular varicosities, and varicose veins are similar but exhibit distinct variations in caliber. Telangiectasias are very small intradermal venules that are too diminutive to demonstrate reflux. These structures measure less than 3 mm. Without associated symptoms and stigmata of other venous disease, they are idiopathic in nature and are not medically necessary to treat. However, although not of concern from a venous standpoint, leg telangiectasias of multiple causes may be a manifestation of a systemic disease. Some of these disorders include autoimmune diseases (such as lupus erythematosus and dermatomyositis), exogenous causes, and xeroderma pigmentosum. Reticular veins are vein branches that enter the tributaries of the main axial, perforating, or deep veins. The axial veins, the great and small saphenous veins, represent the largest caliber veins of the superficial venous system.

Pathology

The precise pathophysiologic mechanism of venous insufficiency has yet to be elucidated. This describes some of the areas in which research has started to reveal its multifactorial pathogenesis.

Mechanical abnormalities. Anatomic differences in the location of the superficial veins of the lower extremities may contribute to the pathogenesis. Primary venous insufficiency may involve both the axial veins (great and small saphenous), either vein, or neither vein. Perforating veins may be the sole source of venous pathophysiologic changes, perhaps because the great saphenous vein is supported by a well-developed medial fibromuscular layer and fibrous connective tissue that bind it to the deep fascia. In contrast, tributaries to the small saphenous vein are less supported in the subcutaneous fat and are superficial to the membranous layer of superficial fascia (Fig. 64-4). These tributaries also contain less muscle mass in their walls. Thus, these veins, and not the main trunk, may become selectively varicose.

When these fundamental anatomic peculiarities are recognized, the intrinsic competence or incompetence of the valve system becomes important. For example, failure of a valve protecting a tributary vein from the pressures of the small saphenous vein allows a cluster of varicosities to develop. Furthermore, communicating veins connecting the deep with the superficial compartment may have valve failure. Pressure studies have shown that there are two sources of venous hypertension. The first is gravitational and is a result of venous blood coursing in a distal direction down linear axial venous segments. This is referred to as hydrostatic pressure and is the weight of the blood column from the right atrium. The highest pressure generated by this mechanism is evident at the ankle and foot, where measurements are expressed in centimeters of water or millimeters of mercury.

The second source of venous hypertension is dynamic. It is the force of muscle contraction, usually contained within the compartments of the leg. If a perforating vein fails, high pressures (range, 150 to 200 mm Hg) developed within the muscular compartments during exercise are transmitted directly to the superficial venous system. Here, the sudden pressure transmitted causes dilation and lengthening of the superficial veins. Progressive distal valvular incompetence may occur. If proximal valves such as the saphenofemoral valve become incompetent, systolic muscular contraction is supplemented by the weight of the static column of blood from the heart. Furthermore, this static column becomes a barrier. Blood flowing proximally through the femoral vein spills into the saphenous vein and flows distally. As it refluxes distally through progressively incompetent valves, it is returned through perforating veins to the deep veins. Here, it is conveyed once again to the femoral veins, only to be recycled distally.

Regardless of the precise source of the elevated hydrostatic pressure, the ultimate end result is increased ambulatory hypertension. The inflammatory processes that occur throughout the venous circulation have been demonstrated within the vein wall as well as within the vein valves. It is unclear as to which abnormality occurs first, that is, whether the vein wall becomes distended from increased pressure and then causes vein wall abnormalities, or vice versa. The resulting increased ambulatory venous pressure affects the endothelium as well as the venous microcirculation. This activation is again caused by changes in shear stress and mechanical stress of the vein wall and vein valves. Altered shear stress causes the endothelial cells to release a variety of agents, including chemokines and inflammatory molecules, which precipitates the inflammatory cascade. In particular, cytokines and metalloproteinases play a prominent role in the mechanical and inflammatory process of venous hypertension. The inflammatory process involves many different pathways that result in elevations of inflammatory modulators and cytokines, growth factors, and metalloproteinase activity.[2] Fundamental defects in the strength and characteristics of the venous wall have been identified. Varicose vein walls demonstrate decreased amounts of elastin and collagen, suggesting a contributing role toward venous pathophysiology.[3]

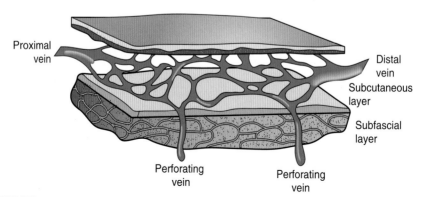

FIGURE 64-4 Dilation of superficial venous tributaries caused by increased transmission of pressure by the perforating veins.

Risk Factors

Risk factors for the development of varicose veins include advancing age, female gender, multiparity, heredity, and history of trauma to the extremity. Additional risk factors include obesity and a positive family history. Advancing age appears to be the most significant risk factor. Venous function is undoubtedly influenced by hormonal changes. In particular, progesterone liberated by the corpus luteum stabilizes the uterus by causing the relaxation of smooth muscle fibers.[4] This directly influences venous function. The result is passive venous dilation, which in many cases causes valvular dysfunction. Although progesterone is implicated in the first appearance of varicosities in pregnancy, estrogen also has profound effects. It produces the relaxation of smooth muscle and a softening of collagen fibers. Furthermore, the estrogen-to-progesterone ratio influences venous distensibility. This ratio may explain the predominance of venous insufficiency symptoms on the first day of a menstrual period, when a profound shift occurs from the progesterone phase of the menstrual cycle to the estrogen phase. Autosomal dominant penetrance has been identified as the underlying genetic risk factor for subsequent development of varicose veins.

Symptoms

Venous valvular dysfunction causes venous hypertension, and as such, patients' symptoms are attributed to excess venous pooling. The patient with symptomatic varicose veins commonly reports heaviness, discomfort, and extremity fatigue. The pain is characteristically dull, does not usually occur during recumbency or early in the morning, and is exacerbated in the afternoon, especially after periods of prolonged standing. Swelling is commonly described. The discomforts of aching, heaviness, and fatigue are usually relieved by leg elevation or elastic support. Cutaneous burning, termed venous neuropathy, can also occur in patients with advanced venous insufficiency. Pruritus occurs from excess hemosiderin deposition and tends to be located at the distal calf or in areas of phlebitic varicose branch segments. Patients may report cramping pain that occurs during or after exercise and is relieved with rest and leg elevation. This syndrome is termed venous claudication and is a clinical manifestation of venous outflow obstruction, secondary venous insufficiency. Predominant causes of venous claudication include a prior deep venous thrombosis (DVT) and May-Thurner syndrome.

Multiparous female patients in their childbearing years may report a constellation of symptoms that involve varicosities of the leg in conjunction with chronic pelvic pain. The lower extremity symptoms may or may not be present. Additional symptoms include a feeling of bladder fullness with standing, dyspareunia, and chronic pelvic pain. This clinical picture suggests pelvic congestion syndrome. As the differential diagnosis for pelvic pain is extensive, the diagnosis of pelvic venous congestion tends to be one of exclusion; diagnostic modalities to confirm its presence include magnetic resonance venous imaging (MRVI) of the pelvis and conventional pelvic venography, which can be both diagnostic and therapeutic.

Physical Examination

A comprehensive examination includes assessment of the arterial circulation. Briefly, palpation of the femoral, popliteal, dorsalis pedis, and posterior tibialis pulses is performed. Nonpalpable pulses necessitate further evaluation. Auscultation of pulse flow is indicated when a thrill or widened pulse is appreciated. Decreased hair, dependent rubor, pallor on elevation, and tissue loss are all indicative of advanced arterial ischemia.

The venous examination includes assessment of the patient in the standing and supine positions. The examination room must be well lighted and warm so that vasospasm does not occur, limiting a comprehensive evaluation. Standing increases venous hypertension and dilates veins, thereby facilitating examination. Patients with superficial axial incompetence commonly exhibit palpable great saphenous veins (Fig. 64-5).

Visual inspection is critical. Location of varicosities can commonly identify a "blown valve" or the axial vein from which the varicosities developed. For example, medial thigh varicose veins are likely to develop from an incompetent great saphenous vein, whereas posterior calf or lateral calf varicose veins tend to originate from the small saphenous vein. In addition, the location of varicose veins can be a diagnostic predictor of a larger process. Varicosities of the scrotum can be associated with gonadal vein incompetence, otherwise termed the nutcracker syndrome (compression of the left renal vein between the aorta and the superior mesenteric artery). Perineal or vulvar varicosities can be a sign of ovarian or pelvic venous insufficiency, or iliac vein obstruction.

The physical examination can provide the physician with important information on the history of the venous disease that the patient might have neglected or forgotten to mention during the history. For example, signs of a chronic or resolved thrombophlebitis may include a partially thrombosed varicosity; a brownish discoloration around a varicosity or along a palpable segment of the axial veins, consistent with hemosiderin deposition; and palpable segments of axial vein, suggesting partially or completely occluded axial vein segments.

Signs of advanced venous insufficiency include hyperpigmentation in the distal calf or gaiter distribution, secondary to hemosiderin deposition, and lipodermatosclerosis. Lipodermatosclerosis develops over time because of prolonged ambulatory venous hypertension and chronic inflammation. Physical examination findings that reflect lipodermatosclerosis are brawny edema of the distal calf, "champagne bottle leg," fibrotic and hypertrophic skin, and hyperpigmentation. Advanced lipodermatosclerosis may

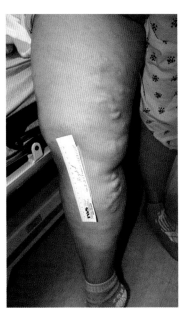

FIGURE 64-5 Varicose veins.

involve fibrosis of the Achilles tendon, impairing motor function of the extremity. Therefore, examination should include motor function at the ankle. Atrophie blanche is an area of pale hue, visualized around the medial malleolus; it is commonly mistaken for a healed ulcer because of its lighter pigmentation (Fig. 64-6). Corona phlebectatica is a term used to describe an accumulation of tiny telangiectasias or venous flare, usually located at the medial malleolus or the dorsum of the foot. Skin changes from chronic venous insufficiency (CVI) can mimic other dermatologic phenomena; both dermatitis and eczematous changes can be seen from venous disease.

Venous stasis ulcers exhibit pathognomonic features that distinguish them from their arterial or neuropathic counterparts. Venous ulcers are not generally painful and appear at the medial malleolus, not in the mid to distal foot. Lack of arterial pulses in patients with a venous ulcer is unusual.

Venous stasis dermatitis is visualized at the distal ankle and can mimic eczema or dermatitis of another cause. It is this important attention to supporting features of the physical examination and history as well as confirmation with duplex reflux examination that will distinguish advanced venous stasis disease from dermatologic conditions.

Diagnostic Evaluation of Venous Dysfunction

The Perthes test for deep venous occlusion and the Brodie-Trendelenburg test of axial reflux have been replaced by in-office use of the continuous-wave, hand-held Doppler instrument supplemented by duplex ultrasound evaluation. The hand-held Doppler instrument can confirm an impression of saphenous reflux, which in turn dictates the operative procedure to be performed in a given patient. A common misconception is the belief that the Doppler instrument is used to locate perforating veins. Instead, it is used in specific locations to determine incompetent valves, for example, the hand-held, continuous-wave, 8-MHz flow detector placed over the great and small saphenous veins near their terminations. With distal augmentation of flow and release,

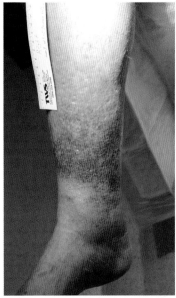

FIGURE 64-6 Lipodermatosclerosis, atrophie blanche, and brawny edema.

normal deep breathing, and performance of a Valsalva maneuver, valve reflux is accurately identified. Formerly, the Doppler examination was supplemented by other objective studies, including photoplethysmography, mercury strain-gauge plethysmography, and photorheography. These are no longer in common use.

Another instrument reintroduced to assess physiologic function of the muscle pump and venous valves is air displacement plethysmography.[5] Its use was discontinued after the 1960s because of its cumbersome nature. Computer technology has now allowed its reintroduction, as championed by Christopoulos and colleagues.[6] It consists of an air chamber that surrounds the leg from knee to ankle. During calibration, leg veins are emptied by leg elevation, and the patient is then asked to stand so that leg venous volume can be quantitated and the time for filling recorded. The filling rate is then expressed in milliliters per second, thus giving readings similar to those obtained with the mercury strain-gauge technique.

Today, duplex imaging is the first and best modality to assess for the normal function and presence of venous insufficiency of the lower extremities. Duplex technology more precisely defines which veins are refluxing by imaging the superficial and deep veins. The duplex examination is commonly done with the patient supine, but this yields an erroneous evaluation of reflux. In the supine position, even when no flow is present, the valves remain open. Valve closure requires a reversal of flow with a pressure gradient that is higher proximally than distally. Thus, the duplex examination needs to be done with the patient standing or in the markedly trunk-elevated position.[7]

There are many advantages of ultrasound imaging. The ultrasound examination is noninvasive, requires no contrast material, and can be performed in the office as well as in the hospital. Drawbacks to the modality include interobserver variability and limitations in imaging in patients with an elevated body mass index and extensive dressings. Imaging is obtained with a 7.5- or 10-MHz probe; the pulsed Doppler consists of a 3.0-MHz probe. The examination begins with the probe placed longitudinally on the groin. First, all of the deep veins are examined. Next, the superficial veins are evaluated. There are four basic components of the examination that should be included to complete a comprehensive venous evaluation of the lower extremity veins: compressibility, venous flow, augmentation after reflux, and visibility. Reflux can be demonstrated with the patient performing a Valsalva maneuver or by manual compression and release of the extremity distal to the point of the examination. A Valsalva maneuver is performed for the proximal extremity, that is, the thigh and groin, whereas compression is used for the calf. Reflux times of 500 milliseconds or longer are considered significant. Perforator veins can be visualized well with the duplex examination. Significant perforator reflux is defined as a diameter of more than 3.5 mm and a reflux time of 500 milliseconds or longer. Demonstration on duplex images of to-and-fro flow, with the presence of dilated segments, constitutes findings compatible with a refluxing perforator. In addition, Doppler studies can provide the clinician with information about the deep system. Widespread use of duplex scanning has allowed a comparison of findings between standard clinical examinations and duplex Doppler studies.[8,9]

Phlebography and venography. In general, phlebography is unnecessary in the diagnosis and treatment of primary venous insufficiency. In cases of secondary CVI, phlebography has specific usefulness. Ascending phlebography is performed by injection of contrast material into a superficial pedal vein after a tourniquet is applied at the ankle to prevent flow into the superficial venous system. Observation of flow defines anatomy and regions of thrombus or obstruction. Therefore, ascending phlebology differentiates primary from secondary venous insufficiency. Descending phlebography is performed with retrograde injection of contrast material into the deep venous system at the groin or popliteal fossa (femoral vein or popliteal vein). This diagnostic modality identifies specific valvular incompetence suspected on B-mode scanning and clinical examination. These studies are performed only as preoperative adjuncts when deep venous reconstruction is being planned.

Magnetic resonance venous imaging. MRVI is a diagnostic imaging modality reserved for evaluation of the abdominal and pelvic venous vasculature. MRVI, unlike venography, is noninvasive and does not require intravenous (IV) administration of contrast material. Studies have documented similar rates of specificity and sensitivity compared with venography. MRVI is used to evaluate pelvic venous outflow obstruction, providing information from the IVC through the iliac venous system. Furthermore, it is an excellent test to evaluate for pelvic congestion syndrome. In some institutions, the computed tomography scan has applications that can be used similar to the MRVI scan.

Classification Systems

In 1994, the American Venous Forum devised the CEAP classification system, which is a scoring system that stratifies venous disease on the basis of clinical presentation, etiology, anatomy, and pathophysiology (Table 64-3). It is useful in helping the physician assess a limb afflicted with venous insufficiency and then arrive at an appropriate treatment plan. A revised CEAP classification was introduced in 2004 that included a Venous Disability Score to document a patient's ability to perform activities of daily living.[10] Although the CEAP classification is a valuable tool to grade venous disease, assessment of outcomes after intervention cannot be realized. As a result, two additional scoring systems, the Venous Clinical Severity Score and the Venous Segmental Disease Score, enhance the CEAP score with the increased ability to plot outcome. These three classification modalities now provide clinical researchers with invaluable tools to study treatment outcomes.[11]

Treatment of Superficial Venous Insufficiency

Nonoperative management. Symptoms of primary venous insufficiency are manifestations of valvular incompetence. Therefore, the objective of conservative management is to improve the symptoms caused by venous hypertension. The first measure is external compression using elastic hose, 20 to 30 mm Hg, to be worn during the daytime hours. Although the exact mechanism whereby compression is of benefit is not entirely known, a number of physiologic alterations have been observed with compression. These include reduction in ambulatory venous pressure, improvement in skin microcirculation, and increase in subcutaneous pressure, which counters transcapillary fluid leakage. Patients are instructed to wear the hose during the day only, but to put the stockings on as soon as the day begins; swelling with standing will make stocking placement difficult. Care must be taken with patients who have concomitant arterial insufficiency because the compression stockings may exacerbate arterial outflow to the foot. Therefore, these patients require less compression—in some cases, no compression whatsoever—depending on the severity of the arterial disease. In general, an ankle-brachial index of less than 0.7 contraindicates the use of 20 to 30 mm Hg compression

stockings.

The second part of conservative therapy is to practice lower extremity elevation for two brief periods during the day, instructing the patient that the feet must be above the level of the heart, or "toes above the nose." With good compliance, these measures may ameliorate symptoms so that patients may not require further intervention. Third, patients are encouraged to participate in activities that activate the calf musculovenous pump, thereby decreasing ambulatory venous hypertension. These activities include frequent ambulation and exercise.

Patients who exhibit venous stasis ulceration will require local wound care (Fig. 64-7). A triple-layer compression dressing, with a zinc oxide paste gauze wrap in contact with the skin, is used most commonly, from the base of the toes to the anterior tibial tubercle with snug graded compression. This is an example of what is generally known as an Unna boot. A 15-year review of 998 patients with one or more venous ulcers treated with a similar compression bandage demonstrated that 73% of the ulcers healed in patients who returned for care (Fig. 64-8). The median time to healing for individual ulcers was 9 weeks. In general, snug, graded-pressure, triple-layer compression dressings result in more rapid healing than with compression stockings alone.

For most patients, well-applied, sustained compression therapy offers the most cost-effective and efficacious therapy in the healing of venous ulcers. After healing, most cases of CVI are controlled with elastic compression stockings to be worn during waking hours. On occasion, older patients and those with arthritic conditions cannot apply the compression stocking required, and control must be maintained by triple-layer zinc oxide compression dressings, which can usually be left in place and changed once a week. In addition to compression, wound care, and surgery, large chronic venous ulcers may benefit from venoactive medications, in particular, pentoxifylline and micronized purified flavonoid fraction.

Indications for interventional treatment are symptoms refractory to conservative therapy, recurrent superficial thrombophlebitis, variceal bleeding, and venous stasis ulceration. After clinical and objective criteria have established the presence of symptomatic varicose veins, the next step is to plan a course of therapy.

The efficacy of conservative versus surgical treatment for varicose veins was studied in the Randomised Clinical Trial, Observational Study and Assessment of Cost-Effectiveness of the Treatment of Varicose veins (REACTIV) trial. The authors concluded that surgical treatment was more cost-effective and patients had a higher quality of life benefit than the group who had maintained conservative management alone with compression therapy.[12,13]

Treatment options for telangiectasias. By definition, telangiectasias, as they are structures with diameters smaller than 3 mm, are not appropriate for surgical treatment. Asymptomatic telangiectasias are of cosmetic concern only. In these asymptomatic patients with only C_1 disease, a reflux examination is not indicated. However, if the patient describes symptoms consistent with possible venous insufficiency or has concomitant varicosities or more advanced disease on physical examination, a reflux examination is indicated. Treatment options for telangiectasias (spider veins and reticular veins) include injection sclerotherapy and transdermal laser treatment (Fig. 64-9).

Injection sclerotherapy is a technique that involves direct injection of a sclerosant agent into the feeding vein (reticular vein) or spider vein. This procedure is performed in the office setting. There is no preprocedural preparation of the patient. However,

TABLE 64-3 Classification of Chronic Lower Extremity Venous Disease

C	Clinical signs (grade$_{0-6}$), supplemented by A for asymptomatic and S for symptomatic presentation
E	Classification by cause (etiology)—congenital, primary, secondary
A	Anatomic distribution—superficial, deep, or perforator, alone or in combination
P	Pathophysiologic dysfunction—reflux or obstruction, alone or in combination

Clinical Classification (C$_{0-6}$)

Any limb with possible chronic venous disease is first placed into one of seven clinical classes (C$_{0-6}$), according to the objective signs of disease.

Clinical Classification of Chronic Lower Extremity Venous Disease*

CLASS	FEATURES
0	No visible or palpable signs of venous disease
1	Telangiectasia, reticular veins, malleolar flare
2	Varicose veins
3	Edema without skin changes
4	Skin changes ascribed to venous disease (e.g., pigmentation, venous eczema, lipodermatosclerosis)
5	Skin changes as defined above with healed ulceration
6	Skin changes as defined above with active ulceration

*Limbs in higher categories have more severe signs of chronic venous disease and may have some or all of the findings defining a less severe clinical category. Each limb is further characterized as asymptomatic (A)—for example, C$_{0-6,A}$—or symptomatic (S)—for example, C$_{0-6,S}$. Symptoms that may be associated with telangiectatic, reticular, or varicose veins include lower extremity aching, pain, and skin irritation. Therapy may alter the clinical category of chronic venous disease. Limbs should therefore be reclassified after any form of medical or surgical treatment.

Classification by Cause (E$_c$, E$_p$, or E$_s$)

Venous dysfunction may be congenital, primary, or secondary. These categories are mutually exclusive. Congenital venous disorders are present at birth but may not be recognized until later. The method of diagnosis of congenital abnormalities must be described. Primary venous dysfunction is defined as venous dysfunction of unknown cause but not of congenital origin. Secondary venous dysfunction denotes an acquired condition resulting in chronic venous disease—for example, deep venous thrombosis.

Classification by Cause of Chronic Lower Extremity Venous Disease

Congenital (E$_c$)	Cause of the chronic venous disease present since birth
Primary (E$_p$)	Chronic venous disease of undetermined cause
Secondary (E$_s$)	Chronic venous disease with an associated known cause (e.g., post-thrombotic, post-traumatic, other)

Anatomic Classification (A$_s$, A$_d$, or A$_p$)

The anatomic site(s) of the venous disease should be described as superficial (A$_s$), deep (A$_d$), or perforating (A$_p$) vein(s). One, two, or three systems may be involved in any combination. For reports requiring greater detail, the involvement of the superficial, deep, and perforating veins may be localized by use of the anatomic segments.

Segmental Localization of Chronic Lower Extremity Venous Disease

SEGMENT NO.	VEINS
Superficial veins (A$_{s1-5}$)	
1	Telangiectasia/reticular veins
	Greater (long) saphenous vein
2	Above knee
3	Below knee
4	Lesser (short) saphenous vein
5	Nonsaphenous
Deep veins (A$_{d6-16}$)	
6	Inferior vena cava
	Iliac
7	Common
8	Internal
9	External
10	Pelvic: gonadal, broad ligament
	Femoral
11	Common
12	Deep
13	Superficial

TABLE 64-3	Classification of Chronic Lower Extremity Venous Disease—cont'd	
14	Popliteal	
15	Tibial (anterior, posterior, or peroneal)	
16	Muscular (gastrointestinal, soleal, other)	
17	Thigh	
18	Calf	

Pathophysiologic Classification (P$_{r,o}$)

Clinical signs or symptoms of chronic venous disease result from reflux (P$_r$), obstruction (P$_o$), or both (P$_{r,o}$).

Pathophysiologic Classification of Chronic Lower Extremity Venous Disease

Reflux (P$_r$)

Obstruction (P$_o$)

Reflux and obstruction (P$_{r,o}$)

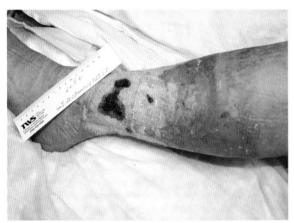

FIGURE 64-7 Venous stasis ulcer.

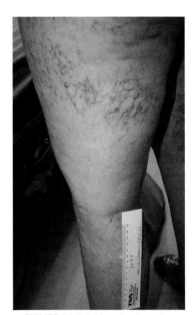

FIGURE 64-9 Spider telangiectasias.

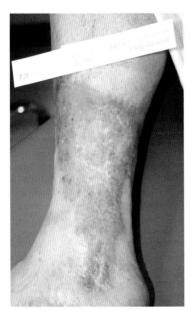

FIGURE 64-8 Healed venous stasis ulcer.

patients are asked not to shave or to apply lotions to the extremity before the treatment. Patients leave the office and are able to perform regular activities immediately. Direct sunlight exposure to the treatment area is avoided for a few weeks after the injection. Although it is a safe technique, injection sclerotherapy is contraindicated in the following situations: pregnancy, patients receiving anticoagulation, patients with acute superficial thrombophlebitis, patients with acute DVT, and patients with a history of severe allergy or severe asthma.

Sclerosants act to disrupt the venous endothelium, causing a periphlebitic reaction, which acts to obliterate the vein segment. There are many sclerosants available, and there are particular categories of sclerosants. They include osmotic, detergent, chemical, and corrosive. Hypertonic saline, in various concentrations, was long considered the agent of choice; however, it can be painful with injection (despite the addition of lidocaine) and appears to exhibit a higher incidence of hyperpigmentation after treatment. Therefore, varying concentrations of sodium tetradecyl sulfate (Sotradecol) and polidocanol (Aethoxysklerol) are now the preferred agents.

The procedure should be performed in a well-lit room. Dilute solutions of sclerosant (e.g., 1% to 3% sodium tetradecyl sulfate; polidocanol 0.5%, 1%, 1.5%) can be injected directly into the venules. Care must be taken to ensure that no single injection dose exceeds 0.1 mL but that multiple injections completely fill all feeding vessels. Larger spider veins should be injected first. Injection should begin proximally and proceed distally. When the session is complete, a pressure dressing is applied, consisting of cotton balls at each injection site, and then covered with compression stockings. Patients are advised to ambulate frequently during the first 24 hours and to abstain from direct sun exposure and airline travel for 2 weeks. On occasion, entrapped blood may form, and patients report significant discomfort. Needle drainage is performed at the site, which facilitates healing and cosmesis and rapidly improves discomfort. This liberation of entrapped blood is as important to success as the primary injection. This therapy is remarkably successful in achieving an excellent cosmetic result. C_1 larger than 1 mm and smaller than 3 mm can also be injected with a sclerosant of slightly greater concentration, but the amount injected at one site needs to be limited to less than 0.5 mL. A total volume of sclerosant should not exceed 4 mL during a treatment session. If one is using hypertonic saline, maximum treatment volume can be 10 mL. Although injection sclerotherapy has met with significant success, complications do occur. They include hyperpigmentation, venous matting, postsclerotherapy necrosis, and an allergic reaction to the sclerosant. In addition, telangiectasia formation after injection sclerotherapy treatment tends to occur. Patients will commonly observe return of spider veins 8 to 12 months after treatment. Although patients may report localized discomfort, sclerotherapy of telangiectasias is considered cosmetic and does not influence the venous circulation of the extremity.[14]

Laser treatment of spider telangiectasias has been performed with a variety of wavelengths and varying techniques, such as high-intensity pulsed light, fiber-guided laser coagulation, and neodymium:yttrium-aluminium-garnet (Nd:YAG) laser with a wavelength of 1064 nm. Evaluation of all existing laser modalities has suggested that the Nd:YAG laser has the most success. However, to date, there have not been any prospective randomized trials to support this presumption. Laser treatment does tend to be more painful. Laser treatment in most centers will be used in conjunction with injection sclerotherapy, that is, injection treats the feeding venules; laser treatment will be used to treat the extremely small branches not adequately addressed with the injection technique. Most patients are satisfied with the injection-only method.

Surgery for axial venous incompetence

Vein stripping. It has been more than a century since surgeons began to develop techniques to treat superficial axial venous reflux. Keller introduced saphenous vein invagination and stripping, and Mayo pioneered use of an external stripper to remove the saphenous vein. Babcock described stripping the saphenous vein intraluminally from the ankle to groin. High ligation of the great saphenous vein briefly gained popularity as a method for treating venous reflux without removing the great saphenous vein. Enthusiasm for high ligation of the great saphenous vein quickly faded as it proved to be ineffective because the reflux in the axial vein was not eliminated. Today, traditional surgical treatment of superficial venous reflux involves high ligation as well as stripping of the great saphenous vein from the knee to the groin. Stripping at the ankle has been largely abandoned because of a high incidence of saphenous nerve injury.

High ligation and vein stripping usually require general or spinal anesthesia. A transverse or oblique groin incision is made just medial to the femoral artery pulse and inferior to the inguinal crease. Sharp dissection allows identification of the proximal great saphenous vein and other venous tributaries that can be ligated and divided. A brief exploration to identify the presence of a duplicate saphenous system should be performed. The great saphenous vein can then be brought up into the surgical field with gentle traction on the saphenofemoral junction. This maneuver affords further visualization of any missed tributaries that require ligation. The great saphenous vein should be ligated with a nonabsorbable suture and transected near its confluence with the femoral vein.

Attention is then directed to the below-knee segment of the great saphenous vein by making a small transverse incision on the proximal, medial calf. The great saphenous vein is identified, ligated distally, and transected. The Codman stripper is then advanced proximally through the great saphenous vein to exit the transected vein in the groin incision. The bulb is attached to the end of the Codman stripper that exits the groin incision, and a handle is attached to the other end (exiting the calf incision). The saphenous vein should be secured to the bulb of the stripper and inverted onto itself. Forcefully pulling on the handle of the Codman stripper removes the great saphenous vein from the groin to the knee. Before stripping, the lower extremity should be wrapped circumferentially to aid in hemostasis and to prevent postoperative edema and permanent hyperpigmentation due to blood extravasation.

Small saphenous vein stripping requires placing the patient in the prone position to optimize surgical exposure. The procedure starts with a proximal dissection involving the saphenopopliteal junction and follows the same techniques used in stripping of the great saphenous vein. Stripping of the small saphenous should be done only to the level of the midcalf to avoid injury to the closely aligned sural nerve.

Complications. Neovascularization refers to the development of new venous tributaries and varicose veins around the previously ligated and divided saphenofemoral junction. The incidence of neovascularization after high ligation and stripping of the great saphenous vein exceeds 30% according to some reports. Interestingly, neovascularization does not occur after endovenous ablation procedures, which obviate the need for a groin dissection or venous tributary ligation. This observation challenges the long-held tenet of varicose vein surgery that stressed the importance of a thorough groin dissection with ligation of all visible venous tributaries. Rather than being beneficial, surgical dissection and tributary ligation may actually trigger neovascularization and varicose vein recurrence. Monitoring for this complication usually involves periodic duplex ultrasound examination.

Saphenous nerve injury is a well-documented complication that occurs more frequently when the great saphenous vein is stripped from the ankle to the groin. The saphenous nerve runs close to the great saphenous vein in the calf compared with the thigh, where the nerve and vein have more separation. This anatomic detail may explain why stripping from the knee to the thigh only reduces the risk of nerve injury (Fig. 64-10).[15]

Although axial venous stripping was considered the "gold standard" of therapy for several decades, several disadvantages to the technique have been realized. Patients required general anesthesia and a hospitalization. In addition, once discharged, patients experienced a prolonged convalescence before resuming baseline activity. Also, the problems of nerve injury and neovascularization were

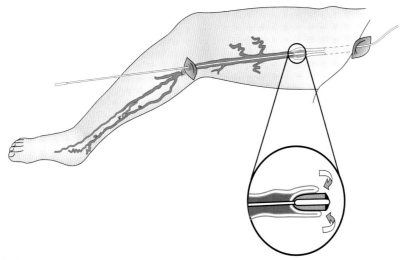

FIGURE 64-10 Inversion stripping of the saphenous vein for superficial venous reflux caused by an incompetent saphenofemoral junction.

frustrating to surgeons and patients.

In an effort to address and to correct these limitations, endovenous techniques have been developed. They are discussed in the next section. As a result of their efficacy, stripping is now considered only in select cases.

Endovenous thermal ablation

Percutaneous vein ablation. Percutaneous endovenous ablation of the superficial axial veins revolutionized the treatment of superficial venous insufficiency. As a minimally invasive alternative to surgical vein stripping, percutaneous endovenous ablation can be performed on an outpatient basis with local anesthesia. Advantages of this technique include less discomfort of the patient and a more rapid recovery. Patients now actively seek treatment for varicose veins, prompting the proliferation of outpatient vein treatment centers. There are three types of endovenous thermal therapy for the superficial axial veins: radiofrequency ablation, laser ablation, and ultrasound-guided sclerotherapy (UGS).

Endovenous thermal ablation requires minimal preprocedure preparation. Healthy patients with no medical history do not require laboratory work, whereas standard laboratory evaluation is usually obtained for patients with significant medical comorbidities. Patients who are receiving anticoagulation should remain on their standard regimen. The risk of bridging therapy is greater than the risk of keeping patients on their baseline anticoagulation as long as the international normalized ratio (INR) is 3 or less. Guidelines for periprocedural DVT prophylaxis remain unclear. The author gives a single preprocedure dose of low-molecular-weight heparin (LMWH) to patients with two or more risk factors for DVT. All antiplatelet medications can be continued throughout the procedural course. The author does not routinely administer prophylactic antibiotics. Patients with advanced CVI and skin changes usually receive a preprocedure dose of cefazolin.

Anesthesia for endovenous thermal ablation procedures can range from local injections to conscious sedation. Many patients tolerate the procedure with minimal anesthesia consisting only of tumescent infusion of dilute lidocaine around the great saphenous vein. Ideally, these patients can be treated in an office setting. Moderate sedation requires hemodynamic monitoring equipment

and is more suited for an outpatient surgical center. The choice of anesthesia ultimately depends on the preferences of the patient and physician as well as the available resources and practice environments.

The venous duplex ultrasound examination plays an essential role in planning of endovenous thermal ablation procedures. The ultrasound examination should provide the treating physician with the following information: patency of the deep venous system, location of normal and refluxing axial veins, areas of communication between the varicosities and the axial vein, and presence of duplicate or accessory refluxing vein segments.

An acute occlusive DVT is an absolute contraindication to endovenous thermal ablation, whereas a chronically recanalized deep venous system in the extremity to be treated is a relative contraindication. In patients who harbor secondary venous insufficiency, the superficial veins play a more important role in venous drainage compared with patients with a pristine deep venous system and primary venous insufficiency. Care must be taken to ensure that superficial venous ablation will not compromise the venous outflow of the post-thrombotic limb.

The site of percutaneous access depends on the patient's symptoms and the location of the varicose vein tributaries. If endovenous thermal ablation of the great saphenous vein is planned in a patient with painful varicosities on the proximal calf, it is helpful to evaluate these branches with ultrasound. Percutaneous access on the distal calf just inferior to the varicose veins will ensure that maximum resolution of the tributary branches is achieved with endovenous thermal treatment.

Radiofrequency ablation and laser energy deliver two different types of energy to the vein lumen. Radiofrequency heat is delivered at a temperature of 120° C. The radiofrequency directly injures the vein wall endothelium, resulting in collagen contraction and thrombosis of the treated vein. Laser energy delivers energy to the blood itself. Steam bubbles are generated with the laser energy, and coagulation occurs after completion of laser energy delivery. Radiofrequency catheters vary in length but not in temperature delivered. In contrast, laser energy catheters come in different wavelengths ranging from 810 nm to 1470 nm. The type of laser catheters continues to develop, and as such, many laser catheters are frequently introduced into the evolving therapeutic armamentarium. Investigators have demonstrated that the higher wavelength fibers appear to be associated with less postprocedural discomfort.

Technique. In most cases, the extremity should be placed in a position of external rotation with the knee slightly flexed. A sheet "bump" may help the patient maintain this position. Placing the patient in reverse Trendelenburg can help dilate the vein to be accessed. After the standard sterile preparation and draping, the ultrasound probe is brought onto the field in a sterile transducer cover. The author reexamines the vein to be treated along its entire course, noting areas of aneurysmal dilation or tortuosity that may affect catheter placement. Ideally, the puncture site should be distal to the lowest level of truncal reflux and provide unobstructed access to the refluxing vein segment.

At the chosen site of percutaneous access, the ultrasound probe is positioned to obtain a stable gray-scale image of the vein in either the transverse or sagittal plane. After puncture of the skin, limited, small movements of the 21-gauge needle help identify its tip on the ultrasound image. On real-time imaging, the needle is guided into the vein lumen and exchanged over a wire for a 6 Fr or 7 Fr sheath using the modified Seldinger technique. With ultrasound guidance, the radiofrequency catheter or laser catheter is then advanced through the sheath, and the ultrasound probe is positioned in the groin to visualize the catheter tip, the saphenofemoral junction, and the deep system. Using ultrasound guidance, the tip of the ablation catheter is placed 2 to 3 cm distal to the saphenofemoral junction to minimize the chance of heat transmission into the femoral vein. Definitive positioning of the therapeutic catheter must be completed at this point, before the administration of local anesthesia during the next stage of the procedure. Imaging artifacts from the tumescent anesthesia tend to impede visualization of the catheter tip, making it difficult to adjust its position.

Before tumescent anesthesia is begun, the patient should be placed in the Trendelenburg position to help empty the vein. Tumescent anesthesia is the infusion of a large volume of dilute local anesthetic. Although there are many recipes for tumescent solution, the main components are lidocaine, epinephrine, and sodium bicarbonate diluted with lactated Ringer solution or normal saline. During laser treatment and radiofrequency ablation procedures, tumescent anesthesia performs three functions: it provides anesthesia over a large area; it compresses the vein around the therapeutic catheter; and it acts as a protective barrier to prevent heating of nontarget tissues, including skin, nerves, arteries, and the deep veins.

For great saphenous vein procedures, the target of tumescent anesthesia is the saphenous sheath. When it is viewed in the transverse plane, the saphenous canal resembles an eye, and the ultrasound image is often referred to as the "saphenous eye." Administration of tumescent anesthesia starts distally on the lower extremity and progresses proximally. Real-time ultrasound imaging guides a 21- to 25-gauge needle into the saphenous canal to deliver the tumescent anesthesia. When it is injected into the proper perivenous tissue plane, the tumescent anesthesia will track up and around the target vein. A long-axis ultrasound view gives the best image of fluid spreading up the saphenous canal. Multiple skin punctures and injections are performed until the vein has a 10-mm halo of tumescent anesthesia along its entire course. The targeted vein segment is then reinspected by ultrasound to ensure that the vein is compressed around the therapeutic catheter and adequately separated from the overlying skin.

Radiofrequency energy or laser energy is then applied to the vein segment by activating and slowly withdrawing the therapeutic catheter. The specifics of retrograde pullback depend on the type of catheter. Radiofrequency energy involves a segmental pullback governed by hash marks on the catheter and a timed activation on the accompanying generator. Laser energy catheters are variable; some have a slow continuous pullback, whereas others require a segmental pullback. Gray-scale ultrasound images can often detect steam bubbles generated by the laser fiber.

Regardless of the type of energy delivered, once the vein has been completely treated, the sheath and accompanying catheter are removed. Ultrasound imaging resumes, confirming the patency of the femoral vein as well as successful occlusion of the great saphenous vein. Color Doppler imaging is often the only way to assess patency at this point because of the distortion caused by the ablation and the surrounding tumescent anesthesia. It is also important to verify retrograde epigastric venous flow into the proximal segment of the great saphenous vein. This provides a "protective flush" of the great saphenous vein. It is believed by many venous experts that this flow pattern prevents postprocedural development of endovenous heat-induced thrombus.

Postprocedural instructions vary by practitioner. The patient's extremity is usually wrapped in a layered compression dressing, or a 20 to 30 mm Hg compression stocking is applied. The patient is instructed to walk every hour until bed. Regular activity except for vigorous cardiovascular exercise can be resumed the following day. After a satisfactory postprocedural duplex examination, all activity restrictions are lifted.

All follow-up protocols should include a duplex ultrasound examination 2 to 5 days after the procedure. The duplex ultrasound examination ensures that the deep venous system remains patent and confirms the ablation of the great saphenous vein. Reported rates of DVT after endovenous ablation range from 0% to 16% after radiofrequency ablation and 0% to 7.7% after laser ablation. Although the incidence of postablation DVT is extremely low, duplex ultrasound examination can detect thrombus in the proximal great saphenous vein that can extend into the common femoral vein. Lowell Kabnick coined the term *endovenous heat-induced thrombus* (EHIT) to describe this ultrasound finding. He classified EHIT into four different levels based on of the size of the thrombus and its extension into the deep venous system.

The mechanism of EHIT formation remains unclear. General consensus assumes that heat-triggered thrombus in the great saphenous vein propagates into the saphenofemoral junction and encroaches on the deep venous system. EHIT and acute DVT differ in their sonographic characteristics and natural history. EHIT becomes sonographically echogenic quickly (<24 hours), whereas acute DVT usually remains hypoechoic for several days after its initial detection. Although EHIT appears to have a low propensity to propagate or to embolize, pulmonary embolism has been reported after venous ablation procedures. Follow-up ultrasound examinations usually demonstrate retraction or complete resolution of EHIT within 7 to 10 days. Given this benign natural history, most practitioners do not treat class 1 and class 2 EHIT. Class 3 EHIT, which involves partial, nonocclusive extension into the deep venous system, usually warrants anticoagulation therapy, the duration of which can vary on the basis of the physician's discretion. Because class 4 EHIT represents occlusive DVT, it requires a 3-month course of anticoagulation.

The choice of whether to use radiofrequency ablation or laser as the energy source for venous ablation procedures remains a matter of the physician's preference. Randomized prospective studies comparing the two techniques have detected few differences. Patients treated with laser ablation tended to have more discomfort in the very early postprocedural period; however, all other outcome variables were similar.[16,17]

Ultrasound-guided sclerotherapy. UGS was first described in 1989 as a treatment for the superficial axial system. Since then, the use of UGS has expanded to treatment of incompetent perforator branches and large venous tributaries caused by neovascularization. UGS gained popularity as a simple, minimally invasive technique that allows patients to rapidly return to their baseline activity level. Preparation for UGS requires a comprehensive duplex examination.

The closed needle technique is the most common method for performing UGS. A 25-gauge needle is used as this is the smallest caliber needle that can be visualized with gray-scale ultrasound. The needle is attached to a syringe containing the sclerosant. The vein can be sonographically visualized in a transverse or longitudinal plane, depending on the operator's preference. The frequency of the transducer depends on the depth of the vein to be treated. High-frequency transducers visualize superficial veins better, whereas deeper veins require lower frequency transducers. The needle tip must be visualized immediately as it penetrates the dermis. After entering the vein, the needle should be aspirated to confirm its position within the vein lumen. Injecting a small test dose of sclerosant provides further confirmation of the needle's position. An alternative method of UGS uses a butterfly needle instead of the needle attached to a syringe.

Volumes and concentrations of sclerosant are dependent on the size and length of vein to be treated. In general, UGS requires high concentrations of sclerosant because of the large caliber of the targeted veins. Specific details about sclerosant preparation are outside the scope of this chapter. Early investigational studies reported promising results. Further study using randomized prospective trials with all modalities is necessary before true standards of practice can be formalized.

Nontumescent ablation and future modalities for axial vein incompetence. In addition to the ultrasound-guided foam sclerotherapy, many other newer techniques have been recently introduced into the therapeutic armamentarium. One device is mechanical chemical ablation. The catheter device is composed of two components. A mechanical portion rotates inside the vein lumen and denudes the venous endothelium. The second component is the chemical portion, which involves concomitant injection of a liquid sclerosant as the mechanical rotation inside the vein is taking place. Potential advantages over the endothermal devices are the lack of tumescence because no heat is required and the small profile of the catheter. Access of the vein is similar. The glue and foam injectable category comprises another group of devices that are also "tumescent free." Time will tell as further data are obtained to determine the role of each therapy in superficial axial insufficiency.

Treatment of branch varicosities. There are three techniques to treat secondary branch varicosities: conventional stab phlebectomy, powered phlebectomy (TriVex; InaVein, Lexington, Mass), and foam sclerotherapy. Ambulatory phlebectomy is performed by the stab avulsion technique (Fig. 64-11). The patient's varicosities are marked after standing to allow optimal dilation and visualization of affected veins. A variety of anesthetic methods are used successfully, including local anesthesia with tumescence and IV sedation. First, 1-mm incisions are made along Langer skin lines, and the vein is retrieved with a hook. Continuous retraction of the vein segment affords maximal removal of the vein, and direct pressure is applied over the site. Incisions are made at approximately 2-cm intervals. The extremity is wrapped with a layered compression dressing, and patients are instructed to ambulate on the day of surgery. The postoperative course is brief, and rarely do patients require more than acetaminophen or nonsteroidal antiinflammatory drugs for discomfort. Compression stockings are worn for 2 weeks after the procedure. Complications are unusual but include bleeding, infection, temporary or permanent paresthesias, and phlebitis from retained vein segments. There can be recurrence.

Powered phlebectomy (TriVex) is a modality that can be used to treat extensive secondary branch varicosities. The patient's varicosities are circumferentially marked preoperatively; in the operating room, 2-mm incisions are made at these boundary sites. These incisions permit placement of a transilluminator and resection device. The instruments are inserted through a subcutaneous plane, just deep to the varicosities. The transilluminator not only provides visualization of the veins but also administers tumescent anesthesia. The resector is a rotating blade that

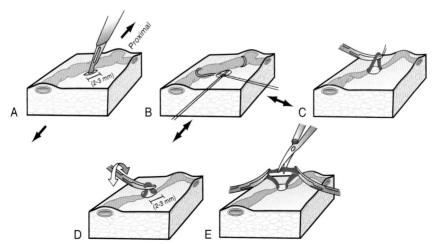

FIGURE 64-11 A-E, Technique of ambulatory phlebectomy (otherwise known as stab avulsions of varicosities).

transects the veins and then removes them through a high-suction tubing system. The extremity is wrapped with a multi-layer compression dressing, and the patient is discharged with instructions to ambulate hourly. The patient returns to the office for a dressing change within 48 hours and usually is changed to standard compression hose. Discomfort is minimal, and over-the-counter analgesia is sufficient. A second-generation TriVex device has been developed; technical issues with the first-generation instrument were revised, and studies now focus on methods to use the TriVex system in an outpatient setting. A steep learning curve occurs with this device, but once it is achieved, experienced physicians can perform most TriVex procedures within 30 minutes. Complications are unusual but can include contained hematoma, bleeding, temporary or permanent paresthesias, and phlebitis.[18]

Secondary Venous Insufficiency

Secondary venous insufficiency is usually caused by a deep venous thrombus. Clinical manifestations of secondary venous insufficiency usually present in a more advanced stage than their primary counterparts. In addition, patients may describe venous claudication, or a bursting pain in the calf, that is classic for secondary venous insufficiency. Conservative treatment regimens are similar to those described in the preceding section for primary insufficiency; however, these patients require a higher grade of compression for efficacy (30 to 40 mm Hg). Interventional treatment focuses on the superficial and deep systems. Diagnostic interrogation of the deep venous system must be more comprehensive in these patients to determine whether they are candidates for deep surgical or endovenous reconstruction.

Treatment

Surgery for deep venous insufficiency. While conservative therapy is being pursued or ulcer healing is achieved, appropriate diagnostic studies generally reveal patterns of venous reflux or segments of venous occlusion so that specific therapy can be prescribed for the individual limb being evaluated. Imaging by duplex ultrasound suffices for the detection of reflux if the examination is carried out while the patient is standing. Such noninvasive imaging may prove the only testing necessary beyond the hand-held, continuous-wave Doppler instrument if superficial venous ablation is contemplated. If direct venous reconstruction by bypass or valvuloplasty techniques is planned, ascending and descending phlebography is required.[19]

Surprisingly, superficial reflux may be the only abnormality present in advanced chronic venous stasis. Correction goes a long way toward permanent relief of the chronic venous dysfunction and its cutaneous effects. Using duplex technology, Hanrahan and associates[20] found that in 95 extremities with current venous ulceration, 16.8% had only superficial incompetence and another 19% showed superficial incompetence combined with perforator incompetence. Another study has demonstrated ulcer healing and decreased ulcer recurrence with perforator reconstruction.[21]

A significant proportion of patients with venous ulceration have normal function in the deep veins, and surgical treatment is a useful option that can definitively address the hemodynamic derangements. Maintaining that all venous ulcers are surgically incurable is not reasonable when data suggest that superficial vein surgery holds the potential for ameliorating the venous hypertension. A randomized controlled trial comparing compression therapy and surgery for superficial reflux versus conservative

management alone has revealed significant improvement in patients who had been treated by the surgical component.[21] Early success in patients with CVI, superficial valvular incompetence, and venous ulceration has been obtained with endovenous radiofrequency and laser therapies.

In the 1938, Linton[22] emphasized the importance of perforating veins, and their direct surgical interruption was advocated. This has fallen into disfavor because of a high incidence of postoperative wound healing complications. However, video techniques that allow direct visualization through small-diameter endoscopes have made endoscopic subfascial exploration and perforator vein interruption the desirable alternative to the Linton technique, minimizing morbidity and wound complications. The connective tissue between the fascia cruris and underlying flexor muscles is so loose that this potential space can be opened up easily and dissected with the endoscope. This operation, done with a vertical proximal incision, accomplishes the objective of perforator vein interruption on an outpatient basis.

The availability of subfascial endoscopic perforator vein surgery has had an impact on the care of venous ulcers in Western countries, albeit not as dramatic as its proponents had hoped. As the limbs of patients with severe CVI were studied accurately, the term *post-thrombotic syndrome* (PTS) had to give way to the term *chronic venous insufficiency;* a link to platelet and monocyte aggregates in the circulation reflected the leukocytic infiltrate of the ankle skin, with its lipodermatosclerosis and healed and open ulcerations.[23]

Data regarding leukocytes in CVI accumulated and were consistent, showing that the activation of leukocytes sequestered in the cutaneous microcirculation during venous stasis was important to the development of the skin changes of CVI. This is reflected in the finding of adhesion markers between leukocytes and endothelial cells and increased production of leukocyte degranulation enzymes and oxygen free radicals. Nevertheless, experimental evidence was still required for decisive proof of the leukocyte hypothesis.

In the United States, several groups have performed perforating vein division using laparoscopic instrumentation. Initial data have suggested that perforator interruption produces rapid ulcer healing and a low rate of recurrence. The North American Registry, which voluntarily recorded the results of perforating venous surgery, has confirmed a low 2-year recurrence rate of ulcers and more rapid ulcer healing.[24]

A comparison of the three methods of perforator vein interruption, including the classic Linton procedure, laparoscopic instrumentation procedure, and single open-endoscope procedure, has revealed that the endoscopic technique produces results comparable to those of the open Linton operation, with much less scarring and a greater tendency toward a fast recovery. More perforating veins were identified with the open technique. However, the mean hospital stay and period of convalescence were more favorable with the endoscope procedures.[25]

In general, registry reports and individual institution clinical experience have shown that patients with true post-thrombotic limbs are disadvantaged by the procedure, enough so that at Leicester (England), the students of the procedure said, "We conclude that perforating vein surgery is not indicated for the treatment of venous ulceration in limbs with primary deep venous incompetence."[25] Nevertheless, studies were reported in which previous superficial reflux was corrected with failures of such treatment. Rescue of these limbs with perforating vein division produced satisfactory results and verified that perforating veins are important in the genesis of venous ulceration and that their division accelerates healing and may reduce recurrence of ulceration.

Part of the difficulty in understanding the need for perforating vein division is the disparity between venous hemodynamics and the severity of cutaneous changes. This is not surprising because the cutaneous changes of CVI are dependent on leukocyte-endothelium interactions, which may not be directly related to venous hemodynamics. However, endoscopic perforator vein division has improved venous hemodynamics in some limbs, as would be expected, by removing superficial reflux and perforating vein outflow. In an effort to eliminate incompetent perforator veins without the associated morbidity described earlier, UGS has been developed as an alternative technique. Early study results are promising and have revealed improved wound healing rates compared with the subfascial endoscopic perforator surgery.[26]

Percutaneous endovenous techniques are also now commonly used modalities to treat incompetent perforator veins. These therapies consist of the same treatments described in the percutaneous vein ablation section. Further study is required to determine the safest and most efficacious technique. For now, the physician has a wealth of varying modalities from which to treat. Interestingly, this may serve the field well; there may be a unique role for each of these techniques.

Direct venous reconstruction. Radiofrequency ablation, laser ablation, and UGS are all commonly used modalities. Historically, the first successful procedures done to reconstruct major veins were the femorofemoral crossover graft of Eduardo Palma and the saphenopopliteal bypass he described, also used by Richard Warren of Boston. These operations were elegant in their simplicity, use of autogenous tissue, and reconstruction by a single venovenous anastomosis.

With regard to femorofemoral crossover grafts, the only group to provide long-term physiologic data on a large number of patients has been Halliday and coworkers from Sydney, Australia. Although phlebography was used in selecting patients for surgery, no other details of preoperative indications were given. These investigators documented that 34 of 50 grafts remained patent in the long term, as assessed by postoperative phlebography. They believed that the best clinical results were achieved in relief of postexercise calf pain but thought that a patent graft also slowed the progression of distal liposclerosis and controlled recurrent ulceration. No proof of this was given in their report. The history of application of bypass procedures for venous obstruction is a fascinating one. Nevertheless, the advent of endovascular techniques has made those operations almost obsolete.[27]

Perforator interruption, combined with superficial venous ablation, has been effective in controlling venous ulceration in 75% to 85% of patients. However, emphasis on failures of this technique led to Masuda and Kistner's[28] significant breakthrough in direct venous reconstruction with valvuloplasty in 1968 and the general recognition of this procedure after 1975. Late evaluations of direct valve reconstruction have indicated good to excellent long-term results in more than 80% of patients.[29] One cannot overestimate Kistner's contributions. The technique of directing the incompetent venous stream through a competent proximal valve by venous segment transfer was his next achievement. After Kistner's studies, surgeons were provided with an armamentarium that included Palma's venous bypass, direct valvuloplasty (of Kistner), and venous segment transfer (of Kistner). Moreover, external valvular reconstruction, as performed by various techniques, including monitoring by endoscopy, has led to renewed

interest in this form of treatment of venous insufficiency. Axillary to popliteal autotransplantation of valve-containing venous segments has been considered since the early observations of Taheri and colleagues.[30] However, long-term verification of the preliminary excellent results has not been accomplished.

DEEP VENOUS THROMBOSIS

Lower Extremity Deep Venous Thrombosis

Acute DVT is a major cause of morbidity and mortality in the hospitalized patient, particularly in the surgical patient. The triad of venous stasis, endothelial injury, and hypercoagulable state, first posited by Virchow in 1856, has held true more than a century and a half later.

Acute DVT poses several risks and has significant morbid consequences. The thrombotic process initiated in a venous segment, in the absence of anticoagulation or in the presence of inadequate anticoagulation, can propagate to involve more proximal segments of the deep venous system, thus resulting in edema, pain, and immobility. The most dreaded sequel to acute DVT is that of pulmonary embolism, a condition of potentially lethal consequence. The late consequence of DVT, particularly of the iliofemoral veins, can be CVI and ultimately PTS as a result of valvular dysfunction in the presence of luminal obstruction.

Thus, understanding the pathophysiology, standardizing protocols to prevent or to reduce DVT, and instituting optimal treatment promptly are critical to reducing the incidence and morbidity of this unfortunately common condition.

Causes

The triad of stasis, hypercoagulable state, and vessel injury is present in most surgical patients. It is also clear that increasing age places a patient at a greater risk, with those older than 65 years representing a higher risk population. In addition, many epidemiologic studies have reviewed additional factors that place patients at risk for the development of deep venous thrombus, including malignant disease, increased body mass index, increasing age (especially >60 years), pregnancy, prolonged immobilization, tobacco use, and prior deep vein thrombus.[31]

Stasis. Labeled fibrinogen studies in patients as well as in autopsy studies have demonstrated convincingly that the soleal sinuses are the most common sites of initiation of venous thrombosis. The stasis may contribute to the endothelial cellular layer contacting activated platelets and procoagulant factors, thereby leading to DVT. Stasis, in and of itself, has never been shown to be a causative factor for DVT.

Hypercoagulable state. Our knowledge of hypercoagulable conditions continues to improve, but it is still in its early stages. The standard array of conditions screened for in searching for a hypercoagulable state is listed in Box 64-1. If any of these conditions is identified, a treatment regimen of anticoagulation is instituted for life, unless specific contraindications exist. It is generally appreciated that the postoperative patient, after major surgery, is predisposed to the formation of DVT. After major operations, large amounts of tissue factor may be released into the bloodstream from damaged tissues. Tissue factor is a potent procoagulant expressed on the leukocyte cell surface as well as in a soluble form in the bloodstream. Increases in platelet count, adhesiveness, changes in coagulation cascade, and endogenous fibrinolytic activity result from physiologic stress, such as major operation or trauma, and have been associated with an increased risk for thrombosis.

Factor V Leiden mutation
Prothrombin gene mutation
Protein C deficiency
Protein S deficiency
Antithrombin III deficiency
Homocysteinemia
Antiphospholipid syndrome
Lupus antibody
Anticardiolipin antibody

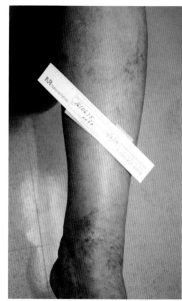

FIGURE 64-12 Edema. Note the loss of ankle definition.

Venous injury. It has been clearly established that venous thrombosis occurs in veins that are distant from the site of operation; for example, it is well known that patients undergoing total hip replacement frequently develop contralateral lower extremity DVT.

In a series of experiments, animal models of abdominal and total hip operations were used to study the possibility of venous endothelial damage distant from the operative site. In these studies, jugular veins were excised after the animals were perfusion fixed. These experiments demonstrated that endothelial damage occurred after abdominal operations and was more severe after hip operations. There were multiple microtears noted within the valve cusps that resulted in exposure of the subendothelial matrix. The exact mechanisms whereby this injury at a distant site occurs and which mediators, cellular or humoral, are responsible are not clearly understood, but that the injury occurs is evident from these and other studies.

Diagnostic Considerations

Incidence. Venous thromboembolism occurs for the first time in approximately 100 persons/100,000 each year in the United States. This incidence increases with increasing age, with an incidence of 0.5%/100,000 at 80 years of age. More than two thirds of these patients have DVT alone, and the rest have evidence of pulmonary embolism. The recurrence rate with anticoagulation has been noted to be 6% to 7% in the ensuing 6 months.

In the United States, pulmonary embolism causes 50,000 to 200,000 deaths annually. A 28-day case-fatality rate of 9.4% after first-time DVT and of 15.1% after first-time pulmonary thromboembolism has been observed. Aside from pulmonary embolism, secondary CVI (resulting from DVT) is significant in terms of cost, morbidity, and lifestyle limitations.

If the consequences of DVT, in terms of pulmonary embolism and CVI, are to be prevented, the prevention, diagnosis, and treatment of DVT must be optimized.

Clinical diagnosis. The diagnosis of DVT requires a high index of suspicion. Most are familiar with Homan sign, which refers to pain in the calf on dorsiflexion of the foot. Although the absence of this sign is not a reliable indicator of the absence of venous thrombus, the presence of Homan sign should prompt one to attempt to confirm the diagnosis. The extent of venous thrombosis in the lower extremity is an important factor in the manifestation of symptoms. For example, most calf thrombi may be asymptomatic unless there is proximal propagation. This is one reason that radiolabeled fibrinogen testing demonstrates a higher incidence of DVT than studies using imaging modalities. Only 40% of patients with venous thrombosis have any clinical manifestations of the condition.

Major venous thrombosis involving the iliofemoral venous system results in a massively swollen leg, with pitting edema (Fig. 64-12), pain, and blanching, a condition known as phlegmasia alba dolens. With further progression of disease, there may be such massive edema that arterial inflow can be compromised. This condition results in a painful blue leg, a condition called phlegmasia cerulea dolens. With this evolution of the condition, venous gangrene can develop unless flow is restored.

PTS is a common and unfortunate manifestation of deep venous thrombus. It occurs in 20% to 50% of patients after a documented episode of DVT. The clinical presentation includes chronic edema, pain, and venous claudication. Venous ulcerations occur. Risk factors for the development of PTS include persistent leg symptoms for months after the acute episode of DVT, an anatomically extensive DVT involving the iliofemoral system, recurrent ipsilateral DVTs, and a prolonged state of subtherapeutic anticoagulation for DVT. Unfortunately, treatment of PTS remains supportive, and compression therapy remains the mainstay of treatment for PTS. Some investigators have advocated the early use of thrombolysis to prevent PTS, but that has not been consistently proven.

Imaging Studies and Laboratory Tests

Venography. Injection of contrast material into the venous system has been long considered the most accurate method of confirming DVT and its location. The superficial venous system has to be occluded with a tourniquet, and the veins in the foot are injected for visualization of the deep venous system. Although this is a good test for finding occlusive and nonocclusive thrombus, it is also invasive, subject to risks of IV administration of contrast material. As a result, this technique has been replaced by less invasive modalities.

Impedance plethysmography. Impedance plethysmography measures the change in venous capacitance and rate of emptying of the venous volume on temporary occlusion and release of the occlusion of the venous system. A cuff is inflated around the upper thigh until the electrical signal has plateaued. When the cuff is deflated, there is usually rapid outflow and reduction of volume. With a venous thrombosis, one notes a prolongation of the outflow wave. It is not useful clinically for the detection of calf venous thrombosis and of patients with prior venous thrombosis.

Fibrin and fibrinogen assays. Fibrin and fibrinogen levels can be determined by measuring the degradation of intravascular fibrin. The D-dimer test measures cross-linked degradation products, which is a surrogate of plasmin's activity on fibrin. In combination with clinical evaluation and assessment, the sensitivity exceeds 90% to 95%. The negative predictive value is 99.3% for proximal evaluation and 98.6% for distal evaluation. In the postoperative patient, D-dimer is causally elevated because of surgery, and as such, a positive result of the D-dimer assay for evaluating for DVT is not useful. However, a negative D-dimer test result in patients with suspected DVT has a high negative predictive value, ranging from 97% to 99%.[32]

Duplex ultrasound. The current test of choice for the diagnosis of DVT is duplex ultrasound, a modality that combines Doppler ultrasound and color flow imaging. The advantage of this test is that it is noninvasive, comprehensive, and without any risk of reaction to contrast angiography. This test is also highly operator dependent, which is one of its potential drawbacks.

Doppler ultrasound is based on the principle of the impairment of an accelerated flow signal caused by an intraluminal thrombus. A detailed interrogation begins at the calf with imaging of the tibial veins and then proximally over the popliteal and femoral veins. A properly done examination evaluates flow with distal compression, which results in augmentation of flow, and with proximal compression, which should interrupt flow. If any segment of the venous system being examined fails to demonstrate augmentation on compression, venous thrombosis is suspected.

Real-time B-mode ultrasonography with color flow imaging has improved the sensitivity and specificity of ultrasound scanning. With color flow duplex imaging, blood flow can be imaged in the presence of a partially occluding thrombus. The probe is also used to compress the vein. A normal vein is easily compressed, whereas in the presence of a thrombus, there is resistance to compression. In addition, the chronicity of the thrombus can be evaluated on the basis of its imaging characteristics, namely, increased echogenicity and heterogeneity. Duplex imaging is significantly more sensitive than indirect physiologic testing. There are many advantages associated with duplex ultrasound: noninvasiveness, portability, and no need for a contrast agent. However, there are significant disadvantages as well; these include interuser variability and skill, body habitus, and suboptimal visualization in regions such as the lower pelvis.

Magnetic resonance venous imaging. With major advances in imaging technology, MRVI has come to the forefront of imaging for proximal venous disease. The cost and the issue of patient tolerance because of claustrophobia limit its widespread application, but this has been changing. It is a useful test for imaging the iliac veins and IVC, an area where the use of duplex ultrasound is limited. MRVI is less invasive than conventional venography and is able to directly visualize the thrombus.

Prophylaxis

The patient who has undergone major abdominal or orthopedic surgery, has sustained major trauma, or has prolonged immobility (>3 days) represents an elevated risk for the development of venous thromboembolism. The specific risk factor analysis and epidemiologic studies detailing the causes of venous thromboem-

bolism are beyond the scope of this chapter. The reader is referred to a more extensive analysis of this problem.[31]

The methods of prophylaxis can be mechanical or pharmacologic. The simplest method is for the patient to walk. Activation of the calf pump mechanism is an effective means of prophylaxis, as evidenced by the fact that few active people without underlying risk factors develop venous thrombosis. A patient who is expected to be up and walking within 24 to 48 hours is at low risk for development of venous thrombosis. The practice of having a patient out of bed into a chair is one of the most thrombogenic positions that could be ordered for a patient. Sitting in a chair, with the legs in a dependent position, causes venous pooling, which in the postoperative milieu could easily be a predisposing factor for the development of thromboembolism.

The most common method of surgical prophylaxis has traditionally revolved around sequential compression devices, which periodically compress the calves and essentially replicate the calf bellows mechanism. This has clearly reduced the incidence of venous thromboembolism in the surgical patient. The most likely mechanism for the efficacy of this device is prevention of venous stasis. Some studies have suggested that fibrinolytic activity systemically is enhanced by a sequential compression device. However, this has not been definitively established because a considerable number of studies have demonstrated no enhancement of fibrinolytic activity.[33]

Another traditional method of thromboprophylaxis has been the use of low-dose unfractionated heparin. The dosage traditionally used was 5000 units of unfractionated heparin every 12 hours. However, analyses of trials comparing placebo versus fixed-dose heparin have shown that the stated dose of 5000 units subcutaneously every 12 hours is no more effective than placebo. When subcutaneous heparin is used on a dosing regimen of every 8 hours rather than every 12 hours, there is a reduction in the development of venous thromboembolism.

More recently, a number of studies have revealed the efficacy of fractionated LMWH for the prophylaxis and treatment of venous thromboembolism. LMWH inhibits factor Xa and IIa activity, with the ratio of anti–factor Xa to anti–factor IIa activity ranging from 1:1 to 4:1. LMWH has a longer plasma half-life and significantly higher bioavailability. The consistent bioavailability and clearance of LMWH do not require monitoring of factor Xa levels, which facilitates use by the patient. Dosing is merely based on the patient's weight. There is a more predictable anticoagulant response than with unfractionated heparin. No laboratory monitoring is necessary because the partial thromboplastin time (PTT) is unaffected. Various analyses, including a major meta-analysis, have shown that LMWH results in equivalent if not better efficacy, with significantly fewer bleeding complications. It was first thought that LMWH results in less bleeding than unfractionated heparin, but no clinical observations have confirmed this. This property may be more a function of dose than an intrinsic drug action.

Comparison of LMWH with mechanical prophylaxis has demonstrated the superiority of LMWH for reduction of the development of venous thromboembolic disease.[34-36] Prospective trials evaluating LMWH in head-injured and trauma patients have also proved the safety of LMWH, with no increase in intracranial bleeding or major bleeding at other sites.[37] In addition, LMWH shows a significant reduction in the development of venous thromboembolism compared with other methods.

Thus, LMWH is considered the optimal method of prophylaxis for moderate- and high-risk patients. Even the traditional reluctance to use heparin in high-risk groups, such as the multiply injured trauma patient and head-injured patient, must be reexamined, given the efficacy and safety profile of LMWH in multiple prospective trials.

Treatment

After a diagnosis of venous thrombosis has been made, a treatment plan must be instituted. Complications of calf DVT include proximal propagation of thrombus in up to one third of hospitalized patients and PTS. In addition, untreated lower extremity DVT carries a 30% recurrence rate.

Any venous thrombosis involving the femoropopliteal system is treated with full anticoagulation. Traditionally, the treatment of DVT has centered around heparin treatment to maintain the PTT at 60 to 80 seconds, followed by warfarin therapy to obtain an INR of 2.5 to 3.0. If unfractionated heparin is used, it is important to use a nomogram-based dosing therapy. The incidence of recurrent venous thromboembolism increases if the time to therapeutic anticoagulation is prolonged. Therefore, it is important to reach therapeutic levels within 24 hours. An initial bolus of 80 units/kg or 5000 units IV bolus is administered, followed by 18 units/kg/hr. The rate is dependent on a target PTT corresponding to an anti–factor Xa level of 0.3 to 0.7 unit/mL.[38] The PTT needs to be checked 6 hours after any change in heparin dosing. Warfarin is started on the same day. If warfarin is initiated without heparin, the risk for a transient hypercoagulable state exists because protein C and protein S levels fall before the other vitamin K–dependent factors are depleted. With the advent of LMWH, it is no longer necessary to admit the patient for IV heparin therapy. It is now accepted practice to administer LMWH on an outpatient basis, as a bridge to warfarin therapy, which is also monitored on an outpatient basis.

The recommended duration of anticoagulant therapy continues to evolve. A minimum treatment time of 3 months is advocated in most cases. The recurrence rate is the same with 3 months versus 6 months of warfarin therapy. If the patient has a known hypercoagulable state or has experienced episodes of venous thrombosis, however, lifetime anticoagulation is required in the absence of contraindications. The accepted INR range is 2.0 to 3.0; a randomized double-blind study has confirmed that a goal INR of 2.0 to 3.0 is more effective in preventing recurrent venous thromboembolism than a low-intensity regimen with a goal INR of 1.0 to 1.9.[39] In addition, the low-intensity regimen did not reduce the risk for clinically important bleeding.

Oral anticoagulants are teratogenic and thus cannot be used during pregnancy. In the case of the pregnant patient with venous thrombosis, LMWH is the treatment of choice; this is continued through delivery and can be continued postpartum, as indicated.

Thrombolysis. The advent of thrombolysis has resulted in increased interest in thrombolysis for DVT. The purported benefit is preservation of valve function, with a subsequently lesser chance for development of CVI. However, there have been few definitive convincing studies to support the use of thrombolytic therapy for DVT.

One exception is the patient with phlegmasia, for whom thrombolysis is advocated for relief of significant venous obstruction. In this condition, thrombolytic therapy probably results in better relief of symptoms and fewer long-term sequelae than heparin anticoagulation alone. The alternative for this condition is surgical venous thrombectomy. No matter which treatment is chosen, long-term anticoagulation is indicated. The incidence of major bleeding is higher with lytic therapy.[27]

Endovascular reconstruction. Chronic proximal venous occlusion of the iliofemoral system is a challenging clinical problem. The presentation is variable, and there is no reliable diagnostic modality to measure proximal iliofemoral venous stenosis and to assess outflow obstruction accurately. The pathophysiologic mechanism is often a combination of primary and secondary venous insufficiency. Therefore, evaluation and treatment can be challenging. Endovascular reconstruction removes the need for surgical bypass and has been used successfully. Recanalization of the occluded iliac vein is performed endovascularly. Balloon dilation of the lesion is then performed, and a stent is placed across the dilated segment. Excellent results have been achieved, thereby obviating an open surgical procedure. Endovascular iliac therapy has evolved to become first-line therapy for iliac occlusions.

Upper Extremity Deep Venous Thrombosis

Upper extremity DVT is much less common than its lower extremity counterpart, constituting only approximately 5% of all documented DVTs. Although not as common, it is a serious problem; pulmonary embolism occurs in up to one third of all patients with an upper extremity DVT. Upper extremity DVT usually refers to thrombosis of the axillary or subclavian veins. The syndrome can be divided into two categories, primary idiopathic and secondary.

Primary causes include Paget-Schroetter syndrome and idiopathic upper extremity DVT. Patients with Paget-Schroetter syndrome develop effort thrombosis of the extremity caused by compression of the subclavian vein, the venous component of thoracic outlet syndrome. A classic presentation involves a young athlete who uses the upper extremity in a repetitive motion, such as swimming, which causes repetitive extrinsic compression of the subclavian vein. In these patients, anatomic anomalies such as a cervical rib or myofascial bands cause the venous compression. Plain films are one of the first diagnostic tests used to confirm thoracic outlet syndrome. Treatment with initial thrombolysis followed by first rib resection is the standard of care. Idiopathic upper extremity DVT is sometimes eventually attributed to an occult malignant neoplasm, and therefore a diagnosis of idiopathic upper extremity DVT warrants evaluation for an undetected malignant neoplasm.

Secondary causes of upper extremity DVT are more common. These include an indwelling central venous catheter, pacemaker, thrombophilia, and malignant disease.

Classic findings on physical examination include unilateral swelling, pain, extremity discomfort, erythema, and a palpable cord. Diagnosis is confirmed by duplex ultrasonography. Because the clavicle obscures the midportion of the subclavian vein, venography or magnetic resonance venography may be required; these are second-line imaging modalities.

Treatment

Treatment of upper extremity DVT involves anticoagulation therapy. Therapeutic dosing parameters are the same as for lower extremity DVT. Treatment should be for 3 months and consist of heparin or LMWH plus warfarin for at least 3 months. Long-term complications of upper extremity DVT include recurrence and PTS. Thrombolysis has not been shown to decrease long-term manifestations from upper extremity DVT and thus PTS. PTS is treated with extremity elevation and graduated elastic compression.[40,41]

Vena cava filter. The most worrisome and potentially lethal complication of DVT is pulmonary embolism. The symptoms of

<table>
<tr><td>

BOX 64-2 Indications for a Vena Cava Filter

Recurrent thromboembolism despite adequate anticoagulation
Deep venous thrombosis in a patient with contraindications to anticoagulation
Chronic pulmonary embolism and resultant pulmonary hypertension
Complications of anticoagulation
Propagating iliofemoral venous thrombus in anticoagulation

</td><td>

BOX 64-3 Indications for Placement of a Retrievable Inferior Vena Cava Filter

Prophylactic placement in a high-risk trauma patient (orthopedic, spinal cord patients)
Short-term duration, contraindication to anticoagulation therapy
Protection during venous thrombolytic therapy
Extensive iliocaval thrombosis

</td></tr>
</table>

pulmonary embolism, ranging from dyspnea, chest pain, and hypoxia to acute cor pulmonale, are nonspecific and require a high index of suspicion. The gold standard remains pulmonary angiography, but increasingly, this has been displaced by computed tomography angiography.

Adequate anticoagulation is usually effective for stabilizing venous thrombosis, but if a patient develops a pulmonary embolism in the presence of adequate anticoagulation, a vena cava filter is indicated. The general indications for a vena cava filter are listed in Box 64-2. Modern filters are placed percutaneously over a guidewire. The Greenfield filter, most extensively used and studied, has a 95% patency rate and a 4% recurrent embolism rate. This high patency rate allows safe suprarenal placement if there is involvement of the IVC up to the renal veins or if it is placed in a woman in her childbearing years.

Device-related complications are wound hematoma, migration of the device into the pulmonary artery, and caval occlusion caused by trapping of a large embolus. In the last situation, the dramatic hypotension that accompanies acute caval occlusion can be mistaken for a massive pulmonary embolism. The distinction between the hypovolemia of caval occlusion and the right-sided heart failure from pulmonary embolism can be made by measuring filling pressures of the right side of the heart. The treatment of caval occlusion is volume resuscitation.

Retrievable vena cava filters. Although they are generally safe, IVC filters are not without risk and significant morbidity. Therefore, permanent placement of a caval filter, particularly in a young patient who may require only short-term caval protection, is not generally accepted. Retrievable filters entered the field as a potential solution for the patient with temporary indications for pulmonary embolus prophylaxis. There are three retrievable IVC filters that have U.S. Food and Drug Administration approval: the Recovery filter (Bard, Helsingborg, Sweden), OptEase filter (Cordis, Johnson & Johnson Gateway, Piscataway, NJ), and Gunther-Tulip filter (Cook Medical, Bloomington, Ind). These filters vary slightly with respect to shape and length. All can be deployed from the internal jugular vein or femoral vein and retrieved from the right jugular vein (Gunther-Tulip and Recovery) or right femoral vein (OptEase). Before retrieval, venography is performed to ensure that there is no nidus of IVC thrombus in the filter. These filters can be placed in an angiography suite or at the bedside using intravascular ultrasound. A major advantage to retrievable filters is that they may be removed when the patient no longer requires pulmonary embolism protection or can undergo anticoagulation. Patient groups that may benefit from retrievable filters include multiple-trauma patients and high-risk surgical patients. Insertion complications reported include vena cava perforation, filter migration, and venous thrombosis at the insertion site. Retrieval complications include failure to retrieve the filter, thrombus embolization from the filter, vein retrieval site thrombus, and groin hematoma. However, the role of retrievable filters

continues to be a work in progress. Further investigation is required before definitive practice guidelines can be established (Box 64-3).[42,43]

SUPERFICIAL THROMBOPHLEBITIS

Superficial thrombophlebitis is a common disorder, diagnosed in the hospital and outpatient setting. In hospitalized patients, superficial thrombophlebitis is usually caused by an indwelling catheter. In the clinic, patients with thrombophlebitis report common predisposing risk factors, such as recent surgery, recent childbirth, venous stasis, varicose veins, or IV drug use. Patients who deny any of these factors may be classified with idiopathic thrombophlebitis. In these cases, care must be taken to ensure that the patient does not harbor an occult hypercoagulable state or occult malignant disease. In 1876, Trousseau identified the phenomenon of migratory thrombophlebitis and malignant disease, particularly involving the tail of the pancreas. Mondor disease involves superficial thrombophlebitis of the superficial veins of the breast. Diagnosis of superficial thrombophlebitis can be easily made by physical examination of an erythematous palpable cord coursing along a superficial vein, usually located along the lower extremities. Duplex ultrasonography is used if there is suspicion of proximal propagation into the deep venous system. With this diagnosis of DVT, anticoagulation is indicated. If, however, thrombus abuts the saphenofemoral junction, treatment of this more elusive condition is controversial. Some authors recommend serial ultrasound examinations and others anticoagulation; another alternative is operative ligation at the junction.

The treatment of localized noncomplicated thrombophlebitis involves conservative therapy, which consists of anti-inflammatory medication and compression stockings. When the thrombophlebitis involves clusters of varicosities, particularly in the lower extremities, excision is indicated. Selective removal of the entire vein along its course is indicated only in the rare case of suppurative septic thrombophlebitis after all other sources of sepsis have been excluded.

CONCLUSION

The spectrum of venous disease is widespread and diverse, providing surgeons who fully understand the unique physiology of veins a rewarding and rich arena for future investigation.

SELECTED REFERENCES

Bergan JJ, Pascarella L, Schmid-Schönbein GW: Pathogenesis of primary chronic venous disease: Insights from animal models of venous hypertension. *J Vasc Surg* 47:183–192, 2008.

This article provides a comprehensive review of the known aspects of venous hypertension pathophysiology.

Caggiati A, Bergan JJ, Gloviczki P, et al: Nomenclature of the veins of the lower limbs: An international interdisciplinary consensus statement. *J Vasc Surg* 36:416–422, 2002.

Revised terminology for the venous anatomy of the lower extremity is outlined.

Eklöf B, Rutherford RB, Bergan JJ, et al: American Venous Forum International Ad Hoc Committee for Revision of the CEAP Classification: Revision of the CEAP classification for chronic venous disorders: Consensus statement. *J Vasc Surg* 40:1248–1252, 2004.

Essential adjunct to the original CEAP document.

Leopardi D, Hoggan BL, Fitridge RA, et al: Systematic review of treatments for varicose veins. *Ann Vasc Surg* 23:264–276, 2009.

Systematic overview of current treatment modalities for superficial venous disease.

Meissner MH, Eklof B, Smith PC, et al: Secondary chronic venous disorders. *J Vasc Surg* 46(Suppl):68S–83S, 2007.
Meissner MH, Gloviczki P, Bergan J, et al: Primary chronic venous disorders. *J Vasc Surg* 46(Suppl):54S–67S, 2007.

These two supplements provide an extremely comprehensive evaluation of venous insufficiency, including pathophysiology, medical and surgical management, and outstanding references.

Wakefield TW, Caprini J, Comerota AJ: Thromboembolic diseases. *Curr Probl Surg* 45:844–899, 2008.

Excellent review of secondary venous disorders.

REFERENCES

1. Caggiati A, Bergan JJ, Gloviczki P, et al: Nomenclature of the veins of the lower limbs: An international interdisciplinary consensus statement. *J Vasc Surg* 36:416–422, 2002.
2. Raffetto JD: Inflammation in chronic venous ulcers. *Phlebology* 28(Suppl 1):61–67, 2013.
3. Kowalewski R, Malkowski A, Sobolewski K, et al: Evaluation of transforming growth factor-β signaling pathway in the wall of normal and varicose veins. *Pathobiology* 77:1–6, 2010.
4. Pascarella L, Schonbein GW, Bergan JJ: Microcirculation and venous ulcers: A review. *Ann Vasc Surg* 19:921–927, 2005.
5. Neglen P, Raju S: A rational approach to detection of significant reflux with duplex Doppler scanning and air plethysmography. *J Vasc Surg* 17:590–595, 1993.
6. Christopoulos D, Nicolaides AN, Szendro G: Venous reflux: Quantification and correlation with the clinical severity of chronic venous disease. *Br J Surg* 75:352–356, 1988.
7. van Bemmelen PS, Bedford G, Beach K, et al: Quantitative segmental evaluation of venous valvular reflux with duplex ultrasound scanning. *J Vasc Surg* 10:425–431, 1989.
8. Gloviczki P, Comerota AJ, Dalsing MC, et al: The care of patients with varicose veins and associated chronic venous diseases: Clinical practice guidelines of the Society for Vascular Surgery and the American Venous Forum. *J Vasc Surg* 53:2S–48S, 2011.
9. Singh S, Lees TA, Donlon M, et al: Improving the preoperative assessment of varicose veins. *Br J Surg* 84:801–802, 1997.
10. Eklof B, Rutherford RB, Bergan JJ, et al: Revision of the CEAP classification for chronic venous disorders: Consensus statement. *J Vasc Surg* 40:1248–1252, 2004.
11. Rutherford RB, Padberg FT, Jr, Comerota AJ, et al: Venous severity scoring: An adjunct to venous outcome assessment. *J Vasc Surg* 31:1307–1312, 2000.
12. Michaels JA, Brazier JE, Campbell WB, et al: Randomized clinical trial comparing surgery with conservative treatment for uncomplicated varicose veins. *Br J Surg* 93:175–181, 2006.
13. Heller JA: Varicose veins. In Gahtan V, Costanza MJ, editors: *Essentials of vascular surgery for the general surgeon*, New York, 2014, Springer, pp 167–183.
14. Franz RW, Knapp ED: Transilluminated powered phlebectomy surgery for varicose veins: A review of 339 consecutive patients. *Ann Vasc Surg* 23:303–309, 2009.
15. Dwerryhouse S, Davies B, Harradine K, et al: Stripping the long saphenous vein reduces the rate of reoperation for recurrent varicose veins: Five-year results of a randomized trial. *J Vasc Surg* 29:589–592, 1999.
16. Raju S, Hollis K, Neglen P: Use of compression stockings in chronic venous disease: Patient compliance and efficacy. *Ann Vasc Surg* 21:790–795, 2007.
17. van den Bos R, Arends L, Kockaert M, et al: Endovenous therapies of lower extremity varicosities: A meta-analysis. *J Vasc Surg* 49:230–239, 2009.
18. Marston WA, Owens LV, Davies S, et al: Endovenous saphenous ablation corrects the hemodynamic abnormality in patients with CEAP clinical class 3-6 CVI due to superficial reflux. *Vasc Endovascular Surg* 40:125–130, 2006.
19. Neglen P, Hollis KC, Olivier J, et al: Stenting of the venous outflow in chronic venous disease: Long-term stent-related outcome, clinical, and hemodynamic result. *J Vasc Surg* 46:979–990, 2007.
20. Hanrahan LM, Araki CT, Rodriguez AA, et al: Distribution of valvular incompetence in patients with venous stasis ulceration. *J Vasc Surg* 13:805–811, 1991.
21. O'Donnell TF, Jr: The present status of surgery of the superficial venous system in the management of venous ulcer and the evidence for the role of perforator interruption. *J Vasc Surg* 48:1044–1052, 2008.
22. Linton RR: The communicating veins of the lower leg and the operative technic for their ligation. *Ann Surg* 107:582–593, 1938.
23. Powell CC, Rohrer MJ, Barnard MR, et al: Chronic venous insufficiency is associated with increased platelet and monocyte activation and aggregation. *J Vasc Surg* 30:844–851, 1999.
24. Gloviczki P, Bergan JJ, Rhodes JM, et al: Mid-term results of endoscopic perforator vein interruption for chronic venous insufficiency: Lessons learned from the North American subfascial endoscopic perforator surgery registry. The North American Study Group. *J Vasc Surg* 29:489–502, 1999.

25. Murray JD, Bergan JJ, Riffenburgh RH: Development of open-scope subfascial perforating vein surgery: Lessons learned from the first 67 cases. *Ann Vasc Surg* 13:372–377, 1999.

26. Masuda EM, Kessler DM, Lurie F, et al: The effect of ultrasound-guided sclerotherapy of incompetent perforator veins on venous clinical severity and disability scores. *J Vasc Surg* 43:551–556, 2006.

27. Sillesen H, Just S, Jorgensen M, et al: Catheter directed thrombolysis for treatment of ilio-femoral deep venous thrombosis is durable, preserves venous valve function and may prevent chronic venous insufficiency. *Eur J Vasc Endovasc Surg* 30:556–562, 2005.

28. Kistner RL: Surgical repair of the incompetent femoral vein valve. *Arch Surg* 110:1336–1342, 1975.

29. Masuda EM, Kistner RL: Long-term results of venous valve reconstruction: A four- to twenty-one-year follow-up. *J Vasc Surg* 19:391–403, 1994.

30. Taheri SA, Lazar L, Elias S, et al: Surgical treatment of post-phlebitic syndrome with vein valve transplant. *Am J Surg* 144:221–224, 1982.

31. Anderson FA, Jr, Spencer FA: Risk factors for venous thromboembolism. *Circulation* 107:I9–I16, 2003.

32. Kovacs MJ, MacKinnon KM, Anderson D, et al: A comparison of three rapid D-dimer methods for the diagnosis of venous thromboembolism. *Br J Haematol* 115:140–144, 2001.

33. Killewich LA, Cahan MA, Hanna DJ, et al: The effect of external pneumatic compression on regional fibrinolysis in a prospective randomized trial. *J Vasc Surg* 36:953–958, 2002.

34. Bernardi E, Prandoni P: Safety of low molecular weight heparins in the treatment of venous thromboembolism. *Expert Opin Drug Saf* 2:87–94, 2003.

35. Couturaud F, Julian JA, Kearon C: Low molecular weight heparin administered once versus twice daily in patients with venous thromboembolism: A meta-analysis. *Thromb Haemost* 86:980–984, 2001.

36. Offner PJ, Hawkes A, Madayag R, et al: The role of temporary inferior vena cava filters in critically ill surgical patients. *Arch Surg* 138:591–594, discussion 594-595, 2003.

37. Mismetti P, Laporte S, Darmon JY, et al: Meta-analysis of low molecular weight heparin in the prevention of venous thromboembolism in general surgery. *Br J Surg* 88:913–930, 2001.

38. Norwood SH, McAuley CE, Berne JD, et al: Prospective evaluation of the safety of enoxaparin prophylaxis for venous thromboembolism in patients with intracranial hemorrhagic injuries. *Arch Surg* 137:696–701, 2002.

39. Kearon C, Ginsberg JS, Kovacs MJ, et al: Comparison of low-intensity warfarin therapy with conventional-intensity warfarin therapy for long-term prevention of recurrent venous thromboembolism. *N Engl J Med* 349:631–639, 2003.

40. Joffe HV, Goldhaber SZ: Upper-extremity deep vein thrombosis. *Circulation* 106:1874–1880, 2002.

41. Martinelli I, Battaglioli T, Bucciarelli P, et al: Risk factors and recurrence rate of primary deep vein thrombosis of the upper extremities. *Circulation* 110:566–570, 2004.

42. Rosenthal D, Wellons ED, Lai KM, et al: Retrievable inferior vena cava filters: Initial clinical results. *Ann Vasc Surg* 20:157–165, 2006.

43. Kearon C, Kahn SR, Agnelli G, et al: Antithrombotic therapy for venous thromboembolic disease: American College of Chest Physicians Evidence-Based Clinical Practice Guidelines (8th Edition). *Chest* 133:454S–545S, 2008.

65 CHAPTER

The Lymphatics

Iraklis I. Pipinos, B. Timothy Baxter

第六十五章　淋巴管疾病

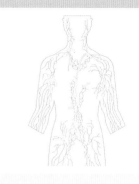

中文导读

　　本章共分为10节：①胚胎学和解剖学；②功能和结构；③病理生理和分期；④鉴别诊断；⑤分期；⑥诊断性检查；⑦治疗；⑧乳糜胸；⑨乳糜腹；⑩淋巴管肿瘤。

　　第一节介绍了淋巴系统在胚胎第6周时开始发育，第8周乳糜池形成，第9周胸导管形成。淋巴系统在发育过程中出现连接和引流障碍，就会形成淋巴管瘤，可分布于颈部、躯干、肠系膜、小肠以及腹膜后。四肢到躯干的淋巴系统发育异常可以导致淋巴水肿。淋巴系统的生长发育受VEGF-C、VEGF-D、VEGFR-3及Nrp2调控。

　　第二节介绍了淋巴系统的构成部分：吸收淋巴液的初始或终端毛细淋巴管、运输淋巴液的集合淋巴管以及过滤淋巴液且具有基础免疫功能的淋巴结。淋巴系统主要功能：吸收大分子及组织液、免疫功能以及脂肪的吸收和运输。

　　第三节介绍了如果现有的淋巴不能调节进入组织间隙的蛋白质和组织液，就会导致淋巴水肿。随着淋巴水肿病情的进展，分为第一期凹陷性水肿，第二期不可凹陷性水肿，第三期皮下过多的纤维化和疤痕形成，可表现为"橡皮肿"。

　　第四节介绍大多数第二期及第三期的淋巴水肿通过特异性的查体结果可以明确诊断。双下肢水肿需与心力衰竭、肾衰竭、肝硬化低蛋白血症、肾病综合征、营养不良、脂肪水肿等一起鉴别。单侧下肢水肿需与静脉疾病相鉴别。

　　第五节介绍淋巴水肿分为原因不明的原发性水肿和已知病因的继发性水肿。原发性水肿根据年龄可以分为早发性和迟发性水肿；继发性淋巴水肿最常见原因是淋巴丝虫病，其他原因包括淋巴结切除术后、消融、放射治疗、肿瘤侵袭、外伤及少见的感染。

　　第六节介绍了淋巴水肿二期、三期诊断较为容易，诊断比较困难的是一期水肿。还介绍了淋巴水肿的几种检查方法，如常用的淋巴闪烁显像（或同位素淋巴管显影）、有创的直接淋巴管造影以及新出现的增强磁共振淋巴管造影。

第七节主要介绍了淋巴水肿的治疗方法，包括一般治疗、佩戴弹力袜、复合减充血物理治疗、空气压力治疗、药物治疗、分子治疗以及手术治疗。绝大部分淋巴水肿病人可以通过抬高患肢、穿弹力袜、物理治疗及空气压缩治疗相结合得到缓解。目前没有有效

药物治疗淋巴水肿。非手术治疗无效、进展期复杂的淋巴水肿可行手术治疗。

第八节介绍了乳糜胸的原因、诊断及处理方法。

第九节介绍了乳糜腹的原因、诊断及处理方法。

第十节介绍了淋巴管良性肿瘤淋巴管瘤的分类、发生部位以及手术治疗，也描述了恶性肿瘤淋巴管肉瘤病因、临床表现、治疗方式及预后。

〔龙　新〕

EMBRYOLOGY AND ANATOMY

The primordial lymphatic system is first seen during the sixth week of development in the form of lymph sacs located next to the jugular veins. During the eighth week, the cisterna chyli forms just dorsal to the aorta, and at the same time, two additional lymphatic sacs corresponding to the iliofemoral vascular pedicles begin forming. Communicating channels connecting the lymph sacs, which will become the thoracic duct, develop during the ninth week.

From this primordial lymphatic system sprout endothelial buds that grow with the venous system to form the peripheral lymphatic plexus (Fig. 65-1). Failure of one of the initial jugular lymphatic sacs to develop proper connections and drainage with the lymphatic system and, subsequently, the venous system may produce focal lymph cysts (cavernous lymphangiomas), also known as cystic hygromas.[1] Similarly, failure of embryologic remnants of lymphatic tissues to connect to efferent channels leads to the development of cystic lymphatic formations (simple capillary lymphangiomas) that, depending on their location, are classified as truncal, mesenteric, intestinal, and retroperitoneal lymphangiomas. Hypoplasia or failure of development of drainage channels connecting the lymphatic systems of extremities to the main primordial lymphatic system of the torso may result in primary lymphedema of the extremities.

Lymphangiogenesis appears to be regulated by the vascular endothelial growth factors C and D (VEGF-C, VEGF-D); their receptor, VEGFR-3; and their binding protein, neuropilin 2 (Nrp2). Consistent with these findings, Nrp2-deficient mice have lymphatic hypoplasia, and heterozygous inactivating mutation of VEGFR-3 is found in Chy mice, an animal model of primary lymphedema, which appears to be the underlying problem in patients with Milroy disease (congenital familial lymphedema).[2] A number of additional genes have recently been found to be related to lymphatic disorders.[3] The best studied at this point are the gene for the forkhead family transcription factor FOXC2 (responsible for the hereditary lymphedema-distichiasis syndrome) and the gene for the transcription factor SOX18 (related

to recessive and dominant forms of hypotrichosis-lymphedema-telangiectasia). As more causal genes are identified, the possibility arises for a classification built on patient phenotypes for which the gene is known.[4]

FUNCTION AND STRUCTURE

The lymphatic system is composed of three elements: (1) the initial or terminal lymphatic capillaries, which absorb lymph; (2) the collecting vessels, which serve primarily as conduits for lymph transport; and (3) the lymph nodes, which are interposed in the pathway of the conducting vessels, filtering the lymph and serving a primary immunologic role.

The terminal lymphatics have special structural characteristics that allow entry not only of large macromolecules but even of cells and microbes. Their most important structural feature is a high porosity resulting from a very small number of tight junctions between endothelial cells, a limited and incomplete basement membrane, and anchoring filaments (4 to 10 nm) tethering the interstitial matrix to the endothelial cells. These filaments, once the turgor of the tissue increases, are able to pull on the endothelial cells and essentially introduce large gaps between them, which then allow very low resistance influx of interstitial fluid and macromolecules in the lymphatic channels. The collecting vessels ascend alongside the primary blood vessels of the organ or limb, pass through the regional lymph nodes, and drain into the main lymph channels of the torso. These channels eventually empty into the venous system through the thoracic duct. There are additional communications between the lymphatic and the venous systems. These smaller lymphovenous shunts mostly occur at the level of lymph nodes and around major venous structures, such as the jugular, subclavian, and iliac veins. Several structures in the body contain no lymphatics. Specifically, lymphatics have not been found in the epidermis, cornea, central nervous system, cartilage, tendon, and muscle.

The lymphatic system has three main functions. First, tissue fluid and macromolecules that undergo ultrafiltration at the level of the arterial capillaries are reabsorbed and returned to the

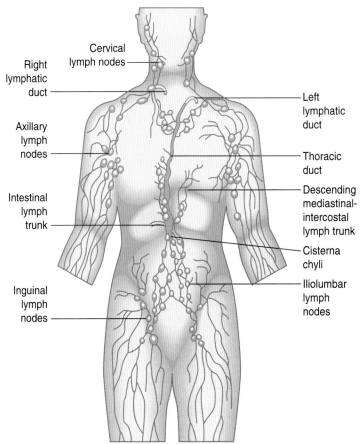

FIGURE 65-1 Major anatomic pathways and lymph node groups of the lymphatic system.

circulation through the lymphatic system. Every day, 50% to 100% of the intravascular proteins are filtered this way in the interstitial space. Normally, they then enter the terminal lymphatics and are transported through the collecting lymphatics back into the venous circulation. Second, antigens, immune cells, microbes, and mutant cells arriving in the interstitial space enter the lymphatic system and are presented to the lymph nodes, which represent the first line of the immune system. Last, at the level of the gastrointestinal tract, lymph vessels are responsible for the uptake and transport of most of the fat absorbed from the bowel. Recent data suggest that a relationship between fat and lymphatics may exist well beyond the gut alone. It appears that peripheral tissue lipid transport and homeostasis may be, in part, determined by lymphatic function, hence the increased fat deposition seen in lymphedema.[3,5]

In contrast to what happens with venous forward flow, lymph's centripetal transport occurs mainly through intrinsic contractility of the individual lymphatic vessels, which in concert with competent valvular mechanisms is effective in establishing constant forward flow of lymph. In addition to the intrinsic contractility, other factors, such as surrounding muscle activity, negative pressure secondary to breathing, and transmitted arterial pulsations, have a lesser role in the forward lymph flow. These secondary factors appear to become more important under conditions of lymph stasis and congestion of the lymphatic vessels.

PATHOPHYSIOLOGY AND STAGING

Lymphedema is the result of an inability of the existing lymphatic system to accommodate the protein and fluid entering the interstitial compartment at the tissue level.[6] In the first stage of lymphedema, impaired lymphatic drainage results in protein-rich fluid accumulation in the interstitial compartment. Clinically, this is manifested as soft pitting edema. In the second stage of lymphedema, the clinical condition is further exacerbated by accumulation of fibroblasts, adipocytes, and, perhaps most important, macrophages in the affected tissues, which culminates in a local inflammatory response. This results in important structural changes from the deposition of connective tissue and adipose elements at the skin and subcutaneous level. In the second stage of lymphedema, tissue edema is more pronounced, is nonpitting, and has a spongy consistency. In the third and most advanced stage of lymphedema, the affected tissues sustain further injury as a result of both the local inflammatory response and recurrent infectious episodes that typically result from minimal subclinical breaks in the skin. Such repeated episodes injure the incompetent, remaining lymphatic channels, progressively worsening the underlying insufficiency of the lymphatic system. This eventually results in excessive subcutaneous fibrosis and scarring with associated severe skin changes characteristic of lymphostatic elephantiasis.

DIFFERENTIAL DIAGNOSIS

In most patients with second- or third-stage lymphedema, the characteristic findings on physical examination can usually establish the diagnosis. The edematous limb has a firm and hardened consistency. There is loss of the normal perimalleolar shape, resulting in a "tree trunk" pattern. The dorsum of the foot is characteristically swollen, resulting in the appearance of the "buffalo hump," and the toes become thick and squared (Fig. 65-2). In advanced lymphedema, the skin undergoes characteristic changes, such as lichenification, development of peau d'orange, and hyperkeratosis.[6] In addition, the patients give a history of recurrent episodes of cellulitis and lymphangitis after trivial trauma and frequently present with fungal infections affecting the forefoot and toes. Patients with isolated lymphedema usually do not have the hyperpigmentation or ulceration one typically sees in patients with chronic venous insufficiency. Lymphedema does not respond significantly to overnight elevation, whereas edema secondary to central organ failure or venous insufficiency does.

The evaluation of a swollen extremity should start with a detailed history and physical examination. The most common causes of bilateral extremity edema are of systemic origin. The most common cause is cardiac failure, followed by renal failure.[7] Hypoproteinemia secondary to cirrhosis, nephrotic syndrome, and malnutrition can also produce bilateral lower extremity edema. Another important cause to consider with bilateral leg enlargement is lipedema. Lipedema is not true edema but rather excessive subcutaneous fat typically found in obese women. It is bilateral, nonpitting, and greatest at the ankle and legs, with characteristic sparing of the feet. There are no skin changes, and the enlargement is not affected by elevation. The history usually indicates that this has been a lifelong problem that "runs in the family."

Once the systemic causes of edema are excluded in the patient with unilateral extremity involvement, edema secondary to venous and lymphatic disease should be entertained. Venous disease is overwhelmingly the most common cause of unilateral leg edema. Leg edema secondary to venous disease is usually pitting and is greatest at the legs and ankles with a sparing of the feet. The edema responds promptly to overnight leg elevation. In the later stages, the skin is atrophic with brawny pigmentation. Ulceration associated with venous insufficiency occurs above or posterior to and beneath the malleoli.

CLASSIFICATION

Lymphedema is generally classified as primary when there is no known cause and secondary when its cause is a known disease or disorder.[8] Primary lymphedema has generally been classified on the basis of the age at onset and presence of familial clustering. Primary lymphedema with onset before the first year of life is called congenital. The familial version of congenital lymphedema is known as Milroy disease and is inherited as a dominant trait. Primary lymphedema with onset between the ages of 1 and 35 years is called lymphedema praecox. The familial version of lymphedema praecox is known as Meige disease. Finally, primary lymphedema with onset after the age of 35 years is called lymphedema tarda. The primary lymphedemas are relatively uncommon, occurring in one of every 10,000 individuals. The most common form of primary lymphedema is praecox, which accounts for approximately 80% of the patients. Congenital and tarda lymphedemas each account for 10%. Worldwide, the most common cause of secondary lymphedema is infestation of the lymph nodes by the parasite *Wuchereria bancrofti* in the disease state called filariasis. In the developed countries, the most common causes of secondary lymphedema involve resection or ablation of regional lymph nodes by surgery, radiation therapy, tumor invasion, direct trauma, or, less commonly, an infectious process.

DIAGNOSTIC TESTS

The diagnosis of lymphedema is relatively easy in the patient who presents in the second and third stages of the disease. It can, however, be a difficult diagnosis to make in the first stage, particularly when the edema is mild, pitting, and relieved with simple maneuvers such as elevation.[8,9] For patients with suspected secondary forms of lymphedema, computed tomography and magnetic resonance imaging are valuable and indeed essential for exclusion of underlying oncologic disease states.[10] In patients with known lymph node excision and radiation treatment as the underlying problem of their lymphedema, additional diagnostic studies are rarely needed except as these studies relate to follow-up of an underlying malignant disease. For patients with edema of unknown cause and a suspicion for lymphedema, lymphoscintigraphy is the diagnostic test of choice. When lymphoscintigraphy confirms that lymphatic drainage is delayed, the diagnosis of primary lymphedema should never be made until neoplasia involving the regional and central lymphatic drainage of the limb has been excluded through computed tomography or magnetic resonance imaging. If a more detailed diagnostic interpretation of lymphatic channels is needed for operative planning, contrast lymphangiography may be considered.

Lymphoscintigraphy (or isotope lymphography) has emerged as the test of choice in patients with suspected lymphedema.[10,11] It cannot differentiate between primary and secondary lymphedemas; however, it has a sensitivity of 70% to 90% and a specificity

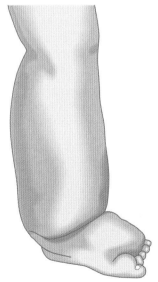

FIGURE 65-2 Lymphedema with characteristic loss of the normal perimalleolar shape, resulting in a "tree trunk" pattern. Dorsum of the foot is characteristically swollen, resulting in the appearance of the "buffalo hump."

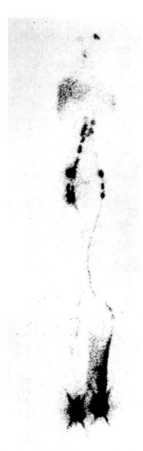

FIGURE 65-3 Lymphoscintigraphic pattern in primary lymphedema. Note area of dermal backflow on the left and diminished number of lymph nodes in the groin. (From Cambria RA, Gloviczki P, Naessens JM, et al: Noninvasive evaluation of the lymphatic system with lymphoscintigraphy: A prospective, semiquantitative analysis in 386 extremities. *J Vasc Surg* 18:773–782, 1993.)

of nearly 100% in differentiating lymphedema from other causes of limb swelling. The test assesses lymphatic function by quantitating the rate of clearance of a radiolabeled macromolecular tracer (Fig. 65-3). The advantages of the technique are that it is simple, safe, and reproducible, with small exposure to radioactivity (approximately 5 mCi). It involves the injection of a small amount of radioiodinated human albumin or technetium Tc 99m–labeled sulfur colloid into the first interdigital space of the foot or hand. Migration of the radiotracer within the skin and subcutaneous lymphatics is easily monitored with a whole body gamma camera, thus producing clear images of the major lymphatic channels in the leg as well as measuring the amount of radioactivity at the inguinal nodes 30 and 60 minutes after injection of the radiolabeled substance in the feet. An uptake value that is less than 0.3% of the total injected dose at 30 minutes is diagnostic of lymphedema. The normal range of uptake is between 0.6% and 1.6%. In patients with edema secondary to venous disease, isotope clearance is usually abnormally rapid, resulting in more than 2% ilioinguinal uptake. Importantly, variation in the degree of edema involving the lower extremity does not appear to significantly change the rate of clearance of the isotope.

Direct contrast lymphangiography provides the finest details of the lymphatic anatomy.[12] However, it is an invasive study that involves exposure and cannulation of lymphatics at the dorsum of the forefoot, followed by slow injection of contrast medium (ethiodized oil). The procedure is tedious, the cannulation often necessitates aid of magnification optics (frequently an operating microscope is needed), and the dissection requires some form of anesthetic. After cannulation of a superficial lymph vessel, contrast material is slowly injected into the lymphatic system. A total of 7 to 10 mL of contrast material is ideal for lower extremity and 4 to 5 mL for upper extremity evaluation. Potential complications include damage of the visualized lymphatics, allergic reactions, and pulmonary embolism if the oil-based contrast agent enters the venous system through lymphovenous anastomoses. Lymphangiography in the present practice of vascular surgery is used infrequently and reserved for the preoperative evaluation of selected patients who are candidates for direct operations on their lymphatic vessels.

New Diagnostic Tests

The field of lymphatic imaging is ever evolving, and we can expect that technologic advances, combined with the development of new contrast agents, will continue to improve diagnostic accuracy.[10] The most promising new test appears to be contrast magnetic resonance lymphangiography.[10,13] The test is performed after intracutaneous injection of gadobenate dimeglumine into the interdigital webs of the dorsal foot. Reported data suggest that the new test is capable of visualizing the anatomy and functional status of lymph flow transport of lymphatic vessels and lymph nodes of lymphedematous limbs.

THERAPY

The majority of lymphedema patients can be treated with a combination of limb elevation, a high-quality compression garment, complex decongestive physical therapy, and compression pump therapy. We currently have no effective medications for the treatment of lymphedema. Operative treatment may be considered for patients with advanced complicated lymphedema for whom management with nonoperative means has failed.

General Therapeutic Measures

All patients with lymphedema should be educated in meticulous skin care and avoidance of injuries.[9,14,15] The patients should always be instructed to see their physicians early for signs of infections because these may progress rapidly to serious systemic infections. Infections should be aggressively and promptly treated with appropriate antibiotics directed at gram-positive cocci. Eczema at the level of the forefoot and toes requires treatment, and hydrocortisone-based creams may be considered. In addition, basic range of motion exercises for the extremities have been shown to be of value in the management of lymphedema in the long term. Finally, the patients should make every effort to maintain ideal body weight.

Elevation and Compression Garments

For lymphedema patients in all stages of disease, management with high-quality elastic garments is necessary at all times except when the legs are elevated above the heart.[16,17] The ideal compression garment is custom fitted and delivers pressures in the range of 30 to 60 mm Hg. Such garments may have the additional benefit of protecting the extremity from injuries, such as burns, lacerations, and insect bites. The patients should avoid standing for prolonged periods and should elevate their legs at night by supporting the foot of the bed on 15-cm blocks.

Complex Decongestive Physical Therapy

This specialized massage technique for patients with lymphedema is designed to stimulate the still functioning lymph vessels, to evacuate stagnant protein-rich fluid by breaking up subcutaneous deposits of fibrous tissue, and to redirect lymph fluid to areas of the body where lymph flow is normal.[18] The technique is initiated on the normal contralateral side of the body, evacuating excessive fluid and preparing first the lymphatic zones of the nonaffected extremity, followed by the zones in the trunk quadrant adjacent to the affected limb, before attention is turned to the swollen extremity. The affected extremity is massaged in a segmental fashion, with the proximal zones being massaged first, proceeding to the distal limb. The technique is time-consuming but effective in reducing the volume of the lymphedematous limbs.[18] After the massage session is complete, the extremity is wrapped with a low-stretch wrap, and then the limb is placed in the custom-fitted garment to maintain the decreased girth obtained with the massage therapy. This kind of therapy is appropriate for patients with all stages of lymphedema.

When the patient is first referred for complex decongestive physical therapy, the patient undergoes daily to weekly massage sessions for up to 8 to 12 weeks. Limb elevation and elastic stockings are a necessary adjunct in this phase. After maximal volume reduction is achieved, the patient returns for maintenance massage treatments every 2 to 3 months.

Compression Pump Therapy

Pneumatic compression pump therapy is another effective method of reducing the volume of the lymphedematous limb by a similar principle to massage therapy. The device consists of a sleeve containing several compartments. The lymphedematous limb is positioned inside the sleeve, and the compartments are serially inflated to milk the stagnant fluid out of the extremity.[19]

When a patient with advanced lymphedema is first referred for therapy, an initial approach with hospitalization for 3 or 4 days involving strict limb elevation, daily complex decongestive physical therapy, and compression pump treatments may be necessary to achieve optimal control of the lymphedema. Patients with cardiac or renal dysfunction should be monitored for fluid overload. After this initial period of intensive therapy, the patients are fitted with high-quality compression garments to maintain the limb volume. Maintenance sessions are then prescribed for the patients on an as-needed basis.

Drug Therapy

Benzopyrones have attracted interest as potentially effective agents in the treatment of lymphedema. This class of medications including coumarin (1,2-benzopyrone) is thought to reduce lymphedema through stimulation of proteolysis by tissue macrophages and stimulation of the peristalsis and pumping action of the collecting lymphatics. Benzopyrones have no anticoagulant activity. The first randomized, crossover trial of coumarin in patients with lymphedema of the arms and legs was reported in 1993.[20] The study concluded that coumarin was more effective than placebo in reducing not only volume but other important parameters, including skin temperature, attacks of secondary acute inflammation, and discomfort of the lymphedematous extremities; skin turgor and suppleness were improved with coumarin. A second randomized, crossover trial was reported in 1999.[21] This study

focused on effects of coumarin in women with secondary lymphedema after treatment of breast cancer. The trial investigators found that coumarin was not effective therapy for the specific group of women. Because of the disagreement between these two major trials, the enthusiasm for use of benzopyrones in the United States has been tempered. Additional trials should be undertaken to clarify the potential effects of the medications on primary and secondary lymphedemas in different extremities and stages.

Diuretics may temporarily improve the appearance of the lymphedematous extremity with stage I disease, leading patients to request continuous therapy. However, other than producing temporary intravascular volume depletion, there is no long-term benefit. Thus, diuretics have no role in the treatment of lymphedema at any stage.

Molecular Lymphangiogenesis

Fundamental discoveries in lymphatic development have pointed to the potential of exciting new treatments for lymphedema. These molecular treatments are based on the activation of the VEGFR-3 pathway by administration of cognate ligands VEGF-C and VEGF-D using a variety of methods.[22] At this point, these treatments have been tested only in animal models, with promising results. Formal clinical trials are now needed to evaluate the therapeutic potential and possible untoward effects (including the possibility of stimulation of dormant tumor cells as a consequence of increased angiogenesis) of therapeutic lymphangiogenesis.[23]

Operative Treatment

Ninety-five percent of patients with lymphedema can be managed nonoperatively. Surgical intervention may be considered for patients with stage II and stage III lymphedema who have severe functional impairment, recurrent episodes of lymphangitis, and severe pain despite optimal medical therapy. Two main categories of operations are available for the care of patients with lymphedema: reconstructive and excisional.

Reconstructive operations[24,25] should be considered for those patients with proximal (either primary or secondary) obstruction of the extremity lymphatic circulation with preserved, dilated lymphatics peripheral to the obstruction. In these patients, the residual dilated lymphatics can be anastomosed either to nearby veins or to transposed healthy lymphatic channels (usually mobilized or harvested from the healthy lower extremity) in an attempt to restore effective drainage of the lymphedematous extremity. Some of the most common candidates for reconstructive procedures are patients with upper extremity lymphedema secondary to axillary lymphadenectomy or patients with leg lymphedema secondary to inguinal or pelvic lymphadenectomy. Treatment of selected lymphedema patients with lymphovenous anastomoses or lymphovenous bypass or lymphaticolymphatic bypass has resulted in objective improvement in 30% to 80% of the patients, with an average initial reduction in the excess limb volume of 30% to 84%.[26-29]

For those patients with primary lymphedema who have hypoplastic and fibrotic distal lymphatic vessels, such reconstructions are not an option. For such patients, a surgical strategy involving transfer of lymphatic-bearing tissue (portion of the greater omentum) into the affected limb has been attempted. This is intended to connect the residual hypoplastic lymphatic channels of the leg to competent lymphatics in the transferred tissue. Omental flap operations have been found to have poor results.[30] Alternatively, a segment of the ileum can be disconnected from the rest of the bowel, stripped of its mucosa, and mobilized to be

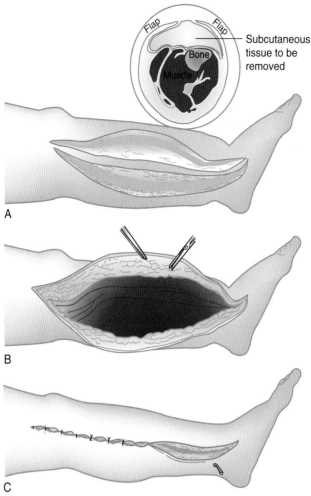

Subcutaneous
tissue to be
removed

Flap   Flap

Bone

Muscle

A

B

C

FIGURE 65-4 A-C, Schematic representation of the Kontoleon or Homan procedure. Relatively thick skin flaps are raised anteriorly and posteriorly, and all subcutaneous tissue beneath the flaps and the underlying medial calf deep fascia are removed along with the necessary redundant skin.

sewn onto the cut surface of residual ilioinguinal nodes in an attempt to bridge the lower extremity with mesenteric lymphatics. When this enteromesenteric bridge procedure was applied to a group of eight carefully selected patients, the outcomes were promising, with six patients showing sustained clinical improvement in long follow-up.[31]

Excisional operations are essentially the only viable option for patients without residual lymphatics of adequate size for reconstructive procedures. For patients with recalcitrant stage II and early stage III lymphedema in whom the edema is moderate and the skin is relatively healthy, an excisional procedure that removes a large segment of the lymphedematous subcutaneous tissues and overlying skin is the procedure of choice. This palliative procedure was introduced by Kontoleon in 1918 and was later popularized by Homan as "staged subcutaneous excision underneath flaps" (Fig. 65-4). The operative approach starts with a medial incision extending from the level of the medial malleolus through the calf into the midthigh.[32,33] Flaps about 1 to 2 cm thick are elevated anteriorly and posteriorly, and all subcutaneous tissue beneath the flaps along with the underlying medial calf deep fascia is removed with the redundant skin. The sural nerve is preserved. After the

first-stage procedure is completed and if additional lymphedematous tissue removal is necessary, a second operation is performed usually 3 to 6 months later. The second-stage operation is performed by similar techniques through an incision on the lateral aspect of the limb. In a recent long-term follow-up study, 80% of patients undergoing staged subcutaneous excision underneath flaps had significant and long-lasting reduction in extremity size associated with improved function and extremity contour. Wound complications were encountered in 10% of the patients.[32]

A minimally invasive version of the Kontoleon procedure is gaining increasing support among lymphedema experts.[34,35] A number of reports have demonstrated that use of liposuction through small incisions is safe and is able to achieve control, at least on a short-term basis, of clinically disabling conditions associated with advanced stages of lymphedema. Surgeons with experience in this technique recommend initial conservative treatment of pitting lymphedema to remove excess fluid, followed by liposuction to remove remaining excess volume bothersome to the patient.[35]

When the lymphedema is extremely pronounced and the skin is unhealthy and infected, the simple reducing operation of

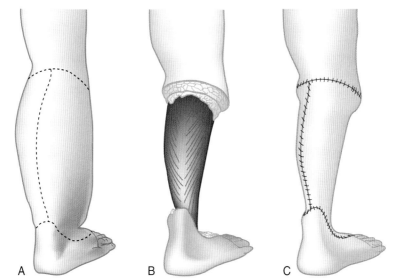

FIGURE 65-5 **A-C,** Schematic representation of the Charles procedure. It involves complete and circum-ferential excision of the skin, subcutaneous tissue, and deep fascia of the involved leg and dorsum of the foot. Coverage is provided preferably by full-thickness grafting from the excised skin.

Kontoleon is not adequate. In this case, the classic excisional operation originally described by Charles in 1912 is performed (Fig. 65-5). The procedure involves complete and circumferential excision of the skin, subcutaneous tissue, and deep fascia of the involved leg and dorsum of the foot.[36] The excision is usually performed in one stage, and coverage is provided preferably by full-thickness grafting from the excised skin. In a follow-up report, patients subjected to the Charles operation had immediate volume and circumference reduction. Skin graft take was 88%, and complications of the operation consisted primarily of wound infections, hematomas, and necrosis of skin flaps. The hospital stay was 21 to 36 days.[37] Although this is a successful and radically reducing operation, the behavior in the healing skin graft is unpredictable. Between 10% and 15% of the grafted segments do not take and can be difficult to manage because of frequent localized sloughing, excessive scarring, focal recurrent infections, and hyperkeratosis or dermatitis. These complications seem to be worse in patients in whom leg resurfacing is performed with split-thickness grafts from the opposite extremity. In advanced cases, the exophytic changes within the grafted skin, chronic cellulitis, and skin breakdown may eventually lead to leg amputation.[38]

CHYLOTHORAX

Chylous pleural effusion is usually secondary to thoracic duct trauma (usually iatrogenic after chest surgery) and rarely a manifestation of advanced malignant disease with lymphatic metastasis.[39] Presence of chylomicrons on lipoprotein analysis and a triglyceride level of more than 110 mg/dL in the pleural fluid are diagnostic. Initially, patients can be treated nonoperatively with tube thoracostomy, medium-chain triglyceride diet or total parenteral nutrition, and octreotide/somatostatin therapy.[40] For patients with thoracic duct injury and an effusion that persists after 1 week of treatment with appropriate diet, octreotide, and thoracostomy drainage, an intervention should be considered to identify and to occlude the thoracic duct above and below the leak. The operative approach of choice has been video-assisted

thoracoscopy or thoracotomy to identify and to ligate the thoracic duct above and below the leak (the site of the leak can be identified if cream is given to the patient a few hours before operation). However, a new endovascular technique has been introduced and is becoming the optimal first approach for the management of persistent postoperative chylothorax. The approach starts with lymphangiography, usually through a groin lymph node access, to identify the location and anatomy of the cisterna chyli and the location of the divided thoracic duct. Once the cisterna chyli is opacified, it is percutaneously accessed with a spinal needle, using radiographic guidance, and is catheterized. The location of the divided thoracic duct is then identified with repeated lymphangiography, and the duct is embolized. In expert hands, this technique has a more than 50% success rate.[41,42] For patients with cancer-related chylothorax and persistent drainage despite optimal chemotherapy and radiation therapy, pleurodesis is highly successful in preventing recurrences.

CHYLOPERITONEUM

In contrast to chylothorax, the most common cause of chylous ascites is congenital lymphatic abnormalities in children and malignant disease involving the abdominal lymph nodes in adults. Postoperative injury to abdominal lymphatics resulting in chylous ascites is rare.[43] Presence of chylomicrons on lipoprotein analysis and a triglyceride level of more than 110 mg/dL are diagnostic. Initial treatment includes paracentesis followed by medium-chain triglyceride diet or total parenteral nutrition. In patients with postoperative chyloperitoneum, if ascites does not respond after 1 to 2 weeks of nonoperative management, percutaneous embolization[41,42] or surgical exploration should be employed to identify and to occlude or ligate the leaking lymphatic duct. Congenital and malignant causes should be given longer periods (up to 4 to 6 weeks) of nonoperative management. If ascites persists in patients with congenital ascites, lymphoscintigraphy or lymphangiography is performed before an attempt is made to control the leak with celiotomy. At the time of exploration, control of the leak can be achieved by ligation of leaking lymphatic vessels or resection of the bowel associated with the leak. Patients with malignant neoplasms should receive aggressive management for their underlying disease, which generally is effective at controlling the chyloperitoneum.

TUMORS OF THE LYMPHATICS

Lymphangiomas are the lymphatic analogue of the hemangiomas of blood vessels. They are generally divided into two types, (1) simple or capillary lymphangioma and (2) cavernous lymphangioma or cystic hygroma.[44] They are thought to represent isolated and sequestered segments of the lymphatic system that retain the ability to produce lymph. As the volume of lymph inside the cystic tumor increases, it grows larger within the surrounding tissues. The majority of these benign tumors are present at birth, and 90% of them can be identified by the end of the first year of life. The cavernous lymphangiomas almost invariably occur in the neck or the axilla and very rarely in the retroperitoneum. The simple capillary lymphangiomas also tend to occur subcutaneously in the head and neck region as well as in the axilla. Rarely, however, they can be found in the trunk within the internal organs or the connective tissue in and about the abdominal or thoracic cavities. The treatment of lymphangiomas should be surgical excision, with care taken to preserve all normal surrounding infiltrated structures.

Lymphangiosarcoma is a rare tumor that develops as a complication of long-standing (usually more than 10 years) lymphedema.[45] Clinically, the patients present with acute worsening of the edema and appearance of subcutaneous nodules that have a propensity toward hemorrhage and ulceration. The tumor can be treated, like other sarcomas, with preoperative chemotherapy and radiation followed by surgical excision, which usually may take the form of radical amputation. Overall, the tumor has a very poor prognosis.[46]

SELECTED REFERENCES

Baumeister RGH: Lymphedema. In Cronenwett JL, Johnston KW, editors: *Rutherford's vascular surgery*, ed 8, Philadelphia, 2014, Elsevier Saunders, pp 1028–1042.

This authoritative treatise provides a succinct summary of the treatment of lymphatic disorders.

Campisi CC, Ryan M, Boccardo F, et al: A single-site technique of multiple lymphatic-venous anastomoses for the treatment of peripheral lymphedema: Long-term clinical outcome. *J Reconstr Microsurg* 2015. [Epub ahead of print].
Granzow JW, Soderberg JM, Kaji AH, et al: Review of current surgical treatments for lymphedema. *Ann Surg Oncol* 21:1195–1201, 2014.

These comprehensive reviews summarize the important elements in the management of patients with lymphedema.

Rockson SG: Diagnosis and management of lymphatic vascular disease. *J Am Coll Cardiol* 52:799–806, 2008.
The diagnosis and treatment of peripheral lymphedema. 2009 Consensus Document of the International Society of Lymphology. *Lymphology* 42:51–60, 2009.

These two reviews illustrate the current knowledge and controversies in the pathophysiology, classification, natural history, differential diagnosis, and treatment of lymphedema.

REFERENCES

1. Levine C: Primary disorders of the lymphatic vessels—a unified concept. *J Pediatr Surg* 24:233–240, 1989.
2. Alitalo K, Tammela T, Petrova TV: Lymphangiogenesis in development and human disease. *Nature* 438:946–953, 2005.
3. Mortimer PS, Rockson SG: New developments in clinical aspects of lymphatic disease. *J Clin Invest* 124:915–921, 2014.
4. Connell FC, Gordon K, Brice G, et al: The classification and diagnostic algorithm for primary lymphatic dysplasia: an update from 2010 to include molecular findings. *Clin Genet* 84:303–314, 2013.
5. Dixon JB: Lymphatic lipid transport: Sewer or subway? *Trends Endocrinol Metab* 21:480–487, 2010.
6. Browse NL, Stewart G: Lymphoedema: Pathophysiology and classification. *J Cardiovasc Surg (Torino)* 26:91–106, 1985.
7. Cho S, Atwood JE: Peripheral edema. *Am J Med* 113:580–586, 2002.
8. Radhakrishnan K, Rockson SG: The clinical spectrum of lymphatic disease. *Ann N Y Acad Sci* 1131:155–184, 2008.
9. Rockson SG: Diagnosis and management of lymphatic vascular disease. *J Am Coll Cardiol* 52:799–806, 2008.
10. Barrett T, Choyke PL, Kobayashi H: Imaging of the lymphatic system: New horizons. *Contrast Media Mol Imaging* 1:230–245, 2006.
11. Szuba A, Shin WS, Strauss HW, et al: The third circulation: Radionuclide lymphoscintigraphy in the evaluation of lymphedema. *J Nucl Med* 44:43–57, 2003.
12. Weissleder H, Weissleder R: Interstitial lymphangiography: Initial clinical experience with a dimeric nonionic contrast agent. *Radiology* 170:371–374, 1989.
13. Liu NF, Lu Q, Jiang ZH, et al: Anatomic and functional evaluation of the lymphatics and lymph nodes in diagnosis of lymphatic circulation disorders with contrast magnetic resonance lymphangiography. *J Vasc Surg* 49:980–987, 2009.
14. The diagnosis and treatment of peripheral lymphedema. 2009 Consensus Document of the International Society of Lymphology. *Lymphology* 42:51–60, 2009.
15. Kerchner K, Fleischer A, Yosipovitch G: Lower extremity lymphedema update: Pathophysiology, diagnosis, and treatment guidelines. *J Am Acad Dermatol* 59:324–331, 2008.
16. Yasuhara H, Shigematsu H, Muto T: A study of the advantages of elastic stockings for leg lymphedema. *Int Angiol* 15:272–277, 1996.
17. Badger CM, Peacock JL, Mortimer PS: A randomized, controlled, parallel-group clinical trial comparing multilayer bandaging followed by hosiery versus hosiery alone in the treatment of patients with lymphedema of the limb. *Cancer* 88:2832–2837, 2000.
18. Franzeck UK, Spiegel I, Fischer M, et al: Combined physical therapy for lymphedema evaluated by fluorescence microlymphography and lymph capillary pressure measurements. *J Vasc Res* 34:306–311, 1997.

19. Richmand DM, O'Donnell TF, Jr, Zelikovski A: Sequential pneumatic compression for lymphedema. A controlled trial. *Arch Surg* 120:1116–1119, 1985.

20. Casley-Smith JR, Morgan RG, Piller NB: Treatment of lymphedema of the arms and legs with 5,6-benzo-[alpha]-pyrone. *N Engl J Med* 329:1158–1163, 1993.

21. Loprinzi CL, Kugler JW, Sloan JA, et al: Lack of effect of coumarin in women with lymphedema after treatment for breast cancer. *N Engl J Med* 340:346–350, 1999.

22. Nakamura K, Rockson SG: Molecular targets for therapeutic lymphangiogenesis in lymphatic dysfunction and disease. *Lymphat Res Biol* 6:181–189, 2008.

23. Tervala T, Suominen E, Saaristo A: Targeted treatment for lymphedema and lymphatic metastasis. *Ann N Y Acad Sci* 1131:215–224, 2008.

24. Campisi C, Boccardo F: Lymphedema and microsurgery. *Microsurgery* 22:74–80, 2002.

25. Gloviczki P: Principles of surgical treatment of chronic lymphoedema. *Int Angiol* 18:42–46, 1999.

26. Damstra RJ, Voesten HG, van Schelven WD, et al: Lymphatic venous anastomosis (LVA) for treatment of secondary arm lymphedema. A prospective study of 11 LVA procedures in 10 patients with breast cancer related lymphedema and a critical review of the literature. *Breast Cancer Res Treat* 113:199–206, 2009.

27. Nagase T, Gonda K, Inoue K, et al: Treatment of lymphedema with lymphaticovenular anastomoses. *Int J Clin Oncol* 10:304–310, 2005.

28. Baumeister RG, Frick A: [The microsurgical lymph vessel transplantation]. *Handchir Mikrochir Plast Chir* 35:202–209, 2003.

29. Campisi CC, Ryan M, Boccardo F, et al: A single-site technique of multiple lymphatic-venous anastomoses for the treatment of peripheral lymphedema: Long-term clinical outcome. *J Reconstr Microsurg* 2015. [Epub ahead of print].

30. Goldsmith HS: Long term evaluation of omental transposition for chronic lymphedema. *Ann Surg* 180:847–849, 1974.

31. Hurst PA, Stewart G, Kinmonth JB, et al: Long term results of the enteromesenteric bridge operation in the treatment of primary lymphoedema. *Br J Surg* 72:272–274, 1985.

32. Miller TA, Wyatt LE, Rudkin GH: Staged skin and subcutaneous excision for lymphedema: A favorable report of long-term results. *Plast Reconstr Surg* 102:1486–1498, discussion 1499-1501, 1998.

33. Wyatt LE, Miller TA: Lymphedema and tumors of the lymphatics. In Moore W, editor: *Vascular surgery, a comprehensive review*, Philadelphia, 1998, WB Saunders, pp 829–843.

34. Espinosa-de-Los-Monteros A, Hinojosa CA, Abarca L, et al: Compression therapy and liposuction of lower legs for bilateral hereditary primary lymphedema praecox. *J Vasc Surg* 49:222–224, 2009.

35. Brorson H, Ohlin K, Olsson G, et al: Controlled compression and liposuction treatment for lower extremity lymphedema. *Lymphology* 41:52–63, 2008.

36. Dellon AL, Hoopes JE: The Charles procedure for primary lymphedema. Long-term clinical results. *Plast Reconstr Surg* 60:589–595, 1977.

37. Dandapat MC, Mohapatro SK, Mohanty SS: Filarial lymphoedema and elephantiasis of lower limb: A review of 44 cases. *Br J Surg* 73:451–453, 1986.

38. Miller TA: Charles procedure for lymphedema: A warning. *Am J Surg* 139:290–292, 1980.

39. Platis IE, Nwogu CE: Chylothorax. *Thorac Surg Clin* 16:209–214, 2006.

40. Bender B, Murthy V, Chamberlain RS: The changing management of chylothorax in the modern era. *Eur J Cardiothorac Surg* 49:18–24, 2016.

41. Lee EW, Shin JH, Ko HK, et al: Lymphangiography to treat postoperative lymphatic leakage: A technical review. *Korean J Radiol* 15:724–732, 2014.

42. Lyon S, Mott N, Koukounaras J, et al: Role of interventional radiology in the management of chylothorax: A review of the current management of high output chylothorax. *Cardiovasc Intervent Radiol* 36:599–607, 2013.

43. Aalami OO, Allen DB, Organ CH, Jr: Chylous ascites: A collective review. *Surgery* 128:761–778, 2000.

44. Ha J, Yu YC, Lannigan F: A review of the management of lymphangiomas. *Curr Pediatr Rev* 10:238–248, 2014.

45. Nakazono T, Kudo S, Matsuo Y, et al: Angiosarcoma associated with chronic lymphedema (Stewart-Treves syndrome) of the leg: MR imaging. *Skeletal Radiol* 29:413–416, 2000.

46. Sordillo PP, Chapman R, Hajdu SI, et al: Lymphangiosarcoma. *Cancer* 48:1674–1679, 1981.

SPECIALTIES IN GENERAL SURGERY

第十三篇　普通外科相关的专科

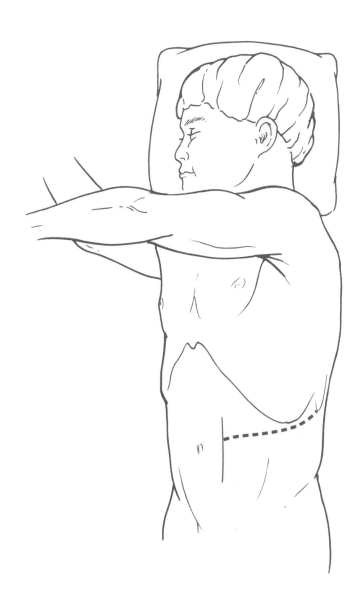

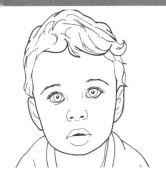

Pediatric Surgery

Dai H. Chung

第六十六章　小儿外科

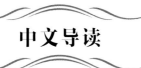

中文导读

本章共分为14节：①新生儿生理；②液体、电解质和营养；③头颈病变；④体外循环；⑤先天性膈疝；⑥肺部畸形；⑦消化道疾病；⑧肝胆疾病；⑨腹壁疾病；⑩胸壁畸形；⑪泌尿生殖系统疾病；⑫小儿实体肿瘤；⑬小儿创伤；⑭胎儿手术。

第一节讲述了新生儿出生时各器官系统功能不成熟是外科疾病管理过程中的重要挑战，着重强调了心血管系统、呼吸系统和免疫系统。

第二节是关于小儿水电解质平衡及营养支持治疗，需根据液体丢失量、摄入量和电解质失衡情况确定补液量，对小儿能量、糖类、蛋白质和脂肪的需求进行了详细的阐述，并进一步介绍了全肠外营养。

第三节颈部疾病包括皮样囊肿和表皮样囊肿、病理性淋巴结、淋巴管瘤、甲状舌管囊肿、鳃裂囊肿、斜颈，从定义、临床表现、诊断、治疗等方面进行进一步阐述。

第四节主要讲述了体外循环的适应证、生理功能

及相关并发症。

第五节先天性膈疝是小儿外科最难治疗的疾病之一，介绍了其发病机制、临床表现、诊断和治疗，并详细介绍了手术修补时机及修补方式的历史演变。

第六节肺部畸形主要包括支气管源性囊肿、先天性肺呼吸道畸形、肺隔离症、先天性肺气肿，并详细介绍了相关发病机制、诊断与产前诊断、治疗预后等。

第七节消化道疾病是本章重点介绍的部分，代表性疾病有食管闭锁和气管食管瘘、胃食管反流、肥厚性幽门狭窄、肠闭锁、肠旋转不良伴中肠扭转、坏死性小肠结肠炎、短肠综合征、胎粪性肠梗阻、先天性

巨结肠、肛门直肠畸形、肠套叠、梅克尔憩室。本节对上述疾病从病理生理、临床表现和分型、诊断、治疗预后等方面分别进行了详细介绍。

第八节重点讲述了胆道闭锁和胆总管囊肿的发病机制、临床表现、诊断和治疗预后等内容，并描述了遗传性胰腺炎和胰腺分裂症、胆囊运动障碍疾病。

第九节主要讲述了腹壁缺损（包括脐膨出和腹裂）和疝（包括腹股沟疝和脐疝）。

第十节胸壁畸形主要包括漏斗胸和鸡胸，讲述了其临床表现和诊断治疗。

第十一节主要讲述了隐睾、睾丸扭转、睾丸肿瘤

的临床表现、诊断治疗和预后。

第十二节小儿实体肿瘤主要包括神经母细胞瘤、Wilms瘤、横纹肌肉瘤、肝脏肿瘤、畸胎瘤和卵巢肿瘤，对各肿瘤的临床表现、基因组学、诊断和分期、治疗和预后进行了详细的介绍。

第十三节主要讲述小儿外伤后的ABC急救处理，小儿头和脊柱外伤、胸外伤、腹部外伤、胰腺损伤和肾损伤后的临床表现、诊断及治疗。

第十四节主要讲述了胎儿手术的适应证及研究进展。

〔冯杰雄　李　宁〕

Pediatric surgery is the last bastion of a true general surgical specialty, delivering comprehensive surgical care covering a broad scope of conditions in infants, children, and young adults. Pediatric surgeons are challenged with the evaluation and management of a wide spectrum of surgical pathologic processes ranging from head and neck lesions to thoracic and gastrointestinal (GI) tract anomalies, oncologic disorders, and trauma. This chapter highlights common and unique pediatric surgical conditions.

NEWBORN PHYSIOLOGY

The newborn physiology is unique in many ways. The smaller size of the patient, volume capacities, and functional immaturity of various organ systems present unique physiologic challenges in the management of surgical disease. Newborns are at risk for cold stress and must be maintained in an ideal thermal environment to reduce oxygen consumption and metabolic demands. The major contributing factors for hypothermia in infants include their relatively large body surface area, lack of hair and subcutaneous tissue, and greater insensible losses. Infants also respond to cold ambient temperature by a mechanism of nonshivering thermogenesis, whereby increases in metabolism and oxygen consumption occur. For radiant and evaporative heat loss to be avoided, the use of overhead radiant heaters and warming lights is a common practice, but a caution for significant insensible water losses should be made.

Cardiovascular

In fetal circulation, arterial blood from the placenta bypasses the lungs through the patent foramen ovale and ductus arteriosus. With the newborn's first breath, the foramen ovale closes, along with a precipitous drop in pulmonary vascular resistance, thereby increasing pulmonary blood flow. Decreased blood flow along with a higher oxygen content also promotes spontaneous closure of the ductus arteriosus. A variety of physiologic factors, such as hypoxemia, acidosis, and sepsis, can contribute to persistent

pulmonary hypertension (PPHN) with right-to-left shunt. Prematurity is also significantly associated with persistent ductus arteriosus. Nonsteroidal anti-inflammatory drugs, such as indomethacin, induce closure of a patent ductus arteriosus in premature infants. If this treatment is unsuccessful, surgical ligation may be necessary. An infant heart has a limited capacity to increase the stroke volume, and therefore cardiac output is largely heart rate dependent. As such, bradycardia can significantly diminish cardiac output. Capillary refill is a sensitive indicator of adequate cardiac perfusion. A prolonged capillary refill longer than 1 to 2 seconds may represent substantial shunting of blood from the peripheral tissues to the central organs, as may occur with cardiogenic or hypovolemic shock.

Pulmonary

The infant lungs are considered immature at birth, and they continue to develop new terminal bronchioles and alveoli until about 8 years of age. Immature lungs have fewer type II pneumocytes and hence a lower production of surfactant. Surfactant regulates alveolar surface tension and thereby increasing functional residual capacity. Therefore, premature infants are at significant risk for alveolar collapse, hyaline membrane formation, and barotrauma. Surfactant is a lipoprotein mixture of phospholipid, protein, and neutral fats. Lecithin, the most predominant phospholipid, can be measured in amniotic fluid, and the lecithin-to-sphingomyelin ratio is used to determine fetal lung maturity. In addition to parenchymal disease, the newborn airway is small (tracheal diameter of 2.5 to 4 mm) and easily plugged with secretions. The respiratory rate for a normal newborn may range from 40 to 60 breaths/min, with a tidal volume of 6 to 10 mL/kg. Nasal flaring, grunting, intercostal and substernal retractions, and cyanosis constitute symptoms of respiratory distress. Infants are obligate nasal and diaphragmatic breathers, and therefore any condition that obstructs the nasal passages (including the nasogastric tube) or interferes with diaphragmatic function may result in severe respiratory compromise. Exogenous surfactant therapy has had a major impact on the management of premature infants.

This has resulted in improved survival and decreased incidence of bronchopulmonary dysplasia, a condition characterized by oxygen dependence, radiologic abnormality, and chronic respiratory symptoms beyond the first 28 days of life. The administration of nitric oxide gas, a potent inducer of vascular smooth muscle relaxation, has also proved useful in infants with PPHN.

Immunology

Infants have lower levels of immunoglobulins (A, G, and M) and of the C3b component of complement at birth. As such, premature infants are at higher risk for systemic infection. The evaluation of sepsis in neonates requires an extensive workup of surveillance cultures of blood, urine, and cerebrospinal fluid as well as a complete blood count with platelet count, differential smear, and plain radiography. Sepsis may result from various invasive devices and therapies that are essential to the care of premature infants, such as prolonged endotracheal intubation, umbilical catheters, and bladder catheterization. Based on subtle clinical changes (e.g., decreased tolerance of enteral feeding, temperature instability, reduced capillary refill, tachypnea, irritability), implementation of empirical antibiotic therapy targeted at common bacterial pathogens, such as group B beta-hemolytic streptococcus, methicillin-resistant *Staphylococcus aureus,* and *Escherichia coli,* may be lifesaving.

FLUIDS, ELECTROLYTES, AND NUTRITION

Fluid and Electrolytes

Fluid and electrolyte therapy requires careful assessment of total fluid intake and losses and electrolyte imbalances before initiation of fluid administration. It also requires frequent monitoring during the course of therapy to ensure the proper response. Accurate estimation of intravenous (IV) fluid and electrolytes is critical, especially in small infants with a narrow margin for error. Because of higher insensible water losses through a thin immature skin barrier, fluid requirements for premature infants are substantial. Insensible water losses are directly related to gestational age, ranging from 45 to 60 mL/kg/day for premature infants weighing less than 1500 g to 30 to 35 mL/kg/day for term infants. Radiant heat warmers, phototherapy for hyperbilirubinemia, and respiratory distress can result in additional fluid loss. In the first 3 to 5 days of life, there is a physiologic water loss of up to 10% of the body weight of the infant. As such, fluid replacement volumes are less during the first several days of life. These fluid volumes are regarded as estimates and may change according to differing clinical conditions.

Fluid requirements are calculated according to body weight (Table 66-1). During the first few days of life, the fluid recommendations are conservative; however, infants require 100 to 130 mL/kg/day for maintenance fluids by the fourth day of life. Infants with conditions that are associated with excessive fluid losses (e.g., gastroschisis) can require as much as 1.5 times maintenance volume. The best indicators of sufficient fluid intake are urine output and osmolarity. The minimum urine output in a newborn and young child is 1 to 2 mL/kg/day. Although adults can concentrate urine in the range of 1200 mOsm/kg, an infant responding to water deprivation is able to concentrate urine only up to approximately 700 mOsm/kg. Clinically, this indicates that greater fluid intake and urine output are necessary to excrete the solute load presented to the kidney during normal metabolism. In general, the daily requirements for sodium and potassium are 2 to 4 and 1 to 2 mEq/kg, respectively. These requirements are usually met with 5% dextrose in 0.45% normal saline with 20 mEq/liter of potassium at the calculated maintenance rate. Fluid losses from gastric drainage, ostomy output, or diarrhea should also be carefully assessed and replaced with an appropriate solution. Gastric losses should be replaced in equal volumes with 0.45% normal saline with 20 mEq/liter of potassium. Diarrheal, pancreatic, and biliary losses are replaced with isotonic lactated Ringer solution. Hypovolemia due to acute hemorrhage should be corrected with rapid transfusion of blood products at a bolus of 10 to 20 mL/kg of packed red blood cells, plasma, or 5% albumin.

Nutrition

Calorie Requirements

Energy requirements vary significantly from birth to childhood and also under different clinical conditions (Table 66-2). The parameter that is most indicative of sufficient delivery of calories in neonates is appropriate weight gain. Total daily calorie requirements and the weight growth curve plateau with age. Nearly 50% of the energy used in term infants younger than 2 weeks and 60% of energy intake in premature infants weighing less than 1200 g is devoted to growth. A general guideline for the enteral calorie requirement of infants is 120 calories/kg/day to achieve an ideal weight gain on average of about 1% of body weight/day. The standard infant formulas as well as breast milk contain 20 calories/ounce. Formulas with higher calorie density are available for those who are unable to consume sufficient volumes to meet their calorie requirements or require fluid restriction. Breast milk or a protein hydrolysate formula (e.g., Pregestimil, Alimentum) should be considered when initiating enteral feedings in infants with compromised gut functions, such as necrotizing enterocolitis or short bowel syndrome. In general, continuous feedings are initiated for infants with a stressed gut and later transitioned to bolus feedings. The enteral feeding tolerance is carefully monitored by assessing for abdominal girth, gastric residuals, and stool output.

TABLE 66-1 Daily Fluid Requirements

WEIGHT	VOLUME
Premature infants <2 kg	140-150 mL/kg/day
Infants, 2-10 kg	100 mL/kg/day
Toddler, 10-20 kg	1000 mL + 50 mL/kg/day for weight 10-20 kg
Children >20 kg	1500 mL + 20 mL/kg/day for weight >20 kg

TABLE 66-2 Average Calorie and Protein Requirements

AGE	CALORIES (kcal/kg/day)	PROTEIN (g/kg/day)
0-1 year	90-120	2.0-3.5
1-7 years	75-90	2.0-2.5
7-12 years	60-75	2.0
12-18 years	30-60	1.5
>18 years	25-30	1.0

Carbohydrate

Carbohydrates are stored mainly as glycogen in the liver and muscles. Because newborn liver and muscle masses are disproportionately smaller than those of the adult, infants are susceptible to hypoglycemia with risks for seizure and neurologic impairment. The minimum glucose infusion rate for neonates is 4 to 6 mg/kg/min. This rate must be calculated daily while the infant is receiving parenteral nutrition. For total parenteral nutrition (TPN), the glucose infusion rate is increased in daily increments of 1 to 2 mg/kg/min to a maximum of 10 to 12 mg/kg/min. Ultimately, the amount of weight gain should dictate the need to continue advancing glucose calories. Furthermore, hyperglycemia from too rapid advancement or underlying sepsis should be avoided because it can lead to rapid hyperosmolarity and dehydration.

Protein

The average intake of protein represents approximately 15% of the total daily calories and ranges from 2 to 3.5 g/kg/day in infants. This protein requirement is reduced in half by the age of 12 years and approaches the adult requirement (1 g/kg/day) by 18 years of age (see Table 66-2). The provision of greater amounts of protein relative to nonprotein calories will result in rising blood urea nitrogen levels. The nonprotein calorie (carbohydrate plus fat calories)–to–protein calorie ratio (when expressed in grams of nitrogen) is therefore not less than 150 to 1. For infants receiving parenteral nutrition, protein administration usually starts at 0.5 g/kg/day and advances in daily increments of 0.5 g/kg/day to the target goal of approximately 3.5 g/kg/day.

Fat

Fat is the other major source of nonprotein calories. Linoleic acid, an 18-carbon chain with two double bonds, is considered an essential fatty acid; its deficiency results in dryness, rash, and desquamation of skin. In pediatric patients, fat is provided as a major source of calories to prevent the development of essential fatty acid deficiency. The lipid requirements for growth are significant, and fat is a robust calorie source. Similar to protein, fat infusions are started at 0.5 g/kg/day and advanced up to 2.5 to 3.5 g/kg/day. In infants with unconjugated hyperbilirubinemia, fat is administered with caution because fatty acids may displace bilirubin from albumin. The free unconjugated bilirubin may then cross the blood-brain barrier and can lead to kernicterus, resulting in mental retardation.

Total Parenteral Nutrition

TPN is reserved for infants for whom GI delivery of adequate daily calories is not feasible for various reasons. Deposition of body fat occurs in the later stages of fetal development, leaving premature infants poorly equipped to deal with periods of starvation as rapid as 2 to 3 days. Thus, an infant's need for parenteral nutrition should be addressed early. Unlike in adults, the key to prescribing pediatric TPN is that the IV infusion rate remains the same, whereas the concentration of nutrients is gradually increased daily until nutritional goals are met. Infants with surgical conditions often become cholestatic, usually caused by prolonged TPN support; however, other causes should be ruled out. Serum bile acid levels are usually elevated first, then direct bilirubin concentration, followed by liver enzyme levels. The ideal treatment for TPN-associated cholestasis is enteral feeding. The use of omega-3 fat emulsion (Omegaven) has helped infants with TPN-induced cholestasis. A medium-chain triglyceride–containing formula is used, and if an infant is receiving total enteral nutrition, fat-soluble vitamins should be supplemented.

HEAD AND NECK LESIONS

Dermoid and Epidermoid Cysts

Dermoid and epidermoid cysts are slow-growing benign lesions that typically occur in the scalp and the skull of infants and children. These cysts usually arise from part of the dermal or epidermal tissues, forming a small cyst filled with normal skin components. Dermoids may contain hair, teeth, and skin glands. Epidermoids typically contain only epidermal tissue and keratin debris. They commonly occur on the forehead, lateral corner of the eyebrow, or anterior fontanelle or in the postauricular space. They are generally asymptomatic but may slowly increase in size over time. Cysts may erode into the skull and in the extremely rare situation may even penetrate into the brain. Most scalp lesions can be accurately diagnosed by physical examination alone. However, imaging studies may be important for those at midline to rule out a communicating cephalocele. Surgical excision is recommended.

Lymphadenopathy

Enlarged lymph nodes are one of the most common pediatric conditions resulting in referral to a pediatric surgeon for evaluation, biopsy, or excision. They occur usually along the sternocleidomastoid muscle border, often in clusters. The cause is unknown but thought to be multifocal. A detailed history and physical examination are sufficient to determine surgical indications. The use of ultrasound has become prevalent recently. In most healthy children, cervical lymphadenopathy presents as a small, mobile, rubbery, palpable mass in the anterior cervical triangle. However, relatively fixed, nontender, progressively enlarging nodes in the supraclavicular region should raise suspicion for more serious underlying conditions. Other symptoms, such as night sweats and recent weight loss, should also prompt a thorough investigation. Chest radiography can be a helpful screening modality to detect mediastinal adenopathy. Patients with acute, bilateral cervical lymphadenitis from respiratory viral infectious causes (e.g., adenovirus, influenza virus, respiratory syncytial virus) are observed alone. *S. aureus* and group A streptococcus are responsible for the majority of acute pyogenic lymphadenitis. When nodes become fluctuant because of central areas of liquefying necrosis, a needle aspiration or incision and drainage should be performed.

Cat-scratch disease is a self-limited infectious condition characterized by painful regional lymphadenopathy. *Bartonella henselae*, a gram-negative bacillus, is responsible for most cases. A history of exposure to cats is helpful but not always present. Indirect immunofluorescent antibody testing has only moderate specificity, and therefore polymerase chain reaction assay of a lymph node biopsy specimen is more useful for diagnosis. There is no specific treatment for cat-scratch disease because it is usually self-limited. A less common infectious cause of cervical lymphadenitis is nontuberculous mycobacterial infection. The nodes are fluctuant, with a violaceous appearance of the overlying skin. The diagnosis is made by positive cultures for nontuberculous acid-fast bacilli along with a tuberculin skin test. Surgical excision is usually indicated because most nontuberculous mycobacteria are resistant to conventional chemotherapy.

Cystic Hygroma

Cystic hygroma is a multiloculated cystic space lined by endothelial cells occurring as a result of lymphatic malformation. Most cystic hygromas involve the lymphatic jugular sacs and present in the posterior neck region. The other common sites are the axillary, mediastinal, inguinal, and retroperitoneal regions, and approximately 50% of these cystic lesions are present at birth. Cystic hygromas are soft cystic masses that distort the surrounding anatomy, including the airway. A large cystic mass of the neck in the fetus can impose a significant risk to the airway at birth and may be associated with chromosomal abnormalities. Prenatal ultrasound and fetal magnetic resonance imaging (MRI) studies allow careful coordination of surgical intervention at the time of delivery. Cystic hygromas are prone to infection and hemorrhage within the mass. MRI can be helpful in preoperative planning. In general, complete surgical excision is the preferred treatment. However, this may be difficult because of the intimate involvement with surrounding vital structures. Surgical resections are generally tedious, requiring careful isolation and ligation of lymphatic branches. Aggressive blunt and electrocautery dissections can result in incomplete control of lymphatics, leading to recurrence or infection caused by accumulation of the lymphatic leak. Radical resection with sacrifice of vital structures must be avoided. Injection of sclerosing agents, such as bleomycin, doxycycline, or OK-432 derived from *Streptococcus pyogenes,* has been reported to be effective in the nonoperative management of cystic hygromas.[1]

Thyroglossal Duct Cyst

A thyroglossal duct cyst is a midline neck lesion that originates at the base of the tongue at the foramen cecum and descends through the central portion of the hyoid bone. Although thyroglossal duct cysts may occur anywhere from the base of the tongue to the thyroid gland, most are found at or just below the hyoid bone (Fig. 66-1A). A thyroid diverticulum develops as a median endodermal thickening at the foramen cecum in the embryonic stage of development. The thyroid diverticulum descends in the neck and remains attached to the base of the tongue by the thyroglossal duct. Also, as the thyroid gland descends to its normal pretracheal position, the ventral cartilages of the second and third branchial arches form the hyoid bone—hence the intimate anatomic relationship of the thyroglossal duct remnant with the central portion

of the hyoid bone. The thyroglossal duct normally regresses by the time the thyroid gland reaches its final position. When the elements of the duct persist despite complete thyroid descent, a thyroglossal duct cyst may develop. Failure of normal caudal migration of the thyroid gland results in a lingual thyroid, in which no other thyroid tissue is present in the neck. Ultrasound or radionuclide imaging may provide useful information to identify the presence of an ectopic thyroid gland in the neck. The standard operation for thyroglossal duct cysts has remained unchanged since it was described by Sistrunk in 1928, which involves complete excision of the cyst in continuity with its tract, the central portion of the hyoid bone, and the tract interior to the hyoid bone extending to the base of the tongue (Fig. 66-1B). Failure to remove these tissues entirely will likely result in recurrence because multiple sinuses have been histologically identified in these locations.

Branchial Cleft Remnants

The branchial cleft remnants typically present as a lateral neck mass on a toddler. The structures of the head and neck are derived from six pairs of branchial arches, their intervening clefts, and pouches. Congenital cysts, sinuses, or fistulas result from failure of these structures to regress, persisting in an aberrant location. The location of these remnants generally dictates their embryologic origin and guides the subsequent operative approach. Failure to understand the embryology may result in incomplete resection or injury to adjacent structures. All branchial remnants are present at the time of birth; however, they are often not recognized until later in life. These lesions can be manifested as sinuses, fistulas, or cartilaginous rests in infants (Fig. 66-2). However, they present more commonly as cysts in toddlers and older children. The clinical presentation ranges from a continuous mucoid drainage from a fistula or sinus to the development of a cystic mass that may become infected. Branchial remnants may also be palpable as cartilaginous lumps or cords corresponding with a fistulous track. Dermal pits or skin tags may also be present.

First branchial remnants are typically located in the front or back of the ear or in the upper neck near the mandible. Fistulas typically course through the parotid gland, deep or through

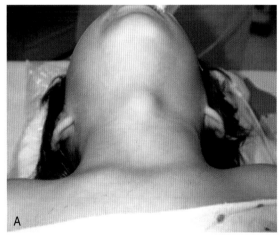
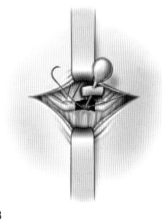

A   B

FIGURE 66-1 A, Thyroglossal duct cyst presents as a midline neck mass. **B,** Sistrunk procedure consists of excision of the thyroglossal duct cyst up to its origin at the foramen cecum, including the central portion of hyoid bone. (From Josephs MD: Thyroglossal duct cyst. In Chung DH, Chen MK, editors: *Atlas of pediatric surgical techniques*, Philadelphia, 2010, Elsevier Saunders, pp 28–33.)

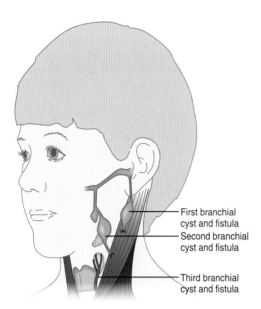

FIGURE 66-2 Branchial cleft cyst and fistula. First branchial cleft sinus occurs along the line extending from the auditory canal to the angle of the mandible. Second branchial cleft sinus is the more common type, typically along the anterior border of the sternocleidomastoid muscle. Third and fourth branchial cleft sinuses are rare in the more inferior aspect of the neck. (From Wesley JR: Branchial cysts, sinuses, and fistulas. In Spitz LS, Coran AG, editors: *Operative pediatric surgery*, London, 2006, Edward Arnold Ltd, p 60.)

branches of the facial nerve, and end in the external auditory canal. The second branchial cleft remnants are the most common type. The external ostium of these remnants is located along the anterior border of the sternocleidomastoid muscle, usually in the vicinity of the upper half to lower third of the muscle. The course of the fistula must be anticipated preoperatively because stepladder counterincisions are often necessary to excise the fistula track completely. Typically, the fistula penetrates the platysma, ascends along the carotid sheath to the level of the hyoid bone, and turns medially to extend between the carotid artery bifurcations. The fistula then courses behind the posterior belly of the digastric and stylohyoid muscles to end in the tonsillar fossa. Third branchial cleft remnants usually do not have associated sinuses or fistulas and are located in the suprasternal notch or clavicular region. These most often contain cartilage and present clinically as a firm mass or subcutaneous abscess.

Torticollis

Torticollis is a state of abnormal muscle tone in the neck, causing the head to twist and turn to one side. It may be congenital or acquired and can occur at any age. In infants with congenital torticollis, the head is typically tilted toward the side of the affected muscle and rotated in the opposite direction. Congenital torticollis presents within a few weeks after birth as an isolated condition. However, acquired torticollis may be associated with a range of conditions, including acute myositis, brainstem tumors, atlantoaxial subluxation, and infectious causes, such as retropharyngeal abscess, cervical adenitis, or tonsillitis. The diagnosis is typically based solely on the clinical examination findings. Treatment is physical therapy involving passive range of motion stretching of the affected muscle for several months. Surgical resection or division of the involved muscle is rarely indicated.

EXTRACORPOREAL LIFE SUPPORT

Extracorporeal life support (ECLS) is a cardiopulmonary bypass that provides temporary support for the critically ill patient with acute refractory respiratory or cardiac failure. In general, ECLS delivers sufficient gas exchange and maintains circulatory support, thus allowing physiologic recovery. The largest experience with ECLS has been for respiratory failure in newborns. Since its first reported neonatal case in 1976, ECLS has become a standard therapeutic option for refractory cardiopulmonary failure in infants and children. There are 226 centers around the world contributing registry data to the Extracorporeal Life Support Organization database (ELSO registry data; July 2015). In 2014 alone, 6510 pediatric and adult patients were supported on ECLS.

Indications

The major indications for neonatal extracorporeal membrane oxygenation (ECMO) include meconium aspiration, respiratory distress syndrome, PPHN, sepsis, and congenital diaphragmatic hernia. Neonates with complex congenital cardiac defects may be supported with ECMO perioperatively. Meconium aspiration is the most common application for neonatal ECMO with the highest survival rate (>90%) among all conditions. Inclusion criteria for the neonatal ECMO vary somewhat among institutions. In general, ECMO is justified when an infant's overall condition deteriorates to a point of roughly 80% predicted mortality. Two guidelines have been historically used as a means to predict survival without ECMO. The alveolar-arterial difference in the partial pressure of oxygen ($PAO_2 - PaO_2$ [also known as $AaDO_2$]) is calculated as

$$AaDO_2 = (\text{atmospheric pressure} - 47) - (PaO_2 + PaCO_2)$$

$AaDO_2$ above 610 for longer than 8 to 12 hours and $AaDO_2$ above 620 for 6 hours, associated with extensive barotrauma and severe hypotension requiring inotropic support, are considered to be criteria for ECMO. The oxygen index is calculated as the fraction of inspired oxygen (usually 1.0) multiplied by the mean airway pressure × 100 divided by PaO_2. An 80% mortality is observed with an oxygen index above 40. Exclusion criteria include gestational age of less than 34 weeks, birth weight of less than 2 kg, intracranial hemorrhage, and a nonreversible pulmonary disease such as congenital alveolar dysplasia. However, with recent advances, gestational age of less than 34 weeks and weight of less than 2 kg are now considered only relative contraindications at many centers. Additional exclusion criteria are presence of cyanotic congenital heart disease or major genetic defects that preclude survival, intractable coagulopathy or hemorrhage, sonographic evidence of a significant intracranial hemorrhage (higher than a grade I intraventricular hemorrhage), and more than 10 to 14 days of high-pressure mechanical ventilatory support. Before ECMO, infants must be evaluated with echocardiography and cranial ultrasound for cyanotic heart defect and significant intracranial hemorrhage, respectively.

Physiology

The basic principle of ECLS is to drain desaturated venous blood, to exchange carbon dioxide and oxygen through the membrane oxygenator, and then to return oxygenated warmed blood into the circulation. Venoarterial bypass is used most commonly for full cardiopulmonary support. The right internal

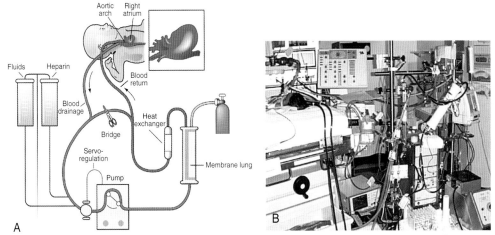

FIGURE 66-3 A, Extracorporeal life support circuit. A venoarterial circuit diagram is shown here. (From Shanley CJ, Bartlett RH: Extracorporeal life support: Techniques, indications, and results. In Cameron JL, editor: *Current surgical therapy,* ed 4, St. Louis, 1992, Mosby Year Book, pp 1062–1066.) **B,** A photograph of ECMO circuit supporting an infant with congenital diaphragmatic hernia.

jugular vein and common carotid artery are typically chosen for cannulation because of their vessel sizes, accessibility, and collateral circulation. The ECLS circuit is composed of a silicone rubber bladder that collapses when venous return is diminished, roller pump, membrane oxygenator, heat exchanger, tubing, and connectors. Venous blood from the right atrium drains through the venous cannula to the bladder and is pumped to the membrane oxygenator, where carbon dioxide is removed and oxygen is added (Fig. 66-3). The oxygenated blood then passes through the heat exchanger and is returned to the patient through the arterial cannula. Systemic anticoagulation to prevent clotting of the ECLS circuit puts patients at risk for bleeding complications. Hematocrit, platelet counts, and fibrinogen levels are closely monitored and maintained within acceptable parameters. An ultrasound examination of the head is performed for the first few days of ECLS to monitor for onset of intracranial hemorrhage. Extracorporeal flow is gradually weaned as native cardiac or pulmonary function improves. Indicators of lung recovery include an increasing PaO$_2$, improved lung compliance, and clearing of the chest radiograph. Once the extracorporeal flow rate reaches minimal levels, the patient is trialed off bypass by temporary clamping of the cannulas. If this is tolerated, the patient is taken off ECLS on moderate conventional ventilatory settings. Venovenous bypass support by a double-lumen cannula has the advantages of avoiding carotid arterial cannulation. Often, perfusion of well-oxygenated blood through venovenous ECMO restores hemodynamic stability.

Complications

Bleeding, the most common complication of ECLS, can occur at any invasive catheter sites, such as cannulas in the neck or an arterial line, and in the head, leading to devastating intracranial hemorrhage. Birth weight and gestational age are the most significant correlates of intracranial hemorrhage on ECLS; infants weighing less than 2 kg and younger than 34 weeks of gestational age are at highest risk. Other complications associated with ECLS include seizures, neurologic impairment, renal failure requiring hemofiltration or hemodialysis, hypertension, infection, and mechanical malfunction (e.g., failure of the membrane oxygenator, pump, and heat exchanger).

CONGENITAL DIAPHRAGMATIC HERNIA

Congenital diaphragmatic hernia (CDH) remains one of the most challenging conditions to treat in pediatric surgery. The overall incidence is 1 in 2000 to 5000 live births. Most CDH defects occur on the left side (80%); bilateral defects are extremely rare. A hernia sac is present 20% of the time. Despite recent innovative treatment strategies, such as fetal tracheal occlusion, ECMO, inhaled nitric oxide, and permissive hypercapnic management protocol, the overall survival rates have not changed significantly and remain in the 70% to 90% range. Accurate determination of true survival rate is distorted by the fact that many infants with CDH are stillborn, and many reports tend to exclude infants with complex associated anomalies from survival calculations.

Pathogenesis

CDH is thought to result from failure of closure of the pleuroperitoneal canal in the developing fetus. Normally, the pleuroperitoneal cavities become separated by the developing membrane during weeks 8 to 10 of gestation. When this process fails, the pleuroperitoneal canal does not close, and a posterolateral diaphragmatic defect results. The posterolateral location of this hernia is known as Bochdalek hernia; it is distinguished from a CDH of the anteromedial location known as Morgagni hernia. As a result of the defect, abdominal contents herniate into the thoracic cavity, compressing the ipsilateral developing lung. These lungs have smaller bronchi, with less bronchial branching and less alveolar surface area than lungs in normal infants. The ipsilateral lung is affected more severely; however, both lungs are affected by pulmonary hypoplasia. In addition to the abnormal airway development, the pulmonary vasculature is also significantly affected by increased thickness of arteriolar smooth muscle. Also, arteriolar vasculature is extremely sensitive to the multiple local and systemic vasoactive factors. Hence, the severity of pulmonary hypoplasia and pulmonary hypertension significantly affect the overall morbidity and mortality in CDH infants.

Clinical Presentation and Diagnosis

Most infants with CDH experience respiratory distress at birth. The initial symptoms and signs may include grunting respiration, chest retractions, dyspnea, and cyanosis with scaphoid abdomen. Decreased breath sounds along with bowel sounds may be auscultated over the chest with CDH. The shifting of heart sounds to the right (for left-sided CDH) is common. A significant differential of preductal and postductal pulse oximetry indicates the right-to-left shunting due to PPHN. The diagnosis of CDH is frequently made prenatally as early as 15 weeks of gestation during a routine ultrasound evaluation. Infants who have a late onset of CDH (beyond 25 weeks of gestation) have been reported to have better overall survival. The herniation of the stomach and liver, polyhydramnios, and associated anomalies have been associated with poor outcome. The delivery of a fetus with CDH should be carefully planned and take place at an institution capable of providing advanced neonatal care, including ECMO. The chest radiograph demonstrates multiple bowel loops in the thoracic cavity along with mediastinal shift (Fig. 66-4A). The differential diagnosis includes congenital cystic adenomatoid malformation, bronchogenic cyst, diaphragmatic eventration, and cystic teratoma. In Morgagni hernia, the diagnosis is often delayed until childhood because most infants are asymptomatic. Typically, the infant does well for several hours after delivery during the so-called honeymoon period and then begins to demonstrate worsening respiratory function. Therapeutic interventions are aimed at stabilizing and treating PPHN. In approximately 10% to 20% of cases, CDH is diagnosed beyond the first 24 hours of life, at which time infants present with various symptoms of feeding difficulties, respiratory distress, and pneumonia.

Treatment

The open fetal surgery for CDH failed to show an overall survival advantage and therefore has been abandoned. However, laparoscopic occlusion of the fetal trachea, resulting in accumulation of lung fluid to stimulate lung growth, has gained increasing interest. External tracheal clips or endotracheal balloons can be placed laparoscopically (often referred to as fetoscopy) to occlude the fetal trachea. The Tracheal Occlusion To Accelerate Lung growth (TOTAL) trial is led by several European centers.[2] However, this intervention is not available in the United States because of lack of a Food and Drug Administration–approved device. The postnatal management of CDH is directed toward stabilization of the cardiorespiratory status while minimizing iatrogenic injury from therapeutic interventions. Immediate securing of the airway with endotracheal intubation is critical. Excessive mean airway pressure ventilation can result in pneumothorax and compromised venous blood return to the heart. An orogastric tube is placed to prevent gastric distention, which may worsen the lung compression, mediastinal shift, and ability to ventilate. The major focus in gentler ventilatory management with permissive hypercapnia has resulted in a significantly higher survival rate for CDH infants. Inhaled nitric oxide is used widely for its pulmonary vasodilatory effect. Pharmacologically, the use of tolazoline, a nonselective α-adrenergic blocking agent, as a pulmonary vasodilator has not produced clinically significant results. Sildenafil, a phosphodiesterase type 5 inhibitor, works by inducing pulmonary vascular smooth muscle relaxation and has been used in many centers with various results. A retrospective cohort study showed an increasing trend for the use of a variety of vasodilators for CDH patients.[3]

Surgical Repair

For infants with relatively stable pulmonary status, CDH repair can be safely performed on the second to fourth day of life after the potential honeymoon period. However, the ideal timing of CDH repair on ECMO remains controversial and highly debated; some advocate early operative repair on ECMO, whereas others recommend repair at the time of weaning from ECMO or even after decannulation. There are no clear prospective data to endorse an exact timing of CDH repair for those requiring ECMO support. However, recent reports suggest that CDH repair after ECMO is associated with improved survival compared with repair while on ECMO.[4] At operation, the preferred approach for a posterolateral CDH is through a subcostal abdominal incision. The viscera are reduced into the abdominal cavity, and the posterolateral defect in the diaphragm is approximated with interrupted nonabsorbable sutures. When present (10% to 15% of cases), a hernia sac should be excised. Typically, the hernia defect is large, with only a small leaflet of diaphragmatic tissue present anteromedially. Although primary repair of the defect is ideal, closure with excessive tension must be avoided to prevent hernia recurrence. Some surgeons advocate the use of pledgeted sutures. A number of reconstructive techniques and materials are available for the repair of large hernia defects. The surgical technique of abdominal or thoracic muscle flaps can be considered, but the use

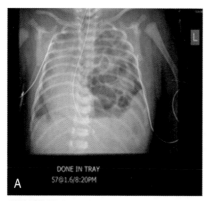
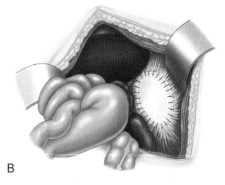

FIGURE 66-4 A, Congenital diaphragmatic hernia. Multiple gas-filled bowel loops are located in the left hemithorax, and the mediastinum is shifted to the right. **B,** Diagram depicting repair of a left congenital diaphragmatic hernia with Gore-Tex patch graft. (From Frischer JS: Congenital diaphragmatic hernia and eventration of the diaphragm. In Chung DH, Chen MK, editors: *Atlas of pediatric surgical techniques,* Philadelphia, 2010, Elsevier Saunders, pp 83–96.)

of prosthetic material, most commonly Gore-Tex patch, has become widespread (Fig. 66-4B). The advantages of a prosthetic patch are shorter operative time and a tension-free repair. However, the major potential problems with prosthetic patches are the risks of infection and recurrence of the hernia. Recently, the use of regenerative extracellular matrix biomaterials has garnered significant interest as an ideal biodegradable patch (e.g., Surgisis [Cook Medical Bloomington, Ind]; AlloDerm [LifeCell, Branchburg, NJ]) to repair diaphragmatic hernia defects. At times, the abdominal cavity may be too small to accommodate the reduced viscera from the thoracic cavity. A temporary abdominal silo may be considered, but allowing an incisional hernia with skin-only closure until the definitive fascia closure can be performed is an alternative surgical option. When CDH is repaired on ECMO, particular attention must be paid to achieve hemostasis. However, despite the use of careful surgical techniques with diligent hemostasis, postoperative bleeding is a common major complication. Beyond the immediate postoperative period, many infants with CDH experience significant morbidity because of PPHN and respiratory dysfunction. For example, infants who survive aggressive management of severe respiratory failure may manifest neurologic problems, such as motor and cognitive deficits, developmental delay, seizures, and hearing loss. Other problems include gastroesophageal reflux (GER) disease and foregut dysmotility. Other morbidities associated with CDH survivors include chronic lung disease, scoliosis, growth retardation, and pectus excavatum deformities.

BRONCHOPULMONARY MALFORMATIONS

Bronchopulmonary malformations are congenital abnormalities of the airway, such as bronchogenic cysts, intralobar and extralobar sequestrations, congenital pulmonary airway malformations, and congenital lobar emphysema.[5] Their natural histories vary widely. In the perinatal period, these lung lesions can result in pleural effusions, polyhydramnios, hydrops, and pulmonary hypoplasia with subsequent respiratory distress and airway obstruction. If severe enough, fetal demise can ensue. With increasing importance placed on prenatal care, many of these lesions are being diagnosed prenatally with imaging. Fetal surgery has been pursued when fetal viability is at risk. Although these congenital abnormalities are often asymptomatic and may even spontaneously regress, there is concern that these anomalies may cause recurrent infections and exhibit long-term malignant potential.

Bronchogenic Cyst

Bronchogenic cyst is the most common cystic lesion of the mediastinum. The cyst wall consists of fibroelastic tissue, smooth muscle, and cartilage, whereas the cyst itself is lined with respiratory tract epithelia (ciliated columnar cells). It can also contain mucus-producing cuboidal cells, which contribute to enlargement of the cyst with mucus. They may occur anywhere along the tracheobronchial tree but are usually found near the carina and right hilum. Less frequently, they present in the neck, lung, pleura, or pericardium or below the diaphragm. When the cysts are large, they can compress the airway or other vital structures. Infants are particularly at risk because of their narrow, easily compressible trachea and bronchus. Cysts can also cause dysphagia, pneumothorax, cough, and hemoptysis or become infected, especially when presenting later in life. Often identified on a routine chest radiograph, the diagnosis is confirmed by computed

tomography (CT) as a spherical nonenhancing, mucus-filled cystic mass, although an air-fluid level can be seen if the cyst communicates with the airway. Cysts within the pulmonary parenchyma typically communicate with a bronchus, whereas those in the mediastinum usually do not. Bronchogenic cysts are resected even if asymptomatic, although some argue otherwise. Rare cases of malignant transformation have been reported. Resection can be performed either thoracoscopically (i.e., by video-assisted thoracic surgery) or open (by minithoracotomy).

Congenital Pulmonary Airway Malformation

Congenital pulmonary airway malformations (CPAMs) have been described as hamartomatous lesions in which a multicystic mass replaces normal lung tissue. They are connected to the tracheobronchial tree, and the blood supply is pulmonary. Although they are usually unilateral and unilobar, they can present in the immediate perinatal period with life-threatening respiratory distress. The majority of CPAMs are asymptomatic at infancy; however, unrecognized CPAMs can present with chronic cough or recurrent pneumonia at a later time. CPAMs can undergo malignant transformation; rhabdomyosarcoma has been reported. They are classified on the basis of their appearance on imaging, and confirmation is made by pathologic examination. According to the Stocker classification, type I lesions account for almost 75% of all cases and consist of a small number of large, 2- to 10-cm cysts that can compress normal lung parenchyma. Type II lesions have numerous cysts, usually measuring less than 1 cm in diameter. Type III lesions are rare and appear to be only a few millimeters in diameter.[6] However, they are associated with mediastinal shift, hydrops, and a poor prognosis.

Prenatal fetal MRI can be used to differentiate CPAM from other congenital thoracic abnormalities. When fetal distress occurs in utero, options include fetal thoracotomy and thoracoamniotic shunting (if the fetus is <32 weeks), but this is extremely rare. Most fetuses with a prenatally diagnosed CPAM experience partial regression in the third trimester and can be treated with expectant management.[5] Some report favorable outcomes with the use of steroids prenatally, which may help promote spontaneous regression or stabilize disease progression in utero.[7] CPAM is generally asymptomatic at birth. However, on rare occasion, infants present with acute respiratory distress requiring emergent open resection. A chest radiograph is usually diagnostic, revealing a cystic thoracic mass with air-fluid levels occasionally; however, ultrasound and CT examinations are frequently obtained for confirmation (Fig. 66-5A). The management of asymptomatic patients is somewhat controversial with respect to ideal timing of the operation. It is generally agreed that they should be resected, given the risk of infection and malignant transformation, such as pleuropulmonary blastoma. Most advocate surgical resection around 6 months of age.

Pulmonary Sequestration

Bronchopulmonary sequestrations (BPSs) are nonfunctional nests of microcystic pulmonary tissue that have no connection to the tracheobronchial tree but are fed by an aberrant systemic artery. There are two types, intralobar and extralobar; the intralobar type is contained within normal lung parenchyma, and the extralobar type is separate and encased by its own pleura.[5] Extralobar sequestrations (ELSs) occur predominantly in males, and in 40% of cases, other congenital anomalies, such as posterolateral diaphragmatic hernia, pectus excavatum and carinatum, and enteric duplication cysts, can be found.

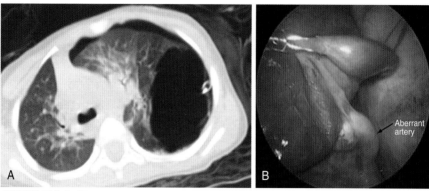

FIGURE 66-5 A, CT scan demonstrating a large left lung CPAM lesion. **B,** Anomalous arterial vascular pedicle to extralobar pulmonary sequestration. The arterial branch comes directly off the thoracic aorta.

Lacking a communication to the airway, sequestrations do not form enlarged cysts or cause spontaneous pneumothoraces. They can, however, infarct, become infected, and cause hemoptysis. It has been reported that ELSs can undergo torsion as well. Because of their aberrant systemic vascular supply (Fig. 66-5B), BPSs can result in significant left-to-right shunting in infants, who are then susceptible to high-output cardiac failure. For an initial evaluation, Doppler ultrasound may reveal a systemic arterial supply from the infradiaphragmatic or thoracic aorta. The lesion itself may appear solid, but it can also be cystic. CT or MRI can aid in further defining the vascular anatomy. Accounting for 75% of all BPSs, intralobar sequestrations (ILSs) are found within the medial or posterior segments of the lower lobes, more on the left side. Most ELSs are found posteromedially in the left lower chest but can occur within or below the diaphragm. Air within an ILS usually signifies infection, whereas the same finding in an ELS suggests the presence of a fistulous connection with the esophagus.[5]

If a BPS is identified on prenatal ultrasound, the fetus is observed with serial ultrasound monitoring for enlargement and potential pleural effusion, polyhydramnios, or hydrops. BPS has been reported to spontaneously regress. In fact, it is estimated that 68% of BPSs undergo spontaneous regression in utero as they become isodense with the surrounding lung. The involution may occur as the lesion outgrows its blood supply. Because of the risk for infection and bleeding, ILSs are usually resected by segmentectomy or lobectomy. ELSs are usually asymptomatic, and because there is generally no tracheobronchial communication, the risk of infection is low. As such, many of these lesions can be observed.

Congenital Lobar Emphysema

Congenital lobar emphysema (CLE) describes a progressively distended, hyperlucent lobe caused by abnormal bronchopulmonary development. Air trapping in the emphysematous lobes occurs with intrinsic or extrinsic obstruction, which includes endobronchial obstruction from mucosal proliferation and extrinsic compression from vascular anomalies. In more than 90% of cases, it involves the left upper or right middle lobe. CLE is rarely diagnosed prenatally, and its prevalence is only 1 in every 20,000 to 30,000 deliveries. It tends to be manifested in the first few days of life and as late as 6 months after birth. On ultrasound examination, CLE appears as an echogenic homogeneous lung mass. When CLE is discovered incidentally, observation is recommended because these lesions can regress spontaneously. A chest

radiograph is customarily diagnostic, revealing overdistention of the involved lobe. Importantly, the lucency should not be mistaken for a pneumothorax, and positive pressure ventilation should be used with caution because of the propensity of these patients to undergo auto–positive end-expiratory pressure; auto–positive end-expiratory pressure is defined as the end-expiratory intrapulmonary pressure that develops as a result of dynamic airflow resistance during mechanical ventilation. When the CLE progresses to cause mediastinal shift and worsening symptoms, an open lobectomy is indicated.

ALIMENTARY TRACT CONDITIONS

Esophageal Atresia and Tracheoesophageal Fistula

Esophageal atresia is a congenital condition of esophageal discontinuity that results in proximal esophageal obstruction. A tracheoesophageal fistula (TEF) is an abnormal fistula communication between the esophagus and trachea. Esophageal atresia and TEF can occur alone or in combination. The incidence of this anomaly is 1 in 1500 to 3000 live births, with a slight male predominance. Approximately one third of infants are born with low birth weight, and 60% to 70% have associated anomalies. During the fourth week of gestation, the esophagotracheal diverticulum of the foregut fails to divide completely to form the esophagus and trachea. In 10% of patients, there is a nonrandom, nonhereditary association of anomalies referred to by the acronym VATER (vertebral, anorectal, tracheal, esophageal, renal or radial limb); an alternative acronym is VACTERL (vertebral, anorectal, cardiac, tracheal, esophageal, renal, and limb). Five anatomic variants of esophageal atresia are depicted in Figure 66-6. In the most common type (C lesion) of proximal esophageal atresia with distal TEF, the proximal blind pouch ends approximately the distance of one or two vertebral bodies from the distal TEF. The distal TEF is typically located approximately 1 cm above the carina in the membranous portion of the trachea.

Clinical Presentation and Diagnosis

The diagnosis of esophageal atresia is considered in an infant with excessive salivation along with coughing or choking experienced at the first oral feeding. A maternal history of polyhydramnios is common, more often in isolated proximal atresia (86%). In an infant with proximal esophageal atresia with distal TEF, acute gastric distention may occur as a result of air entering the distal esophagus and stomach with each inspired breath. Reflux of gastric contents into the distal esophagus will traverse the TEF

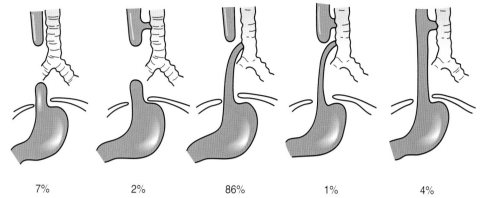

7%   2%   86%   1%   4%

FIGURE 66-6 Anatomic variants and incidence of esophageal atresia with tracheoesophageal fistula.

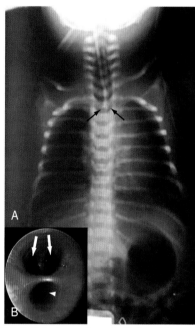

FIGURE 66-7 **A,** Plain chest radiograph of infant with proximal esophageal atresia with distal tracheoesophageal fistula. The distal tip of the orogastric tube is noted, with a surrounding gas-filled proximal esophagus *(arrows)*. The distal tracheoesophageal fistula is indicated by the presence of gastric air. **B,** Rigid bronchoscopy inspection of distal tracheoesophageal fistula. The luminal size of the fistula *(arrowhead)* is equal to that of either main bronchus *(arrows)*.

and spill into the trachea, resulting in cough, tachypnea, apnea, or cyanosis. The clinical presentation of isolated TEF without esophageal atresia may be subtle, often beyond the newborn period. In general, these infants experience choking and coughing associated with feedings. The inability to pass a nasogastric tube into the stomach is a cardinal feature for the diagnosis of esophageal atresia. If gas is present below the diaphragm, an associated TEF is confirmed (Fig. 66-7A). Conversely, the inability to pass a nasogastric tube in an infant with absent radiographic evidence of air in the GI tract is virtually diagnostic of an isolated esophageal atresia. The use of isotonic contrast medium to demonstrate the presence or level of the proximal esophageal atresia is strongly discouraged because of risk for aspiration. The diagnostic

evaluation includes screening for other associated anomalies. Echocardiography and renal ultrasound are routinely performed to evaluate for congenital heart defects (including aortic arch anomaly) and genitourinary malformations.

Management

Initial management includes decompression of the proximal esophageal pouch with a sump tube (e.g., Replogle tube) placed on continuous suction. The infant is positioned in an upright prone position to minimize GER and to prevent aspiration. Broad-spectrum IV antibiotic coverage is started empirically. Routine endotracheal intubation is avoided because positive pressure ventilation may be inadequate to inflate the lungs as air is directed into the TEF through the path of least resistance (Fig. 66-7B). Ventilation may be compounded further by the resultant gastric distention. Gastrostomy to decompress the distended stomach should be avoided because it may abruptly worsen the ability to ventilate the patient. In these circumstances, manipulation of the endotracheal tube advanced distal to the TEF (e.g., right mainstem intubation) may minimize the leak and permit adequate ventilation. The placement of an occlusive balloon (Fogarty) catheter into the fistula through a rigid bronchoscope may also be useful. As a last resort, emergent thoracotomy with ligation of the fistula alone may be required. A preoperative chest radiograph and echocardiogram provide sufficient information to determine the aortic arch anatomy. A right thoracotomy is performed for the operative repair in patients with a normal left-sided aortic arch. However, for infants with a right-sided arch, a left thoracotomy would be preferred. A higher incidence of aortic arch anomalies (e.g., vascular rings) and postoperative complications has been reported with a right-sided aortic arch.[8]

The surgical approach for the most common type of proximal esophageal atresia with distal TEF is an open thoracotomy with an extrapleural dissection. Recently, thoracoscopic repair has been described by several pediatric surgical centers. Some advocate routine rigid bronchoscopy at the start of the operation to exclude the presence of a second fistula or placement of a catheter through the fistula to aid in identifying TEF. However, this technique may be more useful for recurrent fistula repairs. After exposure of the posterior mediastinum, the azygos vein is divided to reveal the underlying TEF. The TEF is dissected circumferentially, and its attachment to the membranous portion of trachea is taken down. The tracheal opening is approximated with interrupted nonabsorbable sutures. The proximal esophageal pouch is then mobilized as high as possible to facilitate a tension-free esophageal

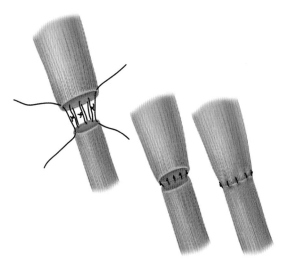

FIGURE 66-8 A single-layer end-to-end anastomosis is performed with nonabsorbable sutures. Two corner stitches are placed, and a back row anastomosis is completed first. Just before completion of the anterior row of the anastomosis, a nasogastric tube is placed across it.

anastomosis. The blood supply to the upper esophageal pouch is generally robust from arteries derived from the thyrocervical trunk. However, the lower esophageal vasculature is more tenuous and segmental, originating from intercostal vessels. As such, extensive mobilization of the lower esophagus should be avoided to prevent ischemia. The esophageal anastomosis is performed with a single- or double-layer technique (Fig. 66-8). The anastomotic leak rates are slightly higher with the single-layer anastomosis, whereas the esophageal stricture rates are higher with the double-layer technique.

In case of a long gap between the two ends of the esophagus, there are several options. A circular or spiral esophagomyotomy of the upper pouch can be performed to gain additional length for a primary anastomosis. Another option is to suture the divided closed end of the distal esophagus to the prevertebral fascia and mark the area with a hemoclip. Over time, the proximal esophageal pouch will lengthen so that a subsequent primary esophageal anastomosis can be considered. In infants with pure esophageal atresia, primary anastomosis in the newborn period is not feasible because of a long gap between the esophageal stumps. Gastrostomy is initially placed for enteral feeding access. Traditionally, a cervical esophagostomy is performed for drainage of oral secretions, and then an esophageal replacement operation using either right or left colon is carried out at approximately 1 year of age. Alternatively, proximal esophageal pouch secretion can be managed with an indwelling orogastric tube (Replogle tube) without cervical esophagostomy until adequate esophageal lengthening takes place, as assessed by a fluoroscopic study. Then, a primary intrathoracic segmental esophageal replacement using a colonic segment can be performed around 4 to 6 months of age. The stomach has also been used as an esophageal replacement but with much less frequency. Small intestinal free graft is another option, but this requires microvascular anastomosis and has poor results. In patients with pure TEF, without esophageal atresia, the TEF is usually near the thoracic inlet. In this case, the surgical approach is made through a cervical incision. At operation, rigid bronchoscopy and cannulation of the TEF with a guidewire can be helpful.

The mortality rate is directly related to associated anomalies, particularly cardiac defects and chromosomal abnormalities. In the absence of associated anomalies, an overall survival greater than 95% is expected. Postoperative complications unique to esophageal atresia or TEF include esophageal motility disorders, GER (25% to 50%), anastomotic stricture (15% to 30%), anastomotic leak (10% to 20%), and tracheomalacia (8% to 15%).

Gastroesophageal Reflux

Infants normally experience some degree of vomiting, thought to be the result of an incompetent lower esophageal sphincter. This physiologic response usually resolves spontaneously around 6 to 12 months of age. Pathologic GER can be manifested with a spectrum of clinical scenarios. Although diagnostic studies are valuable in identifying pathologic reflux, the patient's symptoms remain equally important in deciding the surgical treatment of GER. Neurologically impaired children who are in need of enteral feeding access also have to be evaluated for concomitant reflux before gastrostomy placement. A laparoscopic approach has become a standard for fundoplication with gastrostomy in pediatric patients.

Clinical Presentation

The symptoms of pathologic GER vary considerably, depending on the age of the patient and underlying associated medical conditions. Although vomiting is a common feature, failure to thrive from calorie deprivation is one of the most serious complications of persistent GER. Aspiration of gastric contents can also result in recurrent bronchitis or pneumonia, leading to chronic cough or wheezing. Reflux may stimulate vagal reflex, producing laryngospasm or bronchospasm and leading to an asthma-like clinical presentation.[9] The significant airway spasm caused by reflux can result in apnea or choking spells and may contribute to near-miss sudden infant death syndrome (SIDS). Irritability and crying in infants may also represent pain because of esophagitis induced by chronic reflux. Chronic acid insult to the lower esophagus can progress to the formation of stricture from chronic scarring and produce obstructive symptoms. Although it is rare in pediatric patients, chronic progressive esophagitis can lead to metaplasia of lower esophageal squamous mucosa to columnar epithelium. This condition, known as Barrett esophagus, requires close surveillance to detect the progression of premalignant dysplastic changes.

Many infants and children with neurodevelopmental disabilities require permanent feeding access, such as a gastrostomy. Hence, some are also considered for antireflux surgery at the time of the gastrostomy placement, especially patients who are unable to protect their airway reliably or who already have significant vomiting associated with intragastric tube feeding. However, prophylactic fundoplication in neurologically impaired children is no longer a routine procedure at the time of gastrostomy placement. Some surgeons advocate studies to evaluate for GER disease before gastrostomy, but others rely on clinical judgment, such as tolerance of enteral feeding through an indwelling nasogastric tube. These patients are also at high risk for delayed gastric emptying because of upper gastroduodenal dysmotility. However, fundoplication alone may result in enhanced gastric emptying function, and a gastric emptying procedure is rarely indicated.

Diagnosis

A detailed clinical history will provide valuable information to determine the severity of GER. A near-miss SIDS episode or progressive neurologic disorders may indicate the desirability of an antireflux procedure, regardless of diagnostic study results. There are various diagnostic tools to objectively assess the presence of pathologic GER. Contrast esophagography is used most frequently to acquire anatomic and functional data. Esophageal stricture or mechanical evidence of gastric outlet obstruction, such as antral, duodenal web, or intestinal malrotation, can also be identified. In addition, motility of the esophagus and gastric emptying function can be estimated. However, one drawback is the lack of specificity. A 24-hour esophageal pH probe study remains the "gold standard" for diagnosis of GER. It can measure the frequency and duration of acid reflux episodes along with reflux patterns, such as the total length of acid (pH < 4) reflux, duration of each episode, and longest continuous period of acid reflux. A combined multichannel intraluminal impedance pH test, in which reflux is detected by changes in intraluminal resistance determined by the presence of liquid or gas and pH changes, has become a more reliable comprehensive diagnostic modality. A gastric emptying scan is obtained when a radionuclide-labeled (technetium Tc 99m sulfur colloid) liquid or semisolid food is used to quantitatively assess gastric emptying. In general, approximately 50% of the isotope-labeled meal is normally emptied from the stomach within 60 minutes and approximately 80% by 90 minutes. Delayed gastric emptying may improve simply after an antireflux procedure alone.

Esophageal manometry measures the esophageal body and lower esophageal sphincter pressures and helps identify abnormal esophageal motility. Although it is relatively simple to perform, manometry is infrequently used to evaluate GER disorders in pediatrics. The severity of GER in infants does not always correlate with an incompetent lower esophageal sphincter mechanism. There is also considerably less experience with manometric studies in pediatric patients. However, identifying esophageal dysmotility may be important for choosing the appropriate antireflux procedure. Children with poor esophageal motility are prone to development of refractory dysphagia after complete wrap fundoplication. Endoscopic evaluation of the esophageal mucosa provides a gross and microscopic assessment of mucosal injury secondary to GER. Patients who present with hematemesis or dysphagia may have significant underlying esophagitis. Esophagoscopy can determine the spectrum of esophagitis, from inflammation to ulceration to stricture, and is also helpful in identifying Barrett esophagus. The prevalence of eosinophilic esophagitis in the pediatric population has become more recognized in recent years.[10] Because of inflammation and edema, patients with eosinophilic esophagitis can often present with dysphagia and pain mimicking GER disease. The diagnosis of eosinophilic esophagitis can be made by histologic evaluation of esophageal biopsy specimens obtained at the time of endoscopic evaluation.

Treatment

Conservative management of significant GER includes thickening of formula with cereal, reducing the volume of feeding, and postural maneuvers. In addition, pharmacologic acid suppression may be useful. Indications for surgical intervention include severe GER that is unresponsive to aggressive medical management. Surgery is generally warranted for patients with life-threatening near-miss SIDS episodes, failure to thrive, or esophageal stricture. Other relative indications include those requiring complex surgical airway reconstruction, neurologic impairment requiring permanent feeding access, and a history of recurrent pneumonias or persistent asthma. The gold standard surgical procedure for infants and children with pathologic GER is Nissen fundoplication

(360-degree esophageal wrap). It is the most effective method to control the symptoms of GER; however, the undesirable side effect of gas bloat or dysphagia is more likely to occur after a full fundic wrap than after a partial one. A partial wrap (e.g., Toupet, 270 degrees; Thal, 180 degrees) has been reported to produce fewer complications of dysphagia but is less effective in controlling the reflux symptoms as well. Regardless of which type of fundoplication is performed, a laparoscopic approach has become the standard technique.

Hypertrophic Pyloric Stenosis

Hypertrophic pyloric stenosis (HPS) is a disease of newborns, with an incidence of 1 in 300 to 900 live births. It is most common between the ages of 2 and 8 weeks. Boys are affected four times more often than girls, with first-born male infants being at highest risk. Hypertrophy of the circular muscle of the pylorus results in constriction and obstruction of the gastric outlet, leading to nonbilious, projectile emesis, loss of hydrochloric acid with the onset of hypokalemic hypochloremic metabolic alkalosis, and dehydration. Although the exact cause of HPS remains unknown, a lack of nitric oxide synthase in pyloric tissue has been implicated.

Clinical Presentation

Infants with HPS generally present with progressively worsening nonbilious emesis. Over time, the emesis becomes more frequent, forceful, and projectile in nature. On occasion, visible gastric peristalsis may be observed as a wave of contractions from the left upper quadrant to the epigastrium. Shortly after emesis, infants usually crave additional feedings. A plain abdominal radiograph can show an enlarged gastric gas bubble. Palpation of the pyloric "olive" tumor in the epigastrium by an experienced examiner is pathognomonic for HPS. If the olive is confirmed, no additional diagnostic testing is necessary. When the olive is not appreciated, an ultrasound study should be obtained. Pyloric muscle thickness of more than 3 to 4 mm or a pyloric length greater than 15 to 18 mm in the presence of functional gastric outlet obstruction is diagnostic. With an equivocal clinical presentation, an upper GI contrast study may be useful to evaluate for other causes of vomiting.

Management

The Ramstedt pyloromyotomy remains the standard operation for HPS. Preoperatively, it is imperative that the infant be fully resuscitated with IV fluids to establish an adequate urine output and to restore normal electrolyte balance. If not, there is a high risk for postoperative apnea because the infant with metabolic alkalosis has a propensity to compensate by retaining respiratory carbon dioxide. Thus, the serum bicarbonate level needs to be normalized before surgery, at least to a value of less than 30 mEq/L. Pyloromyotomy involves incising the thickened pyloric musculature while preserving the underlying mucosa. This is performed through a right upper quadrant or periumbilical incision. A laparoscopic approach (Fig. 66-9) has gained popularity because of its smaller incision. However, the general principle of pyloromyotomy is the same regardless of laparoscopic or open procedures, with equivalent outcomes.[11] Postoperatively, infants are allowed to resume enteral feedings gradually. There are various feeding protocols, which range from immediate full ad lib feedings to volume-based incremental advancement. Vomiting after surgery occurs frequently but is generally self-limited. Potential complications include incomplete myotomy and mucosal perforation.

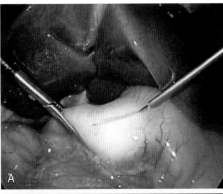

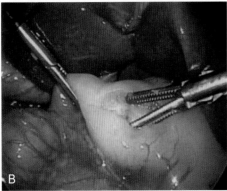

FIGURE 66-9 **A,** Laparoscopic Ramstedt pyloromyotomy is started with a retractable blade. **B,** A spreader with grooves on the outer surface is used to complete the pyloromyotomy. Intact mucosal bulging along with independent muscle wall motion is confirmed. (From St. Peter SD, Ostlie DJ: Laparoscopic and open pyloromyotomy. In Chung DH, Chen MK, editors: *Atlas of pediatric surgical techniques*, Philadelphia, 2010, Elsevier Saunders, pp 253–265.)

Intestinal Atresia

Duodenal atresia is thought to result from failure of vacuolization of the duodenum from its solid cord stage. The range of anatomic variants includes duodenal stenosis, mucosal web with intact muscle wall (so-called windsock deformity), two ends separated by a fibrous cord, and complete separation with a gap within the duodenum. It is associated with several conditions, including prematurity, Down syndrome, maternal polyhydramnios, malrotation, annular pancreas, and biliary atresia. Other anomalies, such as cardiac, renal, esophageal, and anorectal anomalies, are also common. In most cases, the duodenal obstruction is distal to the ampulla of Vater (85%); therefore, infants present with bilious emesis. In patients with a mucosal web, the symptoms of postprandial emesis may occur later in life.

Infants with duodenal obstruction are generally first detected during a prenatal ultrasound evaluation. Immediately after birth, a plain abdominal radiograph shows a typical double-bubble sign if it is obtained before orogastric tube decompression of swallowed gastric air (Fig. 66-10*A*). If distal air is present, an upper GI contrast study should be considered not only to confirm the diagnosis of duodenal stenosis or atresia but also to exclude midgut volvulus, which would constitute a surgical emergency.

The management is by surgical bypass of the duodenal obstruction as a side-to-side or proximal transverse to distal longitudinal (diamond-shaped) duodenoduodenostomy (Fig. 66-10*B*). At the time of anastomosis, additional intestinal atresia should be ruled out by injecting saline into a distal limb using a soft red rubber catheter. When the proximal duodenum is markedly dilated, a tapering duodenoplasty with staples or sutures should be considered to narrow the duodenal caliber to lessen dysmotility. In patients with a duodenal mucosal web, the web is excised transduodenally; caution must be exercised to avoid injury to the ampulla.

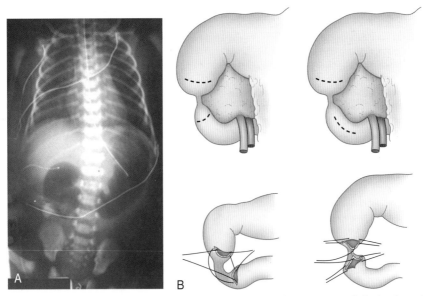

FIGURE 66-10 **A,** Plain abdominal radiograph shows double-bubble appearance of duodenal atresia. **B,** Proximal transverse to distal longitudinal (diamond-shaped) or side-to-side duodenoduodenostomy is performed for congenital duodenal obstruction. (From Duodenal obstruction. In O'Neill JA Jr, Grosfeld JL, Fonkalsrud EW, et al, editors: *Principles of pediatric surgery*, ed 2, St. Louis, 2003, Mosby, p 474.)

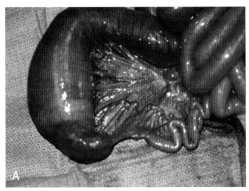

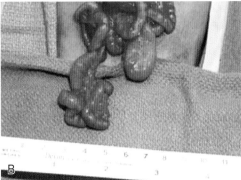

FIGURE 66-11 Jejunoileal Atresia. **A,** Massively dilated jejunum with narrow distal bowel segment. **B,** Apple peel type of atresia with a large mesenteric gap.

Jejunoileal atresia is the most common GI atresia; it occurs in 1 in 2000 live births. It is thought to result from an intrauterine mesenteric vascular accident. Atresias are slightly more common in the jejunum than in the ileum. Jejunoileal atresias are classified as type I, a mucosal web or diaphragm (Fig. 66-11A); type II, with an atretic cord between two blind ends of bowel with intact mesentery; type IIIa, a complete separation of the blind ends of the bowel by a V-shaped mesenteric gap; and type IIIb, an apple peel or Christmas tree deformity with a large mesenteric gap (Fig. 66-11B), in which the distal bowel receives a retrograde blood supply from the ileocolic or right colic artery. This tenuous blood supply has implications for anastomotic failures and the potential for ischemic necrosis from volvulus. Thus, many of these infants with this type of atresia are born with reduced intestinal length. In type IV, there are multiple atresias, with a string of sausage appearance.

Infants present with bilious emesis, abdominal distention, and failure to pass meconium. The clinical presentation varies by the location of the atretic obstruction. In proximal atresia, abdominal distention is less, but significant bilious emesis is present. Abdominal radiographs can show air-fluid levels with absent distal gas. In distal atresias, abdominal distention is more common. A contrast enema study can demonstrate a narrow caliber of colon and may also be useful to exclude multiple atresias, which may be present in 10% to 15% of cases. Jejunoileal atresia is generally not associated with other anomalies except cystic fibrosis in approximately 10% of patients.

Infants are managed for neonatal bowel obstruction. An orogastric tube is placed, and appropriate IV fluid resuscitation is implemented. At operation, the main objective is to establish intestinal continuity while preserving as much intestinal length as

possible. In multiple atresias, multiple anastomoses over an endoluminal stent may be necessary. If the proximal intestine is significantly dilated, prolonged dysmotility may persist, and therefore a tapering enteroplasty of the dilated segment should be considered. However, in cases of adequate bowel length, resection of the dilated segment can result in faster recovery. The overall survival for infants with jejunoileal atresia is more than 90%.

Colonic atresia is the least common, accounting for only 5% to 10% of intestinal atresia; the incidence is 1 in 20,000 live births. Infants usually present with failure to pass meconium, abdominal distention, and bilious vomiting. A plain radiograph shows multiple dilated bowel loops, but differentiation between small and large bowel is not feasible in this age group because of lack of well-developed haustra and semicircularis landmarks. Contrast enema study can confirm the diagnosis, but the clinical picture of bowel obstruction may be enough evidence to proceed with operative intervention of diverting end colostomy.

Intestinal Malrotation and Midgut Volvulus

The actual incidence of rotational anomalies of the midgut is difficult to determine but is estimated to be 1 in 6000 live births. The midgut normally herniates out of the coelomic cavity through the umbilical ring at approximately the fourth week of fetal development. By the tenth week of gestation, the intestine begins to migrate back into the abdominal cavity in a counterclockwise rotation around the axis of the superior mesenteric artery (SMA) for 270 degrees. The duodenojejunal segment returns first and rotates beneath and to the right of the SMA to fix in the left upper quadrant at the ligament of Treitz. The cecocolic segment also rotates counterclockwise around the SMA to rest in its final position in the right lower quadrant. By week 12, this process of intestinal rotation is complete, and the colon becomes fixed to the retroperitoneum. An interruption or reversal of any of these coordinated movements implies an embryologic explanation for the range of anomalies seen.

Abnormal Intestinal Rotation

Complete nonrotation of the midgut is the most common anomaly and occurs when neither the duodenojejunal nor the cecocolic limb undergoes correct rotation. Consequently, duodenojejunal and ileocecal junctions lie close together and the midgut is suspended on a narrow SMA stalk, which can twist in a clockwise fashion to result in midgut volvulus. Nonrotation of the duodenojejunal limb, followed by normal rotation and fixation of the cecocolic limb, results in duodenal obstruction by abnormal mesenteric bands (Ladd bands) that extend from the colon across the anterior duodenum. In this anomaly, the risk of midgut volvulus is low because there is a relatively broad mesenteric base between the duodenojejunal junction and cecum. Normal rotation of the duodenojejunal limb with nonrotation of the cecocolic segment carries the same risk for midgut volvulus as a complete nonrotation anomaly. In this case, the risks for volvulus are high because of a narrow mesenteric base.

Clinical Presentation

The clinical presentation varies, depending on the specific mechanism of obstruction and whether it involves compromised bowel. The major symptoms are related to the presence of midgut volvulus, duodenal obstruction, or intermittent or chronic abdominal pain, or it is an incidental finding in an otherwise asymptomatic patient. Most patients develop symptoms during the first month of life. Midgut volvulus is a true surgical emergency because of evolving ischemic bowel loops. The acute onset of bilious emesis in a particularly somnolent or lethargic newborn is an ominous sign. Midgut volvulus may also be incomplete or intermittent. Toddlers and children may present with chronic abdominal pain, intermittent episodes of emesis (which may be nonbilious), early satiety, weight loss, failure to thrive, or malabsorption and diarrhea. With partial volvulus, the resultant mesenteric venous and lymphatic obstruction may impair nutrient absorption and produce protein loss into the gut lumen as well as mucosal ischemia and melena as a result of arterial insufficiency.

Diagnosis

Abdominal radiographs may demonstrate upper intestinal obstruction or a gasless abdomen; however, these findings are nonspecific. The upper GI contrast series remains the diagnostic study of choice; it demonstrates an abnormal position of the ligament of Treitz along with the appearance of a bird's beak in the third portion of the duodenum, which indicates an obstruction. The ultrasound examination has proved to be a useful tool for the diagnosis of intestinal malrotation with midgut volvulus, in which the normal relationship of the superior mesenteric vessels (the vein is to the right of artery) is reversed or altered.[12] In the acutely ill child with midgut volvulus and obstruction, immediate operative correction is indicated, and little time is available for IV fluid resuscitation, catheterization, or administration of broad-spectrum antibiotics. Time is critical if intestinal salvage is to be achieved.

Surgical Management

Midgut volvulus is a surgical emergency. Once the diagnosis is made, the abdomen must be promptly explored. The Ladd procedure is the operation of choice for rotational anomalies of the intestine (Fig. 66-12). On entering the peritoneal cavity, chylous

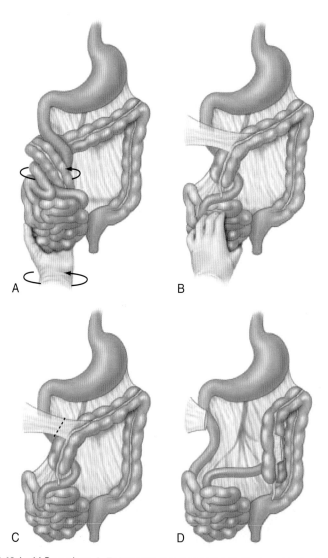

FIGURE 66-12 Ladd Procedure. **A,** Twisted bowel is eviscerated. **B,** The bowel is derotated in a counterclockwise fashion. **C,** The peritoneal attachment between the cecum and retroperitoneum (Ladd band) is divided. **D,** The base of the mesentery is widened, and an appendectomy is performed. (From Warner BW: Imperforate anus. In Chung DH, Chen MK, editors: *Atlas of pediatric surgical techniques*, Philadelphia, 2010, Elsevier Saunders, pp 138–142.)

ascites from obstructive lymphatics is frequently seen. The volvulus is untwisted in a counterclockwise fashion. After detorsion, the intestine may be congested and edematous, and some areas may appear necrotic. Placement of warm sponges and observation for a time may improve the appearance of the intestine when the vascular integrity has been compromised. Necrotic segments are resected; however, marginally ischemic segments may be left in place and a second-look laparotomy performed after 24 to 36 hours. Ladd bands are divided as they extend from the ascending colon across the duodenum to the posterior aspect of the right upper quadrant. In dividing the medial bands, the cecum is mobilized and the mesenteric base is broadened to prevent recurrent volvulus. Securing the cecum or duodenum to the abdominal wall by sutures has no proven benefit. In addition, an intraluminal duodenal obstruction may coexist, and therefore an orogastric tube may be advanced into the distal duodenum to exclude any associated anomaly. An incidental appendectomy is performed because the cecum will ultimately lie on the left side of the abdomen after the Ladd procedure. The intestine is replaced into the abdominal cavity with the small bowel loops on the right side; the colon is positioned on the left. Recurrent volvulus has been reported in up to 10% after the Ladd procedure. The more common cause of postoperative obstruction is adhesive bands. Prolonged ileus is common, particularly if a volvulus has progressed to necrosis, requiring extensive resection. Midgut volvulus accounts for approximately 18% of cases of short gut syndrome in the pediatric population. Urgent recognition and treatment are the most important factors in preventing this complication.

Necrotizing Enterocolitis

Necrotizing enterocolitis (NEC) is the most common GI surgical emergency in the neonatal period. Although several contributing factors, such as ischemia, bacteria, cytokines, and enteral feeding, have been established, prematurity is the single most important risk factor. Recent medical advances in the management of premature infants have led to improved overall survival, hence resulting in more premature infants at risk for development of NEC. However, the overall incidence appears to have decreased because of implementation of a gradual feeding regimen as well as promotion of the use of breast milk. Yet, the exact cause of NEC remains unknown, and research advances have been hampered by the fact that a correlative animal model for NEC does not exist.

Clinical Presentation and Diagnosis

The clinical presentation of NEC can be variable and unpredictable. Acute abdominal distention, tenderness, and feeding intolerance with gross or occult blood in the stool are hallmark features for NEC. Other nonspecific signs include irritability, temperature instability, and episodes of apnea or bradycardia. NEC typically occurs in the first few days of life with the initiation of enteral feedings. In approximately 80% of cases, however, it occurs within the first month of life. As NEC progresses, sepsis develops with hemodynamic deterioration and coagulopathy. The pathognomonic radiographic feature of NEC is pneumatosis intestinalis (Fig. 66-13A). Pneumatosis is composed of hydrogen gas generated by the bacterial fermentation of luminal substrates. Other radiographic findings may include portal venous gas, ascites, fixed loops of small bowel, and free air. The distal ileum and ascending colon are the usual affected areas, although the entire GI tract can be affected as in NEC totalis.

Medical Management

Initial medical management consists of orogastric tube decompression, fluid resuscitation, blood product transfusion, and broad-spectrum antibiotics. NEC can be successfully treated medically in approximately 50% of cases with a 10- to 14-day course of an IV antibiotic regimen and bowel rest. Serial abdominal examinations are performed to closely monitor for any subtle signs for surgical abdomen. The absolute indication for operative management of NEC is the presence of intestinal perforation, as revealed by free air on plain abdominal radiographs (Fig. 66-13B). Other relative indications for surgery include clinical deterioration, abdominal wall cellulitis, palpable abdominal mass, and a persistent fixed radiographic bowel loop.

Surgical Management

The general principles of surgical management of NEC include resection of all nonviable intestinal segments with ostomy diversion. Every effort must be made to preserve maximum intestinal length. Thus, it may be necessary to resect multiple intervening necrotic segments of bowel, preserving all viable intestine. In cases in which the bowel is ischemic but not frankly necrotic, a second-look operation may be performed after 24 to 48 hours. Bowel resection with primary anastomosis may be considered in the rare stable infant with a focal isolated perforation and minimal

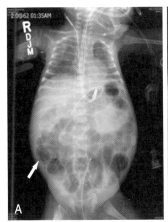
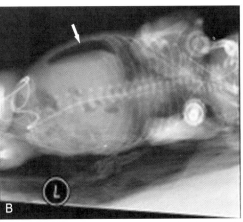

FIGURE 66-13 A, Pneumatosis intestinalis *(arrow),* a pathognomonic radiographic sign for necrotizing enterocolitis. **B,** Pneumoperitoneum *(arrow)* on lateral decubitus radiograph.

peritoneal contamination; however, the serious risks for anastomotic leak and stricture have tempered enthusiasm for this approach.

For infants of extremely low birth weight with perforated NEC, a bedside peritoneal drain placement is an alternative temporizing measure. Drainage of the contaminated peritoneal fluid may improve ventilation and halt the progression of sepsis in select critically ill preterm infants. Surprisingly, drain placement turned out to be the only intervention in some infants. However, percutaneous drain was reported to have poor outcomes in infants of extremely low birth weight (<1000 g). Evidence to support peritoneal drainage as an accepted mode of treatment for NEC was established in a multicenter, randomized prospective clinical trial.[13] In this study, survival, need for parenteral nutrition, and length of hospital stay were similar for NEC infants weighing less than 1500 g treated by peritoneal drainage or laparotomy. The overall mortality rate for surgically managed NEC ranges from 10% to 50%. NEC remains the most common cause of short gut syndrome. Intestinal strictures may develop after medical or surgical management of NEC in approximately 10% of infants. Because of the risk for post-NEC stricture, most notably in splenic flexure of the colon, a contrast enema study is done routinely before stoma reversal. Neurodevelopmental delay is also a frequent long-term complication.

Short Bowel Syndrome

Short bowel syndrome (SBS) is a clinical condition in which there is inadequate length of functional intestine to sustain normal enteral nutrition as a result of massive small bowel resection. Common conditions that can lead to SBS are intestinal atresia, midgut volvulus, NEC, and gastroschisis. In SBS, intestinal

function depends on a number of factors, such as total bowel length, presence of the ileocecal valve, and residual segments of intestine. The jejunum is the site of absorption of most macronutrients and minerals. GI hormones that are critical for gut function, such as cholecystokinin and secretin, are produced in the jejunum. The ileum is essential for the absorption of carbohydrates, proteins, fluids, and electrolytes. Bile acids, vitamin B_{12}, and the fat-soluble vitamins (A, D, E, K) are primarily absorbed in the ileum. Ileocecal valve function is particularly important in SBS, in which intestinal transit time can be significantly altered. The colon is important in SBS patients for absorption of water and electrolytes. After massive small bowel resection, a physiologic process known as intestinal adaptation occurs to compensate for the loss of intestinal length. Many factors are involved in this adaptive process to enhance the absorptive function of the residual intestine. Medical treatment of SBS includes the use of an elemental diet, glutamine and various growth factors, and careful delivery of TPN.[12] Several surgical techniques (excluding small bowel transplantation) aimed at slowing intestinal transit time or increasing the mucosal surface area for enhanced absorption have been described.[14] These include reversed intestinal segment, recirculating loop, artificial intestinal valve, colon interposition, and intestinal pacing. Two procedures that are generally used are the Bianchi procedure and serial transverse enteroplasty (STEP).

Surgical Management

Bianchi procedure. Bianchi[15] originally described an intestinal lengthening procedure in which the mesenteric vascular bed is separated into two systems; the dilated small intestine is split into two parallel segments, each with its own blood supply, and the ends are approximated (Fig. 66-14A). This resulted in a 50%

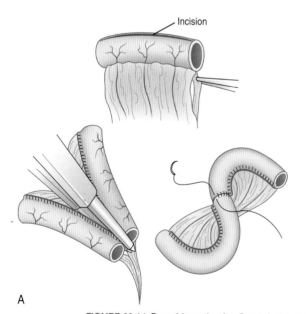
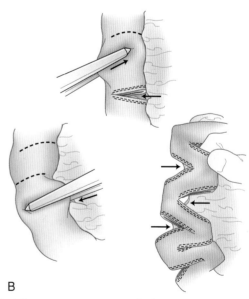

A   B

FIGURE 66-14 Bowel-Lengthening Procedures. **A,** Bianchi technique separates two mesenteric planes. A dilated segment of bowel is stapled longitudinally to create two narrower segments for sequential anastomosis. **B,** Serial transverse enteroplasty (STEP) involves stapling a dilated bowel into V shapes on alternating sides, decreasing width and increasing length. (**A** adapted from Abu-Elmagd KM, Bond G, Costa G, et al: Gut rehabilitation and intestinal transplantation. *Therapy* 2:853–864, 2005. **B** from Kim HB, Fauza D, Garza J, et al: Serial transverse enteroplasty [STEP]: A novel bowel-lengthening procedure. *J Pediatr Surg* 38:425–429, 2003.)

decreased diameter of the small intestine and increased length by 200%. The Bianchi procedure has been shown to be an effective surgical option for treating patients with SBS.

Serial transverse enteroplasty. Since its description in 2003,[16] the STEP procedure has garnered significant interest by the pediatric surgical community. In contrast to the Bianchi procedure, dilated small intestine is serially stapled in a transverse fashion to create a narrower lumen and longer intestinal length (Fig. 66-14*B*). The STEP procedure improved enteral feeding tolerance, resulting in significant catch-up growth, and was not associated with increased mortality.[17] A recent study reported improved enteral tolerance in the majority of 20 patients observed for more than a 7-year period after STEP procedures.[18]

Meconium Ileus

Meconium ileus is a unique form of neonatal obstruction that occurs in infants with cystic fibrosis (CF), an autosomal recessive disorder resulting from a mutation in the CF transmembrane regulator gene *(CFTR)*. It is estimated that 3.3% of the white population in the United States are asymptomatic carriers of the mutated *CFTR* gene. The abnormal chloride transport in patients with CF results in tenacious viscous secretions with a protein concentration of almost 80% to 90%. It affects a wide variety of organs, including the intestine, pancreas, lungs, salivary glands, reproductive organs, and biliary tract. Meconium ileus is classified as simple or complicated.

Clinical Presentation

Meconium ileus in the newborn represents the earliest clinical manifestation of CF; it affects approximately 10% to 15% of patients with this inherited disease. The incidence of CF ranges from 1 in 1000 to 2000 live births. Infants present with three cardinal signs in the first 24 to 48 hours of life: (1) generalized abdominal distention; (2) bilious emesis; and (3) failure to pass meconium. Maternal polyhydramnios occurs in approximately 20% of cases. In simple meconium ileus, the terminal ileum is dilated and filled with thick, tarlike, inspissated meconium. Smaller pellets of meconium are found in the more distal ileum, leading into a relatively small colon. In patients with simple meconium ileus, important plain abdominal radiographic findings include dilated and gas-filled loops of small bowel, absence of air-fluid levels, and a mass of meconium in the right side of the abdomen mixed with gas to give a ground-glass or soap bubble appearance.

Simple Meconium Ileus

Abdominal radiographs show dilated bowel loops with relatively absent air-fluid levels because of thick viscous meconium. A ground-glass appearance is noted in the right lower quadrant corresponding to bowel loops filled with thick meconium mixed with air. The initial diagnostic study of choice is contrast enema using a water-soluble ionic solution. In simple meconium ileus, a Gastrografin contrast enema study can demonstrate a small narrow-caliber colon and inspissated meconium pellets in the terminal ileum (Fig. 66-15*A*). Gastrografin is a hypertonic solution that can aid in the evacuation of meconium. However, it is imperative that the infant be well hydrated and vital signs carefully monitored after the Gastrografin study. Contrast enema is successful in relieving the obstruction in up to 75% of cases, with a bowel perforation rate of less than 3%. The pilocarpine iontophoresis sweat test revealing a chloride concentration higher than 60 mEq/L is the most reliable and definitive method to confirm the diagnosis of CF. A more immediate test is detection of the mutated *CFTR* gene.

Surgical management. Operative management of simple meconium ileus is required when the obstruction is persistent despite contrast enema, along with 5 mL of 10% *N*-acetylcysteine (Mucomyst) solution administered every 6 hours through a nasogastric tube. Historically, the dilated terminal ileum was resected and various types of stomas were created, allowing intestinal

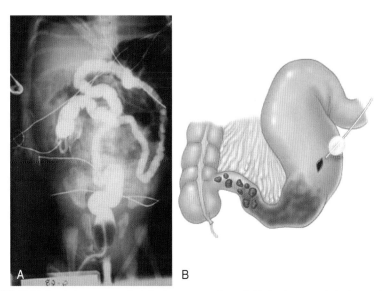

FIGURE 66-15 Surgical management of simple meconium ileus. **A,** Contrast enema study shows microcolon with soap bubble appearance in the right lower quadrant. **B,** Removal of meconium can be facilitated by gentle use of a catheter along with a 2% to 4% *N*-acetylcysteine solution. (From Brandt ML: Meconium disease. In Chung DH, Chen MK, editors: *Atlas of pediatric surgical techniques*, Philadelphia, 2010, Elsevier Saunders, pp 44–53.)

decompression and recovery. However, enterotomy, irrigation with warmed saline solution or 4% N-acetylcysteine, and simple evacuation of the luminal meconium without a stoma has also been advocated (Fig. 66-15B). N-Acetylcysteine serves to break the disulfide bonds in the meconium to facilitate separation from the bowel mucosa. The meconium is manipulated into the distal colon or removed through the enterotomy. After the obstruction is relieved, the enterotomy is closed in standard fashion. If meconium evacuation is incomplete, a T tube may be left in place in the ileum to facilitate continued postoperative irrigation.

Complicated Meconium Ileus

Meconium ileus is considered complicated when perforation of the intestine has taken place in utero or in the early neonatal period. Extravasation of meconium can result in severe peritonitis, with a dense inflammatory response and calcification. The variable clinical presentation includes a meconium pseudocyst, adhesive peritonitis with or without secondary bacterial infection, and ascites. Abdominal radiographs can demonstrate calcifications, bowel dilation, mass effect, and ascites. A distal ileal obstructive syndrome, formerly known as meconium ileus equivalent, may develop as a consequence of noncompliance with oral enzyme replacement therapy or bouts of dehydration. This is managed nonoperatively in most patients with enemas or oral polyethylene glycol purging solutions. Other diagnoses must also be considered, including simple adhesive intestinal obstruction. Furthermore, with the introduction of enteric-coated, high-strength pancreatic enzyme replacement therapy, a fibrosing cholangiopathy has been described. Resection of the inflammatory colon stricture may be necessary.

Meconium Plug Syndrome

Meconium plug syndrome is unrelated to meconium ileus and in most cases is not a sequela of CF. However, it is a frequent cause of neonatal intestinal obstruction and is associated with a number of conditions, including Hirschsprung's disease, maternal diabetes, and hypothyroidism. Infants present with significant abdominal distention and failure to pass meconium in the first 24 hours of life. Contrast enema shows a microcolon extending up to where the colon is dilated, filled with a thickened meconium plug. Often, a contrast enema study is also therapeutic. Although most children with meconium plug syndrome are normal, follow-up studies should be performed to rule out Hirschsprung's disease and CF.

Hirschsprung's Disease

Hirschsprung's disease is a developmental disorder characterized by an absence of ganglion cells in the myenteric (Auerbach) and submucosal (Meissner) plexus. It occurs in 1 in 5000 live births, with boys being affected four times more frequently than girls. This neurogenic parasympathetic abnormality is associated with muscular spasm of the distal colon and internal anal sphincter, resulting in a functional obstruction. Hence, the abnormal bowel is the contracted distal segment, whereas the normal bowel is the proximal dilated portion. Aganglionosis begins at the anorectal line, and the rectosigmoid is affected in approximately 80% of cases, the splenic or transverse colon in 17%, and the entire colon in 8%. The area between the dilated and contracted segments is referred to as the transition zone. Here, ganglion cells begin to appear, but in reduced numbers. Of these patients, 3% to 5% have Down syndrome, and the risk for Hirschsprung's disease is greater if there is a family history. An abnormal locus on chromosome 10 has been identified in some families and is associated with the *RET* oncogene.[19]

Clinical Presentation

Most infants (>90%) present with abdominal distention and bilious emesis with failure to pass meconium within the first 24 hours of life. Infants whose Hirschsprung's disease is not recognized early may present with a chronic history of poor feeding, abdominal distention, and significant constipation. Enterocolitis is the most common cause of death in patients with uncorrected Hirschsprung's disease and may be manifested as diarrhea alternating with periods of obstipation, abdominal distention, fever, hematochezia, and peritonitis.

Diagnosis

The diagnostic test of choice in a newborn with radiographic evidence of a distal bowel obstruction is a contrast enema study. In a study with normal findings, the rectum is wider than the sigmoid colon. In patients with Hirschsprung's disease, spasm of the distal rectum usually results in a narrow caliber with a transition zone and dilated proximal sigmoid colon (Fig. 66-16). Failure to evacuate the instilled contrast medium completely after 24 hours strongly suggests Hirschsprung's disease. An important goal of the study is to exclude other causes of constipation, such as meconium plug, small left colon syndrome, and atresia. The manometric finding of high internal sphincter pressure when the rectum is distended with a balloon can also be useful information in older children, but this is rarely performed. A rectal biopsy is the gold standard for the diagnosis of Hirschsprung's disease. In the newborn period, this is performed at the bedside using a suction rectal biopsy kit. It is important to obtain biopsy specimens at least 2 cm above the dentate line to avoid sampling the normal aganglionated region of the internal sphincter. In older children, a full-thickness biopsy specimen is obtained under general anesthesia because the thicker rectal mucosa is not amenable to suction biopsy technique. Absent ganglia, hypertrophied nerve trunks, and robust immunostaining for acetylcholinesterase are the histopathologic criteria. Recently, calretinin immunostaining has become more widely used and is considered superior

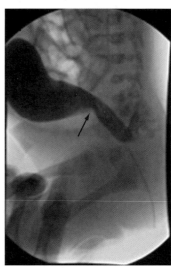

FIGURE 66-16 Contrast enema demonstrating transition point *(arrow)* in Hirschsprung's disease.

to acetylcholinesterase staining to confirm the diagnosis of Hirschsprung's disease.[20]

Surgical Management

Historically, a leveling colostomy was performed initially through a left lower quadrant surgical incision. The location of the transition zone is confirmed by frozen section evaluation of multiple seromuscular biopsy specimens. A diverting colostomy (end or loop) is then performed in the region of normal ganglionated bowel, and a definitive procedure is performed at a later age. There are definitive surgical options for Hirschsprung's disease. In the Swenson procedure, the aganglionic bowel is removed down to the level of the internal sphincters and a coloanal anastomosis is performed. In the Duhamel procedure, the aganglionic rectal stump is left in place and the ganglionated normal colon is pulled behind the stump. A stapler is then inserted through the anus, with one arm within the normal ganglionated bowel posteriorly and the other in the aganglionic rectum anteriorly. Stapling results in the formation of a neorectum that empties normally because of the posterior patch of ganglionated bowel. The Soave technique involves an endorectal mucosal dissection within the aganglionic distal rectum. The ganglionated normal colon is then pulled through the remnant muscular cuff, and a coloanal anastomosis is performed. The laparoscopy-assisted Soave procedure has become popular; it is performed on newborns and has the advantages of primary definitive operation without an initial colostomy. The Soave procedure is also performed entirely through a transanal approach. Postoperatively, the stool dysfunction can persist and be difficult to manage, requiring intermittent rectal decompression in some cases. Constipation is a common postoperative problem along with frequent soiling, incontinence, and postoperative enterocolitis.

Anorectal Malformation

The incidence of imperforate anus is 1 in 5000 live births, and boys are more affected (58%). The spectrum of anorectal malformations ranges from simple anal stenosis to the persistence of a cloaca. The most common defect is an imperforate anus with a fistula between the distal colon and urethra in boys or the vestibule of the vagina in girls.

Embryology

By the sixth week of gestation, the urorectal septum moves caudally to divide the cloaca into the anterior urogenital sinus and posterior anorectal canal. Failure of this septum to form results in a fistula between the bowel and urinary tract (in boys) or vagina (in girls). Complete or partial failure of the anal membrane to resorb results in an anal membrane or stenosis. The perineum also contributes to the development of the external anal opening and genitalia by the formation of cloacal folds, which extend from the anterior genital tubercle to the anus. The perineal body is formed by fusion of the cloacal folds between the anal and urogenital membranes. Breakdown of the cloacal membrane anywhere along its course results in the external anal opening being anterior to the external sphincter (i.e., anteriorly displaced anus).

Classification

An anatomic classification of anorectal anomalies is based on the level at which the blind-ending rectal pouch ends—low, intermediate, or high in relationship to the levator ani musculature. A more therapeutic and prognostic classification is depicted in Box 66-1. An invertogram, a lateral pelvic radiograph taken after the

---

BOX 66-1 Classification of Congenital Anomalies of the Anorectum

Female	Male
Cutaneous (perineal fistula)	Cutaneous (perineal fistula)
Vestibular fistula	Rectourethral fistula
Imperforate anus without fistula	Bulbar
Rectal atresia	Prostatic
Cloaca	Recto–bladder neck fistula
Complex malformation	Imperforate anus without fistula
	Rectal atresia

---

infant is held upside-down for several minutes, was used in the past to determine the most distal point of the rectal pouch. In most cases, a careful inspection of the perineum alone can predict the pouch level. If an anocutaneous fistula is observed anywhere on the perineal skin of a boy or external to the hymen of a girl, a low lesion can be assumed. Most other types of lesions are high or intermediate. Rectal atresia refers to an unusual lesion in which the lumen of the rectum is completely or partially interrupted, with the upper rectum being dilated and the lower rectum consisting of a small anal canal. A persistent cloaca is defined as a defect in which the rectum, vagina, and urethra all fuse to form a single common channel. In girls, a single orifice in the perineum indicates a cloaca. If two perineal orifices are seen (i.e., urethra and vagina), the defect represents a high imperforate anus or, less commonly, a persistent urogenital sinus comprising one orifice and a normal anus as the other orifice. Anorectal malformation often coexists with other lesions, and the VACTERL association must be considered during evaluation. Bone abnormalities of the sacrum and spine, such as absent vertebrae, accessory vertebrae, or hemivertebrae or an asymmetrical or short sacrum, can occur in approximately one third of patients. Absence of two or more vertebrae is associated with a poor prognosis for bowel and bladder continence. Occult dysraphism of the spinal cord may also be present; this consists of a tethered cord, lipomeningocele, or fat within the filum terminale.

Evaluation

Aside from physical examination, plain radiography of the spine and ultrasound of the spinal cord are performed. Genitourinary abnormalities other than the rectourinary fistula occur in 25% to 60% of patients. Vesicoureteral reflux and hydronephrosis are the most common, but other conditions, such as horseshoe, dysplastic, or absent kidney as well as hypospadias or cryptorchidism, must be considered. In general, the higher the anorectal malformation, the greater the frequency of associated urologic abnormalities. In patients with a persistent cloaca or rectovesical fistula, the likelihood of a genitourinary abnormality is approximately 90%. In contrast, the frequency is only 10% with low defects (e.g., perineal fistula). Renal ultrasound and voiding cystourethrography are obtained to assess the urinary tract. If a cardiac defect is suspected, echocardiography is performed before any surgical procedure. Esophageal atresia can also be ruled out with an orogastric tube placement. The decision algorithms for the management of male and female newborns with anorectal malformation are shown in Figures 66-17 and 66-18.

Surgical Management

Low lesions. A newborn with a low lesion can undergo a primary single-stage repair without colostomy. For anal stenosis

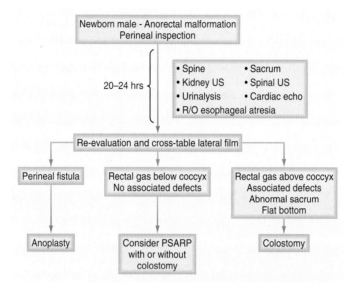

FIGURE 66-17 Decision algorithm for the management of male patients with anorectal malformation. *PSARP,* Posterior sagittal anorectoplasty. (From Levitt M, Peña A: Imperforate anus. In Chung DH, Chen MK, editors: *Atlas of pediatric surgical techniques,* Philadelphia, 2010, Elsevier Saunders, pp 185–205.)

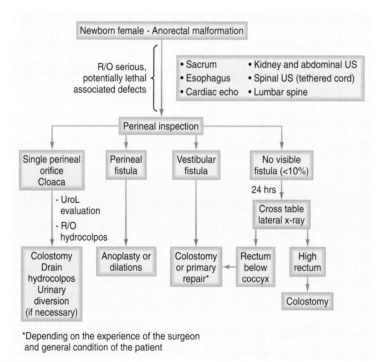

FIGURE 66-18 Decision algorithm for the management of female patients with anorectal malformation. (From Levitt M, Peña A: Imperforate anus. In Chung DH, Chen MK, editors: *Atlas of pediatric surgical techniques,* Philadelphia, 2010, Elsevier Saunders, pp 185–205.)

in which the anal opening is in a normal location, serial dilation alone is usually sufficient. Dilations are performed daily with gradual size increase over time. If the anal opening is anterior to the external sphincter (i.e., anteriorly displaced anus), with a small distance between the opening and the center of the external sphincter, and the perineal body is intact, a cutback anoplasty may be performed. This consists of an incision extending from the ectopic anal orifice to the central part of the anal sphincter, thus enlarging the anal opening. Alternatively, if there is a significant distance between the anal opening and central portion of the external anal sphincter, a transposition anoplasty is performed in which the aberrant anal opening is transposed to the normal position within the center of the sphincter muscles, and the perineal body is reconstructed.

Intermediate or high lesions. Newborns with intermediate or high lesions generally require a diverting colostomy as the first part of a three-stage reconstruction. The colon is completely divided, and an end sigmoid colostomy with a mucous fistula is constructed to minimize fecal contamination into the area of a rectourinary fistula. Furthermore, the distal mucous fistula limb can be used later for a contrast study to determine the rectourinary fistula. The second-stage procedure usually is performed at 3 to 6 months of age. The operation consists of dividing the rectourinary or rectovaginal fistula with a pull-through of the terminal rectal pouch into the normal anal position. A posterior sagittal anorectoplasty, as first described by deVries and Peña, is the procedure of choice.[21] This consists of determining the location of the central position of the anal sphincter by electrical stimulation of the perineum. An incision is then made in the midline, extending from the coccyx to the anterior perineum and through the sphincter and levator musculature until the rectum is identified. The fistula from the rectum to the vagina or urinary tract is divided. The rectum is mobilized and the perineal musculature reconstructed. The third and final stage is colostomy reversal, which is performed several weeks later. Anal dilations begin 2 weeks after the anorectoplasty and continue for several months after the colostomy closure.

A laparoscopically assisted posterior sagittal anorectoplasty has significant advantages as a minimally invasive approach for anorectal malformation with good outcomes.[22] This technique offers the theoretical advantages of placing the neorectum within the central position of the sphincter and levator muscle complex under direct vision and avoids the need to cut across these structures. The long-term outcome of this new approach compared with the standard posterior sagittal method is presently unknown.

Morbidity in patients with anorectal malformations relates to associated anomalies. Fecal continence is the major goal regarding correction of the defect. Prognostic factors for continence include the level of the pouch and whether the sacrum is normal. In general, 75% of patients have voluntary bowel movements. However, 50% of this group still soils their underwear occasionally; the other 50% is considered totally continent. Constipation is the most common sequela. A bowel management program consisting of daily enemas is an important postoperative plan to reduce the frequency of soilage and to improve the quality of life for these patients.

Intussusception

Intussusception is a telescoping of one portion of the intestine into the other; it is usually idiopathic, without an obvious anatomic lead point. It occurs predominantly at the ileocecal junction. Invariably, there is marked swelling of the lymphoid tissue in the region of the ileocecal valve. It is unknown whether this represents the cause or effect of the ileocolic intussusception. The incidence of intussusception is associated with a history of recent episodes of viral gastroenteritis, upper respiratory infections, and even administration of rotavirus vaccine, implying lymphoid swelling in the pathogenesis of intussusception. In older children, the incidence of a pathologic lead point is up to 12%, and Meckel's diverticulum is found to be the most common lead point for intussusception. However, other causes, such as intestinal polyps, inflamed appendix, submucosal hemorrhage associated with Henoch-Schönlein purpura, foreign body, ectopic pancreatic or gastric tissue, and intestinal duplication, must also be considered. Postoperative small bowel intussusception in the absence of

a lead point can also occur; this represents up to 5% of all pediatric cases of intussusception.

Clinical Presentation and Diagnosis

Intussusception produces severe cramping abdominal pain in an otherwise healthy child from 3 months to 3 years. Two thirds of children presenting with intussusception are younger than 1 year. The child often draws the legs up during the pain episodes and is usually quiet during the intervening periods. Other symptoms include vomiting, passage of bloody mucus (currant jelly stool), and a palpable abdominal mass. In approximately 50% of cases, the diagnosis of ileocolic intussusception can be suspected on plain abdominal radiographs by the presence of a mass, sparse colonic gas, or complete distal small bowel obstruction. Currently, abdominal ultrasound is used as an initial diagnostic test. The characteristic sonographic findings of the "target sign" of the intussuscepted layers of bowel on a transverse view or the "pseudokidney sign" when seen longitudinally should prompt air-contrast enema study.

Management

Hydrostatic reduction by enema using contrast material or air is the therapeutic procedure of choice. Contraindications to this approach include the presence of peritonitis and hemodynamic instability. Furthermore, an intussusception located entirely within the small intestine is unlikely to be reduced by an enema and more likely to have an associated lead point. Hydrostatic reduction by air enema is the standard modality. Successful reduction is accomplished in more than 80% of cases and confirmed by resolution of the mass, along with reflux of air into the terminal ileum. For those refractory to air enema attempts, many centers will try a delayed, repeated air enema study a few hours later with some success.[23] The recurrence rate after hydrostatic reduction is approximately 11%, and it usually occurs within the 24 hours after the reduction. When it recurs, it is usually managed by another air enema reduction. A third recurrence is an indication for operative management.

Surgical management. The operative indications with intussusception include peritonitis or bowel obstruction at initial presentation and failed hydrostatic enema reduction or multiple recurrences. The intussusceptum is delivered through a transverse incision in the right side of the abdomen and reduced in a retrograde fashion by pushing the mass proximally. Once it is reduced, warm lap pads may be placed over the bowel, and a period of observation may be warranted in cases of questionable bowel viability. The lymphoid tissue in the ileocecal region is thickened and edematous and may be mistaken for a tumor within the small bowel; therefore, great caution should be exercised before committing to surgical resection. Recurrence rates are extremely low after surgical reduction. Bowel resection is required in cases in which the intussusception cannot be reduced, the viability of the bowel is uncertain, or a lead point is identified. An ileocolectomy with primary anastomosis is usually performed. An appendectomy is an essential component, irrespective of bowel resection. Laparoscopic reduction of intussusception has recently gained some popularity.

Meckel's Diverticulum

Meckel's diverticulum is the most common congenital anomaly of the GI tract and occurs in approximately 2% of the population. More than 70% of symptomatic patients have heterotopic gastric mucosa and another 5% have pancreatic tissue. The rule of 2s is often cited in association with Meckel's diverticulum. Aside from its 2% incidence and two types of heterotopic mucosa, it is located within 2 feet of the ileocecal valve, approximately 2 inches in length, and usually symptomatic by 2 years of age. Meckel's diverticulum is caused by a failure of normal regression of the vitelline duct that occurs during weeks 5 to 7 of gestation. Meckel's diverticulum is a true diverticulum containing all normal intestinal layers.

Diagnosis

The clinical symptoms are related to hemorrhage, obstruction, or inflammation; the most common presenting symptom is a painless, massive, lower GI bleeding in children younger than 5 years. Diagnosis of a persistent vitelline duct remnant may be established by umbilical ultrasound or lateral contrast radiography. Bleeding Meckel's diverticulum may be confirmed by a ^{99m}Tc-pertechnetate isotope scan to detect gastric mucosa. Of note, ectopic gastric mucosa can also be present in patients with intestinal duplication.

Surgical Management

Surgical resection is the definitive therapy for Meckel's diverticulum. A simple V-shaped diverticulectomy with transverse closure of the ileum is an acceptable technique. In patients in whom there is ulceration or inflammation at the base of the diverticulum, a segmental resection of the involved ileum with a primary end-to-end anastomosis is preferred.

HEPATOBILIARY CONDITIONS

Extrahepatic Biliary Atresia

Biliary atresia (BA) is a rare disease of neonates characterized by the inflammatory obliteration of intrahepatic and extrahepatic bile ducts. The incidence is estimated to be 1 in 5000 to 12,000 infants, depending on region. It may be associated with other congenital malformations, particularly splenic abnormalities (e.g., asplenia, double spleen), absence of the inferior vena cava (IVC), and intestinal malformation. If BA is left untreated, progressive cirrhosis and death occur by 2 years of age.

Pathophysiology

The exact mechanism whereby BA develops is unknown, but several theories exist. One theory suggests that the ductal injury is immune mediated—inflammatory cells infiltrate and obliterate the bile ducts. Proinflammatory cytokines, such as interleukin-2, interferon-γ, and tumor necrosis factor, are present. CD4$^+$/CD8$^+$ T cells and natural killer cells are also prominent.[24] However, it remains unclear how the inflammatory process is initiated and progresses. Another theory is that a viral insult, group C rotavirus infection, triggers the immune-mediated fibrosclerosis and obstruction of the extrahepatic bile ducts. Interestingly, animal studies have shown that infection of newborn mice with rotavirus leads to a similar presentation as in infants, with the onset of hyperbilirubinemia, jaundice, and acholic stools. On histologic examination, inflammation and obstruction of the extrahepatic bile ducts are observed. However, this theory has yet to be proven in human newborns because many lack serologic evidence of viral infection. Another hypothesis is that there are genetic components that contribute to the development of BA. There may be an association with human leukocyte antigen (HLA) type. Patients with BA have a significantly high frequency of HLA-B12. It is unclear whether this is causal, but some have argued that abnormal

expression of HLA makes biliary ductal epithelial cells a susceptible target for immunologic assault. Another putative gene, *CFC1*, encodes a protein important in the embryonic differentiation of the left-right axis; when mutated, it is thought to predispose to the development of BA. On histopathologic evaluation, there is significant extrahepatic biliary obstruction with portal tract fibrosis, inflammatory cell infiltration, bile duct proliferation, and cholestasis with bile plugging.

Clinical Presentation and Diagnosis

The disease is classified according to the level of the most proximal biliary obstruction. Type 1 BA has patency to the level of the common bile duct; type 2 has patency to the level of the common hepatic duct; and type 3, which accounts for more than 90% of cases, occurs when the left and right hepatic ducts at the level of the porta hepatis are involved. This aids in the differentiation between correctable BA and others. Correctable BA requires that patent hepatic ducts exist to the porta hepatis. Types 1 and 2 may be amenable to a direct extrahepatic biliary duct–intestinal anastomosis.

Infants present shortly after birth with jaundice, pale stools, and dark urine. Older infants may have failure to thrive and present with hepatomegaly and ascites suggestive of cirrhosis. If, in the postnatal period, the jaundice persists after 14 days in a term infant, an evaluation for liver disease should be initiated. This consists of determining direct or conjugated bilirubin level, which will be elevated (>2.0 mg/dL) in those with liver disease. Liver function test results should also be monitored because derangements are typically seen. Coagulopathy is not generally encountered early because hepatic synthetic function is relatively intact. Other exclusion studies include serologic testing for TORCH (toxoplasmosis, rubella, cytomegalovirus, and herpes) and hepatitis B and C infections, α$_1$-antitrypsin, and CF. Metabolic disorders, such as galactosemia and tyrosinemia, and endocrine abnormalities must also be ruled out.

Evaluation of the biliary anatomy often begins with ultrasound. The gallbladder may be atrophic or absent, and intrahepatic ducts may also be notably absent. The liver may appear echogenic. Other imaging modalities, such as hepatobiliary iminodiacetic acid (HIDA) scintigraphy, magnetic resonance cholangiopancreatography (MRCP), and endoscopic retrograde cholangiopancreatography (ERCP), have been used, with varying success. An HIDA scan would reveal uptake of the technetium isotope but an absence of emptying into the duodenum. MRCP or ERCP can better define the biliary anatomy, but because of the relatively small size of the ducts, it is difficult from a technical and resolution standpoint. Although these are useful adjuncts, liver biopsy is the gold standard for the diagnosis of BA and can safely be done percutaneously.

Surgical Management

Once the diagnosis is suspected, an operative exploration is warranted along with intraoperative cholangiography. Once the diagnosis is confirmed, a Kasai hepatoportoenterostomy is the surgical procedure of choice. Here, the extrahepatic biliary tree is dissected proximally to the level of the liver capsule, where the porta hepatis (portal plate) is transected. The reconstruction is performed by a Roux-en-Y hepaticojejunostomy (Fig. 66-19). Some advocate the use of ursodeoxycholic acid and phenobarbital to promote biliary drainage, but it is uncertain whether these actually improve outcomes. The use of steroids after the Kasai procedure has been advocated by many and thought to promote biliary drainage with

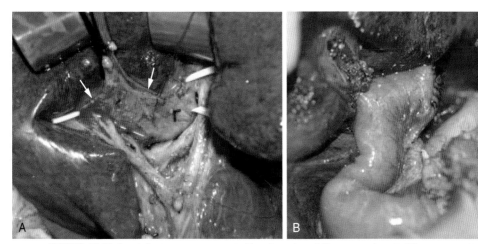

FIGURE 66-19 Kasai Portoenterostomy. **A,** The dissection of fibrous extrahepatic biliary remnant is continued up to the capsular surface of the liver within the bifurcation of the portal vein (*arrows* indicate fibrous portal plate; yellow vessel loops mark lateral dissection margins). **B,** Completed Roux-en-Y portoenterostomy. (From Nathan JD, Ryckman FC: Biliary atresia. In Chung DH, Chen MK, editors: *Atlas of pediatric surgical techniques*, Philadelphia, 2010, Elsevier Saunders, pp 220–231.)

shorter hospital stay.[25] However, the Biliary Atresia Clinical Research Consortium's recent randomized, double-blinded, placebo-controlled trial of steroid therapy (the START trial) after the Kasai procedure demonstrated that high-dose steroid therapy after the procedure did not result in significant treatment differences in bile drainage at 6 months.[26] Furthermore, steroid treatment was associated with earlier onset of serious adverse events.[26] However, steroid pulse therapy remains a treatment option for post-Kasai cholangitis. Antibiotics are also continued postoperatively because the risk of cholangitis is high (45% to 60%) as a result of the ease with which intestinal bacteria can ascend and colonize the bile ducts. Unfortunately, if the Kasai procedure is unable to reestablish bile flow and liver failure or cirrhosis ensues, liver transplantation is indicated.

Kasai hepatoportoenterostomy does not cure BA, which will inevitably progress in more than 70% of infants who undergo this procedure. The rate with which the disease progresses, as evidenced by cirrhosis and portal hypertension, is variable, but it may be expedited by recurrent cholangitis. It is estimated, however, that 80% of those who have successfully undergone a Kasai procedure can live up to 10 years before liver transplantation is needed. In those infants who undergo transplantation, outcomes are good, with 10-year graft survival and overall patient survival of 73% and 86%, respectively.[27]

Choledochal Cyst

Choledochal cysts are cystic dilations of the common bile duct (CBD). They have an incidence of 1 in 100,000 to 150,000 live births, with a 3 to 4:1 female-to-male preponderance. They are classified on the basis of location, and their frequency varies (Fig. 66-20). Type I (50% to 80%) is a simple cyst that can involve any portion of the CBD, and type II (2%) describes a diverticulum arising off the CBD. Choledochoceles represent type III cysts (1.4% to 4.5%), consisting of dilation confined to the distal intrapancreatic portion of the CBD. Although type IV (15% to 35%) involves intrahepatic and extrahepatic bile ducts, type V (20%) is limited to the intrahepatic ducts only. Choledochal cysts can be associated with other congenital anomalies, including duodenal and colonic atresia, imperforate anus, pancreatic arteriovenous malformation, and pancreatic divisum.[28] Moreover, choledochal cysts are considered premalignant lesions.

Pathogenesis

The pathogenesis of choledochal cysts remains unknown, but one hypothesis is that pancreaticobiliary reflux allows the activation of pancreatic enzymes within the duct. The subsequent inflammatory response compromises the integrity of the duct wall, which eventually results in dilation. In support of this theory, amylase and trypsinogen levels in the bile from patients with choledochal cysts are often elevated.[28] Another theory is that these cysts arise from CBD obstruction, which can occur with functional obstruction at the sphincter of Oddi.

Clinical Presentation and Diagnosis

The classic triad of jaundice, a palpable right upper quadrant mass, and abdominal pain is seen in less than 20% of patients, but 85% of children have at least two of these symptoms on presentation. Patients younger than 12 months generally present with obstructive jaundice and abdominal masses, whereas older patients complain of pain, fever, nausea with vomiting, and jaundice. Common complications include cholangitis, pancreatitis, and bile peritonitis secondary to cyst rupture.[28] Abdominal ultrasound can reveal a cystic mass that is separate from the gallbladder and also allows anatomic assessment of the biliary tree. When a diagnosis is uncertain, an HIDA scan should be considered, demonstrating absent filling of the cyst initially, followed by uptake in the cyst and finally delayed emptying into the duodenum. CT is a useful modality for defining the intrahepatic biliary anatomy and evaluating the distal CBD and pancreatic head. Moreover, it has better resolution with regard to confirming continuity of the cyst with the CBD. MRCP is obtained with increasing frequency and can be helpful. However, ERCP is rarely indicated.

Treatment

Prompt excision of the cysts is recommended. After cyst excision, a Roux-en-Y hepaticojejunostomy is performed for

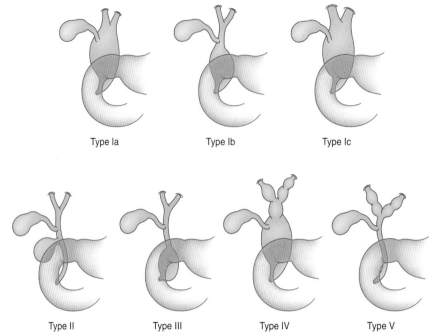

Type Ia   Type Ib   Type Ic

Type II   Type III   Type IV   Type V

FIGURE 66-20 Classification of choledochal cyst. (From O'Neill JA: Choledochal cyst. In Grosfeld JL, O'Neill JA, Fonkalsrud EW, et al, editors: *Pediatric surgery*, ed 6, Philadelphia, 2006, Mosby Elsevier, pp 16–21.)

reconstruction. Complete excision is important because the risk of a primary malignant neoplasm is as high as 6% with a retained choledochal cyst. If the cyst cannot be completely excised because of scarring from chronic inflammation, the cyst should be enucleated. These patients should be monitored by ultrasound examination. Postoperative anastomotic strictures are a common complication and probably arise from chronic intrahepatic cholelithiasis and recurrent cholangitis. Aside from this, outcomes are generally good.

Hereditary Pancreatitis and Pancreas Divisum

Hereditary pancreatitis is an autosomal dominant disorder with a high degree of penetrance. It is rare, representing less than 1% of instances of chronic pancreatitis. The disease results from a mutation in the cationic trypsinogen gene *(PRSS1)*, which leads to an increase in the autoactivation of trypsin and resistance to deactivation.[29] The gene has been mapped to chromosome 7q35; the two most common allelic mutations are *R122H* and *N29I*.[29] Recurrent bouts of pancreatitis usually begin in childhood, between 5 and 10 years of age, with no identifiable cause. Aside from the age at onset, the presentation, natural history, diagnosis, and treatment of this disease are similar to those for other causes of pancreatitis.

Hereditary pancreatitis should be suspected in any patient who experiences at least two bouts of acute pancreatitis without obvious risk factors, such as trauma, hyperlipidemia, gallstones, or pancreas divisum. It should also be considered in any child with acute pancreatitis and a family history of this disease and in children. Making the correct diagnosis is important because there is an extremely high lifetime risk of malignant transformation. It is estimated that these patients have a 50- to 70-fold increase in the risk for development of pancreatic adenocarcinoma within 7 to 30 years of disease onset. The cumulative lifetime risk is estimated

to be 40% by the age of 70 years. Therefore, screening by endoscopic ultrasound is recommended, starting at the age of 30 years.

Pancreas divisum is a congenital anatomic anomaly in which the ventral pancreas and dorsal pancreas fail to fuse. The resultant pancreas has dual drainage, with the dorsal pancreas draining through the duct of Santorini and the ventral pancreas (head and uncinate process) draining through the duct of Wirsung. The onset of symptoms is variable, ranging from early childhood to adulthood. Although ultrasound and CT are usually performed, ERCP is frequently used to confirm the diagnosis. However, MCRP has been touted as more advantageous because it can delineate the dorsal pancreatic duct in its entirety, as opposed to ERCP, which can assess only the ventral duct on cannulation of the major duodenal papilla. The significance of pancreas divisum and its predisposition to chronic pancreatitis remains controversial. Some have suggested that it may result in pancreatitis because all pancreatic output is forced to empty through the smaller lesser papilla. The result is an outflow obstruction that leads to ductal dilation. Treatment consists of transduodenal sphincteroplasty or a Puestow procedure (pancreaticojejunostomy); a Puestow procedure is preferred if the dorsal pancreatic duct is dilated or obstructed.

Biliary Dyskinesia

Obesity has also become a major health problem for adolescents. Along with that, we are seeing an increasing number of pediatric patients with cholelithiasis and biliary colic due to dyskinesia of the gallbladder. Biliary dyskinesia has become more prevalent and should be considered on evaluation of a teenager with epigastric pain. Pediatric surgeons are often consulted to evaluate for the appropriateness of performing a cholecystectomy based on a low ejection fraction from a cholecystokinin-stimulated HIDA scan. When an ejection fraction of less than 35% to 40% correlates with characteristic biliary colic, a cholecystectomy can be therapeutic.[30] However, in patients with vague symptoms, inconsistent with biliary colic, the beneficial role of cholecystectomy is seriously questioned.

ABDOMINAL WALL CONDITIONS

Abdominal Wall Defects

Anterior abdominal wall defects are a relatively frequent neonatal surgical condition in pediatric surgery. During normal development of the human embryo, the midgut herniates outward through the umbilical ring and continues to grow. By the eleventh week of gestation, the midgut returns to the coelomic cavity and undergoes proper rotation and fixation, along with closure of the umbilical ring. If the intestine fails to return, the infant is born with the abdominal contents protruding directly through the umbilical ring, with an intact sac covering the abdominal viscera, termed an omphalocele (Fig. 66-21A). In contrast, gastroschisis represents the abdominal wall defect, which is always to the right of an intact umbilical cord, without sac covering the abdominal viscera (Fig. 66-21B).

Omphalocele

Omphalocele is recognized as a central defect of the abdominal wall. Its defect is generally more than 4 cm in diameter with an intact membranous sac, which is composed of an outer layer of amnion and an inner layer of peritoneum. Defects less than 4 cm in diameter are arbitrarily designated hernias of the cord. Infants with an omphalocele have an approximately 50% incidence of associated anomalies. Beckwith-Wiedemann syndrome is a combination of gigantism, macroglossia, and an umbilical defect, either hernia or omphalocele. Chromosomal abnormalities, trisomies 13, 15, 18, and 21, have also been associated with omphalocele. Other major associated anomalies include exstrophy of the bladder or cloaca and the pentalogy of Cantrell—omphalocele, anterior diaphragmatic hernia, sternal cleft, ectopia cordis, and intracardiac defect, such as ventricular septal defect.

The treatment of omphalocele begins with the preservation of the intact sac with sterile, moistened, saline gauze or transparent bowel bag. IV fluid should be promptly started, along with gastric tube decompression and IV antibiotics. Great care should be taken to prevent hypothermia. A thorough diagnostic workup should be performed to identify associated anomalies. Primary surgical closure of the small to medium-sized defect is preferred. Alternative options to primary closure include prosthetic patch closure (e.g., Gore-Tex), porcine small intestinal submucosa–derived biomaterial (e.g., Surgisis), skin flap closure, and placement of a silo for sequential reduction and staged closure. Giant omphaloceles may be treated by topical application of escharotic agents such as povidone-iodine (Betadine) ointment, merbromin (Mercurochrome), or silver nitrate, allowing the sac to thicken and to epithelialize gradually. The overall survival for infants with omphalocele depends on the size of the defect and the severity of associated anomalies.

Gastroschisis

The gastroschisis defect is usually just to the right of the umbilical cord, at the site of the obliterated right umbilical vein. The fascial defect is typically approximately 4 cm in diameter. Because of the absence of a sac and direct exposure of the intestine to amniotic fluid in utero, the intestine is often thickened, edematous, and foreshortened. Associated anomalies are rare, but intestinal atresia is present in up to 15% of cases. Infants born with gastroschisis should be carefully handled to avoid injury to exposed bowel loops and to minimize fluid losses. In general, infants are placed in a warm, saline-filled plastic organ bag up to the nipple line. This allows gross inspection of eviscerated bowel at all times and also lessens fluid losses. One should be cautious for potential volvulus of eviscerated malrotated intestine. IV fluids are started at 1.5 times maintenance along with IV antibiotics. In general, fluid requirements are greater than those required for omphalocele because of increased fluid losses. An orogastric tube is placed to decompress the stomach.

For primary closure, bowel loops are reduced, and the fascia and skin are approximated. For defects requiring a prosthetic patch closure, a Gore-Tex patch can be used and the skin closed over it. Other biomaterial substitutes (e.g., AlloDerm, Surgisis) have been used with variable success.[31] If the viscera cannot be reduced into the abdomen, a silo is placed at the bedside and the eviscerated intestines are reduced serially during 5 to 7 days, followed by operative fascial closure. During the immediate postoperative period, if the abdominal wall closure is tight, patients may require aggressive fluid resuscitation to maintain adequate tissue perfusion and to prevent metabolic acidosis. Patients are maintained on TPN until they gain bowel function. In cases of associated intestinal atresia or stenosis, inflammation of the bowel may preclude an immediate repair. Then, the abdominal wall is repaired in a usual fashion and intestinal atresia is addressed in 6 to 8 weeks, when the inflammation resolves. Late occurrence of NEC has been reported in up to 20% of patients after gastroschisis

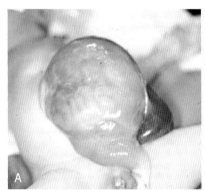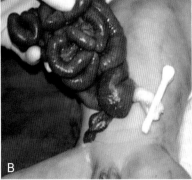

FIGURE 66-21 Abdominal Wall Defects. **A,** Omphalocele with intact sac. **B,** Gastroschisis with eviscerated multiple bowel loops to the right of the umbilical cord.

repair.[32] Undescended testes are also present in 10% to 20% of infants born with gastroschisis. When found outside the coelomic cavity, the testes should be placed into the abdominal cavity at the time of abdominal wall closure or silo bag placement. They are observed for a time to assess for spontaneous descent into the scrotum. If not, orchidopexy is performed. The majority of infants have prolonged ileus. Although TPN has been a lifesaving maneuver, it is associated with a high incidence of cholestasis and cirrhosis. One of the most difficult challenges in the management of gastroschisis remains managing dysfunctional intestine or short gut syndrome.

Hernias
Inguinal Hernia
Inguinal hernia repair is one of the most common surgical procedures in pediatric surgery. The incidence of inguinal hernia, which is almost all indirect and congenital in nature, is approximately 3% to 5% in term infants and 9% to 11% in premature infants. It affects boys approximately six times more often than girls. Sixty percent of inguinal hernias occur on the right side, 30% are on the left side, and 10% are bilateral. The processus vaginalis is an elongated diverticulum of the peritoneum that accompanies the testicle on its descent into the scrotum; it generally is obliterated during the ninth month of gestation or soon after birth. The variable persistence of the processus vaginalis results in a spectrum of clinical presentations, including a scrotal hernia with protrusion of intestine, ovaries, omentum, or communicating hydrocele, with intermittent accumulation of peritoneal fluid. All communicating hydroceles are repaired in the same manner as an indirect inguinal hernia.

Clinical presentation. Diagnosis is established by clinical history and examination alone, especially when the contents of the hernia reduce into the peritoneal cavity. Communicating hydroceles can be difficult to reduce at times and therefore can be misdiagnosed as simple hydroceles. Transillumination of the scrotum to differentiate a hydrocele from a hernia can be misleading because a herniated, thin-walled bowel loop can easily be transilluminated. Palpation of the cord may elicit a "silk glove sign," which is produced by rubbing the opposing peritoneal membranes of the empty sac. At times, palpation of a thickened cord in comparison to the contralateral side and a reliable history are sufficient to derive a diagnosis. The acute development of hydrocele may also be associated with the onset of other conditions, such as epididymitis, testicular torsion, and torsion of testicular appendage. In these clinical settings, ultrasound may be helpful to determine the diagnosis. The major risk factor of inguinal hernia is bowel incarceration, with potential strangulation. The incidence of incarceration is higher in premature infants in the first year of life.

Surgical management. Although early hernia repair may be associated with a higher risk for injury to the cord structures, recurrence rate, and postoperative apneic episodes, most pediatric surgeons advocate operative repair before discharge from the hospital for premature infants because of their significant risks for incarceration. However, for those infants diagnosed after hospital discharge, elective hernia repair may be deferred until the infant is beyond a safe postconceptional age of 52 to 55 weeks, when postoperative apnea risk decreases. In patients presenting with incarcerated inguinal hernia, unless there is clinical evidence of peritonitis, attempts are made to reduce the hernia. Manual reduction is successful in up to 70% of cases. Once the hernia is reduced, the patient is admitted for observation, and hernia repair is performed at 24 to 48 hours, when local tissue edema resolves. A nonreducible incarcerated hernia should be promptly explored in the operating room. Routine contralateral inguinal exploration at the time of symptomatic hernia repair for infants is standard practice based on the high incidence of contralateral patent processus vaginalis (4% to 65%). However, the issue regarding the routine exploration of the asymptomatic contralateral side in toddlers remains unresolved. Most pediatric surgeons routinely explore the asymptomatic contralateral side in children 2 years of age or younger; some surgeons extend the routine contralateral exploration criteria to those up to 5 years of age.

Umbilical Hernia
In general, umbilical hernia has a tendency to close on its own in approximately 80% of cases, and therefore elective repair should be deferred until approximately 5 years of age. The umbilical hernia rarely presents with complications, but there are unique exceptions to this general rule for which an earlier elective repair should be considered. Although rare, a history of incarceration clearly warrants prompt surgical repair, irrespective of age. Enlarging umbilical hernia over time, in particular with a large skin proboscis more than 3 cm or a significantly large umbilical fascial defect (>2 cm), is unlikely to resolve spontaneously; therefore, surgical repair should be considered at an early age.

CHEST WALL DEFORMITIES

The two major types of congenital chest wall deformities are pectus excavatum and pectus carinatum. Pectus excavatum is more prevalent, five times more common than pectus carinatum (Fig. 66-22*A*). Its incidence is estimated at approximately 1 in 100 children, with a male-to-female ratio of 3 to 4 : 1. The deformity is usually present at birth and steadily becomes more prominent. It can become more pronounced between 8 and 10 years of age and later again during puberty. It is also common to have associated kyphosis and scoliosis. Although the exact cause is unknown, abnormalities of costal cartilage development have been implicated. Pectus excavatum can be associated with congenital heart disease, including mitral valve prolapse, Ehlers-Danlos syndrome, and Marfan syndrome, and therefore thorough preoperative evaluation, such as ophthalmologic evaluation and echocardiography, should be considered.

To determine the severity of pectus excavatum and to assess the indications for surgery, two or more of the following criteria should be met: (1) Haller index (ratio of width of chest wall to depth of sternum to vertebral body) of more than 3.2; (2) abnormal pulmonary function test result; (3) mitral valve prolapse, murmurs, or conduction abnormalities on echocardiography; and (4) documentation of progression of deformity. Regardless of these objective measurements, one must carefully assess for the psychosocial burden caused by the pectus deformities. This is a critical issue, particularly for adolescents with significant concerns about body image and development of self-esteem. A multicenter study has shown that surgical repair of pectus excavatum significantly improves body image and perceived ability for physical activity.[33]

Patients are encouraged to perform exercises to strengthen the chest and back muscles and to maintain proper posture. Standard two-view chest radiographs are essential to assess for Haller index and to detect the presence of thoracic scoliosis. Pulmonary function tests may be indicated to document restrictive or obstructive

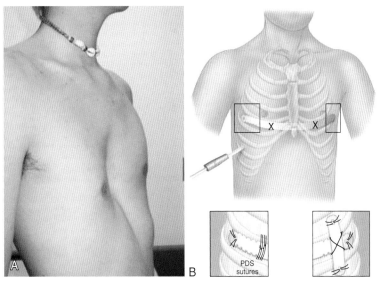

FIGURE 66-22 A, Pectus excavatum. **B,** A bar is placed beneath the sternum and secured onto the chest wall with stabilizers. (From Goretsky MJ, Nuss D: Surgical treatment of chest wall deformities: Nuss procedure. In Chung DH, Chen MK, editors: *Atlas of pediatric surgical techniques*, Philadelphia, 2010, Elsevier Saunders, pp 97–103.)

abnormalities. Aside from plain chest radiographs, a limited CT scan has been used to determine Haller index.

Surgical Management

The optimal age for pectus excavatum repair is 10 to 14 years because the chest wall is still soft and malleable. Also, recovery seems faster in this age group. After puberty, the chest wall is more rigid, thus requiring a longer period of bar support, even with the insertion of two bars. The Ravitch procedure, originally described in 1949, can be performed for pectus excavatum or carinatum deformities. It consists of a transverse inframammary skin incision overlying the deformity, bilateral subchondral resection of abnormal costal cartilages, sternal osteotomy, and anterior fixation of the sternum with a temporary retrosternal stainless metal bar, which is removed at a later time.

In the Nuss procedure, which was developed for pectus excavatum, a curved metal bar, contoured to elevate the sternum, is passed in a retrosternal plane from one hemithorax into the other through two lateral intercostal incisions (Fig. 66-22*B*). The Nuss bar is then flipped so that the convexity is outward, and the chest wall defect is immediately corrected. The bar is left in place for approximately 2 years. In contrast to the Ravitch procedure, a minimally invasive Nuss procedure involves less surgical tissue trauma and thus significantly less surgical morbidity. A multicenter prospective study has demonstrated that surgical repair for pectus excavatum can be performed safely with adequate pain management.[33]

Pectus carinatum occurs less frequently than pectus excavatum. Preoperative considerations are similar to those for pectus excavatum. Despite some compliance issues, a reasonably good outcome can be expected with the use of an external chest brace, especially when patients wear the brace for 14 to 16 hours daily.[34] It can also be surgically repaired by costal cartilage resection and sternal fixation, similar to that for pectus excavatum. However, this operation is becoming obsolete.

GENITOURINARY TRACT CONDITIONS

Cryptorchidism

Cryptorchidism is a condition in which one testis or both testes fail to descend into the scrotum before birth. Up to 30% of preterm infants can present with an undescended testis, but it also occurs in approximately 3% of full-term infants. Some undescended testes eventually descend by 1 year of age, but they are unlikely to descend after this time. The undescended testis is associated with histologic and morphologic changes as early as 6 months of age; atrophy of Leydig cells, decrease in tubular diameter, and impaired spermatogenesis can occur by 2 years of age. An undescended testis has had its descent halted somewhere along the path of normal descent and is most commonly located in the inguinal canal. A retractile testis is a normally descended testis that retracts into the inguinal canal but can be brought down into the scrotal sac during the examination. It is thought to result from a hyperreflexive cremasteric muscle contraction and does not require operative intervention. Nonpalpable testes may include an intra-abdominal, absent, or vanishing testis. Ectopic testes have had an aberrant path of descent; these can be found in perineal, femoral canal, and suprapubic regions.

Diagnosis and Treatment

Although ultrasound has been used increasingly to evaluate for undescended testes, an examination by an experienced surgeon has a higher sensitivity for locating an undescended testis in the inguinal canal. For a unilateral palpable testis in the inguinal canal, standard dartos pouch orchidopexy is performed. The recommended timing for this procedure is 6 months to 1 year of age. A general management algorithm for nonpalpable testes is shown in Figure 66-23. When an undescended testis is not palpable in the inguinal canal, a diagnostic laparoscopy is useful. If the testicular vessels are seen exiting the internal ring, an open inguinal orchidopexy is performed. For an intra-abdominal testis, a

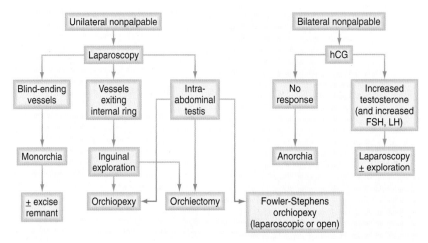

FIGURE 66-23 Algorithm for the management of nonpalpable undescended testes. (Adapted from Lee KL, Shortliffe LD: Undescended testis and testicular tumors. In Ashcraft KW, Holcomb GW, Holcomb GW III, et al, editors: *Pediatric surgery*, ed 4, Philadelphia, 2005, Elsevier Saunders, pp 706–716.)

two-stage Fowler-Stephens orchidopexy can be considered, in which testicular vessels are ligated as a first stage to allow collateral circulation to develop for 6 months before orchidopexy is performed as a second stage of the procedure. However, single-stage laparoscopic orchidopexy is also an ideal option for intra-abdominal testes. If both testes are nonpalpable, a human chorionic gonadotropin (hCG) stimulation test is carried out to confirm the presence of functioning testes. If present, diagnostic laparoscopy is performed to identify the testes and to determine surgical therapy. The risk of malignant transformation has been reported to be significantly greater for men with a history of undescended testes. Although orchidopexy does not decrease the malignancy risk associated with undescended testes, it allows earlier detection. Nonseminomatous germ cell tumors are usually associated with undescended testes.

Testicular Torsion

Torsion of the testis is the most common genitourinary tract emergency of childhood. On diagnosis, a prompt surgical detorsion with testicular fixation should be performed to relieve acute testicular ischemia. Extravaginal torsion is more common in neonates, in whom there can be torsion of the spermatic cord along its course outside the tunica vaginalis. Intravaginal torsion is associated with bell clapper deformity, in which the suspended testis can twist to torsion. Torsion of the testis occurs most frequently in early adolescence with a peak incidence at 14 years of age. Scrotal pain that is abrupt or gradual in nature is the primary symptom. On examination, the testis that has undergone torsion may be high-riding, edematous, and significantly tender. Urinary tract symptoms, such as frequency, urgency, dysuria, and fever, tend to occur more frequently with infectious or inflammatory conditions, such as epididymitis; however, in no way does this rule out testicular torsion. In most cases, a careful history and examination are sufficient to confirm the diagnosis of testicular torsion. However, if the diagnosis is uncertain, prompt ultrasonography may be helpful to determine vascular flow to the testicles. Radioisotope scanning is the most specific diagnostic test, but it can be time-consuming to obtain. The time for diagnosis and surgical repair directly correlates with the testicular salvage rate. Immediate surgical detorsion through

a scrotal medial raphe approach is the appropriate treatment. After detorsion of the affected testis, it is assessed for viability and fixed to the scrotum. In all cases, the contralateral testis should also be fixed in the scrotum. For torsion of less than 6 hours, 90% of testes can be salvaged. However, this salvage rate significantly decreases to less than 10% with more than 24 hours of symptoms.

Testicular Tumors

Testicular cancer accounts for less than 2% of all pediatric solid tumors. The peak incidence is 2 years of age, with a second peak during puberty. These tumors typically are manifested as a painless scrotal mass, often discovered incidentally. An ultrasound examination is useful, but CT scan is critical to evaluate for retroperitoneal lymphadenopathy as well as potential metastatic disease. Serum tumor markers are useful for diagnosis and for follow-up. α-Fetoprotein (AFP) is a glycoprotein produced by the fetal yolk sac, and its level is elevated in yolk sac tumors of the testes; β-hCG is produced by embryonal carcinomas and mixed teratomas. The most common prepubertal testicular cancer is of germ cell origin; yolk sac tumor, also known as endodermal sinus tumor, and embryonal carcinomas account for almost 40%. Children with yolk sac tumors present with elevated serum AFP levels, and tumors are typically localized to the testis. The standard surgical approach is radical inguinal orchiectomy. The role of retroperitoneal lymph node dissection with yolk sac tumor is controversial. Tumors with microscopic node involvement or nodal disease require systemic chemotherapy, with modified retroperitoneal lymphadenectomy. The overall survival from yolk sac tumors is approximately 70% to 90%.

PEDIATRIC SOLID TUMORS

Solid tumors in infants and children represent a challenging therapeutic problem, but with advances in diagnosis, staging, and treatment, outcomes are steadily improving. However, those with advanced-stage disease remain difficult to cure despite multimodality therapy. It is this population of patients that stands to gain the most with cancer biology discoveries.

Neuroblastoma

Neuroblastoma is the most common extracranial solid tumor in infants and children, accounting for 8% to 10% of all childhood cancers and 15% of all cancer-related deaths in the pediatric population.[35] There are approximately 600 new diagnoses reported annually. Although 90% of cases are diagnosed before the age of 5 years, 30% of those are diagnosed in the first year of life. The median age at diagnosis is 22 months.

Clinical Presentation

Arising from neural crest cells, neuroblastoma is a malignant neoplasm of the sympathetic nervous system and therefore occurs in sympathetic ganglia. Approximately 65% are found in the abdomen, with 50% localized to the adrenal medulla. They can also occur in the neck (5%), chest (20%), or pelvis (5%), and 1% of patients have no detectable primary. A patient's clinical presentation is dictated by tumor location, size, extent of invasion, and metabolic activity and presence of paraneoplastic symptoms. Many patients are asymptomatic, although it is not uncommon for some to present with constitutional symptoms (e.g., malaise, fevers, weight loss), an enlarging mass, pain, abdominal distention, lymphadenopathy, or respiratory distress. Pelvic masses may cause constipation or bladder dysfunction, whereas thoracic lesions can cause dysphagia or dyspnea. For cervical tumors, a patient may develop Horner syndrome or stridor, and in up to 15% of patients, epidural involvement may result in neurologic deficits, which, when progressive, can lead to paralysis.

At diagnosis, 50% of patients have localized disease and 35% have regional lymph node involvement. Metastasis to distant organs (e.g., liver, bone, skin) occurs by hematogenous and lymphatic routes. For bone marrow invasion, patients may become anemic, bruise easily, and complain of weakness. Bone metastasis can result in pain, swelling, limp, and pathologic fractures. The orbits are frequently involved, which is manifested as periorbital swelling and proptosis (raccoon eyes). Blue subcutaneous nodules represent skin dissemination of tumor associated with the blueberry muffin syndrome. Neuroblastomas can secrete catecholamines, resulting in early-onset hypertension and tachycardia. Patients may also experience paraneoplastic syndromes, which include intractable diarrhea caused by vasoactive intestinal peptide secretion, encephalomyelitis, and neuropathy. Opsoclonus-myoclonus syndrome—rapid, conjugate eye nystagmus with involuntary spasms of the limbs—although rare, occurs when antibodies cross-react with cerebellar tissue.

Genomics

Neuroblastoma occurs as whole chromosome gains, which result in hyperdiploidy and are associated with a favorable prognosis, or segmental chromosomal aberrations, which encompass *MYCN* amplification and gains or losses that tend to be associated with worse outcomes. The *MYCN* oncogene, which is amplified at chromosome 2p24 in 25% of cases, is overexpressed in 30% to 40% of stage 3 and stage 4 neuroblastomas but only in 5% of localized or stage 4S tumors. Therefore, it is used as a biomarker for disease stratification. It has been shown that deletion of the 1p36 region occurs in 70% of tumors and is usually associated with *MYCN*-amplified, high-stage tumors that confer a poor prognosis.[36] Conversely, a whole chromosome 17 gain is associated with a good prognosis. Deletions of chromosome 11q have been identified in 15% to 22% of neuroblastomas and are also associated with unfavorable patient outcomes and a reduced time of progression-free survival.

Diagnosis

An initial workup includes basic serum tests, imaging, and determination of urine levels of catecholamines or their metabolites (e.g., dopamine, vanillylmandelic acid, homovanillic acid). Patients may have elevated levels of nonspecific biomarkers, such as lactate dehydrogenase (>1500 U/mL), ferritin (>142 ng/mL), and neuron-specific enolase (>100 ng/mL), which are associated with advanced stage or relapse. Ultrasonography may be used to initially characterize the mass, but CT scan is essential to localize the tumor and to determine the degree of involvement (Fig. 66-24*A*). MRI may have advantages if there is concern for spinal extension. Although it is not routinely used, a [131]I- metaiodobenzylguanidine (MIBG) scan is valuable in the detection of primary tumor and metastases because a norepinephrine analogue is selectively concentrated in sympathetic tissue. The ^{131}I-MIBG scan is also used for the surveillance of treatment response and recurrence. The diagnosis is confirmed by demonstrating undifferentiated small round blue cells on histologic section (Fig. 66-24*B*).

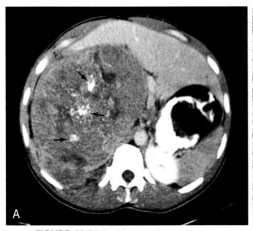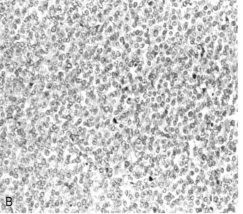

FIGURE 66-24 A, CT scan of neuroblastoma demonstrating areas of calcification *(arrows).* **B,** Small blue round cells of undifferentiated hyperchromatic neuroblasts. (From Kim S, Chung DH: Pediatric solid malignancies: Neuroblastoma and Wilms' tumor. *Surg Clin North Am* 86:469–487, 2006.)

Stage 1 or stage 2 disease can be resected primarily, but advanced-stage neuroblastomas generally require a tissue biopsy specimen from the unresectable tumor first or bone marrow. Molecular studies, such as fluorescent in situ hybridization, can be performed on tissue specimens to assess ploidy, *MYCN* amplification, and other chromosomal abnormalities. This information is required to outline specific risk category–based therapy for individual patients.

Staging

Neuroblastoma can be classified on the basis of the degree of neuroblastic differentiation and mitosis-karyorrhexis index (low, intermediate, or high). On histologic evaluation, neuroblastoma has limited Schwann cell production, is stroma poor, and has abundant neuroblasts.[37] The modified Shimada classification, on which the International Neuroblastoma Staging System (INSS; Table 66-3) is based, has been used to predict prognosis by the histopathologic features of the tumor and age of the patient. This system takes into account the degree of cell differentiation, mitosis-karyorrhexis index, and presence of Schwann cells. The Children's Oncology Group currently stratifies patients into low-, intermediate-, or high-risk categories on the basis of the patient's age at diagnosis, INSS stage, tumor histopathology, DNA index, and *MYCN* amplification status.[38] Thus, treatment recommendations depend on the stage to which the patient is assigned.

Treatment

The standard multimodality therapy is based on disease risk classification and treatment stratification (Table 66-4). Induction chemotherapy consists of a multidrug regimen, including but not limited to cyclophosphamide, doxorubicin, cisplatin, carboplatin, etoposide, and vincristine. However, high-risk group neuroblastomas frequently acquire resistance to chemotherapeutics and thus have high disease relapse. This usually necessitates autologous hematopoietic stem cell transplantation. Complete surgical resection correlates with a lower local recurrence, especially in combination with induction chemotherapy and local radiation therapy. Thus, some advocate that surgical resection should be considered only after adjuvant therapy. Primary surgical resection is recommended for stages 1 to 2B tumors. For more advanced stages 3 and 4, only the incisional biopsy specimen is obtained initially for tumor biology studies. The role of aggressive surgical resection of the primary tumor site for metastatic stage 4 neuroblastoma in patients 18 months or older has recently been questioned.[39] For infants with stage 4S disease, surgical resection is not recommended because of the high rate of spontaneous differentiation and regression.

For high-risk patients, radiation therapy is often needed for local and metastatic control. Radiation is contraindicated for intraspinal tumors because it can lead to vertebral damage, growth arrest, and scoliosis. However, it may be necessary for palliation in the setting of pain, hepatomegaly with respiratory compromise, or acute neurologic symptoms caused by tumor compression of the cord. It is further indicated when there is minimal residual disease after induction chemotherapy and resection. The overall outcomes in patients with neuroblastoma have improved steadily during the past decades, with 5-year survival rates rising from 52% to 74%.[38] The low-risk group has shown significant improvement in survival rates of up to 92%. It is estimated that 50% to 60% of the high-risk group relapse after standard therapy. However, immunotherapy with granulocyte-macrophage colony-stimulating factor and interleukin-2 improved survival in children with high-risk disease in remission after myeloablative therapy and stem cell rescue.[40]

Wilms Tumor

Wilms tumor (WT), also known as nephroblastoma, is an embryonal renal neoplasm consisting of metanephric blastema; it accounts for 85% of cases.[41] It represents 5.9% of all pediatric malignant tumors and has an annual incidence of 7.6 cases/million children younger than 15 years. There are 500 reported new cases annually, and approximately 75% of WT cases are diagnosed in children younger than 5 years. The peak incidence

TABLE 66-3 International Neuroblastoma Staging System

STAGE	DEFINITION
1	Localized tumor with complete gross excision, with or without microscopic residual disease; representative ipsilateral lymph nodes negative for tumor microscopically (nodes attached to and removed with the primary tumor may be positive)
2A	Localized tumor with incomplete gross excision; representative ipsilateral nonadherent lymph nodes negative for tumor microscopically
2B	Localized tumor with or without complete gross excision, with ipsilateral nonadherent lymph nodes positive for tumor; enlarged contralateral lymph nodes must be negative microscopically
3	Unresectable unilateral tumor with contralateral regional lymph node involvement or midline tumor with bilateral extension by infiltration (unresectable) or by lymph node involvement
4	Any primary tumor with dissemination to distant lymph nodes, bone, bone marrow, liver, skin, or other organs (except as defined for stage 4S)
4S	Localized primary tumor (as defined for stage 1, 2A, or 2B), with dissemination limited to skin, liver, or bone marrow (limited to infant <1 year of age)

TABLE 66-4 Risk Group Categories for Neuroblastoma

RISK GROUP	STAGE	FACTORS
Low	1	
	2	<1 yr
		>1 yr, low N-*myc*
		>1 yr, amplified N-*myc*; favorable histology
	4S	Favorable biology*
Intermediate	3	<1 yr, low N-*myc*
		>1 yr, favorable biology*
	4	<1 yr, low N-*myc*
	4S	Low N-*myc*
High	2	>1 yr, all unfavorable biology*
	3	<1 yr, amplified N-*myc*
		>1 yr, any unfavorable biology*
	4	<1 yr, amplified N-*myc*
		>1 yr
	4S	Amplified N-*myc*

*Favorable biology denotes low N-*myc*, favorable histology, and hyperdiploidy (infants).

occurs at 2 to 3 years. Of all patients, 13% can present with a bilateral tumor, which is usually synchronous in 60% of cases.

Genomics

Divided into overgrowth and nonovergrowth disorders, a number of syndromes can predispose to the development of WT. These include Beckwith-Wiedemann (macroglossia, macrosomia, midline abdominal wall defects, and neonatal hypoglycemia), Li-Fraumeni (*p53* germline mutation with predisposition to various cancers), and Denys-Drash (gonadal dysgenesis, nephropathy, and WT) syndromes and neurofibromatosis. In 10% of patients, WT can be associated with other congenital anomalies, collectively known as WAGR syndrome (aniridia, hemihypertrophy, genitourinary malformations, and mental retardation).[42]

The WT suppressor gene *WT1* is located on chromosome 11p13, which contains genes responsible for the development of the kidney, genitourinary tract, and eyes. Mutations in *WT1* result in genitourinary abnormalities, such as cryptorchidism and hypospadias, but also increase the risk for development of WT. Aniridia is found in 1.1% of WT patients, and when *WT1* deletions are found in these patients, there is a 40% rate of WT development. Moreover, mutations in *WT2*, located at 11p15, have been linked to Beckwith-Wiedemann syndrome, and there is a 4% to 10% risk for development of WT in those who also have hemihypertrophy. A study has determined that the X-linked tumor suppressor gene *WTX* can be inactivated in up to one third of WT cases.

Clinical Presentation

WT is typically discovered incidentally during a physical examination or because parents palpate an abdominal mass. Other presenting symptoms include abdominal pain and hematuria, which may signify tumor invasion into the collecting system or ureter. Another 25% develop hypertension, which is thought to occur secondary to disturbances in the renin-angiotensin feedback loop. Less than 10% of patients have atypical presentations; these include varicocele, hepatomegaly caused by hepatic vein obstruction, ascites, and congestive heart failure. WT may also be associated with predisposing syndromes, and the index of suspicion in these cases should be high, with a low threshold to obtain a screening ultrasound study.

Diagnosis

Ultrasonography is initially performed to determine whether the tumor is actually of renal origin, is cystic or solid, or extends into the renal vein or IVC. A CT scan is useful to delineate WT from neuroblastoma (Fig. 66-25) and also to evaluate for regional adenopathy, contralateral kidney involvement, and distant metastasis. MRI is also a useful adjunct for evaluating intravascular invasion; however, an ultrasound study may be preferred. Lung metastases, which are present in 8% at the time of diagnosis, can be identified on an initial chest radiograph, but CT scan is obtained routinely.

Pathology

The histology of WT is categorized as favorable or unfavorable. Favorable histology is more common, characterized by the presence of three elements—blastemal, stromal, and epithelial cells. WT with predominantly epithelial differentiation behaves less aggressively and tends to be stage I when it is diagnosed early. Blastemal-predominant tumors tend to be clinically aggressive and are associated with advanced disease. Outcomes are correlated with histopathologic features and tumor stage. Unfavorable

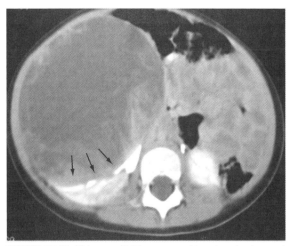

FIGURE 66-25 CT image of Wilms tumor with a claw sign *(arrows).* (From Kim S, Chung DH: Pediatric solid malignancies: Neuroblastoma and Wilms' tumor. *Surg Clin North Am* 86:469–487, 2006.)

histology is defined by the presence of anaplasia, clear cell sarcoma, or rhabdoid tumor. Anaplastic WT can be focal or diffuse and is synonymous with unfavorable histology whenever it is encountered; it is associated with an increased risk of tumor recurrence and resistance to standard chemotherapy. Nephrogenic rests are precursor lesions found in 25% to 40% of kidneys with WT but do not have oncologic potential. Instead, they can undergo differentiation and spontaneously regress through unclear mechanisms.

Staging

Tumor staging is one of the most important criteria in the therapeutic and prognostic consideration of WT. The International Society of Pediatric Oncology (SIOP) staging system is based on preoperative chemotherapy but is applied after resection. The presence of metastases is evaluated at presentation, relying on imaging studies, and chemotherapy is instituted before operative intervention. The National Wilms Tumor Study Group (NWTSG) has also developed a staging system that incorporates the clinical, surgical, and pathologic information that was obtained at the time of resection but stratifies patients before the initiation of chemotherapy (Table 66-5). The advantage of this system is that it favors stage-based therapy, thereby avoiding unnecessary chemotherapy in patients who might not otherwise benefit from it.[43]

Treatment

The mainstay of therapy for WT is surgery and chemotherapy. Surgical exploration is necessary for formal staging, and a radical nephrectomy is the standard. Utmost care must be taken to ensure en bloc resection with tumor-free margins because contamination and tumor spillage result in local recurrence. Vascular tumor extension into the IVC constitutes stage III disease and is managed accordingly. Sampling of the hilar, para-aortic, and paracaval lymph nodes is critical. Nephron-sparing surgery is usually reserved for children with a solitary kidney or bilateral WT. In these patients, preoperative chemotherapy may be used to induce tumor shrinkage to allow a more complete resection. However, there is an increased risk of positive surgical margins and local tumor recurrence. Partial nephrectomy may be considered if the tumor involves only one pole of the kidney, there is no evidence

TABLE 66-5   National Wilms Tumor Study Group Staging System

STAGE	DEFINITION
I	Tumor limited to the kidney and completely excised without rupture or biopsy. Surface of the renal capsule is intact.
II	Tumor extends through the renal capsule but is completely removed, with no microscopic involvement of the margins. Vessels outside the kidney contain tumor. Also placed in stage II are cases in which the kidney has undergone biopsy before removal or where there is local spillage of tumor (during resection) limited to the tumor bed.
III	Residual tumor is confined to the abdomen and of nonhematogenous spread. Includes tumors with involvement of the abdominal lymph nodes, diffuse peritoneal contamination by rupture of the tumor extending beyond the tumor bed, peritoneal implants, and microscopic or grossly positive resection margins.
IV	Hematogenous metastases at any site
V	Bilateral renal involvement

BOX 66-2   Treatment Regimens for Wilms Tumor*

- Stage I (FH, focal anaplasia): Surgery, VA × 18 wk, no XRT
- Stage II (FH): Surgery, VA × 18 wk, no XRT
- Stage II (focal anaplasia): Surgery, VDA × 24 wk, XRT to tumor bed
- Stage III (FH, focal anaplasia): Surgery, VDA × 24 wk, XRT to tumor bed
- Stage III (focal anaplasia): Surgery, VDA × 24 wk, XRT to tumor bed
- Stage IV (FH; focal anaplasia): Surgery, VDA × 24 wk, XRT to tumor bed according to local tumor stage and lung or other metastatic sites
- Stages II-IV (diffuse anaplasia): Surgery, VDEC × 24 wk, XRT to whole lung and abdomen
- Stages I-IV (clear cell sarcoma): Surgery, VDEC × 24 wk, XRT to abdomen; XRT to whole lung for stage IV only
- Stages I-IV (rhabdoid tumor): Surgery, ECCa × 24 wk, XRT

A, Dactinomycin; *C*, cyclophosphamide; *Ca*, carboplatin; *D*, doxorubicin; *E*, etoposide; *FH*, favorable histology; *V*, vincristine; *XRT*, radiation therapy.
*National Wilms Tumor Study. Infants younger than 11 months are given half the recommended dose of all drugs.

of collecting system or vascular involvement, clear margins exist between the tumor and surrounding structures, and the involved kidney demonstrates appreciable function. Unfortunately, less than 5% of patients meet these criteria, and it is uncertain whether this approach provides any long-term benefit. According to NWTSG recommendations (Box 66-2), the typical chemotherapy regimen consists of vincristine and dactinomycin, with the addition of doxorubicin (Adriamycin) or radiation therapy based on tumor stage and histologic favorability. The SIOP advocated the use of preoperative chemotherapy to improve cure and disease-free survival rates at 5 years. The overall survival for children with WT has improved from 30% to almost 90% 5- to 7-year survival. Stage I or stage II favorable histology or stage I unfavorable histology has nearly 95% survival rate. For WT with unfavorable histology, stages II, III, and IV are associated with 70%, 56%, and 17% 4-year survival rates, respectively.

Rhabdomyosarcoma

Derived from embryonic mesenchymal cells that can later differentiate into skeletal muscle, rhabdomyosarcoma is a soft tissue malignant neoplasm that accounts for approximately 4% of all pediatric cancer. The incidence is 4.3 cases/million children, with approximately 350 new cases diagnosed annually.[44] With a bimodal peak incidence, children are affected between the ages of 2 and 5 years and again from 15 to 19 years. Almost 50% are diagnosed before the age of 5 years. Most cases occur sporadically, with no recognizable risk factors, although rhabdomyosarcoma is known to occur with increased frequency in patients with neurofibromatosis type 1 and Li-Fraumeni and Beckwith-Wiedemann syndromes.

Pathology

Rhabdomyosarcoma has been pathologically classified into three types: embryonal, alveolar, and pleomorphic. Embryonal rhabdomyosarcoma is the most common, accounting for more than two thirds of all rhabdomyosarcomas. Two subtypes of embryonal rhabdomyosarcoma, botryoid and spindle cell, appear to be associated with a better prognosis than others of similar histology. On examination of a sample, characteristic rhabdomyoblasts may be present; immunohistochemical staining for muscle-specific proteins, such as myosin and actin, desmin, and myoglobin, can bolster the diagnosis.

Clinical Presentation

Rhabdomyosarcoma can appear at any site in the body, including those that do not typically contain skeletal muscle. The most common sites in children are the head and neck (35%), genitourinary tract (25%), and extremities (20%). Less common primary sites are the trunk, GI tract, and intrathoracic and perineal regions. Head and neck lesions tend to occur in the parameningeal region, orbits, and pharynx. Other specific sites include the bladder, prostate, vagina, uterus, liver, biliary tract, paraspinal region, and chest wall. These tumors are typically asymptomatic, although most symptoms are related to compressive effects and can result in pain. Orbital tumors can produce proptosis, decreased visual acuity, and ophthalmoplegia. Those arising from parameningeal sites frequently produce headaches and nasal or sinus obstruction that can be accompanied by a mucopurulent or bloody discharge. Moreover, these tumors can invade intracranially to produce cranial nerve palsies. For genitourinary rhabdomyosarcoma, paratesticular tumors may present as painless swelling in the scrotum, which may be confused with a hernia, hydrocele, or varicocele. Bladder tumors, commonly located at the base and trigone, result in hematuria and urinary obstruction. Vaginal tumors in girls present with a protruding mass or vaginal bleeding and discharge. Biliary tract tumors represent 0.8% of all rhabdomyosarcomas, and as with other causes of biliary obstruction, patients present with jaundice, abdominal swelling, fever, and loss of appetite. In the extremities, rhabdomyosarcomas involve the distal limb more commonly, and the lower extremities are affected more often. At the time of diagnosis, almost 50% of patients have regional lymph node metastasis. Retroperitoneal tumors can be quite large at presentation. Symptoms arise secondary to invasion of adjacent structures, and the associated pain and distention are typical late features of disease.

Diagnosis and Staging

There are no specific serum tumor markers for diagnosis. Depending on tumor location, MRI or CT should be used to characterize

BOX 66-3   Staging for Rhabdomyosarcoma

Group I: Localized disease that is completely resected, with no regional node involvement

Group II

   A. Localized, grossly resected tumor with microscopic residual disease but no regional nodal involvement

   B. Locoregional disease with tumor-involved lymph nodes with complete resection and no residual disease

   C. Locoregional disease with involved nodes, grossly resected, but with evidence of microscopic residual tumor at the primary site and/or histologic involvement of the most distal regional node (from the primary site)

Group III: Localized, gross residual disease including incomplete resection or biopsy only of the primary site

Group IV: Distant metastatic disease present at time of diagnosis

the mass and to evaluate for adjacent structural invasion, vessel encasement, metastasis, and adenopathy. One of the most critical aspects of the diagnostic evaluation is obtaining tissue samples for histologic confirmation, which is usually accomplished by an incisional or core needle biopsy. A complete surgical resection is ideal, but a large tumor may necessitate preoperative chemotherapy for preoperative tumor shrinkage. Botryoid (cluster of grapes) and spindle cell rhabdomyosarcomas are noted to have a favorable prognosis, whereas embryonal and pleomorphic histology confers an intermediate prognosis, and alveolar and undifferentiated histology exhibits a poor prognosis.

Pretreatment staging serves to stratify patients, to determine the most appropriate treatment regimen, and to compare outcomes. Because it relies on preoperative imaging, this is technically clinical staging, although it is still based on TNM criteria (Box 66-3). Intraoperative or pathologic results from resected samples should have no bearing on stage. This is reserved for what is known as clinical grouping, which consists of selection into a group depending on operative findings, pathology, margins, and node status. Taken together, clinical grouping and pretreatment staging have been shown to correlate with outcomes. For example, low-risk patients have an estimated 3-year failure-free survival rate of 88%, intermediate-risk patients have an estimated 3-year failure-free survival rate of 55% to 76%, and high-risk patients have a 3-year failure-free survival rate of less than 30%.

Treatment

The main goal of multimodality therapy is to achieve cure or, at a minimum, to obtain local control. Equally important is the need to minimize the short- and long-term effects of therapy. Currently, all patients with rhabdomyosarcoma receive some combination chemotherapy because it improves progression-free and overall survival. The recommended regimen depends on the risk stratification, with low-risk patients in subgroup A receiving vincristine and dactinomycin. For patients in the low-risk subgroup B and higher, cyclophosphamide is added to this therapy. Radiation therapy has been found to be effective for the local control of rhabdomyosarcoma, especially in patients who have microscopic disease after resection. It has also been successfully used in patients in whom surgery could result in significant disfigurement, such as with head and neck lesions. However, complications of radiation therapy are not negligible, including the potential development of secondary malignant neoplasms.

As is the case with most surgical approaches, a complete resection with negative margins and nodal sampling is the mainstay of treatment. The specific operative guidelines depend on the location of the tumor. For example, for head and neck tumors that are superficial and nonorbital, wide excision of the primary tumor with sampling of ipsilateral cervical lymph nodes is acceptable. Parameningeal lesions are particularly difficult to resect completely, given their degree of extension into critical structures. In these patients and in patients with tumors that are considered unresectable, chemotherapy and radiation therapy are first-line treatment. For extremity lesions, it is imperative to achieve complete wide local excision. Amputation is rarely necessary, except for distal tumors in the hand or foot that involve neurovascular structures. Given that trunk and extremity lesions have a high incidence of lymph node metastasis, sentinel lymph node mapping is being increasingly used. Re-excision may also be considered with evidence of minimal residual disease after initial resection. Patients with extremity tumors receive combination chemotherapy, but because of the high incidence of the alveolar histology, radiation therapy is also often used. For genitourinary tumors, preservation of bladder function is the key in resection of tumors involving the bladder or prostate. If this goal cannot be met, preoperative chemoradiation is usually recommended. If residual disease remains despite this, more aggressive measures can be considered, including a partial cystectomy, prostatectomy, or anterior (rectum-sparing) exenteration. Patients with paratesticular rhabdomyosarcoma should undergo a radical inguinal orchiectomy, with a retroperitoneal lymph node dissection in boys younger than 10 years because of the frequent prevalence of metastasis. When the tumor is clearly fixed to scrotal skin, resection is required. Chemotherapy is standard, whereas radiation therapy is indicated only with positive nodes. For patients with vaginal or vulvar rhabdomyosarcoma, vaginectomy and wide local excision, respectively, and multiagent chemotherapy are recommended. Approximately 15% of children present with metastatic disease, and their prognosis remains poor. Nearly 30% will experience disease relapse, and 50% to 95% of them will die as the disease progresses. Median survival from the first recurrence is 0.8 year, with an estimated 5-year survival rate of only 17%. Despite these harrowing data, however, rhabdomyosarcoma is a curable disease in most children, with more than 60% surviving 5 years after diagnosis. Survival for children with this malignant neoplasm has improved secondary to a number of factors, including better imaging and pathologic classification, use of multiagent chemotherapy, and appropriate use of radiotherapy.

Liver Tumors

Primary tumors of the liver are rare in the pediatric population but are malignant in approximately 60% of cases. The two most common tumors are hepatoblastoma and hepatocellular carcinoma (HCC). Hepatoblastoma represents 80% of all malignant liver tumors and 1% of all pediatric cancer. The peak incidence of hepatoblastoma is at 3 years of age; the median age for children with HCC is 10 to 11.2 years. More than 90% of patients younger than 5 years with primary liver tumors have hepatoblastoma, whereas 87% of those between 15 and 19 years have HCC.[45] Patients with familial adenomatous polyposis, Gardner, and Beckwith-Wiedemann syndromes are at increased risk for development of hepatoblastoma. HCC is associated with acquired hepatitis B and C and has been observed in children with several types of congenital diseases, including tyrosinemia, glycogen storage disease type I, α_1-antitrypsin deficiency, and cholestasis caused by biliary atresia.

Clinical Presentation

Hepatoblastoma typically is manifested as a painless palpable abdominal mass. Other symptoms are nonspecific and include anorexia, weight loss and failure to thrive, abdominal pain, anemia, and abdominal distention. Jaundice is not commonly encountered because liver function remains relatively normal except in a very advanced tumor. Some patients present with tumor rupture, resulting in intra-abdominal bleeding and peritonitis. HCC is manifested similarly, although stigmata of cirrhosis, such as jaundice, spider angiomas, ascites, and splenomegaly, may be encountered. Almost 25% of patients have metastatic spread to abdominal and mediastinal lymph nodes, lung, bone marrow, and brain.

Diagnosis and Staging

Basic blood tests usually reveal normal liver function in hepatoblastoma, whereas there will be abnormalities in HCC. Anemia, thrombocytopenia, or pancytopenia can be found with splenomegaly caused by sequestration. AFP levels are elevated in more than 70% of hepatoblastoma patients. However, an elevated AFP level is not pathognomonic, and depending on the age of the patient, other disease processes must be ruled out. For example, in infants younger than 6 months, elevated AFP levels may also be seen in sarcomas, yolk sac tumors, and hamartomas. All children being evaluated for HCC should be tested for exposure to hepatitis B and C viruses.

Abdominal ultrasonography is an excellent initial diagnostic study. Doppler ultrasound can also detect the presence of tumor extension into or thrombosis of major vessels, namely, the hepatic veins, IVC, and portal vein. A CT scan is essential in assessing the relationship of the tumor to adjacent vital structures, such as bile ducts and vessels, and excluding intra-abdominal tumor extension beyond the liver. MRI can similarly be used in this setting but does not necessarily provide significant advantages over CT. Because hepatoblastoma frequently spreads hematologically to the lungs, chest CT should also be performed. Bone scintigraphy is recommended for staging in children with HCC because of the high incidence of bone metastases. Hepatoblastoma characteristically appears as a unifocal mass surrounded by a pseudocapsule; it may be a pure epithelial type that contains fetal or embryonal cells or a mixture of the two histologic subtypes, which contains mesenchymal tissue in addition to epithelial components. On the other hand, HCC is characterized by large, pleomorphic epithelial cells that appear much like mature hepatocytes. In gross appearance, HCC forms multifocal nodules that lack a fibrous tumor and often lead to diffuse intrahepatic involvement. Unlike in adults, there has been no indisputable evidence that histopathologic type has any bearing on prognosis.

A standard TNM system has been used for staging purposes, but much effort has been put into the development of a pretreatment staging system, known as the PRE-Treatment EXTent of disease (PRETEXT) definition system (Table 66-6).[46] The PRETEXT system was developed by the International Childhood Liver Tumor Strategy Group (SIOPEL) for staging and risk stratification of liver tumors. It divides the liver into four sections based on segmental anatomy of the liver, and the tumor is subsequently classified by the number of tumor-free sections of liver (Fig. 66-26). This system takes caudate lobe involvement, tumor rupture, ascites, extension into the stomach or diaphragm, tumor

TABLE 66-6 PRETEXT Definition for Hepatoblastoma

PRETEXT GROUP	DEFINITION
I	One section involved; three adjoining sections are tumor free
II	One or two sections involved; two adjoining sections are tumor free
III	Two or three sections involved; one adjoining section is tumor free
IV	Four sections involved

focality, lymph node involvement, presence of distant metastases, and vascular involvement into further consideration. Patients are considered at high risk if they have a serum AFP level above 100 ng/mL, extension beyond the liver, distant metastases, intraperitoneal hemorrhage, and invasion of the hepatic veins, IVC, or portal vein. For PRETEXT I and II, hepatoblastoma may be resected by segmentectomy or anatomic lobectomy.

Treatment

Liver transplantation is a potential surgical option for patients with a massive unresectable tumor. Neoadjuvant chemotherapy is used for tumor shrinkage and potential complete resection. Interestingly, some advocate the use of preoperative chemotherapy to treat what would otherwise be residual microscopic disease left behind after resection. They argue that doing so eliminates tumor cells that could respond to hepatotrophic factors during liver regeneration, thereby decreasing the risk of recurrence. There are two current approaches to hepatoblastoma: (1) tumor resection followed by chemotherapy and (2) tumor biopsy followed by chemotherapy and delayed resection. Patients with stage I tumors with pure fetal histology usually do not require postoperative chemotherapy. However, patients with stage II or higher tumors and tumors of any other type of histology do require chemotherapy consisting of cisplatin, 5-fluorouracil, and vincristine. For patients with residual tumor after resection, chemotherapy should be coupled with an evaluation for transplantation.[45] Criteria for transplantation include having no more than three tumors smaller than 3 cm in diameter and no evidence of extrahepatic disease or vascular invasion. When relapses occur, doxorubicin, irinotecan, and ifosfamide have been used, often with some success. Another modality being used with variable success in children whose tumors are unresponsive to systemic chemotherapy is direct arterial chemotherapy or chemoembolization. Long-term outcomes have yet to be determined. Long-term disease-free survival of more than 85% to 90% can be achieved for resectable hepatoblastoma, although similar estimates have been noted for patients with unresectable hepatoblastoma treated by liver transplantation. The same cannot be said for HCC, in which survival rates with partial hepatectomy remain poor because of relapse. In the past decade, early transplantation has been shown to result in better outcomes in some centers.

Teratoma

Teratomas are typically benign neoplasms that contain elements derived from more than one of the three embryonic germ layers, endoderm, mesoderm, and ectoderm. They are composed of tissue that is foreign to the anatomic site in which they are found. Although teratomas may occur anywhere along the midline, they

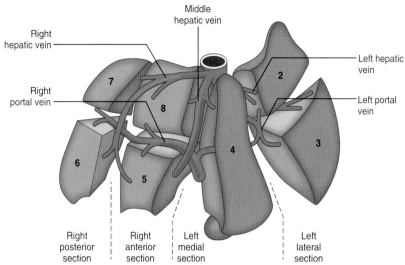

FIGURE 66-26 A diagram of PRETEXT definition system for hepatoblastoma. The liver is divided into four sections based on segmental anatomy of the liver, and the tumor is subsequently classified by the number of tumor-free sections of liver. (From Roebuck DJ, Aronson D, Clapuyt P, et al: 2005 PRETEXT: A revised staging system for primary malignant liver tumors of childhood developed by the SIOPEL group. *Pediatr Radiol* 37:123–132, 2007.)

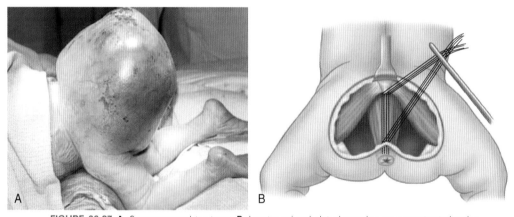

FIGURE 66-27 **A,** Sacrococcygeal teratoma. **B,** Levator ani and gluteal muscles are reconstructed and a drain is left in place. (**B** from Dicken BJ, Rescorla FJ: Sacrococcygeal teratoma. In Chung DH, Chen MK, editors: *Atlas of pediatric surgical techniques*, Philadelphia, 2010, Elsevier Saunders, pp 364–373.)

are usually found in sacrococcygeal, mediastinal, retroperitoneal, and gonadal locations. Teratomas may be solid, cystic, or mixed and are classified as mature or immature. Although immature teratomas can be potentially malignant, the incidence of malignant transformation in mature teratomas is low. There is a preponderance based on gender; almost 80% of all teratomas occur in females. Moreover, location has been associated with age, as evidenced by the fact that extragonadal tumors occur primarily in neonates and young children, whereas gonadal tumors are more commonly noted in adolescents.

Sacrococcygeal Teratomas

Sacrococcygeal teratomas (SCTs) account for 60% of all teratomas and can be manifested as large exophytic masses in utero. In such cases, they are detected on prenatal ultrasound. Complications include polyhydramnios and fetal hydrops, which can result in

fetal demise caused by a tumor-induced vascular steal syndrome that leads to high-output heart failure. Symptoms can include weakness, paralysis, bowel or bladder dysfunction, and other neurologic symptoms that may indicate intradural spinal extension. The diagnosis can be made clinically, especially with exophytic SCTs (Fig. 66-27*A*). If the AFP or β-hCG level is elevated, yolk sac or choriocarcinoma components, respectively, make up the teratoma. Ultrasonography, CT, or MRI may be necessary to detect intra-abdominal lesions or to determine whether there is pelvic or abdominal extension.

Surgical resection is the standard of care and should be performed promptly because of the risk of hemorrhage and tumor rupture. Operative planning must take into account the degree of intra-abdominal extension. Most tumors can be resected by a posterior approach, in which a chevron incision allows the division of the gluteal muscles, ligation of the blood supply, and en bloc resection of the tumor and coccyx (Fig. 66-27*B*). It is important to preserve the anorectal complex to maintain long-term continence. External tumors with significant intra-abdominal extension require a combined abdominal and posterior approach, whereas teratomas that are entirely intra-abdominal may be approached through laparotomy or laparoscopy. Outcomes are favorable with respect to survival and quality of life. The age at diagnosis is the most important factor; those diagnosed at less than 30 weeks of gestation or after 2 months postnatally tend to have a poor prognosis. The risk of malignant transformation associated with embryonal histology is 15% to 20%. Risk of local recurrence ranges from 4% to 11%, although failure to resect the coccyx is associated with a 37% risk of recurrence. AFP levels should be monitored at 3-month intervals for 3 to 4 years. For recurrence, re-excision should be considered.

Ovarian Neoplasms

Approximately 50% of all ovarian lesions in children are neoplastic but are rarely malignant. It is estimated that ovarian malignant neoplasms represent 10% of all ovarian masses but only 1% of childhood cancers. Primary ovarian malignant neoplasms can be classified as germ cell, epithelial cell, and sex cord stromal tumors. Germ cell tumors include teratomas and choriocarcinoma; sex cord stromal tumors consist of granulosa (thecal) and Sertoli (Leydig) cells. Epithelial cell tumors encompass serous and mucinous cystadenomas and cystadenocarcinomas.[47] Symptoms are usually pain related because of mass compression. The presence of ascites, omental masses, peritoneal or diaphragmatic implants, adherence to surrounding organs, aortoiliac adenopathy, size larger than 8 cm, or contralateral ovarian mass should raise suspicion for malignancy.

Germ cell tumors. An ovarian teratoma is the most common ovarian germ cell tumor. It also represents the most common pediatric ovarian neoplasm and accounts for 25% of all childhood teratomas. These tumors occur with equal frequency in either ovary and may even be bilateral in 10% of patients. They typically are manifested with abdominal or pelvic pain and may involve ovarian torsion in approximately 25% of patients. Germ cell tumors account for 7% to 80% of all neoplastic ovarian masses. Dysgerminomas are the least differentiated of the germ cell tumors and are bilateral in 10% to 15% of cases. Although pure dysgerminomas are malignant, they tend to present while still localized and are highly responsive to chemoradiation. Survival is almost 90% with complete surgical resection.

Sex cord tumors. Sex cord tumors arise from the stromal elements of the ovary, producing hormones that may result in precocious puberty. Interestingly, these tumors have been associated with Peutz-Jeghers syndrome. Abnormal menstruation, swelling, and pain are common chief complaints. Outcomes after resection are good in this group because most lesions are still limited to the ovary. Advanced-stage tumors are responsive to platinum-based chemotherapy. Granulosa cell tumors account for 1% to 10% of ovarian malignant neoplasms in females younger than 20 years, whereas Sertoli-Leydig cell tumors account for 20% of ovarian sex cord stromal tumors. Because they are androgenic, serum testosterone metabolite levels can be elevated. With estrogen excess, patients develop early sexual characteristics, such as breast or labial enlargement, axillary and pubic hair growth, and galactorrhea.

Epithelial tumors. Less than 20% of ovarian tumors in childhood are epithelial in nature, given that they are rare before menarche. The two main histologic subtypes are serous and mucinous tumors, which can be further described as benign,

malignant, or borderline malignant. It is possible to classify the subtypes as adenoma or adenocarcinoma; adenocarcinoma is extremely rare but is associated with a poor prognosis.

Diagnosis

AFP and β-hCG levels help provide information about tumor biology and can be used to measure treatment response. Although nonspecific, the lactate dehydrogenase level may also be elevated. Also, if there is any evidence of menstrual abnormalities or precocious puberty, luteinizing hormone and follicle-stimulating hormone levels should also be checked. Abdominal ultrasound is performed to evaluate the tumor and contralateral ovary. A CT scan can provide information on tumor extension, regional adenopathy, and distant metastasis.

Treatment

Surgery is the mainstay of therapy and aims to ensure complete resection, with preservation of reproductive function when possible. Definitive treatment is oophorectomy or salpingo-oophorectomy. Care should be taken to resect the tumor without disrupting the capsule or spilling tumor contents to avoid upstaging of malignant lesions. Ascites, if present, should be tested for cytology evidence of tumor. At operation, liver, diaphragm and peritoneal surfaces, and omentum are examined for ovarian implants, which, when present, should be biopsied for staging and treatment purposes. Bilateral retroperitoneal, iliac, para-aortic, and perirenal lymph nodes should be sampled for appropriate staging. Ascites or peritoneal washings should be sent for cytology. Chemotherapy is indicated for any ovarian tumor with extension beyond the affected ovary, which is often the case with germ cell and epithelial cell tumors. The combination of low-dose bleomycin, etoposide, and cisplatin treatment in patients with stage II disease has resulted in event-free and overall survival rates of 87.5% and 93.8%, respectively.

PEDIATRIC TRAUMA

Traumatic injury, intentional or unintentional, results in more deaths in children and adolescents than all other causes combined. Most pediatric trauma is a result of blunt trauma, although penetrating injury accounts for 10% to 20% of all pediatric trauma admissions with the increase in violence among 13- to 18-year-olds. It must be stressed that the pediatric patient is different physiologically from an adult counterpart, but the basic principles remain the same.

ABCs of Trauma

Evaluation of the pediatric patient's airway is of utmost importance. A child who is crying or able to verbalize is able to protect his or her airway. If a patient is drooling, gurgling, or wheezing, one must rule out correctable causes of airway obstruction, such as a retrievable foreign object in the oropharynx. The threshold for endotracheal intubation, especially with excessive sedation, should be low. The appropriate endotracheal tube size can be estimated as being equivalent to the diameter of the child's fifth digit. Alternatively, the endotracheal tube inner diameter can be calculated (4 + the patient's age in years divided by 4). The trachea is also shorter and narrower in children.

After the airway is secured, a rapid assessment should be made of the respiratory status by determining the presence of flail chest, dyspnea, tachypnea, or unequal breath sounds. Caution should be exercised in using pulse oximetry because it does not reflect proper ventilation. Next, circulation should be assessed to ensure adequate oxygen delivery. The patient should be examined for general color, capillary refill, and presence of peripheral pulses. A weak and thready pulse along with hypotension indicates hypovolemic shock. Blood transfusion should be considered in those with hypovolemic shock unresponsive to two boluses of 20 mL/kg crystalloid. In children younger than 6 years, intraosseous access may be considered when it is difficult to establish peripheral IV lines. After the initial ABCs, a secondary survey should be performed. Hypothermia must be avoided to prevent complications of coagulopathy and acidosis. A detailed examination should be performed of the head and neck, including palpation of the posterior neck beneath the C-collar, and of the torso, back, and extremities.

Head and Spine Injuries

Traumatic brain injury (TBI) is the leading cause of death among injured children. In toddlers 2 years or younger, physical abuse, such as that seen in shaken baby syndrome, is the most common cause of serious head injury. This may be manifested as retinal, subdural, or subarachnoid hemorrhages. In children aged 3 years and older, falls and motor vehicle, bicycle, and pedestrian accidents are responsible for most TBIs. The initial CT scan may demonstrate diffuse edema, and with time, the brain injury may evolve with evidence of diffuse axonal injury, hemorrhage, or parenchymal damage. Children with a mild head injury usually complain of headache and nausea or exhibit amnesia, impaired concentration, and behavior disturbances. Up to 20% of children who sustain mild TBIs can have an intracranial hemorrhage, and approximately 3% will eventually require operative intervention. There is no consensus on how to approach the child with a mild TBI; many advocate the use of a screening head CT scan with close clinical examination. When appropriate, cerebral perfusion pressure must be monitored. Because of its transient effect and propensity to induce vasospasm, prophylactic hyperventilation should be avoided unless there is imminent concern for herniation. Aside from diuretics and hypertonic saline, a barbiturate-induced coma and hypothermia are other maneuvers that can be used to lower the intracranial pressure. Intracranial bleeding causing focal neurologic symptoms or mass effect should be surgically addressed.

Although relatively infrequent, motor vehicle accidents account for most traumatic spinal cord injuries in children. Fractures of the C1 and C2 vertebrae are commonly seen in younger children, whereas compression and chance fractures, frequently associated with improper seat belt use, are seen in older children. Spinal cord injury without radiologic abnormality is a clinical condition in which a child (<8 years of age) can present with transient neurologic deficits. It is thought to occur because incomplete vertebral ossification and ligament laxity allow the cord and nerve roots to stretch or to impact on the opposing bone surfaces of the spinal canal.

Thoracic Trauma

Thoracic injury is the second leading cause of death in pediatric trauma and accounts for 5% of trauma-related hospital admissions. Blunt trauma, particularly from motor vehicle accidents, is responsible for most thoracic injuries. Rib cages in children are primarily cartilaginous and therefore more pliable. Thus, a child may present with a significant intrathoracic injury (e.g., pulmonary contusion, pneumothorax, hemothorax) without obvious evidence of rib fractures. Pulmonary contusions result in an inflammatory response with edema, atelectasis, and subsequent consolidation. Hypoxemia, hypercarbia, and tachypnea can be significant and necessitate intubation. Radiographic findings are variable and unreliable. Nonetheless, most patients respond to conservative management without long-term sequelae. Traumatic asphyxia is a rare presentation after blunt trauma, but sudden compression or crushing of the thorax can result in airway obstruction and retrograde high-pressure flow in the superior vena cava. When this occurs, patients present dramatically with head and neck cyanosis, subconjunctival hemorrhaging, and petechiae. Rib fractures in children younger than 3 years should be approached with a high index of suspicion for child abuse. Surgical exploration of the chest may be indicated for an acute bloody chest tube output of more than 20% of the patient's blood volume or chest tube blood drainage of 2 mL/kg/hr. Intercostal artery bleeding is a common cause.

Tracheobronchial injuries usually occur near the carina and are thought to result from anteroposterior compression of the pliable pediatric chest. The patient can present with pneumothorax, pneumomediastinum, and subcutaneous emphysema. Tracheobronchial disruption results in massive air leak with potential tension pneumothorax, compromising respiratory function and venous return. Aside from hemodynamic instability, primary repair is indicated if the injury involves more than one third of the diameter of the bronchus or if nonoperative management fails. A widened mediastinum on the chest radiograph is rare in children. Most of these injuries result from blunt trauma and are found at the ligamentum arteriosum. Traumatic diaphragmatic rupture with herniation of the stomach and bowel occurs in approximately 1% of children with blunt chest trauma. Left-sided rupture is more common because the liver protects against right-sided rupture.

Abdominal Trauma

When a seat belt sign, a bruising of the midanterior abdominal wall after a motor vehicle accident, is present on a child, the CT scan should be reviewed for any subtle signs of bowel injury or presence of free peritoneal fluid. Intra-abdominal fluid on a CT scan without a solid organ injury should raise the index of suspicion for a hollow viscus injury. Blunt injuries to the stomach are generally seen in children who are struck by a vehicle or who fall across bicycle handlebars and present as blowout or perforation of the greater curvature. Usually seen in restrained children involved in motor vehicle accidents, intestinal injury secondary to blunt trauma is estimated to be less than 15%. Several mechanisms can explain the injury pattern, such as rapid deceleration causing the lap belt to compress the intestines against the spine. The increase in intraluminal pressure may predispose to perforation or rupture. Small intestinal injuries occur predominantly in areas of fixation, such as at the ligament of Treitz or ileocecal valve. A duodenal or mesenteric hematoma may ensue and cause obstruction, with subsequent nausea and bilious emesis. It is not uncommon to encounter retroperitoneal injuries as well.

Treatment of Solid Organ Injuries

The intra-abdominal solid organs are particularly vulnerable to blunt trauma in children. Nonoperative management is the standard therapy for hemodynamically stable children with blunt solid organ injury. Those who fail to respond to nonoperative management usually do so within the first 12 hours. The American Pediatric Surgical Association has detailed guidelines regarding the

TABLE 66-7	Classification of Intra-abdominal Solid Organ Injuries		
GRADE	**LIVER**	**SPLEEN**	**KIDNEY**
I	Hematoma: <10% subcapsular surface area Laceration: capsular tear <1 cm	Hematoma: <10% subcapsular Laceration: capsular tear <1 cm	Contusion: microscopic or gross hematuria Hematoma: subcapsular, nonexpanding, no parenchymal tear
II	Hematoma: 10%-50% subcapsular surface area, <10 cm intraparenchymal hemorrhage Laceration: capsular tear 1-3 cm deep, <10 cm length	Hematoma: 10%-50% subcapsular surface area, <5 cm intraparenchymal hemorrhage Laceration: capsular tear, 1-3 cm parenchymal depth not involving a trabecular vessel	Hematoma: nonexpanding perirenal hematoma confined to retroperitoneum Laceration: <1 cm parenchymal depth of renal cortex without collecting system rupture or urinary extravasation
III	Hematoma: >50% expanding subcapsular surface area, ruptured subcapsular hematoma with active bleeding, or intraparenchymal hematoma ≥2 cm or expanding Laceration: >3 cm parenchymal depth	Hematoma: ruptured subcapsular or parenchymal hematoma; intraparenchymal hematoma >5 cm or expanding Laceration: >3 cm parenchymal depth involving trabecular vessels	Laceration: >1 cm parenchymal depth of renal cortex without collecting system rupture or urinary extravasation
IV	Hematoma: ruptured parenchyma with active bleeding Laceration: parenchymal disruption involving 25%-75% of hepatic lobe	Hematoma: ruptured parenchyma with active bleeding Laceration: hilar vessels with major devascularization (>25% of spleen)	Laceration: parenchymal laceration extending through the renal cortex, medulla, and collecting system Vascular: main renal artery or vein injury with contained hemorrhage
V	Laceration: parenchymal disruption involving >50% of hepatic lobe Vascular: juxtahepatic venous injuries (retrohepatic vena cava, central major hepatic veins)	Laceration: completely shattered spleen Vascular: hilar vascular injury with total devascularization	Laceration: completely shattered kidney Vascular: avulsion of renal hilum with devascularization of kidney
VI	Vascular: hepatic avulsion		

management of isolated liver and spleen injuries based on initial CT findings; these have been shown to reduce the length of hospital stay significantly, without adverse outcomes (Table 66-7). Splenic injuries are relatively common in pediatric trauma. Splenic injuries are managed conservatively unless there is evidence of hemodynamic instability. CT scan can delineate the extent of splenic injury. The role of splenic artery embolization in the treatment of pediatric blunt splenic injury remains uncertain, unlike in adult patients. An isolated hepatic injury without involvement of the hepatic vein, IVC, or portal vein can also be managed conservatively. Some have reported that 85% to 90% of patients can successfully be treated with nonoperative management. However, those who fail to respond do so because of hemodynamic instability, changes in clinical examination findings, or transfusion requirements of more than half of blood volume (roughly 40 mL/kg/day). Delayed bleeding after liver injury has been reported as late as 6 weeks after injury and may be seen in 1% to 3% of patients. As is the case with splenic lacerations, one should proceed with definitive surgical treatment whenever there is hemodynamic instability despite adequate resuscitation.

Pancreatic Injury

Pancreatic injuries occur from blunt trauma, such as falling into bicycle handlebars. An elevated amylase or lipase level is present. CT scan is a useful diagnostic modality for evaluation of most pancreatic trauma, although it is not as sensitive or specific for determination of pancreatic ductal injuries. There is little role for ERCP in acute settings of pediatric pancreatic injury. When presented acutely, transection of pancreas from blunt trauma is best managed with operative intervention of distal pancreatectomy. For those with delayed presentation, a conservative management is more appropriate. This may include TPN and bowel rest. ERCP

is considered to evaluate for ductal injuries. External drainage procedure may be required.

Renal Injury

The nonoperative management of organ injury also applies to renal injuries. Retroperitoneal injuries are frequently seen with direct blows to the back or flank, and the kidney is involved in 10% to 20% of cases. In children, there is a lack of perinephric fat, which makes the kidney a susceptible target. Contusion is the most common renal injury encountered in children, whereas fracture of the renal pelvis occurs in children who have congenital renal abnormalities. Interestingly, the presence of hematuria does not correlate with the severity of renal injury. Conservative management is standard for low-grade renal injuries (grades I to III), and there is no consensus on the controversial management of high-grade renal injuries (grades IV and V). An absolute indication for renal exploration is an expanding or pulsatile hematoma. Relative indications include urinary extravasation, necrosis, and arterial injury. In the case of urinary extravasation, ureteral stenting can be attempted. Grade V injuries usually require operative management, but the salvage rate is poor.

FETAL SURGERY

With modern prenatal care, many congenital conditions are diagnosed before birth. Although these anomalies rarely progress in such a way that fetal survival is threatened, there are cases in which an intervention is warranted. Fetal surgery is a progressive field that aims to alter the natural progression of congenital disease in utero. Many of these anomalies have severe complications associated with fetal demise if they are left untreated. However, given the high-risk nature of the procedures themselves, selection of which patients would benefit most and how best to manage them is the key. Indications for fetal surgery include myelomeningocele, hydrops caused by CPAM, steal syndrome and cardiac failure from SCTs, and oligohydramnios with renal failure from lower urinary tract obstruction. Although initial outcomes were disappointing, recent improvements have been made in selection criteria based on outcomes research, which aims to identify patients with malformations who would see reasonable benefit from prenatal intervention. Ultrasonography continues to be the primary prenatal imaging modality because it is noninvasive and without radiation exposure. However, ultrafast MRI has become a useful imaging adjunct, particularly when the diagnosis is unclear or needs further evaluation.

One of the most significant advances in fetal surgery was made in the treatment of myelomeningocele, the most common form of spina bifida. In a multicenter randomized trial, prenatal surgical repair for myelomeningocele was shown to reduce the need for shunting by the age of 12 months and improved motor outcomes at 30 months compared with standard postnatal surgical repair.[48] Several fetal centers have continued to experience successful outcomes with prenatal repair for myelomeningocele. In contrast, fetal surgery was attempted in the treatment of CDH, but with dismal results because of premature births and other complications. In high-risk fetuses with CDH complicated by thoracic herniation of the liver, reduction of the liver back into the abdomen was associated with kinking of the umbilical vein and subsequent fetal demise. In recent years, the fetal intervention for CDH has focused on reversible tracheal occlusion with clips or endoluminal balloons to induce intrauterine lung growth. Initial outcome data have been variable without significant improvement in survival, with premature rupture of membranes being a frequent complication of the procedure itself.[49] However, the TOTAL trial led by several European centers showed some promising results.[2]

Procedures involving tracheal occlusion have led to the development of the ex utero intrapartum treatment (EXIT) procedure, which is a delivery technique used for fetuses with airway compression that may be caused by the presence of a thoracic mass. To secure the fetus' airway during delivery, the mother is given tocolytics and anesthesia to induce maximal uterine relaxation while maintaining uteroplacental circulation. This allows an airway to be established by endotracheal intubation before the umbilical cord is clamped. After delivery, the newborn can be stabilized for postnatal interventions, when indicated.

SCT is another condition for which fetal surgery may be indicated, but reports of in utero resection are rare. The development of hydrops in a fetus with SCT is caused by high-output cardiac failure from arteriovenous shunting through the tumor. To reduce blood flow to the tumor, coagulation of the arteriovenous shunt, laser photocoagulation, and radiofrequency ablation of the feeding vessels have been used with some success in small studies. Open fetal surgery for SCT is controversial. Because most fetuses with SCT undergo postnatal resection without complication, intrauterine intervention is advocated only for those patients with symptoms related to hydrops. It is unclear whether these interventions change overall survival, given the poor prognosis associated with the development of these symptoms.

CPAM can result in hydrops and pulmonary hypoplasia when it is large enough. One study has found a correlation between the volume of the CPAM and head circumference, which indicated that when the ratio is more than 1.6, the risk for development of hydrops was found to be 80%. It is this subset of patients that

benefits from in utero intervention. Typically, microcystic lesions can be resected with a lobectomy and macrocystic masses can be aspirated or shunted. Outcomes are good; these interventions reverse hydropic symptoms and result in a survival rate of more than 70%.[50]

The application of minimally invasive techniques has been increasing, and its role in fetal surgery is still being explored. It is used for lower urinary tract obstructions, in which oligohydramnios causes pulmonary insufficiency and compression deformities of the face and limbs. These patients may benefit from vesicoamniotic shunting and ablation of posterior valves. Fetoscopic surgery has also been successfully used in the laser ablation of the communicating placental blood vessels in twin-twin transfusion syndrome, characterized by hypovolemia, oliguria, and oligohydramnios in the donor twin and hypervolemia, polyuria, and polyhydramnios in the recipient twin. The procedure is associated with a 75% survival rate of at least one twin.

SELECTED REFERENCES

Adzick S, Thom EA, Spong CY, et al: A randomized trial of prenatal versus postnatal repair of myelomeningocele. *N Engl J Med* 364:993–1004, 2011.

This report details results of a multicenter randomized trial of fetal intervention for myelomeningocele.

Coran AG, Adzick NS, Krummel TM, et al, editors: *Pediatric surgery*, ed 7, Philadelphia, 2012, Elsevier Saunders.

This two-volume set is a comprehensive textbook on pediatric surgery, considered to be the most authoritative textbook for pediatric surgeons.

Holcomb GW, III, Murphy JP, Ostlie DJ, et al, editors: *Ashcraft's pediatric surgery*, ed 6, Philadelphia, 2014, Elsevier Saunders.

This is an excellent single-volume reference. This textbook is easy to read and serves as a good practical resource, especially for young surgical residents, fellows, and medical students.

O'Neill JA, Grosfeld JL, Fonkalsrud EW, et al, editors: *Principles of pediatric surgery*, ed 2, St. Louis, 2004, Mosby.

This is an outstanding textbook for medical students, surgical residents, and pediatric surgical fellows. It is comprehensive yet concisely highlights core elements of pediatric surgical knowledge written by 5 editors and 10 associate editors.

Vandenplas Y: Management of paediatric GERD. *Nat Rev Gastroenterol Hepatol* 11:147–157, 2014.

This is an excellent review for the management of pediatric gastroesophageal reflux disorders.

REFERENCES

1. Perkins JA, Manning SC, Tempero RM, et al: Lymphatic malformations: Review of current treatment. *Otolaryngol Head Neck Surg* 142:795–803, 803.e1, 2010.

2. Deprest J, Brady P, Nicolaides K, et al: Prenatal management of the fetus with isolated congenital diaphragmatic hernia in the era of the TOTAL trial. *Semin Fetal Neonatal Med* 19:338–348, 2014.

3. Hagadorn JI, Brownell EA, Herbst KW, et al: Trends in treatment and in-hospital mortality for neonates with congenital diaphragmatic hernia. *J Perinatol* 35:748–754, 2015.

4. Partridge EA, Peranteau WH, Rintoul NE, et al: Timing of repair of congenital diaphragmatic hernia in patients supported by extracorporeal membrane oxygenation (ECMO). *J Pediatr Surg* 50:260–262, 2015.

5. Parikh DH, Rasiah SV: Congenital lung lesions: Postnatal management and outcome. *Semin Pediatr Surg* 24:160–167, 2015.

6. Masters IB: Congenital airway lesions and lung disease. *Pediatr Clin North Am* 56:227–242, xii, 2009.

7. Derderian SC, Coleman AM, Jeanty C, et al: Favorable outcomes in high-risk congenital pulmonary airway malformations treated with multiple courses of maternal betamethasone. *J Pediatr Surg* 50:515–518, 2015.

8. Berthet S, Tenisch E, Miron MC, et al: Vascular anomalies associated with esophageal atresia and tracheoesophageal fistula. *J Pediatr* 166:1140–1144.e2, 2015.

9. Vandenplas Y: Management of paediatric GERD. *Nat Rev Gastroenterol Hepatol* 11:147–157, 2014.

10. Papadopoulou A, Koletzko S, Heuschkel R, et al: Management guidelines of eosinophilic esophagitis in childhood. *J Pediatr Gastroenterol Nutr* 58:107–118, 2014.

11. Oomen MW, Hoekstra LT, Bakx R, et al: Open versus laparoscopic pyloromyotomy for hypertrophic pyloric stenosis: A systematic review and meta-analysis focusing on major complications. *Surg Endosc* 26:2104–2110, 2012.

12. McMellen ME, Wakeman D, Longshore SW, et al: Growth factors: Possible roles for clinical management of the short bowel syndrome. *Semin Pediatr Surg* 19:35–43, 2010.

13. Moss RL, Dimmitt RA, Barnhart DC, et al: Laparotomy versus peritoneal drainage for necrotizing enterocolitis and perforation. *N Engl J Med* 354:2225–2234, 2006.

14. Jones BA, Hull MA, McGuire MM, et al: Autologous intestinal reconstruction surgery. *Semin Pediatr Surg* 19:59–67, 2010.

15. Bianchi A: Intestinal loop lengthening—a technique for increasing small intestinal length. *J Pediatr Surg* 15:145–151, 1980.

16. Kim HB, Fauza D, Garza J, et al: Serial transverse enteroplasty (STEP): A novel bowel lengthening procedure. *J Pediatr Surg* 38:425–429, 2003.

17. Ching YA, Fitzgibbons S, Valim C, et al: Long-term nutritional and clinical outcomes after serial transverse enteroplasty at a single institution. *J Pediatr Surg* 44:939–943, 2009.

18. Oh PS, Fingeret AL, Shah MY, et al: Improved tolerance for enteral nutrition after serial transverse enteroplasty (STEP) in infants and children with short bowel syndrome—a seven-year single-center experience. *J Pediatr Surg* 49:1589–1592, 2014.

19. Sanchez-Mejias A, Fernandez RM, Lopez-Alonso M, et al: Contribution of RET, NTRK3 and EDN3 to the expression of Hirschsprung disease in a multiplex family. *J Med Genet* 46:862–864, 2009.

20. Kapur RP, Reed RC, Finn LS, et al: Calretinin immunohistochemistry versus acetylcholinesterase histochemistry in the evaluation of suction rectal biopsies for Hirschsprung disease. *Pediatr Dev Pathol* 12:6–15, 2009.

21. Keckler SJ, Yang JC, Fraser JD, et al: Contemporary practice patterns in the surgical management of Hirschsprung's disease. *J Pediatr Surg* 44:1257–1260, discussion 1260, 2009.

22. Bischoff A, Pena A, Levitt MA: Laparoscopic-assisted PSARP—the advantages of combining both techniques for the treatment of anorectal malformations with recto-bladderneck or high prostatic fistulas. *J Pediatr Surg* 48:367–371, 2013.

23. Lautz TB, Thurm CW, Rothstein DH: Delayed repeat enemas are safe and cost-effective in the management of pediatric intussusception. *J Pediatr Surg* 50:423–427, 2015.

24. Bassett MD, Murray KF: Biliary atresia: Recent progress. *J Clin Gastroenterol* 42:720–729, 2008.

25. Lao OB, Larison C, Garrison M, et al: Steroid use after the Kasai procedure for biliary atresia. *Am J Surg* 199:680–684, 2010.

26. Bezerra JA, Spino C, Magee JC, et al: Use of corticosteroids after hepatoportoenterostomy for bile drainage in infants with biliary atresia: The START randomized clinical trial. *JAMA* 311:1750–1759, 2014.

27. Hartley JL, Davenport M, Kelly DA: Biliary atresia. *Lancet* 374:1704–1713, 2009.

28. Singham J, Yoshida EM, Scudamore CH: Choledochal cysts: Part 1 of 3: Classification and pathogenesis. *Can J Surg* 52:434–440, 2009.

29. Rygiel AM, Beer S, Simon P, et al: Gene conversion between cationic trypsinogen (PRSS1) and the pseudogene trypsinogen 6 (PRSS3P2) in patients with chronic pancreatitis. *Hum Mutat* 36:350–356, 2015.

30. Srinath AI, Youk AO, Bielefeldt K: Biliary dyskinesia and symptomatic gallstone disease in children: Two sides of the same coin? *Dig Dis Sci* 59:1307–1315, 2014.

31. Beres A, Christison-Lagay ER, Romao RL, et al: Evaluation of Surgisis for patch repair of abdominal wall defects in children. *J Pediatr Surg* 47:917–919, 2012.

32. Lao OB, Larison C, Garrison MM, et al: Outcomes in neonates with gastroschisis in U.S. children's hospitals. *Am J Perinatol* 27:97–101, 2010.

33. Kelly RE, Jr, Mellins RB, Shamberger RC, et al: Multicenter study of pectus excavatum, final report: Complications, static/exercise pulmonary function, and anatomic outcomes. *J Am Coll Surg* 217:1080–1089, 2013.

34. Colozza S, Bütter A: Bracing in pediatric patients with pectus carinatum is effective and improves quality of life. *J Pediatr Surg* 48:1055–1059, 2013.

35. Irwin MS, Park JR: Neuroblastoma: Paradigm for precision medicine. *Pediatr Clin North Am* 62:225–256, 2015.

36. Brodeur GM: Neuroblastoma: Biological insights into a clinical enigma. *Nat Rev Cancer* 3:203–216, 2003.

37. Ishola TA, Chung DH: Neuroblastoma. *Surg Oncol* 16:149–156, 2007.

38. Maris JM: Recent advances in neuroblastoma. *N Engl J Med* 362:2202–2211, 2010.

39. Simon T, Haberle B, Hero B, et al: Role of surgery in the treatment of patients with stage 4 neuroblastoma age 18 months or older at diagnosis. *J Clin Oncol* 31:752–758, 2013.

40. Yu AL, Gilman AL, Ozkaynak MF, et al: Anti-GD2 antibody with GM-CSF, interleukin-2, and isotretinoin for neuroblastoma. *N Engl J Med* 363:1324–1334, 2010.

41. Vujanic GM, Sandstedt B: The pathology of Wilms' tumour (nephroblastoma): The International Society of Paediatric Oncology approach. *J Clin Pathol* 63:102–109, 2010.

42. Dumoucel S, Gauthier-Villars M, Stoppa-Lyonnet D, et al: Malformations, genetic abnormalities, and Wilms tumor. *Pediatr Blood Cancer* 61:140–144, 2014.

43. Kaste SC, Dome JS, Babyn PS, et al: Wilms tumour: Prognostic factors, staging, therapy and late effects. *Pediatr Radiol* 38:2–17, 2008.

44. Paulino AC, Okcu MF: Rhabdomyosarcoma. *Curr Probl Cancer* 32:7–34, 2008.

45. Otte JB: Progress in the surgical treatment of malignant liver tumors in children. *Cancer Treat Rev* 36:360–371, 2010.

46. Meyers RL, Czauderna P, Otte JB: Surgical treatment of hepatoblastoma. *Pediatr Blood Cancer* 59:800–808, 2012.

47. Kelleher CM, Goldstein AM: Adnexal masses in children and adolescents. *Clin Obstet Gynecol* 58:76–92, 2015.

48. Adzick NS, Thom EA, Spong CY, et al: A randomized trial of prenatal versus postnatal repair of myelomeningocele. *N Engl J Med* 364:993–1004, 2011.

49. Rossi AC: Indications and outcomes of intrauterine surgery for fetal malformations. *Curr Opin Obstet Gynecol* 22:159–165, 2010.

50. Deprest JA, Flake AW, Gratacos E, et al: The making of fetal surgery. *Prenat Diagn* 30:653–667, 2010.

67 | CHAPTER

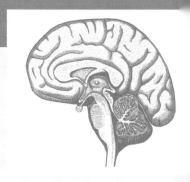

Neurosurgery

Juan Ortega-Barnett, Aaron Mohanty, Sohum K. Desai,
Joel T. Patterson

第六十七章　神经外科

中文导读

　　本章共分为10节：①颅内动力学；②脑血管病；③中枢神经系统肿瘤；④原发性脑肿瘤；⑤颅脑损伤；⑥脊柱退行性疾病；⑦功能和立体定向神经外科；⑧脑积水；⑨小儿神经外科；⑩中枢神经系统感染。

　　第一节介绍了有关大脑的一些基本生理知识，包括颅腔内容物、脑脊液分泌、脑血流供应、颅内压和脑灌注压等相关概念，同时详细阐述了在病理条件下，颅内压和脑灌注压之间的变化和相互作用对脑血流量的影响。详细阐述了颅内压和脑血流以及脑脊液三者之间的相互关系。

　　第二节简要介绍了脑血管疾病的分类以及不同脑血管病，包括动静脉畸形、动脉瘤、烟雾病等。重点介绍了动脉瘤的流行病学、分类、临床特点、并发症以及诊治方法和预后。

　　第三节介绍了根据肿瘤的发生部位、起源和发病

年龄的不同，中枢神经系统肿瘤具有不同的分类，同时作者进一步阐述了中枢神经系统肿瘤的流行病学、临床表现、CT和MRI等影像学技术在肿瘤诊断中的应用以及外科手术对肿瘤的治疗。

　　第四节作者根据肿瘤的分类，分别从疾病的临床表现、治疗和结局等方面介绍了脑实质肿瘤，包括星型细胞瘤、少突胶质细胞肿瘤、室管膜瘤、脉络丛乳头状瘤或癌、儿童脑干胶质瘤；神经元和神经胶质混合成分的肿瘤，包括神经节胶质瘤、神经节细胞瘤和中央神经细胞瘤，胚胎发育不良性神经上皮瘤和副神经节瘤；松果体区肿瘤包括松果体细胞瘤、松果体

母细胞瘤和松果体区乳头状瘤以及原始神经外胚层肿瘤。作者采用同样的方式介绍了颅神经和脊髓神经的肿瘤，包括神经鞘瘤、脑膜和硬脊膜肿瘤、淋巴瘤和造血系统的肿瘤、生殖细胞瘤、鞍区肿瘤和中枢神经系统转移瘤。

第五节作者详细阐述了颅脑损伤的临床流行病学特征，原发性脑损伤以及继发性脑损伤的病理生理机制、院前和急诊救治原则（包括气道管理、血压监测、GCS评分以及影像学评估）和治疗原则（包括手术、药物以及ICP监测、镇静镇痛、感染预防和营养等）。

第六节首先介绍了脊柱的相关解剖和椎间盘的组织学结构，阐述了脊柱退行性病变的病理生理机制，最后作者根据脊柱的解剖部位，从疾病的临床表现、诊断和治疗逐一介绍了颈椎间盘突出、颈椎病和颈椎管狭窄、腰椎间盘突出症与腰椎退行性病变等临床常见脊柱退行性病变。

第七节首先简要地介绍了功能神经外科和立体定向的相关概念、治疗方式、涉及的领域和疾病谱，随后阐述了脑刺激（包括脑刺激、脊髓电刺激和迷走神经电刺激）在运动障碍性疾病、慢性疼痛以及癫痫中的应用以及可植入泵和病变毁损技术的临床应用。同时以癫痫和三叉神经痛两类功能性疾病为例，详细阐述了上述疾病的临床特点、临床诊断以及功能和立体定向神经外科在疾病治疗中的应用。

第八节介绍了脑积水分类，不同分类脑积水的临床症状、体征和诊断。作者详细介绍了作为脑积水的主要治疗方式，脑脊液分流术和内镜技术的临床应用以及相关并发症，同时简要地介绍了一些特殊脑积水病人的临床诊治。

第九节介绍了小儿神经外科的疾病谱，同时从分类、临床表现、治疗方式、预后等方面详细介绍了小儿先天性畸形疾病，包括脑脊膜闭合不全、Chiari畸形和颅缝早闭。

第十节作者按照解剖结构将中枢神经系统感染性疾病划分为颅内感染和脊髓内感染，随后着重阐述了硬膜外脓肿、硬膜下积脓、脑脓肿和脑膜炎等颅内感染和脊柱感染（包括脊柱脊髓炎和免疫获得性感染性疾病）的临床特点、临床表现、治疗和预后。

〔雷　霆，万学焱〕

Neurosurgery is surgery of the brain, spinal cord, peripheral nerves, and their supporting structures, including the blood supply, protective elements, spinal fluid spaces, bony cranium, and spine. This chapter is intended for non-neurosurgeons who want to initiate a framework on which to add further knowledge and experience. It is hoped that it will also help personnel in a community hospital emergency department or a medical student on the ward for the first time communicate patient problems efficiently to neurosurgeons. The chapter first provides an overview of the underlying principles of neurosurgery, with a focus on intracranial dynamics. The remaining sections include a discussion of the following: cerebrovascular disorders, which include subarachnoid hemorrhage, intracerebral hemorrhage, aneurysm, and arteriovenous malformation (AVM); central nervous system (CNS) tumors, which include neoplasms of the brain, skull base, cranial nerves, spinal cord, meninges, and peripheral nerves; traumatic brain injury; degenerative diseases of the spine; functional neurosurgery, which includes stereotactic radiosurgery (SRS), epilepsy surgery, and surgery for the management of pain and movement disorders; hydrocephalus; pediatric neurosurgery; and neurosurgical management of CNS infections. The field of neurosurgery is simply too broad to make a detailed encyclopedic overview realistic, but some introduction to these issues will be useful to the reader.

INTRACRANIAL DYNAMICS

It is essential at the outset to grasp a few basic principles concerning intracranial dynamics, cerebrospinal fluid (CSF), cerebral blood flow (CBF), and intracranial pressure (ICP), and these are summarized here for quick review. Some of these principles are obvious, whereas others might be considered counterintuitive.

The first principle is obvious. The cranial cavity has a fixed volume composed of brain tissue (parenchyma), CSF, and blood vessels and intravascular blood. According to the Monro-Kellie doctrine, the sum of these components within the fixed volume of the cranial cavity implies that an increase in one component must be accompanied by an equal and opposite decrease in one or both of the remaining components.[1] If this does not occur, the ICP will rise, and at some point, the increase in pressure per unit increase in volume becomes asymptotic, approaching levels close to the systemic blood pressure, producing a reverberating blood flow pattern with no net flow. As a consequence, if there is an elevation in the volume of any one compartment, there is a stage of compensation in which the volume of one or more of the other compartments can be reduced to avoid elevations in the ICP. Table 67-1 summarizes and simplifies some of the excess volume syndromes and specific treatment for each.

The second principle is not obvious and may seem counterin-

TABLE 67-1	Intracranial Excess Volume Syndromes and Therapy	
COMPONENT	**EXCESS VOLUME SYNDROME**	**SPECIFIC TREATMENT**
Brain tissue	Edema: cytotoxic, vasogenic, perineoplastic, inflammatory	Diuretics: mannitol, furosemide, hypertonic saline; steroids for perineoplastic and inflammatory vasogenic edema
Vascular	Elevated PCO_2: hyperperfusion state with loss of autoregulation as in severe hypertension, after trauma or AVM removal; relative venous obstruction	Increased ventilation; diuretics (in hyperperfusion state, avoid mannitol), barbiturates; clear venous obstruction; elevate head of bed (to reduce venous volume)
Cerebrospinal fluid	Impaired absorption with congenital, posthemorrhagic, or postinfectious hydrocephalus, communicating or obstructive; loculations; arachnoid or periventricular cysts; rare increased production of CSF with choroid plexus papilloma	Ventricular external drainage (or lumbar drainage only if no threat of herniation) or shunt; with flocculation, or with some types of obstructive hydrocephalus, endoscopic fenestration or third ventriculostomy may be possible; acetazolamide and steroids may temporarily decrease CSF production
Mass lesion	Tumor, cyst, abscess, hematoma, radiation necrosis, or cerebral infarction necrosis	Remove, fenestrate, aspirate lesion (often with stereotactic guidance); less commonly, it might be useful to enlarge intracranial volume by decompression

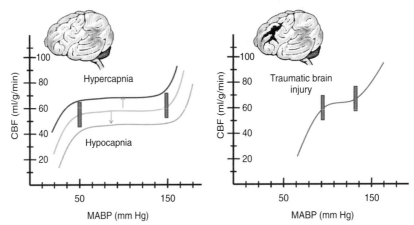

FIGURE 67-1 Cerebral blood flow (CBF) as a function of mean arterial blood pressure (MABP). Note the upward and downward shifts with hypercapnia and hypocapnia, respectively. In traumatic brain injury, the curve is steeper, with large CBF changes occurring with small pressure changes. (Adapted from Rangel-Castilla L, Gasco J, Nauta HJ, et al: Cerebral pressure autoregulation in traumatic brain injury. *Neurosurg Focus* 25:E7, 2008.)

tuitive. Spinal fluid is produced at a constant rate (≈15 to 20 mL/hr), by an energy-dependent, physicochemical process, mainly by the choroid plexus of the ventricles. It is essential to understand that production is little affected by any intracranial backpressure; thus, CSF production continues unabated, even to lethal elevations of ICP. Because production is almost always constant, it follows that derangement of CSF dynamics almost always involves some aspect of impeding CSF absorption through obstruction along the CSF pathways inside the brain, subarachnoid spaces at the basal cisterns or cerebral convexity, or arachnoid granulations from which most absorption occurs. In the following discussions on tumors, infection, intracranial hemorrhage, and trauma, many examples will become apparent whereby impaired CSF absorption contributes to the pathologic condition. The only exceptions to the almost constant CSF production are the excess production associated with the rare choroid plexus papilloma tumor and the occasional decreased CSF production seen with some gram-negative bacterial meningitis with ventriculitis.

The third basic principle is that the CBF normally varies over a wide range (30 to 100 mL/100 g of brain tissue per minute), depending on metabolic demand from neuronal activity within a particular area of the brain. The blood flow to any brain area is generally abundant, exceeding demand by a wide margin, so that

oxygen extraction ratios are often low. The brain vasculature matches the blood flow to tissue metabolic demand, and the CBF generally maintains what is needed, despite wide variations in systemic blood pressure, by a phenomenon known as autoregulation. Factors such as an elevated or decreased arterial PCO_2 shift the curve as indicated. In the setting of traumatic brain injury, the curve becomes more pronounced (i.e., smaller changes in blood pressure or PCO_2) and affects the CBF dramatically (Fig. 67-1). If tissue demand exceeds autoregulation, or if CBF declines for pathologic reasons, the first defense is that the oxygen extraction will increase (i.e., arteriovenous oxygen difference). The tissue begins to experience dysfunction at levels below 0.25 mL per gram of brain tissue per minute. With levels between 0.15 and 0.20, the brain tissue may undergo reversible ischemia; however, infarction will occur when levels range between 0.10 and 0.15 (Fig. 67-2). The metabolic consumption of oxygen in the brain is decreased after traumatic brain injury to levels between 0.6 and 1.2 μmol/mg/min. Complete loss of blood flow to any brain area results in infarction (irreversible damage) within a few minutes. Swelling of the infarcted tissue takes days to peak and weeks to resolve.[2]

An important implication is that if brain dysfunction is occurring clinically because compensatory mechanisms (e.g., autoregu-

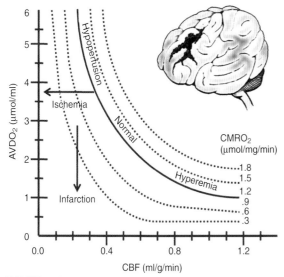

FIGURE 67-2 Relationships among cerebral flow, metabolism, and oxygen extraction in normal and pathologic circumstances. *AVDO₂*, arteriovenous oxygen difference; *CBF*, cerebral blood flow; *CMRO₂*, cerebral metabolic rate of oxygen consumption. (From Rangel-Castilla L, Gasco J, Nauta HJ, et al: Cerebral pressure autoregulation in traumatic brain injury. *Neurosurg Focus* 25:E7, 2008.)

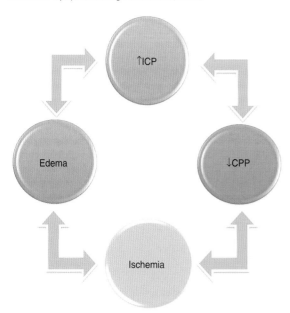

FIGURE 67-3 Relationship among increased intracranial pressure (ICP), reduced cerebral perfusion pressure (CPP), development of ischemia and infarction, and cerebral edema.

lation changing the vascular resistance, capacity to elevate mean systemic arterial pressure, ability to increase oxygen extraction) have been exceeded, the tolerance for further decline in blood flow is low, and there is a serious threat for tissue damage. Therapy to increase blood pressure or to decrease ICP may be urgently needed. When time permits because the dysfunction fluctuates chronically, it may sometimes be appropriate to measure oxygen extraction ratios as one index of the overall adequacy of the CBF. At a low CBF, oxygen extraction is increased with a lower venous PO_2. The variations in CBF and extraction ratios related to neu-

ronal activity are said to underlie the ability to image function by functional magnetic resonance imaging (MRI), a technique that is finding wider use in the clinical neurosciences.

A fourth principle derives from the other three and the fact that injured tissue swells, making obvious the potential for a cascading injury by a vicious circle mechanism (Fig. 67-3). If the stage of compensation (see earlier), even with therapy, is exceeded, and ICP is elevated high enough by some mechanism so that cerebral perfusion pressure (CPP) declines, CBF can decline to levels at which tissue injury occurs.

CPP = mean arterial pressure (MAP)-ICP

Brain edema (swelling) within the closed cranium will lead to further increases in ICP with even further decreases in CPP in a stage of decompensation. When the capacity for autoregulation is exceeded or damaged so that it can no longer play a role, CBF is linked directly to the CPP.

In the management of intracranial disease, ICP and CPP are easy to measure continuously and thus serve as highly practical surrogates for the more fundamental but much more difficult to measure CBF. However, these are not equivalent, and the limitations of these parameters for guiding therapy need to be remembered. Regardless of causation, when concern arises about the possibility of cascading injury, every effort is made to keep the CPP in the realm of 60 mm Hg (range, 50 to 70 mm Hg) and ICP below 20 mm Hg if possible. Routinely using pressors and volume expansion to maintain CPP higher than 70 mm Hg is not supported on the basis of systemic complications.[3]

A fifth principle concerns focal mass effect and its progression in regard to the complex anatomy of the cranial cavity. The cranial cavity is not just a hollow spherical space but contains several almost knifelike projections of folded dura, the falx and tentorium, which divide the cavity into a right and left supratentorial compartment and an infratentorial compartment, the posterior fossa. The sphenoid wing is a prominent, mostly bony ridge that separates the anterior fossa containing the frontal lobe from the middle fossa containing the temporal lobe. A narrow opening, the incisura, edged by the tentorium, surrounds the midbrain and is the only passage between the supratentorial and infratentorial compartments. Apart from the small openings for the cranial nerves and arteries, the foramen magnum is the only sizable opening from the cranial cavity as a whole.

The condition that classically illustrates the expanding mass lesion is the acute epidural hematoma, seen after trauma with skull fracture. Regardless of the source, however, the progression can be similar and has been termed rostrocaudal decay to reflect the early and late stages, as listed in order here:
- Focal distortion only
- Effacement of gyri and sulci
- Compression of the lateral (or other) ventricle
- Midline shift
- Subfalcial herniation
- Temporal lobe tentorial herniation
  - Third nerve compression (unilateral dilated pupil)
  - Obliteration of basal cisterns
  - Midbrain compression
  - Midbrain infarction, Duret hemorrhages (both pupils dilate, with irreversible damage to midbrain)
- Further brainstem compression
  - Loss of brainstem reflexes: progression from flexor posturing to extensor posturing; vestibulo-ocular and oculocephalic reflexes; corneal reflexes

- Medullary compression syndrome: respiratory reflexes; vasomotor reflexes, Cushing reflex with elevation of the systolic blood pressure, widening of the pulse pressure, bradycardia
- Foramen magnum herniation

At stages beyond tentorial herniation, it is unusual for focal mass effects not to be accompanied by an overall increase in ICP. The point at which focal mass effect evolves to include a rise in overall ICP depends largely on the compliance within the cranial cavity. Young patients with so-called tight brains can develop raised ICP, even with relatively small volumes of mass that produce only effacement of the cortical gyri. On the other hand, patients with advanced cerebral atrophy can, for example, tolerate large frontal intracerebral hematomas or chronic subdural hematomas with compression of the lateral ventricle and midline shift while maintaining a tolerable ICP and a surprising degree of intact neurologic function.

Normal ICP varies over a wide range, with generally accepted values between 0 and 20 mm Hg. Diffuse raised ICP, in the fully evolved pure form, results in a clinical picture that may include symptoms of headache, nausea and vomiting, double vision, and obscuration of vision. The accompanying clinical signs may include papilledema and sixth cranial nerve palsy with lateral rectus weakness and side-by-side diplopia, initially worse on far vision or gaze directed toward the side of the palsy. The papilledema is a mostly chronic phenomenon and is not seen acutely. The sixth nerve palsy of raised ICP can occur regardless of its cause and does not imply direct involvement by a mass lesion, large or small, on the sixth nerve. In this situation, the sixth nerve palsy is a false localizing sign. With raised ICP, there may also be obscurations of vision, in which patients report that their vision temporarily fades or becomes gray, in combination with headache. Again, these obscurations are caused by the effect of diffusely increased ICP on the sensitive optic nerves. They do not imply the presence of a focal mass lesion directly affecting the optic nerves or pathways. Intuitively, it seems that if there is a slow increase in a process raising ICP, the pressure would also rise slowly and evenly, in pace with the evolving process. However, as first shown by Lundberg in 1960,[4] the intermediate stages of decompensation are characterized by transient pronounced elevations in ICP (to 60 mm Hg) that characteristically plateau for up to 45 minutes and then transiently cycle down again to a more normal range.

CEREBROVASCULAR DISORDERS

Cerebrovascular disorders encompass a host of disorders: congenital, acquired, and idiopathic (Box 67-1).

Arteriovenous Malformations

An AVM is an abnormal collection of blood vessels wherein arterial blood flows directly into draining veins without the normal interposed capillary beds. AVMs are congenital lesions that can enlarge somewhat with age, recruiting new vascular supply, and often progress from low-flow lesions at birth to higher flow lesions in adulthood. They present with hemorrhage, ischemia of the brain parenchyma around the lesion due to a vascular "steal" phenomenon, or seizures. They have a prevalence of 15 to 18/100,000 and typically are manifested before the age of 40 years. The risk of hemorrhage rate is up to 4% per year,[5] and once they bleed, they may be even more prone to hemorrhage. They are typically composed of one or more feeding arteries; a nidus of varying size, shape, and compactness that is composed of abnormal vessels; and draining veins. They are sometimes associated with high-flow related aneurysms of the feeding arteries.

Patients typically present with headaches, neurologic deficit, seizures, or varying combinations of the three. Workup generally includes computed tomography (CT) and MRI, demonstrating the lesion (Fig. 67-4). Catheter angiography is then performed to define the vascular anatomy of the lesion and is used for treatment planning.

Treatment options include craniotomy with surgical resection of the lesion, embolization, and SRS. Commonly, more than one modality is used. SRS is usually reserved for compact lesions less the 2.5 cm in diameter. It can take up to 3 years for irradiated AVMs to shut down after SRS. The Spetzler-Martin grading system was developed 30 years ago and continues to be used to help make treatment decisions (Table 67-2).[6]

Cavernous Malformations

A cavernous malformation is a well-circumscribed, benign vascular lesion consisting of irregular thin-walled sinusoidal vascular channels located within the brain but lacking intervening neural parenchyma, large feeding arteries, or large draining veins. Characterized by McCormick in an autopsy series,[7] these lesions have a prevalence of approximately 0.5%. There are three familial forms described. Because these are low-pressure, low-flow lesions, hemorrhage is typically not catastrophic unless it is in a highly eloquent area of the brain.

Patients usually present with hemorrhage or headaches with or without a history of new-onset seizures. Although it is often evident on CT, MRI is the imaging modality of choice and demonstrates a characteristic dark hemosiderin ring. Treatment for symptomatic lesions includes seizure control and surgical excision. Radiosurgery has not been shown to significantly alter the natural history of these lesions.

BOX 67-1 **Cerebral Vascular Disease**

Congenital
Arteriovenous malformation and fistula
Cavernous malformation
Telangiectasis
Venous anomaly (angioma)

Acquired
Traumatic
    Some arteriovenous fistulas (type I carotid-cavernous fistula)
    Traumatic aneurysm
Degenerative
    Atherosclerotic, occlusive disease
    Most cerebral (berry) aneurysms
    Some arterial dissections
    Spontaneous intracerebral hemorrhage
Infectious
    Mycotic aneurysms

Idiopathic
Moyamoya
Some arteriovenous fistulas: dural AVM–like or type II carotid-cavernous fistulas

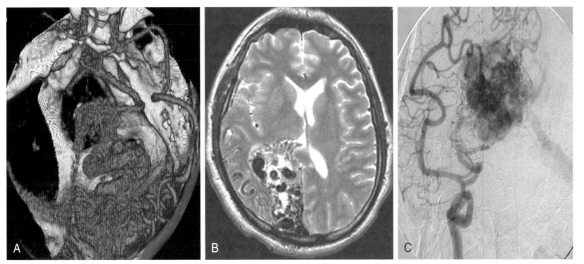

FIGURE 67-4 CT angiography with three-dimensional reconstruction **(A)**, MRI **(B)**, and conventional angiogram **(C)** of a large AVM with supply from the middle and posterior cerebral arteries and ill-defined nidus. Complex deep and superficial venous drainage is present.

TABLE 67-2   Spetzler-Martin Grading System

FEATURE	POINTS
Nidus size (cm)	
Small (<3)	1
Medium (3-6)	2
Large (>6)	3
Eloquence of adjacent brain	
Noneloquent	0
Eloquent (sensorimotor, language, visual, thalamus, hypothalamus, internal capsule, brainstem, cerebellar peduncles, deep cerebellar nuclei)	1
Pattern of venous drainage	
Superficially only	0
Deep	1

Capillary Telangiectasia

This lesion is composed of vascular channels with extremely thin walls similar to those of dilated capillaries. These are usually grouped in small clusters, generally with prominent intervening brain tissue. They are often clinically silent and generally do not appear on imaging studies. They are not evident on conventional catheter angiography unless they are large, and then only in the capillary venous phase. They clearly differ from an AVM in that flow through the lesion is not fast enough to demonstrate arteries and veins in the same conventional angiographic image. These lesions are typically not treated surgically.

Developmental Venous Anomaly: Venous Angioma

These lesions are composed of an abnormally configured venous drainage system converging on a single, enlarged venous outflow channel. The typical appearance is that of a hydra, with radially converging veins. A characteristic feature of this lesion appears to be that the abnormal venous bed is poorly collateralized. The abnormal venous drainage may or may not be fully adequate to

the needs of the brain tissue supplied. Slowly evolving degenerative changes in the brain tissue supplied can occur as a result, but unfortunately, this is not helped by any known intervention. However inadequate, the venous anomaly represents the only venous drainage available to that area of brain, and therefore removal of the venous anomaly is not recommended. Doing so could lead to a venous infarction with swelling and hemorrhage, the consequences of which are particularly dangerous in the posterior fossa.

Traumatic Fistula

Both the internal carotid artery and vertebral artery enter the cranial cavity immediately after passing through a venous network. The internal carotid artery passes through the cavernous sinus, which communicates with the superior ophthalmic vein, petrosal sinus, and sphenoparietal sinus. The vertebral artery passes through a venous plexus at the occipital-C1 epidural space, which communicates with the jugular vein, epidural venous plexus, and paraspinal venous plexus. Trauma leading to a tear in the carotid or vertebral artery at its tether point passing through the skull base can lead to fistula with the surrounding venous plexus. The consequences may vary in severity and suddenness but typically include periorbital swelling, with proptosis and scleral edema in the case of the carotid-cavernous fistula (CCF) and prominent pulsatile bruit in the case of the vertebral-jugular fistula. Intraocular pressure measurement by tonometry can guide the urgency in treating CCF. On radiologic examination, dilation of the superior ophthalmic vein is characteristic (Fig. 67-5). These lesions are usually treated by endovascular techniques. A catheter is advanced through the tear in the artery into the venous side of the fistula. The high flow and large fistulous channel facilitate this process. Embolic material, a coil, or a detachable balloon is then used to occlude the venous side of the fistula. When conventional transvenous routes fail, a direct approach through transorbital puncture may be required to provide endovascular therapy.[8]

Aneurysms

Aneurysms are an excessive localized enlargement of a vessel due to a weakening and subsequent defect in the wall of the artery.

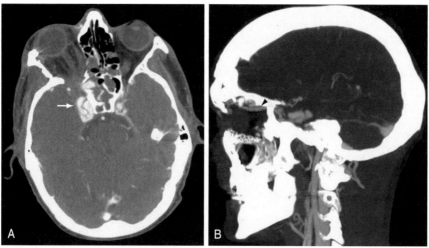

FIGURE 67-5 Right internal carotid–cavernous sinus fistula (**A**, *arrow*) with dilation of the superior ophthalmic drain (**B**, *arrowhead*), a typical imaging finding of this pathologic process.

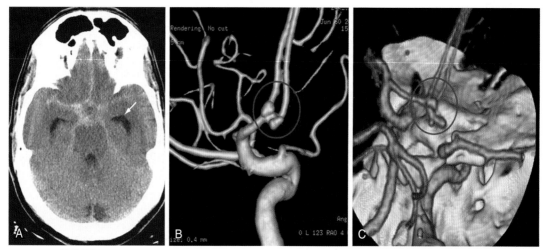

FIGURE 67-6 A, CT scan of brain showing subarachnoid blood in the basal cisterns. Dilated temporal horns *(arrow)* indicate the presence of hydrocephalus. **B**, Cerebral angiogram shows two aneurysms located at the junction of the A1 and A2 segments of the anterior cerebral artery *(circle)*. **C**, CT angiography with three-dimensional reconstruction showing the relationship of the aneurysms *(circle)* with the skull base.

There is an adult prevalence of 2% (this varies according to the study) with an annual incidence of aneurysmal subarachnoid hemorrhage of 6 to 8/100,000 with peak age at 50 years. Modifiable risk factors for subarachnoid hemorrhage include hypertension, smoking, and excessive alcohol. Aneurysms may be further divided into saccular, fusiform, dissecting, infectious, and traumatic aneurysms.

Saccular Aneurysms

As the name implies, these aneurysms, also referred to as berry aneurysms, are usually saccular in form and come off the vessel wall or at a bifurcation. Many of these are found incidentally, given the frequency of neuroimaging, but many present with hemorrhage.[9] The classic presentation of subarachnoid hemorrhage due to a cerebral aneurysm is that of sudden onset of a headache, described as the "worst headache of my life." Workup typically includes a CT scan, demonstrating a typical distribution of blood (Fig. 67-6). Between 10% and 15% of subarachnoid hemorrhages from saccular aneurysms are fatal before the hospital

---

BOX 67-2   Treatment of Vasospasm

Prevention of Arterial Narrowing
Subarachnoid blood removal
Prevention of dehydration and hypotension
Calcium channel blockers (nimodipine)

Reversal of Arterial Narrowing
Intra-arterial calcium channel blockers
Transluminal balloon angioplasty

Prevention and Reversal of Ischemic Neurologic Deficit
Hypertension, hypervolemia, hemodilution

---

is even reached. Of those individuals who reach a medical facility, one third do not survive (usually because of rebleeding), one third will survive with varying degrees of neurologic disability, and one third return to their baseline level.

TABLE 67-3   Risk of Rupture During 5 Years (%) According to International Study of Unruptured Intracranial Aneurysms

TYPE OF ANEURYSM	<7 mm AND NO PRIOR SAH	<7 mm AND PRIOR SAH	7-12 mm	13-24 mm	>24 mm
Carotid-cavernous	0	0	0	3.0	6.4
Anterior circulation	0	1.5	2.6	14.5	40.0
Posterior circulation	2.5	3.4	14.5	18.4	50.0

SAH, subarachnoid hemorrhage.

TABLE 67-4   Hunt and Hess Clinical Grading Scale

DESCRIPTION	GRADE	GOOD OUTCOME
Asymptomatic or minimal headache and slight nuchal rigidity	1	≈70
Moderate to severe headache, nuchal rigidity, ± cranial nerve palsy only	2	≈70
Drowsy, confusion, or mild focal deficit	3	≈15
Stupor, moderate to severe hemiparesis, possibly early decerebrate rigidity	4	≈15
Deep coma, decerebrate rigidity, moribund appearance	5	≈0

TABLE 67-5   World Federation of Neurological Surgeons Clinical Grading Scale

GRADE	GCS SCORE	MOTOR DEFICIT
I	15	No
II	13-14	No
III	13-14	Yes
IV	7-12	Yes or no
V	3-6	Yes or no

GCS, Glasgow Coma Scale.

TABLE 67-6   Fisher Grading for Appearance of SAH on Computed Tomography

GRADE	CT FINDINGS
I	No hemorrhage evident
II	Diffuse SAH with vertical layers < 1 mm thick
III	Localized clots and/or vertical layers of SAH > 1 mm thick
IV	Diffuse or no SAH, but with intracerebral or intraventricular hemorrhage

SAH, subarachnoid hemorrhage.

The major complications of subarachnoid hemorrhage include rebleeding, hydrocephalus (which is observed in around 15% to 20% of cases), cardiac events in around 50% of patients, vasospasm, hyponatremia, and seizures. Rebleeding is a major cause of death in patients who reach medical care after their initial episode of bleeding. Hydrocephalus is caused by disruption in the function of the arachnoid granulations and is commonly treated with an external ventricular drain. Vasospasm is a narrowing of the cerebral arteries thought to be caused by smooth muscle dysfunction related to blood breakdown products in the spinal fluid. When present, it can contribute to significant ischemia of the brain and, as such, be a significant cause of morbidity. Treatment of symptomatic vasospasm is typically multimodality and includes the use of hypervolemia and induced hypertension, endovascular procedures, and a variety of pharmacologic agents (Box 67-2).[10-12]

A classic study of cerebral aneurysms and their treatment documents the risk for rupture according to size and location as demonstrated in Table 67-3.[13] As a means of predicting possible vasospasm and overall outcomes, the Hunt and Hess clinical grading scale[14] and the World Federation of Neurological Surgeons clinical grading scale[15] were developed (Tables 67-4 and 67-5). Another method of classifying subarachnoid hemorrhage is described by Fisher and colleagues[16] and is based on CT scan imaging (Table 67-6).

Treatment of saccular aneurysms consists of coiling, coiling through a stent, or surgical clipping (Figs. 67-7 and 67-8) with subsequent intensive critical care unit management of potential vasospasm and comorbidities. Once the standard of care in the treatment of cerebral aneurysms, open craniotomy and clipping is now typically reserved for those lesions believed not to be amenable to endovascular techniques.[13,17,18] It is generally believed that treatment of ruptured aneurysms is best accomplished as soon as possible after the initial hemorrhage.

Spontaneous Intracerebral Hemorrhage

Spontaneous intracerebral hemorrhages into the brain parenchyma are common, accounting for approximately 10% of all strokes. They generally occur in older patients, usually because of degenerative changes in the cerebral vessels that are often associated with chronic hypertension (Box 67-3). In younger patients, they are more likely related to drug abuse or vascular malformation. They can occur anywhere in the cerebral circulation or brainstem but are classically described in association with small degenerative aneurysms (microaneurysms; also known as Charcot-Bouchard aneurysms) at the junctions of the perforating vessels and larger vessels at the skull base. They are typically on the middle cerebral artery junctions with the small perforating lenticulostriate vessels, leading to hemorrhage into the putamen. The clinical presentation is with a stroke pattern of sudden-onset neurologic signs and symptoms that depend on the area of brain affected. Symptoms are more likely to include headache than ischemic stroke. The diagnosis is with CT, usually done in an emergency department setting. The size and location of the acute hematoma are well visualized with CT, as is any associated brain shift or hydrocephalus (Figs. 67-9A and 67-10). In older patients with a known history of hypertension and classic CT appearance of a hematoma in the putamen, thalamus, cerebellum, or pons, further diagnostic studies are generally not indicated. Rehemorrhage is unlikely in that setting. However, further investigation might be warranted with an atypical hematoma location or appearance, especially if there is any component of subarachnoid

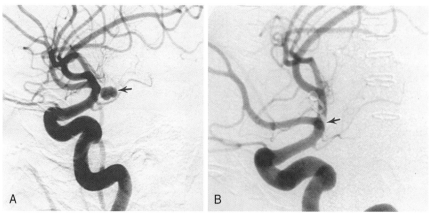

FIGURE 67-7 A, Subtraction carotid angiogram shows a 4 × 6-mm berry aneurysm *(arrow)* originating from the distal internal carotid artery. **B,** Postoperative carotid angiogram shows clip placement *(arrow),* with total obliteration of the aneurysm.

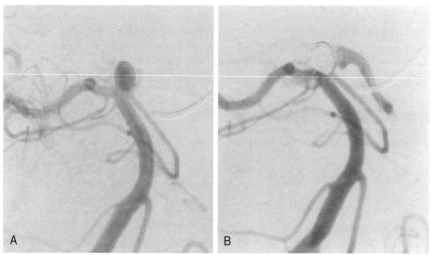

FIGURE 67-8 A, Subtraction vertebral angiogram shows a basilar tip aneurysm. **B,** Subtracted vertebral angiogram after the placement of coils demonstrates excellent obliteration of the aneurysm and preservation of adjacent vessels.

BOX 67-3   Causes of Spontaneous Intracerebral Hemorrhage

Hypertension	Cerebral amyloid angiopathy
Vascular anomaly	Coagulopathy
Cerebral aneurysm	Tumors
Arteriovenous malformation	Drug abuse
Cavernous malformation	Other
Cerebral infarction (stroke) transformation	

---

blood. Also, investigation is usually recommended for younger patients without known hypertension and those with a potential underlying cause for hemorrhage (e.g., history of neoplasm, blood dyscrasias, bacterial endocarditis).

Further investigation is generally done with contrast MRI or magnetic resonance angiography. Any suggestion of aneurysm or AVM is followed by conventional catheter angiography. In older patients with a history of early dementia and multiple episodes of more peripherally located intracerebral hematomas, the diagnosis of amyloid angiopathy needs to be considered.

Most cases of spontaneous intracerebral hemorrhage do not require an operative procedure. Many hemorrhages are small enough to be well tolerated and do not require surgery. Others are so large at the outset that surgery is of little benefit. Relief of any obstructive hydrocephalus by ventricular drainage is usually offered, except in the most impossible cases. Patients who obey commands and can be monitored by changes in their neurologic examination can generally be managed conservatively with hospital observation for at least 5 to 7 days. Peak swelling and decompensation are probably most likely to occur within that time frame. Surgery for evacuation of the hematoma may be appropriate in a small group of patients with intermediate-sized hemorrhages in accessible locations who appear to tolerate the hematoma initially but then deteriorate in a delayed fashion with edema, despite medical therapy. Steroids have not demonstrated benefit. Attempts to predict which patients will deteriorate solely on the basis of hematoma volume have been frustrated by the broad spectrum of intracranial compliance exhibited by different

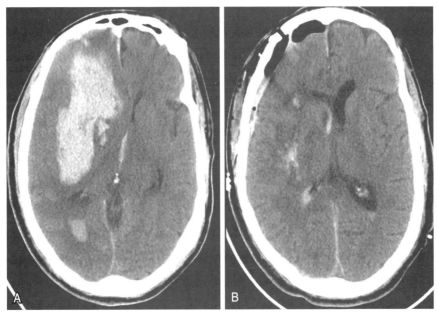

FIGURE 67-9 Nonenhanced CT scan of the head. **A,** Spontaneous hypertensive intracerebral hematoma in the right basal ganglia, with extension to the frontal and temporal lobes. **B,** Immediate postoperative CT scan shows near-total removal of the intracerebral hematoma.

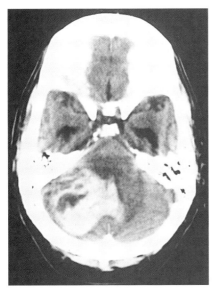

FIGURE 67-10 Nonenhanced CT scan of the brain shows a large, hypertensive, intracerebellar hematoma with obstruction of the fourth ventricle and enlargement of the temporal horns, indicating obstructive hydrocephalus.

patients. In general, younger patients with smaller ventricles and small subarachnoid spaces have a lower compliance, with lower tolerance, than older patients with cerebral atrophy and generous ventricles and subarachnoid spaces.

The Surgical Trial in Intracerebral Hemorrhage has noted a lack of clinical outcome difference in comparing early surgery with conservative management.[19] If indicated, surgical evacuation is usually done by craniotomy over the most accessible part of the hematoma (Fig. 67-9B). Intraoperative ultrasound is often

helpful in finding hematomas that do not quite come to the cortical surface and in monitoring the progress of the evacuation. The goal of surgery is decompression more than complete removal, but it is generally done as far as safely practical. The wall of the hematoma cavity is inspected for any underlying cause, and a biopsy specimen is taken, if indicated. Putamen hemorrhage can sometimes be evacuated with minimal surgical damage to the overlying brain by a trans–sylvian fissure–transinsular approach. Stereotactic aspiration and methods with fibrinolytic agents are being developed and may be a consideration for patients with hematomas in deep locations that are otherwise difficult to access.

A special situation to consider is the patient with cerebellar hemorrhage (Fig. 67-10). Surgery is offered more readily in these cases because the danger of sudden deterioration from brainstem compression is more of a concern and because even extensive damage to the cerebellum itself is generally survivable, with good functional outcome. Patients with fourth ventricular obstruction and hydrocephalus from cerebellar hemorrhage can sometimes be treated with ventricular drainage alone but are usually offered surgical evacuation of the hematoma by suboccipital craniotomy because of the risk for brainstem compression.

Mycotic Aneurysms

These aneurysms are associated with a systemic infection capable of showering small particles of bacteria-infected material into the cerebral vascular bed. Subacute bacterial endocarditis and some pulmonary infections can do this. A distinguishing feature of these aneurysms is that they are generally found more distal in the cerebral vascular bed, as opposed to berry aneurysms, which are usually found on larger vessels near the circle of Willis. There can also be many of them. When the bacterial emboli lodge in distal cerebral arterial branches, they can erode through the wall of these smaller vessels, often creating a hemorrhage contained by the perivascular tissue. Maximal antibiotic treatment is essential at the outset. The presence of an intracerebral hematoma may force immediate craniotomy for evacuation. Operation on the aneurysm at this early stage often reveals a component of subarachnoid hemorrhage and an early inflammatory reaction in the subarachnoid space, with only a blood collection covering the erosion defect in the wall of the small artery. Attempts to dissect and to define a neck are frustrated by a lack of developed fibrous tissues, and intraoperative hemorrhage is then common. Typically, the diseased arterial segment must be occluded and resected when it is operated on in this early stage. The need for arterial bypass to maintain blood flow to critical cerebral areas should be anticipated, but this is not always possible.

If the mycotic aneurysms are discovered or treated at some later stage, a fibrous wall to the aneurysm may have had time to develop, and clipping can then be a possibility. However, the surgeon needs to be forewarned that it may be difficult to find the aneurysm in a distal location, often buried deep in a cerebral sulcus thickened with reactive fibrous scar tissue.

Moyamoya Disease

Moyamoya disease is a cerebrovascular disorder that is characterized by an idiopathic nonatherosclerotic narrowing or occlusion of major intracranial blood vessels with the development of a conspicuous compensatory collateral rete vessel network, which allows continued cerebral perfusion around the occluded or severely narrowed segment. The disorder is usually bilateral, although not necessarily exactly symmetrical. Although generally rare, the disease is more common in persons of Asian ancestry and was first recognized from cases studied with angiography in Japan before the advent of CT and MRI. The term *moyamoya* comes from the Japanese word for "puff of smoke" or mist. The actual disease is sometimes confused with the less conspicuous collateral vascular networks seen around severe narrowing of common atherosclerotic origin in persons of Western origin. In the juvenile form, moyamoya typically is manifested as cognitive decline, with deteriorating school performance and evidence of multiple infarcts. Angiography reveals the internal carotid artery, proximal middle cerebral artery, or proximal anterior cerebral artery with severe narrowing or occlusion and, generally, multiple clusters of fine collateral vessels. In the adult form of moyamoya disease, the rete vessels cause subarachnoid or basal ganglia hemorrhage, the most common presentations. The hemorrhage can usually be treated conservatively. Some form of extracranial to intracranial bypass is generally attempted to take the load off the collateral vascular network. In younger patients, the results are good, with an onlay interposition of the superficial temporal artery sewed into the dura after a strip craniotomy. A feature of the disorder is the vigor with which collaterals form from the onlay transposed vessel. In the adult form, a microvascular anastomosis with the superficial temporal artery or grafted vessel may be preferred.

Dural Arteriovenous Malformations

Dural AVMs (type II CCF is a subtype) are not often seen in younger patients. The lesions seem to occur only in adults and are probably acquired lesions that follow a dural sinus thrombosis, usually of the cavernous sinus or sigmoid-transverse sinus junction area. With subsequent healing, the thrombosed segment triggers a neovascular response that evolves to an AVM configuration with fistulous channels that can gradually enlarge. Usually, there is associated stenosis of the affected dural segment, suggesting the earlier thrombosis. The lesions are generally not dangerous unless they cause retrograde venous drainage into the cerebral circulation.

The risk for intracranial hemorrhage is then fairly high; it is important at least to separate the dural AVM drainage from the cerebral circulation when that occurs. In the case of transverse-sigmoid sinus dural AVM, the patient usually complains of a bruit, and embolization or resection is optional, depending on symptom tolerance. In the case of type II CCF, the problem is usually intraocular and intraorbital venous hypertension, with proptosis, chemosis, and sometimes threatened vision. Ocular tonometry can help determine the extent of the threat to vision. Treatment of type II CCF involves endovascular embolization of prominent feeders, followed by occlusion of the affected venous dural sinus. As long as the dural AVM drainage is separated from the cerebral circulation, occlusion of the affected venous drainage is safe and curative. The affected stenotic transverse-sigmoid sinus segment can be reached by endovascular techniques through the jugular vein. The cavernous sinus can be reached by the petrosal sinus or, with neurosurgical assistance, through the superior orbital vein.

CENTRAL NERVOUS SYSTEM TUMORS

Intracranial Tumors

Intracranial tumors can be classified as primary versus secondary, as pediatric versus adult, by cell of origin, or by location in the nervous system. Primary tumors arise from tissues in the nervous system, whereas secondary tumors originate from tissues outside the nervous system and metastasize secondarily to the brain. They may represent local extension of regional tumors, such as chordoma or scalp cancer, but usually reach the nervous system through the hematogenous route.

In general, the incidence of primary brain tumors is higher in whites than in blacks, and mortality is higher in males than in females. According to the Central Brain Tumor Registry of the United States (CBTRUS), the overall incidence of primary brain tumors was 14.8/100,000 person-years between 1998 and 2002 (CBTRUS statistical report, 2005-2006). On the other hand, secondary tumors outnumber primary brain tumors by 10:1 and occur in 20% to 40% of cancer patients.[20] Because no national cancer registry documents brain metastases, the exact incidence is unknown, but it has been estimated that 98,000 to 170,000 new cases are diagnosed in the United States each year.[21]

Clinical Presentation

The clinical manifestations of various brain tumors can be divided into those caused by focal compression and irritation by the tumor itself and those attributed to secondary consequences, namely, increased ICP, peritumoral edema, and hydrocephalus. Usually, symptoms are caused by a combination of these factors.

The clinical presentation does not differ much by tumor histology; rather, rate of growth and location of the tumor contribute to the clinical features. A meningioma peripherally located in a relatively silent area of the brain, with a slow rate of growth, may enlarge to a significant size in a neurologically intact patient because the brain can accommodate to a slowly growing lesion. On the other hand, a small metastatic lesion at the foramen of Monro or in the sensorimotor strip can cause acute hydrocephalus or seizures, respectively.

Headache occurs in 50% to 60% of primary brain tumors and in 35% to 50% of metastatic tumors. It is classically described as being worse in the morning, probably because of hypoventilation during sleep, with consequent elevation of the PCO_2 and cerebrovascular dilation. The headache is associated with nausea and vomiting in 40% of patients and may be temporarily relieved by vomiting as a result of hyperventilation. Seizures may be the first symptom of a brain tumor. Patients older than 20 years presenting with a new-onset seizure are aggressively investigated for a brain tumor.

Infratentorial lesions may be manifested with headache, nausea and vomiting, gait disturbance and ataxia, vertigo, cranial nerve deficits leading to diplopia (abducens nerve), facial numbness and pain (trigeminal nerve), unilateral hearing deficit and tinnitus (vestibulocochlear nerve), facial weakness (facial nerve), dysphagia (glossopharyngeal and vagus nerves), and CSF obstruction causing hydrocephalus and papilledema. Supratentorial lesions may be manifested with different symptoms, depending on the location. Frontal lobe lesions are manifested as personality changes, dementia, hemiparesis, or dysphasia. Temporal lobe lesions may be manifested with memory changes, auditory or olfactory hallucinations, or contralateral quadrantanopia. Patients with parietal lobe lesions may develop contralateral motor or sensory impairment, apraxia, and homonymous hemianopia, whereas those with occipital lobe lesions may show contralateral visual field deficits and alexia.

Imaging Studies

The initial workup generally involves a relatively inexpensive diagnostic tool, a CT scan of the brain. CT provides a rapid means of evaluating changes in brain density, such as calcifications, hyperacute hemorrhages (<24 hours old), and skull lesions. MRI of the brain, however, is the "gold standard" modality for diagnosis, presurgical planning, and post-therapeutic monitoring of brain tumors. Gadolinium contrast enhancement with MRI is more sensitive in demonstrating defects in the blood-brain barrier and localizing small metastases (up to 5 mm). It can be used in patients allergic to iodine and those with renal failure. Advances in MRI techniques have evolved from strictly morphology-based imaging to a modality that encompasses function, physiology, and anatomy. Diffusion-weighted imaging can help distinguish between gliomas and abscesses, and perfusion-weighted imaging can predict response to radiotherapy in low-grade gliomas. Functional MRI can be used in planning of surgery for tumors in eloquent areas of the brain to enable radical resection with less morbidity. Diffusion tensor imaging can demonstrate the effect of a tumor on white matter tracts. Magnetic resonance angiography is used more routinely as a noninvasive modality to evaluate the vascularity of a tumor or anatomic relationship of a tumor to normal cerebral vasculature.[22]

Surgery

Dexamethasone is recommended for the management of brain tumors because of its propensity to reduce peritumoral edema by stabilizing the cell membrane. An antiepileptic drug is also recommended for tumors close to the sensorimotor strip. Mannitol is often administered before dural opening and operative resection.

Technical advances have made tumor surgery safer and more effective. The intraoperative microscope provides superior illumination and magnification, thereby allowing the surgeon to resect tumors from critical areas through small cranial openings. The cavitational ultrasonic surgical aspirator simultaneously breaks up and sucks away firm tumors while protecting vital neural and vascular structures. Intraoperative ultrasonography provides real-time imaging of tumors and cysts in subcortical and deep areas of the brain. Intraoperative CT or MRI is standard practice in some centers, enabling on-table imaging of the extent of resection (Fig. 67-11A). CT and MRI also allow real-time visualization of

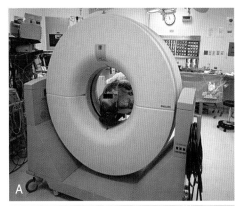
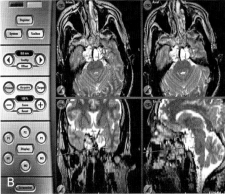

FIGURE 67-11 Technologic advances in the operating room. **A,** Intraoperative CT scanner. **B,** Computer-guided surgical navigation showing real-time location of a surgical probe tip on the preoperative MRI study during resection of clival chordoma.

a biopsy needle within a target. Image-guided (CT or MRI) frameless surgical navigation allows instant and accurate localization of the tip of a probe during a craniotomy by displaying that point on a preoperative CT or MRI scan (Fig. 67-11B).

The primary goals of surgery include histologic diagnosis and reduction of mass effect by removal of as much tumor as is safely possible to preserve neurologic function. The decision between a needle biopsy and more radical surgical resection depends on the location and size of the tumor, its sensitivity to radiation or chemotherapy, the preoperative Karnofsky performance score of the patient, and the systemic status of the primary cancer in case of metastatic brain lesions.

PRIMARY BRAIN TUMORS

Primary tumors of the brain are divided into intra-axial (those arising from within the brain parenchyma) and extra-axial (those arising from outside the brain parenchyma).

Intra-Axial Brain Tumors

Intra-axial brain tumors develop from the glia, or supportive structures, of the neurons and are collectively called gliomas. Total surgical resection of gliomas is extremely rare because of their ability to infiltrate widely along the white matter tracts and to cross the corpus callosum into the contralateral hemisphere. Radiation therapy and chemotherapy options vary according to the histology of the brain tumor. Therapy involving surgically implanted carmustine-impregnated polymer combined with postoperative radiation therapy has a role in the treatment of de novo and recurrent high-grade gliomas. Biologic therapies are currently under evaluation for patients with brain tumors and include dendritic cell vaccination, tyrosine kinase receptor inhibitors, farnesyltransferase inhibitors, virus-based gene therapy, and oncolytic viruses. An ideal therapy will target rapidly growing malignant glioma cells along with infiltrating tumor cells, with minimal toxicity to normal cells. This requires that the therapeutic vehicle of choice have access to all cells in the brain and be able to distinguish invasive or quiescent tumor cells from normal cells.[23]

The current histopathologic classification of brain tumors was recently updated by the World Health Organization (WHO).[24] WHO classifies intra-axial brain tumors by cell type and grades them on a scale of I to IV based on light microscopy characteristics that include the degree of cellularity, pleomorphism, mitotic figures, endothelial proliferation, and necrosis. The higher the grade, the more aggressive and malignant is the tumor.

An exhaustive review of neuro-oncology is beyond the scope of this chapter. What follows is an overview of the most commonly encountered and unique tumors of the central and peripheral nervous systems.

Astrocytic Tumors

Glioblastoma multiforme. A WHO grade IV tumor, this is the most commonly encountered primary brain tumor in adults. Presentation can include headache, seizures, focal deficits, and personality changes. Imaging usually demonstrates a ring enhancing lesion with surrounding edema and mass effect (Fig. 67-12). Treatment of accessible lesions involves attempted gross total resection and postoperative radiation therapy and chemotherapy.

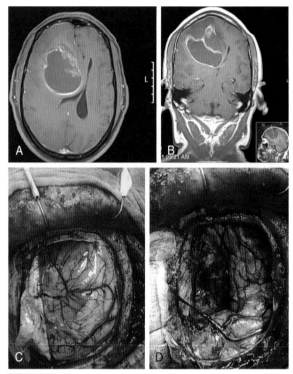

FIGURE 67-12 MRI and intraoperative pictures of a patient with a glioblastoma multiforme. Gadolinium-enhanced axial **(A)** and coronal **(B)** MRI scans show a large tumor with ring enhancement causing a 1-cm subfalcine shift of midline structures. Intraoperative pictures show the yellowish tumor surrounded by normal brain gyri **(C)** and the surgical field after resection of the tumor **(D)**.

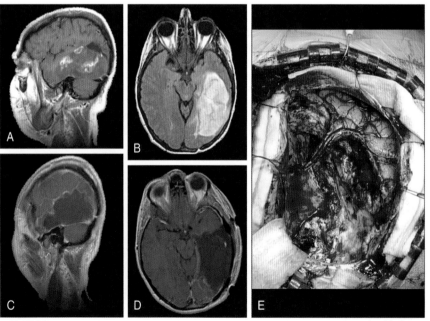

FIGURE 67-13 Radiographic and intraoperative images of a patient with a left temporal anaplastic astrocytoma. **A,** A partially enhancing tumor is noted in the left temporal lobe on this gadolinium-enhanced sagittal MRI study. **B,** Fluid-attenuated inversion recovery sequence axial MRI shows the extent of the tumor. The postoperative gadolinium-enhanced sagittal **(C)** and axial **(D)** MRI scans show near-total resection of the tumor. **E,** Intraoperative illustration of the surgical field after resection of the tumor.

Temozolomide is the current drug of choice and has been shown to improve both survival and quality of life. Recurrence is common, and repeated surgical resection is often deemed reasonable.

Anaplastic astrocytoma. A WHO grade III tumor, this presents much the same as glioblastoma multiforme, with similar treatment but slightly better long-term prognosis (Fig. 67-13).

Pilocytic astrocytoma. Pilocytic astrocytomas are typically classified as WHO grade I gliomas. When arising in the posterior fossa, they can cause obstructive hydrocephalus and cerebellar signs on examination. Surgical resection is the treatment of choice for these posterior fossa lesions. However, for lesions in the hypothalamus or optic tract, biopsy and chemotherapy or radiation therapy should be considered.

Oligodendroglioma

These tumors originate from oligodendroglial cells and represent 25% of all glial tumors; they occur with a male to female predominance of 3:2, observed at an average age of 40 years. They often present clinically with seizures or hemorrhage and nonspecific mass effect. A 5-year survival rate can be observed between 40% and 70%, depending on the grade, with an overall median survival of 3 years. Another form known as oligoastrocytoma behaves like oligodendroglioma, and both have aggressive anaplastic forms.

Treatment consists of surgical resection followed by chemotherapy. A particularly favorable response rate is associated with tumors that show allelic losses of chromosomes 1p and 19q. Radiation therapy is considered for tumors with anaplastic transformation.

Ependymoma

These tumors constitute around 5% of all intracranial gliomas across all ages. In the pediatric population, they may constitute up to 70% of all intracranial gliomas; the peak age at presentation is between 10 and 15 years. In children, ependymomas will typically be found in the fourth ventricle floor. A variant known as subependymoma is a rare form that is generally found incidentally in older patients and rarely requires surgical excision.

An ependymoma typically is manifested as a slowly growing posterior fossa mass that may cause obstruction of CSF flow, leading to hydrocephalus and symptoms of increased ICP with nausea, vomiting, and intense headaches. Up to 80% will have a 5-year survival in treated young patients; however, in the anaplastic variety, the presentation is much more aggressive and outcome is poor.

Treatment consists of maximal possible resection because extent does affect survival, followed by fractionated radiation. Recommendations for spinal MRI plus a lumbar puncture for cytology to rule out subarachnoid drop metastases are required for possible spinal radiation should these be positive.

Ependymomas of the spinal cord and cauda equina are also infrequently seen. Cauda equina lesions are of the myxopapillary variant.

Choroid Plexus Papilloma and Carcinoma

These intraventricular tumors represent 1% of all intracranial tumors, and up to 70% are seen in children 2 years of age or younger. The majority are benign papillomas. They typically are manifested with hydrocephalus. The 5-year survival rate is around 85% with benign lesions; however, only 40% of patients with

choroid plexus carcinoma survive 5 years or more. The atypical papilloma variant has an intermediate prognosis.

Treatment entails total surgical excision and adjuvant chemotherapy in the case of benign lesions. Radiation therapy, in addition to gross total resection, should be used when carcinoma is observed.

Pediatric Brainstem Gliomas

These tumors represent around 10% to 20% of all pediatric brain tumors; the mean age at presentation is 7 years. Midbrain gliomas (tectal and tegmental) usually have better survival rates than pontine gliomas. Tectal gliomas typically are manifested with hydrocephalus but have up to an 80% 5-year progression-free survival rate. Focal tegmental mesencephalic tumors may be manifested with hemiparesis that slowly progresses. The diffuse pontine glioma will usually present with multiple cranial nerve palsies and ataxia with increased ICP and have a poor overall median survival of less than 1 year.

Treatment of tectal gliomas requires vigilant follow-up and frequently CSF diversion or shunting. Focal tegmental mesencephalic tumors might be surgically resected and require adjuvant chemotherapy and radiation therapy if they recur. In the case of diffuse pontine gliomas, treatment is with radiation with or without experimental chemotherapy or palliative care.

Neuronal and Mixed Neuronal-Glial Tumors
Ganglioglioma and Gangliocytoma

These represent less than 12% of all intracranial tumors; presentation is generally before the age of 30 years, with a peak at 11 years. They typically are manifested with seizures and are benign and slow growing. With treatment, the survival rate between 5 and 10 years is 80% to 90%. Treatment should include complete resection when possible, and radiation therapy should be considered for rare anaplastic ganglioglioma.

Central Neurocytoma

These tumors are rare and represent around 10% of all intraventricular tumors and are rarely found extraventricularly. Most cases, around 75%, are found between the ages of 20 and 40 years and present typically with hydrocephalus, increased ICP, and seizures. They are usually slow growing and benign and rarely hemorrhage; they have a survival rate of more than 80%. Treatment with complete resection usually cures, requiring only SRS or chemotherapy should a rare recurrence happen.

Dysembryoplastic Neuroepithelial Tumor

Typically, dysembryoplastic neuroepithelial tumors represent less than 1% of all primary brain tumors, affecting primarily children and young adults younger than 20 years. Patients also typically present with history of seizures, and these tumors are generally benign with very slow or even no growth. Treatment consists of surgical resection of tumor and possible neighboring epileptogenic foci.

Paraganglioma

This tumor is manifested as a slow-growing mass with systemic features of catecholamine release and carcinoid-like syndrome with cranial nerve palsies related to its location. These tumors are commonly slow growing and benign, with a 5-year survival rate of around 90%; they rarely bleed.

Depending on their location, paragangliomas can be named. When the paraganglioma is located at the carotid bifurcation, it is designated a carotid body tumor; at the superior vagal ganglion, glomus jugulare tumor; at the auricular branch of the vagus, glomus tympanicum; at the inferior vagal ganglion, glomus intravagale; and finally, in the adrenal medulla and sympathetic chain, pheochromocytoma. Treatment includes medical therapy to prevent blood pressure lability and arrhythmias with alpha and beta blockers. Surgical resection is preferred, and embolization before resection can sometimes reduce the intraoperative blood loss. When surgery is not possible, radiation therapy will be used.

Other neuronal and mixed neuronal-glial tumors include dysplastic cerebellar gangliocytoma (also known as Lhermitte-Duclos disease), desmoplastic infantile ganglioglioma, cerebellar liponeurocytoma, papillary glioneuronal tumor, and rosette-forming glioneuronal tumor of the fourth ventricle.

Pineal Region Tumors
Pineocytoma

These represent less than 1% of all primary brain tumors; they are observed mainly in children and young adults with a peak incidence between 10 and 20 years of age. As the tumors enlarge, they will typically present with hydrocephalus, increased ICP, and Parinaud syndrome (which is a supranuclear vertical gaze disturbance caused by compression of the tectal plate). Pineocytomas are usually stable and slow growing, with a 5-year survival rate of around 90%, and they rarely hemorrhage. When they are symptomatic or enlarging, the treatment is surgical. Stereotactic biopsy is considered by many to be high risk because of the surrounding venous vasculature.

Pineoblastoma

This tumor also represents less than 1% of all brain tumors. All pineocytomas, pineoblastomas, and those tumors that are intermediate of both (that have features of both) account for 15% of the pineal region tumors. Most are seen in children at a peak age of 3 years and predominantly in females with a ratio of 2:1. Like pineocytomas, pineoblastomas present with increased ICP, hydrocephalus, and Parinaud syndrome. Up to 50% will have CSF seeding, giving a median survival of 2 years from the time of diagnosis. Treatment should consist of surgical resection plus irradiation of the cranial vault and entire spinal axis. If the patient is older than 3 years, chemotherapy should also be considered.

Papillary Tumor of the Pineal Region

This is a rare tumor of children and young adults. It will typically be manifested with hydrocephalus and will behave like a grade II or grade III tumor according to the WHO classification. It can recur and require surgical resection followed by focal irradiation.

Primitive Neuroectodermal Tumors

Medulloblastomas are found to be 15% to 20% of all brain masses and up to one third of all posterior fossa tumors in the pediatric population. They are rarely seen in adults; most are diagnosed by the age of 5 years, with a male to female ratio of 3:1. They tend to have a rapid presentation with hydrocephalus, increased ICP, and cerebellar signs. These tumors tend to disseminate through the CSF and are often found to involve the spinal subarachnoid space in a sizable number of patients at the time of diagnosis. Treatment consists of attempted gross total resection followed by adjuvant chemotherapy and radiation therapy if the child is older than 3 years.

Tumors of Cranial and Spinal Nerves
Schwannoma

Schwannomas make up around 8% of all intracranial tumors. When located within the parenchymal region, they will clinically be manifested with seizures or focal deficit before the age of 30 years. Vestibular schwannomas will usually have sensorineural hearing loss with tinnitus and dizziness and typically present at an age older than 30 years. They are usually slow growing, with an average of 10% recurrence after total resection. When vestibular schwannomas are present bilaterally, the diagnosis of neurofibromatosis type 2 should be ruled out.

Treatment should entail audiology assessment to determine baseline status. Lesions less than 3 cm can be observed with clinical examinations, symptoms, radiographic evaluations, and audiology every 6 months. Some authors will recommend SRS for growing tumors less than 3 cm in diameter; 90% of tumor control is possible with rare facial palsy, and up to 50% to 90% hearing preservation is obtained. When surgical resection is performed on tumors less than 3 cm, this adds the benefit of tumor removal with 80% normal or near-normal facial nerve preservation and between 40% and 80% hearing preservation overall, depending on literature reviewed. When tumors are larger than 3 cm, surgical resection is always recommended, but it is usually accompanied with total loss of hearing and a greater risk of facial palsy.

Neurofibroma

Neurofibromas are rarely found intracranially and can be associated with neurofibromatosis type 1. When located in the head, they can be found as plexiform neurofibromas often in the orbit from cranial nerve V1, scalp, or parotid (cranial nerve VII). Along the spinal canal, they can develop into dumbbell-shaped masses as they exit the neuroforamina or on occasion into large peripheral nerve sheath tumors. They typically are manifested as a painless mass with slow growth that is histologically benign, but between 2% and 12% can degenerate into malignant peripheral nerve sheath tumor with a high recurrence rate. Treatment consists of surgical resection; however, most neurofibromas will encompass nerve fibers, and total resection results in nerve sacrifice as opposed to schwannoma resection, which usually can be achieved without nerve sacrifice.

Tumors of the Meninges
Meningiomas

Meningiomas are observed in between 15% and 20% of all primary intracranial tumors, second only to glioblastoma multiforme. The prevalence is in females (2:1), and it is rare in childhood unless it is associated with neurofibromatosis type 1. The presentation is usually incidental in up to 50% of cases; they are typically slow growing, and overall 5-year survival is greater than 90%.[25] Meningiomas can recur, depending on the resection obtained at surgery as described on the Simpson grading system for meningioma resection (Table 67-7) as well as the atypical histology. Overall, less than 1% will have malignant histology. Surgical resection is the treatment of choice if the patient is neurologically symptomatic. Many small, asymptomatic tumors can be observed.

Hemangioblastoma

Hemangioblastomas are observed in 1% to 2% of all primary intracranial tumors; between 25% and 40% are associated with von Hippel–Lindau syndrome (VHL). When they are associated with VHL, hemangioblastomas typically occur in young adults with a slight male predominance. However, in general, heman-gioblastomas make up around 10% of posterior fossa tumors; when they are not associated with VHL, they have a sporadic peak at the age of 50 years. They tend to present with mass effect because of cyst expansion and typically are slow growing and histologically benign. They have an 85% 10-year survival postresection rate with a 15% recurrence.

Lymphomas and Hematopoietic Tumors
Primary Central Nervous System Lymphoma
The incidence of primary CNS lymphomas has increased to 10% of all primary intracranial tumors, and they are observed in 2% to 6% of patients with AIDS. The mean age at presentation is 60 years in immunocompetent patients and 35 years in patients with acquired immunodeficiency with a slight male predominance. The presentation can be with symptoms from a mass effect and, depending on location, sometimes with neuropsychiatric changes. The median survival is 1 to 4 months without treatment, 1 to 4 years when the patient is treated, and 2 to 6 months in patients with AIDS. There is a dramatic but short-lived response to steroids. Treatment consists of stereotactic biopsy followed by radiation therapy and chemotherapy because of their chemosensitivity to methotrexate. Intrathecal methotrexate will usually be advised for young patients.

Plasmacytoma
Plasmacytoma will usually involve the skull when it is found intracranially. It will often mimic meningioma and is considered at high risk for development of multiple myeloma within 10 years of diagnosis. Treatment consists of ruling out systemic multiple myeloma with urinalysis for protein and serum protein electrophoresis. Complete surgical excision should be followed by radiation therapy.

Germ Cell Tumors
Germinomas compose 1% to 2% of all primary CNS tumors; 50% are found in the pineal region and have most frequently been described in the Japanese population. The peak age at presentation is around 10 years, with more than 90% being found in the population younger than 20 years. The male to female ratio is 10:1 for the pineal region, whereas suprasellar germinomas are more common in females.

When located in the pineal region, they can become large and are present with hydrocephalus and Parinaud syndrome. This consists of paralysis of upward gaze, convergence, and accommodation and is associated with lid retraction, creating the so-called setting sun sign.

When located in the suprasellar region, they may produce compression of the hypothalamus and cause hypothalamic-pituitary dysfunction with diabetes insipidus and visual decline from compression of the optic tracts. Tumor markers help confirm diagnosis and a favorable prognosis when low secretion of human chorionic gonadotropin is observed. There is a 5-year survival rate greater than 90%, and they are usually sensitive and responsive to radiation therapy and chemotherapy. The first line of treatment consists of biopsy, then radiation therapy plus chemotherapy and treatment of hydrocephalus with either placement of a ventricular peritoneal shunt or a third ventriculostomy.

Nongerminomatous germ cell tumor is found most frequently between the ages of 0 and 3 years. These tumors are generally associated with a worse prognosis than germinomas are, with a 5-year survival rate of less than 50%. Embryonal carcinoma (malignant germ cell tumor) represents less than 1% of all CNS tumors and affects prepubertal children but is rarely found in children younger than 4 years; it is associated with Klinefelter syndrome and is considered malignant and invasive. Yolk sac tumors are also known as endodermal sinus tumors; they are usually found in infants or adolescents and are aggressive and malignant. Choriocarcinomas, which are also malignant and highly hemorrhagic, are another variety. Teratomas can be subdivided into mature and immature. The mature variety can be curable when complete resection is obtained. However, in the subtypes, the treatment algorithms, which include attempted resection plus chemotherapy and radiation therapy versus primary chemotherapy plus radiation therapy, are unclear; none of these has shown any significant survival difference. Mixed germ cell tumor is also a variety of the nongerminomatous germ cell tumors.

Tumors of the Sellar Region
Pituitary adenomas (Fig. 67-14) make up 10% of all intracranial tumors, with an equal male to female incidence; the peak incidence is in the third and fourth decades. The tumors can be associated with multiple endocrine neoplasia syndromes. Around 50% present as macroadenomas that are larger than 1 cm in diameter. Symptoms develop from mass effect on the optic tract or hypothalamic-pituitary disturbance with endocrine abnormalities and rarely apoplexy. Typically, when it is a hormone-producing tumor, symptoms will appear at earlier stages in tumor growth than when nonfunctioning adenomas are found.

Treatment consists of endocrine laboratory workup and evaluation with ophthalmology and visual fields. Prolactin levels of 25 ng/mL or less are considered normal; if the prolactin level is between 25 and 150 ng/mL, it is generally considered "stalk effect," although levels above 100 ng/mL should be considered suspicious. However, when the level is higher than 150 ng/mL, it is considered diagnostic for prolactinoma. In the case of apoplexy presentation, rapid administration of corticosteroid and possible surgical decompression must be considered. Surgical options include a trans-sphenoidal approach with microscope or endoscope, open craniotomy, and combination of these two procedures, which would be the case in large extensive suprasellar lesions. Focal or stereotactic radiation is usually reserved for refractory cases. It is always important for an endocrinologic follow-up.

The classic presentation and associated treatment for pituitary adenomas are as follows.

Prolactinoma will be manifested with amenorrhea and galactorrhea in females and impotence in males. Infertility will be

TABLE 67-7 Simpson Grading System for Meningioma Resection

GRADE	EXTENT OF RESECTION	RECURRENCE RATE*
I	Complete including dural attachment and abnormal bone	10%
II	Complete with cauterization of dural attachment	15%
III	Complete without dural attachment	30%
IV	Incomplete resection	Up to 85%
V	Biopsy	100%

*Length of follow-up varies around 5 years; numbers may increase with longer follow-up.

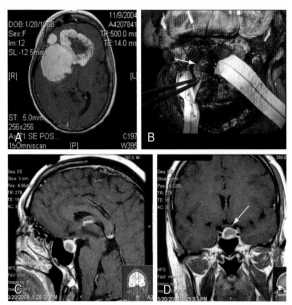

FIGURE 67-14 A, A large enhancing meningioma can be seen in this gadolinium-enhanced axial MRI study. **B,** Intraoperative picture showing dissection of the meningioma *(arrow)* from the surrounding gyri. Gadolinium-enhanced sagittal **(C)** and coronal **(D)** MRI scans of a patient with a pituitary macroadenoma show impingement on the optic chiasm *(arrow)*.

present in both. The treatment consists of dopamine agonist (e.g., bromocriptine) and generally provides complete control.

Adrenocorticotropin adenoma will be manifested as Cushing disease and classic hyperpigmentation of the skin and mucous membranes, ecchymoses, and purple striae, especially in the flanks, breast, and lower abdomen. Generalized muscle wasting with complaints of easy fatigability are among the other well documented signs and symptoms. The first line of treatment is surgery.

Growth hormone secreting tumors will produce acromegaly in adults and gigantism in prepubertal children. Surgery is the first line of treatment. Some patients may respond to octreotide, and others may show improvement with dopamine agonist.

Thyroid-stimulating hormone secreting tumors may present as hyperthyroidism, anxiety, and palpitations (due to atrial fibrillation). Patients have heat intolerance, hyperhidrosis, and thyrotoxicosis, for which the treatment will require surgery.

For both gonadotropin-secreting and nonfunctional adenomas, clinical presentations will be due to mass effect and stalk compression. If the tumor extends to the suprasellar region and compresses the optic chiasm, this will cause bitemporal hemianopia and may also have cranial nerve deficits. Treatment for these last two is also surgical resection.

Craniopharyngiomas are tumors that represent between 2% and 5% of all intracranial tumors; 50% are in children, with a peak incidence between 5 and 10 years of age. Their clinical presentation is similar to that of suprasellar masses with compression of the surrounding structures. The tumor is histologically benign but may sometimes have local aggressive and relentless behavior. Craniopharyngiomas have a 5-year survival rate of 55% to 85%, but recurrences typically happen within 1 year from surgery. The most frequent postoperative complications include diabetes insipidus and hypothalamic injury with 5% to 10%

mortality. Treatment requires medical optimization before surgical resection because if there is adrenal cortical insufficiency, hydrocortisone coverage will often be needed perioperatively. Attempts to obtain total gross resection should be sought if appropriate. It is when subtotal resection is encountered that possible postoperative radiation therapy might be beneficial, but it does add to the morbidity.

Central Nervous System Metastasis

Cerebral metastases are the most common brain tumor in adults and make up more than 50% of all brain tumors across all ages. However, they account for only 6% of all pediatric brain tumor cases.[26] Approximately 20% to 40% of patients with cancer develop brain metastases during the course of their illness.[27] More than 550,000 patients die of cancer in the United States each year, and around 20% of these patients will have brain metastasis.[26,27] It is well known that most brain metastases arise from lung, breast, and renal cell tumors; however, melanoma, followed by lung, breast, and renal cell carcinoma, has the greatest propensity to develop brain metastasis. What is observed frequently is that breast and renal cell carcinoma tends to present as a single metastasis within the brain, whereas melanoma and lung cancers have an increased incidence of multiplicity.[27] The highest incidence of brain metastasis is seen in the fifth to seventh decades of life, and it is equally common among men and women. Lung cancer is the most common source of brain metastasis in men, and breast carcinomas are the most common source of metastases in women. Men with melanoma are more likely to develop brain metastasis than are women. The interval or time period between the diagnosis of the primary cancer and the development of brain metastasis depends on the histology of the primary cancer; breast cancer generally exhibits the longest interval (mean, 3 years) and lung cancer the shortest (mean, 4 to 10 months).[28]

Metastatic lesions tend to cause significant brain edema that initially will respond well to steroids. Typically, dexamethasone is used and will reduce the vasogenic edema. Anticonvulsants are used to reduce the likelihood of seizure but are generally given if the patient has had a seizure. When the lesion is initially encountered and no primary tumor is known, recommendations for stereotactic biopsy or excision should be given. However, if the disease is widespread, with a short life expectancy, and the patient has a poor preoperative status, consideration should be given to possible biopsy or radiotherapy and palliation.[29,30] If, on the other hand, a solitary metastasis is encountered, total surgical excision should be attempted, followed by whole brain radiotherapy. SRS generally will be recommended if surgery is not feasible.[31] When multiple metastases are encountered, consideration should be given to excision of the symptomatic lesion or multiple lesions (but this is controversial), followed by brain therapy or radiotherapy alone, and SRS will usually be considered if surgery is not feasible[32,33] (Fig. 67-15).

TRAUMATIC BRAIN INJURY

The goal of this section on traumatic brain injury is not to present a comprehensive review of the epidemiology, basic science research, and outcome studies on brain injury but to give a practical, common-sense approach to the management of injuries of the brain. There is bound to be overlap between this section and other parts of this text. Guidelines for the management of severe head

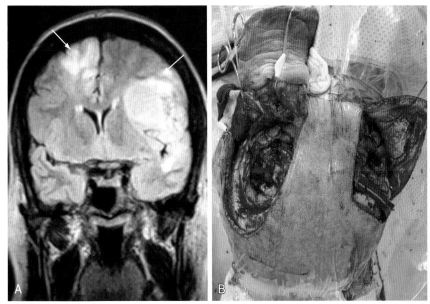

FIGURE 67-15 **A,** Fluid-attenuated inversion recovery sequence coronal MRI of a patient with two simultaneous metastatic tumors along the right and left frontal lobes *(arrows)*. **B,** Simultaneous right and left frontal craniotomies for resection of both metastatic lesions.

injury were first published by the Brain Trauma Foundation in 1995 and last reviewed in 2007.[34] These evidence-based guidelines have been a tremendous aid to the physician caring for brain-injured patients. The following discussion on the management of severe traumatic brain injury is based largely on these guidelines. As with all practice guidelines, they can and need to be modified, as dictated by the experience of the treating physician and in accordance with the needs of the patient. This report and the protocols laid out in the advanced trauma life support guidelines, published by the American College of Surgeons Committee on Trauma, are also invaluable resources for the student and physician.

We first present the epidemiology, pathophysiology, prehospital and emergency management, and definitive treatment of severe traumatic brain injury.

Epidemiology

Depending on the source of information, it is estimated that there are anywhere from 500,000 to well above 1 million cases of head injury every year. Most of these are classified as mild injuries, with approximately 20% classified as moderate to severe. Approximately 50% of the 150,000 trauma deaths every year are caused by head injury. The social, medical, and economic implications are profound. Fortunately, prevention programs appear to be decreasing the incidence of severe traumatic brain injury.

Pathophysiology

Traumatic brain injury can be classified into primary and secondary injuries. Primary injury occurs at impact and is considered first. It includes bone fracture, intracranial hemorrhage, and diffuse axonal injury (DAI). Fractures of the cranial vault and skull base are indicative of the forces applied to the skull at the time of impact. Fractures of the skull base may be associated with cranial nerve deficit, arterial dissection, and CSF fistula formation. Fractures of the cranial vault are classified as follows:

Open or closed
Depressed or nondepressed
Linear or comminuted

Any fracture of the cranial vault can cause disruption of the underlying meningeal arteries or dural venous sinuses, which can lead to intracranial bleeding. Intracranial hemorrhage can be classified as epidural, subdural, subarachnoid, and intraparenchymal or intracerebral. Epidural hemorrhage occurs between the dura and skull and is usually the result of a skull fracture causing the laceration of a meningeal artery.

Rarely, a fracture crossing a dural venous sinus can cause a venous epidural hematoma, especially in children. Subdural hemorrhage occurs in the potential space between the dura and arachnoid. This is often the result of shearing of the bridging veins between the brain and the dural venous sinuses. Sometimes, it comes from injury to cortical vessels, which then bleed into the subdural space. Subarachnoid hemorrhage from trauma consists of bleeding into the spinal fluid spaces surrounding the blood vessels feeding the cerebral cortex. Trauma is the most common cause of subarachnoid hemorrhage. Rupture of an intracranial aneurysm is the second most common cause of subarachnoid hemorrhage and is generally distinguished from traumatic subarachnoid hemorrhage by history and sometimes by the distribution of blood on a CT scan. Intraparenchymal or intracerebral hemorrhage is bleeding into the brain itself. This can run the spectrum from small contusions (bruises of the brain) to large intracerebral clots (which usually are the result of coup and contrecoup injuries) that require emergent surgical evacuation. Although often small and nonsurgical at first, these can blossom and become life-threatening during a period of hours to days. DAI is a rotational acceleration-deceleration injury to the white matter pathways of the brain. This results in a functional or anatomic disruption of these pathways and is cited as the cause of loss of consciousness in patients without mass lesions. DAI can occur with or without other primary injuries, such as an epidural or subdural hematoma (Fig. 67-16). In addition to being one of the many primary injuries seen in severe traumatic brain injury, DAI can also be considered a secondary injury.

Secondary injury to the brain occurs as a result of decreased oxygen delivery to the brain, which in turn sets off a cascade of events that causes even more damage than the initial injury. With severe traumatic brain injury, there can be an alteration in cerebral vessel autoregulation. Systemic hypotension in the presence of this altered autoregulation results in decreased CBF and decreased oxygen delivery. This ischemia is exacerbated even further by systemic hypoxemia; intracranial hypertension, which decreases CBF even further, and a cascade of events involving mediators of inflammation, excitotoxicity, calcium influx, and Na^+,K^+-ATPase dysfunction lead to neuronal cell dysfunction and death. The prevention of secondary injury is therefore thought to lead to increased cell survival and improved outcome. This is achieved by preventing hypotension and hypoxia while taking measures to control ICP and to maintain CPP.

Prehospital and Emergency Department Management

The prehospital and emergency department management of the traumatized patient is reviewed elsewhere in this and other texts. Here we deal more specifically with issues critical to the patient with severe brain injury. The ABCs must always be addressed first, regardless of the severity of the patient's injury. Attention is first paid to securing a patent airway, establishing adequate ventilation and oxygenation, and maintaining adequate circulation. By doing this, one may avoid hypotension and hypoxia and, in so doing, avoid or minimize secondary brain injury. In patients with severe traumatic brain injury, a systolic blood pressure less than 90 mm Hg or a PaO_2 less than 60 mm Hg is a predictor of poor outcome. Appropriate spine precautions are observed in the initial resuscitation of the patient with a severe traumatic brain injury.

Once airway, breathing, and circulation have been addressed, neurologic evaluation may proceed. The Glasgow Coma Scale (GCS) is a simple and reproducible method of neurologic assessment. It is also used to grade traumatic brain injury as mild,

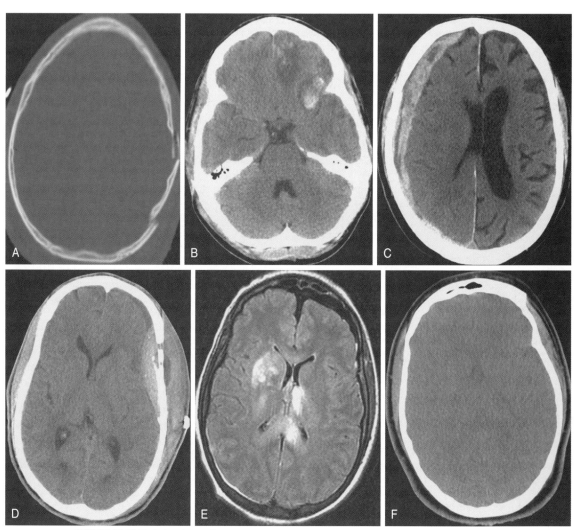

FIGURE 67-16 Typical radiologic findings in traumatic brain injury. **A,** Skull fracture shown on CT. **B,** Intra-parenchymal contusions. **C,** Subdural hematoma. **D,** Epidural hematoma. **E,** Diffuse axonal injury. **F,** Intra-cranial hypertension. Note the effacement of sulci and gray-white matter differentiation.

moderate, or severe. The GCS consists of three components—intensity of stimulus required to cause eye opening, verbal response, and motor response (Table 67-8). Pupillary size and reactivity are also essential components of the initial neurologic examination. Hypoxia, hypotension, alcohol, and drugs may all contribute to abnormal findings on the neurologic examination. In the absence of hypotension and hypoxia, an abnormal finding on examination is considered to be a primary brain injury until proven otherwise. Once all life-threatening injuries have been addressed and stabilized, the patient with a suspected traumatic brain injury undergoes CT. The CT scan is used to evaluate the presence or absence of fracture, epidural and subdural hematomas, intracerebral hematomas and contusions, shift of the midline structures, and appearance of the basal and perimesencephalic cisterns. In many centers with multislice scanners, routine scanning of the cervical spine is also performed to rule out acute fractures or traumatic dislocations. If life-threatening injuries elsewhere necessitate immediate transport of the patient to the operating room and the patient has a suspected intracranial hematoma (e.g., unilateral fixed and dilated pupil on one side, with a contralateral hemiparesis), exploratory burr holes may be performed in the operating room concurrently with the laparotomy or thoracotomy.

Not infrequently, trauma patients with brain injury will require transfer to a hospital equipped to provide those patients with a higher level of care. In preparing these patients for transfer, the physician needs to follow the advanced trauma life support guidelines and secure the airway, ensure adequate ventilation, and maintain circulation. Anemia is treated with transfusion, as necessary. Hypoxia and hypotension need to be avoided. Adequate immobilization with a backboard and cervical collar is mandatory. In patients with obvious intracranial hypertension or mass lesions, treatment with mannitol may be considered after neurosurgical consultation. Vigilance and attention to detail as well as communication between the transferring and accepting physicians are key to the successful transfer and treatment of these patients.

Treatment

When the workup of a patient reveals an intracranial mass lesion and deficits thought to be related to that lesion, operative intervention is indicated. In general, any clot or contusion more than 30 mL is thought to be operable. Epidural and subdural hematomas (Fig. 67-16) are addressed with similar approaches, with the craniotomy centered on the clot. Intracerebral hematomas are addressed through appropriately located craniotomies. ICP monitors are often placed at operation. These can be intraventricular drains, intraparenchymal monitors, or devices placed in the epidural or subdural spaces. The decision about when to place an ICP monitor depends on the patient's preoperative examination findings, appearance of the brain at operation, and potential risk for deterioration. In general, all patients with a GCS score of 8 or less have ICP monitors placed. Some patients with moderate traumatic brain injury may also benefit from ICP monitoring. Postoperatively, the patient is managed similarly to those with nonoperable traumatic brain injury.

The following is a simplified algorithm for the management of intracranial hypertension in the intensive care setting. The head of the bed is elevated to 30 degrees, with the head placed in a neutral position. Care is taken to ensure that any cervical spine immobilization device is not obstructing jugular venous flow because this can increase ICP. The goal of treatment is to try to keep the ICP below 20 mm Hg and to maintain CPP at or above 70 mm Hg (remember that CPP is MAP minus ICP). If the ICP is persistently elevated above 20 mm Hg, it is treated. CSF drainage is now the first line of therapy in decreasing ICP. This is accomplished by an external ventricular drain, or ventriculostomy, which is a drain placed in the operating room or at bedside in the intensive care unit in an appropriately monitored patient. If ICP remains persistently elevated despite CSF drainage, the patient can be sedated and even paralyzed pharmacologically to keep the ICP down. The physician is dependent on the pupillary examination and ICP reading in this situation. If the ICP changes rapidly or the pupillary examination findings change (i.e., blown pupil), emergent CT of the head is indicated. Sedation and paralysis can occasionally be discontinued to allow an adequate neurologic evaluation in this situation.

If the ICP remains persistently elevated despite these interventions, mannitol and other diuretic agents may be used. Mannitol is administered as an intravenous (IV) bolus of 0.25 to 1 g/kg every 4 to 6 hours. Serum osmolality is followed closely when mannitol is being given, and the drug is withheld if the serum osmolality exceeds 320 mOsm/kg. It is also important to maintain euvolemia in these patients. If ICP is still elevated, hyperventilation to a $PaCO_2$ of 30 to 35 mm Hg may be used judiciously. At this point, second-tier therapeutic interventions (e.g., hypertonic saline, high-dose barbiturate therapy, decompressive craniectomy) may be considered.[35,36] Serial CT scans are critical throughout this treatment algorithm, and their use is tailored to the individual patient.

Several comments regarding nutrition, steroids, anticonvulsants, and $PaCO_2$ are appropriate here. Energy requirements after traumatic brain injury are increased. The nonparalyzed patient requires replacement of 140% of his or her resting metabolism expenditure, and the paralyzed patient requires 100%. Of this, 15% is protein. Feeding begins within 7 days of injury. Steroids have no proven benefit in the management of traumatic brain injury and are not used. Prophylactic use of anticonvulsant drugs (e.g., phenytoin, carbamazepine, phenobarbital) is not indicated

TABLE 67-8 Neurologic Assessment Using the Glasgow Coma Scale					
EYE OPENING RESPONSE		VERBAL RESPONSE		MOTOR RESPONSE	
SCORE	RESPONSE	SCORE	RESPONSE	SCORE	RESPONSE
4	Spontaneous	5	Oriented	6	Obeys commands
3	To speech	4	Confused	5	Localizes to painful stimulus
2	To pain	3	Inappropriate responses	4	Withdraws to painful stimulus
1	No response	2	Incomprehensible responses	3	Flexion to painful stimulus
		1	No response	2	Extension to painful stimulus
				1	No response

TABLE 67-9	**Brain Trauma Foundation Recommendations for Traumatic Brain Injury**
PARAMETER	**GUIDELINE**
Hyperosmolar therapy	Mannitol effective for control of raised ICP (0.25-1 g/kg)
Prophylactic hypothermia	Preliminary data suggest that mortality could be decreased when target temperatures are maintained >48 hours
Infection prophylaxis	Routine external ventricular catheter exchange not recommended; indicated if GCS score = 3-8 on admission and abnormal CT; in severe traumatic brain injury and normal CT, indicated with two or more of the following: age >40 years, unilateral posturing, hypotension with systolic blood pressure <90 mm Hg
ICP monitoring	Ventricular catheters are most reliable and cost-effective method; ICP should be kept <20 mm Hg
CPP threshold	CPP <50 mm Hg should be avoided; aggressive interventions to maintain it above 70 mm Hg have a considerable risk of acute respiratory distress syndrome
Brain oxygen monitoring and thresholds	Jugular venous saturation (50%) and brain tissue oxygen tension (15 mm Hg) are treatment thresholds
Blood pressure and oxygenation	Blood pressure should be monitored, hypotension (systolic blood pressure = 90 mm Hg) avoided; hypoxia (saturation <90% or PO_2 <60 mm Hg) should be avoided
Nutrition	Should be initiated within 7 days of injury
Sedatives	High-dose barbiturates recommended to control refractory ICP in the hemodynamically stable patient; propofol recommended for ICP control but does not improve mortality
Seizure prophylaxis	Decreases early post-traumatic seizures (<7 days after injury)
Hyperventilation	Recommended as temporizing measure; PCO_2 below 25 mm Hg not recommended; avoid in first 24 hours after injury
Steroids	Not recommended, contraindicated

TABLE 67-10	**Clinical Findings in Common Lumbar Disc Herniations**				
DISC	**INCIDENCE (%)**	**ROOT**	**PAIN DISTRIBUTION**	**MUSCLE INVOLVED**	**SENSORY DEFICITS**	**REFLEX LOSS**
L3-4	3-10	L4	Anterior thigh	Quadriceps femoris	Medial malleolus and medial foot	Knee jerk
L4-5	40-45	L5	Posterolateral thigh and leg	Tibialis anterior; extensor hallucis longus	Large toe web, dorsum of foot	None
L5-S1	45-50	S1	Posterolateral thigh and leg down to ankle	Gastrocnemius	Lateral malleolus, lateral foot	Ankle jerk

TABLE 67-11	**Clinical Findings in Common Cervical Disc Herniations**				
DISC	**INCIDENCE (%)**	**ROOT**	**PAIN DISTRIBUTION**	**MUSCLE INVOLVED**	**REFLEX LOSS**
C4-5	2	C5	Shoulder	Deltoid	Deltoid
C5-6	19	C6	Upper arm, thumb, radial forearm	Biceps, extensor carpi radialis	Biceps, brachioradialis
C6-7	69	C7	Fingers 2 and 3, all fingertips	Triceps	Triceps
C7-T1	10	C8	Fingers 4 and 5	Hand intrinsics	Finger jerk

for the prevention of late post-traumatic seizures. Anticonvulsants may, however, be used to prevent early post-traumatic seizures, primarily in patients at high risk for early seizures who may suffer adverse effects if they were to seize early in their hospital course. These can usually be tapered after 1 week of therapy. Hyperventilation causes a decrease in ICP by lowering $PaCO_2$, which causes vasoconstriction and decreases intracranial blood volume. Unfortunately, it also causes decreased CBF. If hyperventilation to a $PaCO_2$ of less than 30 mm Hg is required for the maintenance of an acceptable ICP and CPP, monitoring of CBF is strongly recommended by some. Jugular venous oxygen saturation and cerebral oxygen extraction may also be useful in this clinical scenario. Table 67-9 presents a summary of the recommendations of the 2007 guidelines provided by the Brain Trauma Foundation for traumatic brain injury.

DEGENERATIVE DISORDERS OF THE SPINE

Relevant Spinal Anatomy

In adults, the spinal cord terminates at the lower border of L1. The filum terminale, a relatively fibrous structure, extends from the lower border of the spinal cord to attach at the S2 level. On both sides at each level, anterior and posterior nerve roots exit and traverse toward the nerve root foramen and enter the root canal to join and form the spinal nerve. The first spinal nerve roots (C1) exit above the atlas, the C2 roots exit between C1 and C2, and the C8 nerve exists between C7 and T1 (thus, there are only seven cervical vertebrae, whereas there are eight pairs of cervical nerve roots). This is significant in localization of the spinal nerve involvement by a prolapsed disc as a C5-6 disc will involve the C6 nerve root. In the thoracic and lumbar region, the corresponding thoracic nerve root exits below the corresponding vertebra; thus, the L4 nerve root exits between the L4 and L5. However, in the lumbar region, an extreme lateral course of the nerve root while exiting predisposes the next root to be involved in disc prolapse at the corresponding level. For example, in L4-5 disc prolapse, the L5 nerve root is commonly involved as the L4 root crosses the L4-5 disc space at the extreme lateral edge, thus escaping compression. The L5 root courses across the L4-5 disc space more medially, thus being involved in the process. Hence, although prolapsed discs commonly involve the lower level root in both the cervical and lumbar regions, the causes are different in both regions. The motor, sensory, and reflex distribution of the nerve roots are summarized in Tables 67-10 and 67-11.

Pathophysiology of the Degenerative Diseases of the Spine

The intervertebral disc essentially consists of three parts: the annulus fibrosus, which is the tough outer ring composed of 10 to 12 layers of fibrous tissue and fibrocartilage; the central nucleus pulposus, which is initially gelatinous but becomes more fibrous with advancing age; and end plates, which are thin plates of hyaline cartilage attaching the disc to the upper and lower vertebral body. Although the nucleus pulposus can herniate in any direction, posterior and posterolateral herniations cause compression of the adjacent nerve roots and give rise to clinical symptoms. Superior and inferior herniations into the vertebral body are known as Schmorl nodes and are incidental findings. The intervertebral disc herniation is most common in the lower cervical and lower lumbar levels, although it can occur at any level from C2 to L5.

Apart from the soft disc herniations as mentioned before, degeneration of the disc results in small annular tears and mild protrusion of the fragments outside the confines of the disc. This, during a prolonged period, leads to hypertrophy of the adjacent bone edges known as osteophytes. The osteophytes projecting posteriorly can compress on the adjacent nerve root or the spinal cord. Associated hypertrophy and infolding of the ligamentum flavum can cause reduction in the intraspinal space with predominant posterior compression. Facet hypertrophy can result in reduction in the lateral recess of the spinal canal, causing lateral recess stenosis. Most often, these coexist with compression of the neural structures from multiple directions. Severe degeneration of the facets and laxity of the ligaments result in degenerative spondylolisthesis, which is common at L4-5 and L5-S1 levels in the lumbar region and C3-4 and C4-5 levels in the cervical region. This listhesis can result in compression of the spinal cord and adjacent roots.

Cervical Disc Prolapse, Cervical Spondylosis, and Cervical Stenosis

Approximately 90% of the herniated discs in the neck are located at C5-6 and C6-7 levels. An acutely herniated disc (soft disc; Fig. 67-17) typically presents with local pain and tenderness, with the pain radiating in the distribution of the affected nerve root. The symptoms may be precipitated by a minor trauma. Initial local pain often precedes the radiating pain by several weeks. Movement of the cervical spine usually aggravates the pain. Features of nerve root dysfunction in the form of motor weakness or sensory numbness usually follow the initial pain. Large disc prolapse can cause spinal cord compression, resulting in spasticity and weak-

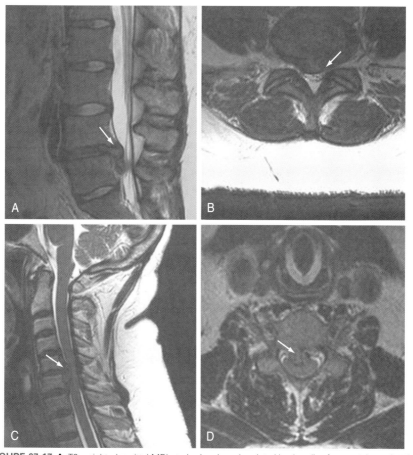

FIGURE 67-17 A, T2-weighted sagittal MRI study showing a herniated lumbar disc fragment *(arrow)* at the L4-5 level. **B,** T2-weighted axial MRI showing the same fragment *(arrow)* compressing the thecal sac. **C,** T2-weighted sagittal MRI of a patient with a large anterior disc prolapse at C5-6 level *(arrow)*. **D,** Axial images showing the disc compressing the spinal cord *(arrow)*.

ness of the lower limbs. In severe cases, there may be accompanying urinary retention.

On the other hand, the presentation of the cervical spondylosis (hard disc) is usually more subtle, with waxing and waning neck pain and paresthesias in the upper limbs. Spondylotic lesions compressing the spinal cord can result in progressive spasticity and weakness of the lower limbs (spondylotic myelopathy) apart from the radiculopathic changes in the upper limbs. The presence of myelopathy is of considerable clinical significance as it usually necessitates a surgical intervention for the patient.

Stenosis of the cervical spinal canal may be either congenital or acquired. Congenital stenosis often presents in young adults with progressive myelopathy and gait disturbances. Acquired stenosis is most commonly due to cervical spondylosis with hypertrophy of the ligamentum flavum (Fig. 67-17).

Diagnosis

The symptoms of acutely herniated disc are so characteristic that the diagnosis is apparent during the clinical evaluation. The diagnostic studies confirm the level and the nature of the disc prolapse. On occasion, nerve root tumors (schwannoma) may present similarly. MRI of the cervical spine will demonstrate the location and extent of the disc bulge as well as if there are any signal changes in the spinal cord. Myelomalacia of the cord suggests chronic significant spinal cord compression and often is prognostic of potential residual deficits after adequate decompression of the spinal cord. In patients with spondylotic changes, MRI demonstrates the degree of osteophyte formation, associated ligamentous hypertrophy, and number of segments involved. Associated cervical spinal stenosis is also identified. CT myelography is often indicated in patients who cannot have MRI scans or when anatomic bone details are essential in making a management decision. Electromyography and nerve conduction studies are sometimes required to exclude other causes like plexopathies and peripheral nerve involvement.

Management Options

Acute *cervical radiculopathy* is often well managed conservatively with rest, analgesics, muscle relaxants, and a short course of steroids. Surgery is considered in patients with persistent pain and persistent neurologic deficits while they are receiving conservative therapy. The aim of the surgery is nerve root decompression. However, with presence of *cervical myelopathy* suggesting spinal cord compression, surgery is indicated to decompress the spinal canal and to relieve the compression on the spinal cord. Although improvement can be anticipated, an arrest of the progression of the myelopathy is often achieved (Fig. 67-18).

With a predominant anterior pathologic process and compression of the neural structures (e.g., compression from bulging disc, osteophytes, or spondylotic bars), the anterior cervical approach with discectomy is usually considered (Fig. 67-19). The osteophytes can be drilled out to decompress the spinal cord and the nerve roots. For a single-level discectomy, an interbody fusion with bone graft may or may not be considered. However, for multilevel discectomies, anterior interbody fusion with bone graft and instrumentation is considered the standard of care. Often with extensive pathologic processes across the vertebral body, the surgeon considers drilling out the vertebral body and replacing it with an iliac crest bone graft or a metallic/synthetic cage. Although the anterior approach is relatively safe and has a quick recovery period, injuries to the adjacent structures like esophagus and recurrent laryngeal nerve are the unique complications.

The posterior approaches to the cervical spine include foraminotomy and decompression, decompressive laminectomy, decompressive laminectomy with fusion, and cervical laminoplasty. *Cervical foraminotomy* is usually indicated for cervical radiculopathy with a lateral osteophyte or a soft disc. The other three approaches are usually considered for patients with a predominant posterior compression of the spinal cord (e.g., ligamentum flavum hypertrophy, degenerative canal stenosis with facet hypertrophy, congenital canal stenosis). *Cervical decompressive laminectomy* during a prolonged follow-up period often predisposes to kyphotic deformity (swan neck deformity) of the cervical spine and is often avoided in younger patients. In these patients, cervical decompressive laminectomy is usually combined with *posterior fusion with instrumentation* and bone graft. In *cervical laminoplasty*, the cervical laminae are fractured and displaced outward by spacers to increase the spinal canal diameter in the anterior-posterior plane. In patients with complex pathologic processes due to chronic spondylotic changes, an anterior and posterior approach can be combined in a single or staged manner.

Lumbar Disc Prolapse and Lumbar Degenerative Conditions
Lumbar Disc Prolapse

Like cervical disc prolapse, approximately 90% of the lumbar disc prolapse occurs at either the L4-5 or L5-S1 level, with the remainder at the L3-4 level. Lumbar disc prolapse at other levels is distinctly uncommon. There are two common presentations of the lumbar disc prolapse: acute radiculopathy and chronic low back pain. The first presentation, acute radiculopathy, usually involves a patient with a prior history of back discomfort manifested with acute back pain precipitated by an episode of lumbar strain, such as bending forward and lifting heavy objects. The

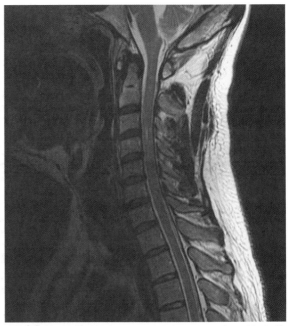

FIGURE 67-18 T2-weighted sagittal MRI scan of a patient with significant cervical canal stenosis. Note the hyperintensity in the cervical spinal cord at the C3-4 level, suggesting myelomalacic changes. This may be indicative of permanent residual deficits.

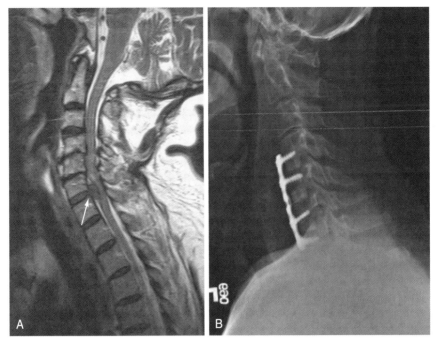

FIGURE 67-19 A, T2-weighted sagittal MRI study of a patient with advanced cervical spondylosis and stenosis from C3-4 down to C6-7 with an acute herniated disc fragment at C6-7 *(arrow)* after cervical spine manipulation. **B,** Postoperative lateral radiograph showing C4-5, C5-6, and C6-7 anterior cervical discectomy and fusion using a bone allograft and titanium plate and screws.

pain is usually in the low back region and often radiates to one of the lower limbs aggravated by coughing or straining. These patients will have restricted straight leg raising; they may have numbness in the dermatomal distribution and associated weakness that may appear a few days later. In severe cases, there may be bladder dysfunction. These patients usually have an annular rupture with herniation of the disc material into the spinal canal compressing the nerve root (see Fig. 67-17). The second category of patients have a long history of chronic backache with intermittent aggravations and remissions, with recent occurrence of leg pain and intermittent paresthesias in the lower limbs that are often poorly localized.

Lumbar Canal Stenosis

Narrowing of the canal diameter can be present congenitally (primary lumbar canal stenosis, congenital lumbar canal stenosis) or be secondary to degenerative changes (secondary lumbar canal stenosis). Advanced degenerative changes leading to arthrosis, facet hypertrophy, and ligamentum hypertrophy result in canal stenosis. Apart from stenosis of the thecal sac, foraminal stenosis can be due to extension of the stenosis to the neural foramen causing radiculopathic changes. Lumbar canal stenosis classically presents as claudication pain in both the legs that is precipitated by walking and occasionally even by standing for a prolonged period. This neurogenic claudication is relieved by maneuvers causing flexion of the spine (e.g., sitting down or bending forward) in addition to stopping the activity, as opposed to vascular claudication, which is relieved by stopping of the activity. The neurologic evaluation often does not elicit any gross deficits unless coexistent pathologic changes are present.

Localization and Diagnosis

The clinical localization is well apparent in the patients who present with radicular pain as the dermatomal distribution of the pain suggests the involved nerve root (Tables 67-10 and 67-11). The radiologic evaluation, in addition to confirming the disc bulge, demonstrates the degree of the bulge and associated additional pathologic change (canal stenosis, adjacent level disc disease, and spondylolisthesis).

Management

The initial management usually involves adequate bed rest, analgesics, muscle relaxants, and minor tranquilizers like diazepam. Most patients will experience benefit with this regimen and will be able to resume activity in a reduced capacity in a few weeks. The second line of treatment is by oral steroids and epidural steroid injection, which often reduces pain. Physical therapy is also useful during the recovery phase.

Certain symptoms and signs indicate the need for hospitalization. Presence of significant motor deficits (e.g., footdrop or occurrence of bladder involvement in the form of retention or urgency) is usually an indication for hospitalization. Surgical intervention is usually considered under these circumstances. The conventional surgical treatment includes a midline approach, partial laminectomy, and excision of the protruded disc with decompression of the nerve root. Radiographic identification of the correct level is essential. The herniated fragment is removed, and the nerve root is traced to the neural foramen to exclude associated foraminal stenosis, which if present would require foraminal decompression. A minimally invasive microscopic approach and an endoscopic approach using paramedian incisions have also been used. The recovery is usually quick, and patients are often discharged on the same evening or the next day. A 10% recurrence rate at the same level is reported with microsurgical discectomy.

The surgical approach is often tailored to the associated conditions. Associated canal stenosis requires a decompressive laminectomy and decompression of the neural foramen. Lumbar fusion and instrumentation are considered for failed surgery, associated spondylolisthesis, or extensive decompression, which can precipitate future instability. Some of the common lumbar fusion techniques include posterolateral fusion with pedicle screws, posterior lumbar interbody fusion, and anterior lumbar interbody fusion. A bone fusion between the adjacent segments is ideally achieved by interposition of cadaveric or autologous bone graft aided with additions like demineralized bone matrix or recombinant bone morphogenic protein. Instrumentation of the adjacent segments helps keep the ends apposed and immobilized.

FUNCTIONAL AND STEREOTACTIC NEUROSURGERY

Functional neurosurgery is concerned with the anatomic or physiologic alteration of the nervous system to achieve a desired effect. This can be done with focal electrical stimulation procedures, ablative procedures, or implantation of pumps to deliver drugs, usually to the CSF but possibly also to the parenchyma. The field of functional neurosurgery deals primarily with the treatment of pain, movement disorders, epilepsy, and some psychiatric disorders when they are refractory to conventional treatments. These disorders all have in common hyperfunction or deranged function of some part of the CNS. Sometimes, the hyperfunction results from a loss of function in some other part of the brain, such as in the output pathways of the globus pallidus when the dopamine system in the brain degenerates, as in Parkinson disease. The transmitter of the overactive globus pallidus output system is inhibitory; the overall effect on the motor system is also inhibitory. The physiology of each functional disorder is often complex and only partly understood. It is not our focus here to detail what is known about the mechanism underlying each of these disorders;

we focus on the surgery, especially the stereotactic techniques and possible interventions at the target site. This section also discusses SRS in general terms.

In considering brain stimulation, if the reader could image the consequences of placing two electrodes on the central processing unit of a computer and running a pulsatile stimulating current across it, not many would expect that the functioning of the computer would be enhanced. Rather, we would expect part of the computer not to work at all as a result. Although we talk about neuroaugmentation as if it were always adding something to the function of the nervous system, most of the interventions are actually effective because they stop certain unwanted activity in the brain. It may be a surprise to many, but in most situations, brain stimulation results in a temporary lesion of the stimulated structure. In almost all cases in the older neurosurgical literature in which a focal lesion was found to be effective, modern stimulation of that same structure is also effective. The difference is that a lesion is permanent and static in size and location. The advantage of stimulation is that it can be turned on or off, increased or decreased, and, in the case of an implanted electrode array, changed in location, depending somewhat on which of the several contacts are activated. Thus, stimulation provides a reversible, scalable, and somewhat movable functional lesion.

There are exceptions to the concept that stimulation is equivalent to a functional lesion. The frequency of stimulation can determine its overall effect, and the neurotransmitters at the site of stimulation can also have an effect. The cerebral cortex, with its high concentrations of excitatory neurotransmitters, may actually be turned on with stimulation. Thus, certain crude visual prostheses may be effective on that basis.

Stereotaxis, as applied to neurosurgery, is concerned with the localization of a target in three-dimensional space. The target deep in the brain is not seen directly at surgery. This can be a tumor, white matter pathway, cranial nerve, vascular malformation, or nucleus deep within the brain. The field has evolved using frame-based and frameless systems, but in each case, a calculated inference is used to reach the target accurately.

Frame-based systems use a rigid frame attached to the skull by pins that penetrate the outer table of the skull (Fig. 67-20). This can easily be done under local anesthesia, with the patient wide awake. The patient is then taken for CT or MRI with a localizer

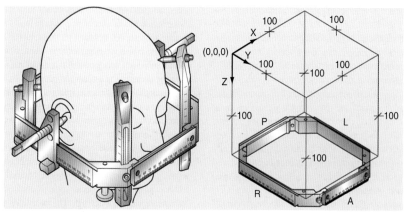

FIGURE 67-20 The Leksell stereotactic coordinate frame is rigidly attached to the head by four threaded pins. The fiducial box is mounted on the frame during the imaging study (MRI or CT). The x, y, and z coordinates are determined directly from the imaging study. The center of the frame is arbitrarily given the coordinates 100, 100, 100. (Courtesy Elekta, Stockholm, Sweden.)

on the frame. Using cartesian coordinates, the x, y, and z coordinates of the target can then be determined. In other words, the position of the target in relation to the frame is known. Using an arc system, which is mounted on the frame, the target can be accessed by different trajectories. When the target is a vascular lesion, arteriography can be performed with a localizing frame, and the position of the vascular lesion in three-dimensional space can be determined. Frame-based systems are used for brain biopsies, deep brain stimulation, ablative procedures, and SRS.

SRS involves the delivery of a concentrated dose of radiation to a defined volume in the brain. The dose of radiation delivered would be toxic if given in a broad field to the entire brain. When it is delivered in multiple collimated beams from numerous different angles or in arcs at different angles, the effect on the surrounding brain is minimized. Two methods of frame-based SRS are currently used widely. The gamma knife uses cobalt-201 radiation sources focused on one point. Once the target is localized in three dimensions, it is placed at this point, and different collimators are used to focus the radiation. Modified linear accelerators deliver the radiation dose in multiple arcs, thereby minimizing the effect on surrounding brain tissue. Both systems use multiple isocenters for the treatment of irregularly shaped lesions. SRS has been used in the treatment of almost every intracranial lesion but is commonly used in the treatment of metastatic tumors, benign lesions of the cranial nerves, AVMs, and trigeminal neuralgia.[37-41] The primary risks of SRS are radiation necrosis and radiation injury to surrounding structures.

Frameless stereotactic techniques use advanced imaging techniques, fiducials, and reference markers in place of a fixed frame. Robotic arms, infrared reflectors, and light-emitting diodes provide the surgeon with real-time information about the anatomy at hand. This technology can also be fused with a display from the operating microscope, aiding in the operative dissection. It is useful for the planning of incisions and craniotomies and, when combined with intraoperative ultrasound, may be of use in determining the extent of tumor resection. Frameless stereotactic radiosurgical devices are commercially available.[37-41]

Brain Stimulation

Electrical stimulation of the nervous system is used in the treatment of movement disorders, pain, and epilepsy. Stimulation involves placement of an electrode, which is then connected to a subcutaneously placed generator. Here we discuss neurostimulation as it applies to the treatment of movement disorders, chronic pain states, and epilepsy.

Parkinson disease is the most common movement disorder for which patients have surgery. Stereotactic techniques developed in the 1950s were used to create lesions in the pallidum and thalamus. These ablative procedures fell by the wayside for a time with the introduction and widespread use of L-dopa (L-3,4-dihydroxyphenylalanine). In the early 1990s, there was a renewed interest in the use of surgical techniques for Parkinson patients who had become unresponsive to pharmacologic agents or intolerant of their side effects. Lesions of the internal segment of the globus pallidus saw a tremendous resurgence. With improvements in imaging and intraoperative microelectrode recording, deep brain stimulation soon replaced ablative procedures in the surgical treatment of these patients. Stimulation induces a reversible inhibition of neuronal activity, which can be adjusted as the clinical situation demands. The subthalamic nucleus has replaced the globus pallidus as the target of choice. Subthalamic nucleus stimulation is most effective for the treatment of rigidity and akinesia.

Tremor is best addressed with stimulation of the ventralis intermedius nucleus of the thalamus.

Spinal cord stimulation is used for the treatment of chronic pain, dystonia, and bladder dysfunction. Patients typically undergo a trial of stimulation in which wire electrodes are placed percutaneously and attached to an external generator. If symptoms improve, permanent wire electrodes or paddle electrodes are placed and connected to a programmable generator placed subcutaneously. The precise mechanism of action is unknown. The most common indication is that of the so-called postlaminectomy syndrome, especially when leg pain is worse than back pain. There is also some benefit for those patients with chronic regional pain syndrome. It has not been found to be routinely effective in the treatment of cancer pain.

Vagal nerve stimulation has been approved by the U.S. Food and Drug Administration for the treatment of intractable seizures and severe depression. The mechanism of action is not clear but is thought to be the result of afferent stimulation of higher cortical centers in the hypothalamus, amygdala, insular cortex, and cerebral cortex through the nucleus of the solitary tract. Stimulation of the left vagus nerve decreases seizure frequency by approximately 50% but rarely makes patients seizure free.[42]

Implantable Pumps

Implantable pumps are used for the treatment of chronic pain and spasticity. An intrathecal catheter is inserted into the lumber spinal canal and a trial infusion used to gauge response. Many patients with cancer pain will respond favorably to intrathecal administration of narcotics through a programmable pump. Baclofen is the agent of choice for the treatment of spasticity with this modality.

Destructive Lesions

Ablative lesioning of the CNS for the treatment of pain, movement disorders, epilepsy, and psychiatric diseases has a long history. Before the advent of antipsychotic drugs, the most efficient way of curing and controlling some patients with severe psychiatric disease was thought to be institutionalization and psychosurgery. Before the development of the technologies described earlier, lesioning of different pathways in the brain and spinal cord was the only method for treating patients with chronic pain and movement disorders. Even though neuroaugmentive procedures and drug infusion technology have replaced many of the neuroablative procedures formerly in widespread use, a few ablative procedures still retain their clinical usefulness.

Dorsal root entry zone lesions are particularly useful for patients with deafferentation pain related to brachial plexus injury and, to a lesser extent, patients with spinal cord injury who have so-called end zone pain. In these conditions, deafferentation of the spinothalamic tract neurons results in spontaneous firing and the sensation of pain. The procedure creates lesions of the dorsal horn of the affected levels using a thermocouple probe. Extension of this concept has been applied to the caudal nucleus of the trigeminal nerve for the treatment of facial pain syndromes.

Myelotomy has traditionally been used in the treatment of bilateral cancer pain. It involves sectioning of the anterior commissure at and above the involved levels, which interrupts pain fibers on their way to the contralateral spinothalamic tract. A modified technique that interrupts only the median raphe of the dorsal columns has been described.[43] This presumably interrupts the second-order visceral pain pathway demonstrated to travel up the mammalian dorsal funiculus.[44]

Cordotomy involves lesioning of the anterolateral quadrant of the spinal cord at cervical levels, thereby eliminating input from the spinothalamic tract on the contralateral side of the body. Historically, it was most useful in the treatment of unilateral cancer pain. Bilateral lesioning increases the risk for neurologically mediated sleep apnea (Ondine's curse). It can be performed percutaneously or as an open procedure.

Sympathectomy involves surgical interruption of the sympathetic chain at the high thoracic or lumbar level. A variety of endoscopic, thoracoscopic, radiofrequency, and open techniques are used. It is primarily used in patients with hyperhidrosis, sympathetically mediated pain, causalgia, chronic regional pain syndrome, and Raynaud disease.

Nerve block or neurectomy uses local anesthetic, sometimes with corticosteroids, which can be injected into the tissues surrounding a peripheral nerve, blocking conductivity and relieving pain. This can result in a long-lasting effect but typically is short-lived. Neurolytic agents (phenol or absolute alcohol) can also be used. Nerves can also be surgically divided or interrupted by radiofrequency techniques. There is a significant risk for recurrence with ablative neurectomy. Local nerve blocks are generally used in diagnostic procedures but can be repeated as necessary for the relief of pain. Ablative neurectomy is usually reserved for short-term relief in patients with a poor prognosis and short life expectancy.

Epilepsy

Epilepsy is not a distinct clinical entity with an identifiable cause but rather a complex collection of disorders of the brain that all share seizures as part of the complex. Seizures are classified as partial, generalized, or unclassified. Partial seizures are simple (consciousness not impaired) or complex (consciousness impaired). Generalized seizures are convulsive or nonconvulsive. Incidence rates in developed countries (40 to 70/100,000) are lower than those in developing countries (100 to 190/100,000). Approximately 20% to 40% of patients with seizures do not respond to anticonvulsant therapy. Failure to respond to three anticonvulsant medications prompts referral to a center specializing in epilepsy

evaluation and treatment, and approximately 1.33% to 4.50% of those patients are candidates for surgical intervention.[45]

The goal of the workup of the patient who is a potential candidate for the surgical treatment of epilepsy is to identify the cortical area responsible for the onset of the seizure. When the radiographic workup (MRI, CT, or both) reveals an obvious lesion causing the seizure (e.g., tumor, vascular malformation), the treatment is relatively straightforward and involves removal of the lesion. In other cases, the offending lesion is not as obvious on imaging, and intensive and often invasive monitoring is necessary to determine the epileptogenic focus. It is also important to determine language dominance and areas of the brain that are functionally abnormal during the interictal period. Noninvasive techniques that have become more widely available and better characterized include magnetoencephalography, positron emission tomography, single-photon emission CT, and functional MRI. Invasive modalities used in the evaluation of patients for seizure surgery include the Wada test for language dominance, stereotactically implanted depth electrodes, implanted strip electrodes, and implanted grid electrodes (Fig. 67-21). Any or all of these techniques may be useful in brain mapping. It has long been possible to map critical speech and limb movement areas in awake, locally anesthetized craniotomy patients at the time of seizure focus resection.

On the basis of the information obtained in a noninvasive workup, the patient may be taken to surgery. Dominant hemisphere lesions are often operated on with the patient awake to allow intraoperative confirmatory brain mapping. This is accomplished by stimulating the cortex and observing and monitoring the patient's response, looking for speech arrest, anomia, or limb weakness or numbness. The most common surgical procedures performed for epilepsy are anterior temporal lobectomy, focal cortical resection, multiple subpial transection, hemispherectomy, and corpus callosotomy.

Anterior temporal lobectomy is the most common operation for seizures. An entirely unilateral interictal focus is the ideal indication (Fig. 67-22). The anterior temporal lobe, anterior hippocampus, and amygdala are excised. If the epileptogenic focus is not completely excised, the patient may continue to experience

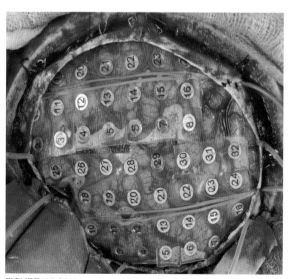

FIGURE 67-21 Intraoperative view of grid electrode placement for epilepsy surgery. (Courtesy Dr. Nitin Tandon, University of Texas, Houston.)

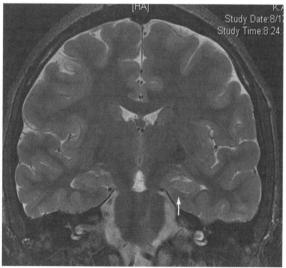

FIGURE 67-22 T2-weighted coronal MRI study shows gliosis and atrophy of the left mesial temporal structure *(arrow).*

intractable seizures. If too much temporal lobe is resected, it can result in a contralateral superior quadrantanopia or, in dominant hemisphere lesions, speech and language dysfunction.

Focal cortical resection is usually performed in the frontal cortex. The results are more variable than those with temporal lobectomy.

Multiple subpial transection is used in more eloquent areas of the brain and involves making cortical incisions perpendicular to the surface of the gyrus in question. This presumably preserves descending fibers and function while interrupting spread of any epileptogenic activity within the cortical mantle itself.

Corpus callosotomy is used to prevent the rapid spread of seizures rather than to eliminate the focus. It is primarily useful in seizures that suddenly generalize, resulting in atonic drop attacks, as in Lennox-Gastaut syndrome.

Hemispherectomy is usually reserved for young children with seizures restricted to one hemisphere but threatening the good hemisphere by secondary effects of repeated seizures, as in Rasmussen syndrome. There is usually some abnormality of cellular migration. In the past, the entire cortex was removed, leaving the basal ganglia intact. Even though there was a significant decrease in seizure activity, the procedure led to a high complication rate, with ex vacuo brain shifts. A newer technique now involves preservation of portions of the cortex and its blood supply while disconnecting them from the rest of the brain by extensive undercutting of the adjacent white matter.[46]

Trigeminal Neuralgia

Trigeminal neuralgia affects approximately 4 in 100,000 individuals and is characterized by brief episodes of severe, lancinating pain in one or more of the three divisions of the trigeminal nerve, usually V2 and V3. Patients often describe that it is precipitated by touch or extremes of temperature. In extreme cases, a patient may refuse to eat or shave to avoid triggering the severe jolts of pain. Sensation usually remains intact, and significant numbness or jaw weakness leads to suspicion of a compressive mass lesion, such as tumor. Often, patients are referred with an already estab-

lished diagnosis. It is reassuring if the patient has responded at some point to carbamazepine or an appropriate medication. MRI is used to rule out posterior fossa tumors and multiple sclerosis, which can present with related symptoms. Most patients respond to the oral administration of carbamazepine. Baclofen and gabapentin also have some clinical usefulness in medical treatment. The most common mechanism is presumed to be related to vascular compression of the fifth cranial nerve as it enters the brainstem (Fig. 67-23). With aging, the arteries elongate and can then begin to loop against the cranial nerves. At its entry to the pons, the fifth nerve has lost its peripheral nerve supportive architecture, the reticulin and mesenchymal elements that toughen the nerve more peripherally. Focal pulsatile pressure of the artery against this vulnerable part of the nerve results in ephaptic transmission from large myelinated fibers to small myelinated (A delta) and unmyelinated fibers.

Surgical therapy is usually reserved for patients who fail to respond to medical treatment. Microvascular decompression involves a small suboccipital craniotomy for microsurgical exploration of the dorsal root entry zone of the trigeminal nerve on the affected side. The offending vessel, usually the superior cerebellar artery, is then dissected off the nerve, and a barrier (Teflon or polyvinyl alcohol sponge) is placed between the vessel and nerve to prevent continued pulsatile focal compression. In especially favorable situations, the offending artery can be dissected free to loop away from the nerve, without the need for padding. A small sling of arterial patch graft material can also be sewn to hold the artery loop away from the nerve.

Percutaneous trigeminal rhizotomy techniques generally involve radiofrequency heat lesioning of the trigeminal ganglion, glycerol injection (Fig. 67-24) into the spinal fluid of Meckel cave (which causes an osmotic damage preferentially to the smaller pain-carrying nerve fibers), or mechanical trauma to the nerve or ganglion by transient inflation of a No. 4 Fogarty catheter balloon. Each method has its proponents along with advantages and disadvantages.

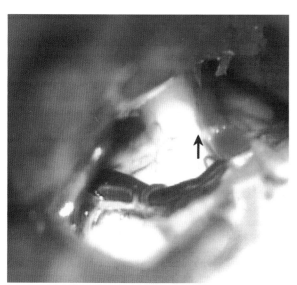

FIGURE 67-23 Intraoperative photograph of a patient with typical trigeminal neuralgia. The left trigeminal nerve is compressed superiorly by an arterial branch of the superior cerebellar artery *(arrow)*.

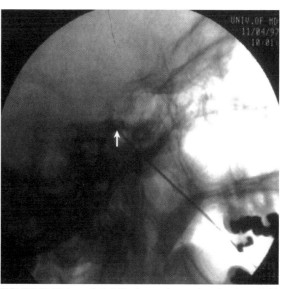

FIGURE 67-24 Lateral skull film in a patient undergoing glycerol rhizotomy for typical trigeminal neuralgia. A 20-gauge spinal needle is directed to the foramen ovale and nonionic contrast agent is injected to outline the trigeminal ganglion *(arrow)*.

SRS has been described for the treatment of trigeminal neuralgia.[37] Although initial results have been encouraging, long-term efficacy has yet to be determined.

HYDROCEPHALUS

Hydrocephalus denotes an excessive accumulation of the CSF in the intracranial compartment. The accumulation of fluid can be in either the intracerebral (ventricular) or extracerebral (subarachnoid spaces and cisterns) compartment.

Normally there exists a fine balance between the CSF production by the choroid plexus and the absorption at the arachnoid villi along the superior sagittal sinuses. The CSF production has been found to be 0.33 mL/kg/hr (20 mL/hr). Almost all the fluid produced is absorbed within 8 hours. Any imbalance in this will lead to excessive accumulation of CSF, causing hydrocephalus. Thus, it can be due to excessive production, decreased absorption, or obstruction anywhere in the pathways.

Communicating and obstructive hydrocephalus. This distinction was made several decades ago to explain whether the obstructed ventricular CSF communicated with the subarachnoid CSF. In obstructive hydrocephalus, the obstruction is at or proximal to the fourth ventricular outlet foramina (foramen of Magendie and Luschka). However, if the obstruction is beyond the fourth ventricular outlet foramina (cisterns or arachnoid granulations), it is classified as communicating hydrocephalus. Common examples of obstructive hydrocephalus are aqueductal stenosis and hydrocephalus associated with tumors. When the term was initially coined, it took into account the findings of the ventriculogram and pneumoencephalogram. However, with the arrival of CT and MRI, in most cases, these investigations are no longer necessary, and the terms *communicating* and *obstructive* were no longer clinically important. However, as we will see later, the advent of endoscopic third ventriculostomy has generated renewed interest in these terms.

Acute and chronic hydrocephalus. Hydrocephalus developing within days or a few weeks (e.g., hydrocephalus due to tumor) is manifested with rapid progression of symptoms known as acute hydrocephalus. It requires early attention and treatment. On the other hand, CSF accumulation during months (or even years) presents with subtle signs of memory impairment, walking difficulty, or urinary incontinence and is termed chronic hydrocephalus. A classic example of chronic hydrocephalus is normal-pressure hydrocephalus, which is seen usually in the geriatric population. At times, chronic hydrocephalus can present acutely because of a change in the pathophysiologic mechanism of the CSF absorption or flow.

Congenital and acquired hydrocephalus. Hydrocephalus present at birth is known as congenital hydrocephalus. At times, congenital hydrocephalus is apparent a few weeks or months after birth, even though the process started while the child was in utero. Although congenital hydrocephalus is commonly obstructive in nature, it can be communicating, as seen in intrauterine toxoplasmosis or cytomegalovirus infections. In acquired hydrocephalus, the pathologic process starts after birth and includes post-traumatic hydrocephalus, hydrocephalus associated with tumors, and normal-pressure hydrocephalus.

Hydrocephalus ex vacuo or compensatory hydrocephalus. Here the ventricles enlarge compensatory to overall shrinking of the brain tissue. This can mislead an inexperienced physician to diagnose hydrocephalus, whereas really the enlargement of the ventricles is due to the shrinkage of the brain tissue. This is commonly seen in advanced age with brain atrophy, after diffuse head injury or stroke, and with various neurodegenerative conditions. The most important condition that is usually confused with hydrocephalus ex vacuo is normal-pressure hydrocephalus, unfortunately also seen in the geriatric age group.

Porencephaly. Porencephaly (or porencephalic cyst) commonly refers to a condition in which a focal brain substance has suffered some loss of volume (e.g., stroke, postsurgical change in volume) leading to collection of CSF in the cavity. Porencephalic cyst is usually differentiated from hydrocephalus ex vacuo by its localized nature.

Arrested hydrocephalus. This represents a condition in which the ventricles are large with the patient having no significant symptoms to require a surgical procedure. However, this term should be used with caution as it is well known that these patients may develop symptoms during a prolonged period or may present acutely after a precipitating event like minor trauma or infection that alters the CSF dynamics.

Clinical Features of Hydrocephalus

In hydrocephalus, CSF retained inside the cranial compartment results in increased ICP and dilation of ventricles, causing compression of the adjacent brain. The symptoms differ considerably in different age groups. In infants, a thin and relatively nonrigid skull allows an overall cranial expansion, whereas in older children and adults, the rigid fused skull prevents its enlargement. Considering this, in *infantile hydrocephalus,* either the infant is born with a large head or the head abnormally grows during the first few months of life. The anterior fontanelle is usually full; it may or may not be bulging. In extreme cases, a relatively higher ICP causes the blood to be diverted from the intracranial to the extracranial compartment, resulting is prominent and dilated scalp veins. A late feature is the classic "sunset sign" manifested with downward deviation of the eyeballs (like a setting sun). This is due to compression of the midbrain tectum by the posterior part of the dilated third ventricle. In later stages, the child will be irritable and fussy and may not accept feeds. There may be associated vomiting. There usually is no associated fever or diarrhea. Lethargy, drowsiness, and, in extreme cases, lapsing into the comatose state will follow if the child remains untreated.

In *older children and adults,* fusion of the skull bones no longer permits the cranium to enlarge. The enlarging ventricles result in raised ICP and cause compression of the adjacent brain. There are two common modes of presentation: rapidly progressive hydrocephalus and chronic hydrocephalus. In *rapidly progressive hydrocephalus,* the increasing accumulation of CSF increases the ICP, presenting with new-onset headache and vomiting. These are commonly known as features of raised ICP. If untreated, these symptoms worsen and blurring of vision is often experienced. In patients with long-standing raised pressure, papilledema can result in secondary optic atrophy. If still untreated, drowsiness and progression to coma follow. Focal neurologic deficits are not experienced, although walking difficulty or the sensation of "giving away" at the knees can happen.

In *chronic hydrocephalus,* the CSF accumulates more slowly, thus gradually compressing the brain. This type of presentation is predominantly seen in the elderly age group, although it can happen in younger age. The patient becomes progressively dull, apathetic, and uninvolved with the surroundings. Memory impairment for recent events is commonly seen; the remote memory is usually well preserved. A short stepped gait with a wide stance with unsteadiness is evident. Urinary incontinence and urgency are also common findings. Although it is uncertain why most of these patients do not have significant headache, it is assumed that slow dilation of the ventricles compresses the adjacent brain to accommodate the CSF without causing raised pressure.

Although seizures due to hydrocephalus are uncommon, they may be caused by the process that initiates the hydrocephalus. A phenomenon seen in late stages of untreated hydrocephalus is known as cerebellar fits or hydrocephalic attacks. Preceded by progressively severe headache, the patient lapses into transient sudden unconsciousness associated with decerebrate or decorticate response, downward deviation of the eyeballs, and respiratory distress. The recovery is usually spontaneous. These episodes recur until CSF diversion is instituted. This is due to acute transtentorial herniation resulting in compression of brainstem. The condition is associated with significant morbidity and can be uniformly fatal unless prompt CSF drainage is instituted. This is a true medical emergency, and under no circumstances should the treatment be delayed. The survivors often develop permanent hemianopia due to occipital infarcts resulting from compression of the posterior cerebral arteries against the tentorial edge during the herniation.

Investigations

The common investigation used for diagnosis of hydrocephalus is a CT scan often accompanied by an MRI scan. Cranial ultrasound evaluation has been used predominantly in the newborn and infants with open fontanelle. The CT scan shows dilated ventricles and often indicates the pathologic process and the site of obstruction. The ventricular system dilates proximal to the obstruction, whereas the CSF pathways distal to the obstruction are not visualized well. As all the ventricles are usually well visualized on the CT scan, one can infer the level of obstruction from the CT scan. Most tumor disease can be well visualized also on the CT scan. However, the CT scan cannot delineate the exact site or nature of the obstruction. Probably the greatest utility of the CT scan in managing hydrocephalus has been in assessing patients with shunt malfunction. An obstructed shunt commonly *but not always* leads to dilation of the ventricles, which can be easily identified on the CT scan. In addition, the radiopaque shunt tube is well visualized on the CT scan.

MRI has been the imaging modality of choice in newly diagnosed hydrocephalus. The ability of MRI to obtain images in three different planes (coronal, sagittal, and axial) has been of considerable value in diagnosing the exact cause of hydrocephalus and the site of obstruction. With a properly done MRI study, the site of obstruction can be well visualized in most patients with obstructive hydrocephalus (Fig. 67-25). This is of considerable importance as small tumors or cysts causing hydrocephalus can be visualized, and when these are removed, the hydrocephalus can be relieved. Also, MRI is considered essential before considering endoscopic third ventriculostomy and aqueductoplasty, which are exciting alternatives in the management of hydrocephalus, and in assessing the effectiveness of endoscopic third ventriculostomy during the follow-up.

Treatment

The ultimate goal in the treatment of hydrocephalus is to reverse the neurologic damage caused by the raised ICP. Reconstitution of the cerebral mantle to allow normal intellectual development and avoidance of shunt dependency should be considered addi-

tional goals in management. In a previous study, cerebral mantle thickness of 2.8 cm or more was found to be associated with good outcome. It was also found that the cortical mantle reconstitution was not satisfactory if the treatment was delayed for more than 5 months.

Surgery for hydrocephalus involves diversion of the accumulated CSF by reopening the obstruction to allow the CSF to flow in its natural pathway, creation of a diversion before the obstruction to let the CSF drain into the intracranial pathways distal to the block, or diversion of the CSF into another cavity to have it absorbed into the bloodstream. Examples of reopening of the obstructed pathway include endoscopic aqueductoplasty and excision of the tumor causing hydrocephalus, whereas endoscopic third ventriculostomy falls into the second category. Ventriculoperitoneal shunts, which have been the mainstay of treatment in hydrocephalus, belong to the third group.

Although shunts have been the mainstay of treatment for several decades, endoscopic procedures have become more popular. These include endoscopic third ventriculostomy, endoscopic aqueductoplasty, and endoscopic aqueductal stenting. Although these alternative procedures appear exciting, strict criteria for selection of patients are required.

It is often difficult for a pediatric neurosurgeon to decide if the patient with ventriculomegaly needs a CSF diversion procedure. Imaging studies and invasive procedures like ICP monitoring have not been able to reliably predict the patients who are likely to develop intellectual deterioration as a result of hydrocephalus. Children younger than 5 years with moderate to severe hydrocephalus without any symptoms often are considered for a CSF diversion procedure as it is often difficult to assess the intellectual development in this age group. It is also considered that mere attainment of developmental milestones is not indicative of adequate development of intellectual function. Insertion of a shunt protects these children against effects of persistent ventriculo-

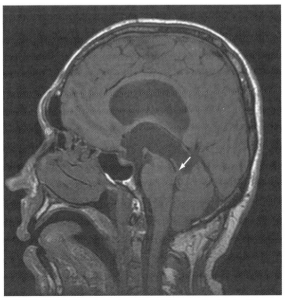

FIGURE 67-25 T1-weighted sagittal MRI scan of patient with gross obstructive hydrocephalus caused by aqueductal stenosis *(arrow)*.

megaly and ascertains an optimal environment for future intellectual development. However, children older than 5 years and adults with asymptomatic ventriculomegaly often are closely watched with frequent assessment of intellectual development before a shunt insertion is considered.

Medical management has not proved to be very useful in hydrocephalus. It is often used as a temporary measure and in conjunction with the surgical management. Acetazolamide has been commonly used as it has been found to reduce the CSF production. However, the benefits are minimal, and high doses of the drug causing metabolic acidosis are required to achieve the effect.

Cerebrospinal Fluid Shunts

Although initially the concept of shunt appeared to be simple, it has proved to be more complex over the years. Being purely mechanical devices, shunts have not been able to effectively manage the complexity of the CSF dynamics associated with hydrocephalus. Basically, CSF shunts are tubes with valves that drain the CSF out from one compartment to another. The shunt contains three parts: the ventricular end, the valve complex, and the distal end. The distal end is usually named after the organ where it is inserted (e.g., in ventriculoperitoneal shunts, it is known as the peritoneal end; in ventriculoatrial shunts, the atrial end). Antisiphon devices preventing the CSF siphoning effect (which can result in overdrainage when the person is erect) are often included in the valve complex.

Shunt malfunction, infection, overdrainage, brain injury, seizures, and distal complications are the major complications associated with shunts. Of these, shunt malfunction is the predominant complication of shunt procedures. The malfunction is so common that sometimes it is not considered a complication but a part of natural history of shunt surgery. Of the several predisposing factors for shunt malfunction, age has been found to be a significant factor. In a multicenter study involving 38 neurosurgical centers and 773 patients, 29% of the shunts failed in the first year, requiring reoperation. About half of the shunts (47%) inserted in children younger than 6 months failed compared with 14% of shunts that failed in children older than 6 months. It was also found that shunts placed as emergency procedures failed more often (34%) than shunts placed electively (29%).[47] Shunt components also can become disconnected at the junctions and migrate to either of the cavities. In the event that the distal end of the tube migrates into the abdominal cavity, the tube is usually left behind. It usually freely floats in the abdominal cavity and does not precipitate bowel obstruction. Some neurosurgeons, however, would prefer to remove the abdominal catheter with laparoscopic devices. As in the subcutaneous tissue, the catheter has to be removed if the shunt is infected or with other abdominal infection.

The incidence of shunt infection, the second significant complication, ranges between 4% and 7%. The common organisms include *Staphylococcus epidermidis* (50% to 60%), *Staphylococcus aureus* (20% to 30%), gram-negative bacilli, and *Propionibacterium* species. Most of the shunt infections occur within 3 months of insertion, with a small percentage occurring as late as 6 months. Most of the shunts are inoculated at the time of insertion, although uncommonly it can be a hematogenous spread. *S. epidermidis* forms a biofilm and adheres to the shunt tube, which protects the bacteria against orally or intravenously administered antibiotics. The colonization permits the bacteria to stay quiescent for weeks or sometimes a few months before the infection is manifested. The clinical picture depends on the severity of the infection, the

time of diagnosis, and the site of infection. Shunt infections can be infection of the shunt tube either in its subcutaneous track or in the wound (wound infection), infection of the CSF spaces (meningitis) or ventricles (ventriculitis), or infection of the abdominal space (peritonitis). Early subcutaneous infections are manifested with low-grade fever, redness along the shunt tube, and purulent discharge from the incision. Wound breakage and exposure of the shunt tube can occur. Later, as the infection involves the CSF and ventricles, it may be associated with decreased sensorium, seizures, and neurologic deficits. If the infection involves the abdominal cavity, it can present with features of peritonitis. A high degree of suspicion for infection in the postoperative period is the key for an early diagnosis. The possibility of a shunt infection should be considered in any patient with a shunt; however, on the contrary, occasionally only the shunt is related to the fever. The diagnosis is confirmed by shunt tap and CSF culture. Complete removal of the shunt tube is recommended with reinsertion of a new shunt once the infection clears. The incidence of shunt infection is reduced by use of catheters impregnated with rifampicin and clindamycin, which are effective against the gram-positive bacteria.

It is imperative that the general surgeon be acquainted with the *distal complications of ventriculoperitoneal shunts* as they may be encountered not infrequently in general surgical practice. The two common distal complications are ascites and pseudoperitoneal cyst. Reduction in the absorption of the CSF causing generalized fluid accumulation in the peritoneal cavity results in *ascites*. The common causes include reduced absorbing surface (premature infants), high protein content of the CSF, peritoneal scarring from previous infections, and elevated venous pressure. Although usually sterile, ascites can be infected in as high as 15% of cases. Not uncommonly, ascites can present as shunt malfunction due to backpressure and reduction in CSF drainage from the intracranial compartment. In infected ascites, there will be associated signs of local and systemic infection. The shunt is usually removed and placed in another cavity like the atrium. In infected ascites, the shunt is externalized and is replaced into an alternative site (atrium, pleura) after the infection is cleared. In premature infants with a reduced absorptive surface, it is not uncommon to find that the peritoneum often functions satisfactorily after a few years.

In *pseudoperitoneal cyst,* there is a loculated pocket of CSF in the peritoneal cavity walled off by bowel and omental tissue. This results in a cystic fluid collection, which often presents as a mass in the abdomen. Most of the time, this is associated with a low-grade infection of either the shunt tube or the abdomen or a previous infection or surgery of the abdominal cavity that has resulted in scarring and reduced absorption. This is usually easy to diagnose as the shunt tube is seen lying inside a fluid filled cavity in the abdomen. The occurrence of pseudoperitoneal cyst often presents with shunt malfunction with abdominal distention. The surgery involves exteriorizing the shunt tube, treating the infection if present, and then reinserting the shunt either in another compartment (i.e., converting it into a ventriculoatrial shunt) or in another place in the abdominal cavity. Surprisingly, the second approach works in most of the patients.

The distinction between ascites and pseudoperitoneal cyst is significant as pseudoperitoneal cyst is associated with a higher infection rate than ascites. In addition, in ascites, the shunt needs to be removed from the peritoneal cavity as the entire peritoneal cavity has not been able to absorb fluid; in pseudoperitoneal cyst, it usually suffices to remove the shunt and to replace it in another region of the peritoneal cavity.

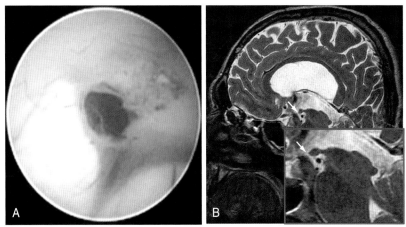

FIGURE 67-26 **A,** Endoscopic view of the third ventricular floor after the third ventriculostomy. **B,** Follow-up MRI scan 4 years later demonstrating good flow at the fenestration site *(arrow).*

Alternatives to Shunting

Advances in endoscopic neurosurgery have opened several alternative options to placement of shunts. Endoscopic third ventriculostomy, endoscopic aqueductoplasty, endoscopic aqueductal stenting, and endoscopic septostomy are available as alternatives to shunt procedures. However, all these alternative procedures are currently effective only in certain types of obstructive hydrocephalus, and not all procedures are effective in all types of obstructive hydrocephalus. In *aqueductoplasty,* the obstructed aqueduct is recanalized with the help of a 3 Fr Fogarty catheter under direct endoscopic vision, whereas *in aqueductal stenting,* a stent is placed in the aqueduct to prevent further reclosure. The stent is usually attached to a subcutaneous reservoir to prevent its migration. Both these procedures are indicated only in obstructive hydrocephalus with short-segment aqueductal stenosis where an adequate reopening can be performed without risking injury to the adjacent midbrain. *Endoscopic third ventriculostomy* involves creation of a fenestration in the floor of the third ventricle to bypass the obstructed CSF into the basal cisterns. Endoscopic third ventriculostomy (Fig. 67-26) is effective in obstructive hydrocephalus associated with obstruction at or beyond the aqueduct (aqueductal stenosis, tumors of fourth ventricle, and fourth ventricular outlet obstruction). However, the effectiveness of these alternative procedures varies with age; the procedure is least efficacious in neonates (20% to 40% success rate) and 80% effective in older children and adults. Although the cause for this is uncertain, failure of absorption of CSF by the normal absorptive process (arachnoid granulations) has been the most common explanation.

Special Types of Hydrocephalus

Two common but distinct types of hydrocephalus seen in two very different age groups need further mention: benign external hydrocephalus, seen in infants; and normal-pressure hydrocephalus, seen in the geriatric population.

Benign external hydrocephalus. Seen exclusively in children, this is often mistaken for subdural hematoma or hygromas in infants. A relative immaturity of the arachnoid villi, which fail to absorb the required amount of CSF into the bloodstream, is postulated as the cause. With the obstruction at the level of the arachnoid villi, a communicating type of hydrocephalus develops. The child usually presents with a macrocrania with mild delayed milestones. The CT or the MRI scan usually reveals evidence of a prominent ventricular system with prominent subarachnoid spaces. Usually a self-limited condition, this is corrected by 2 years of age and uncommonly may require a subduroperitoneal shunt.

Normal-pressure hydrocephalus. This is another form of communicating hydrocephalus seen in elderly patients, with excessive accumulation of the CSF in the intracranial compartment leading to dilation of ventricles and the subarachnoid spaces. The clinical picture is classic of an elderly patient who presents with the triad of gait ataxia, dementia, and urinary incontinence.

Unfortunately, most of the patients with normal-pressure hydrocephalus are either underdiagnosed or misdiagnosed in clinical practice. Although the exact cause is not known, reduction in absorption of CSF by the arachnoid granulations has been postulated. It is also known in these patients that the brain parenchyma is less stiff (more compliant) to allow it to be compressed by the developing ventriculomegaly and thus does not result in increased ICP; but this is not always true as intermittent increases in ICP have been detected by several investigators. However, hydrocephalus developing after several primary insults (trauma, infection, and previous neurosurgical procedures) can present as normal-pressure hydrocephalus. The diagnosis is usually a combination of clinical features associated with prominent ventricles seen on CT and MRI with no other abnormalities. A therapeutic trial of CSF drainage has been used in patients suspected of normal-pressure hydrocephalus to predict response to treatment. Diversion of CSF, commonly by a ventriculoperitoneal shunt or from the lumbar space by a lumboperitoneal shunt, has been the mainstay of treatment. Variable pressure programmable shunt valves have been found to be extremely useful in regulating the flow to avoid complications of overdrainage while optimizing the overall outcome. An early diagnosis and treatment are associated with higher success rates, justifying an early recognition of this treatable form of dementia.

Shunts and Intra-Abdominal Surgeries

Patients with ventriculoperitoneal shunts often require other surgical procedures. It is not uncommon for the neurosurgeon to be asked about the safety of the procedure before it is contemplated.

The circumstances can be broadly divided into the following: surgeries on patients in whom the shunt tube is not exposed; and surgeries on patients in whom the shunt tube will be exposed or may be exposed.

Surgeries on patients in whom the shunt tube is not exposed. These procedures should not cause any mechanical obstruction to the shunt. However, the risk of shunt infection is a potential concern, and the risk is higher if the surgery is performed through a contaminated field with a predisposition to bacterial dissemination (lower gastrointestinal tract; e.g., colonoscopy, colorectal biopsy).

Surgeries on patients in whom the shunt tube will be exposed or may be exposed. This group presents some concerns for the functioning of the shunt in the postoperative period as the shunt tube is expected to be exposed during the procedure. Exposure of the shunt tube also increases the likelihood of shunt infection due to either direct contamination or dissemination during the surgery. Such procedures include abdominal surgeries with an indwelling ventriculoperitoneal shunt and thoracic surgeries with a ventriculopleural shunt. Preoperative discussion with a neurosurgeon and the presence of the neurosurgeon in the operating room is considered ideal under such circumstances.

Shunts and Appendicitis

Appendicitis is a common condition in the general population and it is not uncommon to find patients with shunts attending the emergency department with a diagnosis of appendicitis. Diagnostic errors are not uncommon and often can cause delay in initiating appropriate treatment. Uncomplicated appendicitis often can be effectively managed by the protocols followed conventionally. If the shunt tube is seen during the appendectomy, this often can be managed by replacing the catheter away from the operative site. These patients need to be followed up closely to assess for any chronic abdominal infection that may present several weeks after the initial surgery. Patients with ruptured appendicitis most often need their shunt to be externalized with intravenous antibiotics, and once the peritoneal infection is settled, another site in the peritoneal cavity can be chosen to insert the shunt. Alternatively, a ventriculoatrial or a ventriculopleural shunt can be considered.

Hernia, Hydrocele, and Shunts

It is not uncommon to see an infant with a shunt developing hydrocele or hernia a few months after insertion of the shunt. A prior study reported 15% of shunted children developing inguinal hernias, and hydroceles were seen in another 6% of boys. Persistence of the peritoneovaginal canal causes the CSF to track from the peritoneal cavity into the scrotum, thus causing hydrocele. If the communication is large, bowel loops can migrate into the scrotal sac, which results in inguinal hernia. The collection is usually lax and supple. Uncommonly, the distal end of the shunt tube can migrate into the sac. In most cases, these spontaneously reduce in size and do not need any surgical intervention. However, tense or growing collections need a repositioning of the catheter with correction of the defect.

PEDIATRIC NEUROSURGERY

Neurosurgical conditions in infants and children are significantly different from those in adults. Congenital malformations, hydrocephalus, neoplasms, and pediatric trauma are the major neuro-

surgical disorders commonly encountered by a pediatric neurosurgeon. Hydrocephalus, pediatric brain tumors, and pediatric trauma have been discussed earlier. Here, we discuss the following congenital malformations: spinal and cranial dysraphism, Chiari malformation, and craniosynostosis.

Spinal Dysraphism

Of the three embryonic layers (ectoderm, mesoderm, and endoderm), the neural structures develop from the ectoderm. The neural tube forms from the neural placode at approximately 21 days of gestation. Failure of the neural tube to form results in neural tube defects, such as spinal dysraphism. Neural tube defects have already formed by the time pregnancy is diagnosed; thus, prevention of these defects by the administration of folic acid has to commence before 21 days of gestation.

The spinal dysraphic state can be classified as spina bifida aperta (open defects, usually apparent) and spina bifida occulta (closed defects, commonly missed by an untrained observer; Fig. 67-27). The most common forms of spina bifida aperta are myelomeningocele and meningocele. The common forms of the spinal bifida occulta include simple spina bifida occulta, spinal dermal sinus, lipomyelomeningocele, diastematomyelia, and tethered spinal cord. Some of these may coexist with each other.

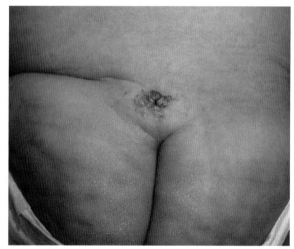

FIGURE 67-27 Child with lumbar cutaneous hemangioma. This often accompanies an underlying spina bifida (spina bifida occulta) during clinical evaluation.

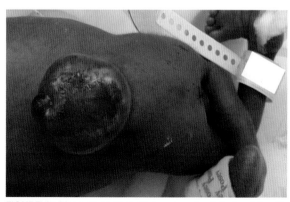

FIGURE 67-28 Myelomeningocele in a neonate. Note the deformity of the lower limbs.

Spina Bifida Aperta

Myelomeningocele. Myelomeningocele, the most common type of spina bifida aperta, has an average incidence of 1/1000 live births. In this disorder, there is protrusion of a varying amount of spinal neural tissue outside the spinal canal confines. It has been associated with folate deficiency in the mother; intake of folate during pregnancy has reduced the incidence considerably. There is a deficiency of the skin, muscle, and bone elements, with the open neural placode exposed anywhere from the thoracic to the sacral level (Fig. 67-28). Varying degrees of motor and sensory deficits with autonomic (bladder and bowel) dysfunction accompany this defect. The degree of the deficit is directly related to the level of the defect, which often determines the child's ability to ambulate in the future. Hence, thoracic defects have the highest incidence of weakness, and sacral defects often have only bladder involvement. Hydrocephalus is also present in 80% of patients and sometimes is manifested after surgical closure of the defect. The incidence of hydrocephalus is also directly related to the level of the defect; thus, thoracic defects have the highest incidence and low sacral defects the lowest. The other significant association is the Chiari II malformation, which occurs in 90% to 95% of cases. Associated brain anomalies include corpus callosal anomalies, fused tectal plates, and thalamic fusion.

Surgical closure of the myelomeningocele is undertaken within 24 to 48 hours of birth to avoid CNS infection (e.g., meningitis, ventriculitis). Before the closure, the child is usually nursed prone, with the defect covered by moist sterile dressings, and given prophylactic antibiotics. All exposed neural tissue is considered viable unless otherwise proven. During the closure, adequate care is taken to separate the neural tissue (placode) from the cutaneous element to prevent an inclusion dermoid. The dura is closed in a watertight fashion and is supplemented by myofascial closure. Skin grafts often are required for large defects. The child is usually also nursed in the prone position in the postoperative period. Ventricular shunts, if indicated, are placed concurrently with myelomeningocele closure or at a later date. Of children with myelomeningocele, 60% to 70% will ultimately require a shunt insertion, whereas only 15% to 30% of children will require a Chiari decompression.

Serum and amniotic fluid α-fetoprotein screening and prenatal ultrasound have been significantly helpful in diagnosing open neural tube defects in the prenatal period. Prenatal counseling should include a discussion of overall long-term mortality (24% during a 25-year period),[48] cognitive development (75% have an IQ higher than 80 if adequately treated for hydrocephalus), future ambulatory assistance (depending on the level of the defect), and presence of incontinence. A 20% to 65% incidence of latex allergies in this population has led to universal latex allergy precautions for this group of children.

Meningocele. Here, there is a protrusion of dura and arachnoid outside the confines of the spinal canal, with neural tissue remaining within the spinal canal confines. Because no neural elements are present, there are no associated neural deficits and repair is simpler. Meningoceles occur less commonly than myelomeningoceles and can be at any location in the spine, although they are most common in the lumbar region.

Spinal Bifida Occulta

Simple spina bifida occulta. A posterior lumbar bone defect is often present in 5% to 10% of the normal population, without any symptoms or deficits. However, association of other markers, such as a tuft of hair, cutaneous hemangioma, or sinus track, should be viewed with suspicion and warrants further investigation.

Dermal sinus. Occurrence of a dermal sinus track from the skin to the spinal subarachnoid space is often associated with a cutaneous dimple or pit. These are most common in the lumbosacral region but can be seen in the cervical and thoracic regions. Although initially asymptomatic, it can cause ascending infection or be symptomatic, with tethering of the cord. It may be associated with intraspinal inclusion tumors, such as dermoids. MRI is helpful for assessing the course of the track and its termination. The track is usually excised surgically, with care taken to untether the cord.

Diastematomyelia. In diastematomyelia, the spinal cord is split into two hemicords, often by a bone or fibrous band that tethers the cord, preventing its free movement and ascent. It is often associated with a hairy patch on the back at the defect level. This needs to be repaired surgically.

Lipomyelomeningocele. In lipomyelomeningocele, there is a varying amount of fatty tissue in the spinal cord and in the spinal canal tethering the cord. Often associated with a large dural defect, these are complex congenital anomalies. Associated neurologic deficits, although uncommon at birth, usually develop later because of the tethering. Almost all lipomyelomeningoceles have a well-developed skin cover, which allows these children to be operated on electively at a later date. The relatively high incidence of postsurgical neurologic deficits (16% to 47%) in otherwise neurologically intact patients has triggered a controversy about the appropriate timing for the surgery; some favor early surgery, and others consider surgery only when the child has developed deficits.

Cranial Dysraphism

Cranial dysraphism includes encephalocele, meningocele, and cranial dermal sinus. The encephalocele can be in the cranial vault or cranial base. The occipital encephalocele is the most common, followed by anterior encephalocele and then basal encephalocele. Encephaloceles may be associated with other developmental anomalies, such as polydactyly, retinal dysplasia, microphthalmia, and orofacial clefts. Cranial vault encephaloceles present with an observable swelling at birth and have brain tissue and blood vessels contained in the sac. Although the brain tissue is thought to be dysplastic, large encephaloceles often contain functional brain. The usual surgical treatment is excision and repair of the defect in the first few days of life. Cranial expansion may be required for patients with functional brain tissue in the sac. The outcome is generally directly proportional to the amount of neural tissue in the sac, with poorer outcomes seen in encephaloceles with a large amount of brain tissue. Basal encephaloceles present with a CSF leak from the nose or ear or as a polyp.

Chiari Malformation

Abnormal descent of the cerebellar tonsils below the level of the foramen magnum is known as a Chiari malformation. A descent of one tonsil of more than 5 mm or a 3-mm descent with associated syringohydromyelia is suggestive of Chiari malformation. Often, the tonsils are peg shaped and associated with crowding of the craniocervical subarachnoid space. Usually, they are classified as Chiari I, II, and III malformations. These are grouped together, but there is a significant difference in cause among these three types. An isolated descent of the tonsils below the rim of the foramen magnum without any spina bifida is known as Chiari I malformation. Chiari II is invariably associated with open spina bifida and has several other diagnostic features, such as descent of the brainstem and fourth ventricle into the upper spinal canal. In the uncommon Chiari type III malformation, there is an associated high cervical encephalocele containing herniated cerebellar and brainstem tissue. We limit the discussion here to the most common types, Chiari I and II malformations.

Chiari I Malformation

Descent of the cerebellar tonsils more than 5 mm below the rim of the foramen magnum is considered Chiari malformation. The 5-mm classification is somewhat arbitrary because many have tonsillar descent and are asymptomatic. The descended tonsils are usually peg shaped, and the descent is associated with crowding of the soft tissue, obstructing CSF flow (Fig. 67-29). There may or may not be associated syringomyelia. Occipital headache, precipitated or aggravated by maneuvers that increase the intrathoracic pressure (e.g., cough, headaches), is typical. There may be associated tingling or numbness in the extremities and impairment of joint position. In patients with advanced compression, cavitation of the spinal cord (syringomyelia) can occur and can be associated with wasting and weakness of the extremities, scoliosis, and varying degrees of sensory impairment. Coexistent hydrocephalus is seen in 10% of cases.

The aim of surgery is to decompress the region of the foramen magnum and to establish CSF flow. Removal of the rim of the foramen magnum and posterior arch of C1 and duraplasty are the most commonly performed procedures. Some also decompress the cerebellar tonsils. Associated hydrocephalus requires ventriculoperitoneal shunt placement or an endoscopic third ventriculostomy. Rescarring is a concern during follow-up and may require repeated surgery.

Chiari II Malformation

Chiari II malformation is characterized by elongation and caudal displacement of the brainstem and cerebellar tonsils and by association with myelomeningocele. Hydrocephalus is common and syrinx occurs frequently. Although it is a common accompaniment of myelomeningocele, surgery is reserved for children who are symptomatic with lower cranial nerve paresis, weakness, respiratory distress, or syrinx.

Craniosynostosis

Craniosynostosis involves premature fusion of the cranial sutures. This results in restricted growth of the skull bones at the involved suture and compensatory growth at the adjacent patent sutures, causing disfigurement of the cranial shape. In multisutural synostosis, restriction of the cranial growth at various sutures can cause impairment of growth of the developing brain. The incidence of nonsyndromic craniosynostosis varies from 0.25 to 0.6/1000 live births. The most common suture involved is sagittal suture (50% to 60%), followed by coronal suture (30% to 35%), metopic suture (5%), and lambdoid suture (2%). Lambdoid suture synostosis has to be distinguished from positional plagiocephaly, which is common and does not require surgical intervention. Genetic patterns are found in 8% of patients with isolated coronal synostosis and 2% of those with sagittal synostosis. However, more complex disorders, such as Crouzon, Apert, and Pfeiffer syndromes, have a genetic predisposition. The clinical picture is recognized by the abnormal skull shape associated with each sutural fusion—sagittal, elongated skull, or scaphocephaly; coronal, brachycephaly; and metopic, trigonocephaly—and is confirmed by skull radiographs and CT scans. Three-dimensional reconstruction of the calvaria is often beneficial (Fig. 67-30). Surgical

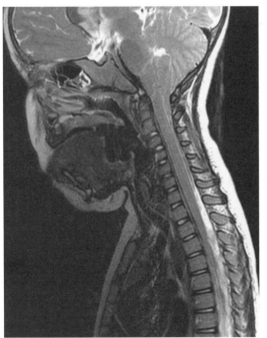

FIGURE 67-29 T2-weighted sagittal MRI scan of a child with a significant type I Chiari malformation. Note the tonsillar descent below the rim of foramen magnum.

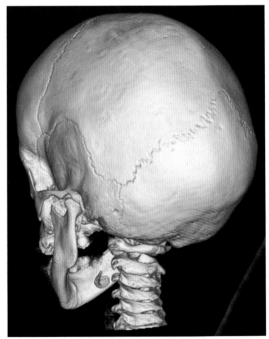

FIGURE 67-30 Three-dimensional reconstruction CT scan of a child with sagittal synostosis. The coronal and lambdoid sutures are well visualized.

correction involves a wide suturectomy and placement in a cranial remodeling helmet in children younger than 4 months and a craniotomy and cranial vault reconstruction in older children. In recent years, simple suturectomies have been performed in children younger than 6 months under endoscopic guidance with a small incision.[49] Patients with coronal craniosynostosis will usually require advancement of the orbital rim in addition to the cranial remodeling.

CENTRAL NERVOUS SYSTEM INFECTIONS

Broadly, CNS infections can be grouped as intracranial infections and spinal infections. The intracranial infections can occur in the epidural space (epidural abscess), in the subdural space (subdural empyema), in the subarachnoid space (meningitis), intracerebrally (cerebral abscess), or in the ventricles (ventriculitis).

Intracranial Infections
Cranial Epidural Abscess

As there is no preexisting epidural space, in epidural abscess, the pus essentially dissects itself in the potential epidural space between the dura and the bone. Cranial epidural abscess accounts for about 2% of all intracranial infections. Epidural abscess is commonly located either in the frontal region associated with frontal sinusitis and osteomyelitis or in the temporal region associated with mastoiditis and chronic ear infection. It can also be seen with nontreated or poorly treated compound depressed skull fractures. Clinically, there is associated local swelling, erythema, and tenderness with signs of localized or systemic infection. The infection, which is contained by the dura if it extends intradurally, can lead to development of meningitis and neurologic deterioration. Cranial CT scan usually shows the infection with osteomyelitis. The treatment is surgical evacuation, débridement of the osteomyelitic bone, drainage of the adjacent infected sinuses, and prolonged antibiotic therapy. A cranioplasty may be required in the future after the infection heals. The outcome is usually good with low morbidity or mortality.

Subdural Empyema

Collection of pus in the subdural space is termed subdural empyema. Usually seen in older children and young adults, it is most commonly related to contiguous spread from the paranasal sinuses or ear infection. Alternatively, infection can enter by retrograde thrombophlebitis of the veins communicating between the mucosal veins of the infected sinuses and dural venous sinuses or by hematogenous spread. About 60% of subdural empyemas occur from the frontal or ethmoid sinuses and about 20% from the inner ear infections. The infection can be on the cerebral convexities, in the hemispheric fissure, or over the tentorium.

Patients with subdural empyema can present with fever, meningeal signs, headache, seizures, focal neurologic deficits, and altered mental status. The most significant complication is cortical venous thrombosis leading to cerebral infarction. It is often heralded by seizures and rapid clinical deterioration. Diagnosis is made by noting presence of a subdural fluid collection adjacent to a known focus of sinus infection. The margins of the collection often enhance with contrast material. Appropriate treatment includes prompt institution of surgical drainage with antibiotic therapy. Anticonvulsants are indicated even in the absence of seizures as there is high risk of seizures. Steroids are often administered with antibiotic to cover life-threatening situations. The

overall prognosis depends on the extent of infection, the neurologic status at the time of diagnosis, the association of cortical venous thrombosis, and the response of infection to treatment. The overall outcome has been as high as 82% of patients who underwent combined medical and surgical management. Craniotomy with evacuation of the pus has better overall outcome than burr hole evacuation.

Meningitis

Acute bacterial meningitis is an infection of the subarachnoid spaces and meninges. Symptoms and signs include fever, malaise, altered mental status, neck stiffness, and headache. These result from leptomeningeal irritation and increased ICP. The causative organism varies with the patient's age. Neonatal meningitis is caused by group B streptococcus, *Escherichia coli*, or *Listeria* spp. infection. Late neonatal meningitis can be caused by any of these organisms as well as by staphylococci or *Pseudomonas aeruginosa*. In children, *Streptococcus pneumoniae* (pneumococcus) and *Neisseria meningitidis* (meningococcus) are the most common causative organisms. In the past, *Haemophilus influenzae* was a common cause of meningitis in children, but its prevalence has decreased secondary to vaccination. Pneumococci and meningococci are the most common causative organisms in adults. Treatment consists of prompt CSF culture and immediate IV administration of antibiotics. Altered mental status secondary to communicating hydrocephalus may necessitate placement of an external ventricular drain and eventual placement of a ventriculoperitoneal shunt once the CSF is sterilized. Recurrent episodes of bacterial meningitis prompt investigation into abnormal communication between the CNS and the exterior environment (dermal sinus or CSF fistula).

Brain Abscess

Accumulation of pus in the cerebral tissue (cerebral abscess) usually is seen in children and young adults. About 25% of children with brain abscess have congenital heart disease with tetralogy of Fallot. Contiguous spread of infection from paranasal sinuses, middle ear, or mastoid is the most common cause, accounting for about 50% of all cases. Hematogenous dissemination from lungs or other parts of the body (dental caries, subacute bacterial endocarditis, diverticulitis) accounts for about 25% of patients. In about 20% of cases, the cause is undetermined. Frontal abscesses along the orbital base are often the result of contiguous spread from the frontal sinuses, whereas temporal or cerebellar abscesses are otogenic in origin. Cardiac malformations with polycythemia resulting in increased blood viscosity, sluggish circulation, and cerebral infarction predispose to development of brain abscess. Brain abscesses can be solitary or multiple. Causative organisms are extremely varied and include aerobic and anaerobic organisms, fungi, and uncommonly parasites.

Abscesses are manifested with signs and symptoms related to a rapidly expanding mass lesion with often subtle signs of infection. Patients can present with headache, nausea and vomiting, seizures, focal neurologic deficit, and altered mental status. Features of infection are present in around 60% of patients. Contrast-enhanced CT and MRI reveal a ring enhancing lesion, usually at the gray-white interface, with surrounding edema (Fig. 67-31). This can be confused with glioblastoma multiforme or metastatic tumor. Diffusion-weighted imaging (abscesses are hyperintense) and magnetic resonance spectroscopy (elevated lactate, low choline peaks) can distinguish between the abscess and tumor disease. Acute deterioration of patients can occur when the abscess ruptures into the ventricle or subarachnoid space, with resultant

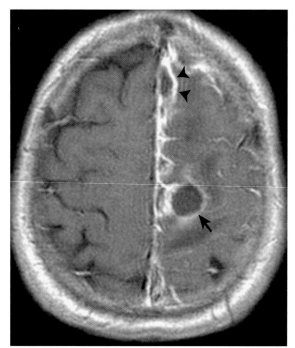

FIGURE 67-31 Brain abscess *(arrow)*, with an area of frontal subdural empyema in the convexity *(arrowheads)*.

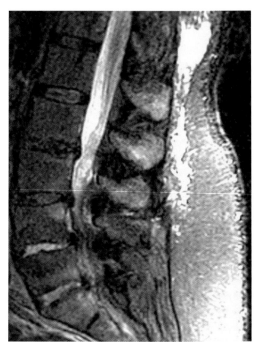

FIGURE 67-32 MRI with gadolinium short T1 inversion recovery sequence revealing disc osteomyelitis in the L4-5 and L5-S1 interspaces suggestive of an infectious process.

ventriculitis or meningitis. Principles of treatment revolve around accurate identification of the causative organism, relief of mass effect, administration of appropriate antibiotic therapy, and treatment of the underlying cause. Prophylactic anticonvulsants are usually indicated, and steroids often can be given with antibiotic cover. Controversy exists as to whether surgical excision or aspiration of the abscess yields better results. The overall morbidity and mortality depend on the neurologic status at the time of diagnosis.

Ventriculitis

Infection of the ventricles is usually a result of spread of infection from either a ruptured cerebral abscess or other intracranial infection. Shunt infections are the most common cause of ventriculitis. Systemically administered antibiotics often do not penetrate significantly into the ventricle spaces. Drainage of infected CSF with intraventricular instillation of vancomycin, gentamicin, or amikacin (depending on the organisms and sensitivity) is often necessary for adequate treatment of the infection.

Postoperative Infections

Infections of the CNS occurring after neurosurgical procedures are typically caused by staphylococci. Enteric organisms and pseudomonal and streptococcal pathogens can also be problematic. As with any infection, treatment involves identification of the causative organism and appropriate antibiotic administration. Postoperative abscesses are addressed with drainage, surgery, or both, as dictated by the clinical situation.

Post-Traumatic Meningitis

Meningeal infection after head injury is typically related to CSF fistula. Most post-traumatic fistulas stop spontaneously within days of injury. The incidence of meningitis increases if a leak persists for longer than 7 days. Clinically obvious leaks are manifested as CSF rhinorrhea or otorrhea. The prophylactic antibiotic treatment of CSF fistula is controversial and needs to be tailored to the clinical situation. A persistent post-traumatic CSF fistula is addressed surgically to prevent the risks associated with recurrent bouts of meningitis.

Spinal Infections

Spinal infections can be grouped into those affecting the bone (vertebral osteomyelitis), disc space (discitis), and epidural space (spinal epidural abscess). On occasion, infectious processes can involve more than one or even all three.

Vertebral Osteomyelitis

Osteomyelitis of the bone is generally seen in IV drug users, diabetic patients, hemodialysis patients, and older adults. The causative organism is usually *S. aureus,* and spread is hematogenous, although postoperative infections are also seen. These infections can and do affect the integrity of the bone, resulting in collapse. This in turn can result in pain and neurologic compromise. Treatment consists of organism identification, appropriate long-term antibiotics, and maintenance of anatomic spinal alignment, with or without surgical intervention.

Discitis

Infection of the disc (discitis) often occurs concomitantly with osteomyelitis and is seen in the same population of patients. Fever, back pain, and an elevated sedimentation rate or C-reactive protein level are often seen. The white blood cell count may or may not be elevated. It may occur spontaneously or postoperatively. Treatment may or may not be surgical. Long-term antibiotic therapy is usually indicated (Fig. 67-32).

Spinal Epidural Abscess

This usually occurs in the setting of an infectious process elsewhere in the body. Spread occurs hematogenously or by direct extension. Patients present initially with localized back pain and possible radiculopathy. Spinal cord compromise can follow rapidly, with paraplegia or quadriplegia. Predisposing factors are the same as those for osteomyelitis and discitis. Diagnosis is made with contrast-enhanced MRI. When spinal cord compression is evident, surgery is usually performed for decompression and diagnosis. Spinal epidural abscess can sometimes be managed medically, with close neurologic observation and imaging studies. This is usually reserved for cases in which the causative organism is known, the abscess is small, and there is no neurologic compromise. As in all fields of medicine, treatment must be tailored to the individual patient.

Acquired Immunodeficiency Syndrome

The most common CNS opportunistic infection in patients with AIDS is toxoplasmosis caused by *Toxoplasma gondii*. The lesions usually present with ring enhancement on contrast-enhanced imaging studies and are usually in the basal ganglia. They may be solitary or multiple. Primary CNS lymphoma occurs in approximately 10% of AIDS patients and presents as an irregularly enhancing mass (target lesion). Progressive multifocal leukoencephalopathy presents with hypodense, nonenhancing white matter lesions. Fungal abscess and viral encephalopathy are not uncommon in this population of patients. Even though the incidence of CNS opportunistic infections has decreased with the widespread use of highly active antiretroviral therapy, the treatment of these problems remains a challenge.

SELECTED REFERENCES

Benzel EC: *Spine surgery: Techniques, complication avoidance, and management*, ed 2, Philadelphia, 2004, Churchill Livingstone.

A nice review of spine surgery and biomechanics in two volumes; thorough explanation and details from an authority in the field.

Brain Trauma Foundation; American Association of Neurological Surgeons; Congress of Neurological Surgeons; Joint Section on Neurotrauma and Critical Care, AANS/CNS, Bratton SL, Chestnut RM, et al: Guidelines for the management of severe traumatic brain injury. *J Neurotrauma* 24:S1–S106, 2007.

Accepted guidelines commonly used in the management of patients with traumatic brain injury.

Guidelines for the management of acute cervical spine and spinal cord injuries. *Neurosurgery* 72:S1–S259, 2013.

Recently published guidelines concerning the care and management of patients with traumatic injuries of the cervical spine and spinal cord.

Quinones-Hinojosa A: *Schmidek and Sweet: Operative neurosurgical techniques*, ed 6, Philadelphia, 2012, Elsevier Saunders.

Atlas of neurosurgical techniques.

Winn RH, editor: *Youmans neurological surgery*, ed 6, Philadelphia, 2011, Elsevier Saunders.

A traditional resource for neurosurgery residents and faculty.

REFERENCES

1. Stern WE: Intracranial fluid dynamics: The relationship of intracranial pressure to the Monro-Kellie doctrine and the reliability of pressure assessment. *J R Coll Surg Edinb* 9:18–36, 1963.
2. Rangel-Castilla L, Gasco J, Nauta HJ, et al: Cerebral pressure autoregulation in traumatic brain injury. *Neurosurg Focus* 25:E7, 2008.
3. Bratton SL, Chestnut RM, Ghajar J, et al: Guidelines for the management of severe traumatic brain injury. IX. Cerebral perfusion thresholds. *J Neurotrauma* 24(Suppl 1):S59–S64, 2007.
4. Lundberg N: Continuous recording and control of ventricular fluid pressure in neurosurgical practice. *Acta Psychiatr Scand Suppl* 36:1–193, 1960.
5. Ondra SL, Troupp H, George ED, et al: The natural history of symptomatic arteriovenous malformations of the brain: A 24-year follow-up assessment. *J Neurosurg* 73:387–391, 1990.
6. Spetzler RF, Martin NA: A proposed grading system for arteriovenous malformations. *J Neurosurg* 65:476–483, 1986.
7. McCormick WF, Hardman JM, Boulter TR: Vascular malformations ("angiomas") of the brain, with special reference to those occurring in the posterior fossa. *J Neurosurg* 28:241–251, 1968.
8. Ong CK, Wang LL, Parkinson RJ, et al: Onyx embolisation of cavernous sinus dural arteriovenous fistula via direct percutaneous transorbital puncture. *J Med Imaging Radiat Oncol* 53:291–295, 2009.
9. Winn HR, Richardson AE, Jane JA: The long-term prognosis in untreated cerebral aneurysms: I. The incidence of late hemorrhage in cerebral aneurysm: A 10-year evaluation of 364 patients. *Ann Neurol* 1:358–370, 1977.
10. Vajkoczy P, Meyer B, Weidauer S, et al: Clazosentan (AXV-034343), a selective endothelin A receptor antagonist, in the prevention of cerebral vasospasm following severe aneurysmal subarachnoid hemorrhage: Results of a randomized, double-blind, placebo-controlled, multicenter phase IIa study. *J Neurosurg* 103:9–17, 2005.
11. Kern M, Lam MM, Knuckey NW, et al: Statins may not protect against vasospasm in subarachnoid haemorrhage. *J Clin Neurosci* 16:527–530, 2009.
12. Wong GK, Poon WS, Chan MT, et al: Intravenous magnesium sulphate for aneurysmal subarachnoid hemorrhage (IMASH): A randomized, double-blinded, placebo-controlled, multicenter phase III trial. *Stroke* 41:921–926, 2010.
13. Molyneux A, Kerr R, Stratton I, et al: International Subarachnoid Aneurysm Trial (ISAT) of neurosurgical clipping versus endovascular coiling in 2143 patients with ruptured intracranial aneurysms: A randomised trial. *Lancet* 360:1267–1274, 2002.
14. Hunt WE, Hess RM: Surgical risk as related to time of intervention in the repair of intracranial aneurysms. *J Neurosurg* 28:14–20, 1968.

15. Report of World Federation of Neurological Surgeons Committee on a universal subarachnoid hemorrhage grading scale. *J Neurosurg* 68:985–986, 1988.

16. Fisher CM, Kistler JP, Davis JM: Relation of cerebral vasospasm to subarachnoid hemorrhage visualized by computerized tomographic scanning. *Neurosurgery* 6:1–9, 1980.

17. Kulcsar Z, Wetzel SG, Augsburger L, et al: Effect of flow diversion treatment on very small ruptured aneurysms. *Neurosurgery* 67:789–793, 2010.

18. Szikora I, Berentei Z, Kulcsar Z, et al: Treatment of intracranial aneurysms by functional reconstruction of the parent artery: The Budapest experience with the pipeline embolization device. *AJNR Am J Neuroradiol* 31:1139–1147, 2010.

19. Mendelow AD, Gregson BA, Fernandes HM, et al: Early surgery versus initial conservative treatment in patients with spontaneous supratentorial intracerebral haematomas in the International Surgical Trial in Intracerebral Haemorrhage (STICH): A randomised trial. *Lancet* 365:387–397, 2005.

20. Patchell RA: The management of brain metastases. *Cancer Treat Rev* 29:533–540, 2003.

21. Levin VA, Leibel SA, Gutin PH: Neoplasms of the central nervous system. In De Vita VT, Jr, Hellman S, Rosenberg SA, editors: *Cancer: Principles and practice of oncology*, Philadelphia, 2001, Lippincott Williams & Wilkins, pp 2100–2160.

22. Gupta A, Shah A, Young RJ, et al: Imaging of brain tumors: Functional magnetic resonance imaging and diffusion tensor imaging. *Neuroimaging Clin N Am* 20:379–400, 2010.

23. Kew Y, Levin VA: Advances in gene therapy and immunotherapy for brain tumors. *Curr Opin Neurol* 16:665–670, 2003.

24. Louis DN, Ohgaki H, Wiestler OD, et al: The 2007 WHO classification of tumours of the central nervous system. *Acta Neuropathol* 114:97–109, 2007.

25. Simpson D: The recurrence of intracranial meningiomas after surgical treatment. *J Neurol Neurosurg Psychiatry* 20:22–39, 1957.

26. Jemal A, Tiwari RC, Murray T, et al: Cancer statistics, 2004. *CA Cancer J Clin* 54:8–29, 2004.

27. Gavrilovic IT, Posner JB: Brain metastases: Epidemiology and pathophysiology. *J Neurooncol* 75:5–14, 2005.

28. Sawaya R, Bindal R, Lang FE: Metastatic brain tumors. In Kaye AH, Laws ER, editors: *Brain tumors: An encyclopedic approach*, New York, 2001, Churchill Livingstone, pp 999–1026.

29. Hart MG, Grant R, Walker M, et al: Surgical resection and whole brain radiation therapy versus whole brain radiation therapy alone for single brain metastases. *Cochrane Database Syst Rev* (1):CD003292, 2005.

30. Kalkanis SN, Kondziolka D, Gaspar LE, et al: The role of surgical resection in the management of newly diagnosed brain metastases: A systematic review and evidence-based clinical practice guideline. *J Neurooncol* 96:33–43, 2010.

31. Iwadate Y, Namba H, Yamaura A: Significance of surgical resection for the treatment of multiple brain metastases. *Anticancer Res* 20:573–577, 2000.

32. Paek SH, Audu PB, Sperling MR, et al: Reevaluation of surgery for the treatment of brain metastases: Review of 208 patients with single or multiple brain metastases treated at one institution with modern neurosurgical techniques. *Neurosurgery* 56:1021–1034, discussion 1021-1034, 2005.

33. Muacevic A, Wowra B, Siefert A, et al: Microsurgery plus whole brain irradiation versus Gamma Knife surgery alone for treatment of single metastases to the brain: A randomized controlled multicentre phase III trial. *J Neurooncol* 87:299–307, 2008.

34. Brain Trauma Foundation; American Association of Neurological Surgeons; Congress of Neurological Surgeons; Joint Section on Neurotrauma and Critical Care, AANS/CNS, Bratton SL, Chestnut RM, et al: Guidelines for the management of severe traumatic brain injury. *J Neurotrauma* 24(Suppl 1):S1–S106, 2007.

35. Ogden AT, Mayer SA, Connolly ES, Jr: Hyperosmolar agents in neurosurgical practice: The evolving role of hypertonic saline. *Neurosurgery* 57:207–215, discussion 207–215, 2005.

36. Kakar V, Nagaria J, John Kirkpatrick P: The current status of decompressive craniectomy. *Br J Neurosurg* 23:147–157, 2009.

37. Kondziolka D, Lunsford LD, Flickinger JC, et al: Emerging indications in stereotactic radiosurgery. *Clin Neurosurg* 52:229–233, 2005.

38. Chang SD, Adler JR, Jr: Current treatment of patients with multiple brain metastases. *Neurosurg Focus* 9:e5, 2000.

39. Flickinger JC, Barker FG, 2nd: Clinical results: Radiosurgery and radiotherapy of cranial nerve schwannomas. *Neurosurg Clin N Am* 17:121–128, vi, 2006.

40. Kuo JS, Yu C, Petrovich Z, et al: The CyberKnife stereotactic radiosurgery system: Description, installation, and an initial evaluation of use and functionality. *Neurosurgery* 62(Suppl 2):785–789, 2008.

41. Romanelli P, Schaal DW, Adler JR: Image-guided radiosurgical ablation of intra- and extra-cranial lesions. *Technol Cancer Res Treat* 5:421–428, 2006.

42. Groves DA, Brown VJ: Vagal nerve stimulation: A review of its applications and potential mechanisms that mediate its clinical effects. *Neurosci Biobehav Rev* 29:493–500, 2005.

43. Nauta HJ, Soukup VM, Fabian RH, et al: Punctate midline myelotomy for the relief of visceral cancer pain. *J Neurosurg* 92:125–130, 2000.

44. Willis WD, Jr, Westlund KN: The role of the dorsal column pathway in visceral nociception. *Curr Pain Headache Rep* 5:20–26, 2001.

45. Zimmerman RS, Sirven JI: An overview of surgery for chronic seizures. *Mayo Clin Proc* 78:109–117, 2003.

46. Devlin AM, Cross JH, Harkness W, et al: Clinical outcomes of hemispherectomy for epilepsy in childhood and adolescence. *Brain* 126:556–566, 2003.

47. Di Rocco C, Marchese E, Velardi F: A survey of the first complication of newly implanted CSF shunt devices for the treatment of nontumoral hydrocephalus. Cooperative survey of the 1991-1992 Education Committee of the ISPN. *Childs Nerv Syst* 10:321–327, 1994.

48. Bowman RM, McLone DG, Grant JA, et al: Spina bifida outcome: A 25-year prospective. *Pediatr Neurosurg* 34:114–120, 2001.

49. Jimenez DF, Barone CM: Multiple-suture nonsyndromic craniosynostosis: Early and effective management using endoscopic techniques. *J Neurosurg Pediatr* 5:223–231, 2010.

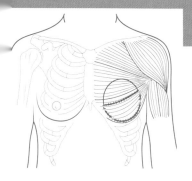

CHAPTER 68

Plastic Surgery

Mary H. McGrath, Jason H. Pomerantz

第六十八章　整形外科

中文导读

本章共分8节：①修复重建技术；②儿童整形；③头颈部整形；④躯干整形；⑤压力性溃疡；⑥下肢修复重建；⑦形体塑形；⑧总结。

第一节介绍了整形外科学的基石——修复重建技术：原位缝合切口、皮片移植、局部或邻位皮瓣移植、游离皮瓣移植，复杂程度逐级上升构成"重建阶梯"。最理想的修复术式，是根据缺损的情况而定的，最简单、安全，并兼顾外形和功能的术式。近年来，在穿支皮瓣、显微外科、组织扩张技术和假体植入材料学上的进展，为修复重建外科带来了新的突破和更多的选择。

第二节儿童整形介绍了先天性颅颌面畸形、耳畸形、唇腭裂畸形、脉管畸形和色素痣等多种儿童先天性疾病的临床表现、诊断方式及手术进展。

第三节介绍了头颈部畸形或缺损的修复，包括急性颌面外伤、头部外伤、颌面骨折的救治原则，损伤后的头皮重建、面部重建和最新的面部移植等技术；以及面部美容技术，包括面部提升术、重睑术、鼻整形术、面部皮肤美容技术和软组织填充术等。

第四节躯干部整形，包括先天性或后天性的胸壁、腹壁和会阴部缺损的重建、乳房重建、隆乳术、巨乳缩小术、乳房下垂矫正、男性乳腺增生等乳房整形技术，以及腹壁松弛整形术。

第五节着重介绍臀髋部缺损的常见致病因素——压力性溃疡的预防和修复技术。

第六节下肢修复重建，包括从足趾到腹股沟的下肢部位，创伤后的创面修复、外观和功能重建，涉及复杂的皮瓣、骨、血管和神经移植技术。

第七节形体塑形是应时而生的新兴技术，是为修复肥胖人群在迅速减肥后所致的全身皮肤软组织冗余松垂的畸形外观。形体塑形手术通常需分阶段地切除多余的皮肤组织，或在脂肪抽吸术后切除多余的皮肤，更重要的是恢复缺陷部位的容积，加强薄弱的组织防治继发性疝，警惕切口难愈和静脉血栓的风险。

第八节总结了整形外科学的进展和未来的发展趋势。整形外科是一门修复人体各种先天性或后天性的缺陷，以达到修复形态、重建功能的外科专业。追寻最理想的修复、重建、再生技术，是整形外科医生的终极目标。随着医学诊疗技术的进展，新的科研成果、组织工程、基因治疗和干细胞技术在整形外科学的应用，整形外科将迎来划时代的变革。

〔吴毅平〕

Challenged by complex clinical problems, the pace of innovation in plastic surgery has accelerated steadily during the past 30 years. The specialty benefits from the absence of anatomic or organ system boundaries and from the collaboration with other surgical specialists who discover new reconstructive and aesthetic challenges even as they make medical progress. With growing sophistication, plastic surgery has matured into areas of specialization, including surgery for congenital abnormalities, maxillofacial surgery, breast surgery, hand surgery, head and neck surgery, skin and soft tissue surgery, aesthetic surgery, body contouring, wound care, microsurgery, and burn care. Plastic surgeons, in a relatively small specialty, stay aware of innovations in each of these areas and are quick to adopt new ideas developed through the clinical and research experience of other plastic surgeons. With the breadth of exposure that this collaboration brings, it is not surprising that unique solutions for perplexing clinical problems sustain the momentum of innovation.

RECONSTRUCTIVE TECHNIQUES

The concept of a reconstructive ladder is used to guide surgical reconstruction. Ascending the rungs of the ladder represents moving from simple to complex reconstructive techniques in a systemized way that considers the requirements of the defect to be repaired. Direct closure is the simplest and most straightforward technique. This may be precluded by the size of the wound or consequences of wound tension at the closure site, including distortion of the surrounding tissue. In this case, a more complex closure technique, such as a skin graft that brings in additional tissue from a distant site, is required. A wound with exposed structures that do not accept a skin graft mandates a step up to a local flap for coverage. A local flap with no distant donor site may not be an option if the surrounding area is within the zone of injury, in which case a regional flap from an adjacent body region is needed. Microvascular free tissue transfer represents the most complex flap option and is usually the top rung on the reconstructive ladder.

When the concept of the reconstructive ladder is used, the triad of form, function, and safety is the basis for setting the reconstructive goals for any given defect. For example, in reconstructing the face, awareness of form would suggest a more complex technique, such as tissue expansion, instead of the simpler technique of skin grafting because it is optimal to restore with skin and soft tissue of the same thickness, texture, and color. For any specific reconstructive situation, this matrix of going from simple to complex, considering form and function and keeping safety paramount, provides direction.

Primary Wound Closure

Good suture technique starts with an incision with the scalpel at right angles to the skin and continues with careful handling of tissue to avoid devitalizing the skin margins, débridement of skin edges if needed, eversion of the wound margin, and precise approximation without tension. The skin edges need to be lined up at the same level, and wound edges should just touch each other. Postoperative edema is predictable and will create additional tension.

Minimizing tension is essential to reduce scarring. This can be done by using buried deep dermal and subdermal sutures to lessen tension on the skin sutures. It is also accomplished by aligning skin incisions along relaxed skin tension lines. These lines of minimal tension, also called natural skin lines, wrinkle lines, or lines of facial expression, run at right angles to the long axis of the underlying muscles. When underlying muscles contract, the lines of facial expression deepen. For example, transverse forehead furrows appear when the eyebrows are raised by the frontalis muscle, and if an incision is placed in one of these furrows, it will be under minimal tension and will heal with minimal scarring.

Skin Grafts

A skin graft is a segment of dermis and epidermis that is separated from its blood supply and donor site and transplanted to another recipient site on the body. Survival of the skin graft in the new site requires a vascularized wound recipient bed. Graftable beds with adequate blood supply include healthy soft tissues, periosteum, perichondrium, paratenon, and bone surface that is perforated to encourage granulation tissue growth. Poor graft surfaces with inadequate blood supply include exposed bone, cartilage, and tendon and fibrotic chronic granulation tissue. The wound must be free of infection and debris interposed as a barrier between the graft and bed.

Skin grafts are classified in the following manner: autograft, self; allograft, other person; homograft, same species; heterograft, different species. Partial-thickness skin grafts consist of the epidermis and a portion of the dermis and are called split-thickness skin grafts (STSGs). Full-thickness skin grafts (FTSGs) include the epidermis and entire dermis, with portions of the sweat glands, sebaceous glands, and hair follicles. The STSG is harvested with a dermatome, which is an air- or electric-powered instrument that can be adjusted for width and depth to cut uniformly thick grafts, usually in strips of 0.006 to 0.024 inch in thickness. The STSG can be meshed by cutting slits into the sheet of graft and expanding it, usually in a 1:1.5 or 1:2 ratio. Meshed grafts are useful when there is a paucity of available donor skin, the recipient bed is bumpy or convoluted, or the recipient bed is suboptimal, as with exudate. An STSG can be taken from anywhere on the body; donor site considerations include color, texture, thickness, amount of skin required, and scar visibility. The STSG takes readily on the recipient site, and the donor site reepithelializes quickly. Its disadvantages are contracture over time, abnormal pigmentation, and poor durability if subject to trauma. The FTSG is removed with a scalpel and is necessarily small in size because the donor site must be sutured closed. Containing skin appendages, the FTSG can grow hair and secrete sebum to lubricate the skin, has the color and texture of normal skin, and has the potential for growth. In general, FTSGs are taken from areas at which the skin is thin and can be spared without deformity, such as the upper eyelids, postauricular crease, supraclavicular area, hairless groin, or elbow crease. The greater thickness makes the FTSG more durable than the STSG, but this thickness also means that the graft take is not as predictable because more tissue must be revascularized from the recipient bed.

The take of either type of skin graft occurs in three phases:

Plasmatic circulation, also called serum imbibition, during the first 48 hours nourishes the graft with plasma exudate from host bed capillaries.

Revascularization starts after 48 hours with two processes. The primary is neovascularization, in which blood vessels grow from the recipient bed into the graft; and the secondary is inosculation, in which graft and host vessels form anastomoses.

Organization begins immediately after grafting with a fibrin layer at the graft-bed interface holding the graft in place. This is replaced by postgraft day 7 with fibroblasts; in general, grafts are securely adherent to the bed by days 10 to 14.

Sensibility returns to the graft over time, with reinnervation beginning at approximately 4 to 5 weeks and being completed by 12 to 24 months. Pain returns first, with light touch and temperature returning later.

The most common cause of skin graft failure is hematoma under the graft, where the blood clot is a barrier to contact of the graft and bed for revascularization. Similarly, shearing or movement of the graft on the bed will preclude revascularization and cause graft loss. Additional causes are infection, poor quality of the recipient bed, and characteristics of the graft itself, such as thickness or vascularity of the donor site. Dressings can prevent some impediments to graft take. A light pressure dressing minimizes the risk of fluid accumulation. A bolster or tie-over dressing left in place for 4 or 5 days improves survival by maintaining adherence of the graft to the bed, minimizing shearing, and preventing hematoma or seroma. A vacuum-assisted compression device can be placed on the grafted surface to stabilize the graft in place; this is especially useful for larger wounds with an irregular three-dimensional surface.

Skin grafts composed of tissue-cultured skin cells are used for the treatment of burns or other extensive skin wounds. Human epidermal cells in a single-cell suspension are grown in monolayers in vitro during a period of 3 to 6 weeks. Concerns with tissue-cultured skin are fragility, sensitivity to infection, length of time for cultivation, and potential risk of malignancy caused by mitogens present during culturing.

Skin Flap Surgery

A surgical flap consists of tissue that is moved from one part of the body to another with a vascular pedicle to maintain blood supply. The vascular pedicle may be kept intact, or it can be transected for microvascular anastomosis of the flap vessels to vessels at another site. Flap defines the tongue of tissue; pedicle is used to describe the base or stem with the vascular supply.

Skin-bearing flaps are classified according to three basic characteristics—composition, method of movement, and blood supply. Composition refers to the tissue contained within the flap, such as cutaneous, musculocutaneous, fasciocutaneous, osseocutaneous, and sensory flaps. The method of movement is local transfer, as with advancement or rotation flaps, or distant transfer, as with pedicle flaps from the abdomen to the perineum or microvascular free flaps.

With regard to blood supply, arteries perfusing the surgical flap reach the skin component in two basic ways. Musculocutaneous arteries travel perpendicularly through muscle to the overlying skin. Septocutaneous arteries arising from segmental or musculocutaneous vessels travel with intermuscular fascial septa to supply the overlying skin. With either of these patterns, the flap can have a random pattern, which means that it derives its blood supply from the dermal and subdermal vascular plexus of vessels supplied by perforating arteries. Alternatively, it can be an axial flap designed to include a named musculocutaneous or septocutaneous vessel running longitudinally along the axis of the flap to penetrate the overlying cutaneous circulation at multiple points along the course of the flap's length to provide greater length and reliability.

Skin Flaps

Local skin flaps contain tissue lying adjacent to the defect that usually matches the skin at the recipient site in color, texture, hair, and thickness. Flaps should be the same size and thickness as the defect and be designed to avoid distortion of local anatomic landmarks, such as the eyebrow or hairline. They can be planned so that the donor site can be closed directly and usually are elevated with incision lines placed in relaxed skin tension lines. Local flaps rely on the inherent elasticity of skin and are most useful in the older patient whose skin is looser. In some cases, the site from which the flap is raised is closed with a skin graft. Commonly used local skin flaps include the following:

Rotation flaps are semicircular flaps of skin and subcutaneous tissue that revolve in an arc around a pivot point to shift tissue in a circle.

Transposition flaps are rectangular or square and turn laterally to reach the defect.

Advancement flaps move directly forward and rely on skin elasticity to stretch and to fill a defect.

V-Y advancement flaps advance skin on each side of a V-shaped incision to close the wound with a Y-shaped closure.

Rhomboid flaps rely on the looseness of adjacent skin to transfer a rhomboid-shaped flap into a defect that has been converted into a similar rhomboid shape.

Z-plasty transposes two interdigitating triangular flaps without tension to use lateral skin to produce a gain in length along the direction of the common limb of the Z.

Failure of a skin flap usually involves necrosis of the most distal portion of the transferred tissue. This could be caused by a flap design in which the size of the flap exceeds its inherent vascular supply, or it could be a result of extrinsic mechanical compromise of the flap pedicle by pressure from a hematoma, compressive dressings, or twisting or kinking of the flap. Measures to optimize viability include proper flap design and avoidance of extrinsic pedicle compression, undue tension with wound closure, and venous congestion caused by excessive flap dependency.

Muscle and Musculocutaneous Flaps

Consideration of a muscle as a potential flap is possible because muscles have independent, intrinsic blood supply. The motor nerves of a muscle are accompanied by an arteriovenous system that often is the major source of blood supply to that muscle. This vascular pedicle may be a dominant one, capable of sustaining the entire muscle independently. A minor pedicle, regardless of the size of the vessel, is defined as one that maintains only a lesser portion of the muscle. Many muscles have multiple unrelated sources of blood supply so that each nourishes only a segment of the muscle, thus called segmental pedicles. Some muscles have both a dominant pedicle and segmental blood supply. One example is the latissimus dorsi muscle with a dominant pedicle, the thoracodorsal artery in the axilla, and additional segmental perforating branches from the intercostal and lumbar vessels posteriorly. In these muscles, the dominant pedicle can be ligated and the muscle moved on the secondary vessels as a reverse muscle flap.

Muscle flaps are classified according to their principal means of blood supply and the patterns of vascular anatomy (Fig. 68-1):

Type I: Single pedicle (e.g., gastrocnemius, tensor fascia lata)
Type II: Dominant pedicle with minor pedicles (e.g., gracilis, trapezius)
Type III: Dual dominant pedicles (e.g., gluteus maximus, serratus anterior)
Type IV: Segmental pedicles (e.g., sartorius, tibialis anterior)
Type V: Dominant pedicle, with secondary segmental pedicles (e.g., latissimus dorsi)

In terms of reliability of the vascular anatomy and usefulness as a flap, large muscles with a recognized dominant pedicle supplying most of a flap (types I, III, and V) are most useful. The territory of the pedicles in type II muscles may vary, and type IV muscles are useful only when smaller flaps are needed. Connections between regions within a given muscle supplied by more than one pedicle are through small-caliber choke vessels with bidirectional flow. An example of a flap depending on these choke vessels is the transverse rectus abdominis musculocutaneous (TRAM) flap, in which the superior epigastric pedicle alone can support the lower half of the muscle normally supplied by the inferior epigastric vessels below the watershed level at the umbilicus. In muscle, venous territories are in parallel with arterial vessels. This means that venous outflow is adjacent to and in a direction opposite from flow in the major arterial pedicles. In a pattern analogous to that of the bidirectional choke vessels, venous flow from one territory to another occurs through oscillating veins that are devoid of valves.

Compared with skin flaps, muscle flaps are less bulky, less stiff, and more malleable to conform to wounds with irregular three-dimensional contours. They have more robust blood supply and demonstrate superiority in wounds compromised by irradiation or infection. The vascular anatomy is predictable and easily identifiable, and the muscle can be put into use as a functional unit for a dynamic tissue transfer. A major consideration with muscle flaps is whether the loss of function is acceptable. In an effort to limit the functional loss associated with use of an entire muscle, methods of functional preservation have been devised. If some

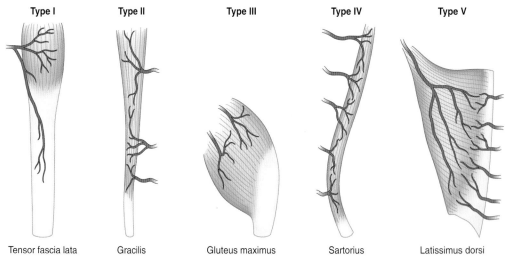

FIGURE 68-1 Classification of muscle and musculocutaneous flaps according to their vascular supply: type I, one vascular pedicle; type II, dominant pedicle and minor pedicles; type III, two dominant pedicles; type IV, segmental vascular pedicles; type V, one dominant pedicle and secondary segmental pedicles. (From Mathes SJ, Nahai F: Classification of the vascular anatomy of muscles: Experimental and clinical correlation. *Plast Reconstr Surg* 67:177–187, 1981.)

portion of the muscle chosen as the flap is left innervated and attached at its insertion and origin, function is preserved after transfer of the remainder of the muscle. This can be done by splitting the muscle into segments, provided each is supplied by a different dominant pedicle. An example is the gluteus maximus, which extends and rotates the thigh laterally. This is not an expendable muscle, but the superior or inferior half of the muscle can be elevated as a flap, with function of the intact half of the muscle preserved.

A musculocutaneous flap, also called a myocutaneous flap, is a muscle flap designed with an attached skin paddle. Each superficial skeletal muscle carries blood supply to the skin lying directly over it through musculocutaneous perforators. The number and pattern of these musculocutaneous perforators vary with each specific muscle; this means that the extent of the skin territory is different for each muscle unit. Through dissection of injected cadaver specimens, the number, size, and location of musculocutaneous perforators have been described; this information, combined with clinical experience, is used to predict the cutaneous territories on the superficial muscles.

In addition to the musculocutaneous branches supplying the overlying skin, source vessels, also called mother vessels, branch within muscle into channels that perforate the deep fascia to anastomose within the subdermal plexus and nourish the skin. The source vessel and its perforating muscular branches can be dissected out of the muscle without jeopardizing skin perfusion. This requires intramuscular dissection to separate the perforators from the muscle and is the basis for the development of muscle perforator flaps. This makes the retention of muscle unnecessary for the survival of the skin paddle; thus, its inclusion serves a passive role, primarily to avoid tedious intramuscular dissection of the vascular tree. To spare the muscle unit, a growing number of muscle perforator flaps have been described, including the deep inferior epigastric perforator flap, which carries the same skin and subcutaneous tissue as the TRAM flap for breast reconstruction. By sparing of the rectus muscle, abdominal wall bulging and other complications are less likely. The superior gluteal artery perforator flap carries the skin territory of the gluteus maximus musculocutaneous flap and preserves the muscle.

Fascia and Fasciocutaneous Flaps

Growing knowledge about musculocutaneous skin circulation has led to the identification of vascular pedicles emerging between muscles, traveling in the intermuscular septum, and entering the deep fascia. Termed septocutaneous perforators, these vessels supply the fascial plexus, which gives off branches to an overlying cutaneous territory. Some state that a fasciocutaneous flap, by definition, should include a specific known septocutaneous perforator. Others accept a less strict definition of a fasciocutaneous flap as a skin flap including the deep fascia.

The anatomic features of a fasciocutaneous flap are the fascial feeder vessels, also called the fascial perforators, which are branches of source vessels to a given angiosome. An angiosome is the three-dimensional block of tissue supplied by a source artery; the entire surface of the body is composed of a multitude of angiosome units. The fascial feeder vessels do not perforate the deep fascia but terminate within the fascial plexus. The fascial plexus is not a structure but a confluence of multiple adjacent vascular intercommunications that exist at the subfascial, fascial, suprafascial, subcutaneous, and subdermal levels (Fig. 68-2).

The concept of fasciocutaneous flaps arose from the observation that the size of a skin flap could be increased if it were ori-

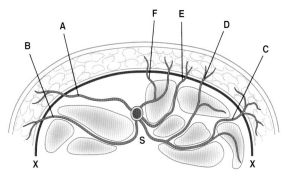

A Direct cutaneous
B Direct septocutaneous
C Direct cutaneous branch of muscular vessel
D Perforating cutaneous branch of muscular vessel
E Septocutaneous perforator
F Musculocutaneous perforator
S Source vessel
X Deep fascia

FIGURE 68-2 Pathways of the various known cutaneous perforators that pierce the deep fascia to supply the fascial plexus. (From Hallock GG: Direct and indirect perforator flaps: The history and the controversy. *Plast Reconstr Surg* 111:855–865, 2003.)

ented along a longitudinal axis on the extremity and if the deep fascia were included. Subsequent anatomic studies have confirmed the presence of septocutaneous pedicles supplying a regional fascial vascular system. The larger septocutaneous pedicles tend to be fairly constant in location, and a number of specific fasciocutaneous flaps have come into wide use (e.g., anterior lateral thigh flap, radial forearm flap, scapular flap).

The design of fasciocutaneous flaps has been learned by experience, and the limits of these flaps still remain to be discovered. There are no set rules because deep fascial perforators are frequently anomalous in caliber and location, not only among individuals but also on opposite sides of the same person. The expected range of flap size is learned through the experience of other surgeons.[1,2]

One of the most useful features of a fasciocutaneous flap is that it can be distally based. Unlike in a muscle flap, in which the dominant pedicle is closest to the heart, blood flow in the fascial plexus is multidirectional. The flow to the corresponding angiosome is equivalent for a distal fascial perforator and proximal fascial perforator. This means that a flap pedicle can be distally based with a reliable skin territory and transposed to cover a defect located at the end of an extremity. For example, the distal-based sural flap uses the skin of the calf, based on a distal perforator of the peroneal artery, for transfer to cover the foot and ankle. Obviating the need for a free microvascular transfer, this has become a standard for foot coverage.

In addition to the advantages provided by a distally based flap design, a fasciocutaneous flap can confer sensibility if a sensory nerve is included. Compared with musculocutaneous flaps, they are accessible on the surface of the body and have the great advantage that no functioning muscle is expended. The comparative disadvantages are the anatomic anomalies in the fascial vascular system and the unanswered question as to whether they are as effective as muscle in the irradiated or infected wound.

Perforator Flaps

Perforator flaps evolved as an improvement over musculocutaneous and fasciocutaneous flaps. They rely on evidence that neither a passive muscle carrier nor the underlying fascial plexus of vessels is necessary for flap survival, provided the musculocutaneous or fasciocutaneous vessel is carefully dissected out and preserved. Advantages of perforator flaps include preservation of functional muscle and fascia at the donor site and versatility of flap design with regard to including as little or as much bulk tissue as required. Disadvantages are the difficult dissection needed to isolate the perforator vessels, longer operating time associated with this dissection, anatomic variability of position and size of perforator vessels, short pedicle length available, and fragile nature of these small blood vessels.

A perforator is a blood vessel passing through the deep fascia and contributing blood supply to the fascial plexus. Perforators arise from a source or mother vessel to a given angiosome. There are direct and indirect perforators. Direct perforators are those that travel directly from the mother vessel to the plexus; these include septocutaneous and direct cutaneous branches. Indirect perforators supply other deep structures on their route from the mother vessel to the plexus (e.g., the musculocutaneous perforator passing through muscle).

The nomenclature of perforator flaps is not yet standardized. They are named variably by location (anterolateral thigh flap), arterial supply (deep inferior epigastric artery perforator flap), and muscle of origin (gastrocnemius perforator flap). They are described as cutaneous, musculocutaneous, septocutaneous, fasciocutaneous, composite, and chimeric; the last is a perforator flap with two separate muscular components with a common vascular source. Several suggestions for an ordering nomenclature have been made.

Because of the small size of the vessels and their anatomic variability, Doppler ultrasound is used routinely to locate the perforators before perforator flap elevation. This is not highly accurate, and other technologies, such as color flow duplex scanning and thermography, may be useful in the future. Technical recommendations for harvesting of a perforator flap include identification of at least one vessel with a diameter of 0.5 mm or more, inclusion of at least two or more perforators, sufficient pedicle length for the procedure, and preservation of a subcutaneous vein to use for venous outflow in situations in which the deep system of perforator veins proves anomalous.

The use of perforator flaps continues to evolve. Current work includes flap thinning, a technique for removing excess adipose tissue from the perforator flap as it is raised. This would provide a large delicate segment of vascularized skin for reconstruction in areas such as the ear, in which contour is important. Another innovation is the discovery of new flaps based on perforators smaller than 0.8 mm in diameter found superficial to the fascial plane. By eliminating the dissection needed to trace a perforator through the muscle, operating time is shortened and there is potential for developing a much larger number of suitable flaps. The challenge with these suprafascial free flaps is the supermicrosurgery needed for anastomoses in such small vessels.[3]

Microvascular Free Tissue Transfer

A microvascular free tissue transfer, also called a free flap, brings distant tissue with a pedicled arterial and venous supply from another part of the body to be anastomosed to vessels at the recipient site to reestablish blood flow. The transferred tissue may be skin, fat, muscle, fascia, bone, nerves, small bowel, large bowel, or omentum as needed to reconstruct a given defect. Selection of tissue for transfer depends on the size, composition, and functional capabilities of the tissue needed; technical considerations, such as vessel size and pedicle length; and donor site deformity that will be created with regard to function and aesthetic appearance.

Preoperative planning starts with selection of the patient and analysis of the defect. Environmental factors, such as previous surgery and prior irradiation, which impair the quality of tissue and vessels, may be an indication for angiography to assess the available vasculature. Muscle does not tolerate warm ischemia for longer than 2 hours; skin and fasciocutaneous flaps can tolerate ischemia times of 4 to 6 hours. Planning is the most important factor to minimize the effects of ischemia, and all structures at the recipient site should be ready for the tissue transfer when the donor pedicle is divided. Sound technique requires healthy vessels of reasonable size with good outflow for the anastomosis, which must be made without tension. This may require mobilization of the vessels to gain more length. Vein grafts have been shown to reduce the success rate and are not a primary choice but may be needed if the pedicle is short or the vessels in the field are damaged. Vein grafts can be obtained from the saphenous vein, dorsum of the foot, volar forearm, or donor site. Adventitia is removed from the vessel ends to improve visualization of the vessel walls for accurate suture placement. Both end-to-end and end-to-side arterial anastomoses have similar patency rates, although end-to-side anastomosis is preferred if there is vessel size or wall thickness discrepancy or the continuity of the recipient vessel must be preserved. Dissection and manipulation of the microvessels frequently cause vasospasm. This can be relieved with topical lidocaine or papaverine, stripping the adventitia to remove sympathetic nerve fibers, or mechanical dilation of the vessels. Failure of reperfusion in an ischemic organ after reestablishment of blood supply is termed the no-reflow phenomenon. The causative mechanism is thought to be endothelial injury, platelet aggregation, and leakage of intravascular fluid. The severity of this effect correlates with ischemia time.

Postoperative anticoagulation is not a uniform practice for elective microvascular transfers. If pharmacologic agents are part of postoperative care, aspirin is generally used, followed by dextran and low-molecular-weight heparin. Surveys of microsurgical centers have shown equal success rates for transplants with and without anticoagulation; the concern with the use of anticoagulants is an increased chance of hematoma at donor and recipient sites. Postoperative monitoring of free tissue transfers is critical because rapid identification of postoperative free flap ischemia permits intervention and flap salvage. Most free flap thromboses occur in the first 48 hours after surgery, and salvage rates are high. Clinical evaluation includes observation of skin color, capillary refill, fullness, and color of capillary bleeding, which can be determined by pinprick testing of the flap. If a flap is buried, a temporary skin island can be added for monitoring purposes, or an implantable monitoring device can be used. Many devices are available for flap monitoring, including temperature probes, pulse oximetry, photoplethysmography, hand-held pencil Doppler probes (low-frequency continuous ultrasonography), and implantable Doppler probes.

Tissue survival rates for free tissue transfers exceed 95%. Reexploration rates range from 6% to 25%, and thrombosis of the arterial anastomosis is the most common finding at reoperation. This is termed primary thrombosis when technical faults lead to anastomotic failure. These faults include narrowing of the lumen; sutures tied too loosely so that media of the vessel is exposed in the gap and clot forms; sutures tied too tightly that tear through the vessel; too many sutures with subendothelial exposure and clot formation; and sutures that inadvertently take a bite of the back wall of the vessel, which obstructs the lumen. Secondary thrombosis refers to kinking or compression of vessels by hematoma or edema, which leads to decreased inflow. With reexploration, salvage rates have been seen to vary from 54% to 100% in different series.[4]

The principles and techniques of microvascular surgery are under continual refinement. An area of current emphasis is the identification of tissue transfers that better suit the needs of the recipient site and minimize donor site sequelae, which has led to minimally invasive and endoscopic techniques for harvesting of flap tissue through smaller incisions. It has also led to the development of tissue transfers such as perforator flaps, which preserve functional muscle and fascia at the donor site, and suprafascial free flaps, which require supermicrosurgery techniques.

Supermicrosurgery

The introduction of supermicrosurgery, which allows the anastomosis of smaller caliber vessels and microvascular dissection of vessels ranging from 0.3 to 0.8 mm in diameter, has led to the development of new reconstructive techniques. Free perforator-to-perforator flaps using suprafascial vessels can be transferred more quickly and the tissue can be obtained from better concealed parts of the body.[5] If a discrete perforator can be identified anywhere on the body, a flap can be designed around it. This has been called a freestyle flap. The constraints of using only described territories can be disregarded and the donor site selected solely on the basis of the best possible match for color, contour, and texture at the recipient site. Disadvantages are the anatomic variation of the perforators and the need for supermicrosurgical technique. The supermicrosurgical technique includes the use of 12-0 nylon sutures with 50- to 30-μm needles; the surgeons who pioneered "freestyle reconstruction" have noted that it is difficult to learn and can be tedious.[6]

Tissue Expansion

Tissue expansion is a technique that uses a mechanical stimulus to induce tissue growth so as to generate soft tissue for reconstructive use. It involves placing a prosthesis that is gradually enlarged by the addition of saline, which causes an increase in the surface area of the overlying soft tissue. Initially, the expanded skin is the result of stretching as interstitial fluid is forced out of the tissue, elastic fibers are fragmented, viscoelastic changes (termed creep) occur in the collagen, and adjacent mobile soft tissue is recruited. Over time, it is not just stretching but actual growth of the skin flap that creates an increase in the surface area, with accompanying increases in collagen and ground substance. Histologic changes in the skin include dermal thinning, epidermal thickening, subcutaneous fat atrophy, and no effect on the skin appendages.

Tissue undergoing expansion must have the capacity for growth. Prior irradiation or scar formation may slow the rate of expansion or make it impossible. Expanders perform poorly under skin grafts, under very tight tissue, and in the hands and feet. Contraindications include expansion near a malignant neoplasm, hemangioma, or open leg wound.

Expanders come in various styles, and sizes range from a few cubic centimeters to 1 liter or more. They can be round, square, rectangular, or horseshoe shaped. The injection ports can be remote or integrated into the wall of the expander so that no dis-

section of a pocket for the remote port is required. The envelope can be smooth or textured for better stabilization at one location in the tissue pocket.

Expanders should be placed under tissue that best matches the lost tissue (Fig. 68-3). Normal landmarks, such as the eyebrow or hairline, should not be distorted. The incision to insert the expander can be placed at the edge of the defect that later will be excised because a scar in this position will be removed at the time of the next surgery. The most common reason for expander failure is construction of a pocket that is too small for the device. An expander with a curled edge may later protrude through the incision or erode through the overlying tissue. Filling of the expander is initiated approximately 2 weeks after surgery and continued at weekly or biweekly intervals. The rate of expansion is limited by the relaxation and growth of the tissue overlying the expander. Pain and palpable tightness over the expander are clinical indicators that guide the rate of expansion. The patient is ready for the second surgical procedure when the expanded tissue is adequate to produce the desired effect. If the flap is to be advanced, it must be measured to ensure that it is large enough and has the correct geometry to cover the defect. At the second surgery, the skin is incised through the old scar, the capsule around the expander is opened, the expander is removed, and the expanded flap is advanced over the defect. It is important to confirm that the expanded tissue will replace the defect before the defect is excised. If it is not sufficient, this is handled by subtotal resection of the defect and leaving the expander in place for a second round of expansion.[7]

Tissue expansion can be combined with other reconstructive techniques. Expander placement in the subcutaneous or submuscular plane can facilitate later repair of abdominal wall hernias. Preexpansion of transposition or rotation flaps increases the amount of tissue, enhances the flap's blood supply, and lessens donor site morbidity. Preexpansion of free flaps increases the surface area and augments the blood supply of the future flap, may make primary closure of the free flap donor site possible, and thins the flap, which may be desirable for reconstructions calling for thinner and more pliable coverage. A disadvantage of the preexpansion of free flaps is the time needed for the expansion process because delay may not be acceptable for oncologic defects and complex wounds. In addition, the preexpanded free flap procedure is technically more difficult because of distortion of the vascular pedicle.

The advantages of expansion are the provision of matching tissue for reconstruction, normal sensibility of the transferred tissue, negligible donor defect, and enhanced success of preexpanded traditional flaps because of enhanced vascularity.

Alloplastic Materials

An alloplastic material is a synthetic substance implanted in living tissue. Its advantages are availability when autologous tissue is not available and the absence of donor site morbidity or scarring. Nonbiodegradable alloplastic materials do not undergo resorption, as do bone or cartilage grafts. In addition, the implant can be manufactured to meet special needs, such as for controlled-release drug delivery systems.

The tissue response to different implants varies with the chemical composition and the microstructure and macrostructure of the synthetic material; these differences are used clinically. For example, the vigorous tissue ingrowth with polypropylene mesh in a hernia repair provides strong and lasting support, whereas the fibrous encapsulation around a silicone tendon prosthesis ensures

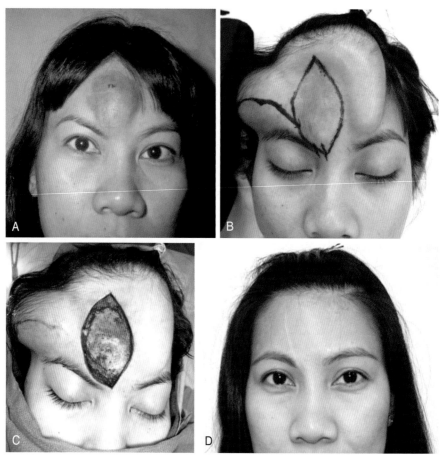

FIGURE 68-3 The use of tissue expansion to generate new soft tissue to restore the forehead and hairline. The expanders are placed under tissue that best matches the lost tissue. **A,** Young woman with an arteriovenous malformation. **B,** Crescent-shaped expander in the central forehead and rectangular expander in the right forehead were expanded gradually with saline during 1 month. **C,** The vascular lesion is excised, and the expanders will be removed with mobilization of the forehead to close the defect. **D,** Postoperative result 1 year after surgery.

free gliding of a tendon graft. However, certain properties (noncarcinogenic, nontoxic, nonallergenic, nonimmunogenic) and concerns (mechanical reliability, biocompatibility) are common to all implants.

Categorization by chemical composition is the most useful framework for the description and comparison of surgical implants. This materials science approach recognizes that the commonality of different groups of materials arises more from their composition than from the organ systems in which they are used. Chemically, there are three major classes of biomaterials: metallic, ceramic, and polymeric. Although they are polymers, biologic materials such as collagen need to be classified separately because they introduce new considerations of protein antigenicity.

Metals in clinical use are stainless steel, Vitallium (cobalt-chromium-molybdenum alloy), and titanium. The general requirements for a metal device are mechanical strength, suitable elastic modulus, density and weight comparable to those of the surrounding tissue, and resistance to corrosion. Very few metals have sufficient corrosion resistance to be used in the hostile environment of the living organism. Corrosion results from the elec-trochemical activity of unstable metal ions and electrons in physiologic salt solutions; corrosion products can be cytotoxic, leading to pain, inflammation, allergic reactions, and loosening of the device.

Ceramic materials have high stability and resistance to chemical alteration and include carbon compounds such as hydroxyapatite, which is capable of bonding strongly to adjacent bone. Used to augment the facial skeleton or as a bone graft substitute, it is a permanent microporous implant that undergoes osseointegration by providing a matrix for the deposition of new bone from adjacent living bone.

Polymers are large, long-chain, high-molecular-weight macromolecules made up of repeated units, or mers. There are a vast number of these synthetic implants in surgical use. To a large extent, this is because of the ease and low cost of fabrication and because they can be processed easily into tubes, fibers, fabrics, meshes, films, and foams. Polymers vary across an enormous range of chemical compositions, degree of polymerization, cross-linking between chains, and presence of chemical additives such as plasticizers to increase flexibility or resins to catalyze polymerization.

With the exception of resorbable polymers, most surgical polymers are relatively inert and stimulate fibrous encapsulation. The physical form of the implant, solid versus mesh or smooth versus rough, will determine whether the entire structure is encapsulated as a whole or whether fibrous tissue will penetrate the interstices. Tissue reaction to the implant is influenced also by the chemical composition, factors such as hydrophilicity and ionic charge, and the chemical durability of the polymer. Silicone rubber, polytetrafluoroethylene, and polyethylene terephthalate polyester (Dacron) are among the most stable of polymers, whereas polyamide (nylon) is vulnerable to hydrolytic reaction and undergoes substantial degradation.

PEDIATRIC PLASTIC SURGERY

Craniofacial Surgery

Craniosynostosis refers to the premature fusion of one or more of the cranial sutures, leading to characteristic deformities of the skull and face. It occurs at an overall frequency of approximately 1 in 2500 live births and is usually sporadic. Any suture may be involved in craniosynostosis, and skull growth is restricted perpendicular to the affected suture. Treatment of craniosynostosis is indicated to correct the deformity and to normalize the shape of the head, to protect the eyes by restoring brow projection, and to minimize the risk for development of increased intracranial pressure and associated developmental and visual sequelae. The timing of treatment is based on which suture is fused and on the protocol at a given center, but correction during the first 6 months of life appears to be associated with better neurodevelopmental outcomes.

Surgical treatment of craniosynostosis is generally done with a coronal approach; techniques differ, but all involve release or excision of the fused suture. The cranium then expands and remodels. Residual bone defects reossify secondarily, a process that is robust in the infant up to 2 years of age (Fig. 68-4).

Other less common congenital abnormalities of the head include agenesis of one or a number of layers of scalp or cranium.

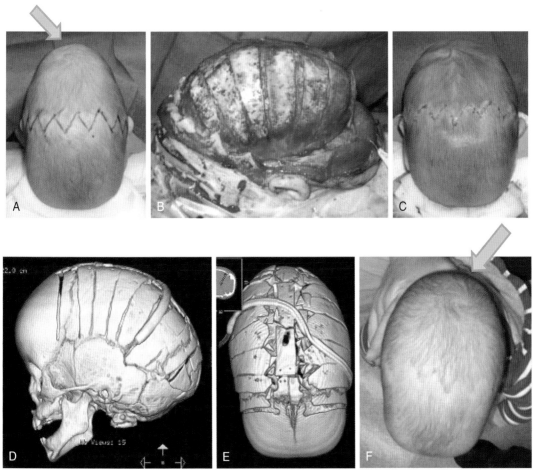

FIGURE 68-4 Infant with sagittal suture craniosynostosis. **A,** Preoperative view showing scaphocephalic head shape. The baby is in a prone position with the face resting on foam. Note the narrow biparietal dimension of the head, typical for this condition *(arrow)*. A zigzag coronal incision is designed to be better hidden once hair grows. **B,** Intraoperative lateral view. The sagittal suture has been removed and reshaped, and lateral barrel stave osteotomies are created to reshape the cranial vault and to relieve growth restriction. **C,** On-table view immediately after the procedure. The biparietal area is widened. **D** and **E,** Lateral and superior views of the postoperative CT scan. **F,** One month after surgery, the skull continues to remodel and the head shape normalizes *(arrow)*.

Aplasia cutis congenita usually refers to a focal defect of skin on the vertex. The defect may include any proportion of skin, bone, or dura. Treatment depends on the size of the defect and layers involved and may encompass local wound care or surgical reconstruction with flaps or grafts in infancy. The cause of this rare condition is unknown and likely varies from case to case. A classification system for aplasia cutis congenita has been developed and is related to the presence of other associated anomalies.

Congenital Ear Deformities

Congenital anomalies of the external ear may occur in isolation or as part of craniofacial microsomia. Common external ear deformities include prominent ears, constricted ears, cryptotia (failure of the upper pole of the ear to stand out from the head), and microtia (a small or abnormally formed outer ear). The most common type of microtia is a malformed vestigial cartilaginous structure associated with a soft tissue component of lobule. In cases of isolated microtia, there is often conductive hearing loss associated with absence of the external auditory canal. This is most important in bilateral cases in which a bone-anchored hearing aid is required.

Reconstruction of typical microtia can take two general approaches, autologous or nonautologous. Nonautologous reconstruction involves placement of a high-density polyethylene implant under the skin. This approach results in good form without the need to harvest tissue from another site or the requirement of shaping a framework. Disadvantages include the presence of a foreign body that may become exposed through the thin skin envelope, is susceptible to infection, and is difficult to salvage in case of complications. The second approach is preferred. This involves the use of autologous tissue (rib cartilage) to shape an ear framework, which is then buried in a subcutaneous pocket. The meticulous shaping of the framework, creation of a thin skin pocket, and use of drains allow the skin to contour around the intricate framework. The procedure requires multiple stages but results in a reconstructed ear that has good form and is capable of responding to trauma and infection like other parts of the body. The disadvantage is the need to harvest cartilage from the rib.

Craniofacial Microsomia

Craniofacial microsomia, also known as hemifacial microsomia, is a constellation of abnormalities involving deficient development of parts of the face related to the first and second branchial arches.[8] Deformity can be unilateral or bilateral and can involve the orbit, mandible, external ear, facial nerve, and facial soft tissue. Each or all of the structures may be involved and to varying degrees. The cause is unknown but is thought to be related to in utero vascular compromise of the stapedial artery. Treatment of craniofacial microsomia is complex, and the approach has to be tailored for individual patients. Functional problems, such as airway compromise or eye exposure, are treated in childhood; reconstruction of other structural defects is delayed until the patient is almost full-grown.

For patients with craniofacial anomalies such as those described as well as for those with cleft lip and palate, the current standard is team care at an established craniofacial center. With referral to a craniofacial center at birth, the craniofacial team can make a diagnosis, carry out genetic testing, educate the family, and outline short- and long-term plans in a coordinated manner, bringing in multiple specialists (e.g., plastic surgeons, neurosurgeons, oral surgeons, orthodontists, speech pathologists, otolaryngologists, ophthalmologists, social workers, nurse practitioners, developmental psychologists, and pediatricians).

Cleft Lip and Palate

Cleft lip and palate are relatively common congenital anomalies. They may be unilateral or bilateral. Most are isolated anomalies, but many syndromes have clefts as one of the features. The genetics of cleft lip and palate is complex, and the condition is multifactorial. The pathophysiologic mechanism of cleft lip and palate is incompletely understood, but the deformity and its variations are well described. A minimum of three operations, and usually four, will be required to correct the deformity. These are performed at specific times corresponding to the developmental stage of the patient:

- Cleft lip repair at 3 months
- Cleft palate repair before 1 year or before speech development begins
- Alveolar bone graft when permanent dentition begins and after orthodontic preparation
- Possible septorhinoplasty in the late teenage years
- Possible lip and nose revision
- LeFort I maxillary advancement, if indicated
- Secondary procedures for speech improvement in 15% of cases

A cleft lip is characterized by a partial or complete lack of circumferential continuity of the lip. Most cleft lips occur at a typical location in the upper lip where one of the philtral columns normally lies, and they extend into the nose. The deformity involves the mucosa, orbicularis oris muscle, and skin. The nasal deformity is characterized by a slumped and widened ala (nostril) that is posteriorly misplaced at its base. The nasal floor is nonexistent in complete clefts and the nasal septum is deviated.

There are many techniques for repair of a cleft lip, but most are a variation of the rotation-advancement repair. Millard introduced this technique of downward rotation of the medial portion of the lip and advancement of the lateral portion into the defect created by the rotation. The repair is based on the principle that existing elements need to be returned to their normal position to restore the normal anatomy while remaining cognizant of future growth and the effects of surgery on growth (Fig. 68-5).[9]

Cleft palate can also be complete or incomplete. The goals of palatal repair are the development of normal speech and prevention of regurgitation of food into the nose. Normal speech requires velopharyngeal competence to close the oral cavity off from the nasal cavity to produce pressure consonants. This requires static physical separation of the two cavities in the region of the hard palate and dynamic closure of the soft palate against the posterior pharyngeal wall with a functioning levator veli palatini muscle. In a cleft palate, the levator veli palatini muscle fibers are oriented abnormally along the cleft. Thus, all modern techniques of cleft palate repair involve repair of the nasal lining and oral mucosa and reorientation and repair of the levator veli palatini muscle. The primary measure of outcome of cleft palate repair is normal speech. The third procedure necessary in most cases is alveolar bone grafting. Cancellous bone, usually from the ilium, is used to restore bone continuity along the dental arch as a foundation for dental implants for missing teeth associated with the cleft, to close a nasolabial fistula (if present), and to produce support for the nose.

Other procedures are indicated for some patients, but this generally cannot be predicted in infancy. Approximately 15% of patients will continue to demonstrate velopharyngeal insufficiency after initial palate repair, and secondary palatal lengthening or other approaches to promote velopharyngeal closure are indicated, typically after 3 years of age.[10] Septorhinoplasty is usually necessary to correct residual nasal deformity in the teenage years

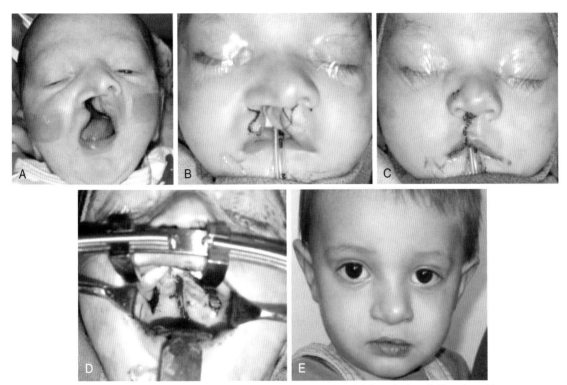

FIGURE 68-5 Infant boy with a wide right-sided unilateral complete cleft lip and palate. **A,** There is a wide cleft with absence of the nasal floor, malrotated central lip element, twisted premaxilla, and severe nasal deformity. **B,** Intraoperative markings for rotation-advancement cleft lip repair at age 3 months. **C,** Immediate postoperative view. **D,** Postoperative views at 11 months of age taken at the time of cleft palate repair. **E,** After primary repair of cleft lip, nose, and palate.

after final dental restoration and orthodontics. A subset of unilateral cleft lip and palate patients will develop maxillary hypoplasia that is iatrogenic and related to scarring and growth retardation from lip and palate surgery. Depending on the degree of maxillary hypoplasia, LeFort I maxillary advancement in the teenage years may be indicated. In sum, treatment of a child born with a cleft lip and palate does not end after palate repair but rather requires observation by a craniofacial team throughout development into adulthood and must be tailored for each individual.

Vascular Anomalies

Vascular anomalies are divided into two major groups, tumors and malformations. Vascular tumors are characterized by increased abnormal proliferation of endothelium. Hemangioma is the most common vascular tumor; others include hemangioendotheliomas, tufted angiomas, hemangiopericytomas, and malignant tumors, such as angiosarcoma. Vascular malformations are the result of abnormal development of arterial, capillary, venous, or lymphatic components of the vascular system. They may involve only one component or may be mixed and are named for the component vessels. They can be high flow, low flow, or mixed. Correct diagnosis depends on the history (e.g., hemangiomas develop in infancy and are usually not visible at birth), physical examination (e.g., malformations with an arterial component may have a palpable pulse or thrill), and imaging to determine the extent of disease and to assist with making the diagnosis.

The natural histories of the different anomalies are diverse. Hemangiomas typically involute spontaneously; 50% involute completely by the age of 5 years. This natural history reduces the indications for surgery to those lesions that are affecting vision or the airway or are large enough that even after involution, the abnormal remaining skin will require surgical modification. In contrast, capillary malformations start as patches, but over time, they typically enlarge and become thick and verrucous; for these lesions, early treatment is indicated. Some vascular malformations or tumors have systemic effects, depending on their mass, status as high or low flow, and thrombosis and consumption of coagulation factors. Treatment of these lesions involves complete resection, when feasible, or debulking if complete resection is not possible. Sclerotherapy is the mainstay of treatment of venous malformations. For arteriovenous malformations, sclerotherapy is useful as an adjunct to surgery but insufficient alone because of the development of collaterals. For these malformations, sclerotherapy and embolization are followed immediately by surgical resection.

Pediatric Neck Masses

Neck masses in the pediatric patient are most likely infectious or congenital noncancerous lesions. In addition to vascular malformations, other common pediatric neck masses include dermoid cysts, teratomas, branchial cleft anomalies, thyroglossal duct cysts, thymic cysts, ranulas, cartilaginous rests, heterotopic neuroectodermal tissue, neurofibromas, ectopic salivary tissue, lymphadenopathy, and malignant tumors. Branchial cleft anomalies may be cysts, sinuses, or fistulas. Cysts and sinuses are located in the anterior cervical triangle and are derived from the first cleft (near the external auditory meatus) and second cleft (below the hyoid) 98% of the time. The treatment of these lesions is surgical excision. Thyroglossal duct cysts may arise anywhere along the course of the thyroglossal duct, from the foramen cecum at the base of the tongue to the thyroid gland. Thyroglossal duct cysts usually present in the first or second decade of life as painless anterior neck masses, and there may be an associated sinus track. Indications for surgery include recurrent infection, tissue diagnosis, and improved cosmesis. Thyroid scan is indicated before excision to rule out a functioning ectopic thyroid gland.

Melanocytic Nevi

Congenital melanocytic nevi are hamartomas consisting of nevus cells. Nevi are classified by size as small (<1.5 cm), medium (1.5 to 19.9 cm), large (>20 cm), and giant (>50 cm). The classification dictates the prognosis and reconstructive approach. Risk of melanoma occurring in a melanocytic nevus varies by report but is estimated to be less than 5% in small or medium-sized lesions and typically presents after puberty. In large and giant nevi, the reported risk of melanoma development is up to 10%.[11] Unlike the case for small or medium-sized nevi, malignancy in large and giant nevi typically occurs in the first 3 years of life. Large and giant nevi also have an increased incidence of leptomeningeal involvement that can be diagnosed by magnetic resonance imaging (MRI). In addition, psychosocial and developmental issues associated with larger nevi are significant, so early excision and reconstruction are recommended for large and giant nevi.

Options for removal of larger nevi include serial excision, excision and grafting, excision and closure with distant flaps, and tissue expansion. Replacement with like tissue is the goal, and therefore tissue expansion is the mainstay approach.

PLASTIC SURGERY OF THE HEAD AND NECK

Maxillofacial Trauma

Facial trauma has decreased in frequency in the United States, and this is attributed in part to the advent of seat belt laws and improved collision safety. However, it remains part of multisystem trauma from motor vehicle accidents, assaults, and combat injuries. Improvements in body armor have resulted in better survival of combat injuries but proportionally more facial injuries.

Emergent Management

Surgical emergencies in the facial trauma patient include airway compromise, life-threatening hemorrhage, and reversible structural injury to the eye or optic nerve. Other injuries, such as lacerations or extraocular muscle entrapment, are treated within the first 24 hours. Fractures are treated within the first 2 weeks. Evaluation of the facial trauma patient follows the advanced trauma life support protocol and includes looking for intracranial trauma and cervical spine injury. Acute airway compromise usually occurs in the setting of combined mandibular-maxillary trauma, with hemorrhage and soft tissue swelling. Endotracheal intubation should be attempted and need not be avoided because of concern about the facial injury. Nasotracheal intubation is contraindicated in the case of severe naso-orbitoethmoid and skull base fractures. Cricothyroidotomy is performed if oral or nasal endotracheal intubation is unsuccessful and should be converted to tracheostomy after the patient has been stabilized. Maxillomandibular fixation by itself is not an indication for tracheostomy because endotracheal intubation may be maintained through the nasal or oral route using an armored tube that can be routed behind the molars without kinking. An alternative technique is to exit the endotracheal tube through a submental incision, which alleviates some of the practical difficulties of working around an oral tube.

Life-threatening hemorrhage, defined as 3 units of blood loss or hematocrit below 29%, occurs in a small percentage of facial trauma patients. In most cases, bleeding is effectively controlled with pressure, packing, and, in the case of significant soft tissue avulsion, rapid placement of temporary bolster sutures. Blind attempts to clamp and ligate vessels should be avoided because this is usually unnecessary and may result in injury to critical structures, such as the facial nerve. With penetrating trauma, hemorrhage is controlled in the operating room with vessel identification and ligation and, if that is unsuccessful, by angiographic selective embolization. With blunt trauma, severe hemorrhage is usually from the internal maxillary artery. The most effective way to control bleeding, especially when it is associated with midfacial fractures, is fracture reduction and stabilization. This can be accomplished quickly by temporary placement in maxillomandibular fixation using rapid techniques such as fixation screws. Severe hemorrhage from skull base and nasoethmoid fractures can often be controlled with anteroposterior nasal packing. Placement of Foley balloon catheters in each nasal airway serves to tamponade the bleeding and also stabilizes the packing. Current protocols for control of hemorrhage in blunt facial trauma settings involve selective angiography if these measures fail (Fig. 68-6).[12] Angiographic embolization is effective but is associated with significant morbidity, including the possibility of stroke or necrosis of midfacial structures, such as the palate. In unstable patients, fracture reduction and nasal packing may be attempted on the angiography table to be followed immediately with embolization, if necessary.

Injuries to the orbit and contents can result in blindness; it is critical to recognize promptly and to treat reversible injuries that

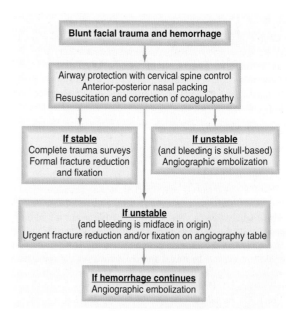

FIGURE 68-6 Algorithm for the management of life-threatening hemorrhage in the setting of blunt facial trauma. (Adapted from Ho K, Hutter JJ, Eskridge J, et al: The management of life-threatening haemorrhage following blunt facial trauma. *J Plast Reconstr Aesthet Surg* 59:1257–1262, 2006.)

are vision threatening. Conditions that require emergent intervention include increased intraocular pressure, globe rupture, and optic nerve impingement. Acute increased intracranial pressure is manifested by pain and vision loss and can result from causes such as hematoma or decreased orbital volume because of fracture or a foreign body. Treatment involves rapid alleviation of intraocular hypertension by lateral canthotomy and administration of mannitol, acetazolamide (Diamox), and steroids. Urgent ophthalmology consultation is indicated. Vision loss may result from mechanical compression of the optic nerve. Computed tomography (CT) will diagnose the presence of a bone fragment or foreign body; such a finding should prompt emergent surgical decompression to preserve vision. Extraocular muscle entrapment presents as the inability to move the eye on the trajectory controlled by the entrapped muscle and is associated with pain on attempted motion. Especially in children, the pain may be severe and accompanied by nausea or vomiting. Muscle entrapment should be treated by surgical release of the entrapped contents. This should be done fairly soon after injury because delaying the treatment of entrapment for 1 week or longer after injury typically results in failure of the entrapped muscle to regain excursion.

Evaluation and Diagnosis

The primary diagnostic studies for facial injury are physical examination and CT. Systematic physical examination can detect deformity, soft tissue injury, cerebrospinal fluid leak, and facial nerve injury. Palpation is used to identify bony stepoffs or midface instability. The eyes are examined for proptosis or enophthalmos, extraocular muscle function, and visual acuity. In patients who cannot cooperate with a physical examination and for whom there is reasonable suspicion of periorbital injury, a forced duction test should be performed. The occlusion is evaluated for subjective or objective malocclusion. Extraocular muscle entrapment, acute enophthalmos, and malocclusion are indications that surgical treatment of facial fractures will be required. Fine-cut CT of the face with direct or reformatted coronal and sagittal views is used to diagnose facial trauma and to direct nonsurgical and surgical treatment. With current CT scanning technology, plain films are not necessary and provide less information. An exception is the Panorex, which is used by many physicians as an adjunct or primary study for mandible fractures and to assess teeth and their roots in particular.

Soft Tissue Injuries

Because of its rich blood supply, even questionable tissue should be salvaged in treating facial lacerations and avulsions. The robust perfusion of facial tissue provides resistance to infection, and repair can be done after a longer delay than would be safe elsewhere on the body. Although there is no strict cutoff, primary repair is generally done up to 24 hours after injury. Even grossly contaminated wounds or those from animal bites are irrigated extensively, débrided, and closed primarily. If there is the possibility of facial nerve injury, this is confirmed by the physical examination finding of weakness or absence of function of a portion of the muscles of facial expression. It is important to recognize a facial nerve laceration so that the distal cut ends can be identified with a nerve stimulator and tagged if they are not to be repaired immediately. Identification of distal stumps by nerve stimulation is not possible after a few days because conduction ceases. Parotid duct injuries should be identified and treated acutely to prevent the formation of sialocele or salivary fistula. In a sharp laceration or penetrating injury to the cheek, a parotid duct injury can be confirmed by direct visualization or injection of dye. This is done by cannulating Stensen duct on the mucosal surface of the cheek and injecting a small amount of methylene blue dye. Extravasation of the dye into the wound indicates a parotid duct laceration, and repair over a stent should be done in the operating room.

Craniofacial Fractures

Current concepts in facial fracture treatment rest on craniofacial techniques to provide surgical exposure of the craniofacial skeleton, anatomic reduction of fractures, and rigid bone fixation with low-profile titanium plates and bone grafting techniques. Failure to reconstruct the bony facial skeleton invariably results in shrinkage and tightening of the facial soft tissue envelope, a sequela that is almost impossible to correct secondarily.

Treatment of forehead fractures involves assessment of the frontal sinus and cranial base. The approach is dictated by injury to the anterior or posterior table of the frontal bone or skull base and whether there is a dural injury or injury to the nasofrontal ducts that drain the frontal sinuses into the nose. Fractures of the upper midface include malar (zygoma) fractures, naso-orbitoethmoid fractures, and orbital fractures. There is considerable overlap in this region. For example, malar fractures occur in association with orbital fractures to a varying degree because the zygoma, in addition to producing cheek projection and determining facial width, is also part of the orbit. Treatment of fractures of the lower midface, the maxilla, focuses on the restoration of the preinjury dental occlusion. It is important to determine the patient's preoperative occlusion; the relationship of the upper and lower teeth is described by the Angle classification.

Maxillary fractures are classified using the LeFort system based on the level at which the midface is separated from the rest of the craniofacial skeleton. Repairs focus on the restoration of facial height and projection. With significant comminution or bone loss, bone grafting may be required to maintain the appropriate position of the maxilla in space. Rigid plate and screw fixation obviates the need for prolonged maxillomandibular fixation. Fractures of the mandible are treated by reduction and rigid fixation using restoration of occlusion as the principle intraoperative and postoperative goal. Many mandibular fractures are treated with open reduction and internal fixation, which may make maxillomandibular fixation unnecessary.[13] Certain fractures, however, are best treated closed, and the decision to pursue an open or closed approach depends on the fracture location and orientation.

The same principles of fracture repair apply in the pediatric patient, with some differences. Early treatment within 1 week is necessary, given the rapid healing in children, and fixation is complicated by the presence of permanent teeth embedded in the maxilla and mandible that are easily damaged by hardware. Resorbable hardware is frequently used for children but does not have the mechanical strength required for most adult fractures.

Scalp Reconstruction

The scalp is composed of skin, subcutaneous tissue, an aponeurotic fascial layer continuous with the frontalis and occipital muscles, a loose areolar layer, and periosteum. Small defects up to a few centimeters in size may be closed primarily, depending on location of the defect and mobility of the surrounding scalp. A skin graft can be placed on intact periosteum. If periosteum is absent, the outer calvarial table can be opened with a burr to expose the diploic space, from which granulation tissue will develop to support a skin graft. In the irradiated scalp or in the case of an open wound with alloplastic material at the base, secondary healing or grafting will not provide stable, durable coverage and a flap will be needed.

Scalp flaps are elevated at the subgaleal level, and many possible designs exist. In theory, defects as large as 30% of the scalp can be closed with scalp flaps elevated on major vessels. Incising, or scoring, the inelastic galea can extend the reach of a scalp flap. Tissue expansion also can be used for the reconstruction of larger defects with hair-bearing tissue.

For large scalp defects not amenable to closure by local remaining scalp, distant flaps may be used. Pedicled flaps with usefulness for scalp coverage include the trapezius, latissimus, and pectoralis major muscle flaps. Pedicled flaps are limited by their arc of rotation, so free microvascular tissue transfer offers more flexibility. The free latissimus dorsi muscle flap is preferred for coverage of near-total or total scalp defects because of its flat contour and ability to cover a large surface area. Traumatic scalp avulsions occur in the subgaleal plane and replantation may be based on a single dominant vessel, with good results.

Facial Reconstruction

Defects of the face are usually the result of tumor resection or trauma. STSG coverage of facial defects has limited application because the tissue match is imperfect. FTSGs are taken from donor sites in the preauricular, postauricular, and supraclavicular areas for the best color match. Local flaps provide tissue of appropriate thickness and have the color and texture of the defect.

Nasal defects up to approximately 1.5 cm in size can be closed with local nasal flaps. For larger defects, the forehead flap is preferred. The forehead flap is based on the supratrochlear vessels, and the reconstruction is performed in a staged fashion. The forehead may be expanded before elevation for closure of larger defects and to assist with primary closure of the donor defect. With nasal defects, different components may be lost, and restoration of skin, mucosal lining, and cartilage may be required. Composite grafts from the ear that contain skin and cartilage are useful for defects of the nasal ala. Reconstruction of total nasal defects is complex and may require bone grafting and free tissue transfer (Fig. 68-7).

In the eyelid, FTSGs are a good option for skin loss alone. For a small, full-thickness lid defect, creating a V-shaped wedge can permit primary closure in layers. Adding a lateral canthotomy helps mobilize the lid margin for closure of larger defects, and in some cases, the incision can be carried out into the temporal skin to mobilize the lid further. Eyelid defects can be repaired with flaps rotated from the other lid; this is useful to provide similar tissue. Extensive eyelid defects require support, typically in the form of a chondromucosal graft obtained from the nasal septum or external ear. The graft is placed and covered with a regional skin flap.

For reconstruction of the cheek, a number of different, smaller local flaps can be designed. For larger defects, cervicofacial rotation flaps mobilize skin from the neck and side of the face for transposition to the more central areas of the face.

In the lip, precise alignment of the vermilion border is critical, as is repair of the orbicularis oris muscle to maintain lip competence. Defects are closed in layers, and direct closure is possible for defects up to one third of the transverse width of the lip. Repair of larger defects requires mobilization of the surrounding tissue to reconstruct the oral sphincter. Central defects of the upper lip are best reconstructed using an Abbe flap, which is a mucosal musculocutaneous flap from the lower lip based on the labial artery. The flap is transferred in a staged fashion, with the

donor pedicle divided 2 to 3 weeks after flap inset. Large defects of the lower lip are reconstructed with mucosal musculocutaneous flaps from the surrounding area. These reconstructions should preserve motor function of the orbicularis muscle, thus ensuring oral competence. Microstomia may be produced but is often temporary because the tissues will stretch over time.

Facial Transplantation

The first successful face transplantation was done in November 2005 in Amiens, France. Since then, there have been more than 28 additional reports of successful facial composite tissue transplantation. All were done for devastating defects and were complex three-dimensional reconstructions, with variable amounts of skin, muscle, nerve, bone, and parts, such as eyelids, noses, and lips. As of early 2015, all the recipients had experienced at least one episode of acute graft rejection of variable severity within the first year of transplantation, and three of the recipients have died—one from sepsis, a second after noncompliance with his immunosuppressive program, and a third with tumor recurrence in an HIV-positive person who had previously had cancer resection. Functional recovery in the faces has been satisfactory in the long-term cases, with sensory function recovering at 3 to 8 months and acceptable motor recovery between 9 and 12 months with ongoing improvement over the years. Psychological outcomes have been positive, and this is related to the psychosocial support provided for these patients. Aesthetic outcomes have been variable.[14]

The benefit of facial transplantation is that for a select number of severely disfigured individuals, it can provide a better functional and aesthetic outcome than conventional reconstructive methods and, in doing so, improve their quality of life. The immediate risks associated with surgery to transplant facial tissues are essentially the same as those for conventional reconstructive procedures. The important difference is the risk posed by the lifelong, multidrug immunosuppression required to prevent rejection of the transplanted facial tissue. It is also assumed that there would be risks associated with the process of facial tissue rejection itself should that occur in any of these patients. At present, no cases of chronic rejection have been reported.

Facial Aesthetic Surgery

Aesthetic surgery starts with an initial patient consultation for discussion and evaluation of the patient's perceptions and wishes, current health and past medical history, and realistic assessment of the benefits and risks of surgery to change appearance. The motivation to have aesthetic surgery is often psychological and involves body image, so the key to achieving success is selection of patients. The core value of the surgery lies not in the objective beauty of the visible result but in the patient's opinion of and response to the change. Thus, being able to predict the likelihood that a patient will be satisfied with the surgical result is critical. Persons who consider their deformities greater than they actually are, who harbor unrealistic expectations, or who have substance abuse or mental health problems are not good candidates for aesthetic surgery because the surgery is unlikely to meet their needs.

Forehead and Brow Lift

With aging, the eyebrow descends below its youthful location at or above the superior orbital rim. This ptosis is accompanied by a wrinkled brow, excess tissue hooding of the upper eyelids (especially in the temporal brow area), and creasing at the outer canthi (crow's feet) and over the dorsum of the upper nose. These changes

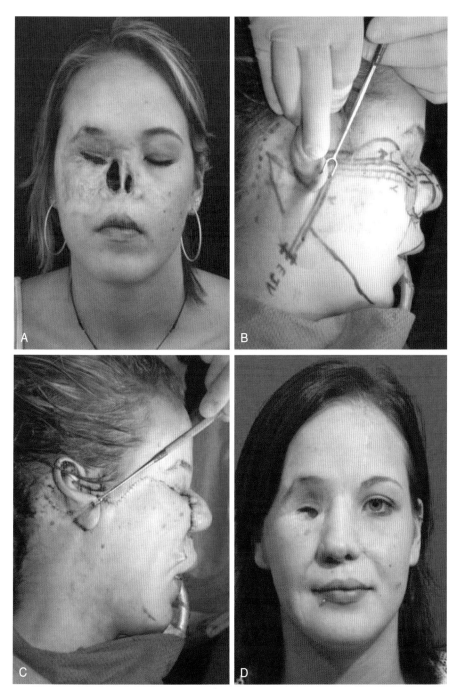

FIGURE 68-7 **A,** This teenager's nose, orbit, and right cheek were obliterated by a shotgun blast. **B,** A cheek flap with a triangular cervical extension is designed. **C,** The cheek skin component is advanced to resurface the anterior cheek. **D,** The result after facial and nasal repair. Surgical procedures included skin grafting of the right cheek and eyelids, a radial forearm microsurgical free tissue transfer for nasal lining, rib grafts to provide nasal skeletal structure, a three-stage pedicle forehead flap for total external nasal reconstruction, and two cheek skin flaps. (From Menick FJ: Discussion: Simplifying cheek reconstruction: A review of over 400 cases. *Plast Reconstr Surg* 129:1300–1303, 2012.)

can be corrected with a forehead or brow lift done as an open or endoscopic procedure. With an open lift, a bicoronal or modified anterior hairline incision is made. The forehead is elevated as a flap with the plane of dissection between the galea and pericranium and drawn taut, and the excess tissue in the frontal scalp is excised. An endoscopic forehead lift is done through several small incisions within the hairline, extensive subperiosteal dissection to include the orbital rim and root of the nose, release and resection of the corrugator and procerus muscles, preservation of the supratrochlear and supraorbital nerves, and forehead elevation and fixation with percutaneous screws or other devices to reattach it in a higher position. The advantages of an endoscopic forehead lift are minimal scarring and no scalp resection; it is especially useful for patients with frontal baldness.

Blepharoplasty

Blepharoplasty, derived from the Greek *blepharon,* meaning "eyelid," is done for dermatochalasis and corrects bagginess, fatty protrusions, and lax hanging skin around the eyes. If the eyelid itself is drooping, this is termed blepharoptosis and is corrected with a different procedure, a ptosis repair.

Upper eyelid blepharoplasty is done through an incision in the crease of the lid after marking the degree of excess skin to prevent overresection and resultant lagophthalmos (inability to close the eye completely). A strip of orbicularis oculi muscle can be taken, and if excess postseptal fat is present, this protruding orbital fat is resected. Lower eyelid blepharoplasty requires elevation of skin or skin–orbicularis oculi muscle flaps, with removal of skin, muscle, and fat. A transconjunctival approach to the lower eyelid is used for removal of lower lid fat or orbital septum tightening, with little or no skin resection. If the lower lid is lax and poorly adherent to the globe, a lateral canthopexy is done for mild laxity and a lateral canthoplasty is performed for significant laxity.

Complications after blepharoplasty include dry eye syndrome, scleral show, and ectropion. All patients should be tested preoperatively for preexisting dry eye, and a Schirmer test may be predictive of this outcome in those who are prone to this. Scleral show is a complication after lower eyelid blepharoplasty in which the white sclera below the colored iris of the globe is exposed when the patient is in forward gaze. Scleral show is caused by lower eyelid retraction, with shortening of the middle lamella of the orbital septum; patients with preoperative laxity of the lower eyelids are predisposed to this complication if the laxity is not addressed at the time of surgery. Ectropion is eversion of the eyelid with exposure of the conjunctiva and is fairly common in the postoperative period, when the lower eyelid is edematous. Persistent ectropion requires surgery to increase lower lid support, possibly with the addition of skin grafts to augment the lower lid tissue.

Facelift

A facelift, or rhytidectomy, derived from the Greek *rhytis,* meaning "wrinkle," is designed to correct the appearance of facial aging by removing lax, redundant facial and neck tissues. Facial aging is characterized by midface infraorbital flattening, prominent nasolabial folds, deepening of the labiomental crease, downturn of the lateral commissures of the mouth, deepening grooves at the outer corners of the mouth (marionette lines), jowl formation, vertical banding of the platysma muscles in the neck, and laxity of the neck skin. The traditional facelift is a subcutaneous dissection to elevate and to redrape the skin of the face and neck. This has been eclipsed by procedures that also correct the effects of aging and gravity on the deeper tissues and structures of the face.

In addition to skin undermining and redraping, the superficial musculoaponeurotic system (SMAS) of the facial and neck fascia can be tightened by plication. With a lateral SMASectomy, a strip of SMAS is excised along the anterior border of the parotid and the mobile SMAS is brought up and sutured to the fixed SMAS at the malar prominence, which produces durable elevation of the superficial fascia and facial fat. It is effective for patients with a wide variety of anatomic differences and is reproducible and safe.

With deep plane rhytidectomy, the facelift flap includes everything down to the fat over the zygomaticus muscles. This procedure corrects midface descent and ptosis but is associated with prolonged facial edema and long recovery.

A number of ancillary procedures are available to enhance the outcome with facelift. Submental lipectomy removes the subcutaneous fat under the chin to improve the contour of the cervical portion of the facelift. Platysmaplasty corrects vertical banding by incising the platysma muscles at the level of the thyroid cartilage and suturing them together in the midline of the upper neck. Fat injection to selected areas under the facelift flaps before closure can fill hollows caused by subcutaneous fat atrophy in areas such as the temple.

Hematoma is the most common complication after facelift; other complications include scarring, alopecia, skin slough, and nerve injury. The most common nerve injury during facelift, occurring at a rate of 3% to 5%, involves the greater auricular nerve, which provides sensation to the lower ear.

Rhinoplasty

Rhinoplasty is a difficult operation because it is a composite of procedures on a number of anatomic structures. When a patient describes a large nose or a long nose, this global description may encompass a dozen contributing structures. Laying the groundwork for a rhinoplasty starts with analysis of the facial proportions, followed by systematic analysis of the nasal components. Starting superiorly, the nasal frontal angle height and depth are noted. The bony pyramid, upper lateral cartilages, and supratip are evaluated for their height, width, and symmetry. The nasal tip is analyzed in terms of its projection, rotation, symmetry, and position of the tip-defining points. The alae are inspected for increased width, collapse, or retraction. The columella is examined for increased or decreased show, and the columellar-labial angle is measured. An internal nasal examination determines whether there is functional deformity by evaluating the septum, turbinates, and internal nasal valves. The soft tissue envelope and thickness of the skin are studied so the effect of underlying changes can be predicted.

Once thorough analysis is complete, this is converted into a surgical plan of action. The initial decision is whether to use an open or endonasal approach. The open rhinoplasty affords excellent exposure and makes it possible to manipulate the osteocartilaginous framework under direct vision. The closed rhinoplasty avoids a visible scar. After the surgical approach is decided on, the rest of the strategy involves choosing techniques based on location-specific criteria. These could include an osteotomy for changing the bony contour of the upper third of the nose, spreader grafts and dorsal resection of the upper lateral cartilages for internal valve collapse and dorsal contour in the middle third of the nose, resection and interdomal sutures for tip refinement and symmetry in the lower third of the nose, and columellar resection or a strut graft for overprojection or loss of tip support at the base of the nose.

The most common surgical complication with rhinoplasty is bleeding, which occurs in up to 3.6% of patients. A more challenging issue is that approximately 5% to 10% of patients require revision or a secondary rhinoplasty for aesthetic or functional reasons. The goal in rhinoplasty is to produce reliable, long-lasting, and natural-appearing results with consistency. It is thought that the key to achieving this goal is component analysis and management of the dorsal, tip, base, and internal nasal structures.[15]

Skin Resurfacing

Several modalities are available to improve the texture, tone, and color of the skin. These include chemical peeling and dermabrasion, but the most rapidly growing technique for skin rejuvenation is laser technology. The use of light as a medical treatment was introduced in the 1960s with the development of the laser (light amplification by stimulated emission of radiation). Ablative lasers (CO_2 and erbium:YAG) have proved highly effective for skin treatment. Removing the epidermis and upper layers of the dermis, this ablation, combined with thermal coagulation of the dermis, heals with robust dermal remodeling that translates into clinical improvement. The problem was resultant scarring in some patients, prolonged edema and erythema, permanent pigmentation abnormalities, and increased risk of infection. Thus, a new concept of fractional photothermolysis was introduced in 2003, which has revolutionized laser surgery. Fractional CO_2 laser resurfacing represents a new class of therapy by delivering dermal coagulative injury without confluent epidermal damage. Distinct lesions of thermal damage are surrounded by larger zones of undisturbed normal skin; this combination allows complete reepithelialization within 24 to 48 hours while producing enough coagulation of the dermal collagen to stimulate connective tissue synthesis and to produce skin tightening. With the fractional approach, results are comparable to those with full-surface ablative lasers without the associated side effects.[16]

The indications for laser resurfacing are facial rhytides, sun-damaged skin, and acne scarring. Benefits of treatment include softening or disappearance of mild to moderate wrinkles, improved skin texture and tone, decreased pore size, and reduction of skin laxity. The entire face, neck, and chest can be treated. Clinical improvement is seen with one or two treatments, scarring and hypopigmentation are rare, and the risk of infection in patients given prophylactic antiviral and antibiotic medications is low because the epidermal layer is restored promptly. When used to treat scars, fractional photothermolysis can flatten out and smooth hypertrophic scars and increases collagen production beneath depressed, atrophic scars, which summate in smoothing of the skin topography. For scarring, a series of treatments at 6- to 12-week intervals may be needed.

Injectable Fillers

In the last few years, there has been more appreciation for the role that loss of volume plays in the contours of the aging face. Contrasting the youthful and aging face shows that areas such as the upper and lateral cheek, temple, nasojugal groove under the eye, and perioral area become atrophic, flat, and hollow in appearance. Restoring volume to reverse the atrophic changes in these areas produces a surprising rejuvenative change.

Volume restoration procedures can include lipotransfer of autologous fat or the use of an increasing number of materials, temporary or permanent, for soft tissue augmentation. Fat grafting is a technique-dependent procedure in which atraumatic handling and methodic layering of the autologous fat is emphasized for long-lasting results. An unexpected finding is that in addition to the volume restoration, fat grafting appears to have rejuvenative effects on the skin itself. The quality of the skin appears to be improved, with softening of wrinkles, decreased pore size, and more even pigmentation.[17] Similar observations are made when fat is injected beneath depressed scars; not only the indentation but the character of the skin itself appears to improve. With reports of the transformative power of fat grafted in areas of radiation damage, chronic ulcers, and other defects, there is much

interest in documenting the extent and identifying the mechanism of these effects.[18]

In addition to autologous material, a number of biologic and synthetic products are available for use as soft tissue fillers. Biologic materials derived from organic sources offer the benefits of ready off-the-shelf availability and ease of use but introduce issues of sensitization to foreign animal or human proteins, transmission of disease, and immunogenicity. Also, as the tissue is processed to reduce these untoward side effects, the molecular structure is destabilized so that lack of persistence at the recipient site becomes the rule. The search during the last few years has been for new materials that are better tolerated and have greater longevity. The two major types of biologic tissue fillers are collagen products and hyaluronic acid products.[19]

Synthetic materials can offer permanence. Many injectable and surgically implantable synthetic products have been used over the years, and many have been condemned for complications such as granulomas, acute and delayed infections, migration or displacement, and deformity, which can result from complications or if the material is removed. Thus, only a limited number of synthetic materials are marketed in the United States for facial augmentation.

PLASTIC SURGERY OF THE TRUNK

Reconstruction of the Chest Wall

New techniques for repair of increasingly complex chest wall defects have accompanied advances in surgical and medical treatment of thoracic disease. Indications for chest wall reconstruction include defects arising from oncologic resection, irradiation ulceration, infection, trauma, and congenital defects. Considerations with reconstruction are the status of the pleural cavity, requirement for skeletal support, and provision of soft tissue coverage.

For management of the pleural cavity, principles include adequate débridement and the introduction of well-vascularized tissue to obliterate intrathoracic dead space. Extrathoracic muscles can be transposed to obliterate empyema spaces after pneumonectomy and to close bronchopleural or tracheoesophageal fistulas. Combined with adequate débridement and resection of poorly vascularized tissue, these muscle flaps can be passed through a thoracotomy incision with a two-rib resection and sutured into the defect, with thoracostomy drainage. The choice of muscle depends on the location of the defect; options include the latissimus dorsi, serratus anterior, and pectoralis major muscle flaps. Other muscle flaps with limited but specific uses are the trapezius and superiorly based rectus abdominis. The greater omentum can be transposed on the right gastroepiploic artery as a pedicle flap to provide well-vascularized tissue with the bulk and pliability to obliterate dead space, but it is a secondary choice because of the risks of intra-abdominal complications.

In evaluation of a chest wall defect, a number of variables influence the decision about whether skeletal reconstruction or stabilization is required. These include the site of the chest wall defect, number of ribs resected, extent of resection of other bony structures of the chest wall, history of irradiation, and whether there is wound contamination or infection. The goals of skeletal reconstruction are protection of underlying vital structures, chest wall stability to preserve pulmonary function, and structural support for shoulder and upper limb function.

The number of resected ribs is accepted as the primary clinical determinant of the need for skeletal reconstruction. Stabilization is recommended with resection of four or more consecutive ribs, or 5 cm or more of lateral chest wall, because the resulting flail segment may impair respiratory mechanics. However, there are no conclusive data about the critical size for flail segment reconstruction, and studies of pulmonary ventilation deficits from skeletal chest resection are controversial, particularly in the case of sternal resection.[20] Some of this lack of clarity may be caused by the presence of other factors that influence chest wall stability. Prior irradiation changes affect chest wall stability because soft tissues with radiation fibrosis have the rigidity and stiffness to limit chest wall motion. Location of the defect is relevant because lateral defects are more prone to flail chest deformity than those stabilized by proximity to the sternum or spine. Pancoast tumor resections are stabilized by scapular support, and upper chest wall defects above the fourth rib generally can be closed with soft tissue only.

In the past, reconstruction of the chest skeleton with rib bone grafts or fascia lata was constrained by the limited availability of autologous tissue. One of the important advances in chest wall reconstruction has been the availability of suitable synthetic materials. The ideal characteristics of prosthetic material for chest wall reconstruction are semirigidity, flexibility, biocompatibility, and radiolucency. Several mesh materials are available, including polypropylene (Prolene), crystalline polypropylene and high-density polyethylene (Marlex), and polytetrafluoroethylene (Gore-Tex). Manufactured in a thick sheet, or doubled by folding, these materials provide support and malleability when sutured under tension. If additional rigidity is desired, methyl methacrylate glue can be sandwiched between sheets of mesh and allowed to harden into a rigid shell incorporated within the mesh. These synthetic materials provide good support and stability and perform well, provided they are covered with well-vascularized tissue to prevent infection. Chest wall infections in the presence of synthetic materials can be managed with drainage and antibiotic therapy; if removal of the foreign material can be delayed, a thickened fibrous layer will form to furnish some chest wall stability. In situations in which a chest defect is contaminated or infected at the outset, consideration can be given to the use of a temporary absorbable mesh, but this may have to be replaced when the infection has cleared.

Soft tissue coverage is the final stage of chest wall reconstruction. If a chest wall defect is limited to the skin and subcutaneous tissues, a skin graft is a reconstructive option. Its drawbacks are the eventual contraction that makes it a less attractive form of coverage than a flap and the poor success with graft healing on an irradiated bed. Thus, for chest wall defects with a radiation ulcer or osteoradionecrosis, there is little indication for a skin graft. The healing of skin grafts on the chest wall has been enhanced by the use of the vacuum-assisted closure device, which improves graft stabilization on a bed that is in motion with respiration.

In chest wall reconstruction, vascularized soft tissue flaps are used to close larger defects, to control infection, to obliterate dead space, to cover synthetic materials, and to close wounds with radiation necrosis. Although skin flaps or fasciocutaneous flaps are of some use, the muscle or musculocutaneous pedicle flap is preferred for its robust blood supply. The latissimus dorsi muscle is used frequently for its reliability, large area, and ability to reach almost any chest wall defect on the ipsilateral thorax. Other muscle flaps used for anterolateral soft tissue reconstruction include rectus abdominis, pectoralis major, external oblique, and serratus anterior. Trapezius muscle flaps are useful for defects of the upper third of the back, midback, and shoulders. Free flaps that transfer distant tissue with microvascular anastomoses are not often used and are reserved for situations in which regional flaps are unavailable or have failed or for very large defects. In one series in which aggressive resections of oncologic disease left chest wall defects as large as 300 to 400 cm², up to four muscle flaps and free flaps were required to achieve wound closure.[21]

One series of 200 chest wall reconstructions reported a mortality of 6%, with complete or partial flap loss in 5% of patients and pneumonia, respiratory distress, infection, hematoma, and delayed wound healing in 27% of patients. Results were better in patients having immediate reconstruction at the time of resection than in those having delayed reconstruction.[22]

Sternotomy Wounds: Treatment and Prevention

Sternal wound infection and mediastinitis after median sternotomy often require reoperation for débridement and reconstruction. Risk factors include diabetes, smoking, chronic obstructive pulmonary disease, immunosuppression, harvest of internal mammary artery grafts, and use of assist devices. Primary rigid plate fixation of the sternum decreases the incidence of serious complications, and there is current enthusiasm for introducing this surgical method for prevention in high-risk situations.

For sternal instability or infection, débridement, use of wound vacuum-assisted closure devices, muscle and omental flaps, and fixation of the sternum have been described. Although minimal débridement may be needed in the wounds without costochondritis or osteomyelitis, single-stage or serial débridement bridged by vacuum-assisted closure as a sole or adjunct measure for definitive closure of the sternum may be required.[23] Fixation of the separated remaining sternal bone with plates before soft tissue coverage is advocated for earlier extubation, shorter length of stay, a more stable base for an overlying flap, and less long-term chest or shoulder pain. The pectoralis major muscle is the flap of choice for reconstruction of median sternotomy wounds. It is mobilized through the midline incision by detaching it from the sternum, ribs, clavicle, and humeral insertion while preserving the thoracoacromial pedicle (Fig. 68-8). It is advanced medially and, because of its size and arc of rotation, can cover almost the entire sternum. If an aortic vascular graft is exposed, the muscle is mobile enough to wrap around the graft and fill the mediastinum. Another option with the pectoralis major muscle is a turnover flap, in which one or both muscles are left attached on either side of the midline on the perforating branches of the internal mammary artery, dissected free from the remainder of the chest wall, and turned over like a book page to cover the sternum. If the pectoralis muscles are not sufficient, which is sometimes the case over the lower third of the sternum, the rectus abdominis muscle can be mobilized. This is based on the superior epigastric artery and rotated 180 degrees to cover the sternum. If this is done in a patient in whom the ipsilateral internal mammary artery has been harvested for bypass grafting, the rectus abdominis muscle flap can be based on the eighth intercostal vessel; but with this as the pedicle, the distal third may be poorly vascularized. With muscle flap reconstruction, the rates of successful sternal closure are approximately 85%.[24]

The greater omentum has been used for 40 years for the closure of sternal defects and provides reliable coverage. It has been claimed that omentum controls median sternotomy infection more successfully than pedicle muscle flaps, but it has been less commonly used because of exposure of the peritoneal cavity to infection, possibility of later intraperitoneal adhesions, and unavailability of omentum in some patients with previous abdominal surgery. Bringing the omentum into the anterior medi-

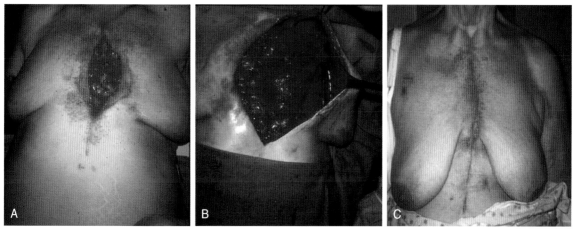

FIGURE 68-8 **A,** 62-year-old woman 1 month after coronary artery bypass procedure with an open infected median sternotomy incision. **B,** The sternal wound was extensively débrided and covered with bilateral pectoralis major muscle flaps. Because the blood supply to the internal mammary perforators was damaged, each pectoralis major muscle was based on its thoracoacromial vascular pedicle after the insertion on the humerus and origin from the ribs was divided to permit muscle transposition. **C,** Postoperative result at 3 months.

astinum through a transdiaphragmatic opening has been recently described.[25]

Breast Surgery

Reduction Mammaplasty

Hypertrophy or overgrowth of the breast is excessive development without any pathologic process. It can be familial, with a typical onset during puberty and pregnancy, when hormonal changes exert an abnormal influence on growth in some individuals. Reduction mammaplasty is the resection of excess fat, breast tissue, and skin to achieve a breast size proportional to the body. The principles guiding reduction mammaplasty for breast hypertrophy are to improve the patient's symptoms, to decrease the volume of the breast, to reshape the breast to correct ptosis, to elevate the breast tissue to an anatomically correct position on the chest wall, to reposition the nipple and areola on the reduced and reshaped breast, to preserve the nerve supply to the skin and nipple-areola complex, to maintain blood supply to the breast tissue, and to minimize scars. Surgical techniques are described by the location of the block of tissue to which the nipple and areola are left attached and by the pattern of incisions and subsequent scars.

The pedicle is the portion of the breast tissue preserved with its blood and nerve supply while the surrounding breast tissue is removed. An inferior pedicle technique is used most often, but there are central, superior, medial, lateral, and doubly attached vertical and horizontal pedicles. All variants are designed to maximize blood supply while allowing adequate tissue removal. Suction-assisted lipectomy is used with excision techniques to remove excess fat laterally, and there are a small number of patients with mild to moderate hypertrophy, fatty breasts, good skin tone, no ptosis, and good breast shape for whom liposuction alone will reduce volume, with small scars. In the very large pendulous breast, in which the pedicle would be exceptionally long, the nipple-areola complex is removed and transplanted as a graft. This technique is useful also for patients with vascular disorders or impaired wound healing.

Before reduction mammaplasty, breast cancer screening with examination and mammography usually is done in patients 35 years of age and older. A small number of breast cancers are discovered at the time of reduction by identifying a suspicious area or during routine pathologic study of the tissue; all breast tissue removed surgically should be sent for histopathologic study. There is no set lower age limit, but for the adolescent with breast hypertrophy, reduction is deferred until the breasts have stopped growing and are stable in size for at least 12 months before surgery. Secondary or repeated breast reduction has a higher complication rate because problems associated with a damaged blood supply, such as delayed wound healing, fat necrosis, and loss of the nipple and areola, are seen when a pedicle is developed again in a previously reduced breast. Wound healing is impaired in the previously irradiated breast because of radiation-induced vascular changes. Recommendations in these patients include the following: delay between radiation and mammaplasty to allow some of the vascular changes to subside; and technical modifications using pedicles that are broader and shorter than usual and minimizing adjustments to the breast tissue. Obese patients are poor candidates for breast reductions, with more local and systemic complications. Smoking is a contraindication to breast reduction.

Sequelae of reduction mammaplasty include changes in the sensibility of the nipple and areola in 20% to 25% of cases, usually a decrease but occasionally an increase in sensation. Lactation and breastfeeding are not always possible after breast reduction. Complications with reduction mammaplasty include wound dehiscence, skin slough, loss of tissue, hematoma, infection, and fat necrosis with palpable nodules of poorly vascularized fat. Fat necrosis may prompt later investigation or biopsy to distinguish these lumps from breast neoplasms.

Outcome studies after reduction mammaplasty have shown that patients gain relief from symptoms, can engage more in activities of daily life, and are happy with the results. In one study of 185 women, 97% reported improvement in back, shoulder, and neck pain; 95% said they were happy or very happy with the results of surgery, and 98% said they would recommend it to others.[26]

Breast Augmentation

Augmentation mammaplasty is a cosmetic procedure done to resolve the dissatisfaction that some women feel with small breasts, either because their breasts never developed to a desired size or because their breasts lost volume after pregnancy or weight loss or with aging. With the development of the sealed silicone gel breast implant in 1962, breast augmentation became widely accepted. All U.S. Food and Drug Administration–approved breast implants, regardless of filling material, have an outer shell or envelope constructed of silicone elastomer. Silicone gel–filled implants are polymerized to a consistency similar to that of breast tissue. Newer gel implants have a thicker, more viscous gel than previous generations of these devices. Called cohesive gel, the material tends to stay in place, even if the shell of the implant is damaged. Gel implants are prefilled and sealed and cannot be adjusted in size in the operating room. Saline-filled implants are silicone rubber shells filled in the operating room. Advantages of the saline implants are the benign nature of saline, some flexibility in adjusting size by varying the amount of fluid put in the implant, and smaller incisions because the implants are inserted while empty. The primary disadvantage is a higher incidence of visible rippling or wrinkling of the implant under the skin, particularly in thin patients.

Breast augmentation requires an incision in the skin and subcutaneous tissue, with creation of a pocket in which a breast implant is placed and positioned. There are a number of technical variations. One of three incisions can be used, each with advantages and drawbacks. The inframammary incision provides excellent access and does not require dissection within the breast parenchyma; the disadvantage is a scar that may be noticeable in the smaller breast. A periareolar incision is camouflaged in the areola and heals with little visible scarring but has the disadvantage of possible changes in sensation in the nipple-areola area. An axillary incision leaves no scars on the breast, but it is more difficult to create the pocket with this approach. The pocket into which the implant will be placed can be in one of two positions relative to the breast tissue and pectoralis major muscle. Subglandular placement superficial to the pectoralis muscle fascia provides more ability to control the shape of the breast and is associated with a more rapid postoperative recovery. With submuscular placement of the implant, the contour of the breast may be smoother because the edges of the implant are blunted by the muscle, there is less chance for development of capsular contracture (hardened scar around the implant), nipple sensation is protected, and mammogram interpretation may be more accurate when the breast tissue is lifted up and away from the implant by the muscle. Disadvantages include more postoperative discomfort and longer recovery, movement of the implant when the muscle is flexed, and less ability to lift the parenchyma in a breast with some degree of ptosis.

In considering potential problems that can develop after augmentation mammaplasty, it is useful to distinguish between operative complications and implant concerns. Perioperative complications are relatively low, with bleeding or hematoma in 1% to 3%, wound infections in 1% to 2%, and some degree of diminished sensibility of the nipple-areola complex in approximately 15% of patients, depending on the incision used and position of the implant relative to the muscle. More numerous and more serious are the sequelae presenting weeks or years after the surgery. These include capsular contracture, implant deflation, implant rupture, and implant displacement.

Capsular contraction occurs when the normal envelope of fibrous tissue around an implant becomes thicker or tighter so that the implant no longer feels soft and pliant. If the degree of capsular contracture is great, there can be pain, distortion, and palpability or distortion of the implant. Capsular contracture occurs in approximately 15% of patients, and it is not possible to predict who will develop it or to take preventive measures. Treatment involves removing the fibrous capsule surgically and replacing the implant, but this often results in recurrence of the capsular contracture. The only permanent correction is removal of the implant.

Saline-filled implants can deflate when the fluid leaks out of the implant through the valve or implant shell. This occurs in approximately 7% of patients within the first 5 years after surgery. Causes include damage from handling at the time of surgery, pressure from capsular contracture, compression of the implant due to trauma, and other reasons that remain unknown.

Silicone gel implants can rupture, releasing the gel material; its frequency is similar to that of deflation of saline implants. However, there is an important difference in how the rupture is detected. When a gel implant ruptures, the breast volume will not change because the gel remains in the area; in many cases, the rupture remains undiagnosed—a silent rupture. Thus, it is recommended that gel implants be studied by MRI at intervals of 3 to 5 years so that silent ruptures can be detected and treated. Mammography is not a reliable diagnostic tool for rupture, and surveillance with MRI is the standard.[27]

Three areas of extensive study have been the questions of whether breast implants are associated with breast cancer, whether a type of anaplastic large cell lymphoma (ALCL) is associated with breast implants, and whether the silicone material in breast implants is associated with connective tissue disease. No study has ever suggested that the presence of a breast implant is a cause of breast cancer. The primary question has been whether the presence of an implant is responsible for delayed detection or poorer prognosis because of compromise of screening mammography. Standard mammograms in a woman with breast implants show only approximately 75% of the breast tissue because the remainder is obscured by the implant. Displacement techniques are used to address this, and additional views are needed. Studies have shown no significant difference between women with and without implants who develop breast cancer in terms of the size or stage of the tumor when it is diagnosed. One series of 3182 women observed for 18.7 years after breast augmentation has shown no increased risk, no delay in diagnosis, and no worse prognosis for these patients compared with a comparable group of women without implants.[28]

There is substantial evidence that a type of ALCL is associated with breast implants. As of 2015, there are reports of 173 patients with breast implants who developed ALCL in the breast. The clinical course seems to be unusually benign compared with other systemic ALCL, but many of the patients are treated with radiation therapy or chemotherapy.[29] Work to standardize an approach to diagnosis, staging, and treatment is currently under way.

Concern about the association of breast implants with the development of autoimmune or connective tissue diseases, such as lupus, scleroderma, or rheumatoid arthritis, arose because of cases reported in the literature in the early 1980s. A number of subsequent epidemiologic analyses failed to support this association, and a committee of the Institute of Medicine of the National Academy of Sciences reviewed more than 2000 peer-reviewed studies and 1200 data sets. In 1999, the Institute of Medicine concluded that there was no definitive evidence linking breast implants to cancer, immunologic disease, or neurologic disease and that women with breast implants were no more likely to develop these disorders than those in the rest of the population.

Breast Ptosis and Mastopexy

Breast ptosis describes the downward displacement of the glandular tissue of the breast. Sagging and drooping develop when lax skin with poor elasticity cannot support and shape the underlying breast parenchyma and the fascial attachments, the suspensory ligaments of Cooper, lose elasticity and become attenuated. These changes are seen with significant weight loss, postpartum atrophy, postmenopausal involution, and the continual gravitational pull associated with aging. Breast ptosis is classified by the position of the nipple-areola complex relative to the inframammary fold and breast mound; the degree of ptosis is considered in choosing the technique for surgical correction. There are numerous options for mastopexy, and these draw on both breast reduction and breast augmentation techniques. The key elements are the removal and tightening of redundant skin and breast tissue and the possible addition of a breast implant. The primary intention when introducing a breast implant is not increased size; rather, the implant adds volume to the flattened upper pole of the breast and provides support and lift for a soft, involuted breast with thin, inelastic skin. The challenge with mastopexy is balancing tightening with restoration of volume. The effects of surgery are only temporary, and ptosis recurs with the passage of time, depending on the age of the patient, the cause of the ptosis, the size of the breast, and whether an implant was used.

Fat Grafting to the Breast

Autologous fat injection into the breast has been used successfully for breast enlargement, correction of breast deformities, additional coverage to disguise breast implants, and treatment of radiation damage to the chest. Historically, there was concern that injected fat would not survive and fat necrosis or calcification might impede breast cancer screening. However, drawing on experience with fat grafting in the face, techniques for harvesting fat with minimal trauma and injecting it into the breast in small aliquots were described. By taking care to avoid placing large amounts of fat at one site, the incidence of fat necrosis is lower, and lipografting in the breast is being done much more commonly. Adjunctive techniques include expanding the skin envelope and generating a recipient matrix before serial seeding with micrografts, placing the grafts outside the breast parenchyma itself, and layering the fat into different levels. With evidence that technical performance is critical, excellent long-lasting results are being reported.[30] An area of intense interest and scrutiny is the use of adipose stem cells in fat grafting for breast enlargement. Still largely theoretical in clinical practice, the possibility of stimulating permanent fat survival in the breast is being weighed against the risk of introducing growing cell lines into tissue that will develop malignancy in some percentage of the treated population.

Gynecomastia

Male breast enlargement occurs bilaterally in 50% to 55% of cases; most patients are asymptomatic or report some tenderness, soreness, or sensitivity. Caused by an increased estrogen to androgen ratio, the incidence is increased with generalized obesity because of increased conversion of testosterone to estradiol in adipose tissue. On histologic evaluation, variable degrees of ductal proliferation and stromal hyperplasia present in three patterns, described as florid, intermediate, or fibrous. The florid pattern shows ductal hyperplasia surrounded by loose cellular connective tissue. The fibrous pattern has extensive fibrosis of the stroma with little ductal proliferation and is seen with gynecomastia longer than 1 year in duration. The intermediate pattern represents a transition between the florid and fibrous types.

There are physiologic, pathologic, and pharmacologic causes. Physiologic or idiopathic gynecomastia, with no pathologic basis, develops transiently in more than 60% of newborns because of exposure to transplacental estrogens. During puberty, estrogen and testosterone shifts result in a prevalence of 50% to 60%, with presentation during midpuberty (14 years) and a self-limited average duration of 1 to 2 years. With increasing age, the prevalence gradually increases to more than 70% in the seventh decade. Pathologic gynecomastia is associated with cirrhosis, malnutrition, hypogonadism, Klinefelter syndrome, renal disease, hyperthyroidism, hypothyroidism, and neoplastic disease. Tumors that may lead to gynecomastia are testicular tumors (e.g., Leydig cell and Sertoli cell tumors, choriocarcinomas), adrenal tumors, pituitary adenomas, and lung carcinoma. Gynecomastia is not associated with male breast cancer except in patients with Klinefelter syndrome, in whom the incidence of mammary carcinoma is 20 to 60 times greater than in men without this chromosomal aberration. Pharmacologic gynecomastia is caused by drugs from a number of classes, including antiandrogens, antibiotics, chemotherapeutic agents, cardiovascular disease drugs, and drugs of abuse (e.g., alcohol, heroin, amphetamines, marijuana).

For the patient presenting with gynecomastia, pertinent history includes duration, concomitant disease, and medication use. The breasts, thyroid, abdomen, testes, and overall degree of virilization are examined. Laboratory studies include determinations of hormone levels and, as indicated, additional selected studies, such as checking karyotype, testicular ultrasound, hepatic or renal function tests, mammography, and imaging studies of the chest or adrenals. Treatment of an underlying disorder may lead to regression of gynecomastia, especially when an offending medication can be identified and withdrawn in drug-related cases or when testosterone is administered for testicular failure. However, gynecomastia of long duration, with a fibrous pattern, is unlikely to resolve spontaneously.

Indications for surgery include symptomatic gynecomastia, enlargement persisting for more than 18 to 24 months in adolescent boys, gynecomastia of long duration that has progressed to fibrosis, and gynecomastia in patients at risk for breast cancer (e.g., those with Klinefelter syndrome). Surgical approaches depend on the degree of enlargement and whether there is associated ptosis (drooping) of the breasts. For patients with mild to moderate gynecomastia with minimal drooping, there are several options, including suction-assisted liposuction, ultrasound-assisted liposuction, direct excision through a small incision confined to the areola, and a combination of these techniques. For the patient with moderate to large gynecomastia and associated laxity and descent of the breast, skin resection and transposition of the nipple-areola complex superiorly to an appropriate position on the chest wall are required. This necessitates additional incisions, with resultant scarring; there are various techniques to minimize the appearance of these scars. For the patient with massive gynecomastia, an en bloc resection of excessive skin and breast tissue is needed, with free nipple grafting or repositioning of the nipple-areola complex on a pedicle flap.[31]

The challenge with surgical excision of gynecomastia is achieving perfect symmetry of the two breasts and producing a smooth contour, without indentations or irregularities. Suction-assisted lipectomy is helpful to smooth the contours and to taper the area of resection into the surrounding subcutaneous tissue on the chest wall to make it undetectable. Postoperative complications include hematoma or seroma caused by the extensive dissection and undermining of the skin through a small incision; these can be mitigated with good hemostasis and the use of drains and compression garments. Less common complications include infection and tissue loss, including loss of a portion of the nipple-areola complex.

Congenital and Developmental Deformities

Breast and chest wall deformities range from hyperplastic anomalies, such as polymastia and polythelia, to hypoplastic deformational anomalies characterized by a paucity of breast tissue, as seen in Poland syndrome. Described by Alfred Poland in 1841, this syndrome is a severe form of chest wall and breast hypoplasia that occurs in approximately 1 in 25,000 live births. It occurs sporadically, is generally unilateral, and affects males more frequently than females (3:1). The syndrome includes a spectrum of deformities, the most consistent of which is absence of the sternocostal head of the pectoralis major muscle. Other features can include absence of the ipsilateral pectoralis major and minor muscles, absence of the anterior portions of ribs 2 to 5, loss of the latissimus dorsi and serratus anterior muscles, absence of axillary hair, limited subcutaneous chest wall fat, and brachysyndactyly of the ipsilateral hand. There can be absence of the breast or a varying degree of hypoplasia, and the nipple can be absent or displaced.

Treatment options for Poland syndrome include autologous tissue, alone or in combination with synthetic implant materials, to correct the contour deformity of the chest wall and to reconstruct the breast. Because of its proximity, a pedicled latissimus dorsi muscle flap is preferred if the muscle itself is not involved; as an alternative, the rectus abdominis muscle can be introduced as a pedicle or free flap. The timing of surgery requires careful consideration. In general, reconstruction is deferred until late adolescence to avoid the risk of growth inhibition with early operative trauma and to minimize the need for multiple revisions to keep pace with chest wall and breast growth.

Abdominal Wall Surgery
Components Separation and Flap Coverage

Acquired abdominal wall defects are caused by incisional hernia, tumor resection, infection, irradiation, and trauma. The goals of abdominal wall reconstruction are protection of the abdominal contents, restoration of the integrity of the musculofascial wall, and provision of dynamic muscle support. Treatment is selected on the basis of a number of factors, including the medical status of the patient, wound bed preparedness, size of the defect, position of the defect, and whether there is loss of stable skin and subcutaneous tissue or loss of myofascial tissue. If skin coverage and myofascial continuity are absent, the defect is a complete, full-thickness loss, and both layers will have to be restored by more complex approaches.

The timing of immediate versus delayed reconstruction depends on the clinical situation. Assessment of the patient includes body mass index and pulmonary evaluation because postoperative loss of domain may decrease vital capacity, total lung capacity, and functional residual capacity.[32] Nutritional status, tobacco use, and fluid and electrolyte imbalance are corrected. Assessment of the wound bed includes identification of bacterial contamination, exposed viscera, adherent bowel, enterocutaneous fistulas, previous irradiation, prosthetic material used in previous operations, and previous incisions or scars that interrupt the abdominal circulation. The presence of inflammation and edema, even in a clean wound, limits local tissue advancement; significant inflammation may be present after dehiscence, traumatic defects, fistulas, or recent infection.

Immediate and one-stage reconstruction of a wall defect is the approach of choice for a patient who is medically stable, with a clean wound bed and reliable reconstructive options. This approach is suitable for patients having ventral herniorrhaphy or tumor extirpation requiring concomitant reconstruction. Definitive repair is delayed if the patient is unstable, the wound is contaminated, further explorations are planned, or there is abdominal distention or inflammation. In these cases, the wound is managed with skin grafts, prosthetic mesh, or vacuum-assisted closure device as a temporary measure until reconstruction can be done.

STSGs have a high rate of success (even in colonized wounds), provide stable coverage to protect from infection, and prevent continued fluid and protein loss from granulation tissue. In addition, they aid in eventual closure by reducing the size of the wound through contracture. The problem is that STSGs become fixed to the viscera on which they are placed; the consequences of skin grafting include hernia, abdominal wall bulge, and possible trauma to the viscera. Later reconstruction involving removal of the skin grafts should be delayed for a minimum of 6 months, until the wound has matured. This will decrease the density of the adhesions and scar tissue and help control the rate of inadvertent enterotomy, which converts a clean case in which prosthetic mesh could be used into a contaminated one.

If temporary fascial support of a contaminated wound is needed to prevent evisceration and to maintain domain, an absorbable mesh can be used while the acute problems are addressed. Absorbable mesh made from polyglycolic acid can remain in place for 3 to 4 months, protecting the intra-abdominal contents and providing support while granulation tissue develops and is skin grafted. This type of mesh undergoes hydrolytic degradation, so its usefulness is temporally limited because of loss of structural strength, with ulceration and delayed hernia formation. If it is left in place, there will be eventual loss of support, but there will be no difficulty in removing the prosthetic material 6 to 12 months later in a patient undergoing definitive repair of the defect.

The vacuum-assisted closure device is effective for temporary closure of an abdominal wall defect by providing the support of a nondistensible dressing, limiting fascial retraction by applying constant medial tension, and stimulating granulation tissue growth. With modification of the standard vacuum pack dressing, visceral adherence to the abdominal wall can be limited, whereas fascial closure is encouraged. Studies in a laboratory model have shown that the vacuum-assisted closure device results in a fourfold increase in vascularization to the wound, decreased bacterial colonization, increased formation of granulation tissue by 103%, and increased flap survival by 21% compared with controls.[33]

In planning of definitive repair, reconstructive options are considered in terms of the type of abdominal wall defect, which can be broadly classified into one of three categories:

Loss of skin and subcutaneous tissue only. These partial defects are closed primarily if small, with skin grafting, random or local flaps, fasciocutaneous flaps, vacuum-assisted closure device, or tissue expander before primary closure.

Loss of musculofascial tissue, with intact skin coverage. These partial defects are repaired with prosthetic mesh or with

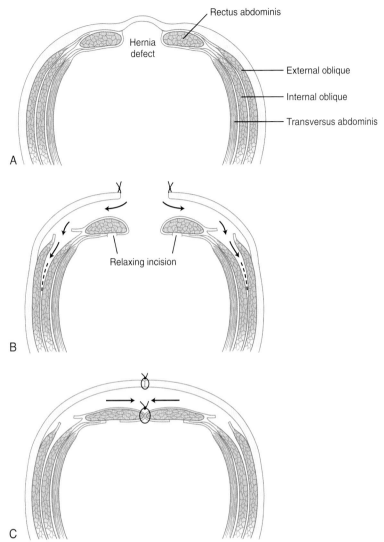

Rectus abdominis

Hernia defect

External oblique

Internal oblique

Transversus abdominis

A

Relaxing incision

B

C

FIGURE 68-9 Components separation to mobilize the musculofascial tissue for closure of a midline abdominal wall defect. **A,** Anterior midline abdominal wall defect. **B,** Anterior rectus sheath separated from the external oblique aponeurosis. Longitudinal relaxing incisions are made anteriorly along the linea semilunaris and posteriorly in the posterior rectus sheath. **C,** Relaxing incisions in anterior and posterior rectus sheath. These allow stretching of the rectus muscle as the anterior rectus wall is pulled medially to correct the defect. (From Nozaki M, Sasaki K, Huang TT: Reconstruction of the abdominal wall. In Mathes SJ, editor: *Plastic surgery*, ed 2, Philadelphia, 2006, Saunders Elsevier, p 1182.)

autologous tissue reconstruction. Autologous techniques include primary repair, open or endoscopically assisted components separation, or local flap and distant flaps selected on the basis of the location of the fascial defect on the trunk.

Loss of both the skin and fascial layers, with a full-thickness open defect. These complete defects can be approached with staged reconstruction to close the skin and return later to provide fascial replacement. Alternatively, a local or distant muscle flap, musculocutaneous flap, fasciocutaneous flap, or free tissue transfer can supply well-vascularized tissue with the use of prosthetic material for fascial support as needed.

Components separation is a technique in which a series of fascial incisions are used to separate the structural components of the abdominal wall and to mobilize the musculofascial tissue for closure of a midline abdominal wall defect (Fig. 68-9). The anterior rectus sheath is separated from the external oblique aponeurosis by making a longitudinal relaxing incision along the linea semilunaris. This allows the anterior rectus sheath and muscle to move medially while maintaining its neurovascular supply, which comes from between the internal oblique and transversus abdominis in a segmental fashion. Posteriorly, the rectus muscle is released from its posterior sheath with medial advancement of 5 cm in the epigastric region, 10 cm at the umbilicus, and 3 cm in the suprapubic region. With the modification of also dividing the internal oblique component of the anterior rectus sheath, unilateral advancement increases to 8 to 10 cm in the epigastrium, 10 to 15 cm in the midabdomen, and 6 to 8 cm in the suprapubic region. With the components separation technique, the reported rate of hernia recurrence is variable, from below 5% to more than 30%, presumably dependent on a number of factors, including the dimensions of the defect. To address this, techniques for augmenting but not bridging the fascial closure with prosthetic mesh have been described, with good results for larger, more complex hernias.[34] The components separation technique eliminates the need for prosthetic material in many patients, restores the dynamic abdominal wall function, and results in improvement in back pain and postural abnormalities. A common complication with this technique is wound breakdown caused by devascularized skin flaps consequent to the wide undermining required. Attention to preserving the periumbilical perforators can reduce the number of wound healing complications; the use of endoscopically assisted components separation has been described as a means to preserve midline perforators to the skin during release of the external oblique. In contrast to midline defects, components separation has limited use in lateral defects, in which the achievable advancement decreases by 50%. In addition, use of components separation in lateral repairs can result in loss of fascial congruity of the abdominal wall, with hernia formation at the donor site.

Various prosthetic materials are available for use as structural support of the abdominal wall. A number of trials have shown that the recurrence rate is halved after repair of incisional hernias more than 5 to 6 cm in size when the use of prosthetic mesh is compared with primary suture repair.[35] From this has come the consensus that prosthetic materials are useful in the presence of adequate skin and subcutaneous coverage and adequate wound bed. The incidence of infection is higher with the use of prosthetics than with primary repair; excessive wound tension, poor wound status, and a history of infection are associated with prosthetic material failure. The materials are classified as meshed or nonmeshed and absorbable or nonabsorbable. There is less fibrous ingrowth with a nonmeshed material such as Gore-Tex, which minimizes adhesions between the prosthesis and viscera; reopening of the abdominal cavity through nonmeshed material is easier. Alternatively, meshed material such as Marlex permits the effusion of fluid for a reduced incidence of seroma and promotes fibrous ingrowth, which enhances tissue strength. Although mesh is preferred, complications can include infection, extrusion of the prosthetic material, and bowel erosion when folds and wrinkles in the mesh exert pressure against the bowel wall. Softer, smoother mesh, made from Prolene, is more pliable, and erosion into bowel is less common. In an effort to avoid these complications of infection, extrusion, abdominal wall stiffness, pain, and fistula formation that are associated with nonabsorbable materials, biomaterials derived from human and animal sources have been developed. These bioprostheses are absorbable; they include human acellular dermis (AlloDerm), porcine acellular dermis (Permacol), and porcine small intestinal submucosa (Surgisis). These materials have an acellular collagen matrix that promotes host tissue remodeling and replacement. Although they are resistant to infection, biocompatible, and mechanically stable over the short term, their disadvantages are high cost and few long-term studies establishing outcomes with regard to hernia recurrence.

Several techniques are used to place prosthetic material—mesh onlay, mesh inlay, retrorectus placement, and intraperitoneal underlay. For onlay grafts, the material is cut larger than the fascial defect, placed superficially to the anterior rectus sheath, and anchored at its margins with sutures. With inlay grafts, the prosthetic material is cut to the same size as the fascial defect, placed in the defect, and anchored to the edges with sutures. With these techniques for mesh repair, recurrence is not uncommon. This is caused not by intrinsic failure of the prosthetic material but by herniation at the suture line of the graft-fascia interface. Therefore, underlay techniques are preferred. With the retrorectus approach, the material is placed in the preperitoneal space between the rectus muscle and posterior rectus sheath. Alternatively, the underlay graft can be placed intraperitoneally, using an endoscopic approach in selected cases, and secured with sutures, tacks, or staples (Fig. 68-10). In an underlay location, intra-abdominal pressure bolsters the repair by holding the graft in apposition to the fascia; at least 4 cm of contact at the margins between the mesh and fascia is desirable to increase the surface area for fibrous ingrowth at the material-fascia interface. When possible, the viscera are protected by interposing omentum between the mesh and abdominal contents. With use of these measures, secure and physiologic repairs with recurrence rates below 10% have been reported.

A number of autologous tissue flaps are available for defects with absent or unstable skin coverage. These include skin flaps, muscle flaps, fasciocutaneous flaps, musculocutaneous flaps, and free tissue transfers. Flap selection depends on the location and size of the defect, and there are guidelines for matching the defect with the flap of choice.[36] For lower abdominal wall reconstruction, the tensor fascia lata musculofasciocutaneous flap based on the lateral circumflex femoral artery is the flap of choice. A dense, strong sheet of vascularized fascia and its overlying skin can be transferred from the lateral thigh in a single stage to resurface the suprapubic region, the lower abdominal quadrants, or as high as the upper quadrant on the ipsilateral abdomen. It is useful in irradiated and contaminated fields because it provides autologous fascia and conveys protective sensation when the lateral femoral cutaneous nerve is included. The rectus femoris musculocutaneous flap, based on the descending branch of the lateral circumflex femoral artery, is another choice for repair of the lower half of the abdomen or ipsilateral abdominal wall. Its drawback is the donor site morbidity of weakened quadriceps function in the leg associated with loss of the muscle. This flap can be extended by incorporating adjacent fascia lata, and this "mutton chop" modification has been used to reconstruct into the epigastrium. Additional flaps for lower abdominal coverage include the anterior thigh flap, external oblique muscle, and rectus abdominis musculocutaneous flap, based inferiorly on the inferior epigastric vessels, which is also the flap of choice for lateral defects of the lower two thirds of the abdomen. In the upper half of the abdomen, the superiorly based vertical or transverse abdominis musculocutaneous flap, based on the superior epigastric artery, is useful for central defects, and the latissimus dorsi musculocutaneous flap, based on the thoracodorsal vessels, is suitable for reconstruction of the lateral parts of the upper abdomen. Free flaps are considered when local tissues are not available or when a pedicle flap cannot reach or is too small to cover a defect. In the case of a free tissue transfer to the abdomen, suitable recipient vessels are required. Usually, the inferior epigastric, deep circumflex iliac, superior epigastric, internal thoracic, or saphenous vein graft may be used. Because it contains fascia, the tensor fascia lata flap is the most commonly used free flap, but use of an innervated free latissimus dorsi flap has been described as a means to bring contractile function and strength to the lost abdominal wall.

Abdominoplasty

Abdominoplasty removes fat and skin from the abdominal wall and repairs fascial laxity or dehiscence to produce an abdominal profile that is smoother and firmer. It is most effective in persons of normal weight who have loose, sagging skin because of heredity,

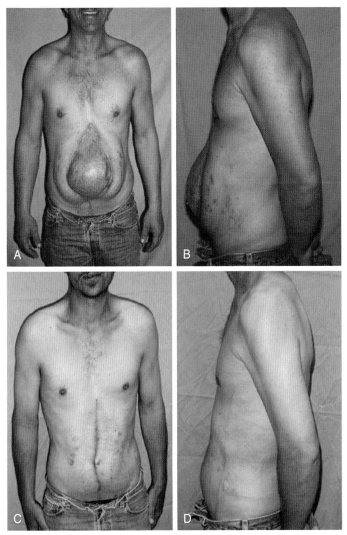

FIGURE 68-10 Abdominal defect with skin graft coverage in a man who sustained major visceral injuries in a motor vehicle accident. **A,** Abdominal compartment syndrome required release of the abdominal closure and split-thickness skin grafts for coverage. **B,** Lateral view of ventral hernia with skin grafts on viscera. **C** and **D,** Postoperative view 1 year after peritoneal mesh reconstruction of abdominal wall.

multiple pregnancies, fluctuations in weight, or significant weight loss. The basic technique includes a horizontal skin incision low on the abdominal wall between the umbilicus and pubic hairline; elevation of the skin and subcutaneous tissue from the deep fascia up to the level of the xiphoid and costal margins; incision around the umbilicus, leaving it attached to the underlying fascia as an isolated island; repair of a diastasis or plication of the muscle fascia; drawing of the flap inferiorly under mild tension; excision of excess skin and subcutaneous tissue; securing of the flap inferiorly to Scarpa or deep fascia; creation of a new opening in the flap for exteriorization of the umbilicus; and placement of multiple drains under the abdominal flap.

In addition to the traditional abdominoplasty, there are several variations. A miniabdominoplasty is a limited abdominoplasty, useful when the excess skin and fat are primarily below the umbilicus. Fleur-de-lis abdominoplasty refers to an inverted T type of abdominoplasty, which is useful for individuals with large amounts of excess skin. An umbilical float may be used in con-

junction with a miniabdominoplasty to avoid the incision and scarring around the umbilicus. Here, the umbilicus is left attached to the skin, cut loose from the underlying abdominal fascia, and allowed to descend or float toward the pubic area as the skin is tightened. This shortens the distance between the umbilicus and pubic bone, so it is not suitable if the distance will be shortened greatly.

Complications, most frequently surgical site infection, hematoma, seroma, marginal skin loss, and minor wound separation, occur in 12% to 32% of abdominoplasty patients.[37] Major complications are reported in 1.4% of cases and include major skin loss, deep venous thrombosis, and pulmonary embolus. Risk factors include diabetes, hypertension, and smoking. Complications are magnified dramatically in obese patients, with reports of complications in 80% of obese patients. Adherence to the guideline that a patient should be at or near his or her ideal body mass index results in fewer serious complications and higher patient satisfaction. Preoperative smoking cessation is mandatory.

Reconstruction of the Perineum

The indications for perineal wound reconstruction have escalated rapidly in the last few years. This is a consequence of more radical surgical resections, in which abdominoperineal resection (APR) may be combined with vaginectomy, sacrectomy, or exenteration of pelvic organs, and of the expanded role for adjuvant radiotherapy in the treatment of rectal cancer. When APR follows chemoradiotherapy, perineal wound complications, including nonhealing wounds, abscess, dehiscence, and fistula, have been reported in 41% of primary perineal wound closures.[38] These complications are caused by the presence of a wide cavity with dead space, poor vascularity of the surrounding tissue, use of irradiated skin in the closure, and bacterial contamination with bowel resection. Musculocutaneous flap reconstruction of a pelvic soft tissue defect introduces well-vascularized nonirradiated tissue with enough bulk to obliterate dead space, brings in a skin paddle for cutaneous wound closure, and provides functional restoration after vaginectomy.

Immediate flap reconstruction has been readily accepted for large perineal defects when the skin cannot be closed primarily or a massive dead space is present. More recently, there has been interest in extending the role of a flap into situations in which a skin paddle is not essential for cutaneous closure of the perineal wound or a large amount of tissue bulk is not needed to fill pelvic dead space. Early results using a musculocutaneous flap to reconstruct irradiated APR defects that could alternatively be closed primarily have shown a reduced incidence of major perineal wound complications. Comparing the outcomes of immediate vertical rectus abdominis musculocutaneous (VRAM) flap reconstruction with outcomes of primary closure in patients with similar irradiated APR defects has shown a 4-fold reduction in major perineal wound dehiscence and a 10-fold reduction in perineal abscess formation associated with flap use.[39]

Flap reconstruction is preferably accomplished at the time of the original extirpative procedure rather than in a delayed manner. Functional issues can be addressed at the same time; in the pelvic area, this typically involves vaginal or penile reconstruction, ideally using the same flap for reparative and functional purposes. Clinical indications for flap reconstruction of the perineum include the following:

- Repair after APR with extensive skin resection
- Repair after APR following chemoradiation of the pelvis to bring in well-vascularized tissue, even when skin is sufficient
- Repair after extended APR with wide tissue resection
- Repair after pelvic exenteration for urologic and gynecologic cancer
- Reconstruction after partial or complete vaginectomy
- Repair of a radical sacrectomy defect
- Repair of the perineum in severe, perianal Crohn's disease
- Neovaginal reconstruction in congenital absence of the vagina
- Repair of postirradiation ulcerated wounds of the perineum
- Pelvic excisions with intraoperative radiation therapy

Commonly used flaps for perineal reconstruction include the rectus abdominis musculocutaneous, gracilis musculocutaneous, posterior thigh fasciocutaneous, and gluteus maximus musculocutaneous flaps. An omental flap is an option in select cases. In the past, thigh-based flaps were regarded as most useful, and unilateral or bilateral gracilis musculocutaneous flaps were preferred for many applications. Today, an abdominal musculocutaneous flap has become the technique of choice.

A pedicled rectus abdominis flap based inferiorly on the inferior epigastric vessels can be designed with a skin paddle oriented obliquely (Taylor flap), horizontally (TRAM flap), or vertically (VRAM flap) along the muscle. This last design, the VRAM flap, is particularly well suited for perineal reconstruction (Fig. 68-11). The VRAM flap has bulk for filling dead space, adequate length to reach to the perineum and sacrum, reliable blood supply, and consistent anatomy and can be designed with a large, sturdy skin paddle 5 to 10 cm wide for perineal skin reconstruction or vaginal reconstruction. In one study of surgical outcomes and complications in patients undergoing immediate reconstruction of the perineum, VRAM flaps performed well, with a 15% rate of major complications versus 42% with thigh flaps.[40] Although harvesting of a VRAM flap results in greater tension on the abdominal wall fascial closure, higher rates of abdominal wound separation and incisional hernias have not been reported. Reinforcement of the donor site with synthetic mesh material is helpful, but other options include using a components separation technique to close the abdominal wall on the donor side and the development of perforator flaps to spare the muscle and fascia.

Use of the VRAM flap requires careful planning because taking one of the rectus abdominis muscles with the flap has implications for ostomy placement. If one rectus muscle is used, a colostomy can be brought out through the opposite rectus muscle. However, if a second ostomy is required for an ileal conduit for urinary diversion after pelvic exenteration or for colostomy relocation to treat a parastomal hernia, there will be no intact, untouched rectus muscle remaining through which the second ostomy can be placed. This can be addressed by placing the new ostomy through the abdominal wall on the flap donor side, lateral to the empty rectus sheath. This is successful in some series, but others have found it problematic, with localized wound infections, abdominal wound dehiscence, and malposition of the associated stoma.

There may be situations encountered that limit the use of a VRAM flap. These include situations in which the rectus muscle or inferior epigastric pedicle has been divided by previous abdominal incisions and scarring, prior elevation of an abdominal flap (as with ventral hernia repair or cosmetic abdominoplasty), and preexisting stomas for fecal and urinary diversion exiting through the rectus muscles. In addition, transfer of the VRAM flap into the pelvis typically requires a laparotomy. Therefore, in cases that can be approached from the perineum alone, a thigh-based flap might be preferable to avoid a transabdominal procedure.[41]

The pedicled gracilis muscle or musculocutaneous flap is a suitable alternative if the need to fill dead space is relatively small. The gracilis muscle originates from the pubis symphysis and inserts on the medial tibial condyle. Its blood supply is from the medial circumflex branch of the profunda femoris vessel and can be found 8 to 10 cm from its origin. This distal location of the dominant vascular pedicle, at the junction of the proximal and middle thirds of the thigh, means a restricted arc of rotation and limits how far the flap can reach onto the perineum and into the pelvis. When gracilis flaps are used for vaginal reconstruction, the depth of the reconstructed vault may be limited. In addition, the skin paddle is smaller and less reliable than the VRAM flap, and flap-specific complications, with wound healing and flap loss, are significantly higher with the gracilis flap.

Another alternative is the posterior thigh flap, a fasciocutaneous flap based on the descending branch of the inferior gluteal artery. This flap can provide an abundant and reliable amount of soft tissue for transfer from the posterior thigh, and because the vascular pedicle is proximal, the flap can easily reach high into the pelvis. The skin is innervated by the posterior femoral cutaneous nerve (S1-3), so the flap can provide sensate soft tissue for perineal

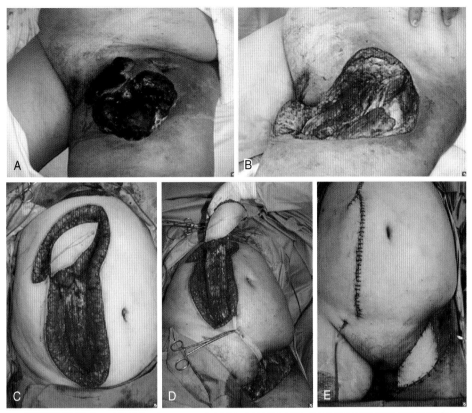

FIGURE 68-11 **A** and **B,** Extensive recurrent melanoma in the groin of a patient previously treated with surgery and irradiation. Resection of the tumor left a large defect with exposed femoral vessels. **C,** An obliquely oriented VRAM flap is elevated on the contralateral side of the abdomen. **D** and **E,** The flap is passed through a subcutaneous tunnel into the groin and used to cover the femoral triangle. A skin graft is placed on the lateral portion of the groin wound where the fascia lata was intact and there were no exposed neurovascular structures.

or vaginal reconstruction, although this is dysesthetic in some patients. There is a relatively high rate of wound healing complications with this flap, but it is a suitable choice when other flaps are unavailable or unsuitable for an individual patient.[42]

A pedicled gluteus maximus musculocutaneous flap based on the inferior gluteal artery has application for some anorectal wounds but will not reach deep into the pelvis. Similarly, flaps of the greater omentum can protect abdominal contents and reach the sacrum but do not provide vascularized skin for tension-free perineal wound closure. However, both these flaps have been shown to improve perineal healing in certain settings. This highlights the importance of preoperative planning for flap selection in clinical practice. Flap choice depends on previous scars, where new incisions will be made, planned location of stomas, vascular patency, and availability of donor sites. Whichever flap is preferred, comparative studies have shown that immediate reconstruction can result in significant improvements in wound healing after radical perineal surgery.

Surgery of Back Defects

Posterior trunk defects result from traumatic wounds; defects after oncologic resection, with or without radiation necrosis; wound breakdown or infection after spinal surgery, with or without exposed orthopedic hardware; and congenital deformities (e.g.,

spina bifida with myelomeningocele). Posterior trunk reconstruction must provide coverage for exposed major neurovascular structures; coverage for exposed bone and skeletal prostheses; and stable soft tissue to obliterate dead space, to protect dura, to control infection, and to permit tension-free wound closure. To meet these needs, reconstruction generally involves muscle or musculocutaneous flaps to provide bulky, durable, well-vascularized tissue. Depth and location are the two wound parameters that determine flap selection. Deep wounds of the spine can be repaired with paraspinal muscle flaps, whereas more superficial wounds are treated with surface muscle flaps. The length of the back means that various regional muscle units can treat different areas of the posterior trunk.

Preparation for surgical coverage depends on the pathogenesis of the defect. Although exposed meninges must be covered promptly, necrotic or infected tissue may require débridement over time, treatment with antibiotic-impregnated materials for exposed hardware, and negative pressure wound therapy to promote granulation tissue. As spine surgery has become more sophisticated, the need has grown for immediate, complex, soft tissue coverage and for strategies for salvage of postoperative complications. Techniques for covering the spine, exposed dura, and any exposed implants rely on mobilization, advancement, and midline closure of the bilateral paraspinous muscles that run the

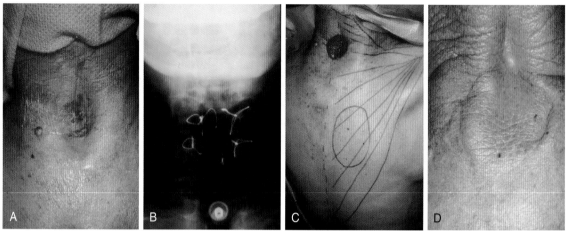

FIGURE 68-12 A, Posterior neck with a chronic open wound, with exposed bone and unstable surrounding soft tissue. **B,** Radiographs show surgical hardware in the cervical vertebrae. **C,** The defect is débrided back to healthy margins, and the skin paddle on the posterior trapezius musculocutaneous flap is planned. **D,** Postoperative view at 6 months with the healed flap in place. The donor site for the flap was closed primarily.

length of the vertebral column deep to the thoracolumbar fascia. This is done as a precautionary measure in patients with multiple previous operations, irradiation, attenuated skin, or stiff and heavily scarred soft tissue.

Conceptually, the posterior trunk is divided into upper, middle, and lower thirds. Each has muscle flap options that are best suited for that part of the posterior trunk. Posterior cervical and upper back defects are reconstructed with the pedicled trapezius muscle or musculocutaneous flap or with the dorsal scapular artery perforator flap (Fig. 68-12). The trapezius flap is reliable and versatile and can include a large skin paddle. It is based on the transverse cervical artery, which has two major branches. The trapezius thus offers two separate muscular territories; the lower portion of the muscle can be elevated and transposed superiorly to cover the cervical spine. Alternatively, a trapezius turnover flap is an easily elevated, reliable solution for cervicothoracic wounds. For the midback, latissimus dorsi muscle and musculocutaneous flaps can be mobilized on the thoracodorsal branch of the subscapular vessels to be rotated for broad, reliable coverage. To extend coverage to the midline farther inferiorly, the latissimus flap can be raised as a reverse turnover flap based on secondary segmental intercostal and lumbar artery perforators. The upper portion of the lower third of the back is the most difficult to cover. More inferiorly on the back, the gluteus maximus muscles provide excellent coverage for the sacrum (see later, "Pressure Sores"). However, in the lumbar area, where it is difficult for the more conventional muscle flaps to reach, perforator flaps, latissimus dorsi with a thoracolumbar fasciocutaneous extension, or vein grafting to the thoracodorsal vessels may be required. The pedicled omental flap also is used for the coverage of lumbar defects. The omentum can be transferred, based on the right or left gastroepiploic artery, by dividing attachments to the transverse colon, ligating one gastroepiploic artery, mobilizing the omentum off the greater curvature of the stomach, and passing it through the retroperitoneum and lumbar fascia to cover the spinal column while the back wound is closed with cutaneous advancement flaps.[43]

With partial or total sacrectomy, extensive soft tissue defects are created by oncologic ablation for chordoma, osteogenic sarcoma, or extension of pelvic carcinoma. An anterior and posterior approach is generally used for resection of the tumor, which creates a large communication between the abdominal cavity and gluteal area. These ablations often require large amounts of hardware for bone repair by the orthopedic surgeon; the hypogastric and gluteal vessels are divided during resection, which eliminates the use of potential local back flaps for repair. Successful reconstruction in these cases calls for well-vascularized tissue to fill the defect, to cover the orthopedic appliances, to close the abdominal cavity to prevent herniation, and to close the skin on the posterior trunk. Initial efforts with gluteal flaps and omentum and the placement of synthetic mesh to prevent herniation had some usefulness. More recently, an inferiorly based, pedicled VRAM flap passed transabdominally has proven effective. With no need for mesh, the VRAM flap has a high success rate, with a low incidence of complications and low morbidity.[44]

Meningomyelocele

Meningomyelocele is a congenital spinal malformation that results from failure of the neural tube to close during the first month of gestation. The most common of the four types of spina bifida, meningomyelocele is a cystic herniation of the meninges and neural tissue that presents as a defect on the surface of the lumbosacral skin. The open meningomyelocele defect should be closed soon after birth to prevent meningitis and to protect the exposed neural structure from desiccation and further damage. Early closure has been shown to be a determinant in the neurosurgical outcome. Approximately 75% of meningomyelocele defects are small enough that soft tissue closure can be achieved by simple undermining of the skin edges and tension-free closure in the midline after dural repair. For defects larger than 5 to 8 cm in diameter, a number of techniques have been described.

The surgical options for closing a meningomyelocele defect include skin grafting, local flaps, musculocutaneous flaps, and fasciocutaneous flaps. Local skin flaps including advancement flaps, bipedicle flaps, transposition flaps, double Z-plasty, bilobed flaps, rhomboid flaps, and V-Y advancement flaps have all been used successfully. For larger defects, latissimus dorsi and gluteus maximus musculocutaneous flaps have been described.[45] For all of these, the first criterion is reliable wound healing so that the defect is closed securely and definitively to avoid cerebrospinal fluid leakage and its accompanying morbidity. (See "Pediatric Neurosurgery" in Chapter 67.)

PRESSURE SORES

Prolonged weight bearing, as in an immobilized or paralyzed patient, can elevate tissue pressure above arterial capillary perfusion pressure (32 mm Hg) and result in compromised oxygenation, ischemia, and eventual tissue necrosis. In models of ischemia, external pressure higher than 60 mm Hg for 2 hours leads to irreversible tissue damage, and clinical studies have confirmed this. The clinical sequelae of this damage are pressure sores with ulceration, infection, and exposure of bone. In order of occurrence, the surfaces most commonly involved are those over the sacrum, calcaneus, ischium, and greater trochanter (Fig. 68-13).

Extrinsic and intrinsic factors contribute to the pathogenesis of pressure ulcers. Extrinsic factors include unrelieved pressure seen in debilitated or spinal cord injury patients and factors that worsen the local wound environment, such as moisture in the perineal area, incontinence, and shearing forces from repositioning of the patient. Intrinsic factors include underlying conditions that lead to poor wound healing, such as advanced age, diabetes, malnutrition, and edema. The Braden Scale for Predicting Pressure Sore Risk is a widely used nursing assessment tool to help predict patients' risk for development of pressure sores. Although there is no clear evidence that using risk assessment scales decreases the incidence of pressure ulcers, the Braden Scale has reasonable predictive capacity, with high interrater reliability. This scale accounts for several extrinsic and intrinsic causative factors by scoring six subscales—sensory perception, moisture, activity, mobility, nutrition, and friction and shear.

Stages of Pressure Ulcers

The National Pressure Ulcer Advisory Panel has defined the stages of pressure ulcers, including an original four stages and adding two stages in 2007:

Stage I: Skin intact but reddened for longer than 1 hour after relief of pressure. This stage represents intact skin with various degrees of erythema that does not blanch when it is compressed. This wound is potentially reversible if extrinsic forces and intrinsic wound healing factors are optimized.

Stage II: Blister or other break in the dermis with or without infection. Here, the skin has broken down, with a partial-thickness loss of dermis. By maintenance of coverage over the wound, these wounds often can generate granulation tissue and undergo wound contraction to heal by secondary intention. Because there is violation of skin, the local environment must be monitored carefully for moisture and soiling to allow this stage to heal. Stage I and stage II pressure ulcers are the most prevalent.

Stage III: Full-thickness tissue loss with visible subcutaneous fat but no exposed bone, tendon, or muscle. In the absence of bone exposure, these sores can heal and contract over a bone prominence. However, this is usually a temporally brief stage because muscle is the most oxygen-sensitive tissue and is most sensitive to ischemic necrosis, quickly reaching the final stage of exposed bone.

Stage IV: Exposed bone, joint, muscle, or tendon, with or without infection, often including undermining and tunneling. This is the most common stage that prompts a surgical consultation because the ulcer is down to the causative bone prominence.

Suspected deep tissue injury: Purple or maroon localized area of discolored intact skin or blood-filled blister caused by damage of underlying soft tissue from pressure or shear. This stage identifies clinically suspicious deep tissue injury.

Unstageable: Full-thickness tissue loss in which the base of the ulcer is covered by slough (yellow, tan, gray, green, or brown) or eschar (tan, brown, or black) in the wound bed. Until enough slough or eschar is removed to expose the base of the wound, the true depth and stage cannot be determined.

Swab cultures of the surface of a pressure sore invariably are positive because of local contamination, so culture samples must be taken from biopsy specimens of soft tissue and bone deep to the surface. Infections generally are polymicrobial, with *Proteus, Bacteroides, Pseudomonas,* and *Escherichia coli* accompanying staphylococcal and streptococcal species. More than 50% of long-term care patients harbor methicillin-resistant *Staphylococcus aureus* organisms. In stage IV pressure ulcers with bone exposure, the desiccation and bacterial colonization of the surface of the bone is termed osteitis. If the deep bone has good blood supply and the patient is not immunocompromised, the bone inflammation of osteitis can be tolerated for protracted periods as long as wound care can contain the zone of injury. Osteomyelitis is infection of the bone requiring long-term systemic antibiotics; definitive diagnosis is made with bone biopsy and bacterial culture. Imaging modalities to diagnose osteomyelitis include radiography, tagged white blood cell scans, and MRI. Appropriate imaging is useful to evaluate the extent of bone involvement and to identify the source of infection in pressure sores associated with perianal fistulas or spinal hardware abscesses.

The management of a pressure sore starts with the correction of causative factors. Surgical interventions will not heal and the sores will recur unless the cause is addressed with pressure-relieving cushions and beds, relief of spasticity, correction of joint contractures, incontinence aids, nutritional support, and infection control.[46] Surgical treatment involves drainage of collections, wide débridement of devitalized and scarred soft tissue, excision of sinus tracks and the bursa-like lining of the chronic wound, ostectomy of involved bone, hemostasis with suction drainage, and obliteration of all residual dead space with well-vascularized tissue introduced to cover bone, to provide padding, and to close the open wound without tension.

Intraoperative débridement of superficial bone is carried out by visual assessment of avascular bone versus bleeding bone. Using rongeurs and rasps to smooth jutting prominences or to excise heterotopic bone accomplishes the second purpose of bone resection, reducing the physical prominence of bone that causes pressure and predisposes to recurrence of the sore. After adequate bone débridement, a biopsy specimen of the deeper, healthy-appearing bone is sent for bone culture. If the culture is positive, the remaining bone is still infected and the patient will need a long-term course of intravenous antibiotics to treat the osteomyelitis. Bone resection must be approached thoughtfully because resecting one of a paired set of pressure points, such as the ischia, shifts the patient's weight to the contralateral side, increasing the risk of a new pressure sore on the second side.

Reconstruction with a flap is necessary for most pressure sores because less complex options, such as primary closure or skin grafting, have limited usefulness. Primary closure places the surgical suture line directly over the area of pressure, whereas a flap shifts the closure and scar away from the pressure point. A skin

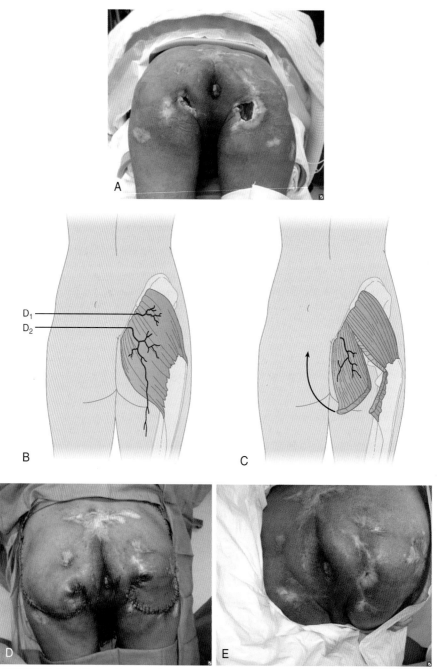

FIGURE 68-13 A 51-year-old paraplegic patient has bilateral stage IV ischial pressure sores with bone exposure in the wounds. **A,** Preoperative view shows bilateral defects and scarring of the surrounding tissue from previous pressure sores and surgical repairs. After débridement and bilateral ischiectomy, well-vascularized tissue will be needed to cover bone, to provide padding, and to close the wound without tension. **B,** The gluteus maximus muscle has blood supply from two branches of the hypogastric artery—the superior gluteal artery to the upper half and the inferior gluteal artery to the lower half. **C,** Based on these two separate upper and lower pedicles, the muscle can be divided into upper and lower halves. **D,** The lower half of the gluteus muscle on each side is detached from the greater tuberosity of the femur and transposed inferiorly with the overlying buttock skin to fill the ischial defects. **E,** Three-month postoperative view shows coverage of both defects. The superior half of the gluteus maximus muscle is preserved.

graft is a thin and fragile coverage option, subject to the shearing forces that created the ulcer in the first place. In addition, a skin graft requires a clean, healthy recipient site, with good blood supply and no exposed bone. Only the most superficial of pressure sores meets these requirements for a base that can be covered successfully with a skin graft. Transferring healthy tissue with its own blood supply to fill the pressure sore can be accomplished with cutaneous, fasciocutaneous, musculocutaneous, muscle-only, and free microvascular flaps.

Sacral pressure sores develop in supine or semireclining patients, and because of the broad pointed shape of the sacrum and thinness of the overlying soft tissue, most ulcers have exposed bone. The soft tissues surrounding the sacrum receive their blood supply from perforators from the superior and inferior gluteal arteries, which are also the arteries supplying the gluteus maximus muscle. This muscle extends and rotates the thigh laterally and is required for ambulation, so the gluteus maximus is not considered expendable except in the spinal cord injury patient. However, the gluteus maximus can survive on either vascular pedicle alone, and using only the superior or inferior half of the muscle will preserve function. Muscle or musculocutaneous flaps of the superior half of the muscle are constructed and moved in two primary ways, a rotational flap or V-Y advancement flap. A rotational flap can be an advancement or with a musculocutaneous skin island. The V-Y advancement technique involves creating a triangular skin island over the muscle, with one side being the defect and the other two sides forming a V. The central V is shifted into the open wound, and the defect is closed in a Y configuration. To get extended coverage of the sacrum, bilateral V-Y advancement flaps can be used, one based on the right and one based on the left gluteal area.

The ischial tuberosities are under high pressure in a seated patient. Unilateral or bilateral ischial sores develop in individuals who are seated for protracted periods without adjusting their position and weight distribution. Ischial ulcers are challenging for several reasons. The pressure points are bilateral, which means that unweighting one side for pressure-reducing purposes shifts increased pressure onto the contralateral ischium. Resecting bone on both sides runs the risk of shifting weight bearing onto the perineal soft tissues, which can cause later scrotal or urethral sores. There can be fistulas involving the rectum or urethra; these may require diversion and control before the ischial ulcers are addressed. Finally, because of the strong hip flexors, there can be flexion contractures with varying degrees of deformity, which reduce mobility and the capacity for normal weight distribution in the sitting or lying position. Because the ischium has a number of surrounding muscles, various flaps suitable for coverage have been described. These include the inferior gluteus maximus rotational, inferior gluteal fasciocutaneous thigh, V-Y hamstring advancement, gracilis muscle, tensor fascia lata rotational, and rectus abdominis rotational flaps.

Because of the mobility of the hip, pressure sores over the greater trochanter characteristically have extensive bursa formation with smaller areas of skin loss. After resection of the trochanter, flaps available for the repair of trochanteric pressure sores include local fasciocutaneous rotational, tensor fascia lata musculocutaneous, and inferior gluteal thigh fasciocutaneous flaps and muscle flaps incorporating the vastus lateralis, rectus femoris, or rectus abdominis muscles.

On the feet, pressure sores can present over the heels, malleoli, and plantar surfaces. Unlike other pressure sores, foot ulcers lack a thick subcutaneous layer, are often modest in size and depth,

and may respond favorably to conservative treatment. Stable (dry, adherent, intact, without erythema or fluctuance) eschar on the heels acts as a biologic dressing and need not be removed. In non–weight-bearing areas requiring a less durable surface, pressure sores may be treated conservatively because a scar left by wound contraction and epithelialization may suffice. For larger wounds, débridement and STSG may be useful. If the ulceration involves a large portion of the weight-bearing surface or if osteomyelitis of the calcaneus is present, débridement of devitalized bone with flap coverage is needed. Muscle flaps of the abductor digiti minimi, abductor hallucis, and flexor digitorum brevis have been described. Fasciocutaneous flaps based on the dorsalis pedis, medial plantar, and lateral plantar arteries can also provide coverage.

Postoperative protocols call for 2 to 6 weeks of strict pressure precautions because a newly transferred flap is vulnerable to pressure necrosis. When weight bearing is resumed in the area of the previous pressure sore, the transition is planned with progressive increases in time each day and frequent wound checks.

RECONSTRUCTION OF THE LOWER EXTREMITY

The goal of lower extremity reconstruction is restoration or maintenance of function. For functionality, there must be a stable skeleton to support weight, muscle to power motion and joint movement, neural supply for proprioception and plantar sensibility, blood supply to sustain the underlying structures, and soft tissue to provide a stable skin envelope. Based on these needs, reconstruction may be needed for open fractures, defects from sarcoma resections, radiation wounds, chronic traumatic wounds of the distal third of the leg, diabetic ulcers, venous ulcers, osteomyelitis of the tibia, unstable scars, and infected vascular grafts. Many reconstructions are complex because they need to contribute more than one element, such as vascularized bone grafts or composite flaps with sensory potential, and many require a multidisciplinary surgical team.

Soft Tissue Coverage of Traumatic Wounds

The loss of soft tissue cover over a fracture, particularly when interrupted endosteal blood supply is combined with periosteal damage, demands coverage of the exposed bone with vascularized tissue after thorough débridement of devitalized tissue (Fig. 68-14). Determinants of outcome after open fractures are wound size, degree of soft tissue injury, and amount of contamination. The Gustilo classification system is used to categorize open fractures of the leg into subtypes predictive of prognosis:

Gustilo I: Open fractures with wound <1 cm
Gustilo II: Open fractures with wound 1-10 cm with moderate tissue damage
Gustilo III: Open fractures with wound >10 cm and extensive tissue damage, making it difficult to cover bone or hardware
Gustilo IIIA: Adequate soft tissue coverage of bone with extensive soft tissue laceration or flaps
Gustilo IIIB: Inadequate soft tissue with periosteal stripping and bone exposure
Gustilo IIIC: As above, with vascular injury and ischemia requiring repair

Gustilo grade I and most grade II fractures can be closed primarily after débridement and orthopedic fixation are applied. However, larger grade II and most grade III fractures require advanced reconstructive techniques. When flap coverage is required, it can be done at the time of fracture stabilization or as

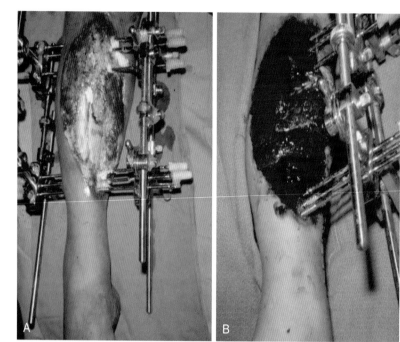
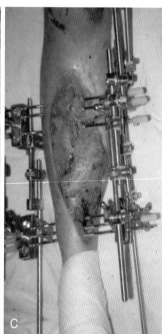

FIGURE 68-14 Soleus muscle flap for coverage of traumatic open fracture of the tibia in the middle third of the leg. **A,** Soft tissue defect with 10 cm of exposed bone after fracture fixation. **B,** The broad flat muscle deep to the gastrocnemius muscle has been mobilized on its proximal pedicles from the posterior tibial and peroneal arteries. It is transposed medially to cover the middle third of the tibia. **C,** Postoperative result. The muscle flap has been covered with a split-thickness skin graft to provide stable wound coverage.

a secondary procedure. Early coverage of exposed bone, tendons, and neurovascular structures decreases the risk of infection, osteomyelitis, nonunion, and ongoing tissue loss. Although the advantages of radical débridement and early wound closure have been accepted, the definition of the duration of the early phase varies. Earlier bone healing and reduced infection rates have been demonstrated if coverage is completed within 72 hours of fracture stabilization; others have shown comparable results when the wounds are closed within the first 6 days after injury. Early reconstruction may be precluded by other injuries or when severely contaminated wounds require serial débridement before delayed reconstruction.[47]

For many years, muscle flaps have been the choice for traumatic lower limb defects. The gastrocnemius and soleus are accessible as local flaps to cover the upper and middle thirds of the leg, and smaller muscles such as the tibialis anterior, extensor digitorum longus, and peroneus brevis can be used for more distal small defects. For larger defects of the distal third of the leg, ankle, and foot, microvascular free tissue transfers of muscles such as the latissimus dorsi, gracilis, serratus anterior, or rectus abdominis are preferred. These free tissue transfers provide more bulk, have longer pedicles for greater flexibility in positioning, and are not dependent on blood supply within the injured area. Most series of lower extremity reconstructions have reported flap failure rates just below 10%. This is higher than at other sites on the body because of associated vascular injuries and preexisting vascular disease in these patients.

More recently, novel wound technologies, combined with growing experience with local fasciocutaneous flaps, are creating new options for reconstruction. Use of the vacuum-assisted closure device reduces edema, decreases wound area, and stimulates granulation tissue, making it possible in some cases to close previously large wounds with local or regional flaps. Fasciocutaneous flaps can cover small to moderate-sized defects, and use of the reverse sural, perforator, and bipedicle flaps is decreasing the need for free microvascular transfers. Clinical advantages of this shift from free flaps to a wider use of skin grafts and local flaps include shorter operations in the trauma patient and elimination of the need for anastomosis to a major leg artery, which may not be available in some traumatic cases.

In injuries with bone loss and a soft tissue defect, the options for skeletal reconstruction include autogenous bone grafts, vascularized bone transfer (pedicle or free), and the Ilizarov technique for osteosynthesis. Bone grafts generally are delayed for approximately 6 weeks after soft tissue reconstruction while orthopedic hardware holds the fracture fragments at length across the gap. The size and location of the bone defect will determine bone graft technique, with a vascularized procedure preferred for larger losses. An alternative to delayed bone grafting is immediate one-stage reconstruction of the bone and soft tissue with an osteocutaneous free tissue transfer.

There are contraindications to salvage of a Gustilo grade IIIC injury of the lower extremity. The most important element in considering primary amputation is disruption of the sciatic or posterior tibial nerve. With laceration of the posterior tibial nerve, the plantar surface is insensate, which results predictably in recurrent ulceration, infection, and osteomyelitis. Other elements include severe infection or contamination, tibial bone loss of more than 8 cm, multilevel severe injury, ischemia time longer than 6 hours, and preexisting severe medical illness. There are several scoring systems to assist in making a decision about limb salvage versus amputation, but these tend to identify patients with good potential for salvage rather than those who will need eventual amputation. The Mangled Extremity Severity Score is used widely but should not be the sole criterion on which an amputation decision is made.[48] Replantation of a severed lower limb is rarely done in the adult because of the inability to restore neurologic function to the foot. A nonfunctional or marginally functional lower extremity is a greater liability than a prosthetic limb capable of allowing high-level function. Absolute contraindications to replantation are older age, poor baseline health, multilevel injury that results in immobility of the knee or ankle, and warm ischemia time longer than 6 hours.

Soft Tissue Reconstruction in the Groin and Thigh

The groin is the most common site of distal extremity prosthetic graft infections. Traditional treatment included removal of the graft material or a salvage attempt at graft preservation with secondary intention healing and its attendant risks of thrombosis, superinfection, and anastomotic disruption. Today, muscle flaps are the mainstay for managing vascular graft infections. Healthy muscle increases tissue oxygen tension in the wound, augments the delivery of antibiotics to the site, and eliminates dead space. Muscle flaps are useful to aid graft salvage in the presence of established infection, when there is increased dead space after drainage of a seroma or hematoma, or in situations in which the tissue bed is compromised by previous surgeries and scarring.

Several muscle flaps are useful for coverage of the femoral vessels. The sartorius muscle is used as first-line treatment because of its proximity, expendability, and relative ease of elevation. The muscle originates on the anterior superior iliac spine, inserts at the medial tibial condyle, and has a segmental blood supply with five or six direct branches from the superficial femoral artery. The muscle is mobilized by dividing the origin and two proximal vascular pedicles, which frees the proximal end of the muscle to be transposed medially and sutured to the inguinal ligament to provide vascularized muscle coverage of the femoral vessels. Disadvantages of the sartorius flap are that it is divided by some surgical incisions in the groin and that division of more than two adjacent pedicles results in devascularization of the muscle. Another local flap option is the rectus femoris muscle; distant pedicled muscle flaps for groin coverage are the gracilis and rectus abdominis.

Defects after oncologic surgery in the thigh and groin are distinctive because extirpation of lower extremity tumors, typically sarcomas, often necessitates wide or radical margins combined with adjuvant radiation therapy. There is a higher incidence of infection and dehiscence after limb-sparing surgery in the thigh and groin than in more distal parts of the lower extremity because of greater dead space, exposure of neurovascular structures, difficulty in keeping the wound clean and dry, and tension with ambulation and hip abduction. For these larger irradiated defects, flap reconstruction is necessary. A number of thigh muscles can be used as a local flap, with or without skin grafts or a skin paddle; these include gracilis, tensor fascia lata, and vastus lateralis flaps. Fasciocutaneous flaps, such as the medial thigh, lateral posterior thigh, and anterior lateral thigh, are also available. In some cases, these local options are no longer useful because of inclusion in the field of radiation, so distant or free flaps are needed for coverage. Reported outcomes after reconstruction of these difficult wounds with a VRAM flap have been promising, with a 9.4% incidence of postoperative wound complications with immediate reconstruction but a significantly higher incidence of 47% in patients with delayed reconstruction.[49]

Soft Tissue Coverage of the Knee, Leg, and Foot

Wounds around the knee can result from trauma, tumor extirpation, or exposure of an infected knee endoprosthesis after total knee replacement. For each of these defects, durable soft tissue coverage is required; a pedicled medial gastrocnemius muscle or musculocutaneous flap based on the medial sural artery is preferred for genicular soft tissue reconstruction. The gastrocnemius muscle has a medial head and lateral head originating from the medial and lateral condyles of the femur, respectively; the two heads share a common insertion on the calcaneus through the Achilles tendon. As a result, one head can be detached from the Achilles tendon independently and transposed with its robust blood supply and vascular drainage without impairing foot dorsiflexion. Because the medial head is longer, it is preferred for knee wounds and can be transposed with or without a skin paddle. In situations in which a pedicled gastrocnemius flap has failed or is unavailable, free tissue transfer of a latissimus dorsi or rectus abdominis muscle flap has led to a high rate of salvage of limbs and knee prostheses.

Options for soft tissue coverage of the leg are determined by the position of the defect relative to the tibia:

Proximal tibia: medial gastrocnemius, lateral gastrocnemius, fasciocutaneous flap

Middle tibia: soleus, gastrocnemius, extensor digitorum longus, tibialis anterior, fasciocutaneous flap

Distal tibia: peroneus brevis, extensor brevis, distal-based soleus, reverse sural artery flap, lateral supramalleolar flap, dorsalis pedis fasciocutaneous flap, free flap

Foot: flexor digitorum brevis, abductor hallucis, abductor digiti minimi, reverse sural flap, medial plantar artery flap, lateral calcaneal artery flap, V-Y advancement, free flap

Muscle flaps are often unreliable in treating distal-third leg wounds. Except for the soleus and gastrocnemius muscles, local muscles on the lower leg are only adequate to cover small defects. This, along with several other factors, means that treatment of the distal tibia, ankle, and foot is difficult. The area is vulnerable to injury because the distal portion of the leg has poor skin elasticity, has bone lying in the subcutaneous space, and may be edematous. The distal third of the leg has little muscle but many tendinous structures, and they support skin grafts poorly. Finally, the foot and ankle require especially durable integument because they are exposed continually to friction and shear with walking and footwear. Any transferred flap may slip or slide at the interface with the underlying structures because the transferred tissue lacks the glabrous quality of the native plantar skin. If the transferred tissue is insensate, it will be at significant risk for eventual breakdown.

For larger defects, reconstruction in the distal third of the leg relies on free tissue transfer techniques. The vascular status of the extremity and recipient vessel selection are key factors for success. Guidelines for the use of free flaps in the lower extremity include making anastomoses to healthy recipient vessels outside the zone of injury and using end-to-side arterial anastomoses, whereas venous anastomoses can be end to side or end to end. Free tissue transfer remains the best option for large defects, for wounds with trauma (e.g., crush injury to the surrounding vicinity that damages blood supply to all local tissues), and when the transfer of vascularized bone with the free flap is desirable. Free fibula flaps with skin paddles are preferred for lower extremity wounds with bone and soft tissue deficits.

More recently, the advent of local fasciocutaneous flaps has begun to change the treatment of difficult lower leg wounds.

Recognition that the vascular plexus accompanying cutaneous sensory nerves can supply overlying skin and soft tissue has allowed the development of many useful, axial pattern fasciocutaneous flaps.[50] Currently, one of the most versatile of these is the distally based, or reverse, sural fasciocutaneous flap. One to three arteries accompany the sural nerve as it travels subcutaneously in the posterior calf. A skin paddle as large as 14 cm in diameter can be elevated on the proximal posterior calf as part of a distally based sural nerve flap; this tissue may be transposed to cover distal leg and foot wounds. Because the sural nerve flap is supported by perforators from the peroneal artery, the patency of this vessel must be ensured for flap success.

BODY CONTOURING

Body Contouring After Bariatric Surgery

With the advent of bariatric surgery and successful treatment of severe obesity, a new deformity has emerged. After massive weight loss, the patient is left with excess skin and subcutaneous tissue that fails to retract and hangs from the torso, abdomen, and extremities. More than a cosmetic issue, this extreme skin redundancy can be painful, limits mobility, and is susceptible to recurrent infection in the intertriginous areas hooded by overhanging tissue. Patients seek body contouring surgery because many are deeply distressed by their appearance. These patients should be no less than 12 to 18 months after bariatric surgery, be stable in weight for 3 to 4 months, have a body mass index of less than 30, and be well-nourished, with no protein or vitamin deficiencies. Proceeding before these criteria are met can result in recurrent skin laxity and delayed wound healing and may be inconsistent with the patient's health insurer's requirements.

Body contouring after bariatric surgery is different from similar procedures in those who have not been obese. The deformity after bariatric surgery is more severe because the skin damage and associated loss of tone and elasticity do not recover, and the laxity is global. A number of procedures may be required; some of these involve restoring volume to areas of deficiency rather than removing tissue. When surgery is done in multiple stages, the procedures are separated by 4 to 6 months to optimize wound healing. The procedures are lengthy, and deep venous thrombosis prophylaxis is required. Abdominal wall hernias, particularly at surgical port sites, are found frequently and are repaired during the course of abdominal contouring. Except for large ventral hernias, these repairs are accomplished easily because the fascia can be approximated readily after massive weight loss (Fig. 68-15). Various techniques are used for contouring:

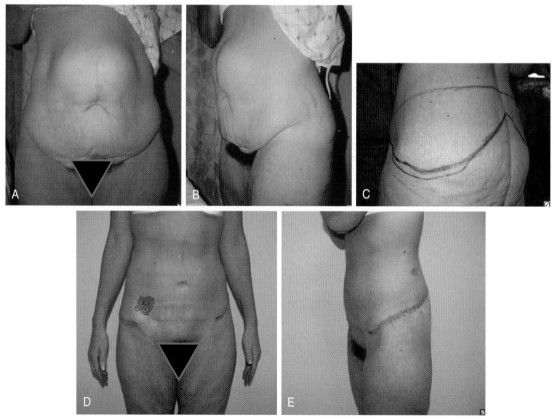

FIGURE 68-15 After gastric bypass, this 40-year-old woman lost 195 pounds. **A** and **B,** The patient presented with a 10-cm ventral hernia, a 2-cm umbilical hernia, and redundant soft tissue. Hernia repair, abdominoplasty, and belt lipectomy were planned. **C,** The planned excision of the redundant soft tissue over the sides and back is shown. **D** and **E,** The postoperative result after primary repair of the ventral hernia in a vertical direction, plication of the rectus fascia inferior to the herniorrhaphy for contour improvement, umbilical hernia repair, modified vertical abdominoplasty, and circumferential resection of soft tissue. A total of 3733 g of soft tissue was resected.

Panniculectomy is removal of excess skin and soft tissue from the abdominal wall without umbilical transposition. It is limited to removal of the overhanging pannus without mobilizing surrounding soft tissue.

Abdominoplasty includes panniculectomy with wide undermining of the upper abdominal flap and umbilical transposition. Unlike in a traditional abdominoplasty, a vertical ellipse or fleur-de-lis pattern of excision often is necessary to remove significant excess skin in the horizontal dimension superior to the umbilicus.

Reverse abdominoplasty uses incisions in the inframammary crease to remove rolls of excess skin from the upper quadrants of the abdomen.

Belt lipectomy is also termed a lower body lift; it corrects the circumferential roll of excess tissue found in most patients by extending the abdominal resection around the sides of the abdomen to include the lower back. In the course of resecting this circumferential ring of tissue, the lateral thighs and buttocks are also lifted.

An upper body lift removes excess skin from the lateral sides of the chest and upper back through a horizontal incision across the back.

A medial thigh lift is excision of a long ellipse of excess tissue parallel to the long axis of the thigh to remove hanging skin on the inner thigh.

A mastopexy is a breast lift for ptosis. No breast tissue is removed because the volume of breast tissue may be small in the drooping, deflated, pancake breast after massive weight loss. The breast skin is resected as the breast is reshaped, and the nipple-areola complex is elevated and centralized. In some cases, augmentation with breast implants is done to restore volume. Alternatively, excess folds of skin under the arms can be deepithelialized and rotated anteriorly to augment the volume of the breast.

Male mastopexy removes excess drooping skin to reduce fullness, with superior elevation of the nipple-areola complex as a flap or with free nipple grafting.

Brachioplasty is the excision of a long ellipse of excess tissue parallel to the long axis of the arm to correct the excess skin, or "bat wing," hanging from the proximal half of the arm.

A minibrachioplasty excises an ellipse of tissue just distal to the axilla perpendicular to the long axis of the arm to remove a mild excess of tissue. The scar is placed in the axilla.

Body contouring after bariatric surgery is a component in the treatment of the obese patient and is well accepted by patients, despite the extensive scarring with all of the surgical procedures. There is evidence that post–bariatric surgery patients who have subsequent body contouring surgery maintain their weight loss. This could merely be a reflection of the motivation of this cohort of patients, but ongoing work is focused on better understanding of the psychological impact of extreme body contouring.

Suction-Assisted Lipectomy

Suction-assisted lipectomy, also termed liposuction, lipoplasty, or liposculpture, was introduced in the late 1970s and early 1980s when plastic surgeons developed the concept of inserting a blunt-ended hollow cannula under the skin and connecting it to a vacuum pump, which generates negative pressure to aspirate the fatty tissue. Before a small opening is made in the skin to introduce the cannula, the area to be treated is injected with a wetting solution, which is saline supplemented with local anesthetic and low concentrations of epinephrine. Terms used to describe variations in this fluid infiltrate are based on the amount of fluid used; these are *dry, wet, superwet,* and *tumescent.* Although the more generous use of saline, lidocaine, and epinephrine results in less blood loss, greater ease of fat removal, and decreased postoperative pain, it also raises concerns about fluid overload and drug toxicity, which call for close intraoperative monitoring of ventilation, circulation, and cardiac function.

The areas usually treated with liposuction are the neck, abdomen and waist, back, and hips and thighs. Good results can be obtained, provided the volume of fat is not too great and there is good skin elasticity. Large-volume liposuction is associated with hemodynamic instability and a risk of damaging the blood supply to the overlying skin, causing skin necrosis. Elastic rebound of the skin after the underlying fat is removed is essential to the success of liposuction. In general, even when large amounts of fat are removed, skin has good elasticity and will conform to the new underlying volume. However, skin that is flaccid or sagging will not retract, and therefore good results are more difficult to achieve in areas such as the face, arms, and inner thighs. The looseness of the skin and the likelihood that it will exhibit poor adaptability means that liposuction will exacerbate the drooping and leave significant surface irregularities.

Suction-assisted lipectomy is a useful surgical treatment for several medical disorders. It is a treatment of choice for gynecomastia when combined, as needed, with resection of any glandular tissue. The skin of the chest wall tends to retract well, and liposuction is particularly useful for tapering the boundaries of the treated area for a smooth contour. Liposuction alone is less often useful to reduce the size of the female breast because the large breast will become droopy if volume is removed without lifting and tightening the skin. The greater benefit of liposuction is in combination with surgical breast reduction techniques, in which it is used to smooth the contours under the arms and at the margins of the breast. For patients with a buffalo hump, liposuction makes it possible to reduce fat deposits on the upper back and lower neck that previously could not be removed without extensive surgery. For patients with HIV infection, lipodystrophy is a syndrome of abnormal fat distribution associated with the therapeutic use of protease inhibitors. The lipodystrophy may be in the form of a neck and upper back fat pad, fat deposition in the trunk and lower face, or increase in the adipose tissue of the breasts. All these respond well to treatment with liposuction.

The most common complications with suction-assisted lipectomy are contour deformity, excessive blood loss, hematoma, seroma, fluid overload, and asymmetry. Less commonly, overlying skin loss, skin burns, deep venous thrombosis, and pulmonary embolus are seen. There have been infrequent reports of fat embolus, cannula penetration of the abdominal cavity, lidocaine toxicity, and surgical shock. A national survey conducted in 2001 found that combining liposuction with other procedures such as abdominoplasty increased the mortality risk almost fivefold. This is presumably related to the longer length of the surgery, greater blood loss, and larger fluid shifts. On the basis of this information, subsequent technical and practice guidelines include limiting of concomitant procedures performed at the time of liposuction, stricter criteria for selection of patients with regard to obesity and general health factors, removal of less fat in one operative session, placement of limits on the length of the surgery, modifications in anesthetic techniques, and additional patient monitoring.

CONCLUSIONS

Plastic surgery continues to evolve with the development of new approaches for the care of people with congenital and acquired deformities. With therapeutic advances in medicine and surgery, new problems have emerged that call for novel reconstructive techniques. Challenged by these difficult problems, plastic surgery continues to look for ways to treat life- and limb-threatening problems and, at the same time, to restore form and function. Chest wall, abdominal wall, and perineal reconstruction are progressing rapidly, and defects that were incapacitating a decade ago are now correctable. Lower extremity salvage after devastating injury is now commonplace. With advances in other surgical specialties such as bariatric surgery, entirely new areas requiring plastic surgery have emerged. Old techniques, such as perforator flaps, continue to evolve and supply better ways to reconstruct defects. New techniques, such as fat grafting, which may revolutionize clinical practice, have come from empirical observations. Developed from new research studies, tissue engineering, gene therapy, and stem cell work will change reconstruction in unforeseeable ways in the future. The search continues for the most reliable, durable, and aesthetic ways to "restore, repair, and make whole those parts … which fortune has taken away" (Gaspare Tagliacozzi [Italian surgeon who became famous for his skill in reconstructive surgery], *De Curtorum Chirurgia per Insitionem*, Venice, 1579).

SELECTED REFERENCES

Hashim PW, Patel A, Yang JF, et al: The effects of whole-vault cranioplasty versus strip craniectomy on long-term neuropsychological outcomes in sagittal craniosynostosis. *Plast Reconstr Surg* 134:491–501, 2014.

This multicenter study compares long-term cognitive outcomes in children with sagittal craniosynostosis treated with either total cranial vault reconstruction or endoscopic sagittal suturectomy. It shows that children having early (before 6 months of age) whole vault cranioplasty attain higher intelligence quotients and achievement scores. It is the first comparative analysis establishing the effects of technique and timing on long-term intellectual functioning in these children.

Kiwanuka H, Bueno EM, Diaz-Siso JR, et al: Evolution of ethical debate on face transplantation. *Plast Reconstr Surg* 132:1558–1568, 2013.

This article examines the evolution of the debate in the scientific literature about the ethics of face transplantation. It notes changes in the dialogue since 2002 as experience-based practical issues have arisen and outlines 15 major ethical concerns that need to be considered to ethically advance the field of face transplantation.

Koshima I, Yamamoto T, Narushima M, et al: Perforator flaps and supermicrosurgery. *Clin Plast Surg* 37:683–689, 2010.

The introduction of supermicrosurgery, the microvascular anastomosis of vessels ranging from 0.3 to 0.8 mm in diameter, opens up a wide array of new reconstructive options. Free perforator flaps can be obtained from anywhere on the

body and provide thinner, more pliant tissue for repair of extremity and facial defects. This paper reviews these new options as well as the technical challenges of supermicrosurgery.

Pannucci CJ, Bailey SH, Dreszer G, et al: Validation of the Caprini risk assessment model in plastic and reconstructive surgery patients. *J Am Coll Surg* 212:105–112, 2011.

This study of the incidence of venous thromboembolism (VTE) in 1126 plastic surgery patients at five tertiary referral centers found that the Caprini Risk Assessment Model effectively risk stratifies plastic and reconstructive surgery patients for VTE risk. Among patients with Caprini score higher than 8, 11.3% have a postoperative VTE when chemoprophylaxis is not provided. In higher risk patients, there was no evidence that VTE risk is limited to the immediate postoperative period.

Walmsley GG, Maan ZN, Wong VW, et al: Scarless wound healing: Chasing the holy grail. *Plast Reconstr Surg* 135:907–917, 2015.

This article on regenerative medicine reviews the stages of wound healing, the differences between adult and fetal wound healing, and the various mechanical, genetic, and pharmacologic strategies to reduce scarring. It discusses the biology of skin stem/progenitor cells that may hold the key to scarless regeneration and concludes that the characterization of functional cell lineages in the integument will follow from increased understanding of signaling molecules, growth factors, and lineage-specific cell origin and function.

REFERENCES

1. Tamai M, Nagasao T, Miki T, et al: Rotation arc of pedicled anterolateral thigh flap for abdominal wall reconstruction: How far can it reach? *J Plast Reconstr Aesthet Surg* 68:1417–1424, 2015.
2. Buchanan PJ, Kung TA, Cederna PS: Evidence-based medicine: Wound closure. *Plast Reconstr Surg* 134:1391–1404, 2014.
3. Hong JP, Koshima I: Using perforators as recipient vessels (supermicrosurgery) for free flap reconstruction of the knee region. *Ann Plast Surg* 64:291–293, 2010.
4. Wei F, Tay SKL: Principles and techniques of microvascular surgery. In Nelligan PC, editor: *Plastic surgery*, ed 3, London, 2013, Elsevier Saunders, pp 587–621.
5. Koshima I, Yamamoto T, Narushima M, et al: Perforator flaps and supermicrosurgery. *Clin Plast Surg* 37:683–689, 2010.
6. Hong JP: The use of supermicrosurgery in lower extremity reconstruction: The next step in evolution. *Plast Reconstr Surg* 123:230–235, 2009.
7. Marks MW, Argenta LC: Principles and applications of tissue expansion. In Nelligan PC, editor: *Plastic surgery*, ed 3, London, 2013, Elsevier Saunders, pp 622–653.
8. Gougoutas AJ, Singh DJ, Low DW, et al: Hemifacial microsomia: Clinical features and pictographic representations of the OMENS classification system. *Plast Reconstr Surg* 120:112e–120e, 2007.

9. Stal S, Brown RH, Higuera S, et al: Fifty years of the Millard rotation-advancement: Looking back and moving forward. *Plast Reconstr Surg* 123:1364–1377, 2009.

10. Sullivan SR, Marrinan EM, LaBrie RA, et al: Palatoplasty outcomes in nonsyndromic patients with cleft palate: A 29-year assessment of one surgeon's experience. *J Craniofac Surg* 20(Suppl 1):612–616, 2009.

11. Tromberg J, Bauer B, Benvenuto-Andrade C, et al: Congenital melanocytic nevi needing treatment. *Dermatol Ther* 18:136–150, 2005.

12. Ho K, Hutter JJ, Eskridge J, et al: The management of life-threatening haemorrhage following blunt facial trauma. *J Plast Reconstr Aesthet Surg* 59:1257–1262, 2006.

13. Ellis E, 3rd, Miles BA: Fractures of the mandible: A technical perspective. *Plast Reconstr Surg* 120:76S–89S, 2007.

14. Khalifian S, Brazio PS, Mohan R, et al: Facial transplantation: The first 9 years. *Lancet* 384:2153–2163, 2014.

15. Janis JE, Rohrich RJ: Clinical decision-making in rhinoplasty. In Nahai F, editor: *The art of aesthetic surgery: Principles and techniques*, St. Louis, 2005, Quality Medical, pp 1515–1533.

16. Carniol PJ, Hamilton MM, Carniol ET: Current status of fractional laser resurfacing. *JAMA Facial Plast Surg* 17:360–366, 2015.

17. Mojallal A, Lequeux C, Shipkov C, et al: Improvement of skin quality after fat grafting: Clinical observation and an animal study. *Plast Reconstr Surg* 124:765–774, 2009.

18. Marino G, Moraci M, Armenia E, et al: Therapy with autologous adipose-derived regenerative cells for the care of chronic ulcer of lower limbs in patients with peripheral arterial disease. *J Surg Res* 185:36–44, 2013.

19. Carruthers JD, Glogau RG, Blitzer A: Advances in facial rejuvenation: Botulinum toxin type A, hyaluronic acid dermal fillers, and combination therapies—consensus recommendations. *Plast Reconstr Surg* 121:5S–30S, 2008.

20. Netscher DT, Baumholtz MA: Chest reconstruction: I. Anterior and anterolateral chest wall and wounds affecting respiratory function. *Plast Reconstr Surg* 124:240e–252e, 2009.

21. Chang RR, Mehrara BJ, Hu QY, et al: Reconstruction of complex oncologic chest wall defects: A 10-year experience. *Ann Plast Surg* 52:471–479, 2004.

22. Losken A, Thourani VH, Carlson GW, et al: A reconstructive algorithm for plastic surgery following extensive chest wall resection. *Br J Plast Surg* 57:295–302, 2004.

23. Preminger BA, Yaghoobzadeh Y, Ascherman JA: Management of sternal wounds by limited debridement and partial bilateral pectoralis major myocutaneous advancement flaps in 25 patients: A less invasive approach. *Ann Plast Surg* 72:446–450, 2014.

24. Davison SP, Clemens MW, Armstrong D, et al: Sternotomy wounds: Rectus flap versus modified pectoral reconstruction. *Plast Reconstr Surg* 120:929–934, 2007.

25. Vyas RM, Prsic A, Orgill DP: Transdiaphragmatic omental harvest: A simple, efficient method for sternal wound coverage. *Plast Reconstr Surg* 131:544–552, 2013.

26. Dabbah A, Lehman JA, Jr, Parker MG, et al: Reduction mammoplasty: An outcome analysis. *Ann Plast Surg* 35:337–341, 1995.

27. Handel N, Garcia ME, Wixtrom R: Breast implant rupture: Causes, incidence, clinical impact, and management. *Plast Reconstr Surg* 132:1128–1137, 2013.

28. Deapen D, Hamilton A, Bernstein L, et al: Breast cancer stage at diagnosis and survival among patients with prior breast implants. *Plast Reconstr Surg* 105:535–540, 2000.

29. Gidengil CA, Predmore Z, Mattke S, et al: Breast implant–associated anaplastic large cell lymphoma: A systematic review. *Plast Reconstr Surg* 135:713–720, 2015.

30. Largo RD, Tchang LA, Mele V, et al: Efficacy, safety and complications of autologous fat grafting to healthy breast tissue: A systematic review. *J Plast Reconstr Aesthet Surg* 64:437–448, 2014.

31. Petty PM, Solomon M, Buchel EW, et al: Gynecomastia: Evolving paradigm of management and comparison of techniques. *Plast Reconstr Surg* 125:1301–1308, 2011.

32. Agnew SP, Small W, Jr, Wang E, et al: Prospective measurements of intra-abdominal volume and pulmonary function after repair of massive ventral hernias with the components separation technique. *Ann Surg* 251:981–988, 2010.

33. Morykwas MJ, Argenta LC, Shelton-Brown EI, et al: Vacuum-assisted closure: A new method for wound control and treatment: Animal studies and basic foundation. *Ann Plast Surg* 38:553–562, 1997.

34. Butler CE, Campbell KT: Minimally invasive component separation with inlay bioprosthetic mesh (MICSIB) for complex abdominal wall reconstruction. *Plast Reconstr Surg* 128:698–709, 2011.

35. den Hartog D, Dur AH, Tuinebreijer WE, et al: Open surgical procedures for incisional hernias. *Cochrane Database Syst Rev* (3):CD006438, 2008.

36. Althubaiti G, Butler CE: Abdominal wall and chest wall reconstruction. *Plast Reconstr Surg* 133:688e–701e, 2014.

37. Hurvitz KA, Olaya WA, Nguyen A, et al: Evidence-based medicine: Abdominoplasty. *Plast Reconstr Surg* 133:1214–1221, 2014.

38. Bullard KM, Trudel JL, Baxter NN, et al: Primary perineal wound closure after preoperative radiotherapy and abdominoperineal resection has a high incidence of wound failure. *Dis Colon Rectum* 48:438–443, 2005.

39. Butler CE, Gundeslioglu AO, Rodriguez-Bigas MA: Outcomes of immediate vertical rectus abdominis myocutaneous flap reconstruction for irradiated abdominoperineal resection defects. *J Am Coll Surg* 206:694–703, 2008.

40. Nelson RA, Butler CE: Surgical outcomes of VRAM versus thigh flaps for immediate reconstruction of pelvic and perineal cancer resection defects. *Plast Reconstr Surg* 123:175–183, 2009.

41. Wong DS: Reconstruction of the perineum. *Ann Plast Surg* 73(Suppl 1):S74–S81, 2014.

42. Friedman JD, Reece GR, Eldor L: The utility of the posterior thigh flap for complex pelvic and perineal reconstruction. *Plast Reconstr Surg* 126:146–155, 2010.

43. O'Shaughnessy BA, Dumanian GA, Liu JC, et al: Pedicled omental flaps as an adjunct in the closure of complex spinal wounds. *Spine (Phila Pa 1976)* 32:3074–3080, 2007.

44. Glatt BS, Disa JJ, Mehrara BJ, et al: Reconstruction of extensive partial or total sacrectomy defects with a transabdominal vertical rectus abdominis myocutaneous flap. *Ann Plast Surg* 56:526–530, discussion 530–531, 2006.

45. Zakaria Y, Hasan EA: Reversed turnover latissimus dorsi muscle flap for closure of large myelomeningocele defects. *J Plast Reconstr Aesthet Surg* 63:1513–1518, 2010.

46. Cushing CA, Phillips LG: Evidence-based medicine: Pressure sores. *Plast Reconstr Surg* 132:1720–1732, 2013.

47. Ong YS, Levin LS: Lower limb salvage in trauma. *Plast Reconstr Surg* 125:582–588, 2010.

48. Shawen SB, Keeling JJ, Branstetter J, et al: The mangled foot and leg: Salvage versus amputation. *Foot Ankle Clin* 15:63–75, 2010.

49. Parrett BM, Winograd JM, Garfein ES, et al: The vertical and extended rectus abdominis myocutaneous flap for irradiated thigh and groin defects. *Plast Reconstr Surg* 122:171–177, 2008.

50. Parrett BM, Talbot SG, Pribaz JJ, et al: A review of local and regional flaps for distal leg reconstruction. *J Reconstr Microsurg* 25:445–455, 2009.

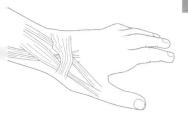

CHAPTER 69

Hand Surgery

David Netscher, Kevin D. Murphy, Nicholas A. Fiore II

第六十九章　手外科

中文导读

　　本章共分为12节：①基础解剖；②检查和诊断；③治疗原则；④创伤；⑤感染；⑥筋膜室综合征、高压注射损伤和外渗损伤；⑦腱鞘炎；⑧周围神经卡压综合征；⑨肿瘤；⑩先天性畸形；⑪骨关节炎和类风湿关节炎；⑫挛缩。

　　第一节介绍了手部的局部解剖，着重描述了手部肌肉的起始点、肌肉收缩所产生的运动及其神经支配、肌腱的走行及其体表投影和手部重要神经的解剖和支配范围。

　　第二节介绍了手的一般检查方法、神经血管及骨骼肌肉的检查及特殊检查方法，例如：影像学检查（X线片、CT、MRI）、腕关节镜检查、超声检查等。

　　第三节阐述了手外伤的治疗原则是修复重要组织结构包括骨、肌腱、神经、血管及皮肤损伤。分别介绍了麻醉方法的选择、止血带的应用、手术切口的设计以及术后绷带和夹板的使用。

　　第四节分别阐述了急诊止血、切割伤、指尖损伤、复杂软组织损伤的处理方法。并重点介绍了屈指肌腱和伸指肌腱损伤的处理原则及修复方法、神经损伤的修复、血管损伤的修复、再植或截肢的适应证及各部位骨折、脱位的治疗原则。

　　第五节主要介绍手部感染性疾病的病因、临床表现和治疗，包括甲沟炎、手部间隙感染、深部感染、慢性或不典型感染、病毒（疱疹）感染和动物或人类咬伤。

　　第六节分别介绍了高压注射损伤、药物外渗损伤和筋膜室综合征的病因、临床表现、体征和处理原则，强调了早期诊断、早期处理、避免并发症的产生。

第七节主要介绍了桡骨茎突腱鞘炎、扳机拇和弹响指以及其他部位腱鞘炎的可能病因、典型症状和治疗方法。

第八节从局部解剖、病因、临床表现和治疗原则等方面介绍了腕管综合征、旋前圆肌综合征、腕尺管和肘管综合征、桡神经卡压和胸廓出口综合征等神经压迫综合征。

第九节主要介绍了手部各类常见软组织肿瘤、皮肤恶性肿瘤和骨肿瘤。

第十节讲述了复杂手部畸形患儿，常常合并有身体其他重要组织器官畸形。手部先天性畸形的手术时机、手术方法因人而异。

第十一节主要阐述了骨关节炎和类风湿关节炎的发病机制、临床表现及影像学特征、治疗方法。

第十二节主要介绍缺血性肌挛缩、创伤后挛缩和掌腱膜挛缩的发病机制、临床表现和疾病不同阶段的治疗方法。

〔康　皓〕

Although hand surgery fellowships traditionally receive trainees primarily with backgrounds in orthopedic surgery or plastic surgery, fellowship training in hand surgery may also be undertaken by those having completed a residency in general surgery. Basic tenets of hand surgery must be acquired by all general surgeons. Depending on the practice locale (rural or urban), type of hospital, and residency rotations (e.g., surgical intern covering the emergency department) or even for the purposes of board examinations, the ability to evaluate and to manage hand injuries and problems is a necessary skill for the general surgeon. The purpose of this chapter is not to provide the general surgeon with an exhaustive study of hand surgery, because specialty texts are more appropriate, but to provide an overview of pathologic processes of the hand encountered more commonly by the general surgeon and especially to emphasize basics in anatomy, physical examination, and treatment of common hand and upper extremity emergencies.

Interestingly, there is a modest amount of recent literature on the quality and duration of hand fellowship training. In a recent survey to which 80% of program directors responded, the majority thought that a 1-year fellowship was still sufficient training despite the increasing breadth of knowledge in the field and new technologic developments.[1] However, programs needed to evaluate their own training to highlight areas that may need enhancement. Nonetheless, many training programs admittedly remain deficient in areas, especially shoulder and elbow, replantation, brachial plexus, congenital, and flap surgery.[2]

BASIC ANATOMY

The arm and hand are divided into volar or palmar and dorsal aspects. Distal to the elbow, structures are termed radial or ulnar to the middle finger axis rather than lateral and medial, respectively, because with forearm pronation and supination, the latter terms become confusing. The nomenclature of digits has become standardized. The hand has five digits, namely, the thumb and four fingers (the thumb is not called a finger). The four fingers are respectively termed the index, long (middle), ring, and small (little) fingers. The use of numbers to designate digits is no longer

accepted (Fig. 69-1). Within the hand, those structures close to the fingertips are termed distal, whereas those farther up toward the wrist are termed proximal. Motion in a palmar direction is flexion, whereas dorsal motion is termed extension. Finger motion away from the long finger axis is termed abduction, whereas motion toward the axis of the long finger is termed adduction. The description of the motion of the thumb is sometimes confusing. Extension of the thumb is in the plane of the palm of the hand, whereas palmar abduction of the thumb is the motion that occurs at 90 degrees away from the plane of the palm. Finally, side to side motion of the wrist is termed radial and ulnar deviation.

Intrinsic muscles of the hand are those that have their origins and insertions in the hand, whereas the extrinsic muscles have their muscle bellies in the forearm and their tendon insertions in the hand. The intrinsic muscles that make up the thenar eminence are the abductor pollicis brevis, flexor pollicis brevis, opponens pollicis, and adductor pollicis. There are four dorsal interossei that arise from adjacent sides of each metacarpal and provide abduction of the metacarpophalangeal (MP) joints of the index, middle, and ring fingers. There are three palmar interossei that adduct the index, ring, and little fingers toward the middle finger. Four lumbricals originate on the flexor digitorum profundus (FDP) tendons in the palm and insert on the radial sides of the extensor mechanisms of the four fingers. Together with the interossei, these bring about flexion of the MP joints and extension of the interphalangeal (IP) joints of the fingers (Fig. 69-2). The flexor pollicis brevis flexes the thumb at the MP joint, in contrast with the extrinsic flexor pollicis longus (FPL), which flexes the thumb IP joint.

The hypothenar muscles consist of the flexor digiti minimi, which flexes the little finger at the MP joint, and the abductor digiti minimi and opponens digiti minimi. A small muscle called the palmaris brevis is located transversally in the subcutaneous tissue at the base of the hypothenar eminence. It is innervated by the ulnar nerve, puckers the skin, and helps in cupping the skin of the palm during grip (Table 69-1).

The extrinsic muscles originate proximal to the wrist and comprise the long flexors and extensors of the wrist and digits. The extensors are located dorsally and are divided into three subgroups. The radialmost subgroup is termed the mobile wad and

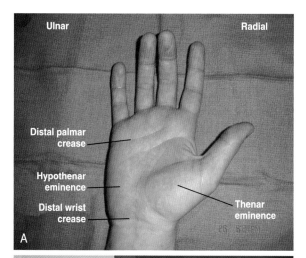

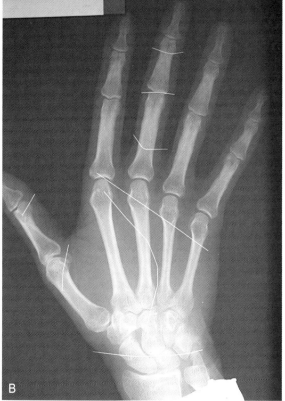

FIGURE 69-1 Surface Anatomy of the Hand. A, Hand surfaces and nomenclature. **B,** Skin creases of the hand superimposed on the skeletal structures.

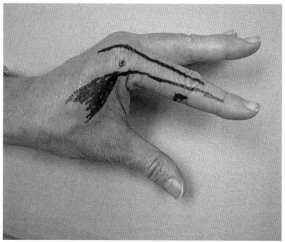

FIGURE 69-2 Outline of first dorsal interosseous muscle on the index finger shows how it passes volar to the fulcrum of flexion of the meta-carpophalangeal joint and dorsal to the interphalangeal joints. Interossei flex metacarpophalangeal joints and extend proximal and distal inter-phalangeal joints. The long extrinsic extensor tendon passes dorsal to all joints.

TABLE 69-1	Intrinsic Muscles of the Hand	
MUSCLE	**INNERVATION***	**FUNCTION**
Abductor pollicis brevis	Median	Abducts the thumb
Flexor pollicis brevis	Median	Flexes the thumb
Opponens pollicis	Median	Opposes the thumb
Lumbricals	Median and ulnar	Flex MP joints and extend IP joints
Palmaris brevis	Ulnar	Wrinkles the skin on the medial (ulnar) side of the palm
Adductor pollicis	Ulnar	Adducts the thumb
Abductor digiti minimi	Ulnar	Abducts the small finger
Flexor digiti minimi	Ulnar	Flexes the small digit
Opponens digiti minimi	Ulnar	Opposes the small finger
Dorsal interossei	Ulnar	Abduct the fingers; flex MP joints and extend the IP joints
Palmar interossei	Ulnar	Adduct the fingers; flex MP joints and extend the IP joints

IP, interphalangeal; *MP,* metacarpophalangeal.
*All the thenar intrinsic muscles are supplied by the median nerve except the adductor pollicis; all the remaining intrinsic muscles are supplied by the ulnar nerve except the two radial lumbricals.

comprises the brachioradialis, extensor carpi radialis longus (ECRL), and extensor carpi radialis brevis (ECRB). The ECRL and ECRB extend the wrist and deviate it radially. The second group is located in a more superficial layer and comprises three muscles, namely, the extensor carpi ulnaris (ECU), extensor digiti minimi (EDM), and extensor digitorum communis (EDC). The ECU deviates the wrist in an ulnar direction and extends the wrist, whereas the EDM and EDC extend the MP joints of the fingers. The third and deeper subgroup comprises four muscles, three of which act on the thumb; the remaining muscle influences the index finger. The abductor pollicis longus (APL), extensor pollicis longus (EPL), and extensor pollicis brevis (EPB) provide function to the thumb, and the extensor indicis proprius (EIP) extends the MP joint to the index finger. Last of the deep muscles is the supinator, which is located proximally in the forearm (Table 69-2).

The extensor tendons pass through six compartments deep to the extensor retinaculum at the dorsum of the wrist. From radial to ulnar side, these tendons and compartments are arranged as follows. The first compartment contains the APL and EPB, which also forms the radial boundary of the so-called anatomic snuffbox. The second compartment consists of the ECRL and ECRB, and the third compartment (which also forms the ulnar boundary of the anatomic snuffbox) contains the EPL. The EIP and EDC pass through the fourth compartment and the EDM passes through the fifth compartment, where they overlie the distal radioulnar joint. The sixth compartment contains the ECU (Fig. 69-3).

At the level of the MP joints, the long extrinsic extensor tendons broaden out to form the extensor hood. The proximal part of the hood at this level is called the sagittal band. It loops

around the MP joint and blends into the volar plate, thus forming a lasso around the base of the proximal phalanx, through which it extends the MP joint. The insertions of the interossei and lumbricals enter into the extensor hood as the lateral bands. These lateral bands insert distally and dorsally to the axis of the proximal interphalangeal (PIP) joint, and it is through this distal insertion that the intrinsic muscles (the interossei and lumbricals) are flexors of the MP joints and yet extensors of the IP joints. The extensor hood inserts to the base of the middle phalanx, which is termed the central slip, and finally proceeds on to the base of the distal phalanx, where it inserts through the terminal slip, thus extending the distal interphalangeal (DIP) joint (Fig. 69-4).

The extrinsic flexor muscles are located on the volar aspect of the forearm and are arranged in three layers. The superficial layer comprises four muscles—pronator teres, flexor carpi radialis (FCR), flexor carpi ulnaris (FCU), and palmaris longus. The palmaris longus muscle may be absent in as many as 10% to 12% of individuals. These muscles originate from the medial humeral epicondyle in the proximal forearm and function to flex the wrist and to pronate the forearm. The intermediate layer consists of the flexor digitorum superficialis (FDS), which allows independent flexion of the PIP joints of the fingers. In the deep layer, there are three muscles: the FPL, which flexes the IP joint to the thumb; the FDP, which flexes the DIP joints of the fingers; and a distal quadrangular muscle that spans between the radius and ulna, termed the pronator quadratus, which helps in pronation of the forearm (Table 69-3).

Nerve supply to the hand is by three nerves, the median, ulnar, and radial nerves. A knowledge of the surface anatomy of nerves helps in evaluation of specific lacerating injuries (Fig. 69-5). The ulnar attachment to the flexor retinaculum is to the pisiform and hook of the hamate, and the radial attachment is to the scaphoid and ridge of the trapezium. The median nerve passes through the carpal tunnel between these landmarks. It gives sensation to the thumb, index finger, middle finger, and radial half of the ring finger. The palmar cutaneous branch of the median nerve originates from its radial side 5 to 6 cm proximal to the wrist, providing sensation to the palmar triangle. The ulnar nerve travels to the radial side of the pisiform and passes to the ulnar side of the hook of the hamate in its passage through Guyon canal. It gives

TABLE 69-2 Extrinsic Muscles of the Dorsal Forearm

MUSCLE	INNERVATION*	FUNCTION
Extensor pollicis brevis	Radial	Abducts the hand and extends the thumb at the proximal phalanx
Abductor pollicis longus	Radial	Abducts the hand and thumb
Extensor carpi radialis longus	Radial	Extends and radially deviates the hand
Extensor carpi radialis brevis	Radial	Extends and radially deviates the hand
Extensor pollicis longus	Radial	Extends the distal phalanx of the thumb
Extensor digitorum communis	Radial	Extends the fingers and the hand
Extensor indicis proprius	Radial	Extends the index finger
Extensor digiti minimi/ quinti	Radial	Extends the small finger
Extensor carpi ulnaris	Radial	Extends and ulnarly deviates the wrist
Supinator	Radial	Supination
Brachioradialis	Radial	Flexes the forearm

*All muscles of the dorsal forearm are innervated by the radial nerve and its respective branches.

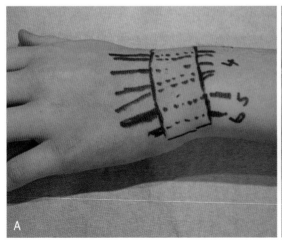 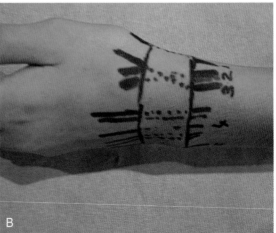

FIGURE 69-3 **A** and **B,** Surface anatomy of the six dorsal extensor compartments at the wrist. Note that the first (abductor pollicis longus and extensor pollicis brevis) and third (extensor pollicis longus) compartments form the radial and ulnar boundaries, respectively, of the anatomic snuffbox.

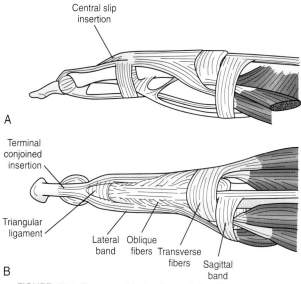

Central slip
insertion

A

Terminal
conjoined
insertion

Triangular
ligament

Lateral   Oblique
band   fibers Transverse
fibers Sagittal
band

B

FIGURE 69-4 Extensor Mechanism of the Fingers. A, Lateral view. B, Dorsal view.

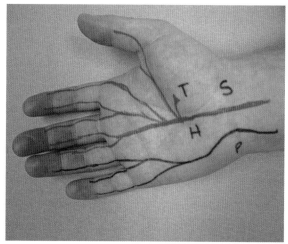

FIGURE 69-5 Surface anatomy of median *(red)* and ulnar *(black)* nerves. *H,* hook of hamate; *P,* pisiform; *S,* scaphoid; *T,* trapezium.

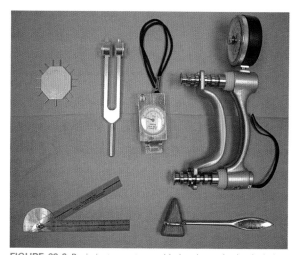

FIGURE 69-6 Basic instruments used in hand examination include a tuning fork, pinch meter, grip dynamometer, two-point discriminator (paperclip also suffices), goniometer, and patella hammer.

TABLE 69-3 Extrinsic Muscles of the Volar Forearm

MUSCLE	INNERVATION*	FUNCTION
Pronator teres	Median	Pronation
Flexor carpi radialis	Median	Flexion and radial deviation of the wrist
Palmaris longus	Median	Flexion of the wrist
Flexor carpi ulnaris	Ulnar	Flexion and ulnar deviation of the wrist
Flexor digitorum superficialis	Median	Flexion of the proximal interphalangeal joint
Flexor digitorum profundus	Median and ulnar	Flexion of the distal interphalangeal joint
Pronator quadratus	Median	Pronation
Flexor pollicis longus	Median	Flexion of the thumb

*All muscles of the volar forearm are innervated by the median nerve and its branches except the two ulnar digits of the flexor digitorum profundus and flexor carpi ulnaris, which are innervated by the ulnar nerve.

sensation to the little finger and ulnar half of the ring finger; the dorsal branch of the ulnar nerve (arising proximal to the wrist and curving dorsally around the head of the ulna) supplies the same digits on their dorsal aspects. The superficial radial sensory nerve emerges from under the brachioradialis in the distal forearm, dividing into two or three branches proximal to the radial styloid that then proceed in a subcutaneous course across the anatomic snuffbox, innervating the skin of the dorsum of the first web space. The number of fingers served by each nerve is variable. However, as an absolute rule, the palmar surfaces of the index and little fingers are always served by the median and ulnar nerves, respectively.

With regard to the motor supply of these nerves, the ulnar nerve supplies the hypothenar muscles, interossei, ulnar two lumbricals, adductor pollicis, and deep head of the flexor pollicis brevis. The median nerve supplies the abductor pollicis brevis,

opponens pollicis, radial two lumbricals, and superficial head of the flexor pollicis brevis. In summary, the median nerve thus supplies all the extrinsic digit flexors and wrist flexors (except the FDP to the ring and little fingers and the FCU, which are supplied by the ulnar nerve) and all the thumb intrinsic muscles (except the adductor pollicis, innervated by the ulnar nerve). The ulnar nerve supplies all the interossei, all the lumbricals (except the radial two, supplied by the median nerve), and the adductor of the thumb. The radial nerve innervates all of the wrist, finger, and thumb extrinsic long extensors.

EXAMINATION AND DIAGNOSIS

Evaluation

Basic instruments used in hand examination are shown in Figure 69-6. Examination of the resting posture of the hand can provide valuable information; for example, if a finger flexor tendon is severed, that affected finger does not assume its normal resting position in line with the natural flexion cascade of the adjacent digits (Fig. 69-7). Extensor tendon injuries may be indicated by a droop at the affected joint. A clawed posture of the little and ring fingers may be characteristic of an ulnar nerve injury (Fig. 69-8). Absence of sweating at the fingertips may imply a nerve injury in that particular distribution. Swelling and erythema may indicate a hand infection, and a purulent flexor tenosynovitis always results in a flexed posture of the digits. Rotational and angular digital deformities may occur when there are underlying fractures.

Neurovascular Examination

The Allen test confirms patency of the ulnar and radial arteries. Two-point sensory discrimination is the most sensitive method of testing for sensory loss and is easily done by using a bent paperclip (Fig. 69-9). The paperclip ends are set to a distance of approximately 5 mm apart for fingertip pulp sensory testing. The points are aligned along the axis of the finger. If this test is not reproducible because of an uncooperative patient, suspicion of a nerve injury can be confirmed by the tactile adherence test, in which a plastic pen is passed back and forth gently across the pulp on either side of each finger. Adhesion, because of the presence of sweat, is shown by slight but definite movement of the finger being examined (anesthetized finger pulp will not sweat).

There are two muscle tests that may provide the examiner with an absolute diagnosis of median or ulnar nerve injury. The motor function of the abductor pollicis brevis tests the median nerve. With the hand flat and facing palm up, the patient is asked to use his or her thumb to touch the examiner's finger, which is held directly over the thenar eminence (Fig. 69-10). The flexor digiti minimi muscle function will test the motor supply of the ulnar nerve. In the same hand position, the patient raises her or his little finger vertically, flexing the MP joint to a 90-degree angle, with the IP joint held straight. Tests for function of the radial nerve and its branches require wrist extension, thumb extension, and finger extension at the MP joint.

Musculoskeletal Examination

The integrity of the tendons is individually tested (Fig. 69-11). Flexion at distal joints of the thumb and fingers confirms that the FPL and FDP, respectively, are intact. Testing of FDS tendons is more complex. It is not possible to flex the DIP joints independently of one another because of a common origin of the FDP tendons. Thus, the other fingers are fixed in extension by the examiner, and the patient is asked to flex the remaining digits. Movement is produced by the FDS and occurs at the PIP joint. In approximately one third of patients, the FDS cannot produce little finger flexion. In 50% of these, in turn, there is a common origin with the ring finger, so flexion will occur if the ring finger is permitted to flex simultaneously. More uncommonly, there is no profundus tendon to the little finger and the superficialis inserts into the middle and distal phalanges. The long and short extensors (EPL and EPB) and long abductor of the thumb are tested by asking the patient to extend his or her thumb against resistance while these tendons are individually palpated. Long extensors of the fingers are tested by asking the patient to extend them against resistance applied to the dorsum of the proximal phalanx.

A closed boutonnière jamming injury may be difficult to initially diagnose. In this type of injury, the central slip insertion is disrupted from the middle phalanx and the triangular ligament on each side of the central slip is stretched or disrupted. The lateral bands then migrate volar. It takes time for this deformity to evolve. Initial presentation may not be immediately obvious until the lateral bands subluxate volarly and create the obvious boutonnière problem with PIP joint flexion and DIP joint hyperextension. The Elson test may help make this diagnosis. Normally, with the PIP joint blocked in flexion, one cannot actively extend the DIP joint because of slack in the lateral bands (Fig. 69-12).

Special Investigations

Radiographs are necessary in almost every case. These help in the diagnosis and evaluation of fractures and also in the investigation of foreign bodies. Multiple radiographic views of the affected part are required to define the precise pathologic process or fracture pattern. Glass is often seen on plain radiographs, and if it is not seen but suspected, it may be visualized by computed tomography (CT) or magnetic resonance imaging (MRI). If plastic is painted, it may be seen on routine radiographs; it is generally poorly visualized with CT but can be clearly seen with MRI. Wooden foreign bodies may be seen by CT or MRI but not by routine radiography.

Various stress radiographic views and cineradiography may be useful for demonstrating dynamic wrist instability patterns, especially scapholunate separation. Arthrography may detect ligamentous tears by extravasation of contrast material between the radiocarpal, distal radioulnar, and midcarpal joints. This is best combined with MRI, especially for the detection of triangular fibrocartilage tears at the ulnocarpal joint. Radionuclide bone scanning may help diagnose osteomyelitis, but in the hand, a false-positive result may occur because of the proximity of soft tissue infections to the bones. Occult wrist fractures may be localized by increased radionuclide uptake, but a false-positive result on evaluation for a fracture may also occur with ligamentous injuries. CT is a helpful modality for diagnosis of suspected carpal fractures (e.g., a scaphoid fracture that may not be seen on routine radiography), although most prefer MRI.

Wrist arthroscopy is useful as a diagnostic and therapeutic modality for a number of wrist problems, especially for disorders of the triangular fibrocartilage. Minimally invasive surgery with arthroscopic guidance has added a new dimension to the treatment of acute wrist disorders, such as scaphoid and distal radius intra-articular fractures.

Patients with ischemic problems often require noninvasive vascular studies. Doppler pressure measurements help localize the site of a vascular lesion. Angiography in the upper extremity is always carried out in the presence of a vasodilator (e.g., tolazoline [Priscoline], nitroglycerin) or an axillary block to differentiate apparent vessel occlusion from vasospasm. Subtraction radiographs with magnification help improve the detail and definition of the vascular study, especially in the distal forearm and hand.

PRINCIPLES OF TREATMENT

In the case of injuries, treatment is directed at the specific structures damaged—skeletal, tendon, nerve, vessel, integument.[3,4] In emergency situations, the goals of treatment are to maintain or to restore distal circulation, to obtain a healed wound, to preserve motion, and to retain distal sensation. Stable skeletal architecture is established in the primary phase of care because skeletal stability is essential for effective motion and function of the extremity. This also reestablishes skeletal length, straightens deformities, and corrects the compression or kinking of nerves and vessels. Arteries

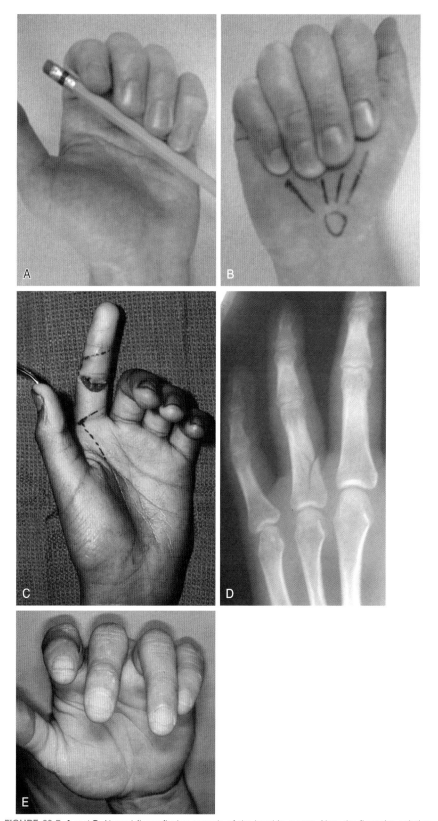

FIGURE 69-7 A and **B,** Natural finger flexion cascade of the hand in repose. Note the fingertips pointing to the distal pole of the scaphoid. **C,** With flexor tendon injury, the affected digit does not adopt this resting flexed posture. **D** and **E,** Spiral finger fractures produce a rotational deformity, which is also noted as an interruption in the finger flexion cascade.

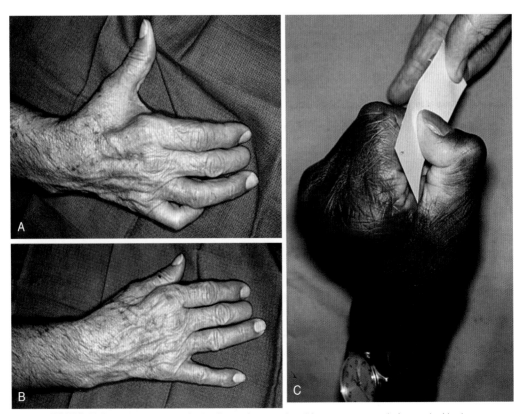

FIGURE 69-8 A, Marked atrophy in the first web space dorsal interosseous muscle is noted with ulnar nerve palsy, with clawing of the little and ring fingers. **B,** The little finger assumes an abducted position and cannot be adducted to the adjacent fingers (Wartenberg sign). **C,** Because thumb adduction is weak, attempts to grasp a piece of paper between the adducted thumb and index finger produce compensatory thumb interphalangeal joint flexion (Froment sign).

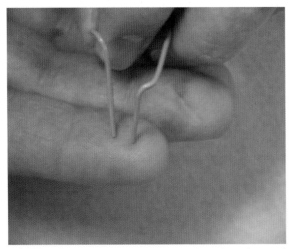

FIGURE 69-9 Two-point discrimination on the fingertip can be tested with a bent paperclip, with the tips of the paperclip set specific distances apart.

are also repaired in the acute phase of treatment to maintain distal tissue viability. Extrinsic compression on arteries must also be released emergently, such as with compartment pressure problems. In clean-cut injuries, tendons can be repaired primarily. In situations in which there is a chance that tendon adhesions may

form, such as when there are associated fractures, it is nonetheless better to repair tendons primarily with preservation of their length and to perform tenolysis, if necessary, at a later date. However, when there are open and contaminated wounds or a severe crushing injury, it is best to delay repair of tendon and nerve injuries.

In clean-cut sharp wounds, primary nerve repair lessens the possibility of nerve end retraction and therefore the need for later nerve grafting. However, primary nerve repair must not be performed in situations in which there is contusion of the nerve (e.g., gunshot wounds, power saw injuries, blunt crushing trauma) because the extent of proximal axonal injury may not be immediately evident. If nerve repair is performed before this is apparent, it may result in abnormal nerve ends being reattached, negating the chance for functional return.

In severe soft tissue injuries, wound closure may not be possible immediately. Initial open treatment of the wound is directed to prevent an infection and to protect critical deep structures by proper dressing and wound management (Fig. 69-13). Adequate débridement is essential, but appropriate soft tissue coverage must be achieved as soon as possible thereafter. The sooner the soft tissue coverage can be achieved, the less likely there will be a secondary deformity caused by fibrosis and joint contractures. The more rapidly hand therapy can be started, the better the chance for maximizing functional return. The treatment regimen must consist of débridement, rigid skeletal fixation, and early soft tissue resurfacing, possibly even requiring microvascular soft tissue

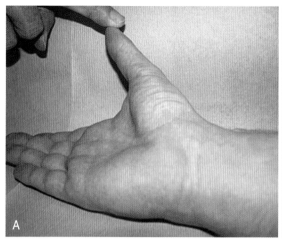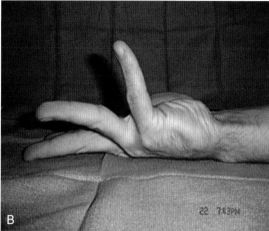

FIGURE 69-10 Motor Innervation of Muscles of the Hand. **A,** Thumb abduction tests median motor nerve function. **B,** Little finger flexion at the metacarpophalangeal joint with simultaneous interphalangeal joint extension tests ulnar motor nerve function.

reconstruction, followed by protected range of motion exercises as soon as possible. It has been shown that early soft tissue reconstruction results in improved function, decreased morbidity, and shortened hospital stay.

Appropriate treatment of upper extremity problems requires a thorough knowledge of local and regional anesthesia, use of a tourniquet to provide a bloodless field, correct placement of incisions to minimize later scar contracture, and appropriate use of dressings and splints to reduce edema and to maintain a functional position. Above all, a clear knowledge of the unique anatomy of the hand and upper extremity not only aids in obtaining an accurate clinical diagnosis but also enables the safe performance of surgery.

Anesthesia

The choice of general, regional (e.g., intravenous Bier block, brachial plexus block that might be a supraclavicular or axillary block), or local anesthesia is governed by the extent and length of the operation. An upper arm or forearm tourniquet can be used in the unanesthetized extremity with only local anesthetic field infiltration or digital block for 30 to 45 minutes in a relaxed, cooperative patient, provided the arm is well exsanguinated. After this time, tourniquet pain will not permit more extensive local anesthetic procedures. If one has to operate in other areas, such as for harvesting of bone, nerve, tendon, or skin graft, or if more extensive surgical procedures are planned, general anesthesia will be required.

A digital block or median, ulnar, or radial wrist nerve block may be useful, especially for more limited emergency department procedures (Fig. 69-14). Digital nerve blocks usually do not include epinephrine, which could lead to vasospasm, but evidence has indicated the safety of distal blocks using an epinephrine solution. A maximum safe dose of lidocaine is 4 mg/kg.

Tourniquet Application

The tourniquet is used to provide a bloodless field so that clear visualization of all structures in the operative field is obtained. Penrose drains, rolled rubber glove fingers, or commercially available tourniquets can be used on digits. Great care must be taken when any constrictive device is used on digits because narrow

bands cause direct injury to underlying nerves and digital vessels. With the use of an arm tourniquet, the skin beneath the cuff must be protected with several wraps of cast padding. During skin preparation, this area must be kept dry to prevent blistering of the skin under an inflated cuff over moist padding. The cuff selected needs to be as wide as the diameter of the arm. Standard pressures used are 100 to 150 mm Hg higher than systolic blood pressure. The cuff is deflated every 2 hours for 15 to 20 minutes (5 minutes of reperfusion for every 30 minutes of tourniquet time) to revascularize distal tissues and to relieve pressure on nerves locally before the cuff is reinflated for more extensive procedures.[5] Exsanguination of the extremities is performed by wrapping the extremity with a Martin bandage in all cases, except those involving infection or tumors. In these latter cases, because of the possibility of embolization by mechanical pressure, exsanguination by bandage wrapping needs to be avoided. Simple elevation of the extremity for a few minutes before tourniquet inflation suffices.[3]

Incisions

Incisions are of the Bruner zigzag or midaxial type, or combinations of these, to avoid longitudinal motion-restricting scars that cross palmar flexion creases (Fig. 69-15). The marginal edge of a skin graft with healthy skin is also a potential scar line, so the margin of the skin graft is designed to be in these same lines to prevent contractures across flexion creases. Palmar incisions follow the pattern of skin creases. Dorsal incisions on the fingers and wrist and incisions on the forearm may follow longitudinal straight lines.

Dressings and Splints

The purposes of dressings are to protect wounds, to absorb drainage, and to help splint repaired structures. The first layer consists of a nonadherent dressing and may contain an antibiotic. The next layer is soft and bulky and is usually followed by a firmer, more conforming external wrap. Conforming compression is useful, but constriction is harmful. Splints are made to protect only the part necessary to be immobilized and must not prevent motion in the remainder of the extremity. Often, patients keep the injured, operated, or infected hand in a flexed wrist position, which

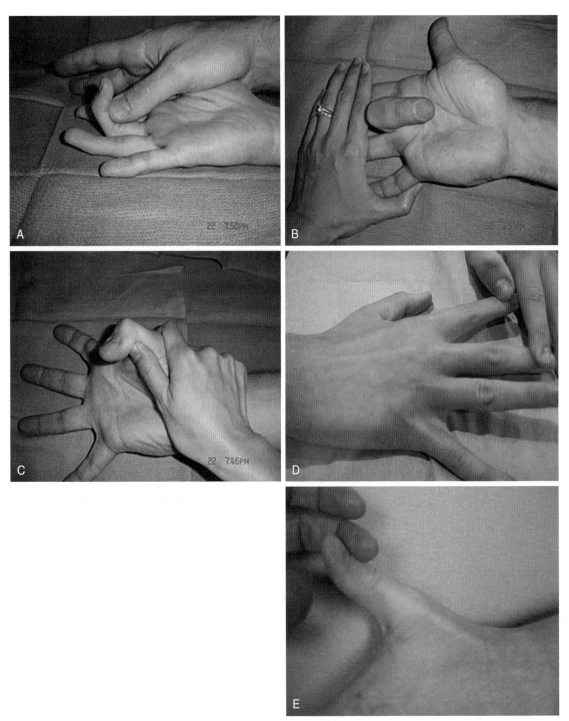

FIGURE 69-11 Individual clinical testing of the flexor digitorum profundus **(A)**, flexor digitorum superficialis **(B)**, flexor pollicis longus **(C)**, finger extensors **(D)**, and thumb extensors **(E)**.

automatically causes the MP joints to extend, thereby placing the collateral ligaments in their shortest lengths. Edema fluid collects dorsally, and the resulting dorsal hand swelling causes stiff joints. Thus, a splint that keeps the hand in the protected position extends the wrist 40 to 50 degrees, maintaining the MP joints at 70 degrees of flexion and the IP joints in a neutral position (Fig. 69-16). Postoperative hand elevation is essential to reduce edema.

TRAUMA

Emergency Control of Bleeding

Bleeding in the extremity can often be profuse when it is first encountered. A reasoned and controlled assessment of the situation almost invariably results in the control of bleeding and minimization of further blood loss and facilitates necessary stabilization of the patient and appropriate assessment of the upper limb injury. Bleeding in the upper extremity often results when vessels lie in a superficial location, such as at the wrist. Bleeding can originate from superficial veins that bleed more profusely when poorly applied dressings result in venous engorgement. The thicker media of transected arterial walls contracts strongly, resulting in hemostasis. Partially lacerated arteries continue to bleed profusely.

If necessary, one may have no fear of using sympathomimetic medications and their potential vasoconstricting effect to support blood pressure, even if free flap reconstruction or microvascular

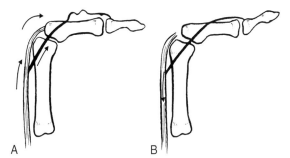

FIGURE 69-12 **A,** Maximal passive flexion of the proximal interphalangeal (PIP) joint causes slack in the lateral bands because they are pulled distally by their interconnections to the extensor hood proximally as the central slip and extensor tendon are pulled forward. Thus, normally, one cannot actively extend the distal interphalangeal (DIP) joint when the PIP joint is passively flexed. **B,** Central slip injury eliminates the lateral band slack that is normally produced by passive PIP joint flexion and allows extensor tension on the DIP joint because of proximal migration of the extensor apparatus. The ability to extend the DIP joint is pathologic.

repair has been done. A study evaluated four sympathomimetic medications and actually showed that both dobutamine and norepinephrine have a beneficial effect on flap skin blood flow, with the maximal beneficial improvement from norepinephrine. This is the optimal pressor to use in patients who may need blood pressure support after free flap surgery. Elevation and accurately placed point pressure over bleeding points result in hemostatic control in almost all cases. Brief use of tourniquets may be a useful adjunct to allow temporary control of blood loss in the emergency department. Poorly applied dressings may be removed, bleeding points identified, point pressure dressings applied, and the hand elevated. This should take no more than 5 to 10 minutes. Extended tourniquet application results in hyperemic bleeding on deflation and subsequently hinders the surgeon. Tourniquets should not be applied for any significant period of time before definitive repair in the operating room, except for control of torrential hemorrhage caused by major amputation in the field. Misguided attempts to control upper extremity bleeding with clamps, ligatures, and cauterization in the emergency department frequently result in additional avoidable injury to adjacent uninjured structures and to vessels that may need to be repaired for adequate limb perfusion. Fracture reduction and stabilization will improve distal perfusion and facilitate hemorrhage control by restoring the limb to its correct anatomic alignment.

Lacerations, Fingertip Injuries, and Complex Soft Tissue Injuries

Although it is tempting to look within a wound to determine whether any tendon or nerve injuries exist, the same information can be obtained by careful physical examination without further violating a potential operative field and causing the patient extreme discomfort. A combination of knowledge of anatomy,

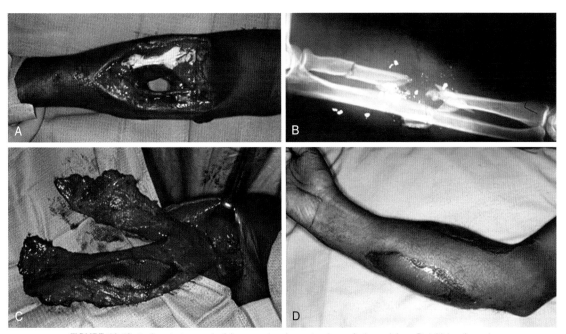

FIGURE 69-13 **A,** Gunshot wound of forearm showing extensive soft tissue injury. **B,** Initial radiograph. **C,** Microvascular reconstruction using a bilobed latissimus dorsi musculocutaneous flap was done in association with fracture fixation. **D,** Long-term follow-up of reconstructed forearm that also required sural nerve grafting to a segmental injury of the median nerve.

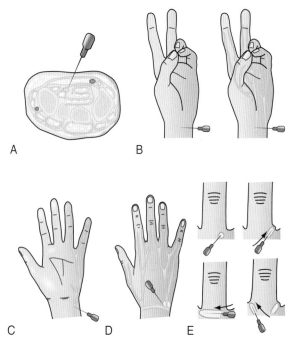

A   B

C   D   E

FIGURE 69-14 A, Median nerve block is done at the wrist, where the median nerve is superficial to all the flexor tendons in the carpal tunnel. **B,** At the wrist, when a median nerve block is performed, the needle is directed between the palmaris longus and flexor carpi radialis tendons. **C,** Ulnar nerve block at the wrist is done by passing the injecting needle around the ulnar deep aspect of the flexor carpi ulnaris tendon just proximal to the pisiform. Intravascular injection into the immediately adjacent ulnar artery is avoided by first aspirating before injection. **D,** Dorsal branches of the ulnar nerve and superficial sensory radial nerve are anesthetized by raising a broad weal of local anesthetic across the dorsum of the wrist. **E,** A dorsal approach to the finger can be used for digital nerve block.

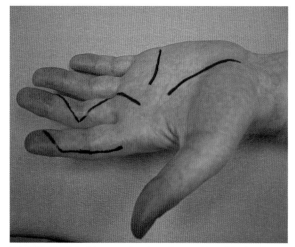

FIGURE 69-15 Incisions used on the palmar surface of the hand must respect the creases. These may be zigzag Bruner incisions or midaxial incisions of the digits.

presence of sensory or motor deficits, and presence or absence of radial or ulnar pulses can narrow the differential diagnosis of injured structures to a minimum. Control of bleeding is attempted by direct pressure with dressings and not by blind clamping of vessels because vital structures may be inadvertently injured in the

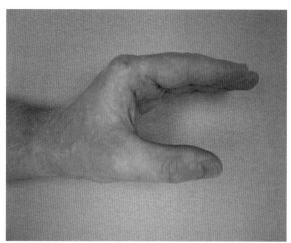

FIGURE 69-16 The safe or protected position of the wrist, hand, and digits for application of a splint and dressings. The thumb is palmar abducted.

depths of the wound. However, a tourniquet may be used if the initial pressure measures fail. Tourniquets are generally not used initially because the entire limb will be ischemic during transport of the patient. If the trauma has caused complete obliteration of anatomy, incisions can be extended into nonviolated areas in which control of bleeding vessels and delineation of injured tendons and nerves may be easier, using the guidelines presented earlier for extremity incisions.

All patients who present with extremity injuries undergo radiography. Fractures of the distal phalanx are among the more commonly encountered hand fractures.[6] A distal phalangeal fracture is appropriately splinted, reduced to improve alignment, or occasionally fixated internally if the fracture is unstable. Internal fixation is usually provided by simply placing a longitudinal 0.028-inch Kirschner wire. Appropriate antibiotics are administered because, technically, these are open fractures.

The least severe injury of the dorsum of the fingertip is a nail bed hematoma. When it is seen early, the hematoma can be decompressed by perforating the nail plate after the administration of a digital local anesthetic block. Fingertip and nail bed injuries can be managed with digital block anesthesia and a Penrose drain at the base of the finger as a tourniquet. After the nail plate has been stripped, simple gentle removal of the nail to examine the underlying nail bed is done, and suture repair of the nail bed is performed using loupe magnification and a 6-0 catgut suture. Once the nail bed has been repaired, it is best to place the thoroughly cleansed nail back under the nail fold, where it serves as a rigid splint for an underlying distal phalangeal fracture and prevents adhesions from forming between the adjacent surfaces of the nail fold, which might lead to an unsightly split nail deformity. If there is a piece of nail bed missing, the undersurface of the avulsed nail plate is examined. Frequently, the missing piece may still be adherent to the nail, and it can be gently removed and replaced as a nail bed graft. Some fingertip injuries may be so severe that amputation revision may be the most sensible and functional solution.

Volar fingertip injuries range from simple to more complex. Multiple digits may be involved, such as with lawnmower injuries. If bone is not exposed and a soft tissue defect of the finger pulp is smaller than 1 cm, the wound is best left open and managed

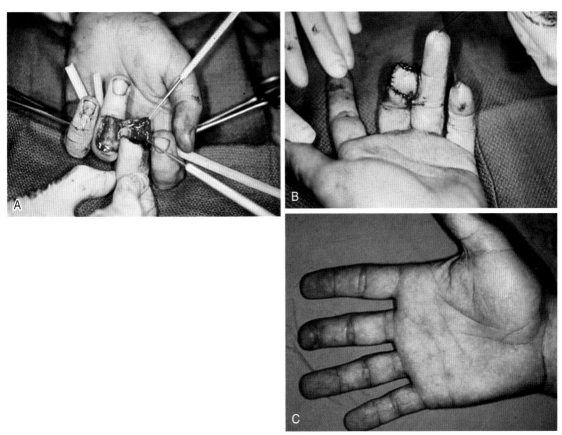

FIGURE 69-17 A and **B,** Volar angulated fingertip injury with loss of pulp pad and bone exposed was treated with a traditional cross-finger flap from the dorsum of the adjacent finger. **C,** Excellent healing is seen in the long term after flap division.

with dressings. Such an injury will heal with excellent functional and cosmetic results. Larger soft tissue defects of the fingertip pulp are more appropriately treated with a small, full-thickness skin graft. However, if bone is exposed and the soft tissue wound is larger, flap coverage or revision of amputation by trimming back exposed bone to obtain soft tissue coverage should be considered. In a dorsally angulated fingertip amputation, soft tissue coverage can be achieved by a neurovascular V-Y advancement flap. If the soft tissue loss is angulated in a more volar direction, a cross-finger flap, adjacent finger digital island flap, or homodigital flap may be performed (Figs. 69-17 to 69-19).

This algorithm for fingertip soft tissue coverage based on the geometry of the wound was previously time honored. However, with the larger homodigital flaps now available, that algorithm has changed because these flaps can be mobilized much more and are less restricted by their pedicle and have a wider arc of rotation. For example, the retrograde homodigital island flap can pivot to cover either volar or dorsal fingertip wounds.

Tendon Injuries
Flexor Tendons
Flexor tendon injuries usually result from lacerations or puncture wounds on the palmar surface of the hand, although flexor tendons can be avulsed from their distal bone insertions by sudden violent contractions. These are best treated by a surgeon experienced in the treatment of such injuries. Flexor tendon injuries are

divided into five zones (Fig. 69-20). In zones 1, 2, and 4, each tendon is surrounded by a synovial sheath and contained within a semirigid fibro-osseous canal, either the flexor tendon sheath of the digit or the carpal tunnel. In the other zones, the flexor tendons are surrounded by loose areolar (paratenon) tissue. Those parts devoid of a fibrous sheath usually heal well because of the good blood supply from the paratenon. Tendons in the carpal tunnel (zone 4) have their rich blood supply provided by the mesotenon; however, zones 1 and 2 have a precarious blood supply through the vincula; complementary nutritional support is provided by the synovial fluid in these two zones. For tendon gliding to occur, the mesotenon has disappeared in the digital flexor sheath except at the sites of the vincula that carry the vessels from the periosteum to the tendons (Fig. 69-21). Tendon zones to the thumb are T1 through T3.

Primary tendon repair undertaken within a few hours of injury is generally reserved for cleanly cut tendons. Delayed primary repair is performed from several hours up to 10 days after injury and is indicated for tidy but potentially contaminated wounds to allow prophylaxis against infection before the tendon repair. Relative contraindications to immediate tendon repair include the following:
- Injuries more than 12 hours old
- Crush wounds with poor skin coverage
- Contaminated wounds, especially human bites
- Tendon loss of more than 1 cm

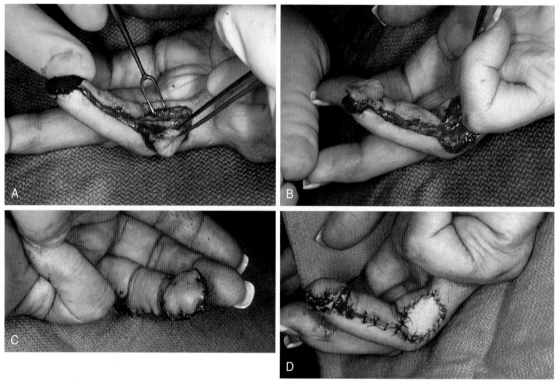

FIGURE 69-18 A-D, More recent understanding of the vascular skin territories of the finger and hand enables intrinsic flap coverage of fingertip injuries and avoids the cumbersome tethering of adjacent fingers, as is done with cross-finger flaps. In this patient, a distally based turnover vascular island flap reconstructs an avulsed fingertip. The reverse-flow perforating vessels at the proximal interphalangeal joint cross from the opposite side to nourish this flap.

- Injury at multiple sites along the tendon
- Destruction of the pulley system

After 4 weeks, a later secondary repair is generally not possible because of retraction of the musculotendinous unit so that reapproximation of the tendon ends produces undesirable joint flexion. In this situation, tendon graft repair may be required. The surgeon's endeavors are directed at avoiding the four major complications that interfere with smooth gliding and the integrated action of tendons—adhesions, attenuation of the repair, repair rupture, and joint and soft tissue contractures. Prerequisites for tendon repair are aseptic conditions in the operating room with good lighting and good instruments, adequate anesthesia, and loupe magnification. A well-performed technical operation can be futile without proper postoperative hand therapy, splinting, and excellent compliance of the patient.[7]

Appropriate treatment of partial flexor tendon injuries is necessary to produce a smooth juncture at the injury site. Prevention of complications requires exploration of all wounds likely to cause partial flexor tendon lacerations. A partial tendon injury of 50% or less is treated by simple trimming of the lacerated portion. Those injuries greater than 50% are repaired. Failure to diagnose a partial flexor tendon laceration at the time of primary repair may lead to delayed tendon rupture, entrapment between the tendon laceration and the laceration in the flexor sheath, or trigger finger.

Zone 2 flexor tendon injuries require special attention. This zone is also called Bunnell's no man's land. There are three tendons—the profundus and two slips of superficialis—that traverse zone 2, and they constantly interchange their mutual spatial relationships. Tendon injury in this region requires opening of the existing laceration in the flexor tendon sheath by making a longitudinal trap door so that a flap of tendon sheath can be elevated. Care must be taken to avoid excising excessive portions of the flexor tendon sheath because bowstringing may result in ineffective finger flexion, although portions can be vented or excised to facilitate repair or to prevent postoperative triggering. Total preservation of the A2 and A4 pulleys, previously thought to be essential, is no longer believed to be critical to success. One can excise up to 50% of the A2 and A4 pulleys without creating unnecessary tendon bowstringing if this is thought to be prudent to avoid the tendon repair's impinging under the pulley.[8] It has also been shown that one can incise the full length of the A4 pulley (but not excise it) without any biomechanical consequences.[9] This is especially helpful when the zone 2 repair occurs proximate to the A4 pulley, the narrowest part of the flexor tendon sheath. Finally, wide-awake anesthesia, which is local anesthetic infiltration using a solution of lidocaine with epinephrine, enables flexor tendon repair without the use of a tourniquet and ensures full cooperation of the patient during the procedure.[10] This was previously thought to be unwise, but this has been proved to be unsubstantiated. Thus, one can determine intraoperatively that there is full flexor tendon excursion at the repair site without impingement under the pulleys as the patient flexes and extends his or her fingers before the skin incision is finally closed. All these novel and revolutionary concepts challenge previously accepted dogma with regard to zone 2 flexor tendon repairs and the

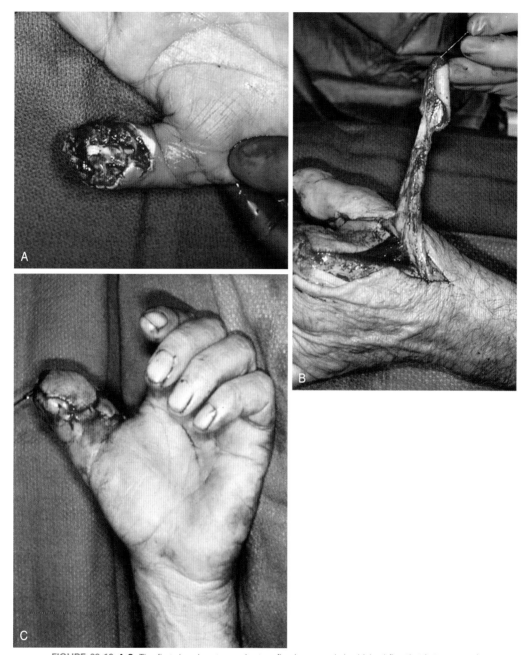

FIGURE 69-19 **A-C,** The first dorsal metacarpal artery flap is a vascularized island flap that is transposed
from the dorsoradial aspect of the index finger to the distal pulp of the thumb after a crushing injury.

significance of the various annular pulleys. It is often difficult to
repair profundus and superficialis tendons if they are injured in
zone 2. Nonetheless, both can be repaired because resection of the
superficialis reduces overall grip strength, predisposes to a recur-
vatum and swan neck deformity at the PIP joint, and damages
the vincula supply to the profundus.

Skin wounds usually have to be extended proximally and distally in a zigzag fashion to display the retracted divided tendon
ends. Tendon ends are handled with a fine-toothed forceps, and
the tendon surface is never touched. The wrist is flexed, and a
small Keith needle is passed transversely through the proximal

tendon, approximately 2 cm from the end, transfixing it to the
skin and tendon sheath. In this way, immobilization of the tendon
end facilitates a tension-free repair. Ragged tendon ends may be
squared off sharply, but no more than 1 cm is resected or permanent finger contracture will result. The tendon ends are brought
together by a single tension-holding, locking, core suture. Various
locking core suture techniques have been described, but a modified Kessler-type suture is usually placed. A specifically placed
locking loop increases the ultimate tensile strength of the tendon
repair by 10% to 50% compared with a simple mattress suture.
If this is not done, tension on the suture line can open up the

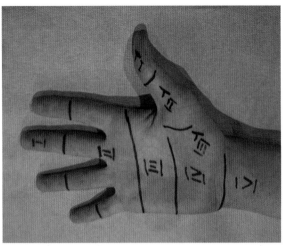

FIGURE 69-20 Zones of flexor tendon injuries on the fingers, thumb, and hand.

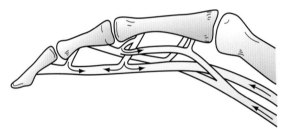

FIGURE 69-21 Complex arrangement of flexor digitorum superficialis and flexor digitorum profundus tendons in the flexor sheath of the fingers. Blood supply to the tendons travels through the vincula from the dorsal aspects of the tendons.

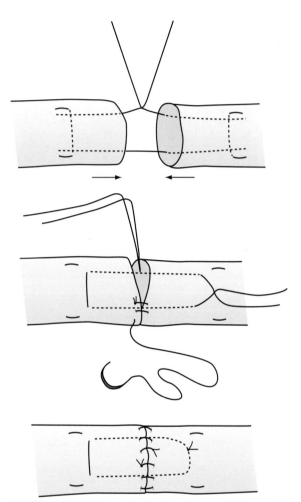

FIGURE 69-22 Technique of performing a four-strand flexor tendon core suture repair is demonstrated in association with a peripheral running suture.

repair, increasing the propensity for tendon gapping at the repair site. The ideal suture material for tendon repairs has not been found. In a study comparing a six-strand flexor tendon repair, braided polyblend (FiberWire) fared best compared with braided cable nylon (Supramid Extra II) and braided polyester (Tendo-Loop) for both ultimate tensile strength and gap force. Tendon repair gapping is important because the exposed tendon ends, although not disrupted totally, lead to increased adhesion formation. However, the knot security of FiberWire remains a concern, requiring at least five-throw knots to minimize unraveling. Thus, FiberWire is generally not used for repair of tendons within the flexor tendon sheath because of the necessary bulkiness of the knots.

A 4-0 coated polyester or braided nylon suture is the best material for the core suture. Increasing the number of suture strands that cross the tendon repair site and obtaining suture bites of at least 0.7 cm will increase the overall tensile strength of the actual repair.[11] However, the more suture strands that are added, the greater will be the friction and edema within the flexor tendon sheath. A four- or six-strand core repair appears to provide optimum repair strength and does not increase stiffness and friction at the repair site excessively. Some perform a four-strand core repair by simply using a double-strand type of suture material, whereas others place a second core suture with a single-strand material. A four-strand core repair permits a light, protected, composite grip for the duration of postoperative healing. A running circumferential epitenon suture repair is also placed (Fig.

69-22). This not only helps smooth the repair but also adds to the ultimate tensile strength at the repair site and reduces gap formation. A peripheral 6-0 nylon suture serves this purpose.

The forces generated on FDP flexor tendons are 600 g during passive finger flexion and 2000 g during active finger flexion; with strong active finger flexion, they are 8000 g. However, after tendon repair, the effects of wound healing, changes in elasticity, and added friction between the flexor tendons and their surrounding tissues will affect the overall work of flexion. There will be added frictional forces caused by edema, the presence of suture material, and the pulley system. The estimated work of flexion (resistance) increases by a factor of 50% after tendon repair. Thus, the estimated forces on repaired tendons, with 50% added for the work of flexion, are 900 g for passive finger flexion, 3000 g for active finger flexion, and 12,000 g for strong active flexion. The ultimate tensile strengths of various repairs are 2600 g for two-strand and simple epitendinous repair, 4600 g for four-strand and simple epitendinous repair, and 6800 g for six-strand and simple epitendinous repair. The strength of the initial tendon repair decreases by approximately 25% during the first 3 weeks and then steadily increases thereafter to 6 weeks. Hence, if one is to undertake a postoperative active finger flexion protocol, at least a four- or six-strand core suture tendon repair is needed.[12]

A variety of interventions have a potential of enhancing tendon repair and healing. Active tendon motion protocols tend to attenuate the weakening of repair strength that we used to believe was an obligatory part of normal tendon repair site healing in the first 3 weeks.[13] In addition, therapy with stem cells can enhance strength of tendon repair because of their regenerative potential. Mechanical stimulation of active motion protocols may potentially act in this by stimulating stem cells.[14] Zone 1 flexor tendon injury may be caused by a penetrating injury. However, closed-traction injury may also cause profundus tendon avulsion, which most frequently involves the ring or middle finger. In the repair of a zone 1 injury, a pullout suture is necessary if the distal tendon length is insufficient to repair the tendon securely (Fig. 69-23), although suture bone anchors have facilitated this mode of tendon repair into bone at the base of the distal phalanx.

Postoperatively, hand elevation is important to reduce edema. The wrist is placed in approximately 20 degrees of flexion and the MP joint at approximately 60 to 70 degrees of flexion. The splint is molded against the fingers, with the IP joints fully extended. A system of rubber band dynamic traction may be used after the repair of flexor tendons in zone 2, with good results obtained in more than 80% of cases. Differential excursion between the two digital flexors is dramatically increased by a synergistic splint that allows wrist extension and finger flexion. This position of wrist extension and MP joint flexion produces the least tension on a repaired flexor tendon during active digital flexion; thus, we have come to use the flexor hinge brace technique and the so-called place-and-hold protocol (Fig. 69-24). Of all the postoperative flexor tendon protocols, this enables the greatest overall tendon excursion of each of the FDS and FDP tendons and the most significant differential tendon gliding between the FDS and FDP repair sites, which theoretically would then reduce the risk of adhesion formation between the two tendons. A tenodesis brace with a wrist hinge is fabricated to allow full wrist flexion, wrist extension of 30 degrees, and maintenance of MP joint flexion of at least 60 degrees. After composite passive digital flexion, the wrist is extended and passive finger flexion is maintained. The patient actively maintains digital flexion and holds that position for approximately 5 seconds. The patient is instructed to use the lightest muscle power necessary to maintain digital flexion. Wrist flexion and finger extension follow. This protected motion postoperative protocol is continued for 6 weeks.

Extensor Tendons

Proper diagnosis of extensor tendon injuries requires full knowledge of the relatively complex anatomy of the extensor mechanism of the dorsum of the finger. The subcutaneous location of extensor tendons makes them susceptible to crush, laceration, and avulsion injuries. The presence of juncturae tendinum prevents proximal retraction of the EDC tendons. Extensor tendon injuries have been divided into nine zones, which ascend numerically from the dorsum of the DIP joints to the forearm. The odd-numbered zones begin at the DIP joint and are located over the joints; the even-numbered zones are located between the joints.

Extensor tendons are thinner than flexor tendons and, over the dorsum of the digits, are spread out to form the extensor hood. It may occasionally be possible to use conventional tendon repair techniques in the proximal parts of the tendons, but this is usually not the case in the extensor hood region. Here, horizontal mattress sutures or figure-of-eight mattress sutures may be needed. All lacerations are repaired if 50% or more of the tendon is divided.

Extensor tendon avulsions are most likely to occur at the DIP joint from a jamming type of injury that results in a mallet finger deformity (Fig. 69-25). If a bone fragment representing 50% or more of the articular surface is involved or if there is volar subluxation of the DIP joint, an open reduction with internal fixation is performed. If there is a tendon rupture only or a small piece of bone is avulsed with the tendon, good results can be obtained by 6 weeks of continuous splinting with the DIP joint in extension (Fig. 69-26). After this period of splinting, the DIP joint is further protected during sleep for 2 more weeks.

Closed tears through the triangular ligament may be caused by PIP joint subluxation or a jamming type of injury that results in a boutonnière deformity. The central slip attachment at the base of the middle phalanx is disrupted, so that extension of that joint is altered. The lateral bands lose their support dorsal to the PIP joint axis and slip volar and become flexors at the PIP joint and extensors of the DIP joint. The consequent deformity is one of

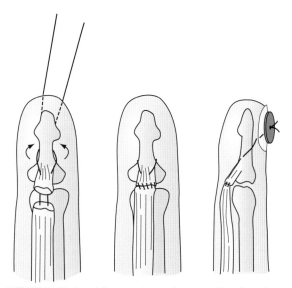

FIGURE 69-23 Zone 1 flexor tendon repair to reattach tendon to bone.

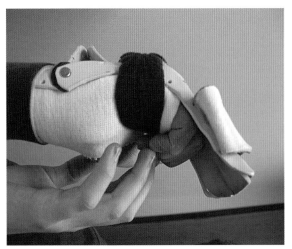

FIGURE 69-24 Flexor hinge brace with place-and-hold technique of finger mobilization is one of the preferred methods for postoperative rehabilitation after flexor tendon repair.

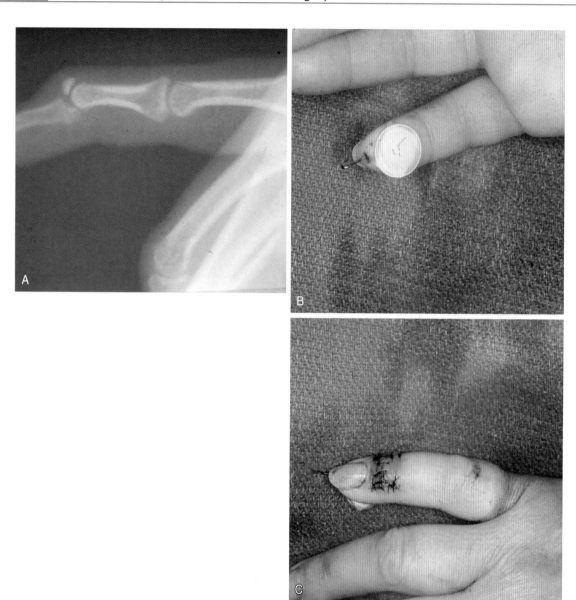

FIGURE 69-25 A-C, Mallet fracture with avulsed bone fragment involving more than 50% of the articular surface with volar subluxation of the distal phalanx. The bone fragment is reapproximated with a tie-over volar suture and a longitudinal pin traversing the distal interphalangeal joint.

flexion at the PIP joint and hyperextension at the DIP joint. Within 6 weeks of injury, these can be treated satisfactorily by extension splinting at the PIP joint, maintaining the DIP joint free for active flexion and extension (Fig. 69-26).

A recently described novel way of splinting and treating closed boutonnière injuries of the finger is to use the relative motion splint shown in Figure 69-27 but to have the proximal phalanx of the injured digit blocked from fully extending. This has been shown to realign the lateral bands dorsally over the PIP joint.

If there is an open laceration to the central slip mechanism and adjacent triangular ligament, direct suture repair or reinsertion into bone by means of bone anchor minisutures is performed, followed by the same postoperative protocol.

Extensor tendon injuries proximal to the PIP joint result in a drop finger (Fig. 69-28). These are repaired and splinted for 4 weeks. Common extensor tendon injuries over the dorsum of the hand and at the wrist must be repaired and then treated postoperatively by various different controlled motion protocols. One is a dynamic rubber band extension outrigger brace or use of a relative motion splint, in which the affected digit is kept at a more dorsal pitch to the adjacent fingers, thus relaxing the repaired tendon. The relative motion splint causes minimal interference with daily activities during rehabilitation (Fig. 69-29).[15]

Nerve Injuries

Sunderland's classification, the most widely used classification, describes five types of nerve injury: neurapraxia (grade I), axonotmesis (grades II to IV), and neurotmesis (grade V). Neurapraxia is a physiologic block of impulse conduction without anatomic destruction of nerve fibers. This might occur with a

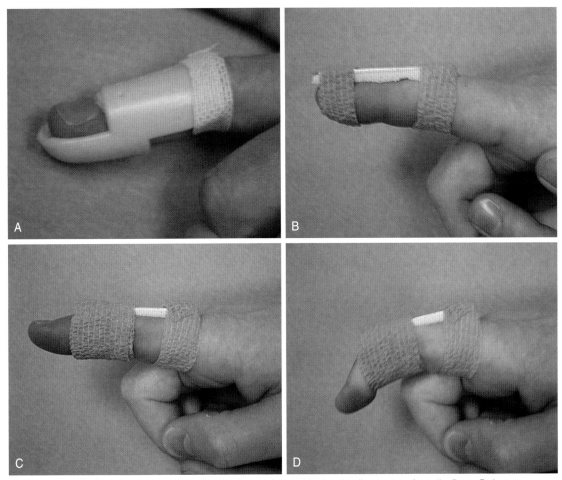

FIGURE 69-26 **A,** Prefabricated stack splint may be used for the closed treatment of a mallet finger. **B,** A simple dorsal aluminum splint may serve equally well for mallet finger treatment. **C** and **D,** Dorsal splinting across the proximal interphalangeal joint enables closed treatment of a boutonnière injury. The distal interphalangeal joint is left free for flexion and extension.

closed injury, such as a radial nerve injury in the spiral groove associated with a midshaft humerus fracture. Neurapraxia may occur because of prolonged pressure in a tight anatomic location (e.g., carpal tunnel) or prolonged application of a tourniquet. Provided the offending cause is promptly removed, spontaneous recovery is generally the rule but can take as long as 3 months. In axonotmesis, axonal fibers are completely ruptured, generally from traction on the nerve (II). With higher energy injuries, the endoneurial (III) and perineurial (IV) nerve sheaths that support and nourish the axons and fascicles are progressively injured, leading to poorer nerve recovery, with increasing damage to intraneural architecture. Neurotmesis refers to complete transection of a nerve and is the most severe degree of nerve injury. It may result from direct sharp trauma or a violent traction injury. Accurate approximation of the cut nerve ends and meticulous repair are required for the best possible recovery. Axonal regeneration after axonotmesis or successful nerve repair after neurotmesis occurs at a rate of 1 mm/day. Traction injuries may result in a combination of all grades of nerve injury, but with intact external nerve sheaths, grades II to IV may be difficult to distinguish from one another clinically.

Severance of a peripheral nerve involves an acute loss of sensory, motor, and sympathetic functions. Knowledge of the motor and sensory distribution of the nerve is essential for clinical evaluation. However, associated injuries, such as fractures and muscle and tendon lacerations, may complicate the evaluation. Loss of pseudomotor activity occurs within 30 minutes of the nerve injury. Clinically, loss of sweating can sometimes be observed, and denervated skin will not wrinkle if it is placed in water. Sensory denervation can also be demonstrated with a ninhydrin test. Nerve conduction studies are not immediately helpful but become valuable 3 weeks after injury, when fibrillation and denervation potentials can be measured in completely denervated muscles. In a closed injury, they may differentiate between neurapraxia and neurotmesis. Later, nerve conduction studies may help monitor nerve regeneration after repair.

Primary nerve repair is done within 72 hours of injury, delayed primary repair from 72 hours to 14 days, and secondary nerve repairs 14 days or longer after injury. Primary neurorrhaphy is recommended in the following situations:
• The nerve is sharply incised.
• There is minimal wound contamination.

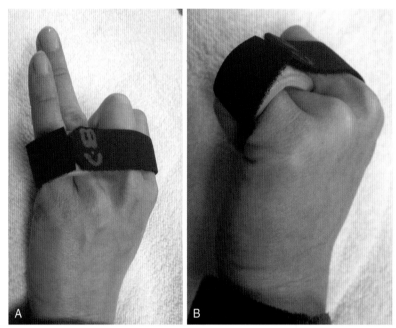

FIGURE 69-27 A and **B,** Relative motion splint can also be used to "depress" and to block extension of the proximal phalanx of a digit affected by boutonnière deformity. This encourages dorsal repositioning of the lateral bands over the dorsum of the proximal interphalangeal joint.

- There are no injuries that preclude obtaining skeletal stability or adequate skin cover.
- The patient is medically stable to undergo an operation.
- Appropriate facilities and instrumentation are available.

In a completely severed nerve, wallerian degeneration occurs in the entire segment distal to the injury and 1 to 2 cm proximal to it. In closed injuries, when the severity of the nerve injury is unknown, repeated clinical evaluation and electrical studies every 3 to 6 weeks help distinguish between neurapraxia and axonal injury. In most cases, surgical exploration with repair is indicated after 3 months if no clinical recovery is detected.

The nerve repair must be tensionless. Stretching a nerve more than 10% compromises epineurial blood flow and thus its recovery. With sharp nerve lacerations, an epineurial repair provides as good a functional recovery as fascicular (perineurial) repair, provided anatomic landmarks such as the vasa nervorum are accurately realigned to provide precise matching of fascicles at the severed nerve ends.

Traditionally, microsuture of lacerated nerve ends has been performed, and epineurial suturing has been the most common technique. In addition to the foreign body reaction to the suture material, it may be difficult to suture the nerve repair in confined anatomic locations. Fibrin glue is an acceptable alternative for nerve repair. Nerve ends still do need to be precisely aligned. However, the use of fibrin glue for nerve repairs is not yet approved by the U.S. Food and Drug Administration. A nerve gap may exist because of segmental nerve loss or when a crushed nerve segment is unsuitable for repair and must be resected. This may be overcome by proximal and distal mobilization of the nerve ends or, in the case of the ulnar nerve, by transposition of the nerve to the front of the elbow. If there is too much tension on the repair (it cannot be held with an 8-0 nylon suture), a nerve conduit or nerve graft must be used.

It has been suggested that optimal nerve regeneration and appropriate matching of axons in proximal and distal nerve segments result from a combination of paracrine-mediated neurotropism and contact guidance of sprouting proximal axons. Experimental evidence has suggested that the neurotropic chemical gradient can effectively guide regenerating axons at least 14 mm through a hollow nerve conduit in the rat model. The conduit allows diffusion of the neurotropic signal while preventing a mechanical fibrous block between the proximal and distal nerve segments. However, large-gap animal models (30 mm) have shown poor or no recovery with use of nerve conduits, suggesting that a finite limit exists for this technique. Although the gap length that can be bridged successfully in humans is still uncertain, many surgeons consider the use of bioresorbable nerve conduits for gap lengths up to 2 cm to be appropriate for small peripheral nerves. Nerve grafting remains the "gold standard" for large or mixed nerves and the brachial plexus. Appropriate conduits are polyglycolic acid tubes and semipermeable collagen tubes, which have shown similar experimental outcomes (Fig. 69-30).[16]

With nerve grafting, fascicular matching, when chosen by the surgeon, may not always be appropriate. However, the additional contact guidance provided to regenerating axons makes successful nerve regeneration possible over longer distances than with conduits. Donor sources for nerve grafting usually include the terminal sensory portion of the posterior interosseous nerve and the medial antebrachial cutaneous nerve for small digital nerves. The sural nerves are used for nerve gaps involving larger nerves.

Processed nerve allografts hold great promise for longer nerve defects of major peripheral nerves where synthetic nerve conduits have failed and then may avoid donor morbidity of autografts or even enable more extensive nerve grafting where insufficient autograft is available. Decellularized nerve allograft is becoming an off-the-shelf option for median and ulnar nerve injuries, and

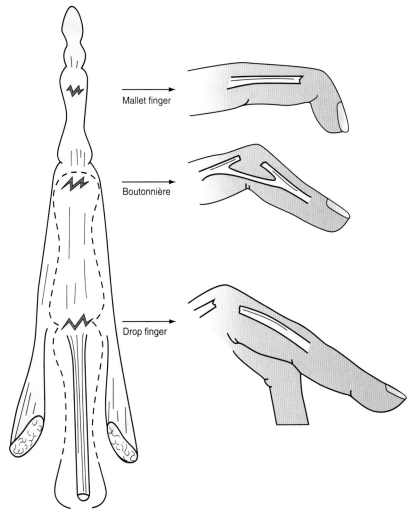

FIGURE 69-28 Extensor Tendon Injuries on the Dorsum of the Finger. Injury at the distal insertion causes a mallet finger, and injury at the central slip over the proximal interphalangeal joint causes a boutonnière deformity. Proximal to the proximal interphalangeal joint, over the proximal phalanx, injury results in a drop finger.

results may be equal to those of nerve autografts. After nerve repair, the affected part is splinted for 3 weeks to protect the repair site in the position of least tension. Tinel sign indicates the position of axonal regrowth; advancing distal progression of Tinel sign with time indicates successful repair and nerve regeneration.

Nerve Transfers

If there may be a long distance between the site of nerve injury and the distal muscle target, primary nerve repair may be fruitless because muscle degeneration would have occurred by the time distal neural growth occurs. Muscle recovery is unlikely after an 18-month lapse. Thus, if nerve growth occurs at the rate of approximately 1 mm/day, a proximal motor nerve lesion more than 540 mm proximal to the hand will be doomed to failure. Hence, for proximal arm nerve and brachial plexus injuries, nerve transfers may result in a nerve repair that is closer to the muscle target. The donor nerve must be chosen so as to minimize morbidity from loss of the donor nerve. The donor nerve must be closely related to the denervated muscle so that the repair is performed

much closer to the muscle target. Nerve transfers have revolutionized the repair of proximal nerve injuries so that distal muscle atrophy is minimized. For example, the classic Oberlin transfer uses part of the ulnar nerve (usually a single fascicle) for transfer to the musculocutaneous nerve and to the brachialis in the upper arm to restore elbow flexion.[17] It is technically easy, quick, and effective. No significant motor or sensory deficits result in the territory of the ulnar nerve. This technique has become popular and is indicated for C5-6 brachial plexus lesions when C8-T1 is intact. It can also be used to neurotize a functioning free muscle transfer that may be required if the native muscles have already sustained atrophy because of prolonged denervation.

Vascular Injuries

Acute vascular injuries may follow closed or penetrating trauma or iatrogenic injury. Fractures or dislocations may cause vascular injury. Indirect vascular trauma may be caused by traction injuries, which can avulse vessels, or by intimal damage or repetitive microtrauma from vibratory tools, which can lead to thrombosis.

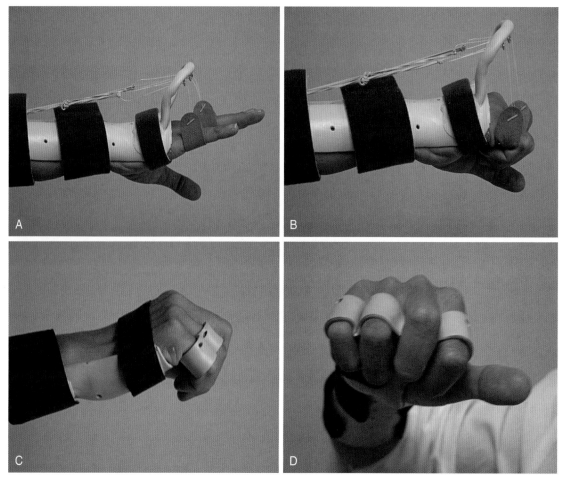

FIGURE 69-29 A and **B,** Extension outrigger dynamic splint commonly used for extensor tendon injuries postoperatively (extension and flexion views). **C** and **D,** Relative motion splint has the advantage of being low profile and causes minimal interference with daily activities and yet provides protection to the freshly repaired extensor tendon.

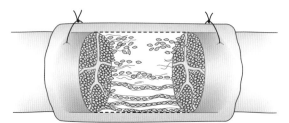

FIGURE 69-30 Nerve conduits may be an appropriate treatment for short nerve gaps in the hand.

The latter usually affects the ulnar artery in Guyon canal at the wrist and is called the hypothenar hammer syndrome. Regardless of the cause, vascular injuries may lead to a critical compromise of circulation in the extremity. With a closed injury, the onset of symptoms may be delayed because swelling, hypotension, and intimal injury combine and result in late thrombosis and vascular insufficiency.

After an acute arterial injury, symptoms result from a combination of the adequacy of collateral circulation, post-traumatic sympathetic tone, and vasomotor control mechanisms. Patients with an upper extremity arterial injury who have adequate collateral circulation and normal vasomotor control may have minimal symptoms, so reconstruction is not necessarily mandatory and the injury can be treated with simple arterial ligation. If there is a noncritical arterial injury, such as to the radial artery alone, reconstruction may be advocated to restore parallel flow in case of future arterial injury, to enhance nerve recovery, to facilitate healing, and to prevent cold intolerance. However, the reported patency rate, even with microvascular techniques for single-vessel repairs, varies from 47% to 82%. The following injuries are optimally managed by vascular repair and reconstruction: axillary or brachial artery injury; combined radial and ulnar artery injury; and radial or ulnar artery injury associated with poor collateral circulation. Relative indications for repair of a noncritical vascular injury are extensive distal soft tissue injury, technical ability to achieve repair without compromising the patient's well-being, and a combined vascular and neural injury. The need for arterial reconstruction necessitates assessing the adequacy of collateral circulation; this is based primarily on initial clinical judgment. However, the final decision regarding arterial reconstruction is often made in the operating room after exploration. Once the injured structures have been isolated, potential bleeding sites have been controlled, and hematoma has been evacuated, the distal extremity can be assessed more adequately. At this time, lacerated vessel ends are controlled by atraumatic vascular clamps and a tourniquet can be released. Capillary refill and perfusion of the distal extremity can then be assessed, as can backflow from the distal lacerated vessel ends. Digital blood pressure can be quantified with a sterile Doppler probe and cuff; a digital brachial index of 0.7 or greater suggests adequate perfusion. If there is poor collateral flow, arterial reconstruction is performed. At this time, standard of care does not require arterial repair of isolated noncritical vessels. In combined radial and ulnar artery injuries, one or both vessels are reconstructed. If possible, both vessels are repaired.[18]

Muscles often swell after prolonged periods of ischemia. This can lead to an increase of pressure within the closed compartment of the forearm, resulting in a compartment syndrome. It is thus the practice of most surgeons to perform a routine fasciotomy to decompress the forearm compartment after a true revascularization procedure has been performed. During the period of ischemia to the muscles, there may be a buildup of lactic acid. Furthermore, myonecrosis might occur. Restoration of circulation to such a limb can cause a sudden flooding of the circulation with myoglobin, lactic acid, and other toxic substances. This is called reperfusion syndrome and can lead to multiorgan failure, especially affecting the renal and cardiac systems.

Replantation and Amputations

It can often be frustrating for the novice general surgeon to be told by a replantation surgeon in the middle of the night that a consultation was obtained inappropriately or not soon enough. There are general indications for the replantation of amputated parts, but the overriding decision is still to save life before limb. Although patients and family members may desire replantation, and in some cases have even been promised it by members of the primary team, it is not performed in patients with severe associated medical problems or injuries. Replantation is also generally not considered under the following circumstances[4,19]:

- Severe crush or multilevel injury of the amputated part
- A psychotic patient who has willfully self-amputated the part
- Amputation of a single digit proximal to the FDS distal insertion (zone 2), except for single-digit amputations in children or those with a demanding profession (e.g., a musician)
- Amputation in patients with severely atherosclerotic arteries (sometimes this can be determined only when the vessels are explored in the operating room)

Indications for replantation of amputated parts are as follows:
- Whenever possible, for a thumb amputation (it provides >40% of the overall hand function)[19]
- Single digits that have been amputated distal to the FDS insertion (e.g., a manual worker may likely desire revision of amputation and desires to return to work quickly)
- Multiple injured digits
- Most amputations in children, including single-digit amputations
- Guillotine-sharp clean amputations at the hand, wrist, or distal forearm

Replantation is the reattachment of the part that has been completely amputated. Revascularization requires reconstruction of vessels in a limb that has been severely injured or incompletely severed in such a way that vascular repair is necessary to prevent distal necrosis, but some soft tissue (e.g., skin, tendon, nerve) is still intact. Revascularization generally has a better success rate

than replantation because venous and lymphatic drainage may be intact.

Minor replantation is a reattachment at the wrist, hand, or digital level, whereas major replantation is performed proximal to the wrist. This clinical distinction exists because in the case of a major replantation, ischemic time is crucial to the viability of muscle and to functional outcome. Ischemic muscle may result in myonecrosis, myoglobinemia, and infection, which may threaten the patient's life (as well as limb). There are three types of amputations:
- Guillotine amputation, whereby the tissue is cut with a sharp object and is minimally damaged
- Crush amputation, in which a local crushing injury can be converted into a guillotine injury simply by débriding back the edges, although this may not be possible in a diffusely crushing amputation
- Avulsion amputation, which is the most unfavorable type for replantation because structures are injured at different levels

Avulsion amputation may occur, for example, with a so-called ring avulsion injury. The extensor tendons are shredded, flexor tendons are often avulsed at the musculotendinous junctions, and nerves are stretched and may be ripped from end organs.

Ischemia time is also an important consideration in evaluating a patient for replantation. For amputated digits, more than 12 hours of warm ischemia is a relative contraindication. Promptly cooling the part to 4° C dramatically alters the ischemia factor, but even ischemia exceeding 24 hours does not necessarily preclude successful digital replantation. Ischemia is more crucial for replantation above the proximal forearm, and reimplantation is not considered after more than 6 to 10 hours of warm ischemia time. Single digits in adults, other than the thumb in zone 2, are generally not reattached because of the consequent adverse overall functional result on the hand, with a single stiff finger.[19]

Amputation is not an outmoded operation; rather, it is necessary in a patient in whom replantation might not be indicated. When primary amputation is performed, the stump is preserved with as much length as possible. An exception might be made if there is only a very short segment of proximal phalanx. A short proximal phalangeal remnant at the index finger position may serve as an impediment for thumb to middle finger prehension, and one might consider a formal ray amputation in this case to improve overall hand function. The ends of the cut nerve are cut sharply and allowed to retract to minimize the occurrence of painful neuromas at the amputation tip. Tendons are also divided sharply and allowed to retract. The practice of suturing flexor and extensor tendons over the ends of the middle, ring, or small finger stump seriously impairs the motion of the uninjured fingers because of the common origin of the flexors. There will be an active flexion deficit in the uninjured digits, the quadriga syndrome; this is corrected simply by release of the flexor tendon remnant at the injured amputated digit.

If it is anticipated that the amputated part will be considered for replantation, it is critical to transport the patient and the part in an appropriate manner. The amputated part is placed in a clean, dry, plastic bag, which is sealed and placed on top of ice in a Styrofoam container. This keeps the part sufficiently cool at 4° C to 10° C without freezing. The amputated part is wrapped in a lightly moistened saline gauze to prevent tissue drying.

With only a few minor variations, the sequence of replantation has been standardized. Preliminary exploration of the distal amputated part under a microscope by an initial surgical team not only determines whether a replantation is technically feasible but also can be started while the patient is being prepared for the operating room. Bone shortening allows skin to be débrided back to where it is free of contusion and direct tension-free closure can be achieved. In the thumb, bone shortening is minimized to less than 10 mm. The order of repair is usually bone, tendons, muscle units, arteries, nerves, and finally veins. Establishment of arterial flow before venous flow clears lactic acid from the replanted part. The functional veins can now also be detected by spurting bleeding. However, blood loss must be closely monitored.

For major replantations, reestablishing arterial circulation as rapidly as possible is crucial to limiting ischemia time. A dialysis shunt or carotid shunt may be placed between the arterial ends. Intermittent clamping of the shunt may be necessary to restrict blood loss. In the upper extremity, bone shortening can be aggressive to achieve primary skin closure and primary nerve repair. Judicious use of anticoagulants may enhance the success of replantation. Topical application of 2% lidocaine or papaverine may help relieve vasospasm. Postoperative dressings consist of nonadherent mesh gauze, loose flap gauze, and a plaster splint, with postoperative elevation to minimize edema and venous congestion. The patient's room must be kept warm, and smoking is forbidden postoperatively. Aside from antibiotics and analgesics, one aspirin tablet daily for its retarding effect on platelet aggregation is suggested. Postoperative monitoring is done hourly to assess color, pulp turgor, capillary refill, and digital temperature.

Fractures and Dislocations

Pain, swelling, limited motion, and deformities suggest the presence of a fracture or dislocation. Standard anteroposterior and lateral radiographs may miss some fractures and dislocations, and multiple views may be necessary to establish the exact diagnosis. Fractures may be rotated, angulated, telescoped, or displaced. Angulation is described by the direction in which the apex of the fracture is pointing, and displacement is described by the direction of the distal fragment. Fractures may be open or closed, depending on whether a wound is involved. They may also be complete, incomplete, or comminuted (more than two pieces). Fractures are also described by their pattern; they may be transverse, longitudinal, oblique, or spiral. Open fractures need to be thoroughly irrigated and débrided urgently. Displaced fractures or dislocations are repositioned as soon as possible. A dislocation is described according to the direction of displacement of the distal bone in the involved joint. The separation of joints may be complete or incomplete (subluxed), depending on the severity of the capsular injury.[6,20,21]

Displaced fractures or dislocations are repositioned as soon as possible to decrease soft tissue injury, to decompress nerves that might be stretched, and to relieve kinking of blood vessels. Good bone contact and stability are necessary for fractures to heal. Some fractures are stable and require only external support in a splint or cast, whereas others are unstable and require internal support, which can be provided by Kirschner wires, internal wire sutures through drill holes in the fracture fragments, screws, plates, or even external fixation devices (Table 69-4). The more complicated the fixation, the more dissection is required to apply that fixation and therefore the greater the potential for scarring around adjacent tendons and consequential stiffness. Plates and screws, however, can nonetheless establish a degree of rigid fixation that allows early motion of the part and thus potentially reduces the risk for cicatricial stiffness. Intra-articular fractures require accurate reduction to preserve motion and to minimize the risk for later development of arthrosis. Persistent rotational and significant lateral angular deformities generally do not remodel with time; these can be avoided by observing the alignment of the injured fingers compared with adjacent digits while passively and gently flexing them into a fist after reduction is attained. If they do not fit comfortably adjacent to each other and do not point toward the distal pole of the scaphoid, a fresh attempt at reduction must be performed. A thorough neurovascular examination is always performed before and after fracture reduction has been completed.

Distal Phalangeal Fractures

Fractures of the distal phalanx are the most frequent hand fractures, representing 50% of all hand fractures. Most result from crush injuries with associated nail bed injuries. Precise reduction is generally not required, and treatment typically consists of splinting alone. However, unstable shaft fractures with overriding fragments are indications for reduction and longitudinal Kirschner wire fixation.

Most closed mallet fractures can be managed by splinting the DIP joint in extension, provided the fracture involves less than 50% of the joint surface and is not associated with DIP joint subluxation. If fixation is required, the fracture fragment is held in place with a monofilament wire or nonabsorbable suture passed through to the palmar aspect of the finger through the distal phalanx. A transarticular longitudinal Kirschner wire is used to keep the joint in neutral position. A so-called jersey finger is an avulsion fracture of the insertion of the FDP tendon into the distal phalanx. It occurs after a pull of the FDP against resistance,

TABLE 69-4   Comparison of Methods of Skeletal Fixation

METHOD OF FIXATION	ADVANTAGES	DISADVANTAGES
Kirschner wires	Come in varying diameters	Pins can loosen
	Can be applied percutaneously or open	Cannot provide rigid fixation
	Second surgery not required for removal	Soft tissue may be transfixed (but can be avoided by careful placement)
	Require less soft tissue dissection than plates and screws	Infection can occur along pin tracks
Screws	Have high stability	Frequently require open approach (although not always)
	Allow early finger mobilization	
Plates	Can be used when fracture line is not oblique enough for screws	Require open approach
	Allow early finger mobilization	Require extensive soft tissue dissection
		Have relatively high profile and may be palpable through the dorsum of fingers and hand
		May promote extensor tendon adhesions by their relative bulk and dissection required for placement

as can occur when a footballer catches onto the jersey of an opponent. On occasion, the avulsed fragment may lie as far proximally as the palm. This fracture fragment generally requires open reduction and internal fixation.[6]

Middle Phalanx and Proximal Phalanx Fractures

Fractures may involve the head, neck, shaft, or base of the respective bone. Head and base fractures may be intra-articular. A middle phalangeal shaft fracture is displaced according to the forces exerted by the insertions of the FDS and central slip mechanism. If the fracture lies distal to the FDS insertion, the proximal fragment is flexed by this muscle, resulting in a volar angulation. In contrast, if the fracture is proximal to the FDS insertion, the proximal fragment is extended by the central slip, whereas the distal part is flexed by the FDS. This results in a dorsal angulation. Most shaft fractures of the proximal phalanx tend to angulate volarward because the interossei reflect the proximal fragment and the central slip, through the PIP joint, extends the distal fragment. Displaced and unstable shaft fractures require open reduction followed by fixation with Kirschner wires, plates, or screws.

Metacarpal Fractures

Stable metacarpal fractures may be treated with splinting alone. Fractures with dorsal or volar angulation can be stabilized by percutaneous insertion of intramedullary fixation pins. If they are displaced or unstable, such as oblique, spiral, or multiple metacarpal fractures, open reduction and internal fixation of these metacarpal fractures are performed. The internal fixation can be achieved with Kirschner wires, lag screws, or plate and screws, depending on the fracture pattern configuration. Dorsally angulated fractures at the neck of the little finger metacarpal, the so-called boxer fracture, do not require reduction if the dorsal angulation is less than 30 degrees. The mobility of the carpometacarpal joint will compensate for this degree of angulation. The index and middle finger metacarpals are less mobile than the ring and little finger metacarpals. Therefore, a maximum of 15 degrees of angular deformity can be tolerated in the index and middle finger metacarpals.

Oblique fractures at the base of the thumb metacarpal (Bennett fracture) result in the small proximal fragment's being held in position by the volar oblique ligament to the trapezium. The remaining portion of the thumb metacarpal is displaced dorsally and radially because of the pull of the APL tendon (Fig. 69-31). These fracture fragments must be properly reduced and secured

with internal fixation with Kirschner wires or a screw. Comminuted fractures at the base of the thumb metacarpal (Rolando fracture) are infrequently treated by closed reduction. If the fragments are large and badly displaced, an open reduction is indicated to ensure accurate restoration of the joint surface at the base of the thumb metacarpal. Fractures of the shaft of the thumb metacarpal tend to become displaced by the opposing muscle forces of the abductor and adductor on the proximal and distal fragments, respectively. Even undisplaced fractures may become progressively more displaced and angulated over time, necessitating an internal fixation. If initial splint immobilization is chosen for an undisplaced thumb metacarpal fracture, close follow-up is required to detect the earliest signs of displacement and instability. Fracture at the base of the little finger metacarpal is analogous to Bennett fracture of the thumb and is sometimes called a reverse Bennett fracture. This results in a fracture-dislocation, with the deforming force being the insertion of the extensor carpi ulnaris tendon.

Scaphoid Fractures

The scaphoid is the most common carpal bone fracture and accounts for approximately 60% of all carpal injuries. Clinical examination shows tenderness over the anatomic snuffbox and over the scaphoid tubercle. If a scaphoid fracture is suspected, the initial radiographic examination includes not only the standard three views of the wrist but also a scaphoid view, which is a posteroanterior image with the wrist in full ulnar deviation (Fig. 69-32). Frequently, immediate postinjury radiographs may not reveal a fracture. CT or MRI may help in these cases, or one may elect to apply a splint and to repeat the radiographs in 2 weeks.[22]

Treatment of a nondisplaced scaphoid fracture is with a long arm cast that includes the thumb. The thumb spica cast is maintained for 6 weeks, followed by a short arm cast until radiographic healing has occurred. There has been a trend toward percutaneous screw fixation of even, undisplaced scaphoid fractures.

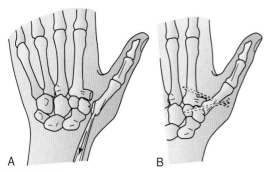

FIGURE 69-31 A, Fracture-dislocation at the base of the thumb metacarpal is called Bennett fracture. The deforming force is produced by the pull of the abductor pollicis longus muscle. B, Open reduction and pinning of the fracture are frequently required.

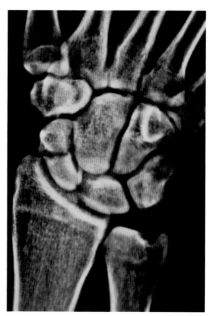

FIGURE 69-32 Anteroposterior radiograph of the wrist demonstrating a fracture of the waist of the scaphoid, the bone in the hand that is usually fractured.

Displaced scaphoid fractures require open reduction with internal fixation, generally using a compression screw. Complications with inadequately treated scaphoid fractures are notorious. The blood vessels enter the scaphoid mainly through its distal half, and fractures through the waist of the scaphoid may deprive the proximal half of its blood supply, leading to avascular necrosis of the proximal pole of the scaphoid. Nonunion also occurs with relative frequency, and these cases need to be treated with cancellous bone grafting or even a pedicle vascularized bone graft. Early diagnosis of scaphoid fractures is essential so that appropriate treatment can be instituted to reduce the risks for these complications. Modern cannulated compression screws, intraoperative fluoroscopy, and arthroscopy have allowed minimally invasive percutaneous fixation of some of these scaphoid fractures, resulting in a trend toward more aggressive surgical treatment of these fractures.

Fractures in Children

The Salter-Harris classification describes five types of epiphyseal injuries (Fig. 69-33). Pediatric bones are still growing and thus permit a greater degree of remodeling. Hence, moderate angular and translational displacement of fractures tends to correct with age. However, rotational deformities never correct in the hand and are totally unacceptable, even in children. Implants that cross the epiphysis must have minimal potential for damage. Hence, smooth Kirschner wires are generally used for the fixation of pediatric skeletal injuries, and threaded screws are usually avoided.

Dislocations

Dislocations are more frequently seen at the PIP joint. A closed dislocation of the PIP joint can frequently be managed by closed reduction and splinting. If the joint is unstable after reduction, it needs exploration for collateral ligament repair. The most common type of PIP joint dislocation is a dorsal dislocation. A PIP joint volar dislocation is often associated with a tear in the triangular

ligament of the extensor mechanism through which the head of the proximal phalanx protrudes and becomes trapped. Attempts at closed reduction fail because they tighten the fibers of the lateral bands and central slip around each side of the protruding proximal phalangeal neck; these injuries often require open reduction with repair of the extensor tear.

Palmar dislocations of the head of the index finger metacarpal often require open reduction. The head of the metacarpal becomes trapped between the superficial transverse metacarpal ligament, flexor tendons, and lumbrical muscles, whereas the volar plate becomes trapped between the metacarpal head and base of the proximal phalanx. Attempts at closed reduction are fruitless because of the entrapment resulting from this arrangement.

MP joint dislocation of the thumb often results from jamming it in a radial direction, thus tearing the ulnar collateral ligament. The ulnar collateral ligament may pull proximally and come to rest dorsal to the extensor hood (Stener lesion; Fig. 69-34). It cannot heal spontaneously because the ulnar collateral ligament is prevented from reattaching to bone. This so-called ski pole injury may then require operative repair. Stress radiography, sometimes able to be performed only after the digit is anesthetized with a metacarpal block, may be required to facilitate diagnosis of a complete ulnar collateral ligament injury of the thumb metacarpal joint.

INFECTIONS

Hand infections commonly present to the surgical resident covering the emergency department. When the infection is diagnosed

SALTER-HARRIS CLASSIFICATION

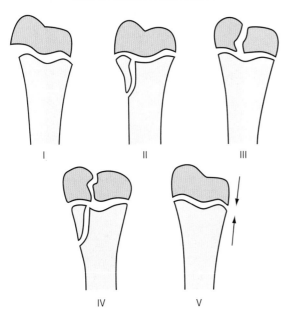

FIGURE 69-33 Salter-Harris fracture patterns involving the epiphysis in children.

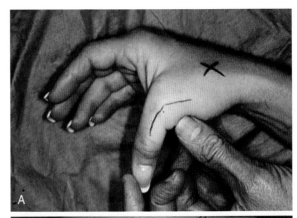

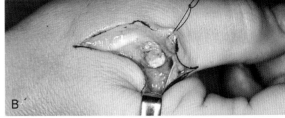

FIGURE 69-34 A, Instability of the ulnar collateral ligament of the metacarpophalangeal joint of the thumb. **B,** Stener lesion shows that the distal insertion of the collateral ligament has avulsed proximal to the extensor hood and is thus blocked from spontaneous reattachment. Open operation is required to reanchor the collateral ligament insertion to the base of the proximal phalanx.

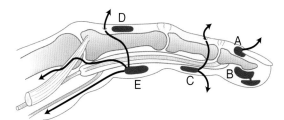

FIGURE 69-35 Spread of soft tissue infections in the hand occurs through loss of containment from the original site and erosion into and spread through contiguous anatomic compartments. **A,** Paronychium. Infecting organisms access periungual tissues through fissures in the eponychial or paronychial tissues and often are discharged spontaneously in these areas. **B,** Infection of pulp tissues (felon). Fibrous septa within the pulp create collar stud abscesses within the pulp. **C,** Volar subcutaneous infections in the digit may be discharged percutaneously on either surface of the digit or penetrate dorsally and spread along the sheaths of the flexor or extensor tendons. **D,** Subcutaneous infections on the dorsum of the digit are usually discharged percutaneously because of the thin and areolar nature of the soft tissues. **E,** Proximally located digital infections or web space infections may rupture into the palmar spaces by tracking along tendon sheaths, palmar fascia, or lumbrical canal. The continuous sheaths of the thumb and little fingers (radial and ulnar bursae) are continuous with the carpal tunnel and space of Parona at the wrist.

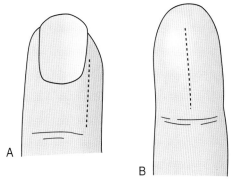

FIGURE 69-36 Incisions for paronychia **(A)** and felon **(B)**.

and treated properly initially, most patients do well. The extent of deep palmar infections may often be underestimated during the early phases because the volar aspect of the hand does not show edema as readily as the dorsal aspect of the hand. Thus, if infections in the hand are not diagnosed at an early stage, infections may spread from one anatomic compartment to another along natural tissue planes. Hand infections can then result in significant morbidity and severe functional compromise if they are not appropriately diagnosed and treated (Fig. 69-35). Some of the more common types of infections are discussed here.

Superficial Paronychial Infections

Paronychia is the most common infection of the hand; it usually results from trauma to the eponychial or paronychial region. The infection localizes around the nail base, advances around the nail fold, and burrows beneath the base of the nail. If pus is trapped beneath the nail, pressure on the nail evokes exquisite pain. The most common causative organism is *Staphylococcus aureus.* Early treatment is with antibiotics, preferably penicillin in combination with a β-lactamase inhibitor such as sulbactam or clavulanic acid. However, there has now been an increasing incidence of methicillin-resistant *S. aureus* in community-acquired infections. After an abscess develops, surgical drainage is required. The surgical approach to an acute paronychia depends on the extent of the infection. Incisions may not be necessary. A Freer elevator is used to lift approximately 25% of the nail adjacent to the infected perionychium, extending proximally to the edge of the nail. This portion of the nail is transected, and gauze packing is inserted beneath the nail fold. A single incision to drain the affected perionychium also allows elevation of the eponychial fold when both eponychium and paronychium are involved (Fig. 69-36).[23-25]

Infections of Intermediate-Depth Spaces

Infections of intermediate-depth spaces are pulp space infections (felons) and deep web space infections. The pulp space infections may involve the terminal, middle, or proximal volar pulp spaces

and may result from direct implantation with a penetrating injury or may represent spread from a more superficial subcutaneous infection. The volar pulp of the distal digital segment is a fascial space closed proximally by a septum joining the distal flexion crease to the periosteum, where the long flexor tendon is inserted. This space is also partitioned by fibrous septa. Tension in the distal digital segment can become so great that the arteries to the bone are compressed, resulting in gangrene of the fingertip and necrosis of the distal 75% of the terminal phalanx. With infection of the digital pulp space, one must not wait for fluctuance before making the decision for surgery because of the danger of ischemic necrosis of the skin and bone. Clinical diagnosis is made by the rapid onset of throbbing pain, swelling, and exquisite tenderness of the affected pulp space. Surgical drainage is required. A single volar or unilateral longitudinal incision may be used (Fig. 69-36). Postoperative care includes packing of the wound and elevation of the extremity. Use of antibiotics is guided by the results of Gram staining. Similar to a paronychia, *S. aureus* is the most common causative agent. Spread from a pulp space infection may move into a joint space or underlying bone or burst through the septum proximally to involve the rest of the finger. More proximally, a pulp space infection at the base of the finger can travel through the lumbrical canal into the palm to create a deep palmar space infection.[25]

Web space abscesses result from direct implantation or spread from a pulp space. An inflamed and tender mass in the web space separates the fingers. There is loss of the normal palmar concavity, with a widened space between the fingers. Dorsal swelling is present and must not be mistaken for the infection site. A surgical incision is placed transversely across the web space, and a longitudinal counterincision may be placed dorsally between the bases of the proximal phalanges; a generous communication is established between these two incisions (Fig. 69-37).

Deep Infections
Palmar Space Infections

These infections are localized to the deep space of the hand between the metacarpals and palmar aponeurosis. A transverse septum to the metacarpal of the middle finger divides the deep space into an ulnar midpalmar and radial thenar space. The transverse head of the adductor pollicis partitions the thenar space from the retroadductor space. There may be ballooning of the palm, thenar eminence, or posterior aspect of the first web space, depending on which of the affected spaces is involved with an abscess. The dorsal subaponeurotic space of the hand deep to the extensor tendons may also be affected by an isolated infection,

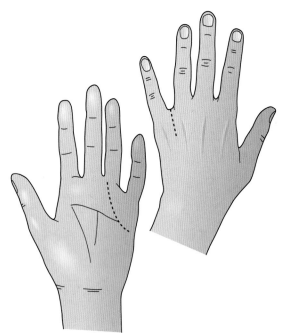

FIGURE 69-37 Incisions for web space abscess between the little and ring fingers.

generally as the result of direct implantation (Fig. 69-38A). For a thenar space infection, the preferred approach to surgical drainage is a dual volar and dorsal incision (Fig. 69-38B). On the volar side, an incision is made adjacent and parallel to the thenar crease. Great care is taken to avoid injury to the palmar cutaneous branch of the median nerve in the proximal part of the incision and the motor branch of the median nerve in a deeper plane. A second, slightly curved longitudinal incision is made on the dorsum of the first web space. Dissection is continued more deeply into this area between the first dorsal interosseous muscle and adductor pollicis. A drain is placed in the incision after thorough exploration of the respective spaces. With midpalmar space infections, dorsal swelling of the hand will be present, as is the case with all palmar infections, and must not be mistaken for the infection site. Motion of the middle and ring fingers is limited and painful. A longitudinal curvilinear incision is the preferred approach for drainage of this space (Fig. 69-38C).

Infection of Parona space occurs in the potential space deep to the flexor tendons in the distal forearm and superficial to the pronator quadratus muscle. It is usually the result of spread from the adjacent contiguous midpalmar space or from the radial or ulnar bursa. Swelling, tenderness, and fluctuation will be present in the distal volar forearm. A midpalmar infection may be associated. Active digital flexion is painful, as is passive finger extension. A surgical incision must be planned to leave the median nerve adequately covered with soft tissue.

Pyogenic Flexor Tenosynovitis

Kanavel's four cardinal signs include the following: (1) the finger is held flexed because this position allows the synovial sheath its maximum volume and eases pain; (2) symmetrical fusiform swelling of the entire finger is present, with edema of the back of the hand; (3) the slightest attempt at passive extension of the affected digit produces exquisite pain; and (4) the site of maximum

tenderness is at the proximal cul-de-sac of the index, middle, and ring finger synovial sheaths in the distal palm or, in the case of infection of the sheaths of the thumb and little finger, more proximally in the palm (Fig. 69-38). The radial and ulnar bursae communicate in approximately 80% of cases and may be simultaneously infected. Bursal infections may spread into the forearm space of Parona, deep to the flexor tendons in the distal part of the forearm, creating a horseshoe abscess.

Pyogenic flexor tenosynovitis may be aborted with parenteral antibiotics, extremity elevation, and hand immobilization if the patient is seen within the first 24 hours of onset of infection. If this course is unsuccessful or if the patient is seen more than 48 hours after onset of infection, surgical drainage is undertaken. The preferred surgical approach is through two separate incisions. The first incision is a midaxial incision made on the finger, usually on the ulnar side of the digit (on the radial side of the thumb or little finger); the digital artery and nerve remain in the volar flap, with the dissection proceeding directly to the tendon sheath. The synovium between the A3 and A4 pulleys is incised, and cloudy fluid is encountered. A second incision is made in the palm over the tendon to drain the cul-de-sac. A 16-gauge polyethylene catheter is inserted beneath the A1 pulley into the sheath, and the sheath is flushed manually with sterile saline every 2 hours after surgery. A bulky hand dressing absorbs the drainage. Studies have found that postoperative catheter drainage may not always be necessary.[26,27]

Chronic and Atypical Infections

Chronic paronychia is generally the result of *Candida albicans* (>95%) infection and is not bacterial. When bacteria are involved, they are more commonly atypical mycobacteria or gram-negative organisms. Chronic paronychia generally responds to treatment with topical antifungal agents, although oral antifungal agents are sometimes used. On occasion, surgical treatment by means of marsupialization of the eponychial fold is required. If the lesion is refractory to treatment, the possibility of a malignant neoplasm is entertained.

Chronic tenosynovitis can occur in the flexor tendons or in the dorsum of the wrist and extensor tendons. It is usually of a granulomatous type and is caused by mycobacteria or fungi. Treatment includes surgical excision of the involved synovium and prolonged treatment with the appropriate antimicrobial agents. Chronic infected tenosynovitis must be differentiated from other causes of chronic granulomatous synovitis, such as sarcoidosis, amyloidosis, gout, and rheumatoid arthritis.

Herpetic Whitlow

Herpetic whitlow is caused by type 1 or type 2 herpes simplex virus and may be confused with a paronychia. Infection begins with the appearance of small clear vesicles with localized swelling, erythema, and intense pain. The vesicles may subsequently appear turbid and coalesce over the next few days before ulcerating. Diagnosis is confirmed by culturing the virus from the vesicular fluid, assessing immunofluorescent serum antibody titers, or performing a Tzanck smear. However, these measures are rarely required because clinical diagnosis is usually sufficient. Infection can occur from autoinoculation from an oral or genital lesion or exposure as a health care worker. Pain is often out of proportion to the physical findings. Treatment is generally nonoperative because this infection is usually self-limited. Antivirals such as acyclovir or famciclovir may be of some benefit if started within the first 48 hours of symptom onset. Surgical incision and

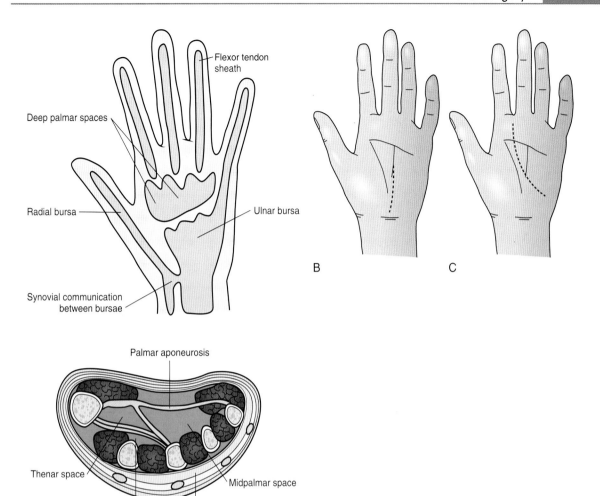

FIGURE 69-38 A, Deep spaces of the hand and synovial bursae. Infections may be bound by these spaces or may track along anatomic dissection planes between these spaces. **B,** Incision for thenar space infection. A dorsal first web space incision is also often required. **C,** Incision for midpalmar space abscess.

drainage can lead to systemic involvement and possible viral encephalitis.

Animal and Human Bites

The most striking difference in the microbial flora of human and animal bite wounds is the higher number of bacterial isolates per wound in human bites, the difference being mostly caused by the presence of anaerobic bacteria. Human bites can occasionally transmit other infectious diseases, such as hepatitis B, tuberculosis, syphilis, or actinomycosis. The incidence of *Eikenella corrodens* in human bite infections of the hand has been reported to vary between 7% and 29%. Usually, isolated organisms from infected human bite wounds are, as in animal bites, alpha-hemolytic streptococci and *S. aureus,* β-lactamase–producing strains of *S. aureus,* and *Bacteroides* spp. Anaerobic bacteria, including *Bacteroides, Clostridium, Peptococcus,* and *Veillonella,* are more prevalent in human bite infections than previously recognized. Most studies of animal bite wounds have focused on the isolation of *Pasteurella multocida,* disregarding the role of anaerobes. However, more recent studies have shown that dog bite wounds indicate multiple organisms, with *P. multocida* being isolated from only 26% of dog bite wounds in adults. Most animal bites cause mixed infections of aerobic and anaerobic bacteria.

Pyogenic joint infections usually result from trauma, such as a bite wound from a tooth when the assailant's hand strikes the jaw. A tooth struck by the clenched fist of an attacker penetrates the skin, tendon, joint capsule, and metacarpal head. Once the finger is extended, the four puncture wounds separate from each other to create a closed space within the joint. All these so-called fight bite wounds of the MP joint need to be explored surgically, débrided, and thoroughly lavaged. Human bite wounds are not closed primarily and are treated with appropriate antibiotics.

COMPARTMENT SYNDROME, HIGH-PRESSURE INJECTION INJURIES, AND EXTRAVASATION INJURIES

High-Pressure Injection Injuries

High-pressure injection injuries to the hand are relatively uncommon, but consequences of a misdiagnosis are serious. Urgent treatment is required. High-pressure injection guns are used for painting, lubricating, cleaning, and farm animal vaccinations. Materials that may be injected with these devices include paint, paint thinners, oil, grease, water, plastic, vaccines, and cement. These high-pressure injection guns may generate pressures ranging between 3000 and 12,000 psi. Injection injuries can also be caused by other sources, such as defective lines and valves, pneumatic hoses, and hydraulic lines. The type of material injected is the most important prognostic factor. Oil-based paints and paint thinners can generate significant early inflammation, leading to severe fibrosis. Because tendon sheaths at the index, middle, and ring fingers end at the level of the MP joints, material injected at the DIP or PIP flexion creases will remain within these digits. However, tendon sheaths at the thumb and little finger extend all the way into the radial and ulnar bursae. Thus, material injected at the little finger or at the IP flexion crease of the thumb may

potentially extend all the way into the forearm and even cause a compartment syndrome.

Initial presentation of a patient with a high-pressure injection may be benign and subtle. This may result in mismanagement by minimizing the patient's complaints. The break in the skin may be a benign-looking, pinhole-sized puncture site. However, within several hours, the digit becomes increasingly more painful, swollen, and pale. Prompt recognition and realization of the severity of injury are paramount. Radiographs may help determine the extent and dispersion of the injected material, either in the form of subcutaneous emphysema or, with lead-based paints, appearing as radiopaque soft tissue densities. The entire digit must be surgically decompressed and all foreign material and necrotic tissue débrided (Fig. 69-39). Wounds are closed loosely over Penrose drains or in a delayed manner. Appropriate antibiotics must be administered. Despite prompt recognition and

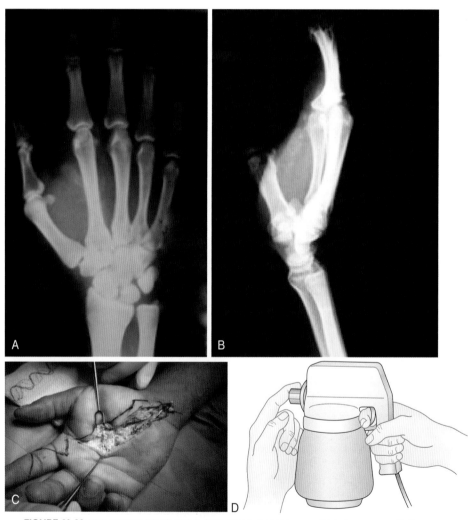

FIGURE 69-39 High-pressure injection injury from paint gun appears completely innocuous, with tiny puncture wound on presentation. **A** and **B,** Anteroposterior and lateral radiographs of the right hand show widely disseminated radiopaque foreign material in soft tissues of the palm and thenar eminence. **C,** Intraoperative photograph of left-handed man with palmar high-pressure injection injury from a paint gun on the nondominant palm. The tissues are extensively infiltrated by paint from the base of the finger to the wrist and require urgent débridement and decompression. **D,** Removal of the guard allows the nozzle to come into close contact, exponentially increasing the pressure delivered to soft tissues.

treatment, many such injuries ultimately result in surgical amputation of the digits.

Extravasation Injuries

In the past, extravasation injuries of chemotherapeutic agents frequently affected the upper extremity. However, subcutaneously tunneled central lines have now reduced the incidence of these injuries. If extravasation is suspected, infusion must be stopped immediately. Cold packs are applied for 15 minutes four times a day, and the extremity is elevated during the next 48 hours. This treatment is generally effective for most extravasation injuries. However, if blistering, ulceration, and pain occur in the damaged tissue, progressive necrosis to the limits of the extravasation will follow, and surgical excision of all damaged tissue is necessary. Most subsequent wounds can generally be treated with delayed split-thickness skin grafting, although the options for wound coverage after débridement depend on the extent of the débridement that was required.

Compartment Syndrome

Compartment syndrome results in symptoms and signs caused by increased pressure within a limited space that compromises circulation and function of the tissues in that space. Volkmann ischemic contracture is the sequel of untreated compartment syndrome; it results in muscle that is fibrosed, contracted, and functionless and nerves that are insensible. Various injuries are known to cause compartment syndrome:

- Decreased compartment volume (e.g., from externally applied tight dressings or casts, lying on a limb in a comatose state)
- Increased compartment content (e.g., from bleeding or trauma with fractures or finger injuries; increased capillary permeability, such as reperfusion after ischemic injury; electrical burn injuries)
- Other injuries (e.g., snakebites, high-pressure injection injuries)[28]

The diagnosis of compartment syndrome is based primarily on clinical evaluation. Although it is possible to measure intracompartment pressure, the decision to perform fasciotomy is based on a high degree of clinical suspicion. Compartment ischemia may be severe and still not affect the color or temperature of the distal fingers, and the distal pulses are rarely obliterated by compartment swelling. However, circulation in the muscle and nerve may be greatly reduced. Muscle ischemia that lasts for more than 4 hours leads to muscle death and may also cause significant myoglobinuria. After 8 hours of total ischemia, irreversible nerve changes are complete. The hallmark of muscle and nerve ischemia is pain, which is progressive and persistent. The pain is accentuated by passive muscle stretching; this is the most reliable clinical test for diagnosis of compartment syndrome. The next most important clinical finding is diminished sensation, which indicates nerve ischemia. The closed compartments of the forearm and hand are also palpated and found to be tense and tender, confirming the diagnosis of compartment syndrome. A passive muscle stretch test elicits severe pain in the presence of compartment syndrome. An arterial injury and nerve injury need to be distinguished in the differential diagnosis of compartment syndrome. All three of these injuries produce paresthesias and paresis; pain with passive stretch is present in compartment syndrome and arterial occlusion, but not in neurapraxia; and pulses are intact in compartment syndrome and neurapraxia, but not with arterial occlusion. In situations in which the patient cannot cooperate because of inebriation or unconsciousness and the

clinical diagnosis is difficult, compartment pressure can be measured.

Release of a forearm compartment syndrome always requires carpal tunnel release (Fig. 69-40). The palmar incision starts in the valley between the thenar and hypothenar muscles, and the incision then curves transversely across the flexion crease of the wrist at the ulnar border. This incision must avoid the palmar cutaneous branch of the median nerve and prevent flexion contracture across the wrist crease. It also provides an opportunity to release Guyon canal. The incision then extends proximally up the forearm before curving back in a radial direction so as to have a large skin flap that will cover the median nerve and distal forearm tendons. At the elbow, the incision for the flap then curves again across the antecubital fossa, providing cover for the brachial artery and median nerve and preventing linear contracture across the antecubital fossa. The dorsal and so-called mobile wad compartments of the forearm are readily released through a straight incision, as needed. Appropriate release of the various intrinsic compartments of the hand may also be required. Most wounds can be partially closed at 5 days. If the skin cannot be closed secondarily within 10 days, a split-thickness skin graft can be applied.

TENOSYNOVITIS

de Quervain Disease

de Quervain disease is a stenosing tenosynovitis of the first dorsal compartment of the wrist and is a common cause of pain and disability. Diagnosis is easily made from a history of pain localized to the radial side of the wrist and aggravated by movement of the thumb. There is frequently a history of chronic overuse of the wrist and hand. Other features are local tenderness and swelling over the first dorsal compartment of the wrist and a positive Finkelstein test result—the patient clasps the thumb and brisk ulnar deviation to the hand elicits extreme pain. Crepitus may be palpable. This condition must be differentiated by radiographic and physical examination from arthritis of the thumb carpometacarpal joint.

Nonoperative treatment includes local steroid injection, thumb and wrist immobilization, local heat, and systemic anti-inflammatory medications. If these nonoperative measures fail, surgical decompression of the first dorsal compartment at the wrist is performed. Care must be taken to protect the radial sensory nerve branches during the course of the operation because these branches traverse just under the skin in this area, and trauma or transection may lead to painful disabling neuromas.

Intersection Syndrome

This condition is not well understood but is characterized by pain and crepitus at the point at which the APL and EPB tendons cross over the tendons of the second dorsal compartment (ECRL and ECRB; Fig. 69-41). Initial treatment is by splinting, local corticosteroid injection, and anti-inflammatory medications. Refractory cases require surgical release at the second dorsal compartment and excision of involved tenosynovial membranes.

Trigger Thumb and Fingers

Trigger finger is a constricting tenosynovitis of the flexor tendons, generally at the level of the A1 pulley. The patient can flex the digit, but an apparent nodule catches at the proximal edge of the A1 pulley, locking the PIP joint (or the IP joint of the thumb) in this flexed position. Attempts at extending the digit cause it to

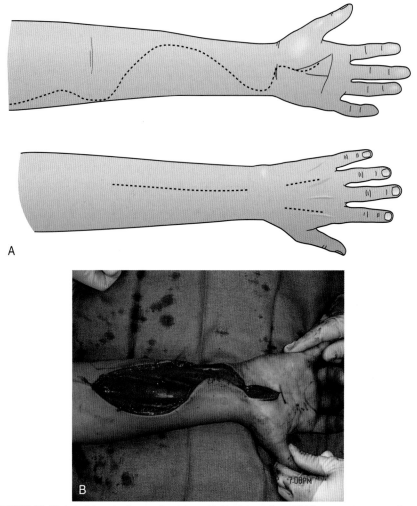

FIGURE 69-40 A, Incisions for forearm fasciotomy. **B,** Fasciotomy in a child for compartment syndrome after a snakebite.

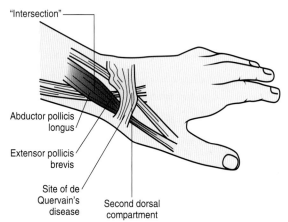

"Intersection"

Abductor pollicis longus

Extensor pollicis brevis

Site of de Quervain's disease

Second dorsal compartment

FIGURE 69-41 Anatomic locations for de Quervain stenosing tenosynovitis and intersection syndrome.

snap back suddenly, much like the trigger of a gun. Often, the patient needs to use the opposite hand to unlock and to extend the digit. In its most severe form, the constriction is so tight that the patient cannot flex the digit or it becomes fixed in a flexed position and can no longer be fully extended. A congenital form of trigger thumb or finger presents in infants, but most cases resolve by the time the child reaches 1 year of age; if not, an operation is indicated.

Nonoperative treatment in adults includes local injection of corticosteroids. If this regimen fails, the A1 pulley is longitudinally divided by surgery.[29]

Other Sites of Tenosynovitis

Other sites include the FCR and FCU tendons. They can frequently be treated by splinting and local corticosteroid injection, although surgery occasionally may be required. Inflammation of the ECU may also be an enigmatic cause of ulnar-sided wrist pain. Diagnosis is made by eliciting tenderness along the ECU tendon, pain on active resisted extension, and ulnar deviation of the wrist.

NERVE COMPRESSION SYNDROMES

Along the length of the upper extremity, nerves pass through a number of anatomic bottlenecks. These are all possible sites of nerve entrapment and lead to characteristic distal sensory and motor deficits. The most common sites of nerve compression, from proximal to distal along the length of the extremity, are at the nerve root secondary to cervical disc disease or cervical degenerative arthritis, thoracic outlet compression at the level of the clavicle, ulnar nerve entrapment at the elbow (cubital tunnel syndrome), entrapment of the posterior interosseous nerve in the proximal forearm (radial tunnel syndrome, posterior interosseous syndrome), entrapment of the median nerve and its branches in the proximal forearm (so-called pronator syndrome, anterior interosseous nerve syndrome), and, finally, entrapment of the median nerve at the wrist (carpal tunnel syndrome) and of the ulnar nerve in Guyon canal (ulnar tunnel syndrome).

In most cases of nerve entrapment, no specific aggravating causative factor is found. An increasing incidence of compression neuropathy is reported in patients whose work involves chronic repetitive stress (e.g., assemblers, chicken cutters). In some, there may be a clearly defined extrinsic compressive problem on the nerve or an aggravating factor. These include the following:

- Trauma that can produce bone compression, for example, carpal tunnel after carpal dislocations or a distal radius malunion (median) and supracondylar humerus fractures that increase the elbow carrying angle (ulnar nerve at the elbow)
- Synovial thickening of the bursa in rheumatoid arthritis in the carpal tunnel (median) or at the elbow (posterior interosseous)
- Tumors such as giant cell tumor in Guyon canal (ulnar) or a lipoma in the radial tunnel (posterior interosseous)
- Developmental, with anomalous muscles present in the carpal tunnel (median), Guyon canal (ulnar), or forearm (median)
- Metabolic, in which disturbances of fluid balance cause increased pressure on the nerve, particularly at the carpal tunnel (e.g., myxedema, pregnancy)

Carpal tunnel syndrome is the most common peripheral nerve entrapment syndrome, followed by ulnar nerve entrapment at the elbow.[30] The other entrapment syndromes are less common.

Diabetes mellitus is recognized as a risk factor for carpal tunnel syndrome, and the response to treatment has previously been unclear. However, studies suggest that patients with diabetes do similarly well to normoglycemic patients after carpal tunnel release.

Carpal Tunnel Syndrome

The carpal tunnel is a packed fibro-osseous tunnel at the wrist that is traversed by the median nerve and nine long extrinsic digital flexor tendons (Fig. 69-42). Its floor is formed by the carpal bones and roofed by the flexor retinaculum (transverse carpal ligament). Normal pressures in this tunnel are 20 to 30 mm Hg. A rise in pressure above this causes a chronic compressive ischemic injury to the nerve segment, resulting first in demyelination and eventually in axonal death. There is progressive conduction block in the nerve, with subsequent sensory and motor dysfunction. The earliest symptoms are pain and paresthesias, which are characteristically more obvious at night, after prolonged activity, and with positional postural changes at the wrist, such as when driving, using a hand-held hair dryer, or reading a book. The patient may complain of clumsiness and a tendency to drop objects. The paresthesias characteristically follow the distribution of the median nerve, including the thumb and index and middle fingers.

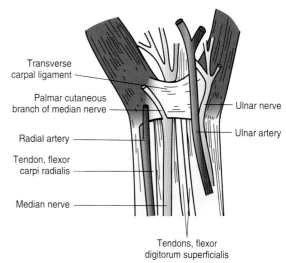

FIGURE 69-42 Anatomy of the Carpal Tunnel. The transverse carpal ligament (flexor retinaculum) is divided longitudinally during a carpal tunnel release.

Physical examination consists of compressing the carpal canal, percussing the median nerve, and hyperflexing the wrist to produce paresthesias (Durkan sign, Tinel sign, and Phalen test, respectively). Sensory evaluation reveals hypoesthesia in the distribution of the median nerve and may reveal a widened two-point sensory discrimination. Thenar weakness or muscle wasting is a late finding. Nerve conduction studies and electromyography are useful adjuncts to the clinical examination.

Initial treatment of carpal tunnel syndrome includes use of wrist splints (especially at night), occasional local corticosteroid injections, and modification in work patterns. If symptoms persist, or if the initial presentation shows severe carpal tunnel syndrome, surgical decompression is required. This is performed by longitudinally dividing the flexor retinaculum by open or endoscopic means. Both the Agee (single-portal) and Chow (two-portal) procedures have shown similar efficacy to the open approach.[31] Synovectomy and removal of any mass lesion may also be required if that is the cause of the problem.[32]

Pronator Syndrome

In the proximal forearm, the median nerve may be compressed at the fibrous arch between the two heads of the FDS, two heads of the pronator teres, lacertus fibrosus (bicipital aponeurosis at the elbow), and ligament of Struthers. Compression at any or all of these sites is loosely grouped under the pronator syndrome. The symptoms produced are similar to those of carpal tunnel, although nocturnal symptoms are uncommon. The palm may also feel numb because the palmar cutaneous branch is involved, but it is specifically spared in carpal tunnel syndrome because that nerve branch passes superficial to the flexor retinaculum and arises proximal to the retinaculum. Symptoms may be reproduced or worsened by attempting pronation against resistance and by resisted flexion of the middle finger. However, it may be difficult to locate the compressive cause in the pronator syndrome precisely, and surgical decompression often involves release of all four potential sites of compression.

The anterior interosseous nerve branch of the median nerve may occasionally be compressed in isolation. This does not produce any sensory symptoms but specifically targets the three

Labels in figure: Transverse carpal ligament; Palmar cutaneous branch of median nerve; Radial artery; Tendon, flexor carpi radialis; Median nerve; Ulnar nerve; Ulnar artery; Tendons, flexor digitorum superficialis

muscles innervated by the anterior interosseous nerve—FPL, FDP to the index and middle fingers, and pronator quadratus.

Ulnar Nerve Compression

The ulnar nerve may be compressed in Guyon canal at the wrist or in the so-called cubital tunnel at the elbow and distal upper arm.

Guyon Canal Compression

This canal is bounded by the hook of the hamate, pisiform, pisohamate ligament, and palmar carpal ligament. Compression by mass lesions may occur at this site, including a ganglion, giant cell tumor, ulnar artery thrombosis, and ulnar artery aneurysm, as in the hypothenar hammer syndrome. Compression at this site may also be idiopathic. Distal ulnar deficits may be in the motor or sensory distribution or both, depending on where in the canal the compression occurs relative to the takeoff of the deep motor branch of the ulnar nerve. Tinel sign may be present, and there may be worsening of symptoms by direct compression over Guyon canal. Treatment is surgical; it consists of dividing the palmaris brevis muscle and palmar carpal ligament as well as removing any offending mass in this region.

Cubital Tunnel Syndrome

The cubital tunnel is a long tunnel starting in the distal upper arm and extending into the proximal forearm. As the ulnar nerve passes into the forearm, it curves tightly around the grooved posterior and inferior surfaces of the medial epicondyle of the humerus. This groove is bridged by the aponeurosis between the two heads of the FCU, the leading edge of which may be thickened and fibrosed, called Osborne ligament. More proximally, the ulnar nerve passes from the anterior compartment of the arm into the posterior compartment, which may be bridged by a long tunnel called the arcade of Struthers. The medial intermuscular septum in the upper arm may also cause ulnar nerve compression. The most distal fibro-osseous tunnel is more accurately termed the cubital tunnel. However, compression on the ulnar nerve can occur at any of these sites, proximal to distal, starting in the upper arm and extending into the forearm. Motor and sensory symptoms develop in the distribution of the ulnar nerve and are worsened by adopting a flexed position at the elbow. Examination reveals Tinel sign over the tunnel. Paresthesias are described in the distribution of the ulnar nerve to the little and ring fingers and ulnar border of the hand. A differential diagnosis includes thoracic outlet syndrome, compression of the ulnar nerve in Guyon canal, and nerve root compression in the neck.

Initial treatment consists of splinting the elbow in extension at night. Use of soft extension elbow pads prevents elbow flexion and direct pressure on the nerve. Failure of nonoperative measures and significant changes in electrodiagnostic studies are indications for surgical decompression. Usually, all the fibrous restraints on the ulnar nerve around the elbow are released, and the nerve is transposed anteriorly to the medial epicondyle into a subcutaneous or submuscular position. There have been preliminary reports of success with endoscopic in situ decompression of the ulnar nerve at the elbow.

Radial Nerve Compression

The radial nerve may be compressed proximally in the triangular space in the axilla (specifically involving the axillary branch), spiral groove posterior to the humerus in the arm, and lateral intermuscular septum proximal to the elbow. More distally in the forearm, the posterior interosseous nerve, the principal motor division of the radial nerve, can be compressed in the so-called radial tunnel, starting at the leading fibrous edge of the supinator (ligament of Frohse). There may be a variable degree of interosseous nerve paresis, or there may be pain radiating down the dorsoradial aspect of the forearm (called radial tunnel syndrome). Initial treatment is nonoperative with splinting, but if this fails, surgical decompression may occasionally be required.

Thoracic Outlet Compression

The thoracic outlet is a narrow space at the base of the neck bounded by the first rib medially, scalenus anterior muscle and clavicle anteriorly, and scalenus medius muscle posteriorly. All elements of the brachial plexus as well as the subclavian artery and vein pass through this narrow space and can be potentially compressed at this site. A Tinel sign can often be elicited at the supraclavicular and infraclavicular regions. A Roos test is performed by asking the patient to hold both arms overhead in a surrender position while opening and closing the fists. This reproduces symptoms within 1 minute and, if continued, the arm collapses at the side. Adson test involves palpating the radial pulse while the patient turns the chin toward the same side, inhales deeply, and holds his or her breath. The radial pulse disappears or diminishes. The costoclavicular compression test involves sustained downward pressure on the clavicle, and the symptoms are reproduced. Radiographic evaluation may reveal a cervical rib. Results of nerve conduction studies are often normal.

Thoracic outlet compression may occur in association with other peripheral sites of nerve compression, a condition termed double-crush syndrome. Treatment is primarily nonoperative, involving posture-improving exercises and avoidance of aggravating activities. If symptoms persist, especially if they are associated with vascular compression, the thoracic outlet may be surgically decompressed. This is accomplished by a transcervical or transaxillary resection of the first rib, often with release of the scalene muscles.

TUMORS

Ganglions and mucous cysts represent 60% to 70% of hand tumors, followed in frequency by inclusion cysts, warts (verrucae), giant cell tumors in tendon sheaths, foreign body granulomas, lipomas, hemangiomas, and pyogenic granulomas (Table 69-5). Benign tumors account for 95% of hand neoplasms. Squamous cell carcinoma is the most frequent primary malignant neoplasm of the hand, basal cell carcinoma is rare, and melanoma is relatively uncommon in the upper extremity. Acral lentiginous melanoma (e.g., in the palm, sole, nail bed) has a tendency for early metastasis. Primary bone tumors of the hand are generally benign; the most common are enchondromas and osteochondromas. Giant cell tumors of bone are rare in the hand, occurring usually in the distal radius. They are locally aggressive and may occasionally metastasize. Of malignant bone tumors, only 1.2% affect the hand. Although bone metastases in other parts of the body are relatively common, bones of the hand are rarely affected by metastases from other sites.[33,34]

Soft tissue sarcomas are rare, representing 1% of all malignant neoplasms of the body, excluding skin tumors. Although uncommon, certain types predominate in the hand. Epithelioid, synovial, and clear cell sarcomas are relatively rare in other sites but by comparison are more common in the hand.

TABLE 69-5 Benign Connective Tissue Tumors of the Hand

SOFT TISSUE TUMORS	PRESENTATION	MOST COMMON LOCATIONS	TISSUE OF ORIGIN AND APPEARANCE	TREATMENT	RADIOGRAPHIC APPEARANCE
Ganglion	Swelling, sometimes painful; DIP mucous cyst may spontaneously drain clear gelatinous fluid; 70% of hand swellings	Volar and dorsal wrist, flexor tendon sheath, dorsum of DIP joint	Synovial cyst containing thick gelatinous fluid	No treatment versus aspiration versus excision	No radiographic alterations; mucous cyst at DIP joint may have osteophytes associated with osteoarthritis
Giant cell tumor of tendon sheath	Progressive enlargement, painless, deeply adherent; potential recurrence after excision; second most common hand tumor	Any synovial site, including tendon sheath, joint, palmar plate, usually in a digit	Synovium and histiocytes; bosselated and yellow-brown color from hemosiderin pigmentation	Excision	Pressure resorption of bone
Lipoma	Painless enlarging mass, usually on volar surface of hand or finger; may reach very large size; seldom nerve compression symptoms	Volar hand and finger	Mature fat cells	Excision (shell out)	Characteristic water-clear appearance on radiograph
Inclusion cyst (implantation dermoid)	Painless, enlarging lesion, adherent to overlying dermis; more common in laborers and those subject to minor hand trauma; may become infected	Palm and fingertips	Implanted epidermis cyst containing keratinous debris	Excision of entire epithelium-lined sac	May cause pressure resorption of bone
Neurofibroma	May be localized, diffuse, or plexiform; may be associated with von Recklinghausen disease; painless enlargement, but pain arouses suspicion of malignant change	Less common on hand than elsewhere; seen more frequently on palm	Perineurial fibroblasts	Excision if noncritical nerve; biopsy if malignancy suspected; possible nerve grafting	Characteristic MRI lobulated appearance
Schwannoma	Painless small mass in a peripheral nerve that is laterally mobile; may be an incidental finding at time of carpal tunnel surgery; occasional distal dysesthesias	Median and digital nerves	Schwann cells	Microneural surgery can shell the tumor out of the nerve without leaving neurologic deficit	No changes on plain radiograph
Pyogenic granuloma	Often at site of previous trivial skin injury on the fingers; friable and bleeds easily; grows rapidly	Fingers	Granulation tissue	Small lesions can be cauterized; excise larger lesions	No radiographic changes
Glomus tumor	Very small lesions; exquisitely painful, localized tenderness, cold sensitive; patients sometimes labeled as malingering	Subungual or volar fingertip; may be multiple	Neuromyoarterial apparatus	Excision; repair nail bed if subungual	May show indentation of distal phalanx

Within the spectrum of benign and malignant tumors, there is a group with intermediate malignancy. Giant cell and desmoid tumors (of soft tissue) have a propensity for local recurrence after surgical excision. Their histologic patterns may belie their behavior. Juvenile aponeurotic fibroma and nodular fasciitis may appear histologically more aggressive than desmoid tumors but are self-limited. The tiny glomus tumor is uncommon but has a propensity for the fingertips and subungual regions. It may be an enigmatic cause of severe and exquisite pain at the fingertips and can be recognized by a pinpoint site of extreme local tenderness and a violaceous hue deep to the nail plate. MRI may occasionally detect these tiny lesions at the fingertip.

If a lesion is thought to be benign, excision without further workup, except perhaps for routine radiographs, is appropriate. However, if a primary malignant neoplasm of bone or soft tissue is suspected, additional studies must be undertaken before biopsy. CT may help delineate tumor boundaries. Desmoid tumors have radiographic density identical to that of muscle and are better demonstrated by MRI.

Soft Tissue Tumors
Ganglion Cysts
Ganglions are formed by an outpouching of the synovial membrane from a joint or tendon sheath and contain thick, jelly-like, mucinous material similar in composition to synovial fluid (Fig. 69-43). Of ganglions, 60% occur on the dorsal aspect of the wrist, arising in the region of the scapholunate ligament. Other sites for ganglions in the hand are at the volar wrist, arising from one of the scaphoid articulations; at the flexor tendon sheath at the area of the A1 pulley; and at the dorsum of the DIP joint, called a mucous cyst, where they are often associated with osteoarthritis of that DIP joint. In the last location, the ganglion cyst can exert pressure on the germinal matrix of the nail bed, resulting in a deformed or grooved nail.

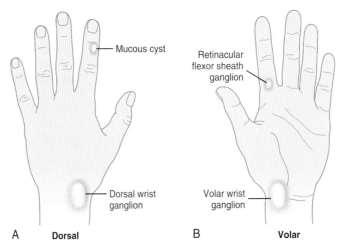

FIGURE 69-43 Dorsal (**A**) and volar (**B**) aspects of the hand and wrist showing common types of ganglions, including the dorsal wrist ganglion, volar wrist ganglion, flexor sheath ganglion (volar retinacular cyst), and mucous cyst.

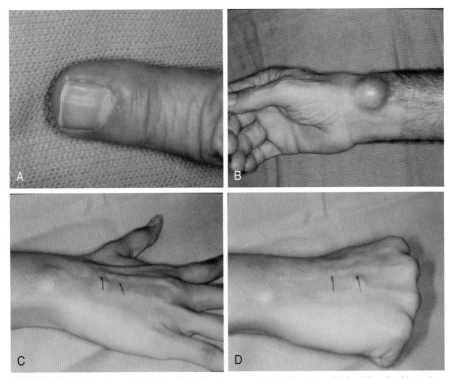

FIGURE 69-44 Ganglions in the Hand. **A,** Ganglion associated with osteoarthritis of the distal interphalangeal joint (mucous cyst), causing longitudinal linear groove in the nail plate from pressure on the germinal matrix. **B,** Volar wrist ganglion on the radial side of the flexor carpi radialis tendon is closely related to the radial artery and should not be aspirated. **C,** Ganglion arising from the extensor digitorum communis tendon of the ring finger located at the level of the proximal skin marking with fingers extended. **D,** Movement of ganglion 2 cm to the level of the more distal skin marking when the fist is clenched. Distal movement of the swelling with the gliding extensor tendon confirms its attachment to the tendon.

Ganglions are most common in women in the third decade of life. They are innocuous and can often be left alone. However, treatment may be required for cosmetic purposes or to relieve pressure effects on adjacent structures (Fig. 69-44). The dorsal wrist ganglion can sometimes be painful as a result of pressure on the posterior interosseous nerve at that location. A very small impalpable dorsal wrist ganglion can become quite painful, the so-called occult ganglion, and on occasion may best be diagnosed by MRI. Treatment of a dorsal wrist ganglion may be performed by aspiration of the mucinous substance with a large-bore needle. If this fails, the ganglion can then be surgically excised. Care must be taken to trace and to resect the pedicle of the ganglion all the way down to the joint or tendon sheath from which it arises.[35] A volar wrist ganglion may often be closely related to the radial artery. Aspiration of volar wrist ganglions is seldom advised because of the potential risk of injury to the radial artery. At the level of the DIP joint, optimal treatment includes not only meticulous excision of the ganglion but also the removal of associated osteophytes from the joint. Arthroscopic decompression of dorsal wrist ganglions has been described.

Giant Cell Tumor

Giant cell tumor, also called pigmented villonodular synovitis, is the second most common hand tumor. It occurs in soft tissues (e.g., synovial membrane of joints, tendon sheaths) and, less commonly, in bone. This yellow-brown multilobular tumor is composed of multinucleated giant cells. Although usually benign, the tumor pushes deeply into the soft tissues of the digits and extends along tendon sheaths and around neurovascular structures. It is frequently asymptomatic and is often larger than suspected clinically. Radiologic notching of bone may be evident in larger, soft tissue giant cell tumors. Complete surgical excision is the treatment of choice. Failure to discern and to remove each lobule substantially increases the reported local recurrence rate of almost 10%. Synovectomy of the joint of origin may be necessary (Fig. 69-45; see also Fig. 69-47B).

Epidermal Inclusion Cysts

Epidermal inclusion cysts, also called implantation dermoids, frequently occur after trauma as keratin-producing epidermal cells

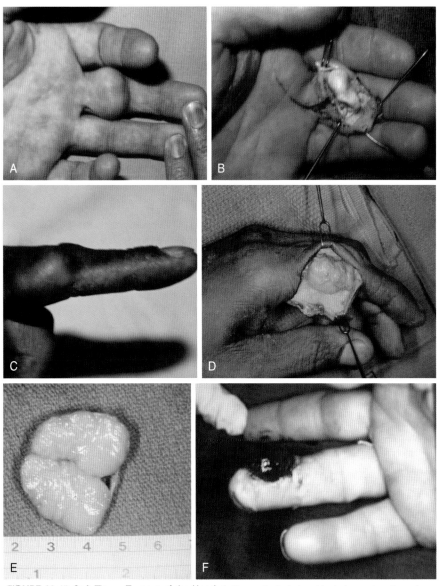

FIGURE 69-45 Soft Tissue Tumors of the Hand. A, Traumatically induced inclusion cyst on the palmar aspect of the middle finger in a manual worker. B, Intraoperative photograph demonstrates cyst filled with toothpaste-like gel derived from keratin. C, Firm, progressively enlarging swelling on the radial side of the left index finger. D, Firm, lobulated, yellow-brown giant cell tumor insinuating onto the dorsal and volar aspects of the finger is noted intraoperatively. E, Giant cell tumor is the most common solid soft tissue tumor encountered in the hand. F, Fleshy friable pyogenic granuloma bleeds easily on contact.

become lodged in the subcutaneous tissues (Fig. 69-45). The resulting cystic mass contains a thick toothpaste-like material. They occur more commonly in men, especially in manual laborers, and most frequently involve the palm of the hand and fingertips. They may also occur in previous surgical scars. Treatment is surgical excision, and recurrence is rare.

Lipoma

Lipomas are small, benign, soft, fluctuant, fatty tumors (Fig. 69-46). In the hand, they usually occur on the thenar eminence. Although generally painless, they may enlarge significantly, insinuating into deep palmar spaces and causing pain by compression on adjacent nerves. Intracarpal lipoma is a rarer cause of carpal

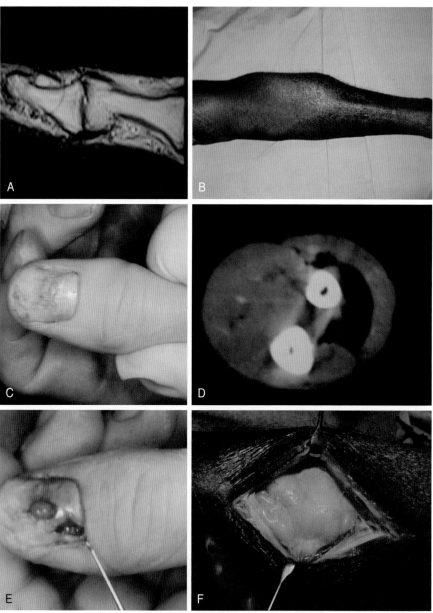

FIGURE 69-46 Soft Tissue Tumors of the Hand. A, Patient presenting with pain in tip of thumb, exacerbated in cold weather. Exquisite pain on palpation of the thumb nail plate is typical of a subungual glomus tumor that can be demonstrated by MRI. **B,** Occult subungual glomus tumor may be difficult to appreciate, even after removal of the nail plate, but it can often be identified by a surface bulge of the nail bed. **C,** Excised glomus tumor sitting on nail bed. A nail bed defect requires repair with fine absorbable sutures. **D,** Man with swelling of left dorsoradial forearm and weakness of finger and thumb extension. **E,** MRI reveals a dorsal forearm mass compressing the posterior interosseous nerve. **F,** Dorsal approach over the mass reveals intramuscular benign lipoma when extensor muscles are split.

tunnel syndrome. Resection of symptomatic lipomas is curative, although 1% to 2% may recur.

Pyogenic Granuloma

Pyogenic granuloma is a misnomer for an exuberant outburst of highly vascular granulation tissue at the site of previous relatively trivial trauma. These lesions are friable, bleed easily, and may grow rapidly. They respond to curettage or simple excision. They usually occur on the fingertips. Histologic confirmation of the diagnosis is necessary because of occasional confusion with aggressive malignant lesions, such as ulcerated, amelanotic, malignant melanomas.

Verruca Vulgaris

Verrucae vulgaris are common contagious warts associated with human papillomavirus type 1. They occur usually as hyperkeratotic filiform lesions on the digits or about the nail bed. The most effective topical treatments are salicylates, liquid nitrogen cryotherapy, and especially curettage. Recalcitrant lesions respond to oral cimetidine given for 6 to 8 weeks and to imiquimod, an immunomodulator that increases interferon production.[36] Their incidence, like that of squamous cell carcinomas, is increased in immunocompromised patients, such as in those after transplantation. Recurrence is relatively common.[37]

Seborrheic Keratoses

Seborrheic keratoses are benign, hyperkeratotic, scaly lesions. They are frequently pigmented and common on the dorsum of the hand in older adults. Occasional confusion occurs with pigmented basal cell carcinomas. When necessary, these superficial scaly lesions are best treated by shave excision, and sutures are unnecessary. Rapid reepithelialization occurs.

Keratoacanthoma

Keratoacanthoma occurs on exposed body parts such as the dorsum of the hand. It grows rapidly during approximately 3 weeks into a nodule with a central umbilicated keratotic plug, often followed by spontaneous resolution in many weeks or months. The resulting scar is often worse than if the lesion had been excised initially.[38] There may be diagnostic uncertainty in regard to well-differentiated squamous cell carcinomas. Hence, most authors recommend surgical excision.

Dermatofibroma

A dermatofibroma arises from fibrous dermal tissue as a firm erythematous plaque, sometimes having central umbilication. It is often adherent to the overlying epidermis. Surgery is required primarily for diagnosis.

Vascular Malformations and Hemangiomas

Hemangiomas are hamartomas that are rarely visible at birth and are usually noticed weeks to months later. Rapid proliferation occurs in the first year of life. On histologic evaluation, proliferation of endothelial cells with increased mitotic activity is seen in conjunction with pericytes and dendritic and mast cells. Hemangiomas occur 10 times more commonly than vascular malformations, and approximately 70% involute by the age of 7 years, leaving a fibrofatty scar with redundant skin. Excision is seldom required and, after involution, is usually cosmetic. On occasion, oral or injectable steroids may be necessary to control rapidly proliferating lesions that cause pain or interfere with function. Propranolol, which reduces basic fibroblast growth factor and

vascular endothelial growth factor expression, is sometimes added in conjunction with steroids for problematic hemangiomas.[39]

By contrast, vascular malformations show normal endothelial growth characteristics and normal mast cell counts. They are often noted at birth, and growth is usually commensurate with the child for low-flow lesions. They do not undergo spontaneous involution.

Vascular malformations are subclassified into low-flow lesions; capillary, venous, and lymphatic lesions predominate. Arterial and arteriovenous fistulas predominate in high-flow lesions, and accelerated growth may occur relative to the patient. Pressure effects, ulceration, bleeding, and high-output cardiac failure can occur in severe cases. Enlarging lesions hinder hand function. Compression garments can provide symptomatic relief in some cases. Pain is often caused by vascular engorgement, phlebitis, or intralesional coagulation. D-dimer levels may be elevated, and some patients obtain relief from aspirin. Combined surgical excision[40] and radiologic embolization[41] are most effective in preventing recurrence caused by dilation of collateral vascular channels after simple excision.

Lymphaticovenous malformations may also be associated with generalized hypertrophy of an extremity. Vascular malformations and isolated macrodactyly are seen in Klippel-Trénaunay syndrome.

Malignant Skin Tumors
Basal Cell Carcinoma

Basal cell carcinoma is rare on the hand and is generally located on the dorsum. It is usually an ulcer with raised pearly edges. Treatment consists of excision with a margin of normal adjacent tissue. Nail bed lesions can be mistaken for paronychial infection, and amputation at the DIP joint may be required.[42]

Squamous Cell Carcinoma

Squamous cell carcinoma may arise de novo from ultraviolet light exposure because of occupation or climate, usually on the sun-exposed dorsum of the hand. Approximately 16% of actinic keratoses may progress to squamous cell carcinoma. Arsenical keratoses may develop secondary to exposure to inorganic arsenic compounds but have a predilection for the palm.

Bowen disease is an intraepidermal squamous cell carcinoma (carcinoma in situ).[43] It is a plaquelike lesion with crusting. Complete surgical excision with a margin of normal tissue is curative. When the nail matrix is involved, amputation at the DIP joint may be necessary.

For squamous cell carcinoma lesions smaller than 2.5 cm in diameter, wide excision with approximately a 6-mm clear margin is recommended. However, for larger lesions, more radical excision may be required, which may even include ray or segmental amputation for deeply adherent and invasive lesions. Mohs micrographic surgery and three-dimensional histologic reconstruction with a pathologist at the time of radical resection help ensure complete excision. Routine prophylactic lymphadenectomy is not beneficial.[44] However, lymphadenectomy may be advised for recurrent tumors, even though lymph nodes may not be clinically palpable. Malignant degeneration may occur in cicatricial tissue and chronic ulcers (e.g., Marjolin ulcer) and, in particular, in burn scars. Prognosis tends to be poorer.[45]

Malignant Melanomas

Melanoma of the hand is cutaneous or subungual. There is an almost equal distribution of cases between the two types.[46]

Frequently, there is a delay in treatment, particularly with subungual melanomas. Suspicious lesions should be biopsied.

Any subungual pigmented lesions should generally be biopsied. Under tourniquet control and with loupe magnification, the nail plate is atraumatically removed, and a longitudinal, elliptical, full-thickness excision of the lesion is performed. Careful nail bed repair is done after biopsy by the advancement of adjacent tissues and using fine absorbable sutures. The nail plate is then reapplied to act as a splint.

Benign melanocytic hyperplasia, without evidence of atypia, is completely treated by this form of biopsy. If there is any evidence of melanocytic atypia, absolute confirmation of complete excision is required. In the absence of a clear margin or with recurrence of such a lesion, total nail bed excision and reconstruction with a full-thickness skin graft are required. Melanoma in situ is similarly treated. Invasive melanoma of the nail bed is treated by amputation at the next most proximal joint. Acral lentiginous melanoma of the palm may sometimes be mistaken for a wart, which may also delay diagnosis. These tumors are aggressively treated with wide local excision and potential sentinel node biopsy, as they might be treated anywhere else on the body.

Bone Tumors
Osteoid Osteoma
This may occur in the hand and classically causes pain that is worse at night and unrelated to use or motion of the hand (Table 69-6). Osteoid osteomas produce prostaglandins; symptoms are relieved by nonsteroidal anti-inflammatory drugs (NSAIDs). On radiologic examination, a round lucent tumor with sclerotic edges is seen (Fig. 69-47A). Conservative treatment with NSAIDs may be considered, but definitive treatment is surgical.

Aneurysmal Bone Cyst
This is an expansile osteolytic bone lesion with a thin wall. It is usually derived from a preexisting bone tumor, usually a giant cell tumor (20% to 40% of cases). Of these, 25% occur in the upper extremity, causing pain that peaks during 2 to 3 months. A bone swelling may be detectable, with increased overlying skin temperature.

Enchondroma
Enchondromas usually occur in the hand and are the most common bone tumor of the hand. Peak incidence is in the second decade, with equal gender distribution. They are frequently asymptomatic and noted incidentally as lytic lesions on plain radiology. Pain, bone swelling, or pathologic fracture may occur as these cartilaginous intraosseous cysts compromise bone structural integrity (Fig. 69-47D). Treatment is by curettage and bone grafting of the osseous defect. Multiple enchondromatosis occurs in Ollier disease and is associated with angiomas in Maffucci syndrome.

Primary Bone Sarcomas
These malignant tumors are rare in the hand.

Secondary (Metastatic) Bone Tumors
Metastatic tumors, even those with a tendency to metastasize to bone, usually occur in the axial skeleton and long bones. They are very rare in the hand.

CONGENITAL ANOMALIES

The causes of congenital hand anomalies may be genetic, teratogenic, or idiopathic and may also have a syndromic association

TABLE 69-6	Bone Tumors of the Hand				
TUMOR	PRESENTATION	MOST COMMON LOCATIONS	TISSUE OF ORIGIN AND APPEARANCE	TREATMENT	RADIOGRAPHIC APPEARANCE
Enchondroma	Often incidental finding on routine hand radiograph; presents as pain secondary to pathologic fracture; most common bone tumor of hand	Proximal and middle phalanges and metacarpals	Fragments of cartilage nests; multiple (Ollier disease); when associated with hemangiomas (Maffucci syndrome), may undergo malignant change	Curettage, filling of defect with cancellous bone if structural bone integrity is compromised	Lesion eccentric in bone shaft with calcific stippling
Osteochondroma	Benign bone prominence (capped with cartilage); rare in hand; may cause angular growth and interfere with joint motion	Fingers and wrist; growth stops after skeletal maturity reached	Aberrant focus of cartilage; multiple osteochondromatosis is autosomal dominant; malignant change may occur	Surgery may be necessary, generally after epiphyseal closure	Exostosis, often at base of proximal phalanx; often shortening of parent bone
Osteoid osteoma	Aching pain, greatest at night, sometimes responding specifically to aspirin; patient may be labeled as malingerer	Phalanges, metacarpals, carpals	Nidus composed of loose fibrovascular connective tissue between bars of osteoid and bone trabeculae	Surgical excision to include the nidus	Very small lesion; some not seen on plain radiographs and require CT scan; cortical sclerosis surrounding a radiolucent area of nidus
Giant cell tumor of bone	Expansile bone swelling at distal radius or in phalanx	Distal radius most common site	May be locally aggressive and even metastasize	Curettage for low-grade lesions, but en bloc resection for high-grade lesions; do not irradiate because it could induce sarcomatous change	Expansile soap bubble lesion in bone; high-grade lesions break through cortex

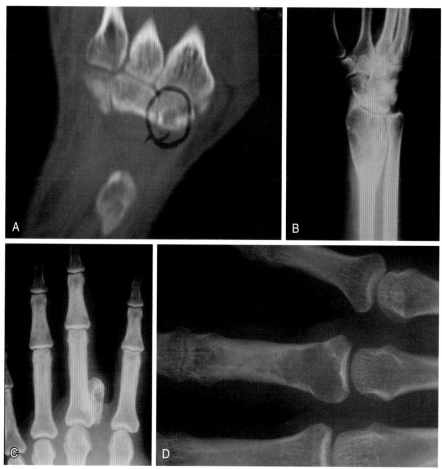

FIGURE 69-47 Plain radiographs of the upper extremity. **A,** Osteoid osteoma of carpus. **B,** Soap bubble appearance of giant cell tumor expanding the metaphysis of the distal radius. **C,** Osteochondroma of proximal phalanx of middle (long) finger. **D,** Patient with finger pain after trivial injury. This is a pathologic fracture of the base of the proximal phalanx through an enchondroma that has replaced most of proximal metaphysis and medulla.

with anomalies elsewhere in the body. Knowledge of these associations is important because the more life-threatening associated problems frequently need to be treated first, before the hand and upper extremity reconstruction can be performed. Such an association is found in a constellation of problems that occur in the VACTERL association of congenital defects (vertebral anomalies, anal atresia, cardiac abnormalities, tracheoesophageal fistula, renal agenesis, and limb anomalies). A number of factors must be considered in optimizing the timing of each surgical procedure to the upper extremity, including the psychosocial development of the child, presence of other illnesses, size of the structures to be operated on, and normal growth and development of the hand. Modern technologic advances have allowed us to operate on smaller structures; the timing of the procedure can now be guided by knowledge of the anatomy and development of the growing hand. Optimal function is the primary goal of surgery. Principles of treatment of congenital hand anomalies recognize that an infant's immunity to infection develops over time, early surgery prevents the emotional scarring associated with a child's awareness of the deformity, and some congenital problems may not be apparent in the neonate. The hand surgeon must work closely with the pediatrician to identify general conditions that

may affect the child's health. Some congenital anomalies of the extremities, especially those with the radial ray, may be associated with bone marrow failure (Fanconi syndrome) or heart defects that may not be immediately apparent in the neonate. Children with congenital anomalies will attempt to keep up with their peers and often develop successful hand substitution techniques. However, once a child experiences the cruel ridicule of playmates or the unintentional but sometimes overly solicitous supervision of a teacher, his or her deformity becomes important. In general, plans for surgical reconstruction are designed to be completed by school age, so that the child may adapt to and fully use the reconstructed limb.[47]

The rationale for early surgery includes the avoidance of deformity and malfunction and optimal use of infantile tissue plasticity. Because hand length almost doubles during the first 2 years of life, a digit tethered to another digit that fails to grow can produce a major deformity during the early growth spurt. For example, with separation of syndactyly that involves the border digits of the hand, because of adjacent tethering to a digit of unequal length, surgical separation of the syndactyly is required at an early age, as early as 6 months, to avoid secondary angular deformity of the digits.

In rare circumstances, urgent treatment in the neonate is required. The distal lymphedema of a severe constriction band syndrome may be so marked as to inhibit function totally or even to threaten distal viability. This may require urgent release. The unusual clinical entity of aplasia cutis may result in exposure of vital structures, requiring urgent soft tissue coverage, even in the neonatal period.

Early operation, although not urgent, may be required not only because of the rapid growth that occurs in the first 2 years of life but also because of functional consequences. Surgery at a young age is considered mandatory in children with malformations in which hand function may be altered by surgery or in those who are at risk for development of certain grasping habits that would have to be unlearned after corrective surgery. An older child, 12 to 14 years of age, has developed grasp patterns that would have to be altered by prolonged periods of physical therapy after corrective surgery.[47,48]

The ability to place the upper limbs in space (a cortical function) and development of a strong grasp are established by 1 year of age, as are grasp and pinch maneuvers between the thumb and fingers. Accuracy of prehension and refinement of coordination continue until 3 years of age. Surgery must be performed early to allow the affected parts to develop differently when the function of the parts of the hand is altered by transposition (e.g., pollicization of an index finger for thumb aplasia). Duplicated thumb correction is carried out before 1 year of age, well in advance of the development of integrated thumb grasp patterns.

Finally, the physical ability of infant bone and soft tissues to adapt to change produced by surgery is also a key factor in deciding when to operate. In the early pollicization of the index finger, the first dorsal interosseous muscle hypertrophies to form a thenar eminence and the first metacarpal (formerly known as the proximal phalanx of the index finger) broadens. If centralization of the wrist for radial dysplasia (formerly known as radial club hand) has been undertaken early, the head of the ulna broadens to resemble the distal end of the radius.

Thus, a number of issues are taken into consideration when deciding on the optimum time for surgical reconstruction of congenital hand and upper extremity anomalies. The more common hand anomalies include syndactyly, polydactyly, constriction band syndrome, and absent or hypoplastic thumb.

Syndactyly results from the failure of programmed cell death (apoptosis) between the individual finger rays. Consequently, there is a resulting fusion of adjacent digits. It can involve part or all of the length of the digits (incomplete or complete) and may be limited to skin and soft tissue only (simple syndactyly) or can also involve skeletal fusion (complex syndactyly). Apert syndrome also involves craniofacial anomalies and is a severe form of bilaterally symmetrical complex syndactyly. Surgical treatment involves digit separation using a local flap to reconstruct the depths of the commissure between the fingers and release of the finger borders with zigzag incisions and the use of full-thickness skin grafts (Fig. 69-48A).

Polydactyly is the presence of extranumerary digits on the hand. Preaxial (radial) polydactyly involves the thumb. It is not as common as postaxial (ulnar) polydactyly, which is the most frequent congenital hand anomaly in African Americans. Polydactyly can be as simple as the presence of a skin tag–like structure or may have a complex arrangement of shared vessels, nerves, and bones. Thumb polydactyly is not merely a duplication but a splitting of a single digit, with variable degrees of development in each of the separate parts. It is typically classified into seven subtypes by the Wassel classification, which is based on the specific duplication,

progressing from distal to proximal in which the odd numbers are at distal and proximal phalanx and metacarpal, and even numbers are at IP, MP and CMC joints respectively. Type IV is the most common type, with total duplication of proximal and distal phalanges and a shared MP joint. Type VII refers to associated triphalangia with a duplication. Reconstructive goals include stabilization without sacrificing mobility, proper alignment of joints along the longitudinal axis of the thumb, balanced motor units, and a cosmetically acceptable nail plate (Fig. 69-48B and C).

The Blauth classification categorizes thumb hypoplasia from type I, which represents minor hypoplasia, to type V, which is a total thumb absence. Surgical correction ranges from reconstruction of the existing hypoplastic thumb to pollicization (creating a thumb from the index finger) for complete absence or for the more severe types of hypoplasia (Fig. 69-49).

Clinodactyly is a curving of the digits in a radial or ulnar direction. It is common, particularly involving the little finger in many individuals, but a curvature of more than 10 degrees is considered abnormal. The distal phalanx is usually affected and a delta phalanx may be associated. A delta phalanx occurs when the epiphysis forms a C shape around the metaphyseal core in the middle phalanx. Most patients present with little or no functional or cosmetic deformity, and operative intervention is seldom required. If there is a functionally impairing deviation of the finger, corrective osteotomy can be done.

Camptodactyly is a congenital flexion deformity of digits. It usually occurs in the little finger PIP joint. The exact cause is unclear, but it has been attributed to a variety of different structures around the PIP joint, including a skin pterygium, collateral ligaments, volar plate, flexor tendon, abnormal insertions of lumbrical or interosseous muscles, and size and shape of the head of the proximal phalanx. Treatment is generally nonoperative and may involve serial splinting. If no improvement occurs and the flexion deformity is sufficient to cause a functional problem, surgical intervention may be required; this includes correction of the deformity with Z-plasty and possibly grafts. One author has reported that all his patients who had reconstructive surgery on one hand did not ask for corrective surgery on the opposite affected hand.

Constriction band syndrome is secondary to intrauterine amniotic bands (Fig. 69-48D). These can act like tourniquets and threaten the viability of digits and even limbs, resulting in congenital amputation. Infants may suffer from a similar problem from the external ligature effect of cotton strands coming off protective booties and even from a human hair, termed the hair-thread tourniquet syndrome.

OSTEOARTHRITIS AND RHEUMATOID ARTHRITIS

Osteoarthritis may be primary or post-traumatic (secondary). Primary osteoarthritis is a degenerative joint disease occurring in later life. An injury that leaves articular surfaces of a joint incongruous can precipitate secondary osteoarthritis. Osteoarthritis begins with biochemical alteration of the water content of articular cartilage. The cartilage weakens and develops cracks, called fibrillation. Progressive erosion and thinning of the cartilage result, and the subchondral bone becomes sclerotic, termed eburnation. New bone forms around the edges of the articular cartilage, and these outcroppings are called osteophytes (Fig. 69-50).

The joints usually affected in the hand are the DIP and PIP joints of the fingers and carpometacarpal joint at the base of the thumb. Osteophytes at the DIP joint are called Heberden nodes,

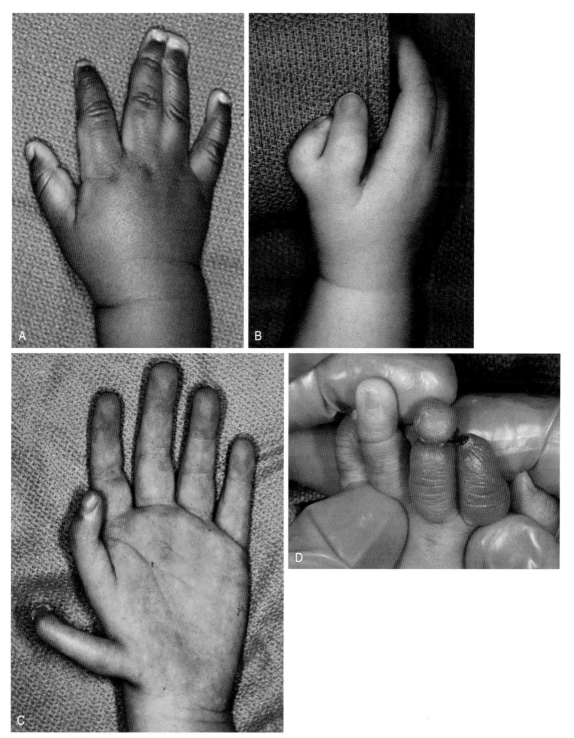

FIGURE 69-48 Congenital hand anomalies include syndactyly **(A),** Wassel type IV thumb polydactyly **(B),** Wassel type VI polydactyly **(C),** and constriction band **(D).**

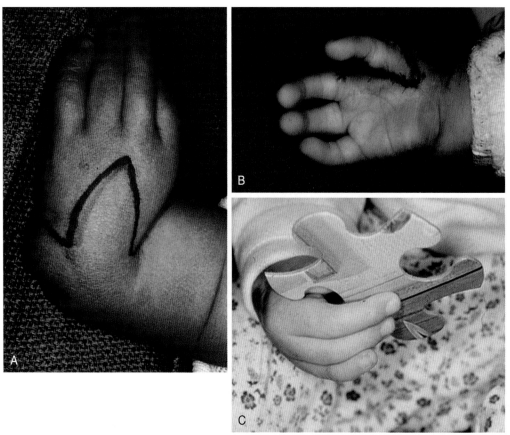

FIGURE 69-49 **A,** Patient with radial dysplasia and absent thumb. **B,** After centralization of the wrist on the distal ulna, pollicization of the index finger is performed. **C,** Natural prehension has been restored to this three-finger hand with a reconstructed wrist and thumb.

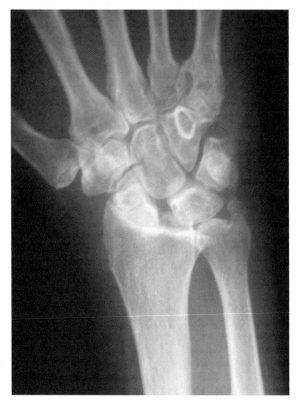

FIGURE 69-50 Radiograph of a hand with a scapholunate advanced collapse wrist showing post-traumatic osteoarthritis at the radioscaphoid junction. This is many years after a wrist sprain in which the scapholunate ligament was torn; a wide scapholunate gap is visible on the radiograph.

and those at the PIP joint are known as Bouchard nodes. The involved joints may be painful, stiff, deformed, or subluxated. Radiographs reveal narrowing of the joint space, sclerosis of subchondral bone, and presence of osteophytes.

Initial treatment may be symptomatic and may include splinting and even local corticosteroid injections. NSAIDs may be helpful, and chondroprotective medications such as glucosamine and chondroitin sulfate can reduce symptoms. In advanced cases, the DIP joints respond best to arthrodesis. The PIP joints may be surgically treated by replacement arthroplasty or by arthrodesis (Fig. 69-51). The thumb carpometacarpal joint may be treated by arthrodesis, which is favored particularly for the young patient who might have post-traumatic arthritis after, for example, an improperly treated Bennett or Orlando fracture. In an older patient with primary osteoarthritis at the thumb base, excision of the trapezium followed by tendon suspension (interposition) arthroplasty may be preferred. This uses local tendons for construction of a sling arthroplasty, with interposition of tendon material.

Rheumatoid arthritis is an autoimmune process whereby destruction of the musculoskeletal system may occur. Synovial inflammation results in pain, joint destruction, tendon ruptures, and characteristic deformities. Some of the more common deformities associated with rheumatoid arthritis include a swan neck deformity (hyperextension of the PIP joint with concurrent flexion at the DIP joint), boutonnière deformity (flexion at the PIP joint, with concurrent hyperextension at the DIP joint), joint subluxation, radial deviation of the wrist, and ulnar deviation and flexion of the fingers (Fig. 69-52). Rheumatoid arthritis is primarily a medical illness for which a number of medications are currently available. Thus, there must be excellent lines of communication between the rheumatologist and surgeon. NSAIDs as well as disease-modifying antirheumatoid drugs are used. Rheumatoid arthritis is a progressive disorder, and ongoing slow destruction may be anticipated despite surgery (Fig. 69-53). Some of the more common surgical procedures include joint synovectomy, tenosynovectomy, tendon transfers, joint replacements (especially at the MP and PIP joints), and arthrodesis (more commonly at the wrist and thumb MP joint).[49]

CONTRACTURES

Volkmann ischemic contracture develops as a result of myofascial contractures in response to prolonged ischemia. This most common contracture results from untreated compartment syndrome of the forearm and hand. Muscle necrosis occurs, and the muscles become replaced by fibrous scar tissue. The FDP and FPL muscles are usually affected, being in the deepest forearm volar compartment, and digits are characteristically flexed, with passive

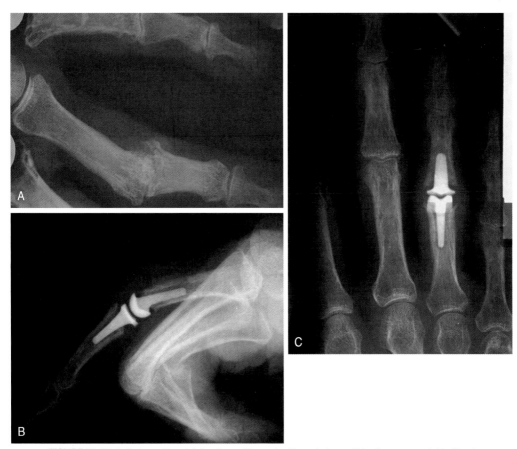

FIGURE 69-51 A, Patient with painful and unstable proximal interphalangeal joint from osteoarthritis. **B** and **C,** Reconstruction is performed by implant arthroplasty. An advantage over arthrodesis is that motion is retained, although there remains the potential for future recurrent joint instability and wear of the artificial joint.

extension of the wrist worsening the flexion deformity of the digits. Intrinsic contractures can occur in the hand; these can be investigated using Bunnell test, in which passive extension of the MP joint makes passive flexion of the PIP joint more difficult.

In the milder forms of Volkmann ischemic contracture, serial splinting and passive stretching exercises may resolve the problem. In more severe contractures, Z-type lengthening of tendons may be required. A flexor pronator muscle slide—subperiosteal elevation of the common flexor origin from the medial epicondyle of the humerus and from the ulna—allows the muscles to slide distally until the contracture is corrected. In the most severe form, all the muscles of the volar forearm may be affected, requiring tendon transfers, even microvascular functional muscle transfers to provide some functional return.

Post-traumatic contractures are the most common type of contracture. These can be prevented by appropriate treatment of the primary injury, especially with attention to detail in how the hand and upper extremity are splinted and immobilized. Once contractures have developed, if they are mild, they may be able to be stretched out by exercises and hand therapy. If these contractures are severe and functionally deforming, surgical release of joint contractures and release of tendon adhesions may be required.

Dupuytren contracture is a disease process of contracting collagen affecting the palmar fascia; it can also affect the dorsum of the fingers (knuckle pads), soles of the feet, and penis (Peyronie disease). It is thought to be a hereditary mendelian dominant disorder and is bilateral in 65% of cases. It is six times more frequent in males and predominantly involves the ring and little fingers (Fig. 69-54).

The process of Dupuytren contracture occurs in the normal bands of collagen tissue that form the palmar fascia, natatory ligaments, and digital sheaths. Nodules containing myofibroblasts and immature collagen (type III) develop in these tissues or in the dermis. The nodules progressively increase in size, leading to thickened contractures and shortened fascial bands that develop into cords extending up the digits. Treatment is surgical excision; it is indicated in MP contractures of 30 degrees or more, when the patient fails the so-called tabletop test and cannot place the palm of the hand flat on a surface, and whenever there is a PIP joint contracture. Careful surgical technique is necessary to avoid complications such as skin necrosis, hematoma, and digital nerve

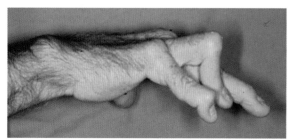

FIGURE 69-52 Patient with inflammatory arthritis has both boutonnière deformity and swan neck deformity on the same hand.

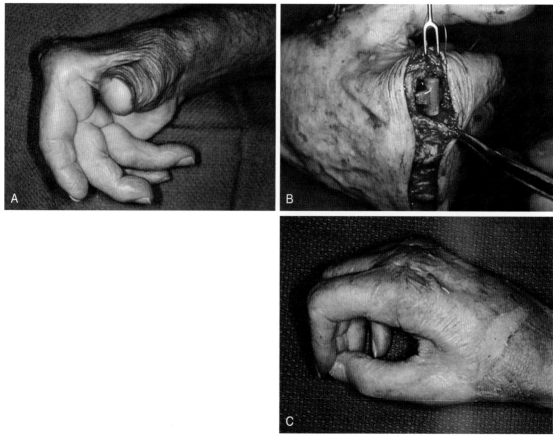

FIGURE 69-53 A, Patient with rheumatoid arthritis showing the characteristic finger deformities. **B** and **C,** Implant arthroplasty at the metacarpophalangeal joints restores function and aesthetics to the hand

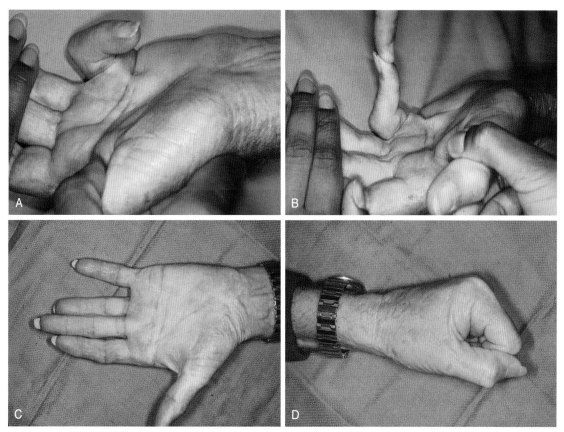

FIGURE 69-54 A-D, Patient with Dupuytren contracture is treated by regional palmar and digital fasciectomy, and good hand function is restored.

injuries. Collagenase injections using enzyme derived from *Clostridium histolyticum* have been attempted and have shown some promise in the treatment of Dupuytren contracture. However, long-term follow-up in patients who had these injections is still necessary.[50-52]

Percutaneous needle fasciotomy is also a reasonable option for treatment of Dupuytren disease and seems to be effective for MP joint contractures but less effective for the PIP joint.[53] An extension external fixation torque device may also preliminarily reverse the PIP contracture before excision of the diseased tissue.[54]

CONCLUSION

The specialty of hand surgery is exhaustive, and a number of specialty textbooks are available. Although general surgeons may be responsible for the basic tenets of hand surgery, knowledge of minute details is often not necessary; thus, most details have been omitted from this chapter because its purpose has been to see the big picture in regard to hand surgery. Those topics of hand surgery that the general surgeon is most likely to encounter have been emphasized, particularly with regard to principles of anatomy, physical examination, and emergency treatments. Taking this into consideration, Table 69-7 includes some high-yield facts relevant to hand surgery that have been compiled from various general surgery review books as well as topics discussed in the American Board of Surgery In-Training Examination (ABSITE).[55,56] This list

is provided for the convenience of general surgeons preparing for ABSITE or board examinations.

SELECTED REFERENCES

General
Bruen KJ, Gowski WF: Treatment of digital frostbite: Current concepts. *J Hand Surg [Am]* 34:553–554, 2009.

> *Experience with tissue plasminogen activator is reported. It shows promise in decreasing rates of digital amputation.*

Cordill LL, Schubkegel T, Light TR, et al: Lipid infusion rescue for bupivacaine-induced cardiac arrest after axillary block. *J Hand Surg [Am]* 35:144–146, 2010.

> *Successful resuscitation of a hand surgery patient after inadvertent intravascular injection of bupivacaine during administration of an axillary block is discussed.*

Harness NG: Digital block anesthesia. *J Hand Surg [Am]* 34:142–145, 2009.

> *The optimum techniques for providing digital block anesthesia are discussed.*

TABLE 69-7　American Board of Surgery Review Topics

TOPIC	ANSWER
Fracture of the distal radius	Injury to the median nerve
Innervation of flexor digitorum profundus to the ring and small fingers	Ulnar nerve
Injury to the ulnar nerve at the elbow	Weakness in abduction and adduction of the index finger through small digits
Midshaft humeral fracture	Associated with radial nerve injury
Distal phalanx fractures	>50% of all hand fractures
Joint involved in Bennett fracture	Carpometacarpal joint of the thumb
Common name for metacarpal fracture of the small finger	Boxer fracture
Most frequently fractured carpal bone	Scaphoid
Complications associated with displaced fractures	Avascular necrosis and nonunion of the scaphoid
Axonal nerve growth rate	1 mm/day
Common maximum intraoperative tourniquet time in hand surgery	2 hours
Single digits that are primarily replanted	Thumbs in adults and children, all digits whenever possible in children
Maximal period of anoxia compatible with replantation	Finger—8 hours (warm ischemia), but longer times have been anecdotally reported; upper and lower extremity—6 hours
Proper method for transportation of an amputated body part to maximize replantation success	Cleaned of debris, wrapped in sterile towel or gauze, moistened with sterile lactated Ringer solution, placed in sterile plastic bag, transported in insulated cooler with ice water (ideal temperature, 4° C)
Complications if nerve repair is delayed >2 weeks	Retraction of nerve's ends resulting in need for nerve grafting
Zone 2, no man's land	Area of flexor tendon injury between metacarpophalangeal joint and flexor digitorum superficialis insertion
Mallet finger	Injury to extensor mechanism at level of distal interphalangeal joint
Gamekeeper thumb	Rupture of ulnar collateral ligament of thumb metacarpophalangeal joint, with resultant instability of the joint to radial-directed force
Most common organism causing hand infections	*Staphylococcus aureus*
Classic symptoms of carpal tunnel syndrome	Paresthesias in median nerve distribution, often waking the patient at night
Most effective therapy for full-thickness burns of the hand	Early excision and grafting
Most common location of ganglion cysts	Scapholunate interosseous ligament at the dorsal wrist
Treatment of de Quervain stenosing tenosynovitis after failed nonoperative management	Surgical release of first extensor compartment
Cause of trigger finger	Stenosing tenosynovitis in the region of the metacarpophalangeal joint, A1 pulley
Late findings of rheumatoid arthritis	Subluxation of involved joints resulting in deformity
Swan neck deformity	Hyperextension of proximal interphalangeal joint with flexion of distal interphalangeal joint
Boutonnière deformity	Flexion of proximal interphalangeal joint with hyperextension of distal interphalangeal joint
Nonoperative measures for Dupuytren contracture	Exercise, local steroid injections, collagenase injections, radiotherapy
Digits usually affected in Dupuytren contracture	Ring and small fingers
Cause of Dupuytren contracture	Proliferation and fibrosis of the palmar fascia
Fractures likely to cause compartment syndrome, Volkmann ischemic contracture	Supracondylar fracture of the humerus
Artery and nerve compromised in Volkmann ischemic contracture	Median nerve and anterior interosseous artery
Complication of cast placement for supracondylar fractures of the humerus	Volkmann ischemic contracture

Omer GE: Development of hand surgery: Education of hand surgeons. *J Hand Surg [Am]* 25:616–628, 2000.

This article traces the development of hand surgery from the publication, in 1916, of Kanavel's classic book on infections of the hand, through the recognition of the specialty of hand surgery, to the training of modern-day hand surgeons and their educational requirements. The article contains historical vignettes and mentions many giants in hand surgery.

Patel MM, Catalano LW: Bone graft substitutes: Current uses in hand surgery. *J Hand Surg [Am]* 34:555–556, 2009.

Bone grafts are used for structural support and biologic properties. The use of bone graft substitutes limits donor morbidity and also shortens operative time.

Slutsky DJ, Nagle DJ: Wrist arthroscopy: Current concepts. *J Hand Surg [Am]* 33:1228–1244, 2008.

Wrist arthroscopy has grown from a diagnostic procedure to a valuable treatment modality for a variety of wrist disorders, such as degenerative arthritis, acute carpal and metacarpal fractures, wrist instability, and ganglions.

Soft Tissue

Foucher G, Khouri RK: Digital reconstruction with island flaps. *Clin Plast Surg* 24:1–32, 1997.

New information of the intrinsic flaps of the hand enables ingenious soft tissue reconstructions using local tissues from the hand and fingers as pedicled, vascularized, island flaps. A thorough knowledge of the vasculature of the hand is required in addition to that in standard anatomy texts.

Godina M: Early microsurgical reconstruction of complex trauma of the extremities. *Plast Reconstr Surg* 78:285–292, 1986.

This paper emphasizes the concept of primary repair and reconstruction of all damaged tissues (including microvascular soft tissue coverage) acutely after major trauma.

Martin D, Bakhach J, Casoli V, et al: Reconstruction of the hand with forearm island flaps. *Clin Plast Surg* 24:33–48, 1997.

Knowledge of the vascular anatomy of the forearm enables an array of pedicled flaps to be used for soft tissue reconstruction of the hand, thus avoiding the need to use microvascular anastomoses.

Flexor Tendons

Hunter JM, Salisbury RE: Flexor tendon reconstruction in severely damaged hands: A two-stage procedure using a silicone-Dacron reinforced gliding prosthesis prior to tendon grafting. *J Bone Joint Surg Am* 53:829–858, 1971.

This paper introduces the concept of two-stage flexor tendon repair in patients in whom the flexor tendon sheath is scarred in a late repair. A tendon spacer is placed as a preliminary procedure to later tendon grafting. This remains a time-honored way of dealing with late flexor tendon reconstructions.

Kim HM, Nelson G, Thomopoulos S, et al: Technical and biological modifications for enhanced flexor tendon repair. *J Hand Surg [Am]* 35:1031–1037, 2010.

An up-to-date current concept on technical essentials to enhance outcome and the potential for future biologic manipulation of the tendon repair site.

Kleinert H, Kutz JE, Atasoy E, et al: Primary repair of flexor tendons. *Orthop Clin North Am* 4:865–876, 1973.

This article was the first substantive evidence that flexor tendons could be safely and effectively repaired in no man's land, emphasizing the importance of postoperative controlled mobilization of the fingers.

Strickland JW: Development of flexor tendon surgery: Twenty-five years of progress. *J Hand Surg [Am]* 25:214–235, 2000.

This excellent review article describes the current state of the art for treatment of flexor tendon injuries.

Extensor Tendons

Merritt WH: Relative motion splint: Active motion after extensor tendon injury and repair. *J Hand Surg [Am]* 39:1187–1194, 2014.

This publication has excellent accompanying videos that demonstrate how this very practical splinting technique can be used for rehabilitation of extensor tendon lacerations, boutonnière deformity, and sagittal band injury.

Nerve Injuries

Cho MS, Rinker BD, Weber RV, et al: Functional outcome following nerve repair in the upper extremity using processed nerve allograft. *J Hand Surg [Am]* 37:2340–2349, 2012.

Nerve repair using decellularized allograft for a nerve gap gives results comparable to nerve autograft for median and ulnar nerve. Off-the-shelf nerve allografts have become a helpful addition to nerve repair.

Isaacs T: Treatment of acute peripheral nerve injures: Current concepts. *J Hand Surg [Am]* 35:491–497, 2010.

Although outcomes after nerve repair are not always excellent, this article assesses well-established basic principles and also includes a number of strategies for repair techniques for small and large traumatic nerve gaps.

Lundborg G: A 25-year perspective of peripheral nerve surgery: Evolving neuroscientific concepts and classical significance. *J Hand Surg [Am]* 25:391–414, 2000.

This excellent article establishes the experimental basis and neuroscience behind nerve repair and nerve regeneration. The rationale for nerve conduits is discussed.

Millesi H, Meissl G, Berger A: The interfascicular nerve-grafting of the median and ulnar nerves. *J Bone Joint Surg* 54:727–750, 1972.

This landmark article emphasizes the importance of tension-free nerve repair, matching of proximal and distal fascicular groups, and use of nerve grafts in cases of a large nerve gap injury.

Weber RV, Mackinnon S: Nerve transfers in the upper extremity. *J Am Soc Surg Hand* 4:200–213, 2004.

The innovative use of nerve transfers is described to bypass and to overcome long nerve gaps after nerve injury to hasten and to improve functional recovery.

Replantation

Buncke HJ: Microvascular hand surgery—transplants and replants—over the past 25 years. *J Hand Surg [Am]* 25:415–428, 2000.

This article traces the history of microvascular surgery as it applies to the upper extremities and of the milestones achieved. It discusses the many microvascular reconstructive options available for free tissue transfer and microvascular toe to hand transfers and also evaluates anticipated survival and functional outcomes for replantation surgery.

Fractures

Carlsen BT, Moran SL: Thumb trauma: Bennett fractures, Rolando fractures and ulnar collateral ligament injuries. *J Hand Surg [Am]* 34:945–952, 2009.

Recent advancements for the treatment of these common injuries are discussed.

Kawamura K, Chung KC: Treatment of scaphoid fractures and non-unions. *J Hand Surg [Am]* 33:938–997, 2008.

Scaphoid fractures are a common injury presenting with unique challenges because of a tenuous scaphoid blood supply. This article updates the reader about diagnostic imaging and current treatment strategies for displaced and nondisplaced acute scaphoid fractures, scaphoid nonunions, and avascular necrosis.

Russe O: Fracture of the carpal navicular: Diagnosis, non-operative, and operative treatment. *J Bone Joint Surg Am* 42:759–768, 1960.

Although new innovations of cannulated compression screw and minimally invasive surgery have changed the management of scaphoid fractures, this article is still relevant in regard to understanding and treatment of scaphoid fractures and their complications.

Stern PJ: Management of fractures of the hand over the last 25 years. *J Hand Surg [Am]* 25:817–823, 2000.

Fluoroscopic imaging has greatly facilitated the operative management of hand fractures. The evolution from Kirschner wires to plates and screws is discussed. Innovations included self-tapping screws, low-profile plates, and cannulated screws, with the goal of achieving rigid bone fixation to enable restoration of early digital motion to minimize the risk for tendon adhesions and joint contractures.

Infections

Kanavel AB: An anatomical, experimental, and clinical study of acute phlegmons of the hand. *Surg Gynecol Obstet* 1:221–259, 1905.

This classic paper described the anatomic spaces of the hand. It changed the course of infection treatment and also saw the origins of hand surgery. The clinical outcome was changed from amputation to surgical management, which preserved the function of structures, emphasizing that hand surgery is founded on a sound knowledge of anatomy. The basic principles of this article, written in the preantibiotic era, still remain true.

Compartment Syndrome

Mubarak SJ, Hargens AR: Acute compartment syndromes. *Surg Clin North Am* 63:539–565, 1983.

This excellent article describes the pathogenesis of acute compartment syndrome, including the diagnosis and surgical management in the upper extremity.

Entrapment Neuropathy

Bickel KD: Carpal tunnel syndrome. *J Hand Surg [Am]* 35:147–152, 2010.

This is the most common compressive neuropathy in the upper extremity. Evidence-based guidelines for diagnosis and treatment are provided.

Koo JT, Szabo RM: Compression neuropathies of the median nerve. *J Am Soc Surg Hand* 4:156–175, 2004.

This comprehensive article gives excellent anatomic descriptions of all the anatomic sites in the upper extremity in which chronic compression of the median nerve can occur. Non-surgical and surgical management guidelines are outlined for each.

Palmer BA, Hughes TB: Cubital tunnel syndrome. *J Hand Surg [Am]* 35:153–163, 2010.

This up to date article provides current concepts in diagnosis and treatment strategies for cubital tunnel syndrome.

Phalen GS: The carpal-tunnel syndrome: Seventeen years' experience in diagnosis and treatment of six hundred fifty-four hands. *J Bone Joint Surg Am* 48:211–228, 1966.

This is a classic paper written by a founder and past president of the American Society for Surgery of the Hand. It presents an understanding of median nerve compression at the wrist that is surgically treated by decompression and release of the transverse carpal ligament. The most common procedure performed by hand surgeons today is median nerve decompression.

Vascular Tumors

Mulliken JB, Glowacki J: Hemangioma and vascular malformations in infants and children: A classification based on endothelial characteristics. *Plast Reconstr Surg* 69:412–422, 1982.

The authors attempted to unify the classification of hemangiomas and vascular malformations. Suggested classifications fall into six broad categories—embryology, histology, clinical features, dynamics of growth, hemodynamic patterns, and cell biology. A classification is useful only if it has diagnostic applicability and aids in planning therapy and understanding pathogenesis.

Congenital Anomalies

McCarroll HR: Congenital anomalies: A 25-year overview. *J Hand Surg [Am]* 25:1007–1037, 2000.

This excellent review discusses the more commonly treated congenital hand anomalies. It also identifies some of the newer (at that time) developments in surgical treatment, which include distraction lengthening, pollicization, microvascular surgery, and potential for in utero interventions. Useful classifications for treatment management are provided.

Netscher DT, Scheker LR: Timing and decision making in the treatment of congenital upper extremity deformities. *Clin Plast Surg* 17:113–131, 1990.

This review describes commonly treated congenital hand anomalies and provides a rational basis for timing surgical interventions to meet critical hand functional milestones.

Osteoarthritis

Burton RI, Pellegrini VD: Surgical management of basal joint arthritis of the thumb. Part II. Ligament reconstruction with tendon interposition arthroplasty. *J Hand Surg [Am]* 11:324–332, 1986.

An excellent description of the pathogenesis and surgical management of basilar joint osteoarthritis of the thumb. This is the usually performed surgical procedure for carpometacarpal joint osteoarthritis of the thumb.

Eaton RG, Littler JW: Ligament reconstruction for the painful thumb carpometacarpal joint. *J Bone Joint Surg Am* 55:1655–1666, 1973.

One of the most common joints affected by osteoarthritis is at the base of the thumb. This operation, originally described by these authors for surgical management, still forms the basis of surgical treatment today, with few modifications in technique.

Rheumatoid Arthritis

Brasington R: TNF-α antagonists and other recombinant proteins for treatment of rheumatoid arthritis. *J Hand Surg Am* 34:349–350, 2009.

Disease-modifying antirheumatic drugs are discussed that specifically target individual molecules. Medical treatment of rheumatoid conditions has changed dramatically in recent years.

Swanson AB: Flexible implant arthroplasty for arthritic finger joints: Rationale, technique, and results of treatment. *J Bone Joint Surg Am* 54:435–455, 1972.

A landmark article that changed the course of treatment for rheumatoid arthritis. In this paper, Swanson introduced small joint arthroplasty.

Contractures

Curtis RM: Capsulectomy of the interphalangeal joints of the fingers. *J Bone Joint Surg Am* 36:1219–1232, 1954.

This classic article changed the course of treatment of the stiff hand and promoted interest in the complex anatomy of the proximal interphalangeal joint. The author was meticulous in technique and insisted on rigid postoperative therapy.

Eaton C: Percutaneous fasciotomy for Dupuytren's contracture. *J Hand Surg Am* 36:910–915, 2011.

Percutaneous needle fasciotomy is a less invasive treatment than surgery. This article describes that technique.

McFarlane RM: Patterns of the diseased fascia in the fingers in Dupuytren's contracture: Displacement of the neurovascular bundle. *Plast Reconstr Surg* 54:31–44, 1974.

This article clearly outlines the pathology, anatomy, and proposed surgical treatment of Dupuytren's contracture. The author describes the patterns of diseased fascia in the palm and fingers and how displacement of the digital neurovascular bundle may occur.

Meals RA, Hentz VR: Technical tips for collagenase injection treatment for Dupuytren contracture. *J Hand Surg Am* 39:1195–1200, e2, 2014.

Collagenase injection has become an increasingly popular method of treating Dupuytren contracture. This article outlines the technique involved for this seemingly less invasive treatment.

REFERENCES

1. Kakar S, Bakri K, Shin AY: Survey of hand surgeons regarding their perceived needs for an expanded upper extremity fellowship. *J Hand Surg [Am]* 37:2374–2380, e1-3, 2012.
2. Sears ED, Larson BP, Chung KC: A national survey of program director opinions of core competencies and structure of hand surgery fellowship training. *J Hand Surg [Am]* 37:1971–1977, e7, 2012.
3. Green DP: General principles. In Hotchkiss RN, Pederson WC, Wolfe SW, et al, editors: *Green's operative hand surgery*, ed 5, Philadelphia, 2005, Elsevier, pp 3–24.
4. Idler RS, Manktelow RT: *The hand: Primary care of common problems*, ed 2, Philadelphia, 1990, Churchill Livingstone.
5. Klenerman L: Tourniquet time—how long? *Hand* 12:231–234, 1980.
6. Netscher DT, Cohen V: Phalangeal fractures. In Evans GRD, editor: *Operative plastic surgery*, New York, 2000, McGraw-Hill, pp 979–991.
7. Hunter JM, Salisbury RE: Flexor-tendon reconstruction in severely damaged hands. A two-stage procedure using a silicone-Dacron reinforced gliding prosthesis prior to tendon grafting. *J Bone Joint Surg Am* 53:829–858, 1971.
8. Tomaino M, Mitsionis G, Basitidas J, et al: The effect of partial excision of the A2 and A4 pulleys on the biomechanics of finger flexion. *J Hand Surg [Br]* 23:50–52, 1998.
9. Tang JB: Indications, methods, postoperative motion and outcome evaluation of primary flexor tendon repairs in zone 2. *J Hand Surg Eur Vol* 32:118–129, 2007.
10. Lalonde DH: Wide-awake flexor tendon repair. *Plast Reconstr Surg* 123:623–625, 2009.
11. Tang JB, Zhang Y, Cao Y, et al: Core suture purchase affects strength of tendon repairs. *J Hand Surg [Am]* 30:1262–1266, 2005.
12. Williamson DT, Richards RS: Flexor tendon injuries and reconstruction. In Mathes SJ, Hentz VR, editors:

Plastic surgery, ed 2, Philadelphia, 2006, Elsevier, pp 351–391.

13. Matarrese MR, Hammert WC: Flexor tendon rehabilitation. *J Hand Surg [Am]* 37:2386–2388, 2012.

14. Ahmad Z, Wardale J, Brooks R, et al: Exploring the application of stem cells in tendon repair and regeneration. *Arthroscopy* 28:1018–1029, 2012.

15. Netscher DT: Extensor tendon injuries. In Goldwyn RM, Cohen MN, editors: *The unfavorable result in plastic surgery*, Philadelphia, 2001, Lippincott Williams & Wilkins, pp 751–770.

16. Cheng CJ: Synthetic nerve conduits for digital nerve reconstruction. *J Hand Surg [Am]* 34:1718–1721, 2009.

17. Oberlin C, Beal D, Leechavengvongs S, et al: Nerve transfer to biceps muscle using a part of ulnar nerve for C5-C6 avulsion of the brachial plexus: Anatomical study and report of four cases. *J Hand Surg [Am]* 19:232–237, 1994.

18. McClinton MA, Wilgis EFS: Ischemic conditions of the hand. In Mathes SJ, Hentz VR, editors: *Plastic surgery*, ed 2, Philadelphia, 2006, Elsevier, pp 791–822.

19. Soucacos PN: Indications and selection for digital amputation and replantation. *J Hand Surg [Br]* 26:572–581, 2001.

20. Netscher DT, Cohen MN: Metacarpals and phalanges. In Evans GRD, editor: *Operative plastic surgery*, New York, 2000, McGraw-Hill, pp 959–978.

21. Stern PJ: Fractures of the metacarpals and phalanges. In Hotchkiss RN, Pederson WC, Wolfe SW, et al, editors: *Green's operative hand surgery*, ed 5, Philadelphia, 2005, Elsevier, pp 277–342.

22. Kumar S, O'Connor A, Despois M, et al: Use of early magnetic resonance imaging in the diagnosis of occult scaphoid fractures: The CAST Study (Canberra Area Scaphoid Trial). *N Z Med J* 118:U1296, 2005.

23. Clark DC: Common acute hand infections. *Am Fam Physician* 68:2167–2176, 2003.

24. Rockwell PG: Acute and chronic paronychia. *Am Fam Physician* 63:1113–1116, 2001.

25. Stevanovic MV, Sharpe F: Acute infections in the hand. In Hotchkiss RN, Pederson WC, Wolfe SW, et al, editors: *Green's operative hand surgery*, ed 5, Philadelphia, 2005, Elsevier, pp 55–93.

26. Lille S, Hayakawa T, Neumeister MW, et al: Continuous postoperative catheter irrigation is not necessary for the treatment of suppurative flexor tenosynovitis. *J Hand Surg [Br]* 25:304–307, 2000.

27. Mollitt DL: Infection control: Avoiding the inevitable. *Surg Clin North Am* 82:365–378, 2002.

28. Kare JA: *Volkmann contracture*, 2010. Available at: <http://emedicine.medscape.com/article/1270462-overview>.

29. Patel MR, Bassini L: Trigger fingers and thumb: When to splint, inject, or operate. *J Hand Surg [Am]* 17:110–113, 1992.

30. Trumble TE: Compressive neuropathies. In Trumble TE, editor: *Principles of hand surgery and therapy*, Philadelphia, 2000, WB Saunders, pp 324–342.

31. Trumble TE, Diao E, Abrams RA, et al: Single-portal endoscopic carpal tunnel release compared with open release: A prospective, randomized trial. *J Bone Joint Surg Am* 84-A:1107–1115, 2002.

32. Mackinnon SE, Novak CB: Compression neuropathies. In Hotchkiss RN, Pederson WC, Wolfe SW, et al, editors:

Green's operative hand surgery, ed 5, Philadelphia, 2005, Elsevier, pp 999–1046.

33. Athanasian EA: Bone and soft tissue tumors. In Hotchkiss RN, Pederson WC, Wolfe SW, et al, editors: *Green's operative hand surgery*, ed 5, Philadelphia, 2005, Elsevier, pp 2211–2265.

34. Netscher DT, Hildreth DH, Kleinert HE: Tumors of the hand. In Georgiade GS, Riefkohl R, Levin LS, editors: *Plastic, maxillofacial, and reconstructive surgery*, Baltimore, 1997, Williams & Wilkins, pp 1046–1070.

35. Cohen V, Netscher DT: Excision of ganglion cysts. In Evans GRD, editor: *Operative plastic surgery*, New York, 2000, McGraw-Hill, pp 924–935.

36. Glass AT, Solomon BA: Cimetidine therapy for recalcitrant warts in adults. *Arch Dermatol* 132:680–682, 1996.

37. Shenefelt PD: *Warts, nongenital*, 2010. Available at: <http://emedicine.medscape.com/article/1133317-overview>.

38. Kopf AW: Keratoacanthoma: Clinical aspects. In Andrade R, Gumport SL, Popkin GL, et al, editors: *Cancer of the skin*, Philadelphia, 1976, WB Saunders, pp 755–781.

39. Buckmiller LM, Munson PD, Dyamenahalli U, et al: Propranolol for infantile hemangiomas: Early experience at a tertiary vascular anomalies center. *Laryngoscope* 120:676–681, 2010.

40. Sofocleous CT, Rosen RJ, Raskin K, et al: Congenital vascular malformations in the hand and forearm. *J Endovasc Ther* 8:484–494, 2001.

41. Koman LA, Ruch DS, Paterson SB: Vascular disorders. In Hotchkiss RN, Pederson WC, Wolfe SW, et al, editors: *Green's operative hand surgery*, ed 5, Philadelphia, 2005, Elsevier, pp 2265–2313.

42. Butler ED, Hamill JP, Seipel RS, et al: Tumors of the hand. A ten-year survey and report of 437 cases. *Am J Surg* 100:293–302, 1960.

43. Bowen JT: Pre-cancerous dermatosis. *J Cutan Dis* 33:787–802, 1915.

44. Johnson RE, Ackerman LV: Epidermoid carcinoma of the hand. *Cancer* 3:657–666, 1950.

45. Novick M, Gard DA, Hardy SB, et al: Burn scar carcinoma: A review and analysis of 46 cases. *J Trauma* 17:809–817, 1977.

46. Glat PM, Shapiro RL, Roses DF, et al: Management considerations for melanonychia striata and melanoma of the hand. *Hand Clin* 11:183–189, 1995.

47. Netscher DT: Congenital hand problems. Terminology, cause, and management. *Clin Plast Surg* 25:537–552, 1998.

48. McCarroll HR: Congenital anomalies: A 25-year overview. *J Hand Surg [Am]* 25:1007–1037, 2000.

49. Feldon P, Terrono AL, Nalebluff EA: Rheumatoid arthritis and other connective tissue diseases. In Hotchkiss RN, Pederson WC, Wolfe SW, et al, editors: *Green's operative hand surgery*, ed 5, Philadelphia, 2005, Elsevier, pp 2049–2136.

50. Hurst LC, Badalamente MA: Nonoperative treatment of Dupuytren's disease. *Hand Clin* 15:97–107, vii, 1999.

51. Reilly RM, Stern PJ, Goldfarb CA: A retrospective review of the management of Dupuytren's nodules. *J Hand Surg [Am]* 30:1014–1018, 2005.

52. Saar JD, Grothaus PC: Dupuytren's disease: An overview. *Plast Reconstr Surg* 106:125–134, 2000.

53. van Rijssen AL, Werker PM: Percutaneous needle fasciotomy for recurrent Dupuytren disease. *J Hand Surg [Am]* 37:1820–1823, 2012.

54. Agee JM, Goss BC: The use of skeletal extension torque in reversing Dupuytren contractures of the proximal interphalangeal joint. *J Hand Surg [Am]* 37:1467–1474, 2012.

55. Blecha M, Brown A: Orthopedic and hand surgery pearls. In Blecha M, Brown A, editors: *General surgery: Pearls of wisdom*, Lincoln, Mass, 2004, Boston Medical, pp 217–224.

56. Deziel DJ, Witt TR, Bines SD: Hand surgery. In Deziel DJ, Witt TR, Bines SD, et al, editors: *Rush University review of surgery*, ed 3, Philadelphia, 2000, WB Saunders, pp 579–589.

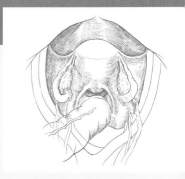

Gynecologic Surgery

Howard W. Jones III

第七十章　妇科

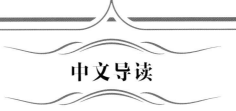

中文导读

　　本章共分为6节：①盆腔脏器的胚胎学及解剖学；②生殖生理学；③临床评估；④非手术治疗选择；⑤手术治疗的技术问题；⑥妊娠期手术。

　　第一节涵盖外生殖器（包括阴阜、大阴唇、小阴唇、阴蒂、阴道前庭、尿道口及附属腺体及结构的开口）和内生殖器（包括卵巢、输卵管、宫体、宫颈、阴道及相关的血供和淋巴回流系统）的胚胎学来源和发育过程、解剖学结构和功能以及外科手术技巧和注意事项。

　　第二节介绍了女性生殖系统的正常生理过程，如卵巢周期、子宫内膜周期的动态过程及相关生理变化、受孕过程及其中的干扰因素、闭经及月经异常的病因、病理生理改变及检查方式等。

　　第三节介绍了妇产科急症的疾病类型、临床表现和鉴别诊断。在疾病的诊断及治疗过程中，需结合病史（年龄、孕产史、月经史、性生活史、避孕史、既

往妇科疾病及治疗经过、现病史等）、体格检查及辅助检查（影像学检查、妊娠试验、性激素检测、宫颈和阴道分泌物微生态分析或病原学检测、下生殖道细胞学检测）等进行综合全面的考虑。

　　第四节介绍了异常子宫出血、自然流产、异位妊娠、盆腔感染、功能性卵巢囊肿、子宫肌瘤、子宫内膜异位症及子宫腺肌瘤等疾病的定义、诊断标准，以及对这些疾病进行非手术治疗的原则、适应证及治疗方案。

　　第五节介绍了月经过多或异常子宫出血、前庭大腺囊肿或脓肿、卵巢囊肿、输卵管或异位妊娠、盆腔肿物等疾病手术方式选择及宫颈锥切术、子宫切除术、广泛性子宫切除术等手术操作步骤、适应证及并

发症。

第六节涵盖妊娠期母体的生理学变化（心血管系统、呼吸系统、消化系统、凝血系统、肾脏），妊娠期常用诊断及评估的检查手段，妊娠期常见外科并发症（阑尾炎、胆囊结石、肠梗阻、卵巢肿物等）及出现腹痛的产科并发症（胎盘早剥、妊娠相关的肝脏并发症、外伤）的诊断及治疗方案、常见产科手术（剖宫产、会阴切开缝合术）的操作过程及并发症处理方案。

〔王世宣〕

 Please access ExpertConsult.com to view the corresponding videos for this chapter.

Gynecologic surgery involves the operative treatment of benign and malignant conditions of the female genital tract. Because of the hormonal responsiveness of these tissues and organs during the menstrual cycle and during the premenarchal, reproductive, and postmenopausal periods of life, the diagnosis, management, and even surgical approach may differ because of the hormonal milieu and the patient's desire for future fertility. All these factors may be even further complicated in pregnant women, in whom the surgical and anesthetic approach must consider the pregnant uterus and fetus. The surgeon who understands and is able to consider the physiology, endocrinology, and anatomy of the female pelvis is most prepared to select the most appropriate and successful operative procedure. In addition, by knowing the alternatives to surgery and risks and advantages of several possible management approaches, a treatment most likely to correct the problem and to be consistent with the patient's desires for fertility preservation, a minimally invasive surgical approach, or even no surgery at all can be accomplished with the best opportunity for a good outcome.

The general surgeon may be called on to assist the gynecologic surgeon when endometriosis or ovarian cancer involves the sigmoid colon, when a diverticular abscess or carcinoma of the colon involves the ovary, in the pregnant woman with acute appendicitis or cholecystitis, or in smaller communities in which there is no gynecologist at all.

A full discussion of gynecologic surgery is beyond the scope of a single chapter. I address the basics of pelvic anatomy, reproductive physiology, clinical evaluation of common gynecologic symptoms, surgical technique for several common operations, and surgical approach to the pregnant patient.

PELVIC EMBRYOLOGY AND ANATOMY

Embryology

The female external genitalia are derived embryologically from the genital tubercle, which, in the absence of testosterone, fails to undergo fusion and devolves to the vulvar structures. The labial structures are of ectodermal origin. The urethra, vaginal introitus, and vulvar vestibule are derived from uroepithelial entoderm. The lower third of the vagina develops from the invagination of the urogenital sinus.

The internal genitalia are derived from the genital ridge. The ovaries develop from the incorporation of primordial germ cells into coelomic epithelium of the mesonephric (wolffian) duct, and the tubes, uterus, cervix, and upper two thirds of the vagina develop from the paramesonephric (müllerian) duct. The embryologic ovaries migrate caudad to the true pelvis. Primordial ovarian follicles develop but remain dormant until stimulation in adolescence by gonadotropins. The paired müllerian ducts migrate caudad and medially to form the fallopian tubes and fuse in the midline to form the uterus, cervix, and upper vagina. The wolffian ducts regress. Failure or partial failure of these processes can result in distortions of anatomy and potential diagnostic dilemmas (Table 70-1).

Anatomy
External Genitalia
The external genitalia consist of the mons veneris, labia majora, labia minora, clitoris, vulvar vestibule, urethral meatus, and ostia of the accessory glandular structures (Fig. 70-1). These structures overlie the fascial and muscle layers of the perineum. The perineum is the most caudal region of the trunk; it includes the pelvic floor and those structures occupying the pelvic outlet. It is bounded superiorly by the funnel-shaped pelvic diaphragm and inferiorly by the skin covering the external genitalia, anus, and adjacent structures. Laterally, the perineum is bounded by the medial surface of the inferior pubic rami, obturator internus muscle below the origin of the levator ani muscle, coccygeus muscle, medial surface of the sacrotuberous ligaments, and overlapping margins of the gluteus maximus muscles (Fig. 70-2).

The pelvic outlet can be divided into two triangles separated by a line drawn between the ischial tuberosities. The anterior or urogenital triangle has its apex anteriorly at the symphysis pubis, and the posterior or anal triangle has its apex at the coccyx.

The urogenital triangle contains the urogenital diaphragm, a muscular shelf extending between the pubic rami and penetrated by the urethra and vagina, and the external genitalia, consisting of the mons pubis, labia majora and minora, clitoris, and vestibule. The mons pubis is a suprapubic fat pad covered by dense skin appendages. The labia majora extend posteriorly from the mons, forming the lateral borders of the vulva. They have a keratinized, stratified squamous epithelium with all the normal skin appendages and extend posteriorly to the lateral perineum. Within the confines of the labium are fat and the insertion of the round ligament. Medial to the labia majora are interlabial grooves and

TABLE 70-1	Selected Anatomic Abnormalities as a Result of Disrupted Embryogenesis
ORGAN	**ABNORMALITY**
Ovary	Duplication of ovary; secondary ovarian rests; paraovarian cysts (wolffian remnants)
Tube	Congenital absence; paratubal cyst (hydatid of Morgagni)
Uterus	Agenesis; complete or partial duplication of the uterine fundus
Cervix	Agenesis; complete or partial duplication of the cervix
Vagina	Agenesis; transverse or longitudinal septum; paravaginal (Gartner duct) cyst
Vulva	Fusion; hermaphroditism; cyst of the canal of Nuck (round ligament cyst)

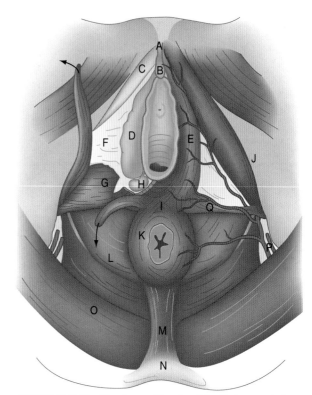

FIGURE 70-2 The Muscles and Fascia of the Perineum. A, Suspensory ligament of clitoris; B, clitoris; C, crus of clitoris; D, vestibular bulb; E, bulbocavernosus muscle; F, inferior fascia of urogenital diaphragm; G, deep transverse perineal muscle; H, Bartholin gland; I, perineal body; J, ischiocavernosus muscle; K, external anal sphincter; L, levator ani muscle; M, anococcygeal body; N, coccyx; O, gluteus maximus muscle; P, pudendal artery and vein; Q, superficial transverse perineal muscle.

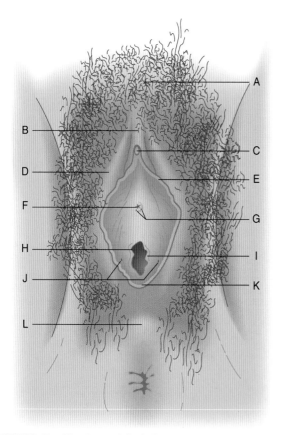

FIGURE 70-1 The External Genitalia. A, Mons pubis; B, prepuce; C, clitoris; D, labia majora; E, labia minora; F, urethral meatus; G, Skene ducts; H, vagina; I, hymen; J, Bartholin glands; K, posterior fourchette; L, perineal body.

the labia minora, of similar cutaneous origin but devoid of hair follicles. The labia minora are richly vascularized, with an erectile venous plexus. The bilateral roots of the clitoris fuse in the midline to form the glans at the lower edge of the pubic symphysis. The labia minora fuse over the clitoris to form the hood and, to a variable degree, below to create the clitoral frenulum.

Contiguous to the medial aspect of the labia minora, demarcated by Hart line, is the vulvar vestibule, extending to the

hymenal sulcus. The vestibular surface is a stratified, squamous mucous membrane that shares embryology with and has similar characteristics to the distal urethra and urethral meatus. Bartholin glands at 5 and 7 o'clock, the paraurethral Skene glands, and minor vestibular glands positioned around the lateral vestibule are all under the vestibular bulb, subjacent to the bulbocavernosus muscle. The ostia of these glands pass through the vestibular mucosa, directly adjacent to the hymenal ring.

The muscles of the external genitalia consist of the deep and superficial transverse perineal muscles; paired ischiocavernosus muscles that cover the crura of the clitoris; and bulbocavernosus muscles lying on either side of the vagina, covering the vestibular bulbs.

The anal triangle contains the anal canal, with surrounding internal and external sphincters; ischiorectal fossa, filled with fatty tissue; median raphe; and overlying skin.

Blood supply to the perineum is predominantly from a posterior direction from the internal pudendal artery, which, after arising from the internal iliac artery, passes through Alcock canal, a fascial tunnel along the obturator internus muscle below the origin of the levator ani muscle. On emerging from Alcock canal, the internal pudendal artery sends branches to the urogenital triangle anteriorly and to the anal triangle posteriorly. Anteriorly, there is blood supply to the mons pubis from the inferior epigastric artery, a branch of the femoral artery. Laterally, the external pudendal artery arises from the femoral artery and supplies the lateral aspect of the vulva. Venous return from the perineum accompanies the arterial supply and therefore drains into the internal iliac and femoral veins. It is important for the surgeon dissecting the external genitalia to be cognizant of the variability of direction from which the blood supply of the operative field is derived.

The major nerve supply to the perineum comes from the internal pudendal nerve, which originates from the S2 to S4 anterior rami of the sacral plexus and travels through Alcock canal, along with the internal pudendal artery and vein. Anterior branches supply the urogenital diaphragm and external genitalia, whereas posterior branches, the inferior rectal nerve, supply the anus, anal canal, ischiorectal fossa, and adjacent skin. Branches of the posterior femoral cutaneous nerve from the sacral plexus innervate the lateral aspects of the ischiorectal fossa and adjacent structures. The mons pubis and anterior labia are supplied by the ilioinguinal and genitofemoral nerves from the lumbar plexus; they travel through the inguinal canal and exit through the superficial inguinal ring. All these paired nerves routinely cross the midline for partial innervation of the contralateral side. The visceral efferent nerves responsible for clitoral erection are derived from the pelvic splanchnic nerves and reach the external genitalia along with the urethra and vagina as they pass through the urogenital diaphragm.

Surgical injury to the pelvic nerve plexus can result in neuropathic pain and diminished sexual, voiding, and excretory function.

The lymphatic drainage of the perineum, including the urogenital and anogenital triangles, travels for the most part with the external pudendal vessels to the superficial inguinal nodes. The deep parts of the perineum, including the urethra, vagina, and anal canal, drain in part through the lymphatics that accompany the internal pudendal vessels and into the internal iliac lymph nodes.

The fascia and fascial spaces of the perineum are important in the spread of extravasated fluids and superficial and deep infections. Fascia covers each of the muscles bounding the perineum, including the deep surface of the levator ani, obturator internus, and coccygeus, as well as other perineal muscles, such as the urogenital diaphragm. The fascia of the levator ani muscles fuses with the obturator internus fascia and pubic rami, creating well-defined fascial spaces, the ischiorectal fossae. Beneath the skin of the external genitalia is a layer of fat; deep to this is Colles fascia, which is attached to the ischiopubic rami laterally and the posterior edge of the urogenital diaphragm. Anteriorly, Colles fascia of the vulva is continuous with Colles fascia of the anterior abdominal wall.

Infections or collections of extravasated urine deep to the urogenital diaphragm are usually confined to the ischiorectal fossa, including the anterior recess, which is superior to the urogenital diaphragm. Collections of fluid or infections superficial to the urogenital diaphragm may pass to the abdominal wall deep to Colles fascia. Because of various fascial fusions, infections spreading from the vulva to the anterior abdominal wall do not spread into the inguinal regions or the thigh.

Internal Genitalia

The internal genitalia consist of the ovaries, fallopian tubes, uterus, cervix, and vagina, with associated blood supply and lymphatic drainage (Figs. 70-3 to 70-5).

Ovary. The oblong ovaries, glistening white in color, vary in size, which is dependent on age and status of the ovulatory cycle. In the prepubescent girl, the ovary will appear as a white sliver of tissue smaller than 1 cm in any dimension. The ovary of a woman during her reproductive years will vary in size and shape. The size of the nonovulating ovary will typically be in the range of $3 \times 2 \times 1$ cm. When a follicular or corpus luteum cyst is present, the size may extend up to 5 to 6 cm. A follicular cyst is an asymmetrical, translucent, clear structure. A corpus luteum cyst will generally be characterized by areas of golden yellow and, occasionally, by hematoma. The ovaries are suspended from the lateral side wall of the pelvis below the pelvic brim by the infundibulopelvic ligament and attach to the superolateral aspect of the uterine fundus by the utero-ovarian ligament.

The primary blood supply to the ovary is the ovarian artery. It arises directly from the aorta and courses with the vein through the infundibulopelvic ligament into the medulla on the lateral aspect of the ovary. The right ovarian vein generally drains to the inferior vena cava, and the left ovarian vein drains to the common iliac vein; however, variations commonly occur. There is a rich anastomotic arterial complex arising from the uterine artery that spreads across the broad ligament and mesosalpinx. The venous return accompanies that arterial supply. There is no somatic innervation to the ovary, but the autonomic fibers arise from the lumbar sympathetic and sacral parasympathetic plexuses. Lymphatic drainage parallels the iliac and aortic arteries.

There are three important relationships to be considered in carrying out surgical dissection. The infundibulopelvic ligament, with the ovarian blood supply, crosses over the ureter as it descends into the pelvis. As the surgeon divides and ligates the ovarian vessels, it is critical that this relationship be identified to avoid transecting, ligating, or kinking the ureter. The risk for ureteral injury is greater with a more proximal dissection of the ligament. Also, in its natural position, the suspended ovary drops along the pelvic side wall along the course of the midureter. If there are adhesions between the ovary and peritoneum of the pelvic side wall, careful dissection is necessary to avoid tenting the peritoneum with the attached ureter and causing injury. The third surgical relationship is the complex of external iliac vessels and femoral nerve, which course along the iliopsoas muscle, directly below the course of the ovarian vessels; with anterior adhesions of an ovary, these structures may be subjacent to the malpositioned ovary.

Fallopian tubes. The fallopian tubes are cylindrical structures approximately 8 cm in length. They originate at the uterine cavity in the uterine cornua, with an intramural segment of 1 to 2 cm and a narrow isthmic segment of 4 to 5 cm, flaring over 2 to 3 cm to the funnel of the infundibular segment and terminating in the fimbriated end of the tube. The fimbriae are fine, delicate mucosal projections that are positioned to allow capture of the extruded oocyte to promote the potential for fertilization. The blood supply to the tube is derived primarily from branches of the uterine artery, with a delicate cascade of vessels in the mesosalpinx. There is a secondary supply from the anastomosis with the ovarian vessels.

The surgeon must be aware of the fragility of the fallopian tube and handle this structure delicately, especially in women wishing to preserve their fertility. The mucosa lining the tubal lumen, especially at the fimbriated end, is highly specialized to facilitate transport of the oocyte and fertilized zygote. Traumatic manipulation of the tube can induce tubal infertility or predispose to later tubal pregnancy through damage to the mucosa or distortion of

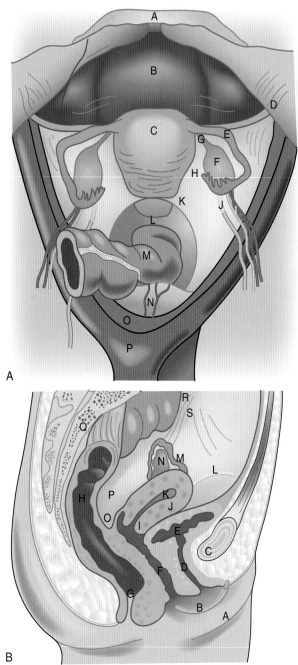

FIGURE 70-3 The Internal Genitalia. **A,** A, Symphysis pubis; B, bladder; C, corpus uteri; D, round ligament; E, fallopian tube; F, ovary; G, utero-ovarian ligament; H, broad ligament; I, ovarian artery and vein; J,
ureter; K, uterosacral ligament; L, cul-de-sac; M, rectum; N, middle sacral artery and vein; O, vena cava; P,
aorta. **B,** A, Labium majus; B, labium minus; C, symphysis pubis, D, urethra; E, bladder; F, vagina; G, anus;
H, rectum; I, cervix uteri; J, corpus uteri; K, endometrial cavity; L, round ligament; M, fallopian tube; N, ovary;
O, cul-de-sac; P, uterosacral ligament; Q, sacrum; R, ureter; S, ovarian artery and vein.

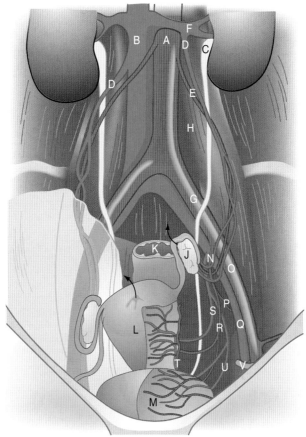

FIGURE 70-4 Blood Supply of the Pelvis. A, Aorta; B, inferior vena cava; C, ureter; D, ovarian vein; E, ovarian artery; F, renal vein; G, common iliac artery; H, psoas muscle; J, ovary; K, rectum; L, corpus uteri; M, bladder; N, internal iliac (hypogastric) artery, anterior branch; O, external iliac artery; P, obturator artery; Q, external iliac vein; R, uterine artery; S, uterine vein; T, vaginal artery; U, superior vesical artery; V, inferior epigastric artery.

the tubal position by adhesions, thereby interfering with the access or transport mechanisms.

Uterus and cervix. The uterus, with the cervix, is a midline, pear-shaped organ suspended in the midplane of the pelvis by the cardinal and uterosacral ligaments. The cardinal ligaments are dense fibrous condensations arising from the fascial covering of the levator ani muscles of the pelvic floor and inserting into the lateral portions of the uterocervical junction. The uterosacral ligaments arise posterolaterally from the uterocervical junction and course obliquely in a posterolateral direction to insert into the parietal fascia of the pelvic floor at the sacroiliac joint. The round ligaments of the uterus arise from the anterolateral superior aspect of the uterine fundus, course anterolaterally to the internal inguinal ring, and insert into the labia majora. The round ligaments are highly stretchable and serve no function in pelvic organ support. The broad ligaments are composed of a visceral peritoneal surface containing loose adventitious tissue. These ligaments also provide no pelvic organ support but do allow access to an avascular plane of the pelvis through which the retroperitoneal vasculature and ureter can be exposed.

The size of the uterus is influenced by age, hormonal status, prior pregnancy, and common benign neoplasms. The normal uterus during the reproductive years is approximately 8 × 6 × 4 cm and weighs approximately 100 g. The prepubertal or postmenopausal uterus is substantially smaller. The mass of the uterus is almost exclusively made up of myometrium, a complex of interlacing bundles of smooth muscle. The uterine cavity is 4 to 6 cm from the internal cervical os to the uterine fundus, shaped as an inverted triangle 2 to 3 mm wide at the cervix and 3 to 4 cm across the fundus, extending from cornua to cornua. It is only a few millimeters deep between the anterior and posterior walls, with no defined lateral walls in the nonpregnant state. The most common reason for variation in size is current pregnancy, followed by uterine fibroids.

If, during a surgical procedure, the surgeon encounters an enlarged uterus, undiagnosed pregnancy must be considered. The morphologic differences between a uterus enlarged by a pregnancy and one enlarged by fibroid include symmetrical enlargement in pregnancy and generally asymmetrical enlargement with fibroids. If enlargement is symmetrical, consider the origin of the round ligaments. With pregnancy, the round ligaments stretch as the uterus grows and continue to originate from the normal site; even with an apparently symmetrical fibroid uterus, the origin of the round ligaments is frequently displaced from the top of the

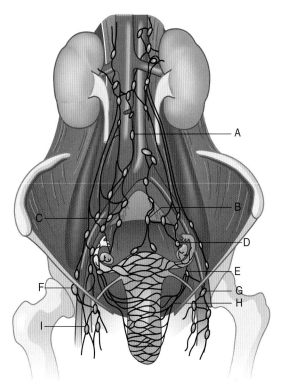

FIGURE 70-5 Lymphatics of the Pelvis. A, Aortic; B, sacral; C, common iliac; D, hypogastric; E, obturator; F, deep inguinal; G, Cloquet node; H, parametrial; I, superficial inguinal.

uterine fundus or in an asymmetrical course through the pelvis. Finally, the pregnant uterus is usually dusky and soft; fibroids, generally firm and nodular masses, can be palpated in the myometrial wall.

The uterine cavity is lined by the endometrium, a complex epithelial-stromal-vascular secretory tissue. The arterial supply to the endometrium is derived from branches of the uterine artery that perforate the myometrium to the inactive basalis layer. There, they form the arcuate vessels, which produce radial branches extending through the functional layer toward the compacted surface layer. There will be further description of the menstrual cycle here, but during the postovulatory phase, these vessels differentiate into spiral arteries, uniquely suited to allow menstruation and subsequent hemostasis.

The uterine cervix is histologically dynamic, with changes in cervical mucus production during the ovarian cycle. In the follicular phase, under estrogen stimulation, copious clear mucus is produced that facilitates the transport of sperm through the cervical canal to ascend through the uterine cavity to the fallopian tubes. During progesterone-dominant states, either luteal phase or with exogenous hormones, the mucus becomes viscous and plugs the cervix. The secretory epithelium of the endocervical canal has a dynamic metaplastic interaction with the stratified squamous epithelium of the portio vaginalis of the ectocervix under hormonal stimulation. Because the cervical canal is continuous with the vagina, surgical procedures involving the uterus and tubes are considered to be clean-contaminated cases.

The major sources of blood supply for the uterus and cervix are the uterine arteries, which are branches of the anterior division of the internal iliac (hypogastric) arteries. Although the origin of the uterine artery is usually a single identifiable vessel, it divides into multiple ascending and descending branches as it courses medially to the lateral margins of the cervicouterine junction. The distance from the uterus at which this division occurs is highly variable. Venous return from the uterus flows into the companion internal iliac vein. Lymphatics from the cervix and upper vagina drain primarily through the internal iliac nodes; but from the uterine fundus, drainage occurs primarily along a presacral path directly to the para-aortic nodes.

The primary surgical consideration for managing the uterine vessels is the proximity of the ureter, which courses approximately 1 cm below the artery and 1 cm lateral to the cervix. If the surgeon loses control of one of the branches of the vessel, it is important to use techniques that avoid clamping or kinking of the ureter. Often, the most prudent way to secure the uterine artery is to expose its origin and place hemostatic clips on the vessel.

Innervation of the uterus and cervix is derived from the autonomic plexus. Autonomic pain fibers are activated with dysmenorrhea, in labor, and with instrumentation of the cervix and uterus.

In the retroperitoneal space lateral to the uterus is the obturator nerve, which arises from the lumbosacral plexus and passes through the pelvic floor by way of the obturator canal to innervate the medial thigh. With relatively normal pelvic anatomy, it is unlikely to be subjected to injury; however, under circumstances in which the surgeon must dissect the retroperitoneal or paravaginal spaces, this relatively subtle structure can be injured, with significant neuropathic residual.

Vagina. The vagina originates at the cervix and terminates at the hymenal ring. The anatomic axis of the upper vagina is posterior to anterior in a caudad direction. The anterior and posterior walls of the upper two thirds of the vagina are normally opposed to each other to create a transverse potential space, distensible through pliability of the lateral sulci. The lower third of the vagina has a relatively vertically oriented caudad lumen. The mucosa of the vagina is nonkeratinized, stratified, squamous epithelium that responds to estrogen stimulation.

The blood supply to the vagina is provided by descending branches of the uterine artery and vein and ascending branches of the internal pudendal artery and its companion vein. These vessels course along the lateral walls of the vagina. Innervation is derived from the autonomic plexus and pudendal nerve, which track with the vessels.

Traumatic lacerations of the vagina are usually located along the lateral side walls, and the degree to which there is major injury to the vessels can be associated not only with significant evident hemorrhage but also with concealed hemorrhage. Spaces in which a hematoma can be concealed are the retroperitoneum of the broad ligaments, paravesical and pararectal spaces, and ischiorectal fossa. Because of the proximity of the pudendal nerve, attempts to ligate the vessels require maintaining orientation to the location of Alcock canal to avoid creating neuropathic injury. In the absence of an accumulating hematoma, the best approach to management is often a bulk vaginal pack to achieve tamponade. To accomplish this requires significant sedation or anesthesia and an indwelling urinary catheter.

The uterus, cervix, and vagina, with their fascial investments, compose the middle compartment of the pelvis. The structures of the anterior compartment, the bladder and urethra, and of the posterior compartment, the rectum, are each invested with a fascial layer. Avascular planes of loose areolar tissue separate the posterior fascia of the bladder and anterior fascia of the vagina and the anterior fascia of the rectum and posterior fascia of the vagina. Anteriorly, the bladder is attached to the lower uterine segment by the continuous visceral peritoneum. This vesicouterine fold can be incised transversely with minimal difficulty to expose the plane and to allow dissection of the bladder from the cervix and vagina. Posteriorly, the proximity of the rectum to the posterior vagina is significant only below the peritoneum of the cul-de-sac of Douglas, unless the cul-de-sac anatomy is distorted by dense adhesions.

Operative techniques for gynecologic procedures are optimized by careful identification of these planes to separate and to protect the adjacent organs from operative injury. The surgeon can create an incidental cystotomy, which may or may not be recognized, or devitalize the bladder wall with a crush or stitch, with delayed development of a vesicovaginal fistula.

In the lower pelvis, the ureter courses anteromedially after it passes under the uterine vessels and progresses toward the trigone of the bladder through a fascial tunnel on the anterior vaginal wall. The fixation of the ureter by the tunnel precludes effective displacement from the operative site by retracting. Although the location of the fascial tunnel is generally 1 to 2 cm safely below the usual site for vaginotomy during hysterectomy, in patients with a large cervix, distorting uterine myoma, prior cesarean birth, or bleeding from the bladder base or vaginal wall, the ureter can be transected, crushed, or kinked with a stitch.

The rectovaginal septum is surgically relevant during the repair of an episiotomy or obstetric laceration, repair of rectovaginal fistula, or pelvic support procedures. Identification of the fascial layers investing the subjacent structures and use of the tissue strength are critical to an optimal repair.

REPRODUCTIVE PHYSIOLOGY

The development of a differential diagnosis of gynecologic complaints is facilitated by an understanding of the reproductive cycle and elicitation of a careful menstrual history. Many conditions are a direct consequence of aberrations in the hypothalamic-pituitary-ovarian cycle and the effects of the hormonal milieu on the endometrium. Others tend to be mere variations in the presentation of different phases of the cycle. A detailed description of the cycle is beyond our scope here, but the surgeon needs to have a basic understanding of the relationships in this complex process to elicit an adequate history, to interpret the findings on physical examination, to use ancillary tests appropriately, and to formulate the differential diagnosis (Fig. 70-6).

Ovarian Cycle

Under the stimulus of hypothalamic secretion of gonadotropin-releasing hormone (GnRH) to the pituitary gland, follicle-stimulating hormone (FSH) is released into the systemic circulation. During this secretory phase of the ovarian cycle, the primordial follicles of the ovary are targeted and stimulated toward growth and maturity. Multiple follicles are recruited each cycle, but generally only one follicle becomes dominant, destined to reach maturity and extrusion at ovulation. The effects of the maturation process include not only the completion of meiotic germ cell development but also the stimulation of the granulosa cells that surround the follicle to secrete estradiol, other estrogenic compounds, and inhibin. As the estradiol level increases in the

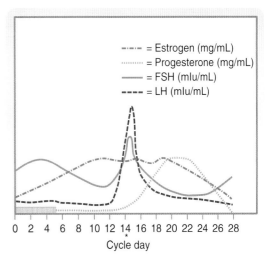

FIGURE 70-6 Hormonal changes during the menstrual cycle. Menses, days 0 to 5; ovulation, day 14.

circulation, it has a positive regulatory effect on GnRH, which in turn stimulates the pituitary gland to release a surge of luteinizing hormone (LH). The LH surge stimulates the release of the oocyte from the follicle. After release, the follicle site converts to the corpus luteum; the dominant hormone secreted during this luteal phase is progesterone. This sequence of hormonal events prepares the cervix, uterus, and tubes for sperm transport into the upper genital tract, fertilization, implantation, and support of the early gestation. In the absence of conception, the corpus luteum undergoes atresia, and the next ovarian cycle begins.

Endometrial Cycle

The hormonal sequence of the ovarian cycle controls the physiologic changes in the endometrium. By convention, each endometrial cycle begins on day 1, defined as the onset of menses. In an idealized cycle, the LH surge and ovulation occur on day 14. Atresia of the corpus luteum occurs on day 28, and menses begin the next day, day 1 of the new cycle.

During the follicular phase of the ovarian cycle, estrogen exerts a stimulatory effect on the endometrium, producing the proliferative phase of the endometrial cycle. The endometrial tissues that are affected include the surface and glandular epithelium, stromal matrix, and vascular bed. The stromal layer thickens, the glandular elements elongate, and the terminal arterioles of the endometrial circulation extend from the basalis toward the endometrial surface. The mucous secretions of the glands of the endometrium and the endocervix become profuse and watery, facilitating the ascent of spermatozoa for potential fertilization.

During the luteal phase of the ovarian cycle, corresponding to the secretory phase of the endometrial cycle, progesterone domination converts the endometrium toward receptivity for implantation of the fertilized oocyte. Several endometrial changes occur under progesterone stimulation. The growth of the endometrial stroma is terminated, the surface layer of the endometrium becomes compacted, the glandular secretions become more viscous, and the terminal arterioles become coiled, creating the spiral arterioles. Cervical mucus similarly becomes more viscous and tenacious, creating a relative barrier between the vagina and uterine cavity.

In the absence of fertilization and with the withdrawal of progesterone because of atresia of the corpus luteum, there is a complex sequence of arteriolar spasm, leading to ischemic necrosis of the endometrial surface and endometrial shedding, or menses. Normal menses, in the absence of structural disease, is an orderly process because these arteriolar changes occur in the entire mucosa simultaneously and universally, with vasospasm and coagulation occluding the terminal vessels. Bleeding associated with normal menses is notable for the absence of clotting because of fibrinolysis within the uterine cavity before flow. With fertilization and implantation, menses are absent (amenorrhea). Alternatively, a disordered ovarian cycle leads to a disordered endometrial cycle and abnormal uterine bleeding patterns.

Early Pregnancy

A brief description of the events leading to pregnancy is useful for understanding the possible complications of early pregnancy. Coitus during the 48 hours before ovulation or during the peri-ovulatory period establishes the conditions for fertilization. As noted, sperm transport is facilitated by the estrogenic environment; the spermatozoa ascend through the cervix and uterine cavity to the fallopian tube. When a mature oocyte and spermatozoa come into contact in the distal fallopian tube, fertilization can occur, usually 3 to 5 days after ovulation. During tubal transport, the zygote undergoes multiple divisions to reach the stage of the morula by the time it reaches the cavity. Implantation generally occurs approximately 5 to 7 days after fertilization.

There are two significant clinical implications to delay in the fertilization-transport sequence. If the zygote has not matured adequately before reaching the endometrial cavity, implantation will not occur, and a preclinical unrecognized pregnancy will be lost. If there is delay in the fertilization-transport sequence, either because of the randomness of coital timing or because of altered tubal structure or function, the zygote can reach the stage at which it is programmed to adhere to genital mucosa while still in the fallopian tube, resulting in an ectopic pregnancy.

Amenorrhea and Abnormal Menses

A disrupted sequence of the hypothalamic-pituitary-ovarian interaction has a profound effect on the endometrium and menses. There are two broad classes of amenorrheic disorders, hypogonadotropic and anovulatory. Although the details of the pathology and evaluation are beyond our scope of this text, hypogonadotropic conditions result from central disruption of the hypothalamic-pituitary axis. Common causes for this condition include stress, hyperprolactinemia, and low body mass (e.g., those with anorexia nervosa, athletes [distance runners, gymnasts, ballerinas]). Because of the hypogonadotropic state, follicles are not stimulated, estrogen is not secreted, and endometrial proliferation does not occur. The result is an atrophic endometrium.

An atrophic endometrium can be identified with ultrasound, measuring the endometrial bilayer. Although local equipment and operator experience will vary, an endometrial bilayer less than 5 mm in a young amenorrheic woman is highly supportive of the diagnosis. This must be followed by a thorough investigation of the entire axis.

Anovulation results from a disrupted sequence of the axis from failure of the feedback loop to trigger the LH surge. The patient may have normal or elevated FSH levels, but FSH continues to stimulate the continuous production of estrogen from the granulosa cells. The chronic unopposed estrogen promotes continuous proliferation of the endometrium, without the maturing sequence induced by progesterone. The proliferation of the endometrium results in excessive thickness. This becomes clinically manifested by prolonged amenorrhea, often followed by prolonged and profuse uterine bleeding (hypermenorrhea, menorrhagia). The most common cause for this presentation is polycystic ovarian disease, but physiologic or social stress can produce a similar clinical scenario.

Ultrasound measurement of the endometrial bilayer can exceed 20 mm. Patients with chronic anovulation with chronic unopposed estrogen are at risk for endometrial hyperplasia and even endometrial cancer. The evaluation of the patient must address the cause for the chronic anovulation and the endometrial consequences. Histologic diagnosis requires an endometrial biopsy or curettage.

After prolonged amenorrhea with excessive proliferation of the endometrial lining, hypermenorrhea and menorrhagia may occur as a result of four parallel mechanisms. The growth of tissue from the basalis to the surface extends beyond the terminal branches of the arterioles, resulting in surface ischemia and necrosis. The volume of endometrial tissue is obviously increased. The normal hemostatic mechanisms of the spiral arterioles in the menstrual cycle are absent. Finally, the shedding of the endometrial surface is not a universal event but is random and leads to multiple foci of bleeding that are dyssynchronous and occur over a prolonged time. Frequently, the rate of bleeding exceeds the capacity of the normal intracavitary fibrinolytic processes, and blood clots are common in the flow.

CLINICAL EVALUATION

Acute life-threatening conditions frequently involve pregnancy, such as a ruptured ectopic pregnancy and heavy vaginal bleeding associated with miscarriage. Therefore, in the acute setting, the possibility of pregnancy must be considered and history focused on this area. It is immediately apparent that many questions in a gynecologic or obstetric history are personal and sensitive, so it may be helpful to conduct the interview or at least part of it in private, without the presence of family members and after attempting to gain the patient's trust and understanding.

Patients will typically present with aberrant bleeding patterns, pelvic-abdominal pain or ill-defined discomfort, or a combination of these symptoms. With a focused history, the differential diagnosis can be constructed with further refinement from physical findings and ancillary tests. The key elements to be elicited are age, pregnancy history, recent and past menstrual history, sexual history, contraception, prior gynecologic disease and procedures, and evolution of the current complaints.

Diagnostic Considerations

Although there are always atypical crossover presentations for any of the possible diagnoses, the most common considerations for the differential diagnosis of symptom complexes are as presented here.

Bleeding Without Pain

- Anovulatory cycle
- Threatened or spontaneous abortion (miscarriage of intrauterine pregnancy)
- Vaginal laceration
- Vaginal or cervical neoplasm

Bleeding Associated With Midline Suprapubic Pain

- Dysmenorrhea
- Threatened or spontaneous abortion (miscarriage of intrauterine pregnancy)
- Endometritis associated with pelvic infection
- Uterine fibroids
- Early presentation of a complication of extrauterine pregnancy
- Vaginal laceration

Bleeding Associated With Lateralized Pelvic Pain

- Extrauterine pregnancy, before rupture
- Functional ovarian cyst
- Ruptured functional ovarian cyst
- Ruptured corpus luteum, with or without an intrauterine pregnancy
- Vaginal trauma

Bleeding Associated With Generalized Pelvic Pain

- Ruptured extrauterine pregnancy
- Ruptured corpus luteum, with or without an intrauterine pregnancy
- Septic spontaneous or induced abortion
- Vaginal trauma

Midline Pelvic Pain Without Bleeding

- Endometritis or pelvic inflammatory disease (PID)
- Endometriosis
- Pelvic neoplasm
- Urinary tract infection
- Constipation

Lateralized Pelvic Pain Without Bleeding

- Extrauterine pregnancy
- Functional ovarian cyst, with or without intraparenchymal hemorrhage
- Functional ovarian cyst with rupture
- Functional or neoplastic ovarian cyst with intermittent torsion
- Pedunculated paratubal or paraovarian cyst with intermittent torsion
- Endometriosis
- Ovarian remnant syndrome
- Ureteritis
- Constipation

Generalized Abdominal Pain Without Bleeding

- Ruptured extrauterine pregnancy
- Ruptured ovarian cyst
- PID with pelvic peritonitis
- Endometriosis

Obstipation

- Cul-de-sac hematoma
- Cul-de-sac adnexal mass
- Posterior uterine fibroid
- Pelvic abscess
- Endometriosis

Flank Pain

- Pyelonephritis
- Ureteral obstruction
- Ovarian remnant syndrome, with or without ureteral obstruction

Other Acute Clinical Presentations
Acute Vulvovaginitis

Acute vulvovaginitis is a common presenting emergency complaint. Presenting symptoms are intense pruritus or cutaneous pain with discharge. The most frequent pathogens are mycotic or herpetic infections. Mycotic infections are generally characterized by a thick, white, cottage cheese–like discharge. Primary herpetic infections often present with profuse watery discharge, inguinal adenopathy, and signs of a viremia. In contrast, other common vaginal infections, such as bacterial vaginosis and trichomoniasis, may cause irritative symptoms and malodorous discharge but rarely cause pain.

Common acute vulvar complaints include infection of skin appendages—folliculitis, furunculosis, and cellulitis. The ostium of the Bartholin gland may become occluded, with or without infection. Sterile cysts are only minimally uncomfortable, but a Bartholin cyst abscess is exquisitely painful.

Necrotizing Fasciitis

Necrotizing fasciitis is a life-threatening infection that can occur in the vulva. It can begin as a cellulitis, from infected skin appendages, or follow biopsy or episiotomy. Once established, it can quickly extend through the fascial planes. Women at risk are patients with obesity, diabetes, and steroid or other immunosuppressive drug use. Treatment is immediate surgical débridement. Patients may require several débridements to determine the extent of the fascial involvement. Skin grafts are often needed to repair large defects. It is important that women with risk factors for necrotizing fasciitis who present with a vulvar cellulitis be admitted for treatment with intravenous (IV) antibiotics and possible surgery.

Pelvic Masses

Masses identified in the pelvis can be functional, congenital, neoplastic, hemorrhagic, or inflammatory and can arise from the ovary or the uterus. Also, the anatomy of the cul-de-sac of Douglas in its dependent position in the pelvis facilitates restriction of pelvic infection as collections or abscesses to that location.

Common ovarian masses include functional cysts, hemorrhagic cysts, paraovarian or paratubal wolffian remnants, endometrioma, and benign or malignant tumors (e.g., epithelial, germ cell, stromal). The most common neoplastic mass in young women is the benign cystic teratoma. Because of the sebaceous content of these lesions, they frequently float to the anterior cul-de-sac between the uterus and bladder. Diagnostic considerations for differentiating among ovarian masses of various causes are discussed in detail in the later section on ovarian cancer.

Common uterine masses include leiomyoma, adenomyoma, and bicornuate uterus. Common inflammatory masses are tubo-ovarian abscesses (TOAs), pelvic collection, and appendiceal or diverticular abscesses.

Inflammatory masses in the anterior cul-de-sac most commonly originate from sigmoid diverticular disease.

History
Age

The patient's age is relevant primarily because of the phases of the reproductive life cycle—menarche at adolescence, perimenopause in middle age, and menopause.

At the time of menarche, the synchrony of the hypothalamic-pituitary-ovarian axis is immature, and the sequence of hypergonadotropic, anovulatory, amenorrhea-hypermenorrhea is common.

Similarly, this is the age group in which emotional stress, anorexia nervosa, and excessive athleticism commonly occur, and the amenorrheic patient may have hypogonadotropic amenorrhea. Finally, however, the young patient may be fertile and sexually active, so pregnancy with complications must always be considered.

In the perimenopausal years, the ovary is less responsive to the gonadotropic stimulus, and anovulation with the amenorrhea-hypermenorrhea sequence is common. In this age group, however, anatomic abnormalities, such as uterine leiomyomas or endometrial polyps, may confound the presentation.

Menopause is defined as cessation of menses for 1 year or more. Any postmenopausal woman who presents with uterine bleeding must be presumed to have uterine disease and needs to undergo an appropriate evaluation for a possible hyperplastic or neoplastic endometrial pathologic process.

Pregnancy History

The commonly used notation for describing pregnancy history is G, T, P, A, L—gravidity (number of pregnancies), term births, preterm births, abortions (spontaneous, induced, or ectopic), and living children. Additional comment is made if there have been recurring spontaneous abortions, ectopic pregnancies, or multiple gestations.

Although any pregnancy can develop complications, the patient with a history of poor outcomes in prior pregnancies will be at higher risk for another adverse outcome. In the acute setting, with pain or bleeding, pregnancy complications must be considered.

Menstrual History

The date of the last menstrual period and the prior menstrual period must be determined as accurately as possible. It is often necessary to elicit menstrual events over several prior months to establish a pattern. In addition, it is important to obtain a description of any variation from the patient's normal pattern of quantity and duration of menstrual flow. One can place the current complaints of bleeding and pain in perspective in the context of this menstrual history.

The amenorrhea-hypermenorrhea sequence has been described earlier. The patient who describes "two periods this month" may merely be describing a normal 28-day cycle beginning early and then late in the same calendar month. Alternating episodes of light bleeding with normal flow may suggest breakthrough bleeding at the time of ovulation or when the patient is taking oral contraceptives. Excessive flow (menorrhagia) associated with regular cycles at normal intervals suggests structural abnormalities of the endometrial cavity, usually submucous leiomyomas or endometrial polyps. Random or intermittent bleeding episodes during the cycle prompt consideration of a lesion of the cervix, endometrial hyperplasia, or, occasionally, adenocarcinoma of the endometrium.

Dysmenorrhea (menstrual cramps) is generally considered to occur only with ovulatory cycles. The patient who typically has dysmenorrhea but who currently denies cramps, even with a current episode of heavy flow, may be having an anovulatory bleeding episode, regardless of the interval between periods. Patients with high-volume flow, with insufficient intracavitary fibrinolysis, may experience cramps as the uterus contracts to expel the clot. Bleeding associated with threatened pregnancy loss or from an extrauterine pregnancy must be considered, whether heavy or light flow, continuous or episodic, preceded by reported normal cycles, or occurring after amenorrhea. Bleeding after menopause demands consideration of endometrial disease and appropriate workup to rule out hyperplasia or carcinoma. Postcoital bleeding suggests cervical lesions, including cervicitis, polyps, and neoplasia.

Sexual History

Sexual activity, a sensitive and personal subject that is often difficult to elicit reliably in the acute setting, may significantly influence the formulation of the differential diagnosis. Beyond the possibility of pregnancy, the patient who will acknowledge unprotected coitus with casual sexual partners is considered to be at high risk for sexually transmitted infections. Reliable reports of the use of barrier contraception reduce but do not eliminate the possibility of a sexually transmitted infection.

Pregnancy must be ruled out in any circumstance in which there is a clinical presentation that is not inconsistent with complications of pregnancy.

Contraception

Reliable use of contraception does not totally preclude the possibility of pregnancy but raises other possible diagnoses to a higher level in the differential diagnosis. Breakthrough bleeding on hormonal contraception is typically low volume and is rarely associated with cramps or pain. In the presence of other symptoms, however, pregnancy complications and genital tract infections need to be considered. Patients with an intrauterine contraceptive device (IUD) may have spotting and cramping, but because use of an IUD increases the risk for endometrial infection and because a disproportionate percentage of pregnancies that are conceived with an IUD are extrauterine, these patients need careful evaluation.

Patients with previous tubal sterilization have a 1% to 3% lifetime risk for pregnancy, with a disproportionate number of extrauterine pregnancies. Irregular bleeding associated with pain mandates careful evaluation.

Prior Gynecologic Diseases and Procedures

The past gynecologic history may indicate recurring conditions suggesting lifestyle issues that create risk for recurrence or raise consideration for complications of previous interventions. Tubal ligation, prior tubal injury from an ectopic pregnancy, endometriosis, and PID all increase the risk for extrauterine pregnancy. Endometriosis with an intraperitoneal inflammatory response may cause significant pain. Patients with a history of functional ovarian cysts, with or without intraparenchymal hemorrhage, have a higher risk for recurrence. Previous pelvic surgery with periovarian adhesions can cause significant pain, even with benign, self-limited ovarian cyst accidents, but it also may predispose to ovarian torsion.

The ovarian remnant syndrome is an interesting and confusing entity. It can cause pelvic pain in ill-defined patterns. The cause of the syndrome is a retained fragment of ovarian capsule after previous ovarian surgery. The fragment is adherent to the peritoneum and remains viable through a parasitic blood supply. Active follicles can be recruited through gonadotropin stimulation, and the dynamics of peritoneal inflammation can be severely symptomatic. These remnants are usually found after resection of a densely adherent ovary with endometriosis or purulent infection of the pelvis. They are frequently located along the course of the ureter and may present with flank pain from urinary obstruction.

History of Present Illness

The surgeon elicits the elements of the history, as described, to determine the evolution of the presenting complaint and to formulate a plan for further evaluation and treatment. This section focuses on the most common emergency presentations, bleeding and pain.

Bleeding

- When did bleeding begin?
- How does the current flow compare with normal? Are there clots in the menstrual flow normally? Currently?
- How did the timing of onset relate to previous menses? Was there any prolongation of the interval between the last period and the onset of the current bleeding event?
- Were recent menses normal? Expected timing, flow, duration?
- Are menstrual periods normally associated with menstrual cramps? Is the current episode associated with similar cramps? No cramps, more intense discomfort?

Pain

- When did the pain begin? Relationship to last menses, ovulatory?
- What is the character of the pain—cramping, sharp, pressure, stabbing, colicky?
- What is the pattern of the pain—constant, intermittent, episodic?
- Where is the pain located—generalized, midline suprapubic, lateralized?
- Does the pain radiate—vagina, rectum, legs, back, upper abdomen, shoulder?
- Were there changes in the character, pattern, or location of the pain over time? For example, did cramping midline pain become acute sharp lateralized pain, followed by relief, evolving to generalized abdominal pain radiating to the shoulder? Did lateralized constant intense pressure evolve to acute sharp pain or intermittent colicky pain?
- Is there exacerbation of the pain with movement, intercourse, coughing?
- Are there any urinary tract symptoms, dysuria?
- Are there any intestinal symptoms, constipation, obstipation, diarrhea?

Physical Examination

The approach to the physical examination of the gynecologic patient must account for the threat to dignity and modesty that a genital examination poses. In the emergency setting, against a background of fear or pain, and especially in young and older patients, the patient must be afforded maximum comfort. This includes an adequate sense of physical privacy, continuous presence of a chaperone, comfortable examination table on which to assume the lithotomy position, and patience by the examiner.

Although the chief complaint might suggest that only a focused pelvic examination is necessary, the examiner will enhance comfort and trust by a more general examination before the pelvic examination. The examiner must remember that the patient cannot see and cannot anticipate what she will experience next; the examiner or assistant informs the patient at every step in the process what the next sensation will be.

At the beginning of the pelvic examination, the examiner encourages relaxation and exposure by having the patient relax her medial thighs to allow the knees to drop out toward laterally placed hands. The knees must never be pushed apart by the examiner. Before contacting the genitalia, gentle touch of the gloved hand on the medial thigh, with gentle pressure and movement toward the vulva, will orient the patient to the progress of the examination. The external genitalia are inspected for lesions and evidence of trauma. This is followed by the insertion of a properly sized, lubricated vaginal speculum. The patient needs to be prepared for the speculum by the examiner's placing a finger on the perineum and exerting gentle pressure with encouragement to relax the introital muscles. The speculum is placed at the hymenal ring at a 30-degree angle from the vertical to minimize lateral or urethral pressure. After the leading edge is through the introitus, the speculum is rotated to the horizontal plane as it is advanced toward the apex of the vagina. The blades are gently separated as the midvagina is approached so that the cervix can be visualized and the blades are spread to surround the cervix. During the advancement and subsequent withdrawal, the walls of the vagina are visualized for lesions or trauma. The cervix is inspected for lesions, lacerations, dilation, products of conception, and purulent discharge. Support of the pelvic structures in the anterior, posterior, and superior compartments is evaluated. Vaginal swabs for microscopic wet mount examination of the vaginal environment, for gonorrhea and chlamydia, and for a Papanicolaou (Pap) test are obtained as indicated.

After the speculum examination, the index and middle fingers of the examiner's dominant hand are inserted into the vagina. Before placing his or her abdominal hand, the examiner's fingers gently palpate the vaginal walls to elicit tenderness or to detect fullness or mass. The cervix is palpated for size and consistency. The examiner's fingers are placed sequentially along the side in all four quadrants of the cervix, and gentle pressure is exerted to move the cervix in the opposite direction to elicit cervical motion tenderness.

Because the major supporting structures for the uterus are the cardinal and uterosacral ligaments that insert at the cervicouterine junction, the junction serves as the fulcrum for leverage. As the cervix is moved in one direction, it is likely that the uterine fundus is being displaced in the opposite direction. Tenderness with cervical motion may be related to traction on the ligamentous attachments, collision of the cervix against a structure in the direction to which the cervix is being displaced, or collision of the fundus against a structure on the opposite side.

The bimanual examination is performed with gentle pressure from the examiner's nondominant hand systematically mobilizing pelvic contents against the vaginal fingers. Except for large masses that are palpable on abdominal examination, the primary information gathered is detected by the examiner's vaginal fingers. The examiner should specifically note lateralized tenderness and masses. The rectovaginal examination provides additional perspective, especially for the cul-de-sac and adnexal structures.

Very young women and some older women will not tolerate the insertion of two fingers or occasionally even one. Under these circumstances, a rectal finger along with the abdominal placement of the other hand can simulate a bimanual examination.

Ancillary Tests

Imaging

The single most effective and efficient modality for assessing pelvic anatomy and pathology is real-time ultrasound, especially with a transvaginal transducer. This technique not only allows assessment of the size and relationship of the pelvic structures but also, by clear delineation of echogenicity, can provide strong suggestion of the nature of the pathologic process. With real-time Doppler flow assessment, blood flow to an organ or mass and fetal heart motion are readily apparent.

Axial tomography and magnetic resonance imaging (MRI) rarely provide additional information for benign pelvic disease but are valuable techniques for assessing malignant neoplasms. IV pyelography may be useful if ultrasound assessment of the urinary tract is inadequate to delineate obstruction or anatomic distortion.

Pregnancy Tests

There are two useful endocrine tests for determining the presence and health of a pregnancy, the β subunit of human chorionic gonadotropin (β-hCG) and progesterone.

Pregnancy tests measure the β-hCG level; the value obtained by the qualitative urine assay can be as low as 20 mIU/mL. This is sufficiently low as almost to exclude all but the earliest of gestations. Unless a viable fetus can be detected clinically or by ultrasound, a positive urine test result in the clinical setting that might suggest an ectopic pregnancy must be followed with a quantitative serum radioimmunoassay. A value lower than 5 mIU/mL is a negative test result. In most laboratories and depending on the quality of the ultrasound equipment and experience of the sonographer, a healthy intrauterine pregnancy that has produced 2000 mIU/mL of β-hCG is generally visualized. In the absence of that threshold, serial β-hCG tests are scheduled at 2-day intervals.[1]

In the so-called typical healthy intrauterine pregnancy, serum β-hCG levels double every 48 hours. However, this description is based on pooled aggregated data; within data sets, there are many patients with successful pregnancies who will have intervals with a lower slope of increase followed by an interval with a steep increase. A decline in value during a 2-day period is always ominous and therefore demands a clinical decision about an intrauterine versus extrauterine failed pregnancy. The greater challenge occurs when the rate of increase is less than 60% during 48 hours. This is ambiguous; if the β-hCG level is below the discriminatory value of 2000 mIU/mL, clinical presentation and clinical judgment are vital to determine whether continued observation or intervention is the appropriate course.[2]

Note that there are three commonly used reference standards for β-hCG as well as significant interlaboratory variation in test results. It is critical to understand the standard used and to be certain that sequential tests are performed in the same laboratory. If a change in laboratories is necessary, repeated parallel testing in the new laboratory using the residual serum from the original sample will resolve the question. Significantly elevated β-hCG levels raise suspicion of a hydatidiform mole or germ cell tumor.

Determining the serum progesterone level can be a useful adjunct in assessing the viability of a pregnancy. The quantitative relationship with pregnancy status is not as discrete, and cutoff values must be established in each laboratory. Progesterone levels lower than 5 ng/mL are rarely associated with successful pregnancies. Studies have demonstrated 100% sensitivity for ectopic pregnancy and 100% negative predictive value for a progesterone level cutoff of 22 ng/mL, but specificity and positive predictive value were poor. The role of the progesterone assay results in the clinical management of the acute patient is not yet clear.

Serum Hormone Assays

Other than the assessment of pregnancy, there is relatively little value to ordering the determination of reproductive hormone levels in the acute setting. These tests are relatively expensive, and the sequence of ordering them is determined by the clinical

findings. The laboratory turnaround time is rarely less than 1 day.

Cervicovaginal Cultures, Gram Staining, and Vaginal Wet Mount

Because the healthy vagina is a polymicrobial environment, there are only four organisms for which cervicovaginal cultures are clinically useful—gonococcus, *Chlamydia trachomatis,* herpes simplex, and, in pregnancy, group B beta-hemolytic streptococci. The tests for gonococcus and chlamydia can be combined in a single-swab medium kit for their molecular analysis.

Gram staining of purulent cervical discharge is useful in the emergency setting for identification of the gram-negative intracellular diplococci, diagnostic of gonococcus. The test may also be useful in helping identify *Trichomonas vaginalis.* Culture and Gram staining of purulent material from an abscess of Bartholin gland may allow the physician to select a narrow-spectrum antibiotic as an adjunct to drainage.

The vaginal wet mount (wet preparation) is useful for diagnosis of the offending organism in acute vaginitis. A sample of discharge is taken from the vaginal pool and by rubbing the vaginal walls with a cotton swab. The swab is placed in 1 to 2 mm of saline in a tube to create a slurry. One drop of the slurry is placed on a slide with a cover slip and examined by low- and high-power light microscopy for polymorphonuclear leukocytes, clue cells, trichomonads, hyphae, and budding yeast forms. If hyphae and budding yeast forms are not identified, a second slide is prepared by mixing one drop of the slurry with one drop of potassium hydroxide, which will lyse the epithelial cells and highlight the fungal organisms.

The clue cell is an epithelial cell with densely adherent bacteria, creating a stippled effect. To make this diagnosis, the density of bacteria must obscure cell margins in a substantial percentage of the cells. These, along with a strong amine (fishy) odor, are diagnostic of bacterial vaginosis. There is rarely a significant white cell response to this condition because it is not an infection but a shift in the normal vaginal ecosystem.

Trichomonads are often obvious as flagellated motile organisms similar in size to white blood cells. The organism is fragile, however, and motility can be inhibited by severe infection or cooling of the specimen during a delay before inspection.

Lower Genital Cytology

The Pap cytology technique has had significant public health impact, reducing the incidence of invasive cervical cancer. Although the processing time for the smear limits usefulness in the acute setting, there are two important reasons to consider obtaining the sample. The first is to take the opportunity of the visit to test a previously noncompliant patient. The second is to satisfy any significant concern about a high-grade cervical lesion before surgical manipulation of the cervix.

There are two fundamental approaches for obtaining and preparing the specimen. In the older technique, a cervical spatula is placed in the cervical os and rotated circumferentially against the cervical epithelium. This is followed by a cotton swab placed in the cervical canal and rotated on its long axis. As each step is completed, the instrument is wiped across a glass slide and spray fixative is applied. In the more recent technique, the specimen from the instrument is swirled in a fluid-based preservative, which is processed to provide a more homogeneous slide for Pap staining. Although the cost of the fluid-based technique is higher, the improved accuracy and reduction of false-positive and false-negative results make this more cost-effective.

ALTERNATIVES TO SURGICAL INTERVENTION

There are valid indications for medical or observational management of many acute gynecologic conditions, even if there is also a surgical option available. Because acute pelvic disease is often accompanied by severe pain or bleeding to a degree that the general surgeon would consider it a surgical emergency in the upper abdomen, some guidance is provided here about the clinical judgment to allow the surgeon to avoid or to defer surgery. Also provided is an overview approach to medical treatment and the points to observe during follow-up observation.

Dysfunctional Uterine Bleeding

Dysfunctional uterine bleeding is uterine bleeding that occurs as a result of abnormal or dyssynchronous pituitary hormonal stimulation of the ovary, abnormal ovarian hormone production, or abnormal response of the endometrium to normal hormonal stimulation.[1-3] If a pregnancy-related condition has been ruled out and the bleeding is not too severe, medical treatment does not require a tissue or even ultrasound diagnosis. Emergency implementation of dilation and curettage is not necessary. The episode can be truncated by inducing acute proliferation and regeneration of the endometrium with high-dose estrogens, followed by induction of a secretory endometrium with a progestin.

An oral or IV bolus of estrogens (e.g., conjugated estrogens, 5 mg orally every 6 hours for four to six doses, or 25 mg IV in two doses 6 hours apart) with simultaneous administration of an active progestin (micronized progesterone, 100 mg orally twice daily, or medroxyprogesterone, 10 mg four times daily) will stabilize the endometrium. The progestin must be continued for at least 7 days and then withdrawn to simulate atresia of the corpus luteum. This will mimic the orderly menses of an ovulatory cycle, although perhaps with heavy bleeding. The patient receives oral contraceptives for several months to stabilize iron stores, to allow orderly evaluation of structural disease, and to initiate a plan to assess underlying hypothalamic-pituitary-ovarian cycle disease.

Spontaneous Abortion

First-trimester pregnancies fail 10% to 15% of the time, often with minimal symptoms. For the patient who presents with pain or bleeding, confirm that this is an early gestation. On inspection of the cervix, observe whether there is placental tissue in the dilated cervical os; if so, it can often be removed with a sponge forceps, which will often resolve the event. The need for acute surgical intervention with curettage is wholly dependent on the amount of blood loss and intensity of pain. The patient who is hemodynamically stable and has pain control may spontaneously complete her miscarriage without any procedural intervention.

Ectopic Pregnancy

Ruptured ectopic pregnancy is a surgical emergency, but there are two other tubal pregnancy scenarios that are amenable to less aggressive treatment for the patient who is hemodynamically stable and has limited intraperitoneal blood loss, tubal abortion and unruptured ectopic pregnancy. A tubal abortion results when the pregnancy is extruded from the fimbriated end of the tube. Pain is often described as lateralized cramping, and the volume of blood identified in the cul-de-sac is approximately 100 mL. These events may be self-limited, and if pain and hemodynamic status are under control during observation, surgery may be avoided.

A patient may present with pain and vaginal bleeding; an intact tubal pregnancy is identified by ultrasound. There are varying sets of criteria for medical management of the unruptured tubal pregnancy, based on gestational size (<3 to 5 cm) and the presence of fetal cardiac activity, but the physician must actively consider medical rather than surgical management.[4]

Surgical procedures for managing an ectopic pregnancy include salpingectomy, salpingostomy, and segmental resection.[5] For the patient desiring to maintain maximal future fertility, preservation of the tube is preferable.

The medical treatment of tubal pregnancy relies on the cytotoxic effect of methotrexate. There are several protocols for dosage (e.g., 1 mg/kg) and follow-up. Consultation with an experienced gynecologist before initiation is advisable.

Pelvic Infection

The diagnosis of PID can be challenging. The differential diagnosis usually includes appendicitis, urinary tract infection, ruptured ovarian cyst, and ectopic pregnancy, all of which share some of the signs and symptoms of PID. The diagnosis of PID is made only when the patient has fever, leukocytosis, purulent discharge from the cervix, bilateral adnexal tenderness on gentle palpation, and peritoneal signs limited to the pelvis. Appendicitis is differentiated by antecedent gastrointestinal symptoms, evolving pain pattern, absence of cervical discharge, and generalized peritonitis. Lower urinary tract infection is distinguished by dysuria and obvious pyuria. Rarely do ovarian cysts or ectopic pregnancy present with significant fever or leukocytosis. In a classic study, Wølner-Hanssen and associates[6] concluded that the sensitivity and specificity of clinical assessment for PID were so poor that laparoscopic inspection of the pelvis is necessary to make a firm diagnosis. Although that may be unduly aggressive in many cases, this diagnosis must be applied cautiously because it is stigmatizing and labels the patient, disproportionately a woman of color, from lower socioeconomic status, or with a counterculture lifestyle.

Acute PID, as a polymicrobial infection, is a medical, not a surgical, disease. The major acute complication of this disease is a TOA. In contrast to abscesses related to the intestine, however, initial management of a TOA is with broad-spectrum IV antibiotics. Indications for surgical intervention are a ruptured TOA with generalized peritonitis and failure to respond to medical therapy.

A pelvic inflammatory collection is a clinical variant of a TOA. Whereas an abscess is an infectious process bounded by an inflammatory response across natural tissue planes, the collection, which may be indistinguishable on ultrasound or computed tomography scan, is bounded by anatomic surfaces of the posterior cul-de-sac, rectum, uterus, and intestine. Pelvic collections are more common than true abscesses and are much more likely to respond to medical therapy than abscesses are.

Functional Ovarian Cysts

Rupture of a follicle or corpus luteum cyst, or intraparenchymal hemorrhage in the corpus luteum, can result in extreme pain, with signs of localized peritoneal irritation. If ultrasound evaluation reveals a simple cyst and does not demonstrate significant intraperitoneal bleeding, and if Doppler flow rules out an ovarian torsion, this acute condition will resolve in 12 to 24 hours. Fluids and analgesic support are all that is necessary.

If the right ovary is affected, the acuity clearly will force the consideration of appendicitis, but prior gastrointestinal symptoms, fever, and leukocytosis are rarely present.

Ovarian torsion is a surgical emergency and sometimes mandates oophorectomy. However, unless the ovary is obviously necrotic at the time of laparoscopic inspection, the surgeon needs to untwist the ovarian pedicle and directly observe for return of blood flow before considering removal.

Uterine Leiomyomas

Uterine leiomyomas are benign myometrial tumors present in up to 40% of women, more prevalent in African American women. With clinical or ultrasound confirmation of the diagnosis, observation for stability over time is indicated. Surgical intervention is warranted if the patient has unresponsive menorrhagia, intolerable pressure symptoms, rapid growth, or change in consistency of palpable masses. Leiomyosarcoma is sufficiently rare that hysterectomy or myomectomy to rule out malignant disease carries a greater statistical risk than the lesion itself.

Observational management is especially valid in women who are approaching menopause because leiomyomas are estrogen dependent, and with the decline in estrogen production, the lesions will typically decrease in size. Continued observation is important after menopause because progressive growth during this period may reflect malignant transformation.

Endometriosis and Endometriomas

Endometriosis is a complex disease created by the presence of ectopic endometrial tissue in the peritoneal cavity or adnexa. The endometrial tissue transforms and bleeds with the ovarian cycle. This process induces a sterile inflammatory response, resulting in pain, pelvic adhesions, and, when it is located in the ovary, a complex hemorrhagic mass known as an endometrioma. First-line therapy for this disease is medical induction of temporary menopause and suppression of ovarian estrogen. Surgical treatment for younger women is conservative, with local destruction of lesions and maximum conservation of reproductive organs. Women who have completed their reproductive plans will benefit from hysterectomy and oophorectomy.

TECHNICAL ASPECTS OF SURGICAL OPTIONS

Surgical Approaches

Similar to all the surgical specialties, minimally invasive surgical approaches have become increasingly adopted in gynecologic surgery during the past decade. Laparoscopy and, more recently, robotically assisted surgery have become more widely used for benign and malignant gynecologic conditions.[7-9] These minimally invasive techniques offer fewer postoperative complications and a shorter postoperative recovery. Postoperative adhesions are markedly reduced in many studies; this translates to a lower risk of infertility, which can be an important consideration after pelvic surgery. Shorter hospitalization and rapid recovery to full function are also major advantages to many patients. Today, most patients are discharged the morning after their hysterectomy if laparoscopy or robotic surgery is used; a 5-day hospitalization with slow return of bowel function is typical for patients managed by a traditional open abdominal hysterectomy.

Although these minimally invasive approaches are popular with patients and surgeons, they often require a longer operative time and definitely require advanced surgical training and skills. They also require significant specialized instrumentation and a well-trained and experienced surgical team. Because of their complexity and special instrumentation required for these approaches, they are not discussed in detail in this chapter. The transvaginal approach is commonly used by gynecologic surgeons and is also highly effective for pelvic disease, especially for the correction of pelvic organ prolapse and various urogynecologic conditions.

These techniques also require special training and experience and are not discussed in this chapter, although they are commonly used by gynecologic surgeons.

Surgery for Menorrhagia or Abnormal Uterine Bleeding

The classic gynecologic procedure for the evaluation and possible therapeutic treatment of menorrhagia, menometrorrhagia, and abnormal uterine bleeding is dilation and curettage. It is now understood that its therapeutic success is 25% or less and is usually temporary. Because it is a blind procedure, it is difficult to ensure that the entire endometrium is curetted uniformly, much like attempting to scoop cake batter out of a bowl with a spoon. Therefore, more commonly now, hysteroscopy is used in conjunction with dilation and curettage so that the cavity can be visualized and any pathologic change seen can be directly resected or removed. The combination of the two adds to the evaluation and therapeutic success.

In addition, ablative techniques are being used for improved therapy for nonstructural bleeding abnormalities. These ablative techniques (e.g., rollerball, thermal balloon, hydrotherapy, cryotherapy, microwave) are advanced techniques best reserved for a surgeon with extensive experience in hysteroscopy and the evaluation and manipulation of the endometrial cavity.

Technique: Dilation and Curettage

A weighted speculum and anterior retracting blade or a bivalve Graves speculum is used in the vagina to visualize the cervix. The cervix is grasped transversely on the anterior lip with a single-toothed tenaculum. A Kevorkian curet is used to curet the endocervix for a specimen. A sound is placed through the cervix and into the uterus and gently tapped on the fundus of the uterus to measure the depth of the cavity. This step is important to help prevent or to recognize uterine perforation for the remainder of the procedure. The cervix is dilated with graduated dilators of increasing diameter. At this time, if hysteroscopy is going to be performed, the hysteroscope is introduced through the cervix and into the uterus for visualization of the endometrial cavity; glycine or saline is commonly used as a distention medium. The curettage phase is performed. A sharp curet, the largest diameter that will easily fit through the cervix, is introduced gently into the cervix and endometrial cavity. This is done without excessive pressure or undue force. The fundus is found, and a firm withdrawal stroke is applied until the curet reaches the cervicouterine junction. This is repeated while moving circumferentially around the uterine cavity, attempting to curet as much of the endometrial cavity as possible. The procedure is then terminated; the instruments are removed with careful attention to the cervix, which may bleed when the tenaculum is removed. The bleeding usually stops with pressure, silver nitrate, or Monsel solution.

Potential Complications

As with any surgical procedure, infection from instrumenting the cavity or bleeding from the denuded endometrial lining can occur. In addition, perforation of the uterine cavity is possible and can occur during any phase of the procedure. However, it usually occurs during the sounding of the uterus, and bleeding from the perforated area can result. The perforation is usually midline and self-limited. In general, observation for 24 hours is all that is required. If there is continued bleeding, as evidenced by a decreasing hemoglobin level or increased abdominal pain, or if other symptoms are present, exploration by laparoscopy or laparotomy may be required. Injury to the bowel is possible, although rare, with perforation.

Treatment of Bartholin Gland Cyst or Abscess

Large, symptomatic Bartholin gland cysts or painful abscesses may not respond to conservative treatment. Surgical treatment options are incision and drainage with Word catheter placement, marsupialization, and excision of the gland itself.

Excision of the gland is rarely indicated. Typically, all that is needed to treat this condition is incision and drainage with appropriate follow-up, with or without marsupialization.

Incision and drainage are generally done on the vestibular side at the hymenal ring in a lower dependent portion of the cyst or abscess using a sharp knife. The cyst is stabilized, and an incision is made into the cyst itself. A small Word catheter is placed into the cyst for drainage and is reevaluated on a weekly basis. Patients with abscesses are pretreated with antibiotics.

To perform a marsupialization, an elliptical incision is made in the vestibular mucosa down to the wall of the gland. The wall of the gland is incised along the entire length of the ellipse. The contents are evacuated, and the wall of the cyst is sutured to the vestibular mucosa with 3-0 synthetic absorbable sutures in an interrupted fashion or using a baseball stitch (Fig. 70-7). The patient is prescribed a regimen of hot sitz baths. If the lesion is an abscess, the patient is given antibiotics. Whether marsupialization or incision and drainage have been performed, sexual intercourse is avoided until the area has completely healed.

Cone Procedure

Conization can be performed with a cold knife or a LEEP. A LEEP (loop electrosurgical excision procedure) conization entails removal of the transformation zone with an ectocervical loop, followed by removal of an endocervical specimen with an endocervical loop. This is called a top hat procedure and allows

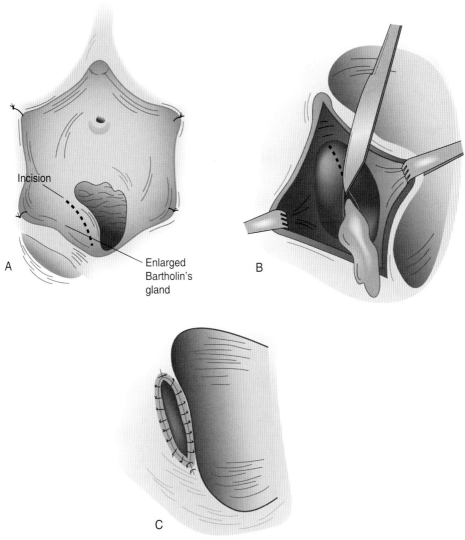

FIGURE 70-7 Bartholin Gland Marsupialization. A, Retraction of the labia and incision over the mucosa of the vagina. **B,** Wall of the gland is excised. **C,** Completed marsupialization. (Adapted from Mitchell CW, Wheeless CR: *Atlas of pelvic surgery*, ed 3, Philadelphia, 1997, Lippincott Williams & Wilkins.)

sampling of the canal. If a cold knife conization is done in the operating room, a single-toothed tenaculum is placed on the anterior lip of the cervix. Figure-of-eight retention sutures of 0-0 Vicryl are placed at 3 and 9 o'clock. A circumferential incision is made around the transformation zone and lesion. The specimen is grasped with Allis clamps to maintain orientation, and a deeper circumferential incision is made in the cervix. The specimen is removed with a scalpel or Mayo scissors. A marking stitch is placed at 12 o'clock on the specimen, and an endocervical curetting is performed above the cone biopsy. Risk for recurrence of dysplasia is dependent on the status of the endocervical and ectocervical margins as well as on whether the endocervical curetting is positive for dysplasia.

Surgery for Ovarian Cysts

Ovarian cysts are common, especially functional cysts. Benign ovarian cysts have been discussed previously. When a cyst is found, it is necessary to determine which type of treatment is most appropriate. It is individualized to each patient, depending on the clinical scenario. When an ovarian cyst is an incidental finding at the time of other surgery, it is important to know what the patient's symptoms are, if any; where the patient is in her menstrual cycle; and what size of follicle is normal for that part of the cycle.

It is critical to remember that whenever surgery is performed on the adnexal structures, there is a risk for adhesion formation that might inhibit fertility. If the patient has been asymptomatic with a small functional cyst, observation, especially for the younger patient, is most appropriate. If the functional ovarian cyst is large (>5 to 6 cm) or symptomatic, aspiration may be considered. If the cyst is larger or is not consistent with a functional lesion, oophorectomy may be considered if the patient is closer to menopause. As an alternative, ovarian cystectomy may be considered. This option removes the cyst but preserves the function of the ovary. It also reduces the risk for recurrence compared with ovarian cyst drainage.

Technique

Ovarian cyst drainage. It is imperative, before considering drainage, to determine that the ovarian cyst is benign and functional in nature. With this being noted, a hollow needle can be used, by laparoscopy or exploratory laparotomy, to pierce the cyst at a 90-degree angle and to suction the fluid from the cyst through tubing and a syringe connected to the needle. Suction is performed until all the fluid is removed. The fluid is sent to pathology to ensure accurate diagnosis. The needle is removed, and the procedure is terminated.

Oophorectomy with or without salpingectomy. When oophorectomy is desired, the infundibulopelvic ligament is identified and isolated. The ipsilateral ureter must be identified and noted to be remote from the area of the infundibulopelvic ligament to be ligated. With the infundibulopelvic ligament isolated, the following strategies can be followed:
1. Clamp, cut, and suture ligate the infundibulopelvic ligament.
2. Ligate the infundibulopelvic ligament with one or two Endoloops and then surgically dissect it.
3. Cauterize the infundibulopelvic ligament with bipolar cautery and sharply dissect it.

If the ipsilateral tube is to be removed, dissection across the mesosalpinx is performed with clamp, sharp dissection, and suture ligation or with bipolar coagulation and sharp dissection. If the

uterus is present, attention is directed to the utero-ovarian ligament. This ligament is dissected in a similar fashion, as described, through bipolar cautery or the clamping technique. The ovary, completely dissected, possibly in conjunction with the fallopian tube, can be removed.

Ovarian cystectomy. To begin an ovarian cystectomy, a surgical line into the ovarian capsule is developed sharply over the area of the cyst, on the antimesovarian side of the ovary. After the incision into the capsule, the cyst is dissected away from the capsule using sharp or blunt dissection. Scissors, knife, Kitner, hydrodissection, or a combination of these may be used for this dissection, taking care to avoid rupture of the cyst. After the cyst is completely removed, the base of the ovarian capsule usually has some bleeding. Hemostasis can be obtained at the base with electrocautery or by suturing. After hemostasis is obtained, most surgeons do not suture the capsule but approximate the edges loosely together to heal spontaneously. It is believed that this reduces the risk for adhesion formation. A Gynecare Interceed absorbable adhesion barrier or another adhesion barrier can be used at this time to reduce adhesion formation.

Potential Complications

Bleeding from the large vascular pedicles is the most dangerous potential risk. If hemostasis is not completely obtained, the large vessels can quickly bleed profusely. The more chronic complication from adnexal surgery is adhesion formation, with infertility or subfertility. Injury to the ureter is always a concern during this procedure if the ureteral course is not monitored appropriately.

Surgery for the Fallopian Tube or Ectopic Pregnancy

There are many options for the treatment of an ectopic pregnancy. Surgical options include salpingostomy, segmental resection, and salpingectomy, depending on the desire for future fertility and whether the tube is salvageable. These procedures can be performed by laparoscopy, laparotomy, or minilaparotomy.

Technique

Salpingostomy. With a salpingostomy, a linear incision is made in the antisalpingetic line over the pregnancy. This is usually performed with a monopolar needle. The pregnancy is removed from the tube. Milking the pregnancy from the tube has been discussed in the past; however, it is no longer recommended because of an increased risk for retained tissue. After the pregnancy is completely removed, hemostasis is achieved with monopolar or bipolar cautery. The tube is not sutured but rather left open to heal spontaneously. This has been shown to improve patency rates and fertility (Fig. 70-8).

Segmental resection. In segmental resection, the portion of the tube encompassing the products of conception is resected, and the proximal and distal ends are left in situ. This gives the option of reanastomosis at a later date if the patient chooses. The mesosalpinx is perforated in an avascular space. Ligatures are placed on each side of the pregnancy. The segment is sharply resected within the ligatures; the vessels of the mesosalpinx are inspected for injury and secured if necessary.

Salpingectomy. In salpingectomy, the tube is grasped and the mesosalpinx is secured using bipolar cautery, an Endoloop, or clamps with a suture ligation. The tube is sharply excised. The area is examined closely for hemostasis (Fig. 70-9).

In rare cases, the ectopic pregnancy is in the abdomen and not in the fallopian tube. In these situations, the fetus is removed with ligation of the umbilical cord near its insertion into the placenta.

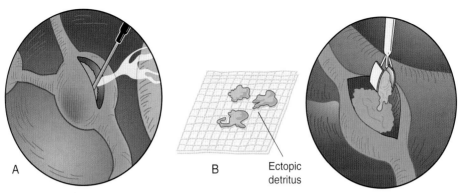

FIGURE 70-8 Salpingostomy. **A,** Fallopian tube is opened in a longitudinal manner. **B,** Trophoblastic tissue is removed in pieces. (Adapted from Mitchell CW, Wheeless CR: *Atlas of pelvic surgery*, ed 3, Philadelphia, 1997, Lippincott Williams & Wilkins.)

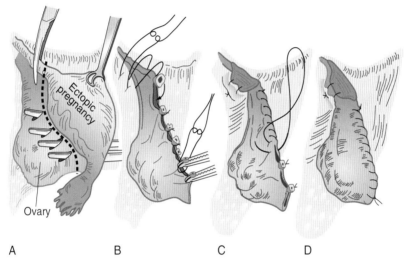

FIGURE 70-9 Salpingectomy. **A,** Tube is excised from the cornual portion across the mesosalpinx to the fimbria. **B,** Pedicles are tied, peritoneal lining is reestablished, and cornual portion of the tube is buried into the posterior segment of the uterine cornu. **C,** Mesosalpinx is reperitonealized. **D,** Mesosalpinx is closed and the procedure completed. (Adapted from Mitchell CW, Wheeless CR: *Atlas of pelvic surgery*, ed 3, Philadelphia, 1997, Lippincott Williams & Wilkins.)

Because of the vascularity of the placenta, the placenta is left in situ, with subsequent medical therapy with methotrexate.

Potential Complications

The vascular supply of the tube in pregnancy is markedly increased; therefore, bleeding is a risk during the surgery and after it is completed. If the tube is preserved, there is a risk for subsequent recurrent ectopic pregnancy. Also, there is a risk for retained placental tissue in the tube and persistent ectopic pregnancy. Adhesions of the affected adnexa are also a significant risk, whether the tube is preserved or removed.

Hysterectomy

Hysterectomy is one of the most common gynecologic procedures performed. The route of hysterectomy depends on the indication for surgery, size of the uterus, descent of the cervix and uterus, shape of the vagina, size of the patient, and skill and preference of the surgeon. Surgical routes for hysterectomy include total abdominal hysterectomy, total vaginal hysterectomy, laparoscopically assisted vaginal hysterectomy, and two more recent techniques—total laparoscopic hysterectomy and laparoscopic supracervical hysterectomy. Robotically assisted total laparoscopic hysterectomy is a popular variation of total laparoscopic hysterectomy.

Because of the significant impact of the transvaginal approach on appreciating anatomic relationships, vaginal hysterectomy and laparoscopically assisted hysterectomy must be performed only by an experienced vaginal surgeon.

Technique

Any lower abdominal incision (vertical, Pfannenstiel, Maylard, Cherney) can be used. The bowel is packed from the pelvis, and the patient is placed in the Trendelenburg position. The ureters are identified, and the following steps are performed bilaterally (Fig. 70-10).

The round ligament is identified, incised between clamps, and ligated with 0-0 absorbable suture. The leaves of the broad ligament are sharply opened anteriorly and posteriorly, with the anterior leaf open to the vesicouterine fold. If the ovary is to be preserved, the proximal tube and utero-ovarian ligament are clamped, incised, and ligated. If the tube and ovary are to be removed, the infundibulopelvic ligament is doubly clamped, incised, and double-ligated with a 0-0 absorbable tie and 0-0 synthetic absorbable suture, as described earlier.

After this has been performed bilaterally, the vesicoperitoneal fold is elevated and incised. The filmy attachments of the bladder to the pubovesical fascia are sharply dissected, mobilizing the bladder off the cervix. The filmy adventitious tissue surrounding the uterine vessels is skeletonized sharply, dissecting the tissue to expose the uterine vessels. The uterine vessels are clamped, incised, and ligated at the level of the lower uterine segment. This is accomplished by placing the tip of the clamp on the uterus at a right angle to the axis of the cervix and sliding or stepping off the uterus. The pedicle is incised, and a simple absorbable 0-0 suture ligature is placed. The cardinal and

uterosacral ligaments are sequentially clamped, incised, and suture ligated with a Heaney double transfixion suture. Each clamp is placed medial to the previous pedicle to allow the ureter passively to retract laterally. The anterior vagina can be entered by a stab incision and cut across with a scalpel or scissors. Alternatively, right-angle clamps can be used to clamp the angle of the vagina, below the distal cervix. The tissue above this angle clamp is then incised and ligated with a Heaney stitch. With the lumen of the vagina now exposed, sharp dissection is used to complete the vaginal transection. The vaginal wall, incorporating perivaginal fascia, muscularis, and mucosal edge, is closed with a series of figure-of-eight 0-0 absorbable sutures, with the angle stitches incorporating the ipsilateral uterosacral ligament. Ligatures need to be snug, but they must not strangulate the vaginal edges. The pelvic peritoneum does not need to be closed. The pelvis is irrigated, hemostasis is ensured, and the abdominal incision is closed routinely.

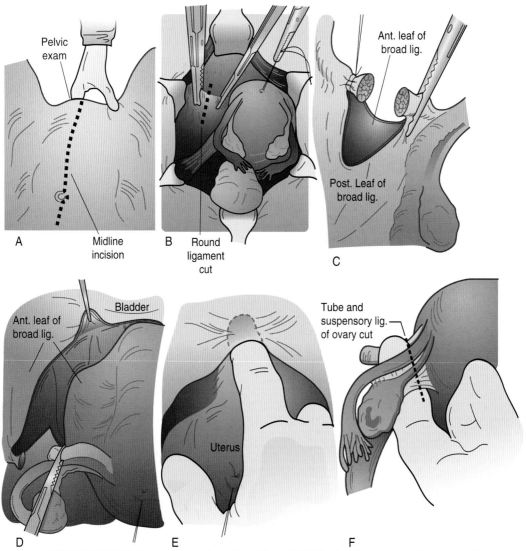

FIGURE 70-10 A-N, Hysterectomy. (Adapted from Mitchell CW, Wheeless CR: *Atlas of pelvic surgery*, ed 3, Philadelphia, 1997, Lippincott Williams & Wilkins.)

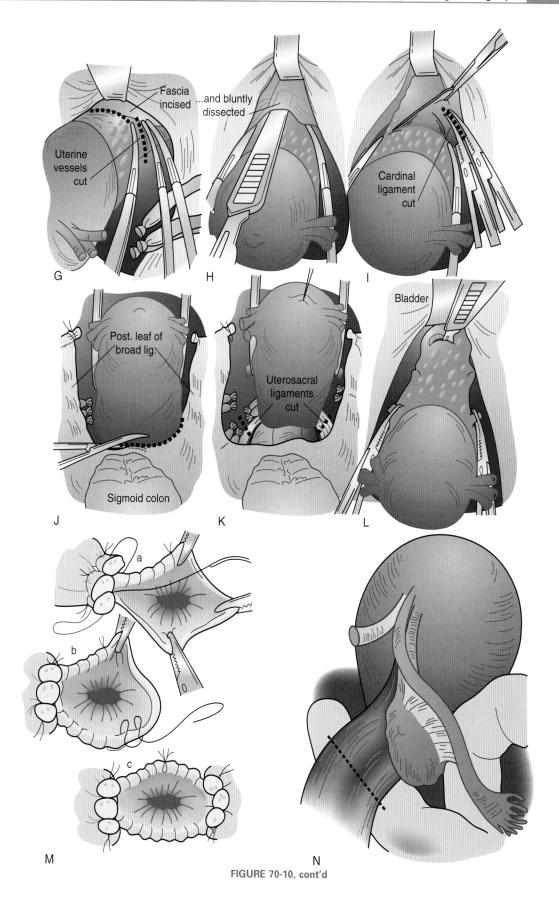

FIGURE 70-10, cont'd

Potential Complications

Because of the proximity of the ureter to the cervix, uterine vessels, and infundibulopelvic ligament, the ureter can be injured during the hysterectomy, and with the dissection necessary between the bladder and cervix, injury to the bladder is similarly a common complication. It is imperative that these injuries be recognized and repaired intraoperatively, if possible. Fistulas, such as vesicovaginal or ureterovaginal, can also form postoperatively secondary to ischemic injury caused by denudation of the bladder muscularis or partial entrapment with a vaginal closure stitch.

The vascular supply to the uterus and ovaries is rich. Intraoperative and postoperative bleeding is a concern. A previously secure pedicle can begin to bleed acutely during the postoperative period. A vaginal stump vessel, missed because of operative vasospasm, can cause a pelvic cuff hematoma. Thromboembolism originating from the pelvic vasculature is also a potential postoperative problem. Hysterectomy is considered a clean-contaminated procedure because of entering the vagina. Pelvic cuff infection is common despite the routine use of prophylactic antibiotics.

There has been discussion about the effect of hysterectomy on the pelvic floor. Failure to reapproximate the endopelvic fascia or failure to heal results in a large, apical, endopelvic fascial defect. This results in an apical enterocele that progresses in size over time. It is estimated that 60% of women have significant pelvic support defects by 60 years of age.

Radical Hysterectomy

Radical hysterectomy can be performed through a vertical, Cherney, or Maylard incision. After the pelvis is entered, the retroperitoneal space is opened, and the paravesical and pararectal spaces are developed. The boundaries of the paravesical space are the symphysis pubis anteriorly, cardinal ligament posteriorly, obliterated umbilical artery medially, and external iliac vein laterally. The boundaries of the pararectal space are the cardinal ligament anteriorly, sacrum posteriorly, ureter medially, and hypogastric artery laterally. The bladder flap is then developed to the level of the vagina. The uterine arteries are isolated back to the origin and ligated. The ureter is then separated from the medial leaf of the broad ligament, and the parametrial tunnel is developed. The ureter is separated from the parametrial tissue and is rolled laterally. The rectovaginal space is then entered, and the uterosacral ligaments are transected two thirds of the way to the sacrum. The amount of postoperative urinary retention is related to how close to the sacrum the uterosacral ligament is ligated. The parametria are then taken at the side wall. The specimen is removed when the vagina is entered 1 cm below the cervix. The angle sutures are secured with 0-0 Vicryl Heaney sutures, and the cuff is closed with 0-0 Vicryl figure-of-eight sutures. More recent surgical techniques for the management of cervical cancer include total laparoscopic radical hysterectomy with lymphadenectomy and fertility-sparing vaginal radical trachelectomy.

Management of a Pelvic Mass

When a pelvic mass is discovered on examination, ultrasound can be helpful in determining characteristics that are worrisome for malignancy. In general, a simple cyst in a premenopausal patient will not be cancerous. However, a mass with complex features, such as septations, papillations, and solid components, is more worrisome. Several benign lesions, such as endometriomas, hemorrhagic corpus luteum, and dermoid cysts, can have these features and must be included in the differential diagnosis (Table 70-2). Inflammatory conditions, including a TOA, can also

TABLE 70-2 Differential Diagnosis of Ovarian Masses

MASS	DIFFERENTIAL DIAGNOSIS
Benign disease	Hemorrhagic corpus luteum, endometrioma, tubo-ovarian abscess, ectopic pregnancy, serous or mucinous cystadenoma, cystadenofibroma, fibroma, Brenner tumor, dermoid
Malignant disease	Serous borderline tumor, mucinous epithelial borderline tumor, invasive cancer (papillary serous, endometrioid, transitional cell, clear cell, neuroendocrine or small cell, malignant mixed müllerian tumor)
Germ cell	Dysgerminoma, endodermal sinus tumor, choriocarcinoma, immature teratoma, embryonal carcinoma, polyembryoma
Stromal	Sertoli-Leydig cell tumor, granulosa cell tumor
Metastasis	Colon cancer, stomach cancer, breast cancer, lymphoma

appear worrisome on ultrasound, so the clinical scenario is important in determining the treatment plan.

In a premenopausal patient with a simple cyst, ultrasound is repeated in 6 to 8 weeks to determine whether it is a hemorrhagic corpus luteum. However, in a postmenopausal patient with a complex adnexal mass, evaluation includes computed tomography to rule out metastatic disease or another site of primary tumor and barium enema study to rule out colon involvement or primary.[10]

Carbohydrate antigen 125 (CA 125) is a glycoprotein produced by certain tumors. Unfortunately, it is not specific for ovarian cancer; its level may be elevated in lung, appendiceal, and signet ring cell carcinomas as well as in other malignant neoplasms. In the premenopausal patient, benign findings such as leiomyomas, endometriosis, menstruation, pregnancy, and PID may elevate the CA 125 level. Other diseases, such as cirrhosis of the liver, may also elevate the value. CA 125 is therefore not checked in the premenopausal patient with a pelvic mass because the false-positive rate is too high. However, in the postmenopausal patient with a pelvic mass and an elevated CA 125 level, ovarian cancer is diagnosed in 80% of these patients. This is the population in which the test is helpful.

Definitive diagnosis of a pelvic mass requires visual inspection and histologic diagnosis. Laparoscopy or laparotomy can be done, depending on the clinical suspicion of malignancy. In patients with potential for carcinomatosis, laparoscopy is not done because of port site metastasis that occurs quickly and can make debulking difficult. At the time of surgery, pelvic washings are done, and the mass is visually inspected to augment prior information from ultrasound. If all indications are that the lesion is benign, ovarian cystectomy or drainage (see earlier, "Technical Aspects of Surgical Options") is indicated, with evaluation of cyst cytology or gross or microscopic evaluation of the tissue to confirm a benign lesion. If there is a higher level of suspicion or the patient is menopausal, oophorectomy is performed and frozen section histologic diagnosis is carried out.[11-13]

Serous and mucinous cystadenomas are common benign tumors of the ovary that can occur in any age group. Treatment can be cystectomy or oophorectomy, depending on the amount of ovary involved. Brenner tumors are benign transitional cell tumors of the ovary that can also be managed in a similar fashion.

If the lesion is an invasive, epithelial ovarian cancer, treatment includes hysterectomy, bilateral salpingo-oophorectomy, and omentectomy, with peritoneal biopsy specimens of the diaphragm, bilateral paracolic gutters, bilateral pelvis, and cul-de-sac and lymph node sampling. If the cell type is mucinous, an appendectomy is also performed to rule out metastasis from the appendix. Attention has turned toward minimally invasive (laparoscopic) and fertility-sparing surgical approaches. Interval laparoscopic staging of newly diagnosed ovarian tumors, with no suspicion of carcinomatosis, may be performed in selected patients.[8]

Extensive disease mandates tumor debulking to remove all possible tumor. Patients who undergo optimal tumor reductive surgery (<2 cm of visible disease) have a survival advantage over patients who cannot be or are not optimally debulked. Complete staging is important because patients who have a grade 1 or grade 2 stage IA ovarian cancer do not require chemotherapy. With other stages, surgery is followed by chemotherapy.

Borderline tumors do not behave like invasive ovarian cancers. Typically, they are treated with surgery alone and do not require chemotherapy. They tend to occur in younger women. If it is found at frozen section and the patient is finished with childbearing, pelvic washings, hysterectomy, bilateral salpingo-oophorectomy, omentectomy, peritoneal biopsies, and lymph node biopsies are performed. If the patient desires future fertility, a unilateral oophorectomy, omentectomy, peritoneal biopsies, and lymph node biopsies on the side of the tumor can be performed. The other ovary can then be monitored with ultrasound. Staging is done in case an invasive ovarian cancer is found at the time of final pathology. Mucinous borderline tumors have also been associated with abnormalities in the appendix. Therefore, an appendectomy is performed in conjunction with other staging.

Other types of ovarian tumors include sex cord stromal tumors, such as granulosa cell and Sertoli-Leydig cell tumors. These typically appear solid but occasionally have a cystic appearance. Hysterectomy, bilateral salpingo-oophorectomy, and staging are performed. For stage I tumors of the adult type, no further therapy is needed. For patients with a higher stage, postoperative chemotherapy or radiation therapy is added.

Germ cell tumors must be considered in girls and young women. The most common cell type is a dysgerminoma; 90% of these are diagnosed at stage I. Conservative surgery with unilateral oophorectomy and staging can be performed, leaving the uterus and other tube and ovary in place. No further treatment is needed.[14] Other germ cell tumors include endodermal sinus tumor, choriocarcinoma, immature teratoma, and embryonal carcinoma. A mixture of these cancers can be present. Tumor markers such as β-hCG, α-fetoprotein, and lactate dehydrogenase may be detected in certain germ cell tumors. Patients who have a gonadoblastoma must be tested by chromosome evaluation. If XY chromosomes are discovered, the gonads are removed to prevent the development of dysgerminoma. This may occur in 20% of patients with gonadoblastoma.

Because these are potentially aggressive tumors, postoperative chemotherapy is implemented with the diagnoses of teratoma (stage IA, grade 2 or grade 3 immature teratoma, or any higher stage), dysgerminoma (stage II and above), any endodermal sinus tumor, or choriocarcinoma.

SURGERY DURING PREGNANCY

Approximately 0.1% to 2.2% of pregnant women require surgery during pregnancy. Changes in maternal-fetal physiology, enlarging gestation, and changes in maternal organ placement can make diagnosis and treatment challenging. This section addresses important issues for the surgeon to consider before proceeding to the operating room.

Physiologic Changes

During pregnancy, multisystem adaptations result in altered physiology.

Cardiovascular System

Blood volume increases by 45% to 50% at term. Placental hormone production stimulates maternal erythropoiesis, which increases red cell mass by approximately 20%. This results in a functional hemodilution manifested by a physiologic anemia. Therefore, pregnancy needs to be considered a hypervolemic state.

The maternal heart rate increases as early as 7 weeks' gestation. In late pregnancy, the maternal heart rate is increased by approximately 20% over antepartum values. Systemic vascular resistance decreases by 20% but gradually increases near term. This results in a decrease in systolic and diastolic blood pressure during pregnancy, with a gradual recovery to nonpregnant values by term. Because there is increased pressure in the venous system, there is decreased return from the lower extremities, resulting in dependent edema.

Respiratory System

In pregnancy, minute volume is increased, whereas functional residual volume is decreased (Table 70-3). Although it seems intuitive that lung volume would decrease during pregnancy, an increase in minute volume in association with an expansion of the anterior and posterior diameter of the chest results in increased tidal volume, thereby also increasing minute ventilation. These changes result in a compensated respiratory alkalosis. Normal PCO_2 values in pregnancy range from 28 to 35 mm Hg. The PO_2

TABLE 70-3 Physiologic Changes of Pregnancy

SYSTEM	CHANGES	RESULT
Cardiovascular, hemodynamic	Blood volume increased by 50%; red cell mass increased by 20%; cardiac output increased by 50%; heart rate increased by 20%; systemic vascular resistance decreased by 20%	High-output cardiac state with a hemodilutional anemia
Respiratory	Minute volume increased by 20%; functional residual capacity decreased by 15%; tidal volume increased by 20% to 30%; oxygen consumption increased by 20%	Compensated respiratory alkalosis
Gastrointestinal	Smooth muscle relaxation; delayed gastrointestinal emptying	Full stomach; constipation
Coagulation	Fibrinogen increased by 30%; protein S decreased by 30% to 40%	Hypercoagulable state regardless of risk factors
Renal	Glomerular filtration rate increased by 50%; serum creatinine decreased by 40%; physiologic hydronephrosis	Increased urination; increased risk for upper tract infection

value is usually 100 mm Hg or higher. Oxygen consumption and basal metabolic rate are also increased during pregnancy by approximately 20%.

These physiologic changes result in less pulmonary reserve for the acutely ill pregnant patient, reducing the time needed for the deterioration of respiratory distress to respiratory failure. Early intervention is mandatory.

Gastrointestinal Tract

During pregnancy, there is a decrease in gastrointestinal motility caused by mechanical changes in the abdomen, with the enlarging uterus and smooth muscle relaxation resulting from the increased production of progesterone in pregnancy. Gastric emptying may be delayed for up to 8 hours. Pregnant women are considered to have a functionally full stomach at all times. In addition, a decrease in large intestine motility may result in constipation severe enough to cause significant abdominal pain.

Coagulation Changes

Pregnancy is a hypercoagulable state. Fibrinogen is increased approximately 30% over baseline values. The hypercoagulable state of pregnancy is associated with an increased risk for deep venous thrombosis and pulmonary embolus. This is particularly compounded when bed rest or immobilization occurs during the gestational period.

Renal Changes

Pregnancy increases blood flow to the renal pelvis by approximately 50%. This results in an increased glomerular filtration rate. Frequent urination is common. The serum creatinine level is approximately 40% less than in a nonpregnant state. Therefore, a creatinine level of 1 mg/dL during gestation is considered abnormal.

Ureteral diameter increases in pregnancy secondary to compression and smooth muscle relaxation. Peristalsis is delayed, and reflux occurs freely from the bladder into the lower ureteral segment. This results in an increased incidence of pyelonephritis during pregnancy. Therefore, asymptomatic bacteriuria must be aggressively treated.

Diagnostic Considerations and Evaluation
Imaging Techniques

The most common imaging technique used during pregnancy is ultrasound, which is considered the safest modality and is used for fetal assessment. In patients with abdominal pain, ultrasound is considered the first-line diagnostic test. During ultrasound, the presence of an intrauterine pregnancy needs to be documented, if possible. In addition, evaluation of the cul-de-sac for fluid, the ureter for dilation or stones, the gallbladder for the presence of gallstones, and the placenta for abnormalities can be carried out.

MRI also can be used during pregnancy. To date, no evidence has suggested an increased risk from this modality; in fact, MRI is used to diagnose fetal abnormalities, especially abnormalities of the central nervous system.

Although there are theoretical risks associated with ionizing radiation, most diagnostic x-ray procedures are associated with minimal or no risk to the fetus. Evidence suggests that there is no increased risk to the fetus with regard to congenital malformations, growth restriction, or abortion from x-ray procedures that expose the fetus to doses of 5 cGy or less. In 1995, the American College of Obstetrics and Gynecology published guidelines regarding diagnostic imaging during pregnancy. Women need to be reassured that concern about radiation exposure must not prevent medically indicated diagnostic procedures. It cannot be stressed enough that maternal well-being is of the utmost importance, and appropriate diagnostic procedures need to be performed to facilitate a rapid diagnosis.

Clinical Evaluation

Abdominal pain during pregnancy can be confusing to the clinician. It is natural for the clinician to attribute most abdominal pain to the pregnancy; however, other organ systems are affected during pregnancy at the rate of the general population. In addition to these diagnoses, diagnosis specific to pregnancy also needs to be considered.

Common Surgical Complications of Pregnancy
Appendicitis

Appendicitis is one of the most common surgical complications of pregnancy, with an incidence of approximately 2/1000 pregnant women. This incidence is no higher than that of the general population; however, appendiceal location during pregnancy changes with the upward displacement of the appendix with advancing gestation (Fig. 70-11). Nevertheless, the most common presenting symptom is pain in the right lower quadrant, which is manifested regardless of gestational age. The diagnosis of appendicitis in pregnancy may be difficult because many of the symptoms of appendicitis are seen during pregnancy. Pain in the right lower quadrant may be mistaken for round ligament pain, and nausea, vomiting, and abdominal discomfort may be mistaken for hyperemesis gravidarum. Because mild leukocytosis is commonly seen in pregnancy, it may confound the diagnosis. However, other symptoms, such as fever and anorexia, can help the clinician establish the diagnosis. Ultrasonography may be used but is of limited value if bowel loops are distended. Computed tomography without contrast enhancement can be used, if needed, to assist in the diagnosis.

Rupture of the appendix during pregnancy increases perinatal morbidity and mortality. This is particularly true when rupture occurs after 20 weeks' gestation. Peritonitis increases the risk for preterm labor and preterm delivery. Therefore, it is prudent that the clinician make an early diagnosis and proceed immediately with surgical intervention.

Cholelithiasis

After appendicitis, biliary tract disease is the second most common general surgical condition encountered during pregnancy. Cholelithiasis of pregnancy usually develops from obstruction of the cystic duct. The clinical presentation ranges from intermittent attacks of biliary colic to persistent pain radiating into the subcapsular area in patients in whom the common bile duct is obstructed by a stone. Ultrasound is helpful for detecting the presence of stones. The differential diagnosis of acute cholelithiasis includes acute pain in the liver of pregnancy, the HELLP (hemolysis, elevated liver enzymes, low platelets) syndrome, and severe preeclampsia. Initial attacks may be treated conservatively with IV fluids, antibiotics, and antispasmodics; however, without prompt resolution of symptoms, surgery needs to be considered. Delay of surgery in a patient with cholecystitis may increase perinatal morbidity. Despite the potential difficulty of operating on a pregnant woman, lower morbidity has been shown in patients managed surgically, particularly in cases involving obstruction. In early gestation, laparoscopic cholecystectomy can be considered.

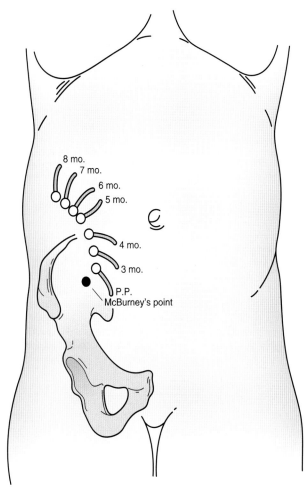

FIGURE 70-11 The approximate location of the appendix during succeeding months of pregnancy is illustrated. In planning an operation, it is better to make the abdominal incision over the point of maximum tenderness unless there is a great disparity between that point and the theoretical location of the appendix. (From Ludmir J, Stubblefield PG: Surgical procedures in pregnancy. In Gabbe S, Neibyl JR, Simpson JL, editors: *Obstetrics: Normal and problem pregnancies*, ed 4, Philadelphia, 2002, Churchill Livingstone, p 617.)

Although rare, pancreatitis may present during pregnancy. The most common cause of pancreatitis in pregnant women is cholelithiasis. However, pancreatitis can be a complication of severe preeclampsia or HELLP syndrome. Pancreatitis caused by milk-alkali toxicity may be seen in patients with an excessive intake of antacids.[15]

Intestinal Obstruction

The incidence of intestinal obstruction in pregnant women is similar to that of the general population. Patients present with classic symptoms of the abdominal colicky pain associated with hyperactive peristalsis. Nausea and vomiting are present in approximately 80% of cases. Bowel distention is marked. Laparotomy needs to be performed before bowel necrosis and perforation occur. If perforation occurs during pregnancy, there is a significant increase in maternal and perinatal morbidity and mortality.

Ovarian Masses

With the frequent use of ultrasound in early pregnancy, the corpus luteum cyst of pregnancy is frequently identified. This is physiologic and, in the absence of symptoms of torsion, requires only follow-up to ensure the diagnosis. The progesterone produced in the first 14 weeks of gestation is necessary to support the pregnancy until placental production of progesterone replaces it. Therefore, if surgery is required for symptoms of torsion or bleeding, every effort must be made to preserve the corpus luteum in the first trimester.[16]

Obstetric Complications Resulting in Abdominal Pain
Placental Abruption

Placental abruption usually occurs in the third trimester and may be associated with excruciating abdominal pain. Contrary to popular belief, overt vaginal bleeding does not need to be present in order for the diagnosis to be made. Ultrasonography is of little use because only 5% to 10% of abruptions can be seen. Therefore, the diagnosis of abruption is clinical. Abruptions are usually associated with uterine hypertonicity, resulting in fetal heart rate abnormalities. It is important for the clinician to diagnose abruption rapidly.

Trauma may increase the risk for abruption. There are three distinct mechanisms for post-traumatic placental abruption:

1. Blunt trauma to the uterus; for example, assault or seat belt placement can cause a direct injury to the placental implantation site.
2. The sudden acceleration-deceleration cycle that occurs in motor vehicle crashes can cause a contrecoup shearing injury.
3. Even in the absence of any overt physical injury, the acute adrenergic reaction to stress can result in sufficient uterine vasospasm to create ischemic necrosis at the implantation site; with reperfusion, a subplacental hematoma can dissect the plane of the implantation site.

The pregnant patient and her fetus who experience trauma need to be monitored for at least 4 hours, with the possibility of prolonged monitoring for 24 hours. Abruption may quickly become a surgical emergency, requiring immediate delivery of the fetus. Laboratory studies that may be helpful in the diagnosis of abruption include a platelet count and measurement of the fibrinogen level. As the retroplacental hematoma expands, clotting factors, especially fibrinogen and platelets, are consumed. This may assist the clinician in the diagnosis in occult cases.

Pregnancy-Related Hepatic Complications

HELLP syndrome and acute fatty liver of pregnancy can present as right upper quadrant pain and nausea and vomiting. HELLP is a form of severe preeclampsia. It is important that the clinician not mistake this for cholelithiasis or some other gastrointestinal pathologic process. Progression of this disease can result in rupture of the hepatic capsule and maternal death if the diagnosis is missed.

Acute fatty liver of pregnancy, which also carries a serious risk for maternal and fetal morbidity and mortality, can present in a similar fashion. Laboratory studies useful in the diagnosis include platelet count and determination of lactate dehydrogenase, aspartate transaminase, creatinine, uric acid, and hematocrit levels. Aspartate transaminase and lactate dehydrogenase levels will be elevated, platelets will be decreased, and the hematocrit value may be increased, especially in association with intravascular volume depletion. In patients with acute fatty liver, the glucose level may also be decreased. It is important that the clinician remember the physiologic changes when interpreting values discussed at the beginning of this chapter.

Trauma

Trauma from accidental injuries occurs in 6% to 7% of all pregnancies. In addition to the risk for placental abruption noted, blunt trauma may increase the risk for preterm labor and preterm rupture of the membranes. It is important that pregnant trauma patients be assessed for the same spectrum of injuries as nonpregnant patients. A number of studies have established that fetal-maternal hemorrhage is increased in women who have suffered trauma. Women who are RhD negative need to have a quantitative assessment of the volume of fetal cells in maternal circulation and an appropriate dose of anti-D immune globulin administered. Peritoneal lavage is not contraindicated in pregnancy and can be performed safely in those patients in whom the possibility of a ruptured viscus is suspected.

Common Obstetric Surgical Procedures

The most common obstetric procedure that the surgeon will perform is cesarean delivery. Most cesarean births are performed through a Pfannenstiel incision; however, a vertical subumbilical midline incision can be used, especially in obese patients and in patients in whom rapid entry into the abdominal cavity is indicated. After the placement of a bladder catheter, entry into the peritoneal cavity can be undertaken. In most cases, the peritoneum of the vesicouterine fold is transected transversely, and the bladder is gently dissected from the lower uterine segment. The lower uterine segment is palpated to check for malrotation to ensure that a transverse uterine incision centers on the midline. The underlying fetal part is palpated. If the presenting part is the fetal head, the incision is marked 1 to 2 cm above the original margin of the bladder. A small transverse incision is made with a scalpel across the midline of the lower uterine segment down to the fetal membranes. The incision may be extended in a transverse fashion using bandage scissors or in blunt fashion. The membranes are then ruptured. The physician's nondominant hand is placed into the cavity below the fetal head to provide leverage that redirects the vertex through the incision. The vertex is delivered through the uterine and abdominal incisions. The remainder of the infant is delivered using gentle fundal pressure. The cord is clamped and cut, and the fetus is handed to the receiving team.

In cases in which the fetus is in a transverse or breech presentation, a low vertical cesarean birth is performed. A vertical incision is made into the lower uterine segment and extended downward toward the bladder and upward toward the fundus using bandage scissors. It is generally preferred that the incision not be taken into the contractile portion of the uterus; however, if head entrapment occurs, extension of the incision in a cephalad direction is appropriate. Although not commonly performed, a classic cesarean birth with an incision over the anterior and superior uterine fundus can be used in patients in whom obstruction of the lower uterine segment occurs secondary to uterine fibroids or in very early gestation.

After the infant is delivered through the incision of choice, closure of the uterine incision may be aided by removing the uterine fundus through the abdominal incision. Delivery of the fundus also facilitates uterine massage. Oxytocin is administered through an IV line. It is recommended that 20 units of oxytocin be placed into a 1-liter bag of IV fluid, with care taken not to run the fluids at a rate of more than 200 mL/hr in most cases. The uterine incision is closed using an interlocking suture of 1-0 Vicryl or a chromic suture. A second imbricating layer may be used to achieve hemostasis. After the uterus incision is reapproximated and completed, care is taken to investigate for bleeding. The abdomen may be irrigated if there is spillage of meconium or vernix outside the operative field. There is no need to reapproximate the peritoneum or rectus muscles. The abdominal wall is closed in the usual fashion with absorbable suture.

It is possible that the surgeon may be called to assist a patient with postpartum hemorrhage. Therefore, it is important to recognize factors that may be unique to pregnancy. As noted at the beginning of the chapter, blood volume is increased during pregnancy. Hemorrhage in pregnancy is defined as blood loss in excess of 1000 mL. Because of the increase in blood volume by term, however, the patient may lose 1500 to 2000 mL of blood before symptoms are manifested. The most common cause of postpartum hemorrhage is uterine atony. Risk factors for uterine atony include prolonged labor, uterine infection, cesarean birth, and overdistention of the uterus. Hemorrhage can also be seen in abruption of the placenta and in patients with placenta previa, before or after delivery. It is recommended that therapy be initiated after the loss of 600 mL.[15,17]

The first step is to assess for vaginal, cervical, or uterine lacerations. If this assessment is negative and uterine atony is the mechanism, manual exploration of the uterus is initiated to ensure complete removal of the placenta, and aggressive fundal massage is begun. If this is unsuccessful, the administration of a solution of oxytocin, 20 units/liter of physiologic saline solution at a rate of 200 mL/hr, may assist with uterine contractility. A rate of as high as 500 mL in 10 minutes can be administered without significant cardiovascular complications; however, maternal hypotension may occur with an IV bolus injection of as low as 5 units.

When oxytocin fails to provide an adequate response, a synthetic 15-methyl prostaglandin $F_{2\alpha}$ (carboprost) is administered intramuscularly or in the uterine wall. In addition, methylergonovine maleate (Methergine), 0.2 mg given intramuscularly, may be administered. Methergine is contraindicated in patients with hypertension. Prostaglandin $F_{2\alpha}$ is contraindicated in patients with asthma. Misoprostol (Cytotec) also has uterotonic properties and can be used at a dose of 1000 µg per rectum.

When pharmacologic measures fail to control hemorrhage, surgical measures are undertaken. If the hemorrhage is secondary to uterine atony, ligation of the uterine vessels may be successful. The first step in ligating the uterine arteries is at the anastomosis of the uterine and ovarian artery high on the fundus, just below the utero-ovarian ligament. A large suture on the atraumatic needle can be passed from the uterus around the vessel and tied. If bilateral utero-ovarian vessel ligation does not stop the bleeding, temporary atraumatic occlusion of the ovarian arteries in the infundibulopelvic ligaments may be attempted. By decreasing perfusion pressure, thrombosis in the vascular bed may produce hemostasis.

If conservative measures are unsuccessful, a cesarean hysterectomy may need to be performed before sequelae of coagulopathy and hemorrhagic shock occur. In the case of postpartum hemorrhage, supracervical hysterectomy is often the procedure of choice. As for the gynecologic hysterectomy described earlier, the superior attachments of the uterus are separated, but after ligation of the uterine arteries, the fundus of the uterus is amputated from the cervix, which is closed with figure-of-eight sutures. This procedure also maintains the integrity of the uterosacral ligaments.

It is difficult to remove the cervix, especially after a vaginal delivery, secondary to dilation of the lower uterine segment. Only surgeons who are skilled in this procedure can proceed without consultation.

Other Procedures

On rare occasions, the surgeon may be consulted to assist with the repair of an episiotomy and extension. Episiotomy is an incision into the perineal body made to help facilitate delivery. Most episiotomies are cut in the midline from the posterior fourchette toward the rectum. Although more comfortable for the patient, these incisions may extend through the anal sphincter (third degree) or through the rectal wall (fourth degree). An inappropriate repair may result in a rectovaginal fistula. These fistulas present with the same symptoms as those seen in other rectal fistulas associated with Crohn's disease but are much easier to repair and have a lower rate of recurrence.

Repair of an episiotomy requires reapproximation of the vaginal tissue and perineal body. Repair of the anal sphincter requires that the fascial capsule that usually retracts posteriorly be identified and reapproximated. If the rectal wall has been compromised, a multilayer closure of mucosa, muscularis, rectovaginal fascia, anal sphincter, vaginal muscularis, and vaginal mucosa

using 2-0 or 3-0 absorbable sutures will provide the best opportunity to avoid a fistula. Because of the increased vascularity associated with pregnancy, with an adequate closure without stitch-induced tissue necrosis, healing is not usually a problem.

ACKNOWLEDGMENT

This chapter is a revision of the chapter written by Stephen S. Entman, Cornelia R. Graves, Barry K. Jarnagin, and Gautam G. Rao for the 18th edition of *Sabiston Textbook of Surgery*. I gratefully acknowledge their contribution and am honored to build on their work.

SELECTED REFERENCES

Baggish MS, Karram MM, editors: *Atlas of pelvic anatomy and gynecologic surgery*, ed 3, Philadelphia, 2011, WB Saunders.

Detailed pelvic anatomy and comprehensive coverage of gynecologic procedures with excellent illustrations are presented.

Edge SB, Byrd DR, Compton CC, et al: *AJCC cancer staging handbook*, ed 7, Philadelphia, 2010, Springer.

Comprehensive staging handbook for gynecologic and other cancers.

Fritz MA, Speroff L: *Clinical gynecologic endocrinology and infertility*, ed 8, Philadelphia, 2011, Lippincott Williams & Wilkins.

This is the classic text that explains the pathophysiology and endocrinology of menstrual abnormalities in practical clinical terms.

Hacker NF, Gambone JC, Hobel CJ, editors: *Hacker and Moore's essential of obstetrics and gynecology*, ed 5, Philadelphia, 2010, WB Saunders.

Excellent coverage of obstetrics and gynecology, with color illustrations and photographs.

Rock JA, Jones HW III, editors: *TeLinde's operative gynecology*, ed 10, Philadephia, 2003, Lippincott Williams & Wilkins.

Encyclopedic coverage addresses all areas of gynecologic surgery, with an expanded oncology section.

REFERENCES

1. Espindola D, Kennedy KA, Fischer EG: Management of abnormal uterine bleeding and the pathology of endometrial hyperplasia. *Obstet Gynecol Clin North Am* 34:717–737, 2007.
2. Goldstein SR: Abnormal uterine bleeding: The role of ultrasound. *Radiol Clin North Am* 44:901–910, 2006.
3. Dimitraki M, Tsikouras P, Bouchlariotou S, et al: Clinical evaluation of women with PMB. Is it always necessary an endometrial biopsy to be performed? A review of the literature. *Arch Gynecol Obstet* 283:261–266, 2011.

4. Barnhart KT: Clinical practice. Ectopic pregnancy. *N Engl J Med* 361:379–387, 2009.

5. Ehrenberg-Buchner S, Sandadi S, Moawad NS, et al: Ectopic pregnancy: Role of laparoscopic treatment. *Clin Obstet Gynecol* 52:372–379, 2009.

6. Wølner-Hanssen P, Mårdh PA, Svensson L, et al: Laparoscopy in women with chlamydial infection and pelvic pain: A comparison of patients with and without salpingitis. *Obstet Gynecol* 61:299–303, 1983.

7. Jonsdottir GM, Jorgensen S, Cohen SL, et al: Increasing minimally invasive hysterectomy: Effect on cost and complications. *Obstet Gynecol* 117:1142–1149, 2011.

8. Subramaniam A, Kim KH, Bryant SA, et al: A cohort study evaluating robotic versus laparotomy surgical outcomes of obese women with endometrial carcinoma. *Gynecol Oncol* 122:604–607, 2011.

9. Paley PJ, Veljovich DS, Shah CA, et al: Surgical outcomes in gynecologic oncology in the era of robotics: Analysis of first 1000 cases. *Am J Obstet Gynecol* 204:551.e1–551.e9, 2011.

10. Guzel AI, Kuyumcuoglu U, Erdemoglu M: Adnexal masses in postmenopausal and reproductive age women. *J Exp Ther Oncol* 9:167–169, 2011.

11. Liu JH, Zanotti KM: Management of the adnexal mass. *Obstet Gynecol* 117:1413–1428, 2011.

12. Gad MS, El Khouly NI, Soto E, et al: Differences in perioperative outcomes after laparoscopic management of benign and malignant adnexal masses. *J Gynecol Oncol* 22:18–24, 2011.

13. Perutelli A, Garibaldi S, Basile S, et al: Laparoscopic adnexectomy of suspect ovarian masses: Surgical technique used to avert spillage. *J Minim Invasive Gynecol* 18:372–377, 2011.

14. Eskander RN, Bristow RE, Saenz NC, et al: A retrospective review of the effect of surgeon specialty on the management of 190 benign and malignant pediatric and adolescent adnexal masses. *J Pediatr Adolesc Gynecol* 24:282–285, 2011.

15. Hull AD, Resnik R: Placenta accreta and postpartum hemorrhage. *Clin Obstet Gynecol* 53:228–236, 2010.

16. Hoover K, Jenkins TR: Evaluation and management of adnexal mass in pregnancy. *Am J Obstet Gynecol* 205:97–102, 2011.

17. Gonsalves M, Belli A: The role of interventional radiology in obstetric hemorrhage. *Cardiovasc Intervent Radiol* 33:887–895, 2010.

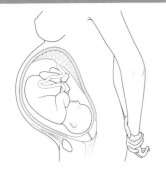

CHAPTER 71

Surgery in the Pregnant Patient

Dean J. Mikami, Jon C. Henry, E. Christopher Ellison

第七十一章 产科

OUTLINE

中文导读

本章共分为14节：①妊娠期的生理变化；②影像诊断注意事项；③麻醉安全问题；④预防早产；⑤腹部疼痛和急性腹痛；⑥微创手术：妊娠的特殊注意事项；⑦乳房肿块；⑧肝胆疾病；⑨内分泌疾病；⑩小肠梗阻；⑪炎症性肠病；⑫结肠和直肠疾病；⑬血管疾病；⑭妊娠期的创伤。

第一节介绍了在妊娠期间，受激素水平和妊娠子宫的机械作用的影响，孕妇全身各器官系统发生的生理变化，涵盖胃肠道、肝胆系统、心血管系统、血液系统、呼吸系统、肾脏系统以及内分泌系统。

第二节介绍了几种影像诊断的注意事项。辐射暴露有造成胎儿畸形或癌变的风险，尤其是放射学检查；而磁共振成像的影响未知；相对面言，超声和内镜检查比较安全。

第三节介绍了麻醉药对母儿的潜在影响。孕妇出现低氧、低血压、流产和致畸风险是主要关注点。在围手术期，外科医生应当与产科医生共同管理，密切

监测胎儿状况，合理控制麻醉镇痛。

第四节阐述了外科手术后存在的早产风险，应按需使用药物预防早产。

第五节总结了孕妇腹痛的常见原因和分类。及时诊断和治疗有助于改善妊娠不良结局。

第六节阐述了妊娠期间进行腹腔镜手术的优缺点，并介绍腹腔镜手术在妊娠期妇女中运用的安全性及注意事项。

第七节详细介绍了妊娠相关乳腺癌的临床特点和诊疗方案。当不存在致畸风险时，不推荐为了治疗乳腺癌而终止妊娠。

第八节介绍了妊娠期几种较常见的肝胆疾病的病因、诊断方法和处理原则，涵盖胆石症、急性胰腺炎、急性脂肪肝、HELLP综合征和肝腺瘤。

第九节内分泌疾病，重点介绍了嗜铬细胞瘤的临床特点、诊断和治疗策略，并列举了Lebeau和Mandel提出的甲状腺功能减退症的指南，阐明了甲状腺功能亢进症的药物疗法。

第十节介绍了小肠梗阻的病因、临床症状、诊断方法和治疗原则。

第十一节简要介绍了溃疡性结肠炎和克罗恩病对妊娠的影响。如发现疾病恶化时，需手术治疗。

第十二节介绍了急性阑尾炎与妊娠生理反应的鉴别难处，进一步说明了急性阑尾炎的常用诊断方法和治疗方式，并简要概括了结肠假性梗阻和结肠癌的治疗原则。

第十三节概述了脾脏动脉瘤破裂对妊娠造成的严重不良后果。阐述了妊娠期急性髂股静脉血栓的形成机理，并推荐清除血栓并在超声引导下置入滤器。

第十四节介绍了妊娠期间受到创伤时的治疗，重点是通过母亲的复苏来改善胎儿的结局。

〔冯　玲，余　俊〕

The pregnant patient presents a complex clinical challenge. An estimated 1% to 2% of pregnant women require surgical procedures, and nonobstetric surgery is necessary in up to 1% of pregnancies in the United States each year. A review by Cohen-Kerem and colleagues[1] evaluated the effects of nonobstetric surgical procedures on maternal and fetal outcomes. These authors reviewed 44 articles and 12,452 patients and reported a maternal death rate of 0.006% and a miscarriage rate of 5.8%. Most indications for surgical intervention are conditions that are common for the patient's age group and unrelated to pregnancy, such as acute appendicitis, symptomatic cholelithiasis, breast masses, or trauma. Changes in maternal anatomy and physiology and safety of the fetus are among the most important issues of which the surgeon must be cognizant. The presentation of surgical diseases in a pregnant patient may be atypical or may mimic signs and symptoms associated with a normal pregnancy, and a standard evaluation may be unreliable because of pregnancy-associated changes in diagnostic tests or laboratory values. Finally, many physicians may be more conservative in diagnostic evaluation and treatment. Any of these factors may result in a delay in diagnosis and treatment, adversely affecting maternal and fetal outcome. Although consultation with an obstetrician is ideal when caring for a pregnant patient, the surgeon needs to be aware of certain fundamental principles when such a consultation is unavailable. This chapter discusses the key points in caring for a pregnant patient who presents with nonobstetric surgical disease.

PHYSIOLOGIC CHANGES OF PREGNANCY

Pregnancy induces many changes to the maternal body through hormonal and mechanical alterations. Normal laboratory and vital sign values differ in the pregnant versus the nonpregnant patient (Table 71-1). Progesterone and estrogen, two of the principal hormones of pregnancy, mediate many of the maternal physiologic changes in pregnancy. Perhaps the greatest hormonal change is seen in smooth muscle tone; elevated progesterone levels and decreased motilin levels lead to relaxation of smooth muscle, which has effects on several body systems. The growing gravid uterus has increasing effects on adjacent maternal organs simply as a result of compression. These changes may also mimic similar pathophysiology that occurs in nonpregnant patients who have cardiac or liver diseases that increase intra-abdominal volumes.

Pregnancy induces multiple changes in the maternal gastrointestinal tract. The gravid uterus expands and displaces the stomach and intestines, which may lead to confusion in diagnoses of intra-abdominal pathology. In the stomach, decreased smooth muscle tone results in diminished gastric tone and motility leading to delayed gastric emptying.[2] The lower esophageal sphincter tone is also decreased; when combined with increased intra-abdominal pressure, this results in an increase in the incidence of gastroesophageal reflux, which may be seen in 80% of pregnant women.[3] Small bowel motility is reduced, increasing small bowel transit time because of compression and decreased smooth muscle tone. However, absorption of nutrients remains unchanged with the exception of iron absorption, which is increased because of increased iron requirements. In women with hyperemesis gravidarum, the severe nausea and vomiting may lead to significant nutrient and electrolyte abnormalities.[4] In the colon, pregnancy-related changes usually manifest as constipation, which is due to a combination of increased colonic sodium and water absorption, decreased motility, and mechanical obstruction by the gravid uterus. An increase in portal venous pressure and in the pressure in the collateral venous circulation results in dilation of the veins at the gastroesophageal junction and in the hemorrhoidal veins leading to hemorrhoids, which are common in many pregnant women.

The liver and biliary systems are also affected by pregnancy. The motility of the gallbladder is decreased, as the chemical composition of bile is altered with increased cholesterol saturation, which leads to more stone and sludge formation during pregnancy. The risk of stones increases with multiple pregnancies. During the second and third trimesters, the volume of the gallbladder may be twice that found in the nonpregnant state, and gallbladder emptying is markedly slower. Up to 11% of pregnant patients have gallstones on routine obstetric ultrasound scans, and

TABLE 71-1   System-Based Physiologic Changes of Pregnancy

Gastrointestinal Tract

Gastric emptying	Decreased
Gastroesophageal reflux	Increased
Small bowel motility	Decreased
Absorption of iron	Increased
Absorption of all other nutrients	Unchanged
Colonic motility	Decreased
Colonic sodium and water absorption	Increased
Portal venous pressure	Increased

Hepatobiliary System

Biliary stasis	Increased
Biliary stone production	Increased
Biliary sludge	Increased
Cholecystitis	Unchanged
Albumin levels	Decreased
Alkaline phosphatase levels	Increased
Bilirubin and hepatic transaminase levels	Unchanged

Cardiovascular System

Heart rate	Increased
Stroke volume	Increased
Mean arterial pressure	Decreased
Vascular resistance	Decreased
Left ventricular mass	Increased

Hematologic System

Plasma volume	Increased
Red blood cell mass	Increased
Hemoglobin/hematocrit	Decreased
White blood cell mass	Increased
Platelet number	Decreased
Coagulation	Increased

Respiratory System

Total lung capacity	Decreased
Functional residual capacity	Decreased
Residual capacity	Decreased
Expiratory reserve capacity	Decreased
Inspiratory capacity	Increased
Vital capacity	Unchanged
Oxygen consumption	Increased
PaO_2	Increased
$PaCO_2$	Decreased

Renal System

Glomerular filtration rate	Increased
Creatinine levels	Decreased
Serum osmolality	Decreased

Endocrine System

Cortisol levels	Increased
T_4	Increased
TSH	Decreased

PaCO$_2$, Partial arterial carbon dioxide tension; *PaO$_2$,* partial arterial oxygen tension; *TSH,* thyroid-stimulating hormone; *T$_4$,* thyroxine.

one third have biliary sludge. However, only 1 of every 1000 pregnant patients develops cholecystitis, which is similar to the incidence in nonpregnant patients. Some changes of pregnancy closely resemble liver disease. These include spider angiomata and palmar erythema from elevated serum estrogen levels. Hypoalbuminemia with decreases in total plasma protein levels is seen, along with elevated serum cholesterol, alkaline phosphatase, and fibrinogen levels. Serum bilirubin and hepatic transaminase levels are unchanged during pregnancy.[3]

In the cardiovascular system, peripheral vascular resistance is decreased by 30% because of diminished vascular smooth muscle tone.[5] Cardiac output increases by 50% during the first trimester of pregnancy and is induced by several factors.[4] There is a gradual increase in maternal heart rate that peaks at 15% to 25% higher in the third trimester. Stroke volume, or the amount of blood pumped during each cardiac cycle, increases 20% to 30% during pregnancy. To accommodate the increased work on the heart, the mass of the left ventricle increases during pregnancy and is 50% larger at term. Despite the decrease in vascular resistance, systolic blood pressure is maintained during pregnancy often with a decrease in diastolic blood pressure, which leads to a slightly lower mean arterial pressure during most of pregnancy.[5]

During the third trimester, cardiac output is dramatically decreased when the mother is lying supine as a result of compromised venous return from compression of the inferior vena cava and impaired arterial perfusion from aortic compression by the gravid uterus.[2] With this decrease in preload, an increase in sympathetic tone usually maintains peripheral vascular resistance and blood pressure. However, 10% of patients may experience supine hypotensive syndrome, in which the sympathetic response is inadequate to maintain blood pressure. During anesthesia induction in the operating room, anesthetic agents may inhibit the compensatory sympathetic response, causing a more precipitous fall in blood pressure. From a surgeon's perspective, it may be necessary to place the patient in a 30-degree left lateral decubitus position during procedures performed during the third trimester, relieving compression on the inferior vena cava by the enlarged uterus.

Venous compression by the gravid uterus has significant effects on the maternal venous system. Compression of the inferior vena cava and iliac veins increases venous pressure to the lower extremities, which leads to increased varicose veins and venous claudication during pregnancy. Inguinal swelling secondary to varicosities of the round ligament also occurs during pregnancy. This swelling is often mistaken for an inguinal or femoral hernia. Appropriate management includes careful physical examination and ultrasound if needed. The varicosities of the round ligament should resolve postpartum, but the lifetime risk of lower extremity varicose veins is increased proportionally to the number of pregnancies for a woman.[6]

Throughout pregnancy, there is a 40% to 50% increase in plasma volume secondary to increased sodium and water retention. There is an increase in red blood cell mass of 30% despite a hemodilutional anemia in pregnancy from the increased plasma volume. Leukocytes progressively increase during pregnancy to 6000 to 16,000 cells/mm³ in the second and third trimesters. Platelet count progressively declines throughout pregnancy, whereas the mean platelet volume tends to increase after 28 weeks of gestation.[4] There is an increase in clotting factors during pregnancy. Fibrinogen levels are elevated to 400 to 500 mg/dL. Plasma levels of factors V, VII, VIII, IX, X, and XII and von Willebrand antigen also progressively increase, whereas levels of factors XI and

XII and protein S decline, and an acquired resistance develops to protein C. Increased venous stasis and a hypercoagulable state lead to a fivefold increase in the rate of venous thromboembolism events during pregnancy.[7]

The respiratory system is affected by both the mechanical and the hormonal changes of pregnancy. The diaphragm can be elevated in pregnancy up to 4 cm by the gravid uterus, and the circumference of the lower chest wall can widen up to 7 cm as a result of ligamentous relaxation of the rib cage. Lung volume changes are also seen with pregnancy. Total lung capacity decreases 5%, but vital capacity is unchanged because the reduction is the functional residual capacity, which is reduced up to 25%. Because of the decrease in functional residual volume, there is a decrease in volume in both the residual and the expiratory reserve volumes. During pregnancy, inspiratory capacity may be increased 10%.[2] Oxygen consumption increases by 30% with a 15% increase in metabolic rate; this leaves pregnant women with smaller oxygen reserves and they are more susceptible to hypoxia. Minute ventilation increases by 50% as a result of an increase in tidal volume and respiratory rate, which appears to be a result of elevated serum progesterone level. The elevated progesterone not only increases the sensitivity of the respiratory centers to carbon dioxide (CO_2) but also acts as a direct stimulant to the respiratory centers. As a consequence of the increased minute ventilation, maternal partial arterial oxygen tension (PaO_2) levels during late pregnancy are 101 to 105 mm Hg, and maternal partial arterial carbon dioxide tension ($PaCO_2$) is 28 to 31 mm Hg. The decreased $PaCO_2$ increases the CO_2 gradient from the fetus to the mother, facilitating CO_2 transfer from the fetus to the mother. The oxygen-hemoglobin dissociation curve of maternal blood is shifted to the right; this, coupled with the increased affinity for oxygen of fetal hemoglobin, results in increased oxygen transfer to the fetus.[4]

In the kidney, the increased systemic vasodilation and increased plasma volume lead to an increase in the glomerular filtration rate of 50%. Urinary glucose excretion increases as a direct consequence of the increased glomerular filtration rate. Blood urea nitrogen decreases by 25% during the first trimester and stays at that level for the remainder of pregnancy. Serum creatinine also decreases by the end of the first trimester from a nonpregnant value of 0.8 mg/dL to 0.7 mg/dL and may be 0.5 mg/dL by term.[2,4] A 5- to 10-fold increase in serum renin occurs with a subsequent 4- to 5-fold increase in angiotensin. Although a pregnant patient is apparently less sensitive to the hypertensive effects of the increased angiotensin, elevated aldosterone levels result in an increase in sodium reabsorption, overcoming the natriuresis produced by elevated progesterone. However, serum sodium levels are decreased because the increase in sodium reabsorption is less than the increase in plasma volume. Serum osmolality is decreased to 270 to 280 mOsm/kg.

Pregnancy has a significant effect on endocrine physiology. Cortisol levels increase to threefold above nonpregnancy levels as a result of estrogen stimulation of corticosteroid-binding globulin release of free cortisol and placental release of corticotropin-releasing hormone.[8] Early in pregnancy, high levels of human chorionic gonadotropin (hCG) stimulate thyroid production and release, causing levels of thyroxine (T_4) to increase and thyroid-stimulating hormone (TSH) to decrease. Estrogen also increases the production of thyroid-binding globulin leading to more T_4 binding and inducing more thyroid hormone production. These factors lead to a 50% increase in overall serum T_4 concentrations. As hCG decreases later in pregnancy, levels of T_4 decrease, and TSH levels increase.[9]

DIAGNOSTIC IMAGING CONSIDERATIONS

Imaging is paramount in diagnosis of many surgical conditions, including in pregnant patients. The use of radiation is a concern in this patient population because of the teratogenic and carcinogenic risk to the fetus from radiation exposure. The consensus acceptable maximum dose of ionizing radiation during the entire pregnancy is 5 rads (0.05 Gy). The fetus is at the highest risk from radiation exposure from the preimplantation period to approximately 15 weeks of gestation; spontaneous abortions and decreased intelligence have been documented at radiation exposures greater than 10 rads. Primary organogenesis occurs during this time, and the teratogenic effects of radiation, particularly to the developing central nervous system, are at their highest. Perinatal radiation exposure has also been associated with childhood leukemia and certain childhood malignancies, especially when the radiation exposure occurs during the first trimester.[10] As shown in Table 71-2, radiation exposure to the fetus with the doses from the more common radiology procedures is well below the maximum threshold of greater than 5 rads. With the increased use of computed tomography (CT) scans to aid in surgical diagnoses, many medical centers are developing pregnancy protocols that use lower doses of radiation with the tradeoff of decreased imaging quality. Fluoroscopic studies may also be used in pregnant patients, but

TABLE 71-2 Fetal Radiation Exposure With Radiographic Imaging

EXAMINATION	FETAL RADIATION EXPOSURE (mGy)
Plain Film Radiographs	
Cervical spine (2-view)	<0.001
Extremities	<0.001
Chest (2-view)	0.002
Thoracic spine (2-view)	0.003
Abdomen (1 view)	1-3
Lumbar spine (2-view)	1
Mammography	0.4
Pelvic	0.6
Fluoroscopy	
Pyelogram	6
Upper GI series	0.05
Barium enema	7
Angiography and interventions	10-60
CT Scans	
Head	0
Chest (PE)	0.2
CT angiography of the aorta	34
Abdomen/pelvis	25
Other Examinations	
Bone scan	6
PET scan	14
MRI	0
U/S	0
HIDA	0.15

CT, Computed tomography; *GI*, gastrointestinal; *HIDA*, hepatobiliary iminodiacetic acid scan; *MRI*, magnetic resonance imaging; *PE*, pulmonary embolism; *U/S*, ultrasound.

attempts must be made to use the minimal amount of radiation possible by using lower doses for shorter periods of time, and the fluoroscopy machine should be set with an alarm when a certain radiation usage threshold is set.[11] Nonetheless, prudence on the part of the clinician is required to avoid unnecessary fetal exposure to ionizing radiation, especially during the first trimester and early second trimester when the risk from exposure is greatest.

Magnetic resonance imaging (MRI) avoids exposure to ionizing radiation but poses an unknown risk to the fetus. Theoretically, the gradient magnetic fields may produce electric currents within the patient, and the high-frequency currents induced by radiofrequency fields may cause local generation of heat. The long-term effect of exposure is unknown. At the present time, the National Radiological Protection Board advises against the use of MRI during the first trimester of pregnancy.[10]

Contrast agents to enhance imaging modalities have been shown to be safe in pregnancy but should be used with extreme care. Iodine-based agents have a theoretical risk of neonatal hypothyroidism that has not been established in the literature. Gadolinium crosses the placental and can stay in the amniotic fluid for a prolonged time, which has led to its use only in extreme conditions for the mother's safety.[10]

Ultrasonography is routinely used by obstetricians during pregnancy. Although tissue heating and mechanical injuries are theoretical effects of ultrasound exposure, such effects have never been reported.[12] Ultrasound may be a helpful alternative diagnostic tool when trying to avoid exposure to ionizing radiation, but it has some limitations: Deeper structures are difficult to visualize, the ultrasound field is limited, and ultrasound is highly operator dependent.

Endoscopy is a commonly used diagnostic modality in pregnant women. Esophagogastroduodenoscopy is the most commonly used endoscopic therapy in pregnancy and has been shown to be safe with very little risk to the fetus. Sigmoidoscopy has been used successfully with little risk to the fetus. An entire colonoscopy is technically very difficult but if necessary can be done safely. Strong indications for the use of endoscopy in pregnancy are upper gastrointestinal bleed, dysphagia for more than 1 week, and possible malignancy. Finally, endoscopic retrograde cholangiopancreatography (ERCP) has been shown to be successful and safe with very few pregnancy complications, although maternal pancreatitis rates of 15% have been reported when ERCP was performed for obstructive jaundice or cholangitis from choledocholithiasis. Therefore, ERCP has been deemed safe as opposed to surgical intervention for obstructive jaundice, which would carry greater risk for the mother and fetus.[13]

ANESTHESIA SAFETY CONCERNS

Anesthesia concerns during pregnancy include the safety of both the mother and the fetus. The primary concerns for the mother during general anesthesia are hypotension, hypoxia, and airway. The airway of the pregnant woman is generally swollen, reducing the glottis opening and making intubation more difficult. These patients are also more prone to aspiration with anesthesia induction because of increased intra-abdominal pressure. The pulmonary reserve is also greatly reduced, so the pregnant patient may become acutely hypoxic very quickly during induction.[14]

The effects of anesthesia on the fetus during pregnancy can be divided into direct, or active, and indirect, or passive, effects. Direct effects are effects that relate to the possible teratogenic or embryotoxic properties of the drugs used for anesthesia, some of which do cross the placenta. Indirect effects are mechanisms by which an anesthetic agent or surgical procedure may interfere with maternal or fetal physiology, such as inducing hypotension, inducing hypoxia, or altering the acid-base balance, and in doing so may potentially harm the fetus. For the most part, the fetus experiences indirect effects as a consequence of anesthetic agents administered to the mother or the effect on the mother of the underlying disease process. The most profound effects on the fetus are related to decreased uterine blood flow or decreased oxygen content of uterine blood. In contrast to circulation to other vital organs, most notably the brain, the uterine circulation is not autoregulated. During the third trimester, uterine circulation represents nearly 10% of cardiac output. When treating maternal hypotension brought about by general anesthesia, pure α-agonists, such as phenylephrine and metaraminol, are most effective at maintaining maternal blood pressure and promoting continuous perfusion to the gravid uterus. Multiple studies support the use of these vasopressor agents in pregnant women during surgery.[14] Other maneuvers, such as fluid bolus, Trendelenburg and left-lateral positions, compression stockings, and leg elevation, have an impact on increasing uterine blood flow.

In addition to the risks related to maternal hypoxia or hypotension, the risks of spontaneous abortion and teratogenesis related to anesthetic agents are of major concern. Labor induction occurs in 5% of all surgical procedures in pregnant women. Many nonhuman studies demonstrated potential teratogenic effects with anesthetic agents, but human studies have not demonstrated such significant effects.

Because of the risks of anesthesia on the fetus and the mother's physiology, elective surgical procedures should be delayed until at least 6 weeks after delivery, when maternal physiology has returned to the nonpregnant state and when the impact on the fetus is no longer a concern. When emergent procedures are required, the life of the mother takes priority, although the anesthesia administered should be altered to optimize fetal well-being. Elective surgery during the first trimester is often avoided because of the potential teratogenic effects of the anesthesia on the developing fetus during organogenesis. However, multiple studies have shown a single exposure to anesthesia during the first trimester to be safe and associated with the same rate of major birth defects as in the population without surgical anesthesia exposure. It is still advisable to limit surgical intervention during the first trimester. The second trimester has classically been assumed safer for nonobstetric surgeries in pregnant patients, but studies have shown that anesthesia may have effects on neuronal development during this trimester, as this is a major period of neural development in the fetus. Although surgery can be performed during this time, it should be done only if necessary. General anesthesia in the third trimester has been studied less frequently but generally has been accepted as safe if surgery is necessary, although it carries a risk for preterm labor induction.[15]

When a pregnant patient requires surgical intervention, consultation with the obstetrician and possibly a perinatologist is essential. These specialists are helpful in determining the optimal technique to monitor fetal status and are able to assist with perioperative management and diagnose and manage preterm labor. Typically, when emergent surgery is performed during the first trimester or early second trimester, fetal heart tones and tachymeter monitoring should be obtained before and after anesthesia exposure. During the late second trimester and third trimester, when the fetus is of viable age, continuous intraoperative monitoring should be performed when possible with electronic fetal monitoring, fetal pulse oximetry, or possibly transvaginal ultrasound when the surgery is on the abdomen.[16] If any signs of fetal distress occur, the team should be prepared for an emergent cesarean section in fetuses who are past 24 weeks. Continuous monitoring should be used to assess fetal well-being if a significant blood loss is possible or anticipated.

Postoperative pain control in pregnant patients should be monitored closely. Nonsteroidal anti-inflammatory drugs should not be used in pregnancy because of the risk of premature labor, fetal renal injury, and premature closure of the ductus arteriosus.[17] Acetaminophen and opioids are the preferred perioperative analgesic choices for pregnant women. Narcotic analgesics have not been found to cause birth defects in humans in normal dosages. A patient-controlled analgesia pump postoperatively may be the best choice because of the low incidence of maternal respiratory depression and drug transfer to the fetus. Postoperative oral narcotic use is generally considered safe in pregnant patients. Long-term use of narcotics during pregnancy may cause fetal dependency at delivery. It is recommended that a pregnant postsurgical patient be weaned off narcotic use as soon as possible.

PREVENTION OF PRETERM LABOR

The incidence of preterm labor associated with nonobstetric surgery is related to both gestational age and the indication for surgery. Studies have suggested the rate of premature labor induced by nonobstetric elective surgical intervention to approach 5%.[18] Elective procedures are usually delayed until later in the postpartum period when the mother is fully recovered from the pregnancy. An exception may be a patient with cancer diagnosed during pregnancy that warrants an earlier surgery. Gestational age at treatment and severity of the underlying disease are the most predictive indicators of patients at risk for preterm labor. The risk of preterm contractions or preterm labor is higher later in gestation. Intraperitoneal operations and disease processes with intraperitoneal inflammation are the most likely to have postoperative courses complicated by preterm contractions and preterm labor. Laparoscopic and open techniques have an equal incidence of preterm labor.

If surgical intervention is necessary, an obstetrician should be consulted. During surgery, measures to avoid maternal hypotension and hypoxia are thought to mitigate against preterm labor. There is no consensus on the use of prophylactic tocolytics after nonobstetric surgery during pregnancy. Tocolytic use varies widely among centers and physicians. Most studies suggest that tocolytics should be used only if contractions are noted during postoperative monitoring or are felt by the patient. Tocolytics used as needed are generally successful at preventing preterm labor and preterm delivery when postoperative contractions are detected. Terbutaline, magnesium, and indomethacin (Indocin) all have been used in different studies with equivalent results. In general, for patients with postoperative contractions before 32 weeks, indomethacin would be a reasonable treatment, whereas terbutaline could be used as a first-line treatment for patients at greater than 32 weeks' gestation. The use of prophylactic tocolytics should be individualized, depending on the patient's gestational age and the underlying disease process and chosen in consultations with the obstetricians. Tocolytics used for postoperative preterm labor are generally successful when used selectively but should not be used as prophylaxis.

ABDOMINAL PAIN AND THE ACUTE ABDOMEN

When a pregnant patient presents with abdominal pain, it may be difficult to distinguish a pathophysiologic cause from normal pregnancy-associated symptoms. Changes in the position and orientation of abdominal viscera from the enlarging uterus as well as alterations in physiology already described may modify the perception or manifestation of an intra-abdominal process. If early in the pregnancy, the woman may not know that she is pregnant. Additionally, some intra-abdominal processes are exclusive to pregnancy, such as ectopic pregnancy, HELLP (hemolysis, elevated liver enzymes, low platelets) syndrome, or acute fatty liver of pregnancy. Moreover, both the patient and the physician may attribute the patient's complaints to normal pregnancy, resulting in a delay in evaluation and treatment. These delays in diagnosis and definitive intervention are the most serious adverse event affecting maternal and fetal outcome. It is usually not the treatment but the delay in diagnosis and severity of the primary disease process that adversely impact outcomes.[3,18] Box 71-1 lists common causes of abdominal pain in pregnant patients, classified according to location. Prompt evaluation and treatment are necessary to avoid maternal and fetal complications.

MINIMALLY INVASIVE SURGERY: SPECIAL CONSIDERATIONS IN PREGNANCY

The field of minimally invasive surgery has advanced tremendously over the last 20 years. The laparoscopic approach, which was previously considered contraindicated in pregnancy, is now

---

BOX 71-1   Common Causes of Abdominal Pain in Pregnant Patients

Right Upper Quadrant
Gastroesophageal reflux
Peptic ulcer disease
Acute cholecystitis
Biliary colic
Acute pancreatitis
Hepatitis
Acute fatty liver of pregnancy
HELLP syndrome
Preeclampsia
Pneumothorax
Pneumonia
Acute appendicitis
Hepatic adenoma
Hemangioma

Right Lower Quadrant
Acute appendicitis
Ectopic pregnancy
Renal or ureteral colic
Pelvic inflammatory disease
Tubo-ovarian abscess
Endometriosis
Adnexal torsion
Ruptured ovarian cyst
Ruptured corpus luteum

Lower Abdomen
Threatened, incomplete, or complete abortion
Abruptio placentae
Preterm labor
Pelvic inflammatory disease
Tubo-ovarian abscess
Inflammatory bowel disease
Irritable bowel syndrome
Pyelonephritis

Flank
Pyelonephritis
Hydronephrosis of pregnancy
Acute appendicitis (retrocecal appendix)

Diffuse Abdominal Pain
Early acute appendicitis
Small bowel obstruction
Acute intermittent porphyria
Sickle cell crisis

HELLP, Hemolysis, elevated liver enzymes, low platelets.

considered a standard approach to many operations done in pregnant patients. Effects of CO_2 pneumoperitoneum on venous return and cardiac output, uterine perfusion, and fetal acid-base status were unknown. Laparoscopy was safely used in several series where the technique was used to evaluate pregnant patients for ectopic pregnancy. Patients with an intrauterine pregnancy had no increase in fetal loss or observed negative effect on long-term outcome.[19] When comparing laparoscopic and open techniques in nonpregnant patients, patients who underwent laparoscopic procedures had decreased postoperative pain, shorter hospital stays, and a quicker return to normal activity.[19,20]

Major concerns of laparoscopy during pregnancy include injury to the uterus, decreased uterine blood flow, fetal acidosis, and preterm labor from increased intra-abdominal pressure. During the second trimester, the uterus is no longer contained within the pelvis. The open technique for abdominal access reduces the risk of injury. Decreased uterine blood flow from pneumoperitoneum remains theoretical because of the significant changes in intra-abdominal pressure that occur normally during pregnancy and during maternal Valsalva maneuvers. The risk of pneumoperitoneum may also be less than the risk of direct uterine manipulation that occurs with laparotomy. Additionally, when comparing laparoscopy and open techniques, no significant difference in preterm labor or delivery-related side effects was observed.[20] Box 71-2 illustrates the general comparison between laparoscopic and open technique.

The Society of American Gastrointestinal Endoscopic Surgeons recommends 23 guidelines for laparoscopic surgery during pregnancy.[21] The guidelines that pertain to laparoscopic surgery are as follows:

- Intraoperative and endoscopic cholangiography exposes the mother and fetus to minimal radiation and may be used selectively during pregnancy. The lower abdomen should be shielded when performing cholangiography during pregnancy to decrease the radiation exposure to the fetus.
- Diagnostic laparoscopy is safe and effective when used selectively in the workup and treatment of acute abdominal processes in pregnancy.
- Laparoscopic treatment of acute abdominal disease has the same indications in pregnant and nonpregnant patients.

BOX 71-2   Advantages and Disadvantages of Laparoscopy Instead of Laparotomy in Pregnancy

Advantages
Decreased fetal depression secondary to decreased narcotic requirement
Lower rates of wound infections and incisional hernias
Diminished postoperative maternal hypoventilation
Decreased manipulation of the uterus
Faster recovery with early return to normal function
Decreased risk of ileus

Disadvantages
Possible uterine injury during trocar placement
Decreased uterine blood flow
Preterm labor risk secondary to increased intra-abdominal pressure
Increased risk of fetal acidosis and unknown effects of CO_2 pneumoperitoneum
Decreased visualization with gravid uterus

CO_2, Carbon dioxide.

- Laparoscopy can be safely performed during any trimester of pregnancy.
- Gravid patients should be placed in the left lateral decubitus position to minimize compression of the vena cava.
- Initial abdominal access can be safely accomplished with an open (Hasson) technique, Veress needle, or optical trocar if the location is adjusted according to fundal height and previous incisions.
- CO_2 insufflation of 10 to 15 mm Hg can be safely used for laparoscopy in pregnant patients.
- Intraoperative CO_2 monitoring by capnography should be used during laparoscopy in pregnant patients.
- Intraoperative and postoperative pneumatic compression devices and early postoperative ambulation are recommended prophylaxis for deep venous thrombosis in gravid patients.
- Laparoscopic cholecystectomy is the treatment of choice in pregnant patients with gallbladder disease, regardless of trimester.
- Choledocholithiasis during pregnancy may be managed with preoperative ERCP with sphincterotomy followed by laparoscopic cholecystectomy, laparoscopic common bile duct exploration, or postoperative ERCP.
- Laparoscopic appendectomy may be performed safely in pregnant patients with appendicitis.
- Laparoscopic adrenalectomy, nephrectomy, and splenectomy are safe procedures in pregnant patients.
- Laparoscopy is safe and effective treatment in pregnant patients with symptomatic ovarian cystic masses. Observation is acceptable for all other cystic lesions, provided that ultrasound is not concerning for malignancy and tumor markers are normal. Initial observation is warranted for most cystic lesions less than 6 cm in size.
- Laparoscopy is recommended for diagnosis and treatment of adnexal torsion unless clinical severity warrants laparotomy.
- Fetal heart monitoring should occur preoperatively and postoperatively in the setting of urgent abdominal surgery during pregnancy.
- Obstetric consultation can be obtained preoperatively or postoperatively based on the severity of the patient's disease, gestational age, and availability of the consultant.

Trocar placement early in pregnancy in a pregnant patient should not differ radically from placement in a nonpregnant patient. Later in pregnancy, the camera port must be placed in a supraumbilical location, and the remaining ports are placed under direct camera visualization. The gravid uterus enlarges superiorly (Fig. 71-1); adjustments in trocar placement must be made to avoid uterine injury and to improve visualization, and an angled scope may aid in viewing over or around the uterus. The uterus should be manipulated as little as possible.

BREAST MASSES

Pregnancy-associated breast cancer is defined as breast cancer that is diagnosed during pregnancy or within 1 year after pregnancy. It has become increasingly more prominent as more women delay childbearing until they are in their 30s and 40s.[22] Overall, pregnancy-associated breast cancer is the most common nongynecologic malignancy associated with pregnancy and has been reported to occur in 1 in 3000 pregnancies; 10% of women with breast cancer younger than 40 years old are pregnant at the time of diagnosis.[22,23] Because pregnancy-related breast cancers occur

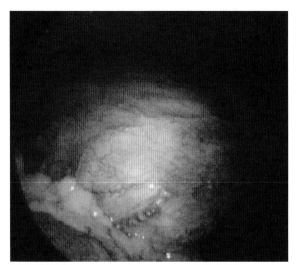

FIGURE 71-1 Intraoperative image of a 24-week gravid uterus taken with a 5-mm, 30-degree, high-definition camera.

at a young age, these women are more apt to have genetic predisposition to breast cancers resulting from *BRAC1* or *BRAC2* mutations. Several studies have demonstrated that pregnancy-associated breast cancer may be more common in women with a genetic predisposition to breast cancer. Patients with *BRCA1*, more than patients with *BRCA2*, were three to four times more likely to develop breast cancer during pregnancy.[24]

Delays in diagnosis and treatment are common. Physiologic changes of breast engorgement, rapid cellular proliferation, and increased vascularity make a reliable physical examination difficult; masses of similar size that would be easily palpable in the nonpregnant state may be obscured, or palpable masses may be attributed to normal pregnancy-related changes. Benign breast lesions, such as galactoceles, mastitis, abscesses, lipomas, fibroadenomas, lobular hyperplasia, and lactational adenomas, account for 80% of breast masses that occur during pregnancy or during lactation. However, any palpable mass that persists for 4 weeks or longer should be evaluated.[23] Most pregnancy-related breast cancers manifest with a painless mass with or without bloody nipple discharge that is often interpreted as a normal pregnancy-related change. Studies have shown that the mean delay of 1 to 2 months in the diagnosis of a breast mass as cancer in a pregnant patient can increase the chance of nodal metastasis from 0.9% to 1.8%.[25]

Compared with age-matched nonpregnant control subjects, women with pregnancy-associated breast cancer are more likely to present with larger primary tumors, increased nodal involvement, and increased inflammatory breast cancer and are more likely to have metastatic disease.[23,26] Most pregnancy-associated breast cancers are poorly differentiated infiltrating ductal carcinomas. Pregnancy-associated breast cancers have estrogen receptor or progesterone receptor expression 25% of the time as opposed to 55% to 60% seen in nonpregnant breast cancers. Her-2 overexpression is seen in 28% to 58% of pregnancy-associated breast cancers, which is slightly higher than in breast cancers with no pregnancy. The pathologic type of breast cancer seen during pregnancy appears to be more aggressive and typically associated with poorer prognosis.[26]

Young age, which would include most pregnant women, has been shown to be an independent risk factor for a worse prognosis

and for increased breast cancer–related mortality.[27] There have been several conflicting studies in regard to the effects of pregnancy on breast cancer and the patient's prognosis. A large meta-analysis of 30 published studies of pregnancy-associated breast cancer demonstrated a clear trend of poorer outcomes in patients with pregnancy-associated breast cancer. The group with the worst prognosis included patients diagnosed immediately postpartum, but patients with breast cancer during pregnancy also had a worse prognosis than similar nonpregnant patients.[22]

Imaging of breast masses in pregnant women is often difficult because pregnancy-related changes result in denser breast tissue. Ultrasound should be the first imaging modality used for the workup of a breast mass in a pregnant woman.[27] The ultrasound scan is able to distinguish solid from cystic lesions in greater than 93% of patients and can be used to evaluate for abnormal axillary lymph nodes. Mammography generally has a high false-negative rate during pregnancy secondary to the increased breast density; this decreases mammographic sensitivity from 63% to 78% for detecting breast cancer in a pregnant woman.[26] Despite the use of radiation, if used with appropriate shielding, mammography carries a limited risk to the fetus and is generally considered safe with 0.02 mGy of radiation exposure. If a lesion is suggestive of cancer by ultrasound, mammography is recommended to rule out multiple lesions or bilateral breast cancers.[27] MRI is a third imaging modality commonly used in young women with breast cancer, but its safety in pregnant patients has not been studied. MRI is a tempting option because it does not use radiation, but MRI requires the use of gadolinium for detection of breast cancer, and gadolinium is listed as a pregnancy category C drug because animal studies have shown that it crosses the placenta and causes fetal abnormalities. Breast MRI is not recommended in pregnancy unless it is necessary for treatment planning. If metastatic disease is suspected, low-dose bone scans or noncontrast MRI scans may be used.[26]

When a suspicious lesion is identified, tissue diagnosis is essential. Core-needle biopsy under local anesthesia with or without ultrasound guidance is a safe and reliable method for obtaining tissue that has a sensitivity rate up to 90%.[23] The major risks are hematoma formation and milk fistula development. A pressure dressing should be applied after the biopsy to minimize the risk of hematoma from the hypervascularity of the breasts. The risk of milk fistula may be reduced by stopping lactation for several days before biopsy and by emptying the breast of milk just before the procedure. If the biopsy is done postpartum, a 1-week course of bromocriptine may also be given before biopsy.[26] Fine-needle aspiration is generally not recommended in pregnant women because hormonal changes of the breast that may lead to cellular proliferation may give false-positive results, as the cellular proliferation is hard to distinguish from cancer. If a core-needle biopsy is not definitive, excisional biopsy of the breast lump should be considered, as this can be done safely and provides adequate tissue.

Treatment of pregnant patients with breast cancer requires a multimodality team comprising a surgeon, oncologist, obstetrician, and perinatologist. The mainstay of therapy for pregnancy-associated breast cancer is surgical resection, and resection can be offered during every trimester. Modified radical mastectomy classically has been the first choice for local control of breast cancer because it eliminates the need for adjuvant radiation and its risk to the fetus, but it is not mandatory especially when performed later in pregnancy. The combination of local control and adjuvant therapy may be tailored to the patient according to the stage of pregnancy as well as the stage of the cancer. Classically, in early pregnancy, mastectomy with axillary dissection is preferred for control and appropriate staging. However, at the present time, most breast surgeons avoid axillary dissection unless there are clinically positive nodes. After the first trimester, sentinel node biopsy poses potential risk to the fetus, but more recently it has been shown to be potentially safe. Supravital dyes, such as isosulfan blue dye, can potentially be used in the first trimester but should be used with extreme caution in pregnancy because of the potential for maternal anaphylaxis and pregnancy compromise.[26] Several studies on the use of technetium sulfur colloid for sentinel lymph node detection have been safely performed in pregnant women. Axillary lymph node dissection can be avoided in most pregnant women, especially after the first trimester, as a sentinel lymph node biopsy using technetium sulfur colloid can be recommended.[23]

Breast-conserving therapy is becoming an option for pregnant patients. In patients in whom breast cancer is diagnosed during the late second trimester or later, immediate breast-conserving lumpectomy and axillary dissection followed with radiation postpartum is a treatment option. If the diagnosis of breast cancer is made in the first or early second trimester of pregnancy, lumpectomy and axillary dissection can be followed by chemotherapy after the first trimester and radiation after delivery. Chemotherapy is indicated for node-positive cancers or node-negative tumors greater than 1 cm. Current chemotherapeutic regimens are relatively safe after the first trimester, when the teratogenic risk is greatest. Generally, treatment regimens are the same as for nonpregnant patients with dose alterations because the increased plasma volume, the hypoalbuminemia, and the fact that almost all chemotherapeutic agents cross the placenta change the pharmacokinetics of the drugs. Cytotoxic chemotherapy in the first 4 weeks of gestation results in no detrimental effect on the fetus or loss of the pregnancy. For the rest of the first trimester, at which time organogenesis is occurring, chemotherapy is thought to have a high risk for fetal malformation and is not recommended during this time. The risk of mutations appears to be worsened with the number of agents from 10% with single agents to 25% with multiagent regimens. During the second and third trimesters, chemotherapy has generally been shown to be safe with the risk of fetal malformations being 1.3%. However, chemotherapy during the last two trimesters is not benign, in that almost half of infants born to mothers undergoing chemotherapy have intrauterine growth retardation, prematurity, and low birth weight. Chemotherapy is generally not recommended after 35 weeks so as to reduce the likelihood of myelosuppression in the newborn after delivery.[24] Antimetabolites such as methotrexate should be avoided because of the high risk of spontaneous abortion even after the first trimester. Multiple studies have demonstrated treatment with fluorouracil, doxorubicin (Adriamycin), and cyclophosphamide to be safe. In general, most systemic chemotherapy regimens have been shown to be safe in pregnant women when administered after the first trimester, but patients with early-stage cancer have been shown to have no adverse outcome in delaying therapy until after birth to prevent the low-birth-weight effects on the fetus. Trastuzumab is not recommended during pregnancy because of increased neonatal death. Tamoxifen has shown increased rates of genital abnormalities in newborns and is not recommended in pregnancy.[23,26]

Radiation is typically not offered during pregnancy because of its teratogenic risk and its risk of induction of childhood malignancies. Although the fetal radiation exposure would be relatively low, there is a potential for adverse outcomes. The risk is directly related to dose and developmental stage. During the preimplantation stage and continuing to 15 weeks after conception, during organogenesis, the rapidly proliferating cells of the fetus are most sensitive to radiation, and exposure greater than 1 Gy during this period has a high likelihood of causing fetal death. The standard therapeutic course of 5000 rads (50 Gy) results in a varying exposure to the fetus, depending on the gestational age and proximity of the gravid uterus to the radiation bed. Even with abdominal shielding, the greatest fetal exposure is due to scatter. Although there are several case reports of healthy infants born after maternal radiation exposure, radiation is not recommended during pregnancy because of the risks to the fetus.[23,26]

Elective termination of the pregnancy to receive appropriate therapy without the risk of fetal malformation is no longer routinely recommended because no improvement in survival has been demonstrated. With the treatment options available to the pregnant patient with breast cancer, a combined approach involving the input of the patient, surgeon, oncologist, and maternal-fetal medicine specialist should ensure optimal treatment of the disease, while minimizing risk to the patient and the fetus. A suggested algorithm for the management of breast masses in pregnancy is shown in Figure 71-2.

HEPATOBILIARY DISEASE

Cholelithiasis

Most pregnant women with gallstones are asymptomatic. Although an estimated 2% to 4% of pregnant women may be found to have gallstones by ultrasound, only 0.05% to 0.1% of those women are symptomatic. The symptoms of biliary colic are the same in pregnant and nonpregnant patients. In patients with symptoms consistent with cholelithiasis, ultrasound is the diagnostic examination of choice. Ultrasound is as accurate in identifying gallstones and signs of inflammation in pregnant patients as it is in nonpregnant patients. Jaundice in pregnancy is usually not related to gallstones; it is associated with hepatitis in 45% of cases, benign cholestasis in 20% of cases, and choledocholithiasis in 7% of cases.[3,18]

Cholecystectomy for symptomatic cholelithiasis is second to appendectomy as the most common nonobstetric surgical procedure performed during pregnancy. Historically, pregnant patients with a clear operative indication, such as obstructive jaundice, gallstone pancreatitis, and choledocholithiasis, underwent cholecystectomy regardless of gestational age. Patients with recurrent biliary colic or acute cholecystitis that responded to medical management were treated expectantly until after delivery, at which time they underwent cholecystectomy. As it has become understood that adverse maternal and fetal outcomes are related more to the disease process and not the surgical intervention, management patterns have changed. Additionally, complications from nonoperative management of gallstone disease result in an increase in maternal and fetal mortality. With gallstone pancreatitis during pregnancy, maternal mortality of 15% and fetal mortality of 60% have been reported. In a study of 63 patients who were admitted with symptomatic cholelithiasis, surgical management reduced the need for labor induction, rate of preterm deliveries, and fetal mortality.[28] Surgical intervention should be considered as primary management of gallstones in pregnancy.

The timing of cholecystectomy for biliary colic depends on the gestational age and the severity of symptoms. A spontaneous abortion rate of 12% with open cholecystectomy during the first trimester decreases to 5.6% and 0% during the second and third

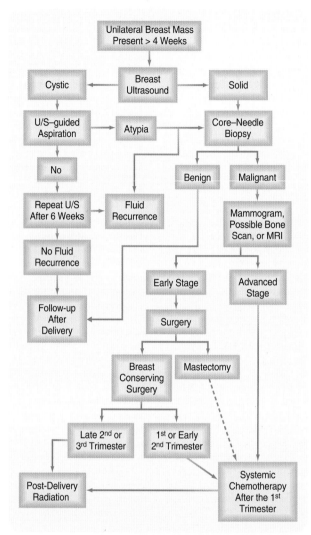

FIGURE 71-2 Algorithm for the management of a breast mass during pregnancy. *MRI*, Magnetic resonance imaging; *U/S*, ultrasound.

trimesters, respectively. The risk of preterm labor is nearly zero during the second trimester and 40% during the third trimester. The optimal time for cholecystectomy is the second trimester, when the risk of spontaneous abortion and preterm labor are the least, unless the patient develops a complication of cholelithiasis.[3]

Acute Pancreatitis

Acute pancreatitis occurs in 3 per 10,000 pregnancies. Gallstone pancreatitis has better outcomes than other causes. Gallstone pancreatitis is managed successfully with the same techniques as in nonpregnant patients, including ERCP with endoscopic sphincterotomy. Cholecystectomy is indicated in the presence of gallstones. The timing of operative intervention for complicated pancreatitis should follow the same guidelines used for nonpregnant patients.[3]

Liver

Liver abnormalities during pregnancy can be classified as occurring exclusively during pregnancy as a direct result of conditions during pregnancy, occurring simultaneously but not exclusively during pregnancy, or developing before the pregnancy. Examples of liver disorders unique to pregnancy include acute fatty liver of pregnancy; intrahepatic cholestasis of pregnancy; and liver disease related to preeclampsia or eclampsia, specifically HELLP syndrome and spontaneous hepatic hemorrhage or rupture. Pre-existing liver disorders that may manifest with complications during pregnancy include hepatic adenoma and hepatocellular carcinoma.

Acute Fatty Liver of Pregnancy

The cause of acute fatty liver of pregnancy is unknown, although it is more common in women with first pregnancies, women with twin pregnancies, and women who are pregnant with a male fetus. Although acute fatty liver of pregnancy has been diagnosed at 26 weeks of gestation, it usually occurs during the third trimester, typically at approximately 35 weeks of gestation. Acute fatty liver of pregnancy carries a 20% maternal and fetal mortality rate. Initial nonspecific symptoms, such as malaise, nausea, vomiting, and right upper quadrant pain, are followed by signs of significant liver dysfunction within 2 weeks of onset of symptoms. Progression to fulminant hepatic failure quickly leads to preterm labor and an increased risk of fetal mortality. Although there is no specific treatment for acute fatty liver of pregnancy, prompt delivery after diagnosis may prevent progression to fulminant hepatic failure and reduce the risk of fetal death. Liver function typically returns to normal after delivery.[3,29]

HELLP Syndrome

Approximately 10% of women with preeclampsia or eclampsia have associated liver involvement, ranging from severe elevation of hepatic enzymes to HELLP syndrome to hepatic rupture.[3] Hepatic hemorrhage or rupture occurs primarily during the third trimester or can develop up to 48 hours after delivery. Right upper quadrant pain is the initial manifestation, followed by hepatic tenderness, peritonitis, chest and right shoulder pain, or the development of hemodynamic instability within a few hours. The diagnosis should be suspected in a pregnant patient with preeclampsia who develops right upper quadrant pain. A CT scan of the abdomen is highly sensitive and specific in diagnosis; ultrasound findings are usually nonspecific and have a higher incidence of false-negative studies. The diagnosis may also be made during cesarean section. Management depends on suspicion of ongoing intraperitoneal hemorrhage or vascular instability. Hepatic hematomas without evidence of ongoing bleeding in hemodynamically stable patients may be managed nonoperatively with serial imaging and close monitoring, and these lesions typically heal without intervention. Hypotension indicates that rupture has occurred. If there is evidence or suspicion of rupture, immediate intervention is required because maternal and fetal mortality from hepatic hemorrhage is 60% and 85%, respectively. Immediate laparotomy with either abdominal packing or hepatic artery ligation reduces maternal and fetal mortality. Coagulopathy should be corrected aggressively. If the patient is relatively stable or abdominal packing has been unsuccessful in controlling hemorrhage, angiography with selective embolization may be performed. Angiography is most useful when the diagnosis is made postpartum.[29]

Hepatic Adenomas

Hepatic adenomas are uncommon, benign lesions that are usually associated with oral contraceptive use in young women.[26] Hepatic adenomas are also associated with glycogen storage disease, diabetes, exogenous steroids, and pregnancy. They are usually solitary lesions but may be multifocal, and they have a low potential for malignant transformation. Although the specific cause is unknown, it has been hypothesized that a change in hormone levels, specifically the sex steroids, leads to hepatotoxicity or exposes a hereditary defect in carbohydrate metabolism that results in hepatocyte hyperplasia and adenoma formation. The observation that adenomas may resolve after cessation of exogenous steroid or oral contraceptive use supports this hypothesis. The association of hepatic adenomas with pregnancy supports the hypothesis that elevated levels of endogenous hormones may contribute to adenoma formation, although no data exist showing regression of a hepatic adenoma after pregnancy. Similarly, the true incidence of hepatic adenomas during pregnancy is unknown. Diagnosis is best made with CT or MRI of the liver.

The major risk of a hepatic adenoma during pregnancy is spontaneous rupture, which carries a mortality rate of approximately 45% for both mother and fetus, even with operative intervention. When spontaneous rupture does occur, the presentation

may be similar to that described previously for hepatic hemorrhage associated with preeclampsia: right upper quadrant pain with referred right shoulder pain with progression to shock. Immediate laparotomy should be performed with cesarean section, control of hemorrhage, and resection of the adenoma if possible.[30]

Because of the high mortality rate associated with rupture of a hepatic adenoma, elective resection may be performed. Resection during the second trimester minimizes operative risk to the mother and fetus and does not interfere with the remainder of the pregnancy or subsequent pregnancies. Because of the unknown recurrence risk; however, subsequent pregnancy and oral contraceptive use may be discouraged in these patients.

ENDOCRINE DISEASE

Adrenal Disorders

Adrenal disorders in pregnancy are uncommon. Diagnosis and management of adrenal disorders are difficult because of the associated physiologic changes seen in pregnancy. Cushing syndrome is a common cause of endocrine dysfunction seen in pregnant patients.[31] The most common cause of Cushing syndrome in pregnancy is an adrenal adenoma. Other causes include pituitary conditions and adrenal carcinoma. Adrenal insufficiency is extremely rare during pregnancy. It is estimated that primary adrenal insufficiency is seen in 1 of 3000 pregnancies.[31]

Pheochromocytomas originate from chromaffin cells in the adrenal medulla or from extramedullary paraganglion cells. They are hormonally active tumors, secreting the catecholamines norepinephrine, epinephrine, and, less commonly, dopamine. Pheochromocytomas are usually described by the "rule of 10," which states that 10% of pheochromocytomas are extra-adrenal, 10% are bilateral, 10% are malignant, and 10% are familial. These tumors can occur sporadically or as part of a syndrome, such as multiple endocrine neoplasia type 2a, multiple endocrine neoplasia type 2b, or von Hippel-Lindau disease.

Although pheochromocytomas are uncommon in pregnancy with an incidence of 0.007%, they have devastating effects for both the mother and the fetus.[32] Pheochromocytomas that remain undiagnosed during pregnancy have a postpartum maternal mortality rate of 15%, with fetal mortality also exceeding 25%. The greatest risk occurs from the onset of labor to 48 hours after delivery. The index of suspicion should be high in any patient with preeclampsia, paroxysmal hypertension, or unexplained fever after delivery. With diagnosis and appropriate treatment, maternal mortality is reduced to nearly 0%, and fetal mortality is decreased to 15%.[32] The diagnosis is made by elevated urine catecholamines; urinary catecholamines in a pregnant patient without a pheochromocytoma are the same as in a nonpregnant patient. Lack of proteinuria also helps eliminate preeclampsia as a cause of hypertension. Metaiodobenzylguanidine imaging is not recommended during pregnancy because the small molecule may cross the placenta; use of metaiodobenzylguanidine imaging has not been evaluated in pregnancy.

Surgical resection should be performed before 20 weeks of gestation, when spontaneous abortion is less likely and the size of the gravid uterus does not interfere with the procedure. If the diagnosis is made late in the second trimester or during the third trimester, medical management followed by combined cesarean section and resection of the pheochromocytoma may be an option. It is unknown if the standard preoperative management in nonpregnant patients with alpha blockade or calcium channel blockade followed by perioperative beta blockade is safe during pregnancy. The long-term effects of the alpha blocker phenoxybenzamine on the fetus have not been determined, although calcium channel blockers are safe to use during pregnancy. Beta blockers are frequently used during pregnancy with close monitoring for intrauterine growth retardation. Consultation with a maternal-fetal medicine specialist is essential to determine the preoperative management that will ensure the optimal postoperative result for the patient and the fetus. In nonpregnant patients, the management approach depends on suspected malignancy, unilateral versus bilateral tumors, extra-adrenal location, size of the tumor, and surgeon's preference and experience. In all series comparing the different approaches, including open versus laparoscopic technique, pregnant patients were not included.

Thyroid

Thyroid diseases during pregnancy can be categorized into three groups: hypothyroidism, hyperthyroidism, and thyroid cancer. Hypothyroidism is found in 3% to 15% of pregnancies.[33] Of these, only 20% to 30% of patients develop symptoms. The first step is to obtain a serum TSH concentration to help categorize primary hypothyroidism versus hypothyroidism resulting from pituitary or hypothalamic causes. Current guidelines from Lebeau and Mandel for treatment of hypothyroidism during pregnancy are as follows:

1. Check serum TSH.
2. Initial levothyroxine dosage is based on severity of symptoms. Levothyroxine should be started at 1.2 mcg/kg/day for subclinical hypothyroidism with TSH less than 4.2 mlIU/L, 1.42 mcg/kg/day with TSH greater than 4.2 to 10, and 2.33 mcg/kg/day for overt hypothyroidism.[33a]
3. For previously diagnosed hypothyroidism, monitor TSH every 3 to 4 weeks.
4. Goal TSH level is less than 2.5 mU/liter.
5. Monitor serum TSH and total every 3 to 4 weeks with each dose change.

The incidence of hyperthyroidism during pregnancy is less than 0.5%.[34] Gestational thyrotoxicosis is a multifactorial phenomenon. High serum concentrations of hCG during pregnancy activate the TSH receptors. Elevated serum-free T_4 and low-serum TSH levels are seen with this form of thyrotoxicosis. Gestational thyrotoxicosis is usually self-limiting and spontaneously resolves by 20 weeks of gestation, when the hCG level declines. Repeat evaluation is warranted if thyrotoxicosis persists. Most cases of hyperthyroidism are a result of Graves disease. When the diagnosis is made, medical treatment with thionamides (propylthiouracil and methimazole) is the mainstay of treatment. Iodides should be avoided except in patients preparing for thyroidectomy during pregnancy. The dosage of methimazole sufficient to control hyperthyroidism is 15-100 mg daily, administered as divided doses 3 times daily. The appropriate dosage of PTU can range from 300 mg daily to a maximum dose of 1200 mg daily in divided doses 3 times daily. Once serum thyroid hormone levels return to normal, it is necessary to decrease the dosage to 5-20 mg daily of methimazole or 50-300 mg daily for PTU in divided doses. When doses of PTU are >300 mg/day or >20 mg/day for methimazole are taken long term, fetal goiter and hypothyroidism may result. Subtotal thyroidectomy for Graves disease should be reserved for patients who are consistently receiving high-dose propylthiouracil (>600 mg/day) or methimazole (>40 mg/day), are allergic to thionamides, are noncompliant, or experiencing compressive symptoms as a result of goiter size. Surgery should be performed during

the second trimester before 24 weeks to minimize the risk of miscarriage. A 2-week course of a β-adrenergic agent, along with potassium iodide, should be implemented before surgery to minimize perioperative complications. Radioactive iodine therapy is contraindicated during pregnancy.

Thyroid nodules may have a higher prevalence during pregnancy as a result of hormonal changes, but thyroid cancers do not. Traditional workup of thyroid cancers should be done during pregnancy. Fine-needle aspiration, along with ultrasound evaluation, remains the cornerstone of diagnosis. If cytology shows thyroid cancer, surgery is recommended during the second trimester, before 24 weeks. If thyroid cancer is found after the second half of pregnancy, surgery can be performed after delivery. Postoperative radioactive iodine therapy should also be delayed until after delivery.

SMALL BOWEL OBSTRUCTION

Intestinal obstruction is the third most common nonobstetric surgical emergency condition in pregnancy, after acute appendicitis and acute cholecystitis. The incidence of small bowel obstruction during pregnancy is estimated at 1 in 4000 live births.[35] Small bowel obstructions usually occur during the second and third trimesters. Adhesions resulting from prior abdominal and pelvic surgeries are the most frequent causes for intestinal obstruction in pregnancy, accounting for 53% to 59% of cases. Other causes of small bowel obstruction in pregnant patients include volvulus, intussusception, malignancy, and hernia, although the displacement of the small bowel out of the pelvis by the enlarging uterus makes this a rare cause.

The symptoms of an obstruction are identical to symptoms in nonpregnant patients and consist of the triad of abdominal pain, vomiting, and obstipation. Pain, present in 85% to 98% of cases, is usually colicky in nature and located in the midabdomen, although the character and duration are highly variable. Nausea and vomiting are seen in 80% of pregnant patients with small bowel obstruction; however, nausea and vomiting are common during the first trimester of normal pregnancy. Nausea and vomiting that persist or begin later in pregnancy should arouse suspicion and be evaluated. Bowel distention may be marked but difficult to assess because of the gravid uterus. The diagnosis is made by serial examination and plain abdominal radiograph.

Treatment for small bowel obstruction in pregnancy is identical to treatment in a nonpregnant patient. Therapy consists of nasogastric decompression and intravenous fluids. However, a lower threshold for operative management is necessary. If there is no satisfactory patient response after 6 to 8 hours of nonoperative treatment, a laparotomy should be performed before perforation or bowel necrosis occurs. Maternal mortality ranges from 6% to 20% because of sepsis and multisystem organ failure, and fetal loss is 26% to 50%.[35] To avoid the risk to the mother and fetus, a more aggressive approach should be used.

Midgut volvulus accounts for 25% of small bowel obstructions in pregnancy, and it is a difficult diagnosis. It should be treated during the postpartum period. Midgut volvulus is usually more common in a pregnant patient if she has undergone previous abdominal surgery; however, spontaneous midgut volvulus may occur. A case of maternal death caused by midgut volvulus after bariatric surgery was reported.[36] The key is increased vigilance for all the individuals involved in the patient's care. Early exploration is warranted if the diagnosis is unclear.

INFLAMMATORY BOWEL DISEASE

Although some studies report adverse obstetric outcomes with inflammatory bowel disease, the effect of ulcerative colitis or Crohn's disease on pregnancy characteristically depends on the severity of the disease at the time of conception. Management differs in pregnancy.[37]

Ulcerative Colitis

Patients in remission at conception are likely to remain so during the pregnancy. Relapse occurs in up to one third of patients usually in the first trimester. Because of the potential for pregnancy-induced exacerbation, pregnancy should be delayed in patients with active disease until they are in remission.

Crohn's Disease

Crohn's disease follows a course similar to ulcerative colitis. Complications are similar to complications in a nonpregnant patient with the exception of the unusual occurrence of an enterouterine fistula. If there is active Crohn's disease, pregnant patients have an increased incidence of premature delivery and infants with low birth weight. Extensive perianal involvement may warrant a cesarean section to avoid a complicated perineal fistula.

Surgery

If there is a significant exacerbation of the disease, surgery may be necessary. The indications for surgery are the same as in nonpregnant patients. Surgery in the second trimester is preferred. If fulminant colitis develops, a proctocolectomy with end ileostomy is preferred. Ileostomy issues may evolve as the patient gains weight, including stomal retraction, prolapse, or hernia. Preoperative consultation with an enterostomal therapist is advisable.

COLON AND RECTUM

Appendicitis

Acute appendicitis is the most common nonobstetric surgical emergency in pregnant patients, occurring in 1 in 1500 pregnancies.[35] Acute appendicitis is more common in the first two trimesters with an incidence of 32%, 42%, and 26% in the first, second, and third trimesters.[38] Timely and accurate diagnosis is challenging because the typical clinical findings of nausea, vomiting, abdominal pain, and mild leukocytosis may be findings in a normal pregnancy. Delay in diagnosis results in an increased perforation rate of 10%; this has significant consequences for the patient and fetus. Fetal mortality increases from 1.5% in acute appendicitis to 35% in perforated appendicitis.[38] Preterm labor and premature delivery rates are 40% in cases of perforated appendicitis compared with a 13% rate of preterm labor and 4% rate of premature delivery in cases of acute appendicitis.[38,39]

In 1932, Baer studied 78 normal pregnant women with radiographic studies at regular intervals from the second month of pregnancy to 10 days postpartum. As the uterus enlarges, the appendix is driven upward with a counterclockwise rotation. Baer concluded that early in pregnancy, pain is low, and that as the gestation progresses, pain is located higher in the abdomen.[40] A review of 45 pregnant patients with acute appendicitis demonstrated that pain in the right lower quadrant is the most common symptom, regardless of gestational age (first trimester, 86%; second trimester, 83%; third trimester, 85%).[39] Despite the inconsistency, acute appendicitis should be included in the differential diagnosis of every pregnant woman who presents with right-sided abdominal pain. The treatment for suspected acute appendicitis in the pregnant patient is emergent appendectomy. Although helical CT scans have demonstrated greater than 90% sensitivity and specificity in the diagnosis of acute appendicitis, few data are available in pregnant patients. In nonpregnant patients, a 10% to 15% negative laparotomy rate is considered acceptable. Because of the increased risk to both the mother and the fetus with appendiceal perforation, a negative rate of 30% to 33% is acceptable during pregnancy. The debate is then between open versus laparoscopic technique. The argument for open appendectomy is that the laparoscopic approach exposes the fetus to the risks of pneumoperitoneum and trocar placement without the benefit of a significantly smaller incision. The laparoscopic technique enables examination of a larger portion of the abdomen with less uterine manipulation and allows localization of the appendix as it is pushed into the right upper quadrant by the enlarging uterus.

Colonic Pseudo-obstruction

Colonic pseudo-obstruction, or Ogilvie syndrome, is a functional obstruction, or adynamic ileus, without a mechanical cause. Postpartum patients account for 10% of all cases of Ogilvie syndrome. It is characterized by massive abdominal distention with cecal dilation. Although neostigmine is an effective first-line therapy in nonpregnant patients, its safety in pregnancy is unknown. It can be used safely in the postpartum period. Colonoscopic decompression has been described in postpartum patients, with laparotomy indicated only in suspected perforation.[41]

Colon Cancer

The incidence of colon cancer is 1 in 50,000 pregnancies. The diagnosis is often delayed. Treatment follows similar guidelines as treatment in nonpregnant patients with the following exceptions. Carcinoembryonic antigen is not helpful. Neoadjuvant treatment of rectal cancer is avoided. In the presence of a large rectal lesion, cesarean section is advisable. Pregnancy does not in itself alter the maternal prognosis of colorectal cancer.[42]

VASCULAR DISEASE

Ruptured splenic artery aneurysm in a pregnant patient is rare, but the rate of maternal and fetal survival is very poor.[43] Ruptures usually occur during the third trimester, and it is typically misdiagnosed as splenic rupture or uterine rupture. Maternal mortality can be 75% with a fetal mortality of 95%. Increased portal pressures, high splenic artery flow as a result of distal aortic compression, and progressive arterial wall weakening are contributing factors. Multiparity may increase the risk. Most patients who survive a rupture experience a "two-stage rupture," in which the lesser sac temporarily tamponades the bleeding aneurysm.

When ruptured splenic artery aneurysm is treated electively in nonpregnant patients, mortality is only 0.5% to 1.3%. When the diagnosis is made in a woman of childbearing age or in a pregnant patient, a splenic artery aneurysm of 2 cm or larger should be treated electively because of the increased risk of rupture during pregnancy.[44]

Acute iliofemoral venous thrombosis is six times more frequent among pregnant patients compared with nonpregnant patients. Pregnancy may increase the risk of thrombosis through many factors, including mechanical obstruction of venous drainage by the enlarging uterus, decreased activity in late pregnancy and at time of delivery, intimal injury from vascular distention or surgical manipulation during cesarean section, and abnormal levels of coagulation factors already described.[45] Additionally, a wide spectrum of pathologic abnormalities, such as the presence of lupus anticoagulant antibodies and deficiencies of proteins C and S, may further increase the risk of thrombotic disease. Protein S serves as a cofactor for activated protein C, which has anticoagulant activity. A deficiency of protein S leads to spontaneous, recurrent thromboembolic complications in nonpregnant adults. Even in normal individuals, protein S levels are substantially reduced during pregnancy.

The management of acute iliofemoral venous thrombosis during pregnancy is controversial because thrombolytic therapy poses hazards to the fetus. The risk of pulmonary thromboembolism with manipulation of the clot during thrombectomy would have catastrophic effects on both the mother and the fetus. Techniques that have been described include interruption of the inferior vena cava via a right retroperitoneal approach or interruption of the inferior vena cava by passage of a Fogarty catheter through the unaffected contralateral femoral vein. The disadvantage of the retroperitoneal approach is that an extensive dissection is required. The disadvantages of the Fogarty catheter are that the catheter may still dislodge clots that have extended into the vena cava and that once the catheter is removed, an inferior vena cava filter must still be placed. However, the most effective technique is filter placement in the inferior vena cava via the internal jugular vein using ultrasound guidance, followed by thrombectomy.[46]

TRAUMA IN PREGNANCY

Trauma is the leading nonobstetric cause of maternal mortality and occurs in approximately 1 in 12 pregnancies.[47] The most common mechanisms of injury are from falls or from motor vehicle crashes.[45] Compared with age-matched pregnant controls, pregnant women who sustained trauma had a higher incidence of spontaneous abortion, preterm labor, fetomaternal hemorrhage, abruptio placentae, and uterine rupture.[48] Multiple studies have attempted to identify risk factors that predict morbidity and mortality in the pregnant trauma patient. The maternal Injury Severity Score, mechanism of injury, and physical findings are unable to adequately predict adverse outcomes such as abruptio placentae and fetal loss. Early involvement of an obstetrician in the care of an injured pregnant patient is important to evaluate both maternal and fetal well-being.

In the management of a pregnant trauma patient, the critical point is that resuscitation of the fetus is accomplished by resuscitation of the mother. Fetal outcomes are directly related and correlate with the state of maternal resuscitation. Therefore, the initial evaluation and treatment of an injured pregnant patient is identical to that of a nonpregnant patient. Maternal and fetal hypoxia is avoided through rapid assessment and a precise primary survey that includes the maternal airway, breathing, and circulation and ensuring an adequate airway. In the later stages of pregnancy, as already described, uterine compression of the vena cava may result in hypotension from diminished venous return, so a pregnant trauma patient should be placed in left lateral decubitus position. Women in late pregnancy may have difficult airways. Prolonged ventilation can significantly increase the risk of aspiration.[45] If spinal cord injury is suspected, the patient may be secured to a backboard and then tilted to the left.

The increased blood volume associated with pregnancy has important implications in a trauma patient. Signs of blood loss such as tachycardia and hypotension may be delayed until the patient loses nearly 30% of her blood volume. As a result, the fetus may be experiencing hypoperfusion long before the mother manifests any signs. Early and rapid fluid resuscitation should be administered even in a pregnant patient who is normotensive. If an emergent blood transfusion is warranted, Rh-negative blood should be administered.[45]

Along with the primary survey, the secondary survey should proceed in a similar fashion as in a nonpregnant patient. Special attention should be given to the abdominal examination. The uterus remains protected by the pelvis until approximately 12 weeks of gestation and is relatively well sheltered from abdominal injury until that time. As the uterus grows, it becomes more prominent and more vulnerable to injury. Measurement of fundal height provides a rapid approximation of gestational age. At 20 weeks of gestation, the fundal height should be at the level of the umbilicus and should be approximately 1 cm above the umbilicus per week of gestation. Intrauterine hemorrhage or uterine rupture may result in a discrepancy in measurement. Fetal monitoring should be done as soon as the primary survey is complete. A pelvic examination should be performed, by an obstetrician if possible to evaluate for vaginal bleeding, ruptured membranes, or a bulging perineum. Vaginal bleeding may indicate abruptio placentae, placenta previa, or preterm labor. Rupture of the amniotic fluid may result in umbilical cord prolapse, which compresses the umbilical vessels and compromises fetal blood flow. Immediate cesarean section is required. If cloudy white or greenish fluid is seen from the cervical os or perineum, the presence of amniotic fluid is confirmed by Nitrazine paper, which changes from green to blue.

The Kleihauer-Betke test for the assessment of fetomaternal transfusion is useful after maternal trauma and should be ordered with the initial laboratory studies that include a type and crossmatch. Because of the sensitivity of the Kleihauer-Betke test, a small amount of fetomaternal transfusion may be undetected. Therefore, all Rh-negative pregnant trauma patients should be considered for Rh immunoglobulin (RhoGAM) therapy.

Diagnostic radiologic testing in a pregnant patient should be completed if clinically indicated. Ultrasound should be the first imaging modality, followed by judicial use of x-rays and CT scans. CT scan should be considered if there are no other modalities to diagnose a suspected injury.

The most common cause of fetal death after blunt injury is abruptio placentae. Deceleration of the fetal heart rate may be the earliest sign of abruption. The uterus should be evaluated for contractions, rupture, or abruptio placentae. Early initiation of cardiotocographic fetal monitoring adequately warns of deterioration in the condition of the fetus.

SUMMARY

Pregnant patients are susceptible to the same surgical diseases as nonpregnant patients of similar age. Maternal physiologic changes and the enlarging uterus may result in atypical presentation of surgical disease, or symptoms may be attributed to normal pregnancy. A delay in diagnosis and treatment of surgical illnesses in pregnancy poses a greater risk to maternal and fetal well-being than the risks of anesthesia or of surgical intervention. Early consultation with an obstetrician, maternal-fetal medicine specialist, and perinatologist can ensure optimal outcomes and avoid pitfalls. Laparoscopy is becoming increasingly accepted in pregnant patients, and it is hoped that future advances will make it even safer for obstetric patients. Prevention of preterm labor should be individualized based on the patient's gestational age and underlying disease process.

SELECTED REFERENCES

Amant F, Loibl S, Neven P, et al: Breast cancer in pregnancy. *Lancet* 379:570–579, 2012.

This current and comprehensive review of breast cancer in pregnancy includes ongoing trends in treatment.

Babler EA: Perforative appendicitis complicating pregnancy. *JAMA* 51:1310, 1908.

This landmark article contains the first description of appendicitis in pregnancy.

Baer JL: Appendicitis in pregnancy. *JAMA* 98:1359, 1932.

This landmark article illustrates the change in appendiceal location during pregnancy.

Brodsky JB, Cohen EN, Brown BW, Jr, et al: Surgery during pregnancy and fetal outcome. *Am J Obstet Gynecol* 138:1165, 1980.

This large series was the first to look at fetal outcomes in nonobstetric surgery.

Cohen-Kerem R, Railton C, Oren D, et al: Pregnancy outcome following non-obstetric surgical intervention. *Am J Surg* 190:3, 2005.

This large series looked at nonobstetric surgical pregnancy outcomes in 12,452 patients reported in 44 articles. The maternal death rate was 0.006%, and the miscarriage rate was 5.8%.

LeBeau SO, Mandel SJ: Thyroid disorders during pregnancy. *Endocrinol Metab Clin North Am* 35:117–136, 2006.

This article is a comprehensive review of all the major thyroid abnormalities that occur during pregnancy.

Mourad J, Elliott JP, Erickson L, et al: Appendicitis in pregnancy: New information that contradicts longheld clinical beliefs. *Am J Obstet Gynecol* 182:1027, 2000.

This article, which retrospectively reviewed more than 66,000 deliveries and found 45 pregnant patients with appendicitis, challenged the original landmark paper by Baer regarding the presentation of acute appendicitis in pregnant patients.

Pearl J, Price R, Richardson W, et al: Guidelines for diagnosis, treatment, and use of laparoscopy for surgical problems during pregnancy. *Surg Endosc* 25:3479–3492, 2011.

This article presents current guidelines from the Society of American Gastrointestinal Endoscopic Surgeons regarding laparoscopy in pregnancy.

Tarraza HM, Moore RD: Gynecologic causes of the acute abdomen and the acute abdomen in pregnancy. *Surg Clin North Am* 77:1371, 1997.

This review accurately describes the increased risk to the mother and fetus resulting from the underlying pathology as opposed to the risk imposed by surgical intervention.

REFERENCES

1. Cohen-Kerem R, Railton C, Oren D, et al: Pregnancy outcome following non-obstetric surgical intervention. *Am J Surg* 190:467–473, 2005.
2. Tan EK, Tan EL: Alterations in physiology and anatomy during pregnancy. *Best Pract Res Clin Obstet Gynaecol* 27:791–802, 2013.
3. Boregowda G, Shehata HA: Gastrointestinal and liver disease in pregnancy. *Best Pract Res Clin Obstet Gynaecol* 27:835–853, 2013.
4. Costantine MM: Physiologic and pharmacokinetic changes in pregnancy. *Front Pharmacol* 5:65, 2014.
5. Melchiorre K, Sharma R, Thilaganathan B: Cardiac structure and function in normal pregnancy. *Curr Opin Obstet Gynecol* 24:413–421, 2012.
6. Lohr JM, Bush RL: Venous disease in women: Epidemiology, manifestations, and treatment. *J Vasc Surg* 57:37S–45S, 2013.
7. ESHRE Capri Workshop Group: Venous thromboembolism in women: A specific reproductive health risk. *Hum Reprod Update* 19:471–482, 2013.
8. Duthie L, Reynolds RM: Changes in the maternal hypothalamic-pituitary-adrenal axis in pregnancy and post-partum: Influences on maternal and fetal outcomes. *Neuroendocrinology* 98:106–115, 2013.
9. Budenhofer BK, Ditsch N, Jeschke U, et al: Thyroid (dys-) function in normal and disturbed pregnancy. *Arch Gynecol Obstet* 287:1–7, 2013.
10. Wang PI, Chong ST, Kielar AZ, et al: Imaging of pregnant and lactating patients: Part 1, evidence-based review and recommendations. *AJR Am J Roentgenol* 198:778–784, 2012.
11. Goodman TR, Amurao M: Medical imaging radiation safety for the female patient: Rationale and implementation. *Radiographics* 32:1829–1837, 2012.
12. Abramowicz JS: Benefits and risks of ultrasound in pregnancy. *Semin Perinatol* 37:295–300, 2013.
13. Friedel D, Stavropoulos S, Iqbal S, et al: Gastrointestinal endoscopy in the pregnant woman. *World J Gastrointest Endosc* 6:156–167, 2014.
14. Reitman E, Flood P: Anaesthetic considerations for non-obstetric surgery during pregnancy. *Br J Anaesth* 107(Suppl 1):i72–i78, 2011.
15. Palanisamy A: Maternal anesthesia and fetal neurodevelopment. *Int J Obstet Anesth* 21:152–162, 2012.
16. Moaveni DM, Birnbach DJ, Ranasinghe JS, et al: Fetal assessment for anesthesiologists: Are you evaluating the other patient? *Anesth Analg* 116:1278–1292, 2013.

17. Bloor M, Paech M: Nonsteroidal anti-inflammatory drugs during pregnancy and the initiation of lactation. *Anesth Analg* 116:1063–1075, 2013.

18. Evans SR, Sarani B, Bhanot P, et al: Surgery in pregnancy. *Curr Probl Surg* 49:333–388, 2012.

19. Corneille MG, Gallup TM, Bening T, et al: The use of laparoscopic surgery in pregnancy: Evaluation of safety and efficacy. *Am J Surg* 200:363–367, 2010.

20. Germain A, Brunaud L: Visceral surgery and pregnancy. *J Visc Surg* 147:e129–e135, 2010.

21. Pearl J, Price R, Richardson W, et al: Guidelines for diagnosis, treatment, and use of laparoscopy for surgical problems during pregnancy. *Surg Endosc* 25:3479–3492, 2011.

22. Azim HA, Jr, Santoro L, Russell-Edu W, et al: Prognosis of pregnancy-associated breast cancer: A meta-analysis of 30 studies. *Cancer Treat Rev* 38:834–842, 2012.

23. Amant F, Loibl S, Neven P, et al: Breast cancer in pregnancy. *Lancet* 379:570–579, 2012.

24. Brewer M, Kueck A, Runowicz CD: Chemotherapy in pregnancy. *Clin Obstet Gynecol* 54:602–618, 2011.

25. Woo JC, Yu T, Hurd TC: Breast cancer in pregnancy: A literature review. *Arch Surg* 138:91–98; discussion 99, 2003.

26. Viswanathan S, Ramaswamy B: Pregnancy-associated breast cancer. *Clin Obstet Gynecol* 54:546–555, 2011.

27. Cardoso F, Loibl S, Pagani O, et al: The European Society of Breast Cancer Specialists recommendations for the management of young women with breast cancer. *Eur J Cancer* 48:3355–3377, 2012.

28. Lu EJ, Curet MJ, El-Sayed YY, et al: Medical versus surgical management of biliary tract disease in pregnancy. *Am J Surg* 188:755–759, 2004.

29. Joshi D, James A, Quaglia A, et al: Liver disease in pregnancy. *Lancet* 375:594–605, 2010.

30. Almashhrawi AA, Ahmed KT, Rahman RN, et al: Liver diseases in pregnancy: Diseases not unique to pregnancy. *World J Gastroenterol* 19:7630–7638, 2013.

31. Lekarev O, New MI: Adrenal disease in pregnancy. *Best Pract Res Clin Endocrinol Metab* 25:959–973, 2011.

32. Abdelmannan D, Aron DC: Adrenal disorders in pregnancy. *Endocrinol Metab Clin North Am* 40:779–794, 2011.

33. Negro R, Stagnaro-Green A: Diagnosis and management of subclinical hypothyroidism in pregnancy. *BMJ* 349:g4929, 2014.

33a. Abalovich M, Vázquez A, Alcaraz G, et al: Adequate levothyroxine doses for the treatment of hypothyroidism newly discovered during pregnancy. *Thyroid* 23:1479–1483, 2013. doi: 10.1089/thy.2013.0024.

34. Lazarus JH: Management of hyperthyroidism in pregnancy. *Endocrine* 45:190–194, 2014.

35. Miloudi N, Brahem M, Ben Abid S, et al: Acute appendicitis in pregnancy: Specific features of diagnosis and treatment. *J Visc Surg* 149:e275–e279, 2012.

36. Loar PV, 3rd, Sanchez-Ramos L, Kaunitz AM, et al: Maternal death caused by midgut volvulus after bariatric surgery. *Am J Obstet Gynecol* 193:1748–1749, 2005.

37. Friedman S, McElrath TF, Wolf JL: Management of fertility and pregnancy in women with inflammatory bowel disease: A practical guide. *Inflamm Bowel Dis* 19:2937–2948, 2013.

38. Gilo NB, Amini D, Landy HJ: Appendicitis and cholecystitis in pregnancy. *Clin Obstet Gynecol* 52:586–596, 2009.

39. Walker HG, Al Samaraee A, Mills SJ, et al: Laparoscopic appendicectomy in pregnancy: A systematic review of the published evidence. *Int J Surg* 12:1235–1241, 2014.

40. Baer JL: Appendicitis in pregnancy. *JAMA* 98:1359, 1932.

41. Kim TH, Lee HH, Chung SH: Constipation during pregnancy: When a typical symptom heralds a serious disease. *Obstet Gynecol* 119:374–378, 2012.

42. Saif MW: Management of colorectal cancer in pregnancy: A multimodality approach. *Clin Colorectal Cancer* 5:247–256, 2005.

43. Nanez L, Knowles M, Modrall JG, et al: Ruptured splenic artery aneurysms are exceedingly rare in pregnant women. *J Vasc Surg* 60:1520–1523, 2014.

44. Aubrey-Bassler FK, Sowers N: 613 cases of splenic rupture without risk factors or previously diagnosed disease: A systematic review. *BMC Emerg Med* 12:11, 2012.

45. Raja AS, Zabbo CP: Trauma in pregnancy. *Emerg Med Clin North Am* 30:937–948, 2012.

46. Koh MB, Lao ZT, Rhodes E: Managing haematological disorders during pregnancy. *Best Pract Res Clin Obstet Gynaecol* 27:855–865, 2013.

47. Mendez-Figueroa H, Dahlke JD, Vrees RA, et al: Trauma in pregnancy: An updated systematic review. *Am J Obstet Gynecol* 209:1–10, 2013.

48. John PR, Shiozawa A, Haut ER, et al: An assessment of the impact of pregnancy on trauma mortality. *Surgery* 149:94–98, 2011.

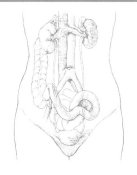

CHAPTER 72

Urologic Surgery

Thomas Gillispie Smith III, Michael Coburn

第七十二章　泌尿外科

OUTLINE

Urologic Anatomy for the General Surgeon
Endoscopic Urologic Surgery
Urologic Infectious Disease
Voiding Dysfunction, Neurogenic Bladder, Incontinence, and Benign Prostatic Hyperplasia
Male Reproductive Medicine and Sexual Dysfunction
Urolithiasis
Urologic Trauma
Nontraumatic Urologic Emergencies
Urologic Oncology

中文导读

　　本章共分为9节：①泌尿系统解剖；②泌尿外科内镜；③泌尿系统感染性疾病；④排尿功能障碍、神经源性膀胱、尿失禁与良性前列腺增生症；⑤男性生殖医学与性功能障碍性疾病；⑥尿石症；⑦泌尿系统损伤；⑧非创伤性泌尿外科急症；⑨泌尿系统肿瘤。

　　第一节介绍了腹膜后及盆腔的泌尿系统各器官的解剖（包括肾上腺、肾脏、输尿管、膀胱、前列腺、尿道、男性生殖器及会阴）。

　　第二节介绍了泌尿外科常用的内镜设备（包括硬性/软性膀胱镜、输尿管硬镜、输尿管软镜、经皮肾镜、导丝和输尿管支架）的各种尺寸以及在临床诊断治疗工作中的具体用途。

　　第三节介绍了泌尿系统各种感染性疾病的诊断及具体治疗方法，包括单纯性尿路感染、复杂性尿路感染、男性生殖系统感染以及非典型性感染（如真菌、结核以及寄生虫）。

　　第四节介绍了神经源性膀胱、膀胱过度活动症、尿失禁和良性前列腺增生症的发病机制，以及各种泌尿外科的具体诊断和治疗方法。

　　第五节介绍了男性不育和性功能障碍的病因（先天性的解剖异常、环境及行为因素的影响和医源性因素）诊断评估、药物治疗及外科治疗的方法。

第六节介绍了尿石症的流行病学、发病机制、结石的分类、临床代谢评估、临床诊断及治疗的各种具体方法（包括药物治疗、体外冲击波碎石、输尿管镜碎石以及经皮肾镜手术）。

第七节介绍了肾脏损伤、输尿管损伤、膀胱损伤、尿道及生殖系统损伤的诊断评估、临床分级、各种手术以及非手术的标准治疗流程、处理原则及最佳手术时机选择的策略。其中重点介绍了在处理各种复杂的泌尿系统急性损伤时泌尿外科医生与普通创伤外科医生之间的合作。

第八节介绍了各种非创伤原因引起的泌尿外科常见急症的处理原则和方法，如睾丸扭转、严重肉眼血尿导致的急性尿潴留以及阴茎异常勃起等。

第九节重点介绍了各种泌尿系统肿瘤（包括肾细胞癌、膀胱癌、前列腺癌及睾丸癌）的流行病学、病理分类、临床分期分级、手术以及非手术治疗方法的选择。其中重点介绍了当肿瘤处于不同时期时该如何选择合适的治疗手段以及不同类型肿瘤的预后。

〔陈志强〕

Urology is the study, treatment, and surgery of diseases of the retroperitoneum, pelvis, and male genitalia. Of the subspecialties, urology shares the most in common with general surgery because of our operative approaches and techniques (both open and minimally invasive) in the abdomen, retroperitoneum, and pelvis. Like general surgeons, urologists treat patients with open, laparoscopic, robotic, and endoscopic techniques. Frequently, urologists and general surgeons collaborate in care of patients across our many interdisciplinary subspecialties. Examples of this include the stress of major trauma surgery, complexity of exenterative surgery for advanced pelvic malignant neoplasms, management of iatrogenic urologic and surgical injury, and challenges of necrotizing infections of the genitalia and perineum.

General surgeons will encounter patients with urologic conditions as either presenting symptoms of or comorbidities to their general surgical diseases. Urology itself has multiple subspecialties and treats a wide range of patients and diseases spanning pediatrics, stone disease, and oncology. The intent of this chapter is to give the practicing surgeon and trainee a broad overview of the field of urology and to impart a fundamental knowledge of our field to assist in our common goal of surgical care of the patient.

UROLOGIC ANATOMY FOR THE GENERAL SURGEON

The organs of the genitourinary system span the entire retroperitoneum, pelvis, inguinal region, and genital region. Because of the close anatomic relationships of the organs in the abdomen and retroperitoneum, general surgeons must be familiar with all of the urologic organ systems to prevent iatrogenic injury and to deal with variations in normal anatomy. These challenges arise in many fields of surgery, including vascular, oncology, and colorectal surgery.

Upper Abdomen and Retroperitoneum
Adrenal

Beginning at the most superior aspect of the retroperitoneum lie the adrenal glands. These small, paired organs have two different embryologic origins and serve a primary endocrine function. The adrenal glands are composed of the cortex and medulla and are fused after development. The cortex is the outer layer of the adrenal gland and is derived from mesoderm.[1] On cross section, the layers, from external to internal, are the zona glomerulosa, zona fasciculata, and zona reticularis. The different zones secrete various steroid-derived hormones including mineralocorticoids (glomerulosa), glucocorticoids (fasciculata), and sex steroids (reticularis).[2] The adrenal medulla is derived from neural crest cells and is directly innervated by presynaptic sympathetic fibers.[1] The medulla is responsible for secreting catecholamines in response to sympathetic stimulation. The adrenal glands lie within Gerota fascia and have an orange-yellow appearance and an area of usually 3 to 5 cm in transverse diameter.[1] The arterial supply is through three sources: superior—inferior phrenic; medial—abdominal aorta; and inferior—ipsilateral renal artery. The venous drainage does not mirror the arterial supply; on the right, the single adrenal vein drains to the vena cava, whereas on the left, the adrenal vein drains into the left renal vein. Supernumerary veins can exist on either side because of anatomic variation. The adrenal glands are anatomically distinct from the kidney, although there are ventral and dorsal fascial investments that connect it to the kidney. The anatomic relations to the right adrenal gland are the vena cava on the anteromedial aspect and the liver and duodenum on the anterior aspect of portions of the adrenal gland. On the left, the pancreas and splenic vein are anterior to the cortical surface.

Kidney

The kidneys are the next paired organs just inferior to the adrenal glands. These organs are completely enveloped within the perirenal fascia (Gerota fascia) and are mobile structures supported only by the perirenal fat, renal vasculature, and abdominal muscles and viscera. Although Gerota fascia separates the kidney capsule and parenchyma from these adjacent organs and reduces the risk of renal injury with local dissection, renal parenchymal injury is possible with abnormal anatomy. The kidneys are approximately the size of a closed fist, measuring 10 to 12 cm in length and 5 to 7 cm in width. The right kidney lies more inferiorly than the left kidney because of the liver. Despite being located in the retroperitoneum, the kidney is well protected from external injury. Posteriorly, each kidney is covered by the diaphragm on the upper third of its surface and is crossed by the twelfth rib. The inferior aspect of the kidney is adjacent to the psoas muscle medially and the quadratus lumborum and transversus abdominis laterally.[1] The anterior surfaces of the kidneys are intimately related to several intraperitoneal structures. On the right, the liver is attached to the kidney by the hepatorenal ligament, and the anterior upper pole is adjacent to the peritoneal surface of the liver.[1] The duodenum lies on the medial aspect of the anterior right kidney, typically on the hilar structures. The hepatic flexure of the colon crosses anterior to the inferior pole of the right kidney. On the left, the superior pole of the kidney lies posterior to the tail of the pancreas and the splenic vessels and hilum. The spleen is situated anteromedial to the kidney and is directly attached to the kidney by the lienorenal ligament. The splenic flexure of the colon is draped over the caudal aspect of the anterior left kidney.

The renal vasculature has significant variability occurring in 25% to 40% of kidneys.[3] The typical vasculature is based on a paired artery and vein supplying the kidney as direct branches of the aorta and vena cava, respectively. The renal artery branches from the aorta inferior to the superior mesenteric artery at the level of the second lumbar vertebra. The renal artery then branches into four or five segments, each being an end artery.[3] The renal arteries are located posterior and slightly superior to the renal veins. The artery initially branches posteriorly into the posterior segmental artery. The anterior branches are variable but include the apical, upper, middle, and lower segmental arteries. These arteries branch multiple times within the cortical kidney, creating a complex filtration mechanism at the capillary level. The venous capillary branches coalesce to mirror the parenchymal arterial system. Renal segmental veins are not end vascular structures and collateralize extensively. The renal vein on the right is short, typically 2 to 4 cm in length, and enters the posterolateral inferior vena cava.[3] The left renal vein is longer, 6 to 10 cm, and travels anterior to the aorta and inferior to the superior mesenteric artery and enters the left lateral vena cava.[3] The left renal vein also is the common entry point for the left adrenal vein, gonadal vein, and a lumbar vein. Renal ectopia is accompanied by markedly variable and unpredictable renal vasculature, with multiple branches arising from the iliac arteries or aortic bifurcation.

Ureter

The upper collecting system begins within the renal parenchyma at the level of the papilla. The papillae coalesce to become the minor calyces which, in turn, become the major calyces. The major calyces converge to form the renal pelvis. The ureter begins at the inferior aspect of the renal pelvis, where it narrows to become the ureteropelvic junction posterior to the renal artery.[2] Each ureter is typically 22 to 30 cm in length, depending on height, and courses through the retroperitoneum into the pelvis, where it connects to the urinary bladder at the ureterovesical junction.[4] At its origin, the ureter courses along the anterior psoas major muscle and is

crossed by the gonadal vessels bilaterally. The ureters cross over the iliac vessels to enter the pelvis, just superior to the bifurcation of the iliac vessels into the internal and external segments. Once in the pelvis, the ureters course medially to enter the bladder. The ureters are divided into three segments, upper, middle, and lower, using this anatomic landmark as a junction point.[4] The upper segment runs from the ureteropelvic junction to the superior margin of the sacrum. The middle segment runs over the bony pelvis. The lower segment begins at the inferior margin of the sacrum and continues into the bladder. The ureteral lumen is not uniform throughout its length and has three distinct narrowing points: the ureteropelvic junction, crossing the iliac vessels, and the ureterovesical junction. The right and left ureters have separate anatomic relationships (peritoneal and retroperitoneal structures). On the right, the ureter is posterior to the ascending colon, cecum, and appendix. The left ureter is posterior to the descending and sigmoid colon. In the male, the ureters are crossed by the vasa deferentia as they emerge from the internal ring before turning medially to join the prostate. The ureteral blood is drawn from multiple vessels throughout its course and within the adventitia; the arterial vessels create an anastomosing plexus. In general, the upper ureteral segments have a medial vascular supply (i.e., renal artery and aorta), and the lower ureteral segments have a lateral vascular supply (i.e., internal iliac and various branches). This unique collateral blood flow allows extensive mobilization of the ureter, outside of its adventitia, without loss of its blood supply.[4]

The ureter is best identified, intraoperatively, in an area of normal anatomy and then followed to the area of concern. This is readily accomplished medial to the lower pole of the kidney or at the iliac bifurcation. After prior surgery or retroperitoneal disease processes, any of these rich collateral blood supply sources may not be contributory; thus, it is critical to avoid unnecessary extensive circumferential dissection of the ureter.

Pelvis

Bladder and Prostate

The bladder, the end reservoir for urine, is located within the inferior pelvis. The bladder, when empty, is located behind the pubic rami; but as the bladder becomes distended, the superior aspect of the bladder extends out of the pelvis and into the lower anterior abdomen.[5] The bladder can be injured on entering of the abdomen through a midline incision in the retropubic space (of Retzius) if the bladder is not displaced posteriorly when the midline rectus fascial incision is extended to the pubis. Superiorly, the bladder is covered by the parietal peritoneum of the pelvis as the peritoneum reflects off the anterior and lateral abdominal walls. The anterior and lateral bladder walls do not have a peritoneal surface but reside within pelvic fat and lie along the musculature of the pelvic side wall or pubis anteriorly. Prior lower abdominal or pelvic surgery can change the anatomic relations of the bladder and cause it to be affixed abnormally within the pelvis. The bladder has a unique cross section with a urothelial lining creating a tight barrier from urine and a central muscular detrusor layer involved in the excretory function of the bladder.[6] Branches of the internal iliac artery, the superior and inferior vesical arteries, supply blood to the bladder. Similar to the ureter, the bladder has a rich collateral vascular network, so ligation or damage to an artery is not detrimental to the bladder. The innervation of the bladder is important because of the excretory function of the bladder. The bladder has autonomic and somatic innervation with a dense neural network to the brain. The sympathetic innervation to the bladder is through the hypogastric nerve, and the parasympathetic supply is through the sacral cord and pelvic nerve.[5] The anatomic relationships of the bladder differ between male and female patients. In the male patient, the posterior bladder wall is adjacent to the anterior sigmoid colon and rectum. Prior pelvic surgery, irradiation, or pelvic trauma can make the plane between these structures difficult to define, resulting in inadvertent injury. In the female patient, the parietal peritoneum becomes contiguous with the anterior uterus, and the superior bladder lies against the lower uterus while the bladder base sits adjacent to the anterior vaginal wall. The spherical bladder funnels caudally into the bladder neck, and this becomes the tubular urethra inferiorly.

In the male patient, the first segment of the urethra is surrounded by and integrated into the prostate. The prostate, an endocrine gland involved with male reproductive function, is located immediately inferior to the bladder and invested in the circular fibers of the bladder neck. The prostate is surrounded by the lateral pelvic fascia on its anterior surface, by endopelvic fascia on its lateral surface, and by Denonvilliers fascia posteriorly.[7] The rectum sits immediately posterior to the prostate and is separated by a second layer of Denonvilliers fascia. This fascia also extends superiorly on the posterior prostate to encompass the seminal vesicles. The seminal vesicles are the reservoirs for seminal fluid that makes up the majority of the ejaculatory fluid. The arterial supply to both structures is through branches of the inferior vesical artery. The venous drainage mirrors the arterial supply, draining through the inferior vesical veins and subsequently into the internal iliac veins. In addition to the rectum, the other major anatomic relationship of the prostate is Santorini plexus, a network of veins derived from the dorsal venous complex of the penis.[7]

Urethra, Male Genitalia, and Perineum

The drainage of urine from the bladder is through the tubular urethra, which begins at the level of the bladder neck. In male patients, the urethra has five distinct segments: prostatic, membranous, penile, bulbar, and glandular (also known as the fossa navicularis). The prostatic and membranous urethra is surrounded by striated muscle, and when the urethra penetrates the genitourinary diaphragm in the perineum, the outer layer becomes spongy vascular tissue. Within the prostate, the ejaculatory duct opens into the urethra and serves as the exit point for seminal emission. The blood supply of the extraprostatic urethra is through the common penile artery, which is a branch of the internal pudendal artery.[5] The venous drainage of the urethra is through the circumflex penile veins and ultimately into the deep dorsal vein of the penis. The major surrounding structure in the proximal male urethra is the rectum, which sits posterior to the proximal bulbar segment. The female urethra is more regular in length and is approximately 4 cm long.[5] The female urethra contains three distinct layers as opposed to the male urethra. The proximal urethra is surrounded by smooth and striated musculature, which forms the urinary sphincter. The arterial and venous blood supply are through the internal pudendal, vaginal, and inferior vesical veins. The only structure adjacent to the female urethra is the anterior vaginal wall.

The male external genitalia consist of the penis, scrotum, and paired testes. The penis consists of three circular erectile bodies: the two dorsal corpora cavernosa and the ventral corpus spongiosum. The corpora cavernosa are responsible for penile erection; the corpus spongiosum provides support and structure to the urethra. Blood supply of the penis is through the external and internal pudendal arteries. The external pudendal artery supplies the penile skin; the internal pudendal artery supplies the urethra and the paired erectile bodies. The venous drainage of the penis is through the superficial and deep dorsal veins and the cavernosal veins. The penis is entirely an external structure, with all three erectile bodies terminating in the perineum. The scrotum is a surprisingly complex structure consisting of a muscular sac covered with a unique epidermal layer with no fat but many sebaceous and sweat glands. The sac is divided into two halves by a midline septum of dartos muscle. The blood supply to the scrotum is through the external pudendal arteries anteriorly and branches of perineal vessels posteriorly. Within the scrotum are the right and left testicles. The testicles have both endocrine and reproductive function in men. Typically, the testes are 4 to 5 cm long and 3 cm wide.[5] The vascular and genital ductal structures leave the testis from the mediastinum in the posterosuperior portion and travel through the scrotal neck into the inguinal canal. The spermatic cord is invested by the internal spermatic fascia, cremaster muscle, and external spermatic fascia, which are derived from the transversalis fascia, internal oblique, and external oblique, respectively. Arterial blood supply is primarily through the testicular or gonadal artery, which is a direct branch from the aorta inferior to the renal artery. Secondary blood supply to the testicle is through the cremasteric and vasal arteries. The venous drainage of the testicle initially begins as a pampiniform plexus coalescing into the gonadal or testicular veins. On the right, the vein drains directly into the vena cava; on the left, the vein drains into the left renal vein. The testicles are also responsible for spermatogenesis. After production, the spermatozoa exit through a series of ductal structures that emerge into the epididymis and ultimately the vas deferens. The epididymis is located posteriorly and slightly lateral to the testis. The spermatic artery, vein, and vas deferens are invested together in the fascial structures of the spermatic cord. The spermatic cord travels through the external inguinal ring through the inguinal canal and then into the pelvis through the internal inguinal ring. The spermatic cord is susceptible to injury during inguinal dissection for hernia repair, especially in redo cases, when it may be encased in fibrosis and injured without recognition. Significant injury to the spermatic cord may put the viability of the testis at risk, even though it is supported by three collateral arteries. The perineum is divided into an anterior and posterior triangle in the male by a line connecting the ischial tuberosities.[5] The posterior perineal triangle contains the anus and internal and external sphincters. The anterior triangle (or urogenital triangle) contains the corpus spongiosum and proximal aspect of the paired erectile bodies, the corpora cavernosa. The layers to the corpus spongiosum consist of the skin, subcutaneous fat, Colles fascia, and bulbospongiosus muscle (surrounding the corpus spongiosum) and ischiocavernosus muscles (surrounding the corpora cavernosa). The blood supply to this region is based on branches of the internal pudendal artery, and drainage is through the internal pudendal vein. The presence of a urethral catheter is helpful in palpating the location of the urethra, but the corpus spongiosum surrounding the bulbar urethra is still vulnerable to injury with dissection in an inflamed or obliterated anatomic plane.

ENDOSCOPIC UROLOGIC SURGERY

Urologists were early adopters of endoscopic surgery and began evaluating the urethra and bladder with cystoscopy in the early part of the 20th century. The first diagnostic and therapeutic endoscopic procedures were performed for treatment of urologic disease processes. Endoscopic procedures are divided on the basis of intervention or evaluation of the lower or upper urinary tract as each has specialized procedure-specific equipment.

Cystoscopy, or cystourethroscopy as it is formally called, is used for evaluation of the urethra, both anteriorly and posteriorly, and the bladder. Cystoscopic procedures are typically performed to evaluate the lower urinary tract in the setting of hematuria, voiding symptoms, or bladder obstruction; for surveillance in the setting of malignant neoplasms; and for removal of genitourinary foreign bodies. Furthermore, cystoscopy can be used to perform diagnostic evaluation of the upper urinary tract with use of ureteral catheters and instillation of contrast material, which is visualized within the collecting system by fluoroscopy. Cystoscopy can be performed with both rigid and flexible endoscopes, each with certain benefits and advantages. Endoscopes are sized with the French size system, which refers to the outer circumference of the instrument in millimeters. The rigid endoscope uses optical lens systems, similar to laparoscopes, and has excellent resolution. The inflexible structure is intuitive and easy to orient. Rigid cystoscopes have a range of sizes typically from 16 Fr to 26 Fr; surgical endoscopes, or resectoscopes, have the largest size of 25 Fr or 26 Fr.[8] Rigid endoscopes have larger luminal diameter, which allows greater irrigation flow, improving visualization, and passage of a number of working instruments. Rigid lower tract endoscopy is more difficult to perform in the awake patient, although it is much better tolerated in the female patient than in the male patient because of the short, straight female urethra. Flexible endoscopes are smaller, 15 Fr or 16 Fr, and better tolerated by patients for examination. Both male and female patients can be examined with local anesthetic. The flexible endoscope does not require any specific patient positioning and can be used supine and at the bedside. Finally, because of the large deflection radius, the bladder is easily evaluated without changing lens or patient position. The optics of flexible endoscopes continue to improve by advancements in camera chip capability, with new digital platforms approaching the resolution of optical lens systems. Pediatric endoscopes are smaller, 8 Fr to 12 Fr, and are typically used in the operating room.

Upper tract evaluation is performed with either a ureteroscope or a nephroscope. The most common reason for either procedure is management of calculous disease, both ureteral and renal. Ureteroscopy can also be used to visualize and to inspect the upper collecting system, ureter, and renal pelvis; for hematuria originating from the upper urinary tract; for surveillance of urothelial carcinoma; and for treatment or biopsy of abnormal findings. Ureteroscopy is performed with both flexible and semirigid endoscopes, each with different benefits and purposes. Semirigid endoscopes are 6 Fr to 7.5 Fr at the tip and gradually enlarge to 8 Fr to 9.5 Fr.[8] The taper at the tip allows introduction into the ureteral orifice at the trigone of the bladder. These endoscopes have larger working channels that allow greater irrigation flow and a larger field of view. Because semirigid ureteroscopes are fairly inflexible, they are used to evaluate and to treat conditions below the level of iliac vessels and mid and distal ureter. Flexible ureteroscopes are 5.3 Fr to 8.5 Fr at the tip and gradually enlarge to 8.4 Fr to 10.1 Fr.[8] The major advantage of flexible ureteroscopes is the deflection of the tip, which ranges from 130 to 250 degrees in one direction and 160 to 275 degrees in the opposite direction, with newer endoscopes approaching 360-degree deflection. In addition, these endoscopes can be advanced through ureteral tortuosity and over external compression, such as the psoas muscle. The working channel on the flexible ureteroscope is typically

smaller because of the fiberoptic system, and introduction of instruments, such as baskets or laser fibers, reduces irrigation flow. These flexible endoscopes can be used throughout the upper urinary tract but are most useful in the proximal ureter and renal pelvis and calyceal system.

The other method of upper tract endoscopy is through direct percutaneous access into the renal collecting system. Similar to retrograde ureteroscopy, nephroscopy is most commonly used to treat large renal calculi. More recently, consideration has been given to management of upper tract urothelial tumors with fulguration and resection. Nephroscopy is performed with both rigid and flexible nephroscopes; however, most intervention is performed with the rigid system. The rigid nephroscope is placed through a percutaneous working access sheath, similar to a laparoscopic trocar, to visualize the stone or tumor. Rigid nephroscopes are usually 25 Fr to 28 Fr, and their appearance is similar to a rigid cystoscope, although they have a fixed lens system rather than an exchangeable lens. Newer rigid nephroscopes are built on a digital platform that allows a larger working channel with comparable optics to a standard endoscope. Various intracorporeal lithotripters are placed through the working channel to fragment large stones into manageable pieces. Flexible nephroscopes are essentially flexible cystoscopes that are dual purposed for evaluation of the kidney. Flexible endoscopy of the upper tract is advantageous because all areas of the upper collecting system (upper, mid, and lower pole calyces) can be inspected regardless of angle or direction of the internal infundibula.

Numerous working elements are used in both upper and lower tract endoscopy. Guidewires are commonly used to access the upper urinary tract collecting system or the bladder and serve as guides to pass catheters, stents, and sheaths. Most guidewires have a flexible tip and a rigid shaft and are constructed of inner core and outer covering, which may hydrophilic or neutral (polytetrafluoroethylene). Guidewires range in size from 0.018 to 0.038 inch and have various lengths. Urethral catheters and ureteral catheters may be placed over wires to assist with direct placement into the lower or upper urinary system, respectively. Ureteral stents are hollow catheters with flexible ends that form a coil on the proximal and distal ends to maintain position within the collecting systems. Stents are placed to ensure drainage of the kidney and to bypass blockages of the ureter from inflammation, stones, or tumors. Most stents are composed of thermodynamic material, which becomes softer at higher body temperatures. Stents range in size from 4.8 Fr to 10 Fr and have various lengths to accommodate variable ureteral lengths. Ureteroscopic baskets are used to remove ureteral and renal calculi and to perform extraction and biopsy of tumors. These range in size from 1.3 Fr to 3.2 Fr and are constructed of flexible material to allow placement into various calyceal locations within the kidney.

UROLOGIC INFECTIOUS DISEASE

Urinary tract infections (UTIs) are a common medical problem, although patients with UTI evaluated and treated by urologists have a complicated or unusual element to their diagnosis. Other infections treated by urologists include infections of the genital skin, a spectrum of disease from cellulitis to necrotizing fasciitis, and reproduction organs in men (i.e., orchitis, epididymitis, or prostatitis). Furthermore, these infections may require simple antibiotic therapy or multimodal treatment with surgical drainage or débridement and management in an intensive care setting.

Urinary tract obstruction with proximal infection may result in sepsis, challenging the skills of the urologist and surgical critical care specialist.

Uncomplicated Urinary Tract Infection

Between the years of 2002 and 2007, UTIs in adult women and men accounted for 39 million office visits and 6 million emergency department visits.[9] In adult patients, more than 50% of women and 12% of men will develop a UTI during their lifetime.[9] Urinary infection is considered uncomplicated when it occurs in the immunocompetent host, without underlying anatomic or physiologic abnormalities of the urinary tract in women. UTI diagnosed in men is always considered complicated. For diagnosis of a UTI, a clean catch, midstream urine specimen is preferred, and on culture, 10^5 colony-forming units must be demonstrated. In catheterized specimens, UTI can be diagnosed with as little as 10^3 colony-forming units. The typical symptoms associated with UTI are dysuria, frequency, urgency to void, and malodorous urine. Because of the inherent differences in etiology, evaluation, and treatment, uncomplicated UTIs are divided into those occurring in premenopausal and postmenopausal women. A third category of uncomplicated UTI, that occurring in pregnant patients, is beyond the scope of this overview. In general, risk factors include genetic, biologic, and behavioral; specific aspects are discussed with each group.

Premenopausal Patients

History and physical examination of patients in this age group presenting with symptoms of UTI are particularly important because of overlapping disease processes. In patients without vaginal discharge, the majority can be expected to have a UTI as the diagnosis. However, in sexually active women, sexually transmitted infections (STIs) must be considered, especially in the setting of a negative urine culture. Furthermore, in patients with vaginal discharge, vaginitis caused by yeast, trichomoniasis, and bacterial vaginosis are possible causes. Risk factors for UTI in this population of patients include frequent sexual intercourse, initial UTI at a young age, maternal history of UTI, and number of pregnancies and deliveries.[10] Important aspects of the physical examination in these patients include palpation of costovertebral tenderness (assessing for ascending infection) and pelvic examination to evaluate for STI. The most common cause of infection in these patients is *Escherichia coli* (80% to 85%), followed by *Staphylococcus saprophyticus* (10% to 15%) and *Klebsiella pneumoniae* and *Proteus mirabilis* (4% each).[10] Empirical therapy is acceptable, although confirmatory urine cultures are useful as the incidence of antibiotic resistance continues to rise. Prevention includes increased hydration and evaluation of hygiene practices.

Postmenopausal Patients

As in younger patients, history and physical examination are important aspects of UTI evaluation in this group of patients. Presenting symptoms are similar in this group, although some elderly patients may simply present with altered mental status. Furthermore, an important component in diagnosis and treatment of postmenopausal women is the change in the vaginal pH levels and change or reduction in lactobacillus in the vaginal flora. The physical examination findings may differ in these patients as STIs are less likely but physical changes, such as pelvic organ prolapse and incomplete bladder emptying, become causative factors. In addition, the pathologic bacterial species are different. *E. coli* continues to be the predominant organism but in this age group, *P. mirabilis, K. pneumoniae*, and *Enterobacter* species become more prevalent pathogens.[10] Again, empirical therapy is acceptable, but urine cultures are important because of increasing antibiotic resistance patterns and differing organisms. Prevention includes increased hydration and evaluation of hygiene practices.

Complicated Urinary Tract Infection

Complicated UTIs require more vigilance on the part of the treating physician because of patient factors that may lead to a more rapid progression or worsening of the infection. By definition, complicated UTIs occur in men and in patients with diabetes, immunosuppression, upper tract infection, resistant organisms, urinary tract anatomic abnormalities, prior surgery, calculous disease, spinal cord injury, or recent or current indwelling Foley catheter. In these patients, similar evaluation is warranted, but the evaluation should not be limited to simply history and physical examination. Empirical treatment of complicated UTI alone is not appropriate, and urine cultures should be performed on all patients with suspected complicated UTI before initiation of antibiotic therapy. In addition, imaging is indicated in these patients because of concern for calculous disease and urinary stasis, so at a minimum, a kidney, ureter, and bladder study and renal ultrasound with cross-sectional imaging should be performed in all patients with equivocal or concerning findings. Finally, antibiotic therapy alone may not be adequate, and these patients may require surgical drainage of obstructed urinary systems or later surgical correction of anatomic abnormalities or removal of urinary stones (once infections are treated) to prevent recurrent UTIs. Consultation with infectious disease specialists may also be indicated in patients with urologic anatomic abnormalities and recurrent UTIs with resistant organisms.

Urinary Tract Infection in Men

Because of the lower incidence of UTI in men, when men present with symptoms of infection, it is always considered complicated, regardless of other patient factors. As in women, younger men (younger than 50 years) and older men (older than 50 years) have different causes of their UTI and symptoms. Common presenting symptoms are urethritis, dysuria, hesitancy, frequency, and urgency of urination. A history and physical examination in these patients are important to delineate different sources of symptoms or UTI. Men can present with these symptoms and have different diagnoses, including UTI, STI, urethritis, and chronic pelvic pain. Furthermore, bacterial infections can extend to other proximal areas of the genitourinary system, such as the prostate and testicle. Men younger than 50 years are more likely to have STI as the cause rather than UTI. These men should have a thorough sexual history, genital examination, and microscopic urinalysis performed. Urethral swab or urine tests for STI should be performed as well. Men older than 50 years often have underlying lower urinary tract symptoms (LUTS), and this can be a contributing factor. Men in this age group more frequently will have UTI as a source of their symptoms, and common urinary pathogens, as in women, should be considered. Furthermore, older men should be questioned about recent surgical procedures, catheterization, or hospitalization. Elderly men can also present with mental status changes as their only symptom of UTI, and this diagnosis must be ruled out in these patients. A lower threshold for imaging and hospital admission is necessary in men with UTI as they may present with more systemic symptoms. Patients who cannot tolerate oral intake, are immunocompromised, or have medical comorbidities should be admitted with cross-sectional imaging performed. Broad-spectrum intravenous antibiotics, based on local resistance patterns, and fluid resuscitation should be initiated in these patients while the initial workup and evaluation are completed. Urinary obstruction or stone disease in these patients constitutes a urologic emergency and must be addressed rapidly.

Specific Complicated Genitourinary Infectious States
Pyelonephritis

Pyelonephritis is a spectrum of infectious or inflammatory processes that involve the kidney collecting system or parenchyma. Pyelonephritis results from a UTI moving proximally upward from the lower urinary tract. In the simple form, pyelonephritis may be treated on an outpatient basis with oral antibiotics for 1 to 2 weeks. In this group of patients, urine culture is necessary to identify the causative organism. If the patient appears more acutely infected, hospitalization may be warranted for broad-spectrum intravenous antibiotic therapy, fluid resuscitation, and cross-sectional imaging. *Emphysematous pyelonephritis* represents an advanced form of pyelonephritis and is considered a urologic emergency. These patients have a significant necrotizing infection of the kidney with gas-forming organisms, with pockets of gas within the parenchyma apparent on imaging (Fig. 72-1). The common bacterial pathogens include *E. coli*, *P. mirabilis*, and *K. pneumoniae*.[11] These patients require either prompt percutaneous drainage of the infection or rapid nephrectomy. Most patients who present with this condition are diabetic or have significant

medical comorbidities, and control of the metabolic abnormalities, aggressive broad-spectrum antibiotic therapy, and supportive critical care are essential. *Xanthogranulomatous pyelonephritis* is a chronic infectious process resulting from renal obstruction, recurrent infection, and renal calculous disease. The disease presents in three forms, focal, segmental, or diffuse, and each is treated in a different manner. The underlying histologic process involves a foamy, lipid-laden, macrophage infiltrate in the renal parenchyma, with extensive inflammation, fibrosis, and loss of renal function. On imaging, there may be indications of collecting system dilation; however, drainage attempts often are unproductive because the material is often solid or too viscous to drain. Patients with focal or segmental disease may be treated with antibiotics, but those with diffuse disease frequently require nephrectomy. The risk of iatrogenic adjacent organ injury is high in these nephrectomies, and the renal hilum may be so inflamed and fibrotic that the renal vessels cannot be individually dissected. These cases may require placement of a vascular pedicle clamp with renal excision and oversewing of the pedicle.

Male Genital Organ Infection

UTIs may ascend into the genital ducts, resulting in infection of the prostate, epididymis, or testicle. Beginning in the urethra, the verumontanum is the exit point of the seminal vesicles and vas deferens into the urinary tract. Prostatitis refers to any inflammatory process affecting the prostate, but the general surgeon more commonly may encounter acute bacterial prostatitis, which results

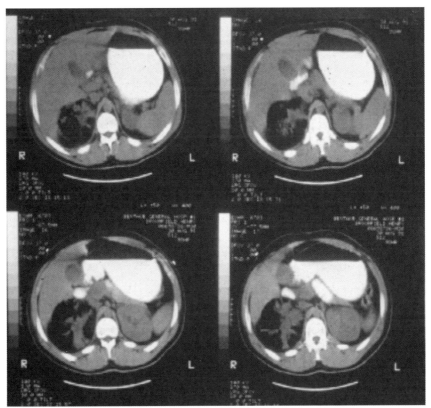

FIGURE 72-1 Emphysematous Pyelonephritis. This CT scan demonstrates extensive destruction of the right kidney with intraparenchymal gas on the right, obliterating the renal architecture. The left kidney is normal.

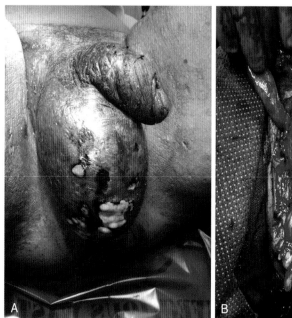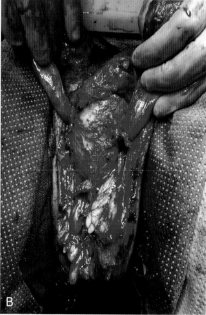

FIGURE 72-2 Fournier Gangrene. **A,** Skin necrosis, purulence, and edema of the scrotum. The skin can also appear normal, with much more subtle physical findings in some cases. **B,** Appearance after extensive débridement of scrotal skin and underlying tissues. The base of the penis is visible centrally; the testes are elevated out of the field, and the spermatic cords are visible anteriorly.

from bacterial infiltration into the prostatic parenchyma. Most infections of the prostate are secondary to gram-negative bacterial infection and typically are associated with UTI. Two important considerations in these patients are physical examination and disease extent. Although a full history and physical examination are warranted, elimination of digital rectal examination (DRE) should be considered as pressure exerted on an infected prostate may lead to hematogenous spread of the bacteria. In addition, patients who do not have reasonably rapid resolution of their symptoms should be evaluated for prostatic abscess. Prostatic abscesses typically do not respond to antibiotic therapy and require transurethral unroofing to allow adequate drainage.

Epididymitis-orchitis results when the UTI ascends through the vas deferens into the epididymis or testicle. Again, the cause is different according to the patient's age; men younger than 35 years typically have an STI as a source, commonly *Chlamydia trachomatis,* whereas men older than 35 years will often have infections related to *E. coli.* Examination of these patients is often difficult because of significant swelling of the affected epididymis or testicle; scrotal ultrasound is useful diagnostically, especially to rule out associated abscess. When infection is advanced, the entire ipsilateral scrotal contents become involved, with overlying skin fixation and edema. It may be difficult to distinguish this entity from late torsion, incarcerated inguinal hernia, or testicular tumor with necrosis and inflammation. Patients without abscess may be managed with antibiotic therapy, rest, and scrotal elevation; however, recovery is slow, with eventual resolution of edema and discomfort. If abscess is present, surgical drainage and often orchiectomy are indicated. A subset of patients may have persistent pain or mass, and on repeated Doppler imaging, signs of testicular ischemia or persistent inflammation may be noted. These patients require exploration and possible orchiectomy to resolve the process.

Fournier Gangrene

Fournier gangrene is a necrotizing infection of the male genitalia and perineum similar to other progressive fasciitis and soft tissue infections (Fig. 72-2). When the genitalia are involved, patients typically present with significant pain and tenderness, scrotal and genital swelling, discoloration or frank necrosis, crepitus, and, at times, foul-smelling discharge. Fournier gangrene is usually a polymicrobial infection with microaerobes, anaerobes, and gram-positive and gram-negative organisms.[12] Risk factors for development include peripheral vascular disease, diabetes mellitus, malnutrition, alcoholism, and other immunocompromised states. This disease represents a urologic emergency. Treatment requires urgent surgical drainage with aggressive débridement of the necrotic tissue, broad-spectrum intravenous antibiotics, and intensive monitoring with supportive care. The magnitude of the débridement depends entirely on the degree of progression of the process. It is rare for the process to involve the testicles or deep tissues of the penis because of the tunica vaginalis and Buck fascia, respectively, so these structures should be preserved. It is uncommon for the urethra to be involved, although a defined urinary tract source may be evident, such as a urethral stricture, with perforation and local infection. Suprapubic tube diversion is generally not necessary; urethral catheter drainage is generally sufficient. Once the active infection is controlled, the predominant management issues become wound care and reconstruction, which may require delayed skin grafting for tissue coverage.

Atypical Urinary Tract Infections
Fungal Infection

Fungal infections in the urinary system are most common in specific populations of patients: diabetics, immunocompromised patients, and the elderly. Fungal infections may not be symptomatic and in an outpatient setting may not require therapy. Most fungal infections are related to the *Candida* species, and it is incumbent on the treating physician to determine which infections require treatment and which represent contamination. Patients who require careful evaluation and treatment include neutropenic patients and intensive care patients, who may need evaluation for an internal source, such as a fungus deposit (ball) in the bladder or kidney. Infectious disease consultation is valuable in these cases because the organisms are atypical and selection of treatment agents may not be straightforward. Renal and bladder imaging with ultrasound may demonstrate a treatable source. These patients may need antifungal bladder or kidney irrigation or occasionally endoscopic removal.

Tuberculosis

The genitourinary tract is the third most common extrapulmonary site for tuberculosis infection. This disease is spread hematogenously from the lungs and into the affected organ system. Most patients with genitourinary tuberculosis are immunocompromised, so assessment of HIV infection status is important. Patients present with various symptoms that include voiding symptoms, sterile pyuria or hematuria, and chronic kidney disease. Not all patients will have a positive PPD test result, and diagnosis is confirmed with acid-fast bacilli smears of urine and mycobacterial culture with sterile pyuria, chest radiograph, and imaging of the genitourinary system to look for anatomic abnormalities. Tuberculosis affecting the kidney may result in segmental or global glomerular dysfunction, and progression antegrade down the urinary system may result in ureteral strictures. Tuberculosis of the epididymis may result in chronic epididymitis or mass. Antibiotic therapy consists of 2 months of a four-drug regimen with a subsequent 7-month treatment with isoniazid and rifampin. Infectious disease consultation is mandatory in treating these patients because of public health concerns. Significant anatomic infection or functional change or loss may ultimately require surgical excision.

Parasitic Infection

With the ease of global transportation and a mobile global population, parasitic infections are considerations in patients with recent travel histories. The main parasitic infections of the genitourinary system are schistosomiasis, echinococcal infection, and filariasis. Each parasite has a different point of entry, systemic spread, and organ infestation. Typically, in schistosomiasis, the parasite enters the body percutaneously and spreads through the venous and lymphatic system. Most infestations affect the bladder, resulting in chronic inflammation and granulomas. These patients present with LUTS or hematuria. Medical therapy (praziquantel) can be used to treat granulomatous disease; however, untreated infections can result in squamous cell carcinoma of the bladder. Echinococcal infections are spread through ingestion of contaminated food, and the parasite penetrates the intestinal walls and infests the liver. On occasion, renal infestation can occur, with the parasite becoming encysted in the parenchyma. Medical therapy can shrink the cysts, but surgical removal by partial or total nephrectomy is required for cure. These cysts must be removed intact as rupture or spillage of internal contents can result in severe anaphylaxis. Filariasis results from direct infection of the lymphatic system through percutaneous entry. The parasite creates noticeable symptoms when it dies, resulting in obstruction of the lymphatics. Only mild infestation can be treated with oral therapy (albendazole); advanced disease requires excision and reconstruction.

VOIDING DYSFUNCTION, NEUROGENIC BLADDER, INCONTINENCE, AND BENIGN PROSTATIC HYPERPLASIA

A central aspect of urology is management of bladder function and evaluation and treatment of bladder dysfunction. The bladder is a large muscular sac responsible for storing and eliminating urine. Common dysfunctions of the bladder include neurogenic problems with bladder function, storage problems, incontinence, and outflow issues related to benign prostatic hyperplasia (BPH) or enlargement. Changes in these functional areas are one of the most common reasons for urologic consultation. Although this is a broad area of urology, concentrating on these core divisions will give the general surgeon an understanding of the complex dynamics of bladder function.

Neurogenic Bladder

Patients with neurogenic bladder dysfunction present with a wide spectrum of neurologic diseases or injuries that affect bladder function on the basis of the location of the injury or disease process. There is a complex interaction between the bladder and brain that primarily regulates bladder storage and bladder emptying. Bladder storage is driven by the sympathetic nervous system, specifically at the level of the adrenergic receptor. α-Adrenergic receptors are the most common adrenergic receptors in the bladder, prostate, and urethra; most are α_1 and α_2, with three subtypes of α_1 identified: α_{1a}, α_{1b}, and α_{1d}.[13] The α_1 receptor is the most common subtype in the lower urinary system. Bladder emptying is driven by the parasympathetic stimulation of cholinergic receptors, specifically the muscarinic receptors. The predominant muscarinic receptors in the bladder are M_2 and M_3.[13] Sensory information is carried away from the bladder by myelinated and unmyelinated afferent nerve fibers traveling through the pelvic and pudendal nerves. Any interruption in the sympathetic or parasympathetic nervous system and its communication with the bladder can result in neurogenic dysfunction. In addition, several centers within the pons, midbrain, and cerebral cortex have direct effect on the storage and emptying of the bladder.[13] Voiding is initiated at the level of the pontine micturition center, which sends out a parasympathetic signal to the bladder to initiate voiding. The pontine micturition center is inhibited by the periaqueductal gray located in the midbrain, and this is connected to the afferent signaling pathways from the bladder. Based on this standard sensory function, specific voiding symptoms or LUTS can be predicted by the location of neurologic disease or injury.

Basic evaluation of these patients includes a through history with neurologic and urologic historical focus, physical examination (focusing on the abdomen, pelvis, and peripheral and central nervous system), and urinalysis. Additional evaluation is tailored to location of injury. Cortical brain disease and injury, such as cerebrovascular accident, are evaluated by history, physical examination, and urinalysis. These disease processes do not directly affect the bladder function, and patients are treated on the basis of symptoms alone. Spinal cord lesions are divided into suprasacral spinal lesions (spinal cord injury, infarcts) and sacral or peripheral spinal cord lesions (pelvic plexus damage from surgery, diabetic neuropathy). Patients with lesions of the suprasacral spinal cord tend to have increased bladder muscle tension, which results in abnormal elasticity of the bladder (poor bladder compliance).[14] In addition, these patients have incoordination of the bladder and urinary sphincter, resulting in detrusor-sphincter dyssynergia. Patients with sacral or peripheral nerve lesions tend to have variable LUTS but typically do not have changes in bladder elasticity.[14] The detrusor muscle is often partially or completely nonfunctional, and the urinary sphincter remains closed. Specialized evaluation of the patients with spinal cord lesions includes upper tract ultrasonography to monitor for evidence of hydronephrosis and urodynamic evaluation. Urodynamic evaluation involves measuring the elasticity of the bladder on filling (compliance), the pressure generated on emptying (detrusor function) by recording the abdominal pressure, and the intraluminal bladder pressure with specialized catheters. Surveillance cystoscopy is indicated in chronic patients to rule out the development of intravesical disease. Treatment for neurogenic bladder has recently been revolutionized by the introduction of onabotulinum toxin. In the past, these patients required complex regimens of antimuscarinic agents and reconstructive surgery. Now, with the use of onabotulinum toxin, most patients are treated with periodic cystoscopic injections and intermittent catheterization.

Problems With Bladder Storage

Overactive bladder (OAB) is the most common storage-related problem of the bladder. It is defined as urinary urgency with or without urgency urinary incontinence in the absence of UTI or other obvious disease.[15] Typical symptoms of this problem include urgency, urinary frequency, nocturia, and urgency urinary incontinence. Urgency refers to the sudden, compelling desire to pass urine that is difficult to defer and replaces the normal urge.[15] Urinary frequency is the complaint of micturition occurring more frequently than previously deemed normal and characterized by daytime and nocturnal voids.[15] Nocturia is the complaint of interruption of sleep one or more times because of the need to urinate.[15] Finally, urgency urinary incontinence is the involuntary loss of urine associated with urgency.[15] A difficult aspect of this disease process is that it occurs in the spectrum of other LUTS and may be the result of long-term bladder outflow obstruction. Other conditions to consider in patients who present with OAB and LUTS are UTI, urinary calculi, diabetes, polydipsia, neurogenic bladder, and malignant disease. OAB has a worldwide prevalence of 11%, and with the aging population, this is presumed to increase over time.[16]

All patients who present with OAB should undergo a thorough evaluation. At the basic level, this includes a thorough history to fully disclose the symptoms and to rule out other causes. Historical elements that may be contributory include caffeine intake, constipation, recurrent UTI, pelvic organ prolapse in women and prostatic enlargement in men, and excessive fluid intake. Physical examination should be directed toward evaluation of the abdomen, pelvis, and neurologic systems. Other findings may include decreased mental status or cognitive function and peripheral edema. The last absolute examination element is urinalysis, which can reveal infection, inflammation, or hematuria that may indicate more serious disease. Simple adjunctive tests that can be performed in the office include measurement of post-void residual urine volume, noninvasive flow test, validated symptom questionnaires, and voiding diaries. Specialized tests and evaluation performed by the urologist may include cystoscopy, ultrasound, and urodynamic testing as appropriate. However, current guidelines do not require any of these specialized tests for initiation of treatment.[17]

Treatment of OAB is directed toward therapy, symptoms, and motivation of the individual patient (Fig. 72-3). As many patients suffering from this problem take multiple medications, pharmacologic therapy is not always offered as an initial treatment.

Behavioral therapies are the first-line treatment for all patients. Behavioral therapies may include lifestyle modifications or specific physical therapies. Typically, this includes fluid intake management and modification with particular attention paid to timing of fluid intake and amounts. For example, in patients who complain of nocturia, limiting nighttime fluid intake can be beneficial. Bladder training is a noninvasive method of physical therapy whereby the patient postpones voiding to lengthen the time intervals between voids. This may be coupled with urgency suppression and timed voids to reinforce retraining of the sensory output from the bladder. Finally, voiding diaries are important to help the patient and urologist quantify the number of voids and voided amount to better target improvement goals and to tailor therapy. Pharmacologic management continues to be a mainstay of treatment and is indicated for patients as an adjunct to behavior therapies or for patients unresponsive to first-line therapy. Classic pharmacologic therapy is antimuscarinic agents that target the parasympathetic muscarinic cholinergic receptors, primarily M_2 and M_3, and block the action of these receptors. Most of the drugs in this category are administered daily and have the common side effects of dry mouth, dry eyes, and constipation. A newer pharmacologic agent, beta agonists (β_3), targets receptors in the detrusor muscle to stimulate bladder relaxation. Treatment options for patients who fail to respond to these therapies fall into the specialized third-line treatments, which include neuromodulation (either peripheral or central), onabotulinum toxin, chronic indwelling catheters, and augmentation cystoplasty.

Urinary Incontinence

Urinary incontinence is the involuntary loss of urine; it can be divided into stress urinary incontinence, urge urinary incontinence, and mixed urinary incontinence.[15] National data indicate that the prevalence of urinary incontinence in America is 49.6% in women older than 20 years.[18] Men are typically affected after the age of 50 years, and incontinence develops as a symptom of LUTS or other problems rather than as a primary complaint as in women. Stress urinary incontinence is defined as the involuntary loss of urine with Valsalva maneuver.[15] Urge urinary incontinence is the involuntary loss of urine associated with a strong urge to void.[15] Mixed urinary incontinence is any combination of these two causes.

Evaluation of these patients includes history, physical examination (including pelvic examination), urinalysis, post-void residual volume measurement, and voiding diaries. The history and physical examination are important to rule out any complicating factors including neurogenic source, anatomic changes (pelvic organ prolapse in the female patient and prostatic enlargement in the male patient), and prior surgical intervention (radical prostatectomy in the male patient or hysterectomy in the female patient) that might affect evaluation and the treatment decision. In the neurologically normal patient with no confounding factors, nonsurgical management is the first step in treatment before any surgical intervention. As with OAB, behavior modification and bladder training are the initial steps. Dietary modification is important for management of urinary incontinence. Patients are counseled to limit fluid intake to around 2 liters per day, depending on body size and activity level. In addition, patients should limit caffeine intake and other bladder irritants including alcohol, carbonated beverages, spicy foods, and citrus juices and fruits. Furthermore, bowel programs should be initiated to ensure that the patient has normal bowel function and is not constipated. Other nonsurgical treatment includes weight loss to a normal body mass index and

DIAGNOSIS & TREATMENT ALGORITHM:
AUA/SUFU GUIDELINE ON NON-NEUROGENIC OVERACTIVE BLADDER IN ADULTS

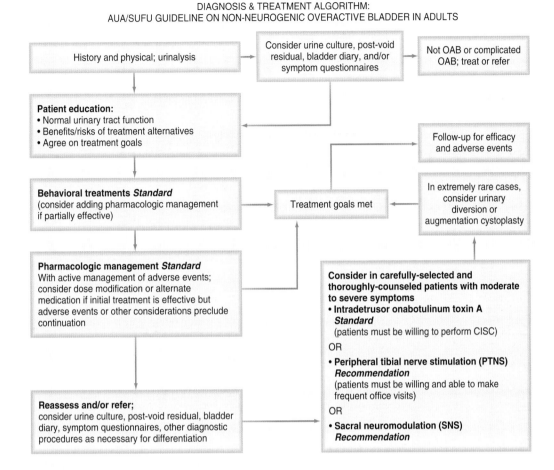

FIGURE 72-3 Algorithm for diagnosis and management of overactive bladder (OAB). (Adapted from Gormley EA, Lightner DJ, Burgio KL, et al: Diagnosis and treatment of overactive bladder [non-neurogenic] in adults: AUA/SUFU guideline. *J Urol* 188:2455–2463, 2012.)

exercise, particularly core muscle exercises. Pelvic floor muscle training and biofeedback have been shown to have acceptable rates in helping patients achieve satisfactory management of their urinary incontinence.

Surgical treatment options for women and men differ because of the inherent mechanism causing the incontinence, typically poor pelvic anatomic support in women and sphincteric in men. In women, treatment options progress from less to more invasive. The simplest treatment is injection of a urethral bulking agent through a cystoscopy. The objective of this treatment is to improve coaptation of the urinary sphincter and to increase the urethral wall volume. Unfortunately, this treatment is not likely to produce long-term cure, and re-treatment or progression to other options is often necessary. The next option is placement of a midurethral sling to resupport the central hammock of the urethra and to provide backing to the urethra during stress maneuvers. These approaches have a higher success rate, and long-term data show cure rates of approximately 90%.[19] With the success and ease of the midurethral sling, fewer open retropubic suspensions are performed. These procedures also work to improve the support of the urethra and to reduce urethral hypermobility. In men, surgical therapy is designed to reinforce the urinary sphincter to increase

bladder outlet resistance. Typically, treatments are divided into male urethral slings, which have a larger surface area for the mesh suspension material, and artificial urinary sphincters. An artificial sphincter is a complex device that is implanted in the patient and opened through a one-way valve contained in the scrotum.

Benign Prostatic Hyperplasia

BPH is the development of nodules within the prostate gland as a result of enlargement of the stromal and epithelial components of the gland.[20] As the BPH progresses, the entire prostate enlarges in a process called benign prostatic enlargement, resulting in compression of the prostatic urethra and development of bladder outflow obstruction (Fig. 72-4).[20] As part of the bladder outflow obstruction, patients can develop LUTS requiring evaluation and treatment by a urologist. BPH is prevalent, affecting approximately 70% of men between the ages of 60 and 69 years, making it one of the most common conditions treated by urologists.[20] The LUTS that result from BPH can be divided into storage, voiding, and post-void symptoms. Interestingly, there is little correlation between the measured volume of the prostate and the symptoms that result. In addition, the degree of bladder outflow obstruction does not necessarily correlate with the severity of LUTS.

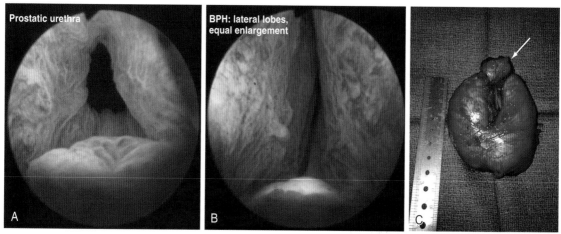

FIGURE 72-4 BPH. A, Normal cystoscopic appearance of the prostate in a young man. **B,** Moderate BPH, viewed cystoscopically. The size of the prostate correlates poorly with the magnitude of voiding symptoms. **C,** Prostatic adenoma after simple open prostatectomy. Note the small medial lobe *(arrow, top center),* with large lateral lobes (130-g specimen).

As with all conditions, evaluation of the patients is centered on the history and physical examination. Key elements of the physical examination include DRE and a focused neurologic examination. Laboratory evaluation includes urinalysis and prostate-specific antigen (PSA) testing in appropriate patients with a life expectancy of more than 10 years. Further evaluation of these patients includes the use of disease-specific validated questionnaires (International Prostate Symptom Score), measurement of post-void residual urine volumes, and noninvasive urinary flow testing.[20] Depending on initial evaluation findings, cystoscopy and urodynamic studies may be appropriate adjunct tests. Practice guidelines for BPH have been produced by the American Urological Association (AUA) to guide providers in the diagnosis and management of BPH (Figs. 72-5 and 72-6).[20] Similar to all voiding-related conditions, behavior and dietary modifications are appropriate first-step treatment measures in all patients. Medical therapy can be used in conjunction with the initial behavior modifications or added subsequently.

The mainstay of treatment for LUTS due to BPH is α_1-adrenergic receptor blockers.[20] As previously discussed, α-adrenergic receptors are the most common adrenergic receptors in the bladder, and α_1 is the most common subtype in the lower urinary system, prostate, and urethra. The action of α_1 blockers is to relax the smooth muscle in the bladder neck and prostate and to reduce outflow resistance. This class of drugs has become progressively more selective to the α_1 subtypes, and many now target the α_{1a} subtype receptor specifically. The most common side effects of these drugs are dizziness related to orthostasis, retrograde ejaculation, and rhinitis. A second category of pharmacologic therapy is the 5α-reductase inhibitors that target the glandular component of the prostate. These drugs block the conversion of testosterone to dihydrotestosterone in the prostate and subsequently reduce the prostate volume, thereby reducing outflow resistance. This class of drugs also alters the serum PSA level (reduces it about 50%), which must be kept in mind with regard to prostate cancer screening. In addition, these drugs can be used in combination because of their differing mechanism of action, and studies show superior results to either drug used independently.

When medical therapy is ineffective, symptoms remain bothersome, or an objective surgical indication arises (e.g., acute urinary retention, bladder calculi, azotemia, recurrent UTI, or recurrent hematuria), surgical intervention is considered. The standard approach to surgical treatment of BPH is transurethral resection of the prostate (TURP) using various electrosurgical options (monopolar, bipolar, or laser). Minimally invasive treatment options, such as microwave thermotherapy and radiofrequency ablation, can be performed in an office setting but do not have equivalent long term outcomes compared to standard surgical procedures. When the adenomatous growth is particularly large, open simple prostatectomy is performed to enucleate the adenoma surgically. Outcomes of the transurethral procedures show dramatic improvement in International Prostate Symptom Score numbers, urinary flow rates, and post-void residual volumes. Procedures such as simple prostatectomy have such a long historical use that objective data have not been measured or compiled, but outcomes are similar to those of TURP. Complications of TURP procedures include persistent bleeding, dilutional hyponatremia from fluid absorption of the glycine irrigation, UTI, urinary incontinence, and urethral stricture. With newer electrosurgical systems (bipolar and laser), normal saline irrigation is used and dilutional hyponatremia has been eliminated. In addition, visualization is improved, with a significant reduction in bleeding complications and a lower incidence of urinary incontinence.

MALE REPRODUCTIVE MEDICINE AND SEXUAL DYSFUNCTION

Male infertility and sexual dysfunction are a specialized area of urologic practice. Diagnostic evaluation, medical treatment, and surgical therapy of male infertility represent sophisticated aspects of urologic care. Male sexual dysfunction is becoming more prominent as the field of men's health continues to evolve. Many patients seen and evaluated by general surgeons may be receiving specific medical therapy or have undergone prosthetic surgical implants for sexual dysfunction management. A basic familiarity

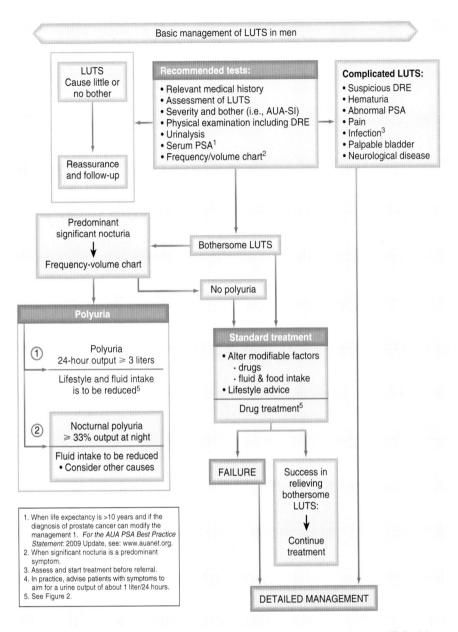

Basic management of LUTS in men

LUTS Cause little or no bother

↓

Reassurance and follow-up

Recommended tests:
- Relevant medical history
- Assessment of LUTS
- Severity and bother (i.e., AUA-SI)
- Physical examination including DRE
- Urinalysis
- Serum PSA[1]
- Frequency/volume chart[2]

Complicated LUTS:
- Suspicious DRE
- Hematuria
- Abnormal PSA
- Pain
- Infection[3]
- Palpable bladder
- Neurological disease

Predominant significant nocturia

↓

Frequency-volume chart

Bothersome LUTS

No polyuria

Polyuria

① Polyuria 24-hour output ≥ 3 liters

Lifestyle and fluid intake is to be reduced[5]

② Nocturnal polyuria ≥ 33% output at night

Fluid intake to be reduced
- Consider other causes

Standard treatment
- Alter modifiable factors
  · drugs
  · fluid & food intake
- Lifestyle advice

Drug treatment[5]

FAILURE

Success in relieving bothersome LUTS:

↓

Continue treatment

1. When life expectancy is >10 years and if the diagnosis of prostate cancer can modify the management 1. *For the AUA PSA Best Practice Statement:* 2009 Update, see: www.auanet.org.
2. When significant nocturia is a predominant symptom.
3. Assess and start treatment before referral.
4. In practice, advise patients with symptoms to aim for a urine output of about 1 liter/24 hours.
5. See Figure 2.

DETAILED MANAGEMENT

FIGURE 72-5 Algorithm for initial diagnosis and management of BPH. (Adapted from McVary KT, Roehrborn CG, Avins AL, et al: Update on AUA guideline on the management of benign prostatic hyperplasia. *J Urol* 185:1793–1803, 2011.)

with these specialized areas is beneficial to general surgeons in their surgical practice.

Male Infertility: Evaluation and Treatment

Infertility affects approximately 8% to 14% of couples; the male factor is the primary or sole factor in 36% to 75% of these cases.[21] Couples are often referred to the urologist after a period of infertility, and referrals are generally from a primary care physician or from the evaluating gynecologic reproductive endocrinologist. Infertility is defined as a couple's inability to achieve pregnancy after 1 year of unprotected intercourse.[21]

The standard male factor evaluation involves a detailed history, physical examination, and basic laboratory and imaging evaluation. The AUA has produced a series of best practice statements on the evaluation of the infertile man with the following objectives: to recognize and to treat reversible conditions, to categorize disorders potentially amenable to assisted reproductive techniques, to identify syndromes and conditions that may be detrimental to the patient's health, and to distinguish genetic abnormalities that can be transmitted to or affect the health of offspring.[22]

The causes of infertility can be divided into anatomic, behavioral and environmental, and iatrogenic. Anatomic causes of male

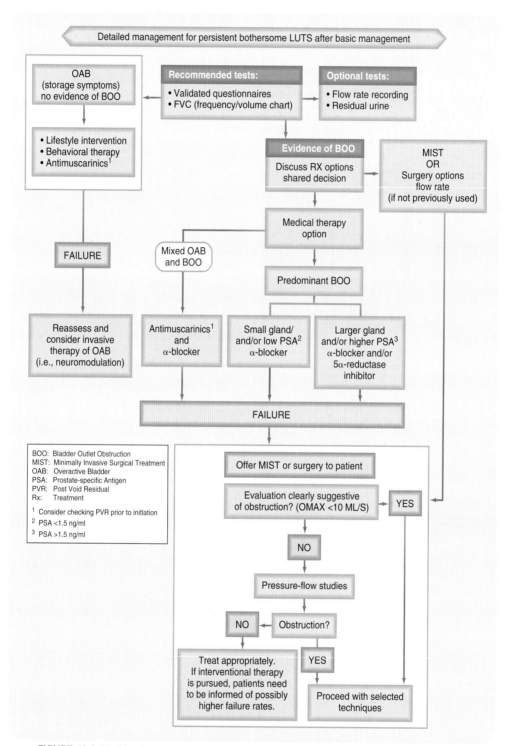

FIGURE 72-6 Algorithm for secondary management of BPH. (Adapted from McVary KT, Roehrborn CG, Avins AL, et al: Update on AUA guideline on the management of benign prostatic hyperplasia. *J Urol* 185:1793–1803, 2011.)

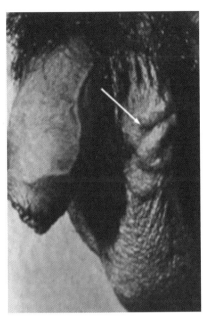

FIGURE 72-7 Varicocele. The bag of worms appearance is visible and palpable through the scrotal skin, representing the dilated branches of the internal spermatic venous system.

infertility are either congenital or acquired.[21] The most significant anatomic cause is congenital absence of the vas deferens, which is a partial or complete agenesis of the vas deferens. Although uncommon, the finding is associated with a cystic fibrosis transmembrane conductance regulator *(CFTR)* gene mutation, making these patients carriers for cystic fibrosis.[22] Other anatomic findings include cryptorchidism, ejaculatory duct obstruction (at the level of the prostate), and varicocele (Fig. 72-7). Behavioral and environmental sources of infertility are more common and easier to reverse than anatomic causes of male infertility. These include obesity, environmental exposures, substance abuse (including exogenous testosterone), and vitamin deficiency. Finally, iatrogenic causes to be considered include prior chemotherapy or radiation therapy, prior inguinal or genital surgery, and current medical treatments. Surgeons must be aware of iatrogenic causes of infertility in groin and pelvic surgical procedures from damage to the spermatic cord vasculature, vas deferens, and ejaculatory duct region or vasal entrapment from mesh used for inguinal hernia repair. The blood supply to the vas deferens or testicle is vulnerable to injury when the groin is explored in reoperative surgery or when the anatomy is obscured because of inguinal trauma as identification of these structures is challenging.

The history should include a discussion of sexual and reproductive history. This includes potential gonadotoxic exposure; urologic infections and STIs; trauma and prior surgery involving the pelvis, groin, and genitalia; and family history of infertility. Physical assessment should include a general evaluation of masculinization and genital findings, including normal meatal location, testicular size and consistency, presence and normalcy of the epididymis and vas deferens, and possible presence of a varicocele. Perineal and rectal examinations are routine parts of this assessment.

Basic Laboratory Assessment

Laboratory evaluation of these patients includes two semen analyses and serum hormone studies. The semen analyses should be separated by 1 month and preceded by 2 to 3 days of abstinence. Semen analysis parameters of importance include semen volume, pH, sperm concentration and total count, total motility, progressive motility, quality of sperm movement, morphology, and presence of red and white blood cells or bacteria.[21] The World Health Organization has defined parameters of normal for routine semen analyses.[21] Semen analysis abnormalities fall into two main categories: azoospermia—the complete absence of sperm from the semen; and abnormal semen parameters—reduced concentration, motility, or morphology and abnormal function. Azoospermia can roughly be divided into three categories: pretesticular, testicular, and post-testicular. Pretesticular azoospermia results from endocrine causes, such as hypogonadotropic hypogonadism, or congenital causes. Testicular causes are the result of primary testicular failure of germinal epithelium of the testis to produce mature sperm. This is often accompanied by normal semen volume and by a markedly elevated serum follicle-stimulating hormone (FSH) level. Post-testicular causes, such as ejaculatory dysfunction and obstruction, account for 40% of cases of azoospermia.[22] Abnormal semen parameters may be indicative of a wide range of disorders that may cause reduced sperm numbers, motility, or morphology, including varicocele, antisperm antibodies, genital duct infection with pyospermia, and prior or current gonadotoxic exposure. Reduced semen volume may be artifactual, indicating incomplete ejaculation or specimen collection, or it may represent true disease, including, for example, congenital absence of the seminal vesicle, ejaculatory duct obstruction, or retrograde ejaculation caused by diabetes or neurologic injury or prior bladder neck surgery or medications.

Serum hormone testing includes determination of levels of FSH, luteinizing hormone, testosterone, free testosterone, and prolactin. Hypogonadotropic hypogonadism may be diagnosed on the basis of serum hormone studies or elevation in the FSH level. A patient with a low testosterone level should have follow-up prolactin levels measured to rule out a prolactinoma of the pituitary gland.

Ultrasound of the scrotum is useful to measure testicular volume and symmetry, to exclude the possibility of testicular neoplasm, to identify epididymal anatomy, and to define or to confirm the presence of a varicocele, which is an abnormal dilation of the pampiniform venous plexus of the internal spermatic venous system (Fig. 72-7). Transrectal ultrasound (TRUS) of the prostate may provide evidence of ejaculatory duct obstruction with seminal vesicle dilation or congenital absence of the seminal vesicle, which may accompany congenital absence of the vas deferens.

Treatment

Treatment of male infertility depends on the identified cause and on the availability and affordability of assisted reproductive technology support options for specific or empirical treatment of failure to conceive. Medical therapy is used to treat hormone deficiencies, hormone excess, thyroid hormone excess, and prolactin excess. The most common medical therapies include hormonal stimulation of spermatogenesis, such as gonadotropin agents and antiestrogen agents, which have been met with mixed results. Anti-inflammatory or antibiotic therapy can be used in patients with findings of pyospermia or concern for genital duct infection. Surgical therapies may include microsurgical reconstruction for vasal or epididymal occlusion (including vasectomy reversal), transurethral resection of the ejaculatory duct for obstructive lesions, and varicocele repair.

Male Sexual Dysfunction and Treatment

Sexual dysfunction in men refers to a range of disorders, including erectile dysfunction (ED), diminished libido, hypogonadism, and ejaculatory dysfunction. Because of the numerous organ system interactions, patients with these conditions may have associated neuropathy, endocrinopathy, vasculopathy, and psychological disorders, and these abnormalities may affect nonurologic patient management and surgery.

Normal erectile function is a complex interaction between the nervous and vascular systems, with unique molecular actions occurring in penile vascular structures. Many medical comorbidities and lifestyle choices can contribute to ED, including age, coronary artery disease, smoking, hypertension, dyslipidemia, atherosclerosis, peripheral vascular disease, obesity, diabetes, spinal cord injury and degenerative neurologic conditions, treatment of pelvic malignant neoplasms, and chronic kidney disease.[23] The causes of ED can be divided into neurologic, vascular, metabolic, medication induced, endocrine, and psychological; importantly, it can be an early marker for coronary artery disease.[23] The initial evaluation of the ED patient centers on the history and physical examination. The history is focused on sexual performance and erectile function; the nonsexual historical aspects center on possible medical and surgical conditions. Social aspects, such as smoking, recreational drug use, and diet, are also important considerations. Validated questionnaires provide objective historical data both for initial treatment and for evaluation of therapy outcomes. The physical examination centers on the genitalia and evaluation of male secondary sexual characteristics. Basic laboratory studies in these patients include morning total testosterone concentration, fasting lipid levels, and hemoglobin A1c level. Important consideration should be given to assessment of cardiovascular function in younger patients because this disease process is considered an early marker for cardiovascular disease, especially in younger patients. Further evaluation is specialized but may include neurologic testing (e.g., biothesiometry) and vascular testing (e.g., penile duplex Doppler ultrasound studies).

Most treatments of ED are based on restoring penile arterial blood flow to achieve or to maintain a satisfactory erection. Lifestyle modifications are an important component of this, and dietary changes and increased regular cardiovascular exercise have been shown to independently improve erectile function. Evaluation and adjustment of offending medications should be considered as well. The basis of medical therapy for ED is phosphodiesterase type 5 inhibitors. These medications improve penile blood flow by limiting the breakdown of cyclic guanosine monophosphate and potentiating penile blood flow. These drugs should be limited in their use in men with known cardiovascular disease, especially those taking oral nitrates. Other forms of nonsurgical treatment include vacuum erection devices, intraurethral suppository therapy with prostaglandin compounds, intracavernosal self-injection, and occasionally psychotherapy. Surgery for ED includes primarily placement of a penile prosthesis and limited vascular reconstruction. Penile implant surgery may involve malleable implants, which have a flexible wire core inside a silicone sleeve, implanted bilaterally in the corpora, or, more commonly, inflatable penile implants. These are fluid-containing, completely internalized systems that may include paired corporal cylinders, a scrotal pumping device, and a fluid reservoir, which is typically positioned in the retropubic space or extraperitoneal lower abdominal quadrant (Fig. 72-8). The general surgeon should be aware that intraperitoneal positioning may also occur, intentionally or

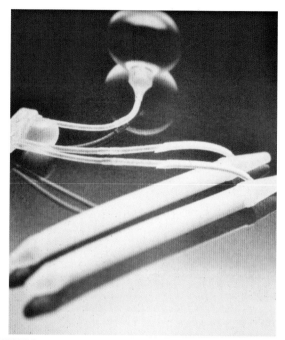

FIGURE 72-8 Inflatable Penile Prosthesis. A three-component device is shown. The reservoir *(top)* is placed retropubically in an extraperitoneal position. The paired cylinders *(right)* are placed within the corpora cavernosa. The pump *(left)* is placed in the scrotum, adjacent to the testes.

through erosion through the peritoneal membrane, and the reservoir or system tubing may be encountered during nonurologic abdominopelvic surgery. Care should be taken not to contaminate any of the implant components or inadvertently injure the tubing or device components. If it is known that an implant is in place and pelvic or inguinal surgery is planned, urologic consultation may be helpful in handling any issues that arise with the implant. Revascularization of the penis to restore erectile function, following arteriography for anatomic documentation, is usually achieved using an inferior epigastric artery pedicle flap, whereby new arterial inflow is brought to the corpora cavernosa. This has limited indications, most relevant in younger patients with traumatic injury to the pelvic blood supply, and national practice guidelines consider this to be controversial.

The other area of male sexual medicine affecting a significant number of patients is testosterone deficiency or hypogonadism. Serum testosterone is produced in the Leydig cells of the testes (90%) and adrenal glands (10%). Testicular synthesis of testosterone is controlled by the hypothalamus and anterior pituitary. This is a condition in which serum testosterone levels decline and are associated with symptoms of fatigue, lack of energy, depressed mood, irritability, reduced motivation, decreased cognitive acuity, decreased strength and stamina, reduced muscle mass and increased fat, and sexual side effects including decreased libido and ED. There is a normal age-related decline in testosterone as men age, and total testosterone declines by 1%, on average, each year after the age of 40 years. The prevalence of this condition is between 2.1% and 39% of men older than 40 years, depending on the criteria used and association of symptoms.[24] The patient's history should elicit information on the specific symptoms of testosterone deficiency, and physical examination is similar to that for ED with evaluation of the genitalia and secondary sexual characteristics. Validated questionnaires are useful to assess and to monitor therapy. Laboratory studies should include free and total morning testosterone, luteinizing hormone, prolactin, hematocrit, and hemoglobin levels.[25] Therapy for testosterone deficiency is based on lifestyle modifications and testosterone supplementation.[25] Many men who suffer from this condition are either obese or have metabolic syndrome. Dietary changes to improve nutritional status and to result in weight loss have been shown to improve not only baseline medical conditions but also serum testosterone levels. Furthermore, moderate-intensity exercise has been shown to improve serum testosterone levels. In addition to lifestyle modifications, many patients are treated with supplemental testosterone. Synthetic testosterone may be administered orally, transdermally, through intramuscular injections, and by subcutaneous pellets. The goal of therapy is maintenance of testosterone levels between 400 and 700 ng/dL and resolution or improvement of presenting symptoms.[25] Whereas there are few absolute contraindications to testosterone administration, many potential adverse side effects exist and should be discussed before administration of these medications as this is the area of greatest controversy with testosterone supplementation. Potential adverse effects include cardiovascular events and mortality, dermatologic changes, polycythemia, diminished spermatogenesis, gynecomastia, LUTS, prostate cancer, and sleep apnea.[25]

UROLITHIASIS

Urinary tract stones are a common cause of visits to the emergency department. The prevalence of renal calculous disease in the United States is increasing, with a lifetime risk of forming a renal stone at 5% in 1994 and 9% in 2010.[26] The incidence of stone disease peaks in the fourth to sixth decades of life and is more common in men than in women by a 2 : 1 margin.[26] Renal calculous disease has several aspects of management and evaluation, including acute stone presentation, metabolic evaluation, and medical and surgical therapy. As most general surgeons will encounter patients either in the acute presentation or around the time of surgical intervention, this section focuses on these areas.

Background

The pathogenesis of calculus formation is governed by the physical chemistry characteristics of the urine in the upper collecting system. Most stones are formed by minerals or stone-forming salts and begin to crystallize when their concentration becomes supersaturated in the urine. Just as certain minerals or salts promote calculus formation, there are many inhibitors of calculus formation, including citrate, phosphate, and magnesium. There are many theories to stone formation, none of which are definitively proven, such as Randall plaque formation, stasis, bacteria, and reactive oxygen species from oxalate excretion.[27] Kidney stones are classified by the stone composition, and the mineral composition directs evaluation, treatment, and nonsurgical management. Kidney stones can be generally classified as calcium based, uric acid stones, struvite stones, and cystine stones.[27] Calcium stones are usually composed of two calcium salts, calcium phosphate and calcium oxalate, and are the most common renal calculi. Risk factors for calcium stone formation include abnormal urine pH; high urine concentration of calcium, oxalate, or uric acid; and low urine concentration of the stone inhibitor citrate. Uric acid stones form in a low pH urine in patients with hyperuricosuria and can be the result of purine metabolism from cellular breakdown

(tumor lysis) or excessive protein intake. These stones are often radiolucent. Struvite stones, also called infection stones or magnesium ammonium phosphate, result from specific bacterial infections (*P. mirabilis, K. pneumoniae, Staphylococcus aureus,* and *Staphylococcus epidermidis*) that contain urease, which converts urea into ammonia. The base properties of ammonia lead to higher urine pH and crystallization with phosphate. Cystine stones are formed from an autosomal recessive defect in the metabolism of the COLA amino acids (cystine, ornithine, lysine, and arginine), which results in elevated urine cystine levels.[27] The other rare cause of calculi is pharmacologically induced, resulting from poor drug metabolite urine solubility and precipitation in the urine. The most notable of these are protease inhibitors (indinavir and ritonavir), which are not visible on noncontrast computed tomography (CT) scans.

Acute Presentation and Management

Patients presenting with an acute stone episode or renal colic typically have characteristic complaints of abdominal, flank, or back pain that waxes and wanes but cannot be resolved with position changes. Often, these patients can localize the most intense center of the pain, giving some indication of stone location. When the ureter is obstructed by a stone, the pressure in the proximal collecting system rises, and with progressive distention, the patient may experience visceral symptoms, including nausea, vomiting, and ileus. Physical examination in these patients should be focused on the back, flank, abdomen, and genitalia. Patients who have specific vital sign findings in combination (temperature higher than 101.5° F, hypotension, or tachycardia) should be assessed for obstructive upper tract UTI with the potential for sepsis. Basic laboratory evaluation should include complete blood count, metabolic panel, and urinalysis with microscopy. Significant findings of leukocytosis or acute kidney injury may direct urgency of therapy and type of intervention. A non–contrast-enhanced CT scan of the abdomen and pelvis is the preferred imaging study because of its superior sensitivity and specificity compared with intravenous urography and plain radiography. Patients with ureteral calculi may benefit from a plain radiograph, as 85% of calculi are radiopaque, to observe for stone passage.

Once the stone is identified and the location established, pain management is the next step. Patients who are diagnosed with renal or ureteral calculi should receive intravenous nonsteroidal anti-inflammatory drugs (ketorolac) or opioid analgesics as initial therapy. A successful attempt at pain control with oral agents determines if the otherwise hemodynamically stable patient can be discharged or requires inpatient treatment for the stone. Those patients who present with upper tract UTI and obstruction should undergo expeditious drainage with either cystoscopic ureteral stent placement or percutaneous nephrostomy tube placement. If one upper tract is totally obstructed by stone, the patient could have a serious infection with pyonephrosis, and the voided urine would be deceptively normal. Patients who are suitable for hospital discharge include those with no evidence of UTI, hemodynamic stability, good oral intake, pain well controlled on oral analgesics, and a stone size with reasonable chance of spontaneous passage. In patients who are discharged from the hospital, medical expulsive therapy, with agents to promote spontaneous stone passage, is the recommended management.[28] The most common drug used is tamsulosin, the α_{1a} blocker that relaxes ureteral smooth muscle.[28] If a patient is discharged for outpatient management, she or he should be observed closely to determine whether the stone has passed. It should not be assumed that because the pain has resolved, the stone has passed. With persistent upper tract obstruction, the pressure in the collecting system eventually declines as renal blood flow diminishes and urine output drops. The patient's pain can disappear and the kidney can remain obstructed, undergoing silent destruction in the weeks and months that follow. Reimaging is necessary if there is no definitive evidence that the stone has been passed (e.g., the patient brings it in for analysis).

Elective Diagnostic Evaluation and Management

Patients who are diagnosed with asymptomatic renal calculi, such as nonobstructing renal calyceal stones found incidentally during a hematuria evaluation, and patients who have convalesced after an acute presentation undergo a basic metabolic screening evaluation. Important historical aspects to obtain include prior stone passage or treatment, family history, bowel disease or malabsorption, gout, hyperthyroidism, obesity, and dietary supplements.[29] Routine laboratory work includes urinalysis, basic metabolic panel with determination of calcium and uric acid levels, urine culture, and stone analysis (if available). A 24-hour urine specimen is also collected to evaluate the urine for specific chemical and mineral content: volume, pH, creatinine, calcium, oxalate, uric acid, citrate, sodium, and potassium.[29] Specific dietary changes and medical therapy can be used for prevention of stone formation in specific populations. These dietary modifications and pharmacologic treatments are based on stone composition and findings on 24-hour urinalysis. The two most common stone types, calcium and uric acid, are discussed.

In patients with calcium-based stone disease (oxalate or phosphate), the single most important treatment or dietary modification is increased fluid intake to achieve more than 2 liters of urine output daily. In addition, there should be no changes in calcium consumption, and patients, in general, should consume the recommended daily allowance of dietary calcium. Dietary levels of sodium, foods high in oxalate, and animal protein should be reduced as each of these can affect urinary oxalate and citrate levels. Pharmacologic therapy is typically based on three different agents—thiazide diuretics, potassium citrate, and allopurinol—each of which has separate effects on calcium urine levels and calcium stone formation. Patients with uric acid stones are treated with drug therapy.[29] There are no dietary recommendations other than to increase fluid intake to raise urine output to 2 liters per day. Pharmacologic therapy in this group consists of potassium citrate and allopurinol. Many uric acid stones can be dissolved by raising urinary pH levels with use of alkalinizing agents.

Elective Surgical Management

Patients who have large stone burdens or continue to have symptomatic stones require surgical treatment of their calculous disease. Surgical treatment of renal and ureteral calculi varies from completely noninvasive, shock wave lithotripsy (SWL), to minimally invasive, percutaneous nephrolithotomy (PCNL). SWL is a transcutaneous procedure using generated shock waves to fragment stones. Shock waves create positive and negative pressure components that are focused on the stone and create fractures in the targeted stones, ultimately resulting in stone fragmentation.[30] The progress of stone fragmentation is monitored during SWL, typically with fluoroscopy, to direct treatment length and location. Nonradiopaque stones, stones larger than 2 cm, and certain ureteral calculi should not be treated with this method. Complications from SWL include renal injury, steinstrasse (street of stones), hypertension, and chronic kidney disease.[30]

Smaller renal stones and ureteral calculi can be managed in an endoscopic fashion using ureteroscopes (Fig. 72-9). As previously mentioned, ureteroscopes are both semirigid and flexible, allowing full upper tract collecting system access. Through the working channel of ureteroscopes, a variety of working instruments can be placed to fragment or to remove stones. The most common stone treatment is laser lithotripsy to completely fragment the symptomatic calculus. Smaller fragments can be removed using different basket and grasping systems to render the patient stone free. Complications of ureteroscopy include acute ureteral perforation or avulsion, UTI, and late ureteral stricture formation.

For larger renal stones or select proximal ureteral stones, PCNL is preferred because of the larger working endoscopes and better instrumentation for stone fragmentation. The basic steps of PCNL are percutaneous renal access, dilation of the nephrostomy track, placement of the working sheath for stone fragmentation and extraction, and postoperative renal drainage. The advantage of PCNL is that numerous intracorporeal lithotripsy devices are available, and large stones can be rapidly fragmented. Flexible nephroscopes can be used as well in this setting. Complications of PCNL are most significant because of the more invasive nature of the procedure; these include sepsis, renal hemorrhage, renal

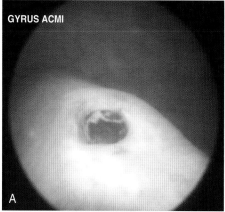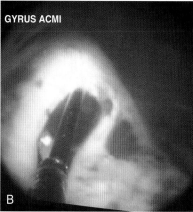

FIGURE 72-9 Ureteral Stone. A, An obstructing calculus is shown crowning within the right ureteral orifice. **B,** Cystoscopic extraction performed with a grasping forceps.

collecting system injury, and damage to adjacent organs and viscera. PCNL may result in hydrothorax or pneumothorax from transpleural or peripleural access tracks that requires evacuation. With the refinement of PCNL, open stone surgery is rarely indicated even for the most complex intrarenal calculi. Laparoscopic and robotic procedures for specific renal calculi have been described.

UROLOGIC TRAUMA

Urologic injury is present in approximately 15% of all abdominal and pelvic trauma patients regardless of mechanism, blunt or penetrating.[31] Renal injuries, for example, are reported to occur in 0.3% to 1.2% of all trauma patients; however, the kidneys are the second most common visceral organ injured, accounting for approximately 24% of injuries.[31] In many trauma centers, injuries are typically initially assessed by an emergency physician or general surgeon and may be addressed without urologic consultation, although, for complex urologic injuries, the input of a urologist can be essential. For example, high-grade, nonreconstructible renal injury can be managed with an expeditious nephrectomy; however, most renal injuries, such as an extensive parenchymal and collecting system laceration, should be repaired with renorrhaphy. Management of trauma patients is the greatest overlap between urology and general surgery and allows numerous areas for collaboration; urologic expertise can enhance the quality of care provided for all urologic injuries, whether they are managed operatively or nonoperatively.

The focus of the following section on urologic trauma is the practical management of a variety of acute urologic injuries and the optimal interaction between the urologist and general trauma surgeon. The management of common injuries throughout the urinary tract, the optimal timing of such interventions, and the role of damage control techniques are discussed.

Core Guideline and Consensus Statements for Urologic Trauma Management

The Organ Injury Scaling system of the American Association for the Surgery of Trauma describes an objective grading system for urologic injuries (Table 72-1 and Fig. 72-10).[32] The staging system for renal trauma has become well established in the urologic literature and has been externally validated. The Organ Injury Scaling system also describes staging for other urologic injuries; however, the subjective criteria applied to these divisions do not practically affect management decisions and treatment (Fig. 72-10).

In 2002, a consensus conference for the diagnosis and treatment of urologic injuries was convened by the World Health Organization and the Société Internationale d'Urologie. The resulting consensus statements were divided by organ site: kidney, ureter, bladder, urethra, and external genitalia.[33-37] These reports still constitute the centerpiece of urologic trauma management. Management guidelines have subsequently been produced by the European Association of Urology and the AUA to create core documents to guide the management of urologic injuries.[38]

Renal Injuries

The majority of renal injuries are the result of blunt trauma (80%); the remainder are the result of penetrating injury (20%).[33] Approximately 70% of all patients who sustain renal injury are male, and most of these patients are younger than 50 years. As

TABLE 72-1   Organ Injury Scaling System: Kidney

GRADE	INJURY DESCRIPTION		AIS-90
I	Contusion	Microscopic or gross hematuria, urologic studies normal	2
	Hematoma	Subcapsular, nonexpanding, without parenchymal laceration	2
II	Hematoma	Nonexpanding perirenal hematoma confined to renal retroperitoneum	2
	Laceration	<1 cm parenchymal depth of renal cortex without urinary extravasation	2
III	Laceration	>1 cm depth of renal cortex, without collecting system rupture or urinary extravasation	3
IV	Laceration	Parenchymal laceration extending through the renal cortex, medulla, and collecting system	4
	Vascular	Main renal artery or vein injury, with contained hemorrhage	5
V	Laceration	Completely shattered kidney	5
	Vascular	Avulsion of renal hilum, which devascularizes kidney	5

Adapted from Moore EE, Shackford SR, Pachter HL, et al: Organ injury scaling: Spleen, liver, and kidney. *J Trauma* 29:1664–1666, 1989.

discussed in the retroperitoneal anatomy section, the kidneys are well protected in the retroperitoneum but are close to intraperitoneal structures. The key points in evaluation, as with any trauma patient, are the ABCs: airway, breathing, and circulation. In patients with a history of blunt trauma, key findings include location of impact, flank ecchymosis, and gross or microscopic hematuria. Other relevant historical information is concomitant injury and mechanism of injury. Close attention to the entry and exit points in penetrating injuries are also important to estimate the trajectory of the missile.

Imaging

There are many well-established indications for renal imaging after blunt or penetrating injury. In patients with blunt trauma, the criteria for imaging include gross hematuria, hemodynamic instability (systolic blood pressure < 90 mm Hg), microscopic hematuria (>5 red blood cells/high-power field), a traumatic mechanism, and suspicion of injury on screening radiographs (Fig. 72-11). In patients with penetrating injury who are hemodynamically stable, imaging is indicated for any degree of hematuria, microscopic or gross (Fig. 72-12).[38] The relevance of imaging to detect and to stage urinary tract injury before abdominal trauma surgery has been debated in the general surgical and urologic literature. Cross-sectional imaging, specifically contrast-enhanced CT scan, is the preferred study to evaluate the renal injuries. Proper imaging should include arteriovenous phases with delayed imaging to evaluate the urinary collecting structures. In those patients who proceed directly to surgery, the "one-shot" intravenous urogram (intravenous administration of 2 mL/kg contrast material followed by a single abdominal radiograph) can provide information concerning the presence or absence of a contralateral kidney. Ultrasound, intravenous urography, and magnetic resonance imaging (MRI) have a limited role in renal imaging for injury staging.

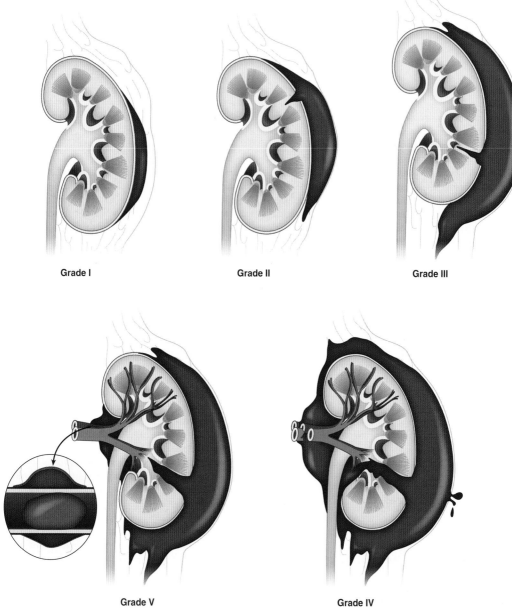

Grade I   Grade II   Grade III

Grade V   Grade IV

FIGURE 72-10 Illustrative diagram showing grade I-V renal injuries from the AAST organ injury scaling system. (From Moore EE, Shackford SR, Pachter HL, et al: Organ injury scaling: Spleen, liver, and kidney. *J Trauma* 29:1664–1666, 1989.)

Management: Operative versus Nonoperative

With better staging of renal injury, management paradigms have changed over time (Figs. 72-11 and 72-12). Furthermore, as urologists learned more from general trauma surgeons in the management of solid organ injury, nonoperative management of renal injuries has become more commonplace. The basis of nonoperative management centers around a properly staged injury with contrast-enhanced cross-sectional imaging (Fig. 72-13). In general, lower grade injuries, grades I to III, in hemodynamically stable patients are managed nonoperatively. Grade IV injuries are more controversial, and many are managed nonoperatively.

High-grade injuries, grades IV and V, particularly in patients with concomitant intraperitoneal injuries, may undergo surgical exploration.

In hemodynamically unstable patients who proceed directly to the operating room, there are absolute and relative criteria for operative exploration. The absolute criteria for exploration are expanding hematoma, pulsatile hematoma, and persistent renal bleeding. Any of these findings are concerning for possible renal pedicle injury.[39] The relative criteria for renal exploration include persistent urinary extravasation, nonviable renal parenchyma, arterial injury, and incomplete renal staging.[39] In the absence of

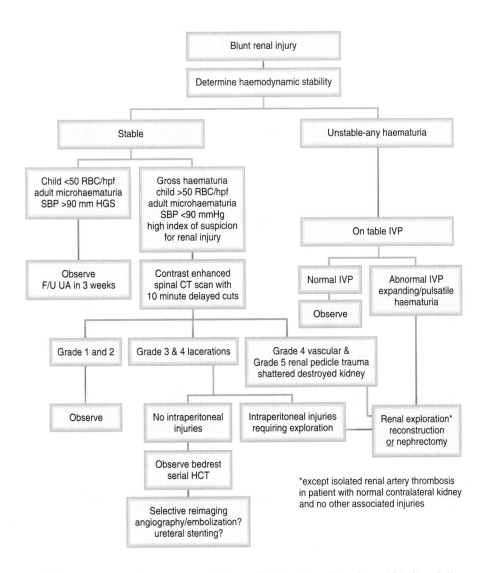

FIGURE 72-11 Algorithm for management of blunt renal injuries. (Adapted from Santucci RA, Wessells H, Bartsch G, et al: Evaluation and management of renal injuries: Consensus statement of the renal trauma subcommittee. *BJU Int* 93:937–954, 2004.)

such findings or in patients in whom a damage control approach is to be implemented, exploration may be avoided if the surgeon is uncomfortable with the potential requirements for reconstructive renal surgery.

Renal vascular injury is uncommon, and the radiologic presentation is variable. On CT imaging, these patients may have either large perinephric hematomas with intravascular extravasation of contrast material (indicating possible renal pedicle injury) or absent renal perfusion (indicating renal artery thrombosis). Segmental renal vascular injuries are usually the result of blunt renal trauma and appear as wedge-shaped defects in the renal parenchyma. These injuries rarely require intervention.

With an increase in nonoperative management of renal injuries, renal arteriography and selective angioembolization have been used with increasing frequency in management of renal trauma (Fig. 72-14). However, only select patients have been shown to benefit from this intervention: those with intravascular

extravasation of contrast material, perirenal hematoma rim distance of more than 25 mm, and medial hematomas.[40] In addition, patients who are assigned to a nonoperative management protocol and have received more than 2 units of red blood cell transfusion should undergo angiography.

Surgical Exploration and Operative Approach

Strict criteria exist for renal exploration. In those patients who proceed directly to the operating room, renal exploration is indicated with an expanding, pulsatile, uncontrolled retroperitoneal hematoma or renal pedicle avulsion. Patients with persistent renal bleeding but who require damage control management may require nephrectomy for hemodynamic stability. Patients with certain intraperitoneal injuries require surgical exploration and repair of renal injuries, including patients with concomitant bowel or pancreatic injury. Patients with renal pelvic laceration or persistent urinary extravasation of contrast material may require

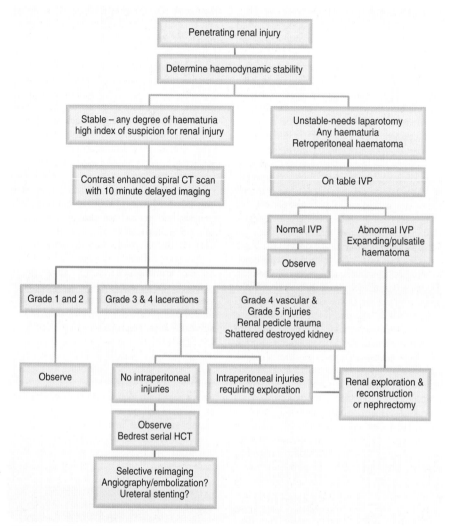

FIGURE 72-12 Algorithm for management of penetrating renal injuries. (Adapted from Santucci RA, Wessells H, Bartsch G, et al: Evaluation and management of renal injuries: Consensus statement of the renal trauma subcommittee. *BJU Int* 93:937–954, 2004.)

surgical repair of the collecting system. Patients with large segments of devitalized renal parenchyma and urinary extravasation may need early partial or total nephrectomy to prevent long-term complications. Trauma patients who have continued urinary extravasation despite percutaneous or endoscopic urinary diversion may require renal exploration and repair, although this may result in nephrectomy.

There are conflicting data concerning early vascular control before renal exploration, although the guidelines recommend vascular control.[33] Urologists are typically trained to approach the injured kidney anteriorly through a midline incision and to obtain vascular control of the renal vessels, before opening Gerota fascia and exposing the kidney, to avoid severe renal bleeding that may necessitate an urgent nephrectomy. In significant anatomic distortion, which may occur in the trauma setting, renal pedicle control can be obtained by bluntly creating a window medial to the lower pole of the kidney and lateral to the aorta (left) or vena cava (right), down to the psoas muscle fascia, which allows a vascular pedicle clamp to be placed if bleeding is encountered on renal exposure

(Fig. 72-15). Once vascular access is achieved, the kidney is exposed through an anterior vertical incision in Gerota fascia, which extends from the upper to the lower pole of the kidney. If there is parenchymal injury, care must be taken to identify the renal capsule in exposing and mobilizing the kidney to avoid stripping the entire capsule from the renal parenchyma and affecting kidney closure after renal reconstruction. The entire kidney should be exposed to reveal any lacerations, to evacuate hematoma, and to facilitate full mobility for repair. In general, if half the kidney can be preserved, renal reconstruction has benefit; however, if there is extensive destruction of the hilar region, successful reconstruction is unlikely. The preferred surgical management is renorrhaphy with suture ligation of bleeding vessels and closure of the collecting system with fine absorbable suture followed by parenchyma and capsular approximation with absorbable suture. For renal reconstruction in the trauma setting, pedicle clamping with a warm ischemia time of less than 30 minutes generally will not have a permanent adverse impact on renal function. The use of hemostatic agents and tissue sealants may aid in the reconstructive effort, and

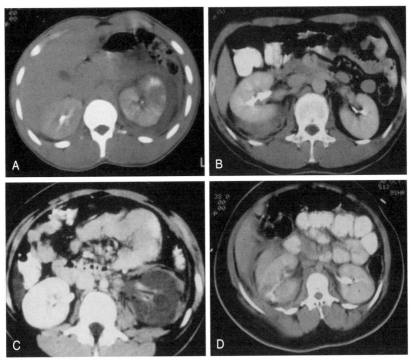

FIGURE 72-13 CT Scans Depicting Renal Trauma. **A,** Left renal contusion with heterogeneous contrast enhancement. **B,** Small right posterior pericapsular renal hematoma. **C,** Nonperfused left kidney after deceleration trauma and intimal disruption, with thrombosis of the renal artery. Vessel cutoff sign and some pericapsular enhancement are demonstrated. **D,** Grade IV laceration to the posterolateral right kidney, with posterolateral extravasation of contrast material.

closed suction drainage is beneficial in the instance of a collecting system injury or significant bleeding.

Ureteral Injuries

Ureteral injuries are uncommon (1% to 2.5% of all urologic injuries) and are rarely life-threatening but occur in the context of complex polytrauma.[39] Ureteral injuries due to external violence are most often the result of penetrating injuries; blunt injuries are the result of injuries with high-energy transfer, such as motor vehicle collision. Up to 5% to 10% of penetrating abdominal or pelvic injuries have ureteral involvement.[39] Management of ureteral injuries is dependent on mechanism of injury, anatomic location, and overall condition of the patient. The ureter is infrequently injured because of its mobility and location in the retroperitoneum protected by large muscle groups and the spine and bony pelvis. Ureteral injuries do not present with specific signs and symptoms, and their diagnosis requires heightened suspicion for injury based on mechanism and injury location.[38] Evaluation of ureteral injuries should be performed in the context of evaluation for more serious or life-threatening injuries.

Imaging

Ureteral imaging should be performed with contrast-enhanced, cross-sectional imaging, preferably CT scan, and must include delayed imaging to evaluate urinary excretion.[38] Findings suggesting ureteral injury include extravasation of contrast material, absence of contrast material distal to the suspected injury, and ipsilateral hydronephrosis. Other forms of imaging, including retrograde pyelography and intravenous urography, are difficult in the acute setting and often of lower quality.

Management

As a general principle, injuries to the ureter are best managed by surgical repair. Endoscopic ureteral stents or percutaneous diversion is generally reserved for missed injuries and for patients for whom reoperation is prohibitively morbid or the timing would make a successful repair unlikely. Ureteral contusions from adjacent penetrating trauma may benefit from ureteral stent placement to reduce progressive edema, occlusion, and ischemia and potentially to diminish the risk of delayed urinary extravasation.

Surgical Exploration and Operative Approach

When a ureteral injury is suspected, the ureter should be identified and directly inspected. The ureter can be approached surgically at any level by finding an area of normal anatomy and proceeding expeditiously to the areas in question. While dissecting around the ureter and mobilizing it from surrounding tissues, it is important to avoid stripping the periureteral tissue, causing devascularization. Ureteral injuries should be managed at the time of initial injury to decrease the chance of complication, such as urinoma, fistula, ureteral obstruction, and renal failure.[34] Repair usually involves minimal débridement of viable tissue. Lacerations are closed perpendicular to the axis of incision and transections with a spatulated, tension-free anastomosis. Injuries of the distal ureter often require reimplantation into the bladder. Gunshot wounds represent a particular concern as the viability of the ureteral stump may be compromised because of local tissue injury from the blast effect of the missile.[34] Fine absorbable suture is used in a running or interrupted fashion. Stent placement is desirable to allow low-pressure drainage, to minimize postoperative urinary extravasation, and to prevent angulation of the healing ureter.

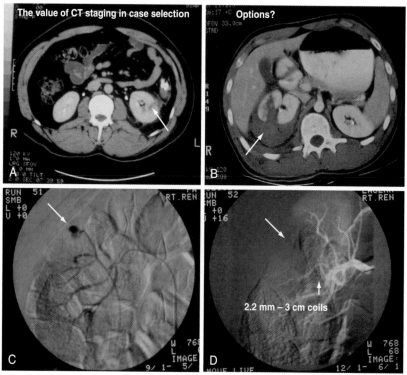

FIGURE 72-14 CT Scans Depicting Penetrating Renal Injury. A, Superficial laceration to the lateral left kidney from a stab wound. Note minimal hematoma and proximity of the posterior descending colon to the track of injury. Nonoperative management was selected and was successful. **B,** Deep laceration to the right kidney following a stab wound. Note the proximity to renal hilar structures and moderate-sized hematoma. **C,** Renal angiography performed for significant postinjury hematuria with hemodynamic instability, demonstrating pseudoaneurysm. **D,** Postembolization appearance of the right kidney showing a wedge-shaped defect after coil placement, which was successful.

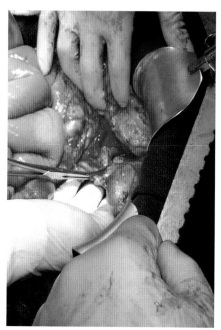

FIGURE 72-15 Placement of a pedicle clamp across renal vasculature.

Ureteral injuries are highly amenable to damage control approaches when repair acutely is not appropriate because of the patient's condition or the need to prioritize the management of other, more critical injuries.[41]

Bladder Injuries

The bladder is the second most commonly injured urologic structure and accounts for 10% of all urologic injuries. The most common source of bladder injury is blunt trauma (80% to 85%) from high-energy transfer, and it is often associated with pelvic fracture (83% to 95%).[35] The most common blunt sources of trauma are motor vehicle collision, falls from height, and industrial injuries. Patients with suspected bladder injuries often present with multisystem trauma and should be evaluated in the context of their presenting trauma. Most of the patients with bladder injury will present with hematuria and pelvic fracture, and in patients with gross hematuria and pelvic fracture, bladder injury is associated in 13% to 55% of cases.[38]

Imaging

Patients with suspected bladder injury should be evaluated with retrograde cystography. Both plain film cystography and CT cystography are acceptable, although CT scan may provide more anatomic detail. A necessary component of appropriate cystography is adequate retrograde filling of the bladder with 300 to

400 mL of contrast material.[38] If plain film cystography is performed, three anterior-posterior images must be obtained: scout, full bladder, and after drainage. CT cystography requires a diluted contrast agent of at least 1 : 6 concentration (Figs. 72-16 to 72-18). In patients with penetrating bladder injuries, imaging should not delay operative exploration as the bladder can be visually inspected at the time of surgery.

Management: Operative versus Nonoperative

Management of bladder injuries is dependent on location of the injury, extraperitoneal or intraperitoneal (Fig. 72-19). In general, intraperitoneal bladder injuries should be surgically repaired at the time of diagnosis. On the other hand, most extraperitoneal bladder injuries can be managed in a nonoperative fashion with simple catheter drainage. Extraperitoneal bladder injuries that should be managed in an operative fashion include penetrating bladder trauma, ongoing hematuria, concomitant pelvic organ injury, foreign body or bone fragment in the bladder, and bladder neck injuries.

Surgical Exploration and Operative Approach

The operative repair of bladder injuries is through a lower midline incision, often extending the midline incision from abdominal exploration to the pubic symphysis. Intraperitoneal injuries are often evident at the dome of the bladder within the overlying peritoneum. The traumatic cystotomy should be extended, if necessary, to fully evaluate the lumen of the bladder. In extraperitoneal injuries, the bladder is often opened through an anterior midline cystotomy to evaluate the lumen. This is especially true in the case of pelvic fracture to avoid disturbing the associated hematoma. If necessary, ureteral catheters can be inserted to confirm efflux of urine and ureteral continuity. Defects in the bladder wall are closed with absorbable 2-0 sutures in two layers to enhance watertightness. Use of a tissue interposition flap (e.g., omental flap) at the time of bladder repair may be necessary in cases of contiguous injuries to the rectum or vagina to prevent fistula formation. Diversion with a large-bore Foley catheter (at least 20 Fr to 24 Fr in the adult) allows bloody urine to drain and manual catheter irrigation, if necessary. Suprapubic cystostomy tubes are used for cases of extensive injuries requiring complex repairs or if prolonged bladder drainage is anticipated, such as with concomitant rectal or vaginal injury or traumatic brain injury. In patients with significant multisystem trauma who are hemodynamically unstable, definitive bladder repair may be delayed as a damage control maneuver.

Urethral Injuries

The urethra is not a common source of urologic trauma, and injury due to external violence accounts for approximately 4% of all genitourinary injuries.[36,42] Broadly, the urethra is divided into the anterior and posterior segments. Each segment has a different cause for injury and different management options based on the mechanism of injury, the involvement of surrounding structures, and the medical condition of the patient. The anterior segment of the urethra most commonly injured is the bulbar urethra, which accounts for 85% of urethral injuries.[36] Approximately 3% to 6% of posterior urethral injuries are associated with pelvic fracture, the so-called pelvic fracture urethral injury. The male anterior urethra may be injured at the time of penile injury, and 40% to 50% of penetrating wounds to the penis have urethral

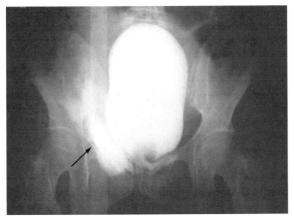

FIGURE 72-16 Static cystogram in patient with pelvic fracture and gross hematuria showing extraperitoneal extravasation of contrast material on the right side.

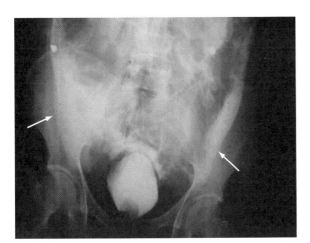

FIGURE 72-17 Static cystogram in patient after blunt injury to the lower abdomen showing the typical contrast material extravasation pattern of intraperitoneal bladder rupture. Note contrast material outlining the left and right colic gutters and present within the peritoneal cavity.

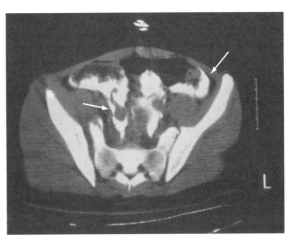

FIGURE 72-18 CT cystogram demonstrating intraperitoneal contrast material extravasation pattern of intraperitoneal bladder rupture. Note contrast material in the colic gutters, within the deep pelvis, and outlining the ovaries.

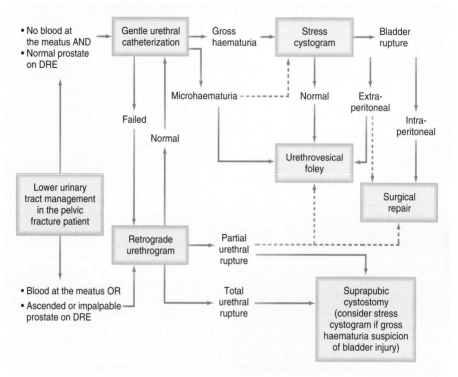

FIGURE 72-19 Algorithm for management of bladder injuries. (Adapted from Chapple C, Barbagli G, Jordan G, et al: Consensus statement on urethral trauma. *BJU Int* 93:1195–1202, 2004.)

involvement. The classic triad of physical examination findings for urethral injury is blood at the urethral meatus, inability to void, and a palpably distended bladder. Blood at the urethral meatus occurs in 37% to 93% of patients with urethral injury. The other physical finding that occurs in urethral trauma is perineal or "butterfly" hematoma due to rupture of Buck fascia; this can spread into the scrotum or up the abdomen along the layers of dartos and Scarpa fascia (Fig. 72-20).

Imaging

In patients with suspected urethral injury, retrograde urethrography should be performed before attempting the insertion of a Foley catheter.[38] Proper performance of retrograde urethrography involves adequate filling of the entire urethra with passage of contrast material into the bladder. Extravasation of contrast material occurs when continuity of the urethra has been lost because of the injury (Fig. 72-21).

Management

The immediate goal in managing urethral injury is to provide urinary bladder drainage and to avoid further injury.[36] Few urethral injuries, barring those resulting in significant ongoing external bleeding, such as with penetrating perineal trauma, require acute operative reconstruction. A delayed approach can almost always be implemented and often produces better outcomes. The surgeon with limited experience with these injuries should perform urinary diversion maneuvers for these cases. Urethral reconstruction is a highly specialized area of urology; definitive

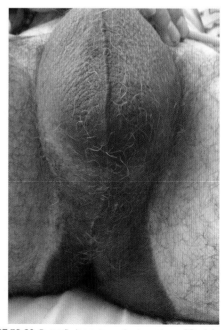

FIGURE 72-20 Butterfly hematoma due to rupture of Buck fascia after urethral injury.

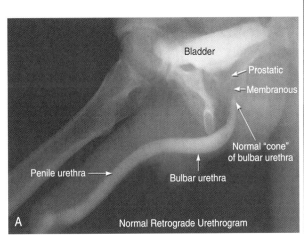
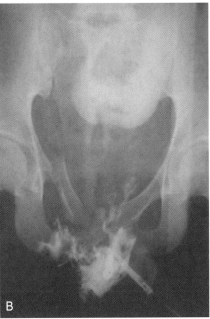

FIGURE 72-21 **Retrograde Urethrograms. A,** Standard technique with patient in an oblique position and complete filling of the anterior and posterior urethra with contrast material. **B,** Posterior urethral disruption in patient with displaced pelvic fracture. Note the deformity of the right superior pubic ramus and extensive extravasation of contrast material, extending above and below the urogenital diaphragm, on retrograde injection into the urethra. The bladder, which is greatly displaced cephalad, is filling with contrast material administered intravenously. The photograph demonstrates the so-called pie in the sky bladder resulting from dramatic displacement by a large pelvic hematoma after the prostatomembranous disruption injury. (**A** from Older RA, Hertz M: Cystourethrography. In Pollack HM, McClennan BL, Dyer R, Kenney PJ, editors: *Clinical urography*, ed 2, Philadelphia, 2000, WB Saunders.)

reconstructive surgery can be performed in a subacute or delayed fashion, with good results.[36]

Surgical Exploration and Operative Approach

Penetrating anterior urethral injuries should be explored and repaired primarily unless the patient is hemodynamically unstable. Urethral repair should be performed in two layers with fine absorbable suture over a catheter, creating a spatulated primary repair. Other anterior and posterior urethral injuries should be managed with suprapubic catheter insertion rather than by instrumentation of the traumatized urethra with risk of further injury. If the bladder is palpably distended and there is no evidence of prior lower abdominal surgery or the bladder can be clearly localized with ultrasound, percutaneous tube placement is appropriate. If these criteria are not met, open surgical cystostomy tube placement is safer and can be accomplished through a small anterior cystotomy. The drainage catheter should be anchored at the anterior bladder wall with absorbable sutures and at the skin exit site.

Immediate operative repair of posterior urethral injuries is not indicated, and management should consist of suprapubic tube placement. Posterior urethral injuries are well suited to damage control maneuvers.[41] Although it is controversial, there has been increased interest in early catheter realignment for posterior urethral disruption in the setting of pelvic fracture within 7 to 10 days of injury (Fig. 72-22). This technique requires substantial expertise in urologic endoscopic procedures, and the risk of creating further injury is substantial. Catheter realignment is performed using the suprapubic access that has been established

acutely, so there is no need to feel a sense of urgency in doing this on the day of injury. The outcomes of this procedure are unclear, but much of the literature indicates that 30% to 50% of patients can avoid urethral reconstruction, although strictures typically develop and require at least endoscopic management.

Genital Injuries

Genital trauma involves a range of anatomic structures, creating a difficulty in classification and standardization of treatment. The injuries are often the result of blunt or penetrating trauma but may include burns, bites, and avulsions and involve the penis, testicles, or scrotum in the male patient and the vulva in the female patient. Injuries to the external genitalia occur in 28% to 68% of patients with injuries to the genitourinary system; however, the incidence of genital trauma varies because of few epidemiologic studies.[43] The majority of external genital trauma is blunt in nature, although 40% to 60% of penetrating injuries to the genitourinary system involve the external genitalia.[43] Genitalia injuries may be the result of a variety of trauma, such as sexual excess in penile fracture, blunt scrotal trauma in testicular injury, or industrial accidents with skin avulsion in scrotal injuries.

Imaging

Imaging may be helpful in further diagnosing injuries in penile and scrotal trauma. In most patients, the genital trauma diagnosis is made on physical examination but can be confirmed with ultrasonography. For equivocal cases of penile fracture injury that results from sudden flexion of the erect penis during sexual

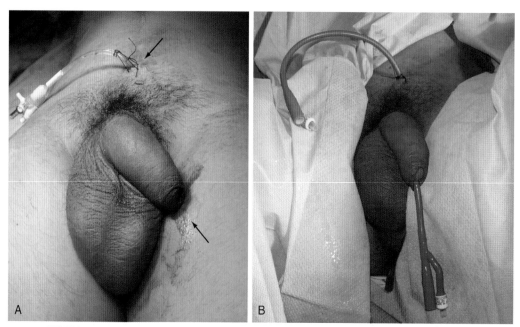

FIGURE 72-22 Posterior Urethral Disruption Injury. A, Patient with blood visible at penile meatus, managed with percutaneously placed suprapubic cystostomy tube. **B,** Patient initially managed similarly has undergone an endoscopic, fluoroscopically guided realignment procedure, with placement of urethral and suprapubic Foley catheters.

activity, penile ultrasound can demonstrate interruption of the corpora cavernosa. For blunt scrotal injuries, scrotal ultrasound may be helpful in determining whether the testis is ruptured. Key findings on ultrasound indicating testicular injury are loss of testicular contour of the tunica albuginea and heterogeneous echotexture of the testicular parenchyma.[38,42] Retrograde urethrography can be performed if there is concern for concomitant urethral injury.

Management

Because of the normal flaccid nature of the penis, the only injury that can occur is fracture of the erect penis. Management of these injuries involves surgical exploration of the penis and identification of the defect in the corporal body.[38,42] This is closed with slowly absorbing suture in a running fashion (Fig. 72-23). Blunt testicular injuries should be explored if ultrasound confirms testicular rupture. Repair of the injury is performed by limited débridement of the seminiferous tubules and closure of the tunica albuginea (Fig. 72-24). Orchiectomy is reserved for those injuries that thoroughly destroy the blood supply to the testis or those parenchymal injuries in which there is no viable parenchyma available to salvage.

Penetrating injuries to the external genitalia warrant surgical exploration in most cases. Functional and structural outcomes are greatly improved by early exploration and repair for penetrating penile, scrotal, and testicular injuries. For penile injuries, the goal is to remove foreign material, to cleanse the wound, to obtain hemostasis, to identify any defects in the tunica albuginea or urethra, and to proceed with appropriate repair while exercising caution not to be excessively aggressive with débridement of tissues of uncertain viability. For testicular injuries, débridement of devitalized parenchyma, closure of the capsule (tunica albuginea of the testis), and repair of the scrotum are key tasks.

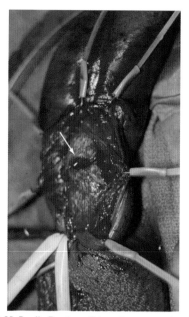

FIGURE 72-23 Penile Fracture. This patient was undergoing surgical exploration for a suspected penile fracture injury sustained during sexual activity. A ventral midline penoscrotal incision is used to expose the transverse laceration in the ventral right tunica albuginea of the corpus cavernosum, shown centrally. The Penrose drain at the bottom was used briefly as a tourniquet to control bleeding during suture repair of the injury. The hook and ring retractor system shown is useful for genital surgery.

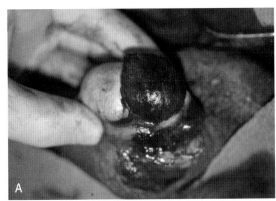

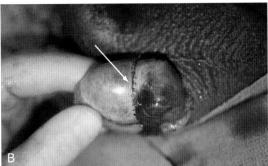

FIGURE 72-24 Testicular Rupture from Blunt Trauma. **A,** Intact tunica albuginea with a large transverse laceration *(left)*; the extruded testicular parenchyma from the upper portion of the testis is also shown *(right)*. **B,** Appearance after repair with running absorbable sutures.

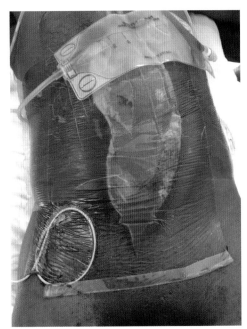

FIGURE 72-25 Damage control management of gunshot wound to right ureter. A diversion stent has been secured into the right ureter and externalized to gravity drainage.

Damage Control Techniques for Urologic Injuries

Many urologic injuries are amenable to initial management by applying damage control strategies. Damage control surgery refers to the concept of limiting the initial operative interventions, in the unstable trauma patient, to those maneuvers that are immediately lifesaving (e.g., control of surgical hemorrhage, control of continued fecal contamination). More time-consuming, definitive reconstructive efforts are delayed until later, after resuscitation, when the patient is more stable and can tolerate such reconstructive efforts. The physiologic rationale for damage control surgery relates to the metabolic consequences of extensive blood loss and blood and fluid replacement. These patients develop progressive hypothermia, acidosis, and coagulopathy (the so-called lethal triad), which can be corrected only when the patient can be brought to the intensive care unit with appropriate warming, fluid resuscitation, and other critical care interventions performed.[41]

Initially described in the military trauma literature, then applied to civilian penetrating abdominal trauma, these principles have now been successfully applied to a wide range of penetrating and blunt injuries. Extensive studies now support the view that appropriately selected patients managed by damage control strategies demonstrate improved survival compared with patients who undergo prolonged surgical efforts during the initial operative period. With the exception of patients with severe renal or bladder bleeding, urinary tract injuries do not directly result in early mortality. In the surgeon's judgment, when the patient would not tolerate the extended reconstructive effort needed to deal definitively with a urologic injury at initial laparotomy—because of pattern of injury, hypothermia, acidosis, coagulopathy, or other

parameters that mandate a damage control approach—certain temporary solutions may be used. The complexity of patient selection for damage control surgery requires a multidisciplinary interaction, with the trauma surgeon and surgical specialists involved, to determine which injuries must be addressed initially and which can be definitively handled in a delayed fashion. Earlier selection of damage control surgery candidates, based on patterns of injury and response to initial resuscitative efforts, results in improved survival when the initial operative procedure can be concluded before significant metabolic deterioration occurs.[41]

Renal injuries that are incompletely staged or unstaged may be approached with delayed assessment and exploration, as long as a determination is made that life-threatening bleeding from the injury is unlikely to occur. In the absence of significant bleeding from the renal fossa into the peritoneal cavity, a large midline hematoma, or an expanding or pulsatile renal hematoma, one can elect to leave the perinephric hematoma undisturbed and fully resuscitate the patient.[41] Appropriate staging studies can be performed and delayed exploration and reconstruction completed at the time of a second-look procedure. If a major reconstructive effort is still needed in the unstable patient, packing the kidney and returning for reconstructive interventions later is also an option.

Ureteral injuries may be managed initially with externalized stents, ligation, or simple local drainage. Of these options, externalized stents are preferred as they allow control of the urinary output, minimize ongoing urinary extravasation, and can be maintained until the patient is stable enough to return to surgery for definitive reconstruction. Any number of medical tubes or catheters can be used, but the ideal solution is a 7 Fr or 8.5 Fr single-J urinary diversion stent placed into the ureter through the injury site, advanced proximally into the kidney, and then externalized through the abdominal wall (Fig. 72-25). The catheter should be tied to the very end of the injured ureter at the injury site so as not to lose ureteral length by ligating it more proximally and making later reconstruction more challenging. The distal ureteral limb is best left undisturbed; ligating it requires subsequent débridement and causes further tissue loss.

A similar approach can be used for extensive bladder injuries; the ureteral orifices can be catheterized, the catheters externalized, and the pelvis packed, leaving bladder reconstruction to be performed at a more suitable time, after appropriate resuscitation. Urethral and genital injuries are also amenable to damage control approaches, generally involving tube diversion, placement of moistened dressings, and tissue preservation until definitive reconstruction after appropriate resuscitation.

NONTRAUMATIC UROLOGIC EMERGENCIES

Within the field of urology are several emergent conditions, although not due to external violence, that represent true emergencies, some of which are life-threatening. These urologic emergencies include obstructed upper tract UTI, hematuria with urinary retention due to blood clots, and the acute scrotum—specifically testicular torsion, priapism, and Fournier gangrene. Some of these conditions have been discussed in other sections of this chapter (Fournier gangrene and obstructed upper tract UTI); the remainder are covered in this discussion.

Testicular Torsion

The most urgent cause of the acute scrotum is testicular torsion. Testicular torsion occurs when arterial blood supply is compromised by a twist of the spermatic cord, creating occlusion of the spermatic cord and loss of vascular supply. In the normal anatomic arrangement, the inferior aspect of the testicle is attached to the scrotum by the gubernaculum, preventing rotation of the testicle within the scrotum. When torsion occurs, the testicle is subjected to warm ischemia; without reversal of the occluded blood supply, irreversible damage begins as soon as 4 hours and is complete by 8 to 12 hours. Although testicular torsion is most common in adolescent males, it may occur in any age group from neonate to adult men. As many other conditions may result in the so-called acute scrotum, a high index of suspicion is necessary on the part of the treating physician to ensure rapid diagnosis and treatment. Differential diagnosis includes trauma, epididymitis, incarcerated hernia, and torsion of the appendix testis or appendix epididymis. Diagnosis is strongly suspected on the basis of history and physical examination. Classic historical findings include sudden onset of intense unilateral scrotal pain, unrelated to trauma, that may be associated with nausea and vomiting. The most consistent physical examination finding is loss of the cremasteric reflex of the testicle; however, in an acute setting, this may be difficult to elicit. The best confirmatory radiologic study is color Doppler ultrasound of the scrotum, which shows absence of arterial flow to the testis in torsion. In patients with suspected testicular torsion, there is no need to delay scrotal exploration to obtain imaging or further laboratory evaluation.

Treatment of testicular torsion involves surgical exploration through a midline or transverse scrotal incision with inspection of the testis with detorsion, if present, of the spermatic cord (Fig. 72-26). For testes that are deemed to be viable, suture orchiopexy or fixation to the interior scrotal wall is performed, followed by a similar orchiopexy on the contralateral side at the same setting to prevent contralateral torsion. Because of the important medicolegal considerations in these cases, urgent exploration is still

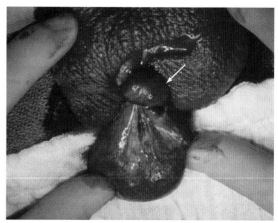

FIGURE 72-26 Testicular Torsion. Exploration through a transverse scrotal incision demonstrates the twisted cord *(top)*. Note the degree of edema, erythema, and ecchymosis present after several hours of torsion.

indicated even in patients who present with a suspected late torsion (e.g., several days of fixed swelling, firmness). Many times, it is difficult to know exactly how long complete ischemia has been present and whether there is still a potentially viable testicle.

Gross Hematuria With Urinary Retention from Blood Clots

Most patients who have hematuria present with either microscopic hematuria or episodic gross hematuria. However, in a subset of patients, onset of gross hematuria is rapid with significant blood loss and development of blood clots within the bladder. This problem is exacerbated in patients who are receiving chronic anticoagulation for underlying cardiovascular disease processes. The blood clots are organized into larger masses; the patient may not be able to expel the clot, leading to urinary retention and a potential surgical emergency (Fig. 72-27). Other causes of significant vesical hemorrhage include postoperative bleeding after TURP or transurethral resection of bladder tumor (TURBT), radiation cystitis, pelvic trauma, upper tract arteriovenous fistula, and iliac arterial fistula to the ureter.

It is difficult to judge the amount of blood that is being lost from the urinary tract with gross hematuria because only a small amount of blood mixed with urine will darken the bladder efflux. If, however, copious amounts of clot are evacuated from the bladder, one should suspect at least moderate blood loss and monitor the patient with vital signs and hemoglobin measurements. If bleeding from these events causes symptomatic anemia, the patient may require multiple urgent blood transfusions. In the patient with a significant amount of blood clot in the bladder, it will be necessary to place a large-bore irrigation catheter (in the adult, often 20 Fr to 26 Fr) and adequately irrigate the clots from the bladder using normal saline irrigation. Special hematuria catheters are designed to allow large-volume irrigation and clot removal, but if this is unsuccessful, the patient may require urgent operative cystoscopy to evacuate the clot and to identify and fulgurate any bleeding source. Typically, this involves rigid cystoscopy with a large working sheath or resectoscope sheath and irrigation performed with a piston syringe or special evacuation devices (Ellik evacuator). After clot evacuation and fulguration, a

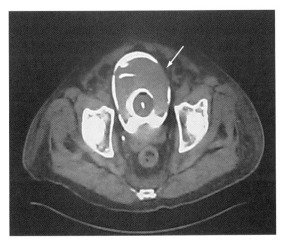

FIGURE 72-27 CT scan of the pelvis with cystography in a patient with urinary clot retention caused by chronic hemorrhagic cystitis after radiation therapy for prostate cancer. A clot may be seen surrounding the Foley catheter balloon, with instilled contrast material outlining the balloon and intact bladder wall.

large three-way catheter is left in place to run continuous irrigation to prevent a recurrent episode of clot retention. Upper tract clot formation may produce a so-called clot colic, with renal pain similar to that experienced from passage of a renal calculus. Supportive care and, in some cases, stent insertion may be helpful to address the underlying problem. If unexplained, significant, gross hematuria occurs after minor trauma, one should suspect an underlying abnormality of the urinary tract, such as a neoplasm, congenital anomaly, or arteriovenous malformation.

Priapism

Priapism is a prolonged, painful penile erection that occurs in the absence of sexual arousal or stimulation. Priapism is typically divided into ischemic and nonischemic priapism. Important causes of ischemic priapism include sickle cell disease or other blood dyscrasias and certain types of drug or medication use, especially drugs for penile erection and hematologic malignant disease. Nonischemic priapism is the pelvic or genital trauma that results in arteriovenous fistula of the penile circulation. Priapism may resolve spontaneously, but if it persists longer than 4 hours, measures should be taken to reverse the process in most cases. Patients with priapism that lasts longer than 12 hours may develop irreversible damage to the penile vascular structure and long-term ED.

Evaluation in cases of ischemic priapism is centered on detailed history for risk factors, corporal blood gas analysis, and color Doppler ultrasound of the corpora cavernosa. Nonischemic priapism is evaluated similarly; however, aspirated blood has an arterial appearance and arterial blood gas parameters.

Ischemic priapism is managed with initial needle aspiration of the corpora cavernosa and irrigation with saline. In patients who do not respond to this step, needle aspiration is repeated with the injection of small, dilute doses of an α-adrenergic agonist substance, such as dilute phenylephrine. For patients who fail to respond to these measures, various shunting procedures can be performed to create shunts between the corpus cavernosum and other vascular structures, like the corpus spongiosum, to induce blood flow. For priapism related to sickle cell disease, medical

treatment of the sickle crisis (e.g., hydration, oxygenation, pain management, and addressing hemoglobin and transfusion status) with hematology support is a mainstay of therapy to resolve priapism. For nonischemic priapism, there is no role for aspiration or irrigation of the erection as this is the result of an abnormality of the vascular system. Compression of the perineum or other injury site can be performed as an initial maneuver. If this fails, the next treatment step is usually superselective angioembolization to occlude the arteriovenous fistula with reversible agents, such as autologous blood clots or Gelfoam. It is important that the general surgeon consult with the urologist about treatment because corporal fibrosis and loss of erectile function are risks that increase with significant delays in therapy.

UROLOGIC ONCOLOGY

Urologic malignant neoplasms account for a significant disease burden in adults in the United States. Cancers of the genitourinary system encompass the full spectrum of malignant neoplasms and are of some of the most common (prostate) and rare (penile) cancers in the United States. Of the 12 most common cancers diagnosed annually in the United States, three are urologic in origin: prostate, bladder, and kidney. Low-stage cancers are typically managed with extirpative surgery or therapeutic radiation. Urologic cancers may involve adjacent viscera, vasculature, and soft tissue and body wall structures so that additional surgical expertise is necessary to complete the extirpative surgery and to support reconstructive efforts. As is the case with other malignant neoplasms, cancers of the genitourinary system are often managed with a multidisciplinary approach. The major anatomic types of urologic cancers are discussed in this section, with a focus on the essential basic background knowledge, the fundamental therapeutic approaches for various stages of cancer presentation, and the basic outcomes for different tumor types.

Renal Tumors

Renal cell carcinoma, the most common type of renal malignant disease, accounts for 2% to 3% of all adult malignant neoplasms.[44] The majority of renal malignant neoplasms are now diagnosed incidentally by cross-sectional imaging or ultrasound evaluation of other nonspecific complaints. Historically, renal cell carcinoma was diagnosed only at an advanced stage because of its location within the retroperitoneum. The classic triad of renal cell carcinoma (flank pain, gross hematuria, and palpable abdominal mass) is now seen in less than 10% of patients. Despite this increase in asymptomatic diagnoses, 30% of patients present with metastatic disease.[45] Other symptoms on advanced presentation include hemorrhage, paraneoplastic syndrome, and symptoms of metastasis, such as pathologic fracture. Paraneoplastic syndromes are present in 20% of patients at diagnosis and include Stauffer syndrome (reversible hepatitis without liver metastasis), constitutional symptoms, polycythemia, and elevated inflammatory markers (erythrocyte sedimentation rate and C-reactive protein).[45] Renal cell carcinoma typically presents in the sixth to eighth decade of life and is more common in men. Risk factors for renal cell carcinoma include smoking, hypertension, obesity, acquired renal cystic disease (in patients with end-stage renal disease), and occupational exposures (aromatic hydrocarbons, asbestos, cadmium, and chemical and rubber industries).[44] These tumors typically arise in the proximal convoluted tubule or collecting duct within the renal parenchyma.[44]

Renal cell carcinoma is classified as follows: clear cell carcinoma, papillary renal cell carcinoma, chromophobe renal cell carcinoma, collecting duct carcinoma, and renal medullary carcinoma; this classification is based on microscopic appearance and cell of origin.[45] The genetics of these malignant neoplasms is fairly well described. The most common tumor, clear cell carcinoma, is the result of chromosome 3 abnormalities; papillary carcinoma is the result of aberrations of chromosome 7, 17, or Y.[45] In addition, clear cell carcinoma and papillary carcinoma are responsible for the two most common familial cancer syndromes, von Hippel–Lindau and hereditary papillary renal cell carcinoma, respectively. Most renal masses are malignant, and only 15% to 20% are benign; the two most common benign masses are oncocytoma and angiomyolipoma.[45]

A final consideration with renal neoplasms is cystic renal masses, which present diagnostic challenges. Depending on specific characteristics of renal cystic lesions, the risk of these lesions representing cystic malignant neoplasms must be considered. The Bosniak classification system describes cystic renal masses according to their malignant risk and CT appearance, ranging from category I (simple cysts) to category IV (cysts associated with enhancing or solid elements).[45] Category III and IV cysts are usually treated as representing cystic renal cell carcinomas.

Staging

Outcomes in renal cell carcinoma are directly tied to clinical stage at time of diagnosis. Evaluation and staging for renal cell carcinoma include history, physical examination, and laboratory testing. Evaluation for renal masses includes imaging of the primary tumor, usually with a contrast-enhanced CT scan or MRI study of the abdomen and pelvis, as well as chest imaging, typically chest radiography. Also, based on clinical suspicion or abnormal results of laboratory studies, bone and brain imaging is performed. A key aspect of abdominal CT or MRI is evaluation of the renal vein and inferior vena cava as renal cell carcinoma commonly forms tumor thrombus in these structures, and this finding is not necessarily correlated with tumor stage. The TNM staging system is listed in Table 72-2. Histologic grading is based on the Fuhrman nuclear grading system on a scale of I to IV.

Management

The management of renal cell carcinoma has evolved in recent years. Historically, renal cell carcinoma was a surgical disease, and patients diagnosed with any renal mass underwent total radical nephrectomy. Now, select patients may undergo renal biopsy and active surveillance protocols. In the past, renal biopsies were fraught with high false-negative rates and low accuracy. Contemporary series show an accuracy rate of more than 90% in experienced centers with low complications.[45] Those patients who are appropriate for renal biopsy are patients considered for either active surveillance or renal ablation therapy. Active surveillance protocols have been developed for patients with incidentally diagnosed, small (<3 cm) renal masses and those patients who would not tolerate extirpative or ablative therapy.[45] The natural history of renal masses is a tendency to grow slowly, on average 0.5 cm/yr, and they do not metastasize. Patients assigned to surveillance protocols undergo imaging every 3 to 6 months; once mass size stability is observed, this interval is extended to 6 to 12 months.[45] Small renal masses (<5 cm) can be considered for percutaneous, laparoscopic, or open ablation using cryotherapy or radiofrequency energy.[44] This treatment should be considered more for patients with significant medical comorbidities and less often in healthy patients.

TABLE 72-2	Staging of Kidney Cancer
Primary Tumor (T)	
TX	Primary tumor cannot be assessed
T0	No evidence of primary tumor
T1	Tumor 7 cm or less in greatest dimension, limited to the kidney
T1a	Tumor 4 cm or less in greatest dimension, limited to the kidney
T1b	Tumor more than 4 cm but not more than 7 cm in greatest dimension, limited to the kidney
T2	Tumor >7 cm in greatest dimension, limited to the kidney
T2a	Tumor >7 cm and ≤10 cm in greatest dimension, limited to the kidney
T2b	Tumor >10 cm in greatest dimension, limited to the kidney
T3	Tumor extends into major veins or perinephric tissues but not into the ipsilateral adrenal gland and not beyond Gerota fascia
T3a	Tumor grossly extends into the renal vein or its segmental (muscle-containing) branches, or tumor invades perirenal and/or renal sinus fat but not beyond Gerota fascia
T3b	Tumor grossly extends into the vena cava below the diaphragm
T3c	Tumor grossly extends into the vena cava above the diaphragm or invades the wall of the vena cava
T4	Tumor invades beyond Gerota fascia (including contiguous extension into the ipsilateral adrenal gland)
Regional Lymph Nodes (N)	
NX	Regional lymph nodes cannot be assessed
N0	No regional lymph node metastasis
N1	Metastasis in regional lymph node(s)
Distant Metastasis (M)	
M0	No distant metastasis
M1	Distant metastasis
Stage Grouping	
Stage I	T1 N0 M0
Stage II	T2 N0 M0
Stage III	T1 or T2 N1 M0, T3 N0 or N1 M0
Stage IV	T4 Any N M0

For renal tumors that are diagnosed in the absence of metastases or for those with a solitary metastasis, extirpative surgery is the standard approach. Resection of solitary synchronous metastatic disease is performed when it is technically feasible. Renal surgery has undergone a significant transformation in the past 10 years, and most renal surgery, both nephron sparing and radical excision, is now performed through either a laparoscopic or robotically assisted approach. The trend in extirpative surgery is to perform nephron sparing or partial nephrectomy for most T1 tumors. Partial nephrectomy is equivalent to radical nephrectomy in this tumor stage and should be considered for all patients with a T1a tumor and most with T1b tumors. Partial nephrectomy surgery may be straightforward in dealing with small, well-encapsulated, superficial, exophytic lesions or complex in dealing with larger, central lesions that involve the renal hilar structures. For partial nephrectomy, a negative margin should be obtained with the parenchymal resection, and only a few millimeters of normal parenchyma around the tumor are considered necessary. The general principles for partial nephrectomy include achievement of a negative surgical margin, identification and suturing of significant segmental renal vessel branches, and collecting system repair when the collecting system is entered or partially resected.

To assist with blood loss, atraumatic vascular clamping of the renal artery and surface cooling of the kidney with iced saline slush are effective. When laparoscopic or robotic approaches are used for partial nephrectomy, local hypothermia is more cumbersome, and rapid tumor resection and clamp times of less than 30 minutes are employed. Tissue sealants, hemostatic agents, and absorbable mesh reconstruction of the kidney are all useful techniques to aid in hemostasis of a partial nephrectomy in the open surgical, laparoscopic, or robotic setting.

Radical nephrectomy is performed in patients with large tumors and those patients in whom a partial nephrectomy is not technically feasible. The primary long-term risk in this surgery is chronic kidney disease and loss of renal function. In comparison to partial nephrectomy, radical nephrectomy has a lower rate of complications. The adrenal gland is no longer removed with radical nephrectomy except in cases of obvious tumor involvement as the rate of synchronous involvement is less than 10%. Typically, radical nephrectomy is performed by either a laparoscopic or open approach. Standard incisions for radical nephrectomy include anterior subcostal, flank, chevron, and midline, although the midline incision has the most difficult vascular access. Regardless of approach, dissection of the renal pedicle with ligation of a renal artery must precede vein ligation to prevent swelling and dangerous bleeding from the kidney. The entire Gerota fascial envelope, containing the perinephric fat as a margin around the kidney parenchyma and tumor, is excised intact. The ureter is ligated and divided where convenient. A regional lymph node dissection is often performed with a radical nephrectomy, although, on the basis of most evidence, it is more helpful as a staging and prognostic procedure than as a therapeutic one. For patients with locally advanced or metastatic disease, immunotherapy and targeted therapy (drugs with action on vascular endothelial growth factor and mammalian target of rapamycin) are used in a neoadjuvant or adjuvant setting. Overall organ-confined disease has an 80% to 100% 5-year survival in T1 tumors and a 50% to 80% 5-year survival in T2 disease.[45] Advanced disease has grim prognosis of 0% to 20% 5-year survival.[45]

Bladder Cancer

Urothelial malignant disease can arise anywhere in the upper or lower collecting system, but the most common site is the bladder. The entire upper and lower urinary tracts, renal collecting system through the prostatic urethra, are lined with surface epithelium called urothelium. The urothelium has a variable thickness of three to six cell layers, and transitional cell carcinoma arises from the basal cell layer. Bladder cancer is the fifth most common adult malignant neoplasm diagnosed in the United States and is more common in men than in women.[46] The tumor arises most frequently in the eighth decade of life, and men older than 70 years have a 3.7% probability for development of bladder cancer.[46] The multiple risk factors for development of bladder cancer include tobacco smoke, arsenic, chronic infections and inflammatory conditions (e.g., schistosomiasis), and occupational exposures (such as arylamines and aromatic hydrocarbons). The most common presenting symptom in bladder cancer is hematuria, microscopic in 1% to 11% and gross in 13% to 35%.[46] The other presenting symptom is irritative voiding—frequency, urgency, and dysuria. Bladder cancer can be divided into non–muscle invasive and muscle invasive, which have different treatments and outcomes. TNM staging is included in Table 72-3; the T stage at diagnosis, specifically non–muscle invasive (T1 or less) or muscle invasive (T2 or greater), is highly predictive of long-term outcome and

TABLE 72-3 Staging of Urothelial Cancer

Primary Tumor (T)

TX	Primary tumor cannot be assessed
T0	No evidence of primary tumor
Ta	Noninvasive papillary carcinoma
Tis	Carcinoma in situ: "flat tumor"
T1	Tumor invades subepithelial connective tissue
T2	Tumor invades muscularis propria
pT2a	Tumor invades superficial muscularis propria (inner half)
pT2b	Tumor invades deep muscularis propria (outer half)
T3	Tumor invades perivesical tissue:
pT3a	Microscopically
pT3b	Macroscopically (extravesical mass)
T4	Tumor invades any of the following: prostatic stroma, seminal vesicles, uterus, vagina, pelvic wall, abdominal wall
T4a	Tumor invades prostatic stroma, uterus, vagina
T4b	Tumor invades pelvic wall, abdominal wall

Regional Lymph Nodes (N)

Regional lymph nodes include both primary and secondary drainage regions. All other nodes above the aortic bifurcation are considered distant lymph nodes.

NX	Lymph nodes cannot be assessed
N0	No lymph node metastasis
N1	Single regional lymph node metastasis in the true pelvis (hypogastric, obturator, external iliac, or presacral lymph node)
N2	Multiple regional lymph node metastasis in the true pelvis (hypogastric, obturator, external iliac, or presacral lymph node metastasis)
N3	Lymph node metastasis to the common iliac lymph nodes

Distant Metastasis (M)

M0	No distant metastasis
M1	Distant metastasis

survival. Ta disease refers to papillary tumors, with involvement of only the mucosa. T1 tumors involve the lamina propria, and T2 disease involves the detrusor muscle. Higher stages of the local tumor reflect involvement of perivesical fat or adjacent organs. Tumors are graded on the basis of histologic appearance from papilloma to high grade.

Non–Muscle Invasive Bladder Cancer

Urothelial tumors that have not invaded the detrusor muscle are termed non–muscle invasive bladder cancers (NMIBCs). Approximately 70% of patients who present with bladder cancer will be diagnosed with NMBIC, which includes T stages Tis (carcinoma in situ), Ta, and T1.[46] Patients who are suspected of having bladder cancer should undergo a thorough evaluation, which includes history, physical examination, basic laboratory tests, upper urinary tract imaging (preferably contrast-enhanced cross-sectional imaging), and office cystoscopy. If bladder cancer is present, characteristic flat, papillary, or bizarre, aggressive-appearing masses will be present on the urothelial surface of the bladder. NMIBCs typically appear as flat (carcinoma in situ) or papillary (Ta or T1) lesions. An adjunct test for equivocal findings is urine cytology, which is either as voided or bladder wash at the time of cystoscopy. Urine cytology is most sensitive for high-grade tumors and can be equivocal or nondiagnostic in the setting of low-grade NMIBCs. Adjunct urine tumor markers exist but are not recommended on consensus guidelines because of cost and low specificity.

Any tumor identified in the bladder should be fully resected by TURBT. TURBT allows pathologic analysis, tumor staging but identification (if present) of muscle invasion, and treatment of noninvasive, low-grade disease. TURBT is performed through a surgical endoscope, called a resectoscope, and uses either monopolar or bipolar energy to shave the tumor from the bladder wall. At the time of TURBT, patients should undergo a bimanual examination of the bladder to identify extravesical extension of disease and palpable mass. Any patient identified with high-grade T1 tumors or absence of muscle in the initial resection should undergo repeated TURBT. All patients who undergo TURBT should receive immediate intravesical chemotherapy within 6 hours of surgery; this treatment has been shown to reduce the tumor recurrence rate by 35%.[46] The agent most commonly used for this purpose is mitomycin C. Six weeks after TURBT, patients with carcinoma in situ or NMIBC with high risk for progression or recurrence should receive intravesical therapy with either immunotherapy or chemotherapeutic agents. Standard immunotherapy for NMIBC consists of serial bacille Calmette-Guérin (BCG) intravesical instillations for induction and periodic maintenance therapy. Intravesical BCG significantly decreases the invasion and progression rate for NMIBCs, compared with transurethral resection alone. Patients with recurrent NMIBC may require regimens of BCG plus interferon for salvage therapy. Maintenance BCG instillations reduce the risk of recurrence and progression and are given at variable intervals for periods of 1 to 3 years. Other salvage intravesical treatments include chemotherapeutic agents such as mitomycin C and gemcitabine. Visual surveillance by office cystoscopy is mandatory in these patients as 15% to 80% of these tumors recur, and in higher grade tumors, 25% to 50% progress to higher stage or muscle invasive tumors.[46]

Muscle Invasive Bladder Cancer

Muscle invasive bladder cancer (MIBC) includes stage T2 or greater bladder cancer at diagnosis. The majority of patients who present with MIBC have invasive disease at diagnosis; approximately 15% to 20% of patients who present with NMIBC progress to MIBC.[46] MIBC is typically urothelial cell carcinoma, but other histopathologic types occur, including squamous cell carcinoma, adenocarcinoma, and small cell carcinoma. The last two have the worst prognostic outcomes. MIBC should be staged in a similar fashion to NMIBC, with cross-sectional imaging of the abdomen and pelvis, but consideration should be given to chest CT rather than plain radiography. Despite adequate staging, 40% of patients are understaged at diagnosis and have extravesical disease on the final pathologic specimen.

Management. Standard management of MIBC is radical cystoprostatectomy. In the male patient, radical cystectomy involves the removal of the entire urinary bladder en bloc with the perivesical fat, prostate, seminal vesicles, and pelvic lymph nodes. In the female patient, radical cystectomy typically involves en bloc removal of the female pelvic viscera, although salvage of these structures may at times be considered, depending on the details of the case. Extended lymph node dissection is performed at the same setting and includes removal of the external and internal iliac lymph nodes, common iliac lymph nodes to the aortic bifurcation, and presacral lymph nodes. Improved survival is associated with extended pelvic lymph node dissection at the time of radical cystectomy. Perioperative complication rates are high, and more than 60% of patients undergoing radical cystectomy and extended

pelvic lymph node dissection have at least one complication within 90 days of surgery.[46] Because of the high rate of extravesical extension at the time of radical cystectomy, many patients are treated with neoadjuvant chemotherapy. Typical regimens for neoadjuvant chemotherapy include MVAC (methotrexate, vinblastine, doxorubicin [Adriamycin], and cisplatin) and GC (gemcitabine and cisplatin). The use of neoadjuvant chemotherapy improves overall survival by 5% to 7%.[46]

The selection of the type of urinary diversion after radical cystectomy must take into account any history of pelvic irradiation, presence of renal insufficiency, liver function abnormalities, and mechanical tasks for which the patient will be responsible. There are various options for urinary diversion, including ileal conduit, orthotopic bladder substitution with anastomosis to the native urethra, and more complex forms of cutaneous catheterizable reservoirs with continence mechanisms. No randomized study has shown one type of urinary diversion to be superior to any other, and the decision is usually directed by the patient's preference or the surgeon's choice. There is an extensive and complex history involving the use of intestinal segments in the urinary tract for urinary diversion after cystectomy and in other reconstructive settings. The surgeon should be familiar with the metabolic, mechanical, and other risk factors associated with the use of intestinal segments in the reconstructed urinary tract, including electrolyte abnormalities, bone demineralization, mucus production, stone formation, chronic infection, diarrhea, vitamin B_{12} deficiency, and increased cancer risk. Patients with organ-confined, node-negative disease have the best overall disease-specific survival at 5 and 10 years at 60% to 85%.[46]

Prostate Cancer

Prostate cancer is the most common cancer diagnosed in men and the third most common cancer diagnosed in the United States, behind breast and lung, with approximately 220,000 men diagnosed annually.[47] Prostate cancer is an adenocarcinoma and arises from the glandular structures within the prostatic parenchyma. Most new prostate cancer cases are diagnosed in men 60 years of age and older, are low grade and low stage, and are diagnosed by routine screening.[48] Screening for prostate cancer is performed with the blood test PSA, a serine protease, and DRE. The most controversial aspect of prostate cancer is screening and determining which patients require treatment. The goal of prostate cancer screening is to detect potentially lethal cancer at an early, treatable stage and to intervene with intent to cure. Because of the controversy surrounding the recent U.S. Preventive Services Task Force recommendation against screening for prostate cancer in 2012, the AUA released its own guidelines for screening in 2013.[49] These recommendations are for screening in men aged 55 to 69 years to be a joint decision between the physician and the patient, with recognition that the mortality of prostate cancer is 1 in 1000 men screened per decade, and a routine screening interval to occur every 2 years.[49] Routine screening is not routinely recommended in men aged 40 to 54 years and in men older than 70 years or younger than 40 years.[49] Furthermore, screening should not be performed in men with a life expectancy of less than 10 to 15 years.

Evaluation

Patients who have either an elevated total PSA level or abnormal findings on DRE or both undergo TRUS-guided biopsy of the prostate. In equivocal cases, other testing, including determination of free PSA level or calculation of PSA velocity, can help guide the decision for biopsy or further evaluation. The standard biopsy template involves 12 cores with a spring-loaded biopsy instrument; tissue is obtained from the base, mid, and apex regions, medially and laterally from the left and right sides. Prophylactic antibiotics are routinely administered, and cleansing enemas are advised. When feasible, patients are asked to stop anticoagulants to help prevent bleeding complications. Common adverse events that follow TRUS biopsy include rectal bleeding, gross hematuria, and hematospermia, all of which are usually self-limited. Fever and urinary infection and retention occur in less than 5% of patients; bacteremia occurs, but it is a rare occurrence in less than 1% of patients.

Prostate cancer is diagnosed histologically by the Gleason grading system, which evaluates the level of abnormality in the patterns of the glandular architecture of the prostate in comparison to normal. The grading system is based on a scale of 1 to 5, with 1 being the most differentiated and 5 being the least differentiated. Most prostate cancers have a Gleason grade of 3 with a sum of 6 or 7. Patients diagnosed with prostate cancer are risk stratified on the basis of PSA level at time of diagnosis, clinical stage based on DRE, and Gleason sum score on the prostate biopsy. Patients with high-risk cancers should undergo cancer staging, which in prostate cancer may include radionuclide bone scan to evaluate for bone metastasis and cross-sectional imaging of the abdomen and pelvis to evaluate for nodal metastasis (Table 72-4).

TABLE 72-4 Staging of Prostate Cancer

Primary Tumor (T)

TX	Primary tumor cannot be assessed
T0	No evidence of primary tumor
T1	Clinically inapparent tumor neither palpable nor visible by imaging
T1a	Tumor incidental histologic finding in 5% or less of tissue resected
T1b	Tumor incidental histologic finding in more than 5% of tissue resected
T1c	Tumor identified by needle biopsy (for example, because of elevated PSA)
T2	Tumor confined within prostate
T2a	Tumor involves one-half of one lobe or less
T2b	Tumor involves more than one-half of one lobe but not both lobes
T2c	Tumor involves both lobes
T3	Tumor extends through the prostate capsule
T3a	Extracapsular extension (unilateral or bilateral)
T3b	Tumor invades seminal vesicle(s)
T4	Tumor is fixed or invades adjacent structures other than seminal vesicles, such as external sphincter, rectum, bladder, levator muscles, and/or pelvic wall

Lymph Nodes (N)

NX	Regional lymph nodes were not assessed
N0	No regional lymph node metastasis
N1	Metastasis in regional lymph node(s)

Distant Metastasis (M)

M0	No distant metastasis
M1	Distant metastasis
M1a	Nonregional lymph node(s)
M1b	Bone(s)
M1c	Other site(s) with or without bone disease

Treatment

The treatment of prostate cancer has changed significantly during the past several years. As most prostate cancer, at diagnosis, is low risk, many patients are now treated with active surveillance rather than with active therapy. In general, men with cancer of low clinical stage (T1c), low grade (Gleason sum ≤ 6), and low volume on biopsy are candidates for active surveillance.[48] Patients assigned to active surveillance protocols undergo DRE and PSA monitoring every 3 to 6 months, with repeated TRUS-guided prostate biopsies every 1 to 3 years.[48] Patients with increase in Gleason sum or increase in tumor volume on biopsy typically shift to an active treatment plan.

Prostate cancer can be treated with either radical surgical excision or definitive radiation therapy. Radical prostatectomy involves the surgical removal of the entire prostate and seminal vesicles with anastomosis of the urethral stump to the bladder neck. Pelvic lymph node dissection is controversial in the management of prostate cancer; some protocols recommend no lymph node dissection for low-risk disease, and others recommend extended pelvic lymph node dissection. For prostate cancer Gleason sum 7 or higher, at a minimum, the external iliac and obturator lymph nodes should be removed. Radical prostatectomy can be performed with an open, laparoscopic, or robotically assisted laparoscopic approach. The majority of radical prostatectomies in the United States are now performed by a robotically assisted laparoscopic prostatectomy (RALP).[47] The advantages of RALP appear to be decreased blood loss, shorter hospital stay, and quicker return to work. When it is technically feasible and oncologically appropriate, a nerve-sparing approach is used, which avoids injury to the cavernous nerves that run posterolateral along the prostate in the neurovascular bundle and mediate penile erection. Important landmarks for radical prostatectomy are the dorsal venous plexus anteriorly, bladder neck cephalad, prostatomembranous urethral junction distally, and rectal wall posteriorly. The correct plane of posterior dissection in radical prostatectomy is just posterior to the Denonvilliers fascia. The primary long-term risks of radical prostatectomy are urinary incontinence and ED. Because of the recent introduction and adaptation of RALP, most long-term survival series are based on historical open radical prostatectomy data. Ten-year cancer progression-free survival is approximately 85% for patients with organ-confined disease, approximately 60% to 70% for extracapsular extension, and approximately 50% for patients with positive surgical margins.

Patients who do not desire surgical extirpation may undergo local therapy with either intensity-modulated radiation therapy (IMRT) or brachytherapy. The typical treatment dose for IMRT-based prostate cancer therapy is 76 to 86 Gy. The most common form of brachytherapy is low-dose ultrasound-guided placement of iodine-125 or palladium-103 radioisotope sources into the prostate. Both treatments are commonly used for low-risk prostate cancer. Intermediate- and high-risk prostate cancer is typically treated with IMRT coupled with androgen deprivation therapy for up to 2 years. Low- and intermediate-risk prostate cancers have outcomes after radiation-based therapy similar to those of radical prostatectomy.[47] In advanced prostate cancer, androgen deprivation therapy may become ineffective, with clinical or PSA progression observed in spite of appropriate hormonal therapy. In these cases, second-line treatment includes antiandrogens, chemotherapy, and investigational agents. Other forms of treatment that can be considered for local treatment of prostate cancer include cryotherapy and proton beam therapy, although long-term results for these modalities are still being reported.

After prostate cancer therapy, patients are monitored for post-treatment morbidities (e.g., continence, erectile function, voiding adequacy) and possible cancer recurrence. The latter involves PSA testing and potentially repeated metastatic evaluation, when indicated. Long-term follow-up for prostate cancer patients should continue at least 10 years, if not permanently, because very late recurrences can occur. If the PSA level becomes significantly detectable or is rising after definitive treatment, it may be appropriate to consider repeated TRUS of the anastomotic region, possibly with biopsy, and repeated metastatic evaluation to decide whether to proceed with local radiation therapy, androgen deprivation therapy, or observation.

Testicular Cancer

Testicular cancer is an uncommon malignant neoplasm; in the United States, the incidence is 5/100,000 men.[50] Most cases of primary testicular cancer are germ cell origin (95%); the remainder are predominantly stromal (Leydig cell) or sex cord (Sertoli cell) tumors.[50] Any solid intratesticular mass is likely to represent a malignant germ cell tumor and is typically treated as such unless there is a strong suspicion to the contrary. Risk factors for testicular tumors include cryptorchidism, family history of testicular cancer, and intratubular germ cell neoplasia.

Germ cell–derived testicular tumors can be broadly divided into seminoma and nonseminoma germ cell tumors (NSGCTs); the division is approximately 50% for each. The majority of seminomas are classic (85%); the remainder are either anaplastic or spermatocytic seminoma.[50] NSGCTs can be divided into numerous histologic types: embryonal carcinoma, yolk sac or endodermal sinus tumors, choriocarcinoma, teratoma, and mixed germ cell tumors. Testicular malignant neoplasms are the most common tumors in men between the ages of 20 and 40 years.[50]

Seminomas, however, present in the fourth or fifth decade of life, and spermatocytic seminomas may present in men older than 50 years.[50] The most common presenting complaint in men with testicular cancer is a painless testicular mass; however, it is not uncommon for men to present with symptoms of metastatic disease, including palpable abdominal mass, shortness of breath, and hemoptysis. In patients who present with a painless testicular mass, scrotal ultrasonography is the diagnostic study of choice. In addition to history, physical examination, and ultrasonography, patients with testicular tumors should have determination of specific tumor markers: α-fetoprotein, β-human chorionic gonadotropin, and lactate dehydrogenase. After treatment, these markers have a characteristic half-life, and appropriate clearance has important prognostic significance.

Treatment

Initial treatment of suspected testicular tumor is radical inguinal orchiectomy, which involves removal of the testicle and spermatic cord at the level of the inguinal ring (Fig. 72-28). Because of the characteristic and well-described lymph drainage of the testicle, there is no role for trans-scrotal biopsy or orchiectomy. If the intrascrotal tissue planes are violated during orchiectomy, the lymphatic drainage can be altered, affecting future treatment. After radical inguinal orchiectomy, the patient should undergo disease staging, including cross-sectional, contrast-enhanced imaging of the abdomen and pelvis and chest imaging, either chest radiography in low-risk patients or cross-sectional chest imaging in patients with high-risk disease.

Clinical staging for testicular cancer includes primary tumor pathology, lymph and metastatic staging on imaging, and postorchiectomy serum tumor markers (Tables 72-5 and 72-6). The half-life of β-human chorionic gonadotropin is 24 to 36 hours,

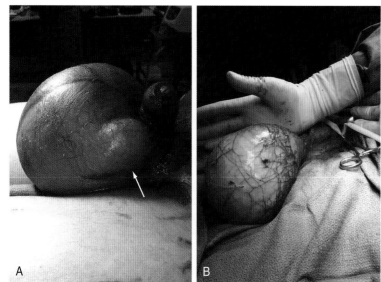
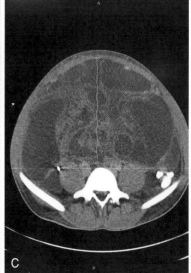

FIGURE 72-28 Advanced Testicular Carcinoma. A, Preoperative appearance of the scrotum in a patient with a large right testis tumor. The normal left testis is seen pushed cephalad by the right-sided mass. **B,** Surgical exploration through right inguinal incision, showing the right testis that has been dissected from the scrotum in an extravaginal plane, still attached by the spermatic cord pedicle to the right. **C,** Massive retroperitoneal lymphadenopathy in the same patient. Note that the descending colon is opacified with contrast material, but all other viscera are pushed cephalad so that no small intestine is seen in this image. The patient was managed with primary chemotherapy followed by retroperitoneal lymphadenectomy for the residual mass.

TABLE 72-5 Staging of Testicular Cancer

Primary Tumor (T)

pTX	Primary tumor cannot be assessed
pT0	No evidence of primary tumor
pTis	Intratubular germ cell neoplasia
pT1	Tumor limited to the testis and epididymis without lymphovascular invasion, may invade tunica albuginea but not tunica vaginalis
pT2	Tumor limited to the testis and epididymis with lymphovascular invasion or tumor involving the tunica vaginalis
pT3	Tumor invades the spermatic cord with or without lymphovascular invasion
pT4	Tumor invades the scrotum with or without lymphovascular invasion

Regional Lymph Nodes (Clinical) (N)

NX	Regional lymph nodes cannot be assessed
N0	No regional lymph node metastasis
N1	Metastasis within one or more lymph nodes less than 2 cm in size
N2	Metastasis within one or more lymph nodes greater than 2 cm but less the 5 cm in size
N3	Metastasis within one or more lymph nodes greater than 5 cm in size

Regional Lymph Nodes (Pathologic) (N)

NX	Regional lymph nodes cannot be assessed
N0	No regional lymph node metastasis
N1	Metastasis within 1-5 lymph nodes; all node masses less than 2 cm in size
N2	Metastasis within a lymph node greater than 2 cm but not greater than 5 cm in size, or more than 5 lymph nodes involved, none greater than 5 cm and none demonstrating extranodal extension of tumor
N3	Metastasis within one or more lymph nodes greater than 5 cm in size

Distant Metastasis (M)

MX	Distant metastasis cannot be assessed
M0	No distant metastasis
M1	Distant metastasis
M1a	Nonregional nodal or pulmonary metastasis
M1b	Distant metastasis at site other than nonregional lymph nodes or lung

Serum Tumor Markers (S)

SX	Tumor markers not available or performed
S0	Tumor markers within normal limits
S1	LDH <1.5× normal, hCG <5000 IU/L, AFP <1000 ng/mL
S2	LDH 1.5-10× normal, hCG 5000-50,000 IU/L, AFP 1000-10,000 ng/mL
S3	LDH >10× normal, hCG >50,000 IU/L, AFP >10,000 ng/mL

AFP, α-fetoprotein; *hCG,* human chorionic gonadotropin; *LDH,* lactate dehydrogenase.

TABLE 72-6 Clinical Staging of Testicular Cancer

STAGE	T	N	M	S
Stage I	pT1-4	N0	M0	SX
IA	pT1	N0	M0	S0
IB	pT2	N0	M0	S0
	pT3	N0	M0	S0
	pT4	N0	M0	S0
IS	Any pT	N0	M0	S1-3
Stage II	Any pT	N1-3	M0	SX
IIA	Any pT	N1	M0	S0-1
IIB	Any pT	N2	M0	S0-1
IIC	Any pT	N3	M0	S0-1
Stage III	Any pT	Any N	M1	SX
IIIA	Any pT	Any N	M1a	S0-1
IIIB	Any pT	N1-3	M0	S2
	Any pT	Any N	M1a	S2
IIIC	Any pT	N1-3	M0	S3
	Any pT	Any N	M1a	S3
	Any pT	Any N	M1b	Any S

distributions may be altered and the metastatic pattern may be unpredictable, potentially leading to involvement of the inguinal or pelvic nodes. Distant metastases are typically seen to the lung, liver, brain, bone, kidney, and adrenal gland.

Second-line treatment is directed by tumor histology and lymph node staging. Further treatment may consist of regular surveillance, retroperitoneal radiation therapy, retroperitoneal lymph node dissection (RPLND), systemic chemotherapy, or a multimodal therapy approach. The treatment decisions are complex, often at the direction of an institutional tumor board, but several general principles apply:

- For seminoma stage IA and IB disease, treatment options include surveillance, radiotherapy to the regional lymph nodes (20 Gy), and one or two cycles of carboplatin-based chemotherapy.[50]
- For seminoma stage IIA and IIB, radiotherapy of the retroperitoneal lymph nodes is standard therapy; for stage IIC or III, platinum-based chemotherapy is standard therapy.[50]
- For NSGCT stage I disease, the options include surveillance, RPLND, and cisplatin-based chemotherapy.[50]
- For NSGCT stage IIA, either primary RPLND (in patients with normal levels of tumor markers) or three or four cycles of cisplatin-based chemotherapy is standard; for stage IIB, three or four cycles of cisplatin-based chemotherapy is standard, followed by RPLND or surveillance.[50]

RPLND involves removal of all lymph nodes in the retroperitoneum from the renal vessels to the aortic bifurcation. An appropriate RPLND should include the lymph tissue surrounding the great vessels and division of the appropriate lumbar vessel to ensure thorough dissection, the split-and-roll technique. The most challenging RPLNDs are after chemotherapy, when the retroperitoneal tissues may be fibrotic or desmoplastic and adherent to the inferior vena cava, aorta, bowel, and mesentery. RPLND is template driven, and the appropriate levels and location of tissue excision are well described. Following the appropriate templates, the sympathetic nerve chain should be uninjured, allowing antegrade ejaculation.

and the half-life of α-fetoprotein is 5 to 7 days; these levels should normalize in the absence of metastatic disease. Metastatic disease from testicular cancer typically follows a predictable retroperitoneal lymphatic path, although choriocarcinoma is notorious for hematogenous spread early to distant sites. From the right testis, initial lymph node metastasis is to the infrarenal interaortocaval nodes, paracaval nodes, and para-aortic nodes; on the left, the para-aortic nodes and then interaortocaval nodes. Retroperitoneal lymph nodes are the primary metastatic site in more than 70% of patients with metastatic testicular cancer.[50] If the patient has had prior groin or pelvic surgery, the natural lymphatic

Many patients undergoing RPLND will have been exposed to bleomycin chemotherapy, which requires meticulous intraoperative anesthetic management because of the exquisite sensitivity of these patients to elevated oxygen exposure; often, the anesthetic is run essentially on room air ventilation in these cases.

After orchiectomy and before any additional therapy for testicular cancer, consideration should be given to preservation of fertility. Patients should be made aware of the potential impact of radiation, chemotherapy, or RPLND on the ability to ejaculate and on spermatogenesis. It is essential that patients be offered sperm cryopreservation before therapies that could adversely affect their reproductive potential. In addition, patients should be made aware that radiation has the potential morbidity of delayed secondary malignant disease as high as 15% within 25 years of treatment.[50]

Curative treatment of testicular cancer is one of the great success stories of modern oncology. Overall, long-term survival for testicular cancer ranges from 98% to 99% for stage I seminoma or NSGCT.[50] In patients with stage II seminoma, radiotherapy yields survival of up to 100%, and stage II NSGCT standard treatments yield survival of 90% to 95%.[50] Even advanced disease, stage III seminoma, has an expected survival of more than 90%, and NSGCTs have long-term survivals of 80% to 90%.[50]

SELECTED REFERENCES

Bhasin S, Cunningham GR, Hayes FJ, et al: Testosterone therapy in men with androgen deficiency syndromes: An Endocrine Society clinical practice guideline. *J Clin Endocrinol Metab* 95:2536–2559, 2010.

The most current reference on the management of male testosterone deficiency. Broad-based consensus statement on evaluation, management, and therapy options.

Brandes S, Coburn M, Armenakas N, et al: Diagnosis and management of ureteric injury: An evidence-based analysis. *BJU Int* 94:277–289, 2004.

This article is a classic reference from the first consensus panel discussing evaluation and management of ureteral injuries.

Carter HB, Albertsen PC, Barry MJ, et al: Early detection of prostate cancer: AUA guideline. *J Urol* 190:419–426, 2013.

The evidence-based response to the U.S. Preventive Services Task Force recommendation to no longer screen men for prostate cancer. This article is a systematic critique of the literature used by the U.S. Preventive Services Task Force to give a grade D to the regular screening of prostate cancer.

Chapple C, Barbagli G, Jordan G, et al: Consensus statement on urethral trauma. *BJU Int* 93:1195–1202, 2004.

This article is a classic reference from the first consensus panel discussing evaluation and management of urethral injuries.

Gomez RG, Ceballos L, Coburn M, et al: Consensus statement on bladder injuries. *BJU Int* 94:27–32, 2004.

This article is a classic reference from the first consensus panel discussing evaluation and management of bladder injuries.

Gupta K, Hooton TM, Naber KG, et al: International clinical practice guidelines for the treatment of acute uncomplicated cystitis and pyelonephritis in women: A 2010 update by the Infectious Diseases Society of America and the European Society for Microbiology and Infectious Diseases. *Clin Infect Dis* 52:e103–e120, 2011.

This document represents the most current guideline for the diagnosis and treatment of outpatient or uncomplicated urinary tract infection in women.

Haylen BT, de Ridder D, Freeman RM, et al: An International Urogynecological Association (IUGA)/International Continence Society (ICS) joint report on the terminology for female pelvic floor dysfunction. *Neurourol Urodyn* 29:4–20, 2010.

This article is the most recent consensus guideline to standardize terminology, diagnosis, and management of pelvic floor dysfunction and incontinence.

Jarow J, Sigman M, Kolettis P, et al: The optimal evaluation of the infertile male. AUA Best Practice Statement, 2010, pp 1–39.

This article represents the best recommendations for evaluation and diagnosis of the infertile male. The AUA recommendations regarding specific aspects of the infertile male workup are highlighted throughout this manuscript, making it easily searchable.

Moore EE, Shackford SR, Pachter HL, et al: Organ injury scaling: Spleen, liver, and kidney. *J Trauma* 29:1664–1666, 1989.

This classic article describes injury grading in the urologic system.

Morey AF, Brandes S, Dugi DD, 3rd, et al: Urotrauma: AUA guideline. *J Urol* 192:327–335, 2014.

The first edition of the urologic trauma guidelines by the American Urological Association provides the best evidence-based recommendations for the management of traumatic urologic injuries.

Morey AF, Metro MJ, Carney KJ, et al: Consensus on genitourinary trauma: External genitalia. *BJU Int* 94:507–515, 2004.

This article is a classic reference from the first consensus panel discussing evaluation and management of genital injuries.

Santucci RA, Wessells H, Bartsch G, et al: Evaluation and management of renal injuries: Consensus statement of the renal trauma subcommittee. *BJU Int* 93:937–954, 2004.

This article is a classic reference from the first consensus panel discussing evaluation and management of renal injuries.

Smith TG, 3rd, Coburn M: Damage control maneuvers for urologic trauma. *Urol Clin North Am* 40:343–350, 2013.

This reference represents the only literature on management of traumatic urologic injuries using damage control principles and organized by urologic organ systems.

REFERENCES

1. Anderson JK, Cadeddu JA: Surgical anatomy of the retroperitoneum, adrenals, kidneys, and ureters. In Wein AJ, Kavoussi LR, Campbell MF, et al, editors: *Campbell-Walsh urology*, ed 10, Philadelphia, 2012, Elsevier Saunders.
2. McNeil BK: Kidney, adrenal, ureter. <https://www.auanet.org/university/core_topic.cfm?coreid=59>. Accessed August 7, 2015.
3. Kim IY, Clayton RV: Surgical renal anatomy. *AUA Update Series* 25:361–368, 2006.
4. Webster GD, Anoia E: Principles of ureteral reconstruction. In Smith JA, Howards SS, Preminger GM, et al, editors: *Hinman's atlas of urologic surgery*, ed 3, Philadelphia, 2012, Elsevier/Saunders.
5. Chung BI, Sommer G, Brooks JD: Anatomy of the lower urinary tract and male genitalia. In Wein AJ, Kavoussi LR, Campbell MF, et al, editors: *Campbell-Walsh urology*, ed 10, Philadelphia, 2012, Elsevier Saunders.
6. Smith PP: Lower urinary tract. American Urological Association. <https://www.auanet.org/university/core_topic.cfm?coreid=131>. Accessed December 18, 2014.
7. Walz J, Graefen M, Huland H: Basic principles of anatomy for optimal surgical treatment of prostate cancer. *World J Urol* 25:31–38, 2007.
8. Duffey B, Monga M: Principles of endoscopy. In Wein AJ, Kavoussi LR, Campbell MF, et al, editors: *Campbell-Walsh urology*, ed 10, Philadelphia, 2012, Elsevier Saunders.
9. Urinary tract infection. In Litwin M, Saigal C, editors: *Urologic diseases in America. U.S. Department of Health and Human Services, Public Health Service, National Institutes of Health, National Institute of Diabetes and Digestive and Kidney Diseases*, Washington, DC, 2012, U.S. Government Printing Office, pp 366–404. NIH Publication No. 12-7865.
10. Gupta K, Hooton TM, Naber KG, et al: International clinical practice guidelines for the treatment of acute uncomplicated cystitis and pyelonephritis in women: A 2010 update by the Infectious Diseases Society of America and the European Society for Microbiology and Infectious Diseases. *Clin Infect Dis* 52:e103–e120, 2011.
11. Lin WR, Chen M, Hsu JM, et al: Emphysematous pyelonephritis: Patient characteristics and management approach. *Urol Int* 93:29–33, 2014.
12. Sorensen MD, Krieger JN, Rivara FP, et al: Fournier's gangrene: Management and mortality predictors in a population based study. *J Urol* 182:2742–2747, 2009.
13. Clemens JQ: Basic bladder neurophysiology. *Urol Clin North Am* 37:487–494, 2010.
14. Gormley A, Stoffel J, Kielb S: Neurogenic bladder. American Urological Association. <https://www.auanet.org/university/core_topic.cfm?coreid=144>. Accessed August 7, 2015.
15. Haylen BT, de Ridder D, Freeman RM, et al: An International Urogynecological Association (IUGA)/International Continence Society (ICS) joint report on the terminology for female pelvic floor dysfunction. *Neurourol Urodyn* 29:4–20, 2010.
16. Irwin DE, Kopp ZS, Agatep B, et al: Worldwide prevalence estimates of lower urinary tract symptoms, overactive bladder, urinary incontinence and bladder outlet obstruction. *BJU Int* 108:1132–1138, 2011.
17. Gormley EA, Lightner DJ, Burgio KL, et al: Diagnosis and treatment of overactive bladder (non-neurogenic) in adults: AUA/SUFU guideline. *J Urol* 188:2455–2463, 2012.
18. Dooley Y, Kenton K, Cao G, et al: Urinary incontinence prevalence: Results from the National Health and Nutrition Examination Survey. *J Urol* 179:656–661, 2008.
19. Ford AA, Rogerson L, Cody JD, et al: Mid-urethral sling operations for stress urinary incontinence in women. *Cochrane Database Syst Rev* (7):CD006375, 2015.
20. McVary KT, Roehrborn CG, Avins AL, et al: Update on AUA guideline on the management of benign prostatic hyperplasia. *J Urol* 185:1793–1803, 2011.
21. Jarow J, Sigman M, Kolettis P, et al: The optimal evaluation of the infertile male. AUA Best Practice Statement, 2010, pp 1–39.
22. Jarow J, Sigman M, Kolettis P, et al: The evaluation of the azoospermic male. AUA Best Practice Statement Revised, 2010, pp 1–25.
23. Bacon CG, Mittleman MA, Kawachi I, et al: A prospective study of risk factors for erectile dysfunction. *J Urol* 176:217–221, 2006.
24. Crawford ED, Barqawi AB, O'Donnell C, et al: The association of time of day and serum testosterone concentration in a large screening population. *BJU Int* 100:509–513, 2007.
25. Bhasin S, Cunningham GR, Hayes FJ, et al: Testosterone therapy in men with androgen deficiency syndromes: An Endocrine Society clinical practice guideline. *J Clin Endocrinol Metab* 95:2536–2559, 2010.
26. Scales CD, Jr, Smith AC, Hanley JM, et al: Prevalence of kidney stones in the United States. *Eur Urol* 62:160–165, 2012.
27. Miller NL, Evan AP, Lingeman JE: Pathogenesis of renal calculi. *Urol Clin North Am* 34:295–313, 2007.
28. Preminger GM, Tiselius HG, Assimos DG, et al: 2007 guideline for the management of ureteral calculi. EAU/AUA Nephrolithiasis Guideline Panel. *J Urol* 178:2418–2434, 2007.
29. Lange JN, Mufarrij PW, Wood KD, et al: Metabolic evaluation and medical management of the calcium stone former. *AUA Update Series* 31, 2012.
30. Weizer AZ, Zhong P, Preminger GM: Shock wave lithotripsy: Current technology and evolving concepts. *AUA Update Series* 24, 2005.
31. Hotaling JM, Wang J, Sorensen MD, et al: A national study of trauma level designation and renal trauma outcomes. *J Urol* 187:536–541, 2012.
32. Moore EE, Shackford SR, Pachter HL, et al: Organ injury scaling: Spleen, liver, and kidney. *J Trauma* 29:1664–1666, 1989.
33. Santucci RA, Wessells H, Bartsch G, et al: Evaluation and management of renal injuries: Consensus statement of the renal trauma subcommittee. *BJU Int* 93:937–954, 2004.
34. Brandes S, Coburn M, Armenakas N, et al: Diagnosis and management of ureteric injury: An evidence-based analysis. *BJU Int* 94:277–289, 2004.

35. Gomez RG, Ceballos L, Coburn M, et al: Consensus statement on bladder injuries. *BJU Int* 94:27–32, 2004.

36. Chapple C, Barbagli G, Jordan G, et al: Consensus statement on urethral trauma. *BJU Int* 93:1195–1202, 2004.

37. Morey AF, Metro MJ, Carney KJ, et al: Consensus on genitourinary trauma: External genitalia. *BJU Int* 94:507–515, 2004.

38. Morey AF, Brandes S, Dugi DD, 3rd, et al: Urotrauma: AUA guideline. *J Urol* 192:327–335, 2014.

39. Voelzke BB, Hudak SJ, Coburn M: Renal, ureter trauma. American Urological Association. <https://www.auanet.org/university/core_topic.cfm?coreid=87>. Accessed August 7, 2015.

40. Charbit J, Manzanera J, Millet I, et al: What are the specific computed tomography scan criteria that can predict or exclude the need for renal angioembolization after high-grade renal trauma in a conservative management strategy? *J Trauma* 70:1219–1227, 2011.

41. Smith TG, 3rd, Coburn M: Damage control maneuvers for urologic trauma. *Urol Clin North Am* 40:343–350, 2013.

42. Myers J, Smith TG, III, Coburn M: Bladder, urethra, genitalia trauma. American Urological Association. <https://www.auanet.org/university/core_topic.cfm?coreid=88>. Accessed August 7, 2015.

43. McGeady JB, Breyer BN: Current epidemiology of genitourinary trauma. *Urol Clin North Am* 40:323–334, 2013.

44. Campbell SC, Novick AC, Belldegrun A, et al: Guideline for management of the clinical T1 renal mass. *J Urol* 182:1271–1279, 2009.

45. Raman JD, Smaldone M, Thompson RH, et al: Renal neoplasms. American Urological Association. <https://www.auanet.org/university/core_topic.cfm?coreid=75>. Accessed August 7, 2015.

46. Inman BA, Lotan Y, Daneshmand S, et al: Bladder neoplasm. American Urological Association. <https://www.auanet.org/university/core_topic.cfm?coreid=76>. Accessed August 7, 2015.

47. Meeks JJ, Lowrance WT, McBride S, et al: Prostate cancer. American Urological Association. <https://www.auanet.org/university/core_topic.cfm?coreid=74>. Accessed August 7, 2015.

48. Thompson I, Thrasher JB, Aus G, et al: Guideline for the management of clinically localized prostate cancer: 2007 update. *J Urol* 177:2106–2131, 2007.

49. Carter HB, Albertsen PC, Barry MJ, et al: Early detection of prostate cancer: AUA guideline. *J Urol* 190:419–426, 2013.

50. Woods M, Castle EP, Stroup SP, et al: Testis neoplasms. American Urological Association. <https://www.auanet.org/university/core_topic.cfm?coreid=77>. Accessed August 7, 2015.

ELSEVIER

Elsevier (Singapore) Pte Ltd.
3 Killiney Road, #08-01 Winsland House I, Singapore 239519
Tel: (65) 6349-0200; Fax: (65) 67

This English Adaptation of Sabiston Textbook of Surgery, 20/E by Courtney M. Townsend, Jr., R. Daniel Beauchamp,
B. Mark Evers, and Kenneth L. Mattoxwas undertaken by Hunan Science & Technology Press and is published by
arrangement with Elsevier (Singapore) Pte Ltd.

Sabiston Textbook of Surgery, 20/E by Courtney M. Townsend, Jr., R. Daniel Beauchamp, B. Mark Evers, and
Kenneth L. Mattox由湖南科学技术出版社进行改编影印，并根据湖南科学技术出版社与爱思唯尔（新加坡）
私人有限公司的协议约定出版。

克氏外科学Sabiston Textbook of Surgery，影印中文导读版，（陈孝平，刘玉村等改编）
ISBN: 978-7-5710-0725-6

图书在版编目（ＣＩＰ）数据

克氏外科学：第 20 版：影印中文导读版：汉、英文 下册 ／［美］考特尼 M. 汤森德
（Courtney M.Townsend）等主编；陈孝平，刘玉村等编译.—长沙：湖南科学技术出版社，
2020.10
（西医经典名著集成）
ISBN 978-7-5710-0725-6

Ⅰ.①克…　Ⅱ.①考…　②陈…　③刘…　Ⅲ.①外科学—汉、英文　Ⅳ.①R6

中国版本图书馆 CIP 数据核字（2020）第 155682 号

著作权合同登记号　18-2020-190

西医经典名著集成
KESHI　WAIKEXUE
克氏外科学　第 20 版　（影印中文导读版）　下册

主　　　编：［美］考特尼 M. 汤森德（Courtney M.Townsend），［美］R. 丹尼尔·比彻姆（R.Daniel Beauchamp），
　　　　　　［美］B. 马克·埃弗斯（B.Mark Evers），［美］肯尼斯 L. 马托克斯（Kenneth L.Mattox）
编 译 者：陈孝平　刘玉村等
责任编辑：李　忠　王　李
出版发行：湖南科学技术出版社
社　　址：长沙市湘雅路 276 号
　　　　　http://www.hnstp.com
印　　刷：湖南天闻新华印务有限公司
　　　　　（印装质量问题请直接与本厂联系）
厂　　址：湖南望城·湖南出版科技园
邮　　编：410219
版　　次：2020 年 10 月第 1 版
印　　次：2020 年 10 月第 1 次印刷
开　　本：787mm×1092mm　1/16
印　　张：70.75
字　　数：4000 千字
书　　号：ISBN 978-7-5710-0725-6
定　　价：950.00 元（上、下册）